COLD SPRING HARBOR SYMPOSIA ON QUANTITATIVE BIOLOGY

VOLUME LXI

COLD SPRING HARBOR SYMPOSIA ON QUANTITATIVE BIOLOGY

VOLUME LXI

Function & Dysfunction in the Nervous System

COLD SPRING HARBOR LABORATORY PRESS
1996

COLD SPRING HARBOR SYMPOSIA ON QUANTITATIVE BIOLOGY VOLUME LXI

©1996 by Cold Spring Harbor Laboratory Press
International Standard Book Number 0-87969-071-2 (cloth)
International Standard Book Number 0-87969-072-0 (paper)
International Standard Serial Number 0091-7451
Library of Congress Catalog Card Number 34-8174

Printed in the United States of America

COLD SPRING HARBOR SYMPOSIA ON QUANTITATIVE BIOLOGY

Founded in 1933 by
REGINALD G. HARRIS
Director of the Biological Laboratory 1924 to 1936

Previous Symposia Volumes

I (1933) Surface Phenomena
II (1934) Aspects of Growth
III (1935) Photochemical Reactions
IV (1936) Excitation Phenomena
V (1937) Internal Secretions
VI (1938) Protein Chemistry
VII (1939) Biological Oxidations
VIII (1940) Permeability and the Nature of Cell Membranes
IX (1941) Genes and Chromosomes: Structure and Organization
X (1942) The Relation of Hormones to Development
XI (1946) Heredity and Variation in Microorganisms
XII (1947) Nucleic Acids and Nucleoproteins
XIII (1948) Biological Applications of Tracer Elements
XIV (1949) Amino Acids and Proteins
XV (1950) Origin and Evolution of Man
XVI (1951) Genes and Mutations
XVII (1952) The Neuron
XVIII (1953) Viruses
XIX (1954) The Mammalian Fetus: Physiological Aspects of Development
XX (1955) Population Genetics: The Nature and Causes of Genetic Variability in Population
XXI (1956) Genetic Mechanisms: Structure and Function
XXII (1957) Population Studies: Animal Ecology and Demography
XXIII (1958) Exchange of Genetic Material: Mechanism and Consequences
XXIV (1959) Genetics and Twentieth Century Darwinism
XXV (1960) Biological Clocks
XXVI (1961) Cellular Regulatory Mechanisms
XXVII (1962) Basic Mechanisms in Animal Virus Biology
XXVIII (1963) Synthesis and Structure of Macromolecules
XXIX (1964) Human Genetics
XXX (1965) Sensory Receptors
XXXI (1966) The Genetic Code
XXXII (1967) Antibodies
XXXIII (1968) Replication of DNA in Microorganisms
XXXIV (1969) The Mechanism of Protein Synthesis
XXXV (1970) Transcription of Genetic Material
XXXVI (1971) Structure and Function of Proteins at the Three-dimensional Level
XXXVII (1972) The Mechanism of Muscle Contraction
XXXVIII (1973) Chromosome Structure and Function
XXXIX (1974) Tumor Viruses
XL (1975) The Synapse
XLI (1976) Origins of Lymphocyte Diversity
XLII (1977) Chromatin
XLIII (1978) DNA: Replication and Recombination
XLIV (1979) Viral Oncogenes
XLV (1980) Movable Genetic Elements
XLVI (1981) Organization of the Cytoplasm
XLVII (1982) Structures of DNA
XLVIII (1983) Molecular Neurobiology
XLIX (1984) Recombination at the DNA Level
L (1985) Molecular Biology of Development
LI (1986) Molecular Biology of *Homo sapiens*
LII (1987) Evolution of Catalytic Function
LIII (1988) Molecular Biology of Signal Transduction
LIV (1989) Immunological Recognition
LV (1990) The Brain
LVI (1991) The Cell Cycle
LVII (1992) The Cell Surface
LVIII (1993) DNA and Chromosomes
LIX (1994) The Molecular Genetics of Cancer
LX (1995) Protein Kinesis: The Dynamics of Protein Trafficking and Stability

Front Cover (Paperback): Living Purkinje neuron deeply embedded in a guinea pig brain slice, filled with fluorescein dextran. Imaging was performed by two-photon excitation laser scanning microscopy using a solid-state mode locked laser as light source. (Photo courtesy of K. Svoboda, W. Denk, W. Knox, and S. Tsuda, Bell Labs.)

Back Cover (Paperback): Atrophic Purkinje cell dendritic tree seen in a cerebellum from a 1-week-old B05 transgenic mouse. (For details, see Orr and Zoghbi, p. 654, this volume.)

All Cold Spring Harbor Laboratory Press publications may be ordered directly from Cold Spring Harbor Laboratory Press, 10 Skyline Drive, Plainview, NY 11803. Phone: 1-800-843-4388 in Continental U.S. and Canada. All other locations (516) 349-1930. FAX: (516) 349-1946. E-mail: cshpress@cshl.org. For a complete catalog of all Cold Spring Harbor Laboratory Press publications, visit our World Wide Web Site http://www.cshl.org/

Symposium Participants

ADAMSON, D. CORY, Dept. of Neuroscience and Neurology, Johns Hopkins University School of Medicine, Baltimore, Maryland

ADELSTEI, ROBERT, Dept. of Molecular Cardiology, National Institutes of Health, Bethesda, Maryland

ALONSO, JOSE-MANUEL, Dept. of Neurobiology, Rockefeller University, New York, New York

ANDERSEN, RICHARD, Dept. of Behavioral Biology, California Institute of Technology, Pasadena, California

ARNOLD, DONALD, Dept. of Molecular Biology, Rockefeller University, New York, New York

ATWELL, CONSTANCE, National Institute of Neurological Disorders, Bethesda, Maryland

AUER, MANFRED, EMBL, Structures and Biocomputing, Heidelberg, Germany

AUSTEN, BRIAN, St. Georges Hospital Medical School Surgery, London, United Kingdom

AXEL, RICHARD, Columbia University, Howard Hughes Medical Institute, New York, New York

BAHN, SABINE, Dept. of Neurobiology, MRC-LMB, Cambridge, United Kingdom

BALDWIN, ANNE, Dept. of Neurobiology, Stanford University Medical Center, Stanford, California

BAO, JUN, Dept. of Neuroscience and Neurology, Johns Hopkins University, Baltimore, Maryland

BAR-PELED, OSNAT, Dept. of Neurology/Neuromuscular, Johns Hopkins University School of Medicine, Baltimore, Maryland

BARDE, YVES-ALAIN, Dept. of Neurobiochemistry, Max-Planck Institute für Psychiatrie, Martinsreid, Germany

BARGMANN, CORNELIA, Dept. of Anatomy, University of California, San Francisco/Howard Hughes Medical Institute, San Francisco

BARINAGA, MARCIA, *Science* Research News, Berkeley, California

BAULIEU, ETIENNE EMILE, INSERM, Le Kremlin-Bicetre France

BENNETT, MICHAEL, Dept. of Neuroscience, Albert Einstein College of Medicine, Bronx, New York

BERG, MARGARET, Dept. of Neurobiology, Northwestern University, Evanston, Illinois

BERRETTINI, WADE, Dept. of Psychiatry and Pharmacology, Thomas Jefferson University, Philadelphia, Pennsylvania

BESSEN, RICHARD, Lab. of Persistent Viral Diseases, National Institutes of Health, Rocky Mountain Laboratory, Hamilton, Montana

BESSEREAU, JEAN-LOUIS, Dept. of Neurobiologie Moleculaire, Institut Pasteur, Paris, France

BLUTHMANN, HORST, Central Research Units, Hoffmann-LaRoche and Company, Ltd., Basel, Switzerland

BODNER, RUTH, Dept. of Biology, University of California at San Diego, La Jolla

BONETTA, LAURA, Picower Institute Press, Molecular Medicine, Manhasset, New York

BORCHELT, DAVID, Dept. of Pathology, Johns Hopkins School of Medicine, Baltimore, Maryland

BOXER, ADAM, Dept. of Biochemistry, New York University Medical Center, Howard Hughes Medical Institute, New York, New York

BRAUN, JOCHEN, Computation and Neural Systems, California Institute of Technology, Pasadena

BRUIJN, LUCIE, Dept. of Cell Biology, Ludwig Institute for Cancer Research, La Jolla, California

BUCHMAN, VLADIMIR, Dept. of Biological and Medical Sciences, University of St. Andrews, Fife, United Kingdom

BUCK, LINDA, Dept. of Neurobiology, Harvard Medical School/Howard Hughes Medical Institute, Boston, Massachusetts

BUERGER, ERICH, Boehringer Ingelheim KG Bio, Research Binger, Ingelheim, Germany

CAHILL, LAWRENCE, University of California, Center for Neurobiology of Learning and Memory, Irvine

CARONI, PICO, Friedrich Miescher Institute, Basel, Switzerland

CASKEY, C. THOMAS, Merck Research Laboratories, West Point, Pennsylvania

CHANG, CHIA-PING, Dept. of Molecular Biology, Bristol-Myers Squibb, Wallingford, California

CHANGEUX, JEAN-PIERRE, Dept. of Neurobiology, Institut Pasteur Molecular, Paris, France

CHASE, THOMAS, Dept. of Experimental Therapeutics, National Institutes of Health, Bethesda, Maryland

CHEN, CHONG, Center for Learning and Memory, Massachusetts Institute of Technology/Howard Hughes Medical Institute, Cambridge

CHEN, HONG, Dept. of Genomics, Millennium Pharmaceuticals, Inc., Cambridge, Massachusetts

CHOI, DENNIS, Dept. of Neurology, Washington University School of Medicine, St. Louis, Missouri

CHRISTINE, CHAD, Dept. of Neurology, University of California, San Francisco

CLARK, ROBERT, Dept. of Psychiatry, Washington University School of Medicine, St. Louis, Missouri
CLEVELAND, DON, Ludwig Institute for Cancer Research, University of California, San Diego
CLINE, HOLLY, Cold Spring Harbor Laboratory, Cold Spring Harbor, New York
COBURN, CARA, Dept. of Anatomy, Howard Hughes Medical Institute, University of California, San Francisco
COOKE, BOB, *Newsday*, Melville, New York
COREY, DAVID, Dept. of Neurology, Massachusetts General Hospital, Boston
CRUMP, GAGE, Dept. of Anatomy, University of California, San Francisco
D'AGOSTARO, GIACOMO, ENEA Biophysics, Roma, Italy
DASH, PRAMOD, Dept. of Neurobiology and Anatomy, University of Texas Medical School, Houston
DE JAGER, PHILIP, Dept. of Molecular Biology, Rockefeller University, New York, New York
DE KOKER, RUDI, Dept. of Chemistry, Stanford University, Stanford, California
DE ARMOND, STEPHEN, Dept. of Neuropathology, University of California, School of Medicine, San Francisco
DEPAULO, J. RAYMOND, Dept. of Psychiatry, Johns Hopkins University, Baltimore, Maryland
DECHARMS, CHRISTOPHER, Dept. of Physiology, University of California, San Francisco
DIAZ-NIDO, JAVIER, Centro De Biologia Molecular, Universidad Autonoma, Madrid, Spain
DIETRICH, PAUL, Roche Bioscience Neurobiology Unit, Palo Alto, California
DODELET, VINCENT, Dept. of Neuroimmunology, Montreal Neurological Institute, Quebec, Canada
DRAGE, JOSEPH S., National Institute for Neurological Disorders and Stroke, National Institutes of Health, Bethesda, Maryland
DREYFUSS, GIDEON, Dept. of Biochemistry and Biophysics, University of Pennsylvania School of Medicine, Howard Hughes Medical Institute, Philadelphia
DU PASQUIER, RENAUD, Neurology Hospital, Cantonal Universitaire, University of Geneva, Switzerland
DUNLOP, THOMAS WILLIAM, Dept. of Molecular Genetics, University of Glasgow, United Kingdom
DWYER, NOELLE, Dept. of Neuroscience, University of California, San Francisco
EDENHOFER, FRANK, Genzentrum Institut Biochemie Der Lmu, Munchen, Germany
EDWARDS, ROBERT, Dept. of Neurology and Physiology, University of California, San Francisco
EICHENBAUM, HOWARD, Center for Behavioral Neuroscience, State University of New York, Stony Brook
ENIKOLOPOV, GRIGORI, Cold Spring Harbor Laboratory, Cold Spring Harbor, New York
EVINGER, CRAIG, Center for Neurobiology and Behavior, State University of New York, Stony Brook
FARHANGRAZI, ZAHRA SHADI, Dept. of Neurology, Center for Study of Nervous System, Washington University, St. Louis, Missouri
FEDOROV, NIKOLAI, Cold Spring Harbor Laboratory, Cold Spring Harbor, New York
FERRARO, TOM, Thomas Jefferson University, Philadelphia, Pennsylvania
FISCHBACH, GERALD, Dept. of Neurobiology, Harvard Medical School, Boston, Massachusetts
FISCHBECK, KENNETH, Dept. of Neurobiology, University of Pennsylvania, Philadelphia
FLEISSNER, ERWIN, Division of Science and Mathematics, Hunter College, CUNY, New York, New York
GALUSKE, RALF, Dept. of Neurophysiology, Max Planck Institute for Brain Research, Frankfurt, Germany
GAMER, JURGEN, BASF Aktiengesellschaft ZHA Pharmaceuticals Research, Heidelberg, Germany
GANDY, SAM, Dept. of Neurology and Neuroscience, Cornell University Medical College, New York, New York
GARDNER, PAUL, Institute of Biotechnology, University of Texas Health Science Center, San Antonio
GASIC, GREGORY, *Cell* Press Editor of Neuron, Cambridge, Massachusetts
GELLIBOLIAN, ROBERT, Institute of Biosciences and Technology, Texas A&M University, Houston
GERBER, DAVID, Center For Cancer Research, Massachusetts Institute of Technology, Cambridge
GIESE, PETER, Cold Spring Harbor Laboratory, Cold Spring Harbor, New York
GILBERT, CHARLES, Dept. of Neurobiology, Rockefeller University, New York, New York
GILLIAM, CONRAD, Dept. of Genetics and Development, Columbia University, New York, New York
GLASS, DAVID, Regeneron Pharmaceutical Discovery, Tarrytown, New York
GOEDERT, MICHEL, Medical Research Council Lab. of Molecular Biology, Cambridge, United Kingdom
GOGOS, JOSEPH, Dept. of Neurobiology and Behavior, Columbia University, New York, New York
GRICE, DOROTHY, Child Study Center Research and Clinical Child Psychiatry, Yale University, New Haven, Connecticut
GUSELLA, JAMES, Dept. of Molecular Neurogenetics, Massachusetts General Hospital, Boston
HAERTEL, MARION, Clinic for Tumor Biology Molecular Medicine, Freiburg, Germany
HALL, ZACH, National Institute of Neurological Dis-

orders and Stroke, National Institutes of Health, Bethesda, Maryland

HAMILTON, BRUCE, Whitehead Institute, Cambridge, Massachusetts

HARMAR, ANTHONY, Medical Research Council Brain Metabolism Unit, Royal Edinburgh Hospital, Scotland, United Kingdom

HARPER, SARAH, Dept. of Pharmacology, Merck Research Laboratories, Harlow, United Kingdom

HEMPERLY, JOHN, Dept. of Neurobiology, Becton Dickinson Company, Research Triangle Park, North Carolina

HEYN, SIETSKE, Dept. of Biological Chemistry, University of California, Davis

HOMAN, RICHARD, Dept. of Neurology, Texas Tech Health Science Center, Lubbock

HONG, KYONSOO, Dept. of Molecular Biology and Biochemistry, Rutgers University, Piscataway, New Jersey

HUDSPETH, JAMES, Dept. of Sensory Neuroscience, Rockefeller University/Howard Hughes Medical Institute, New York, New York

HUGHES, STEPHEN, Dept. of Molecular Biology, Hoechst Marion Roussel Pharmaceuticals, Inc., Somerville, New Jersey

IRONSIDE, JAMES, Pathology Neuropathology Lab., University of Edinburgh, Scotland, United Kingdom

ISENMANN, STEFAN, Max Planck-Institut fur Entwicklungs Biologie I, Tuebingen, Germany

JALONEN, TUULA, Dept. of Neurosurgery, Albany Medical College, Albany, New York

JENNINGS, CHARLES, *Nature*, Washington, D.C.

JOHNSON, EDWIN, Sibia Neurosciences Electrophysiology, La Jolla, California

JOHO, ROLF, Dept. of Cell Biology and Neuroscience, University of Texas Southwestern Medical Center, Dallas, Texas

JONAK, GERALD, Central Nervous System Disease Research, DuPont Merck Pharmaceutical Co., Inc., Wilmington, Delaware

JONES, ELIZABETH, Dept. of Pharmacology, Yale University School of Medicine, New Haven, Connecticut

KANDEL, ERIC, Center for Neurobiology and Behavior, Columbia University/Howard Hughes Medical Institute, New York, New York

KARAYIORGOU, MARIA, Human Neurogenetics Laboratory, Rockefeller University, New York, New York

KATZ, LARRY, Dept. of Neurobiology, Duke University Medical Center, Durham, North Carolina

KAUFMANN, CHARLES, Dept. of Psychiatry, Columbia University, New York, New York

KELNER, KATRINA, *Science*, Washington, D.C.

KIMELBERG, HAROLD, Dept. of Neurosurgery, Albany Medical College, New York

KIORPES, LYNNE, New York University Center for Neural Science, New York, New York

KIRSCH, DONALD, American Cyanamid Company, Molecular Genetics Screen Design, Princeton, New Jersey

KLAR, AMAR, Frederick Cancer Research and Development Center, ABL-Basic Research Program, Frederick, Maryland

KLOMP, LEONARD, Dept. of Pediatrics, Washington University, St. Louis, Missouri

KNEUSSEL, MATTHIAS, Dept. of Pharmacology, University College, London, United Kingdom

KOGAN, JEFFREY, Cold Spring Harbor Laboratory, Cold Spring Harbor, New York

KOLLMAR, RICHARD, Dept. of Sensory Neuroscience, Rockefeller University, New York, New York

KOOTHAN, THILLAI, Cold Spring Harbor Laboratory, Cold Spring Harbor, New York

KRANTZ, DAVID, Dept. of Neurology, University of California, San Francisco

KRETZSCHMAR, DORIS, Zoology Institut für Entwicklungsbiologie, Universitat Regensburg, Germany

KRYLOVA, OLGA, University College of London Anatomy and Developmental Biology, United Kingdom

KUMAR, LALITH, Dept. of Psychiatry, Henry Ford Hospital, Detroit, Michigan

KURODA, YOICHIRO, Dept. of Molecular and Cellular Neurobiology, Tokyo Metropolitan Institute for Neuroscience, Japan

KUWANA, YOSHIHISA, Dept. of Neurology, Kyowa Hakko Kogyo Co., Ltd., Shizuoka, Japan

LAMPE, RICHARD, Dept. of Respiratory, Inflammation, and Neuroscience, Zeneca Pharmaceuticals, Wilmington, Delaware

LAN, NANCY, Scientific Affairs and Intellectual Properties, Cocensys Inc., Irvine, California

LANDIS, STORY, NINDS/National Institutes of Health, Bethesda, Maryland

LEDOUX, JOSEPH, Dept. of Neural Science, New York University, New York, New York

LEGOUIS, RENAUD, Dept. of Biotechnologies, Institut Pasteur, Paris, France

LIEBERMAN, ANDREW, Dept. of Pathology, Hospital of the University of Pennsylvania, Philadelphia

LINTS, THIERRY, Dept. of Physiology and Cellular Biophysics, Columbia University, New York, New York

LIU, QING, Howard Hughes Medical Institute, University of Pennsylvania, Philadelphia

LIVINGSTONE, MARGARET, Dept. of Neurobiology, Harvard Medical School, Boston, Massachusetts

LO ZENECA, MATHEW, Dept. of Biomedical Research,

Pharmaceuticals, Inc., Wilmington, Delaware

LU, SHAO-MING, Hohhs Lab., Dept. of Developmental Neuroscience, Vanderbilt University, Nashville, Tennessee

LUPSKI, JAMES, Dept. of Molecular and Human Genetics, Baylor College of Medicine, Houston, Texas

LUQUE, FRANCISCO, Dept. of Neurology, New York Medical College, Valhalla

MACDONALD, MARCY, Dept. of Genetics, Massachusetts General Hospital, Charlestown

MAGAZIN, MARILYN, Sanofi Recherche Biochemistry, Labege Innopole Labege, France

MALHERBE, F. PARI, Pharma Division, Hoffmann La Roche Ltd., Basel, Switzerland

MANDEL, JEAN-LOUIS, IGBMC, Illkirch, France

MARCHIONNI, MARK, Dept. of Molecular Biology, Cambridge NeuroScience, Inc., Massachusetts

MARGOLSKEE, ROBERT, Dept. of Physiology and Biophysics, Mt. Sinai School of Medicine, New York, New York

MARTINS, VILMA, Fundacao Antonio Prudende Research Center, San Paulo, Brazil

MASKOS, UWE, LMB/NINDS, National Institutes of Health, Bethesda, Maryland

MASTERS, COLIN, Dept. of Pathology, University of Melbourne, Parkville, Victoria, Australia

MAUE, ROBERT, Dept. of Physiology, Dartmouth Medical School, Hanover, New Hampshire

MCGUFFIN, PETER, Dept. of Psychological Medicine, University of Wales College of Medicine, United Kingdom

MCNAMARA, JAMES, Dept. of Medicine, Neurobiology, and Pharmacology, Duke University Medical Center, Durham, North Carolina

MERZENICH, MICHAEL, Dept. of Otolaryngology/Physiology, University of California School of Medicine, San Francisco

MIHALY, ANDRAS, Dept. of Anatomy, Kuwait University, Faculty of Medicine

MIINEA, CRISTINEL, Biochemistry HSC, Houston, Texas

MIZUNO, KEIKO, LDN, NICHD, National Institutes of Health, Bethesda, Maryland

MOBLEY, WILLIAM, Dept. of Neurology, University of California, San Francisco

MOMBAERTS, PETER, Rockefeller University, New York, New York

MOSS, ROBERT, Dept. of Physiology, University of Texas Southwestern Medical Center, Dallas

MOVSHON, J. ANTHONY, New York University Center for Neural Science/Howard Hughes Medical Institute, New York, New York

MULVIHILL, EILEEN, Dept. of Immunology and Molecular Biology, Darwin Molecular Inc., Bothell, Washington

NAEF, ROLAND, Swiss Federal Institute of Technology, Institute of Cell Biology, Zuench, Switzerland

NAEVE, GREG, Dept. of Molecular Biology, Amgen, Thousand Oaks, California

NAKAI, SHIGEYASU, Dept. of Cell Biology, Cancer Institute, Tokyo, Japan

NAKANISHI, SHIGETADA, Dept. of Biological Sciences, Kyoto University, Faculty of Medicine, Japan

NAWA, HIROYUKI, Niigara University, Brain Research Institute, Niigata, Japan

NERI, CHRISTIAN, CEPH Neurogenetic Disorders, Paris, France

NISHI, MAYUMI, Dept. of Biology, New York University, New York, New York

NOEBELS, JEFFREY, Dept. of Neurology, Baylor College of Medicine, Houston, Texas

NORTH, GEOFFREY, *Current Biology*, London, United Kingdom

NOTTEBOHM, FERNANDO, Dept. of Animal Behavior, Rockefeller University Field Research Center, Millbrook, New York

OGILVIE, ALAN, MRC Morningside Brain Metabolism Unit, Royal Edinburgh Hospital, Scotland, United Kingdom

OHSHIMA, KEIICHI, Dept. of Biosciences and Technology, Texas A&M University, Houston

OKUSE, KENJI, Dept. of Anatomy and Developmental Biology, University College of London, United Kingdom

OLIVER, KEVIN, Dept. of Pharmacology, Merck Sharp and Dohme, Essex, United Kingdom

ORR, HARRY, Dept. of Human Genetics, University of Minnesota, Minneapolis

OTOMO, JUN, Advanced Research Laboratory, Hitachi, Ltd., Saitama, Japan

OZSARAC, NESRIN, Dept. of Biochemistry and Molecular Genetics, University of New South Wales, Sydney, Australia

PAGLIUSI, SONIA, Dept. of Neurobiology, Glaxo Institute for Molecular Biology, Geneva, Switzerland

PATIL, NILA, Dept. of Genetics, Stanford University Medical Center, Stanford, California

PEUNOVA, NATALIA, Cold Spring Harbor Laboratory, Cold Spring Harbor, New York

PHAN, MIMI, Dept. of Neuroscience, University of California, Davis

PHILLIPS, HEIDI, Dept. of Neuroscience, Genentech, South San Francisco, California

PICHEL, JOSE, Mammalian Genes and Development, NICHD/National Institutes of Health, Bethesda, Maryland

PLUMIER, JEAN-CHRISTOPHE, Dept. of Anatomy and Neurobiology, Dalhousie University, Halifax, Nova Scotia, Canada

POLLOCK, JONATHAN, Dept. of Biological Sciences, Purdue University, Lilly Hall of Life Sciences, West Lafayette, Indiana
PRICE, DONALD, Dept. of Neuropathology, Johns Hopkins University School of Medicine, Baltimore, Maryland
PRICE, RICHARD, Dept. of Neurology, San Francisco General Hospital, California
PROSSER, HAYDN, Massachusetts Institute of Technology Center for Cancer Research, Cambridge
PRUSINER, STANLEY, Dept. of Neurology, University of California, San Francisco
PULVER, ANN, Dept. of Psychiatry, Johns Hopkins University School of Medicine, Baltimore, Maryland
RAICHLE, MARCUS, Dept. of Radiological Sciences, Washington University School of Medicine, St. Louis, Missouri
RAMACHANDRAN, VILAYANUR, Dept. of Psychology, University of California, San Diego, La Jolla
RAO, TADIMETI, Dept. of Neuropharmacology, Sibia Neuroscience Inc., La Jolla, California
REED, RANDALL, Dept. of Molecular Biology and Genetics, Johns Hopkins University, Baltimore, Maryland
ROBERTSON, MIRANDA, Garland Publishing, Middlesex House, London, United Kingdom
RODRIGUS, ROLAND, I.C.P.U.C.L. Virology, Brussels, Belgium
ROSBASH, MICHAEL, Dept. of Biology, Brandeis University/Howard Hughes Medical Institute, Waltham, Massachusetts
ROSS, CHRISTOPHER, Dept. of Psychiatry and Neuroscience, Johns Hopkins Medical Institutions, Baltimore, Maryland
ROVELLI, GIORGIO, Dept. of Molecular and Cellular Biology, Ciba-Geigy Ltd., Basel, Switzerland
RUIZ-AVILA, LUIS, Dept. of Physiology and Biophysics, Mt. Sinai School of Medicine, New York, New York
RUSANESCU, GABRIEL, Dept. of Neurobiology, State University of New York, Stony Brook
SACHDEV, ROBERT, Dept. of Developmental Neuroscience, Vanderbilt University, Nashville, Tennessee
SAHASRABUDHE, SUDHIR, Dept. of Molecular Neurobiology, Hoechst Marion Roussel Pharmaceuticals, Inc., Somerville, New Jersey
SASSONE-CORSI, PAOLO, CNRS IGBMC, Strasbourg, France
SAYEED, OMER, Dept. of Biology, California Institute of Technology, Pasadena, California
SCHOEPFER, RALF, Dept. of Pharmacology, University College, London, United Kingdom
SCHOFIELD, PETER, Garvan Institute of Medical Research, Sydney, New South Wales, Australia
SCHUMACHER, MICHAEL, Inserm, France
SCOTT, KRISTIN, Dept. of Biology, University of California, San Diego, La Jolla
SELKOE, DENNIS, Dept. of Neurological Diseases, Harvard Medical School, Brigham and Womens Hospital, Boston, Massachusetts
SHAH, NIRAO, Dept. of Biology, California Institute of Technology, Pasadena
SHANK, RICHARD, Dept. of Pharmaceutical Research, R.W. Johnson Pharmaceutical Research Institute Spring House, Pennsylvania
SHEN, JIE, Massachusetts Institute of Technology Center for Cancer Research, Cambridge
SHEN, LIYA, Mammalian Gene and Development/NICHD, National Institutes of Health, Bethesda, Maryland
SIDDIQUE, TEEPU, Northwestern University Medical School, Chicago, Illinois
SIDDIQUI, SHAHID, Dept. of Ecological Engineering, Toyohashi University of Technology, Japan
SIEGEL, VIVIAN, *Cell*, Cambridge, Massachusetts
SILOS, INMACULADA, Dept. of Molecular Oncology, Bristol-Myers Squibb, Princeton, New Jersey
SILVA, ALCINO, Cold Spring Harbor Laboratory, Cold Spring Harbor, New York
SINGLE, FRANK NICOLAI, ZMBH Center for Molecular Biology, University of Heidelberg, Germany
SIOMI, HARUHIKO, Dept. of Biochemistry and Biophysics, University of Pennsylvania School of Medicine, Philadelphia
SMIGA, SUSAN, Dept. of Psychiatry, University of California, San Francisco
SMITH-SWINTOSKY, VIRGINIA, CNS Drug Discovery, R.W. Johnson Pharmaceutical Research Institute, Spring House, Pennsylvania
SPILLANTINI, MARIA GRAZIA, Dept. of Molecular Biology, Medical Research Council, Cambridge, United Kingdom
SQUIRE, LARRY, Veterans Administration Medical Center, La Jolla, San Diego, California
ST. GEORGE-HYSLOP, PETER, Dept. of Medicine, University of Toronto, Ontario, Canada
STEBBINS, MICHAEL, Cold Spring Harbor Laboratory, Cold Spring Harbor, New York
STILLMAN, BRUCE, Cold Spring Harbor Laboratory, Cold Spring Harbor, New York
STRAUB, RICHARD, Dept. of Psychiatry, Medical College of Virginia, Richmond
STRICKLAND, SIDNEY, Dept. of Pharmacology, University Medical Center at Stony Brook, New York
STRITTMATTER, WARREN, Dept. of Neurology, Duke University Medical Center, Durham, North Carolina
STRYKER, MICHAEL, Dept. of Physiology, University

of California Medical School, San Francisco

STUTZMANN, GRACE, Dept. of Neural Science, New York University, New York, New York

SWAIN, AMANDA, Dept. of Developmental Genetics, National Institute for Medical Research, London, United Kingdom

SZEKELY, ANNA, Dept. of Neurology, Yale University Medical School, New Haven, Connecticut

TAKAHASHI, JOSEPH, Dept. of Neurobiology and Physiology, Northwestern University, Evanston, Illinois

TALAN, JAMIE, *Newsday*, Melville, New York

TEKIRIAN, TINA, Dept. of Anatomy and Neurobiology, University of Kentucky, Sanders-Brown Alzheimers Disease Research Center, Lexington

THALER, JOSHUA, Dept. of Biomedical Sciences, Ludwig Institute for Cancer Research, La Jolla, California

THOENEN, HANS, Max Planck Institute for Psychiatry Neurochemistry, Martinsried, Germany

TONEGAWA, SUSUMU, Massachusetts Institute of Technology Center for Learning and Memory, Cambridge

TRANEL, DANIEL, Dept. of Neurology and Psychology, University of Iowa College of Medicine

TREMP, GUNTER, Rhone-Poulene Rorer Central Research 13, Vitry-sur-Seine, France

TROEMEL, EMILY, Dept. of Anatomy, University of California, San Francisco

TSIRKA, STELLA, Dept. of Pharmacology, State University of New York, Stony Brook

TULLY, TIM, Cold Spring Harbor Laboratory, Cold Spring Harbor, New York

URNOV, FYODOR, Dept. of Biology and Medicine, Brown University, Providence, Rhode Island

VALLEE, RICHARD, Dept. of Cell Biology, Worcester Foundation for Experimental Biology, Shrewsbury, Massachusetts

VEZZONI, PAOLO, Consiglio Nazionale delle Ricerche Insituto Di Tecnologie Biomediche Avanzate, Milano, Italy

WALKER, PHILIPPE, Astra Pain Research Unit, Armand Frappier, Laval, Quebec, Canada

WALLIN, JOHAN, Astra Pain Control AB, Preclinical R & D Cellular and Molecular Pharmacology, Novum Unit Halsovagen 7, Huddinge, Sweden

WANG, ZUO-ZHONG, Dept. of Cell Biology, National Institutes of Health, Bethesda, Maryland

WARREN, STEPHEN, Dept. of Biochemistry, Emory University School of Medicine, Atlanta, Georgia

WAXHAM, NEAL, Dept. of Neurobiology and Anatomy, University of Texas Medical School, Houston

WEHR, ROLAND, Dept. of Molecular Cell Biology, Max Planck Institute of Biophysical Chemistry, Gottingen, Germany

WEISSMANN, CHARLES, University of Zurich Institut fur Molekularbiologie/ABT.I Honggerberg, Zurich, Switzerland

WELCHER, ANDREW, Dept. of Immunology, Amgen Inc., Thousand Oaks, California

WESTPHAL, HEINER, National Cancer Institute, Bethesda, Maryland

WEXLER, NANCY, Dept. of Psychiatry, Columbia University, New York, New York

WHITE, FROST, Dept. of Neuroscience, Pfizer Central Research, Groton, Connecticut

WICKELGREN, INGRID, Freelance journalist

WICKNER, REED, NIADDK Lab. of Biochemical Pharmacology, National Institutes of Health, Bethesda, Maryland

WILDENAUER, DIETER, Dept. of Psychiatry, University of Bonn, Germany

WILLE, HOLGER, Dept. of Neurology, University of California, San Francisco

WISHART, WILLIAM, Sandoz Pharma AG, Central Nervous System, Human Genome Group, Basel, Switzerland

WONG, PHILIP, Dept. of Pathology, Neuropathology, Johns Hopkins University School of Medicine, Baltimore, Maryland

WRIGHT, BEVERLY, Dept. of Physiology, University of California, San Francisco

XU, ZUOSHANG, Dept. of Neurobiology, Worcester Foundation for Biomedical Research, Shrewsbury, Massachusetts

YANCOPOULOS, GEORGE, Regeneron Pharmaceuticals, Inc., Tarrytown, New York

YANG, YANMIN, Dept. of Molecular Genetics and Cell Biology, University of Chicago/Howard Hughes Medical Institute, Illinois

YE, WEILAN, Dept. of Neuroscience, Genentech, South San Francisco, California

YOUNG, KATHLEEN, Dept. of Molecular Genetic Screen Design, American Cyanamid Company, Princeton, New Jersey

YOUNG, MICHAEL, Dept. of Genetics, Rockefeller University, Howard Hughes Medical Institute, New York, New York

ZALUTSKY, ROBERT, NINDS, National Institutes of Health, Bethesda, Maryland

ZENG, HONGKUI, Dept. of Biology, Brandeis University, Waltham, Massachusetts

ZOGHBI, HUDA, Dept. of Molecular and Human Genetics, Baylor College of Medicine, Houston, Texas

ZUKER, CHARLES, Dept. of Biology and Neurosciences, University of California, San Diego, La Jolla

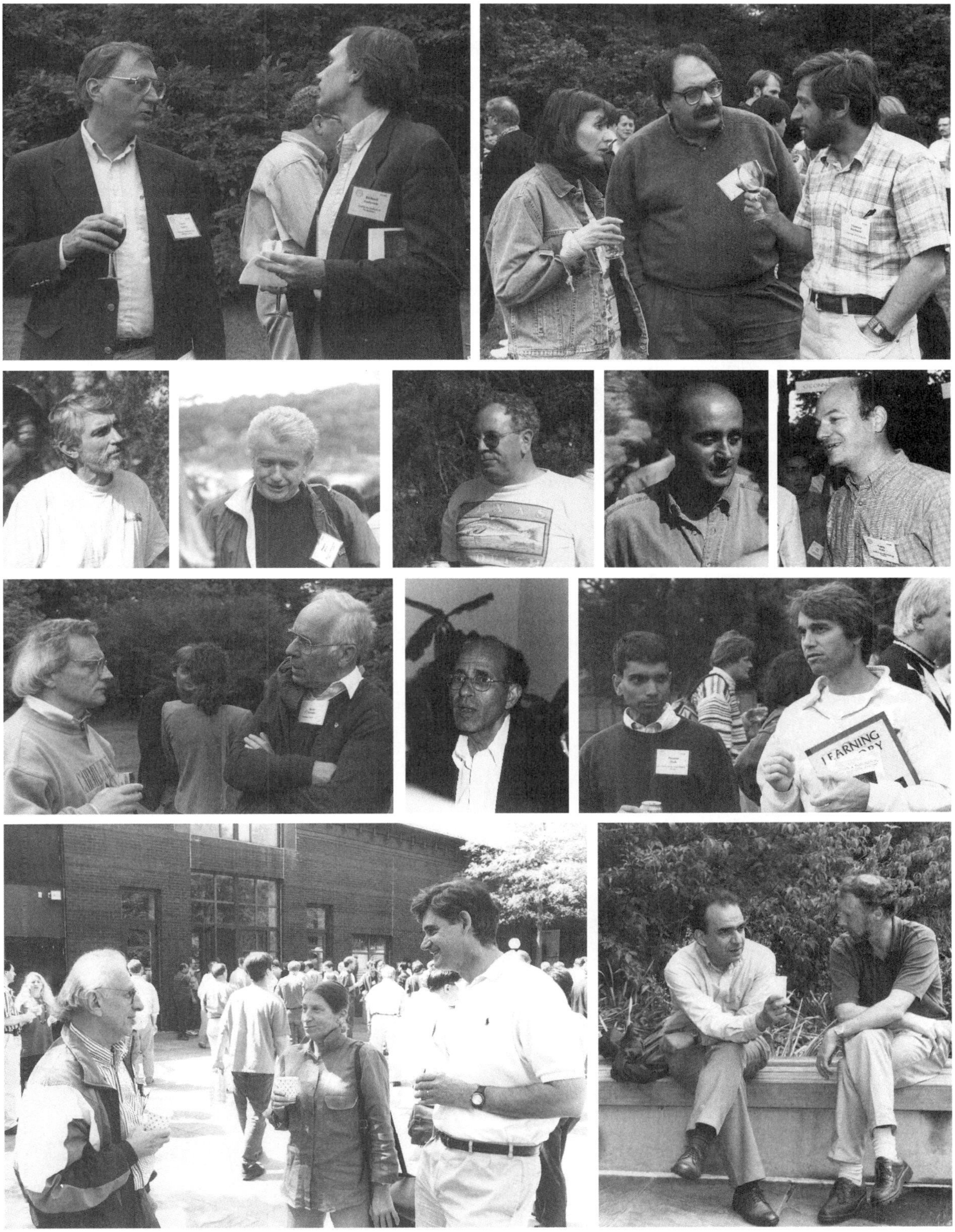

First row: L. Squire, R. Anderson; N. Peunova, G. Enikolopov, V. Buchman
Second row: Z. Hall; D. Price; J. Noebels; J. Witkowski, P. Sassone-Corsi; L. Katz
Third row: H. Blüthmann, H. Westphal; R. Axel; P. Dash, N. Waxham
Fourth row: E. Kandel, M. Robertson, B. Stillman; R. McKay, J. Inglis

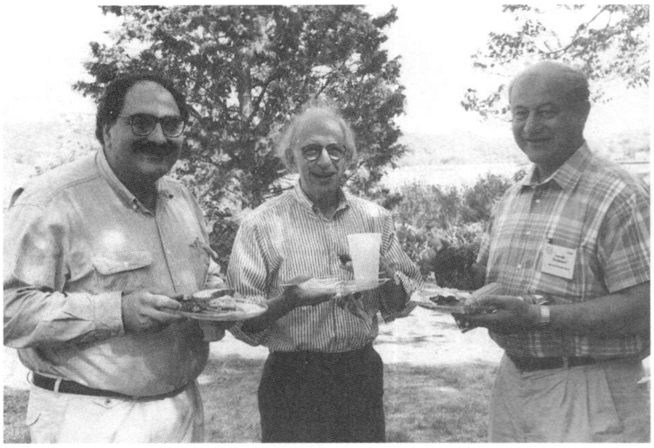
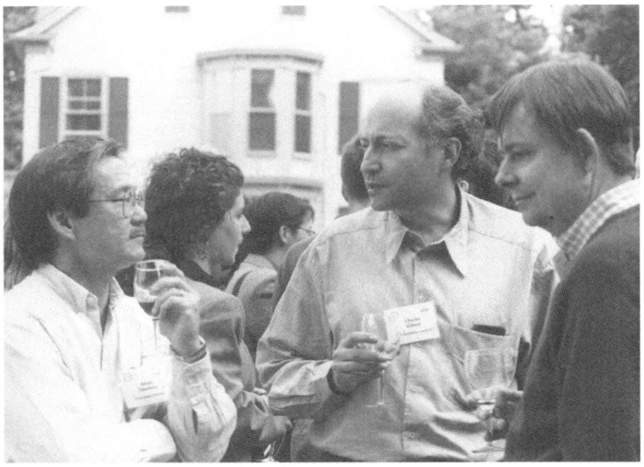
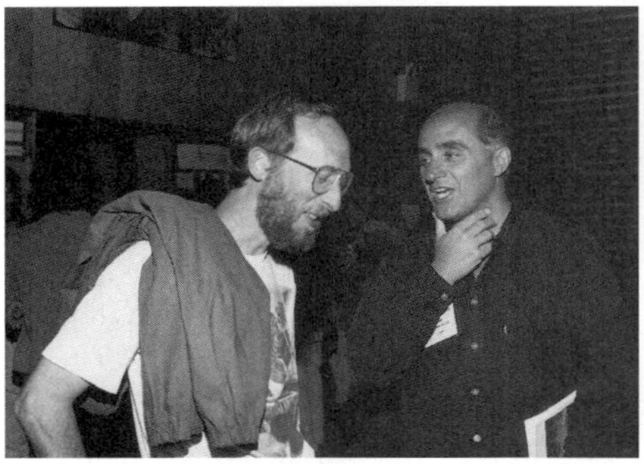
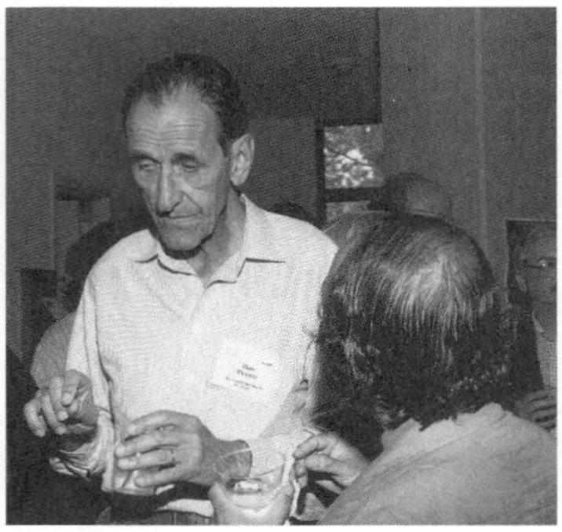
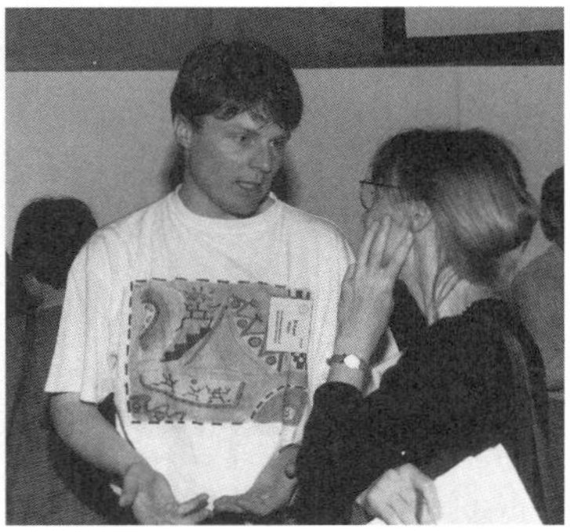
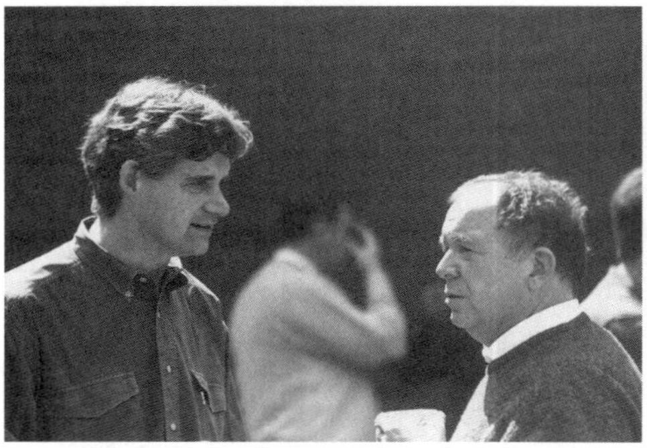
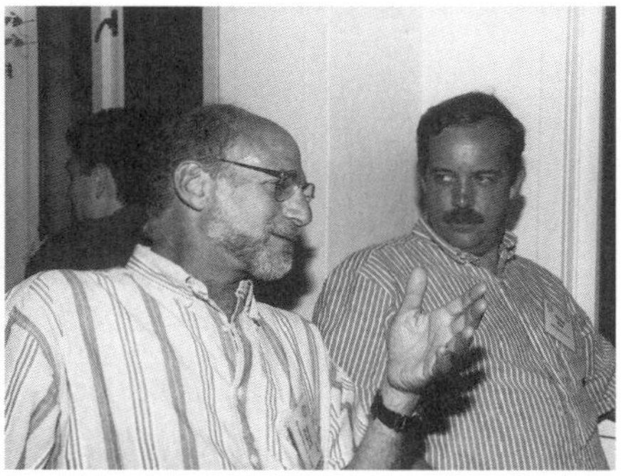
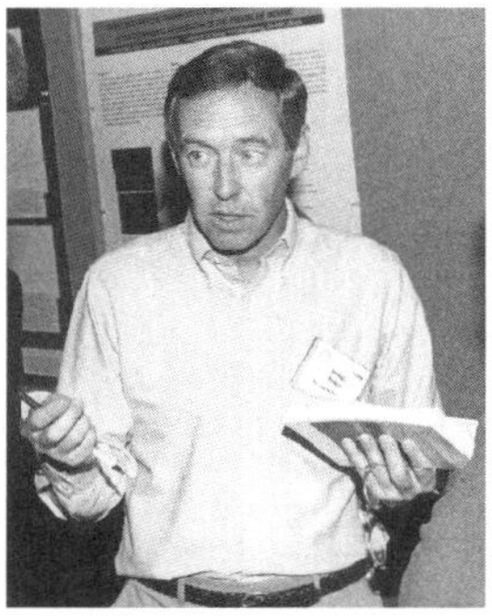
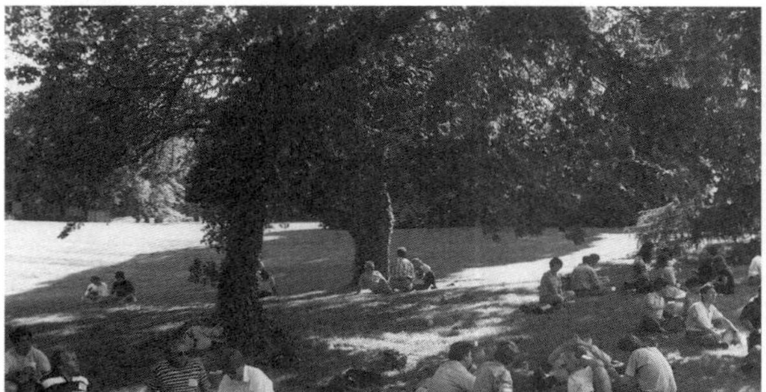
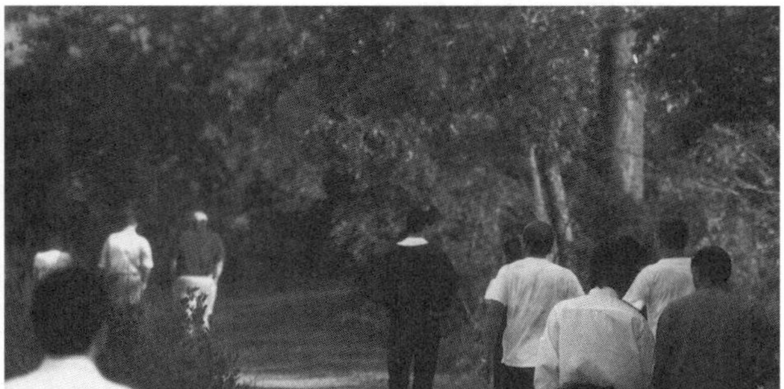

First row: G. Enikolopov, E. Kandel, G. Fischbach; J. Takahashi, C. Gilbert, G. Gasic
Second row: D. Cleveland, P. Sassone-Corsi; H. Thoenen, Y. Kuroda; R. Wehr, M. MacDonald
Third row: B. Stillman, J.P. Changeux; M. Rosbash, R. Reed; D. Selkoe
Fourth row: Picnic

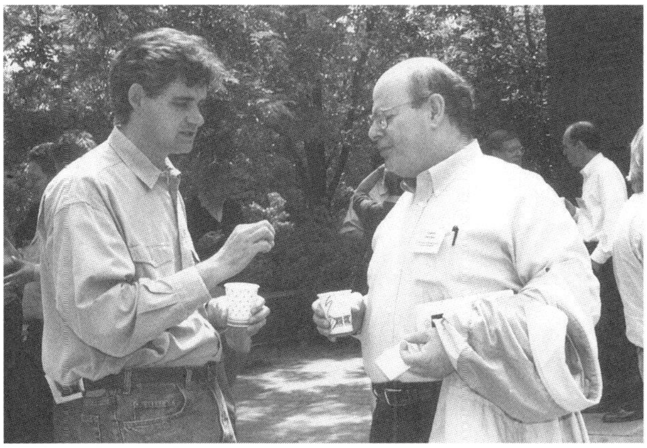
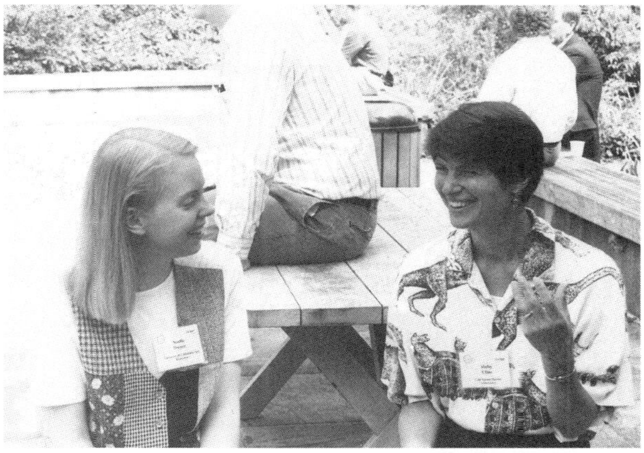
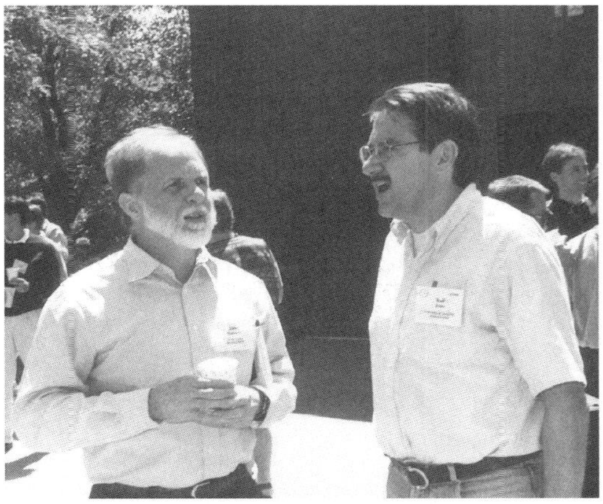
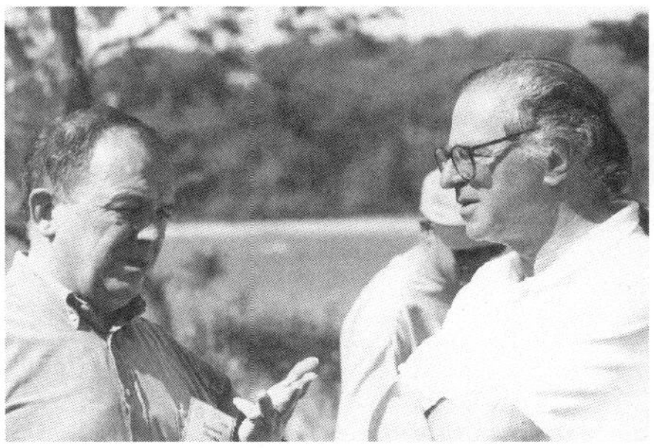
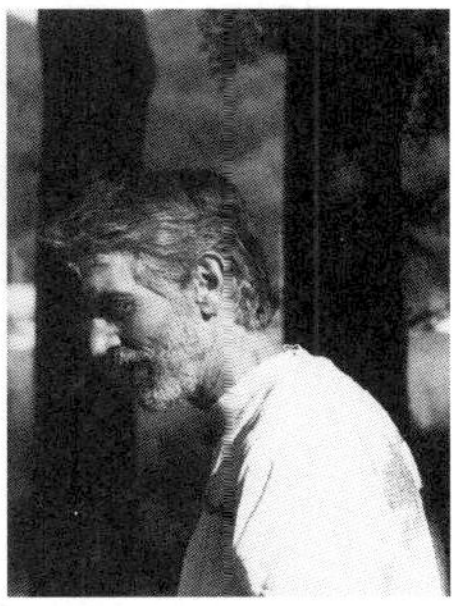
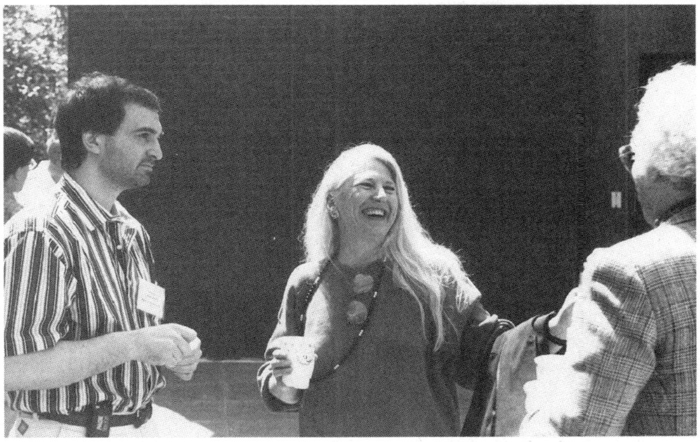
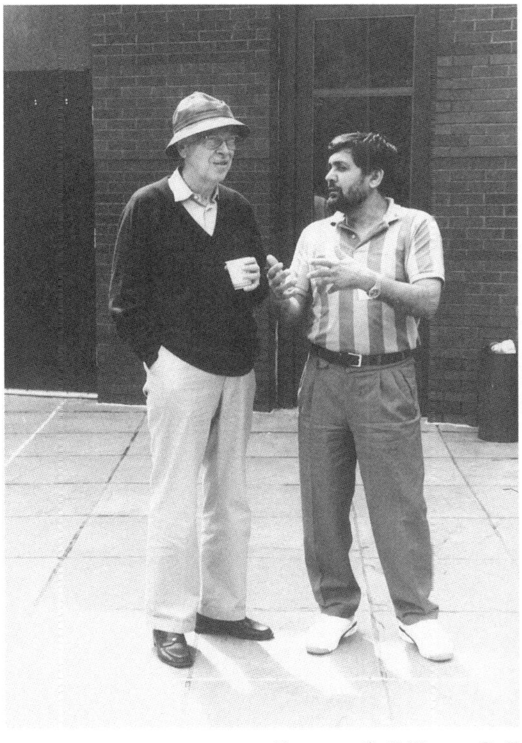
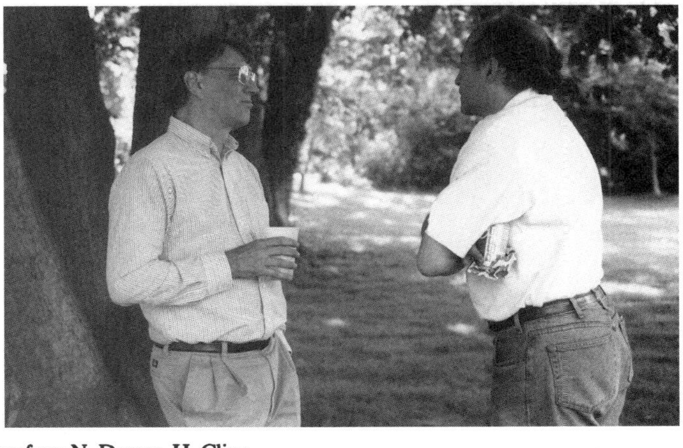

First row: B. Stillman, G. Dreyfuss; N. Dwyer, H. Cline
Second row: J. Hudspeth, R. Joho; J.P. Changeux, C. Weissmann; Z. Hall
Third row: J. Watson, A. Klar; G. Yancopoulos, N. Wexler, S. Prusiner
Fourth row: L. Squire, C. Gilbert

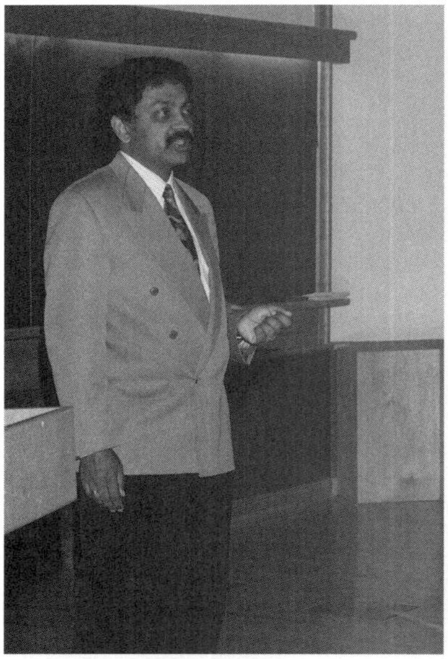
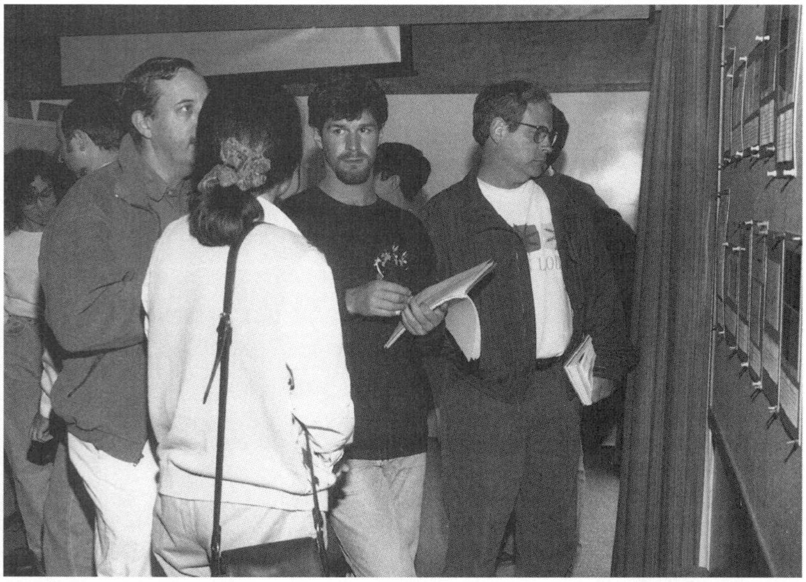
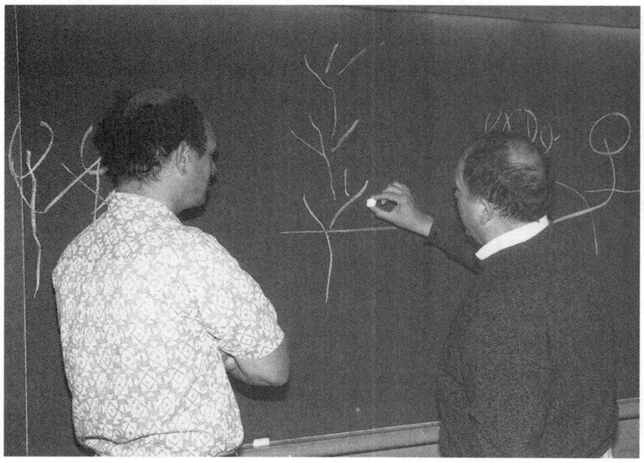
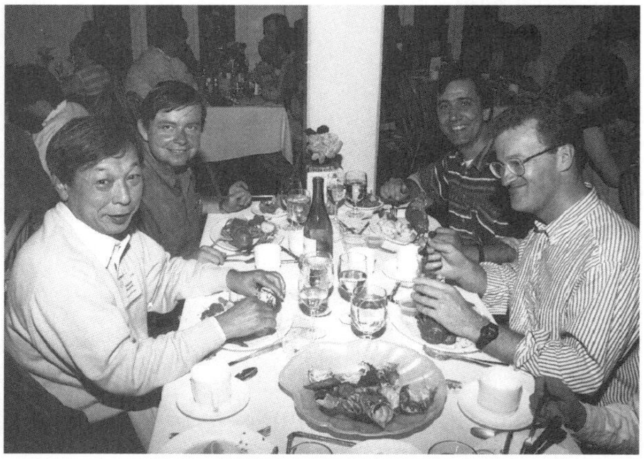
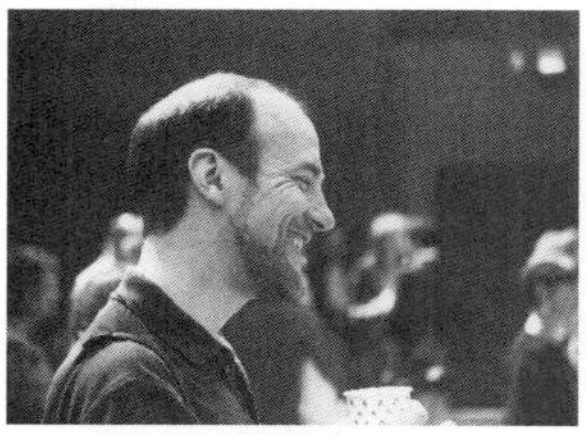
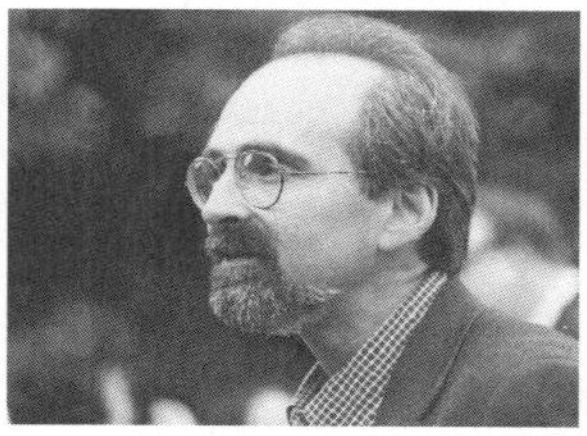
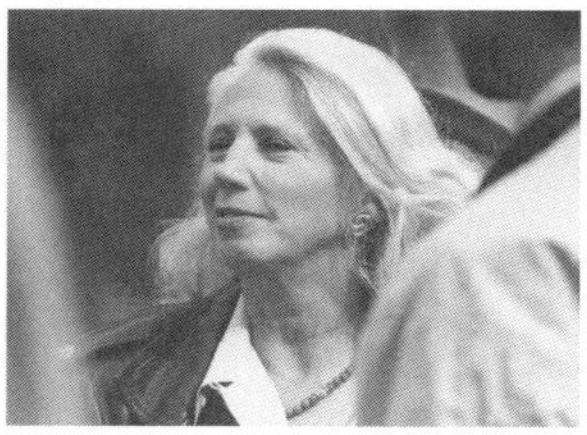
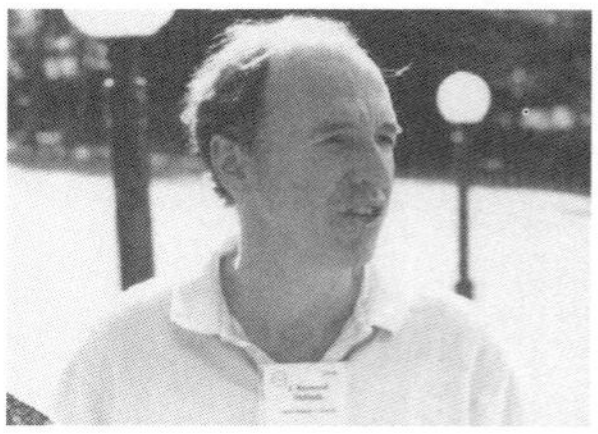
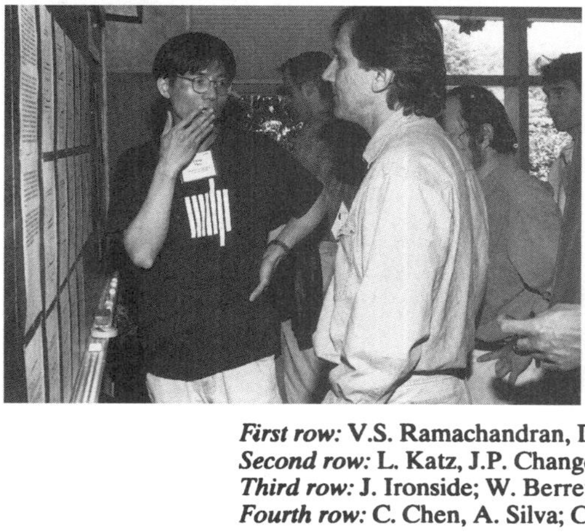
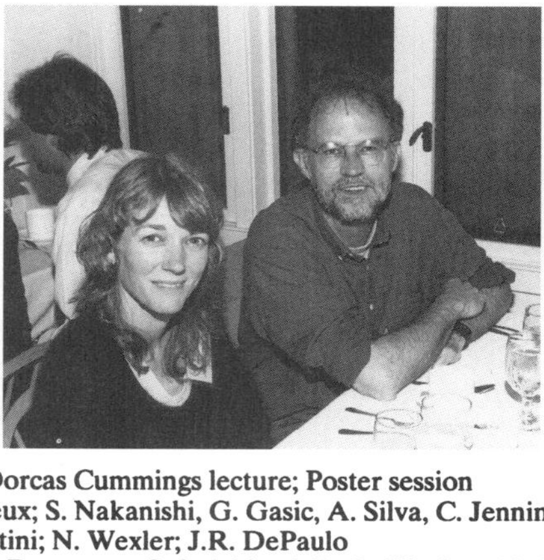
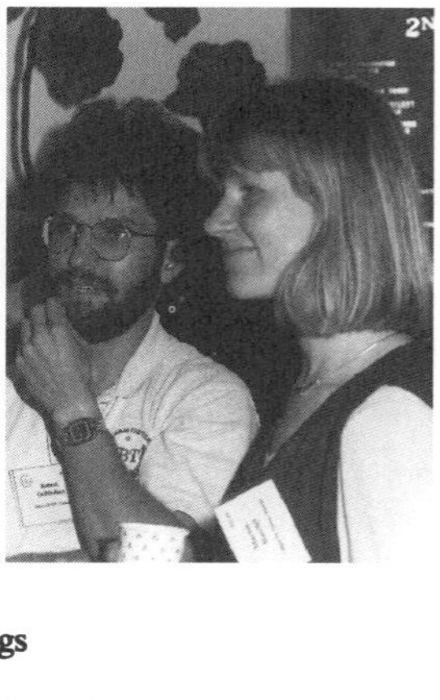

First row: V.S. Ramachandran, Dorcas Cummings lecture; Poster session
Second row: L. Katz, J.P. Changeux; S. Nakanishi, G. Gasic, A. Silva, C. Jennings
Third row: J. Ironside; W. Berrettini; N. Wexler; J.R. DePaulo
Fourth row: C. Chen, A. Silva; C. Bargmann, S. Strickland; R. Gellibolian, M. Haertel

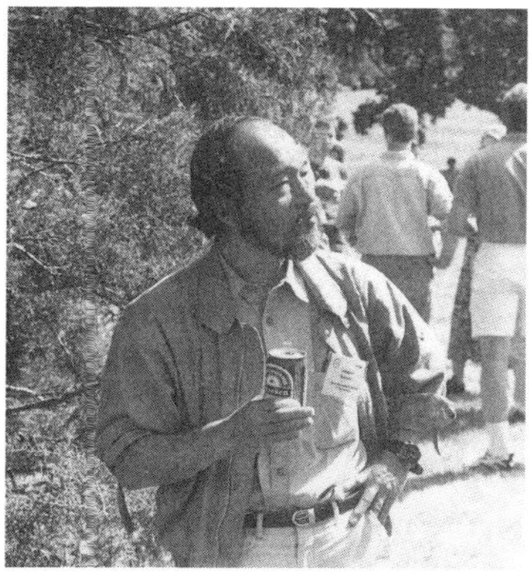
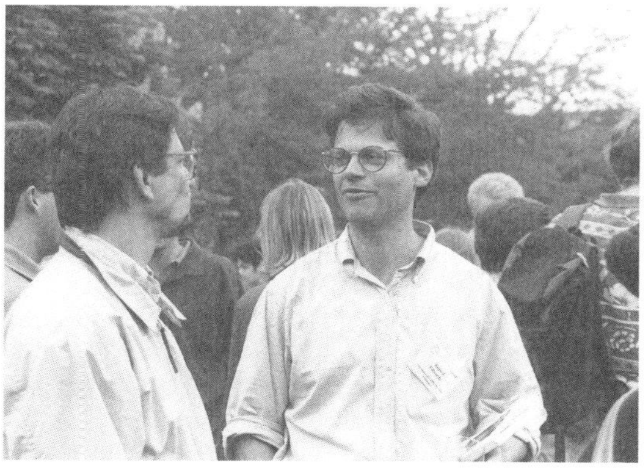
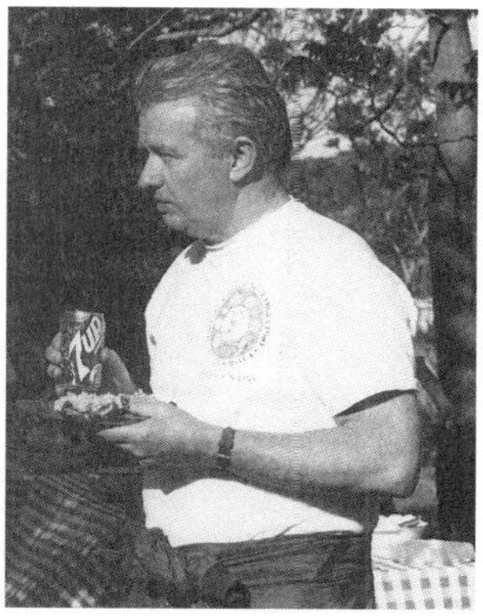
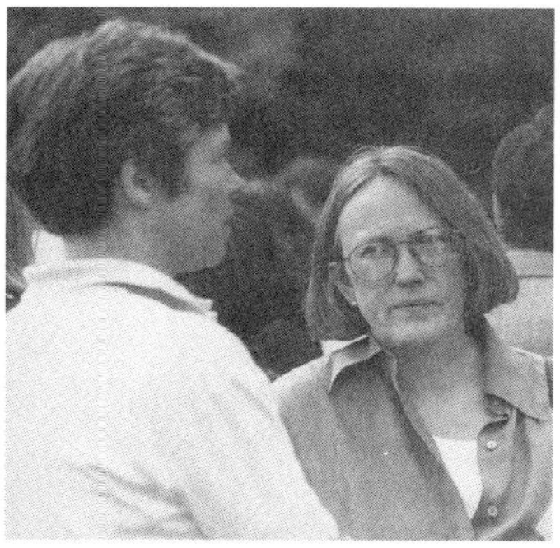
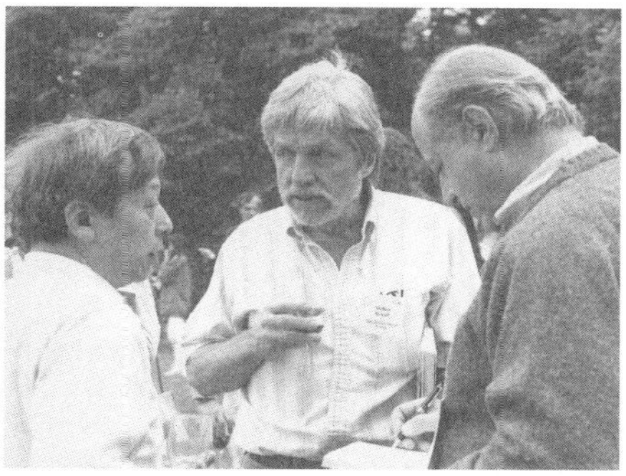
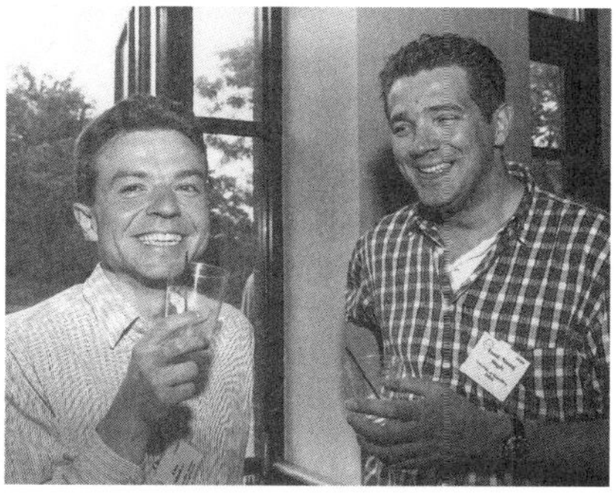
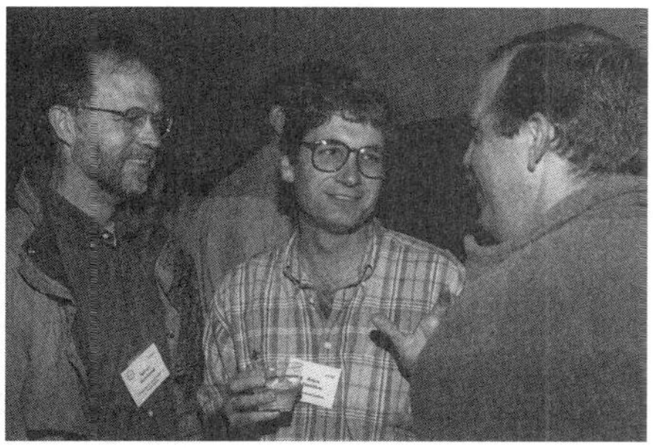
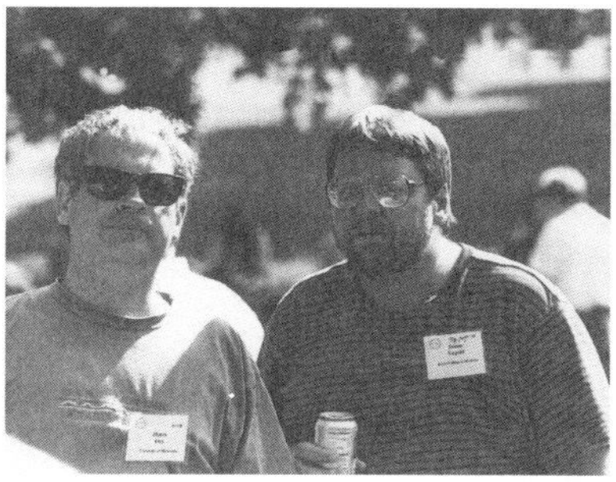
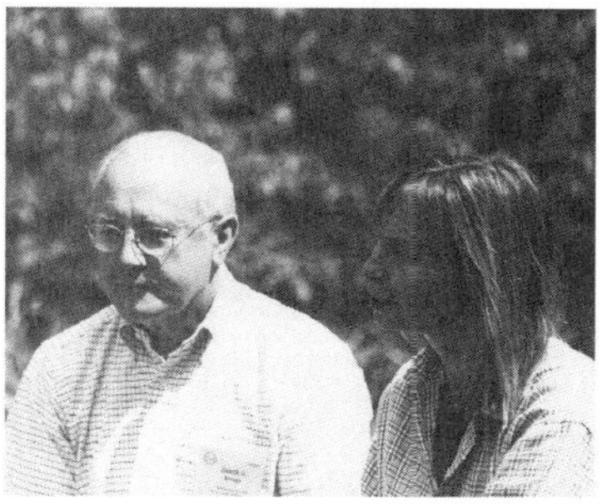
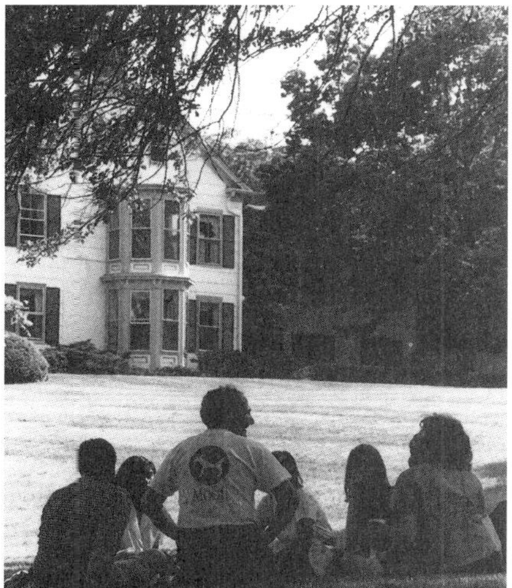
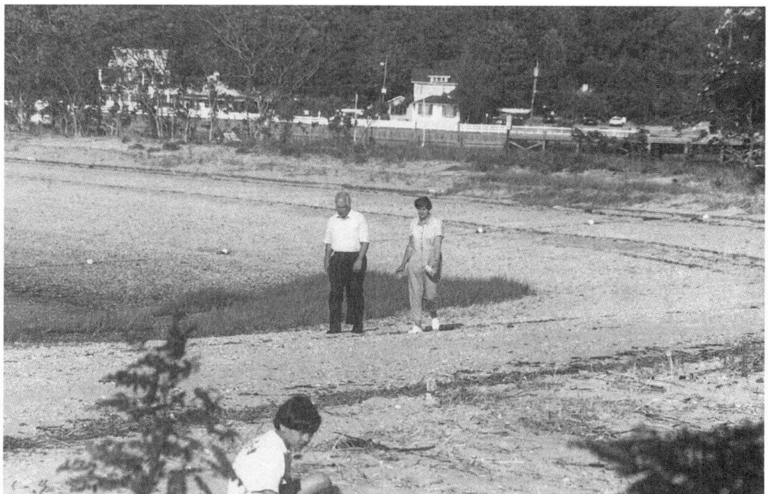

First row: Y. Kuroda; R. Malinow, R. Edwards; D. Price
Second row: M. Livingstone, S. Landis; S. Nakanishi, M. Bennett, G. Fischbach; U. Maskos, F. Nicolai-Single
Third row: S. Strickland, B. Hamilton, R. Reed; H. Orr, J. Lupski; J. Drage, M. MacDonald
Fourth row: Picnic

Foreword

It is inherent in our nature to want to understand all that is wrong, as well as what is right, with the biological systems that we study. Perhaps one of the most fascinating areas of biology where this is applicable is the nervous system. Increasingly, progress in biology is influenced by the diseases and maladies that afflict us. Diseases of the brain and the periphery of the nervous system afflict many millions throughout the world, and the problems are as varied as the biology itself. But as modern techniques allow us to probe ever more deeply, we are able to understand how small changes can greatly influence our health and behavior. By studying the disease processes, we uncover surprising new findings that influence all of biology. For example, the discovery of prions and their unusual inheritance resulted from interest in a infectious disease in the highlands of New Guinea.

The decision to hold the sixty-first Symposium on "Function and Dysfunction in the Nervous System" was driven by the belief that in the near future we will learn an enormous amount about how the nervous system works by simultaneously studying the diseases that affect it. These studies, in parallel with other studies on the normal function of the nervous system, will greatly advance neurobiology in much the same way that genetics of model organisms has hastened unexpected and fundamental discoveries. The goal of this meeting was to intermingle scientists interested in the study of systems neuroscience with those trying to understand how those systems fail, so that an overview of the problems in neurological diseases could be obtained. This was a somewhat risky venture because neurobiology is as varied as biology itself, and the bringing together of investigators with diverse interests can create a hodgepodge of science that does not interest anyone. But the diseases of the nervous system are as fascinating as biology gets and it was well worth the risk.

Some Symposia celebrate past accomplishments in fields of biology, but this one looked mostly to the future, which we hope, and even expect, is an exciting one. I anticipate that this Symposium will provide a stepping stone for future progress. The current meeting could not have been organized without the great help of several colleagues, including Eric Kandel, Stan Prusiner, Richard Axel, Conrad Gilliam, Gideon Dreyfuss, and Tony Movshon. The formal scientific program consisted of 86 speakers and 94 poster presentations, and the meeting attracted 281 participants. Introductory talks on the first evening were from Michael Merzenich, Eric Kandel, Stan Prusiner, Richard Price, and Ann Pulver. The second Reginald G. Harris Lecture was delivered by Richard Axel, who presented his exciting work on olfaction. V.S. Ramachandran gave a fascinating Dorcas Cummings Lecture to our friends and neighbors about the illusions of the body image, and was widely acclaimed.

Essential funds to run this meeting were obtained from the National Institute of Neurological Disorders and Stroke and the Du Pont Merck Pharmaceutical Company. In addition, the financial help from the Corporate Sponsors of our meetings program is essential for these meetings to remain a success, and we are grateful for their continued support. These sponsors are: Alza Corporation; Amgen Inc.; BASF Bioresearch Corporation; Becton Dickinson and Company; Boehringer Mannheim Corporation; Bristol-Myers Squibb Company; Chiron Corporation; Chugal Research Institute for Molecular Medicine, Inc.; Diagnostic Products Corporation; The Du Pont Merck Pharmaceutical Company; Forest Laboratories, Inc.; Genentech, Inc.; Hoechst Marion Roussel, Inc.; Hoffmann-La Roche Inc.; Johnson & Johnson; Kyowa Hakko Kogyo Co., Ltd.; Life Technologies, Inc.; Eli Lilly and Company; Oncogene Science, Inc.; Pall Corporation; The Perkin-Elmer Corporation, Applied Biosystems Division; Pfizer Inc.; Pharmacia & Upjohn, Inc.; Research Genetics, Inc.; Sandoz Research Institute; Schering-Plough Corporation; Sumitomo Pharmaceuticals Co., Ltd.; Wyeth-Ayerst Research; and Zeneca Group PLC.

I thank the staff, in particular Diane Tighe, in our meetings and courses office, under the able direction of David Stewart, for their efficient and outstanding organization of this meeting. Mary Horton competently handled the various grant applications, and Herb Parsons and his staff provided excellent audiovisual assistance. The organization of this meeting relied on the essential work of my assistant Delia King. It was again a pleasure to work with the Laboratory Press, under the direction of John Inglis, particularly Nancy Ford, Patricia Barker, Joan Ebert, and Elaine Gaveglia. This year marks Nancy's retirement from the Cold

Spring Harbor Laboratory Press. She has shepherded the annual Symposium volumes for the past 24 years. Throughout that time, biology has undergone a revolution that has been recorded in these pages, and Nancy Ford played a great role in recording this important story. We wish her all the best.

Bruce Stillman
March 1997

Contents

COLD SPRING HARBOR SYMPOSIA ON QUANTITATIVE BIOLOGY

VOLUME LXI

Cortical Plasticity Underlying Perceptual, Motor, and Cognitive Skill Development: Implications for Neurorehabilitation

M. MERZENICH, B. WRIGHT, W. JENKINS,[1] C. XERRI,[2] N. BYL, S. MILLER,[1] AND P. TALLAL[3]
Keck Center for Integrative Neurosciences, University of California, San Francisco, California 94143-0732

During the past decade, there has emerged a new understanding of how changes in the brain account for perceptual, cognitive, and motor skill learning. Studies have shown that the brain reorganizes its effective inputs and local circuits through the course of learning. With skill mastery, brain representations are demonstrably specialized in the various specific tasks that underlie skill performance. This capacity for brain "remodeling" is lifelong.

To cite a very simple example, we trained New World owl monkeys and squirrel monkeys to pick up small round objects (food pellets) from shallow wells on a flat surface (Nudo et al. 1996a; C. Xerri et al., in prep.). The objects were about 1/3 the diameter of the slender fingers of these monkeys. This task required that a monkey fully extend its arm, differentially control and drop one or two or three fingers into a shallow well, palpate the pellet at the bottom of the well and manipulate it to remove it, grasp the small round object as it was ejected from the well, and carry it up to the mouth.

Performance was invariably initially ragged; the round pellet was usually fumbled and dropped during early attempts. However, performance improved dramatically with practice. In a few days, after a few hundred or thousand "practice trials," small-object retrieval was nearly flawless. Few pellets were dropped. The daily allotment of 100 pellets was picked up in a short working time period. The hand and arm movements were fluid, the grasp of the small objects decisive and secure, and the movement sequence beautifully stereotyped for success.

After skill mastery, examination of several cortical areas revealed a "new" brain that was highly specialized for this simple task (Nudo et al. 1996a; C. Xerri et al., in prep.). Areas of the brain representing somatosensation (SI cortical areas 3b and 1) were elaborated, specifically for that area of skin that the individual monkey used to palpate, manipulate, and control the grasp of these small round objects (C. Xerri et al., in prep.). The much more refined information from this exercised skin derived from this elaborated, far more topographically detailed representation presumably supported the more reliable perception of the surfaces, shapes, and movements of these small round objects as they were palpated and manipulated as a critical part of grasping and retrieving them.

When the region of the brain that represents sensory information from muscles was examined, it was also clearly specialized. The brain representation of sensory information fed back from muscles and joints (SI cortical area 3a) was now more refined, specifically supporting the more precise and differentiated movements that the monkey had to develop to perfect this small-object manipulation and grasping.

When the area represesenting movement output control patterns (cortical area 4) was examined, it was found to be specialized to elaborate and refine the representations of just those special movements and movement combinations that must occur for a reliable, almost-always-successful motor act (Nudo et al. 1996a).

In fact, if you could look all across the brain in a subject trained at a simple sensorimotor skill like this one, studies documenting behavioral specific response properties of neurons in trained monkeys indicate that you would presumably record major changes in neural activity within 15 or 20 cortical areas (Aizawa et al. 1991; Mitz et al. 1991; Germain and Lamarre 1993; Merzenich and Samashima 1993; Aosaki et al. 1994; Merzenich and Jenkins 1994). Each area would have undergone progressive change as it plays its special role in the progressive learning of the simple skill. Tens of millions or hundreds of millions of neurons would have changed the way they respond through the course of learning this skill. Billions of synaptic connections providing extrinsic inputs or linking brain cells to one another will have been changed. Collectively, this dramatic brain remodeling almost certainly *is* the cortical part of the skill acquisition.

Present addresses: [1]Scientific Learning Corp., 417 Montgomery Street, Suite 500, San Francisco, California 94104; [2]Laboratoire de Neurobiologie des Restaurations Fonctionelles, Université de Provence, Centre de Saint-Jérome, 13397 Marseille Cedex 14, France; [3]Center for Molecular and Behavioral Neuroscience, 197 University Avenue, Rutgers, The State University of New Jersey, Newark, New Jersey 07102.

CONSEQUENCES OF "MINISTROKES" INDUCED IN THESE CORTICAL ZONES

Cortical lesions have been introduced into two of these remodeled cortical zones in monkeys trained at this small-object retrieval task (Nudo et al. 1996b; C. Xerri et al., in prep.). A lesion that completely destroyed the behaviorally elaborated representations in cortical area 3b of just those fingertip surfaces that a monkey used to palpate and grasp the small objects resulted in a marked degradation of the earlier-mastered retrieval behavior (C. Xerri et al., in prep.). A New World monkey suffering such a microlesion that destroyed its true primary skin representation behaved as if this fingertip was anesthetic, adopting a strategy of opening the hand to determine whether or not a pellet had been retrieved (it often had not) as a part of every grasp/retrieval trial. Retrieval success was initially substantially maintained, because prior to the lesion the behavior had come to be performed "automatically." However, task performance rapidly degraded, and the monkey began to use a variety of alternative grasping strategies to eject and grasp these small objects. After several days of such practice, the monkey appeared to recover the sensibility on the fingers that had earlier been primarily involved in the behavior. The monkey soon began using those fingers again, in successful pellet retrievals. Over a period of days, it again progressively improved at this task, ultimately usually achieving pre-lesion training performance levels.

When the cortical representations of the skin surfaces of the hand were again reconstructed in these stroke-recovered monkeys, they were found to be dramatically altered once again (C. Xerri et al., in prep.). The representations of the surfaces of the hand were especially strikingly modified in cortical areas 3a and 1, two other SI zones in the anterior parietal cortex that can represent hand surfaces. In both regions, there was now a major elaboration of just those skin surfaces that provided inputs that guided palpation, ejection, and grasping of the small round objects in the retrieval behavior. Before the lesion, the most striking elaboration of the skin representation that was recorded had been in cortical area 3b. After the lesion restricted to just those zones of area 3b and subsequent training and behavioral recovery, there were equally prominent representational elaborations in *alternative* cutaneous response zones in areas 3a and 1 (C. Xerri et al., in prep.).

When the ministroke in cortical area 4 destroyed the representation of movements critical for performing the behavior, as has been studied elegantly by Nudo and colleagues (1996b), the monkey's movement control was again strikingly degraded. Some monkeys neglected their hands; the consequence was a dramatic further degradation of the movement representation of the hand. If the monkey again heavily practiced the behavior and recovered proficiency at this small-object-retrieval task, the representation of movements critical to this task reemerged in cortical area 4 in zones formerly representing other hand or forelimb movements (Nudo et al. 1996b).

These simple ministroke recovery experiments strengthen the argument that these massive, collective cortical representational changes *are* the cortical part of skill acquisition. They clearly manifest a representational plasticity/learning contribution to stroke recovery, consistent with the conclusions of earlier stroke recovery studies (Cole and Glees 1954; Schaefer and Meyer 1974; Lacour and Xerri 1981; Jenkins and Merzenich 1987; Goldberger 1988). They demonstrate that functional recovery can be accounted for by the reemergence of the representation of functions critical for the behavior, in cortical zones that were concerned primarily with other primary activities prior to the lesion.

A DIFFERENT VIEW OF THE ORIGINS OF HUMAN DISABILITY

An emerging understanding of this lifelong "brain plasticity" has led to an important rethinking about the origins, and the treatments, of human ability and disability. In general, most neurological science during the past two decades has focused on molecular or genetic or physical brain defect explanations for human disabilities or neurological illnesses. We now understand that there is a potentially powerful role played by the "functional-self-creation plasticity processes" of the brain. Consider two simple examples: (1) the origins of and a plasticity-based treatment of a developmental disability, specific language impairment; and (2) the origins of and a plasticity-based treatment of an acquired adult disability, occupationally based movement disorders of the hand.

ORIGINS AND THERAPEUTIC REMEDIATION OF SPECIFIC LANGUAGE IMPAIRMENTS

Seven to eight percent of children entering school are identified as specifically language impaired (SLI); i.e., (1) they are delayed in their language learning when they are benchmarked against their chronological age or their nonverbal intelligence and (2) they have no other known neurological deficits (Beitchman et al. 1986; Tomblin 1996). Most of these children will fail to successfully initiate reading in a timely way. There are genetic contributions to the language disabilities of many of these children (Arnold 1961; Tallal et al. 1991; Lewis et al. 1993; Pennington 1995). There are physical differences between the brains of at least some SLI individuals as compared with normals that are arguably related to their language impairment (Flynn et al. 1992; Hagman et al. 1992; Galaburda and Livingstone 1993; Neville et al. 1993; Galaburda et al. 1994; Hari and Kiesila 1996). In general, these genetic factors and these physical differences have been presumed to be "causes" of the specific language impairment and the consequent dyslexia (reading failure) that usually emerges in these children.

At the same time, we also know that functional self-creation processes in the brain are necessarily contributing massively to the processes of language creation in every child. Could they be a contributing cause of this disability? Consider the changes that occur in the brain of a child learning normal or abnormal language skills in terms of our earlier example of a subject learning to pick up small round objects. In an adult brain, picking up small objects a few hundred or thousand times over a period of a few days resulted in a "new" brain in which responses were altered on a wide scale as the brain progressively specialized, parallel with progressive improvements at this simple skill. In achieving that specialization, the basic activities of tens of millions or hundreds of millions of brain cells and the functions of hundreds of millions or billions of synapses are remodeled.

By the time a SLI child enters primary school, he/she has undergone several *million* "practice trials" in the development of language skills. The brain of the child is unquestionably highly specialized at the representation of their defective language. The creation of a functional language is the product of massive brain remodeling inducing enduring changes in hundreds of millions of neurons. Whether these processes are the cause of the disability or not, they must be contributing powerfully to the emergent language phenomenology in these children.

A LANGUAGE-IMPAIRED CHILD IS A SPECIALIST AT A PARTICULAR FORM OF LANGUAGE PROCESSING

Every language-impaired child is heavily "practicing" his/her disabling language skills. Why has the child's progressive learning about language resulted in a debilitating form of language? Why does a child continue to use a marginally successful brain-processing strategy for language? If the brain is so plastic, why doesn't the child simply correct the problem on his/her own? Why is the child apparently ensnared by brain processes that appear to be highly resistant to change?

Studies indicate that more than 10% of children, including most children that fit the clinical definition of "specifically language-impaired," have actually created their early language constructs in an alternative way. Unlike normal children, they integrate sound information over relatively long chunks of time, of the order of one-fifth to one-third of a second (Tallal and Piercy 1974; Merzenich et al. 1993; Tallal et al. 1993; Farmer and Klein 1995; Merzenich and Jenkins 1995; Kraus et al. 1996; McAnally and Stein 1996). If the interferences in their sound input stream are measured in masking experiments, it is seen that most of these children have very consistent *and highly abnormal* temporal integration/segmentation abilities marked by especially strong and prolonged backward masking effects (Wright et al. 1997). What are these children practicing to produce such consistent, abnormal, successive sound event interferences?

Psychophysical studies have led us to the hypothesis that they are simply taking in integrated sound chunks that extend over the period length of syllables without reliably developing the further crucial step of making rapid intrasyllabic distinctions. Furthermore, we hypothesize that they are storing information about speech using this long-time-chunk (approximately syllable-length) representational mode—as contrasted with the normal, intrasyllabic feature-distinguishing (phoneme-based) mode. The brains of these children have not developed the skill of separately segmenting and distinguishing the brief, successive sound features from which syllables are constructed. Consistent with that view, these children have impoverished phonetic reception abilities (Vellutino and Scanlon 1987; Hodgson 1992; Watson and Miller 1993; Bird et al. 1995; Stothard and Hulme 1995; Vellutino et al. 1995).

The cortical plasticity/learning processes in these children *are* working powerfully throughout the period of their language development; they are not "learning disabled" in any general sense. These children have a normal capacity to learn, as is reflected by their normal nonverbal intelligence. In their language learning, they are trained specialists at receiving and interpreting speech using an alternative long-time-chunking aural representational processing mode. Once their special skills have been developed through many hundreds of thousands or millions of "practice events," they hypothetically then get the most information about sound using this—i.e., their special—speech representation mode. Therein lies their trap. These children have evolved an expertise at a language representational system that lacks the symbolic representational power of normal, phonologically based language. Their substantially nonphonologically based language representation does not provide a basis for reliable sound-to-phonologically based orthographic script translation.

OTHER ASPECTS OF THE DEFICITS OF SLI CHILDREN

Three other aspects of the specialization in speech perception in these children contribute importantly to their impairment. First, they are also significantly impaired in the way their brain distinguishes different spectral (tonal) parts of sound (Wright et al. 1997). As noted above, these individuals have massive interferences between fast, successive sounds; e.g., between the successive sound pieces of speech. They also have abnormal interferences between the tonal parts of speech. Like the temporal processing deficit, this "spectral processing deficit" arises, we believe, because of the brain's heavy practice at integrating and chunking sounds over syllable-length time periods. At the same time, the temporal interferences between successive sounds are most powerful when those sounds have more similar spectral (tonal) contents. These spectrally specific interactions have been a source of confusion for speech scientists who have tried to define the "rules" governing errors in speech reception and comprehension in these special children.

Second, the interferences that apply for a given phonetic element in running speech are a very complicated function of the specific context in which it occurs. Perceptual generalization is a critical aspect of our normal phonological represention al schema. For these children, the rules of perceptual generalization that apply for normal children cannot work. Because they are destined to be asked to use generalized, aurally based perceptual constructs as a basis for translating sounds in alphabetic terms, difficulty in initiating reading is a not-surprising outcome.

Third, other coping behaviors and learning consequences can be expected to arise as a consequence of this alternative language representation mode. The perceptual and cognitive skills of different affected children might be expected to progressively elaborate, possibly in manifold ways, in this population.

WHY IS THE TRAP SPRUNG ON THESE CHILDREN?

What underlies the creation of this second form of language representation in so many children? What goes wrong? Hypothetically, anything that degrades the very early treatment of sound by the brain in very early childhood could give rise to this alternative language mode (Merzenich et al. 1993; Merzenich and Jenkins 1995). For example, if sound is consistently perceived as muffled during the first 6 or 8 or 10 months of life, the brain would be expected to adopt this alternative, syllable-based processing mode. In such circumstances, the child cannot make reliable and therefore consistently behaviorally rewardable distinctions between fast, successive phonemic events, but it can learn to make distinctions about the far more powerful signal modulations that distinguish successive syllables. You could think of the child as adopting that alternative language-processing mode as a "fall-back" position for a brain that is having significant difficulty making fine distinctions about intrasyllabic sound inputs.

There are almost certainly multiple causes that could initiate this alternative language learning progression (Merzenich et al. 1993; Merzenich and Jenkins 1995), some of which undoubtedly can be inherited. For example, such a problem could arise from defective or delayed or middle ear infection-impaired hearing. It could arise from a variety of developmental delays in the brain. It could arise in a perfectly normal brain opting to derive information about speech using an alternative strategy. Recent studies have recorded the origins of this problem within the first year of life (Benasich and Tallal 1996). Language learning-impaired children simply do not progress in their development of hearing of fast, successive sounds as do normal children. They are heavily practicing sound processing with syllable length sound chunking by their first birthday.

FUNCTIONAL SELF-CREATION PROCESSES CAN AT LEAST PARTIALLY "CORRECT" THIS DEVELOPMENTAL LEARNING PROGRESSION IN SLI CHILDREN

Brain plasticity studies have shown that a monkey can be trained to make many-fold improvements in its ability to identify rapidly successive sounds with a particular form of practice (Recanzone et al. 1993). A monkey can also be trained to specialize at distinguishing slow events received in long time chunks by an intense regime of practice, again paralleled by major neuronal response remodeling (Beitel et al. 1996). Related scientific experiments conducted by visual and auditory psychophysicists have shown that major improvements in the ability to detect or recognize rapidly successive stimuli can be achieved with practice (Karni and Sagi 1991, 1993; Ahissar and Hochstein 1993). Could this kind of progressive, adaptive training be used to help a SLI child change his/her processing mode from a slow-time-chunk, syllable-based mode to a fast-time-chunk, phonologically based mode? To address that question, a series of training tools for 5- to 9-year-old SLI children were created and were applied in a special 20-day-long, 3-hour per day "summer school" organized by Professor Paula Tallal in her Rutgers University laboratories (Merzenich et al. 1996; Tallal et al. 1996). These training exercises, modeled after exercises applied in earlier monkey and human psychophysical studies, were implemented in the form of CD ROM-mounted audiovisual "games."

The first set of games was designed to train the child to make progressively faster (in speech, progressively more high-speed, natural) accurate distinctions about successive acoustic stimuli. All SLI children improved at these skills. Their abilities to recognize fast consonant sounds invariably improved markedly with training, and at a non-speech, fast-successive-element recognition task, gains in two summer school studies of 7 and 11 children averaged 5-fold and 15-fold, respectively. At the end of training, many children were approaching normal performance abilities at some variations of this task. In parallel with this training, the phonetic reception abilities of these children also improved, and they continued to improve, differentially re control children, after training was completed. These children were initially severely receptively impaired. *By several months after training, all 18 children tested at or above normal in their phonetic reception abilities.*

A second set of exercises was designed to rapidly improve the language skills of these language-delayed children by conducting training exercises that employed synthetically disambiguated speech. This speech was extended in time, and its fast, weak phonetic elements were differentially amplified to make it more intelligible to SLI children. On the average, SLI children improved about two years in their language age by working at these language training tasks over a 20-day period. Moreover, with their parallel fast-element-recognition training, their language training gains generalized to natural speech. Language-processing gains were strongly correlated (r = 0.86 and 0.85) with the number of practice trials that children were able to complete over these 20 days in fast-element-recognition exercises, in two studies of 7 and 11 SLI children.

It seems unlikely that these results can be accounted for by the development of two or more years of cognitive skill training accomplished through this relatively limited period of language training. We hypothesize that the main gains in measured achievement levels actually derive from the fact that the trained child now has a much improved ability to perform on the language measurement tests because of his/her clarified speech signal reception capabilities. By this view, pre-test versus post-test language battery comparisons would be akin to pre-test versus post-test visual test battery comparisons with the "after" battery administered 1 month after corrective lenses were given to a visually impaired child. By this view, widescale performance changes are recorded because the child is receiving a temporally-spectrally clarified acoustic signal, which is now being segmented and analyzed by the brain on a time scale on which critical phonetic distinctions can be accurately processed.

Whatever the ultimate complete explanations for these very large and rapid changes in language processing, these studies show that we *can* train most SLI children to make more accurate distinctions about progressively faster (more natural, higher-speed) speech element sequences. As a consequence, these impaired children developed more competent speech reception. With only 20 days of training, they were apparently able to effectively shift their processing mode from a substantially nonphonological mode to a phonologically more competent mode. With limited parallel practice, other trained language skills were rapidly brought up nearer to age-appropriate levels, although the true origins of these very rapid, large-scale changes in receptive and expressive language measures are not yet completely understood (Merzenich et al. 1996; Tallal et al. 1996).

These results demonstrate that the problem in at least most of these children is not an irreversible one. In functional terms, these individuals do not appear to have substantially defective learning machinery, per se. Differences in brain imaging or brain morphology recorded in these children must at least often reflect *effects* of their peculiar learning histories, rather than their causes. In any event, the powerful functional self-creation powers of the brain can apparently be marshalled quickly and effectively to convert a child's brain from operating as a syllable-based speech processor that is relatively poor at making intrasyllabic distinctions to a more normal and more cognitively powerful phoneme-based speech processor that is making reliable intrasyllabic distinctions.

WHAT DO INTEGRATIVE NEUROSCIENCE STUDIES REVEAL ABOUT THE LEARNING REQUIRED TO REMEDIATE THIS KIND OF PROBLEM?

A scientific understanding of the probable contribution of the brain plasticity-based development of a defective language representation to the language disabilities of these children carries with it a very important precaution: There can be no quick fix for this kind of problem. This developmental disability has been very hard won through years of practice and the functional brain development that it has driven. SLI children are dedicated experts at using their special processing strategies, not just in speech reception, but in the cognitive skills, including special coping skills, that flow directly from it. Only very intensive exercises applied over an extended time period can be expected to generate any real cortical plasticity-based correction.

Cognitive neuroscience studies also reveal the most effective strategies for driving brain change. The subject must be attentive and motivated. The training must be progressive and adapted to each training subject. The training schedule must be repetitious and the training schedule intense. A computer-based adaptive training approach like the one applied in these experimental studies in SLI children is an appropriate way of achieving these requisite conditions for driving rapid neurological change.

THE ORIGINS OF OCCUPATIONALLY BASED MOVEMENT DISORDERS OF THE HAND

A second example of a cortical plasticity/learning-induced disability has been studied intensively by us in monkey and human models: the origins of focal dystonias of the hand (FDh) accompanying a "repetitive strain injury." This second model of a common human disability reveals another interesting aspect of cortical functional-self-creation plasticity processes. Although plasticity in learning usually operates to generate elaborating, differentiating, representational changes that drive progressively more refined behavioral performance, under special circumstances *the same change mechanisms can drive de-differentiating brain remodeling that grossly degrades behavioral performance.*

FDh is a common part of a repetitive strain injury (Sheehy and Marsden 1982; Newmark and Hochberg 1987; Cohen and Hallett 1988; Bureau of National Affairs 1991; Millender et al. 1992). It is usually manifested by the loss of control of digital movements when the hand is brought down into what had been a heavy-use posture, then replicating heavily practiced sensory stimulus events. For example, a pianist or typist can lose the ability to produce rapidly successive movements with two fingers. In the dystonic hand, when either one of the two digits is brought down onto the keyboard, the other moves uncontrollably. Movement from any other digit onto the two offending digits occurs with normal facility, but movement between the two involved digits is frozen.

This condition commonly arises out of a period of heavy hand use that specifically involves the fingers that express the dystonia. It was earlier hypothesized that this common problem is an *expected* negative aspect of input coincidence-based (Hebbian) plasticity mechanisms (Merzenich et al. 1990; Merzenich and Jenkins 1993). That is because an integrative time constant that is at least several tens of milliseconds long governs synaptic effectiveness-change mechanisms. If inputs are driven into the cortex from normally differentiated input sources within these time limits in a learning context, they will be integrated by the plasticity machinery of the brain. The consequent *de*-differentiation of sensory feedback information from the hand would be expected to result in an inability to control previously independent finger movements, because after such training induced integration, the brain would interpret input coming back from either of the two fingers as coming from a single (now integrated, two-finger) input source.

To test this simple hypothesis, adult owl monkeys were trained at a task at which weak but temporally sharp vibratory stimuli were delivered to the hand while it was engaged in a digital grasp. In this simulation of the genesis of a "writer's cramp," the vibratory shocks were meant to simulate stimulus events delivered back to the grasping fingers via the writing instrument. In our model, these weak vibratory events nearly simultaneously engaged wide digital surfaces. The four conditions critical for driving de-differentiating changes in hand representations in the cortex were met by this task: Inputs were generated (1) nearly simultaneously from multiple-digit skin surfaces and muscle and joint afferents, (2) in a highly stereotypic manner, (3) in a repetitive task, and (4) with stimuli delivered under behaviorally attentive conditions.

This training resulted in a profound de-differentiation of the representations of sensory feedback information from the digits of these monkeys, by which the independent representations of sensory feedback information from the fingers were largely destroyed in parallel with the emergence of a dystonic hand (Bly et al. 1995a,1997; Wang et al. 1995). In such a FDh monkey, the normal topographic representation of feedback sensory information that guides hand movement was grossly degraded. Now, (1) many or most neurons representing finger surfaces had receptive fields that were 10 to 20 or more times larger than normal; (2) in sharp contradistinction to the normal condition, receptive fields commonly extended across large surfaces of single or multiple digits; and (3) unlike the normal case, receptive fields commonly extended across large parts of both the dorsal and volar hand. In comparison to normals, input from any given digital location was represented very widely across the most topographic (area 3b) cortical representation of the hand, and now, there could be an equally dramatic de-differentiation of the representation of muscle afferent inputs in cortical area 3a.

This de-differentiation leading to a dystonic hand is of an increasingly wide occurrence because of contemporary workplace demands on human hand use. Why has it not occurred to most medical specialists who treat these individuals that *attended, heavy hand use is learning*, and that learning-induced plasticity could partly underlie the problems that can emerge from hand use? In our view, it is because the common models of the origins or treatments of human disability and disease do not yet acknowledge the powerful, in place, lifelong functional self-creation mechanisms of the brain.

Consider how that understanding could affect the way a complex problem like a "repetitive strain injury" marked by a FDh is treated. What do plasticity studies indicate about the possible treatment of this common condition? First, it has now been demonstrated that these individuals have degraded haptic and small-figure recognition abilities that would be a part of any fine tactually guided movement task (Byl et al. 1995b). There is an increasingly clear concept of what the brain requires to generate progressively more elaborated, differentiated representations of sensory feedback information and movements. The true correction of this problem hypothetically requires a *re*-differentiation, through training, of these cortical representations. Such training has been applied in a qualitative way in human studies by using haptic and stimulus discrimination and recognition tasks, with encouraging initial success. The development of computer-guided training should greatly facilitate the delivery of the heavy requisite schedules of stimuli and should provide a basis for monitoring the progressive refinement of sensory feedback information and movement control.

Second, as these studies are elaborated, they should clarify exactly what use conditions in the workplace account for the genesis of the problem. For a worker at risk, workplace monitoring of potentially destructive behaviors and prophylactic exercises could be constructed into a workday routine.

Third, once it is understood that massive, learning-induced changes in brain representations are occurring in repetitive strain injury patients, it is logical to ask whether or not these brain changes have anything to do with the genesis of the inflammation or pain that are other common aspects of the repetitive strain injury syndrome.

CLOSING COMMENT

Neuroscience is creating an increasingly detailed understanding of the neuroplasticity processes underlying the learning/plasticity-based elaboration of functional abilities. That science is also revealing how normal brain plasticity processes contribute to the expressions of neurological dysfunction and impairment recorded in developmental disabilities, and throughout life, in large human populations. It has also led to new rehabilitation models in which cortical plasticity processes have been marshalled to ameliorate or reverse underlying causes or consequences of severe human disability. Important successes in ameliorating language-learning impairments and occupationally based movement disorders represent the beginnings of an important new era in integrative neuroscience-based neurological rehabilitation, in which brain plasticity-based training methods will be used to attack the fundamental behavioral deficits marking *many* chronic neurological disabilities and "diseases."

REFERENCES

Ahissar, M. and S. Hochstein. 1993. Attentional control of early perceptual learning. *Proc. Natl. Acad. Sci.* **90:** 5718.

Aizawa, H., M. Inase, H. Mushiake, K. Shima, and J. Tanji. 1991. Reorganization of activity in the supplementary motor area associated with motor learning and functional recovery. *Exp. Brain Res.* **84:** 778.

Aosaki, T., H. Tsubokawa, A. Ishida, K. Watanabe, A.M. Graybiel, and M. Kimura. 1994. Responses of tonically active neurons in the primate's striatum undergo systematic changes during behavioral sensorimotor conditioning. *J. Neurosci.* **14:** 3969.

Arnold, G.E. 1961. The genetic background of developmental language disorders. *Folia Phoniatr.* **13:** 246.

Beitchman, J.H., R. Nair, and P.G. Patel. 1986. Prevalence of speech and language disorders in 5-year-old kindergarten children in the Ottawa-Carlton region. *J. Speech Hear. Disord* **51:** 98.

Beitel, R.E., C.E. Schreiner, X. Wang, S.W. Cheung, and M.M. Merzenich. 1996. Amplitude modulated tones: Effects of carrier frequencies on psychophysical discrimination and responses of primary auditory cortical neurons in the owl monkey. *J. Neurosci. Abstr.* **22:** 1623.

Benasich, A.A. and P. Tallal. 1996. Auditory temporal processing thresholds, habituation, and recognition memory over the first year. *Infant Behav. Dev.* **19:** 339.

Bird, J., D.V. Bishop, and N.H. Freeman. 1995. Phonological awareness and literacy development in children with expressive phonological impairments. *J. Speech Hear. Res.* **38:** 446.

Bureau of National Affairs. 1991. *Cumulative trauma disorders in the workplace: Costs, prevention and progress.* Bureau of National Affairs, Washington, D.C.

Byl, N.N., M.M. Merzenich, and W.M. Jenkins. 1995a. A primate genesis model of focal dystonia and repetitive strain injury: I. Learning-induced de-differentiation of the representation of the hand in the primary somatosensory cortex in adult monkeys. *Neurology* **47:** 508.

Byl, N., M.M. Merzenich, S. Cheung, P. Bedenbaugh, S.S. Nagarajan, and W.M. Jenkins. 1997. Primate model for studying focal dystonia and repetitive strain injury: Effects on the primary somatosensory cortex. *Phys. Ther.* (in press).

Byl, N., A. McKenzie, F. Wilson, M. Melnick, P. Scott, A. Oakes, W. Jenkins, and M. Merzenich. 1995b. Discriminative tactile processing in patients with repetitive injury syndromes: Tendinitis or focal dystonia. *J. Orthop. Sports Phys. Ther.* **3:** 234.

Cohen, L. and M. Hallett. 1988. Hand cramps: Clinical features and electromyographic patterns in focal dystonia. *Neurology* **38:** 1005.

Coles, J. and P. Glees. 1954. Effects of small lesions in sensory cortex in trained monkeys. *J. Neurophysiol.* **17:** 1.

Farmer, M.E. and R.M. Klein. 1995. The evidence for a temporal processing deficit linked to dyslexia: A review. *Psychon. Bull. Rev.* **2:** 460.

Flynn, J.M., W. Deering, M. Goldstein, M.H. Rahbar. 1992. Electrophysiological correlates of dyslexic subtypes. *J. Learn Disabil.* **25:** 133.

Galaburda, A. and M. Livingstone. 1993. Evidence for a magnocillular effect in developmental dyslexia. *Ann. N.Y. Acad. Sci.* **682:** 70.

Galaburda, A.M., M.T. Menard, and G.D. Rosen. 1994. Evidence for aberrant auditory anatomy in developmental dyslexia. *Proc. Natl. Acad. Sci.* **91:** 8010.

Germain, L. and Y. Lamarre. 1993. Neuronal activity in the motor and premotor cortices before and after learning the associations between auditory stimuli and motor responses. *Brain Res.* **611:** 175.

Goldberger, M.E. 1988. Partial and complete deafferentation of cat hindling: The contribution of behavioral substitution to recovery of motor function. *Exp. Brain Res.* **73:** 343.

Hagman, J.O., F. Wood, M.S. Buchsbaum, P. Tallal, L. Flowers, and W. Katz. 1992. Cerebral brain metabolism in adult dyslexic subjects assessed with positron emission tomography during performance of an auditory task. *Arch. Neurol.* **49:** 734.

Hari, R. and P. Kiesila. 1996. Deficit of temporal auditory processing in dyslexic adults. *Neurosci. Lett.* **205:** 138.

Hodgson, J. 1992. The status of metalinguitic skills in reading development. *J. Learn. Disabil.* **5:** 96.

Jenkins. W.M. and M.M. Merzenich. 1987. Reorganization of neocortical representations after brain injury. A neurophysiological model of the bases of recovery from stroke. *Prog. Brain Res.* **71:** 249.

Karni, A. and D. Sagi. 1991. Where practice makes perfect in texture discrimination. Evidence for primary visual cortex plasticity. *Proc. Natl. Acad. Sci.* **88:** 4966.

———. 1993. The time course of learning a visual skill. *Nature* **365:** 250.

Kraus, N., T.J. McGee, T.D. Carrell, S.G. Zecker, T.G. Nico, and D.B. Koch. 1996. Neurophysiologic responses and behavioral discrimination deficits in children with learning problems (comments). *Science* **273:** 867.

Lacour, M. and C. Xerri. 1981. Vestibular compensation: New perspective. In *Lesion-induced neuronal plasticity in sensorimotor systems* (ed. H. Flohr and W. Precht), p. 240. Springer-Verlag, Berlin.

Lewis, B.A., N.J. Cox, and P.J. Bayard. 1993. Segregation analysis of speech and language disorders. *Behav. Genet.* **23:** 191.

McAnally, K.I. and J.F. Stein. 1996. Auditory temporal coding in dyslexia. *Proc. R. Soc. Lond. B Biol. Sci.* **263:** 961.

Merzenich, M.M. and W.M. Jenkins. 1993. Reorganization of

cortical representations of the hand following alterations of skin inputs induced by nerve injury, skin island transfers, and experience. *J. Hand Ther.* **6:** 89.

———. 1994. Cortical representation of learned behaviors. In *Memory concepts* (ed. P. Anderson et al.), p. 247. Elsevier, Amsterdam.

———. 1995. Cortical plasticity, learning and learning dysfunction. In *Maturational windows and adult cortical plasticity* (ed. B. Julesz and I. Kovacs), p. 247. Addison-Wesley, Reading, Massachusetts.

Merzenich, M.M. and K. Samashima. 1993. Cortical plasticity and memory. *Curr. Opin. Neurobiol.* **3:** 187.

Merzenich, M.M., G.M. Recanzone, W.M. Jenkins, and K.A. Grajski. 1990. Adaptive mechanisms in cortical networks underlying cortical contributions to learning and nondeclarative memory. *Cold Spring Harbor Symp. Quant. Biol.* **55:** 873.

Merzenich, M.M., C. Schreiner, W. Jenkins, and X. Wang. 1993. Neural mechanisms underlying temporal integration, segmentation, and input sequence representation: Some implications for the origin of learning disabilities. *Ann. N.Y. Acad. Sci.* **682:** 1.

Merzenich, M.M., W.M. Jenkins, P. Johnston, C. Schreiner, S.L. Miller, and P. Tallal. 1996. Temporal processing deficits of language-learning impaired children ameliorated by training. *Science* **271:** 77.

Millender, L.H., D.S. Louis, and B.P. Simmons. 1992. *Occupational disorders of the upper extremity.* Churchill Livingstone, New York.

Mitz, A.R., M. Godschalk, and S.P. Wise. 1991. Learning-dependent neuronal activity in the premotor cortex: Activity during the acquisition of conditional motor associations. *J. Neurosci.* **11:** 1855.

Neville, H.J., S.A. Coffey, P.J. Holcomb, P. Tallal. 1993. The neurobiology of sensory and language processing in language-impaired children. *J. Cogn. Neurosci.* **5:** 235.

Newmark, J. and F. Hochberg. 1987. Isolated painless manual incoordination in musicians. *J. Neurol. Neurosurg. Psychiatry* **50:** 291.

Nudo, R.J., G.W. Milliken, W.M. Jenkins, and M.M. Merzenich. 1996a. Use-dependent alterations of movement representations in primary motor cortex of adult squirrel monkeys. *J. Neurosci.* **16:** 785.

Nudo, R.J., B.M. Wise, F. Sifuentes, G.W. Milliken. 1996b. Neural substrates for the effects of rehabilitate training on motor recovery after ischemic infarct. *Science* **272:** 1791.

Pennington, B.F. 1995. Genetics of learning disabilities. *J. Child Neurol.* (suppl. 1) **10:** 69.

Recanzone, G.H., C.E. Schreiner, M.M. Merzenich. 1993. Plasticity in the frequency representation of primary auditory cortex following discrimination training in adult owl monkeys. *J. Neurosci.* **13:** 87.

Schaefer, K.P. and D.L. Meyer. 1974. Compensation of vestibular lesions. In *Handbook of sensory physiology* (ed. H.H. Kornhuber), p. 463. Springer-Verlag, Berlin.

Sheehy, M.P. and C.D. Marsden. 1982. Writer's cramp—A focal dystonia. *Brain* **105:** 461.

Stothard, S.E. and C. Hulme. 1995. A comparison of phonological skills in children with reading comprehension difficulties and children with decoding difficulties. *J. Child Psychol. Psychiatry Allied Discip.* **36:** 399.

Tallal, P. and M. Piercy. 1974. Developmental aphasia: Rate of auditory processing and selective impairment of consonant perception. *Neuropsychologia* **12:** 83.

Tallal, P., S. Miller, and R.H. Fitch. 1993. Neurobiological basis of speech: A case for the preeminence of temporal processing. *Ann. N.Y. Acad. Sci.* **682:** 27.

Tallal, P., J. Townsend, S. Curtiss, and B. Wulfech. 1991. Phenotypic profiles of language-impaired children based on genetic/family history. *Brain Lang.* **41:** 81.

Tallal, P., S.L. Miller, G. Bedi, G. Byma, X. Wang, S.S. Nagarajan, C. Schreiner, W.M. Jenkins, and M.M. Merzenich. 1996. Acoustically modified speech improves language comprehension in language-learning impaired children. *Science* **271:** 81.

Tomblin, H.B. 1996.. The big picture of SLI: Results of an epidemiological study of SLI among kindergarten children. Paper presented at the 17th Annual Symposium on Research in Child Language Disorders, Madison, Wisconsin.

Vellutino, F.R. and D.M. Scanlon. 1987. Phonological coding, phonological awareness, and reading ability: Evidence from a longitudinal and experimental study. *Merrill-Palmer Q.* **33:** 321.

Vellutino, F.R., D.M. Scanlon, and D. Spearing. 1995. Semantic and phonological coding in poor and normal readers. *J. Exp. Child Psychol.* **59:** 76.

Wang, X., M.M. Merzenich, K. Sameshima, and W.M. Jenkins. 1995. Remodelling of hand representation in adult cortex determined by timing of tactile stimulation. *Nature* **378:** 71.

Watson, B.U. and T.K. Miller. 1993. Auditory perception, phonological processing, and reading ability/disability. *J. Speech Hear. Res.* **36:** 850.

Wright, B.A., L.J. Lombardino, W.M. King, C.S. Puranik, C.M. Leonard, and M.M. Merzenich. 1997. Deficits in auditory temporal and spectral processing in language-impaired children. *Nature* (in press).

What Words Are Telling Us about the Brain

M.E. Raichle
Departments of Radiology, Neurology and Neurobiology, Washington University School of Medicine, St Louis, Missouri 63110

In 1861, Paul Broca described a patient with expressive language difficulty associated with a lesion of the left frontal operculum. This landmark observation was followed a short time later by the observations of Carl Wernicke (1874) relating damage in the left temporoparietal junction to language comprehension. On the basis of these observations and many subsequent data, a general framework for the understanding of language in the human brain has emerged (for review, see Damasio 1992). However, a damaged brain is not simply a normally functioning brain minus the damaged part. Compensatory changes can and do occur in undamaged areas, clouding the interpretation of such findings (see, e.g., Buckner et al. 1996a). Furthermore, lesions (most often strokes) are usually large and, hence, likely to disrupt multiple, functionally distinct areas of the brain simultaneously. It is not surprising that researchers, beginning at the time of Broca and Wernicke and continuing to the present, have recognized these limitations and have sought a safe means of determining the detailed functional anatomy of language and other cognitive functions of the normal human brain.

This scientific quest for the functional anatomy of language in the normal human brain began in earnest with the development of radically new brain imaging tools in the early 1970s. The first of these tools was X-ray-computed tomography (CT) followed by position emission tomography (PET) and magnetic resonance imaging (MRI). These imaging tools have changed dramatically the way in which we approach the study of the normal human brain. It is possible to examine not only the physical anatomy of the living human brain with X-ray CT and MRI, but also its functional anatomy (i.e., the actual areas involved in specific tasks) with PET (for review, see Posner and Raichle 1994) and, more recently, with MRI (Kwong et al. 1992; Ogawa et al. 1992). Combining these imaging techniques with the experimental strategies of psychology and linguistics has produced a new way of approaching an understanding of the organization of language in the normal human brain (Posner and Raichle 1994). As this work has proceeded, new insights into language organization have begun to appear.

It is the purpose of this paper to review briefly the techniques and experimental strategies involved in this work and to give some flavor for the information beginning to appear. It is too early to posit major new organizational schemes for language in the human brain with absolute certainty, but it is not too early to prepare for the inevitable changes that are likely to occur in our understanding of this uniquely human capacity for communication.

IMAGING TECHNIQUES AND STRATEGIES

Measurements of *blood flow* to local areas of the brain are at the heart of assessing brain function with either PET or functional magnetic resonance imaging (fMRI). It is well over a century since the great Italian physiologist Angelo Mosso first noted what has been documented repeatedly since; i.e., a most remarkable and precise coupling of local blood flow to neuronal activity in the normal human brain as well as in the brains of laboratory animals (for review, see Raichle 1987; Posner and Raichle 1994). PET measures blood flow by adapting an autoradiographic technique for laboratory animals developed in the late 1940s by Seymour S. Kety and his colleagues at the National Institutes of Health (for a detailed review, see Raichle 1987). PET relies on water radioactively labeled with oxygen-15. The labeled water, which emits positrons as it decays with a half-life of approximately 2 minutes, accumulates in the brain in less than a minute, forming an accurate image of blood flow.

fMRI measures a complex function of blood flow related to the fact that when blood flow increases in the brain during normal functional brain activation, oxygen consumption does not (Fox and Raichle 1986; Fox et al. 1988). Under these circumstances, more oxygen is present locally in the tissue because the blood flow (i.e., supply) has increased but demand for oxygen has not. The amount of oxygen carried on the hemoglobin molecule affects its magnetic properties (i.e., deoxyhemoglobin disrupts magnetic fields whereas oxyhemoglobin does not). This important fact was first noted by Linus Pauling (Pauling and Coryell 1936) well before the discovery of nuclear magnetic resonance (NMR) and the invention of MRI. Because MRI is based on detecting the unique properties of atoms and molecules in a magnetic field, it can detect a functionally induced change in the local ratio of oxyhemoglobin to deoxyhemoglobin. This change, an actual signal enhancement as this ratio increases, is often referred to as the blood oxygen level-dependent (BOLD) effect (Ogawa et al. 1990).

A distinct *behavioral strategy* for the functional mapping of neuronal activity has emerged during the past 15 years. Initially developed for PET, it has been extended and expanded for fMRI (see, e.g., Buckner et al. 1996b). The strategy is based on a concept introduced by the Dutch physiologist Franciscus C. Donders in 1868 (for a detailed review, see Posner and Raichle 1994). Donders proposed a general method to measure thought process based on a simple logic. He subtracted the time needed to respond to a light (say, by pressing a key) from the time needed to respond to a particular color of light. He found that discriminating color required about 50 msec. In this way, Donders isolated and measured a mental process for the first time by subtracting a *control state* (i.e., responding to a light) from a *task state* of interest (i.e., discriminating the color of the light). One criticism of this approach has been that the time necessary to press a key after a decision to do so has been made is affected by the nature of the decision process itself. By implication, the nature of the processes underlying key press may have been altered. Although this issue has been the subject of continuing discussion in cognitive psychology, it finds its resolution in functional brain imaging, where changes in any process are directly signaled by changes in observable brain states. Events occurring in the brain are not hidden from the investigator as in the purely cognitive experiments. Careful analysis of the changes in the functional images reveals whether processes (e.g., specific cognitive decisions) can be added or removed without affecting ongoing processes (e.g., motor responses).

The current functional imaging strategy compares images of blood flow (PET) or blood flow-related changes (fMRI) taken in a control state to those obtained when the brain is engaged in a task of interest. Great care is taken to choose the control state and the task state so as to isolate as well as possible a limited number of mental operations when subtracting the two states. Subtracting or otherwise comparing blood flow-dependent measurements made in the control state from those made in the task state should isolate those parts of the brain uniquely responsible for the performance of the task. The details of the image manipulations necessary for the accomplishment of such comparisons and the subsequent statistical analysis of the resulting data are subjects beyond the scope of this paper.

STUDIES OF SINGLE WORD PROCESSING

As mentioned above, the manner in which language skills are acquired and organized in the human brain has been the subject of intense investigation for more than a century. From this work, largely based on the study of patients with focal brain lesions, a concept of language organization has emerged which, in broad outline, posits the following: Information flows from visual and auditory reception areas to areas at the junction between the left temporal and parietal lobes for comprehension, and then on to frontal areas for verbal response selection and speech production. The question now is whether this organization, derived from patients with lesions, represents the actual organization in the *normal* human brain?

Beginning in the 1980s, the author and his colleagues Steven E. Petersen, Michael I. Posner, Peter T. Fox, and Mark A. Mintun began a series of experiments (Petersen et al. 1988, 1989, 1990; Raichle et al. 1994) designed to answer this question. We focused our work on the manner in which the human brain processes single words, from perception to speaking. We designed our experiments in an hierarchical manner in which several levels of information processing of increasing complexity were employed. This design was in keeping with the experimental model discussed above. In these experiments, words were presented to the subjects either on a television monitor or through ear phones. The illustrative material focuses on those aspects of our work involving the *visual presentation* of words.

Beginning in the simplest possible manner, we first wanted to know how the brain organizes the task of reading words aloud (in our case common English nouns). We recognize that some would consider this far too complex a beginning, but we believe that however naive our work might have seemed to some, the results have provided useful support for the experimental approach and have provided a number of important new insights into the brain organization of language.

In the initial experiment, normal young adults were scanned with PET in a series of hierarchically organized tasks designed to look at word reading. Because reading aloud in our experiment involved opening the eyes and maintaining visual fixation on a television monitor while lying with the head immobilized in a PET camera, it is useful to illustrate, first, just what areas of brain become active as the result of opening the eyes. As shown in the first row of Figure 1, opening the eyes and maintaining fixation on a blank television monitor (a small cross hair in the middle of the monitor made it easy for subjects to maintain fixation in the middle of the screen throughout the experiments) resulted in significant activation of areas of visual cortex as compared to resting quietly with eyes closed.

With this level of baseline brain activation in mind, it is possible to appreciate the response of the brain when we presented our subjects with common English nouns which appeared just below the fixation cross hair on the television monitor at the rate of 40–60 words per minute. Their only instruction was to maintain fixation on the cross hair. The images in the second row of Figure 1 represent those *additional* areas of the brain that became active as the result of this passive perception of words. Note that these images (row 2, Fig. 1) represent the *difference* between looking at a blank television monitor and looking at the monitor while words are presented.

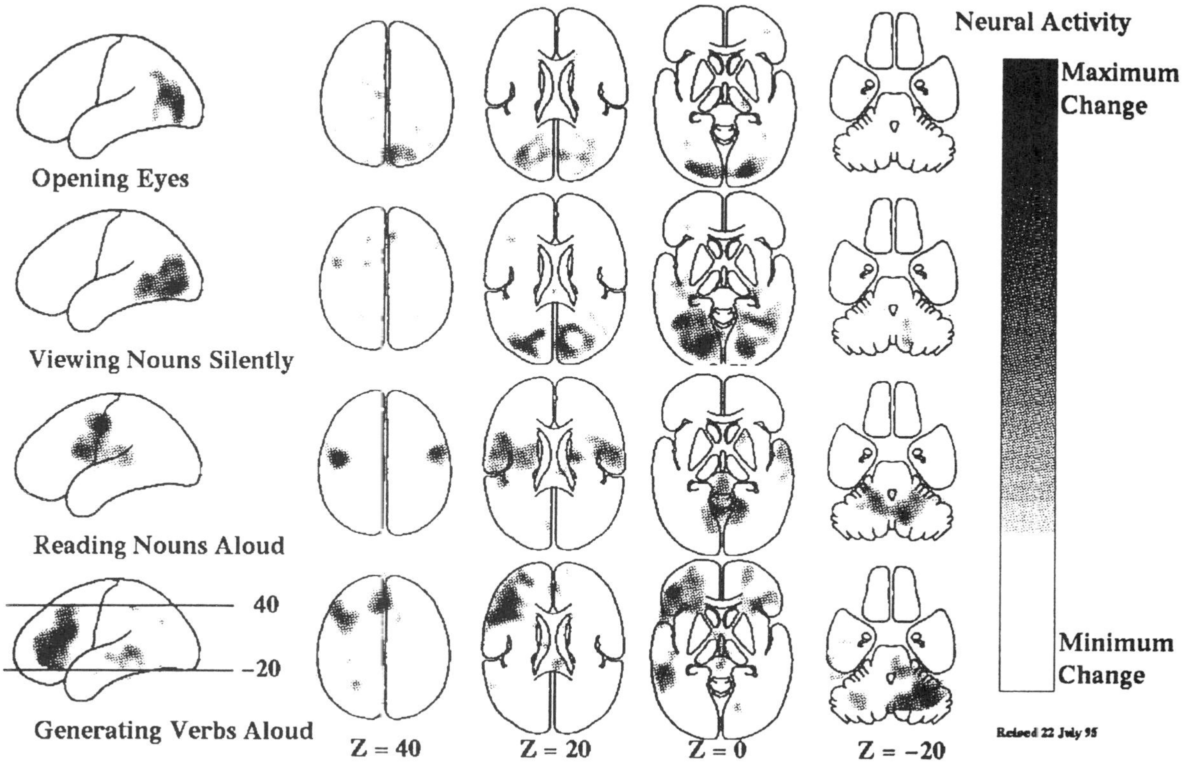

Figure 1. Four different task states are represented in these mean blood flow difference images obtained with PET from a group of normal subjects performing an hierarchically designed set of language tasks. Each row represents the mean difference images between the designated task state and a control state. The images on the left represent projections of the changes as seen through the lateral surface of the brain with the front of the brain to the reader's left. The horizontal lines through these images denote the orientation of the horizontal slices through the same data as seen to the right of this first image. These horizontal images are oriented with the front of the brain on top and the left side to the reader's left. The markings "Z = 40" indicate millimeters above and below a horizontal plane through the brain marked "Z = 0." The *top row* indicates the difference between a control state of lying quietly awake with eyes closed and lying quietly with eyes opening fixating on a small cross hair in the middle of a television monitor. Note the changes in the visual cortices associated with visual fixation on a small dot of light on a television monitor. The *second row* indicates the differences between the control state of lying quietly awake with eyes open fixating on a small cross hair (row *1*) and passively viewing the same television monitor with common English nouns appearing once a second just below the cross hair. Note the increased blood flow, over and above that observed with opening the eyes (row *1*), in the back of the brain in areas known to be concerned with visual perception. The *third row* indicates the differences between the control state of passively viewing the nouns (row *2*) and reading the same nouns aloud as they appeared on the television monitor. Note the changes in primary motor cortices (Z = 40), Sylvian-insular cortices (Z = 20), and cerebellum (Z = –20) associated with speaking aloud words seen on a television monitor. The *fourth row* indicates the difference between the control state of reading nouns aloud (row *3*) and saying aloud an appropriate verb for each noun as it appears on the screen. Note the extensive changes in the left frontal and temporal cortices and the right cerebellar hemisphere. Not shown are increases in the anterior cingulate gyrus and decreases in activity in Sylvian-insular cortices in the areas seen active in reading nouns aloud (row *3*, Z = 20). Taken together, these difference images, arranged in this hierarchical fashion, are designed to demonstrate the spatially distributed nature of the processing by task elements going on in the normal human brain during a language task.

It was clear that even with this rather blurred representation of foci of activity in the brain, there were multiple areas within human visual cortices activated by the passive perception of words. One might postulate several *levels of analysis*. These could include the *visual features* of the words (i.e., lines in various spatial orientations and relationships); actual *letters* themselves; *orthographic regularities* (i.e., relationships among letters that reflect the pronunciation rules of the English language); and, of course, *words* themselves with their unique meanings. A number of attempts have been made to relate these levels of analysis to specific patterns of brain activity (Howard et al. 1992; Price et al. 1994; Fiez et al. 1996a; Price et al. 1996), but the results have been inconclusive. Clearly, we must await further experimentation. It seems reasonable to expect that as further data are accumulated on the human visual system, it will become clearer how this analysis of such things as letters and orthographic regularities are instantiated in networks of areas whose individual components represent much more elemental visual processing operations (i.e., we will not find a single "visual word form area").

Next we asked the subjects to read aloud the same words as they appeared on the television monitor while we again obtained an image of brain blood flow. From this image we subtracted the image obtained during passively viewing the words (row 2, Fig. 1). The resulting difference image (row 3, Fig. 1) should reflect those areas of the brain concerned with the motoric aspects of reading words aloud. Not surprisingly, we observed activity in primary motor cortices bilaterally (Z = 40, row 3, Fig. 1) and in paramedian cerebellum (Z = –20). In addition, there was prominent activity in Sylvian-insular cortices bilaterally (Z = 20, row 3, Fig. 1). Not shown in the selected images in Figure 1 was prominent activity in the supplementary motor area (anterior midline at about Z = 30).

None of the above findings was unexpected, with the possible exception of the bilateral activity in Sylvian-insular cortices. Noteworthy was what was apparently missing; namely, activity in either Broca's or Wernicke's areas. These data clearly suggested that merely reading aloud familiar words does not necessarily activate these traditional components of the human language system as derived from the study of patients with lesions. So, then, when does the human brain make use of Broca's and Wernicke's areas? The answer began to emerge in the next step of our original experiment (Raichle et al. 1994).

To assure ourselves that subjects actually thought about the meaning of the words they were reading aloud (common English nouns), we asked them to inhibit their natural tendency to read aloud the words themselves and, instead, say aloud an appropriate use or verb (e.g., see KNIFE, say "CUT"). Some have argued that semantics was not the only linguistic operation introduced by this rather complex and unusual task. We agree. In retrospect, its importance was not in accessing semantics or meaning so much as in introducing the concepts of *novelty* and *inhibition* (Dempster 1992) to the task of reading words aloud.

Subtracting the PET blood flow images obtained during reading nouns aloud (row 3, Fig. 1) from generating verbs aloud for the same common English nouns revealed activations in the anterior cingulate cortex (Z = 40, row 4, Fig. 1), the left prefrontal cortex and left frontal operculum (Z = 40 through 0, row 4, Fig. 1), the left posterior temporal cortex (Z = 0, row 4, Fig. 1), and the right lateral cerebellar hemisphere (Z = –20, row 4, Fig. 1). Clearly, legitimate candidates for Broca's and Wernicke's areas were now active.

Several general observations are apparent from the data presented in Figure 1. First, reading aloud involves activity in a complex distributed network of areas spatially distributed from the cerebellum to the frontal cortex. Although the more traditional language areas of the left hemisphere (i.e., so-called Broca's and Wernicke's areas) are involved, many additional areas of the brain, not necessarily confined to the left hemisphere, are involved as well. Second, involvement of areas is task-specific. This is particularly unexpected with regard to the classic language areas of Broca and Wernicke. They do not appear to be active during the simple, learned act of reading aloud common English nouns, whereas elements of them become active during verb generation and other more complex verbal tasks (see, e.g., Buckner et al. 1995; Fiez et al. 1996b). Third, the cerebellum appears to contribute significantly not only to the motoric aspects of speech production with activity in paramedian areas (see row 3, Fig. 1), but also to the purely cognitive aspects of word generation with striking activity in the right cerebellar hemisphere (compare Z = –20 in rows 3 and 4 of Fig. 1).

Whereas the first of these three general observations is not particularly surprising, although certainly important to emphasize (i.e., that language is supported by an extensive, distributed network of brain areas), the other two observations regarding the task-specific nature of Broca's and Wernicke's areas and the role of the cerebellum deserve some additional comment.

As indicated above, in anticipation of our initial findings (Petersen et al. 1988, 1989), most would have predicted that reading words aloud would be associated routinely with activation in Broca's and Wernicke's areas. That this was not necessarily the case, indeed, did cause some surprise and concern! Our understanding of the implications of this observation began to emerge from a number of subsequent observations. First, we noted additionally that the areas of Sylvian-insular cortex bilaterally active during reading nouns aloud (row 3, Fig. 1) were not active during verb generation. Second, quite accidentally we noted that when subjects practiced the verb generation task prior to imaging, their resulting images obtained during verb generation could not be distinguished from simply reading nouns aloud (i.e., none of the areas seen active in row 4, Fig. 1 were activated after practice). Prompted by these discoveries, we examined the performance of subjects on the verb generation task with some care. We discovered that there was a significant reduction in response times and the occurrence of stereotyped responses across practice blocks (Raichle et al. 1994). We also confirmed our serendipitous observation that practice-induced changes in behavior were accompanied by major changes in the underlying brain circuitry (Raichle et al. 1994).

The above observations led us to the conclusion that two distinct routes exist between word perception in visual cortices and speech production from motor cortices (Raichle et al. 1994). One route involves the anterior cingulate, left temporal and left prefrontal cortices, and the right cerebellar hemisphere (row 4, Fig. 1), and the other involves areas of the Sylvian-insular cortices bilaterally (row 3, Fig. 1). Furthermore, the use of these two routes reflects the degree to which a given response is novel or practiced. Novelty would appear to require unique neural circuitry to inhibit habitual responses and instantiate new modes of responding. Obviously, the ability of a mature nervous system to benefit from the convenience of smoothly functioning habits yet accommodate changing contingencies is provided for in such an organizational scheme.

One major surprise in our original language work was the apparent role of the *cerebellum* in the purely cognitive aspects of single word processing. This is dramatically demonstrated in Figure 1. The role of the cerebellum in the motoric aspects of speech is clearly shown during reading aloud (Z = –20, row 3, Fig. 1). These areas of the cerebellum can readily be distinguished from the large area of the right cerebellar hemisphere which becomes active when reading aloud is subtracted from verb generation (Z = –20, row 3, Fig. 1). This latter subtraction provides a direct demonstration of an internal mental operation, the motoric aspects of which have been subtracted away. Although others had speculated that the cerebellum might play an important role in human cognition (e.g., for review, see Leiner et al. 1993) the evidence for this assertion was limited. Our imaging data provided that evidence.

This unexpected discovery of a role for the cerebellum in human cognition had three important consequences. First, it greatly expanded our view of the extent of language-critical areas in the human brain. Although neurological clinicians had recognized for many decades the important role of the cerebellum in articulate speech, its role in the cognitive aspects of language had clearly escaped notice. Second, it forced us to think in much broader terms about the role of the cerebellum. Third, it initiated a paradigm shift in the way in which we as neurological clinicians approached patients with brain lesions. Newly armed with the knowledge that a particular area of the *normal* human brain was active in a specific way during the performance of a task, we now approached patients with lesions, in this case in the cerebellum, with a completely new set of questions (Fiez et al. 1992). Patient evaluation was now based on an understanding of normal functional brain anatomy. We quickly discovered (Fiez et al. 1992) that patients with lesions of the cerebellum had, in addition to their traditional motoric deficits, specific cognitive abnormalities that could be clearly demonstrated when tasks were designed around an understanding of the circumstances that utilized that part of the brain. The resulting studies of patient RC1 (Fiez et al. 1992), a patient with a right cerebellar hemisphere infarction, provided our first hint about the role played by the cerebellum in the circuitry underlying a task like verb generation. By combining studies of normal functional anatomy with studies of patients with lesions, we shall certainly enrich our understanding of human brain function more rapidly than when either approach is used in isolation.

A final comment with regard to the study of patients with specific brain lesions should be made. Recovery from stroke, for example, does occur despite the permanence of the lesion in the brain. It is difficult to understand how this process occurs without being able to view the functional anatomy supporting the recovered function in the damaged brain. Functional brain imaging with PET and fMRI provides that opportunity. Often a particular region of the brain may, in varying combinations with other regions, activate across a range of tasks. Armed with this knowledge, it is possible to determine which tasks are irreparably impaired and which appear to be performed normally (i.e., recovered). Imaging the performance of the preserved tasks provides a direct assessment of those areas of the brain that are used to compensate for the damage element in the original circuit. We have pursued just such a strategy in studying a patient with damage to the left frontal operculum and found that for the performance of certain tasks that utilize this area of the brain (e.g., word stem completion), function is preserved; however, the performance of other tasks (e.g., verb generation) is permanently impaired (Buckner et al. 1996a). Imaging studies of the patient with preserved word stem completion revealed activity in the right frontal operculum, strongly suggesting that the adult human brain was able to compensate for some functions but not others by using a homologous region in the undamaged hemisphere. Future studies of this type should improve our understanding of the neurobiological basis of recovery of function in the damaged human nervous system.

SUMMARY

Modern functional brain imaging with PET and fMRI provides a new perspective on the organization of language in the human brain. A better definition of the distributed nature of the brain circuits involved, an appreciation of the flexibility of these circuits in adapting to the different aspects of speech production, an identification of areas not previously associated with the cognitive aspects of language, and a new understanding of the implications of specific brain lesions on the lives and behavior of patients are all early suggestions of the benefits to be derived from this work. Much exciting work lies ahead.

ACKNOWLEDGMENTS

This work has been supported by National Institutes of Health grants NS-06833 and HL-13851, the McDonnell Center for Studies of Higher Brain Function of Washington University, and the Charles A. Dana Foundation.

REFERENCES

Buckner, R.L., M.E. Raichle, and S.E. Petersen. 1995. Activation of human prefrontal cortex across different speech production tasks and gender groups. *J. Neurophysiol.* **74:** 2163.

Buckner, R.L., M. Corbetta, J. Schatz, M.E. Raichle, and S.E. Petersen. 1996a. Preserved speech abilities and compensation following prefrontal damage. *Proc. Natl. Acad. Sci.* **93:** 1249.

Buckner, R.L., P.A. Bandetini, K.M. O'Craven, R.L. Savoy, S.E. Petersen, M.E. Raichle, and B.R. Rosen. 1996b. Detection of transient and distributed cortical activation during averaged single trials of a cognitive task using fMRI. *Proc. Natl. Acad. Sci.* **93:** 14878.

Damasio, A.R. 1992. Aphasia. *N. Engl. J. Med* **326:** 531.

Dempster, F.N. 1992. The rise and fall of the inhibitory mechanism: Toward a unified theory of cognitive development and aging. *Dev. Rev.* **12:** 45.

Fiez, J.A., S.E. Petersen, and M.E. Raichle. 1996a. Identification of two pathways used for verbal response selection. In *Development dyslexia* (ed. C.H. Chase et al.), p. 227. York Press, Baltimore.

Fiez, J.A., S.E. Petersen, M.K. Cheney, and M.E. Raichle. 1992. Impaired nonmotor learning and error detection associated with cerebellar damage: A single case study. *Brain* **115:** 155.

Fiez, J.A., M.E. Raichle, D.A. Balota, P. Tallal, and S.E. Petersen. 1996b. PET activation of posterior temporal regions during auditory word presentation and verb generation. *Cereb. Cortex* **6:** 1.

Fox, P.T. and M.E. Raichle. 1986. Focal physiological uncoupling of cerebral blood flow and oxidative metabolism during somatosensory stimulation in human subjects. *Proc. Natl. Acad. Sci.* **83:** 1140.

Fox, P.T., M.E. Raichle, M.A. Mintun, and C. Dence. 1988. Nonoxidative glucose consumption during focal physiologic neural activity. *Science* **241:** 462.

Howard, D., K. Patterson, R. Wise, W.D. Brown, K. Friston, C. Weiller, and R. Frackowiak. 1992. The cortical localization of the lexicons. *Brain* **115:** 1769.

Kwong, K.K., J.W. Belliveau, D.A. Chesler, I.E. Goldberg, R.M. Weisskof, B.P. Poncelet, D.N. Kennedy, B.E. Hoppe, M.S. Cohen, R. Turner, H.-M. Chen, T.J. Brady, and B.R. Rosen. 1992. Dynamic magnetic resonance imaging of human brain activity during primary sensory stimulation. *Proc. Natl. Acad. Sci.* **89:** 5675.

Leiner, H.C., A.C. Leiner, and R.S. Dow. 1993. Cognitive and language functions of the human cerebellum. *Trends Neurosci.* **16:** 444.

Ogawa, S., T.-M. Lee, A.S. Nayak, and P. Glynn. 1990. Oxygenation-sensitive contrast in magnetic resonance image of rodent brain at high magnetic fields. *Mag. Res. Med.* **14:** 68.

Ogawa, S., D.W. Tank, R. Menon, J.M. Ellermann, S.G. Kim, H. Merkle, and K. Ugurbil. 1992. Intrinsic signal changes accompanying sensory stimulation: Function brain mapping with magnetic resonance imaging. *Proc. Natl. Acad. Sci.* **89:** 5951.

Pauling, L. and C.D. Coryell. 1936. The magnetic properties and structure of hemoglobin, oxyhemoglobin and carbonmonoxyhemoglobin. *Proc. Natl. Acad. Sci.* **22:** 210.

Petersen, S.E., P.T. Fox, A.Z. Snyder, and M.E. Raichle. 1990. Activation of extrastriate and frontal cortical areas by visual words and work-like stimuli. *Science* **249:** 1041.

Petersen, S.E., P.T. Fox, M.I. Posner, M.A. Mintun, and M.E. Raichle. 1988. Positron emission tomographic studies of the cortical anatomy of single word processing. *Nature* **331:** 585.

———. 1989. Positron emission tomographic studies of the processing of single words. *J. Cog. Neurosci.* **1:** 153.

Posner, M.I. and M.E. Raichle. 1994. Images of Mind. W.H. Freeman, New York.

Price, C.J., R.J.S. Wise, and R.S.J. Frackowiak. 1996. Demonstrating the implicit processing of visually presented words and pseudo words. *Cereb. Cortex* **6:** 62.

Price, C., R. Wise, J. Watson, K. Patterson, D. Howard, and R. Frackowiak. 1994. Brain activity during reading: The effects of task and exposure duration. *Brain* **117:** 1255.

Raichle, M.E. 1987. Circulatory and metabolic correlates of brain function in normal humans. In *The handbook of physiology. Second 1: The nervous system,* Vol. V. *Higher function of the brain.* Part 1 (ed. F. Plum and V. Mountcastle), p. 643. American Physiology Society, Bethesda.

Raichle, M.E., J. Fiez, T.O. Videen, P.T. Fox, J.V. Pardo, and S.E. Petersen. 1994. Practiced-related changes in human brain functional anatomy during non-motor learning. *Cereb. Cortex* **4:** 8.

Wernicke, C. 1874. *Der aphasische symptomencomplex.* Cohn and Weigert, Breslau, Germany.

Neural Mechanisms for Heading and Structure-from-Motion Perception

R.A. Andersen, D.C. Bradley, and K.V. Shenoy
Division of Biology, California Institute of Technology, Pasadena, California 91125

Two of the most important perceptual functions of the visual motion system are to compute our direction of heading as we move through the environment, and to deduce the three-dimensional structure of objects and the environment from motion cues. Below, we review experiments that provide insights into how these perceptual phenomena are constructed by the brain. Understanding how the motion system performs these analyses will likely have general applicability to other perceptual functions, both within and outside the motion pathway. For instance, understanding how motion signals are perceived as spatially constant despite eye movements, an important prerequisite for determining heading direction, may lead to a general understanding of spatial-perceptual constancy. Likewise, understanding how three-dimensional form is processed from motion cues in the dorsal visual pathway may provide important suggestions as to how form is derived from other visual cues in the ventral visual pathway.

In the first part of this paper, we discuss how "optic flow" signals, which are generated by translation through the environment, can be used for navigation. In particular, an important question in this area is how flow generated by eye or head movements is subtracted from the flow generated by translation in order to recover the direction of heading. Current studies indicate that the dorso-medial superior temporal area (MSTd) plays a pivotal role in heading computation.

In the second part of the paper, we examine the neural basis of structure-from-motion (SFM) perception. In particular, evidence is reviewed indicating that the middle temporal area (MT) is a site for the extraction of three-dimensional structure from motion cues.

HEADING COMPUTATION BY AREA MSTd

Theories of Heading Computation

Gibson (1950) proposed that observers in motion can use the focus of expansion of the retinal image to determine the direction of heading. If the eyes and head do not move, then the focus of expansion corresponds to the direction of heading, and navigation can be achieved by maintaining that focus in the desired direction of locomotion. Regan and colleagues and other investigators have pointed out that such a solution only works in the special case of no eye or head rotations (Longuet-Higgins and Prazdny 1980; Regan and Beverley 1982; Koenderink and Van Doorn 1986; Royden et al. 1992; Warren 1995). This point is made in Figure 1 for the simple case of moving toward a wall. If the eyes are moving, such as would occur while fixating a feature on the wall that is displaced from the heading direction, then a roughly laminar motion (which is opposite in direction to the eye movement) is added to the expansion component. As a result, the retinal expansion focus is shifted in the direction of eye movement. The true focus of expansion could be recovered by decomposing the flow field into its components due to translation (forward movement) and rotation (eye movement). After decomposition, the focus of the expansion component would indicate the direction of heading (Longuet-Higgins and Prazdny 1980). The same principles apply for scenes with depth variation, although the flow pattern during eye movements can be more complex.

Two general methods can be used to accomplish the decomposition of the translational and rotational components of flow. One uses information from the retinal image, such as local speed differences (motion parallax), and the other uses extra-retinal cues, such as a signal related to pursuit eye movements. There have been several different computational proposals to explain how this decomposition is performed (Longuet-Higgins and Prazdny 1980; Koenderink and Van Doorn 1981; Rieger and Lawton 1985; Hildreth 1992), and all of these models use retinal cues in the flow field to perform this decomposition. In general, these computational models use depth variation in the display to separate the expansion and laminar components of flow. This decomposition is made possible by the fact that translation through the world causes differential retinal motions as a function of depth, whereas rotation of the eyes or head causes laminar motion which is the same across the visual field and does not depend on depth. Therefore, if the image contains depth differences, it is possible to tease apart the flow components due to translation and rotation.

The above, earlier models developed rather general algorithms for solving the optic flow problem, and as such, were generally not specific about how they would be implemented by the brain. Subsequently, several models have been developed to perform the decom-

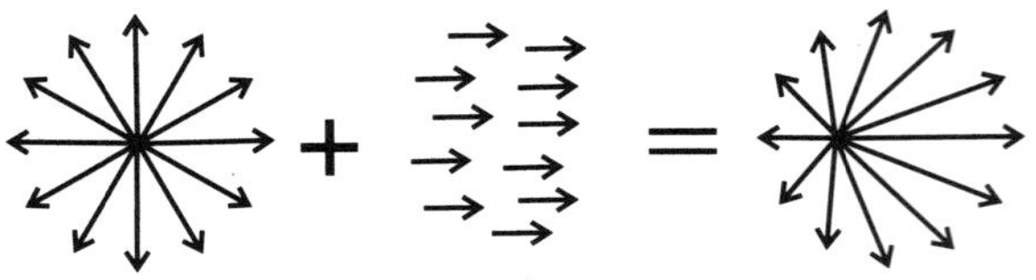

Figure 1. The problem of navigating while our eyes are moving. Moving toward a flat surface, we see an expanding image (*left* panel), and as long as our eyes are still, the focus of this expansion corresponds to our direction of heading. However, if we move our eyes to the left—as we would, e.g., while tracking an object off to the side—this adds rightward laminar flow to the retinal image (*middle* panel). The combined retinal image (*right* panel) is similar to the original expansion but has its focus shifted. Therefore, when the angle of gaze is changing, the retinal focus no longer corresponds to the heading. (Reprinted, with permission, from Bradley et al. 1996a [copyright AAAS].)

position of eye rotation and observer translation components in a biologically realistic manner (Hatsopoulos and Warren 1991; Lappe and Rauschecker 1994; Perrone and Stone 1994; Warren 1995; Stone and Perrone 1996). These are generally referred to as template models because they use receptive fields as templates to match various flow patterns. These models contain many maps (sets of templates) for the many different optic flow conditions that can arise from different eye rotation speeds, translation speeds, and depth variations and structure in the scene. A criticism of this template approach is that it requires too many maps (and neurons) to be biologically plausible. Our findings indicate that optic-flow-sensitive neurons adjust their focus tuning to account for tracking eye movements, which greatly reduces the number of templates required and makes the general template approach more realistic. This adjustment is made using an extra-retinal eye-movement signal, the method for computing heading which has not received much attention in computational models.

Psychophysics

For a long time after Gibson's original proposal, it was believed, on the basis of psychophysical studies, that humans were not very accurate at using flow information for navigation. This issue was later reexamined by Warren and colleagues using more controlled psychophysical techniques. When their stimuli imitated the approach to a wall (i.e., no relative depth cues), they found that heading judgments were very accurate under conditions of no eye or head rotations (for review, see Warren 1995). These judgments remained accurate during pursuit eye movements, even though these add laminar flow to the stimulus and shift the focus away from the heading. However, if the eye movements were simulated by adding laminar flow directly to the stimulus, subjects were unable to compensate for the laminar flow and thus could not accurately judge their heading. These results, later confirmed by Banks and colleagues (Royden et al. 1992, 1994), suggested that an extra-retinal (pursuit) signal is needed to decompose the retinal image into its radial and laminar components.

The psychophysical studies discussed above were based on the simulated approach to a wall. Different results were obtained when stimuli contained motion parallax cues—differential motions created by depth differences in the stimulus. In some cases, these parallax cues allowed observers to correctly judge their heading movements (Warren and Hannon 1988; Warren 1995), whereas in other conditions they could not (Royden et al. 1992, 1994).

Physiology of Area MSTd: Optic Flow and Smooth Pursuit Sensitivity

Area MSTd cells have been found to respond to rotations, expansion/contractions, and laminar motion (Sakata et al. 1985; Saito et al. 1986; Tanaka et al. 1986, 1989; Tanaka and Saito 1989; Duffy and Wurtz 1991a,b; Graziano et al. 1994; Lagae et al. 1994). The observation that many MSTd cells are selective for these types of stimuli led many observers to propose that area MSTd is involved in navigation from optical flow analysis. Moreover, the receptive fields of the expansion-selective neurons are also tuned for the location of the expansion focus, providing additional support for the idea that MSTd plays a role in navigation from optic flow (Duffy and Wurtz 1995). Another important aspect of MSTd neurons is their invariance for location, scale, or form cues (Graziano et al. 1994; Geesaman and Andersen 1996). In other words, a cell preferring an expansion will be tuned best to an expansion stimulus (e.g., as opposed to a rotation stimulus) regardless of its location in the receptive field, its size, or the environmental features conveying the motion signal. This high degree of invariance is important for accomplishing navigation independent of the exact structure of the visual environment and provides strong support for template models.

Several studies have documented activity in the medial superior temporal area (MST) related to smooth pursuit eye movements (Mountcastle et al. 1975; Lynch et al. 1977; Komatsu and Wurtz 1988a,b; Newsome et al. 1988). This coincidence of optic flow selectivity and pursuit selectivity in MSTd suggests that this area is a prime candidate for a brain center involved in heading computation. Area MST also receives angular-rotation vestibular signals, which are generated during head pursuit (Kawano et al. 1980, 1984; Kawano and Sasaki 1984; Thier and Ericksen 1992). The vestibular component during head pursuit has been measured with vestibulo-ocular reflex (VOR) cancellation, a condition in which the monkey maintains fixation on a stimulus that is attached to a rotating vestibular chair in which he is seated. The preferred direction of activity during VOR cancellation typically corresponds to the preferred eye pursuit direction, suggesting that the cells are coding gaze-tracking movements, independent of whether eye or head rotations lead to the gaze pursuit. Thus, area MSTd may also provide heading compensation during head, as well as eye, movements.

Heading Computation during Eye Movements

Recently, we examined the simplest case of heading computation from a physiological perspective, translation of an observer toward a wall (i.e., a frontoparallel plane) (Bradley et al. 1996a,b). Compensation for pursuit in this condition has been shown to occur for human observers when subjects are pursuing, but not when pursuit is simulated with an identical retinal stimulus while the eye is held fixed. We examined the focus tuning of area MSTd neurons with a stimulus on the screen corresponding to observer translation toward a wall; i.e., expansion with no depth variation. If MSTd is involved in heading computation, we would expect focus-tuning curves to shift during pursuit eye movements in order to continue to code the correct heading direction with the eyes moving. We would also expect from the psychophysical results that movement compensation would not be present when the same retinal stimulus is generated as the pursuit condition, but without eye movements. We found that both of these predictions are true, providing strong evidence that area MSTd plays a direct role in heading computation.

In these experiments, monkeys were seated with heads fixed and trained to fixate a spot of light on a projection screen. The spot was stationary or moving at 15.7°/sec in a constant direction. When the spot moved, the monkey was required to pursue it. Neurons were stimulated, during pursuit or stationary fixation, with a visual expansion pattern made up of 600 moving dots. The expansion stimulus was 130° x 130° square, but only a 50° x 50° segment (window) of this larger pattern was shown in a given trial (see Fig. 2).

After isolating an MSTd neuron and mapping its receptive field, we determined the neuron's preferred optic flow pattern, i.e., expansion, contraction, clockwise rotation, or counterclockwise rotation, by showing these patterns in pseudorandom order and noting the strongest response. If the cell responded to expansion, we proceeded with the experiments below. If it responded to one of the other patterns, we proceeded with the experiments outlined in a subsequent section. We then determined the neuron's preferred pursuit direction by requiring the monkey to pursue a dot across the screen in eight different directions: 0°, 45°, . . . , 315°. The direction eliciting the strongest response was taken as the preferred pursuit direction, with the opposite direction being designated the "antipreferred" pursuit direction. Next, nine expanding patterns were shown, in each case shifting the expansion focus (origin) to a new location. The focus varied from

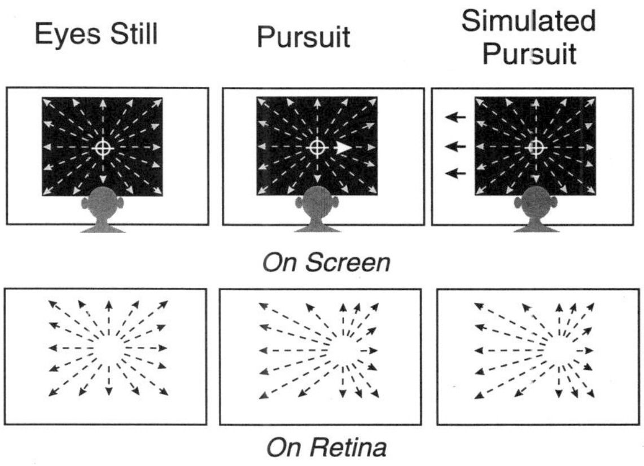

Figure 2. Paradigm to test whether MSTd cells encode the heading. A series of expanding images are shown while the monkey fixates (*top left*), during which time we record single-unit MSTd activity. The expanding patterns differ in terms of their focus position, allowing us to measure each neuron's output as a function of focus position. The focus position is the same on the screen and on the retina with eyes still (*bottom left*). The same series of expansions is also shown while the monkey pursues a moving target over a short distance (*top middle*). The eye position is about the same as in the fixed-eye case, but the eye velocity displaces the retinal focus relative to the screen focus (*bottom middle*). If a given neuron encodes the heading, its activity should be the same for a given screen focus position, regardless of whether the eyes are moving or still. In control experiments, eye movement is simulated by holding the eye still while moving the stimulus (*top right*). Like the pursuit condition (*middle* panels), this shifts the retinal focus (*bottom right*), but now no eye movement signal is available.

-40° to 40° in 10° increments, along an axis parallel to the neuron's preferred-antipreferred pursuit axis. Focus shifts were accomplished by shifting the 130° x 130° pattern behind the 50° x 50° viewable window, which remained at the same screen location. Thus, the stimulus always appeared in the same location on the screen (approximately centered in the neuron's receptive field); only the position of the focus, relative to this window, varied.

While the above stimuli were being shown, the monkey was required to fixate a stationary spot or to pursue a spot moving in the preferred or antipreferred direction for the cell (Fig. 2, left and center panels). Data were collected for the middle 0.5 sec of the stimulus presentation interval (1 sec), and the starting point of the moving spot was set so that the average position of the spot during the data collection interval was the same as the spot's position during stationary fixation. Therefore, the position of the eyes was about the same in both conditions (fixation and pursuit), differing at most by 4° during the data collection period. However, during pursuit, the retinal focus position was shifted relative to the focus position on the screen (Fig. 2, compare lower left and lower center panels). The magnitude of this shift was 30° for all stimuli in the direction of pursuit, since at this eccentricity, dot speeds equal the pursuit speed (15.7°/sec; see above). In other words, a dot moving at the pursuit speed (and in the same direction) was stationary on the retina and thus became the new focus.

For each neuron, we defined three focus-tuning curves: one for stationary fixation, one for pursuit in the neuron's preferred direction, and one for pursuit in the neuron's antipreferred direction. Each curve expressed the neuron's firing rate as a function of the position of the focus. Since each focus position can be expressed in two ways—the position of the focus on the screen, or the position on the retina—our basic task was to find the coordinate frame (screen or retina) in which the three tuning curves are best aligned.

To illustrate, Figure 3 shows the basic result of the experiment. The upper panels show focus-tuning curves for fixation and preferred/antipreferred pursuit eye movements. The left panel expresses these curves in screen coordinates (recall that the screen focus is equivalent to heading), and the right panel expresses the curves in retinal coordinates. All three curves are well aligned in screen coordinates but are shifted relative to each other in retinal coordinates. In other words, this neuron tends to give the same response to a given screen focus position, regardless of whether or not the eyes are moving. In contrast, this neuron's response to a given retinal focus varies considerably, depending on the state of the eyes. Therefore, neurons such as this could compute heading by shifting their retinal tuning curves in such a way as to maintain a constant output for a given screen focus (direction of heading).

Shifts in retinal tuning curves could be caused either

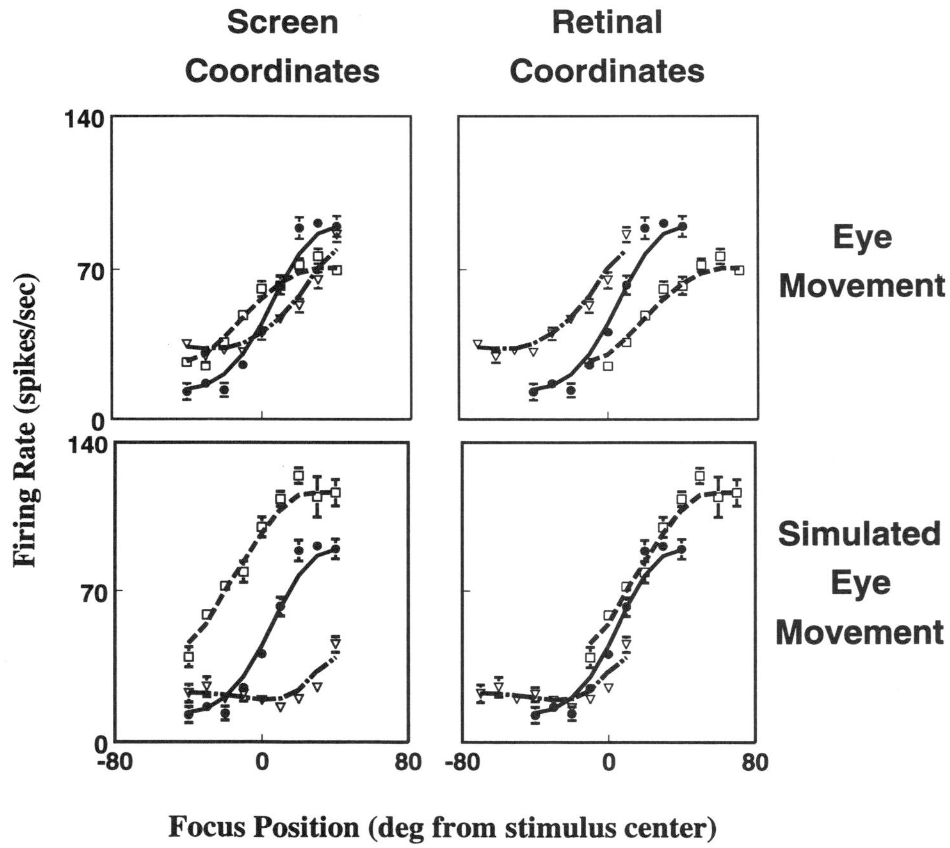

Figure 3. Example of an MSTd "heading cell." In all panels, the solid lines/solid circles represent the fixed-eye focus tuning (identical in all four graphs), dashed lines/open squares are preferred-direction eye movements (real or simulated), and dot-dashed lines/open triangles are antipreferred-direction eye movements (real or simulated). (*Top row*) Pursuit eye movements. (*Bottom row*) Simulated pursuit eye movements. (*Left column*) Screen coordinates. (*Right column*) Retinal coordinates. Data in the left and right columns are the same, except pursuit curves in the right column were shifted by ± 30° relative to screen coordinates to give retinal coordinates. When responses are expressed in screen coordinates (*top left*), activity is roughly constant for a given focus position. Since the screen focus corresponds to the heading, this implies that neurons such as this could encode heading direction. Note that for simulated eye movements, results are quite different (*bottom right*), so an extraretinal signal is essential for computing the heading. Data points are means ± S.E.M for four replicates, where each replicate is the mean firing during the middle 500 msec of the stimulus-presentation interval. (Reprinted, with permission, from Bradley et al. 1996a [copyright AAAS].)

by eye movements directly, or by what the retina sees during that movement. To distinguish these possibilities, we used a simulated eye movement control. For example, to simulate smooth pursuit to the right, we moved the entire stimulus left while holding the eyes still (Fig. 2, upper right panel). Thus, the retinal image was identical for real and simulated pursuit, the only difference being the actual velocity of the eyes (Fig. 2, compare lower center and lower right panels). The lower panels in Figure 3 show simulated eye movement data for the neuron described immediately above In this case, tuning curves are well aligned in retinal coordinates but highly dissimilar in screen coordinates. Thus, the shift in retinal tuning exhibited by this neuron was due to the eye movement itself, not the retinal consequences of the movement.

To quantify results in the MSTd population as a whole, we used cross-correlation techniques to find the shift in retinal focus tuning caused by pursuit. In other words, focus-tuning curves for pursuit and stationary fixation were incrementally shifted relative to each other (in retinal coordinates), in each case correlating the two. The relative shift at which maximal cross-correlation occurs was taken as the "best" shift—that which best aligns relevant features of the two curves, such as maxima, minima, and inflections. These best shifts were then summarized in a frequency histogram for the population.

We have cross-correlation data for 57 expansion-selective MSTd neurons. When eye movements were simulated, the frequency distribution clearly peaks at zero, indicating that in the absence of real eye movements, retinal focus-tuning curves generally do not shift. On the other hand, the histogram for real eye movements was clearly spread out to one side, so that more than half of the neurons have focus-tuning curves shifted by 10° or more, in every case in the direction required to compensate for the retinal focus shift induced by the eye movement (average shift = 11 ± 3° relative to simulated pursuit; 18 ± 3° when shifts are computed based on mean square difference between the curves). Our findings therefore indicate that MSTd cells integrate eye movement signals with optic flow in order to shift their retinal focus sensitivity, thus compensating for retinal focus shifts incurred during eye movements.

These results indicate that many MSTd neurons shift their focus tuning by the right amount, while others do not at all; a third group is intermediate. There are two possible interpretations of these results: (1) Only a portion of the MSTd neurons are involved in heading computation (those with complete compensation), whereas the others are involved in some other function (these being the ones that do not compensate), or (2) the distribution of shifts reflects the transformation from retinal to heading coordinates. In the latter case, we would expect to find cells in different stages of the transformation, i.e., early (non-shifted), intermediate (partly shifted), and final (fully shifted), which is indeed what we found. The following section suggests a mechanism for this transformation.

Gain Effects and a Model for Pursuit Compensation

As mentioned above, results indicate that a fraction of cells in MSTd do not have focus-tuning shifts with pursuit. However, most of these cells do show modulation of their amplitude tuning by pursuit, by an average of 25 ± 3% for the cells in our sample. This finding suggests a possible model of how the shifting might be accomplished using an intermediate step of gain-modulated neurons without shifting fields (Bradley et al. 1996a).

The model for the transformation from retinal to screen coordinates uses two first-stage neurons whose focus tunings are offset, and whose activity is summed by a second-stage neuron that shifts its focus tuning during pursuit (see Fig. 4). The first-stage cells have nonshifting focus-tuning fields which are sine functions. Sine functions are used because different parts of a sine function can approximate either a gaussian or a sigmoid, which are the general shapes of the MSTd focus-tuning curves. Each sine function has three parameters: amplitude, frequency, and phase, as well as two gain parameters that are applied during each of the opposed pursuits. All parameters were adjusted simultaneously, fitting the fixed-eye and two pursuit directions concurrently, using nonlinear least-squares regression. This analysis was performed on the data from all cells that show focus-tuning shifts. This analysis accounted not only for shifts in focus-tuning curves, but also for gain modulation of the magnitude of activity for the shifting neurons. We have performed this analysis on 36 neurons that clearly shift their focus tuning during pursuit. The fits have been extremely good for such a simple model ($r^2 = 0.72 \pm 0.03$) and much better than single-stage models that use nonlinear pursuit modulations of the focus-tuning curves (sigmoids, exponentials, thresholded linear functions).

The above model demonstrates how MSTd can correct for the motions due to eye rotation. However, neither this model nor the experimental results can at this point determine in which coordinate frame MSTd represents the heading. In the above study, the position of the eyes, head, and body were all aligned and we referred to the MSTd response as being converted to "screen coordinates" only as an operational term. Additional experiments will be needed to dissociate these different coordinate frames by performing the experiments with the eyes, head, and body in different positions with respect to one another. One would presume that at some point in the nervous system, heading direction is represented in body and world coordinates in order to permit one to walk or drive through the world.

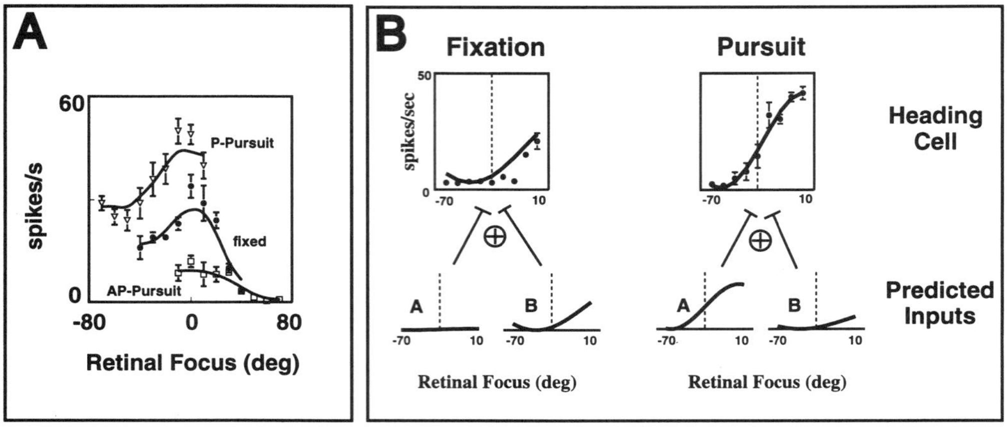

Figure 4. (*A*) Example of a neuron whose focus tuning does not shift during pursuit, but instead changes in amplitude. The three curves, corresponding to stationary fixation and opposite directions of pursuit, all peak near 0°, but their amplitudes vary considerably. Cells like this could serve as input to "heading cells," whose focus tuning does shift during pursuit. (*B*) Example of a heading cell and how it might be constructed from nonshifting, gain-modulated cells. The upper graphs show the neuron's measured focus tuning, during fixation (*left*) and preferred-direction pursuit (*right*). (*Circles*) Mean response; (*curves*) model fit. (*Lower panels*) Predicted input functions. Each function is characterized by three sine-wave parameters and multiplied by a gain; the two functions are summed to make the focus-tuning curve of a heading cell. All parameters were adjusted by nonlinear regression to fit the data (*upper panels*). This neuron's focus tuning shifts leftward during pursuit, and the model recreates this shift by increasing the gain on input function A while decreasing the gain on input function B. The sine-wave parameters (other than gain) were identical for the fixation and pursuit conditions; only the gains were adjusted to simulate the focus-tuning shift. (Reprinted, with permission, from Bradley et al. 1996a [copyright AAAS].)

Heading Computation during Head Movements

The results from the previous section indicate that an eye velocity signal is needed to compensate for smooth pursuit eye movements during heading judgments. A head velocity signal would also enable heading direction to be calculated during head movements. In conjunction, the eye and head velocity signals would permit the computation of heading from optic flow during arbitrary eye and head motions, especially in situations where a part of the gaze pursuit is supported by head movement and part by eye movement. It is presently not known if MSTd neurons compensate during head movements, or even if human subjects can perceive heading direction during pursuit head movements. If head pursuit compensation is present, there are at least three potential sources for the head movement signal: efference copy, the vestibular system, and neck proprioception. As mentioned above, vestibular as well as eye pursuit signals have been recorded in area MSTd. In preliminary experiments in which a monkey is rotated in a vestibular chair, we have found evidence that at least some cells show focus-tuning compensation during head movement as well as eye movement (Shenoy et al. 1996). Since the animals were rotated with fixed head-on-body orientation in the chair, the source of the compensation originates from vestibular canal signals. This result suggests that MSTd may also play a role in heading computation during head movements.

Rotation, Contraction, and Spiral Patterns

Area MSTd contains cells sensitive not only to expansion, but also to rotation, contraction, laminar flow, and spiral motions. During self-motion, these various motion patterns can be generated depending on the structure of the environment and the movement of the eyes. For instance, when fixating a location forward and to the side on the ground plane while translating forward, the motion around the fixation point is in the form of a spiral (Graziano et al. 1994; Warren 1995). Such nonexpansion stimuli can potentially provide information for computing heading. However, nonexpansion stimuli suffer similar problems when the eyes are moving; i.e., their focus shifts on the retina during pursuit movements. Interestingly, these shifts are not in the direction of the eye movement as in the case of expansion. For rotation, the focus shifts orthogonally to the direction of pursuit (see Fig. 5), the contraction focus moves opposite to the direction of pursuit, and spiral foci move in oblique paths that depend on the rotation and expansion/contraction components producing the spiral.

In the previous experiments, we have only discussed expansion stimuli. However, we have also investigated the effects of pursuit eye movements on 36 rotation and 46 contraction neurons. The speed of the dots was the same as the expansion stimuli, although each dot motion was oriented at 90° (rotation) or 180° (contraction) from the expansion case. These cells showed simi-

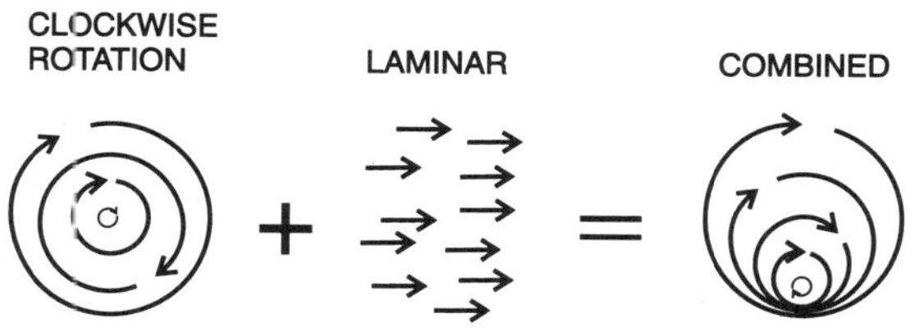

Figure 5. Eye movements across rotating patterns cause an orthogonal shift in the rotation center. For example, the focus in a clockwise rotation shifts downward during a leftward eye movement. To correct for this shift, clockwise-rotation cells must shift their retinal focus-tuning curves downward. (Reprinted, with permission, from Bradley et al. 1996a [copyright AAAS].)

lar focus-tuning curves to the expansion stimuli and compensated the focus tuning in the correct directions (orthogonal to pursuit for rotation and opposite pursuit for contraction). The cross-correlation results on the population data also showed that shifts were similar for all three patterns of motion.

This finding—that pursuit compensation also occurs for rotation- and contraction-sensitive MSTd neurons—has interesting implications for its role in perceptual functions. Fixation of a point straight ahead while moving over a ground plane leads to expansion on the retina. Points tracked farther off to the side lead to increasing amounts of rotation. This is due to the fact that eye-rotation components about an axis orthogonal to the ground plane make the plane appear to rotate. Thus, outward spirals are generally seen (expansion + rotation) when tracking a point on the ground. The focus of such a spiral can in principle tell us the direction of heading, as long as the eye velocity is taken into account. The same arguments pertain to contraction and inward spiral stimuli when looking in a direction opposite to the direction of motion. Thus, the correction of the focus tuning of MSTd neurons for motion patterns other than expansions during eye movements is consistent with their assisting in the mechanism of heading computation.

A second important perceptual function may also be served by the compensation for multiple patterns of motion stimuli. The shifts in focus tuning for all flow stimuli indicate a more general phenomenon of perceptual stability in the face of retinal image motions due to pursuit eye movements. Thus, for instance, when the eyes track across a moving wheel, the wheel does not appear to move up or down. Thus, MSTd may play a general role in compensating for self-induced motion using eye-movement signals. One important outcome of this compensation is the ability to compute heading direction, and another is the perceptual stability of motions in the environment.

Summary

Psychophysical studies have shown that humans use optic flow for heading perception and that heading judgments remain accurate even during smooth pursuit eye movements. In the absence of depth cues, this computation is only possible if eye velocity is taken into account. Recent physiological studies show that area MSTd, whose neurons combine optic-flow and eye-movement information, is central to heading computation. Expansion-selective neurons in this area are tuned for the retinal position of an expansion focus, and during pursuit, their focus tuning shifts in a way that compensates for the flow added by the eye movement. As a result, these neurons encode the direction of heading both when the eyes are still and when they are moving. Preliminary data suggest that MSTd accounts for head movements as well, in this case by integrating a vestibular signal. Surprisingly, nearly identical results were obtained in neurons selective for rotation and contraction. This suggests that a broad class of optic-flow patterns—not just expansion—may contribute to heading computation.

THREE-DIMENSIONAL-SFM PERCEPTION

Position Versus Velocity Cues

There are two broad theories for SFM perception: one that uses velocity measurements (Clocksin 1980; Longuet-Higgins and Prazdny 1980; Koenderink and Van Doorn 1986; Husain et al. 1989; Treue et al. 1993, 1995; Hildreth et al. 1995) and one that uses position measurements (Ullman 1984; Rieger and Lawton 1985; Grzywacz and Hildreth 1987; Grzywacz et al. 1988; Shariat and Price 1990) to derive three-dimensional structure. Perhaps the best-known position-measurement model is the incremental rigidity algorithm originally formulated by Ullman (1984). This algorithm samples position information derived from a few discrete image views of a moving object and attempts to find a rigid three-dimensional interpretation from the two-dimensional sample frames. Velocity-based algorithms measure the local velocities of points on an image and use the global velocity field to compute three-dimensional SFM. In our laboratory, we explored how humans perceive SFM using a novel stimulus designed to differentiate between position- and velocity-based algorithms. The results of these experiments support the use of velocity and not position measurements (Treue et al. 1993, 1995; Hildreth et al. 1995). Monkeys were also trained to perform similar SFM tasks using this stimulus. When area MT was lesioned, the monkeys could no longer perform this task (Siegel and Andersen 1986). Area MT cells are sensitive to the velocity of stimuli (Maunsell and Van Essen 1983a) and would in general be an unlikely area for making precise position measurements. These experiments establish that the brain uses velocity measurements for the SFM computation. They also establish area MT as a likely site for SFM processing.

Surface Reconstruction

Recent studies from our laboratory suggest that part of the SFM process is the reconstruction of surfaces (Husain et al. 1989; Hildreth et al. 1995; Treue et al. 1995). These studies indicate that the brain forms a mental image of a moving surface, based on velocity measurements. We have modeled this reconstruction process with three stages (Hildreth et al. 1995). The first is the measurement of motion signals, which are made independently of each other. The second step, the segregation of surfaces, is important for interpolation over areas with sparse features while still respecting surface borders. In addition, under transparent conditions or at motion borders, there are often motions in different directions that should not be averaged, but rather assigned to separate surfaces. A third stage then assigns three-dimensional depth values across the surface through the use of motion gradient information. As shown below, neurophysiological studies suggest that macaque areas V1, MT, and MST may carry out functions analogous to the proposed model stages. Specifically, V1 neurons have properties suitable for detecting motion signals, whereas MT neurons probably have a role in surface segmentation and integration. Finally, MT neurons, which are selective for motion gradients (Treue and Andersen 1996), or MST neurons, which are sensitive to motion patterns, may compute depth from motion gradients.

Transparency

Motion transparency—the perception of multiple directions of motion in the same location—is an important part of SFM processing. Transparent stimuli have proven invaluable in exploring the surface reconstruction process and SFM perception. It has long been appreciated that motion thresholds are higher under transparent conditions (Snowden et al. 1991). In physiology experiments, we found that direction-selective V1 neurons generally give the same response to a stimulus moving in their preferred direction, whether or not a second stimulus is present and moving in the opposite direction (Snowden et al. 1991; Qian and Andersen 1994). On the other hand, we found strong suppression for MT neurons under these transparent conditions (Snowden et al. 1991). This result supports the idea that the motion pathway contains two stages, one in V1 that measures motion signals, and a second, opponent stage in MT. We proposed that this opponent stage is part of a surface-reconstruction process and functions to suppress noise such as motion flicker.

The two-stage motion-detection hypothesis suggests that there might exist motion stimuli that would be completely "balanced," containing motion signals in opposite directions at every local region in the display, which would completely erase the perception of motion. We developed several displays that all eliminated perceived motion; one of these consisted of two random dot patterns in which the dots moving in opposite directions were all paired with one another. This stimulus produced greater suppression in area MT than in V1, providing strong evidence that area MT is the locus of perception of motion transparency (Qian and Andersen 1994). Furthermore, the degree of suppression of individual MT neurons correlates negatively with their response to visual noise, supporting our proposal that one purpose of the opponency is to suppress noise during surface reconstruction.

Integration of Depth and Stereo

In our psychophysical studies with balanced, nontransparent stimuli, we found that if the two surfaces were separated in depth, the perception of the two surfaces re-emerged (Qian et al. 1994a). Physiological experiments have established that area MT neurons are selective not only to motion, but also to stereoscopic depth (Maunsell and Van Essen 1983b). We reasoned that the improved perception of transparency with stereoscopic depth separation may be a result of the opponent suppression in MT operating primarily within the same stereo planes. Our experiments showed that in fact this is true—inhibition in MT occurs mainly between motion signals with similar disparity (Bradley et al. 1995). This is consistent with opponency operating to minimize random motion signals from a given surface (e.g., due to flicker), whereas stereospecificity prevents opponency between motion signals from different objects at different visual depths. In Figure 6 this basic MT network is shown, with excitatory connections between opponent directions at different stereoscopic depths (D.C. Bradley et al., unpubl.).

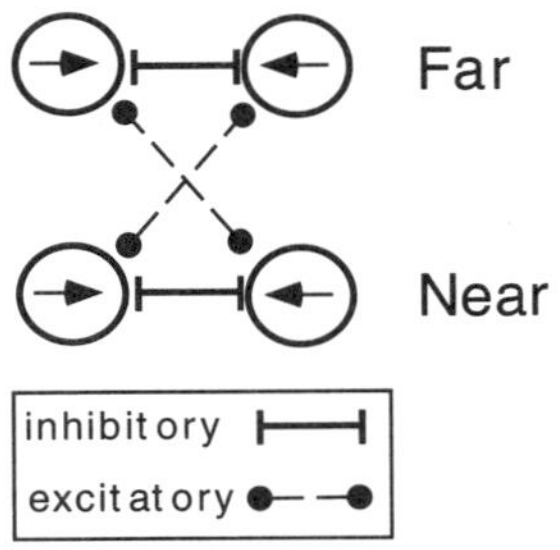

Figure 6. Model of MT motion processing. Neurons tuned to opposite directions inhibit each other within a given disparity channel (*solid lines*) and excite each other between disparity channels (*dashed lines*). Since very few MT neurons are tuned for near-zero disparities, this channel is omitted. However, most near- and far-tuned MT cells respond at least somewhat to zero disparity. What is the predicted response to a stimulus with opposite directions, both at zero disparity? Either direction could be represented in either the near or far channels. However, the preferred configuration would be one in which the two directions occupy *different* disparity channels. Therefore, it is possible that basic depth percepts in SFM stimuli result from depth-specific inhibition and facilitation in MT.

A stereospecific opponency was also proposed in a modeling paper by Nawrot and Blake (1989, 1990) based on psychophysical results showing depth-specific motion adaptation. Another important prediction of the Nawrot and Blake study was that the impression of depth might arise due to these opponent interactions alone (Hiris and Blake 1996). When we see opposite directions at the same disparity, as with two planes or the cylinder stimulus, MT neurons tuned to these opposing motions mutually inhibit each other, possibly driving activity into the near and far channels. This is possible because most MT neurons have broad disparity tuning that extends into the zero-disparity range. The excitatory connections across disparity planes for different motion directions, combined with opponency within stereoplanes, prevent both the near and far cells from representing the same direction (surface). We might thus perceive a depth ordering of the surfaces due to the constraint in MT that different directions must be represented in different disparity channels.

Recent work in our laboratory showed that MT neurons are sensitive to velocity gradients (Treue and Andersen 1996), but the effects are modest. Thus, it is unclear whether MT is also responsible for the depth percept that occurs as a result of motion gradients. Another possible site for this function is MST. Cells in this region, especially MSTd cells, are selective for various types of motion patterns and might be expected to play a role in the third stage of SFM computation; namely, the assignment of three-dimensional shape to surfaces. These MST neurons may be constructed from gradient-selective neurons within MT (Treue and Andersen 1996).

Neural Correlates of SFM Perception in MT

As discussed above, lesions to MT in macaques irreversibly suppress the perception of SFM, suggesting that MT has a major role in SFM computation. However, it could be that MT is needed simply to supply image velocity estimates to another area that computes SFM. To distinguish between these possibilities, we tested for trial-by-trial correlation between MT activities and the percept of SFM in behaving monkeys (Chang et al. 1996). Monkeys were trained to view a revolving cylinder, then make a saccade to indicate the perceived direction of motion of the front surface of the cylinder. Some cylinders contained disparity cues to specify the cylinder's rotation direction, whereas others—the bistable cylinders—contained no disparity and could therefore be seen as turning in either direction. Our preliminary findings suggest that MT responses are indeed correlated with the perceived rotation direction of these bistable cylinders. Therefore, MT's role in SFM perception does not appear limited to velocity estimation, but may in fact be central to the computation of depth from two-dimensional motion signals.

Summary

Humans are able to reconstruct the three-dimensional structure of an object based solely on two-dimensional motion information. This remarkable computation is known as structure-from-motion (SFM). Psychophysical studies have shown that SFM derives from velocity, rather than position, measurements. Moreover, surface interpolation, whereby similar motions are grouped, is a fundamental step in the SFM calculation. Physiological studies suggest that surface movements are computed in a heirarchical fashion, with component motions measured in area V1 and integrated in MT. Recent experiments on the mechanism of this integration have revealed a property of MT cells that may be essential to the SFM percept; namely, opposite directions are mutually inhibitory *within a given disparity channel.* As a result, MT does not readily represent multiple directions at the same depth, and MT neurons may thus be forced to encode opposing directions at different depths. Therefore, it is possible that the basic inference of depth in SFM stimuli stems directly from the stereospecificity of opponent interactions in MT. It is not clear whether MT computes depth veridically in these stimuli using motion gradients. There is evidence for gradient selectivity in MT neurons, but the effect is moderate compared to the cell's selectivity for direction of disparity. It is also possible that MST, which contains neurons sensitive to motion patterns, contributes to perceived depth from motion gradients.

CONCLUSION

Studies on heading and SFM perception have taught us a great deal about how different kinds of information converge on the primate motion pathway, allowing us to extract useful information from the visual world. One important observation is that even early stages of cortical processing are involved in rather specific computations. MT, for example, appears to have a central role in SFM computation, and MST is very likely involved in heading perception. Both of these computations are elaborate and highly relevant to our survival in a changing environment. This is not to say that cortical areas are specialized for a single computation. Indeed, it is probable that MT participates in heading analysis by providing velocity estimates to MSTd, whereas MST itself may help compute SFM. However, as experiments have gone beyond simple, unidirectional stimuli to more realistic displays that provide multiple retinal and extraretinal cues, it has become clear that the cortical motion areas combine these cues in ways that suggest a particular type of computation. Therefore, to understand the function of cortical areas, it is essential that they be studied in the context of a specific computational goal.

ACKNOWLEDGMENTS

We thank Sylvie Gertmenian, Betty Gillikin, and Jason Liao for their excellent technical assistance. This work was supported by the National Eye Institute, the Sloan Center for Theoretical Neurobiology at Caltech, the Office of Naval Research, and the Human Frontiers Scientific Program.

REFERENCES

Bradley, D.C., N. Qian, and R.A. Andersen. 1995. Integration of motion and stereopsis in middle temporal cortical area of macaques. *Nature* **373:** 609.

Bradley, D.C., M. Maxwell, R.A. Andersen, M.S. Banks, and K.V. Shenoy. 1996a. Neural mechanisms for heading perception in primate visual cortex. *Science* **273:** 1544.

———. 1996b. Heading computation during pursuit eye movements in cortical area MSTd. *Soc. Neurosci. Abstr.* **22:** (in press).

Chang, G.C., D.C. Bradley, and R.A. Andersen. 1996. Neural correlate of 3-D structure from motion (SFM) perception in area MT. *Soc. Neurosci. Abstr.* **22:** (in press).

Clocksin, W.F. 1980. Perception of surface slant and edge labels from optical flow: A computational approach. *Perception* **9:** 253.

Duffy, C.J. and R.H. Wurtz. 1991a. Sensitivity of MST neurons to optic flow stimuli. I. A continuum of response selectivity to large-field stimuli. *J. Neurophysiol.* **65:** 1329.

———. 1991b. Sensitivity of MST neurons to optic flow stimuli. II. Mechanisms of response selectivity revealed by small-field stimuli. *J. Neurophysiol.* **65:** 1346.

———. 1995. Response of monkey MST neurons to optic flow stimuli with shifted centers motion. *J. Neurosci.* **15:** 5192.

Geesaman, B.J. and R.A. Andersen. 1996. The analysis of complex motion patterns by form/cue invariant MSTd neurons. *J. Neurosci.* **16:** 4716.

Gibson, J.J. 1950. *The perception of the visual world.* Houghton Mifflin, Boston, Massachusetts.

Graziano, M.S.A., R.A. Andersen, and R.J. Snowden. 1994. Tuning of MST neurons to spiral motions. *J. Neurosci.* **14:** 54.

Grzywacz, N.M. and E.C. Hildreth. 1987. Incremental rigidity scheme for recovering structure from motion-position-based versus velocity-based formulations. *J. Opt. Soc. Am.* **4:** 503.

Grzywacz, N.M., E.C. Hildreth, V.K. Inada, and E.H. Adelsen. 1988. The temporal integration of 3-D structure from motion: A computational and psychophysical study. In *Organization of neural networks* (ed. W. Von Seelen et al.) p. 239. VCH, Weinheim, Germany.

Hatsopoulos, N.G. and W.H. Warren. 1991. Visual navigation with a neural network. *Neural Networks* **4:** 303.

Hildreth, E.C. 1992. Recovering heading for visually-guided navigation. *Vision Res.* **32:** 1177.

Hildreth, E.C., H. Ando, R.A. Andersen, and S. Treue. 1995. Recovering three-dimensional structure from motion with surface reconstruction. *Vision Res.* **35:** 117.

Hiris, E. and R. Blake. 1996. Direction repulsion in motion transparency. *Visual Neurosci.* **13:** 187.

Husain, M., S. Treue, R.A. Andersen. 1989. Surface interpolation in three-dimensional structure-from-motion perception. *Neural Comp.* **1:** 324.

Kawano, K. and M. Sasaki. 1984. Response properties of neurons in posterior parietal cortex of monkey during visual-vestibular stimulation. II. Optokinetic neurons. *J. Neurophysiol.* **51:** 352.

Kawano, K., M. Sasaki, and M. Yamashita. 1980. Vestibular input to visual tracking neurons in the posterior parietal association cortex of the monkey. *Neurosci. Lett.* **17:** 55.

———. 1984. Response properties of neurons in posterior parietal cortex of monkey during visual-vestibular stimulation. I. Visual tracking neurons. *J. Neurophysiol.* **51:** 340.

Koenderink, J.J. and A.J. Van Doorn. 1981. Exterospecific component of the motion parallax field. *J. Opt. Soc. Am.* **71:** 953.

———. 1986. Depth and shape from differential perspective in the presence of bending deformations. *J. Opt. Soc. of Am.* **A3:** 242.

Komatsu, H. and R.H. Wurtz. 1988a. Relation of cortical areas MT and MST to pursuit eye-movements. I. Localization and visual properties of neurons. *J. Neurophysiol.* **60:** 580.

———. 1988b. Relation of cortical areas MT and MST to pursuit eye-movements. III. Interaction with full-field visual stimulation. *J. Neurophysiol.* **60:** 621.

Lagae L, H. Maes, S. Raiguel, D.K. Xiao, and G.A. Orban. 1994. Responses of macaque STS neurons to optic flow components—A comparison of areas MT and MST. *J. Neurophysiol.* **71:** 1597.

Lappe M, and J.P. Rauschecker. 1994. Heading detection from optic flow. *Nature* **369:** 712.

Longuet-Higgins, H.C. and K. Prazdny. 1980. The interpretation of a moving retinal image. *Proc. R. Soc. Lond. B Biol. Sci.* **211:** 151.

Lynch, J.C., V.B. Mountcastle, W.H. Talbot, and T.C.T. Yin. 1977. Parietal lobe mechanisms for directed visual attention. *J. Neurophysiol.* **40:** 362.

Maunsell, J. and D.C. Van Essen. 1983a. Functional properties of neurons in middle temporal visual area of the macaque monkey. I. Selectivity for stimulus direction, speed, and orientation. *J. Neurophysiol.* **49:** 1127.

———. 1983b. Functional-properties of neurons in middle temporal visual area of the macaque monkey. II. Binocular interactions and sensitivity to binocular disparity. *J. Neurophysiol.* **49:** 1148.

Mountcastle, V.B., J.C. Lynch, A. Georgopoulos, H. Sakata, and C. Acuna. 1975. The posterior parietal association cortex of the monkey: Command functions for operations within extrapersonal space. *J. Neurophysiol.* **38:** 871.

Nawrot, M. and R. Blake. 1989. Neural integration of information specifying structure from stereopsis and motion. *Science* **244:** 716.

———. 1990. A neural network model of kinetic depth. *Visual Neurosci.* **6:** 219.

Newsome, W.T., R.H. Wurtz, and H. Komatsu. 1988. Relation of cortical areas MT and MST to pursuit eye-movements. II. Differentiation of retinal from extraretinal inputs. *J. Neurophysiol.* **60:** 604.

Perrone, J.A. and L.S. Stone. 1994. A model of self-motion estimation within primate extrastriate visual-cortex. *Vision Res.* **34:** 2917.

Qian, N. and R.A. Andersen. 1994. Transparent motion perception as unbalanced signals: II. Physiology. *J. Neurosci.* **14:** 7367.

Qian, N., R.A. Andersen, and E.H. Adelson. 1994a. Transparent motion perception as detection of unbalanced motion signals: I. Psychophysics. *J. Neurosci.* **14:** 7357.

———. 1994b. Transparent motion perception as detection of unbalanced motion signals: III. Modeling *J. Neurosci.* **14:** 7381.

Regan, D. and K.I. Beverley. 1982. How do we avoid confounding the direction we are looking and the direction we are moving. *Science* **215:** 194.

Rieger, J.H. and D.T. Lawton. 1985. Processing differential image motion. *J. Opt. Soc. Am.* **A2:** 354.

Royden, C.S., M.K.S. Banks, and J.A. Crowell. 1992. The perception of heading during eye movements. *Nature* **360:** 583.

Royden, C.S., J.A. Crowell, and M.K.S. Banks. 1994. Estimating heading during eye movements. *Vision Res.* **34:** 3197.

Saito H., M. Yukie, K. Tanaka, K. Hikosaka Y. Fukada, and E Iwai. 1986. Integration of direction signals of image motion in the superior temporal sulcus of the macaque monkey. *J. Neurosci.* **6:** 145.

Sakata, H., H. Shibutani, K. Kawano, and T. Harrington. 1985. Neural mechanisms of space vision in the parietal association cortex of the monkey. *Vision Res.* **25:** 453.

Shariat, H. and K.E. Price. 1990. Motion estimation with more than 2 frames. *IEEE Trans. Patt. Anal. Mach. Intell.* **12:** 417.

Shenoy, K.V., D.C. Bradley, and R.A.Andersen. 1996. Heading computation during head movements in macaque cortical area MSTd. *Soc. Neurosci. Abstr.* **22:** (in press).

Siegel, R.M. and R.A. Andersen. 1986. Motion perceptual deficits following ibotenic acid lesions of the middle temporal area in behaving rhesus monkey. *Soc. Neurosci. Abstr.* **12:** 1183

Snowden, R.J., S. Treue, R.G. Erickson, and R.A. Andersen. 1991. The response of area MT and V1 neurons to transparent motion. *J. Neurosci.* **11:** 2768.

Stone, L.S. and J.A. Perrone. 1996. Translat on and rotation trade-off in human visual heading estimation. *Invest. Opthalmol.* **37:** 2359. (Abstr.).

Tanaka, K. and H.A. Saito. 1989. Analysis of motion of the visual field by direction, expansion/contraction, and rotation cells clustered in the dorsal part of the medial superior temporal area of the macaque monkey. *J. Neurophysiol.* **62:** 626.

Tanaka, K., Y. Fukada, and H.A. Saito. 1989. Underlying mechanisms of the response specificity of expansion/contraction and rotation cells in the dorsal part of the medial superior temporal area of the macaque monkey. *J. Neurophysiol.* **62:** 642.

Tanaka, K., K. Hikosaka, H. Saito, M. Yukie, Y. Fukada, and E. Iwai. 1986. Analysis of local and wide-field movements in the superior temporal visual areas of the macaque monkey. *J. Neurosci.* **6:** 134.

Thier, P. and R.C. Ericksen. 1992. Responses of visual tracking neurons from cortical area MST-1 to visual, eye and head motion. *Eur. J. Neurosci.* **4:** 539.

Treue, S. and R.A. Andersen. 1996. Neural responses to velocity gradients in macaque cortical area MT. *Visual Neurosci.* **13:** 797.

Treue, S., R. Snowden, and R.A. Andersen. 1993. The effect of transiency on perceived velocity of visual patterns: A case of "temporal capture." *Vision Res.* **33:** 791.

Treue, S., R.A. Andersen, H. Ando, and E.C. Hildreth. 1995. Structure-from-motion: Perceptual evidence for surface interpolation. *Vision Res.* **35:** 139.

Ullman, S. 1984. Maximizing rigidity: The incremental recovery of 3-D structure from rigid and nonrigid motion. *Perception* **13:** 255.

Warren, W.H. 1995. Self-motion: Visual perception and visual control. In *Perception of space and motion* (ed. W. Epstein and S.J. Rogers), p. 263. Academic Press, San Diego.

Warren, W.H. and D.J. Hannon. 1988. Direction of self-motion is perceived from optical flow. *Nature* **336:** 162.

Visual Responses in V1 of Freely Viewing Monkeys

M.S. LIVINGSTONE, D.C. FREEMAN, AND D.H. HUBEL
Department of Neurobiology, Harvard Medical School, Boston, Massachusetts 02115

We have developed techniques to study the response properties of single units in V1 of alert non-fixating macaque monkeys. We map the orientation preference and the receptive field of each single unit using stimuli that do not require the animal to fixate. We then allow the animal to freely view simple and complex images while we record from these units. For each spike, we record the position of the eyes at a given interval preceding its occurrence; this should reveal the parts of the image that lead to the cell's firing. V1 cells in the alert monkey tend to have higher spontaneous activity than in the anesthetized monkey, and this high background firing usually obscured the specific responses in activity maps for complex images. We found that the response patterns of neurons gave surprisingly poor reflections of what the animal had been viewing, unless we restricted the analysis to bursts of spikes or short intervals of very fast firing.

METHODS

We recorded 31 units from V1 of an alert male macaque monkey. We have recently obtained similar results from a second monkey.

Stimulus Presentation and Data Collection

We first mapped the orientation tuning and receptive-field location using stimuli that did not require the animal to fixate.

Orientation tuning. To determine the orientation selectivity of a unit, the monkey was presented with a series of images such as that of panel a in Figure 1, consisting of 40–60 randomly positioned parallel bars. All orientations, in 10-degree increments, were presented at a rate of 5 or 10 Hz. In a given cycle, each orientation was presented once, in random order. Because many bars were presented in each frame, it did not matter precisely where the monkey looked, but because we were recording from the left hemisphere (and therefore the right visual field), we encouraged the monkey to keep his gaze in the left half of the monitor screen by rewarding him with a drop of water or juice whenever he kept his gaze for 3–4 seconds within 5–15 degrees of a 2- to 5-degree spot on the left side of the monitor. On different days different fixation requirements were used, depending on the monkey's willingness to fixate; the goal was simply to keep his gaze in the left half of the screen. Total spikes were recorded for all except the first 35 msec of each presentation. Tuning curves show polar plots of firing rate versus orientation angle (0 degrees = vertical). For simplicity in viewing the plots, the data points were reflected through the origin. Each curve represents at least 7 cycles of each orientation. At least two tuning curves showing approximately the same optimal orientation curves were required before we went on to the next step with a given cell. Error bars indicate the standard error of the mean.

Receptive-field mapping: Flashing bar stimulus. A single bar of optimal orientation was flashed at random positions on the screen at 10 Hz (for a few cells the stimulus rate was 20 Hz) while the monkey was encouraged to keep his gaze in the left half of the screen (because the electrode was in the right hemisphere) as described above. For each spike, a 200-msec history was recorded of bar positions, eye positions, and preceding interspike intervals. After recording this information for 2000 or more spikes, usually over a period of 10–60 minutes, the record was analyzed by reading back the information for each spike as eye position relative to bar position at various times before the spike occurred (the "delay time"). We could also read back either all spikes in the record or only those events that consisted of two, or more, spikes within a specified time interval (the "burst filter"). When using the burst filter, a dot is plotted at each eye position at a given delay before the first spike in each burst that passed the burst filter. Each panel in the figures represents the entire video monitor, which covered 60 by 45 degrees of visual angle. For each flashing bar record, the bar position is shown only once, plotted at the same location, and the foveal position relative to the bar position is calculated for each spike or burst.

In the gray-scale maps, the number of spikes assigned to each 10 pixel x 10 pixel area was calculated; these values were scaled linearly to fall into seven value ranges and assigned a corresponding gray level (darker corresponds to more spikes per unit area). For each cell studied, we used the flashing bar data to determine the optimum burst filter and delay time for data collection during free viewing.

Free-viewing recording. Static stimuli were put on the video monitor screen and remained there continuously for up to 3 hours; for cells recorded in the left hemisphere calcarine sulcus whose receptive fields were 15–30 degrees to the right of the center of gaze,

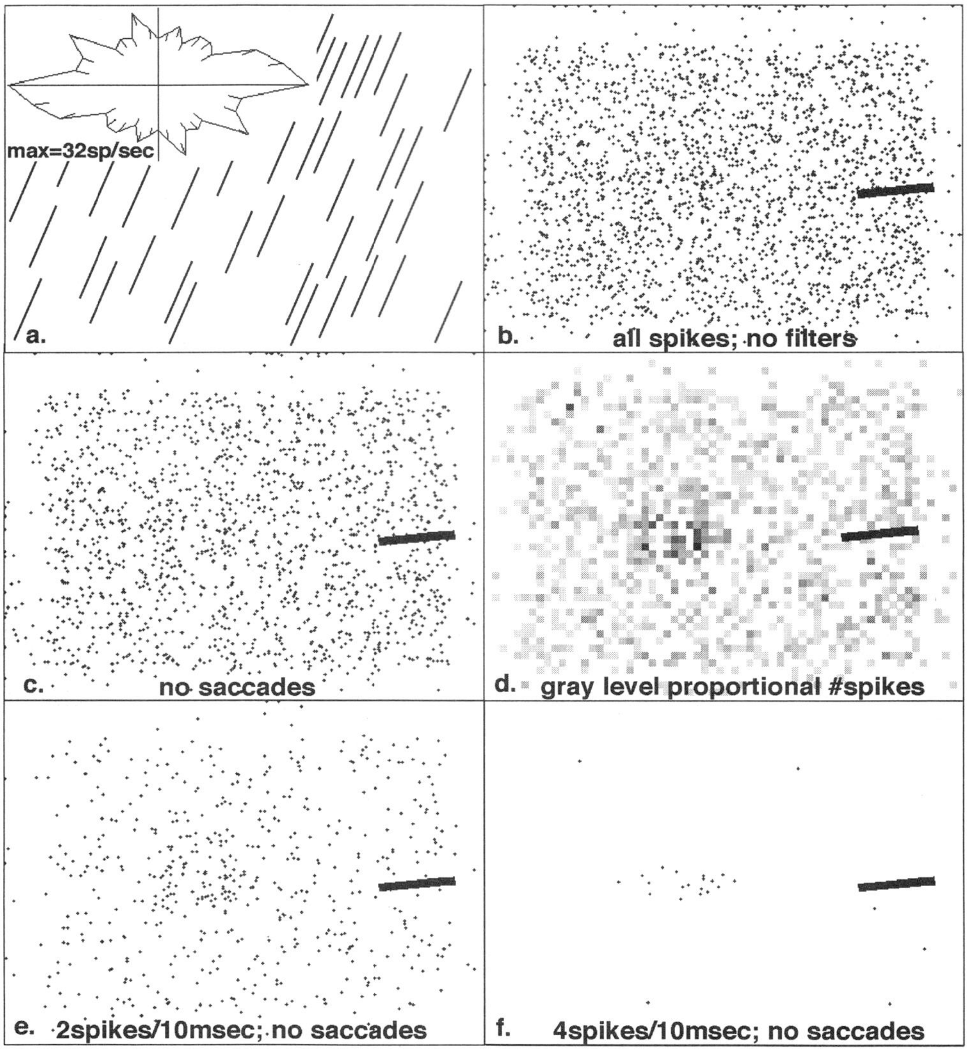

Figure 1. Panel *a* shows one frame of a series of stimuli used to generate the orientation-tuning curve shown in the inset from a single unit from Area V1 in the roof of the calcarine sulcus of the left hemisphere. The inset shows a polar plot of bar orientation vs. average firing rate; error bars indicate standard error of the mean. Panel *b* shows the foveal positions relative to the bar for every spike recorded during the flashing bar stimulus, using a delay time of 35 msec. Total spike number = 2400. There was no clear positional specificity in the response pattern, and it did not become any clearer at any delay time tested between 0 and 100 msec. (We show this particular delay time for the total spike train because a delay of around 35 msec gave the clearest receptive-field maps using the burst filter.) Panel *c* shows the same data, after eliminating all spikes that occurred within 50 msec of an eye movement of more than one-half degree. Panel *d* shows the same data as panel *b*, but with the number of spikes assigned to each unit area represented by a linear gray-scale value. The total spike data, as well as the total minus eye-movement spikes, also showed no clear evidence for a receptive field structure. Panels *e* and *f* show responses to a flashing white bar stimulus using different burst filters for the same unit. From the clear enhancement of the receptive-field map, such a burst filter enables us to restrict data collection predominantly to spikes that occurred in response to the bar stimulus. The receptive field map corresponds to an eccentricity of 30 degrees.

the stimulus was placed on the right half of the screen, and the left half of the screen was left completely blank. A 200 msec-long running buffer of eye position was continuously updated, and whenever an event (spike burst) occurred that satisfied the burst filter, the foveal position at a preset time before the first spike in the burst was recorded, and a pixel was plotted there.

Guided scanning recording. Similar stimuli and data collection as for the free-viewing experiments were used. A fixation spot appeared for 2 seconds at random locations over the image within a designated region, which was sized and positioned so that as the animal's center of gaze followed the fixation spot, the cell's receptive field would be positioned over all parts of the image. The animal was rewarded for following the spot.

Interspike interval distribution calculations. Using a receptive-field map from a flashing bar stimulus set, a rectangle was drawn around an area on the map—either the area that represented the response to the bar, or an area outside the response region. All spikes in the rectangle were tagged, and the time was determined between each tagged spike and the next spike in the train (this second spike did not have to be tagged). Predicted interspike interval distributions for random spike trains having a given rate were predicted using the exponential function:

$$f(t) = \lambda\, e^{-\lambda t}$$

In this expression, t = time, and λ = the rate of firing (Ash 1993). All histograms and curves were calculated for a bin size of 1 msec up to a total maximum interval of 35 msec; all results were normalized to give percentages of the total number of intervals up to 35 msec.

Alert monkey recording methods. Before recording began, under general anesthesia (1.5–2% halothane in 1:1 oxygen in air) and using sterile techniques, we implanted a head post, a scleral search coil, and a recording chamber (Wurtz 1969; Judge et al. 1980). The monkey was given analgesics for 2 days postoperatively (Torbutrol, 0.25 mg/kg, q12 hr) and prophylactic antibiotics 10 days postoperatively (2.5 mg/kg Baytril, bid). The monkey was allowed to recuperate for 2 weeks before recording began.

During recording we took extensive precautions to prevent infections. Anything that came in contact with the inside of the recording chamber, such as instruments, electrodes, guide tubes, and the electrode advancer, was either sterilized or disinfected with Nolvasan before use. The chamber was rinsed daily with sterile saline, and drops of antibiotic/anti-inflammatory solution (Neodecadron) were applied daily. The skin margins around the implants were painted with Nitrofurazone ointment daily.

The monkey was trained to sit in a primate chair with his head fixed, and, during the orientation tuning and receptive-field-mapping parts of the experiment, was rewarded with a drop of water or fruit juice when he kept his gaze within 5–10 degrees of a 1- to 5-degree-diameter spot for 3–4 seconds. Eye position was sampled at 250 Hz. The monitor was 34 cm from the monkey's eyes. Single units were recorded with lacquer-coated electropolished tungsten electrodes. All procedures conformed to National Institutes of Health guidelines for the care and use of laboratory animals.

RESULTS

Figure 1a shows one frame of the stimulus used to determine a cell's orientation preference, and the inset shows the orientation tuning of a typical unit. After the optimal orientation was determined, the unit's receptive-field location was determined by flashing an optimally oriented bar at various positions on the monitor screen, while storing a continuously updated buffer of eye position and bar location for the previous 200 msec. The bar was flashed in a different random position every 100 msec. Every time a spike occurred, the eye positions, bar positions, and preceding interspike intervals for the previous 200 msec were recorded. To analyze these spike trains, the bar was plotted at one position on the screen, and then a dot was plotted at the position the monkey's center of gaze had occupied, relative to the bar, at a designated time before the spike occurred (the delay time). This procedure is similar to a reverse correlation calculation (Jones and Palmer 1987). When all the spikes recorded were mapped in this manner, we could seldom see a very clear reflection of receptive-field organization at any delay time for a narrow bar stimulus (Fig. 1b).

We considered several possible explanations for this unexpected difficulty in seeing the effects of an appropriate visual stimulus on a V1 cell. We thought perhaps that eye movements might result in erroneously assigned eye positions. We therefore programmed the computer to eliminate from the plot all spikes that occurred within 50 msec of an eye movement of more than one-half degree. As shown in panel c, only a very few spikes were eliminated by this procedure, and the receptive field became no clearer.

Next we asked whether increases in firing might be concealed if points from more than one spike were plotted on top of each other during rapid firing. To test this possibility we converted the same spike data to a gray-scale map, assigning a gray level to each 10 pixel x 10 pixel area depending on the number of spikes assigned to that area (darker areas represent the highest spike counts). As shown in panel d, the cell of Figure 1 showed a hint of a receptive field in this gray-scale map, reflecting the fact that on average the cell fired 3 times faster when the bar was somewhere in the cell's receptive field (average rate = 53 spikes/sec) than when it was outside (average rate = 17 spikes/sec). The response was clearer than in the map in panel b, but not nearly as clear as we would have expected from listening to the neuronal activity on the audio monitor, or from our experience with anesthetized animals.

Our failure to produce a clear response map corresponding to the presence of the stimulus in the cell's receptive field surprised us, since we could often hear, and see on the oscilloscope trace, that cells did respond to the flashing bar, often in bursts of action potentials. We therefore tried analyzing the spike trains to display only those events when spikes occurred in bursts of a given number of spikes within a given interval. A clear response map then usually emerged. After collecting several thousand spikes for a particular unit, we could display the data using various burst filters (varying the number of spikes required within a variable time window) and using different delay times. Panels e and f show two maps, using different burst filters, for the same spike train. Restricting the display to responses consisting of 2 or 4 spikes within 10 msec shows an increasingly clear picture of the response to the flashing bar. Different cells showed the clearest maps using different filters, but the optimal delay time was usually between 35 and 50 msec.

For each unit, having first determined the optimal orientation, we used the flashing bar stimulus to determine the receptive-field location and optimal burst filter and delay. We then allowed the monkey to freely view simple black and white images or to scan the images by following a fixation spot that appeared at various positions, while recording spikes and keeping track of eye position. Figure 2 shows results for one cell. The flashing bar stimulus reveals a response map with the unfiltered spike train, but the map is much clearer when only those events where 2 spikes occurred within 10 msec were plotted. The right panels show the cell's responses while the animal viewed a simple circular white spot on a black background with and without this same burst filter. We positioned the white circle as shown, near the right edge of the monitor; thus, for the receptive field of the cell to be over part of the circle, the animal had to be looking at the lower left part of the screen. The animal was encouraged to explore the entire lower left part of the screen by rewarding him for following a fixation spot that appeared at various locations in that part of the screen. In

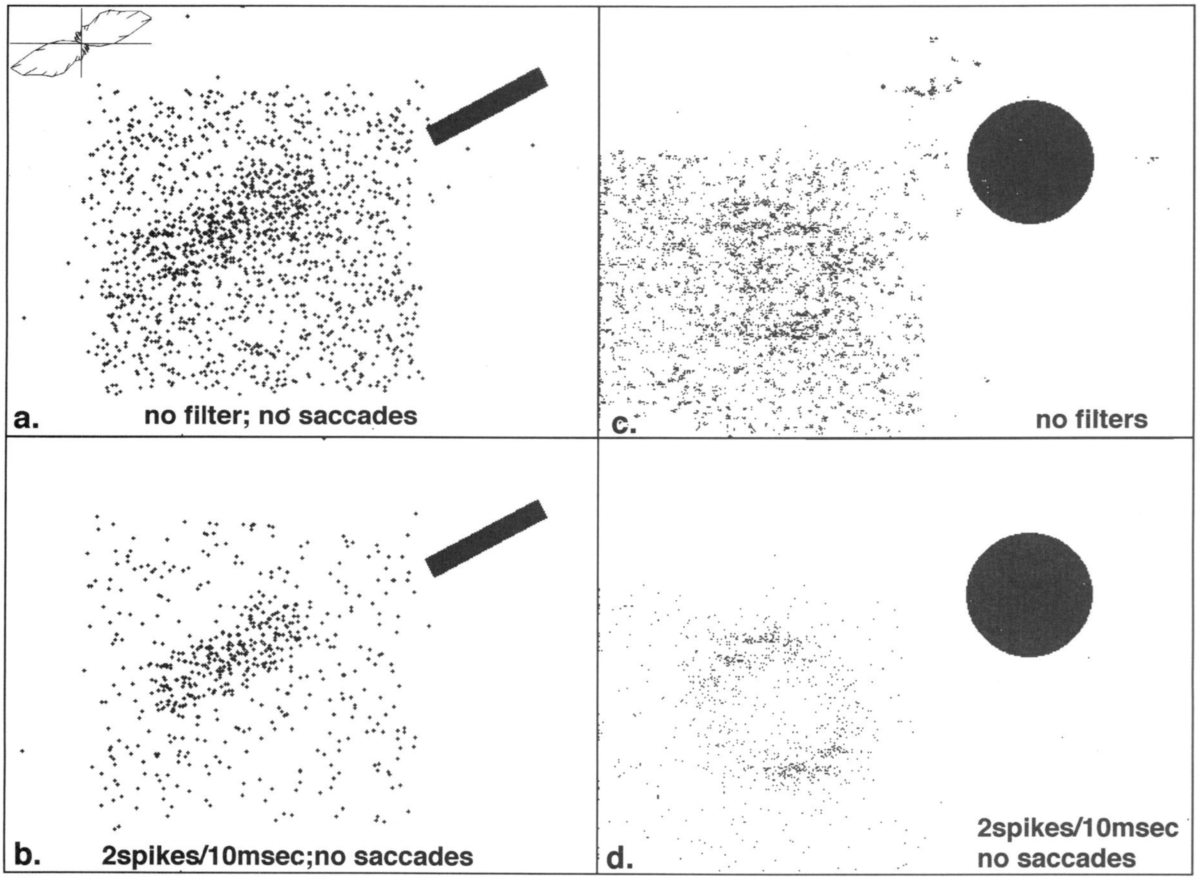

Figure 2. Responses of a cell located in the roof of the calcarine sulcus of the left hemisphere. The inset at the top left shows the cell's orientation tuning. Panel *a* shows the responses to the flashing bar stimulus (a white bar on a black background presented at 20 Hz), using no burst filter, but with spikes that occurred within 50 msec of a one-half degree eye movement eliminated. Total spike number for the flashing bar stimulus = 6300 spikes. Panel *b* shows the same spike train, filtered to show only those events when 2 spikes occurred within 10 msec. In this experiment, the monkey did not freely view the static stimuli, because we wanted to compare the responses with a burst filter to responses without a burst filter, and for technical reasons the two sets of spike trains had to be collected separately. Therefore, we programmed a fixation spot to appear at random locations, changing positions every 2 sec, in the otherwise blank lower left part of the screen, and the monkey was rewarded for following the spot. Panel *c* shows the spikes recorded in response to the white disk, while the monkey followed the fixation spot, without using any burst filter. Panel *d* shows the responses to the same stimulus, but recording only those events when 2 spikes occurred within 10 msec, and no eye movements of more than one-half degree occurred within 50 msec.

the right panels, each dot indicates the foveal position 35 msec before each spike (c), or before each pair of spikes occurring within 10 msec (d). This cell had a spontaneous firing rate of 20 spikes/sec and a visually evoked firing rate of 60 spikes/sec, but this difference in rate was not enough to produce a clear picture of what the animal had been viewing using the total spike record (c). When we filtered the spike train, however, it became clear that the cell tended to fire bursts of action potentials most frequently when its receptive field lay on or near contours of the same orientation as its preferred orientation.

Responses from a different cell are shown in Figure 3. This cell showed a poor response map to the flashing bar stimulus with no filter, even after eliminating spikes that occurred within 50 msec of an eye movement of more than one degree. A clearer response map emerged when we mapped only those events in which 5 spikes occurred within 40 msec. Then the monkey was allowed to freely view the monitor screen with a stationary white spot in the upper right corner. The cell fired bursts predominantly when the eyes were in such a position that the receptive field lay over contours of the preferred orientation. Unlike the cell of the preceding figure, this experiment was done without any guiding fixation spot, although the monkey was encouraged to keep his gaze in the (completely blank) left part of the screen by being rewarded for keeping his gaze in that half of the screen.

We also used slightly more complicated figures to see how cells would respond and how accurately the responses reflected the image the animal had been viewing. For several cells we let the monkey freely view images with multiple contours, without using any fixation spot (Fig. 4). The cells fired bursts not only to the parts of the arcs that had the same orientation as

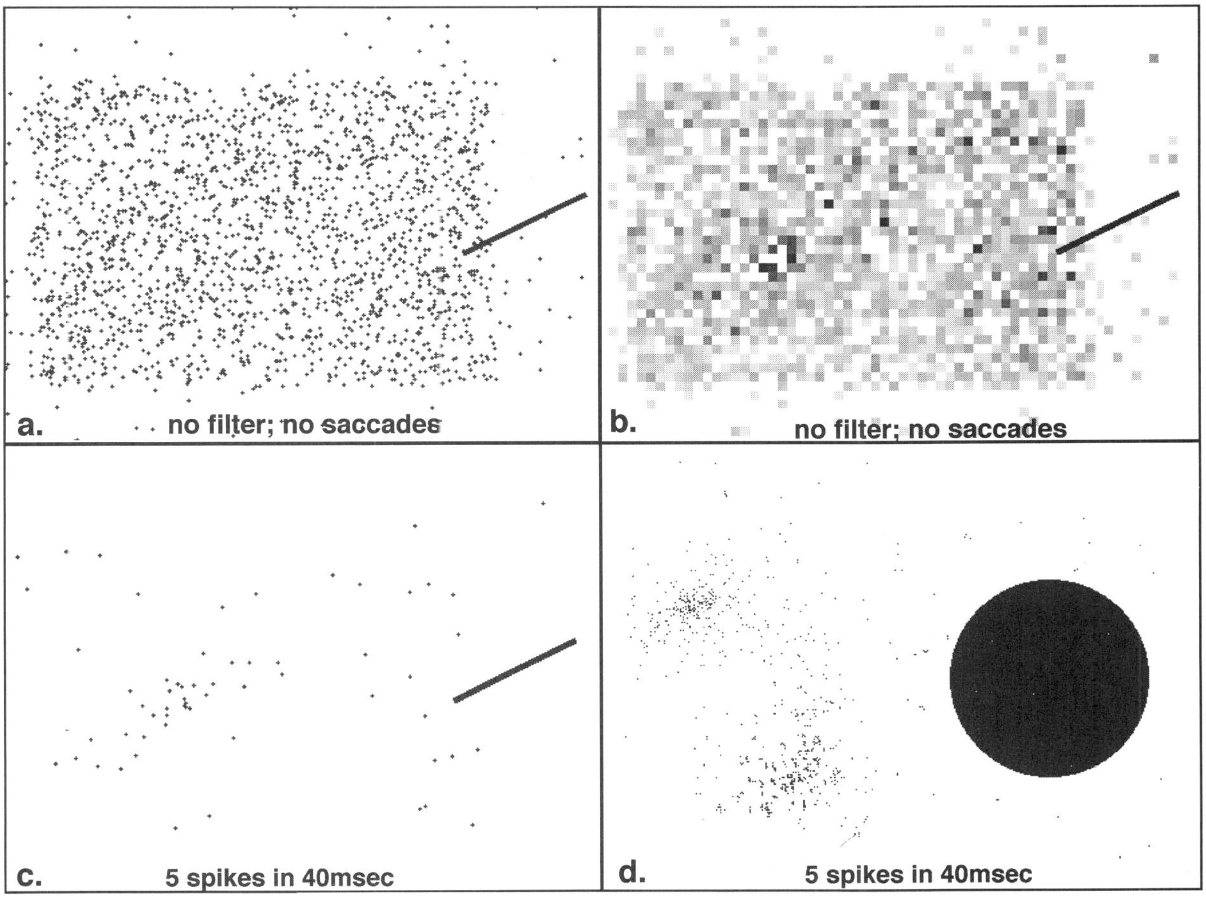

Figure 3. Responses of another cell recorded from V1 in the roof of the calcarine sulcus. Panel *a* shows the responses to the flashing bar stimulus (a white bar on a black background presented at 10 Hz), using no burst filter, but with spikes that occurred within 50 msec of a one-half degree eye movement eliminated. Panel *b* shows the same data, displayed using a gray scale to represent the density of events at each location. Panel *c* shows the same spike train filtered to show only those events when 5 spikes occurred within 40 msec. Panel *d* shows eye positions corresponding to events of 5 spikes within 40 msec while the animal freely viewed a large white spot on a black background. There was no fixation spot; the animal was encouraged to keep his gaze in the blank left half of the screen by juice rewards.

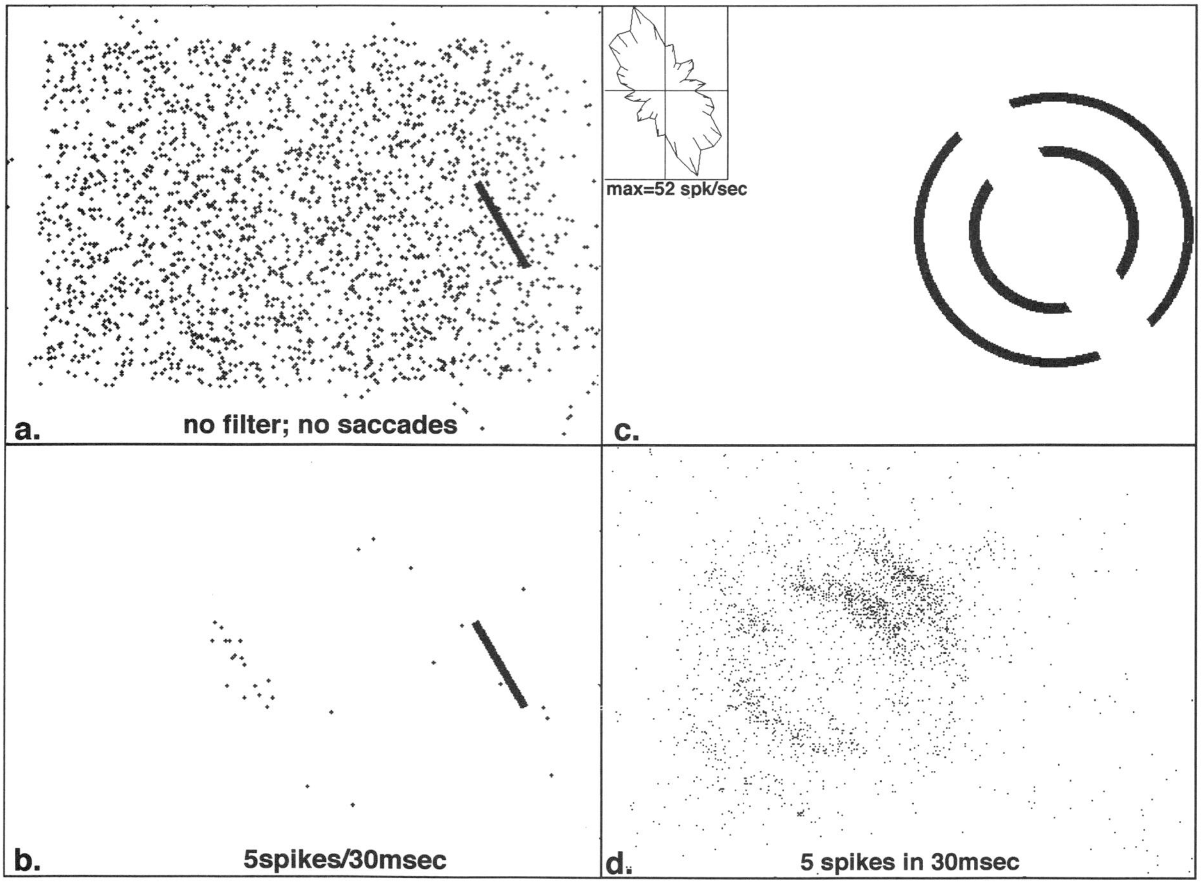

Figure 4. The inset in the upper right panel shows the orientation tuning of a cell recorded in the roof of the calcarine sulcus of the left hemisphere. Panels *a* and *b* show responses to the flashing bar stimulus, without and with a burst filter, as indicated (total spikes = 9600). Panel *c* shows the stimulus used during the free-viewing recording. In this experiment, there was no fixation spot; the animal was rewarded only for keeping his gaze in the blank left half of the screen. Panel *d* shows the foveal positions 35 msec before each event that passed the burst filter during the free viewing. All stimuli for this cell were white on a black background.

the cell's preferred orientation, but also usually to the short terminations of the arcs, which were also of the appropriate orientation. Figure 5 shows responses of another cell, using guided scanning with a similar stimulus.

One could ask whether the burst filter revealed the cells' responses simply because it acted as a temporal cutoff, indicating when cells fired faster than some baseline rate, or whether the responses were characterized by bursts of action potentials, as was our impression from listening to the cells and from looking at the oscilloscope trace. If we define a burst as a pair of spikes occurring within a given interval, t, for a theoretical random spike train, we can calculate the predicted burst rate. The average burst rate will be equal to the average firing rate times the probability that any spike in the train will be followed by a second spike within an interval, t. The probability that a second spike will occur within t is roughly proportional to the rate, as long as the average number of spikes per interval t is small. That is, for low spike rates and short intervals, the ratio of the burst rates is predicted to be approximately the square of the ratio of the two spike rates. For bursts of three events within a short interval, the ratio of burst rates will be roughly the cube of the ratio of the spike rates. For most of the cells we looked at, the average firing rate in response to the flashing bar stimulus was less than 100 spikes/sec. For spike rates below 100 spikes/sec, a burst filter of 2 spikes in 5 msec roughly squares the ratio of evoked to spontaneous firing (see Appendix). The effectiveness of the filter is less for higher rates or longer intervals.

This power relationship at least partly explains how our burst filter increases the evoked-to-spontaneous event ratio. That is, the fact that the burst filter increases the ratio of the rates of evoked-to-spontaneous events does not necessarily mean that a cell would have to show a change in firing pattern, such as an increase in burstiness, during evoked responses. Nevertheless, we do think that for some cells the firing

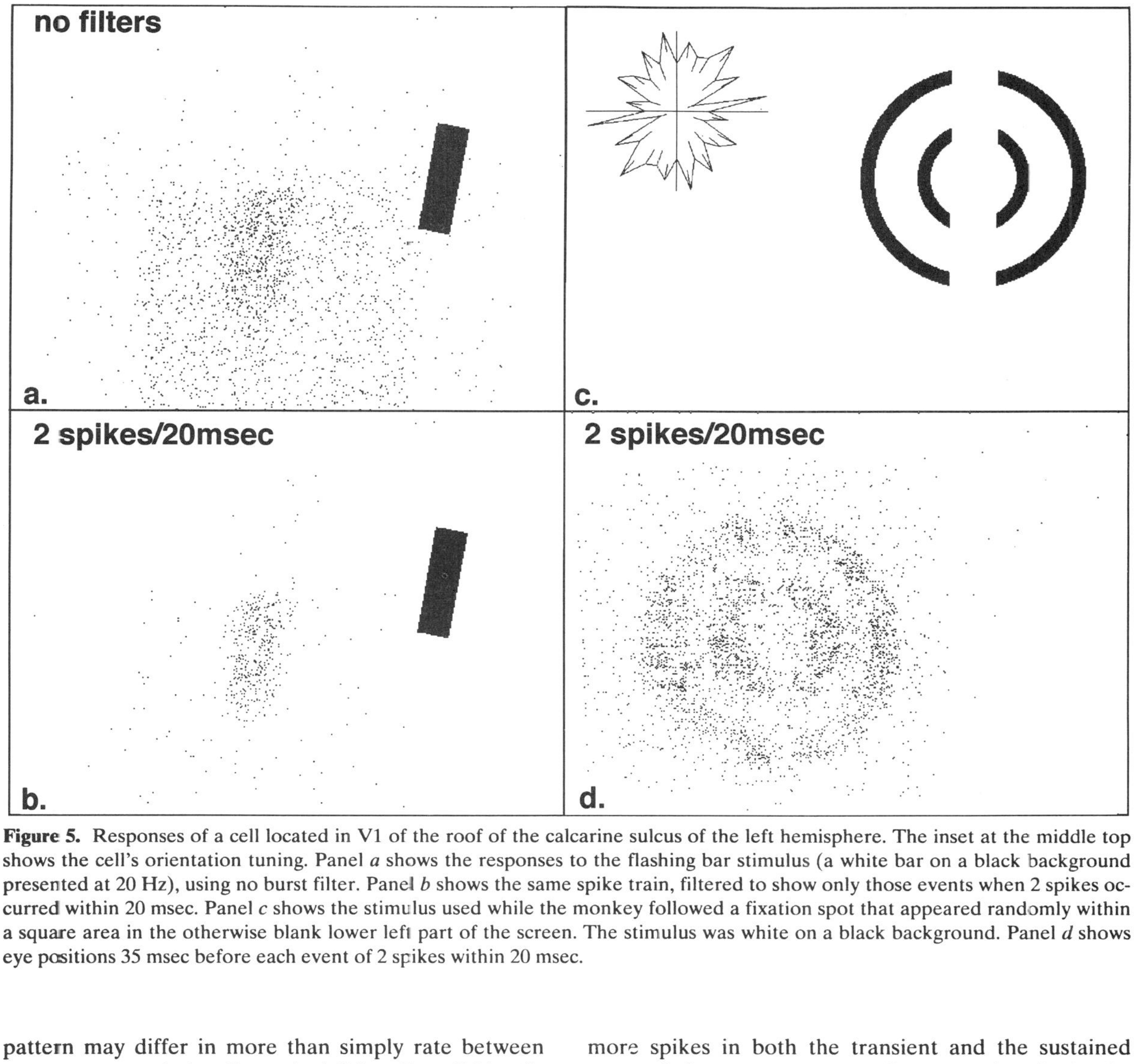

Figure 5. Responses of a cell located in V1 of the roof of the calcarine sulcus of the left hemisphere. The inset at the middle top shows the cell's orientation tuning. Panel *a* shows the responses to the flashing bar stimulus (a white bar on a black background presented at 20 Hz), using no burst filter. Panel *b* shows the same spike train, filtered to show only those events when 2 spikes occurred within 20 msec. Panel *c* shows the stimulus used while the monkey followed a fixation spot that appeared randomly within a square area in the otherwise blank lower left part of the screen. The stimulus was white on a black background. Panel *d* shows eye positions 35 msec before each event of 2 spikes within 20 msec.

pattern may differ in more than simply rate between spontaneous and visually evoked firing. For all 31 cells in this study, we calculated the predicted rate for events of 2 spikes per 10 msec as $\lambda\ (1-e^{-\lambda T})$, where λ is the rate in spikes/sec and $T = 0.01$ sec. Of this population of 31 cells, one third showed evoked-to-spontaneous event ratios that exceeded the prediction by more than 20%, suggesting a difference in firing pattern between evoked and spontaneous activity.

To get some idea of what this difference might be, we looked at raw spike records and calculated interspike-interval histograms for visually evoked and spontaneous firing. Figure 6 shows raster plots of individual responses for the cells illustrated in Figures 1 and 2. The responses of the cell of Figure 1, shown in the top panel of Figure 6, are characterized by a transient increase in firing rate, followed by a sustained response of about twice the background rate, lasting for the length of the stimulus presentation (100 msec). By inspection, there are frequent clusters of two or more spikes in both the transient and the sustained parts of the response, as well as occasionally in the spontaneous firing, shown to the left of time = 0. Interspike interval histograms for visually evoked and spontaneous firing for these two cells are shown in the bottom half of Figure 6. The interspike interval histogram for the first cell indicates that half the spikes in the visually evoked response occurred within 6 msec of another spike, yet the average rate during the visually evoked response was only 53 spikes/sec. For a random spike train with a rate of 53 spikes/sec, only a third of the interspike intervals should be less than 6 msec. This suggests that this cell does tend to respond with pairs or bursts of spikes. Of course, the initial response transient will contribute to the proportion of short intervals in the histogram. We do not know whether there is also a contribution from sustained bursty firing. The second cell responded to visual stimulation with a sustained increase in firing rate that lasted for about 50 msec, which was the duration of the

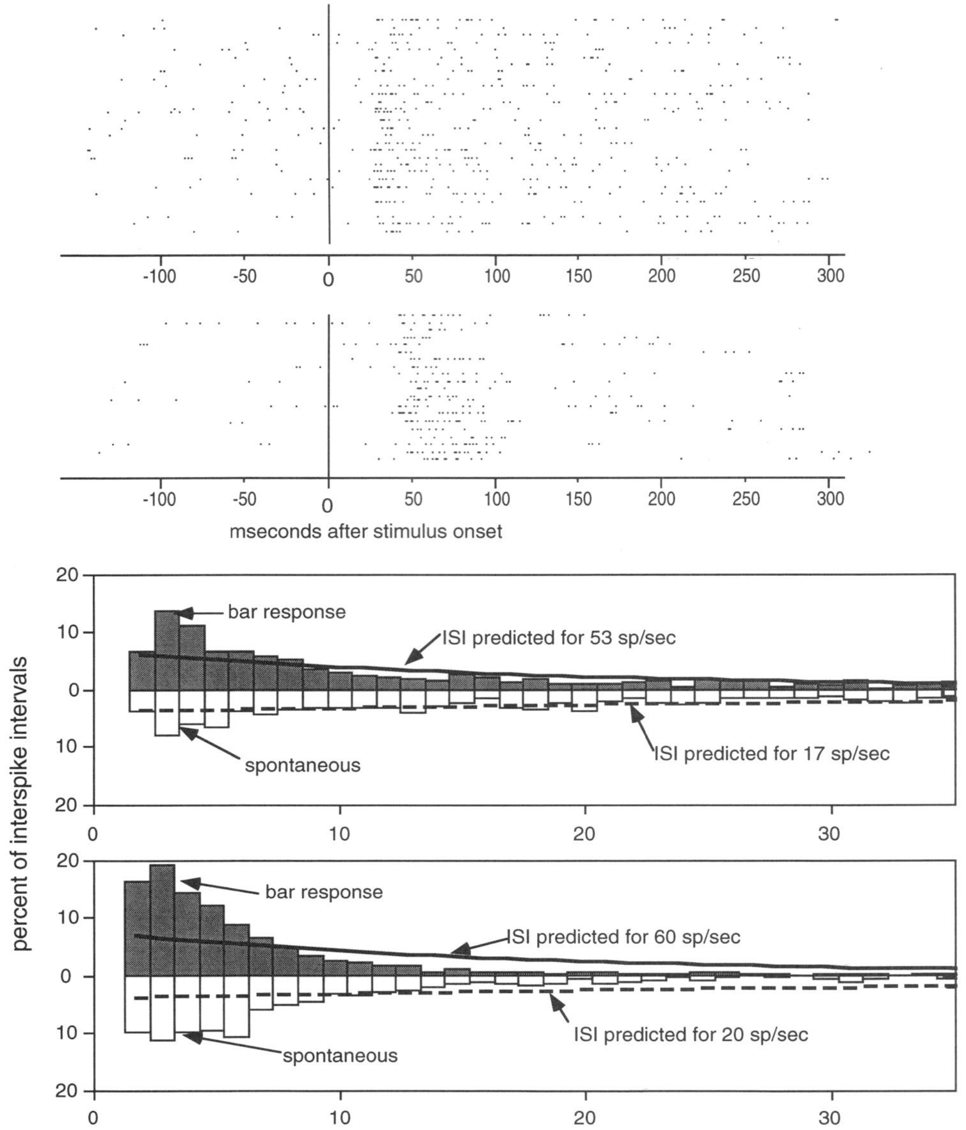

Figure 6. Raster plots and spike interval histograms for the cells shown in Figs. 1 and 2. The top panels show raster plots for a series of consecutive responses aligned so that 0 represents the appearance of the flashing bar in the cell's receptive field. For the cell of Fig. 1 (*top panel*) the stimulus duration was 100 msec; for the second cell it was 50 msec. The bursts do not show any relationship to the refresh rate of the monitor. The lower panels show interspike interval histograms for the same cells. The dark upward-going bars indicate interspike intervals for visually evoked firing, and the white downward-going bars indicate interspike intervals for spontaneous activity. The curves indicate the predicted interspike interval distribution for random spike trains having the same rate as the spontaneous firing (dotted downward-going curves) or the same rate as the average firing rate for that cell during the visual response (solid upward-going curves).

stimulus presentation in this experiment. For this second cell, the interspike interval histogram had 2.2 times as many interspike intervals between 2 and 6 msec as would be predicted for a random spike train with the same firing rate as this cell showed during the visually evoked response (60 spike/sec).

For the 31 cells in this study, the receptive field shape and size did not differ qualitatively with different filter settings; the only differences were in the ratio of visually evoked to background signal. Cells varied in how clear the receptive field was without using any filter; the average ratio of evoked-to-background firing was 4. However, all the cells showed an increase (on average a fivefold increase) in the ratio of visually evoked versus background events using a filter of 2 spikes/5 msec. All cells studied showed interspike interval histograms that were shifted to the left of what would be predicted for a random process, with, on average, twice as many intervals in the 2 to 6 msec bins as would be predicted, for visually evoked firing, and 1.5 times as many short intervals as predicted for spontaneous firing.

DISCUSSION

We find that looking selectively at 2 or more spikes within a short interval greatly increases the evoked-to-spontaneous event ratio. There are at least four contributing factors to the effectiveness of the burst filter in revealing visually evoked responses: (1) Any increase in firing rate is selectively enhanced because of the power relationship of the rate ratios; (2) many cells tend to fire in a bursty pattern, and the burstiness is increased during visual stimulation; (3) most cells show a transient period of very fast firing at the beginning of the response, which is selectively passed by the burst filter; (4) during free viewing or guided scanning, we suspect that small eye movements (Ditchburn and Foley-Fisher 1967) tend to bring the stimulus repeatedly into and out of the receptive field, producing a series of transient responses.

It is not surprising that the firing patterns of cells in V1 of alert, freely viewing macaque monkeys showed position- and orientation-specificity, as these properties have been well documented in anesthetized macaques (Hubel and Wiesel 1968) and in alert fixating macaques (Wurtz 1969; Dow 1974; Schiller et al. 1976; Maunsell and Gibson 1992; Snodderly and Gur 1995). Previous studies on alert fixating macaques of course found that cells do show an overall increase in firing rate to specific stimuli, but in these studies responses are averaged over many identical presentation repetitions, time-locked to stimulus presentation, so even a small increase in overall rate can be clearly distinguished as a specific response. In our experiments, for both the free-viewing situation and with the flashing bar stimulus, the appropriate stimulus falls on the cell's receptive field only a small proportion of the recording time, giving a much lower ratio of signal to noise. Moreover, the response is spatially distributed depending on the geometry of the stimulus. Gallant et al. (1994) recently reported that in V1 and V2 of freely viewing macaque monkeys, neuronal responses were poorly correlated with the cells' receptive-field properties, just as we found for most cells when no burst filter was used.

Our results suggest that, in the freely viewing animal, bursts of spikes, or episodes of very rapid firing, convey more information about the environment than single spikes or overall firing rate. We cannot yet distinguish between the contribution of transient high firing rate at the beginning of a response and genuine bursty firing, although both bursty firing and response transients may be very common in V1: Figures 6 and 7 of Wurtz (1969) show two cells in alert macaque V1 with very bursty responses; in the alert and the anesthetized cat, cells in area 17 frequently respond with bursts (Cattaneo et al., 1981); and responses in more than half the cells of a population of MT cells in the alert macaque showed bursty firing (Bair et al. 1994). In the present study, most of the cells showed transient high firing rates, with elevated average firing rates lasting 30 msec or less, and this transient response is essentially a single burst of spikes.

One might question our assumption that the burst-filtered response patterns, which more accurately reflect the image the animal had been viewing, carry more information than the noisier unfiltered maps. It is not sensible to assume that the function of a cell in the visual cortex is to reproduce as clearly as possible the image the animal was viewing, because this generates the homunculus problem, by implicitly assuming that some (one?) must be viewing this internal image. We do not assume that there is more information in the burst-filtered records because of the clarity of the images, but rather simply because the burst filter increases by severalfold the ratio of evoked-to-spontaneous events.

It seems reasonable to ask whether a method of looking just at bursts of spikes or transient rapid firing may be useful, not only as a technique for the neurophysiologist, but also to the brain. That is, if we find that the information carried by cortical cells (in V1) is carried more by bursts of spikes (or episodes of very fast firing) than by overall firing rate, it would make sense for the brain region receiving inputs from these cells to respond preferentially to bursts of spikes. Indeed, because of synaptic facilitation (Koch and Crick 1994), a postsynaptic cell is more likely to reach threshold when it is bombarded by bursts of spikes than when its input is evenly spaced spikes of the same overall rate. Moreover, if afferent neurons not only burst, but also burst in synchrony (Kreiter and Singer 1992; Softky and Koch 1993; Livingstone 1996), both temporal and spatial summation would make those signals carried by simultaneous bursts of spikes particularly potent at the next stage.

ACKNOWLEDGMENTS

This work was supported by the National Eye Institute, the Human Frontiers Program, and the Office of Naval Research. We thank Gail Robertson and Jason Rosenberg for skilled technical assistance. Ronald J. Bosch helped us with the statistical analyses.

APPENDIX

Prediction of Rate Ratios for Two or Three Events within a Short Interval

We will define a burst as two events occurring within a given interval, t. For a Poisson process, the predicted burst rate is equal to the product of the single event rate times the probability that at least one other event will occur within an interval t. For each single event, the probability of at least one other event occurring within an interval t of the first event is equal to 1 minus the probability that no event will occur within t.

Given a random spike train (Poisson process), the probability of k events occurring in an interval t is

$$e^{-\lambda t}(\lambda t)^{k} / k!$$

where λ = the average rate for the process (Ash 1993). From the above equation, the probability that no event will occur within a given interval ($k = 0$) is

$$e^{-\lambda t}$$

The probability that at least one event will occur within an interval t is

$$1-e^{-\lambda t}$$

So the predicted (2 spike) burst rate will be

$$\lambda\,(1-e^{-\lambda t})$$

For small λt, the function $1-e^{-\lambda t}$ is approximated by the function λt as λt approaches 0. The ratio of these functions, as λt approaches 0, is 1.

$$\lim_{\lambda t \to 0} (1-e^{-\lambda t})/\lambda t = 1$$

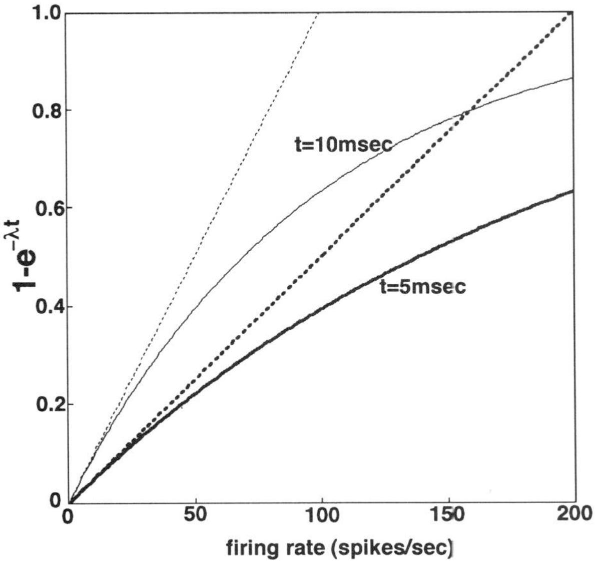

Figure 7. Evaluation of $1-e^{-\lambda t}$ as a function of λ, spike rate, for spike rates from 0 to 200 spikes/sec for intervals, t, of 5 msec (*thick solid line*) and 10 msec (*thin solid line*). The dotted lines show λ versus λt for spike rates from 0 to 200 spikes/sec for $T = 5$ msec (*thick dotted line*) and 10 msec (*thin dotted line*). For low spike rates and short intervals, the value of $1-e^{-\lambda t}$ approaches λt.

So, for low rates and short intervals, the burst rate for bursts of two events within a given interval approaches $\lambda^2 t$. Therefore, the ratio of burst rates for two different spike trains should be the square of the ratio of their rates.

In Figure 7 we have graphed the values of $1-e^{-\lambda t}$ for rates from $\lambda = 0$ to 200 spikes per second for two intervals, $t = 5$ msec and $t = 10$ msec. Figure 7 shows that for an interval of 5 msec, the probability of a second spike occurring within 5 msec of another spike is proportional to the rate for low firing rates, but falls below proportionality above rates around 100 spikes/sec. For a 10-msec interval, the proportionality falls off at lower rates. Thus, for evoked spike rates below 100 spikes/sec, a burst filter of 2 spikes in 5 msec will roughly square the ratio of evoked-to-spontaneous firing. The effectiveness of the filter will be less for higher rates or longer intervals.

By a similar argument, for bursts of three events within a given interval, the ratio of the burst rates will be approximately the cube of the ratio of the spike rates, for low rates and short intervals.

REFERENCES

Ash, C. 1993. Continuous random variables. In *The probability tutoring book*, p. 120. IEEE Press, New York.

Bair, W., C. Koch, W. Newsome, and K. Britten. 1994. Power spectrum analysis of bursting cells in area MT in the behaving monkey. *J. Neurosci.* **14:** 2870.

Cattaneo, A., L. Maffei, and C. Morrone. 1981. Patterns in the discharge of simple and complex visual cortical cells. *Proc. R. Soc. Lond. B Biol. Sci.* **212:** 279.

Ditchburn, R.W. and J.A. Foley-Fisher. 1967. Assembled data in eye movements. *Optica Acta* **14:** 113.

Dow, B.M. 1974. Functional classes of cells and their laminar distribution in monkey visual cortex. *J. Neurophysiol.* **37:** 927.

Gallant, J.L., C.E. Connor, and D.C. Van Essen. 1994. Responses of visual cortical neurons in a monkey freely viewing natural scenes. *Soc. Neurosci. Abstr.* **20:** 838.

Hubel, D.H. and T.N. Wiesel. 1968. Receptive fields and functional architecture of monkey striate cortex. *J. Physiol.* **195:** 215.

Jones, J.P. and L.A. Palmer. 1987. The two-dimensional spatial structure of simple receptive fields in cat striate cortex. *J. Neurophysiol.* **58:** 1187.

Judge, S.J., B.J. Richmond, and F.C. Chu. 1980. Implantation of magnetic search coils for measurement of eye position: An improved method. *Vision Res.* **20:** 535.

Koch, C. and F. Crick. 1994. Some further ideas regarding the neuronal basis of awareness. In *Large-scale neuronal theories of the brain* (ed. C. Kock and J. Davis), p. 93. M.I.T. Press, Cambridge, Massachusetts.

Krieter, A.K. and W. Singer. 1992. Oscillatory neuronal responses in the visual-cortex of the awake macaque monkey. *Eur. J. Neurosci.* **4:** 369.

Livingstone, M.S. 1996. Oscillatory firing and interneuronal correlations in squirrel monkey striate cortex. *J. Neurophysiol.* (in press).

Maunsell, J.H.R. and J.R. Gibson. 1992. Visual response latencies in striate cortex of the macaque monkey. *J.*

Neurophysiol. **68:** 1332.

Schiller, P.H., B.L. Finlay, and S.F. Volman. 1976. Quantitative studies of single cells in monkey striate cortex. II. Orientation specificity and ocular dominance. *J. Neurophysiol.* **39:** 1288.

Softky, W.R. and C. Koch. 1993. The highly irregular firing of cortical cells is inconsistent with temporal integration of random EPSPs. *J. Neurosci.* **13:** 334.

Snodderly, D.M. and M. Gur. 1995. Organization of striate cortex of alert, trained monkeys (*Macaca fascicularis*): Ongoing activity, stimulus selectivity, and widths of receptive field activating regions. *J. Neurophysiol.* **74:** 2100.

Wurtz, R.H. 1969. Visual receptive fields of striate cortex neurons in awake monkeys. *J. Neurophysiol.* **32:** 727.

Amblyopia: A Developmental Disorder of the Central Visual Pathways

L. KIORPES[1] AND J.A. MOVSHON[1,2]
[1]Center for Neural Science and [2]Howard Hughes Medical Institute,
New York University, New York, New York 10003

The primate visual system is organized with remarkable spatial precision. In the central retina, which supports our finest spatial discriminations, signals from each of thousands of photoreceptors are faithfully transmitted into the central visual system along a series of synaptic relays which are so refined that they lose no significant information about spatial precision. This precise order arises during development as a result of visual experience; indeed, visual experience of clearly focused, stable, and binocularly aligned images seems to be required (for review, see Movshon and Kiorpes 1993). If visual experience in early life is abnormal, monkeys and humans commonly develop a disorder of spatial vision called *amblyopia.* Amblyopia has no obvious organic cause. It manifests itself as a deficit in visual acuity that cannot be corrected optically. Amblyopia in humans can be caused by strabismus (misalignment of the eyes), and by other forms of abnormal visual experience such as anisometropia (a difference in the refractive state of the two eyes) and visual deprivation from cataracts, when these conditions are present during infancy and early childhood (see Levi and Carkeet 1993; Movshon and Kiorpes 1993).

The most prominent deficit in amblyopia is in spatial vision, and the condition is commonly characterized by a deficit in spatial resolution, as measured by either Snellen (optotype) acuity or grating acuity. In addition to acuity losses, amblyopes also show decreased contrast sensitivity and visual discrimination ability when tested through their amblyopic eyes. Indeed, studies of human amblyopes often show that the deficits in simple detection tasks (e.g., grating acuity) are relatively small compared to their deficits in visual discrimination (e.g., vernier acuity). Strabismic amblyopes are thought to be particularly severely impaired on a variety of spatial localization tasks like vernier alignment and bisection; they seem to have a distortion of the spatial sense that is not completely captured by measurements of grating acuity. Anisometropic amblyopes, on the other hand, are thought to show localization deficits that are proportional to their deficits in acuity (Levi and Klein 1985). It is, however, difficult to make classification of human amblyopes by the conditions they show at the time of examination, since complete clinical histories are rarely available to verify that these conditions have obtained throughout life. Moreover, we and other investigators have found evidence that strabismus and/or anisometropia may sometimes arise as a *result* of an amblyopia that has a different underlying cause (von Noorden 1980; Almeder et al. 1990; Kiorpes et al. 1993; Kiorpes and Wallman 1995).

To understand the causes, character, and biological basis of amblyopia, it is necessary to study the condition in an animal model. The pioneering work of Wiesel and Hubel (1963a,b; Hubel and Wiesel 1965) on the effects of abnormal early visual experience uncovered many important principles that govern the development of visual function, and the susceptibility of that development to the influence of the visual environment. Their work did not include a detailed analysis of visual function per se and concentrated on forms of visual deprivation that cause large changes in neural function and connectivity. We have developed and studied primate models for strabismic and anisometropic amblyopia. The use of the animal model has the virtue that the visual experience and clinical history of the subjects can be controlled and completely known.

The results of our behavioral experiments reveal that in a series of psychophysical tests, experimentally created amblyopia in monkeys has the same range of characteristics as naturally occurring amblyopia in humans. Physiological recordings show that the neural changes associated with amblyopia are seen in the primary visual cortex but not earlier in the visual pathway. The results suggest that the biological basis of amblyopia is a disruption of the processes responsible for the spatial precision of neuronal connections in the thalamo-cortical pathway.

METHODS

Our general methods for raising infant monkeys under conditions of abnormal visual experience, testing their visual capacities, and studying the properties of neurons in the visual thalamus and cortex have been described in detail elsewhere (Kiorpes et al. 1987, 1993; Kiorpes 1992a,b; Movshon et al. 1987; Levitt et al. 1994). All rearing and experimental procedures were conducted in compliance with the *NIH Guide for the Care and Use of Laboratory Animals.*

The subjects in these experiments were macaque monkeys, *Macaca nemestrina* or *Macaca mulatta*. The monkeys became amblyopic after a controlled period of abnormal early visual experience, either monocular eyelid closure, surgically created strabismus, or unilateral blur created by instillation of atropine or by extended-wear -10D contact lenses. Control data were obtained from eight monkeys raised normally. Monocular lid closure began within a few days of birth. Esotropic strabismus was induced 3–4 weeks after birth and persisted indefinitely; the size of the deviation was typically 5–25 degrees. Blur-rearing was begun 10–25 days after birth; unilateral defocus was imposed for 7–10 months thereafter.

Human data were obtained as part of the Cooperative Amblyopia Classification Study (McKee et al. 1992; Movshon et al. 1996). The data used here were taken from 251 observers aged 8–40 years. Of these, 67 were normal and 184 were amblyopes with a clinical history of anisometropia and/or strabismus.

RESULTS

Characteristics of Experimental Amblyopia in Macaque Monkeys

The spatial capacity of the visual system is commonly measured by the spatial contrast sensitivity function, which relates sensitivity (the inverse of threshold) to the spatial frequency of a sinusoidal grating target. Figure 1A shows the contrast sensitivity functions measured for each eye of a normal monkey (Kiorpes et al. 1993); the functions have a characteristic inverted-U shape. The peak contrast sensitivity of about 100 (corresponding to a contrast threshold of 0.01) is near 3 c/deg, and sensitivity falls to 1 (the lowest possible) slightly above 20 c/deg; this value is the finest spatial frequency resolved by the animal, or its grating acuity.

The visual sensitivity deficit in amblyopia is directly revealed by the contrast sensitivity function. Amblyopic eyes typically show reduced sensitivity to contrast; the loss is typically greatest at moderate and high spatial frequencies. The actual pattern of contrast sensitivity loss varies among individuals but does not vary by etiology: Similar contrast sensitivity deficits are seen in strabismic and anisometropic amblyopes.

Figures 1B and 1C show contrast sensitivity measurements for two amblyopic monkeys, one strabismic and one anisometropic (Kiorpes et al. 1993). In each case, the contrast sensitivity function for the amblyopic eye is shifted down and to the left of the function for the fellow eye, indicating losses in both sensitivity and spatial resolution. The contrast sensitivity of the fellow eye is similar to that of a normal monkey's eye.

Amblyopia is a disorder of development, and spatial vision in amblyopes is in many ways similar to spatial vision in normal infants. The contrast sensitivity function in young monkeys reveals that the infant visual system is less sensitive to contrast and can resolve only relatively low spatial frequencies compared to the adult. Similarly, the amblyopic eye resolves lower spatial frequencies and is less sensitive to contrast than the fellow eye. Figure 1D shows a comparison of contrast sensitivity in the same infant monkey at the ages of 5 weeks and 20 weeks (Boothe et al. 1988). Comparing these data with those of amblyopes (Fig. 1B,C) suggests (and a quantitative analysis of infant and amblyope contrast sensitivity data confirms) that the performance of the amblyopic eye resembles the performance of the eyes of young normal monkeys (Kiorpes 1992a,b, 1996).

As Figure 1D suggests, during the development of spatial contrast sensitivity, the peak of the function moves up and to the right; this happens without important changes in the overall shape of the function (Movshon and Kiorpes 1988). Figure 2 shows that the positions of these contrast sensitivity peaks in young normal animals (Fig. 2A) are similar to those observed in older amblyopes, either strabismic (Fig. 2B) or anisometropic (Fig. 2C).

Grating acuity is the highest spatial frequency that can be resolved at 100% contrast; that is, it is the spatial frequency at which the spatial contrast sensitivity functions in Figure 1 fall to a value of 1. Vernier acuity is another indicator of spatial visual performance and is usually measured by determining the smallest detectable offset between a pair of abutting colinear lines or edges. We studied the development of grating acuity and vernier acuity in normal monkeys and in monkeys with strabismus (Kiorpes and Movshon 1989; Kiorpes 1992a,b). The development of acuities both in normal animals and in the fellow eye of amblyopes follows a regular time course that appears roughly linear when plotted as a function of the logarithm of age. Amblyopia seems to slow the developmental time course for these acuities, rather than arresting development at a particular time or causing a deterioration of visual performance after maturation is complete. In addition, in normal monkeys and humans, vernier acuity is relatively poorer near birth and therefore shows a greater postnatal change than does grating acuity (Shimojo et al. 1984; Kiorpes and Movshon 1989).

In human amblyopes, vernier acuity—a measure of spatial discrimination performance and position sensitivity—is relatively more disrupted than is grating acuity, which is a measure of spatial resolution and sensitivity (Levi and Klein 1985). Figure 3A examines this in amblyopic monkeys by comparing the interocular ratio of vernier acuity and grating acuity for the two eyes. Virtually all the data lie above the diagonal, showing that vernier acuity losses are larger than grating acuity losses. In humans, Levi and Klein (1985) reported that this effect was larger for strabismic than for anisometropic amblyopes, but Figure 3A shows that there is no important difference between the losses shown by the two kinds of monkey amblyopes.

This pattern of a superordinate loss in vernier acuity can be accounted for in terms of the differences in de-

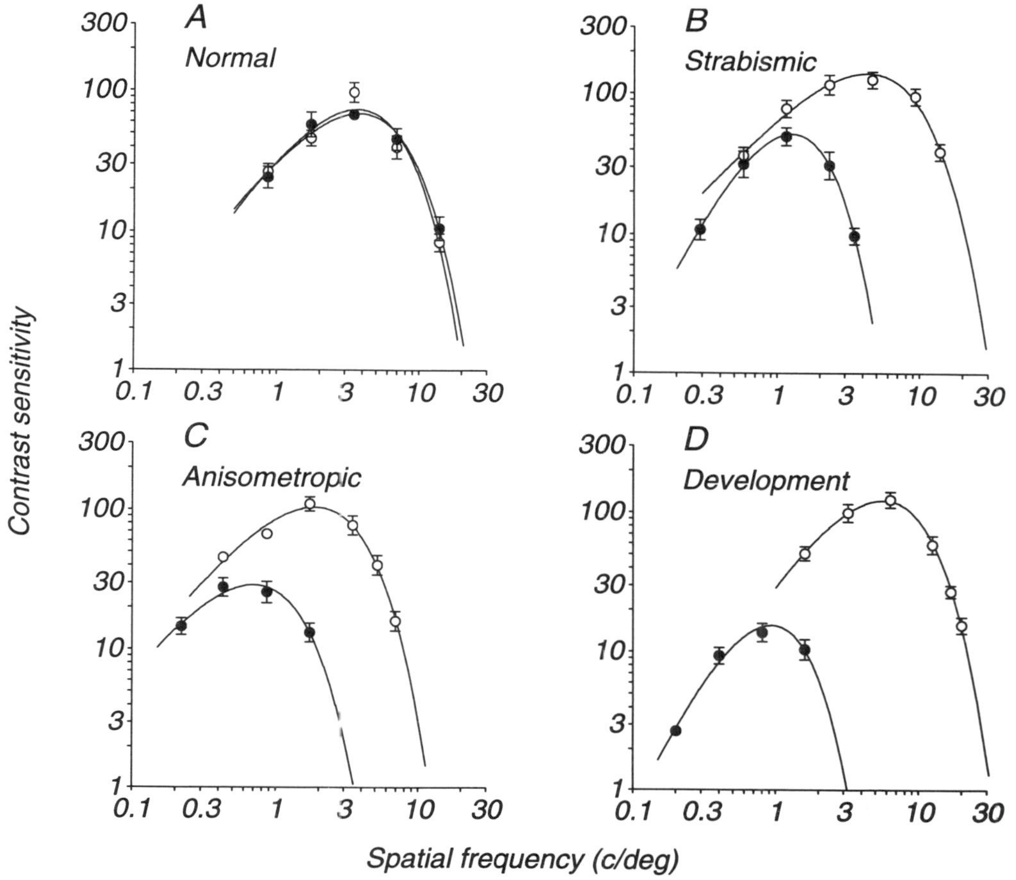

Figure 1. Contrast sensitivity functions measured in four monkeys. (*A*) Data from a normally reared monkey, viewing monocularly; the filled and open symbols show data taken from each eye. (*B*, *C*) Data from two amblyopic monkeys, one strabismic and one anisometropic. Filled symbols show data from the amblyopic eye, open symbols show data from the fellow eye. (*D*) Longitudinal data from one normally reared monkey, measured at the ages of 5 weeks and 20 weeks (*filled* and *open* symbols, respectively).

velopment of the two acuities. In normal animals, vernier acuity is relatively less mature in infants and develops to a greater extent than grating acuity during maturation. The relatively greater disruption of vernier acuity may then be a consequence of the relative immaturity of the visual system, rather than a peculiar deficit in positional acuity. Figure 3B compares the values of grating and vernier acuity for several kinds of monkey observers. Developmental data for normal monkeys are shown by the pluses. If these two acuities developed in lock-step, then the data would lie together along a line of unit slope, but evidently they do not. The filled symbols in Figure 3B show that the data for amblyopic monkeys lie near the data for young normal monkeys, further reinforcing the notion that the disorder in amblyopia can be understood as a failure of normal developmental processes to run their course.

Comparison of Amblyopia in Monkeys and Humans

Our experimentally amblyopic monkeys show many patterns of visual loss that are also characteristic of human amblyopia. To examine this impression quantitatively, we compared our monkey data directly with human data from the Cooperative Amblyopia Classification Study, a recently completed large-scale prospective study of human subjects (McKee et al. 1992; Movshon et al. 1996). We confined our comparison to data from a subset of the subjects in that study: normals, and amblyopes with a documented clinical history of strabismus, anisometropia, or both.

Figure 4 uses the same format as Figure 3 and adds to the monkey data previously shown four additional human data sets: normal observers, "pure" strabismics, "pure" anisometropes, and strabismic-anisometropic observers ("strab/aniso"). Figure 4A shows a comparison of the relative losses in vernier and grating acuity, as in Figure 3A. Almost all the human observers, like the monkeys, show a greater interocular difference in vernier acuity than in grating acuity. In contrast to some earlier reports (see e.g., Levi and Klein 1985), there is no apparent difference in this pattern of loss among the different groups of human amblyopes; this is of course the pattern seen in the

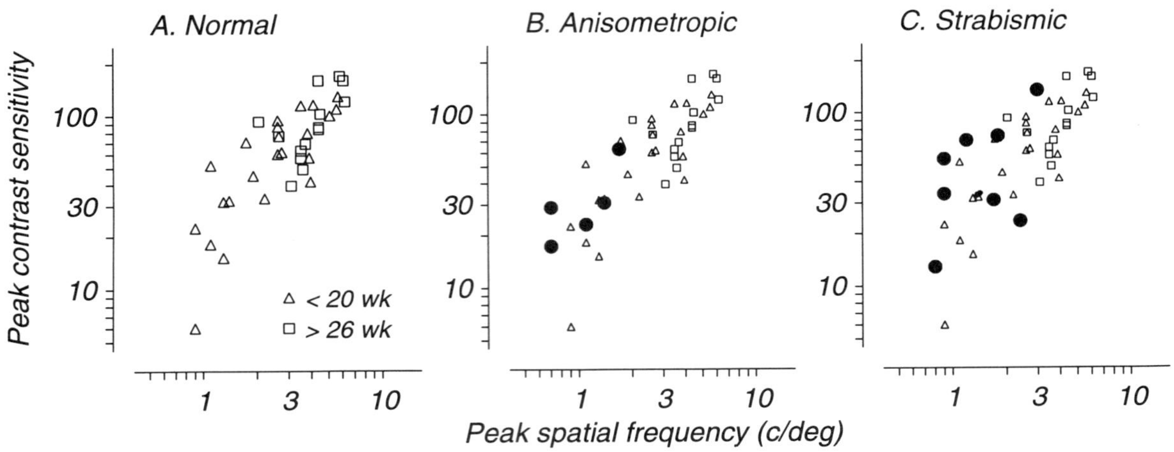

Figure 2. Results of a quantitative analysis of contrast sensitivity data showing how the curve shifts with age and with amblyopia. The relationship between peak spatial frequency and peak contrast sensitivity for normal infants (*triangles*) and adults (*squares*) is shown in *A*. The same data are plotted along with data from strabismic (*B*) and anisometropic (*C*) amblyopes. The data from amblyopes are similar to those from young normal monkeys.

monkey amblyopes as well. Figure 4A does show in humans that individuals with both strabismus and anisometropia tend to be more profoundly amblyopic than those with only one condition; we have not attempted to make this distinction in the monkey data since we classify the animals by the condition we created experimentally. However, we have shown that strabismic animals with more profound amblyopia tend also to develop anisometropia later in life (Kiorpes and Wallman 1995). These monkeys would therefore appear as combined strabismics/anisometropes and would have more severe amblyopias like their human counterparts.

Figure 4B shows the relationship between grating and vernier acuity, as in Figure 3B. Again, the data from monkeys and humans overlap almost completely, excepting only that normal humans achieve values of both grating and vernier acuity that slightly exceed those observed in monkeys. The more profound amblyopia in human strab/anisos is again evident. Thus, both in the pattern of relative interocular differences and in the pattern of relative vernier and grating acuity losses, the monkey data show the same pattern as the human data, and the ranges of the data for humans and monkeys overlap almost completely.

Experimentally strabismic and experimentally anisometropic monkeys are excellent models with which to study the factors that affect the development of amblyopia. In our experimental populations, approximately two-thirds of the monkeys raised with either anisometropia or strabismus subsequently developed amblyopia. This is very close to the prevalence of amblyopia in humans with naturally occurring strabismus or anisometropia, which is typically 40–60%. Strabismic animals that adopted a unilateral (as opposed to alternating) pattern of fixation were most likely to develop amblyopia; a similar association is found in humans. Additionally, the younger the age at which the abnormal visual conditions were imposed, the more likely it was that amblyopia developed (Kiorpes et al. 1989).

Neuronal Changes in Amblyopia

The goal of creating an animal model is to permit an exploration of the neurobiological changes that underlie the condition. There are a number of possibilities. Since amblyopia usually affects one eye, it is natural to wonder whether its effects are seen in the normally monocular portions of the visual pathway, the retina and lateral geniculate nucleus (LGN). Following monocular visual deprivation, Wiesel and Hubel (1963a,b) showed that there were large qualitative changes in the pattern of binocular inputs to cortical neurons but found little discernible effect on the response properties of neurons in the LGN.

We quantitatively examined the spatiotemporal properties and contrast sensitivity of 254 LGN neurons in five monkeys that were deprived of vision from the time of birth by suturing closed the lids of one eye (Levitt et al. 1989). This rearing creates an amblyopia so profound that the deprived eye is effectively left without any spatial vision at all, although rudimentary sensitivity to luminance differences remains (Harwerth et al. 1983). Like Wiesel and Hubel, we found no important differences in visual responsiveness or sensitivity between groups of LGN neurons driven by the deprived and non-deprived eye. There were some subtle differences, the most obvious being that the contrast gain of magnocellular and parvocellular neurons driven by the deprived eye was on average about 20% lower than that of comparable neurons driven by the non-deprived eye. In almost all respects the data for neurons driven by the two eyes were identical, and the few anomalies are far too subtle to account for the complete loss of visual capacity in the deprived eyes.

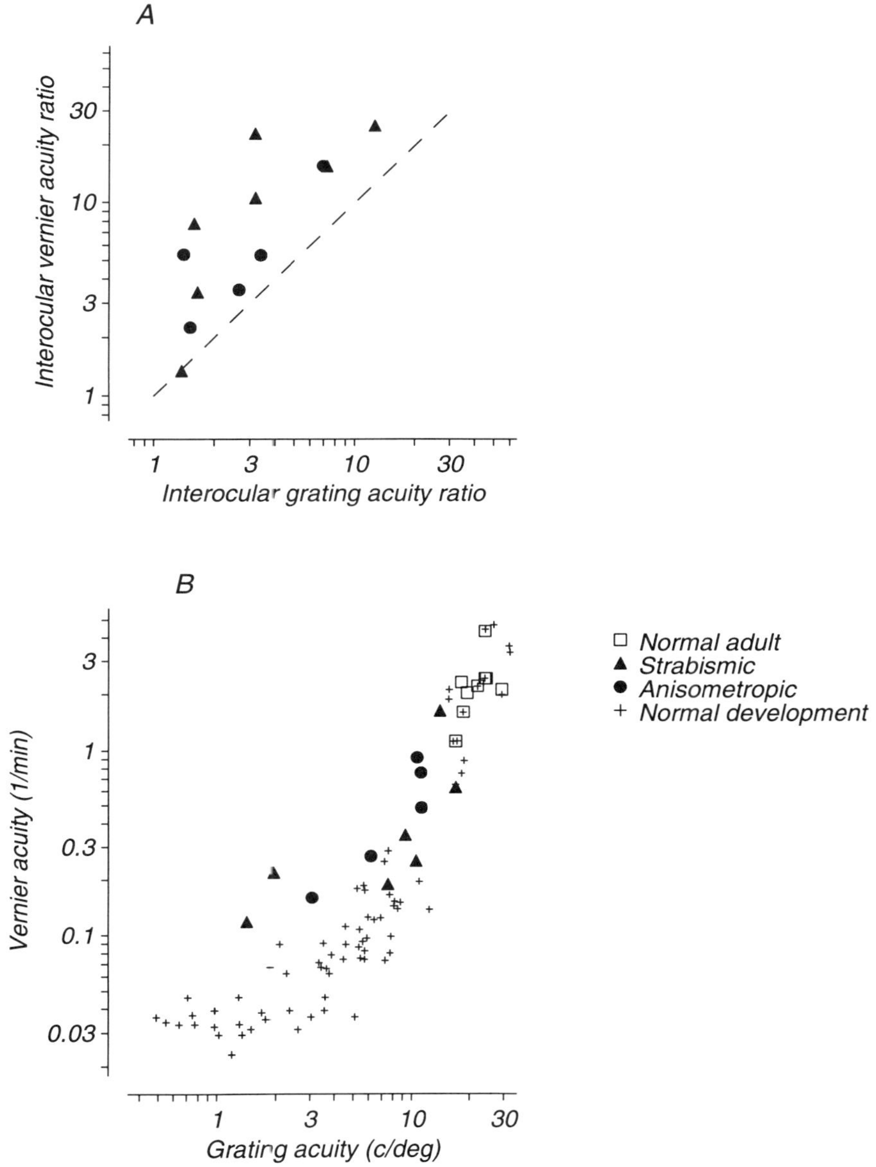

Figure 3. (*A*) Comparison of the magnitude of the vernier and grating acuity deficits for strabismic (*triangles*) and anisometropic (*circles*) amblyopes. The ratio of the vernier acuity values for the two eyes of each monkey is plotted against the ratio of the grating acuity values. In most cases, the vernier acuity deficit is larger than the grating acuity deficit (the data lie mostly above the dashed line, which represents a 1:1 relationship). (*B*) Relationship between vernier acuity and grating acuity in amblyopic monkeys as compared to that during normal development. The normal developmental data (*pluses*) are from animals ranging in age from near birth to 1 year. The performance of the amblyopes resembles that of young normal monkeys, although the data from two severe strabismic amblyopes deviate from the function.

We made similar measurements of the properties of 76 neurons from one monkey that was raised with unilateral blur; again there were no differences in the properties of cells driven by the two eyes (Movshon et al. 1987).

Visual deprivation is a crude manipulation that produces very profound changes in the central visual pathways. Monocular deprivation functionally disconnects the deprived eye from the cortex, so that few neurons there show any influence of visual signals arising in the deprived eye (Wiesel and Hubel 1963b; Hubel et al. 1977; LeVay et al. 1980). This suggests a second possible explanation for amblyopia: Perhaps a smaller-than-normal proportion of cortical neurons can be activated through the amblyopic eye, leading to its reduced visual capacity.

We studied the functional binocular connections and spatiotemporal properties of neurons in the pri-

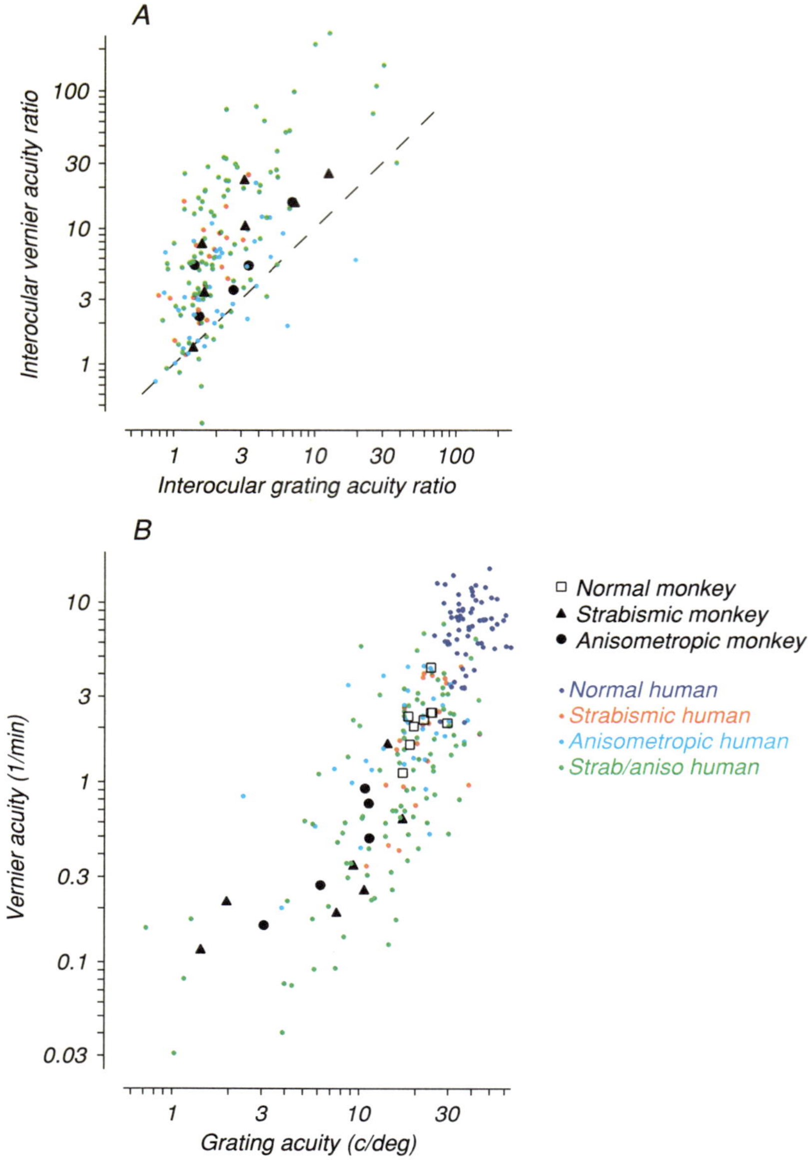

Figure 4. Comparison between monkey and human amblyopia. The format of *A* is the same as Fig. 3A; the format of *B* is the same as Fig. 3B; the monkey data are as shown in those figures. The human data are from 221 subjects classified as indicated in the legend. There is good correspondence between the human and monkey data, although normal humans have finer acuity than normal monkeys (*B*).

mary visual cortex of monkeys made amblyopic by either simulated anisometropia or strabismus. Figure 5 compares the distributions of cortical eye dominance for neurons recorded from these animals with data from normal monkeys, and with data from monocularly deprived monkeys (Hubel et al. 1977). Figure 5A shows the pattern of eye dominance found in 394 neurons recorded from normally reared monkeys. About 70% of cortical neurons are binocularly activated. Figure 5B shows the eye dominance of 600 neurons recorded in the cortex of eight monocularly deprived monkeys (Hubel et al. 1977; LeVay et al. 1980). The deprivation virtually disconnects the deprived eye from the cortex. Figure 5C shows the eye dominance of 316 neurons recorded from four amblyopic monkeys raised with unilateral blur produced by atropine (Movshon et al. 1987). Although the number of binocular neurons in these monkeys is somewhat reduced, there is little evidence of a wholesale shift in cortical eye dominance away from the blurred eye. Figure 5D shows the eye dominance of 225 neurons recorded from two amblyopic monkeys raised with esotropic strabismus (J.A. Movshon et al., unpubl.). Although almost all binocular neurons are lost in these

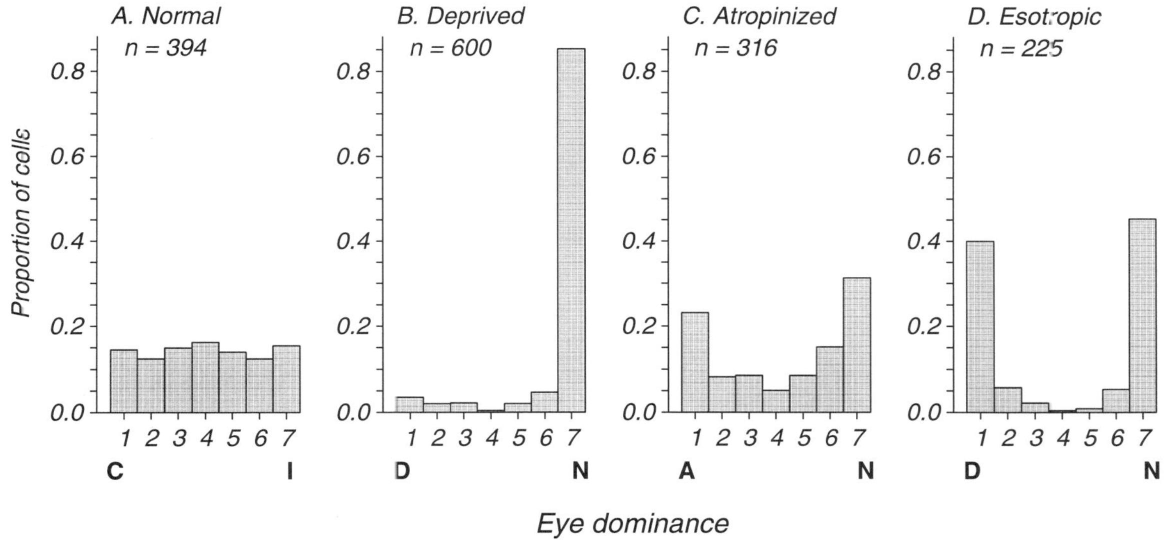

Figure 5. Eye dominance distributions for neurons recorded from the primary visual cortex of four groups of monkeys. The eye dominance scale is based on the traditional 7-point scale, in which groups 1 and 7 represent monocularly driven neurons, group 4 represents neurons equally driven from the two eyes, and groups 2, 3, 5, and 6 represent graded degrees of relative binocularity. (*A*) Data from 394 neurons recorded from normally reared animals. The scale goes from complete dominance by the contralateral eye (group 1, **C**) through complete dominance by the ipsilateral eye (group 7, **I**). (*B*) Data from 600 neurons recorded from eight monocularly deprived animals by Hubel et al. (1977) and LeVay et al. (1980). The data are combined so that the deprived eye (**D**) corresponds to group 1 and the non-deprived eye (**N**) corresponds to group 7. (*C*) Data from 316 neurons recorded from four atropine-treated monkeys by Movshon et al. (1987). The data are combined so that the atropinized eye (**A**) corresponds to group 1 and the untreated eye (**N**) corresponds to group 7. (*D*) Data from 225 neurons recorded from two esotropic strabismic monkeys (J.A. Movshon et al., unpubl.). The data are combined so that the surgically deviated eye (**D**) corresponds to group 1 and the non-deviated eye (**N**) corresponds to group 7. In all atropinized and esotropic monkeys, the treated eye was the amblyopic eye.

animals, each eye's signals control approximately the same number of neurons. Since the animals whose data are shown in Figure 5C and D were all amblyopic, it appears that amblyopia can occur without significant changes in the eye dominance of cortical neurons, although strabismus can cause such changes in some cases (Eggers et al. 1984).

If the *number* of cortical neurons driven by each eye is not changed by amblyopia, perhaps some of their other properties are altered. Because amblyopia is, as we have discussed, a deficit of spatial vision, we studied the spatial properties of the receptive fields of cortical neurons in monkeys raised with strabismus and unilateral blur. Figure 6 shows that the spatial resolution and sensitivity of neurons in the portions of the visual cortex that represent the central visual field are indeed altered in amblyopia. Figure 6A plots the optimal spatial frequency and peak contrast sensitivity of 255 neurons from the four amblyopic monkeys raised with unilateral blur (Movshon et al. 1987). Figure 6B shows in similar format the data for 204 neurons from the two amblyopic monkeys raised with experimental strabismus. It is evident in each part of this plot that the neurons driven through the treated eye had, on average, lower contrast sensitivity and lower peak spatial frequencies than neurons driven through the untreated eye; the magnitude of the effects is between 30% and 41%, and is similar for the two groups of monkeys. We conclude that the visual neuronal disorder associated with amblyopia that arises earliest in the visual process is this modification of the receptive field properties of cortical neurons. As we consider in more detail below, this may not be the only neuronal abnormality in these animals, but it is arguably the most important for understanding the visual resolution and sensitivity losses associated with amblyopia. These changes must arise from a failure of afferent neurons to make their normal precisely patterned connections.

DISCUSSION

The results of our experiments on amblyopic monkeys lead to three main conclusions:

1. Strabismus and simulated anisometropia, when present in the first few months of a monkey's life, create a visual anomaly that seems to be indistinguishable from human amblyopia.
2. Neurophysiological recordings from these monkeys show that there are no significant changes in the visual properties of neurons in the thalamus (and, by deduction, in the retina). The first important changes are seen in the primary visual cortex, V1.
3. Both behaviorally and neurophysiologically, the am-

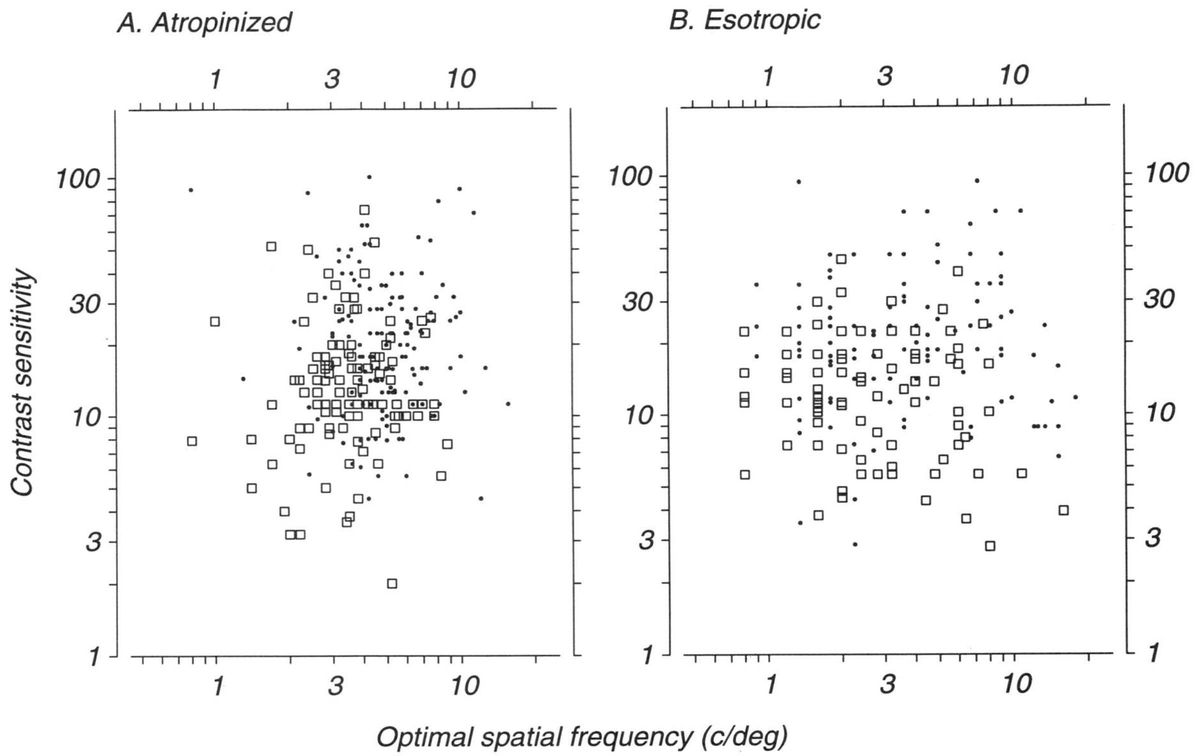

Figure 6. Scatter plots showing the optimal spatial frequency and peak contrast sensitivity of neurons recorded from the representation of the central visual fields in the primary visual cortex of two groups of amblyopic monkeys. Each point represents the two values for a single neuron. Small points represent data for neurons dominated by (and tested through) the untreated eye, and large squares represent data for neurons dominated by (and tested through) the treated eye. (*A*) Data from 255 neurons from four atropine-treated monkeys (Movshon et al. 1987). The geometric mean optimal spatial frequency is 31% lower for neurons driven through the treated eye, and the geometric mean contrast sensitivity is 35% lower. (*B*) Data from 204 neurons from two esotropic strabismic monkeys (J.A. Movshon et al. unpubl.). The geometric mean optimal spatial frequency is 30% lower for neurons driven through the treated eye, and the geometric mean contrast sensitivity is 41% lower.

blyopic eye functions as though its spatial contrast sensitivity has been shifted both down to lower sensitivities and leftward to lower spatial frequencies.

It is interesting to consider how the reduction in spatial resolution and sensitivity might arise biologically. The receptive field structure of neurons in the primary visual cortex is quite heterogeneous. However, those neurons with the highest spatial resolution have receptive fields whose spatial structure consists of subregions only 1–2 min arc in width, which suggests that their main inputs arise from only a few photoreceptors (Hawken and Parker 1991). These inputs are presumably relayed through neurons in the parvocellular layers of the LGN, whose receptive fields are comparably tiny (Blakemore and Vital-Durand 1986). Our measurements of neuronal properties in amblyopic monkeys show that these afferent neurons in the LGN are still present and normal in function, but they are absent in parts of the cortex controlled by the amblyopic eye. Because cortical eye dominance does not change overall, we do not believe that these neurons are lost. Rather, it seems that their connections with afferents from the LGN are disrupted, so that they receive inputs from neurons whose receptive fields are dispersed over a substantial region of the retina. This results in cortical receptive fields whose structures are "blurred." The subregions of the receptive fields are larger, leading to a leftward shift in their spatial contrast sensitivity. It is also conceivable that the regions are also less perfectly segregated from one another than in normal animals, leading to partial cancellation of signals from different regions and a reduction in contrast sensitivity.

If we assume that the usual highly precise topographic representation of the visual field (Blasdel and Fitzpatrick 1984) is not altered in the cortex of amblyopic monkeys, we can make simple calculations to estimate the extent of the spatial disruption. The peak of local cortical magnification in monkeys is around 10 mm/deg (i.e., movement of 1 mm on the cortical surface causes an average movement of the location of visual receptive fields of 0.1 deg; Tootell et al. 1988; Wässle et al. 1990). The spatial blurring of visual receptive fields can be calculated from data like those shown in Figure 6 to be of the order of 0.1 deg, corresponding to a local misrouting of signals over distances of approximately 1 mm. Interestingly, this is the approximate extent of the terminal arborizations of parvocellular LGN afferents to the cortex in neonatal monkeys; perhaps this is the reason that visual cortical receptive fields in neonates show the same reduced spatial resolution as do neurons in amblyopic adults (Blakemore and Vital-Durand 1983; Blasdel and Lund 1983). In the course of normal development with clear, binocularly aligned images, these connections prune down to their adult size of approximately 0.1 mm (Blasdel and Lund 1983; Blasdel and Fitzpatrick 1984). We may suppose that the altered visual conditions that create amblyopia interfere with this pruning, so that afferents from the LGN are randomly misrouted by a distance on the order of 0.5–1 mm in the adult amblyopic visual cortex.

It may be that this misrouting is the basis for the changes seen in the visual sensitivity of amblyopic cortical neurons, and for the abnormal performance of amblyopes themselves. It is important to note, however, that the magnitude of the changes in sensitivity and spatial resolution seen in the neuronal populations (Fig. 6) are probably too small to account for the whole of the visual losses seen in behavioral measurements (Fig. 1). It is also not obvious that these changes can account for the extraordinary loss of vernier acuity seen in some amblyopes (Figs. 3,4) (Levi and Klein 1985). The primary visual cortex is of course only the first in a complex pathway of visual cortical areas (Felleman and Van Essen 1991), and it would be naive to assume that it is the *only* area whose development can be modified by the visual environment. Indeed, we have recently shown that the binocular connections of neurons in MT, an extrastriate visual area, can also be modified by strabismus (Kiorpes et al. 1996). It is thus likely that neurons in other areas are also affected in amblyopia, and we may suppose that a comprehensive account of the biological basis of amblyopia will require examination of the changes in these areas as well as in the primary visual cortex.

ACKNOWLEDGMENTS

The research described in this paper was supported by grants from the National Eye Institute (EY-02017 and EY-05864) and by the Howard Hughes Medical Institute. These experiments would not have been possible without the contributions of Howard Eggers, Martin Gizzi, Daniel Kiper, Dennis Levi, Jonathan Levitt, Suzanne McKee, Lawrence O'Keefe, Murray Sherman, Peter Spear, and Chao Tang. We are also grateful to Patricia Adler, Michael Gorman, and Jasmine Allen Siegel for their expert technical assistance.

REFERENCES

Almeder, L.M., L.B. Peck, and H.C. Howland. 1990. Prevalence of anisometropia in volunteer laboratory and school screening populations. *Invest. Ophthalmol. Visual Sci.* **31:** 2448.

Blakemore, C. and F. Vital-Durand. 1983. Development of contrast sensitivity by neurones in monkey striate cortex. *J. Physiol.* **334:** 18P.

———. 1986. Organization and postnatal development of the monkey's lateral geniculate nucleus. *J. Physiol.* **380:** 453.

Blasdel, G.G.and D. Fitzpatrick. 1984. Physiological organization of layer 4 in macaque striate cortex. *J. Neurosci.* **4:** 880.

Blasdel, G.G. and J.S. Lund. 1983. Termination of afferent axons in macaque striate cortex. *J. Neurosci.* **3:** 1389.

Boothe, R.G., L. Kiorpes, R.A. Williams, and D.Y. Teller. 1988. Operant measurements of spatial contrast sensitivity in infant macaque monkeys during normal development. *Vision Res.* **28:** 387.

Eggers, H.M., M.S. Gizzi, and J.A. Movshon. 1984. Spatial properties of striate cortical neurons in esotropic macaques. *Invest. Ophthalmol. Visual Sci.* (suppl.) **25:** 278.

Felleman, D.J. and D.C. Van Essen. 1991. Distributed hierarchical processing in the primate cerebral cortex. *Cereb. Cortex* **1:** 1.

Harwerth, R.S., E.L. Smith III, R.L. Boltz, M.L.J. Crawford, and G.K. von Noorden. 1983. Behavioral studies on the effect of abnormal early visual experience in monkeys: Spatial modulation sensitivity. *Vision Res.* **23:** 1501.

Hawken, M.J. and A.J. Parker. 1991. Spatial receptive field organization in macaque V1 and its relationship to the cone mosaic. In *Computational models of visual processing* (ed. M.S. Landy and J.A. Movshon). MIT Press, Cambridge, Massachusetts.

Hubel, D.H. and T.N. Wiesel. 1965. Binocular interaction in striate cortex of kittens reared with artificial squint. *J. Neurophysiol.* **28:** 1041.

Hubel, D.H., T.N. Wiesel, and S. LeVay. 1977. Plasticity of ocular dominance columns in monkey striate cortex. *Philos. Trans. R. Soc. Lond. B Biol. Sci.* **278:** 377.

Kiorpes, L. 1992a. The development of vernier acuity and grating acuity in normally-reared monkeys. *Visual Neurosci.* **9:** 243.

———. 1992b. The effect of strabismus on the development of vernier acuity and grating acuity in monkeys. *Visual Neurosci.* **9:** 253.

———. 1996. Development of contrast sensitivity in normal and amblyopic monkeys. In *Infant vision* (ed. F. Vital-Durand et al.), p. 3. Oxford University Press, United Kingdom.

Kiorpes, L. and J.A. Movshon. 1989. Differential development of two visual functions in primates. *Proc. Natl. Acad. Sci.* **86:** 8998.

Kiorpes, L. and J. Wallman. 1995. Does experimentally-induced amblyopia cause hyperopia in monkeys? *Vision Res.* **35:** 1289.

Kiorpes, L., M.R. Carlson, and D. Alfi. 1989. Development of visual acuity in experimentally strabismic monkeys. *Clin. Vision Sci.* **4:** 95.

Kiorpes, L., D.C. Kiper, and J.A. Movshon. 1993. Contrast sensitivity and vernier acuity in amblyopic monkeys. *Vision Res.* **33:** 2301.

Kiorpes, L., P.J. Walton, L.P. O'Keefe, J.A. Movshon, and S.G. Lisberger. 1996. Effects of early-onset artifical strabismus on pursuit eye movements and on neuronal responses in area MT of macaque monkeys. *J. Neurosci.* **16:** 6537.

Kiorpes, L., R.G. Boothe, A.E. Hendrickson, J.A. Movshon,

H.M. Eggers, and M.S. Gizzi. 1987. Effects of early unilateral blur on the macaque's visual system. I. Behavioral observations. *J. Neurosci.* **7:** 1318.

LeVay, S., T.N. Wiesel, and D.H. Hubel. 1980. The development of ocular dominance columns in normal and visually deprived monkeys. *J. Compar. Neurol.* **191:** 1.

Levi, D.M. and A. Carkeet. 1993. Amblyopia: A consequence of abnormal visual development. In *Early visual development: Normal and abnormal* (ed. K. Simons). Oxford University Press, New York.

Levi, D.M. and S.A. Klein. 1985. Vernier acuity, crowding and amblyopia. *Vision Res.* **25:** 979.

Levitt, J.B., D.C. Kiper, and J.A. Movshon. 1994. Receptive fields and functional architecture of macaque V2. *J. Neurophysiol.* **71:** 2517.

Levitt, J.B., J.A. Movshon, S.M. Sherman, and P.D. Spear. 1989. Effects of monocular deprivation on macaque LGN. *Invest. Ophthalmol. Visual Sci.* (suppl.) **30:** 296.

McKee, S.P., C.M. Schor, S.B. Steinman, N. Wilson, G.G. Koch, S.M. Davis, C. Hsu-Winges, S.H. Day, C.L. Chan, J.A. Movshon, M.C. Flom, D.M. Levi, and J.T. Flynn. 1992. The classification of amblyopia on the basis of visual and oculomotor performance. *Trans. Am. Ophthalmol. Soc.* **90:** 123.

Movshon, J.A. and L. Kiorpes. 1988. Analysis of the development of spatial contrast sensitivity in monkey and human infants. *J. Opt. Soc. Am. A* **5:** 2166.

———. 1993. Biological limits on visual development in primates. In *Early visual development: Normal and abnormal* (ed. K. Simons). Oxford University Press, New York.

Movshon, J.A., S.P. McKee, and D.M. Levi. 1996. Visual acuity in a large population of normal, strabismic, and anisometropic observers. *Invest. Ophthalmol. Visual Sci.* **37:** S670.

Movshon, J.A., H.M. Eggers, M.S. Gizzi, A.E. Hendrickson, L. Kiorpes, and R.G. Boothe. 1987. Effects of early unilateral blur on the macaque's visual system. III. Physiological observations. *J. Neurosci.* **7:** 1340.

Shimojo, S., E.E. Birch, J. Gwiazda, and R. Held. 1984. Development of vernier acuity in human infants. *Vision Res.* **24:** 721.

Tootell, R.B.H., E. Switkes, M.S. Silverman, and S.L. Hamilton. 1988. Functional anatomy of macaque striate cortex. II. Retinotopic organization. *J. Neurosci.* **8:** 1531.

von Noorden, G.K. 1980. *Binocular vision and ocular motility.* Mosby, St. Louis, Missouri.

Wässle, H., U. Grünert, J. Röhrenbeck, and B.B. Boycott. 1990. Retinal ganglion cell density and cortical magnification factor in the primate. *Vision Res.* **30:** 1897.

Wiesel, T.N. and D.H. Hubel. 1963a. Effects of visual deprivation on morphology and physiology of cells in the cat's lateral geniculate body. *J. Neurophysiol.* **26:** 978.

———. 1963b. Single-cell responses in striate cortex of kittens deprived of vision in one eye. *J. Neurophysiol.* **26:** 1003.

The Functional Anatomy of Visual Awareness

C. KOCH AND J. BRAUN
Computation and Neural Systems, California Institute of Technology, Pasadena, California 91125

What is the relationship between our subjective world of perceptions, thoughts, and memories and the activity of nerve cells that must somehow be responsible for this experience? The past 5 years have witnessed a transformation in the way the neuroscience community is approaching this complex of problems. As reported below, psychophysical and electrophysiological experiments are being carried out to elucidate the neuronal correlate of sensory awareness. If this aim can be realized and the anatomical structures and neuronal groups representing the contents of sensory awareness[1] can be identified, we will be one step closer to understanding the most mysterious and central aspect of our existence.

In the visual modality, there is a preponderance of evidence, not yet conclusive but certainly persuasive, that visual awareness does not depend equally on all parts of visual cortex. In particular, it seems that visual awareness does not arise from neural activity in striate cortex (area V1, primary visual cortex) but in certain extrastriate cortical areas. The matter is complicated by the fact that an intact and functioning striate cortex is required for most forms of visual awareness (as are the eyes). Evidence pointing to some extrastriate visual areas, but not others, as being necessary for visual awareness is less compelling but certainly deserves a closer look. Here our point of view seems likely to evolve rapidly in the near future.

Once the link between visual awareness and certain visual cortical areas is confirmed, this will open subjective experience to the kind of systematic attack by neuroscience to which other mental functions—perception or language, for example—are already being subjected. How do areas that contribute to subjective experience differ from those that do not? Do these areas contain different cell types that express different proteins? Do they exhibit particular types of connectivity? Are they characterized by particular temporal patterns of neuronal firing?

The possibility that extrastriate, but not striate, cortex is necessary for visual awareness is consistent with a recent prediction to this effect, advanced mostly on theoretical and anatomical grounds (Crick and Koch 1995). The emphasis of this paper is not on these theoretical arguments, however, but on the gratifying amount of supporting evidence that has recently come to light.

We review evidence from patients suffering lesions in striate and extrastriate cortex, from single-cell recordings in nonhuman primates which have attempted to correlate the subjective experience of the animal with neuronal firing, and from psychophysical studies with displays that selectively stimulate early levels of processing and that have succeeded in manipulating visual awareness in normal human subjects.

FUNCTIONAL ANATOMY OF VISUAL AWARENESS

As neuroscientists, our point of departure must be that awareness is a property of the brain and thus, in principle, no more mysterious than other mental functions (for a different point of view, see Chalmers 1996). If this is so, awareness can be expected to depend to different degrees on different parts of the brain; in other words, it can be expected to possess a functional anatomy.

Recently, Crick and Koch (1995) have attempted to deduce some features of this functional anatomy by postulating that visual awareness imposes a dual requirement: (1) an "explicit" neuronal representation of visual information and (2) a representation that is directly available to the "planning stages" of the brain. The distinction between explicit and implicit neuronal representations is best understood from an example: Illusory contours are known to elicit neuronal firing in visual area V2 (but not in striate cortex) (Peterhans and von der Heydt 1991). This activity explicitly represents the presence of illusory contours, whereas firing in the retina, lateral geniculate nucleus, and striate cortex represents such features merely in an implicit manner.

This dual requirement of an explicit representation that is available to the planning stages narrows the range of cortical areas that can contribute to visual awareness. The planning stages that initiate voluntary motor action are generally identified with frontal areas, and visual areas that project directly to frontal areas include all visual cortical areas with the notable exception of striate cortex (Felleman and Van Essen 1990). At least, this is the case in the macaque monkey. Ex-

[1] We use "awareness" to denote subjective sensory experience and make a distinction between this and other forms of consciousness that accompany higher mental functions.

trapolated to humans, this implies that visual information that is explicitly represented only in striate cortex (but not in extrastriate cortex) will not be available to visual awareness (Crick and Koch 1995). This does not in any way question, of course, that striate cortex is crucial for vision and visual awareness (just like the retina). It simply means that an explicit representation in striate cortex *alone* is not sufficient for visual awareness.

Drawing on a series of provocative findings, Milner and Goodale have proposed that different extrastriate visual areas contribute differentially to visual awareness (Milner and Goodale 1995). Specifically, they hypothesize that the ventral extrastriate areas which form the occipito-temporal pathway (areas V2, V3, V4, TEO, and inferotemporal cortex; "what" or "object" pathway) are far more consequential for subjective visual experience than the dorsal extrastriate areas of the occipito-parietal pathway (areas V3a, MT, MST, FST, STP, and posterior parietal cortex; "where," "spatial," or "action" pathway) (Ungerleider and Haxby 1994).

Evidence for this hypothesis comes from patients with lesions in striate cortex (discussed below) and especially from a patient with ventral occipital damage resulting from carbon monoxide poisoning (Goodale et al. 1991). Although this patient exhibits no sign of being aware of visual shapes and orientations, she nevertheless performs visually guided movements such as placing her flat hand into a narrow slot of varying orientation. Thus, information about visual orientation seems to be almost normally represented in the occipito-parietal pathway without contributing subjective visual experience. Another observation supporting the hypothesis of Milner and Goodale is that the familiar effects of size constancy (e.g., Titchner illusion) do not bias visually guided motor behavior in normal subjects, suggesting that size is processed independently in the two pathways and that only the size represented in the occipito-temporal pathway reaches subjective awareness (Milner and Goodale 1995).

SINGLE-CELL RECORDING AND VISUAL AWARENESS

Much of our knowledge about the way visual information is represented in the brain derives from single-cell recordings in cat and monkey (Felleman and Van Essen 1990; Van Essen and Gallant 1994). Unfortunately, whether the information encoded by a particular cell or cell population is actually used by the organism—i.e., whether the cell or population exercises some discernible influence on behavior—is rarely obvious (Britten et al. 1992; Salzman and Newsome 1994). Determining whether a given cell or population contributes not only to behavior, but also to subjective visual experience poses an even greater challenge.

An ideal paradigm to probe the neuronal correlate of visual awareness with single-cell recording is binocular rivalry (Myerson et al. 1981; Sengpiel et al. 1995). Here, constant visual stimulation (e.g., a horizontal grating viewed by the left eye and a vertical grating viewed by the right eye) results in a discontinuously changing visual percept (horizontal and vertical gratings alternating on a time scale of a few seconds). Assuming that one can train the animal to promptly and truthfully report its subjective experience, one may thus ask where in the visual system there are single cells whose activity correlates with the alternating percept rather than the constant visual stimulation.

Earlier experiments with awake macaques viewing rivalrous stimulus motion indicated that up to 40% of the neurons in area MT show either a positive or negative correlation with the direction of motion reported by the animal (Logothetis and Schall 1989). Logothetis and colleagues extended these observations to rivalrous stimulus orientation and found 38% of neurons in area V4 and 18% of neurons in area V1/V2 were significantly modulated by the changing percept, with some neurons being strongly correlated and others strongly anti-correlated with the reported orientation (Leopold and Logothetis 1996). Their results leave open the possibility that the percentage of neurons modulated in this way is even smaller in striate cortex (area V1) alone. The vast majority of the cells whose activity changes with the percept are driven binocularly, rather than monocularly, arguing against the widespread notion (see, e.g., Sengpiel et al. 1995) that binocular rivalry results from the mutual inhibition of left- and right-eye-dominated cells (Logothetis et al. 1996). The most exciting aspect of these results in the present context is that subjective experience appears to correlate far better with activity in extrastriate cortex (area MT, area V4) than with activity in striate cortex (area V1).

Another compelling, if slightly less "clean," situation in which subjective experience can be correlated with neuronal activity has been discovered by Andersen and colleagues (Qian and Andersen 1994; Qian et al. 1994a,b). Working with visual textures composed of two sets of dots moving in opposite directions, these researchers showed that the percept of two transparent, moving surfaces known as "motion transparency" (Adelson and Movshon 1982) is replaced by a percept of incoherent flicker when each dot moving in one direction is "paired" with another dot moving in the other direction. This perceptual breakdown of transparency occurs only when paired dots are in close spatial proximity (less than 0.1° of visual angle). Recording from single-direction-selective cells in areas V1 and MT, they further showed that the pairing of dots moving in opposite directions reduces neuronal responses in area MT far more than responses in area V1, suggesting that responses in area MT, not area V1, are responsible for the percept of motion transparency.

Thus, it again appears that subjective experience correlates better with extrastriate than with striate activity. Yet another instance may be provided by perceptual color constancy, which also seems to correlate better with neuronal responses in area V4 than in area V1 (Zeki 1983; Schein and Desimone 1990; Heywood et al. 1995).

DAMAGE TO STRIATE CORTEX: BLINDSIGHT

Patients who have suffered damage to striate cortex generally believe themselves to be "blind" in all parts of the field of view affected by the lesion. Despite their extremely impoverished subjective experience, visual stimulation of the blind field may nevertheless have a strong influence on the response of such patients in forced-choice situations. This ability to discriminate stimuli without being aware of them has been termed "blindsight" (Pöppel et al. 1973; Weiskrantz et al. 1974). Although it has been suggested that some of these patients may retain islands of intact striate cortex (Fendrich et al. 1994), other patients clearly exhibit blindsight in parts of the field of view no longer represented by striate cortex (Weiskrantz 1986; Cowey and Stoerig 1991). Indeed, there is a strong case for blindsight even in macaque monkeys with complete (hemilateral) ablation of striate cortex (Cowey and Stoerig 1995).

The nature of subjective experience during blindsight may be somewhat variable. In some situations, there appears to be a complete lack of any subjective awareness of a stimulus ("I have no sense of anything. There is nothing at all. I am just guessing"; patient DB [Weiskrantz 1986]). In other situations, there seems to be a reduced form of awareness of a nonvisual character ("I did not see, but I was sure"; patient DB [Weiskrantz 1986]; a "content-less kind of awareness, a feeling of something happening, albeit not normal seeing"; patient GY [Weiskrantz et al. 1995]). The latter state tends to be elicited by more intense stimulation (higher luminance contrast or higher speed of motion), but it does not seem to be comparable to the normal visual awareness that characterizes healthy parts of the visual field (Weiskrantz et al. 1995). This is an important point, because it suggests that blindsight is mediated by visual pathways other than conscious vision.

The retention of visual function after ablation of striate cortex is not as paradoxical as it might appear (Fig. 1a). Although a striate lesion triggers massive retrograde degeneration in the lateral geniculate nucleus and in the retina, the retinal degeneration is incomplete, and approximately 20% of retinal ganglion cells remain functional (Cowey and Stoerig 1993; Stoerig and Cowey 1993). In addition, a striate lesion does not completely deafferentiate extrastriate visual areas: in non-human primates, a striate lesion abolishes visual responsiveness in areas V2, V3, V4, and inferior temporal cortex, but not in areas V3a, MT, and the superior temporal polysensory area (STP) (for review, see Bullier et al. 1994). For example, lesion or inactivation of striate cortex considerably weakens responses in area MT, but leaves selectivity for direction of motion and receptive field size unchanged (Rodman et al. 1989, 1990; Girard et al. 1992). A strong indication that the same is true for humans comes from blindsight patient GY, whose striate cortex and optic radiation were almost completely destroyed hemilaterally, but in whom visual responsiveness of area MT can be discerned with positron emission tomography (PET) (Barbur et al. 1993).

Visual information can bypass striate cortex along a number of known anatomical pathways (Stoerig and Cowey 1993; Bullier et al. 1994). The largest alternative route leads from the retina to the superior colliculus and onward to the lateral and inferior pulvinar nucleus of the thalamus (Fig. 1a). From the pulvinar, information is widely distributed to different striate and extrastriate areas. Another, rather minor, pathway projects directly from the interlaminar and S layers of the lateral geniculate to extrastriate cortex, including inferior temporal cortex (Hernandez-Gonzalez et al. 1994). The existence of tecto-extrastriate pathways bypassing striate cortex finds further support in the fact that a combined lesion of striate cortex and superior colliculus abolishes all visual responsiveness in area MT (Rodman et al. 1990). When only superior colliculus is lesioned, response properties in area MT remain largely unchanged. Behavioral studies with nonhuman primates confirm the superadditive effects of individual and combined lesions of striate cortex and superior colliculus (Mohler and Wurtz 1976).

The importance of blindsight lies in the fact that an anatomically defined lesion impairs visual awareness while sparing a significant degree of visual function. Unfortunately, more specific inferences are complicated by the fact that a striate lesion adversely affects large parts of the visual system outside striate cortex (either by deafferentiation or by triggering retrograde degeneration). Thus, we may put down the disruption of visual awareness either to the striate lesion itself or to the effective deafferentiation of ventral extrastriate areas. The fact that some visual function is retained can be attributed to the continued visual responsiveness of subcortical nuclei and/or of dorsal extrastriate areas. Thus, as argued most prominently by Milner and Goodale (1995), the functional anatomy of blindsight suggests that dorsal and ventral extrastriate areas may contribute differentially to visual awareness. In any case, the question that remains is not why patients without striate cortex retain some faculty of "sight," but why they experience themselves as "blind."

DAMAGE TO EXTRASTRIATE CORTEX

A number of recent cases of "cortical blindness" bear upon the role of extrastriate cortex in visual awareness. One of these concerns two patients with

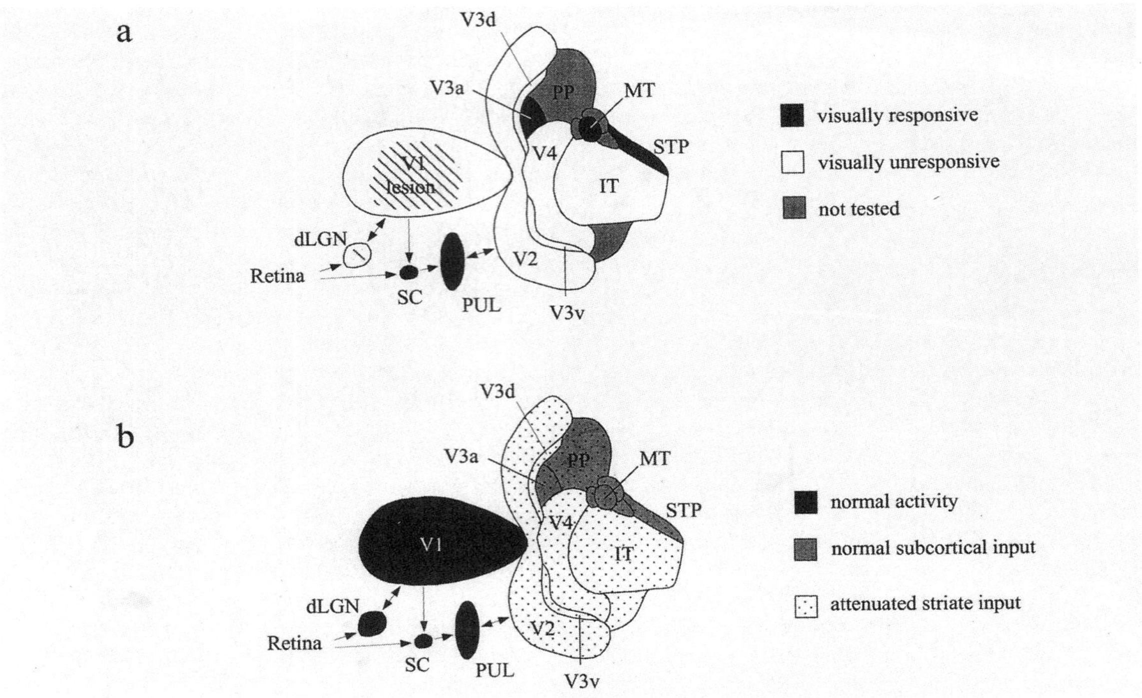

Figure 1. Expected activity distribution for different visual cortical areas during two types of "blindsight" (highly schematic and based on maps of macaque visual cortex of Van Essen and Gallant [1994]). (*a*) When striate cortex (area V1) is ablated or cooled in a monkey, responses are absent in V2, V3v, V3d, V4, and IT (*white*), while (reduced) responsiveness remains in V3a, MT, and STP (*black*). In patients with blindsight, a lesion in striate cortex triggers neuronal degeneration in the lateral geniculate nucleus (*dashed*) and retina, but leaves the superior colliculus, the pulvinar, and several extrastriate cortical areas visually responsive. The responsive areas of cortex form part of the occipito-parietal pathway (areas V3a, MT, STP, and PP) (Bullier et al. 1994; Milner and Goodale 1995). (*b*) Hypothetical activity distribution for conflicting visual displays that induce blindsight in normal observers (Kolb and Braun 1995). Due to opponency, the response to conflicting displays may be significantly reduced in many extrastriate areas (Qian et al. 1994a). Subcortical nuclei and parts of striate cortex are unaffected, possibly triggering extrastriate activity in the occipito-parietal pathway. (dLGN) Dorsal lateral geniculate nucleus; (SC) superior colliculus; (PUL) pulvinar nucleus of the thalamus; (V1) striate cortex; (V2, V3a, V3d, V3v, V4, MT) extrastriate visual cortical areas; (PP) posterior parietal cortex; (IT) inferior temporal cortex; (STP) superior temporal polysensory area. (Reprinted, with permission, from Koch and Braun 1996.)

profoundly impaired vision (due to astrocytoma) in the lower quadrant of the visual field (Horton and Hoyt 1991). The remarkable feature of this "quadrantanopia" is that the defective region ends precisely at the horizontal midline. This, in combination with magnetic-resonance imaging of the occipital lobe, led the authors to argue that the lesion is restricted to areas V2 and V3 (in which the respective representations of upper and lower quadrants are anatomically separate), rather than in striate cortex (where upper and lower quadrant representations are anatomically contiguous). Unless damage to white matter complicates the issue (Pollen 1995), this implies that the intactness of areas V2/V3, rather than that of striate cortex, is critical for normal visual awareness.

Another case of interest is patient PB who, having suffered anoxia, combines profoundly impaired form perception, to the point of being unable to distinguish vertical from horizontal, with relatively preserved color perception (Humphrey et al. 1991, 1995). Remarkably, after adaptation to a grating of alternating red and green stripes, this patient exhibits the orientation-specific McCollough effect, demonstrating that orientation information continues to be processed, presumably in the intact striate cortex. If the presumed sparing of striate cortex can be confirmed, this patient will constitute another instance where visual awareness is impaired by damage to extrastriate rather than to striate cortex.

PSYCHOPHYSICAL MANIPULATIONS OF VISUAL AWARENESS

In normal observers, deficits of visual awareness are necessarily fleeting and are thus difficult to document from an objective, third-person point of view (Merikle 1992; Shacter 1992). To overcome this problem, we need a behavioral measure of visual awareness that is at least as sensitive as the traditional behavioral measures of visual discrimination: Verbal debriefing of observers is not enough. Fortunately, there has been steady progress toward this goal in recent years, largely due to a technique involving a "comment key" (Weiskrantz et al. 1995). In this technique, the observer is asked not only to make a forced choice between stimulus alternatives, but also to comment on his or her subjective experience in every trial. In its most elementary form, the only two comments allowed are whether the stimulus was "seen" or "not seen" (Graves and Jones 1992; Weiskrantz et al. 1995). This technique has even been used to demonstrate blindsight in nonhuman primates, challenging the notion that the inner life of other creatures must remain forever closed to us (Cowey and Stoerig 1995).

A refinement of the comment-key technique involves giving observers a greater choice of comments and, more importantly, correlating comments with the success or failure of individual trials (Kolb and Braun 1995). This last measure establishes whether subjective experience reflects objective performance in a forced-choice task. Of course, this is almost always the case. In a hyperacuity discrimination, for example, subjective experience closely follows objective performance even in the threshold regime, where performance is barely above chance (Fahle and Koch 1996). However, in certain exceptional situations, subjective confidence becomes decoupled from objective performance, and the positive correlation between the two is lost, although objective performance itself remains quite high (Kolb and Braun 1995). In these situations, observers report that they do not see the stimulus and that their forced-choice response is based on guessing.

This "blindsight in normal observers" is of interest in the present context because of the nature of the displays in question. These are ambiguous displays composed of conflicting stimuli in close spatial proximity, and single-unit results from nonhuman primates suggest that such displays stimulate extrastriate visual cortex much less than striate cortex (see below). The deficits of subjective experience observed in such displays thus bear directly on the functional anatomy of awareness.

One example of a situation involving conflicting information is dichoptic stimulation of the two eyes. In the display shown schematically in Figure 2a, each eye views an array of oriented stimuli, and in a small target region these stimuli are oriented orthogonally to the rest of the array. However, at each visual location, left and right eyes view stimuli of *both* orientations, so that neither orientation is clearly perceived. At viewing times of less than about 0.3 seconds, the array is reported to be subjectively uniform without any impression of a target region (at longer viewing times, "binocular rivalry" develops and the target region is perceived by the currently dominant eye). A similar failure to become aware of a target region can be obtained when conflicting information is delivered in other ways; for example, by a (binocularly viewed) dynamic texture of two sets of dots moving in opposite directions.

The surprising finding with these displays is that, although observers claim not to see the target and to guess its location, they report target position quite reliably in a forced-choice situation. To document lack of target awareness, observers comment on their subjective experience by rating their subjective confidence of having correctly located the target on a scale of 1 to 10. For the conflicting displays described above, no significant correlation between subjective confidence and objective performance is obtained, suggesting a complete lack of target awareness (Fig. 2c). In a control situation in which both eyes view consistent stimuli (Fig. 2b), a large positive correlation is observed, indicating normal target awareness (Fig. 2d). Importantly, the contrast between conflicting and consistent displays is not limited to the threshold regime but persists over the entire performance range. This can be demonstrated by varying either presentation time or luminance contrast. In short, consistent displays yield significant correlations even when performance approaches chance, and conflicting displays yield insignificant correlations even when performance approaches ceiling (Kolb and Braun 1995).

It seems clear that the neural response to conflicting displays is to a large extent shaped by "opponent mechanisms," that is, by reciprocal inhibition between conflicting visual features. An important indication as to the neural level of this opponency is that conflicting features must enter into close spatial proximity in order for visual awareness to be suppressed. In fact, the spatial separation of conflicting features must be comparable to a typical receptive field diameter in striate cortex (Qian and Andersen 1994; Kolb and Braun 1995; Braun and Kolb 1996). This is borne out by the single-unit studies with nonhuman primates described earlier. As mentioned previously, these studies suggest that conflicting orientation (viewed dichoptically) reduces orientation-selective responses far more in extrastriate area V4 than in striate cortex (Leopold and Logothetis 1996) and that conflicting motion (viewed binocularly) reduces direction-selective responses far more in extrastriate area MT than in striate cortex (Qian et al. 1994a). Overall, these single-unit results suggest that, at least to a first approximation, conflicting displays elicit a nearly normal response from striate cortex but a relatively poor response from extrastriate areas.

If these inferences are correct, then conflicting displays may create a situation where the major remaining inputs to extrastriate areas derive not from striate cortex but from subcortical nuclei (Fig. 1b), not at all unlike the situation after a striate cortex lesion! Of course, this assumes that subcortical responses are *not* attenuated by opponency. In contrast to the lesion, however, conflicting displays would still be processed by striate cortex, and responses in striate cortex could continue to reach extrastriate cortical areas after being relayed through subcortical areas. This would constitute strong evidence that a neuronal response in striate cortex is not sufficient for visual awareness. Whether or not this scenario corresponds to fact remains to be seen. Nevertheless, we find it intriguing

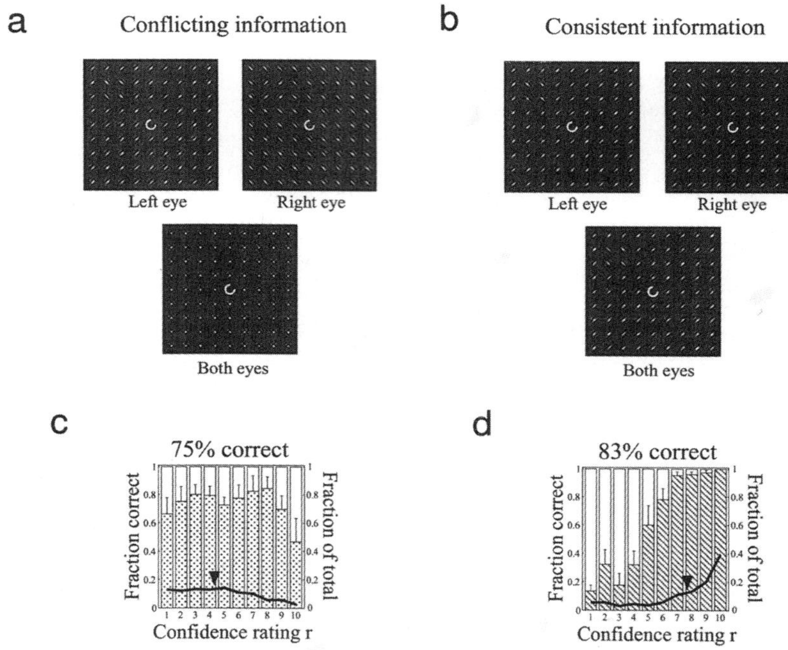

Figure 2. Psychophysical displays (schematic) and results pertaining to blindsight in normal observers. (*a*) Left and right eyes view conflicting displays consisting of oriented stimuli. In a small target region these stimuli are oriented orthogonally to the rest of the array. At each visual location, left and right eyes view stimuli of orthogonal orientations. As a result, the target region is not subjectively apparent. A fixation task (central C) ensures that both eyes fixate the same point of the display. Observers guess the location of the target region, choosing between four possible locations, and rate their confidence on a scale of 1 to 10. (*b*) Control situation in which left and right eyes view identical, consistent, displays. Here the target region is subjectively seen. (*c*) Results from three observers for conflicting displays (Kolb and Braun 1995). Performance is plotted separately for trials with different confidence ratings (e.g., when subjects give the lowest possible confidence rating of 1, performance still is near 65%, far above the chance level of 25%). No correlation between confidence and performance is observed, indicating complete lack of visual awareness of the target region (roughly flat bar graph). The thick line represents the frequency of different confidence ratings, the arrow being the distribution mean. (*d*) Results from the same observers for consistent displays. Confidence and performance are strongly correlated, indicating normal visual awareness of the target region (rising bar graph). (Reprinted, with permission, from Koch and Braun 1996.)

that similar pathways may mediate blindsight in patients with striate damage and in normal observers viewing conflicting displays.

Additional psychophysical evidence that a striate response is insufficient for awareness comes from experiments on the perception of high-frequency gratings (He et al. 1995). Although the orientation of such gratings is not subjectively apparent, they nevertheless induce an orientation-specific aftereffect. The high spatial frequencies involved (>50 cps) are such that only neurons with the smallest receptive fields in striate cortex are likely to respond, and neurons with larger receptive fields in extrastriate cortex remain silent. The contrast between the presumed striate response and the failure to become aware of grating orientation in this experiment is especially glaring.

Yet another instance in which a striate response is not sufficient to ensure visual awareness seems to be provided by visual "crowding" (He et al. 1996). When a single patch of a luminance grating appears on a computer screen (Fig. 3a), the grating is clearly visible and it induces an orientation-specific aftereffect; that is, it raises detection thresholds for any faint grating of similar orientation that may appear afterward. However, when additional gratings appear at either side, the original grating is "masked" and ceases to be visible as a distinct entity (Toet and Levi 1992). Subjectively, one still sees "something" at the location of the original grating but cannot discern its orientation, even when given unlimited viewing time. Yet the aftereffect induced by this "invisible" grating remains strong and orientation-specific (Fig. 3b). The conclusion that can be drawn from these observations, which is foreshadowed by earlier experiments (Blake and Fox 1974), is that visual awareness arises at higher levels of visual processing than orientation-specific adaptation. Since adaptation is thought to be mediated by orientation-selective neurons in striate cortex (Blakemore and Campbell 1969), this implies that visual awareness must arise at a later stage.

Of course, the weakness of purely psychophysical experiments is that the actual anatomical distribution of neuronal activity is unknown and must be inferred from other evidence. Fortunately, the precise mapping

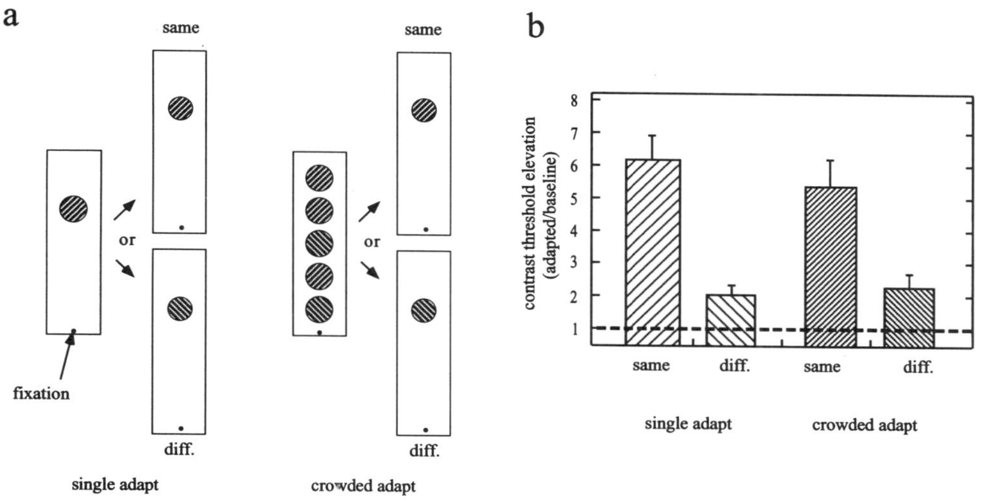

Figure 3. Psychophysical displays (schematic) and results pertaining to adaptation by crowded grating patches. (*a*) Adaptation followed by contrast threshold measurement for a single grating (*left*) and a crowded grating (*right*). In each trial, the orientation of the adapting grating was either the same as or different from the orientation of the test grating. Observers fixated at a distance of approximately 26° from the adapting and test gratings. (*b*) Threshold contrast elevation after adaptation relative to baseline threshold contrast before adaptation. Data are averaged across four subjects. The difference between same and different adapt-test orientations reflects the orientation-selective aftereffect of the adapting grating. The data show that this aftereffect is comparable for a crowded grating (whose orientation is not perceived) and for a single grating (whose orientation is readily perceived). (Reprinted, with permission, from He et al. 1996 [copyright Macmillan].)

of the human visual cortical areas with functional magnetic resonance imaging (Sereno et al. 1995) opens up the very real possibility of repeating these psychophysical experiments while the observer's visual cortex is being scanned.

Experiments on visual imagery are sometimes cited (we think misleadingly) in support of a striate contribution to visual awareness. A recent brain imaging study (Kosslyn et al. 1995) has resolved the debate whether visual imagery can lead to an activation of striate cortex (Roland and Gulyas 1994). Using PET, Kosslyn and colleagues showed that visual imagery can activate visual cortical areas as early as striate cortex (Kosslyn et al. 1995). However, this finding does not address the question of whether V1 activity expresses the phenomenal aspects of visual imagery (indeed, V1 activation may simply be necessary for activity in extrastriate visual cortical areas that would give rise to the phenomenal aspects).

CONCLUSION

The picture that emerges is that neurons in striate cortex, although necessary for almost all forms of phenomenal vision (as are retinal ganglion cells), do not *directly* contribute toward the neuronal correlate of conscious visual experience. Whether or not this has anything to do with the connectivity of area V1, especially its lack of a direct projection to frontal lobe (Crick and Koch 1995), remains an open question. Of course, it would be difficult to establish that none of the neuronal activity in area V1 correlates with the current contents of visual awareness. However, the evidence reviewed here uniformly points to the conclusion that visual awareness correlates far better with extrastriate than with striate neuronal activity. An even more specific hypothesis—that visual awareness correlates with activity in areas of the occipito-temporal rather than the occipito-parietal pathway—is not as well supported at present, but may well be confirmed by future evidence.

Further progress in understanding visual (and indeed all forms of) awareness can only come from precisely localizing the "neural correlate of consciousness" to specific brain areas and neuronal populations. That activity correlated with the changing percept in binocular rivalry in area MT occurs mostly in the deeper layers of cortex (Leopold and Logothetis 1996) constitutes very encouraging news on this front. It is conceivable that the correlate of visual awareness is expressed by a subset of neurons with very specific biophysical, biochemical, and morphological properties, rather than by all neurons in a given cortical area. This raises the fascinating, if distant, prospect of molecular tools that specifically label and manipulate such neurons (Koch 1996). It is by studying the dynamics and projection patterns of these neurons that we will begin our final assault on the age-old puzzle of the relationship between mind and brain.

ACKNOWLEDGMENTS

We thank Francis Crick for very fruitful discussions over the years, and Sheng He and Patrick Cavanagh for making Figure 3 available to us. Our work was supported by the National Science Foundation, by the Center for Neuromorphic Systems Engineering as a part of NSF's Engineering Research Center Program, and by the Beckman Institute at Caltech.

REFERENCES

Adelson, E.H. and J.A. Movshon. 1982. Phenomenal coherence of moving visual patterns. *Nature* **300:** 523.

Barbur, J.L., J.D.G. Watson, R.S.J. Frackowiak, and S.M.Zeki 1993. Conscious visual perception without V1. *Brain* **116:** 1293.

Blake, R. and R. Fox. 1974. Adaptation to invisible gratings and the site of binocular rivalry suppression. *Nature* **249:** 488.

Blakemore, C. and F.W. Campbell. 1969. On the existence of neurones in the human visual system selectively sensitive to the orientation and size of retinal images. *J. Physiol.* **203:** 237.

Braun, J. and F.C. Kolb. 1996. Blindsight in normal observers: A spatial range implicates striate visual cortex. *Invest. Ophthalmol. Visual Sci.* (suppl.) **37:** 1148.

Britten, K.H., M.N. Shadlen, W.T. Newsome, and J.A. Movshon. 1992. The analysis of visual motion: A comparison of neuronal and psychophysical performance. *J. Neurosci.* **12:** 4745.

Bullier, J., P. Girard, and P.-A. Salin. 1994. The role of area 17 in the transfer of information to extrastriate visual cortex. *Cereb. Cortex* **10:** 301.

Chalmers, D. 1996. *The conscious mind: In search of a fundamental theory.* Oxford University Press, New York.

Cowey, A. and P. Stoerig. 1991. The neurobiology of blindsight. *Trends Neurosci.* **14:** 140.

———. 1993. Insights into blindsight? *Curr. Biol.* **3:** 236.

———. 1995. Blindsight in monkeys. *Nature* **373:** 247.

Crick, F. and C. Koch. 1995. Are we aware of neural activity in primary visual cortex? *Nature* **375:** 121.

Fahle, M. and C. Koch. 1996. Performance and confidence in vernier hyperacuity tasks. *Perception* (ECVP Abstr.) (in press).

Felleman, D.J. and D.C. VanEssen. 1990. Distributed hierarchical processing in the primate cerebral cortex. *Cereb. Cortex* **1:** 1.

Fendrich, R., C.M. Wessinger, and M.S. Gazzaniga. 1994. Residual vision in a scotoma: Implications for blindsight. *Science* **258:** 1489.

Girard, P., P.A. Salin, and J. Bullier. 1992. Response selectivity of neurons in area MT of the macaque monkey during reversible inactivation of area V1. *J. Neurophysiol.* **67:** 1.

Goodale, M.A., A.D. Milner, L.S. Jakobson, and D.P. Carey. 1991. A neurological dissociation between perceiving objects and grasping them. *Nature* **349:** 154.

Graves, R.E. and B.S. Jones. 1992. Conscious visual perceptual awareness vs. non-conscious visual spatial localisation examined with normal subjects using possible analogues of blindsight and neglect. *Cogn. Neuropsychol.* **9:** 487.

He, S., P. Cavanagh, and J. Intriligator. 1996. Attentional resolution and the locus of visual awareness. *Nature* **383:** 334.

He, S., H. Smallman, and D.I.A. MacLeod. 1995. Neural and cortical limits on visual resolution. *Invest. Ophthalmol. Visual Sci.* (suppl) **36:** 2010.

Hernandez-Gonzalez, A., C. Cavada, and F. Reinoso-Suarez. 1994. The lateral geniculate nucleus projects to the inferior temporal cortex in the macaque monkey. *NeuroReport* **5:** 2693.

Heywood, C.A., D. Gaffan, and A. Cowey. 1995. Cerebral achromatopsia in monkeys. *Eur. J. Neurosci.* **7:** 1064.

Horton, J.C. and W.F. Hoyt. 1991. Quadrantic visual field defects. *Brain* **114:** 1703.

Humphrey, G.K., M.A. Goodale, and R. Gurnsey. 1991. Orientation discrimination in a visual form agnosic: Evidence from the McCollough effect. *Psychol. Sci.* **2:** 331.

Humphrey, G.K., M.A. Goodale, M. Corbetta, and S. Aglioti. 1995. The McCollough effect reveals orientation discrimination in a case of cortical blindness. *Curr. Biol.* **5:** 545.

Koch, C. 1996. A neuronal correlate of consciousness? *Curr. Biol.* **6:** 492.

Koch, C. and J. Braun. 1996. Towards the neuronal correlate of visual awareness. *Curr. Opin. Neurobiol.* **6:** 158.

Kolb, F.C. and J. Braun. 1995. Blindsight in normal observers. *Nature* **377:** 336.

Kosslyn, S.M., W.L. Thompson, I.J. Kim, and N.M. Alpert. 1995. Topographical representations of mental images in primary visual cortex. *Nature* **378:** 496.

Leopold, D.A. and N.K. Logothetis. 1996. Activity-changes in early visual cortex reflect monkeys' percepts during binocular rivalry. *Nature* **379:** 549.

Logothetis, N.K. and J.D. Schall. 1989. Neuronal correlates of subjective visual perception. *Science* **245:** 761.

Logothetis, N.K., D.A. Leopold, and D.L. Sheinberg. 1996. What is rivaling during binocular rivalry? *Nature* **380:** 621.

Merikle, P.M. 1992. Perception without attention: Results of a new method. *Am. Psychol.* **47:** 792.

Milner, A.D. and M.A. Goodale. 1995. *The visual brain in action.* Oxford University Press, United Kingdom.

Mohler, C.W. and R.H. Wurtz. 1976. Organization of monkey superior colliculus: Intermediate layer cells discharging before eye movements. *J. Neurophysiol.* **39:** 722.

Myerson, J., F. Miezin, and J. Allman. 1981. Binocular rivalry in macaque monkeys and humans: A comparative study in perception. *Behav. Anal. Lett.* **1:** 149.

Peterhans, E. and R. von der Heydt. 1991. Subjective contours: Bridging the gap between psychophysics and physiology. *Trends Neurosci.* **14:** 112.

Pollen, D.A. 1995. Cortical areas in visual awareness. *Nature* **377:** 293.

Pöppel, E., R. Held, and D. Frost. 1973. Residual visual function after brain wounds involving the central visual pathways in man. *Nature* **243:** 295.

Qian, N. and R.A. Andersen. 1994. Transparent motion perception as detection of unbalanced motion signals: II. Physiology. *J. Neurosci.* **14:** 7367.

Qian, N., E.H. Adelson, and R.A. Andersen. 1994a. Transparent motion perception as detection of unbalanced motion signals. III. Modeling. *J. Neurosci.* **14:** 7381.

Qian, N., R.A. Andersen, and E.H. Adelson. 1994b. Transparent motion perception as detection of unbalanced motion signals. I. Psychophysics. *J. Neurosci.* **14:** 7357.

Rodman, H.R., C.G. Gross, and T.D. Albright. 1989. Afferent basis of visual response properties in area MT of the macaque. I. Effects of striate cortex removal. *J. Neurosci.* **9:** 2033.

———. 1990. Afferent basis of visual response properties in area MT of the macaque. II. Effects of superior colliculus removal. *J. Neurosci.* **10:** 1154.

Roland, P.E. and B. Gulyas. 1994. Visual imagery and visual representation. *Trends Neurosci.* **17:** 281.

Salzman, C.D. and W.T. Newsome. 1994. Neural mechanisms for forming a perceptual decision. *Science* **264:** 231.

Schein, S.G. and R. Desimone. 1990. Spectral properties of V4 neurons in the macaque. *J. Neurosci.* **10:** 3369.

Sengpiel, F., C. Blakemore, and R. Harrad. 1995. Interocular suppression in the primary visual cortex: A possible neural basis of binocular rivalry. *Vision Res.* **35:** 179.

Sereno, M.I., A.M. Dale, J.B. Reppas, K.K. Kwong, J.W. Belliveau, and R. Tootell. 1995. Borders of multiple visual areas in humans revealed by functional magnetic resonance imaging. *Science* **268:** 889.

Shacter, D.L. 1992. Implicit knowledge: New perspectives on unconscious processing. *Proc. Natl. Acad. Sci.* **89:** 11113.

Stoerig, P. and A. Cowey. 1993. Blindsight—Neurons and behavior. *Prog. Brain Res.* **95:** 445.

Toet, A. and D.M. Levi. 1992. The two-dimensional shape of spatial interaction zones in the parafovea *Vision Res.* **32:** 1349.

Ungerleider, L.G. and J.V. Haxby. 1994. "What" and "where" in the human brain. *Curr. Opin. Neurobiol.* **4:** 157.

Van Essen, D.C. and J.L. Gallant. 1994. Neural mechanisms of form and motion processing in the primate visual system. *Neuron* **13:** 1.

Weiskrantz, L. 1986. *Blindsight: A case study and implications.* Oxford University Press, United Kingdom.

Weiskrantz, L., J.L. Barbur, and A. Sahraie. 1995. Parameters affecting conscious versus unconscious visual discrimination with damage to the visual cortex (V1). *Proc. Natl. Acad. Sci.* **92:** 6122.

Weiskrantz, L., E.K. Warrington, and M.D. Sanders. 1974. Visual capacity in the hemianoptic field following a restricted occipital ablation. *Brain* **97:** 709.

Zeki, S. 1983. The distribution of wavelength and orientation selective cells in different areas of monkey visual cortex. *Proc. R. Soc. Lond. B Biol. Sci.* **217:** 449.

A Single Locus, *RGHT*, Specifies Preference for Hand Utilization in Humans

A.J.S. KLAR

Gene Regulation and Chromosome Biology Laboratory, NCI-Frederick Cancer Research and Development Center, ABL-Basic Research Program, Frederick, Maryland 21702-1201

It has been a long-standing controversy whether nature or nurture causes individuals to prefer utilization of one hand over the other. A model for a single gene (*RGHT* = *Right*- and *r* = *r*andom-handedness) controlling human hand preference is proposed, and data satisfying two key genetic predictions of the model are presented. First, by calculating the gene frequency from RH (right-handed) x LH (left-handed) families, the model explains the percentage of LH children observed in RH x RH families. Second, the RH children of LH x LH families are evidenced to contain the *r/r* genotype as they produce a higher percentage of LH children, similar to those of LH individuals in the general population. This model also explains discordance of handedness in monozygotic twins due to randomicity in hand preference of *r/r* individuals. It is speculated that the *RGHT* gene/locus functions primarily to specify cerebral laterality such that language is processed in the left brain hemisphere, and secondarily to coordinate left brain dominance with development of the right-hand preference.

Nearly one in ten individuals is left-handed (LH) or ambidextrous (Corballis 1991). Despite dozens, if not hundreds, of studies conducted for many decades, it has not been possible to unambiguously determine how human handedness is specified. Although many interesting hypotheses have been advanced to explain human handedness, no consensus about the correct explanation has yet been reached. A major school of thought proposes that handedness is a learned behavior and that as children develop, they acquire handedness preference by watching their parents and other individuals (Collins 1975; Corballis and Morgan 1978; Morgan and Corballis 1978; Coren 1992) or due to other environmental factors including stress during birth (Bakan 1971; Perelle and Ehrman 1983). This cultural model explains why a higher percentage of children are LH if one or both parents are LH, compared with children of RH x RH parents. In contrast, since the first suggestion by Jordan (1911), many genetic models propose that handedness is controlled by one or more genes with additive or dominant effects (for reviews, see Levy and Nagylaki 1972; Annett 1985; McManus 1991). From the segregation analysis of family data, Risch and Pringle (1985) concluded that either a single-locus model or a polygenic model is consistent with the data, although they cautioned that their analysis could not be taken as evidence of genetic etiology. A more recent study on this subject proposed a gene-culture coevolution model (Laland et al. 1995), in which selection is thought to have eliminated all genetic variation contributing to handedness such that all individuals are predisposed to be right-handed, but cultural influences dictate their hand preference (see also Perelle and Ehrman 1994). Thus, a child with two RH parents would be more likely to be RH than a child with one or two LH parents. Furthermore, much attention has been given to the Geschwind hypothesis (Geschwind and Galaburda 1987) suggesting that fetal testosterone levels relate to handedness and cerebral dominance.

Proponents of environmental models advance three major arguments/observations against genetic models. First, hand preference can be changed, because LH individuals can learn to use certain tools, such as scissors, that are made only for right-hand use. Second, 18.3% of the individual members of monozygotic twins, who obviously share the identical genetic makeup, are discordant such that one member is RH, while the other is LH (Rife 1940). Third, not all of the children of LH x LH parents are LH; about 50% are LH and 50% are RH (Rife 1940).

The genetic human handedness model presented here hypothesizes that a single gene, designated *RGHT* (pronounced as right), confers right-handedness and individuals lacking this gene (*RGHT⁻/RGHT⁻*) display random handedness such that one half are LH and the other half are RH. Tests of the two genetic predictions of the model are presented below.

DEFINITION OF HANDEDNESS

Although it seems trivial to a lay person, a major difficulty in studies of handedness lies with the definition of handedness. There is no general agreement among investigators of hand utilization as to what constitutes right- or left-handedness. Furthermore, a sizable proportion of individuals are neither; they are ambidextrous. For human handedness, defining hand preference only by the criterion of writing is highly problematic, because many cultures discourage left-handed writing by children. Some investigators in this field (see, e.g., Annett 1985) seem to agree that the best criteria and definition are those adopted by Rife

(1940). Rife argued that cultural attitudes do play an important part in the execution of human hand preference. To compensate for these attitudes, Rife chose the following definition of handedness. An individual is considered right-handed if ten acts are routinely done only with the right hand: throwing a ball, using a spoon, sawing, sewing, shooting marbles, bowling, cutting with a knife, cutting with scissors, hammering, and writing. An individual who performs one or more of these acts with the left hand or with either hand is defined as non-right handed. Thus, ambidextrous people are recognized as non-right handed. To simplify the terminology here, all non-right handed individuals are referred to as left-handed (LH).

RIFE'S SURVEY OF HUMAN HAND UTILIZATION

Employing the definition presented above, Rife conducted a survey of the families of 687 students attending Ohio State University. Table 1 presents the results of his survey. Note that approximately half of the children of LH x LH families were LH and the remainder were RH. This result has been a major problem for the genetic model, which predicts that 100% of these children should have been LH. By analogy, for example, all the children of blue-eyed parents are blue-eyed, since both parents lack the gene to produce brown eye color. The following model is proposed to explain this discrepancy.

R = *R*IGHT- AND *r* = *R*ANDOM-HANDEDNESS MODEL

It is proposed here that a gene designated *R* (for *R*ight) specifies right-handed preference and, in the absence of this gene (i.e., for individuals containing the *r*, for *r*andomness allele in the *r/r* homozygous state), the phenotype will be randomly specified such that half will be LH and the other half RH. In human genetic terminology, the gene for right-handedness is designated *RGHT* and the absence of this gene is designated as the *RGHT*⁻ allele. However, in the interest of clarity, these alleles are written in this paper as *R* and *r*, and the right- and left-handedness phenotypes are designated as RH and LH, respectively. The main concept of the model can be appreciated by following the physical analogy presented in Figure 1. Salient features of the model are that there is only a binary choice available for establishing hand preference, that choice is dictated by the dominant *R* gene, and that in the absence of that gene there is random specification of handedness.

Table 1. Rife's (1940) Survey

	Parents		
	RH x RH	RH x LH	LH x LH
	↓	↓	↓
LH children	(7.6%) ~8.0%	(19.5%) ~20%	(54%) ~50%

GENE FREQUENCY DETERMINATION

According to this human handedness model, the gene frequency in RH individuals can be easily calculated from the handedness of the children of RH x LH families from Table 1 (Fig. 2). Note that about 20% of such children are LH. The model requires that they carry recessive alleles with the homozygous *r/r* genotype. In addition, according to the randomness feature of the model (Fig. 1), another 20% of the children will have the same *r/r* genotype, but they will be RH (Fig. 2). In other words, 40% of the children in these families will be *r/r* homozygotes. Since one of the parents is LH in these families, 100% of the gametes from these LH parents will have the *r* allele. Thus, all children will inherit one *r* allele from the LH parent. As we have calculated that 40% of the children contain the *r/r* genotype, it follows that 60% of the children are *R/r* heterozygotes. Therefore, to produce 40% *r/r* plus 60% *R/r* children in the RH x LH families, 40% of the gametes from the RH parents must contain *r*, while 60% contain *R*. Obviously, the RH parents will represent a mixture of *R/R*, *R/r*, and *r/r* genotypes, but collectively in their gene frequency, 40% of their gametes/specific chromosomes are calculated to carry the *r* allele, whereas 60% will carry the *R* allele.

FIRST TEST OF THE MODEL: PREDICTION #1

A major prediction of the model is that the calculated gene frequency of RH individuals must explain the observation of 8% LH children of RH x RH families presented in Table 1. Since the RH individuals are calculated as described above to produce 40% *r*-containing gametes, then 40% x 40% = 16% of their children are predicted to contain the *r/r* genotype. Because only half of these children will be LH due to random specification of phenotype in the *r/r* children, the predicted result of 16% x 1/2 = 8% was observed!

SECOND TEST OF THE MODEL: PREDICTION #2

Another crucial prediction of the genetic model is that all RH children of LH x LH families should have the genetic makeup of *r/r*, since both of their parents are LH, *r/r* homozygotes. For easier reference, these RH children of LH x LH parents are denoted as RH* to distinguish them from RH individuals whose parental handedness is unknown.

How can one test whether RH* individuals are indeed *r/r* homozygotes? Recall that RH x RH families produced 8% LH children in Rife's survey (Table 1). A key test is that RH* individuals should not produce a lower percentage of LH children than found with

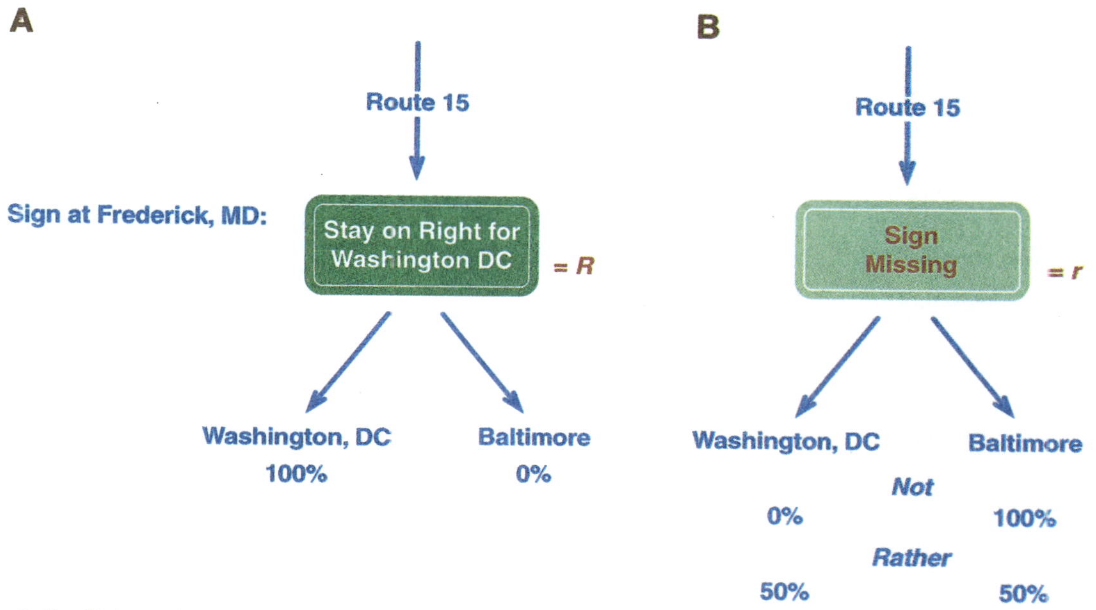

Figure 1. R = Right- and r = $r$andom-handedness model explained via a physical analogy. Imagine that one is driving south on Route 15 and wants to go to Washington, DC. After reading the sign at Frederick, Maryland (as in *A*) indicating that the road on the right at the fork goes to Washington, DC, all individuals would end up in Washington, DC and no one would arrive at Baltimore, Maryland. If that sign were missing, however (as in *B*), then not all of the drivers would go to Baltimore; rather, there would be a random choice so that 50% would reach Washington, DC and 50% would arrive at Baltimore. In this analogy, the individuals containing one (R/r) or two (R/R) copies of the R gene will develop as right-handed because they contain the signpost directing development to make them right-handed. Lacking this signpost (as in *B*), the r/r individuals will develop equally as left- or right-handed. Note that the 50% LH:50% RH phenotype is not due to conventional 50% penetrance of the trait in r/r individuals; rather, a lack of consistent left-right asymmetry due to the absence of the R gene is expected to result in random-handed persons.

other RH individuals in the general population. Rather, they should produce a higher percentage of LH children, similar to LH individuals in the general population. That is, by the cultural model, RH* x RH parents should produce about 8% LH children (Fig. 3; Table 1 [RH x RH families]). (Note, however, that this 8% figure is effectively explained by prediction #1 using our genetic model.) In contrast, by the genetic model, the RH* x RH parents should produce 20% LH children (Fig. 3), equivalent to the percentage observed in the RH x LH families (Table 1).

To test this prediction, a three-generational survey was conducted to identify LH x LH grandparents and their RH* children, and then the proportion of LH children in the RH* x RH families was determined. The survey was conducted with families living only in the United States, and only the data of individuals 6 years or older are reported. These families were identified through advertisements in the local (Frederick, Maryland) paper and in *Lefthander* magazine (Topeka, Kansas), as well as through an article regarding this study printed in the newspapers nationally by the Associated Press. Data collected in response to the questionnaire, following the same criteria used by Rife (1940), showed that 11/48 (~23%) of the children of RH* x RH families are LH. This number is significantly different from the 7.6% observed in RH x RH families (Table 1) predicted by the cultural model (χ^2 = 15.2, df = 1, p = <0.005), but it is a result similar to the RH x LH matings in Table 1.

THIRD TEST OF THE MODEL: PREDICTION #3

Another prediction of the model is that RH* x RH* families should produce 50% LH and 50% RH chil-

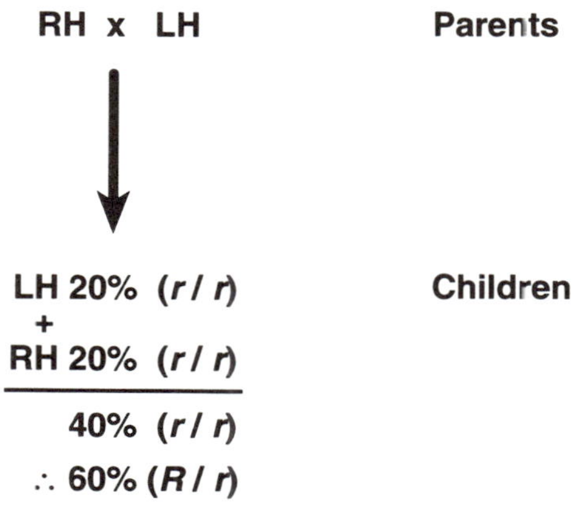

Figure 2. Calculation of the gene frequency of RH individuals. See text for details.

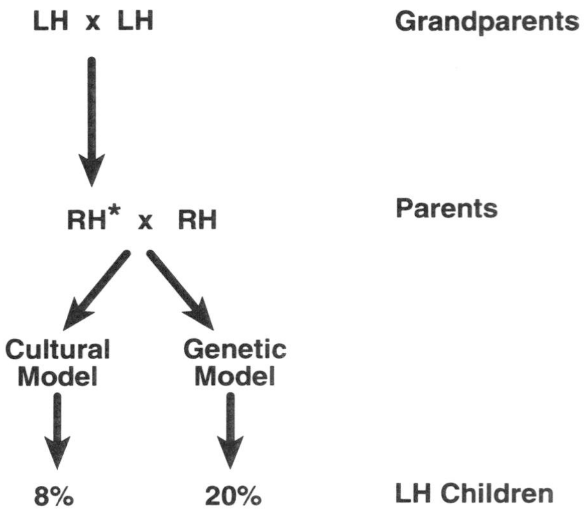

Figure 3. A specific, three-generational survey can distinguish between cultural and genetic models. Predictions of both models are presented. RH* individuals are children of LH x LH parents, whereas the handedness of parents of RH individuals derived from the general population is unknown.

dren. This experiment is nearly impossible to conduct because of the rarity of RH* x RH* couples. However, in the data of our survey we found a low number of RH* people who were married to LH individuals. By the cultural model, they are expected to produce 20% LH children (Table 1 [RH x LH families]), but by the genetic model, 50% of their children are expected to be LH. Although the sample size was small, 7/9 (78%) of their children were observed to be LH. Statistically, this result is more consistent with the 50% expectation of the genetic model ($\chi^2 = 1.4$, df = 1, $p = >0.20$) and not with the 20% expectation ($\chi^2 = 15$, df = 1, $p = <0.005$) of the cultural model.

These genetic results satisfy the key predictions of the R = *R*ight- and r = *r*andom-handedness genetic model and strongly argue against the cultural model which states that hand preference is a learned behavior.

A POSSIBLE ROLE OF THE *R* GENE IN BRAIN HEMISPHERE LATERALIZATION

The left and right hemispheres of the cerebellum seem to specialize in different brain functions, the most prominent of which is speech and language lateralization. An overwhelming majority (97%) of RH individuals have left hemisphere lateralization for speech and language (for review, see Coren 1992); the remaining 3% constitute a mixture of right hemisphere dominance plus bilateral symmetry (i.e., individuals having language development in both hemispheres; Table 2). Thus, in RH individuals, there is a nearly perfect correlation of handedness and brain lateralization, so much so that the same gene affecting handedness can be postulated to be acting in brain development. A

Table 2. Handedness Is Only Partially Correlated with Brain Hemisphere Dominance

		Dominant brain hemisphere[a]	
Handedness	Genotype[b]	left	right or bilateral
RH	*R/R* 33% *R/r* 49% *r/r* 9%	97%	3%
LH	*r/r* 9%	70%	30%

[a]Data from a review (Coren 1992).

[b]Genotype and percentage calculated from the R = *R*ight- and r = *r*andom-handedness model.

major difficulty for this model is that brain lateralization of LH individuals is not a mirror image of that of RH individuals. In fact, a majority (70%) of left-handed people—although not as large a proportion as left-speech RH individuals—also show left-speech lateralization, and 30% of LH individuals show right-speech dominance or bilateral symmetry (Rossi and Rosadini 1967; Warrington and Pratt 1973; for a review, see Coren 1992). In light of the model for handedness presented here, the following postulate can be used to explain brain hemisphere dominance and its complex relation to handedness: The primary function of the R gene is to specify left-brain dominance and the secondary function is to couple it to the development of right-hand preference. Accordingly, in the absence of this gene (i.e., in *r/r* individuals), development of brain hemisphere dominance and hand preference is uncoupled. Consequently, there is a strong correlation in these two attributes of human development in RH but not in LH individuals.

The existing data of 3% of RH individuals developing right hemisphere dominance or bilateral symmetry seem to support this model. According to the calculated *R:r* gene frequency, about 9% of individuals are LH, *r/r* homozygotes (Table 2). The model predicts that another 9% of the general population will also have the *r/r* genotype, although they are RH. Thus, among RH individuals, 9.9% (9/91) have the *r/r* genotype. If these RH, *r/r* individuals also develop their brain hemisphere dominance like the LH (*r/r*) individuals because they have the same genotype, then 9.9% x 30% = 2.9% of RH should develop right hemisphere dominance or bilateral speech. This number is remarkably similar to the 3% reported in the literature (Table 2) (for review, see Coren 1992).

DISCUSSION

The long-standing question of hand preference has been subject to much debate and controversy, and thus far, there is no consensus of how hand preference is established. The genetic human handedness model was postulated to explain the finding that nearly half of the children of LH x LH parents are RH (Rife 1940). In a conventional and simple genetic model, LH individuals that possess a homozygous recessive gene should only produce LH children. The second major problem for genetic models is that a substantial frequency (18.3%) of monozygotic twins are discordant for handedness; i.e., one individual is LH and the other is RH (Rife 1940). Previous genetic models have tried to accommodate these two observations by various postulations: 50% penetrance of the trait or variable expressivity of a gene, genetic heterogeneity such that many loci are required to specify right- or left-handedness, gene function skipping a generation, randomness, genetic modifiers, etc. However, all of these models were based on the available data and did not make predictions to rigorously test such models. Furthermore, each of these models has used a different criterion for handedness; thus, different studies are not sufficiently comparable to arrive at a consensus. Primarily because of problems with the genetic models, most of the literature on behavioral studies concludes that handedness is primarily determined as a learned trait (Perelle and Ehrman 1983, 1994; Coren 1992; Laland et al. 1995).

Two significant findings satisfying key predictions of the R = *R*ight- and r = *r*andom-handedness model and ruling out the cultural model as a major determinant for hand preference are presented in this paper. First, by calculating the gene frequency of the R and r alleles in RH individuals from RH x LH families, derived from the survey by Rife (1940), the predicted percentage of LH children was indeed observed in RH x RH matings. Second, the RH children of LH x LH parents functioned similarly to LH individuals as they produced a predicted equivalently higher percentage of LH children of their own, and thereby established that their genotype is the same as that of LH individuals. These two results strongly support the single-gene model and establish that individuals possessing the recessive nonfunctional allele are random-handed. Both of the observations reported here provide evidence that the R gene functions with 100% penetrance such that both R/R and R/r individuals are right-handed and that R is dominant to the r allele.

Minor differences in handedness between males and females and the influence of maternal effect (Rife 1940; Annett 1985) may be attributed to different sensitivities of males compared to females to social pressures, including parental influence. Encouraged by results of the genetic analysis presented here, we want to map this locus with the ultimate goal of cloning the gene for molecular analysis.

Twin Discordance Is Explained by the Model

A particularly interesting feature of the genetic model is that it rather simply explains discordance of handedness in monozygotic twins despite both individuals in each pair of twins having an identical genetic makeup. With the gene frequency in the general population calculated as 58% R and 42% r from the R = *R*ight- and r = *r*andom-handedness model, approximately 18% of the offspring are expected to be r/r homozygotes in the general population. It was also shown conclusively that left-handedness occurs more frequently in the parents and siblings of RH-LH twins than among these relatives of RH-RH twins (Boklage 1981; Annett 1985). Consequently, there is an increased proportion of the r allele in the parents of RH-LH twins than that found in the general population. Therefore, most, if not all, of the discordance in monozygotic twins can be explained by the genetic model presented here, which proposes randomness of hand preference in r/r individuals of monozygotic twins. With this rationale, the mirror imaging proposed earlier (Newman 1928) may contribute only minimally or not at all to the handedness discordance of twins. This concept explaining discordance in monozygotic twins, along with dizygotic twins, will be further explored in a subsequent publication.

Comparison with Other Genetic Models

Since the model presented here shares some features of the genetic models proposed earlier (see below), it is fair to ask why other models have not been accepted thus far. In this context, it is helpful to compare this model with previous models. The proposed model has incorporated the randomicity feature of recessive homozygotes originally suggested by Trankell (1955). This feature was also incorporated in two other major genetic models used by Annett (1985) and McManus (1991), but major differences exist among all three models both in concepts of function of the gene and in tests of the models. First, Annett suggested that hand preference alone is a truly continuously distributed normal variable, such as an asymmetry of manual strength as a quantitative trait, and the description of right- or left-handedness depends on the empirically defined arbitrary position of a threshold on the normal distribution of skill asymmetry. Thus, Annett's model proposes a description of handedness in terms of a continuous skill asymmetry. However, the model proposed here explains handedness in terms of a binary developmental event, thereby dividing the population into RH and LH. In this regard, ambidextrous individuals are considered here as left-handed, but cultural influences have taught them to use either hand. Second, in Annett's method of model-fitting with the data, the presence of the right-shift (rs^+) gene is proposed to cause most of the individuals to be RH, yet 1.14% rs^+ individuals will be LH, since accidental biases toward the left hand will not always be counteracted by the rs^+ factor (Annett 1985). In the present model, all of the individuals containing the R gene (R/R as well as R/r) are expected to be RH. Third, in early versions of the model, Annett assumed that there existed a complete dominance of rs^+ allele, but to fit the data, later suggested an additive model affecting the extent of the right-shift with rs^+ and rs^- alleles (Annett and Kilshaw 1983). In contrast, in the R= *R*ight- and r = *r*andom-handedness model, R is dominant to the r allele. Fourth, in the model proposed here, the gene frequency for the R gene is calculated directly from the handedness studies, whereas Annett (1985) inferred gene frequency entirely indirectly from association of handedness with speech lateralization in brain hemispheres (see below). In this regard, McManus (1985) previously pointed out that it is premature to interrelate models of handedness and speech dominance. Furthermore, the apparent bimodal distribution of brain laterality is inconsistent with the main tenet of the right-shift model proposing hand preference as due to continuously distributed variable. Fifth, Annett explained discordance in twins by arbitrarily changing the parameters of threshold in comparison to single-borns. McManus (1985) also argued against the right-shift model as it requires different parameters in twins and single-borns. In the present model, discordance is principally explained by the randomness of handedness in *r/r* individuals.

In the data-fitting model proposed by McManus (1991), LH individuals would either be homozygous for the chance allele (C) of the handedness gene or represent a heterozygous genotype with dextral (D) in one allele and C in the other. In the present model, only individuals with the recessive *r/r* allele are expected to be LH. Because of this major difference, the 15.5% population gene frequency of the C allele calculated by McManus is vastly different from the 42% r gene prevalence derived by the present model. However, the idea of bimodality of LH and RH populations is shared between the present model and the McManus model. Levy and Nagylaki (1972) proposed another two-locus model, with one locus determining the lateralization of language and the second deciding contralateral versus ipsilateral motor controls that dictate writing-hand preference.

Major differences thus exist among all of these models and, clearly, none of the previous genetic models has been accepted thus far. In contrast to the other genetic models, which were based on data-fitting and which have not been satisfactorily scrutinized by testing their predictions, the R = *R*ight- and r = *r*andom-handedness model has been subjected to crucial genetic tests.

Why Stress Only Rife's Survey?

The present study is based only on the survey by Rife (1940), although many other surveys have been performed (for reviews, see Annett 1985; McManus 1991) which are purposely not addressed here in the context of the R = *R*ight- and r = *r*andom-handedness model. The main reason for using only Rife's data is the precise definition of handedness discussed above. Many studies have used different criteria and surveyed different cultures and, consequently, are not comparable. Therefore, it is not surprising that the frequency of left-handedness has ranged from 0.7% to 40% in different studies (Perelle and Ehrman 1994). Likewise, most studies report that LH x LH families produce less than 50% LH children, some of which have only used a single writing-hand criterion; adding more tasks to such surveys increases the percentage of LH children in all categories of matings (McGee and Cozad 1980). Accordingly, in our survey using 10 criteria, we find that LH x LH families produce 42% (37/88) LH children and 43% in the McGee and Cozad (1980) study. Note that changing the proportion of LH with changes in number and type of tasks surveyed only changes the ratio of R and r alleles in the population, but it will not affect the major conclusions that handedness is a single-gene trait and that *r/r* homozygotes are random-handed individuals. Trying to fit all disparate surveys with widely varying percentages of LH into one model, we believe, has contributed to past failure to arrive at a consensus model for the inheritance of handedness. For example, the present model does not attempt to explain the low level (0.7%) of individuals in the Chinese population who use their left hand for writing (Teng et al. 1976), which most likely is due to strong cultural influences prohibiting left-hand utilization. Keeping this difficulty in mind, the present three-generational survey used the exact same definition and the North American population used by Rife (1940); therefore, these studies are comparable to each other and not to others.

Right-hand preference seems to be exclusively a human trait (Coren 1992). The best study on nonhumans was conducted by Collins (1969) on the paw preference in mice. He found that individual mice preferred using either the right or left paw, and the population as a whole is random. With further breeding of mice who shared similar preferences, it was observed that the preference of the parents was not inherited by the progeny. Such a comparison with nonhumans leads to an interesting evolutionary question. If other animals do not show handedness/pawed-ness, then why and how do humans develop hand preference? A strong hint for the possible function of hand preference is provided by the finding that 97% of RH humans have speech lateralized in their left-brain hemisphere. Although most (70%) LH humans still contain lateralized speech in the left hemisphere, a significant proportion (30%) contain bilateral or right hemisphere speech localization. Notably, most (70%) *r/r* individuals are still lateralized with left-hemisphere dominance. This intrinsic lateralization in the absence of R gene is proposed to be dictated by other gene(s) partially controlling brain lateralization. We suspect that the primary function of the R gene is for cerebral lateralization, and the secondary function appears to be coordination of that lateral asymmetry with hand preference. The complex correlation of handedness with brain hemisphere dominance has been very well documented in the literature (see, e.g., Levy and Nagylaki 1972; Annett 1975; McManus 1991), and Annett (1975, 1983) used this complex correlation to infer the gene frequency of the right-shift gene and come up with values very similar to ones calculated here directly from handedness data. According to the genetic basis for handedness, the *R* gene may be postulated to have evolved in humans to specify lateralization of speech in one hemisphere, which for some reason may be beneficial for coordinating the functioning of higher brain activity, an attribute presumably not found in nonhuman species.

The finding that handedness is primarily specified genetically has wide-ranging social implications. Although utilization of the right hand is not as strictly enforced in North America and parts of Western Europe as in the past, LH individuals in most other countries, especially in the Eastern hemisphere, are still forced to use their right hand. Now, knowing that there is a genetic/biological basis for LH behavior, (1) superstitions associated with the sinistral handedness should be discouraged, (2) more tools for LH individuals should be designed for this large minority in the world, and (3) children should not be discouraged from using their preferred hand.

ACKNOWLEDGMENTS

I particularly thank the many families who have participated in the hand utilization survey. Informed consent was obtained from them after the nature and possible consequences of the studies were explained. I also thank my colleagues in the Gene Regulation and Chromosome Biology Laboratory for many discussions as well as suggestions to improve the manuscript, J. Hopkins for preparing the manuscript, A. Arthur for editorial assistance, R. Frederickson for the artwork, and K. Kipers and C. Riddle of Lefthanders International for advertising this survey in *Lefthanders* magazine. Research was sponsored by the National Cancer Institute, Department of Health and Human Services, under contract N01-CO-46000 with ABL. The contents of this publication do not necessarily reflect the views or policies of the Department of Health and Human Services, nor does mention of trade names, commercial products, or organizations imply endorsement by the U.S. government.

REFERENCES

Annett, M. 1975. Hand preference and the laterality of speech. *Cortex* **11:** 305.

———. 1983. Hand preference and skill in 115 children of two left-handed parents. *Br. J. Psychol.* **74:** 17.

———. 1985. *Left, right, hand and brain: The right shift theory.* Erlbaum, London, United Kingdom.

Annett, M. and D. Kilshaw. 1983. Right and left-hand skill II: Estimating the parameters of the distribution of L-R differences in males and females. *Br. J. Psychol.* **74:** 269.

Bakan, P. 1971. Handedness and birth order. *Nature* **229:** 195.

Boklage, C.E.. 1981. On the distribution of nonright-handedness among twins and their families. *Acta Genet. Med. Gemellol.* **30:** 167.

Collins, R.L. 1969. On the inheritance of handedness. II. Selection for sinistrality in mice. *J. Hered.* **60:** 117.

———. 1975. When left-handed mice live in right-handed worlds. *Science* **187:** 181.

Corballis, M.C. 1991. *The lopsided ape.* Oxford University Press, New York.

Corballis, M.C. and M.J. Morgan. 1978. On the biological basis of human laterality: I. Evidence for maturational left-right gradient. *Behav. Brain Sci.* **1:** 261.

Coren, S. 1992. *The left-hander syndrome—The cause and consequences of left-handedness.* MacMillan, New York.

Geschwind, N. and A.M. Galaburda. 1987. *Cerebral lateralization.* MIT Press, Cambridge, Massachusetts.

Jordan, H.E. 1911. The inheritance of left-handedness. *Am. Breed. Mag.* **2:** 19-29.

Laland, K.N., J. Kumm, J.D. Van Horn, and M.W. Feldman. 1995. A gene-culture model of human handedness. *Behav. Genet.* **25:** 433.

Levy, J. and T. Nagylaki. 1972. A model for the genetics of handedness. *Genetics* **72:** 117.

McGee, M.G. and T. Cozad. 1980. Population genetic analysis of human hand preference: Evidence for generation differences, familial resemblance, and maternal effects. *Behav. Genet.* **10:** 263.

McManus, I.C. 1985. Right- and left-hand skill: Failure of the right-shift model. *Br. J. Psychol.* **76:** 1.

———. 1991. The inheritance of left handedness. *CIBA Found. Symp.* **162:** 251.

Morgan, M.J. and M.C. Corballis. 1978. On the biological basis of human laterality. II. The mechanism of inheritance. *Behav. Brain Sci.* **1:** 270.

Newman, H. 1928. Asymmetry reversal or mirror imaging in identical twins. *Biol. Bull.* **55:** 298.

Perelle, I.B. and L. Ehrman. 1983. The development and laterality. *Behav. Sci.* **28:** 284.

———. 1994. An international study of human handedness: The data. *Behav. Genet.* **24:** 217.

Rife, D.C. 1940. Handedness, with special reference to twins. *Genetics* **28:** 178.

Risch, N. and G. Pringle. 1985. Segregation analysis of human hand preference. *Behav. Genet.* **15:** 385.

Rossi, G.F. and G. Rosadini. 1967. Experimental analysis of cerebral dominance in man. In *Brain mechanisms underlying speech and language* (ed. F.L. Darley), p. 167. Grune and Stratton, New York.

Teng, E.L., P. Lee, P.C. Yang, and P.C. Chang. 1976. Handedness in a Chinese population: Biological, social and pathological factors. *Science* **193:** 1148.

Trankell, A. 1955. Aspects of genetics and psychology. *Am. J. Hum. Genet.* **7:** 264.

Warrington, E.K. and R.T.C. Pratt. 1973. Language laterality in left handers assessed by unilateral ECT. *Neuropsychologia* **11:** 423.

Functions and Roles of Glutamate Receptors in Synaptic Transmission and Plasticity

S. NAKANISHI, Y. NAKAJIMA, A. NOMURA, M. MASU, H. IWAKABE, Y. HAYASHI, AND M. YOKOI
Department of Biological Sciences, Kyoto University Faculty of Medicine, Kyoto 606, Japan

Glutamate receptors mediate most excitatory synaptic transmission in the central nervous system and play an essential role in neural plasticity, neural development, and neurodegeneration (Nakanishi 1992, 1994; Hollmann and Heinemann 1994; Nakanishi and Masu 1994). There are two general groups of glutamate receptors (Nakanishi 1992, 1994; Hollmann and Heinemann 1994; Nakanishi and Masu 1994). Ionotropic glutamate receptors comprise ligand-gated cation channels and are subdivided into α-amino-3-hydroxy-5-methyl-4-isoxazolepropionate (AMPA)/kainate type and *N*-methyl-D-aspartate (NMDA) type of receptors. Metabotropic glutamate receptors are G-protein-coupled receptors that modulate the production of intracellular second messengers. With the aid of a functional cloning strategy that combines electrophysiology and a *Xenopus* oocyte expression system, we cloned and characterized the NMDA receptor and mGluR (Masu et al. 1991; Moriyoshi et al. 1991). Both receptors exist as diverse members of receptor subunits and subtypes (Fig. 1) (Hollmann and Heinemann 1994; Nakanishi and Masu 1994). The NMDA receptor subunits are classified into two distinct groups. NMDAR1 is a key subunit that possesses all properties of the NMDA receptor-channel complex, whereas four NMDAR2 subunits (NMDAR2A–2D) serve as modulatory subunits that potentiate and differentiate NMDA receptor activity by heteromeric formation with NMDAR1. The mGluRs form a family consisting of at least eight different subtypes (mGluR1–mGluR8) (Fig. 1) (Nakanishi 1994; Pin and Duvoisin 1995). mGluR1 and mGluR5 are coupled to inositol triphosphate/Ca^{++} signal transduction and respond strongly to quisqualate. The other six subtypes are linked to the inhibitory cascade of cAMP formation. mGluR2 and mGluR3 react effectively with (2S, 1′R, 2′R, 3′R)-2-(2,3-dicarboxycyclopropyl)glycine (DCG-IV) (Hayashi et al. 1993), whereas mGluR4, mGluR6, mGluR7, and mGluR8 respond potently to L-2-amino-4-phosphonobutyrate (L-AP4). The mGluR subtypes are thus subdivided into three groups according to their sequence similarities, signal transduction mechanisms, and agonist selectivities (Nakanishi 1994; Pin and Duvoisin 1995). It is thus important to explore roles of diverse members of glutamate receptors in brain function and dysfunction on the basis of the knowledge of the molecular diversity of glutamate receptors. This paper deals with some specialized functions of the diverse members of mGluRs in the central nervous system.

EXPERIMENTAL PROCEDURES

Targeted disruption of the mGluR2 and mGluR6 genes was carried out with the use of an embryonic cell line (Masu et al. 1995; Yokoi et al. 1996). ON and OFF responses were recorded from the superior colliculus with extracellular recording techniques (Masu et al. 1995). GABA-mediated inhibitory postsynaptic currents (IPSCs) at a mitral cell of the accessory olfactory bulb (AOB) were recorded by the slice patch-clamp recording methods after electrical stimulation of a granule cell (Hayashi et al. 1993). Basal synaptic transmission and paired-pulse facilitation at the mossy fiber-CA3 synapses were determined in hippocampal slices (Yokoi et al. 1996). Long-term potentiation (LTP) and long-term depression (LTD) at the mossy fiber-CA3 synapses were induced by tetanic stimulation (100 Hz, 1 sec) and low-frequency stimulation (1 Hz, 15 min), respectively (Yokoi et al. 1996). Immunostaining of mGluR2 and mGluR6 was carried out with use of the mGluR2/mGluR3 antibody and the mGluR6 antibody, respectively (Nomura et al. 1994; Yokoi et al. 1996).

RESULTS AND DISCUSSION

mGluR6 in Visual Information Processing

Visual signals are transmitted from photoreceptors to bipolar cells. A key process of visual information transmission is detecting visual contrasts (Dowling 1987; Shepherd and Koch 1990; Schiller 1992; DeVries and Baylor 1993). Photoreceptors hyperpolarize by light exposure and reduce glutamate release. In turn, ON and OFF bipolar cells depolarize and hyperpolarize, respectively. The opposite reaction occurs by dark stimulus. Thus, the visual signals are segregated into parallel ON-center and OFF-center pathways at the level of bipolar cells (Schiller 1992; Wässle et al. 1991; DeVries and Baylor 1993). Electrophysiological evidence has indicated that a putative L-AP4-sensitive mGluR subtype mediates postsynaptic responses of ON-bipolar cells by enhancing cGMP hydrolysis similar to that of signal transduction in photoreceptors (Nawy and Jahr 1990, 1991; Shiells and Falk 1990). We cloned mGluR6 from a retinal cDNA library. mGluR6

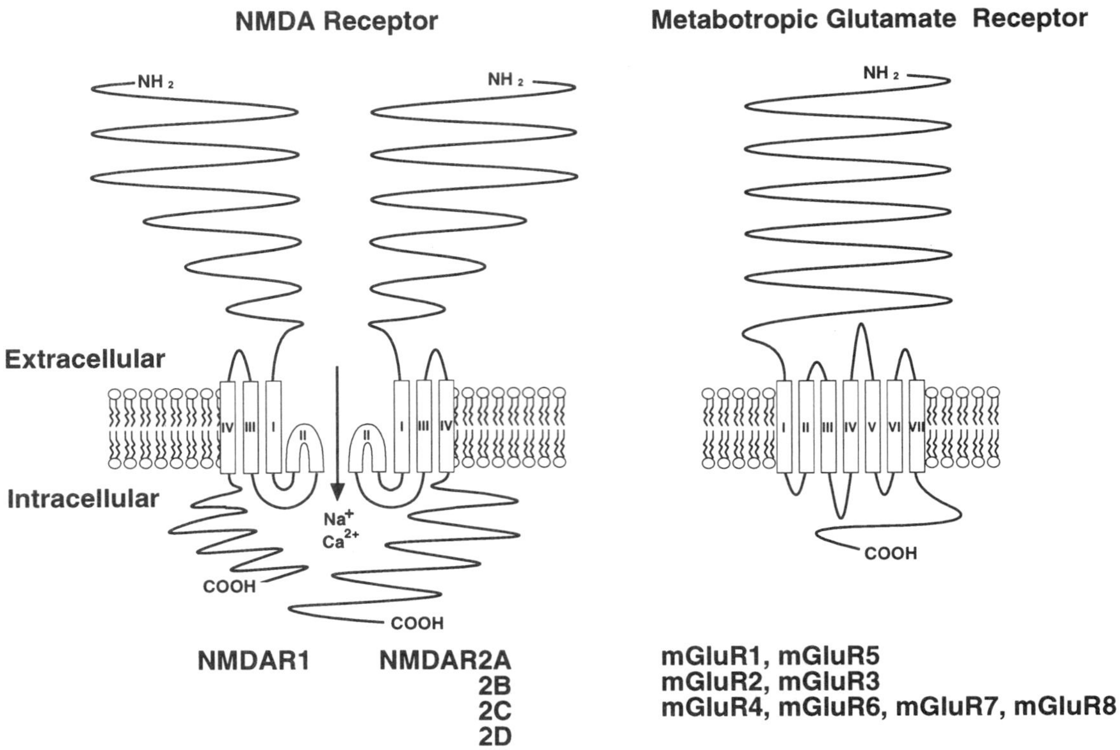

Figure 1. Structural models of NMDA receptors and mGluRs.

is exclusively expressed in the retinal bipolar cell layer and selectively responds to L-AP4 in CHO cells expressing the recombinant mGluR6 (Nakajima et al. 1993). mGluR6 immunoreactivity is restrictedly located at the outer plexiform layer where photoreceptors form synaptic contacts with bipolar cells (Fig. 2A) (Nomura et al. 1994). Furthermore, immunoelectron microscopy disclosed a specific and selective localization of mGluR6 at the postsynaptic site of rod (ON-type) bipolar cells (Nomura et al. 1994). In addition, mGluR6 is localized from the cell body to the postsynaptic site during retinal development, and this change in the mGluR6 subcellular localization agrees well with the synaptic formation between photoreceptors and bipolar cells (Nomura et al. 1994). These observations strongly suggest that mGluR6 functions as an mGluR subtype responsible for ON responses.

Taking advantage of the restricted expression of mGluR6 in retinal ON-bipolar cells, we generated knockout mice lacking mGluR6 expression (Masu et al. 1995). The homozygous mGluR6-deficient mice showed no apparent behavioral abnormality and no gross anatomical changes in the retinal cell organization or in the projection of optic nerve fibers to the brain. When electroretinograms were monitored in mGluR6-deficient mice, the b-wave that represents ON responses never appeared by exposure to any intensities of light (Masu et al. 1995). More direct evidence for the deficit of ON responses in the mGluR6 deficiency was indicated by recording field potentials from the superior colliculus, a major target of the optic nerve fibers. This recording indicated that the mGluR6 deficiency results in a complete loss of ON responses to light stimulus but unchanged OFF responses to dark stimulus (Fig. 2B) (Masu et al. 1995). Thus, mGluR6 is essential for synaptic transmission in the ON pathway.

Despite the lack of light-induced ON responses in mGluR6-deficient mice, they retained the ability to respond to visual inputs as assessed by shuttle box avoidance behavioral analysis in conjunction with light exposure (Masu et al. 1995). Furthermore, the mGluR6-deficient mice were unaltered in a light-dark cycle of daily locomotor activity as well as in light-stimulated induction of Fos immunoreactivity in the suprachiasmatic nuclei (H. Iwakabe et al., in prep.). These results demonstrate that the deficit of ON responses does not completely disrupt responsiveness to visual stimulation and lead to the conclusion that OFF responses also serve as an important signal for transmission of visual information.

We examined possible visual dysfunction that results from the deficit of ON responses (H. Iwakabe et al., in prep.). The pupillary response is controlled by different pretectal neurons that distinctly respond to light and dark stimuli (Clarke and Ikeda 1985). Thus, ON and OFF responses are thought to be critical for the pupillary reflex. Wild-type mice showed light-induced responses of pupillary contraction with an approximately straight-line relationship between the pupil diameter and the logarithmic units of light in-

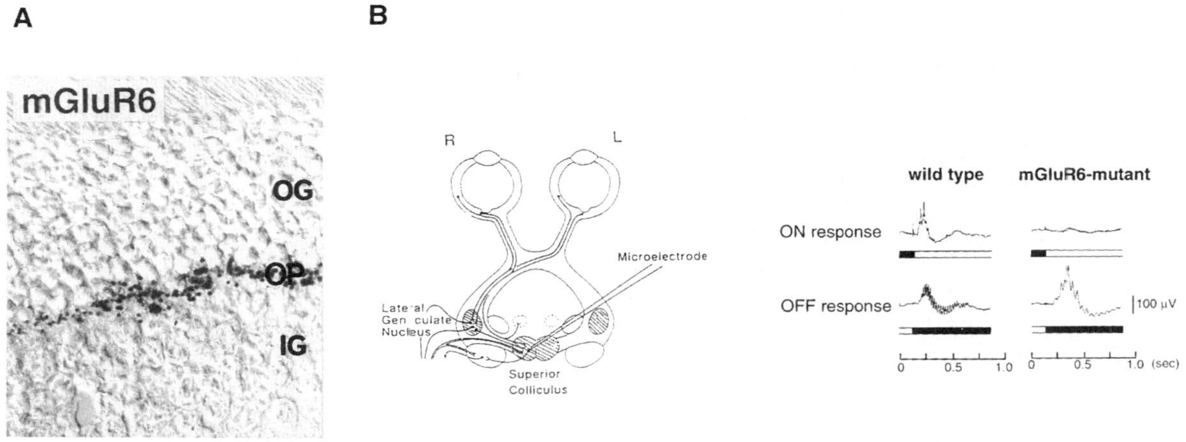

Figure 2. mGluR6 immunostaining in the retina and specific deficit of ON responses in mGluR6-deficient mice. (*A*) Intense punctate mGluR6 immunoreactivity is seen only at the outer plexiform layer (OP) of the wild-type retina (Nomura et al. 1994). (OG) Outer nuclear layer; (IG) inner nuclear layer. (*B*) In mGluR6-deficient mice, ON responses to light stimuli (*open bar*) were abolished without any changes in OFF responses to dark stimuli (*filled bar*) (*right*) when ON and OFF responses were recorded from the superior colliculus (*left*) (Masu et al. 1995).

tensity (H. Iwakabe et al., in prep.). In contrast, mutant mice exhibited little or no pupillary contraction at low luminances, and the pupillary contraction occurred only at high luminance (H. Iwakabe et al., in prep.). The intensity-response relationship in mutant mice was thus shifted toward high luminances by about two logarithmic units. Furthermore, the latency period preceding a pupillary contraction was markedly prolonged in mutant mice (H. Iwakabe et al., in prep.). Thus, the pupils of mutant mice respond to light stimulus, but the sensitivity and rapid responsiveness of light-induced pupillary contraction are markedly impaired in mGluR6-deficient mice. We next examined optokinetic nystagmus (OKN) to address the ability of mutant mice to discriminate visual contrasts (H. Iwakabe et al., in prep.). OKN represents a stereotyped pattern of eye movements that keep a moving subject on the retina. OKN thus provides a useful tool for evaluating the ability of detecting visual contrasts (Fig. 3). Wild-type mice showed robust OKN in response to the rotation of both high-contrast (30:1) and low-contrast (2:1) stripes but did not display OKN

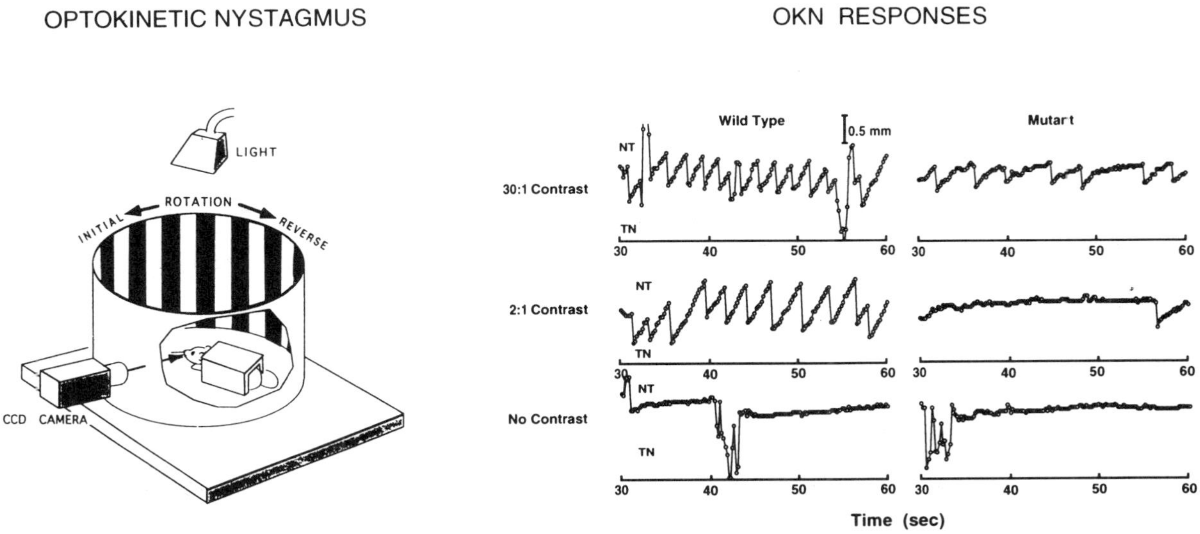

Figure 3. OKN in wild-type and mGluR6-deficient mice. The animal was restrained in the middle of an optokinetic drum with an alternating vertical stripe, and OKN was measured by rotating the optokinetic drum (*left*). mGluR6-deficient mice showed severe impairment in driving OKN in response to a low visual contrast (*right*) (H. Iwakabe et al., in prep.).

in the drum with no contrast. In mutant mice, the high-contrast stimulus did elicit OKN, but with a markedly reduced frequency. Furthermore, OKN was almost abolished in response to the low-contrast stimulus. Thus, the mGluR6 deficiency severely impairs the ability to drive OKN in response to visual contrasts, indicating that mGluR6 is essential for discrimination of visual contrasts (H. Iwakabe et al., in prep.).

On the basis of the characterization of mGluR6 together with the electrophysiological study of ON responses (Nawy and Jahr 1990, 1991; Shiells and Falk 1990), the synaptic mechanism in visual transmission from photoreceptors to ON-bipolar cells can be summarized as follows (Fig. 4) (Nakanishi 1994; Shiells 1994): When photoreceptors respond to light stimulus, cGMP is lowered through the stimulation of phosphodiesterase via transducin (Stryer 1991). This decrease in cGMP hyperpolarizes photoreceptors by closing the cGMP-gated ion channel and reduces glutamate release (Stryer 1991). In the absence of glutamate release, mGluR6 keeps inactive, and a high concentration of cGMP is maintained in ON-bipolar cells and depolarizes these cells by stimulating the cGMP-gated ion channel. Glutamate release from ON-bipolar cells, in turn, increases and excites the subsequent ON pathway.

The key role of mGluR6 in ON-bipolar cells is the conversion of membrane polarization of photoreceptors to an opposite polarization at the postsynaptic bipolar cells. In contrast, OFF-bipolar cells use postsynaptic AMPA receptors and preserve the sign of photoreceptors (de la Villa et al. 1995). Two distinct types of glutamate receptors are thus effectively utilized for evoking ON and OFF responses to the common glutamate transmitter (Fig. 4). Our investigation has provided the compelling evidence that a specific mGluR subtype plays an essential role in synaptic transmission. It is also noted that two G protein-coupled receptors, rhodopsin and mGluR6, are involved in an initial step of visual transmission and are capable of amplifying visual inputs via a second-messenger system (Fig. 4). The peripheral sensory organs receive graded external signals, and these graded signals must be converted to action potentials at an early step of information processing. Thus, the involvement of mGluR6 in visual transmission is important for discrimination and amplification of external signals prior to transmission of these signals to higher centers of the brain.

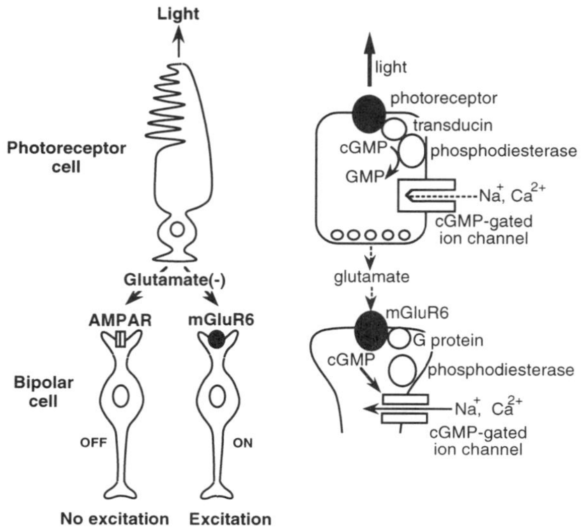

Figure 4. Model for the synaptic mechanism underlying the ON and OFF segregation and for the function of mGluR6 in the ON pathway. (AMPAR) AMPA receptor.

mGluR2 in Olfactory Memory Formation

Most mammalian species possess two olfactory systems, the main olfactory bulb and accessory olfactory bulb (AOB). In both systems, olfactory receptor neurons project axons to glomeruli where they make synaptic contacts with mitral cells (Shepherd and Koch 1990). Granule cells are inhibitory interneurons that form typical dendrodendritic synapses with mitral cells, and these synapses undergo reciprocal regulation (Brennan et al. 1990; Shepherd and Koch 1990); the mitral cell, when activated by olfactory receptor neurons, excites the granule cell via glutamate, and this depolarization in turn releases γ-aminobutyrate (GABA) from the granule cell and hyperpolarizes mitral cells (Fig. 5). The granule cell lacks an axon and forms divergent dendrodendritic synapses not only with an excited mitral cell, but also with a large number of unexcited neighboring mitral cells and is thought to cause both recurrent and lateral inhibition via inhibitory GABA transmission (Shepherd and Koch 1990).

In situ hybridization and immuno-electron-microscopic analysis indicated that mGluR2 is highly expressed and localized at the dendrites of granule cells in the AOB (Hayashi et al. 1993). In contrast, mGluR3 is not appreciably expressed in granule cells. Since DCG-IV was identified as a potent and selective agonist for mGluR2/mGluR3 (Hayashi et al. 1993), we investigated the role of mGluR2 in olfactory transmission by examining the effect of the DCG-IV-induced activation of mGluR2 on GABA transmission from the granule cell to the mitral cell (Fig. 5A) (Hayashi et al. 1993). Whole-cell recording of a mitral cell was performed by the slice patch-clamp recording method. When a granule cell was electrically stimulated, GABA-mediated IPSCs were evoked in a mitral cell. When mGluR2 was activated by the addition of DCG-IV in this system, the GABA-mediated IPSCs were markedly reduced in a reversible manner (Fig. 5A). This observation, as well as others, indicated that glutamate released from an excited mitral cell activates mGluR2 of the granule cell and relieves the mitral cell from the GABA-mediated inhibition (Hayashi et al.

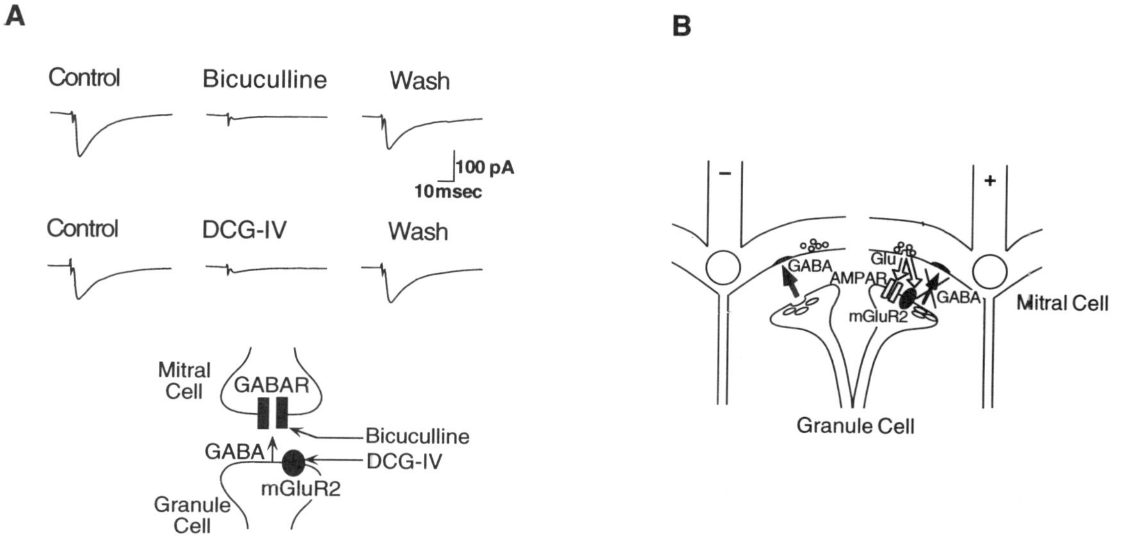

Figure 5. Suppression of GABA-mediated IPSCs by DCG-IV and a model for olfactory discrimination by mGluR2 activation. (*A*) GABA-mediated IPSCs that were blocked by the $GABA_A$ receptor antagonist bicuculline were markedly reduced by DCG-IV in a reversible manner (Hayashi et al. 1993). (GABAR) $GABA_A$ receptor. (*B*) Dendrodendritic synapses between a granule cell and mitral cells are thought to cause both recurrent inhibition and lateral inhibition. This model holds that the mGluR2 activation relieves recurrent inhibition by suppressing GABA release but keeps lateral inhibition. (AMPAR) AMPA receptor; (Glu) glutamate.

1993; Nakanishi 1995). Because this modulatory effect of mGluR2 is thought to be confined to the synapses of excited mitral cells, this modulation would relieve recurrent inhibition of excited mitral cells but keep lateral inhibition of unexcited neighboring mitral cells (Fig. 5B). The mechanism discussed here evidently enhances the signal-to-noise ratio between excited and unexcited mitral cells and would contribute to discrimination of olfactory transmission (Fig. 5). The synaptic circuitry of the second-order neurons is thus crucial for resolving and discriminating external sensory stimuli. Furthermore, AMPA receptors are used for exciting granule cells, whereas mGluR2 functions to relieve excited mitral cells from recurrent inhibition. Thus, the existence of two different types of glutamate receptors is again crucial for sensory information processing in the olfactory system.

The reciprocal dendrodendritic synapses in the AOB are known to have the capacity for the neural plasticity that is involved in the formation of olfactory memory (Brennan et al. 1990; Kaba and Nakanishi 1995). It is thus possible that the persistent activation of mGluR2 by glutamate results in prolonged excitation of olfactory transmission that may enhance synaptic efficacy responsible for memory formation. Female mice form an olfactory memory at mating, thus maintaining pregnancy during exposure to familiar pheromones of the stud male but evoking pregnancy block after exposure to unfamiliar male pheromones of a different strain (Brennan et al. 1990). This olfactory block of pregnancy, known as the Bruce effect, is caused by sustained norepinephrine in the AOB (Fig. 6A) (Brennan et al. 1990). Norepinephrine is enhanced in the AOB after mating and persistently excites mitral cells by reducing GABA transmission from granule cells, thus forming olfactory memory specific to pheromones exposed after mating. The activation of mGluR2 similarly reduces inhibitory GABA transmission and may create olfactory memory formation.

To investigate a possible role of mGluR2 in olfactory memory formation, we carried out the following animal behavioral analysis (Fig. 6B) (Kaba et al. 1994). mGluR2 agonists were infused into the AOB of females during exposure to male pheromones without mating. The females were then mated with a different strain and reexposed to test pheromones of the original strain. Under this protocol, the memory formation by drug infusions can be evaluated by measuring the protection of pregnancy block induced by the test pheromonal exposure. Infusion of DCG-IV, but not phosphate buffer alone, into the AOB during exposure to male pheromones reduced pregnancy block significantly. This formation of memory required the concomitant action of DCG-IV and of pheromonal exposure. More importantly, this memory was specific to the pheromones to which the females were exposed during infusion of DCG-IV. Furthermore, the α-adrenergic receptor antagonist phentolamine had no effect on the DCG-IV-mediated formation of memory, indicating the direct action of DCG-IV on mGluR2 rather than the enhancement of actions of norepinephrine. This study demonstrates that a specific mGluR subtype plays an important role in neural plasticity responsible for recognition memory formation (Kaba et al. 1994). The olfactory bulb is relatively simple in structural organization and synaptic opera-

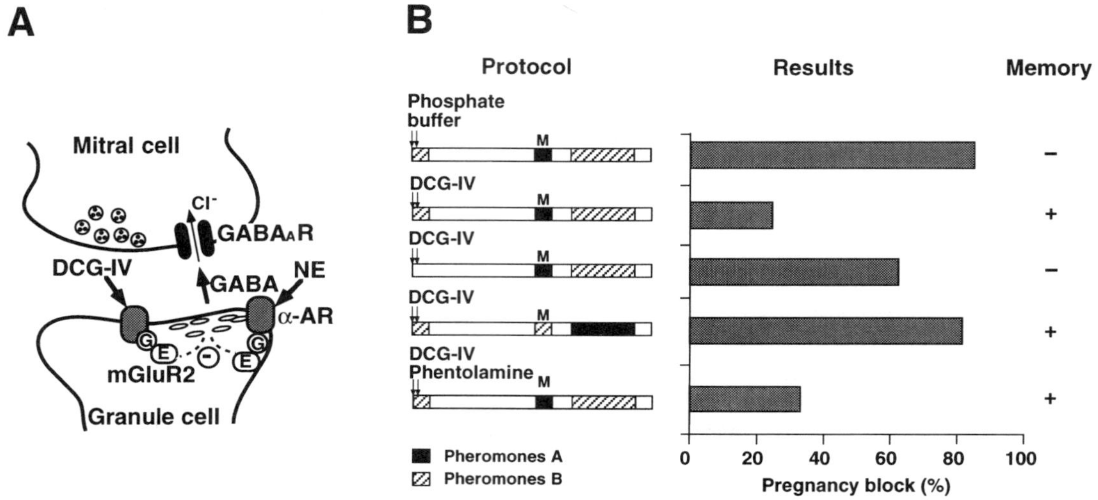

Figure 6. Microcircuitry in dendrodendritic synapses between a mitral cell and a granule cell in the AOB and olfactory memory formation by activation of mGluR2. (*A*) Inhibitory actions of both DCG-IV and norepinephrine (NE) on GABA release are indicated by a minus symbol; ($GABA_AR$) $GABA_A$ receptor; (α-AR) α-adrenergic receptor; (G) G protein; (E) intracellular effector. (*B*) In the protocol of behavioral analysis, shaded and filled boxes indicate exposures to pheromones of two different strains. Arrows show drug injections. (M) Mating. Data are taken from Kaba et al. (1994) and modified.

tion. This system should provide a useful behavioral paradigm for study of the mechanism underlying memory formation.

mGluR2 in Hippocampal Synaptic Plasticity

LTP and LTD at the CA1 region of the hippocampus are mediated by the activation of NMDA receptors at the postsynaptic cell (Bliss and Collingridge 1993; Nicoll and Malenka 1995). It is generally believed that these modifications in synaptic efficacy are of fundamental importance for memory acquisition and learning (Bliss and Collingridge 1993; Nicoll and Malenka 1995). In contrast, both LTP and LTD in hippocampal mossy fiber-CA3 synapses result entirely from changes in the presynaptic cell and are independent of NMDA receptor activation (Zalutsky and Nicoll 1990; Nicoll and Malenka 1995; Kobayashi et al. 1996). In situ hybridization study and immunostaining in combination with lesion analysis indicated that mGluR2 is predominantly expressed in granule cells of the hippocampal dentate gyrus and is distributed to mossy fibers (Shigemoto et al. 1995). Furthermore, immuno-electron microscopy revealed a unique localization of mGluR2 at the preterminal zone rather than the synaptic junction of mossy fibers (Fig. 7A) (Yokoi et al. 1996). To investigate the role of the presynaptic mGluR2 in synaptic transmission and plasticity in the mossy fiber-CA3 synapses, we generated mutant mice lacking mGluR2 (Yokoi et al. 1996).

The mGluR2-deficient mice grew normally and showed no behavioral abnormality, nor any gross anatomical changes in the brain. Neither field excitatory postsynaptic potentials (EPSPs) evoked by stimulation of mossy fibers nor paired-pulse facilitation at the mossy fiber-CA3 synapses was distinguishable between the wild-type and mutant mice (Yokoi et al. 1996). The mGluR2/mGluR3-selective agonist, DCG-IV, markedly and reversibly depressed EPSPs at the mossy fiber-CA3 synapses in wild-type mice, but this depression was greatly reduced in mutant mice (Yokoi et al. 1996). The presynaptic mGluR2 thus plays an important role in presynaptic inhibition. We investigated effects of mGluR2 deficiency on LTP and LTD at the mossy fiber-CA3 synapses. mGluR2-deficient mice showed normal LTP after tetanic stimulation (Yokoi et al. 1996). In contrast, LTD induced by low-frequency stimulation was significantly impaired in mutant mice (Fig. 7B) (Yokoi et al. 1996). In wild-type mice, EPSPs were facilitated during low-frequency stimulation and then decreased below control levels after low-frequency stimulation. This depression lasted for at least 45 minutes. In mutant mice, the facilitation of EPSPs and the subsequent short-term depression were unchanged. However, this depression was transient, and EPSPs returned gradually to control levels. Therefore, the presynaptic mGluR2 is not required for mossy fiber LTP but is essential for mossy fiber LTD.

We tested for the involvement of mossy fiber LTD in spatial learning by performing the Morris water-maze tasks. The wild-type and mutant mice showed no differences in their ability to perform either the visible- or hidden-platform tasks (Yokoi et al. 1996). In a transfer test, the wild-type and mutant mice exhibited no difference in either the time spent or the number of crossings in the trained quadrant. To evaluate spatial learning flexibility, we examined the ability of trained mice to adapt to a new platform location (Yokoi et al. 1996). The wild-type and mutant mice capably adapted to a new platform location with no significant dif-

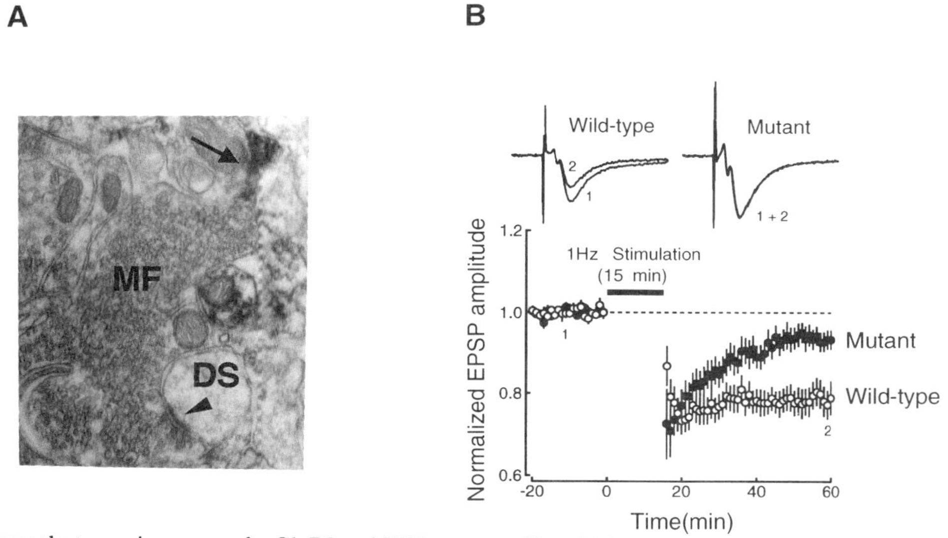

Figure 7. Immunoelectron microscopy of mGluR2 and LTD at mossy fiber-CA3 synapses. (*A*) mGluR2 immunostaining (*arrow*) is seen at the preterminal zone of a mossy fiber terminal (MF). (DS) A dendritic spine; (*arrowhead*) an active zone. (*B*) LTD recorded after low-frequency stimulation was impaired in mGluR2-deficient mice (Yokoi et al. 1996).

ference. These observations demonstrate that impairment of the CA3 LTD does not hinder spatial learning.

Recent evidence has shown that enhancement of calcium entry into the presynaptic terminal of the mossy fiber by tetanic stimulation activates Ca^{++}/calmodulin-sensitive adenylate cyclase 1, and this activation would in turn produce LTP through protein kinase A (Fig. 8) (Huang et al. 1994; Weisskopf et al. 1994; Nicoll and Malenka 1995). mGluR2 is coupled to inhibition of the cAMP cascade (Tanabe et al. 1992). Thus, taken together with the mechanism proposed for LTP induction (Huang et al. 1994; Nicoll and Malenka 1995), a model for induction of LTP and LTD at the mossy fiber-CA3 synapses is illustrated in Figure 8. At the mossy fiber-CA3 synapses, slowly accumulating glutamate during low-frequency stimulation activates the presynaptic mGluR2, and this activation of mGluR2 would inhibit the cAMP cascade and result in induction of LTD. It is thus conceivable that LTP and LTD can occur by up- and down-regulation of the cAMP cascade at the presynaptic site of the mossy fiber-CA3 synapses. Interestingly, the elimination of mossy fiber LTP by gene targeting of protein kinase A has been shown to have no effect on spatial learning (Huang et al. 1995). Thus, contrary to current theories about hippocampal function, neither LTP nor LTD at the mossy fiber-CA3 synapses appears to be required for spatial learning, although they may have a variety of other physiological roles. LTD, for example, may involve a dynamic modulation of information processing; an increase in the flexibility of circuit formation; protection of postsynaptic cells from overexcitation; or cancellation of acquired memory. Thus, the mGluR2-deficient mouse should serve as an interesting model to study the LTD-relevant brain function.

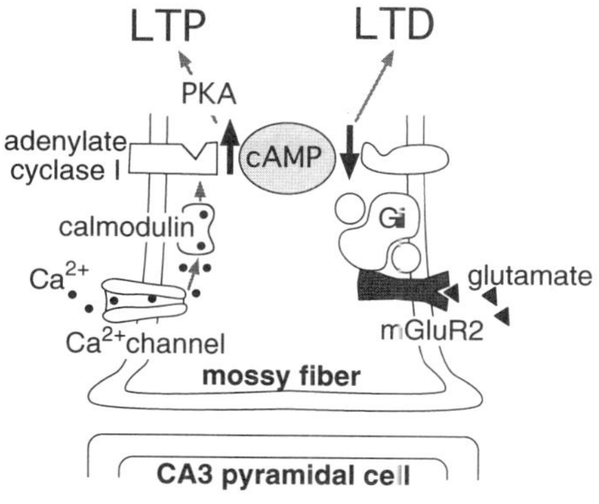

Figure 8. Model for induction of LTP and LTD at the mossy fiber-CA3 synapses.

CONCLUSION

Ionotropic glutamate receptors exert the rapid neuronal excitation characteristic of glutamate transmission. The mGluRs, on the other hand, mediate relatively slow responses by coupling to intracellular signal transduction, and less attention has been paid to the functions of mGluRs. However, glutamate is a common transmitter that acts on both the ionotropic receptors and mGluRs with similar efficacy. Furthermore, G-protein-coupled receptors have the potential to modulate a variety of intracellular signal transduction events. The mGluRs have thus been expected to share important roles in glutamate transmission with the ionotropic receptors. The different subtypes of the mGluR family play critical roles in synaptic transmission, modulation, and plasticity. The ionotropic receptors also consist of diverse members of subunits that form different heteromeric receptors. Further studies of both individual subtypes of the mGluR family and different heteromeric assemblies of the ionotropic receptors will be important for an understanding of implications of glutamate transmission in brain function.

ACKNOWLEDGMENTS

We thank our collaborators, Drs. R. Shigemoto, H. Ohishi, S. Nomura, N. Mizuno, Y. Nakamura, T. Miyoshi, M. Yamashita, Y. Fukuda, H. Sasaki, K. Hiroi, K. Nakamura, K. Nakao, M. Katsuki, H. Kaba, T. Higuchi, K. Kobayashi, T. Manabe, T. Takahashi, I. Sakaguchi, and G. Katsuura, for their invaluable contributions. This work was partly supported by the Ministry of Education, Science and Culture of Japan, the Ministry of Health and Welfare of Japan, the Uehara Memorial Foundation, and the Sankyo Foundation of Life Science.

REFERENCES

Bliss, T.V.P. and G.L. Collingridge. 1993. A synaptic model of memory: Long-term potentiation in the hippocampus. *Nature* **361:** 31.

Brennan, P., H. Kaba, and E.B. Keverne. 1990. Olfactory recognition: A simple memory system. *Science* **250:** 1223.

Clarke, R.J. and H. Ikeda. 1985. Luminance and darkness detectors in the olivary and posterior pretectal nuclei and their relationship to the pupillary light reflex in the rat. I. Studies with steady luminance levels. *Exp. Brain Res.* **57:** 224.

de la Villa, P., T. Kurahashi, and A. Kaneko. 1995. L-Glutamate-induced responses and cGMP-activated channels in three subtypes of retinal bipolar cells dissociated from the cat. *J. Neurosci.* **15:** 3571.

DeVries, S.H. and D.A. Baylor. 1993. Synaptic circuitry of the retina and olfactory bulb. *Neuron (suppl.)* **10:** 139.

Dowling, J.E. 1987. *The retina: An approachable part of the brain.* The Belknap Press of Harvard University Press, Cambridge, Massachusetts.

Hayashi, Y., A. Momiyama, T. Takahashi, H. Ohishi, R. Ogawa-Meguro, R. Shigemoto, N. Mizuno, and S. Nakanishi. 1993. Role of a metabotropic glutamate receptor in synaptic modulation in the accessory olfactory bulb. *Nature* **366:** 687.

Hollmann, M. and S. Heinemann. 1994. Cloned glutamate receptors. *Annu. Rev. Neurosci.* **17:** 31.

Huang, Y-Y., X-C. Li, and E.R. Kandel. 1994. cAMP contributes to mossy fiber LTP by initiating both a covalently mediated early phase and macromolecular synthesis-dependent late phase. *Cell* **79:** 69.

Huang, Y.-Y., E.R. Kandel, L.Varshavsky, E.P. Brandon, M. Qi, R.L. Idzerda, G.S. McKnight, and R. Bourtchouladze. 1995. A genetic test of the effects of mutations in PKA on mossy fiber LTP and its relation to spatial and contextual learning. *Cell* **83:** 1211.

Kaba, H. and S. Nakanishi. 1995. Synaptic mechanisms of olfactory recognition memory. *Rev. Neurosci.* **6:** 125.

Kaba, H., Y. Hayashi, T. Higuchi, and S. Nakanishi. 1994. Induction of an olfactory memory by the activation of a metabotropic glutamate receptor. *Science* **265:** 262.

Kobayashi, K., T. Manabe, and T. Takahashi. 1996. Presynaptic long-term depression at the hippocampal mossy fiber-CA3 synapse. *Science* (in press).

Masu, M., Y. Tanabe, K. Tsuchida, R. Shigemoto, and S. Nakanishi. 1991. Sequence and expression of a metabotropic glutamate receptor. *Nature* **349:** 760.

Masu, M., H. Iwakabe, Y. Tagawa, T. Miyoshi, M. Yamashita, Y. Fukuda, H. Sasaki, K. Hiroi, Y. Nakamura, R. Shigemoto, M. Takada, K. Nakamura, K. Nakao, M. Katsuki, and S. Nakanishi. 1995. Specific deficit of the ON response in visual transmission by targeted disruption of the mGluR6 gene. *Cell* **80:** 757.

Moriyoshi, K., M. Masu, T. Ishii, R. Shigemoto, N. Mizuno, and S. Nakanishi. 1991. Molecular cloning and characterization of the rat NMDA receptor. *Nature* **354:** 31.

Nakajima, Y., H. Iwakabe, C. Akazawa, H. Nawa, R. Shigemoto, N. Mizuno, and S. Nakanishi. 1993. Molecular characterization of a novel retinal metabotropic glutamate receptor mGluR6 with a high agonist selectivity for L-2-amino-4-phosphonobutyrate. *J. Biol. Chem.* **268:** 11868.

Nakanishi, S. 1992. Molecular diversity of glutamate receptors and implications for brain function. *Science* **258:** 597.

———. 1994. Metabotropic glutamate receptors: Synaptic transmission, modulation, and plasticity. *Neuron* **13:** 1031.

———. 1995. Second-order neurones and receptor mechanisms in visual- and olfactory-information processing. *Trends Neurosci.* **18:** 359.

Nakanishi, S. and M. Masu. 1994. Molecular diversity and functions of glutamate receptors. *Annu. Rev. Biophys. Biomol. Struct.* **23:** 319.

Nawy, S. and C.E. Jahr. 1990. Suppression by glutamate of cGMP-activated conductance in retinal bipolar cells. *Nature* **346:** 269.

———. 1991. cGMP-gated conductance in retinal bipolar cells is suppressed by the photoreceptor transmitter. *Neuron* **7:** 677.

Nicoll, R.A. and R.C. Malenka. 1995. Contrasting properties of two forms of long-term potentiation in the hippocampus. *Nature* **377:** 115.

Nomura, A., R. Shigemoto, Y. Nakamura, N. Okamoto, N. Mizuno, and S. Nakanishi. 1994. Developmentally regulated postsynaptic localization of a metabotropic glutamate receptor in rat rod bipolar cells. *Cell* **77:** 361.

Pin, J.P. and R. Duvoisin. 1995. The metabotropic glutamate receptors: Structure and functions. *Neuropharmacology* **34:** 1.

Schiller, P.H. 1992. The ON and OFF channels of the visual system. *Trends Neurosci.* **15:** 86.

Shepherd, G.M. and C. Koch. 1990. Introduction to synaptic circuits. In *The synaptic organization of the brain*, 3rd edition (ed. G.M. Shepherd), p. 3. Oxford University Press, New York.

Shiells, R. 1994. Glutamate receptors for signal amplification. *Curr. Biol.* **4:** 917.

Shiells, R.A. and G. Falk. 1990. Glutamate receptors of rod bipolar cells are linked to a cyclic GMP cascade via a G-protein. *Proc. R. Soc. Lond. B Biol. Sci.* **242:** 91.

Shigemoto, R., E. Wada, S. Nomura, H. Ohishi, M. Takada, S. Nakanishi, and N. Mizuno. 1995. Differential presynaptic and postsynaptic localization of metabotropic glutamate receptor subtypes in rat hippocampus. *IBRO Abstr.* **4:** A3.41.

Stryer, L. 1991. Visual excitation and recovery. *J. Biol. Chem.* **266:** 10711.

Tanabe, Y., M. Masu, T. Ishii, R. Shigemoto, and S. Nakanishi. 1992. A family of metabotropic glutamate receptors. *Neuron* **8:** 169.

Wässle, H., M. Yamashita, U. Greferath, U. Grünert, and F. Müller. 1991. The rod bipolar cell of the mammalian retina. *Visual Neurosci.* **7:** 99.

Weisskopf, M.G., P.E. Castillo, R.A. Zalutsky, and R.A. Nicoll. 1994. Mediation of hippocampal mossy fiber long-term potentiation by cyclic AMP. *Science* **265:** 1878.

Yokoi, M., K. Kobayashi, T. Manabe, T. Takahashi, I. Sakaguchi, G. Katsuura, R. Shigemoto, H. Ohishi, S. Nomura, K. Nakamura, K. Nakao, M. Katsuki, and S. Nakanishi. 1996. Impairment of hippocampal mossy fiber LTD in mice lacking mgluR2. *Science* (in press).

Zalutsky, R.A. and R.A. Nicoll. 1990. Comparison of two forms of long-term potentiation in single hippocampal neurons. *Science* **248:** 1619.

Combination of Gene Targeting and Gene Transfer by Adenoviral Vectors in the Analysis of Neurotrophin-mediated Neuronal Plasticity

O. GRIESBECK,[1] M. KORTE,[2] V. STAIGER,[2] C. GRAVEL,[3] P. CARROLL,[1]
T. BONHOEFFER,[2] AND H. THOENEN[1]

[1]*Department of Neurochemistry and* [2]*Department of Neurophysiology, Max-Planck-Institute for Psychiatry, Martinsried, Germany, 82152;* [3]*Laboratoire de transfert de gènes, Centre de recherche Université Laval Robert-Giffard, Local F-7500, Québec G1J 2G3, Canada*

There is increasing evidence that neurotrophins play an essential role in activity-dependent neuronal plasticity (for review, see Lo 1995; Thoenen 1995; Bonhoeffer 1996). This evidence evolved from the observation that nerve growth factor (NGF), brain-derived neurotrophic factor (BDNF), and neurotrophin (NT)-4/5 dramatically interfere with the well-characterized development of activity-dependent ocular dominance in rats and cats (Maffei et al. 1992; Carmignoto et al. 1993; Cabelli et al. 1995; Fiorentini et al. 1995; Riddle et al. 1995; Galuske et al. 1996). The fact that this interference results not only from the local administration of neurotrophins, but also from blocking anti-NGF antibodies (Berardi et al. 1994; Domenici et al. 1994) and trkB-IgGs (R.J. Cabelli and C.J. Shatz, pers. comm.), which have the same effect as blocking anti-BDNF or anti-NT-4/5 antibodies, suggests that the observed effects are indeed of physiological relevance rather than representing mere pharmacological actions. Although the activity-dependent neuronal plasticity of the visual cortex is well-characterized and can be manipulated experimentally in a very precise manner (see Goodman and Shatz 1993), this system does not lend itself favorably to a direct cellular and molecular analysis (Thoenen 1995). All the neurotrophins, in particular NGF, BDNF, and NT-4/5, are present in the visual cortex at very low levels and, despite great effort, no sufficiently precise information is available to clearly decide which neurons produce the individual neurotrophins, which neurons express the corresponding receptors, where these trk receptors are located (i.e., on soma and/or dendrites), and how these neurons interact with each other (see Thoenen 1995 and references therein). However, complementary information from various in vitro and in vivo systems has recently become available that supports a function of neurotrophins in modifying very specific synapses in an activity-dependent manner. This invited the analysis in a structurally and functionally (relatively) simple system that can easily be manipulated experimentally, namely, the CA3/CA1 system in hippocampal slices. In this paper, we briefly summarize the evidence from different systems supporting the concept of the involvement of neurotrophins in activity-dependent neuronal plasticity and then discuss in more detail the approaches we used to demonstrate that BDNF is involved in the establishment of long-term potentiation (LTP) in the CA3/CA1 hippocampal system, using gene targeting procedures and localized gene transfer by adenoviral vectors.

OBSERVATIONS SUPPORTING THE FUNCTION OF NEUROTROPHINS IN NEURONAL PLASTICITY

Activity-dependent Regulation of Neurotrophin Synthesis

BDNF and NGF synthesis is regulated in a very precise and rapid manner by neuronal activity: Up-regulation by glutamate via *N*-methyl-D-aspartate (NMDA) and non-NMDA receptors and by acetylcholine via muscarinic receptors; and down-regulation, at least in adult animals, by GABA via $GABA_A$ receptors (for review, see Lindholm et al. 1994). This regulation occurs not only in response to very strong artificial stimuli, such as kainic acid administration or kindling procedures, it also becomes apparent when subtle physiological stimuli, such as visual input and osmotic stress (Castrén et al. 1992, 1995) are used. The pattern of regulation shows very characteristic regional differences, such as the differential regulation in the different layers of the visual cortex (Castrén et al. 1992; Bozzi et al. 1995).

Characteristics of Neurotrophin Secretion from Neurons

Both NGF (Blöchl and Thoenen 1995, 1996) and (in preliminary experiments) BDNF (Griesbeck et al. 1995) have been demonstrated to be secreted from hippocampal slices and primary cultures of hippocampal neurons, according to the constitutive and activity-dependent pathway. The activity-dependent secretion shows unconventional features. It depends on extracellular sodium, is independent of extracellular calcium, but depends on intact intracellular calcium stores. Thus, for activity-dependent neurotrophin secretion, the release of calcium from intracellular stores at very specific strategic sites in consequence of sodium influx seems to be required. Moreover, the storage compartments of neurotrophins show the characteristics of an endoplasmic reticulum-like, membrane-confined compartment being located not only in the perikaryon, but also in all neuronal processes of hippocampal neurons (Blöchl and Thoenen 1996). Analyses by confocal microscopy demonstrated a high degree of NGF colocalization with Golgi markers and inositol triphosphate receptors. The latter represent a marker for neuronal endoplasmic reticulum. Interestingly, the activity-mediated release initiated by high potassium, glutamate, or carbachol resulted in the release of neurotrophins from both soma and neurites of cultivated hippocampal neurons, in particular, dendrites (Blöchl and Thoenen 1996). The constitutive, temperature-sensitive (blockade at 15°C) release was largely confined to the cell body and proximal parts of primary dendrites.

Neurotrophins Enhance the Release of Classic Neurotransmitters from Neurons Expressing the Corresponding trk Receptors

In a great variety of systems, including frog neuromuscular junction (Lohof et al. 1993), synaptosomal preparations (Knipper et al. 1994a,b), hippocampal slices (Kang and Schuman 1995), and primary cultures of hippocampal neurons (Lessmann et al. 1994), it has been demonstrated that neurotrophins enhance the release of classic transmitter substances, such as glutamate and acetylcholine, provided they express the trk receptors corresponding to the added neurotrophin. This neurotrophin-mediated transmitter release can be blocked by K252a, a protein kinase inhibitor with relative preference for trk tyrosine kinases (Knüsel and Hefti 1992), the main signal-transducing units of neurotrophin receptors. The neurotrophin-mediated transmitter release is also reflected by instantaneous calcium transients in individual neurons (Berninger et al. 1993), but also in neuronal circuits, exhibiting spontaneous rhythmic activity that is enhanced by the administration of neurotrophins (see Thoenen 1995). Moreover, the local intracerebral injection of neurotrophins initiates characteristic patterns of electrical activity that reflect the transmitter release from specific populations of neurons expressing the corresponding trk receptors. The local injection of BDNF into the hilus of the dentate gyrus in the hippocampus in vivo initiates predominantly glutamatergic effects, whereas NGF initiates predominantly cholinergic effects. They can be blocked by corresponding glutamate or muscarinic receptor antagonists, demonstrating that the observed electrical activity initiated by the local injection of neurotrophins results from the release of classic neurotransmitters (Berzaghi et al. 1995).

CHARACTERIZATION OF A HYPOTHETICAL FUNCTION OF NEUROTROPHINS IN ACTIVITY-MEDIATED NEURONAL PLASTICITY

The integration of all the available information originating from different experimental systems supports the interpretation that, indeed, neurotrophins may play an essential role in neuronal plasticity. In particular, they may stabilize specific synapses in an activity-dependent manner. The highly selective, regionally differential expression of neurotrophins and the corresponding receptors (for review, see Bothwell 1995; Lewin and Barde 1996) precludes a general function as an activity-dependent retrograde messenger, as has been postulated for arachidonic acid, NO, and CO (Williams et al. 1989; Zhuo et al. 1993; Schuman and Madison 1994a,b). The modulatory role of neurotrophins in the function of neuronal circuits would come into play when neurotrophins are released from dendrites in an activity-dependent manner and the presynaptic nerve terminals express the appropriate trk receptors. In this way, neurotrophins might act as selective retrograde messengers, resulting not only in trk receptor-mediated rearrangement of the presynaptic cytoskeleton, but also in an enhancement of transmitter release from these nerve terminals. We have chosen the CA3/CA1 hippocampal system for corresponding functional analyses. Both BDNF and trk-B receptors are widely expressed in this system and, consequently, it is conceivable that BDNF acts as a selective retrograde messenger on presynaptic nerve terminals or in an autocrine manner on postsynaptic sites in the context of LTP modulation.

INACTIVATION OF THE BDNF GENE RESULTS IN A MARKED IMPAIRMENT OF LTP IN ACUTE HIPPOCAMPAL SLICES

In contrast to the peripheral nervous system, there are no gross defects in the CNS of BDNF knockout mice (see Snider 1994; Bothwell 1995; Lewin and Barde 1996). In particular, no reduction of specific populations of neurons in the hippocampus is detectable, and there are no morphological changes at the light microscopic level in the CA3/CA1 region (Korte et al. 1995). In particular, there is no change in number and structure of dendrites and their spines in pyramidal neurons as far as can be judged from Golgi preparations (Fig. 1). The extracellular field potentials from CA1 pyramidal neurons, resulting from the stimulation of the Schaffer collaterals, showed normal characteristics. No changes in paired-pulse facilitation (PPF) and in the pharmacological characteristics of the responses of the different glutamate receptors and their antagonists became apparent in response to the stimulation of the Schaffer collaterals (Korte et al. 1995). However,

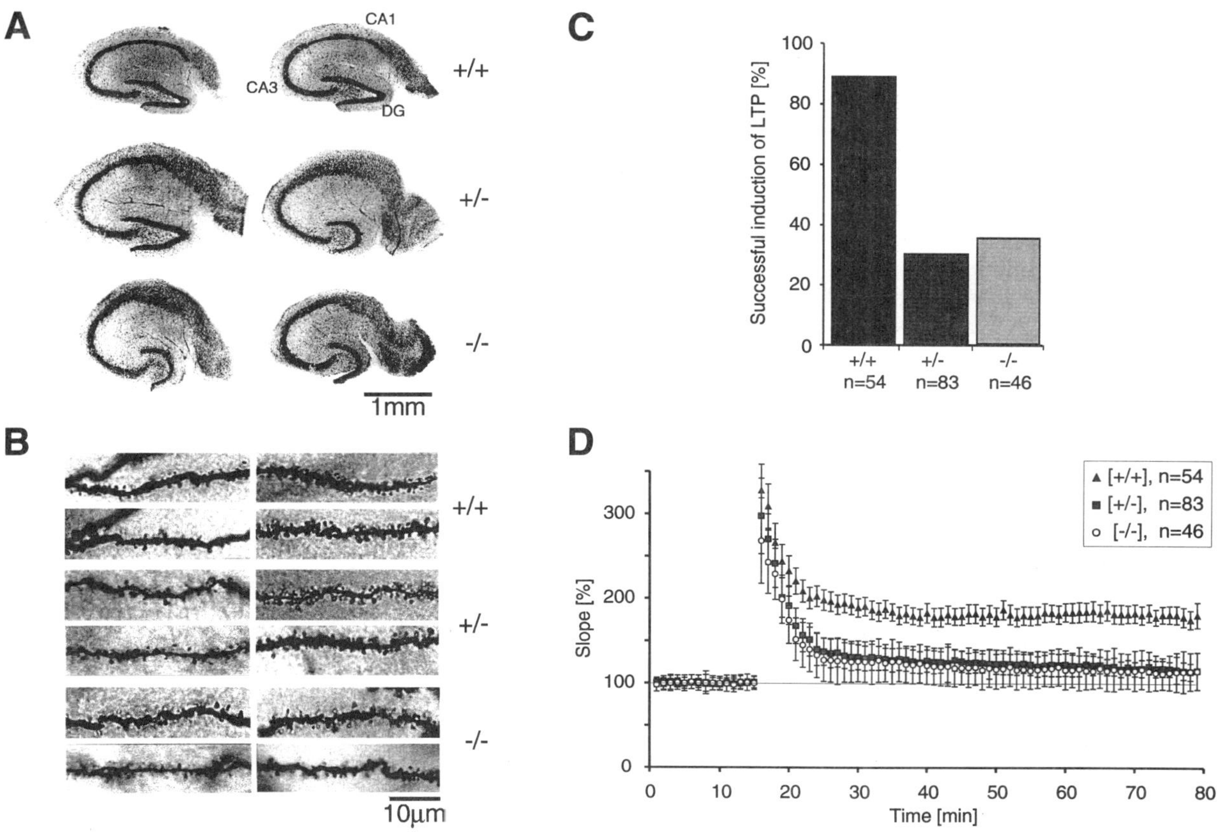

Figure 1. Effect of BDNF gene targeting on morphology and function of hippocampal neurons as evaluated in acute hippocampal slices in the CA3/CA1 system. (*A*) Nissl-stained hippocampal slices of BDNF +/+, +/–, and –/– mice. There is no difference detectable in the overall structure between slices originating from controls (+/+), heterozygote (+/–), and homozygote (–/–) gene-targeted animals. (*B*) Dendritic segments from Golgi-stained CA1 pyramidal neurons in the hippocampus for all genotypes. Although considerable differences in spine densities were observed within the different genotypes (*left* column: low densities; *right* column: high densities), no significant differences in spine density could be observed between the different genotypes ($p>0.05$, t-test, two-tailed). Nissl and Golgi staining were performed according to standard procedures (see Korte et al. 1995). (*C*) Percentage of successful LTP induction for +/+, +/–, and –/– mice older than P16. LTP was judged to be successful if 60 min after the tetanus (3 times 30 pulses at 100 Hz) the slope of the field EPSP was larger than 120% of the baseline value. Hippocampal transverse slices (400 μM thick) were prepared and maintained using standard procedures. (Medium: 124 mM NaCl, 3 mM KCl, 1.25 mM KH_2PO_4, 2 mM Mg_2SO_4, 26 mM $NaHCO_3$, 2.5 mM $CaCl_2$, 10 mM glucose.) Temperature 32 ± 0.2°C; submerged recording. (*D*) Ensemble average for all experiments in +/+, +/–, and –/– mice. The data are presented as mean ± S.E.M.; *n* = number of slices. The abscissa shows the increase of the field EPSP initial slope (in percent). The ordinate displays time. At 15 min, 3 x 30 pulses (100 Hz) were used to induce LTP. (Data from Korte et al. 1995.)

there was a drastic impairment of LTP both in BDNF –/– and BDNF +/– animals. There was not only a marked reduction of the successful initiation of LTP from 90% in wild type to 30% in both –/– and +/– animals, but also a marked reduction in the magnitude of LTP (Fig. 1). The fact that both the degree of potentiation and the characteristics of LTP were virtually the same in both –/– and +/– animals indicates that for the formation of LTP, the presence of BDNF is not an all-or-none phenomenon, but it seems that, in most cases, a threshold level of BDNF is necessary for the formation and maintenance of a fully developed LTP (Fig.1).

GENE TRANSFER INTO PRIMARY CULTURES OF HIPPOCAMPAL NEURONS AND SLICES BY ADENOVIRAL VECTORS

In hippocampal slices of BDNF knockout animals there were, besides the drastic impairment of LTP, no other detectable morphological or functional changes (Korte et al. 1995). However, it cannot be decided with absolute certainty whether the observed impairment of LTP results from the actual absence of BDNF or whether the observed deficits result from (subtle) cumulative developmental defects. Therefore, we set out to distinguish between these two possibilities by reexpressing BDNF at very specific sites in hippocampal slices of BDNF-defective mice.

Of all available procedures for precise local gene transfer, the use of adenovirus vectors seemed to be the most suitable, because there is a favorable ratio between the rapidity and extent of the expression of transduced genes, on the one hand, and the appearance of cytopathic effects, on the other hand. This advantage is particularly important when the adenovirus-mediated gene transfer is used in a limited time frame (Table 1). To date, adenovirus-mediated gene transfer was generally performed with the goal to replace defective inherited genes or the local expression of neurotrophic factors or neurotransmitter synthesizing enzymes (for review, see Kozarsky and Wilson 1993). These experiments aim at a neuroprotective action or neurotransmitter replacement in experimental models, in which neuronal damage results from gene defects or is initiated by mechanical lesion or neurotoxic procedures leading to degenerative changes in specific populations of neurons, as for example, by the administration of 6-hydroxydopamine, 1-methyl-4-phenyl-1,2,3,6-tetrahydropyridine (MPTP), or excitotoxic amino acids. The requirements for the use of adenoviral-vector-mediated gene transfer in these cases are, with respect to possible interference with physiological functions, not very demanding. It can be considered as a success when at least part of the neuronal damages can be prevented or defective neuronal functions are partially restored. This is in distinct contrast to the use of adenoviral vectors for gene transfer with the goal to analyze refined physiological functions. Here it is mandatory to analyze in all details whether the infection procedure as such results in changes of structural and functional parameters unrelated to the transduced gene.

Although the final goal of our experiments was the rapid reexpression of BDNF in hippocampal slices originating from BDNF-deficient mice, we first had to collect information about the efficiency of adenoviral gene transfer on the one hand and the occurrence of possible cytopathic effects on the other hand in primary cultures of hippocampal neurons. For this purpose we used the replication-defective E-1-deleted adenovirus, containing the β-galactosidase gene as a reporter under the control of the (strong) cytomegalovirus (CMV) promoter (Fig. 2). Virus-stock solutions of 3 x 10^9 to 5 x 10^9 pfu/ml were prepared by standard methods (Graham and Prevec 1991). Hippocampal neurons were prepared from embryonic day 17 Wistar rats and cultivated according to the procedure described by Zafra et al. (1990). The neurons were infected with ADCMV-lac-Z. The volume of the culture medium was reduced to 300 μl/cm^2 and exposed to different quantities of ADCMV-lac-Z and stained for β-galactosidase activity at different time points after infection (Table 1). The efficiency of transfection showed a dose-response relationship. Infection of 10^5 neurons by 10^5 pfu resulted in 20% β-gal-positive neurons after 24 hours. Using 10^7 pfu, 90% of the neurons were β-gal-positive after 24 hours and, most importantly, did not show any signs of cytopathic changes. Following infection with the minimum quantity of ADCMV-lac-Z (10^5 pfu/10^5 neurons), the percentage of β-gal-positive

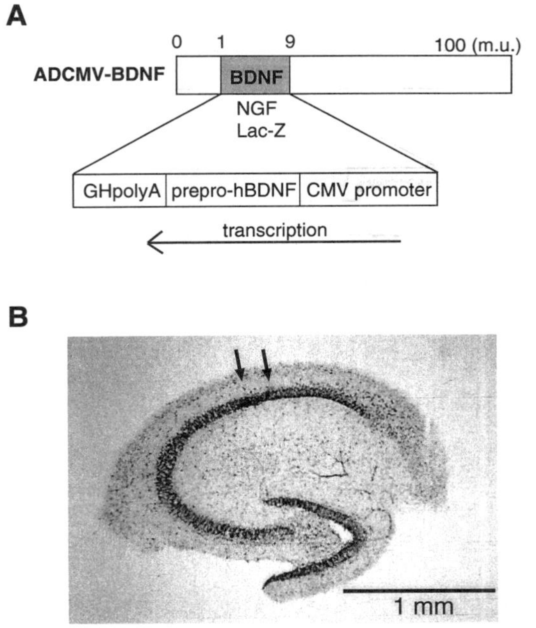

Figure 2. Schematic presentation of the structure of the E1-deleted recombinant adenoviral vector ADCMV-BDNF and a hippocampal slice infected with ADCMV-lac-Z. (*A*) BDNF, NGF, and Lac-Z have been inserted into the ADCMV shuttle vector at a polycloning site. The expression cassette consists of the cytomegalovirus (CMV) promoter, the coding cDNAs, and the growth hormone poly(A) signal. Recombinant virus was produced by homologous recombination in the human embryonic kidney cell line 293. Adenoviral sequences in the E1 region between map units (m.u.) 1 and 9 are deleted in the vector and replaced by the expression construct. (*B*) Example of a hippocampal slice infected (two injection sites) with a Lac-Z-expressing adenovirus in the CA1 region.

Table 1. Comparison between the Time Course of the Infection Efficiency and Occurrence of Cytopathic Effects

Adenovirus titer (pfu/10^5 neurons)	β-Gal-positive neurons % infection (in days) 1	3	5	7	Surviving neurons (%) 3 days after infection
1 x 10^5	21 ± 1	30 ± 4	51 ± 11	52 ± 5	98 ± 6
5 x 10^5	44 ± 7				89 ± 14
1.25 x 10^6	59 ± 0.4				85 ± 15
2.5 x 10^6	65 ± 9				53 ± 6
1 x 10^7	88 ± 2				10 ± 4

Primary cultures of hippocampal neurons were infected with different concentrations of pfu, and the infection efficiency was evaluated by counting β-gal-positive neurons and compared with the occurrence of cytopathic effects. The values given represent the mean ± S.D. of independent observations.

Table 2. Percentage of Successful LTP Inductions in Hippocampal Slices of BDNF +/+, BDNF +/–, and BDNF –/– Mice after Infection with Adenovirus-expressing Lac-Z, NGF, or BDNF

Genotype	ADCMV-lac-Z		ADCMV-NGF		ADCMV-BDNF	
	LTP		LTP		LTP	
	yes	no	yes	no	yes	no
+/+	14 (61%)	9	7 (64%)	4	14 (67%)	7
+/–	6 (20%)	24	2 (25%)	6	16 (52%)	15
–/–	4 (19%)	17	1 (20%)	4	11 (46%)	13

LTP was judged as successful if 60 min after the tetanus (3 times 30 pulses at 100 Hz) the slope of the field EPSP was at least 20% higher than the baseline values. The experiments were performed in a blind fashion; i.e., the person recording from the slices and analyzing the data was not informed on the origin of the slice and the adenovirus-mediated gene transfer used.

neurons increased from 20% after 1 day to 50% after 5 days and remained at this level up to 7 days (Table 1). Although after infection with 10^7 pfu/10^5 neurons there was no detectable cytopathic effect after 24 hours, distinct cytopathic manifestations became apparent in a dosage-dependent manner after 3 days. Up to 1.25 x 10^6 pfu produced no significant cytopathic effects as evaluated by the procedures of Jones and Senft (1985). To obtain more refined functional information on the consequences of adenoviral infection, we analyzed the extent and time course of calcium transients in response to the exposure to 10 μM glutamate. There was no detectable difference between control and infected cultures, neither in the rapidity and extent of the onset nor in the duration of the calcium transients. After infection of hippocampal cultures with ADCMV-NGF or ADCMV-BDNF, a distinct increase in both NGF and BDNF mRNA became apparent as early as 4 hours after infection, and there was a further 10- to 15-fold increase after 12 hours.

After having established the criteria of infection efficiency and occurrence of cytopathic effects in primary cultures of hippocampal neurons, we proceeded to the gene transfer into acute hippocampal slices. It was of particular importance to learn whether adenoviral infection of the transduced gene occurs within a few hours after infection. Using the highest titers of pfu, there was no evidence for cytopathic effects within 24 hours. For gene transfer into acute hippocampal slices, a specific problem arose from the fact that there is a discrepancy between the optimal temperature for infection and the optimal temperature for maintenance of the slices. Optimal adenoviral infection occurs at 37°C, whereas acute hippocampal slices are often prepared and maintained at room temperature and then recorded at 32°C. After no adenoviral infection became apparent at room temperature within 12 hours, we injected the slices with an estimated 25–50 nl of virus stock solution and kept them in the incubation chamber at 35°C for at least 5 hours before they were subjected to the electrophysiological analysis.

RESTORATION OF LTP IN HIPPOCAMPAL SLICES FROM BDNF-DEFECTIVE MICE BY LOCAL REEXPRESSION OF BDNF IN THE CA1 REGION

Before approaching the question whether reexpression of BDNF restores the possibility of inducing LTP in the CA3/CA1 system, it was essential to evaluate whether the infection procedure as such modifies the basic parameters to be analyzed. Indeed, transfected slices were indistinguishable from untreated controls in that (1) equivalent synaptic responses were evoked with similar stimulus strength; (2) the area under the field excitatory postsynaptic potential (EPSP), produced by a single afferent volley, was equal in treated and untreated slices; (3) PPF was normal in all slice preparations tested with 20, 30, 50, and 100 ms. This indicates that the infection procedure with ADCMV-BDNF, ADCMV-lac-Z, or ADCMV-NGF does not alter the basic properties of synaptic transmission in hippocampal slices. These were favorable prerequisites for our restoration experiments and, indeed, when hippocampal CA1 pyramidal cells in slices from BDNF mutant animals were infected with ADCMV-BDNF, the reduction of LTP could largely be restored (Tables 2 and 3). The proportion of successfully induced LTP was increased 2.6-fold for slices originating from +/– BDNF mice and 2.4-fold for BDNF –/– mice in comparison to ADCMV-lac-Z-injected slices. In contrast, in +/+ mice there was no significant difference between ADCMV-BDNF-, ADCMV-NGF-, or ADCMV-lac-Z-injected slices. The average level of potentiation achieved in +/– mice treated with ADCMV-BDNF is significantly higher than in –/– mice treated with the same virus construct ($p < 0.05$ two-tailed t-test). This most likely results from the fact that in +/– mice 50%

Table 3. Comparison of EPSP Slopes 60 Minutes after Tetanic Stimulation Expressed as Percentage of Baseline Values

Genotype	ADCMV-BDNF	ADCMV-lac-Z	ADCMV-NGF	Untreated
+/+	162 ± 10 (n = 23)	156 ± 11 (n = 21)	158 ± 9 (n = 11)	178 ± 8 (n = 78)
+/–	141 ± 9 (n = 31)	112 ± 10 (n = 30)	116 ± 10 (n = 8)	116 ± 14 (n = 94)
–/–	131 ± 6 (n = 24)	110 ± 8 (n = 21)	112 ± 12 (n = 5)	116 ± 12 (n = 59)

The experiments were performed in acute hippocampal slices originating from BDNF +/+, +/–, or –/– mice infected with adenovirus-expressing BDNF, Lac-Z, or NGF, or untreated slices. The values are given as mean ± S.E.M.; n = number of independent experiments.

of the normal levels of BDNF is already expressed in comparison to wild-type mice (Korte et al. 1995). It is therefore reasonable to assume that in rescue experiments a critical threshold level of BDNF is necessary to elicit LTP and that this level is reached more easily in +/– than in –/– mice.

ACKNOWLEDGMENTS

We thank I. Hajjar and E. Hering for secretarial help and J. Cooper for linguistic revisions.

REFERENCES

Berardi, N., A. Cellerino, L. Domenici, M. Fagiolini, T. Pizzorusso, A. Cattaneo, and L. Maffei. 1994. Monoclonal antibodies to nerve growth factor affect the postnatal development of the visual system. *Proc. Natl. Acad. Sci.* **91:** 684.

Berninger, B., D.E. García, N. Inagaki, C. Hahnel, and D. Lindholm. 1993. BDNF and NT-3 induce intracellular Ca^{2+} elevation in hippocampal neurones. *NeuroReport* **4:** 1303.

Berzaghi, M.P., R. Gutiérrez, U. Heinemann, D. Lindholm, and H. Thoenen. 1995. Neurotrophins induce acute transmitter-mediated changes in brain electrical activity. *Soc. Neurosci. Abstr.* **21:** 226.3.

Blöchl, A. and H. Thoenen. 1995. Characterization of nerve growth factor (NGF) release from hippocampal neurons: Evidence for a constitutive and an unconventional sodium-dependent regulated pathway. *Eur. J. Neurosci.* **7:** 1220.

———. 1996. Localization of cellular storage compartments and sites of constitutive and activity-dependent release of nerve growth factor (NGF) in primary cultures of hippocampal neurons. *Mol. Cell. Neurosci.* **7:** 173.

Bonhoeffer, T. 1996. Neurotrophins and activity-dependent development of the neocortex. *Curr. Opin. Neurobiol.* **6:** 119.

Bothwell, M. 1995. Functional interactions of neurotrophins and neurotrophin receptors. *Annu. Rev. Neurosci.* **18:** 223.

Bozzi, Y., T. Pizzorusso, F. Cremisi, F.M. Rossi, G. Barsacchi, and L. Maffei. 1995. Monocular deprivation decreases the expression of messenger RNA for brain-derived neurotrophic factor in the rat visual cortex. *Neuroscience* **69:** 1133.

Cabelli, R.J., A. Hohn, and C.J. Shatz. 1995. Inhibition of ocular dominance column formation by infusion of NT-4/5 or BDNF. *Science* **267:** 1662.

Carmignoto, G., R. Canella, P. Candeo, M.C. Comelli, and L. Maffei. 1993. Effects of nerve growth factor on neuronal plasticity of the kitten visual cortex. *J. Physiol.* **464:** 343.

Castrén, E., H. Thoenen, and D. Lindholm. 1995. Brain-derived neurotrophic factor messenger RNA is expressed in the septum, hypothalamus and in adrenergic brain stem nuclei of adult rat brain and is increased by osmotic stimulation in the paraventricular nucleus. *Neuroscience* **64:** 71.

Castrén, E., F. Zafra, H. Thoenen, and D. Lindholm. 1992. Light regulates expression of brain-derived neurotrophic factor mRNA in rat visual cortex. *Proc. Natl. Acad. Sci.* **89:** 9444.

Domenici, L., A. Cellerino, N. Berardi, A. Lattaneo, and L. Maffei. 1994. Antibodies to nerve growth factor (NGF) prolong the sensitive period for monocular deprivation in the rat. *NeuroReport* **5:** 2041.

Fiorentini, A., N. Berardi, and L. Maffei. 1995. Nerve growth factor preserves behavioral visual acuity in monocularly deprived kittens. *Visual Neurosci.* **12:** 51.

Galuske, R.A.W., D.-S. Kim, E. Castrén, H. Thoenen, and W. Singer. 1996. Brain-derived neurotrophic factor reverses experience-dependent synaptic modifications in kitten visual cortex. *Eur. J. Neurosci.* (in press).

Goodman, C.S. and C.J. Shatz. 1993. Developmental mechanisms that generate precise pattern of neuronal connectivity. *Neuron* **10:** 77.

Graham, F.L. and L. Prevec. 1991. Manipulation of adenovirus vectors. *Methods Mol. Biol.* **7:** 109.

Griesbeck, O., A. Blöchl, J.F. Carnahan, H. Nawa, and H. Thoenen. 1995. Characterization of brain-derived neurotrophic factor (BDNF) secretion from hippocampal neurons. *Soc. Neurosci. Abstr.* **21:** 417.12.

Jones, K.H. and J.A. Senft. 1985. An improved method to determine cell viability by simultaneous staining with fluorescein diacetate-propidium iodide. *J. Histochem. Cytochem.* **33:** 77.

Kang, H. and E.M. Schuman. 1995. Long-lasting neurotrophin-induced enhancement of synaptic transmission in the adult hippocampus. *Science* **267:** 1658.

Knipper, M., L.S. Leung, D. Zhao, and R. Rylett. 1994a. Short term modulation of glutamatergic synapses in adult rat hippocampus. *NeuroReport* **5:** 2433.

Knipper, M., M. Berzaghi, A. Blöchl, H. Breer, H. Thoenen, and D. Lindholm. 1994b. Positive feedback between acetylcholine and the neurotrophins nerve growth factor and brain-derived neurotrophic factor in the rat hippocampus. *Eur. J. Neurosci.* **6:** 668.

Knüsel, B. and F. Hefti. 1992. K-252 compounds: Modulators of neurotrophin signal transduction. *J. Neurochem.* **59:** 1987.

Korte, M., P. Carroll, E. Wolf, G. Brem, H. Thoenen, and T. Bonhoeffer. 1995. Hippocampal long-term potentiation is impaired in mice lacking brain-derived neurotrophic factor. *Proc. Natl. Acad. Sci.* **92:** 8856.

Kozarsky, K.F. and J.M. Wilson. 1993. Gene therapy: Adenovirus vectors. *Curr. Opin. Genet. Dev.* **3:** 499.

Lessmann, V., K. Gottmann, and R. Heumann. 1994. BDNF and NT-4/5 enhance glutamatergic synaptic transmission in cultured hippocampal neurones. *NeuroReport* **6:** 21.

Lewin, G. and Y.-A. Barde. 1996. Physiology of the neurotrophins. *Annu. Rev. Neuroscience* **19:** 289.

Lindholm, D., E. Castrén, M. Berzaghi, A. Blöchl, and H. Thoenen. 1994. Activity-dependent and hormonal regulation of neurotrophin mRNA levels in the brain-implications for neuronal plasticity. *J. Neurobiol.* **25:** 1362.

Lo, D.C. 1995. Neurotrophic factors and synaptic plasticity. *Neuron* **15:** 979.

Lohof, A.M., N.Y. Ip, and M. Poo. 1993. Potentiation of developing neuromuscular synapses by the neurotrophins NT-3 and BDNF. *Nature* **363:** 350.

Maffei, L., N. Berardi, L. Domenici, V. Parisi, and T. Pizzorusso. 1992. Nerve growth factor (NGF) prevents the shift in ocular dominance distribution of visual cortical neurons in monocularly deprived rats. *J. Neurosci.* **12:** 4651.

Riddle, D.R., D.C. Lo, and L.C. Katz. 1995. NT-4-mediated rescue of lateral geniculate neurons from effects of monocular deprivation. *Nature* **378:** 189.

Schuman, E.M. and D.V. Madison. 1994a. Locally distributed

synaptic potentiation in the hippocampus. *Science* **263:** 532.

———. 1994b. Nitric oxide and synaptic function. *Annu. Rev. Neurosci.* **17:** 153.

Snider, W.D. 1994. Functions of the neurotrophins during nervous system development: What the knockouts are teaching us. *Cell* **77:** 627.

Thoenen, H. 1995. Neurotrophins and neuronal plasticity. *Science* **270:** 593.

Williams, J.H., M.L. Errington, M.A. Lynch, and T.V. Bliss. 1989. Arachidonic acid induces a long-term activity-dependent enhancement of synaptic transmission in the hippocampus. *Nature* **341:** 739.

Zafra, F., B. Hengerer, J. Leibrock, H. Thoenen, and D. Lindholm. 1990. Activity dependent regulation of BDNF and NGF mRNAs in the rat hippocampus is mediated by non-NMDA glutamate receptors. *EMBO J.* **9:** 3545.

Zhuo, M., S.A. Small, E.R. Kandel, and R.D. Hawkins. 1993. Nitric oxide and carbon monoxide produce activity dependent long-term synaptic enhancement in the hippocampus. *Science* **260:** 1946.

Neurotrophins in Cortical Development

D.R. Riddle,[1] A.K. McAllister,[2,3] D.C. Lo,[3] and L.C. Katz[2,3]

[1]*Department of Neurobiology and Anatomy, The Bowman Gray School of Medicine, Winston-Salem, North Carolina 27157-1010;* [2]*Howard Hughes Medical Institute, and* [3]*Department of Neurobiology, Duke University Medical Center, Durham, North Carolina 27710*

In addition to acting as target-derived survival factors and regulating cell death, neurotrophins modulate the subsequent growth and differentiation of the surviving neurons and may act as mediators for activity-dependent regulation of circuit formation (Thoenen 1995; Bonhoeffer 1996; Henderson 1996; Lewin and Barde 1996). Neurotrophins are able to serve such diverse functions because their effects at a given point in development are modulated by other factors in the microenvironment. These regulatory factors include other growth-related molecules (see, e.g., Stoop and Poo 1996; Verdi et al. 1996), as well as the patterns and levels of electrical activity experienced by particular neurons (for review, see Lo 1995; Thoenen 1995; Bonhoeffer 1996; Henderson 1996; Lewin and Barde 1996). Thus, to understand all of the functions of the neurotrophins, it is necessary to evaluate their effects within their overall intra- and intercellular context, a context that presumably becomes more complex as development proceeds and cells become increasingly differentiated. We have been able to investigate the potential roles of neurotrophins in the development and plasticity of central neurons using a combination of in vitro and in vivo approaches that have preserved, to a large extent, the natural tissue environment of neurons. These experiments have provided new insight into the roles of neurotrophins in the regulation of neuronal growth and differentiation and in activity-dependent development and plasticity.

DIFFERENTIAL NEUROTROPHIC REGULATION OF THE GROWTH OF CORTICAL NEURONS

The cerebral cortex provides an attractive focus for studies of regulation of neuronal growth in the central nervous system. The diversity of cortical neurons and their consistent organization suggest that a variety of regulatory processes are involved in cortical development. Each of the six cortical layers contains a different assembly of neuronal types, reflected in specific axonal projections, physiological properties, and dendritic arbors. Anatomically, different classes of cortical neurons are most easily recognized on the basis of their dendritic morphology. Since dendrites are the site of most synapses, dendritic development also largely determines the number and pattern of synapses received by each neuron (Hume and Purves 1981; Purves and Hume 1981) and, to a significant degree, its functional abilities. Thus, understanding the control of dendritic development is critical to understanding both the structural and functional development of the cortex.

In general, dendritic growth appears to be regulated by both intrinsic developmental programs (Bartlett and Banker 1984) and a variety of epigenetic cues, including synaptic activity (Valverde 1968; Harris and Woolsey 1981; Katz et al. 1989). Studies of the peripheral nervous system indicate neurotrophins are among the factors that can regulate dendritic growth. Nerve growth factor (NGF), for example, strongly influences dendritic complexity of sympathetic ganglion cells in vivo (Purves et al. 1988; Snider 1988; Ruit et al. 1990; Ruit and Snider 1991). There is reason to suspect a similar role for the neurotrophins in developing cortex, as neurotrophins and their receptors (the Trk family of tyrosine kinase receptors; for review, see Chao 1992) are expressed in discrete layers of neocortex during the time dendrites develop (Merlio et al. 1992; Ringstedt et al. 1993; Allendoerfer et al. 1994; Lindsay et al. 1994). It has been hard, however, to assign specific biological functions to neurotrophins in the cortex due to the difficulty of manipulating neurotrophins and their receptors in vivo and due to the loss of identifying neuronal characteristics, such as laminar identity and cell polarity, in dissociated culture. These problems are largely overcome by the use of organotypic slice cultures in which neurotrophins can be manipulated while preserving much of the local environment of each neuron, including the laminar organization of cortex and many of the connections within and between layers (Bolz et al. 1990; Molnar and Blakemore 1991; Yamamoto et al. 1992).

We recently used this approach to investigate neurotrophin regulation of dendritic development of cortical neurons (McAllister et al. 1995a). Slices of primary visual cortex from postnatal day-14 ferrets were cultured for 36 hours with or without exogenous neurotrophin. Neurons within the slices were visualized using a particle-mediated gene transfer technique that provided complete labeling of the dendritic arbors of many neurons in each slice (Lo et al. 1994). Labeled neurons in each layer were examined, and their dendritic arbors were measured and analyzed to determine the effects of neurotrophin treatment.

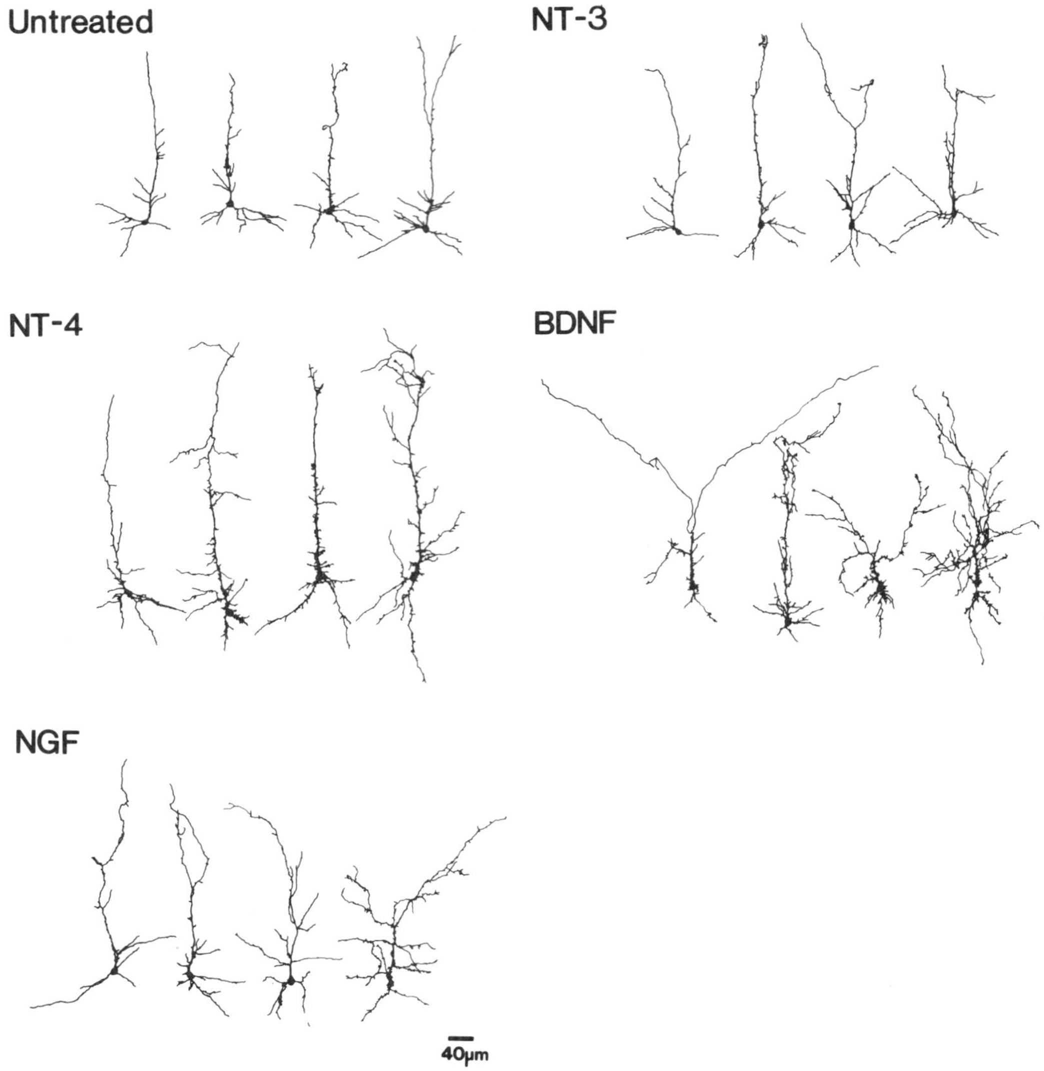

Figure 1. Neurotrophin effects on dendritic growth of pyramidal neurons. These camera lucida reconstructions of neurons are representative of the range of cellular morphologies found in each of the treated populations. All four neurotrophins enhanced dendritic growth of layer-4 pyramidal neurons. BDNF elicited the most extensive increases in dendritic complexity and length, NT-4 and NGF caused smaller increases, and NT-3 had only a minor effect on these cells. (Reprinted, with permission, from McAllister et al. 1995a.)

Each of the four neurotrophins generally caused dendritic arbors to grow longer and more complex (Fig. 1). Quantitative analysis based on a weighted sum of several measures of dendritic complexity (the dendrite modification index or DMI; see Fig. 2) revealed specific effects of each neurotrophin on neurons in each cortical layer. Basal dendrites of neurons in each layer were maximally enhanced by a single factor. The TrkB ligands, brain-derived neurotrophic factor (BDNF) and neurotrophin 4/5 (NT-4/5), caused the most growth of dendrites in all layers. In layer 4, BDNF increased the DMI almost 90% over controls while NT-4/5 produced a smaller but significant increase (Fig. 2). In layer 5, the response to NT-4/5 (90% increase in the DMI) exceeded that of BDNF (36% increase). Layer 6 was similar to layer 5 in that NT-4/5 produced the greatest effect, but, in contrast to its effects on layer-5 dendrites, BDNF *decreased* dendritic growth in layer 6. The effects of the TrkA and TrkC ligands were less dramatic but equally variable. NGF minimally enhanced the DMI in layers 4 and 5 but decreased dendritic growth in layer 6. Neurotrophin 3 (NT-3) elicited modest growth of dendrites in layer 6 but produced no change in the other layers. Clearly, each neurotrophin had a different pattern of effects in each cortical layer, and even NT-4/5 and BDNF, which both bind primarily to TrkB receptors (Lindsay 1994), elicited distinct patterns of growth.

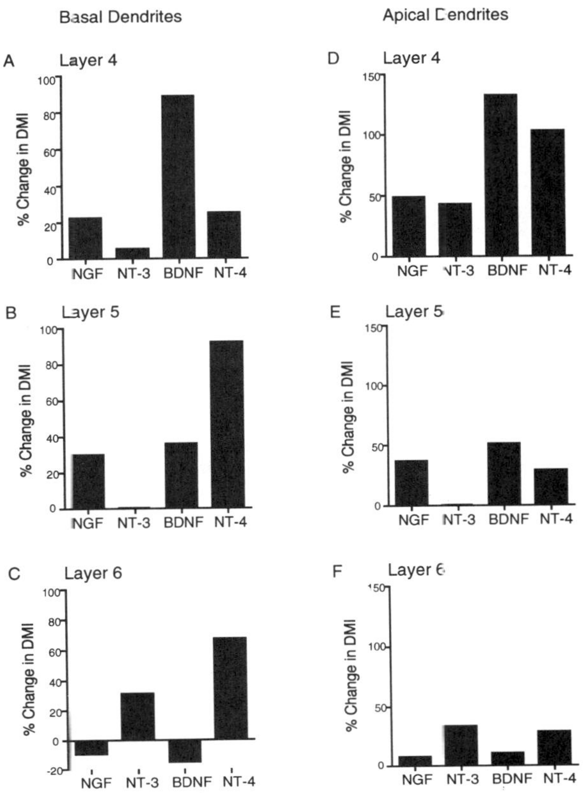

Figure 2. Quantitation of neurotrophin effects on dendritic growth. The effects of neurotrophin treatment on dendritic elaboration were summarized using a dendrite modification index (DMI). The DMI is a weighted sum of the ratios of each of the four parameters of dendritic growth in treated vs. untreated cells (see McAllister et al. 1995). Basal dendrites (*A–C*) responded mainly to a single neurotrophin, with BDNF and NT-4 exerting the greatest effects. Apical dendrites (*D–F*) responded to a wider range of neurotrophins. (Reprinted, with permission, from McAllister et al. 1995a.)

In addition to basal dendrites, cortical pyramidal neurons bear a single, apical dendrite (layer-4 neurons retract this apical neuron, and thus lose their early pyramidal morphology, over the course of cortical development; see Peinado and Katz 1990). Comparison of the growth of these apical dendrites with that of basal dendrites revealed that neurotrophin effects differed between the two dendritic compartments of individual neurons (Fig. 2). In general, apical dendrites responded to a wider range of neurotrophins than their basal dendritic counterparts. The order of efficacy of the four neurotrophins differed between the apical and basal dendrites of some neurons. For example, apical dendrites of layer-5 cells were most strongly enhanced by BDNF, which increased both their length and branching (Fig. 2), whereas basal dendrites of the same cells were strongly enhanced by NT-4/5 and much less so by BDNF (Fig. 2). This difference makes it clear that the growth of distinct dendritic compartments can be differentially regulated and reinforces the conclusion, based on the responses of basal dendrites, that the actions of the two TrkB ligands (NT-4/5 and BDNF) are distinct.

As in the peripheral nervous system (Purves et al. 1988; Snider 1988; Ruit and Snider 1991), neurotrophins enhance dendritic growth and complexity of neurons in developing visual cortex. The effects of neurotrophins are complex, and neurons in each cortical layer respond only to certain neurotrophins. Even within a layer, neurons respond to each neurotrophin with a distinct constellation of dendritic changes, revealed both by measures of overall dendritic size and complexity (like the DMI) and by detailed analysis of individual characteristics of dendritic growth (such as number of primary dendrites and degree of branching; see McAllister et al. 1995a). This specificity apparently extends to differential responses of anatomically and functionally distinct cellular compartments as well, and may be critical for development of the specific dendritic forms and patterns of inputs characteristic of the neurons in each cortical layer.

This initial study revealed little about how the specificity of neurotrophin effects arises. The correspondence between the pattern of neurotrophic effects and the reported patterns of Trk expression is not exact (see McAllister et al. 1995a), indicating that the response of a particular neuron to a given neurotrophin is influenced by aspects of cellular context beyond Trk receptor expression. Other factors that may influence signaling include the expression of alternative splice variants and noncatalytic, truncated forms of Trk receptors (for review, see Barbacid 1994; see also Valenzuela et al. 1993; Biffo et al. 1995), as well as binding of neurotrophins to non-preferred Trk receptors (see, e.g., Clary and Reichardt 1994). In addition, concurrent or recent electrical activity may also regulate neurotrophin responses (see, e.g., Lindholm et al. 1994). A link between neural activity and neurotrophin signaling is of significant interest, since it could help specify neurotrophin effects on neuronal growth and differentiation and is almost certainly fundamental to any role the neurotrophins may play in regulating synapse formation and modification during development and refinement of neural circuits.

COUPLING OF ELECTRICAL ACTIVITY AND NEUROTROPHIN SIGNALING

There are several ways in which the synaptic and electrical activity of neurons might be coupled to neurotrophin signaling. Changes in the level of electrical activity appear to affect the expression of both neurotrophins and their receptors (for review, see Lindholm et al. 1994; Lo 1995; Thoenen 1995; Lewin and Barde 1996). Seizure activity increases the levels of mRNA for NGF, BDNF, TrkB, and TrkC in the hippocampus (Gall and Isackson 1989; Zafra et al. 1990; Ernfors et al. 1991; Bengzon et al. 1993; Mudo et al. 1995) and increases TrkB expression in the striatum

(Salin et al. 1995). Less radical changes in electrical activity, such as the induction of hippocampal LTP and manipulation of visual experience, also modulate neurotrophin and Trk expression (Castren et al. 1992, 1993; Patterson et al. 1992; Schoups et al. 1995; Bramham et al. 1996).

These changes in levels of message cannot, of course, be assumed to reflect absolutely changes in the amount of neurotrophin or receptor available for signaling. Changes in neurotrophin levels may follow different time courses than an associated increase in mRNA levels (Nawa et al. 1995), and neurotrophin levels may increase during periods in which mRNA levels remain stable or even decrease (see Large et al. 1986; J. Johnson, pers. comm.). Neurotrophin signaling could even fluctuate with no change in mRNA or overall protein levels, if activity influenced the release of neurotrophins into the extracellular space (see, e.g., Blöchl and Thoenen 1995). Thus, the influence of activity on neurotrophin signaling is likely to be complex, even considering only the amount of neurotrophin available for signaling and the number of Trk receptors available to mediate that signal.

Activity-dependent regulation of growth by neurotrophins could also be achieved if the cellular response to a given amount of neurotrophin was influenced by the activity state of the neurons; that is, if neurotrophins acted preferentially or differentially on more (or less) active neurons. To test this supposition, we treated organotypic slices of visual cortex from postnatal day-14 ferrets with BDNF alone or in combination with tetrodotoxin (TTX) to block spontaneously generated action potentials and action-potential-evoked synaptic transmission, 6-cyano-7-nitro-quinoxaline-2,3-dione (CNQX) to block non-NMDA-type glutamate receptors, or DL-2-amino-5-phosphonovaleric acid (APV) to block NMDA receptors. Blocking neuronal activity had striking effects on the growth-promoting action of BDNF on neurons in layer 4 of visual cortex (Fig. 3) (McAllister et al. 1995b, 1996). For apical dendrites, all of the activity inhibitors completely prevented the substantial increase in complexity elicited by BDNF alone. For basal dendrites, glutamate-receptor blockade prevented BDNF from inducing dendritic formation and growth, but TTX had only a minor inhibitory influence on the effects of BDNF. Thus, BDNF-induced growth of basal dendrites requires synaptic release of glutamate, but spontaneous release may be sufficient since Na^+-dependent action potentials apparently are not required.

The effects of combined BDNF treatment and activity blockade were not due to an inhibitory effect on dendritic growth arising from the activity blockade itself. Simply inhibiting activity in slices, in the absence of exogenously applied BDNF, *enhanced* basal dendritic growth. This increased growth differed substantially, however, from that elicited by BDNF (Fig. 3). BDNF caused robust sprouting of basal dendrites, increasing their number as well as their length and complexity, whereas inhibiting activity caused elongation and modest branching of existing dendrites with no change in their number. Thus, whereas exogenous BDNF and activity blockade each augment dendritic growth (in different ways) when acting alone, their combined effects are not additive but inhibitory, indicating that synaptic activity is *required* for the growth-promoting effects of BDNF on layer-4 neurons. As noted above, several studies have demonstrated upregulation of neurotrophin mRNA in response to increased synaptic activity. It has never been clear, however, how nonspecific release of neurotrophin in response to activity could produce selective effects on only a subpopulation of the local neurons or on a subset of the synapses formed on a given neuron. Such specificity might be conferred by selective responsiveness to neurotrophins as determined by levels of activity.

Clearly, there is no simple mechanism by which electrical activity and neurotrophic signaling interact. Synaptic activity can alter neurotrophin and Trk receptor production and may also determine whether a neuron responds to a neurotrophin at all. Conversely, neurotrophins may alter ion channels (see, e.g., Berninger et al. 1993; Lesser and Lo 1995), synaptic transmission (Lohof et al. 1993; Kim et al. 1994; Knipper et al. 1994; Kang and Schuman 1995; Levine et al. 1995; Wang et al. 1995; Figurov et al. 1996), and even stimulus-dependent activity in the intact cortex (Prakash et al. 1996). Thus, the mechanisms by which activity modulates neurotrophin signaling, and vice versa, may well involve complex feed-back and feed-forward regulation.

ACTIVITY-DEPENDENT NEUROTROPHIC EFFECTS IN CIRCUIT FORMATION

The approaches described above provide powerful tools for investigating the cell biological mechanisms by which neurotrophins influence neuronal differentiation and growth. If neurotrophins also play a defining role in the development of neuronal connections, however, this function is likely to depend on specific patterns and levels of neural activity that are unlikely to be reproduced in reduced preparations. Experiments within the intact brain are more likely to provide insight into neurotrophin regulation of development and plasticity of neural circuits. Recent experiments have tested the effects of exogenous neurotrophins, delivered in vivo, on activity-dependent development of connections in the visual system.

The development of ocular dominance columns in the primary visual cortex of carnivores and primates is a well-characterized activity-dependent process. In normal development, geniculocortical axons that are driven by either of the two eyes, which initially have overlapping distributions in the visual cortex, segregate and form alternating bands. This segregation is activ-

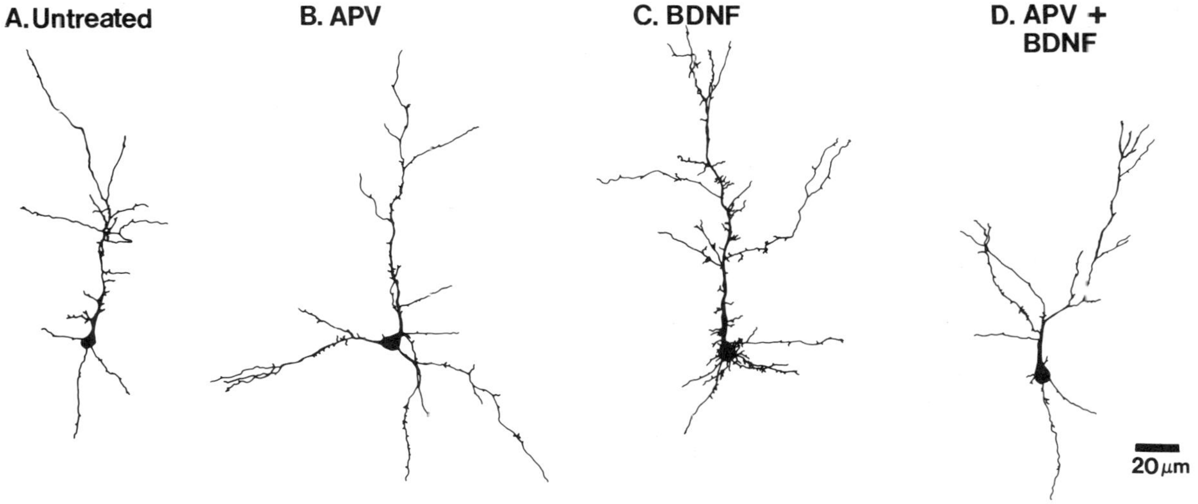

Figure 3. Inhibiting activity blocks the effects of BDNF on pyramidal neurons. These camera lucida reconstructions of layer-4 neurons are from an untreated slice (*A*) and slices treated with 50 μM APV (*B*), 200 ng/ml BDNF (*C*), or APV and BDNF together (*D*). Inhibiting spontaneous activity blocked the strong effects of BDNF on dendritic complexity (*D*). The neuron in *B* shows that activity blockade by itself did not result in a generalized slowing of dendritic growth.

ity-dependent and does not occur if activity is blocked (Stryker and Harris 1986). Recently, Cabelli et al. (1995) showed that segregation is also blocked when either BDNF or NT-4/5 is infused into the visual cortex. These authors suggest that axons from the lateral geniculate nucleus (LGN) normally compete for a TrkB ligand that is present in the visual cortex in limiting supply. By providing exogenous NT-4/5 or BDNF, they have eliminated the competition, and therefore prevented the segregation of axons that causes ocular dominance columns to form. More recent studies have shown that, as one would predict from the initial experiments, blocking TrkB activity has a similar effect (C. Shatz, pers. comm.).

Activity-dependent competition also is thought to underlie the effects of monocular deprivation (MD) in the developing visual system. Altering the balance of activity between the two eyes during the critical period for visual system development changes the competitive interactions among developing neurons in the LGN and primary visual cortex (for review, see Sherman and Spear 1982; Wiesel 1982). Neurons in the LGN and their axons in the visual cortex that are deprived of activity (by closing or silencing one eye) atrophy, presumably as a result of competition with non-deprived neurons for some critical factor(s) present in limiting supply within the cortex. In addition to such anatomical changes, the deprived neurons largely lose their ability to drive responses among the cortical neurons. These changes appear to depend on activity at the level of V1 (Reiter et al. 1986; Bear and Coleman 1990; Bear et al. 1990). A detailed series of experiments indicates NGF may also be involved in regulating the changes that follow MD; NGF injected into the cerebral ventricles blocks both anatomical and functional effects of MD (see, e.g., Berardi et al. 1993; Carmignoto et al. 1993; Domenici et al. 1993). The locus of the NGF effect in these experiments remains unclear, since NGF influences NGF-responsive neurons throughout the brain after ventricular infusion (Holtzman et al. 1995). It seems likely that NGF alters MD through actions outside of the primary visual pathway, since LGN neurons do not express TrkA mRNA or transport NGF when it is injected into V1 (Holtzman et al. 1992; Merlio et al. 1992; Domenici et al. 1994), and since TrkA receptors have not been demonstrated on visual cortical neurons or LGN afferents.

Recently, we reexamined the hypothesis that neurotrophins mediate the intracortical competition of LGN axons using a new method for in vivo delivery of neurotrophins that permits highly localized delivery of the factor to the terminals of those axons within the visual cortex, thereby precluding confounding actions of the factor elsewhere in the brain (Riddle et al. 1995). We monocularly deprived developing ferrets (postnatal day 38–42) and made injections of fluorescent latex microspheres coated with NGF, NT-4/5, NT-3, or BDNF into the contralateral V1 (Fig. 4). Independent experiments in vitro demonstrated that each of the neurotrophins could be delivered with full activity by the microspheres and that active factor continued to be released for several days (data not shown). In addition to labeling the site of application, the microspheres were taken up by nerve terminals and retrogradely transported (Katz et al. 1984; Katz and Iarovici 1990). We could identify, therefore, the projection neurons in the LGN that had axonal terminals which were exposed to neurotrophin (Fig. 4). Within individual animals, adjacent injections of control microspheres

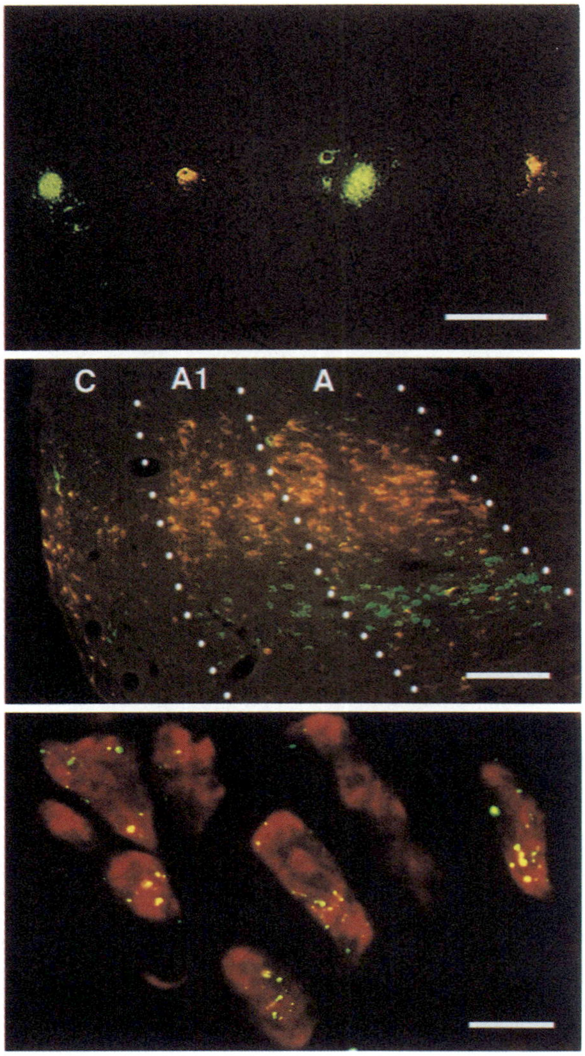

Figure 4. In vivo delivery of neurotrophins. A horizontal section through Area 17 of ferret cortex is shown containing four injection sites, two with red NT-4-coated microspheres (which appear orange in this double exposure) and two with green control microspheres (*top* panel). Columns of retrogradely labeled neurons extend across the A and A1 layers of the LGN after injections in V1 (*middle* panel); laminar borders are indicated by dotted lines (sublaminae are apparent within A and A1). Adjacent regions of red and green labeled cells projected to adjacent injection sites in the visual cortex. At higher magnification, green microspheres are apparent throughout the cytoplasm of several labeled neurons (*bottom* panel, dual-channel confocal micrograph). Bars: top panel, 500 μm; middle panel, 200 μm; and bottom panel, 10 μm. (Reprinted, with permission, from Riddle et al. 1995 [copyright Macmillan].)

permitted comparison of these neurons with others that projected to V1 but were not exposed to neurotrophin. Since the inputs from the two eyes (one open and one closed in these experiments) are segregated within the LGN, we could identify which LGN neurons had been deprived of activity and which had not, and thus measure the effect of activity deprivation on cell body size and determine whether that effect was modulated by neurotrophin exposure.

After 4 days of MD, neurons labeled with control microspheres in the deprived layer of the LGN shrank by 20–30% relative to control neurons in the adjacent region of the nondeprived layer. NT-4/5, but not BDNF, NT-3, or NGF, prevented this shrinkage. The average somal area for NT-4/5-treated cells in the deprived layer of the LGN was only slightly smaller than that of control cells in the nondeprived layer; NT-4/5 prevented the shift in cell size distribution toward smaller somata that followed MD (Fig. 5). Nondeprived neurons that were treated with NT-4/5 were no larger than control neurons (Fig. 5). Thus, NT-4/5 specifically rescued neurons from the effects of MD and did not simply promote growth, suggesting that NT-4/5 plays a specific role in the competition among deprived and nondeprived axons. Further evidence that NT-4/5 may mediate this competition comes from the observation that the shrinkage of LGN neurons in the closed-eye layer was not reversed when NT-4/5-coated microspheres were injected several weeks after the start of MD (Riddle et al. 1995). To prevent the atrophy of deprived neurons, it appears that NT-4/5 must be provided early in the period of deprivation, presumably during the time at which axons are actively competing for the critical trophic factor.

These results suggest that LGN afferents normally compete for NT-4/5 (or a similar endogenous ligand) and the ability of LGN terminals to acquire NT-4/5 is decreased when their activity is reduced relative to neighboring fibers. Injecting NT-4/5-coated microspheres provided an abundant local source of NT-4/5 and maintained trophic support to deprived neurons that would otherwise atrophy. Like the results of Cabelli et al. (1995) with regard to ocular dominance column formation, the data provide support for the hypothesis that activity-dependent, competitive processes that regulate neuronal growth and connectivity in the developing visual system may be mediated through one or more of the neurotrophins.

CONCLUSION

In each of these experiments, manipulating neurotrophins within a largely normal neuronal environment provided information about their effects that would have been impossible to glean from more simplified systems. Had the dendritic growth of cortical neurons been examined using dissociated neurons, the regionally specific nature of the neurotrophin effects would have been obscured. Revealing the differential effects of neurotrophins on the growth of basal and apical dendrites, and the nature of the activity dependence of neurotrophin regulation of their growth, required maintaining neuronal polarity and connections among neurons. Investigating the relationship between

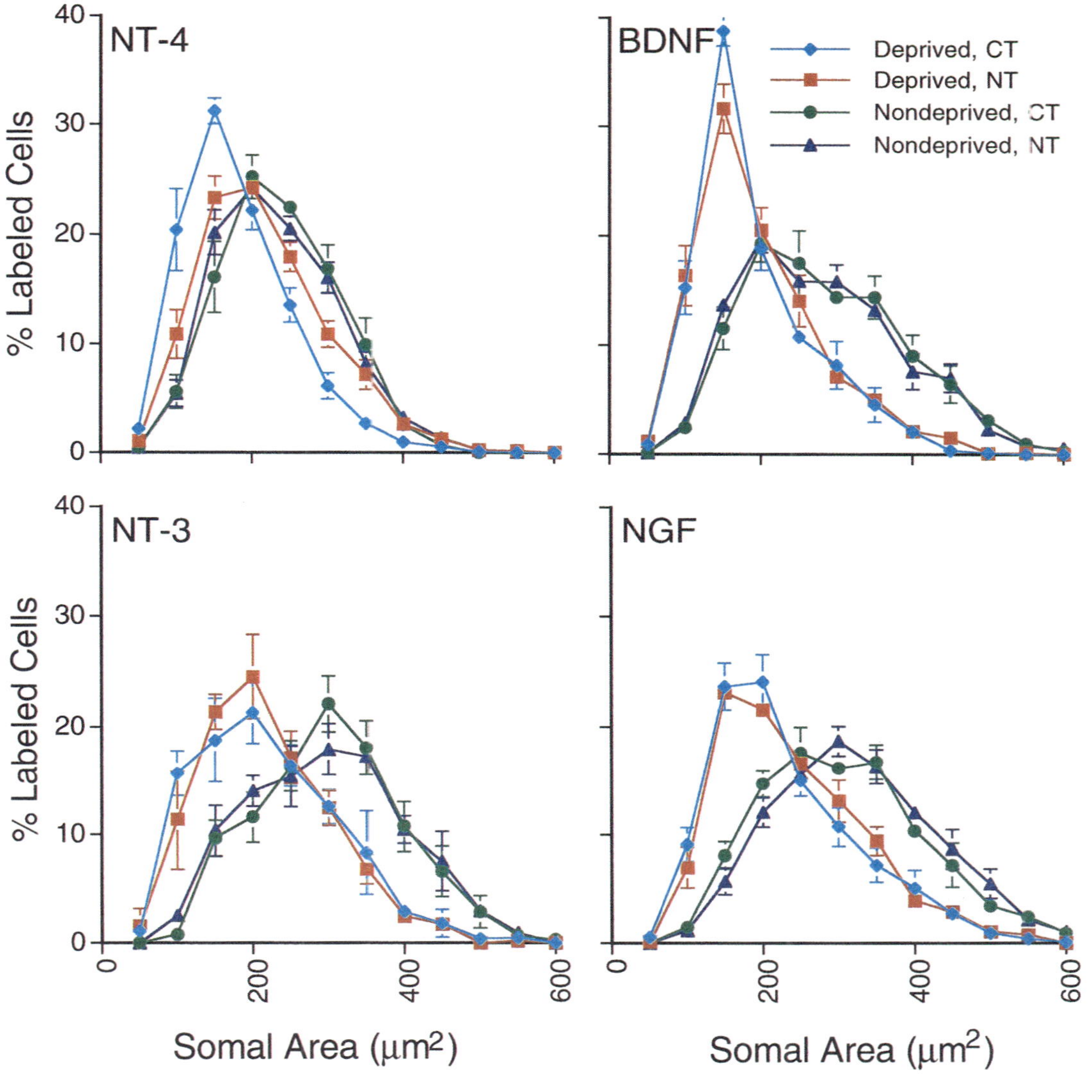

Figure 5. NT-4 prevents the shift in neuronal soma size caused by MD. Histograms for somal area (mean ± S.E.M. percentage per bin) are shown for deprived (closed-eye) and nondeprived (open-eye) layers of the LGN in MD animals injected with neurotrophin-coated (NT) and control (CT) microspheres. For control neurons in all animals, the distribution in the deprived layer (*blue*) is shifted significantly toward smaller cells relative to the distribution in the nondeprived layer (*green*). NT-4 treatment shifted the distribution in the deprived layer (*upper left, red*) back toward that seen in the nondeprived layer. The other neurotrophins had no effect on the distribution in the deprived layer (*red*). None of the neurotrophins affected the size of cells in the nondeprived layer (*purple*).

neurotrophin actions and the changes in neural activity that result from sensory experience clearly was possible only in the intact brain. Studies such as these should continue to play a critical role in understanding how the actions of neurotrophins are integrated with those of the other factors that regulate neuronal growth and the development of neural circuits.

ACKNOWLEDGMENTS

We thank Regeneron Pharmaceuticals for generously providing neurotrophins and the PC12*TrkB* cell line. This work was supported by a Broad Biomedical Research Foundation Fellowship (A.K.M), the Alfred P. Sloan Foundation and Esther A. and Joseph Klingenstein Fund (D.C.L), and National Institutes of Health grants EY-06617 (D.R.R.), NS-32742 (D.C.L.), and EY-07690 (L.C.K.).

REFERENCES

Allendoerfer, K.L., R.J. Cabelli, E. Escandon, D.R. Kaplan, K. Nikolics, and C.J. Shatz. 1994. Regulation of neurotrophin receptors during the maturation of the mammalian visual system. *J. Neurosci.* **14:** 1795.

Barbacid, M. 1994. The Trk family of neurotrophin receptors. *Neurobiology* **25:** 1386.

Bartlett, W.P. and G.A. Banker. 1984. An electron microscopic study of the development of axons and dendrites by hippocampal neurons in culture. I. Cells which develop without intercellular contacts. *J. Neurosci.* **4:** 1944.

Bear, M.F. and H. Coleman. 1990. Binocular competition in the control of geniculate cell size depends upon visual cortical *N*-methyl-D-aspartate receptor activation. *Proc. Natl. Acad. Sci.* **87:** 9246

Bear, M.F., A. Kleinschmidt, Q. Gu, and W. Singer. 1990. Disruption of experience-dependent synaptic modifications in striate cortex by infusion of an NMDA receptor antagonist. *J. Neurosci.* **10:** 909.

Bengzon, J., Z. Kokaia, P. Ernfors, M. Kokaia, G. Leanza, O.G. Nilsson, H. Persson, and O. Lindvall. 1993. Regulation of neurotrophin and trkA, trkB and trkC receptor messenger RNA expression in kindling. *Neuroscience* **53:** 433.

Berardi, N., L. Domenici, V. Parisi, T. Pizzorusso, A. Cellerino, and L. Maffei. 1993. Monocular deprivation effects in the rat visual cortex and lateral geniculate nucleus are prevented by nerve growth factor (NGF). I. Visual cortex. *Proc. R. Soc. Lond. B Biol. Sci.* **251:** 17.

Berninger, B., D.E. Garcia, N. Inagaki, C. Hahnel, and D. Lindholm. 1993. BDNF and NT-3 induce intracellular CA^{2+} elevation in hippocampal neurones. *NeuroReport* **4:** 1303.

Biffo, S., N. Offenhäuser, B.D. Carter, and Y.-A. Barde. 1995. Selective binding and internalization by truncated receptors restrict the availability of BDNF during development. *Development* **121:** 2461.

Blöchl, A. and H. Thoenen. 1995. Characterization of nerve growth factor (NGF) release from hippocampal neurons: Evidence for a constitutive and an unconventional sodium-dependent regulated pathway. *Eur. J. Neurosci.* **7:** 1220.

Bolz, J., N. Novak, M. Gotz, and T. Bonhoeffer. 1990. Formation of target-specific neuronal projections in organotypic slice cultures from rat visual cortex. *Nature* **346:** 359.

Bonhoeffer, T. 1996. Neurotrophins and activity-dependent development of the neocortex. *Curr. Opin. Neurobiol.* **6:** 119.

Bramham, C.R., T. Southland, J.M. Sarvey, M. Herkenham, and L.S. Brady. 1996. Unilateral LTP triggers bilateral increases in hippocampal neurotrophin and Trk receptor mRNA expression in behaving rats—Evidence for interhemispheric communication. *J. Comp. Neurol.* **368:** 371.

Cabelli, R.J., A. Hohn, and C.J. Shatz. 1995. Inhibition of ocular dominance column formation by infusion of NT-4/5 or BDNF. *Science* **267:** 1662.

Carmignoto, G., R. Canella, P. Candeo, M.C. Comelli, and L. Maffei. 1993. Effects of nerve growth factor on neuronal plasticity of the kitten visual cortex. *J. Physiol.* **464:** 343.

Castren, E., F. Zafra, H. Thoenen, and D. Lindholm. 1992. Light regulates expression of brain-derived neurotrophic factor mRNA in rat visual cortex. *Proc. Natl. Acad. Sci.* **89:** 9444.

Castren, E., M. Pitkanen, J. Sirvio, A. Parsadanian, and D. Lindholm. 1993. The induction of LTP increases BDNF and NGF mRNA but decreases NT-3 mRNA in the dentate gyrus. *NeuroReport* **4:** 895.

Chao, M.V. 1992. Neurotrophin receptors: A window into neuronal differentiation. *Neuron* **9:** 583.

Clary D.O. and L.F. Reichardt. 1994. An alternatively spliced form of the nerve growth factor receptor TrkA confers an enhanced response to neurotrophin 3. *Proc. Natl. Acad. Sci.* **91:** 11133.

Domenici, L., A. Cellerino, and L. Maffei. 1993. Monocular deprivation effects in the rat visual cortex and lateral geniculate nucleus are prevented by nerve growth factor (NGF). II. Lateral geniculate nucleus. *Proc. R. Soc. Lond. B Biol. Sci.* **251:** 25.

Domenici, L., G. Fontanesi, A. Cattaneo, P. Bagnoli, and L. Maffei. 1994. Nerve growth factor (NGF) uptake and transport following injection in the developing rat visual cortex. *Visual Neurosci.* **11:** 1093.

Ernfors, P., E.J. Bengzon, Z. Kokaia, H. Persson, and O. Lindvall. 1991. Increased levels of messenger RNAs for neurotrophic factors in the brain during epileptogenesis. *Neuron* **7:** 165.

Figurov, A., L.D. Pozzo-Miller, P. Olafsson, T. Wang, and B. Lu. 1996. Regulation of synaptic responses to high-frequency stimulation and LTP by neurotrophins in the hippocampus. *Nature* **381:** 706.

Gall, C.M. and P.J. Isackson. 1989. Limbic seizures increase neuronal production of messenger RNA for nerve growth factor. *Science* **245:** 758.

Harris, R.M. and T.A. Woolsey. 1981. Dendritic plasticity in mouse barrel cortex following postnatal vibrissa follicle damage. *J. Comp. Neurol.* **196:** 357.

Henderson, C. 1996. Role of neurotrophic factors in neuronal development. *Curr. Opin. Neurobiol.* **6:** 64.

Holtzman, D.M., J. Kilbridge, Y. Li, E.T. Cunningham, N.J. Lenn, D.O. Clary, L.F. Reichardt, and W.C. Mobley. 1995. TrkA expression in the CNS: Evidence for the existence of several novel NGF-responsive neurons. *J. Neurosci.* **15:** 1567.

Holtzman, D.M., Y. Li, L.F. Parada, S. Kinsman, C.K. Chen, J.S. Valletta, J. Zhou, J.B. Long, and W.C. Mobley. 1992. p140trk mRNA marks NGF-responsive forebrain neurons: Evidence that *trk* gene expression is induced by NGF. *Neuron* **9:** 465

Hume, R.I. and D. Purves. 1981. Geometry of neonatal neurones and the regulation of synapse elimination. *Nature* **293:** 469.

Kang, H. and E.M. Schuman. 1995. Long lasting neurotrophin-induced enhancement of synaptic transmission in the adult hippocampus. *Science* **267:** 1658

Katz, L.C. and D.M. Iarovici. 1990. Green fluorescent latex microspheres: A new retrograde tracer. *Neuroscience* **34:** 511.

Katz, L.C., A. Burkhalter, and W.J. Dreyer. 1984. Fluorescent latex microspheres as a retrograde neuronal marker for *in vivo* and *in vitro* studies of visual cortex. *Nature* **310:** 498.

Katz, L.C., C.D. Gilbert, and T.N. Wiesel. 1989. Local circuits and ocular dominance columns in monkey striate cortex. *J. Neurosci.* **9:** 1389.

Kim, H.G., T. Wang, P. Olafsson, and B. Lu. 1994. Neurotrophin 3 potentiates neuronal activity and inhibits gamma-aminobutyratergic synaptic transmission in cortical neurons. *Proc. Natl. Acad. Sci.* **91:** 12341.

Knipper, M., L.S. Leung, D. Zhao, and R.J. Rylett. 1994. Short-term modulation of glutamatergic synapses in adult rat hippocampus by NGF. *NeuroReport* **5:** 2433.

Large, T.H., S.C. Bodary, D.O. Clegg, G. Weskamp, U. Otten, and L.F. Otten. 1986. Nerve growth factor gene expression in the developing rat brain. *Science* **234:** 352.

Lesser, S.S. and D.C. Lo. 1995. Regulation of voltage-gated ion channels by nerve growth factor and ciliary neurotrophic factor in Sk-N-SH neuroblastoma cells. *J. Neurosci.* **15:** 253.

Levine, E.S., C.F. Dreyfus, I.B. Black, and M.R. Plummer. 1995. Brain-derived neurotrophic factor rapidly enhances synaptic transmission in hippocampal sensors via postsynaptic tyrosine kinase receptors. *Proc. Natl. Acad. Sci.* **92:** 8074.

Lewin G.R. and Y.-A. Barde. 1996. Physiology of the neurotrophins. *Annu. Rev. Neuroscience* **19:** 289.

Lindholm, D., E. Castren, M. Berzaghi, A. Blochl, and H. Thoenen. 1994. Activity-dependent and hormonal regulation of neurotrophin mRNA levels in the brain—Implications for neuronal plasticity. *J. Neurobiol.* **25:** 1362.

Lindsay, R.M. 1994. Neurotrophins and receptors. *Prog. Brain Res.* **103:** 3.

Lindsay, R.M., S.J. Wiegand, C.A. Altar, and P.S. DiStefano. 1994. Neurotrophic factors: From molecule to man. *Trends Neurosci.* **17:** 182.

Lo, D.C. 1995. Neurotrophic factors and synaptic plasticity. *Neuron* **15:** 979.

Lo, D.C., A.K. McAllister, and L.C. Katz. 1994. Neuronal transfection in brain slices using particle-mediated gene transfer. *Neuron* **13:** 1263.

Lohof, A.M., N.Y. Ip, and M.-M. Poo. 1993. Potentiation of developing neuromuscular synapses by the neurotrophins NT-3 and BDNF. *Nature* **365:** 350.

McAllister, A.K., D.C. Lo, and L.C. Katz. 1995a. Neurotrophins regulate dendritic growth in developing visual cortex. *Neuron* **15:** 791.

———. 1995b. Neurotrophins and activity interact to modulate dendritic growth in developing ferret visual cortex. *Soc. Neurosci. Abstr.* **21:** 1284.

———. 1996. Neurotrophin regulation of cortical dendritic growth requires activity. *Neuron* **17:** 1057.

Merlio, J.-P., P. Ernfors, M. Jaber, and H. Persson. 1992. Molecular cloning of rat *trk*C and distribution of cells expressing messenger RNAs for members of the *trk* family in the rat central nervous system. *Neuroscience* **51:** 513.

Molnar, Z. and C. Blakemore. 1991. Lack of regional specificity for connections formed between thalamus and cortex in coculture. *Nature* **351:** 475.

Mudo, G., T. Salin, D.F. Condorelli, X.H. Jiang, P. Dell' Albani, T. Timmusk, M. Metsis, H. Funakoshi, and N. Belluardo. 1995. Seizures increase trkC mRNA expression in the dentate gyrus of rat hippocampus. Role of glutamate receptor activation. *J. Mol. Neurosci.* **6:** 11.

Nawa, H., J. Carnahan, and C. Gall. 1995. BDNF protein measured by a novel enzyme immunoassay in normal brains and after seizure: Partial disagreement with mRNA levels. *Eur. J. Neurosci.* **7:** 1527.

Patterson, S.L., L.M. Grover, P.A. Schwartzkroin, and M. Bothwell. 1992. Neurotrophin expression in rat hippocampal slices: A stimulus paradigm inducing LTP in CA1 evokes increases in BDNF and NT-3 mRNAs. *Neuron* **9:** 1081.

Peinado, A. and L.C. Katz. 1990. Development of cortical spiny stellate cells: Retraction of a transient apical dendrite. *Soc. Neurosci. Abstr.* **16:** 1127.

Prakash, N., S. Cohen-Cory, and R.D. Frostig. 1996. Rapis and opposite effects of BDNF and NGF on the functional organization of the adult cortex *in vivo*. *Nature* **381:** 702.

Purves, D. and R.I. Hume. 1981. The relation of postsynaptic geometry to the number of presynatic neurones that innervate autonomic ganglion cells. *J. Neurosci.* **1:** 441.

Purves, D., W.D. Snider, and J.T. Voyvodic. 1988. Trophic regulation of nerve cell morphology and innervation in the autonomic nervous system. *Nature* **336:** 123.

Reiter, H.O., D.M. Waitzman, and M.P. Stryker. 1986. Cortical activity blockade prevents ocular dominance plasticity in the visual cortex. *Exp. Brain Res.* **65:** 182.

Riddle, D.R., D.C. Lo, and L.C. Katz. 1995. NT-4-mediated rescue of lateral geniculate neurons from effects of monocular deprivation. *Nature* **378:** 189.

Ringstedt, T., H. Lagercrantz, and H. Persson. 1993. Expression of members of the *trk* family in the developing postnatal rat brain. *Dev. Brain Res.* **72:** 119.

Ruit, K.G. and W.D. Snider. 1991. Administration or deprivation of nerve growth factor during development permanently alters neuronal geometry. *J. Comp. Neurol.* **314:** 106.

Ruit, K.G., P.A. Osborne, R.E. Schmidt, E.M. Johnson, and W.D. Snider. 1990. Nerve growth factor regulates sympathetic ganglion cell morphology and survival in the adult mouse. *J. Neurosci.* **10:** 2412.

Salin, T., G. Mudo, X.H. Jiang, T. Timmusk, M. Metsis, and N. Belluardo. 1995. Up-regulation of trkB mRNA expression in the rat striatum after seizures. *Neurosci. Lett.* **194:** 181.

Schoups, A.A., R.C. Elliot, W.J. Friedman, and I.B. Black. 1995. NGF and BDNF are differentially modulated by visual experience in the developing geniculocortical pathway. *Dev. Brain Res.* **86:** 326.

Sherman, S.M. and P.D. Spear. 1982. Organization of visual pathways in normal and visually deprived cats. *Physiol. Rev.* **62:** 738.

Snider, W.D. 1988. Nerve growth factor enhances dendritic arborizations of sympathetic ganglion cells in developing mammals. *J. Neurosci.* **8:** 2628.

Stoop, R. and M.-M. Poo. 1996. Synaptic modulation by neurotrophic factors: Differential and synergistic effects of brain-derived neurotrophic factor and ciliary neurotrophic factor. *J. Neurosci.* **16:** 3256.

Stryker, M.P. and W.A. Harris. 1986. Binocular impulse blockade prevents the formation of ocular dominance columns in cat visual cortex. *J. Neurosci.* **6:** 2117.

Thoenen, H. 1995. Neurotrophins and neuronal plasticity. *Science* **270:** 592.

Valenzuela, D.M., P.C. Maisonpierre, D.G. Glass, E. Rojas, L. Nuñez, Y. Kong, D.R. Gies, T.N. Stitt, N.Y. Ip, and G.D. Yancopoulos. 1993. Alternative forms of rat TrkC with different functional capabilities. *Neuron* **10:** 963.

Valverde, F. 1968. Structural changes in the area striata of the mouse after enucleation. *Exp. Brain Res.* **5:** 274.

Verdi, J.M., A.K. Groves, I. Fariñas, K. Jones, M.A. Marchionni, L.F. Reichardt, and D.J. Anderson. 1996. A reciprocal cell-cell interaction mediated by NT-3 and neuregulins controls the early survival and development of sympathetic neuroblasts. *Neuron* **16:** 515.

Wang, T., K. Xie, and B. Lu. 1995. Neurotrophins promote maturation of developing neuromuscular synapses. *J. Neurosci.* **15:** 4796.

Wiesel, T.N. 1982. Postnatal development of the visual cortex and the influence of environment. *Nature* **299:** 583.

Yamamoto, N., K. Yamada, T. Kurotani, and K. Toyama. 1992. Laminar specificity of extrinsic cortical connections studied in coculture preparations. *Neuron* **9:** 217.

Zafra, F., B. Hengerer, J. Leibrock, and H. Thoenen. 1990. Activity-dependent regulation of BDNF and NGF mRNAs in the rat hippocampus is mediated by non-NMDA glutamate receptors. *EMBO J.* **9:** 3545.

In Vivo Development of Neuronal Structure and Function

H.T. CLINE, G.-Y. WU, AND R. MALINOW
Cold Spring Harbor Laboratory, Cold Spring Harbor, New York 11724

The formation of the nervous system requires a coordinated development of neuronal morphology and synaptic physiology. We have used the frog retinotectal system to examine the development of brain structure and function. The retinotectal system of frogs is well known for its developmental and experience-dependent synaptic plasticity. As the animal grows, retinotectal axon arbors migrate considerable distances within the contralateral optic tectum in order to maintain a high degree of refinement in the retinotopic map. The capacity of the arbors to move within the tectal neuropil indicates that the retinotectal synapses and axon arbor branches are dynamic. The maintenance of retinotopy despite the axonal mobility indicates that there must be a mechanism which controls sites of synapse formation and stabilization. Considerable evidence supports the hypothesis that N-methyl-D-aspartate (NMDA) receptor activity is required to maintain the retinotopic map (Cline 1991), but it is still not clear how activity influences the neuronal growth and synaptogenesis required for the development of organized projections. Here, we review two sets of experiments that provide key information on the interaction between morphological and electrophysiological aspects of circuit formation. In one set of experiments, we have performed time lapse in vivo imaging of retinotectal axons in albino *Xenopus* tadpoles to examine the time course and magnitude of morphological changes of the normal retinal axons and those exposed to the NMDA receptor antagonist, APV. In the second set of experiments, we have examined the development of retinotectal glutamatergic synaptic responses using whole-cell patch-clamp recordings of tectal neurons in an isolated whole-brain preparation. Finally, we present a model for "minimal cost" formation of functional circuits in which trial synapses are functionally silent. These silent synapses are maintained only if they are functionally relevant to the developing circuit.

The retinotectal projection is glutamatergic, as are the majority of excitatory synapses within the vertebrate central nervous system (Hollman and Heinemann 1994). This transmission is mediated by two types of postsynaptic ionotropic glutamate receptors, the α-amino-3-hydroxy-5-methyl-4-isoxazole propionic acid (AMPA) and NMDA receptors. AMPA and NMDA receptors can be readily distinguished in electrophysiological recordings based on their pharmacological and biophysical properties (Edmonds et al. 1995). In particular, at hyperpolarized potentials, NMDA receptor channels are largely blocked by Mg^{++}, whereas AMPA receptors are capable of transmission. These receptors are thought to be colocalized within neurons (Hestrin et al. 1990); however, the subcellular distribution of the receptor types at individual synapses is less clear (Bekkers and Stevens 1989; Kullmann 1994; Isaac et al. 1995; Liao et al. 1995).

The role of NMDA receptors in structural plasticity of developing sensory projections prompted several investigations into the relative contribution of NMDA and AMPA receptors to synaptic transmission during postnatal development in mammals. These studies indicate a developmental shift in the component makeup of glutamatergic synaptic responses from a low AMPA/NMDA ratio in younger tissue to a higher AMPA/NMDA ratio in older animals, as well as a change in the kinetics of the NMDA response (Fox et al. 1989; Carmignoto and Vicini 1992; Hestrin 1992; Crair and Malenka 1995).

The initial events during synaptogenesis of excitatory synapses have been more difficult to elucidate. Several studies using slices have shown that neurons exhibit NMDA responsivity soon after differentiation and prior to synaptogenesis (Blanton et al. 1990; LoTurco et al. 1991). In the hippocampus, pure NMDA-receptor-mediated transmission is more prevalent in tissue from younger animals (Durand et al. 1996; Liao and Malinow 1996). Furthermore, new synapses generated during a plastic paradigm in the owl auditory system primarily use NMDA-receptor-mediated transmission (Feldman et al. 1996). These observations raise the possibility that glutamatergic synaptic transmission may be initially mediated solely by NMDA receptors and that the AMPA component of the synaptic response becomes functional as the neuron and synapses mature.

BRANCH DYNAMICS AND GROWTH IN RETINOTECTAL AXONS

Support for an anatomical contribution to neuronal plasticity has long been available from studies in several systems (Bailey and Kandel 1995), including visual projections (Sretavan et al. 1988; Constantine-Paton et al. 1990; Antonini and Stryker 1993; Goodman and Shatz 1993; Darian-Smith and Gilbert 1994; Ghosh and Shatz 1994). However, the time course over which these changes occurred is not known. The expectation that changes in neuronal structure occur slowly suggested that they may represent the outcome of plasticity events rather than contribute to the plasticity itself. Recent studies show that geniculocortical axon arbors can change their structure within days of monocular deprivation (Antonini and Stryker 1993). Retinotectal axons in frog tadpoles also change their structure to a significant degree over a period of hours and days (O'Rourke and Fraser 1990; O'Rourke et al. 1994; Zou and Cline 1996). The rates of structural changes in axon arbors that we have recently reported (Witte et al. 1996) are compatible with the idea that some forms of neuronal plasticity that occur on the time scale of minutes to hours can be mediated by physical changes in the structure of the component neurons.

We used the laser scanning confocal microscope (LSCM) to take repeated images of individual retinal axons labeled with the lipophilic fluorescent carbocyanine dye, DiI, in anesthetized *Xenopus laevis* tadpoles. The LSCM allows reliable resolution of branches of approximately 2 μm in arbors with a complex three-dimensional structure. Axon arbors were observed at 30-minute intervals for a period of 2 hours, or at 2-hour intervals for a total period of 8 hours, in an attempt to gather information on the continuum of morphological changes in the arbor. Between imaging sessions, animals recovered from anesthetic and were put in an incubator with red light to permit visual stimulation. By mounting the animal in the same position for subsequent imaging sessions, stable arbor branches can be identified from observation to observation, and dynamic branches can be detected (Fig. 1).

Arbors observed at 30-minute intervals show relatively modest changes in total arbor structure over the observation period (Fig. 1) that were mainly confined to additions and retractions of shorter branch tips and rearrangements of growth cones. Arbors observed at 2-hour intervals show more obvious changes in structure than those imaged at 30-minute intervals (Fig. 1).

The magnitude and distribution of branch dynamics within two arbors, imaged at 30-minute and 2-hour intervals, are shown in Figure 1. The "stable" portion of the arbor, which is unchanged during the observation period, is shown in pink, and the dynamic portion of the arbor is in white. On average, 50% of the total branch length of the axon remained unchanged over an 8-hour period. The remainder of the arbor structure is remodeled at some point during the 8 hours over which the arbor was observed. The remodeled portion of the arbor includes many higher-order branches tens of microns in length. This contrasts with the degree of remodeling seen over a 2-hour time course, where branches tens of microns in length are only rarely included in the remodeled portion of the arbor.

Comparable numbers of branches are added and retracted at each time point (Fig. 2). Over an 8-hour observation period, the total number of branch additions is slightly greater than branch retractions. This tendency toward net branch addition likely corresponds to the gradual increase in arbor complexity seen when arbors were imaged at daily intervals. More of the branches that were added and retracted at 2-hour intervals were longer than those added and retracted over 30-minute intervals (Fig. 1), reflecting the longer time allowed for branch extension in the 2-hour-interval experiments.

The population of axons examined at both 30-minute and 2-hour intervals had comparable initial numbers of branches; however, the total number of branch additions recorded over 2 hours with the 30-minute observations is significantly greater than the number of branch additions recorded over 2 hours with one single observation. This discrepancy indicates that branches are added and retracted too quickly to be recorded with a single observation over a 2-hour interval. Therefore, observations taken at the shorter time interval provide more accurate data on the numbers of branch additions and retractions.

A principal finding of the imaging experiments is that axon arbor structure can change over a time scale of minutes to hours. Time-lapse images of growing axons taken at 3-minute, 30-minute, and 2-hour intervals show that the rearrangements in arbor morphology are the result of dynamic additions and retractions of branches, as well as extension and shortening of preexisting branches (Witte et al. 1996). Over 8 hours, we observed a modest increase in the total number of branches, but over this same period, an average of 50% of the total branch length in an arbor was modified. Synaptophysin and synapsin 1 immunolocalization within single retinal axons shows that synaptic vesicle proteins are concentrated in discrete puncta which are distributed throughout the axon arbor (Anderson et al. 1993). Therefore, it is likely that the degree of restructuring of the presynaptic axon observed here has an impact on retinotectal synaptic communication.

In the 30-minute observations, branch additions and retractions were distributed throughout the arbor structure without apparent hot spots of dynamic activity. However, in observations taken at 2-hour intervals, some arbors appeared to have net growth concentrated in particular areas or branches within the arbor. This indicates that changes in arbor morphology seen in observations taken at 1- to 2-hour intervals already reflect the selective stabilization and further elongation of some branches, as well as the retraction of other newly sprouted branches.

To examine the effect of blocking NMDA receptors on branch dynamics, single retinal axons were imaged in animals exposed to APV. An initial image of the axon was taken prior to exposure to APV, and four more images were collected of the axons at 30-minute intervals in the presence of 100 μM DL-APV in the rearing solution. Exposure of animals to APV caused a rapid increase in the rate of branch additions, which was statistically significant ($p < 0.05$) even at the first 30-minute time point in APV (Fig. 3). APV exposure did not change the rates of branch retractions. Over the 2-hour observation period, this resulted in a significant increase in branch-tip number in APV-treated

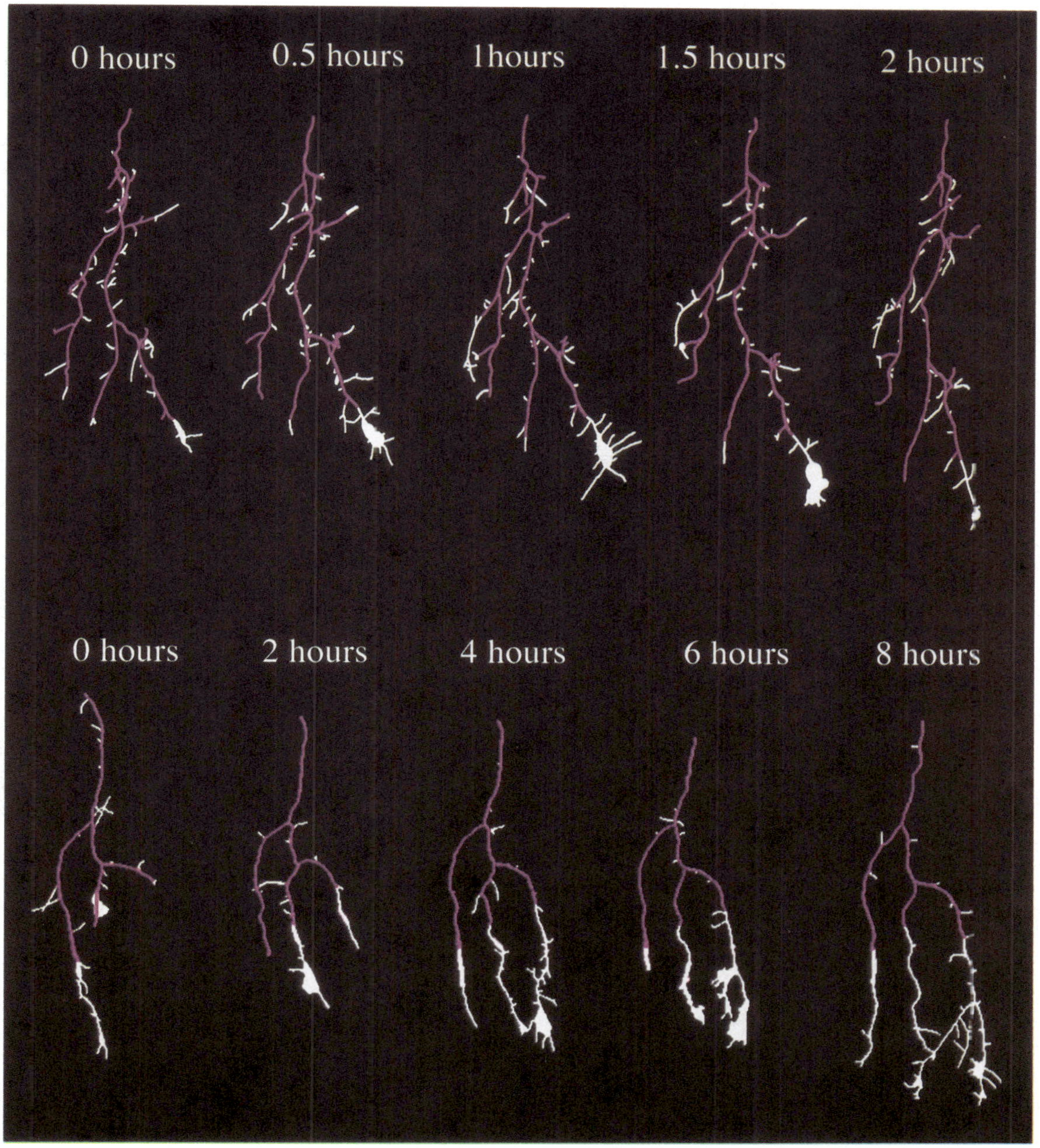

Figure 1. Stable and dynamic portion of axon arbors imaged for 2 hr and 8 hr. The stable portion of an arbor imaged at 30-min intervals over 2 hr (*top*) and one imaged at 2-hr intervals over 8 hr (*bottom*) are colored pink, and the dynamic portion of the arbors is shown in white. For the arbor observed every 30 min, the dynamic portion of the arbor is confined to shorter branch tips and a growth cone. For the arbors observed every 2 hr, half of the total branch length of the arbor changes over the course of the observation period. (Reprinted, with permission, from Witte et al. 1996.)

arbors compared to untreated controls. However, there was no difference between untreated and APV-treated arbors after 24-hour APV exposure, consistent with previous studies showing that APV disrupted topography but not axon arbor morphology (Cline 1991).

The cellular mechanisms controlling arbor complexity are not yet known. One possibility is that branch additions are actively induced at specific sites within the arbor and the new branches have a high probability of being stabilized. A second possibility is that new branches are added in excess throughout the arbor structure. Some of those branches might then be stabilized and the remainder would be retracted. The stabilized branches would be sites of further elaboration as new branches sprouted on these branches and became stabilized themselves. We observe a vast ex-

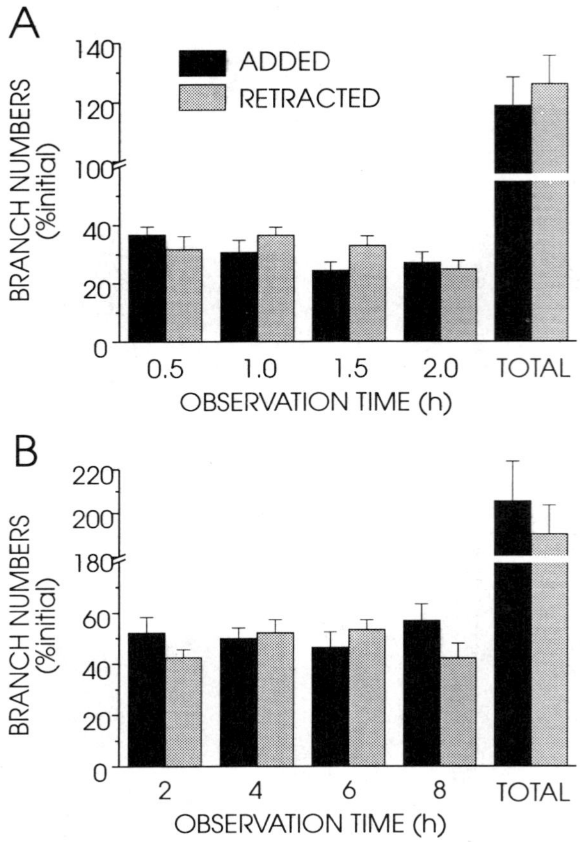

Figure 2. Branch additions and retractions for arbors observed at 30-min and 2-hr intervals. The numbers of branch additions and retractions for each time point for 30-min observations (*A*) and 2-hr observations (*B*) and for the entire observation periods are graphed relative to the initial number of branches per axon arbor.

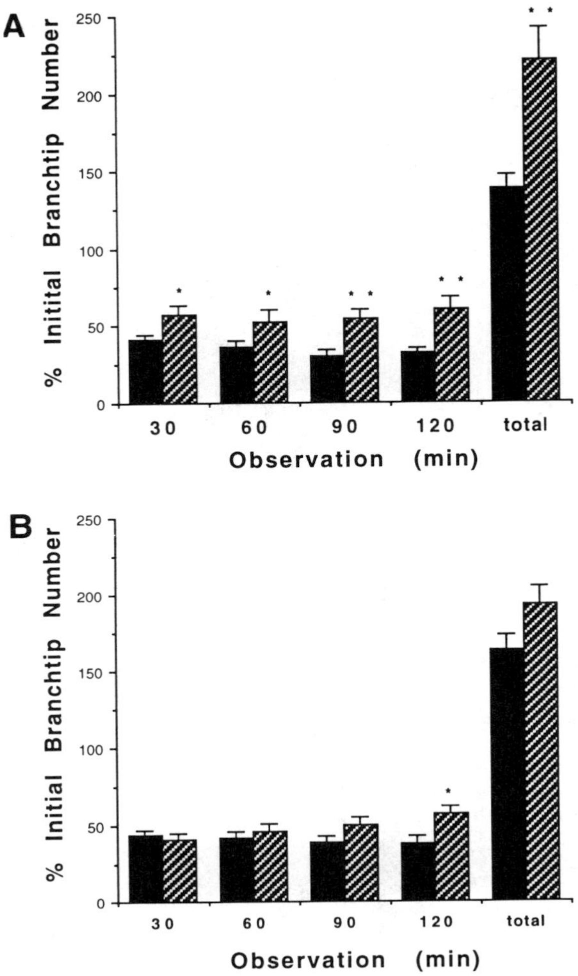

Figure 3. APV increases the rate of branch additions in retinal axon arbors. Rates of branch additions (*A*) and retractions (*B*) for arbors in control (*black* bars) and APV-treated animals (*shaded* bars) observed at 30-min intervals. The branch additions at each time point and over the 2-hr period are greater in arbors from APV-treated animals than in controls.

cess of branch additions to the arbor, apparently added without any spatial order. Blocking NMDA receptor activity increases the rate of branch additions. A small fraction of new branches are maintained, but the majority are rapidly retracted. These data are consistent with the second scenario mentioned above. These data are also consistent with the increasing evidence of a role for branch retraction in structural plasticity (Callaway and Katz 1991; Katz and Callaway 1992; Antonini and Stryker 1993).

THE FIRST THREE DAYS OF A CENTRAL GLUTAMATERGIC SYNAPSE

To examine the development of glutamatergic synaptic transmission in the vertebrate CNS, we developed a preparation of the isolated intact tadpole brain amenable to reliable single-fiber stimulation, whole-cell recording and dye labeling, pharmacological control of the extracellular environment, and transient expression with a recombinant viral vector. The tadpole optic tectum is particularly advantageous for the study of neural development because new neurons are constantly being generated in a proliferative zone in the caudal region of the optic tectum. Neurons from rostral tectum are chronologically older and morphologically more complex than neurons in caudal tectum, so that within a single preparation, there exist neurons over a range of developmental stages arranged along the rostro-caudal (RC) axis of the tectum (Fig. 4).

Retinotectal synaptic currents were evoked by stimulating retinal axons in the optic chiasm. Excitatory postsynaptic currents (EPSCs) recorded from the tectal neurons at different positions along the RC extent of the tectum reveal a developmental progression in the glutamatergic responses. Mature neurons located in the rostral third of tectum exhibit classic

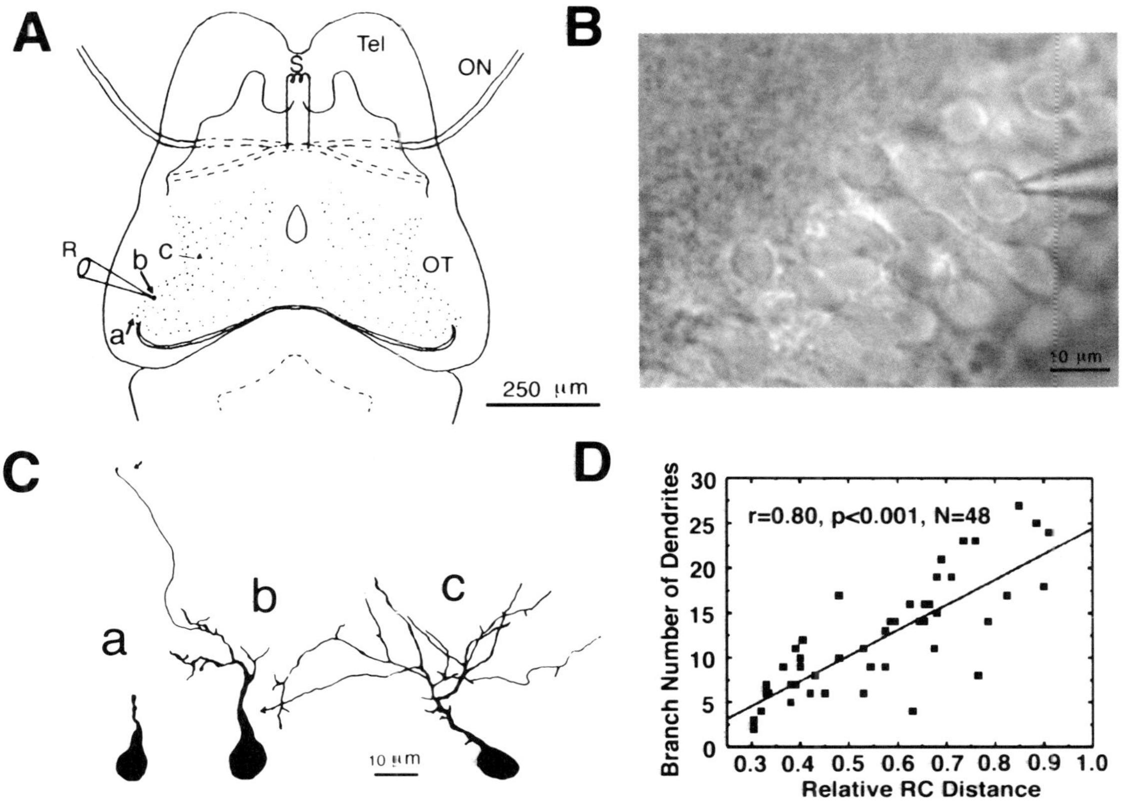

Figure 4. (*A*) Diagram of the rostral portion of the whole-brain preparation. A stimulating electrode (S) is positioned in the optic chiasm on the ventral aspect of the brain to evoke retinotectal synaptic responses. A recording patch pipette (R) is shown in the optic tectal cell body region (OT). Tectal locations (a,b,c) refer to positions of dye-labeled neurons in *C*. (*B*) Optic tectal neurons and a patch pipette positioned close to a tectal neuronal cell body. (*C*) Representative dye-labeled neurons from the caudal (a), middle (b), and rostral (c) regions of optic tectum, corresponding to the designated locations in the diagram in *A*. (*D*) Plot of dendritic branch tip number versus relative distance from the caudal border of the optic tectum. Branch number is highly correlated with the relative position of the neuronal cell body along the RC axis of the tectum.

glutamatergic synaptic transmission (Fig. 5A). EPSCs recorded at -60 mV have rapid onset and decay times and are blocked by the specific AMPA receptor antagonist CNQX. At +55 mV, EPCSs rise rapidly but decay more slowly than at hyperpolarized potentials. CNQX blocks the rapid component, leaving a slow component, which is blocked by APV.

In contrast to the synaptic physiology recorded from more mature neurons in rostral tectum, recordings from younger neurons in caudal tectum showed responses primarily (or even solely) mediated by NMDA receptors. In some neurons from caudal tectum, evoked synaptic responses are only recorded at depolarized potentials and are completely blocked by APV (Fig. 5B). Evoked responses recorded from neurons at different locations along the RC tectal axis show a progressive increase in the amplitude of the AMPA component with no change in the amplitude of the NMDA component as a function of position along the RC axis of the tectum. The AMPA/NMDA ratio is highly correlated with cell body position along the RC axis of the tectum (Fig. 5).

The progressive changes in AMPA-mediated responses with no change in NMDA-mediated responses suggest that synapses initially transmit with only NMDA receptors and acquire AMPA responsivity as they mature. To gain more insight into the nature of responses at individual synapses, we evoked single-fiber transmission and compared amplitude distributions of responses obtained at hyperpolarized and depolarized potentials. Associated with position in the RC axis, we see a significant decrease in failure rate at hyperpolarized potentials, but we see no significant decrease in failure rate at depolarized potentials (Fig. 6). A general increase in presynaptic function (e.g., increase in the number of synapses or probability of release) during development should produce a comparable decrease in failure rate in both hyperpolarized and depolarized potentials. This indicates that there is a change in postsynaptic function.

Evoked responses recorded from (mature) neurons in rostral tectum show comparable levels of failures at depolarized and hyperpolarized potentials (Fig. 6E,F). However, recordings from neurons in caudal tectum show significantly more failures at -60 mV than at +55 mV (Fig. 6A,B). If there are synapses showing only NMDA responses, then the failure rate at hyperpolarized potentials will be greater than at depolarized potentials (Liao et al. 1995). The fraction of synaptic responses mediated solely by NMDA receptors can be

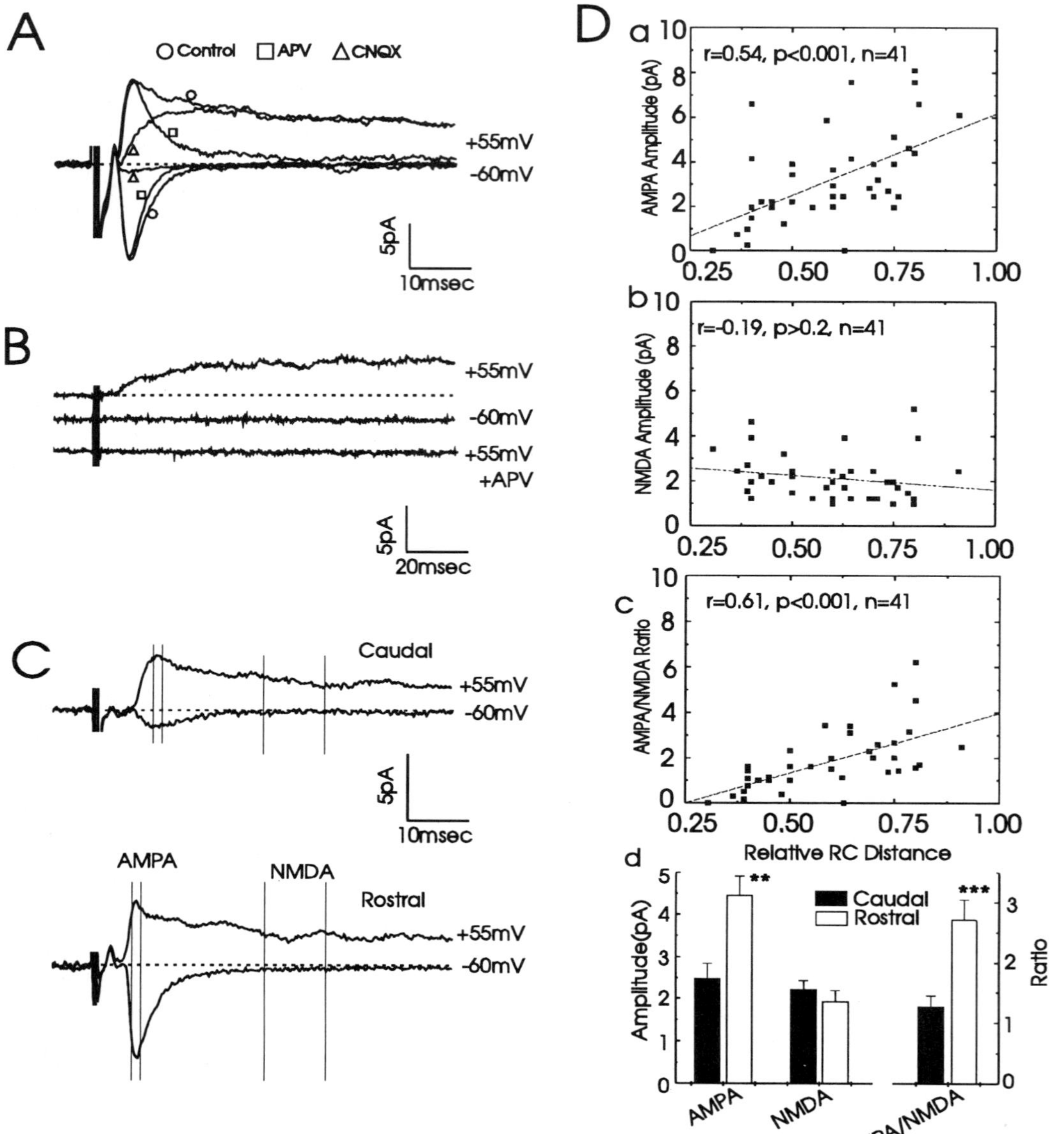

Figure 5. The AMPA component of the synaptic response increases with neuronal development. (*A*) Retinotectal evoked synaptic responses recorded in rostral optic tectum have mixed AMPA and NMDA components. Each trace is the average of 100 consecutive trials. Top 3 traces obtained at +55 mV, bottom 3 traces obtained at –60 mV. Symbols indicate no drugs (control); 100 μM DL-APV (APV); 10 μM (CNQX) in perfusate during recording. (*B*) Evoked synaptic transmission recorded from a neuron in caudal optic tectum with pure NMDA responses. No evoked response is recorded when the neuron is held at –60 mV. The slow response recorded at +55 mV is blocked by APV. (*C*) Evoked responses in 2 neurons, from caudal (*top*) and rostral (*bottom*) tectum. Windows used to measure AMPA (at –60 mV) and NMDA (at +55 mV) components of transmission are indicated. Each trace shown in *A–C* is the average of 10–50 consecutive responses. (*D*) Plots of the amplitudes of the AMPA (*a*) and NMDA (*b*) responses and AMPA/NMDA ratio (*c*) of single-fiber responses for neurons recorded at different positions along the RC axis. (*d*) Values (mean ± S.E.M.) for responses from neurons in caudal (n = 21) or rostral (n = 20) tectum are indicated. The amplitude of the AMPA response increases from an average of 2.4 ± 0.4 pA in neurons from caudal tectum to 4.4 ± 0.4 pA in neurons from rostral tectum, whereas the amplitude of the NMDA response is the same in neurons from caudal (2.2 ± 0.2 pA) and rostral (1.9 ± 0.3 pA) tectum. The average AMPA/NMDA ratio increases from 1.3 ± 0.2 in neurons from caudal tectum to 2.7 ± 0.3 in neurons from rostral tectum.

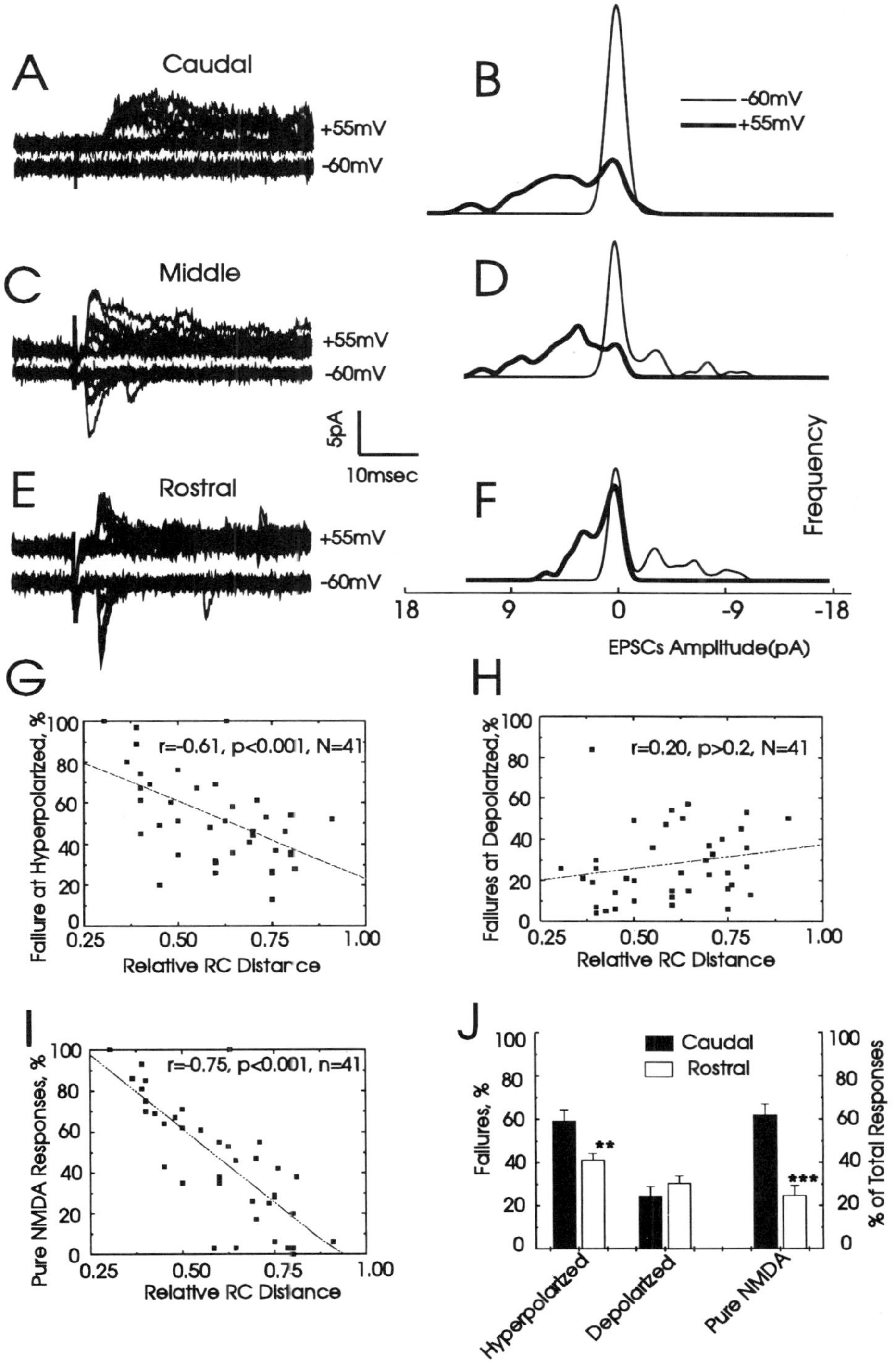

Figure 6. The fraction of pure NMDA responses decreases with neuronal development. Evoked synaptic currents recorded at +55 mV and −60 mV from neurons located in caudal (*A*), middle (*C*), and rostral (*E*) optic tectum. Amplitude distribution histograms of synaptic currents recorded at −60 mV (*light* line) and +55 mV (*dark* line) are shown to the right of each set of recordings (*B*, *D*, *F*). The peaks at 0 amplitude represent synaptic failures. Note that the failure rates at the two potentials are similar in the neuron from rostral tectum, but are successively more disparate in neurons from middle and caudal tectum. Plots of the failure rates at hyperpolarized (*G*) and depolarized (*H*) potentials. The fraction of total events that are mediated purely by NMDA receptors (*I*) for the 41 neurons recorded at different locations along the RC optic tectal axis decreases from ~100% in caudal tectum to ~5% in rostral tectum. (*J*) Failure rates at hyperpolarized potentials decrease significantly from 59 ± 5% in caudal tectum to 41 ± 3% in rostral tectum. Failure rates at depolarized potentials increase from 24 ± 4% in caudal tectum to 30 ± 3% in rostral tectum. The fraction of pure NMDA responses decreases from 62 ± 5% in caudal neurons to 25 ± 4% in rostral neurons (mean ± S.E.M. **, $p < 0.01$; ***, $p < 0.001$).

estimated by comparing the failure rates at hyperpolarized and depolarized potentials. This is because responses mediated by only NMDA receptors are seen as failures at hyperpolarized potentials, but are detected at depolarized potentials. We estimate that pure NMDA responses account for nearly 100% of transmission in (immature) neurons from caudal tectum, and this form of transmission decreases to about 15% as neurons mature (rostral tectum).

Single-fiber responses from cells at more developed stages show a larger synaptic AMPA component. This could be because there is increased presynaptic function (either from increased release probability or increased number of synaptic contacts) or because existing pure NMDA synapses acquire AMPA responses. Our data suggest that there is no net increase in presynaptic function at the connection between a single retinal ganglion cell fiber and a given postsynaptic cell. This is indicated by the observation that there is no increase in the NMDA component of transmission nor in the failure rate at depolarized potentials. If there were an increase in presynaptic function, one would expect an increase in these parameters.

This view is supported by the estimate of pure NMDA responses evoked early and later in development. Responses in caudal tectum show many more failures at hyperpolarized compared to depolarized potentials, indicating a large fraction of responses mediated purely by NMDA receptors. In contrast, in rostral tectum there is little difference in failure rate at depolarized and hyperpolarized potentials, indicating that few responses activate only NMDA receptors. Thus, the simplest model to explain all of our data, including evoked and spontaneous responses at hyperpolarized and depolarized potentials, is that initial synapses have only NMDA receptors and acquire AMPA receptor function as development progresses.

Two additional measures of synaptic physiology that have been previously studied in a developmental context were analyzed: the decay time course (Carmignoto and Vicini 1992; Hestrin 1992) and voltage dependence of NMDA responses (Ben-Ari et al. 1988). As shown previously for NMDA responses from rat cortical neurons (Carmignoto and Vicini 1992; Hestrin 1992), the time to decay was shorter in more mature tectal neurons (Fig. 7A). There was, however, no observable difference in the voltage dependence of NMDA responses obtained from rostral or caudal neurons (Fig. 7B,C).

Recent studies in the hippocampus indicate that a significant fraction of synapses activate only NMDA receptors and that a conversion of synapses from pure NMDA to mixed AMPA/NMDA sensitivity may underlie long-term potentiation (LTP), a form of activity-dependent plasticity (Isaac et al. 1995; Liao et al. 1995; Durand et al. 1996; Liao and Malinow 1996). We have demonstrated that pure NMDA-receptor-mediated transmission occurs at the retinotectal synapses and that a conversion from pure NMDA to mixed AMPA/

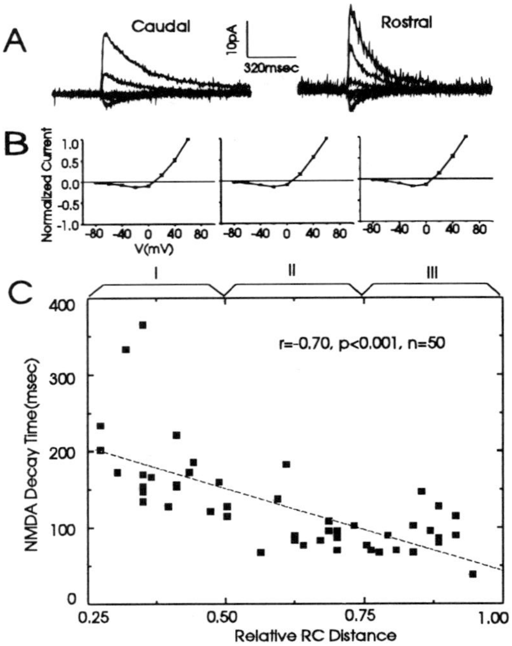

Figure 7. NMDA responses decay more rapidly in mature neurons than in less mature neurons. (*A*) Evoked synaptic NMDA responses recorded at a range of holding potentials (–80 mV to +60 mV, 20-mV steps) in the presence of 10 μM CNQX from neurons in caudal (*left*) and rostral (*right*) tectum. Note faster decays in the caudal neuron. (*B*) Current-voltage relations of evoked NMDA responses for neurons from caudal (n = 17), middle (n = 17), or rostral (n = 16) tectum. For each cell, current is normalized relative to amplitude at +60 mV. (*C*) Plot of the time from peak to 50% amplitude (decay time) of the NMDA component versus the position of the neuronal cell body along the RC axis. Neurons in the caudal tectum have a longer decay time than those in rostral tectum.

NMDA sensitivity occurs with development. This indicates that parallel mechanisms operate during development and LTP to stabilize and strengthen synapses.

We propose a model for minimal cost formation of functional circuits that provides a role for pure NMDA-receptor-sensitive transmission in the development of synaptic physiology (Fig. 8). From our in vivo imaging of the retinal axons, we know that they constantly extend small branches, the majority of which shortly retract. These short branches contain punctate immunostaining for synapsin and synaptophysin. We propose that the small branches form trial synapses that are mediated solely by NMDA receptors. These pure NMDA synapses are silent if the postsynaptic membrane is at resting potential. If the trial synapse is active at the same time that the postsynaptic neuron is depolarized, then there is transmission through the NMDA receptors resulting in an increase in postsynaptic calcium. This calcium signal can then trigger events that lead to the increase in AMPA receptor function at the active synapse. With the addition of AMPA recep-

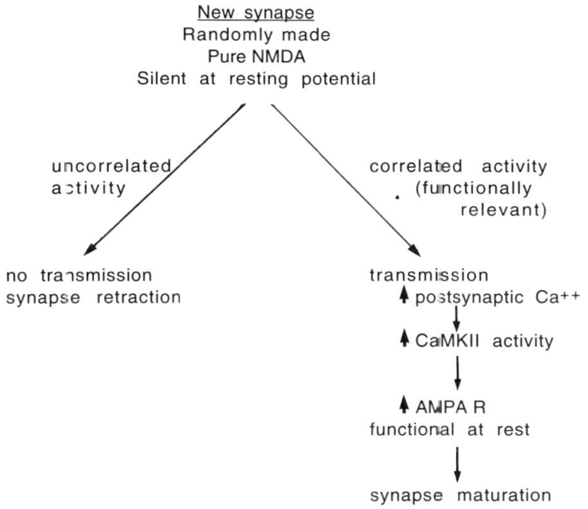

Figure 8. Model for "minimal cost" formation of functional circuits. We propose that new synapses between retinal axons and tectal cell dendrites form on a trial basis. They are mediated solely by NMDA receptors and are silent at resting potentials. The pattern of activity in the trial synapse is likely to be correlated with the activity pattern in the tectal neuron if that retinal ganglion cell body is located in a similar region of retina as the other retinal afferents that terminate on the tectal cell. In such a case, the postsynaptic membrane is depolarized at the same time as the trial synapse is active; there is transmission through the NMDA receptors at the trial synapse, resulting in a transient rise in postsynaptic calcium. One possible outcome of the elevated calcium is to activate calcium-sensitive enzymes, such as CaMKII, which may then increase AMPA receptor function at the trial synapse. The addition of AMPA receptors renders the synapse functional at resting potential. This synapse and the branch on which it is located are then stabilized. In cases where the activity in the trial synapse is not correlated with the pattern of activity in the postsynaptic neuron, no transmission occurs at the trial synapse. After a short period, possibly on the order of minutes, the synapse retracts. This may be followed by the retraction of the axon branch on which the trial synapse had formed.

tor function, the synapse becomes functional at resting potential. If the activity pattern in the trial synapse is not correlated with that in the postsynaptic neuron, there is no transmission through the pure NMDA synapse, and we propose that these silent trial synapses retract after a short time. Such a conditional two-step process for synapse formation and maturation may be beneficial in a system that requires transmission fidelity while new randomly connected synapses are continually formed. These randomly made synapses may transmit information only if other, more mature synapses, are active. Such a mechanism for controlling which synapses mature (i.e., develop an AMPA component) would select for inputs that are correlated with and thus presumably functionally relevant to, other converging inputs.

Such a system could work well in cases where new synapses are forming on neurons that have already developed AMPA responses at other synapses. For instance, the small fraction of pure NMDA responses recorded from rostral neurons may originate from new retinotectal synapses that form as retinal afferents grow into and migrate within the tectum. However, in the most caudal region of tectum, where the neurons can have 100% NMDA responses, the depolarization must come from another source. One potential source for depolarization in caudal tectum is GABAergic inputs. GABAergic synapses mediated by $GABA_A$ receptors develop early in the CNS (Schousboe and Redburn 1995); and in the tectum, we record picrotoxin-sensitive mEPSCs in neurons before they receive any glutamatergic inputs (G.-Y. Wu et al., unpubl.). $GABA_A$ responses are depolarizing in young neurons (Cherubini et al. 1991; Wang et al. 1994) and later become hyperpolarizing due to a shift in the chloride equilibrium (Cherubini et al. 1991). Therefore, depolarizing GABA responses may relieve the voltage-dependent block of the NMDA channel and permit conductance through the NMDA channel prior to addition of the AMPA component. One unexpected consequence of this might be that the first NMDA synapses to develop an AMPA component would be located close to, and be temporally correlated with, GABA inputs.

ACKNOWLEDGMENTS

This work was supported by grants from the National Institutes of Health and the National Science Foundation. Salary support from the National Down Syndrome Society was provided to H.T.C.

REFERENCES

Anderson, M., R.E. Fellows, and H.T. Cline. 1993. Distribution of presynaptic sites within retinal axon arbors of *Xenopus* larvae. *Soc. Neurosci. Abstr.* **19:** 239.

Antonini, A. and M.P. Stryker. 1993. Rapid remodeling of axonal arbors in the visual cortex. *Science* **260:** 1819.

Bailey, C.H. and E.R. Kandel. 1995. Structural changes accompanying memory storage. *Annu. Rev. Physiol.* **55:** 397.

Bekkers, J.M. and C.F. Stevens. 1989. NMDA and non-NMDA receptors are co-localized at individual excitatory synapses in cultured rat hippocampus. *Nature* **341:** 230.

Ben-Ari, Y., E.A. Cherubini, and K. Krnjevic. 1988. Changes in voltage-dependence of NMDA currents during development. *Neurosci. Lett.* **94:** 88.

Blanton, M.G., J.J. LoTurco, and A.R. Kreigstein. 1990. Endogenous neurotransmitter activates *N*-methyl-D-aspartate receptors on differentiating neurons in embryonic cortex. *Proc. Natl. Acad. Sci.* **87:** 8027.

Callaway, E.M. and L.C. Katz. 1991. Effects of binocular deprivation of clustered horizontal connections in cat striate cortex. *Proc. Natl. Acad. Sci.* **88:** 745.

Carmignoto, G. and S. Vicini. 1992. Activity-dependent decrease in NMDA receptor responses during development of the visual cortex. *Science* **258:** 1007.

Cherubini, E., J.L. Gaiarsa, and Y. Ben Ari. 1991. GABA: An excitatory transmitter in early postnatal life. *Trends Neurosci.* **14:** 515.

Cline, H.T. 1991. Activity-dependent plasticity in the visual systems of frogs and fish. *Trends Neurosci.* **14:** 104.

Constantine-Paton, M., H.T. Cline, and E.A. Debski. 1990. Patterned activity, synaptic convergence and the NMDA receptor in developing visual pathways. *Annu. Rev. Neurosci.* **13:** 129.

Crair, M.C. and R.C. Malenka. 1995. A critical period for long-term potentiation at thalamocortical synapses. *Nature* **375:** 325.

Darian-Smith, C. and C.D. Gilbert. 1994. Axonal sprouting accompanies functional reorganization in adult cat striate cortex. *Nature* **368:** 737.

Durand, G.M., Y. Kovalchuk, and A. Konnerth. 1996. Long-term potentiation and functional synapse induction in developing hippocampus. *Nature* **381:** 71.

Edmonds, B., A.J. Gibb, and D. Colquhoun. 1995. Mechanisms of activation of glutamate receptors and the time course of excitatory synaptic currents. *Annu. Rev. Physiol.* **57:** 495.

Feldman, D.E., M.S. Brainard, and E.I. Knudsen. 1996. Newly learned auditory responses mediated by NMDA receptors in the owl inferior colliculus. *Science* **271:** 525.

Fox, K., H. Sato, and N. Daw. 1989. The location and function of NMDA-receptors in cat and kitten cvisual cortex. *J. Neurosci.* **9:** 2443.

Ghosh, A. and C.J. Shatz. 1994. Segregation of geniculocortical afferents during the critical period: A role for subplate neurons. *J. Neurosci.* **14:** 3862.

Goodman, C.S. and C.J. Shatz. 1993. Developmental mechanisms that generate precise patterns of neuronal connectivity. *Cell* **72S:** 77.

Hestrin, S. 1992. Developmental regulation of NMDA receptor-mediated synaptic currents at a central synapse. *Nature* **357:** 686.

Hestrin, S., D.J. Perkel, P. Sah, T. Manabe, P. Renner, and R.A. Nicoll. 1990. Physiological properties of excitatory synaptic transmission in the central nervous system. *Cold Spring Harbor Symp. Quant. Biol.* **55:** 87.

Hollman, M. and S. Heinemann. 1994. Cloned glutamate receptors. *Annu. Rev. Neurosci.* **17:** 31.

Isaac, J.T.R., R.A. Nicoll, and R.C. Malenka. 1995. Evidence for silent synapses: Implications for the expression of LTP. *Neuron* **15:** 427.

Katz, L.C. and E.M. Callaway. 1992. Devolpment of local circuits in mammalian visual cortex. *Annu. Rev. Neurosci.* **15:** 31.

Kullmann, D.M. 1994. Amplitude fluctuations of dual-component EPSCs in hippocampal pyramidal cells: Implications for long-term potentiation. *Neuron* **12:** 1111.

Liao, D. and R. Malinow. 1996. Developmental regulation of glutamatertic synapses and LTP in hippocampal slice. *Learn. Mem.* (in press).

Liao, D., N.A. Hessler, and R. Malinow. 1995. Activation of postsynaptically silent synapses during pairing-induced LTP in CA1 region of hippocampal slice. *Nature* **375:** 400.

LoTurco, J.J., M.G. Blanton, and A.R. Kriegstein. 1991. Initial expression and endogenous activation of NMDA channels in early neocortical development. *J. Neurosci.* **11:** 792.

O'Rourke, N.A. and S.E. Fraser. 1990. Dynamic changes in optic fiber terminal arbors lead to retinotopic map formations: An in vivo confocal microscopic study. *Neuron* **5:** 159.

O'Rourke, N.A., H.T. Cline, and S.E. Fraser. 1994. Rapid remodeling of retinal arbors in the tectum with and without blockade of synaptic transmission. *Neuron* **12:** 921.

Schousboe, A. and D.A. Redburn. 1995. Modulatory actions of gamma aminobutyric acid (GABA) on GABA type A receptor subunit expression and function (Review). *J. Neurosci. Res.* **41:** 1.

Sretavan, D.W., C.J. Shatz, and M.P. Stryker. 1988. Modification of retinal ganglion cell axon morphology by prenatal infusion of tetrodotoxin. *Nature* **336:** 468.

Wang, J., D.B. Reichling, A. Kyrozis, and A.B. MacDermott. 1994. Developmental loss of GABA- and glycine-induced depolarization and Ca^{2+} transients in embryonic rat dorsal horn neurons in culture. *Eur. J. Neurosci.* **6:** 1275.

Witte, S., H. Stier, and H.T. Cline. 1996. In vivo observations of the timecourse and distribution of morphological dynamics in retinal axon arbors. *J. Neurobiol.* **31:** (in press.)

Zou, D.-J. and H.T. Cline. 1996. Expression of constitutively active CaMKII in target tissue modifies presynaptic axon arbor growth. *Neuron* **16:** 529.

Cortical Dynamics and Visual Perception

C.D. GILBERT, A. DAS, M. ITO, M.K. KAPADIA, AND G. WESTHEIMER
The Rockefeller University, New York, New York 10021-6399

Plasticity has traditionally been associated with experience-dependent functional and structural alterations early in development and postnatal life. In the visual system, a measure of plasticity was found to be limited to the critical period, which lasts only for the first few months or years of postnatal life, depending on the species (Hubel and Wiesel 1970). During the critical period it is possible, by altering visual experience, to alter cortical connections, functional architecture, and receptive field properties. Although certain functions may be mutable only early in life, the demands of visual perception entail an ability to store percepts throughout life. The plasticity associated with visual learning has traditionally been associated with the temporal lobe, but there is a growing body of evidence that adult plasticity is a property of the entire cortical visual pathway, extending as far back as the primary visual cortex. Here we attempt to give an overview of the influences on visual cortical plasticity in the adult, which include the global context within which local features are embedded, the previous history of visual stimulation, including deprivation and enrichment of visual experience in a local part of the visual field, and visual attention or expectation. We also address the substrate of the observed plasticity, in terms of the connections and the possible synaptic changes involved.

At the outset, one must make a caveat about the use of the term "plasticity." It tends to be interpreted differently by different people. The clearest use of the term applies to the formation of new connections, perhaps in association with regression of other connections. Another source of functional mutability is the change in strength of existing connections, which may be achieved by a potentiation or depression of excitatory or inhibitory connections. Yet a third way to alter the functional consequences of a given input to a cell is by the concurrent activation of other inputs. Any number of nonlinear mechanisms, such as voltage-dependent sodium conductances, can produce very different properties during the conjoint activation of two inputs from what one would anticipate by the effects generated by either input alone.

CONTEXTUAL EFFECTS

In thinking about the role of context in visual processing, it is important to keep in mind that one important task of the visual system is to link contours associated with the same object and to segregate or segment surfaces and contours belonging to different objects. Using simple stimulus patterns, one can observe the attempt of the visual system to link contours, even in the absence of the appropriate physical stimulus, and to segregate salient contours from their background. Many visual illusions reflect the attempt by the visual system to perform this linkage even in the absence of the complete physical entity. For example, with illusory contours, such as the Kanizsa triangle, one sees a complete figure even though large segments of the figure's sides are missing (Kanizsa 1987). Another example of the visual system's attempt at completion is seen with perceptual fill-in or neon spreading, where one perceives a complete surface, even though the physical stimulus occupies only a part of the surface or even the surrounding area (Yarbus 1957; Krauskopf 1961; Crane and Piantanida 1983; Ramachandran and Gregory 1991).

The physical characteristics of visual scenes obey rules by which we can link contours and differentiate them from their backgrounds. The Gestalt psychologists posited the rules of continuity, contiguity, and saliency, where contours formed out of line segments that are close together and of similar orientation tend to be more easily picked out of their backgrounds (Wertheimer 1938; Grossberg and Mingolla 1985; Ullman 1990; Field et al. 1993). This ability to link contours belonging to the same object reflects rules of connectivity in primary visual cortex (V1). Pyramidal cells in V1 form long-range horizontal connections, running for long distances (6–8 mm) parallel to the cortical surface (Gilbert and Wiesel 1979, 1983; Rockland and Lund 1982, 1983; Martin and Whitteridge 1984). An example of a cortical pyramidal cell forming long-range connections within V1 is shown in Figure 1a. These connections have been identified in nearly every cortical area. In V1 their functional significance can be understood in terms of the functional architecture of V1. With respect to the visuotopic organization of V1, their widespread nature implies that the cells receiving input from the horizontal collaterals integrate input over an area of cortex representing an area of visual field much larger than their own receptive fields, as measured with simple stimuli such as a single line segment of a given orientation. Furthermore, the long-range connections have a distinctive clustered nature, giving off sheaves of axon collaterals approximately every millimeter (Gilbert and Wiesel 1979, 1983, 1989). Using various approaches, the clusters have been shown to relate to the columnar functional architecture

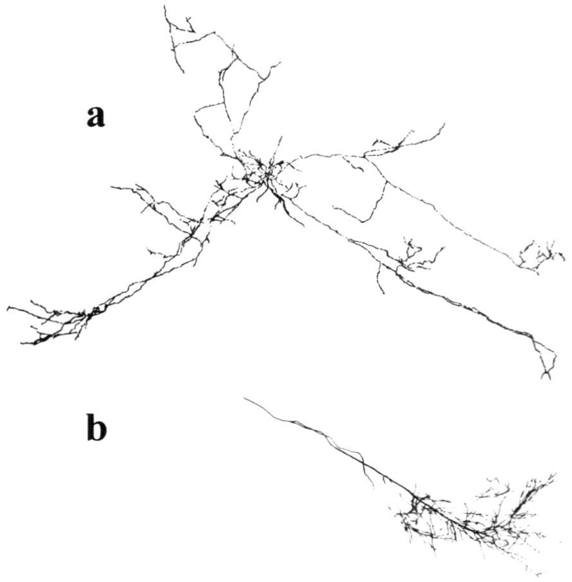

Figure 1. Lateral interactions in cortex are mediated by long-range horizontal connections formed by cortical pyramidal cells. The axonal field of one cell, labeled by intracellular injection of horseradish peroxidase, is shown in surface view in *a*, the axon of a pyramidal cell lying in the superficial layers of V1. It illustrates several characteristics of these cells: The axons extend for up to 8 mm parallel to the cortical surface (this example has an extent in excess of 3 mm), and the axon collaterals are distributed in a series of discrete clusters, separated by distances of ~ 1 mm. The clusters become progressively sparser as they emerge at progressively greater distances from the cell body, which is found near the center of the axonal field. (*b*) The distal portion of an axon, labeled with biocytin, projecting into a region of V1 that has undergone topographic reorganization following binocular retinal lesions. The most distal portions of this axon lie more than 4 mm from the originating cell body, and yet the illustrated cluster is considerably richer in the number and density of axon collaterals than those labeled in normal cortex by intracellular dye injection. The increased density of collaterals and boutons suggested by this example is confirmed in quantitative comparisons of the density of the horizontal plexus in normal and reorganized cortex. (Adapted from Gilbert and Wiesel 1983; Darian-Smith and Gilbert 1994.)

of cortex, the distribution of cells into columns of similar orientation preference. The registration between the axon collateral clusters and the orientation columns was shown by combined retrograde labeling of the horizontal connections and of the orientation columns with 2-deoxyglucose autoradiography (Gilbert and Wiesel 1989). The relationships of receptive field properties between cells interconnected by horizontal connections was shown by the cross-correlation technique (Ts'o et al. 1986; Ts'o and Gilbert 1988).

A new technique, optical recording, also shows the lateral spread of activity mediated by the horizontal connections. Optical recording enables one to visualize the distribution of activity, projected onto the cortical surface, in response to a given stimulus. The images taken were based on an "intrinsic signal," a change in cortical surface reflectance correlated with local activity (Grinvald et al. 1986; Frostig et al. 1990; Ts'o et al. 1990). Using this technique, one can visualize the distribution of orientation columns projected onto the cortical surface (Bonhoeffer and Grinvald 1991) and the patterns of activity resulting from various stimuli. We used the approach to look at the lateral spread of activity from a focus of spiking cells by measuring the optical recorded "point spread," the activity resulting from a point stimulus (McIlwain 1975; Grinvald et al. 1994; Das and Gilbert 1995a). An example of cortical point spread is shown in Figure 2. When the animal is presented with a short line segment, roughly the diameter of the smallest receptive fields in the superficial layers of V1, the optical point spread is approximately 4 mm in diameter. In contrast, the area of spiking activity, measured by multiple closely spaced electrode penetrations, is only 0.5 x 1 mm in diameter. The remaining 95% of the area measured by the optical point spread represents subthreshold activity, including contributions of both excitatory and inhibitory synaptic potentials. This subthreshold activity is likely to represent the postsynaptic effects of the long-range horizontal connections formed by pyramidal cells projecting from the region of the spiking point spread to the surrounding area included within the optical point spread. Hence, a patch of cells with a given orientation preference communicates with distant patches of cells covering an area several millimeters in diameter. This area of cortex represents an area of visual field roughly an order of magnitude greater in diameter than the diameter of the receptive fields of superficial-layer cortical cells, equivalent to the distance covered by the long-range horizontal connections. Furthermore, the orientation preference of the columns receiving the patchy projections, as shown by optical recording, matches that of the columns sending the projections, providing additional evidence that the horizontal connections run between columns of similar specificity (Das and Gilbert 1995a).

The ability for cells in V1 to integrate information over relatively large regions of visual space opens the possibility that the lateral interactions play a role in the linkage of contours, because of both the extent and the specificity of these interactions. Just as the perceptual studies on contour saliency show the strongest pop-out effects for contours made of similarly oriented line segments, the horizontal connections link cells with widely separated receptive fields having similar orientation preference. We explored the role V1 plays in perceptual linkage by doing parallel psychophysical experiments in human subjects and single-cell recordings in alert, fixating primates. Our experiments progressed from examining interactions between lines in a pair to extended contours placed within a complex background. In the psychophysical experiments, we measured the contrast threshold for detecting a line, presented by itself and together with a second, nearby

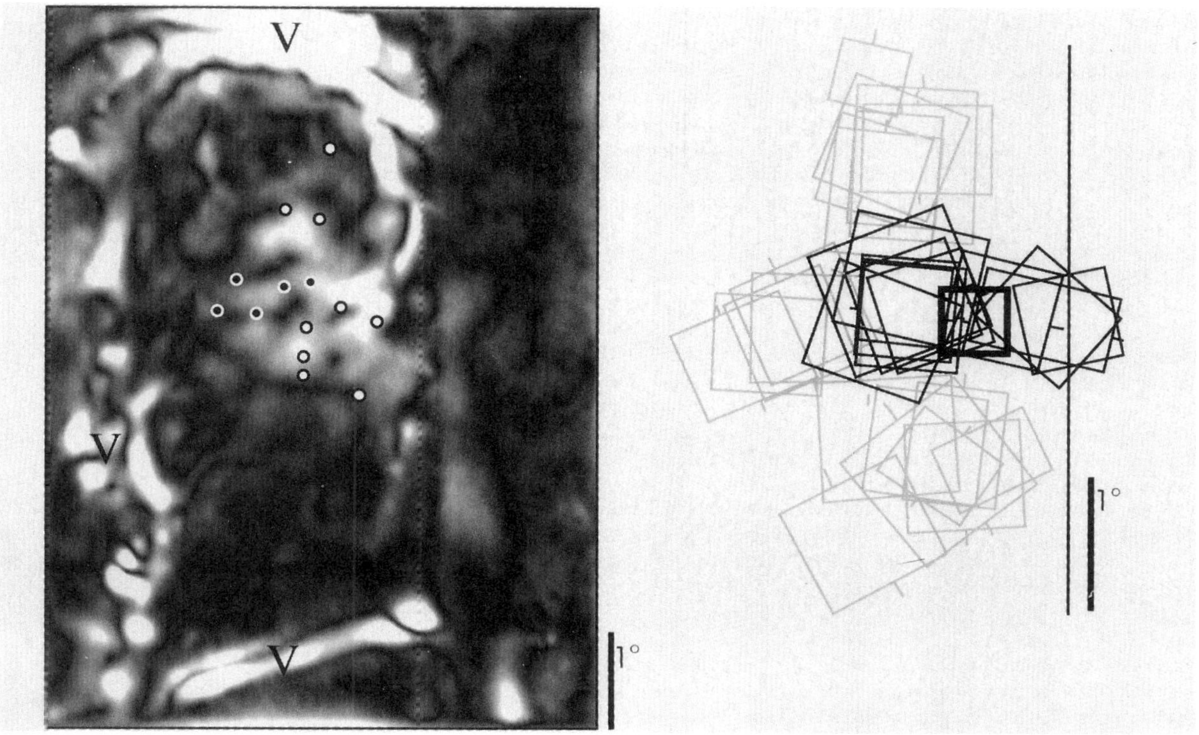

Figure 2. Lateral interactions in cortex visualized with optical recording and multisite electrode recordings. The overall extent of excitation, including suprathreshold and subthreshold activity, is measured by the optical imaging technique, and the area of spiking activity is measured electrophysiologically. The *left* panel shows the intensity of the optical activity induced in cortex by a small 0.5° light bar (optical point spread, PS). The bright patch in the middle of the field is the optical PS (the surrounding bright areas, marked with a V, indicate vascular artifacts around the edges of the imaged region of cortex). The receptive fields (RFs) corresponding to the penetration sites (*dots*) superimposed on the optical image are plotted in outline on the right. The visual stimulus used to generate the optical image was placed within the RF shown in heavy black. Only a small portion of the optical PS contains sites with RFs overlapping with the stimulus (penetrations shown as filled dots, RFs shown with black outlines), an area measuring roughly 0.5 mm x 1.0 mm. The area of spiking activity represents only 5% of the area of activation measuring optically. The remaining sites (penetrations shown as open circles, RFs shown with gray outlines) receive subthreshold activation via the horizontal collaterals of cells projecting from the central core of spiking activity. The visual field representation of this extended area of cortical activation is an order of magnitude larger than the diameter of the stimulus. (Adapted from Das and Gilbert 1995a.)

colinear line. These experiments are summarized in Figure 3. The flanking line had the effect of lowering by approximately 40% the threshold of detection of the target line (Fig. 3A). In the physiological studies, we studied the influence of lines placed outside the receptive field on the response properties of cells. By definition, when a single, isolated line is presented outside the receptive field, it has no influence on the cell's response. When it is shown together with an optimally oriented line placed within the receptive field, however, it can double or triple the response of the cell relative to its response to a single line within the receptive field (Fig. 3B). The facilitatory effects seen psychophysically and physiologically have similar dependencies on the geometric relationships of the lines: The effects disappear as the flanking line is shifted away from the target line along its orientation axis, when the two lines are offset laterally with respect to each other, or when they are tilted away from parallel. The psychophysical and physiological effects also operate over similar spatial scales at a given eccentricity in the visual field. That these facilitatory effects may be related to line continuity is supported by the observation that they disappear when one adds a stimulus to break continuity between the target and flanking lines, such as a cross bar between the two lines.

These facilitatory interactions are likely to play a role in the linkage of contours and the segmentation between contour and background. When an appropriately oriented line is placed within the receptive field of a cell, one obtains a good response as long as the background is blank. Natural scenes bear little relationship, however, to such simple stimuli. If one surrounds the line segment in a complex background of randomly placed and oriented line segments, the response of the cell is often profoundly suppressed, due to the presence of inhibitory surrounds outside the excitatory core of the receptive field. As one shifts ad-

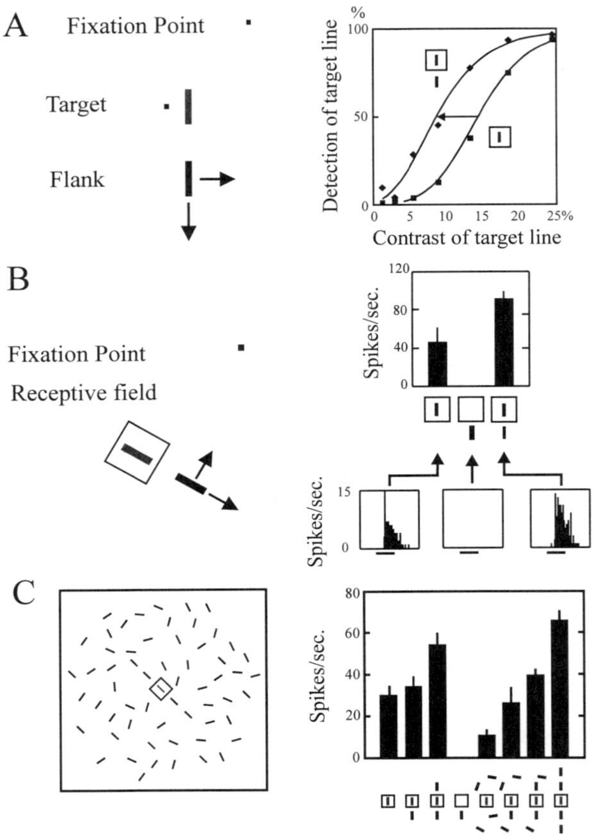

Figure 3. Visual spatial integration and long-range facilitatory interactions in visual cortex. Parallel psychophysical experiments in human subjects and single-cell recordings in superficial layers of monkey primary visual cortex show facilitatory interactions having similar dependencies on stimulus configuration. This is first shown by the influence of a flanking line on the detectability of a target line: The threshold contrast required to detect a single line is obtained by the right of the two psychometric curves shown in *A*. When a second, colinear and parallel line is placed near the target line, the psychometric curve shifts to the left, indicative of a 40% lowering of the threshold for detectability. Similarly, the response of a cell in visual cortex to a line placed within the receptive field is increased when a second, colinear line is added outside the receptive field (*B*). This second line by itself has no influence on the response of the cell, but when the appropriately oriented line is located inside the receptive field, the cell's response can be increased severalfold. The facilitatory effects seen in the psychophysical and physiological experiments show similar dependencies on the spatial relationships between the target and flanking lines, with the facilitation diminishing as the lines are separated along the colinear axis, shifting laterally orthogonally to their axis of orientation, or with changes in their relative orientation. These effects may be related to the saliency of contours embedded within complex visual environments, as shown in *C*. The presence of a context of randomly oriented and placed lines in the example shown has an inhibitory influence on the cell's response. As lines in this pattern are moved into a colinear spatial relationship with the line lying within the receptive field (indicated by the diagram on the left), the cell is lifted out of its inhibitory influence and progressively facilitated in its response as lines are added, ultimately showing a response much greater than that seen to the line within the receptive field presented in isolation. (Adapted from Kapadia et al. 1995.)

ditional line segments within this pattern into alignment with the line lying within the receptive field, the cell is lifted from the inhibition and one often sees a substantial additional facilitation in its response above its response to the single isolated line (Fig. 3C). Thus, cells even in area V1 are highly dependent on the context within which features are presented, and even if the local features within the receptive field are optimal for the cell, the cell will not respond unless the global context has the appropriate geometric relationships for contour saliency.

The context-dependent dynamics in cell responses in itself does not require alterations in synaptic weights, but can be accounted for by nonlinear integration of different inputs to a cell. The horizontally evoked excitatory postsynaptic potential (EPSP), for example, greatly increases when the cell is depolarized by other inputs, even though one is bringing the cell closer to the reversal potential for excitation. This voltage dependency is produced by voltage-dependent sodium conductances (Hirsch and Gilbert 1991). Such mechanisms can explain why a line outside the receptive field has no effect on a cell's firing, because it activates the horizontal inputs without the vertical inputs, but when an additional line is placed within the receptive field, the vertical inputs are activated at the same time, depolarizing the cell and potentiating the horizontally evoked synaptic potential.

EXPERIENCE-DEPENDENT MODIFICATION OF RECEPTIVE FIELDS

Substantial changes in the strength of lateral inputs can be induced by experience. In the visual system, this is seen in rearrangements of cortical topography following retinal lesions. This plasticity is not limited to the critical period, which affects the balance of input coming from the two eyes to the cortex, but is seen throughout life. If one places focal retinal lesions binocularly, so that homologous regions of the two retinas are affected, the portion of visual cortex receiving input from the destroyed parts of retina is silenced. We referred to this silent region as the "cortical scotoma." Over a period of weeks and months, the cortical scotoma regains visually driven activity, with cells shifting their receptive fields to positions outside of the retinal lesion. As a result, there is shrinkage in the cortical representation of the lesioned part of the retina and an expansion in the representation of the parts of the retina surrounding the lesion (Fig. 4) (Gilbert et al. 1990; Kaas et al. 1990; Chino et al. 1991; Heinen and Skavenski 1991; Gilbert and Wiesel 1992).

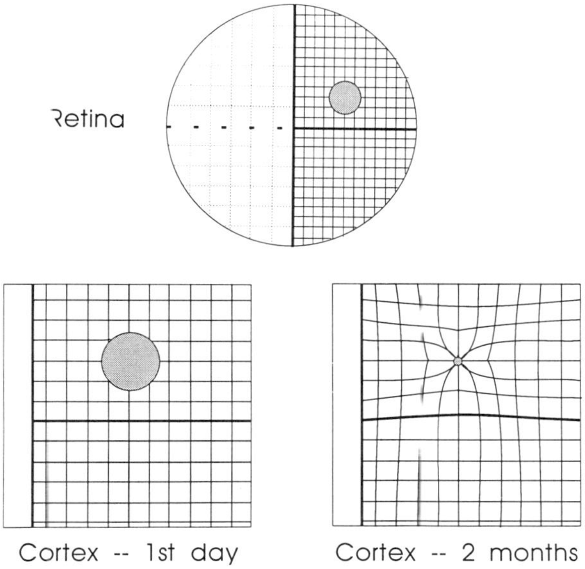

Figure 4. Effect of retinal lesions on cortical topography. The visuotopic axes are represented as the Cartesian grid superimposed on the retina in the corresponding maps on the cortex in surface view. A lesion, made with a diode laser, destroys the photoreceptor layer in a restricted part of the retina (*shaded area, top*), effectively removing visual input from the cortical region representing that retinal area (*lower left*). Over a period of months, the topography of the cortex is reorganized (*lower right*), with a decreased representation of the silenced input and an increased representation of the perilesion retina (Gilbert and Wiesel 1990, 1992; Kaas et al. 1990; Heinen and Skavenski 1991). The area of reorganized cortex is up to 8 mm in diameter. (Reprinted, with permission, from Gilbert 1992 [copyright Cell Press].)

This process can involve a remapping of up to 8 mm of silenced cortex, and the fullest extent of recovery can take several months. To explore the mechanism underlying these extensive changes in cortical topography, we first attempted to pinpoint the stage along the visual pathway at which the changes were initially occurring and to determine the class of connection involved. Recording in the lateral geniculate nucleus, the stage immediately antecedent to area V1, showed the persistence of a large silent region at a time when the cortical reorganization was complete, pointing toward the cortex as the initial site of remapping (Gilbert and Wiesel 1990; Darian-Smith and Gilbert 1995). Within the cortex, several classes of connections were candidates for the source of visual input into the cortical scotoma, including the thalamocortical projections, the long-range horizontal connections, and feedback connections from higher-order cortical areas. The thalamocortical connections could not account for the spatial extent of recovery observed, since they have a lateral spread of only a couple of millimeters. Retrograde labeling of this pathway showed that these connections did not sprout into the cortical scotoma, and thus could not account for the reorganization (Darian Smith and Gilbert 1995). The horizontal connections seemed the most likely candidate, however, since their lateral extent does approximate the maximum amount of recovery observed. Consistent with the involvement of horizontal connections is the close correspondence of the patterns of orientation columns before lesioning and after recovery. Since the horizontal connections run between columns of similar orientation specificity, providing visual input into the cortical scotoma via horizontal connections would produce the same pattern of connections after recovery, despite the substantial shift in receptive field position (Das and Gilbert 1995a).

The match between the extent of horizontal connections and the extent of recovery suggested that cortical plasticity can only operate within the framework of existing connections. Although under ordinary circumstances the plexus of horizontal connections provides a modulatory role, as described above, these connections have to be strengthened sufficiently to provide a suprathreshold, driving influence to bring about remapping of cortical topography. What is the nature of this strengthening, and why does it take so long? One plausible explanation is that a profound morphological change is taking place. To test this idea, we labeled the horizontal connections originating from cells lying at the boundary of the initial cortical scotoma, whose receptive fields end up overlapping with those of cells within the scotoma. We labeled the horizontal fibers with biocytin injections and compared the density of projections into reorganized and into normal cortex (Fig. 1b). The experiments showed roughly a doubling of the density of the projection in the reorganized cortex, and an even greater change in the superficial layers. This shows that even in the adult cortex, there is a capacity for sprouting of axon collaterals and synaptogenesis (Darian-Smith and Gilbert 1994). Compared to the developing brain, however, there seems to be one singular limitation: The connections do not increase their overall extent, but instead add collaterals to existing clusters. This effectively elevates the set point around which the strength of a given input is modulated.

The proximal signal for this sprouting is the imbalance in activity, induced by the retinal lesion, between adjacent patches of cortex. It is of considerable interest to trace the signal transduction cascade that leads from this to the formation of new connections. At this stage we have found that very early (within a few days) following the lesions there is an up-regulation within the cortical scotoma of a number of factors, including neurotrophins and their receptors. We have identified an increase in brain-derived neurotrophic factor (BDNF), neurotrophin 3 (NT-3), and the trkB receptor. There is also an increase in synaptic vesicle associated proteins, such as synapsin 1, reflecting the increased synaptic density. In addition, we observed an elevation of CREB, MAP2, and CaMKII-43 (S. Obata and C.D. Gilbert, unpubl.). These signals remain elevated for more than a year following the lesion. It is intriguing that the stimulus for sprouting appears very early, but the fullest extent of recovery takes many months.

Although a lesion of the central nervous system appears to be a potent stimulus for cortical reorganization, it is undoubtedly not the sole purpose for which this phenomenon has evolved. Rather, it is likely to play a role in the continuing calibration and normalization of, in this case, visual processing, and perceptual learning as well. Perceptual learning has been studied for well over a hundred years, but its cellular basis is poorly understood. It has characteristics, however, that are suggestive of the involvement of early stages in the visual pathway. As an initial stage toward exploring the cortical basis of perceptual learning, we devised a stimulus that would allow us to study it psychophysically in human subjects and physiologically in alert primates (Crist et al. 1996). Our model is a three-line bisection task, in which a subject is asked to determine whether the central of three vertical lines is located nearer the line on the left or that on the right. By repeatedly doing this task, several hundred trials a day, over a number of weeks, there is a substantial improvement (by a factor of three) in the amount of offset required to judge the middle line as being closer to either of the two outer lines. The specificity of this learning indicates a potential involvement of V1: It is specific to the trained position in visual space, with transfer of learning dropping off to within a few degrees of the trained location; it is specific to the trained orientation, showing no transfer when the triad of lines is rotated to the orthogonal orientation. This points toward the involvement of V1, since there the retinotopic organization and orientation specificity is the most refined. There is an additional specificity, however, that suggests the mechanism does not simply involve cortical recruitment, the enlargement of the representation of the trained position in visual space. There is an additional involvement of higher-order influences, since the task does not transfer to other tasks in the same position in the visual field and therefore involving the same area of cortex as the trained task. Thus, one sees no improvement in an orientation discrimination task or in a vernier acuity task, even though the latter involves discriminating the position of the same line in the same position and of the same orientation as in the trained task, but relative to a different line. The dependence on behavioral context and on the spatial configuration of the visual stimulus suggests that the cortical changes might be gated by influences from higher-order cortical areas. We plan to explore the receptive field and architectural changes that correlate with the perceptual improvement.

SHORT-TERM PLASTICITY

Although the fullest extent of the rearrangement discussed above evolves over several months, there are shorter-term changes, evolving over minutes and perhaps even seconds, that are experience-dependent. Within minutes after making a retinal lesion, the receptive fields that were initially located just within the boundary of the lesioned area shift outside the boundary to the unlesioned part of the retina, and they expand in size by an order of magnitude (Chino et al. 1992; Gilbert and Wiesel 1992). The fact that these changes can occur rapidly, and that the lesion involves a destruction primarily of the photoreceptor layer, with an intact retinal ganglion cell layer and presumably normal projections from retina to lateral geniculate nucleus and from the lateral geniculate nucleus to the cortex, it seemed possible to mimic the effects of a lesion simply by patterned stimulation.

We did this by recording from an individual cell, mapping its receptive field, and then providing a visual stimulus that we call an "artificial scotoma." The artificial scotoma consists of a patterned stimulus, such as a series of drifting lines or a dynamic random dot pattern, within which we place a gray mask or occluder (Fig. 5, top left). The occluder is positioned over the receptive field such that the patterned stimulus lies well outside the receptive field. After providing such a conditioning stimulus for a few minutes, we remap the receptive field. Remarkably, within this short period of time the receptive field expands severalfold in diameter. Stimulating within the receptive field then causes it to collapse back down to its original diameter. In this manner, one can expand and contract the receptive field repeatedly (Fig. 5, bottom) (Pettet and Gilbert 1992; Das and Gilbert 1995b; Gilbert et al. 1996). This raises something of an uncertainty problem in sensory physiology analogous to the Heisenberg uncertainty principle in physics, where anything one does to measure the receptive field can change it.

The mechanism underlying the rapid changes in receptive field size once again may involve the long-range horizontal connections. Here, however, rather than formation of new synapses, the strengthening may involve an unmasking of existing connections. The horizontal connections are formed by excitatory, pyramidal cells, but they contact both other pyramidal cells and inhibitory interneurons. Therefore, the unmasking process may involve either a facilitation of the excitatory connections themselves, or a reduction in the strength of the inhibitory connections. In slices of visual cortex it is possible to produce use-dependent changes in the strength of the excitatory component of the horizontal input (Hirsch and Gilbert 1993). In either case, it would be manifest as a change in the effective strength of connections between cells with receptive fields lying within the artificial scotoma. We demonstrated this strengthening using a technique known as cross-correlation analysis, which provides a measure of the strength of interaction between pairs of cells by a histogram of time differences between the occurrence of spikes in the two cells (Fig. 5, top) (Das and Gilbert 1995b).

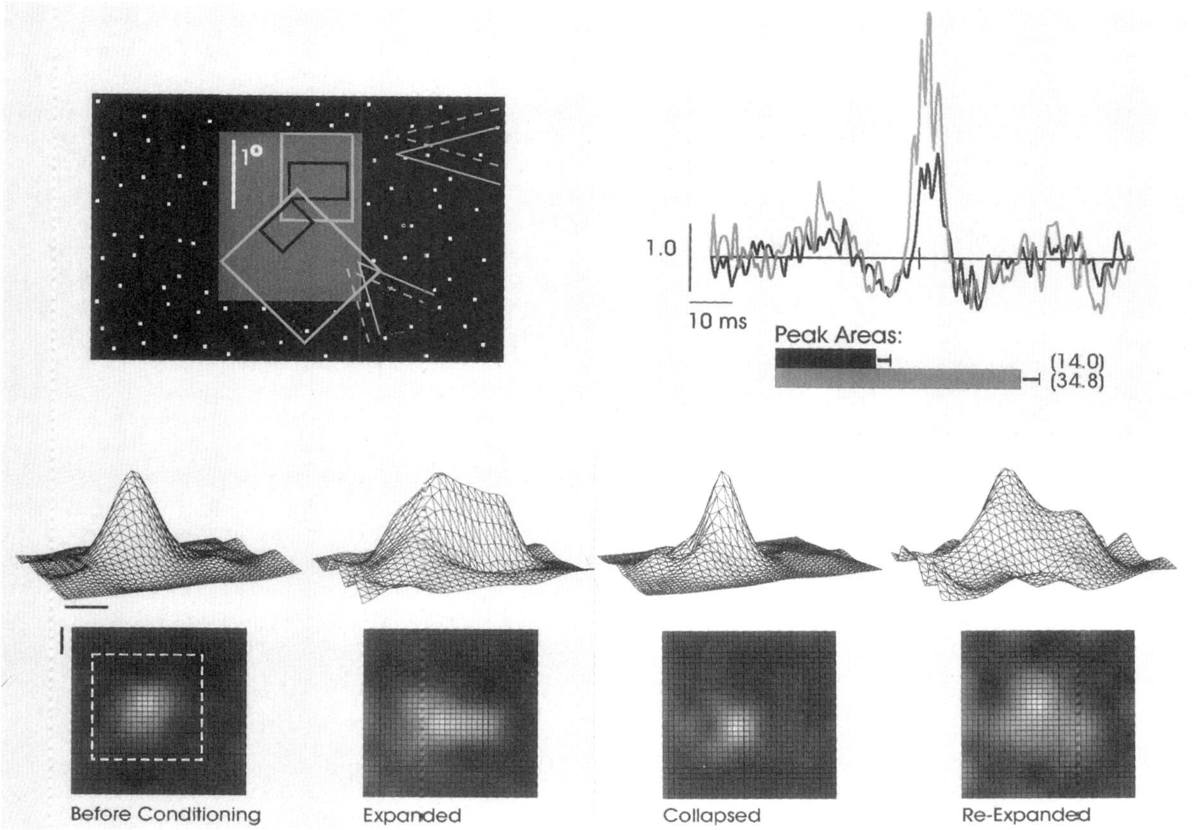

Figure 5. Short-term plastic changes in receptive field (RF) size and the attendant changes in effective connection strength. (*Top left*) Layout of the artificial scotoma stimulus used to induce RF size changes. After isolating a pair of neurons in primary visual cortex (RFs indicated by dark black), the animal was shown a visual stimulus consisting of flashing dots surrounding a region of visual occlusion that enclosed the two RFs isolated. After a period of a few minutes, both RFs are seen to expand (to the boundaries indicated in gray). If the RFs are then stimulated vigorously using an optimal stimulus, their RFs are seen to shrink. The RFs can be made to expand again by showing the animal the artificial scotoma. The progress of one RF through a sequence of expansion, collapse, and re-expansion is shown in the set of four RF profiles in the lower panel. RF profiles were mapped by placing a small bar at different positions in an 8 x 8 grid. In each case, the responses are shown both as three-dimensional perspective plot, above, and as two-dimensional plot, below, where response rate is marked by the brightness of each pixel. Scale bars mark 1° in visual angle. Top right panel shows cross-correlograms of the visually driven activity of the neuron pair shown at top left, before conditioning with the artificial scotoma (*black*) and while both RFs were expanded (*gray*). The correlograms were computed from the visually driven activity using the same test stimulus both before and after expansion, and are shown after normalization by the baseline to compensate for changes in overall neuronal activity. In the expanded state, the two neurons show a 2.5-fold larger cross-correlation peak (as quantified using the area under the peak), indicating an increase in the effective connection strength; i.e., a selective increase in the synaptic inputs common to the two neurons. (Adapted from Das and Gilbert 1995b; Gilbert et al. 1996.)

The perceptual consequences of this short-term plasticity are several. They may relate to the process of establishing continuity between lines and over surfaces. The process of linkage is seen in illusory contours, such as the Kanizsa triangle, where the physical stimulus consists only of a portion of the perceived figure, and the visual system fills in the rest. It is also seen for surfaces in a process known as perceptual fill-in. The artificial scotoma, for example, will fill in after steady fixation for a period of time, such that the twinkling dots lying outside of the occluder eventually appear to be located within the occluder as well. We made a measure of perceptual shifts induced by an artificial scotoma and found that lines lying near the boundary of the scotoma appear to be sucked toward its center like a black hole (Kapadia et al. 1994). These shifts can be explained by the expansion of receptive fields in the artificial scotoma: If a cell represents a labeled line for a position in space centered within its receptive field, when it expands it is stimulated by features farther from its center. Expansions of fields in one part of the visual field and not in the surrounding area then create a false percept of features shifting toward the expanded fields.

The role of short-term receptive field plasticity in normal vision remains to be elucidated. Clearly, the potential function depends heavily on the time course of the change. Long-term changes may be related to perceptual learning, whereas shorter-term changes may be related to the process of linkage, fill-in, and segmentation required for the interpretation of visual scenes.

ATTENTION AND EXPECTATION

A final influence on receptive field properties, which itself may be dynamically tuned, is that of expectation. There are various influences on the perception of local attributes that are dependent on expectation, and these have characteristics once again suggestive of involvement of early visual processes. The ability to discriminate the brightness or contrast of a line is greatly influenced by attention to the visual field location in which the line will appear. The influence of attention to spatial location also manifests training effects. If, for example, an observer is not cued to which of four possible positions a line will appear, the threshold for brightness discrimination gradually decreases with repetitive performance of the discrimination task. The improvement in performance for the unattended condition is specific for the visual field locations of the four stimuli. In addition, the contextual effects described above are influenced by attention to the position at which the target and flanking stimuli are presented (Ito et al. 1996). The fact that attentional influences show considerable positional specificity and affect simple attributes suggests the involvement of early visual processes. This non-retinal influence is in turn gated by context and by learning.

CONCLUSIONS

A growing body of evidence reveals a surprising degree of mutability of function in the visual cortex that is not limited to the first months of life but extends throughout the adult life of animals. We already know from experiments on the recovery of function after lesions, on the context dependency of receptive field properties, and on short-term experience-dependent modification of receptive field structure, that changes can be observed at as early a stage in the visual pathway as the primary visual cortex. Psychophysical evidence shows a mutability in visual perception resulting from perceptual learning and from expectation, the characteristics of which are suggestive of changes also in primary visual cortex. Further experiments will be directed at finding the cellular basis of these changes in terms of the cortical areas in which they are manifest, the underlying alterations in functional architecture and receptive field properties, and the synaptic changes involved. Various classes of connections have been identified as the likely source of the changes. For some of the effects, the horizontal connections appear to be responsible, particularly in view of their relationship to cortical topography and columnar functional architecture. For others, the feedback connections from higher-order cortical areas are likely to be the source, particularly for effects involving expectation and attention. Even when V1 is identified as expressing changes that correlate with perceptual changes, other areas may be responsible for performing the fundamental calculation, with V1 representing a buffer or template to which the result of these calculations is written.

From the evidence now available, it is clear that rather than performing a fixed and stereotyped calculation on its input, the cells in area V1 represent active filters. They dynamically change according to context, which may play a key role in the process of linkage and segmentation. They are altered according to the previous history of visual stimulation, which may provide a continual normalization and calibration of the visual system, as well as a basis for perceptual learning. The perceptual consequence of the history-dependent changes depends on the time scales over which the changes occur. Finally, the functional properties of V1 cells may change according to expectation, which may allow the visual system to test hypotheses about the nature of the incoming sensory input.

ACKNOWLEDGMENTS

This work has been supported by grants from the National Eye Institute (EY-07968), the National Science Foundation (IBN 92-21854), and the McKnight Foundation.

REFERENCES

Bonhoeffer, T. and A. Grinvald. 1991. Iso-orientation domains in cat visual cortex are arranged in pinwheel like patterns. *Nature* **353:** 429.

Chino, Y.M., J.H. Kaas, E.L. Smith III, A.L. Langston, and H. Cheng. 1992. Rapid reorganization of cortical maps in adult cats following restricted deafferentation in retina. *Vision Res.* **32:** 789.

Chino, Y.M., E.L. Smith III, H.Wada, W.L. Ridder III, A.L. Langston, and G.A. Lesher. 1991. Disruption of binocularly correlated input leads to deficits in spatial properties of striate cortical neurons in cats. *J. Neurophysiol.* **65:** 841.

Crane, H.D. and T.P. Piantanida. 1983. On seeing reddish-green and yellowish-blue. *Science* **221:** 1078.

Crist, R.E., M.K. Kapadia, G. Westheimer, and C.D. Gilbert. 1996. Perceptual learning of spatial localization: Specificity for position, orientation and context. *Soc. Neurosci. Abstr.* **22:** 269.

Darian-Smith, C. and C.D. Gilbert. 1994. Axonal sprouting accompanies functional reorganization in adult cat striate cortex. *Nature* **368:** 737.

———. 1995. Topographic reorganization in the striate cortex of the adult cat and monkey is cortically mediated. *J. Neurosci.* **15:** 1631.

Das, A. and C.D. Gilbert. 1995a. Cortical point spreads in normal and reorganized primary visual cortex reflect long range intracortical connections. *Nature* **375:** 780.

———. 1995b. Receptive field expansion in adult visual cortex is linked to dynamic changes in strength of intrinsic cortical connections. *J. Neurophysiol.* **74:** 779.

Field, D.J., A. Hayes, and R.F. Hess. 1993. Contour integration by the human visual system: Evidence for a local "association field." *Vision Res.* **33:** 173.

Frostig, R.D., E.E. Lieke, D.Y. Ts'o, and A. Grinvald. 1990. Cortical functional architecture and local coupling between neuronal activity and the microcirculations revealed by *in vivo* high resolution optical imaging of intrinsic signals. *Proc. Natl. Acad. Sci.* **87:** 6082.

Gilbert, C.D. 1992. Horizontal integration and cortical dynamics. *Neuron* **9:** 1.

Gilbert, C.D. and T.N. Wiesel. 1979. Morphology and intracortical projections of functionally identified neurons in cat visual cortex. *Nature* **280:** 120.

———. 1983. Clustered intrinsic connections in cat visual cortex. *J. Neurosci.* **3:** 1116.

———. 1989. Columnar specificity of intrinsic connections in cat visual cortex. *J. Neurosci.* **9:** 2432.

———. 1990. The influence of contextual stimuli on the orientation selectivity of cells in primary visual cortex of the cat. *Vision Res.* **30:** 1689.

———. 1992. Receptive field dynamics in adult primary visual cortex. *Nature* **356:** 150.

Gilbert, C.D., J.A. Hirsch, and T.N. Wiesel. 1990. Lateral interactions in visual cortex. *Cold Spring Harbor Symp. Quant. Biol.* **55:** 663.

Gilbert, C.D., A. Das, M. Ito, M. Kapadia, and G. Westheimer. 1996. Spatial integration and cortical dynamics. *Proc. Natl. Acad. Sci.* **93:** 615.

Grinvald, A., E.E. Lieke, R.D. Frostig, and R. Hildesheim. 1994. Cortical point-spread function and long-range lateral interactions revealed by real-time optical imaging of macaque monkey primary visual cortex. *J. Neurosci.* **14:** 2545.

Grinvald, A., E.E. Lieke, R.D. Frostig, C.D. Gilbert, and T.N. Wiesel. 1986. Functional architecture of cortex revealed by optical imaging of intrinsic signals. *Nature* **324:** 361.

Grossberg, S. and E. Mingolla. 1985. Neural dynamics of perception grouping: Textures, boundaries and emergent segmentations. *Percept. Psychophys.* **38:** 141.

Heinen, S.J. and A.A. Skavenski. 1991. Recovery of visual responses in foveal VI neurons following bilateral foveal lesions in adult monkey. *Exp. Brain Res.* **83:** 670.

Hirsch, J.A. and C.D. Gilbert. 1991. Synaptic physiology of horizontal connections in primary visual cortex. *J. Neurosci.* **11:** 1800.

———. 1993. Long-term changes in synaptic strength along specific intrinsic pathways in the cat's visual cortex. *J. Physiol.* **461:** 247.

Hubel, D.H. and T.N. Wiesel. 1970. The period of susceptibility to the physiological effects of unilateral eye closure in kittens. *J. Physiol.* **206:** 419.

Ito, M., C.D. Gilbert, and G. Westheimer. 1996. The interaction of visual attention, learning and context on luminance discrimination in humans and monkeys. *Soc. Neurosci. Abstr.* **22:** 269.

Kaas, J.H., L.A. Krubitzer, Y.M. Chino, A.L. Langston, E.H. Polley, and N. Blair. 1990. Reorganization of retinotopic cortical maps in adult mammals after lesions of the retina. *Science* **248:** 229.

Kanizsa, G. 1987. Quasi-perceptual margins in homogeneously simulated fields. In *The perception of illusory contours* (ed. S. Petry and G.E. Meyer). Springer-Verlag, New York.

Kapadia, M.K., C.D. Gilbert, and G. Westheimer. 1994. A quantitative measure for short-term cortical plasticity in human vision. *J. Neurosci.* **14:** 451.

Kapadia, M.K. M. Ito, C.D. Gilbert, and G. Westheimer. 1995. Improvement in visual sensitivity by changes in local context: Parallel studies in human observers and in V1 of alert monkeys. *Neuron* **15:** 843.

Krauskopf, J. 1961. Heterochromatic stabilized images: A classroom demonstration. *Am. J. Psychol.* **80:** 632.

Martin, K.A.C. and D. Whitteridge. 1984. Form, function and intracortical projections of spiny neurones in striate visual cortex of the cat. *J. Physiol.* **353:** 463.

McIlwain, J.T. 1975. Visual receptive fields and their images in superior colliculus of the cat. *J. Neurophys.* **38:** 219.

Pettet, M.W. and C.D. Gilbert. 1992. Dynamic changes in receptive field size in cat primary visual cortex. *Proc. Natl. Acad. Sci.* **89:** 8366.

Ramachandran, V.S. and T.L. Gregory. 1991. Perceptual filling in of artificially induced scotomas in human vision. *Nature* **350:** 699.

Rockland, K.S. and J.S. Lund. 1982. Widespread periodic intrinsic connections in the tree shrew visual cortex. *Brain Res.* **169:** 19.

———. 1983. Intrinsic laminar lattice connections in primate visual cortex. *J. Comp. Neurol.* **216:** 303.

Ts'o, D.Y. and C.D. Gilbert. 1988. The organization of chromatic and spatial interactions in the primate striate cortex. *J. Neurosci.* **8:** 1712.

Ts'o, D.Y., C.D. Gilbert, and T.N. Wiesel. 1986. Relationships between horizontal connections and functional architecture in cat striate cortex as revealed by cross-correlation analysis. *J. Neurosci.* **6:** 1160.

Ts'o, D.Y., R.D. Frostig, E.E. Lieke, and A. Grinvald. 1990. Functional organization of primate visual cortex revealed by high resolution optical imaging. *Science* **249:** 417.

Ullman, S. 1990. 3-dimensional object recognition. *Cold Spring Harbor Symp. Quant. Biol.* **55:** 889.

Wertheimer, M. 1938. *Laws of organization in perceptual forms.* Harcourt Brace Jovanovich, London.

Yarbus, A.L. 1957. The perception of an image fixed with respect to the retina. *Biophysics* **2:** 683.

What Neurological Syndromes Can Tell Us about Human Nature: Some Lessons from Phantom Limbs, Capgras Syndrome, and Anosognosia

V.S. Ramachandran

Brain and Perception Laboratory, University of California, San Diego, La Jolla, California 92093-0109

A recurring theme in the history of neurology is the concept of localization of function; the idea that different mental capacities such as language, seeing, hearing, and memory (maybe even esoteric capacities such as foresight and judgment), may be localized in different parts of the brain which are highly specialized for each of these functions. The most striking evidence for this view comes, of course, from clinical neurology. When a patient sustains a very small lesion in one part of his brain, what is often seen is not an across-the-board reduction in the person's mental abilities—a sort of general blunting of his cognitive capacity. What is seen instead is a highly selective loss of one specific capacity with other functions being relatively intact. This gives some confidence in asserting that that area might be specialized for that function, or at least be necessary for certain components of that function.

I begin with two striking illustrations. My favorite is a curious neurological syndrome called prosopagnosia, where a patient has a stroke that damages the medial-inferior parts of both temporal lobes. After he has sustained the stroke, the patient may be mentally quite lucid, fluent, and attentive, but the surprising thing is that he is unable to recognize people by looking at their faces. There is nothing wrong with his vision, because he can still read a newspaper, and his acuity is normal according to a Snellen chart. His only visual problem seems to be his inability to recognize faces. This has led to the view that this part of the brain is somehow specialized for the recognition of faces (Damasio 1985; Farah 1990). There is also evidence from monkeys showing that this is in fact the case. In recording from cells in the temporal lobes of monkeys, a large proportion of these cells are selectively tuned to faces and relatively unresponsive to other types of stimuli.

Prosopagnosia has been studied extensively, but I now describe a disorder called Capgras syndrome, which is one of the rarest and most colorful syndromes in neurology (Capgras and Reboul-Lachaux 1923; Ellis and Young 1990). The most striking feature of this disorder is that the patient comes to regard close acquaintances, typically either his parents, children, spouse, or siblings, as "imposters," i.e., he may claim that the person in question "looks like" or is even "identical to" his father, but really isn't his father. Although frequently seen in psychotic states, more than a third of the documented cases of Capgras syndrome have occurred in conjunction with traumatic brain lesions, suggesting that the syndrome has an organic basis (Signer 1994). The remarkable thing about these patients is that they are relatively intact in other respects; they are mentally lucid, their memory is normal, their speech is normal, and other aspects of their visual perception are completely unaffected.

Because this is a very bizarre syndrome, it is hardly surprising that many theories have been put forth to explain it. The most popular view of Capgras syndrome, oddly enough, is a Freudian view. The idea goes something like this: The patient, like all of us, felt a strong sexual attraction for his mother in early childhood (the so-called Oedipus complex) and, therefore, strong jealousy toward his father who is a rival for sexual attention. Fortunately, all of this is repressed as the child grows up, so no normal person would ordinarily be attracted to his mother or father. However, as a result of the blow to the head, somehow these latent sexual impulses are unmasked and come to the surface. Suddenly and inexplicably, the patient finds himself sexually attracted to his mother, and he says, "My God, if this is my mother, how come I'm sexually attracted to her? This must be some other strange person."

This argument is ingenious, as indeed most Freudian arguments are. However, there are many cases in the neurological literature where a patient experiences the Capgras delusion not only with his parents, but also with his pet dog (i.e., the patient claims that his pet poodle has been replaced with a duplicate). How does the Freudian argument apply to this particular case? I started thinking about this and realized that there was a much simpler explanation for this syndrome, as follows: Earlier I mentioned prosopagnosia and the so-called face area of the brain. The messages from this area of the brain are usually transmitted to the limbic system, which is composed of clusters of cells concerned mainly with the perception, experience, and expression of emotions. The "gateway" to the limbic system is the amygdala. Thus, the visual centers of the brain in the temporal lobes send their information to the amygdala, which assesses the emotional significance of the incoming visual input and then transmits this to other limbic structures where these emotions are "experienced." Is it possible that in this patient there has been a disconnection between the face area of the temporal lobes and the part of the temporal lobes concerned with the experience of emotion? Perhaps the face area and the amygdala are both intact, but the two areas have been disconnected from each other. As a result of this, the patient can recognize people's faces (this is what makes the syndrome different from prosopagnosia). When he looks at his mother, however, even though he realizes that she resembles his mother, he does not experience the appropriate warmth, and therefore says, "Well, if this is my mother, why is it I'm not experiencing any emotion? This must be some strange person." However bizarre this may seem to you and me, it is the only interpretation, perhaps, that makes sense to him with this peculiar disconnection.

How can a hypothesis of this kind be tested? What Bill Hirstein and I did was to obtain galvanic skin responses from one of these patients. When a normal person looks at something emotionally salient like his mother or father, this message is transmitted from the visual centers of the brain to the amygdala, where the emotional significance of this visual event is judged. The message goes to the limbic system and then to the hypothalamus and from there to the autonomic nervous system. This produces sweating, increase in heart rate, increase in blood pressure, and other signs of noradrenergic activity. It turns out that the sweating can be measured by simply measuring changes in skin resistance. This is the so-called galvanic skin response (GSR), which forms the basis of the lie detection test, and it is a fairly reliable index of emotional arousal. Almost all normal people give a strong GSR when they see their mother, but when we tested our patient, D.S., who had Capgras syndrome, we found that when he looked at a photograph of his mother, there was very little change in GSR, supporting the disconnection hypothesis (Ramachandran 1996; Hirstein and Ramachandran 1997). It is important to emphasize that D.S. had no problem in seeing that the photograph *looked* like his mother and he had no problem with experiencing emotions in general. During the interview he experienced joy, fear, impatience, boredom, and all other emotions that one would normally expect a human being to experience, because his limbic system was unaffected. What was deranged is the *communication* between vision and emotion. (Consistent with this, D.S. never experienced this delusion when talking to his parents on the *phone*.)

I mention Capgras syndrome because it is a striking example of how a completely bizarre, seemingly incomprehensible psychiatric syndrome can be simply explained in terms of the known neuroanatomy of the temporal lobes. This idea can then be tested to show that something like this might in fact be going on in the brain. This is what makes the whole field of cognitive neuroscience so exciting: We can generate these conjectures and then test them not only by using GSR, but also by taking advantage of the new imaging techniques such as positron-emission-tomography (PET) or functional magnetic resonance imaging (fMRI) that have now become widely available.

In the rest of this paper, I consider two other syndromes that we have begun investigating in our laboratory—phantom limbs and anosognosia (denial of paralysis). The experiments on phantom limbs are relatively straightforward and I describe them first. Although the results seemed very surprising when we first reported them, they have now been confirmed by several groups. The second part of this paper (on anosognosia) is much more speculative, and I present some preliminary observations. My purpose in doing this is to raise some new questions about this syndrome and to stimulate the reader's curiosity, rather than to provide any definitive answers.

PHANTOM LIMBS

My experiments on phantom limbs are directly relevant to the theme of this volume. I argue that they provide a valuable probe for studying neural plasticity in the adult human brain.

When I began my career as a medical student nearly 20 years ago, I was taught that no new neural connections can be formed in the adult mammalian brain. Once connections had been laid down in fetal life, or in early infancy, it was assumed that they hardly change later in life. It is this stability of connections in the adult brain, in fact, that is often used to explain why there is usually very little functional recovery after damage to the nervous system and why neurological diseases are so notoriously difficult to treat. In this paper, I present some evidence suggesting that we may need to revise these views radically.

It is known that a complete somatotopic map of the entire body surface exists in the somatosensory cortex of primates (Kaas et al. 1981; Merzenich et al. 1981, 1983, 1984; Wall 1988; Florence and Kaas 1995), including humans (see Fig. 1) (Penfield and Rasmussen 1950). In a series of pioneering experiments, Merzenich et al. amputated the middle finger of adult primates and found that within 2 months, the area in the cortex corresponding to this digit starts to respond to touch stimuli delivered to the adjacent digits; i.e., this area is "taken over" by sensory input from adjacent digits.

Merzenich et al. also made two other important observations:

1. If a monkey "uses" one finger excessively (e.g., if that finger is placed on a revolving corrugated drum) for an hour and a half each day, then after 3 months, the area of cortex corresponding to that finger "expands" at the expense of adjacent fingers; i.e., there is an increase in the cortical magnification factor for the overstimulated finger. The receptive

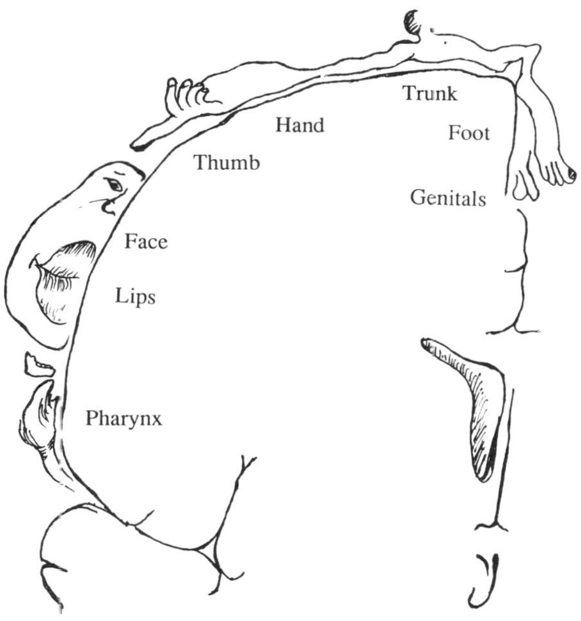

Figure 1. The Penfield homunculus. Notice that the sensory hand area is flanked below by the face and above by the upper arm and shoulder, the two regions where we usually find reference fields in arm amputees. Note that the area representing the genitals is just below the foot representation, a fact that might explain the frequent occurrence of certain foot fetishes even among normal individuals.

fields of neurons in this area also were found to have shrunk so that they were unusually small. Hence, these effects are unlikely to be "epiphenomenal"—they must be *functionally* important.

2. If more than one finger was amputated, there was no takeover beyond about 1 mm of cortex. Merzenich et al. (1984) concluded from this that the expansion is probably mediated by arborizations of thalamo-cortical axons, which typically do not extend beyond 1 mm.

This figure—1 mm—was often cited as the fixed upper limit of reorganization of sensory pathways in adult animals (Calford 1991). A remarkable experiment performed by Pons et al. (1991), however, suggests that this view might be incorrect. They found that after long-term (12 years) deafferentation of one upper limb, the cortical area originally corresponding to the hand is taken over by sensory input from the face; the cells in the "hand area" now start responding to stimuli applied to the lower face region! Since this patch of cortex is more than a centimeter in width, we may conclude that sensory reorganization can occur over at least this distance—an order of magnitude greater than the original 1 mm limit.

These exciting results from animals raise two interesting new questions. First, can a similar reorganization of the Penfield map be observed in the human somatosensory cortex following deafferentation or amputation of an arm? Second, if such reorganization occurred, what would the person actually *feel* if his face was touched? Since the message now (presumably) goes to the original hand area of the cortex, would he also experience touch sensation in his missing (phantom) hand? I now try to answer these two questions.

Magnetoencephalogram Correlates of Cortical Reorganization

Recent advances in magnetoencephalography (MEG) have been made possible with the advent of large array magnetometers (>30 detectors) and with the understanding of the physics and mathematics of the measurements of cortical electrical activity (Mosher et al. 1992). These advances have permitted fine localizations (>3 mm) of processing (Allison et al. 1980; Hari et al. 1984; Okada et al. 1984; Baumgartner et al. 1991; Dale and Sereno 1993). The work of Gallen et al. (1993a,b) and of Yang et al. (1993) is especially relevant, since they have obtained very detailed somatosensory (SI) maps of the hand, face, and several other body parts. They have been able to resolve the cortical areas representing individual digits and even segments of digits.

We realized that MEG studies could also be useful in determining whether remapping effects of the kinds reported in monkeys by Pons et al. would also be seen in human patients following amputation. In collaboration with Yang and Gallen, I began such a study in 1992 and found that reorganization does indeed occur. In all four upper-limb amputees whom we studied, we found that the sensory input from the face had "invaded" the hand territory in SI. (Fig. 2 shows the results from two of the four patients whom we tested.) Thus, it looked as though the famous Penfield map in SI, which every medical student and psychology undergraduate learns about, can be reorganized over a distance of at least 2 or 3 cm even in the adult brain (Ramachandran 1993; Yang et al. 1994a,b). To our knowledge, this is the first demonstration that such large-scale reorganization over several centimeters can occur in the adult human brain.

Perceptual Correlates of Massive Cortical Reorganization

From the MEG studies described above, it was clear that remapping occurs in the human brain, just as it does in monkeys. The sensory input from the face now gets sent to two different cortical areas—the original "face area" as well as the area that previously only signaled information from the arm. We wondered what the perceptual correlates of this reorganization might be. Would a sensory stimulus applied to the face be perceptually mislocalized; i.e., would it appear to come from the hand as well as the face? To explore this, we had initially studied localization of sensations in two patients (V.Q. and D.S.) after upper-limb amputation.

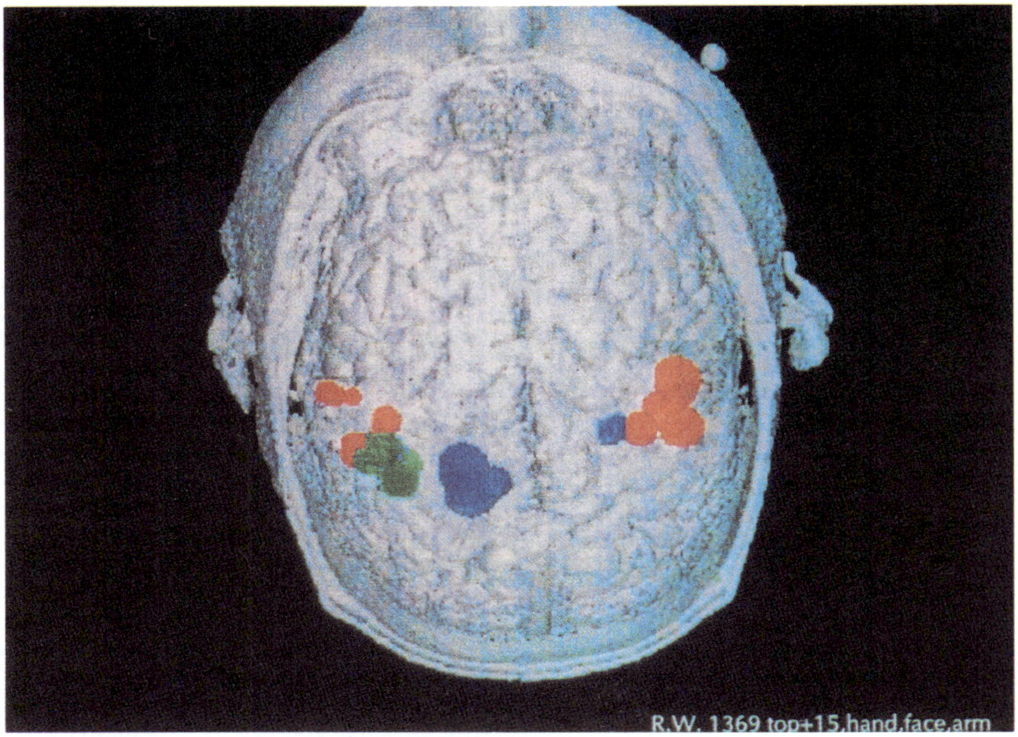

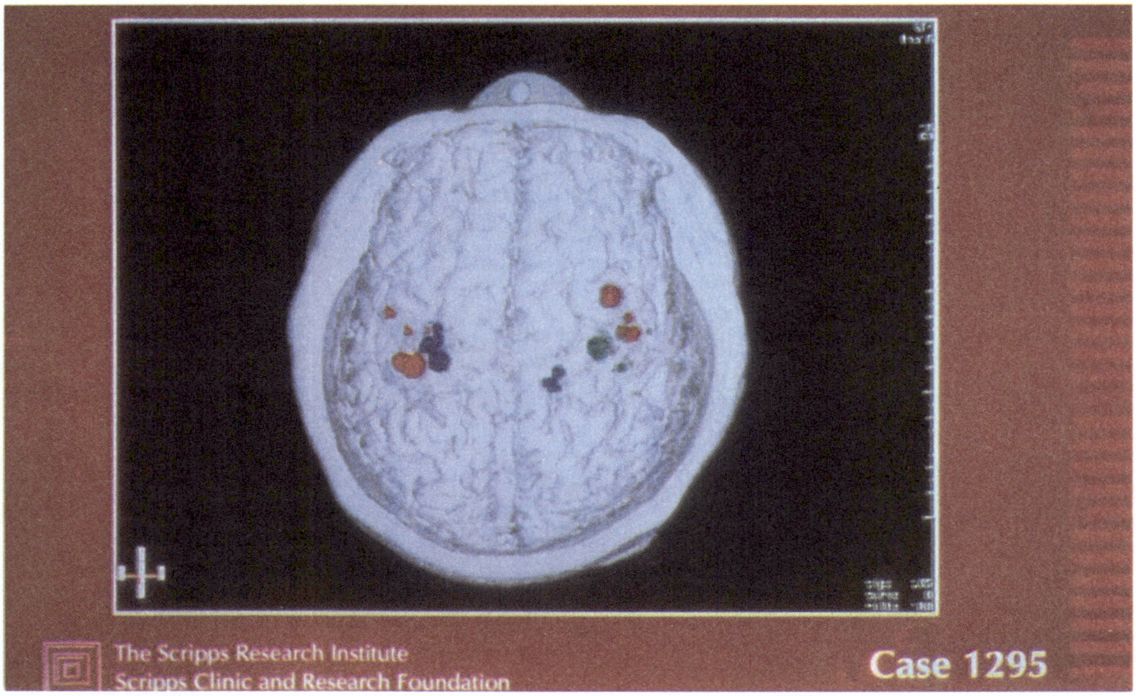

Figure 2. (*A*) Top view of a combined MEG and 3D surface-rendered MRI of an adult whose right arm was amputated below the elbow at age 11. The right hemisphere is normal and shows the primary somatosensory face area (*red*) lateral, anterior, and inferior to the hand localizations (*green*), which are in turn lateral, anterior, and inferior to the upper arm region (*blue*). The left hemisphere shows the face (*red*) and upper arm region (*blue*) extending into the expected hand territory, reflecting reorganization of the sensory map as a result of the amputation. (Adapted from Yang et al. 1994.) (*B*) Combined MEG and 3D surface-rendered MRI of patient F.A. Unaffected right hemisphere shows three spots corresponding to left face (*red*), hand (*green*), and upper arm region (*blue*). This patient's right arm was amputated below the elbow 8 years prior to these recordings (for details, see Ramachandran 1993; Yang et al. 1994).

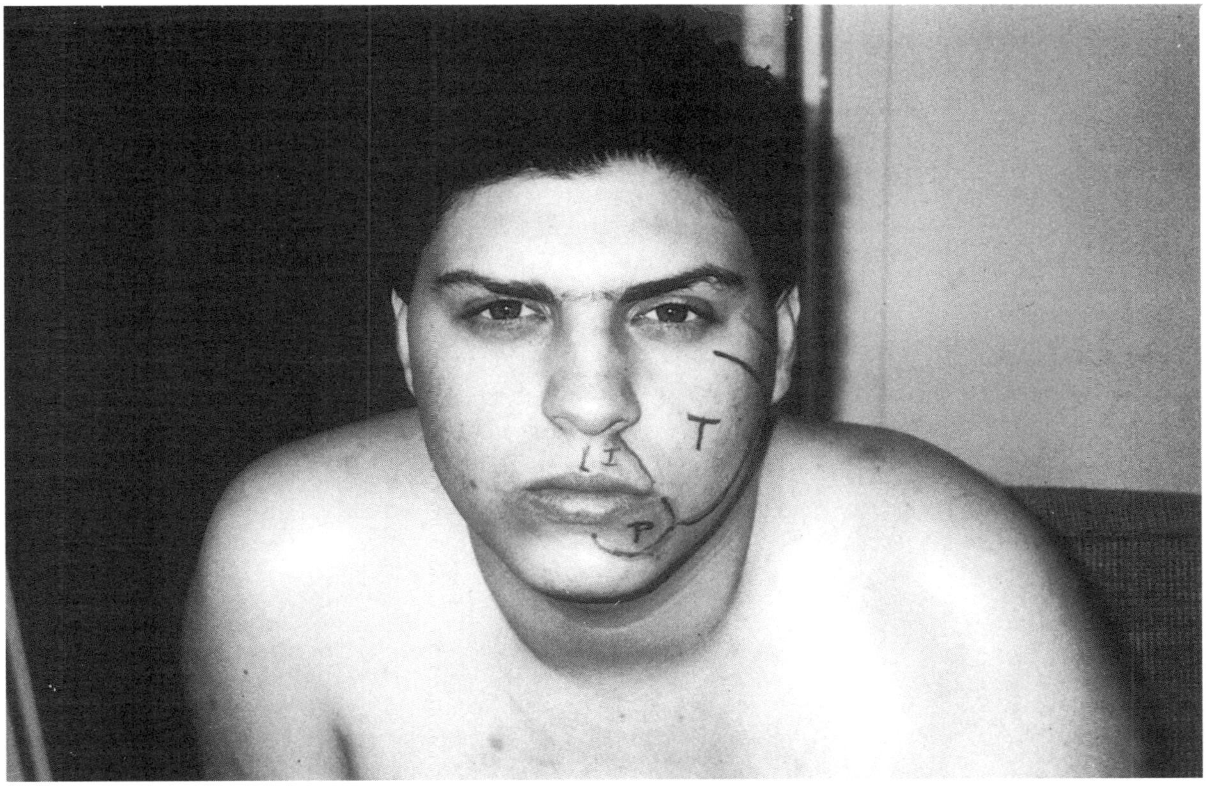

Figure 3. Regions on the left side of the face of patient V.Q. that elicited precisely localized referred sensations in the phantom digits. "Reference fields," regions that evoke referred sensations, were plotted by brushing a cotton swab repeatedly on the face. The region labeled T always evoked sensation from the phantom thumb; P, from the pinkie; I, from the index finger; and B, from the ball of the thumb. This patient was tested 4 weeks after amputation.

Patient V.Q. Patient V.Q. was an intelligent alert 17-year-old whose left arm was amputated 6 cm above the elbow about 4 weeks prior to our testing him. He experienced a vivid phantom hand that was "telescoped," i.e., it felt like it was attached just a few centimeters below his stump. We studied localization of touch (and light pressure) in this patient using a cotton swab that was brushed twice in rapid succession at various randomly selected points on his skin surface. His eyes were shut during the entire procedure and he was simply asked to describe any sensations that he felt and to report the perceived location of these sensations. Using this procedure, we found that even stimuli applied to points remote from the amputation line were often systematically mislocalized to the phantom arm. Furthermore, *the distribution of these points was not random*. They appeared to be clustered on the lower left side of the face (i.e., ipsilateral to amputation), and there was a systematic one-to-one mapping between specific regions on the face and individual digits (e.g., from the cheek to the thumb, from the philtrum to the index finger, and from the chin to the fifth finger or "pinkie"). Typically, the patient reported that he simultaneously felt the cotton swab touching his face and a "tingling" sensation in an individual digit. By repeatedly brushing the swab on his face, we were even able to plot "receptive fields" (or "reference fields") for individual digits of the (phantom) left hand on his face surface (Fig. 3). The margins of these fields were remarkably sharp and stable over successive trials. Stimuli applied to other parts of the body such as the tongue, neck, shoulders, trunk, axilla, and contralateral arm were never mislocalized to the phantom hand.

The second cluster of points that evoked referred sensations was found about 7 cm above the amputation line. Again there was a systematic one-to-one mapping with the thumb being represented medially on the anterior surface of the arm and the pinkie laterally, as if to mimic the pronated position of the phantom hand. Stimulating points halfway between these two elicited referred sensations in the index or ring fingers.

We repeated the whole procedure again after 1 week and found an identical distribution of points. We conclude, therefore, that these one-to-one correspondences are stable over time—at least over the 1-week period that separated our two testing sessions (Ramachandran et al. 1992a,b).

Patient D.S. Patient D.S. had a brachial avulsion following a motorcycle accident, and his arm was amputated a year after the accident. He experienced a vivid phantom that felt "paralyzed"—as if to mimic the

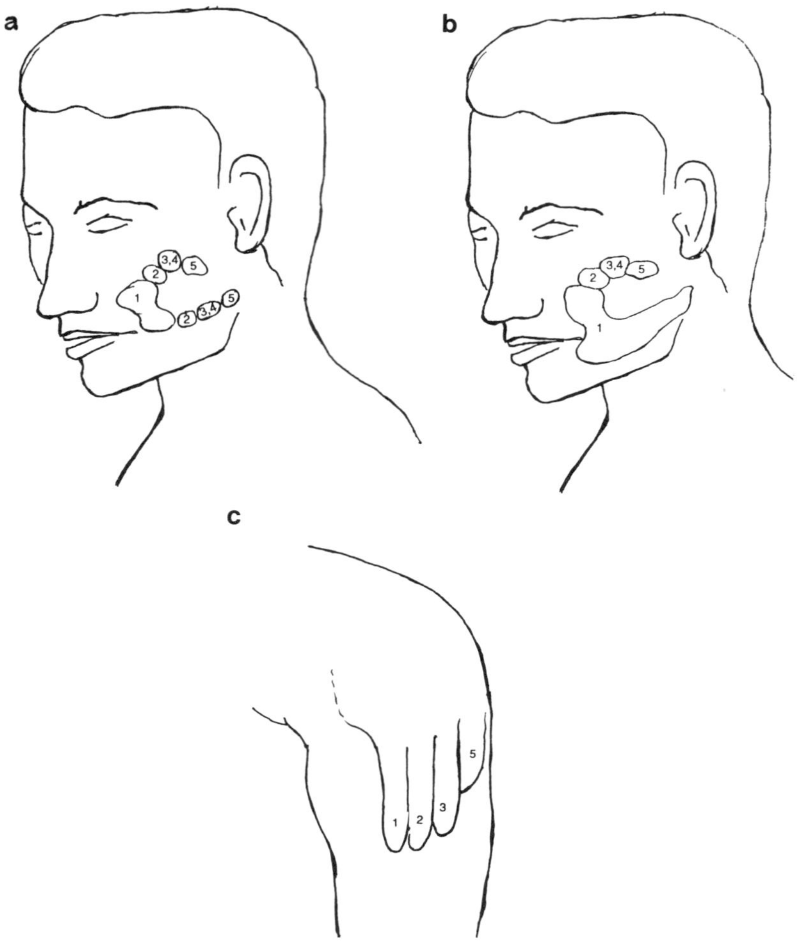

Figure 4. (*A*) Distribution of reference fields in patient D.S. Notice the prominent representation of the thumb (1), which we have seen in several patients, and the roughly topographic arrangement of digits 2, 3, 4, and 5 on the face. This pattern was nearly identical 24 hr later, but after 6 months, the representations of some of the digits had changed noticeably (*B*). This may occur as a result of sensory input and spontaneous activity from the face (and stump) continuously remodeling neural connections in S1. If this interpretation is correct, then phantom limbs might provide a valuable preparation for studying the manner in which sensory maps emerge and change in the adult nervous system. (*C*) The second map in the region of the deltoid muscle. Patient D.S.'s arm always felt completely extended and paralyzed; it was never telescoped into the stump.

paralysis that preceded the amputation. We mapped the distribution of reference fields in this patient extensively on three separate occasions, the first two separated by 24 hours and the third one after 6 months. The arrangement of reference fields is shown in Figure 4a. Notice the topographic arrangement of digits on the face (e.g., digits 1–4 are neatly laid out on the zygoma). The thumb receptive field was especially large, as in some of our other patients. Curiously, there was also a second map of sorts on the mandible, with the digits following approximately the same sequence as on the zygoma. (Stimulating the buccal region between these two maps elicited diffuse tingling on the palm.) Thus, each digit appeared to be represented twice, but the reference field on the zygoma usually corresponded to the distal interphalangeal joint, whereas the field on the mandible elicited sensations from the base of the digit.

The map remained stable during the first two testing sessions, but when we saw the patient again after 6 months, there had been some small but noticeable changes (Fig. 4b). In particular, the thumb region appeared to have expanded to stretch across the entire mandible—the base of the thumb near the ramus and the tip near the symphysis menti. It was unclear why the map had changed in this manner, but it may have occurred as a result of changing patterns of sensory input (and spontaneous activity) from the face and from the stump. It might be interesting to test this hypothesis by actually stimulating a specific region of the map (e.g., the index finger reference field) for a few days to see if this increases the size of that reference field. A second map was found in the region of the deltoid muscle and this, too, was topographically organized. Unlike the face map, however, it remained stable across all three testing sessions (Fig. 4c).

An especially convincing way of demonstrating topography in patient D.S. was as follows. When the cotton swab was moved continuously from the angle of the mandible to the symphysis menti, the referred sensation also felt like "it was moving from the ball of the thumb to the tip in an arclike motion." This observation was replicated several times. Additionally, if a short excursion was made on the jaw, the excursion on the hand was correspondingly short. Curiously, however, if the direction of motion of the cotton swab was reversed, D.S. reported a diffuse tingling in the thumb; there was no reversal of the direction of motion on the thumb. Thus, distance and velocity were accurately referred, but direction was not. A similar effect could also be evoked by moving the cotton swab across the digits' reference fields on the deltoid muscle, and in this case, reversing the direction of the cotton swab also reversed the direction of motion on the phantom hand.

Finally, it was our general impression that in patient D.S. as well as in other patients, the topography was usually much more precise in the map proximal to the stump than on the face. The reason for this difference is not clear (but see Agliotti et al. 1997).

Modality-specific Effects

The neural pathways that mediate the sensations of warmth and cold are quite different from those that carry information about touch from the skin surface to the brain (Landgren 1957, 1960; Emmers 1966; Kreisman and Zimmerman 1971). We wondered, therefore, whether the remapping effects reported by Pons and his collaborators occur separately in each of these pathways or only in the touch pathways. To find out, we tried placing a drop of warm water on V.Q.'s face. He felt the warm water on his face, of course, but, remarkably, he reported (without any prompting) that his phantom hand also felt distinctly warm. On one occasion when the water accidentally trickled down his face, he exclaimed, with surprise, that he could actually feel the warm water trickling down the length of his phantom arm! We have now seen these modality-specific effects in five patients: four patients after upper-limb amputation and one after an avulsion of the brachial plexus.

These results are important, for they imply that even when the new input is "heterotypic," i.e., derived from a foreign source, it is still *modality-specific* and preserves some semblance of topography. The manner in which such new inputs maintain their modality specificity even when innervating a "foreign" territory remains a challenging question for future research.

Discussion

The occurrence of "referred sensations" in the phantom limb is in itself not new. It has been noticed by many previous researchers (Weir-Mitchell 1872; Cronholm 1951) that stimulating points on the stump often elicits sensations from missing fingers, and the great American psychologist William James (1887) once wrote "A breeze on the stump is felt as a breeze on the phantom." Unfortunately, since the results of Pons and his collaborators were not available at the time, these early observations were open to multiple interpretations. For example, the severed nerves in the stump would be expected to reinnervate the stump and this might explain why sensations from this region are referred to the fingers. What is novel about our observations is that we discovered an actual map on the face and also found that relatively complex sensations such as "trickle" were mislocalized from the face to the phantom hand. Obviously, this cannot be attributed to accidental stimulation of nerve endings on the stump. Our observations imply, instead, that highly precise and organized new connections can be formed in the adult brain with extreme rapidity.

We have tried to relate our findings in a systematic way to physiological results—especially the "remapping" experiments of Pons et al. (1991). We have suggested, for example, that the reason we often see two "clusters" of points, one on the lower face region and a second set near or around the amputation line, is that the map of the hand on the sensory homunculus in the cortex and thalamus is flanked on one side by the face and on the other side by the upper arm, shoulder, and axilla (Fig. 1). If the sensory input from the face and from around the stump were to "invade" the cortical territory of the hand, one would expect precisely this sort of clustering of points (Fig. 2).

With regard to our experimental results themselves, what is novel can be summarized as follows:

1. The extreme rapidity of the observed changes. Patient V.Q. was tested 4 weeks after amputation.
2. The strict *one-to-one correspondence* between individual points on the lower face and points on the phantom limb.
3. The *nonrandom* distribution of points that evoke referred sensations. In both patients, the points appeared clustered on the lower ipsilateral face and near or around the line of amputation. This correlates well with the physiological remapping effect described by Pons et al. (1991). Recall, especially, that in the Penfield homunculus the hand area is flanked on one side by the face and on the other side by the areas close to the amputation line (shoulder, upper arm).
4. The presence of well-defined "reference fields" with sharp, stable margins.
5. The disproportionate representation of the hand in general and the digits in particular—especially the thumb. This may be a consequence of cortical magnification.
6. The fact that very specific sensations such as warmth, "pinpricks," or "trickle" could also be mis-

localized. This suggests that referred sensations can be modality-specific.

7. The possible existence of topography. The very fact that adjacent points on the normal skin surface (e.g., the cluster of points on the lower face or near the amputation line) map onto adjacent points in the phantom limb (i.e., hand, digits, etc.) is in itself suggestive of topography, of course. Additionally, in patient D.S., when we moved the swab over the jaw, he experienced an equivalent movement of referred sensation on his phantom arm.

What is the actual neural mechanism underlying the perceptual "remapping" that we have observed? In trying to answer this question we have to bear three facts in mind: (1) The extent of thalamocortical axon arborizations can be quite large—up to 1 cm or more (Jones and Friedman 1982). (2) The distance between the cortical maps for the hand and face is about 1–2 cm. (3) The changes we observed are quite rapid, whereas Pons et al. (1991) recorded from their monkeys nearly 12 years after deafferentation. Taken collectively, these facts suggest that the effects we have shown may arise from the unmasking of occult synapses rather than actual anatomical changes such as "sprouting." This conclusion is consistent with the pioneering physiological observations of Wall (1971) and Calford and Tweedale (1991), who found rapid unmasking of synapses after partial deafferentation. It should be borne in mind, however, that even though the cortical maps had been reorganized, the actual synaptic changes could have occurred anywhere along the somatosensory pathway en route, e.g., the thalamus or the dorsal column nuclei (see, e.g., Florence and Kaas 1995).

Our findings also suggest a novel explanation for the very existence of phantom limbs. We would argue that the effect arises because tactile and proprioceptive input from the face and tissues surrounding the amputated limb "takes over" the brain maps corresponding to the limb. (Such effects might occur not only in 3b, but also in the thalamus, the dorsal column nuclei, and the cortical areas S2 and 3a. Indeed, remapping has been shown to occur even in the motor cortex; see Cohen et al. [1991].) Consequently, spontaneous discharge from these tissues would get misinterpreted as arising from the missing limb and might therefore be felt as a phantom limb. This hypothesis is different from, although not incompatible with, the view that phantom limbs arise from a persistence of a "neurosignature" in a "neuromatrix" (Melzack 1992). We would argue, instead, that the effect arises from mechanisms of a much more specific nature such as the remapping effects reported by Pons et al. (1991).

Whatever the ultimate interpretation of our findings, however, they present a challenge to one of the basic concepts of neuroscience—the relative stability of connections in the adult brain. The extreme rapidity (4 weeks) of the changes that we have observed suggests instead that the adult mammalian brain has the latent capacity for a much more rapid functional reorganization and over a much greater spatial extent than previously suspected; a capacity that could conceivably be exploited for therapeutic purposes.

Intersubject variability. How general are the findings we have reported here? Of the 18 patients we have seen so far, the "map" on the face was seen in 8. The second cluster of points near the line of amputation, on the other hand, was seen in 12 patients.

Why do some patients not have a cluster of points on the face? There are at least four possibilities that are not mutually exclusive. First, the brain maps themselves might vary slightly from patient to patient, and this, in turn, might influence the degree of remapping. Second, some patients may eventually "learn" to ignore the referred sensations from the face by using visual feedback. Third, even without visual feedback the plasticity exhibited by the afferent pathways may be propagated further along the pathways to perception so that the input gets correctly interpreted as originating from the face alone (i.e., the peripheral organ might "specify" the central connections as suggested by Weiss [1939]). Fourth, if the patient uses the stump constantly, the skin corresponding to it may "regain" the territory that was initially lost to the face. Obviously, more extensive testing of a large number of patients is needed before we can distinguish among these possibilities. It is worth noting, in this context, that at least one patient (F.A.) who showed clear evidence of remapping as revealed by MEG (Yang et al. 1993) did *not* refer sensation for his face to his hand, suggesting that the second or third of these hypotheses is correct; i.e., the remapping in the primary sensory areas is not *sufficient* to guarantee the occurrence of referred sensations, although it may be necessary.

Related studies by other groups. Our findings on perceptual referral of sensations from the face to the phantom and the accompanying MEG changes were reported in 1992 (Ramachandran et al. 1992a,b) and 1993 (Ramachandran 1993; Yang et al. 1994a,b). During the last 3 years there have been several follow-up studies by other groups that have confirmed and significantly extended these findings. I now briefly describe some of these studies.

Halligan et al. (1993) studied a patient whose arm had been amputated at the shoulder level. They were able to replicate our basic observation—the occurrence of a map on the ipsilateral lower face. Curiously, they found that although the map was nearly complete and was in many ways quite similar to ours, it lacked an index finger and thumb. Careful questioning of the patient revealed that she had completely lost sensations in her thumb and index finger for over a year preceding the amputation (she had suffered from carpal tunnel syndrome). It was as though this sensory loss had been "carried over" into her phantom!

Our own observations, as well as those of Halligan et al. (1993), do not resolve the issue of whether what we call remapping arises from the sprouting of new axon terminals that invade the hand territory or from unmasking or disinhibition of previously silent inputs (Wall 1971). Since we had seen the face-to-hand referral of sensations 4 weeks after amputation in one patient, we originally suggested that reactivation of previously silent pathways may be involved (Ramachandran et al. 1992a,b), but we had no direct proof.

A recent discovery made by D. Borsook et al. (in prep.) at the Massachusetts General Hospital suggests that such unmasking may indeed be taking place. They examined two patients (one after amputation and one after brachial avulsion) and just 24 hours after the deafferentation found that touch and cold sensations from the lower face were referred to the hand and that the referral was topographically organized. This provides compelling evidence that activation of dormant and ordinarily silent connections can occur, at least in some patients.

The recent MEG results of Flor et al. (1995) are also broadly consistent with what we had found. Flor et al. obtained MEG recordings from 20 arm amputees and found that in all of them, the input from the face and upper arm could now activate the hand territory. In addition, many (but not all) of these patients reported the tactile stimuli on the face were also felt in the phantom, which is essentially identical to what we had reported. Intriguingly, Flor et al. also found a high correlation between the extent of remapping (observed with MEG) and the extent to which the patient reported phantom pain. If these findings hold up, they would imply that cortical remapping can not only lead to referral of neutral sensation, but may also contribute to the genesis of phantom pain.

How massive a deafferentation is required for remapping to occur? This has not been investigated in detail, but an intriguing report by Aglioti et al. (1997) deserves mention. These authors studied a patient who had lost an index finger and found that the patient not only reported referral from adjacent fingers (as we had reported in Ramachandran 1993), but also had a topographically organized referral from the ipsilateral face to the finger. Indeed, there appeared to be a "map" of the finger neatly draped across the cheek and lower jaw. This was seen 5 months after amputation, but when the patient was seen again 3 years later, this map of the finger on the ipsilateral face disappeared and, mysteriously, a scrambled representation of the same finger appeared on a mirror symmetric location on the contralateral face! The referral from the adjacent fingers, however, remained stable and identical to what it had been 3 years earlier. The authors suggest that repeated "use" of the adjacent fingers helps stabilize topography, whereas the map on the cheek disintegrates since it isn't used in a systematic manner. This is an important point and is consistent with some of our own speculations (Ramachandran 1993).

The technique of transcortical magnetic stimulation has been exploited successfully for studying reorganization of the *motor* cortex (Pascua-leone et al. 1996). Recently, these authors attempted to simultaneously track perceptual referral and stimulation-induced referral in the same patient. No change in the cortical map was observed immediately after amputation, but after 5 weeks, stimulation of the original "hand area" of the cortex began to evoke dual sensations—one in the hand and one in the lower face. (The resolution of the technique did not allow them to determine whether motor or sensory strips were being stimulated. In all likelihood, both were.) Interestingly, touch sensations on the lower ipsilateral face were also referred to the phantom, as in our patients. Finally, when the experiment was repeated a third time several months later, magnetic stimulation of the face area of the cortex did *not* evoke sensations in the hand—only face sensations were felt. (Consistent with this, touch stimuli on the face were no longer mislocalized to the phantom.) These findings would explain why referral from face to phantom may be seen only transiently, e.g., during the first few months, and why the phenomenon may disappear after a few years in many patients (Ramachandran 1993).

Finally, the question arises as to what happens after lower-limb amputation. In the Penfield homunculus, the genitals are adjacent to the foot and, as one might expect, we found that two patients reported experiencing sensations in their phantom foot during sexual intercourse. One of these patients, a 60-year-old engineer, reported actually feeling erotic sensations in the foot so that his "orgasm is much bigger than it used to be" (Ramachandran 1993). Agliotti et al. (1994) undertook a more systematic investigation of several lower-limb amputees and found that many of them had topographically organized maps proximal to the stump and, often, a second cluster of points on the genitals that yielded referred sensations in the phantom leg. (One wonders whether foot fetishes, even in normal individuals, may have a similar origin.)

Summary. Taken collectively, these studies suggest that the emergence of referred sensations in amputees is a robust perceptual phenomenon that can be related in a systematic way both to animal studies and to the results of noninvasive imaging experiments. With the advent of inexpensive new imaging techniques such as fMRI, the stage is now set for exploring plasticity in the adult human brain by simultaneously tracking perceptual and anatomical changes in individual patients. This, in turn, may allow us to develop conceptual links between conscious experience and the activity of somatosensory maps in the brain.

ANOSOGNOSIA

In the previous sections, I discussed two very unusual neurological syndromes—phantom limbs and the Capgras syndrome. I turn now to another equally fascinating disorder called anosognosia (Babinsky 1914; Weinstein and Kahn 1950; Critchley 1966; Cutting 1978; Edelman 1989; Kinsbourne 1989; McGlynn and Schacter 1989; Levine 1990; Bisiach and Geminiani 1991; Heilman 1991; Galin 1992; Damasio 1994; Ramachandran 1994, 1995b). When the right hemisphere of the brain is damaged, there is usually complete paralysis of the left side of the body. Of course, most of these patients complain about their paralysis and often ask their physician when they are going to recover. Surprisingly, however, there is a small percentage of these patients who obstinately insist that their left arm is not paralyzed even though they are mentally lucid in other respects. Indeed, on rare occasions they even deny ownership of their left arm, asserting that it belongs to either a spouse or to the examining physician! The syndrome was first noticed at the turn of the century by Babinsky (1914), who coined the term anosognosia: denial of illness. Although this syndrome has been known for almost 100 years, there has been a tendency within the medical community to regard it as an enigmatic clinical curiosity. Surprisingly, there have been almost no attempts to do systematic experiments on these patients.

To familiarize the reader with the syndrome, I briefly describe a patient I saw not long ago. Mrs. F.D. was a patient in her late 70s who had sustained a stroke about 1 week prior to my seeing her in the hospital. The left side of her body was completely paralyzed as a result of her stroke. I walked into the hospital and started chatting with her.

V.S.R.: Mrs. F.D., what is your husband's name?

She answered correctly.

V.S.R.: Mrs. F.D., how many children do you have and what do they do?

Again she answered all these questions correctly. All this was done simply to make sure that she was mentally quite lucid and capable of normal fluent conversation. Following this conversation I asked her,

V.S.R.: Mrs. F.D., why did you come to the hospital?
F.D.: I came here because I had a stroke.
V.S.R.: When did you have the stroke?
F.D.: A week ago.
V.S.R.: How do you know you had a stroke?
F.D.: I know I had a stroke because I fell in the bathroom and my daughter then brought me to the hospital and they did some brain scans and told me I had a stroke.

Clearly, she was aware she had a stroke.

V.S.R.: Mrs. F.D., how are you feeling today?
F.D.: I've got a headache. I've had a stroke so they brought me to the hospital.
V.S.R.: Mrs. F.D., can you walk?
F.D.: Yes.

She had been in a wheelchair for the past week. She could not walk.

V.S.R.: Mrs. F.D. hold out your hands. Can you move your hands?
F.D.: Yes.
V.S.R.: Can you use your right hand?
F.D.: Yes.
V.S.R.: Can you use your left hand?
F.D.: Yes.
V.S.R.: Are both hands equally strong?
F.D.: Yes, of course they are.

At this point an interesting question arises, what if you were to actually confront the patient? What if you were to ask her to perform an action with her left arm? How far can you push the patient along this line of questioning? Clinicians are usually reluctant to do this for fear of precipitating what Kurt Goldstein (1940) has called a "catastrophic reaction." This is simply medical jargon which means, "The patient starts crying because her defenses break down and she falls apart." But I thought I'd try it anyway. (If you empathize with the patient and take her very slowly through the process perhaps you can avoid a catastrophic reaction.)

V.S.R.: Can you point to my nose with your right hand?

She pointed to my nose.

V.S.R.: Point to me with your left hand.

Her hand lay paralyzed in front of her.

V.S.R.: Are you pointing at my nose?
F.D.: Yes.
V.S.R.: Can you clearly see it pointing?
F.D.: Yes, it is about 2 inches from your nose.

At this point the woman produced a frank confabulation, a delusion about the position of her arm. She had no problems with her vision and could see her arm perfectly clearly, yet she created a delusion about her own body image. (I had verified previously that she had no left hemineglect, and I also took the precaution of standing on her right side.) I couldn't resist asking her:

V.S.R.: Can you clap?
F.D.: Of course I can clap.
V.S.R.: Will you clap for me?

She proceeded to make clapping movements with her right hand as if clapping with an imaginary hand near the midline.

V.S.R.: Are you clapping?
F.D.: Yes, I'm clapping.

Thus, here at last, we may have an answer to the Zen master's eternal riddle: What is the sound of one hand clapping? Mrs. F.D. obviously knew the answer!

What we've seen in Mrs. F.D. is unusual. More commonly what the patient does when you keep probing further and further is to finally come up with an excuse, a rationalization, to account for her failure to use her left arm. Consider the following example with another patient, Mrs. L.R.:

V.S.R.: Mrs. L.R., can you use both your right and left arms?
L.R.: Yes.
V.S.R.: Can you use your left arm?
L.R.: I can use my left arm.
V.S.R.: Mrs. L.R., can you point to my nose with your right hand?

She pointed to me with her right hand.

V.S.R.: Mrs. L.R., can you point to me with your left hand?

She doesn't do anything.

V.S.R.: Mrs. L.R., why aren't you using your left arm?
L.R.: Oh, I've got severe arthritis in my shoulder. You know that, Doctor; it hurts.

On another occasion:

V.S.R.: Mrs. L.R., why aren't you using your left arm?
L.R.: Doctor, these medical students have been prodding me all day and I'm sick of it. I don't want to use my left arm.

Sometimes they'll come up with all sorts of ingenious euphemisms to avoid admitting they're paralyzed.

V.S.R.: Mrs. L.R., how come you're not using your left arm?
L.R. I've never been very ambidextrous, Doctor.

When I first started studying this syndrome about 2 years ago, I was struck by the fact that many of the excuses that these patients come up with bear a striking resemblance to what Sigmund and Anna Freud have called "psychological defense mechanisms." Examples of such defense mechanisms are shown in Table 1.

Table 1. Psychological Defenses

1. Denial	denying something that is potentially threatening
2. Repression	blocking access to unpleasant memories
3. Confabulation	fabrication of missing information
4. Reaction formation	asserting the opposite of what one "knows" to be true (e.g., "gay bashing" may signify latent homosexuality)
5. Rationalization	inserting a spurious "reason" or excuse to account for something
6. Projection	attributing a potentially unpleasant trait to someone else
7. Dissociation	being aware of something intellectually but suppressing its emotional overtones
8. Displacement	deflecting attention from the main source of threat to another more harmless target. Sometimes humor can serve as a displacement

A partial list of psychological defense mechanisms used by the mind to restore equilibrium (adapted from S. Freud [1895–1961] and A. Freud [1946]). Examples of each of these were frequently seen in our anosognosia patients, often in comically exaggerated form; e.g., a patient with a terminal right frontal brain tumor displays 7 and 8, often drawing attention to his carbuncle. Patients L.R. and F.D. frequently resorted to 1, 5, and 3, and L.R. also to 2 and 4. Many of the patients also unknowingly used humor as a defense.

The reader will recall that I began this paper by debunking Freud. Indeed "Freud bashing" has become a fashionable intellectual pastime these days. Bear in mind that although Freud wrote a great deal of nonsense, he did have deep insight into the human condition, and specifically with regard to psychological defense mechanisms, I think he was right on the mark.

So, what causes anosognosia? Not surprisingly, there have been dozens of theories, but most of them can be classified into two main categories: first, the cognitive-sensory deficit theory and second, the Freudian/ psychodynamic theory. I think neither of these theories completely accounts for the syndrome, but I describe them anyway. The first theory postulates that even though the patient's left arm is paralyzed, his right hemisphere is continuing to send motor commands to the paralyzed arm. These are monitored elsewhere in the brain, so the patient vividly experiences the arm to be moving even though it's not moving. Together with this, the patient often has visual hemineglect, a general indifference to the left side of the world, and consequently may not notice that the left arm is not adequately responding to his motor command. This may be the basis of anosognosia. Later in this paper, I mention two experiments that directly demolish this view of anosognosia, but suffice it to say here that I don't think this theory adequately explains the syndrome for two reasons: First, neglect and anosognosia are dissociable (we've seen several patients with anosognosia who do not have neglect and conversely several patients who have neglect who do not have anosognosia; also see Bisiach and Geminiani 1991). Second, the motor commands sent to the arm may create the illusion that the arm is moving, but the patient does not merely suffer from the illusion. He does not say, "I have this vivid illusion that my arm is moving but I realize that it is paralyzed." He actually *believes* that the arm is moving, and it is this change in belief that cries out for an explanation. Contrast this with the patients with phantom limbs we discussed earlier in this paper. They often experience vivid movement in their phantom, presumably because they're monitoring the motor outflow to those limbs, and yet they do not say "my arm has actually come back and I am actually moving my arm." They recognize that in fact what they're experiencing is an illusion (Ramachandran and Rogers-Ramachandran 1996b), but this is not true for patients with anosognosia.

According to the second theory (i.e., the Freudian view), this is simply a form of psychological defense. In other words, the patient is paralyzed, and since this is unpleasant, he does not want to confront it and therefore engages in emotional denial of paralysis. The problem with this theory is that it doesn't explain the asymmetry—why the syndrome is seen more often after a right hemisphere stroke. When a patient has a left hemisphere stroke, he also has a paralysis which is presumably just as unpleasant, and yet the patient rarely engages in denial. This asymmetry suggests that you have to look to neurology for an explanation, not psychology. It is precisely this fact that makes this syndrome of anosognosia so fascinating. It sits right at the border between neurology on the one hand and psychiatry on the other hand. In our laboratory, we have a special interest in these types of syndromes, which straddle the boundary between neurology and psychiatry.

Maximizing Fitness: The Coherencing of Consciousness and the Evolution of Freudian Defenses

In this section, we argue that the peculiar remarks made by patients with anosognosia can actually help us understand the evolutionary origins of Freudian defenses in normal human behavior. In particular, there appears to be a need for "coherencing" consciousness and for smoothing over or "filling in" gaps in information that might be potentially distracting to central executive structures. The ultimate purpose of doing this, we suggest, is to stabilize behavior and to optimize resource allocation, given the ever-present need for rapid action (Ramachandran 1995a). The overarching rule seems to be that *any* decision—even one that has a small chance of being flawed—is better than no action at all. A perpetually indecisive organism is unlikely to pass its genes to the next generation.

What is the basis of anosognosia? The best way of formulating the problem, in my view, is to ask two questions. The first question is why normal people engage in these defenses; the phenomenon is certainly not unique to anosognosia. It is surely obvious that normal individuals also frequently engage in the different forms of self-deception, and it is a challenge for evolutionary theory to try to explain this. The second question is why these mechanisms are so grossly exaggerated in these patients. If you have paralysis of your left arm, you might play it down a little bit, but you certainly wouldn't say, "Yes, I can see it touching your nose," or " I can hear it clapping." We have to explain why these defenses are so floridly exaggerated in these patients (Ramachandran 1994, 1995a).

To understand this, we have to look to hemispheric specialization. The left hemisphere is specialized for language, especially for syntactic and expressive aspects of language (Gazzaniga 1992). The right hemisphere, on the other hand, is specialized for holistic aspects of vision and for some aspects of emotion. I submit that there is an even more fundamental distinction between the two hemispheres; one that concerns the manner with which they deal with discrepancies in the sensory input. First consider the left hemisphere. Each person, in his waking life, is confronted with a bewildering array of sensory inputs as he interacts with the world. All this information needs to be put together to create a coherent and internally consistent belief system—what one believes to be true about oneself and the world. (In other words, you need a story.) I'd argue that this construction of a belief system is done primarily by the left hemisphere. When some new information is encountered, this ordinarily is assimilated seamlessly into the preexisting belief system. However, what if the new information that comes in doesn't fit the preexisting scheme? Then there are several options. First, the belief system could simply be completely changed and started from scratch. The trouble is, on most occasions there simply isn't enough time, and if one tried to do this every time a minor discrepancy was encountered, sooner or later the behavior would become completely chaotic and unstable. Therefore, in most instances, a better option would be to either generate an ad hoc auxiliary hypothesis or *simply pretend that the discrepancy doesn't exist*. This is what would correspond roughly to what we call a denial or a repression. Indeed, all of the mechanisms listed in Table 1 would fall into this category. I submit that the main reason these defense mechanisms evolved is to impose stability on behavior; i.e., they should, in essence, be regarded as a by-product of a general coherencing mechanism in the left hemisphere that has evolved mainly to override discrepancies and optimize resource allocation whenever rapid action is required. Clearly, there has to be a limit to this process, for it is only a useful strategy as long as the discrepancy is small. If one were to suddenly encounter a glaring anomaly, it would be foolish to keep ignoring it. To do so would cause one to become progressively more and more delusional and, in fact, get trapped in cul-de-sacs of delusion. I suggest that there is an exactly complementary mechanism in the right hemisphere—a "devil's advocate"—that serves to counterbalance the delusional tendencies of the left hemisphere. Its job is to look for global inconsistencies and when these inconsistencies reach a certain magnitude, to force a complete revision in one's world view—what Thomas Kuhn might call a "paradigm shift." In other words, it requires the right hemisphere's participation to generate a paradigm shift in response to an anomaly. In anosognosia, only the patient's right hemisphere is damaged, so the left hemisphere goes about its job of rationalizing, denying, confabulating, etc. In the absence of a correcting mechanism in the right hemisphere, however, there's no limit to the kinds of delusions that the patient will engage in. "Yes Doctor, I can see my finger touching your nose." "Yes Doctor, I can (actually) clap." This, I think, explains many aspects of the syndrome.

Another intriguing aspect of these patients' behavior is their frequent use of quasi-humorous remarks when talking about their paralyzed arm. For example,

V.S.R.: Mrs. D., do you think you can touch my nose with your left hand?

Table 2. Patients

Patient	Age, sex	Handedness	Major neurological deficits	Site of lesions
L.R.	78, F	R	left hemiplegia and severe neglect	right frontoparietal CVA (CT scan)
Q.S.	65, F	R	left hemiplegia	right temperoparietal infarct (CT scan)
L.H.	77, F	R	left hemiplegia and neglect	right middle cerebral artery and left cerebellar artery infarct (CT scan)
F.D.	77, F	R	left hemiplegia and severe neglect	infarct in the territory of right middle cerebral artery and right cerebellar arteries (CT scan)
D.C.	56, M	R	left hemiplegia and severe neglect	right middle cerebral artery infarct (CT scan)

All five patients who participated in our anosognosia study had recently sustained right hemisphere stroke causing left hemiplegia. No formal neuropsychological tests (such as WAIS-R or CVLT) were administered, but I conducted a routine neurological workup, including a mental status examination, on each patient. At the time when our experiments were conducted, they did not have any obvious signs of dementia, aphasia, or amnesia and were able to clearly understand my instructions. Whenever possible, a CT scan and/or an MRI was obtained. For details, see Ramachandran (1996).

D.: Yes, but watch out! I might poke you in the eye as I am doing it.

On another occasion,

V.S.R.: Mr. C., do you think you are going to be completely okay when you return home from the hospital?

C.: Yeah. I can't wait to get back to two-fisted beer-drinking.

These remarks have the odd implication that at *some* level the patient may be "aware" that he/she is indeed paralyzed. The fact that the remarks are tinged with a perverse sense of humor is especially interesting, and one wonders whether the language areas of the left hemisphere have become especially creative in humorous wordplay as a result of the right hemisphere stroke!

The model of hemispheric specialization I have proposed—the left being a die-hard conservative and the right being a starry-eyed revolutionary—is unashamedly speculative. The idea may help explain not only why normal individuals are so notoriously prone to self-deception, but also why these psychological defenses are so floridly exaggerated in anosognosia. Additionally, notice the similarity between this view and the dialectic that underlies the scientific enterprise as a whole—long periods of humdrum "normal science" punctuated by paradigm shifts or revolutions in response to anomalies. The usual response of the scientific community to an anomaly is, of course, to brush it under the carpet. However, if the anomaly is too glaring, the appropriate response would be to tear down the whole edifice and start from scratch, and this has happened time and again in the history of science. I find it tantalizing that what we see in the scientific enterprise as a whole should find instantiation in the basic architecture of individual human brains.

I turn now to the actual experiments I have been doing on these patients (see Table 2) during the last 2 years. In particular, we can use the theoretical ideas outlined above as a starting point to ask several new questions about the syndrome; questions that have never been asked before. I have so far been able to obtain only partial answers to these questions since the syndrome is quite rare, but I hope this essay will provoke the reader to try to answer them when he/she encounters patients in the clinic.

EXPERIMENTS ON CONFABULATION

Question 1: Does Anosognosia Arise from Monitoring Motor Commands to the Paralyzed Arm?

Does anosognosia arise from simply monitoring the motor commands that are sent to the paralyzed arm, combined with visual hemineglect so that the patient fails to notice that the arm has not moved? If, in addition, the patient has mild dementia (as they sometimes do), it is easy to see how the three factors could conspire to produce anosognosia (see, e.g., Levine 1990).

This account is probably at least partially correct, but it fails to satisfy me for three reasons. First, although some patients with the syndrome display mild dementia, especially in the first few days, an equal number are mentally quite lucid (as we showed above). Second, hemineglect and anosognosia are dissociable, even though they frequently occur together. Last, even when the neglect is overcome and the patient's attention is drawn to the arm, he/she will often continue to deny that it is paralyzed. It is the vehemence of the denial, not merely the indifference to the paralysis, that cries out for our explanation and makes one wonder whether there is an "emotional" component to the syndrome.

To answer the question more decisively, however, I conducted two experiments. The first experiment was conducted on patient Cooper, a friendly, intelligent 56-year-old man who had sustained a RT cerebrovascular accident (CVA) a week prior to my seeing him. After chatting with him informally, I walked out of the room for 5 minutes and then walked back in again. As I approached the bed I looked at him and said, "Mr. Cooper, why did you just move your left arm?" even though his left arm was perfectly still (as, indeed, was his right arm). Any normal person would have responded by saying, "What do you mean? I *wasn't* doing anything with my left arm," or "I don't understand," or "*Did I* move my left arm?" Mr. Cooper looked at me calmly and said, "I was gesticulating to make a point!" On the next day I repeated exactly the same experiment and his response was, "It hurts so I moved it to relieve the pain."

Since there can be no question of Mr. Cooper having sent a "motor command" to the arm at exactly the time when I questioned him, this result suggests that anosognosia is the result of a *deranged belief system* that may involve an emotional component as well. We return to this point in a later section.

Question 2: Does Anosognosia Arise from Neglect?

Can anosognosia really be conceived of as a failure to generate paradigm shifts in response to an anomaly? An alternate interpretation, as we noted earlier, would be in terms of hemineglect of the left side of the body, i.e., the patient's failure to *orient* to the left. I have already noted that I find this idea implausible, but to test the idea more directly, I devised a new experiment. What would happen, I wondered, if one were to temporarily paralyze the *right* arm of a patient who was already suffering from anosognosia in association with left hemiplegia? (Assume the paralysis is achieved by cutting peripheral nerves in the right arm.) Would the anosognosia now encompass his *right* arm as well? Note that my theory of anosognosia, outlined above, makes the counterintuitive prediction that he should now deny that his *right* arm is paralyzed (since his devil's advocate fails to initiate a paradigm shift), whereas the neglect theory makes the opposite prediction, since there is no neglect of his right side.

To "paralyze" the patient's (Mrs. F.D.) right arm, I used a simple optical trick. The technique is similar to one originally developed for studying intersensory conflict in *normal* subjects (Nielsen 1963), but I realized that it might provide a valuable tool for probing the depth of anosognosia in patients with a right parietal lesion.

The "virtual reality box" was constructed out of cardboard and mirrors. The patient's gloved right hand is inserted through a window in front of the box and she peeks into the box from a hole in the top to look at what she thinks is her own hand. Unbeknownst to the patient, an accomplice inserts his gloved left hand through another opening in the box so that its mirror image is optically superimposed on the patient's right hand and she is "tricked" into thinking that she is looking directly at her own right hand. The patient is then instructed to move her right hand up and down to the rhythm of a metronome. The accomplice holds his hand completely steady so that the patient is "fooled" into thinking that her hand is absolutely still, as though it were paralyzed. I repeated the experiment on two consecutive days, and on each day she maintained that she could clearly see her arm moving up and down to the rhythm of the metronome, even though the view afforded to her through the virtual reality box was that of a paralyzed hand!

This simple experiment demolishes all "neglect" theories of anosognosia, since there was certainly no neglect of the right visual (or somatic) field in this patient, and yet she was producing confabulations about her right hand! Clearly, at least in this one patient, what is deranged is the manner in which she deals with a discrepancy in sensory inputs concerning her body image; it is not critical whether the discrepancy arises from the left or from the right side of the body.

Question 3: How Deep Is the Denial?

When thinking about anosognosia, a second question that arises is, How deeply does the patient believe his/her own denials and confabulations? Is it simply a surface facade, or perhaps even an attempt at malingering?

The vehemence of the patient's denials and her quasi-humorous, euphemistic remarks can themselves be taken as evidence that she is "aware" at some level that she is paralyzed (e.g., "Yes, of course, I can use my left hand. In fact, I used it to wash my face this morning," or, "Yeah, I can't wait to get back to two-fisted drinking," or, "I am not very ambidextrous, Doctor").

The question then becomes, For what sorts of behavior is this tacit knowledge available if it exists? For example, would it be available for a spontaneous, nonverbal motor response?

I did two experiments to explore this. In the first experiment, I simply placed a large cocktail tray in front of the patient. (The tray had six plastic glasses containing water.) When normal people reach for the tray to lift it, their right hand goes to the right end of the tray and the left hand to the left side. When I tested hemiplegic patients who did *not* have anosognosia, their nonparalyzed hand went straight for the middle of the tray near its center of gravity as expected, but when I tried the same experiment with patients who had anosognosia, their right hand went to the *right* side of the tray! Obviously, the glasses toppled but they usually made remarks such as, "Oops! How clumsy of me." Thus, even when no direct verbal confrontation is involved, the patient behaves as though his left hand is working normally.

The logic of the second experiment was somewhat different. I gave four patients a choice between a simple unimanual task or a simple bimanual task which would be impossible to perform with one hand; e.g., in one case the choice was to either thread a light bulb into a socket that was mounted on a heavy base (unimanual) or to tie a shoelace (bimanual). If the patient threaded the light bulb, she would receive a $5 reward, and if she tied the shoelace she would receive $10. Remarkably, the patients start trying to tie the laces and keep at it for several minutes without showing any signs of frustration. Even when the patients were then given the same choice 10 minutes later, they *again* went invariably for the bimanual task. In one case (Mrs. L.R.), the tests were repeated on several consecutive occasions—always with the same result. Indeed, it looks as though the patients have no memory of their previous failures, a "selective amnesia" for their previous failed attempts.

Question 4: Does the Patient Also Deny Remote Consequences of Paralysis?

Clearly, then, the patients appear not to have "tacit" knowledge of paralysis, or if such knowledge exists, it is not available for these two tasks—the cocktail tray and the unimanual/bimanual choice. The implication is that the denial runs very deep, it's not just a surface facade at a purely verbal level. This raises another interesting question. Given that the patients deny only the immediate consequences of the paralysis, would they also deny its remote consequences, or are they dimly aware that something is seriously wrong? What if you were to ask them indirect questions? "Are you doing okay? Can you drive home tonight? Can you go back to the same job you were holding before?"

We have not explored this on a systematic basis, but on the four occasions when we have specifically asked this question, the responses indicate that the patients are indeed unaware of the remote consequences of the paralysis, e.g., the patient will, as we have seen, usually state that she can walk. ("I walked to the restroom this morning, Doctor.") We have even seen examples of patients (e.g., Mr. Cooper) whose job requires the use of two hands, and if they are asked, "Can you go back to your job?" they will assert vehemently, "Oh, yes. I don't see a problem there." This is interesting because it suggests, once again, that far from being a more sensory/motor distortion, their whole range of beliefs about such matters has been radically altered to accommodate the denial.

Question 5: How Domain-specific Is Anosognosia?

The next question is, How domain-specific is anosognosia? The patient denies that her left arm is paralyzed; but will she also deny other disabilities that she is currently suffering from? This question has in fact been raised before by other researchers (see, e.g., Kinsbourne 1989; Bisiach and Geminiani 1991). The usual answer is that the patient does not deny other disabilities, so anosognosia seems to be domain-specific. It is confined to matters concerning her left arm, although, as we saw in the previous example, it can also extend to her right arm under appropriate circumstances. To give an example, one of my patients, Ms. B.M., when I offered her some candy as a reward for the bimanual task, vehemently protested, saying "I am diabetic, Doctor, I can't eat candy." Clearly, she was aware of her diabetes. Almost all the patients I have tested are also aware of the fact that they have had a stroke; they certainly don't suffer a global denial. However, the real answer to this question, I think, depends on how far anterior the lesion is in the right hemisphere. When the lesion is confined to the right parietal, confabulations and denials are confined to body image. On the other hand, if the lesion is more anterior, the denial may become more global. I saw a patient not too long ago with a right frontal grade-five malignant astrocytoma who had no more that 6 months to live (statistically speaking). When I saw this patient, he was intelligent and lucid. He had been trained as an engineer, and he was certainly aware at some level that he had been diagnosed as having a terminal brain tumor, yet he seemed to be blissfully unconcerned about having this problem. When I saw him, he would frequently draw attention to a little carbuncle he had on his forehead. He constantly complained that the other doctors hadn't done anything about it and asked if I could do anything to help. When I would return to the topic of the brain tumor, he would avoid talking about it and make assertions such as, "Well, you know how these doctors sometimes incorrectly diagnose things." Here is an intelligent person flatly contradicting the evidence provided by his physicians and somehow playing down the fact that he has a terminal brain tumor. This sort of general indifference is characteristic of right frontal patients. Whether the tendency to cling to status quo pertains only to matters concerning "self" or also to other aspects of the world around them remains to be investigated. For instance, are the confabulations of right hemisphere patients geared mainly toward protecting the integrity of the self, or can they be provoked to confabulate about other abstract matters as well? If you were to ask such a patient, "How many hairs does Clinton have on his head?", would he confabulate or would he admit ignorance?

On the one occasion when I tried this, the patient looked very perplexed (but not amused), and she responded "I don't know." It is possible that more global confabulation of this kind can be provoked only in patients with frontal involvement, but there have been very few systematic studies to specifically explore this.

Question 6: Would the Patient Deny Another Patient's Paralysis?

Another fascinating question concerns the extent to which the patient will admit/deny the paralysis of *another* patient in an adjacent wheelchair. Unfortunately, we have been unable to get a clear-cut answer to this question. Of five densely anosognosic patients we have tested to date, two denied the paralysis of another patient (or "stooge") near them, even when the paralysis was explicitly demonstrated to them by the examining physician. The other three patients, on the other hand, readily acknowledged that the stooge was *not* moving his arm, making remarks such as, "Of course, his left arm is paralyzed" (Ramachandran and Rogers-Ramachandran 1996b). The reason for these differences is obscure, but it is possible that the first two patients had some form of object-centered (or "person-centered") neglect, so that they didn't notice the stooge's failure to move. Alternately, one may need to access one's own body schema in order to make judgments about other peoples' movements, and those patients may have been unable to do so because of their right parietal lesion. Finally, although they had no difficulty following our commands to move their right arm, they may have had a mild apraxia (in addition to the anosognosia), and it is well known that apraxic patients can have difficulty making judgments about other peoples' movements (e.g., see Heilman 1985).

Question 7: Is There an Emotional Component to Denial?

Although clinical experience indicates that anosognosia may have an emotional component, there are many theories that are opposed to this view. For example, as we pointed out earlier, one popular theory of anosognosia is the sensory/cognitive theory, which asserts that anosognosia results from simply monitoring motor commands to the paralyzed arm, combined with neglect and indifference to the contradictory information from the left arm. Consider also that some of the patients may have an element of dementia, and you have three separate factors that may conspire to create the more florid manifestations of anosognosia (Levine 1990). As noted previously, this may be true for some patients, but it doesn't get to the crux of the problem. I now describe an experiment which demonstrates very directly that in anosognosia there is an actual change in the patient's belief system. Here is an intelligent patient denying that his left arm is paralyzed. The question then arises, What if you somehow make this paralysis more acceptable to the patient? Well, how do you do that? To achieve this goal, I began by simply conducting an informal neurological workup on the patient. I then showed a syringe full of saline to the patient and told him, "As part of your neurological exam, I would like to inject your left arm with this anesthetic. And as soon as I do it your left arm will be temporarily paralyzed for a few minutes." After making sure that the patient has understood this, I proceed to "inject" the arm with the saline. The question is, Will the patient suddenly admit that she is paralyzed, now that it has been made more acceptable to her, or will she say, "Your injection doesn't work; I can move my arm fine."? This is a lovely example, because it demonstrates that we can actually do experiments on peoples' belief systems, and I would like to coin a new name for this field of inquiry: experimental epistemology (just to annoy the philosophers)! We have not done this experiment on a systematic basis on a large number of patients, but I briefly describe some preliminary results. I vividly recall one patient, Ms. R., who had complete paralysis of her left side and was in denial. I went through my usual questioning to elicit anosognosia, asking, "Can you use your right or left arm? Are they equally strong?" To which all her answers were "Yes." Then I said, "Ms. R. I am now going to inject your left arm with this local anesthetic and it will be temporarily paralyzed." As soon as she heard this, she looked me straight in the eye, and without batting an eyelid, said, "But Doctor, is that *fair*?" It was as though the patient was playing some sort of game with me and I had suddenly changed the rules and this was forbidden! I did not have the heart to proceed further with the experiment, so I went to the next patient, Mr. C. After conducting a brief neurological exam, I told him, "Mr. C., I am going to inject your left arm with this anesthetic and it's going to be paralyzed for a few minutes." To this he responded, "Okay, I can live with that." I proceeded to inject his left arm and ask him, "Mr. C., can you move your left arm?" Mr. C., "No, it don't seem to want to do nothing. It's not moving." Apparently, my mock injection had worked, and it had allowed him to accept the fact that his left arm was paralyzed!

How could I be sure that this was not simply the result of my persuasive charm? Maybe I was just hypnotizing the patient into accepting that his arm was paralyzed. Therefore, I did the obvious control; I repeated the same procedure with his *right* arm. I went back into the room and, after chatting with him briefly about other irrelevant topics, I said, "As part of the neurological exam I'm going to inject your *right* arm with this local anesthetic, and after I perform the injection, your right arm will be paralyzed for a few minutes." I proceeded to give him the injection (remember he had seen me use the same syringe earlier to "paralyze" his left arm) and asked him if his right arm was moving. As expected, he moved his right arm and replied, "Yes, it's moving doctor." I said, "Well, how is that possible? I just injected you with an anesthetic!" To which he responded, "Well, I don't know, Doctor. I guess it's mind over matter. I have always believed that." As pointed out earlier in this paper, these patients are remarkably creative and ingenious in coming up with quasi-rational explanations to account for the strange discrepancies that they encounter. In fact, I'm sometimes tempted to wonder if the damage to the right hemisphere has actually made them more creative—in the verbal domain—than they used to be before the stroke!

Question 8: Does the Patient Deny Only Negative Attributes or Will He Also Deny Positive Ones?

Clearly, anosognosia entails a change in the patient's belief system, and there appears to be a strong emotional component to the denial, at least in some patients. Earlier in this paper I suggested this arises, at least in part, from the left hemisphere's tendency to cling to the status quo and its refusal to change its world view in response to anomalies of the sensory input. If so, another interesting question arises, Will the patient only deny negative attributes such as paralysis of the left arm, or will he also be tempted to deny positive attributes? Consider the following far-fetched example. What if by some miracle the left arm became stronger—perhaps super-humanly so—compared to the right arm. Would he then deny it was stronger? Obviously there is no simple way to answer this question, but I did have the opportunity to try to answer this question with Mr. C. recently. I did so by simply asking questions such as the following:

V.S.R.: Mr. C., can you use your right arm?
Mr. C.: Yes, I can use my right arm.
V.S.R.: Mr. C., Can you use your left arm?
Mr. C.: Yes.
V.S.R.: Are they equally strong?
Mr. C.: Yes.
V.S.R.: Mr. C., can you lift 100 pounds with your left arm?
Mr. C.: Oh, yes. I can lift 100 pounds.
V.S.R.: Mr. C., can you lift 300 pounds?

My question was, would he be willing to attribute superhuman powers to his left arm? (One recalls one of the Freudian defense mechanisms, reaction formation.)

Mr. C.: No, I don't think I could lift 300 pounds.

Yet on a later occasion when I asked him, "Can you balance this cup on the end of a pencil using your left arm?" he replied without any hesitation, "Yes, of course I can." Clearly this experiment needs to be performed on additional patients, but it looks as though on some trials, at least, the patient was willing to attribute absurd abilities to the left arm!

More commonly, I have seen patients assert that their left arm is actually stronger than their right. For example, when I asked Mrs. M.G. whether her two hands were equally strong, she replied "No; my left hand is stronger." (I made sure, of course, that she had no left/right confusion).

V S.R.: Can you lift a table with your right hand?
Mrs. M.G.: Why yes, I could probably lift it about one inch.
V S.R.: What about your left hand?
Mrs. M.G.: Oh yes, I can lift the table *two* inches with my left hand.

Question 9: Does the Patient Remember His Confessions or Denials?

Some of the experiments we described above seem to indicate that the patient does not have tacit knowledge about his paralysis or that, even if such information exists, it's not available for the types of tasks that we were giving him, e.g., for the unimanual/bimanual choice, or for lifting the cocktail tray. This raises an interesting question. Is it the case that knowledge of paralysis simply doesn't exist in his brain? Or does the knowledge exist somewhere, but access to it is blocked? One hint comes from the kind of euphemistic remarks the patients often make when talking about their left arm. For example, after Mrs. L.R. had unsuccessfully tried performing the bimanual task of tying the shoelace on several trials, one of my students went up to her and asked,

S.: Mrs. L.R., you remember Dr. Ramachandran?
L.R.: Yes, of course, he's that nice Indian doctor.
S.: What did he ask you to do?
L.R.: He gave me a child's shoe and asked me to tie the shoelaces.
S.: Did you do it?
L.R.: Yes, I did it successfully with *both* my hands.

This raises an interesting question. Why would any normal person volunteer that she used both her hands to tie a shoelace? It is a striking example of what Freud called "reaction formation"—asserting the opposite of what you really believe to be true ("Methinks the lady doth protest too much"). Again, it seems to suggest that at some level the patient is actually aware that she is paralyzed, although there are many layers of self-deception masking this knowledge and preventing access to it. (Also recall Mrs. T.'s remark, "But is that fair, Doctor?").

Our next question concerns the patients' memories for their paralysis. As noted above, patients with anosognosia will continue to vehemently deny their paralysis even when confronted with contradictory evidence. There have been some occasions where the patient eventually admits that her left arm is "not working," is "weak," or sometimes even "paralyzed." Interestingly, even having admitted the paralysis, patients sometimes remain unconcerned about it and display a sort of absent-minded indifference. After the patient has finally admitted that the arm is paralyzed, with repeated questioning, what if you were to show up again after 10 minutes and ask her about her left arm? Would she remember her confession? We've tried this experiment on several occasions and the usual answer seems to be "no." In other words, if you can return to the patient 10 minutes later, the patient will once again say, "Oh, yes. My left arm is working fine" (Ramachandran 1994, 1995b). Thus, there seems to be a sort of selective amnesia of the patient's own earlier admissions of her paralysis. Surprisingly, even on the one occasion when the patient had a "catastrophic reaction," she had no recollection of this a few hours later. This is about as close as one can get to a direct demonstration of what Freudians would call "repression."

This amnesia seems to affect only the *actions* of the left hand, but not other aspects of that hand. On one occasion, the patient was surprised to notice that I had slipped a red hair-band on her left hand. After removing the band, I started questioning her about the movements of that hand and, as expected, she vehemently denied the paralysis but, with repeated questioning, she finally admitted that it "wasn't working." Yet, a few minutes later, she had no recollection of this "confession," even though she vividly remembered the hair-band!

My second question concerning memory is the following: Patients with anosognosia very often recover completely after 2 or 3 weeks and stop denying that they are paralyzed. Why this happens is still unclear, but it raises another question. What if you were to go to the patient after she has completely recovered and ask her, "When I saw you earlier this week and I asked you about your left arm, what did you tell me?" Would they admit that they had been denying the paralysis or would they also deny the denial (Ramachandran 1994, 1995b, 1996)?

We have tried this experiment on three patients but, unfortunately, were unable to obtain a clear-cut answer. One patient (Mr. Cooper), interviewed 3 days after recovery from anosognosia, vividly recalled that he had denied his paralysis. "I could see that it wasn't moving but my mind didn't want to acccept it. I guess I was in denial." The second patient (O.S.) vehemently denied her paralysis on the several occasions that I tested her but recovered completely from the anosognosia after a month. Yet, when I questioned her several months later, she denied her denials and added, "If I denied it, I must have been lying and I am *not* a liar." The third patient, Mrs. M.G., developed dense anosognosia 12 hours after a right hemisphere stroke. She asserted repeatedly that her left hand was working fine. (Indeed, she claimed it was stronger than her right hand.) The next day she recovered completely from the denial and admitted paralysis. Yet, when questioned about the previous day she said, "You asked me if I could lift a table, and I said I could lift it one inch." "What about your left arm?" I asked. "I said I couldn't use my left arm," she said confidently. The reason for the difference between Mr. Cooper and the other two patients is unclear, but even after apparently complete recovery from anosognosia, there may be a residual neural defect in the right hemisphere, and the extent to which the patient admits or denies her earlier denials may itself depend on the extent of these residual lesions (Ramachandran 1996).

Despite the variability, however, it is clear from these examples that some patients do indeed "deny their denials," even though they are mentally lucid and remember other details quite clearly. Perhaps there is no simple way for the patient to reconcile her current insight into her paralysis with her previous lack of it, and consequently, her only recourse is to "repress" her denials to match her current beliefs. Further experiments on the patients may therefore allow us to explore the formation of memory traces—caught in flagrante—and to discover how new items of information are incorporated seamlessly into one's preexisting cognitive schemata.

I conclude this section with one final question about memory. What if a patient were to have a peripheral nerve lesion in her left arm so that her left arm was paralyzed for a few months and *then* she develops a right hemisphere stroke rendering her hemiplegic on the left side? Assume, further, that she also had a lesion of the right hemisphere of the kind that normally produces anosognosia. Would she then suddenly say, "Oh, my God, Doctor. My arm that had been paralyzed all along is suddenly moving again." Going back to my theory that the patient tends to cling to his preexisting world view, does he cling to his *updated* world view and therefore say that his left arm is paralyzed, or would he go back to his earlier body image and assert that in fact his arm is moving again? Needless to say, I've yet to see such a patient, but we are hoping that sooner or later someone will encounter a patient with this problem and ask him this question.

Summary

Talking to a patient with anosognosia can be an uncanny experience. With most neurological syndromes, the patient loses some specific mental capacity (e.g., syntax in Broca's aphasia and face recognition in prosopagnosia), but the integrity of the person remains largely intact. What is especially fascinating about anosognosia, on the other hand, is that the very notion of a "person" or "self" is called into question. To listen to a patient deny ownership of her left arm and yet in the same breath admit that it is attached to her shoulder is one of the most perplexing experiences one can have as a neurologist.

My goal, in this paper, has been mainly to ask several new questions about this curious disorder. It is remarkable that although the syndrome has been known since 1910, many of these questions have not even been asked before. Given the relative rarity of the disorder, I have only been able to provide partial answers to some of the questions (e.g., Questions 1, 2, 3, and 7). For example, it seems reasonably clear that there has been an actual change in the patient's *belief* about his arm and that there is an emotional component to this denial. For certain other questions, however, the answers continue to remain elusive, e.g., Would the patient deny another patient's paralysis? If the patient recovers from anosognosia, will she deny her earlier denial? It may be a long time before we get all the answers, but to me the exciting thing is that one can even *begin* to experimentally approach such questions as self-deception or Freudian psychology.

CONCLUSIONS

I began this paper with a mysterious disorder—the Capgras delusion—and suggested that at last some aspects of the syndrome could be explained in a fairly precise manner, taking into account the known anatomy and connections in different parts of the temporal lobes. In the second section, I dealt with a more well known, but equally perplexing, syndrome, phantom limbs. I suggested that far from being a mere clinical curiosity, this syndrome provides a valuable opportunity for tracking plasticity in the adult human brain and for developing conceptual links between perceptual experience and the activity of sensory maps in the cortex. The experiments are relatively straightforward, and most of the basic findings have been replicated by other groups.

The third section is highly speculative and deals with the most enigmatic syndrome of all—anosognosia—in which a lucid mentally alert patient vehemently denies the paralysis of his left arm. In this section I raised several new empirical questions about this curious syndrome and tried to provide partial answers to at least some of them (e.g., How deep is the denial? Is there an emotional component?). I would emphasize, however, that these empirical questions are just the tip of the iceberg. When I began my training as a student of neurology over 15 years ago, I was taught (as indeed most students are taught today!) that there are certain questions about the brain and mind that are best avoided—questions such as, "What is consciousness? What brings about the seamless unity of my conscious experience? What does it mean to "will" an action? What is the neural representation of a "belief?" What is the self? Was Freud right?" And so on and so forth. In other words, we were advised to stay away from all those questions that everyone was interested in! Yet, oddly enough, it is precisely these "taboo" questions that you come face-to-face with each time you encounter one of these patients. I would argue, therefore, that by studying syndromes such as anosognosia or the Capgras delusion we can begin to experimentally approach these elusive and enigmatic aspects of human nature. Indeed, as we have seen, they may even help us answer the Zen master's eternal riddle, "What is the sound of one hand clapping?"

ACKNOWLEDGMENTS

I thank P. Churchland, W. Hirstein, O. Sacks, J. Smythes, E. Altschuller, F. H. C. Crick, D. Galin, M. Kinsbourne, J. Salk, C. Jennings, J. Bogen, and A. Starr for stimulating discussions. The ideas for experiments discussed under Question 5 and Question 6 emerged from conversations I had with numerous colleagues, especially I. Faber, D. Rogers-Ramachandran, and W. Hirstein. I also thank the National Institute of Mental Health for support. This paper is based on the Dorcas Cummings lecture I gave at Cold Spring Harbor in 1996.

REFERENCES

Aglioti, S., A. Bonazzi, and F. Cortese. 1994. Phantom lower limb as a perceptual marker for plasticity in the mature human brain. *Proc. R. Soc. Lond. B Biol. Sci.* **255:** 273.

Aglioti, S., N. Smania, A. Atzei, and G. Berlucchi. 1997. Spatio temporal properties of the pattern of evoked phantom sensations in a left index amputee patient. *Behav. Neurosci.* (in press).

Allison, G., W.R. Goff, P.D. Williamson, and J.C. Van Gilder. 1980. On the neural origin of early components of the human somatosensory evoked potential. *Prog. Clin. Neurophysiol.* **7:** 51.

Babinski, M. J. 1914. Contribution a l'etude des troubles mentaux dans l'hemiplegie organique cerebrale. *Rev. Neurol.* **1:** 845.

Baumgartner, C., W.W. Sutherling, S. Di, and D.S. Barth. 1991. Spatiotemporal modeling of cerebral evoked magnetic fields to median nerve stimulation. *Electroencephalogr. Clin. Neurophysiol.* **79:** 27.

Bisiach, E. and G. Geminiani. 1991. Anosognosia, related to hemiplegia and hemianopia. In *Awareness of deficit after brain injury* (ed. G. Prigatano and D. Schacter), p. 17. Oxford University Press, New York.

Calford, M. 1991. Curious cortical change. *Nature* **352:** 759.

Calford, M. and R. Tweedale. 1991. Immediate expansion of receptive fields of neurons in area 3B of macaque monkeys after digit denervation. *Somatosens. Mot. Res.* **8:** 249.

Capgras, J. and J. Reboul-Lachaux. 1923. L'illusion des "sosies" dans un delire systematise chronique. *Bull. Soc. Clin. Med. Ment.* **2:** 6.

Cohen, L.G., S. Bandinelli, T.W. Findley, and M. Hallett. 1991. Motor reorganization after upper limb amputation in man. A study with focal magnetic stimulation. *Brain* **114:** 615.

Critchley, M. 1966. *The parietal lobes.* Hafner, New York.

Cronholm, B. 1951. Phantom limbs in amputees. A study of changes in the integration of centripetal impulses with special reference to referred sensations. *Acta Psychiatr. Neurol. Scand. Suppl.* **72:** 1.

Cutting, J. 1978. Study of anosognosia. *J. Neurology Neurosurg. Psychiatry.* **41:** 548.

Dale, A.M. and M.I. Sereno. 1993. Improved localization of cortical activity by combining EEG and MEG with MRI cortical surface reconstruction—A linear approach. *J. Cogn. Neurosci.* **5:** 162.

Damasio, A.R. 1985. Prosopagnosia. *Trends Neurosci.* **8:** 132.

———. 1994. *Descartes error.* Putnam, New York.

Edelman, G.M. 1989. *The remembered present.* Basic Books, New York.

Ellis, H.D. and A.W. Young. 1990. Accounting for delusional misidentifications. *Br. J. Psychiatry* **157:** 239.

Emmers, R. 1966. Separate relays of tactile, pressure, thermal, and gustatory modalities in cat thalamus. *Proc. Soc. Exp. Biol. Med.* **121:** 527.

Farah, M. 1990. *Visual agnosia.* MIT Press, Cambridge, Massachusetts.

Flor, H., T. Elbert, S. Knecht, C. Pantev, N. Birbaumer, and E. Taub. 1995. Phantom limb pain. *Nature* **375:** 482.

Florence, N. and J. Kaas. 1995. Large-scale reorganization at multiple levels of the somatosensory pathways follows therapeutic amputation. *J. Neurosci.* **15:** 8083.

Freud, A. 1946. *The ego and the mechanisms of defense.* International Universities Press, New York.

Freud, S. 1895–1961. *The standard edition of the complete works of Sigmund Freud*, vols. 1–23. Hogarth Press, London

Galin, D. 1992. Theoretical reflections on awareness, monitoring and self in relation to anosognosia. *Conscious. Cognition* **1:** 151.

Gallen, C.C., D.F. Sobel, J.A. Sanders, B.L. Hart, L.E. Davis, and W.W. Orrison. 1993a. Magnetic resonance functional mapping. *Radiology* **187:** 863.

Gallen, C.C., D. Sobel, T. Waltz, M. Aung, B. Copeland, B.J. Schwartz, E.C. Hirschkoff, and F.E. Bloom. 1993. Noninvasive pre-surgical neuromagnetic mapping of somatosensory cortex. *Neurosurgery* **33:** 260.

Gazzaniga, M. 1992. *Nature's mind.* Basic Books, New York.

Goldstein, K. 1940. *Human nature.* Harvard University Press, Cambridge, Massachusetts.

Halligan, P., J. Marshall, and N. Wade. 1993. Thumb in cheek. *NeuroReport* **4:** 233.

Hari, R., K. Reinikaimen, E. Kaukoranta, M. Hamalainen, R. Ilmoniemi, A. Penttinen, J. Salminen, and D. Teszner. 1984. Somatosensory evoked cerebral magnetic fields from SI and SII in man. *Electroencephalogr. Clin. Neurophysiol.* **57:** 254.

Heilman, J. 1991. *Awareness of deficits after brain injury* (ed. G. Prigatano and D. Schacter). Oxford University Press, United Kingdom.

Heilman, K. 1985. Appraxia. In *Clinical neuropsychology* (ed. K. Heilman and E. Valenstein). Oxford University Press, United Kingdom.

Hirstein, W. and V.S. Ramachandran. 1997. Capgras syndrome: A novel probe for understanding the temporal "binding" of memories. *Proc. R. Soc. Lond. B Biol. Sci.* (in press.)

James, W. 1887. The consciousness of lost limbs. *Proc. Am. Soc. Psychical Res.* **1:** 249.

Jones, E. G. and P. Friedman. 1982. Projection pattern of functional components of thalamic ventrobasel complex on monkey somatosensory cortex. *J. Neurophysiol.* **48:** 521.

Kaas, J.H., R.J. Nelson, M. Sur, and M.M. Merzenich. 1981. *The organization of the cerebral cortex*, p. 237. MIT Press, Cambridge, Massachusetts.

Kinsbourne, M. 1989. A model of adaptive behavior. *Emotions and the dual brain* (ed. G. Gianotti and C. Caltagrione). Springer-Verlag, Heidelberg.

Kreisman, N. R. and I.D. Zimmerman. 1971. Cortical unit responses to temperature stimulation of the skin. *Brain Res.* **25:** 184.

Landgren, S. 1957. Convergence of tactile, thermal, and gustatory impulses on single cortical cells. *Acta Physiol. Scand.* **40:** 210.

———. 1960. Thalamic neurons responding to cooling of the cat's tongue. *Acta Physiol. Scand.* **48:** 255.

Levine, D.N. 1990. Unawareness of visual and sensorimotor defects: A hypothesis. *Brain Cognition* **13:** 233.

McGlynn, S.M. and D.L. Schacter. 1989. Unawareness of deficits in neuropsychological syndromes. *J. Clin. Exp. Neuropsychol.* **11:** 143.

Melzack, R. 1992. The painful reality of phantom limbs. *Sci. Am.* **266:** 90.

Merzenich, M.M., M. Sur, R.J. Nelson, and J.H. Kaas. 1981. Organization of the SI cortex: Multiple cutaneous representations in areas 3b and 1 of the owl monkey. In *Cortical sensory organization* (ed. C.N. Woolsey), vol. 1, p. 47. Humana Press, Clifton, New Jersey.

Merzenich, M.M., J.H. Kaas, J.T. Wall, R.J. Nelson, M. Sur, and D. Felleman. 1983. Topographic reorganization of somatosensory cortical areas 3b and 1 in adult monkeys following restricted deafferentation. *Neuroscience* **8:** 33.

Merzenich, M.M., R.J. Nelson, M.S. Stryker, M.S. Cynader, A. Schoppmann, and J.M. Zook. 1984. Somatosensory cortical map changes following digit amputation in adult monkeys. *J. Comp. Neurol.* **224:** 591.

Mosher, J.C., P.S. Lewis, and R.M. Leahy. 1992. Multiple dipole modeling and localization from spatio-temporal MEG data. *IEEE Trans. Biomed. Eng.* **39:** 541.

Nielsen, T. 1963. Volition: A new experimental approach. *Scand. J. Psychol.* **4:** 215.

Okada, Y.C., R. Tanenbaum, S.J. Williamson, and L. Kaufman. 1984. Somatotopic organization of the human somatosensory cortex revealed by neuromagnetic measurements. *Exp. Brain Res.* **156:** 197.

Pascual-leone, M., M. Peris, J. Tormos, and D. Catala. 1996. Reorganization of human cortical motor output maps following traumatic amputation. *NeuroReport* **7:** 2068.

Penfield, W. and T. Rasmussen. 1950. *The cerebral cortex of man.* MacMillan, New York.

Pons, T.P., A.K. Garraghty, A.K. Ommaya, J.H. Kaas, E. Taub, and M. Mishkin. 1991. Massive cortical reorganization after sensory deafferentation in adult macaques. *Science* **252:** 1857.

Ramachandran, V.S. 1993. Behavioural and MEG correlates of neural plasticity in the adult human brain. *Proc. Natl. Acad. Sci.* **90:** 10413.

———. 1994. Phantom limbs, neglect syndromes and Freudian psychology. *Int. Rev. Neurobiol.* **37:** 291.

———. 1995a. Anosognosia in parietal lobe syndrome. *Conscious. Cognition* **4:** 22.

———. 1995b. Perceptual correlates of neural plasticity in the adult human brain. In *Early vision and beyond* (ed. T. Papathomas and C. Chubb), p. 227. MIT Press, Cambridge, Massachusetts.

———. 1996. *Decade of the Brain Lecture.* Illusion of body image: What they reveal of human nature. In *The mind brain continuum* (ed. R. Linas and P. Churchland). MIT Press, Cambridge, Massachusetts.

Ramachandran, V.S. and D. Rogers-Ramachandran. 1996a. Denial of disabilities in anosognosia. *Nature* **382:** 501.

———. 1996b. Synaesthesia in phantom limbs induced with mirrors. *Proc. R. Soc. Lond. B Biol. Sci.* **263:** 377.

Ramachandran, V.S., D. Rogers-Ramachandran, and M. Stewart. 1992a. Perceptual correlates of massive cortical reorganization (comments). *Science* **258:** 1159.

Ramachandran, V.S., M. Stewart, and D. Rogers-Ramachandran. 1992b. Perceptual correlates of massive cortical reorganization. *NeuroReport* **3:** 583.

Signer, S.F. 1994. Localization and lateralization in the delusion of substitution. *Psychopathology* **27:** 168.

Wall, J.T. 1988. Variable organization in cortical maps of the skin as an indication of the lifelong adaptive capacities of circuits in the mammalian brain. *Trends Neurosci.* **11:** 549.

Wall, P. 1971. The presence of inaffective synapses and the circumstances which unmask them. *Philos. Trans. R. Soc. Lond. B Biol. Sci.* **278:** 361.

Weinstein, E.A. and R.L. Kahn. 1950. The syndrome of anosognosia. *Arch. Neurol. Psychiatry* **64:** 772.

Weir-Mitchell, S. 1872. *Injuries of nerves and their consequences.* Lippincott, Philadelphia.

Weiss, P. 1939. *Principles of development.* Holt, New York.

Yang, T., C. Galen, and V.S. Ramachandran. 1994a. Noninvasive detection of cerebral plasticity in the adult human somatosensory cortex. *NeuroReport* **5:** 701.

Yang, T., C. Gallen, F. Bloom, V.S. Ramachandran, and S. Cobb. 1994b. Sensory maps in the human brain. *Nature* **368:** 592.

Yang, T.T., C.C. Gallen, B. Schwartz, and F.E. Bloom. 1993. Detailed somatosensory homunculus mapping using a large array biomagnetometer. *Proc. Natl. Acad. Sci.* **90:** 3098.

The Molecular Biology of Olfactory Perception

P. MOMBAERTS,[1] F. WANG, C. DULAC, R. VASSAR,[2] S.K. CHAO, A. NEMES,
M. MENDELSOHN, J. EDMONDSON, AND R. AXEL
Department of Biochemistry and Molecular Biophysics, Howard Hughes Medical Institute, and the Center for Neurobiology and Behavior, College of Physicians & Surgeons, Columbia University, New York, New York 10032

Sensory systems receive information from the environment and transmit these signals to higher cortical centers in the brain, where they are processed to provide an internal representation of the external world. Mammals possess an olfactory system of enormous discriminatory power (for review, see Shepherd 1994; Buck 1996). Humans, for example, are thought to be capable of distinguishing among thousands of discrete odors. The perception of odors in humans is often viewed as an aesthetic sense, a sense capable of evoking emotion and memory leading to measured thoughts and behaviors. Smell, however, is the primal sense and can elicit innate and stereotyped behaviors. For most organisms, olfaction is the central sensory modality allowing communication with the environment.

How are the diversity and specficity of odor recognition accomplished? The initial step in olfactory discrimination requires the interaction of odorous ligands with a family of seven-transmembrane-domain receptors on olfactory sensory neurons. The repertoire of mammalian olfactory receptors is extremely large and consists of about 1000 different genes (Buck and Axel 1991; Levy and Bakalyar 1991; Parmentier et al. 1992; Ben-Arie et al. 1994). Discrimination among odorants requires that the brain determine which of the numerous receptors have been activated. In situ hybridization with olfactory receptor genes suggests that each cell expresses only one or a small number of receptor genes, such that individual olfactory neurons are functionally distinct (Ngai et al. 1993b; Ressler et al. 1993; C. Dulac and R. Axel, unpubl.). The problem of distinguishing which receptor has been activated can therefore be reduced to a problem of distinguishing which neurons have been activated.

How does the brain determine which of the functionally distinct sensory neurons have been activated? In other sensory systems, defined spatial patterns of sensory neurons or their projections are used to indicate the quality of the stimulus. In the somatosensory system, for example, the different somatic sensory submodalities (touch, proprioception, nociception, and thermoreception) result from the activation of distinct sensory cells that project to specific regions of the brain via topographically segregated pathways (Mountcastle 1957; Perl et al. 1962; Dykes et al. 1982; Berkeley 1985). The olfactory system, therefore, may also use spatial segregation of sensory input to encode the identity of the odorant stimulus.

One particularly clear example of the spatial segregation of olfactory neurons responsive to different odorant modalities is provided by the presence of two anatomically distinct olfactory organs in mammals: the main olfactory epithelium (MOE) and the vomeronasal organ (VNO) (for review, see Halpern 1987; Wysocki 1989). The pheromones activate the VNO and elicit a characteristic array of innate reproductive and social behaviors, along with dramatic neuroendocrine responses. The axons from sensory neurons of the MOE project to the main olfactory bulb, and then send most of its fibers to the olfactory cortex which in turn projects higher sensory centers. The vomeronasal system, however, transmits olfactory information via a separate pathway of neuronal projections (Fig. 1). The neurons of the VNO send axons to the accessory olfactory bulb, which projects to a discrete locus within the amygdala (Winans and Scalia 1970; Broadwell 1975; Scalia and Winans 1975). The vomeronasal nucleus in the amygdala in turn sends fibers directly to the hypothalamus (Krettek and Price 1978; Kevetter and Winans 1981). Thus, unlike the MOE, the VNO pathway bypasses higher cognitive centers, resulting in innate and stereotyped behavior in neuroendocrine responses.

What features of the vertebrate olfactory apparatus might form the anatomic basis for a spatial map of olfactory information recognized by the MOE? Odorant stimuli are received from the environment by receptors on olfactory sensory neurons in the olfactory epithelium. Each olfactory neuron projects a single unbranched axon (Fig. 1). As the collection of axons emerge from the olfactory mucosa, they fasciculate to form the olfactory nerve. The axons of the olfactory neurons synapse with dendrites of the mitral and tufted cells in the olfactory bulb, the first relay station for olfactory signaling in the brain. The mitral and tufted cells of the olfactory bulb in turn project axons to higher cortical centers via the olfactory tract (Fig. 1). Thus, the anatomy of the olfactory system affords the opportunity for spatial segregation of afferent sensory input at all levels from the peripheral epithelium to the olfactory cortex.

Present addresses: [1]The Rockefeller University, 1230 York Avenue, New York, New York 10021; [2]AMGEN, 1840 Dehavilland Drive, Thousand Oaks, California 91320-1789.

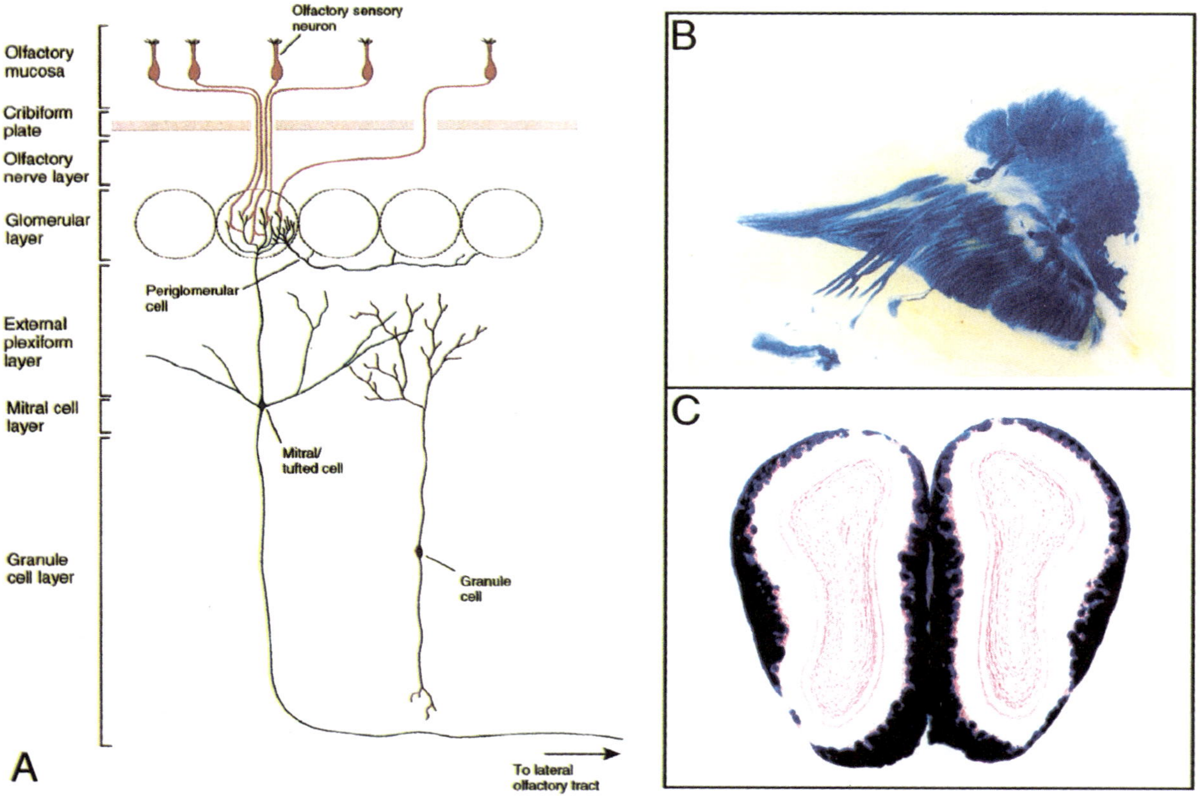

Figure 1. Organization of the mammalian olfactory system. (*A*) Cellular organization of the olfactory bulb. Sensory neurons in the olfactory epithelium (*red*) project axons to spherical regions of neuropil in the olfactory bulb called glomeruli. The sensory neurons synapse with the principal output neurons of the bulb mitral and tufted cells, which project axons to the cortex via the olfactory tract. Granule and periglomerular cells are local inhibitory interneurons. (*B*) Whole-mount view of the olfactory system. Gene targeting was used to generate mice in which the olfactory marker protein gene was replaced by tau-lacZ, allowing visualization of olfactory neurons, along with the axons as they project through the cribriform plate into the olfactory bulb. Three collections of olfactory neurons are visible: the main olfactory epithelium (*right*); the VNO (*bottom left*); and the septal organ. The olfactory bulb is at the top right. (*C*) The olfactory bulb. Coronal section through the olfactory bulbs of OMP tau-lacZ mouse revealing staining in the blue outer nerve layer and glomerular layer, which contain the axons and axon terminals of olfactory neurons. Neutral red stains the cell bodies of periglomerular cells, mitral cells, and granule cells.

We have performed a series of genetic and molecular biological experiments which provide physical evidence that neurons expressing a given receptor, although randomly distributed within a zone of the epithelium, project their axons to one or a few discrete glomeruli within the olfactory bulb. The positions of specific glomeruli are bilaterally symmetric and are conserved in the brains of all animals within a species. These data, together with previous physiological studies (Lancet et al. 1982; Kauer et al. 1987; Imamura et al. 1992; Katoh et al. 1993), support a model of olfactory coding in which the discrimination of odor quality would result from the detection of specific spatial patterns of glomerular activity within the olfactory bulb.

RESULTS

A Multigene Family of Odorant Receptors

Insight into the mechanisms underlying the logic of olfactory perception is likely to emerge from the identification of the genes encoding the odorant receptors, from the analysis of the extent of receptor diversity and specificity, and from an understanding of the pattern of receptor expression in the olfactory epithelium. Several discrete classes of odorant receptors have been identified from both invertebrate (Troemel et al. 1995; Sengupta et al. 1996) and vertebrate species (for review, see Buck 1996). We have identified a large family of genes encoding transmembrane receptors expressed in mammalian olfactory sensory neurons which exhibit an array of properties that render them uniquely suited to their task of recognizing a vast array of odors (Buck and Axel 1991).

What are the expected properties of odorant receptors, and what is the evidence that the multigene family we have identified encodes these receptors? First, the genes we have identified encode a large family of receptors that traverse the plasma membrane seven times and are likely to interact with G proteins. This is in accord with the presumed pathway of olfactory sig-

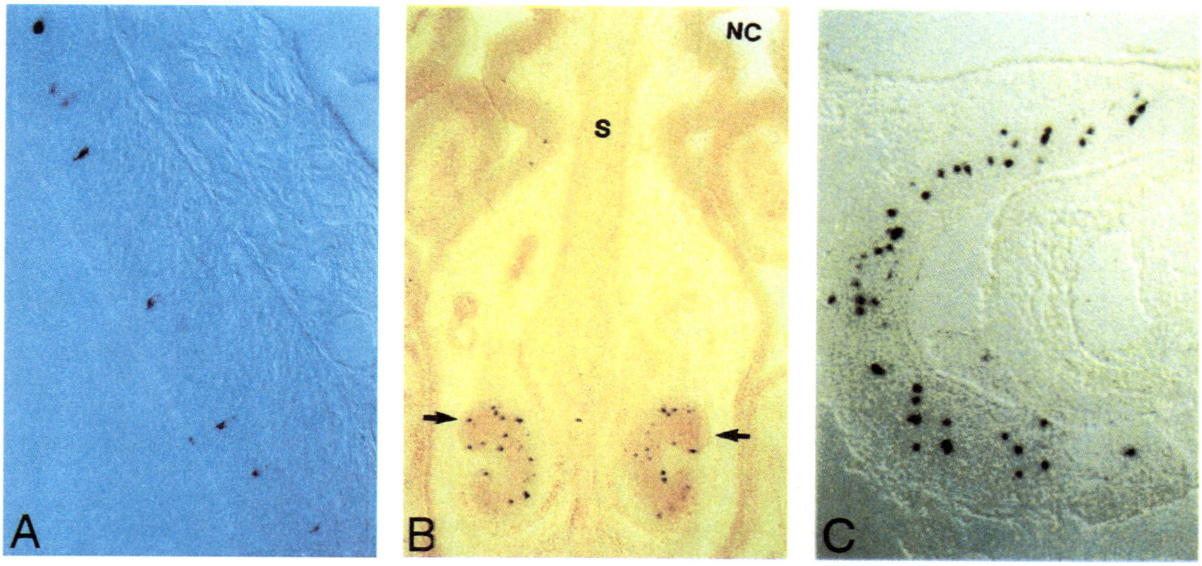

Figure 2. Localization of odorant receptors in the MOE and the VNO. (*A*) In situ hybridization to the main olfactory epithelium. Sections through the main olfactory epithelium were subjected to in situ hybridization with digoxigenin-labeled odorant receptor I7 of the rat. A punctate pattern of hybridization to a subpopulation of cells is observed. (*B*) Pheromone receptor expression is restricted to VNO neurons. A coronal section through the head of an E17 rat shows hybridization of a mix of six putative pheromone receptor probes to neurons within the VNO (*arrows*), but not to neurons within the MOE, nor to other tissues in the nose. (NC) Nasal cavity; (S) septum. Bar, 250 μm. (*C*) In situ hybridization to the VNO. Coronal sections of the VNO were annealed with digoxigenin-labeled antisense RNA probes for the VNO-specific receptor, VN1. Hybridization is observed to the cell bodies of a subpopulation of VNO neurons.

nal transduction in which odorant receptors are thought to transduce intracellular signals by interacting with G_{olf}, which in turn activates second-messenger pathways that ultimately alter the membrane potential of the neuron (Reed 1992). Second, we have shown that the family of olfactory genes we have cloned is expressed in subpopulations of olfactory sensory neurons (Fig. 2A). Hybridizing RNA is not detected in brain nor in a host of nonneural tissues. Third, the family of odorant receptors must be capable of interacting with extremely diverse molecular structures of odorants. The genes we have cloned are members of an extremely large multigene family that exhibits variability in regions thought to be important in ligand binding. Southern blotting experiments, along with polymerase chain reaction (PCR) analysis and screens of genomic libraries, suggest that in rodents this gene family may contain as many as 1000 distinct receptor genes (Buck and Axel 1991; Levy and Bakalyar 1991). The possibility that each member of this large family of seven-transmembrane proteins is capable of interacting with only one or a small number of odorants provides a plausible mechanism to accommodate the diversity of odor perception. Finally, the odorant receptors must bind odorants and transduce an intracellular signal leading to the activation of second-messenger systems. This criterion, at present, is difficult to satisfy experimentally because the diversity of odorants and the large number of individual receptors make it difficult to identify the appropriate ligand for a particular receptor. Nonetheless, the properties of the gene family we have identified suggest that this family is likely to encode a large number of distinct odorant properties.

A Superfamily of Putative Pheromone Receptor Genes

Our initial efforts to identify the genes encoding the pheromone receptors were based on the assumption that the MOE and the VNO might share a common evolutionary origin such that DNA sequence homology may exist between the two receptor families. However, low-stringency hybridization of MOE receptor probes to rat vomeronasal cDNA libraries, as well as PCR using conserved motifs both from the family of odorant receptor genes and from the superfamily of known seven-transmembrane-domain receptors were consistently unsuccessful. Moreover, the components of the olfactory signal transduction cascade in the main olfactory epithelium (the olfactory-specific G-protein, G_{olf}, [Jones and Reed 1989], the olfactory-specific adenylate cyclase [Bakalyar and Reed 1990], and the cyclic nucleotide-responsive ion channel [Dhallan et al. 1990] were not detectable in VNO neurons by in situ hybridization or by screening cDNA libraries (Dulac and Axel 1995). These observations suggest that the pheromone receptors and the signal transduction pathways which they activate may have evolved independently in the VNO and the MOE.

We therefore developed a cloning procedure that made no assumptions concerning the structural class of the receptor molecules. Rather, we only assumed that the expression of the pheromone receptors would be restricted to the VNO, and that individual neurons within the VNO were likely to express different receptor genes. The generation of libraries from individual neurons provided an experimental solution to the problem of detecting a specific mRNA expressed in only a subset of cells in a heterogeneous population of neurons (Dulac and Axel 1995). Reverse transcriptase PCR (RT-PCR) was used to generate double-stranded cDNA, as well as cDNA libraries from individual vomeronasal sensory neurons. A library from a single VNO cell (neuron 1) was screened with cDNA probes from neuron 1 and neuron 2 to identify genes expressed in abundance in only a subset of the VNO cells (Fig. 2B,C).

This experimental approach, differential screening of cDNA libraries constructed from single sensory neurons, has led to the isolation of a novel family of putative pheromone receptor genes. Genomic blot hybridizations, taken together with library screening, suggest that the repertoire of pheromone receptors may consist of 100 distinct genes. Each member of the gene family is expressed in a small subpopulation of neurons. The expression of this gene family is restricted to neurons within the VNO and is not observed in sensory neurons of the MOE, nor in other nonneuronal cells (Fig. 2B,C). This array of properties is consistent with those predicted for the mammalian pheromone receptors. However, proof that these sequences indeed encode pheromone receptors will require the demonstration that these receptor proteins bind pheromones and are able to transduce pheromone binding into alterations in membrane potential.

The sequences of seven different cDNAs from this gene family suggest that each of the seven sequences contains seven hydrophobic stretches that represent potential transmembrane domains. Sequence analysis therefore suggests that these putative receptors are likely to adopt a structure similar to that previously characterized for the superfamily of seven-transmembrane receptors. However, the VNO receptors do not share any of the conserved sequence motifs exhibited by members of the previously identified superfamily. Moreover, the sequences of the odorant receptors of the MOE and the pheromone receptors of the VNO share no apparent homology, indicating that the two olfactory sensory systems of mammals have evolved independently.

What is the evolutionary origin of the VNO? Pheromone-responsive neurons and neurons responsive to the more general class of odorants are likely to have been present throughout vertebrate evolution. With the emergence of terrestrial forms, segregation of the two types of neurons may have occurred, generating a distinct VNO that facilitates the access and binding of the two classes of odorous ligands. Thus, terrestrial vertebrates from amphibians to mammals, including humans, retain two distinct olfactory systems, the VNO and the MOE (Potiquet 1891; Bertmar 1981; Garcia-Velasco and Mondragon 1991; Stensaas et al. 1991; Eisthen 1992; Moran et al. 1991).

One Neuron/One Receptor

The interaction of odorous ligands with a large number of receptors in olfactory sensory neurons provides a mechanism for the specific recognition of a diverse array of odors. Discrimination among odors, however, requires that the brain determine which of the numerous receptors have been activated. The mechanisms employed to discern which receptors have been activated depend on the diversity of receptor expression in an individual sensory neuron. If a sensory neuron expresses only one odorant receptor, then the problem of distinguishing which receptor has been activated reduces to a problem of identifying which neurons have been activated. Perception of an odorant encountered by the organism would then require the identification of that subset of cells responsive to a given odorant. Several lines of experimental evidence suggest that this is indeed the case, that a sensory neuron expresses only one of 1000 possible receptor genes. In situ hybridization studies in mammals with a repertoire of about 1000 genes reveal that a given receptor identifies about 0.1% of the sensory neurons. Moreover, in in situ hybridization experiments, the number of cells detected by a mix of probes approximates the sum of the cells detected by the four probes individually, indicating that the four receptor genes are expressed in different and largely nonoverlapping sets of neurons (Ressler et al. 1993; Ngai et al. 1993a; Vassar et al. 1993).

Finally, we have analyzed the diversity of receptor expression in individual neurons in the MOE by analysis of cDNA prepared from single olfactory sensory neurons (C. Dulac and R. Axel, unpubl.). RT-PCR was employed to analyze receptor genes expressed in cDNA synthesized from individual neurons. Only a single species of receptor mRNA can be detected in cDNA synthesized from a given cell. Moreover, in each of 20 cells analyzed, the receptor genes identified were all different. As a control, when the same procedures are applied to a collection of neurons, multiple different receptor genes are obtained. Taken together, these observations suggest that each cell expresses only one receptor, such that individual olfactory neurons are functionally distinct. The discrimination of odors may therefore be accomplished by determining which of the distinct classes of neurons have been activated.

Topographic Organization of Sensory Projections

How does the brain determine which neurons have been activated in order to decode olfactory information from peripheral sensory neurons? In most sensory systems in vertebrates, the spatial segregation of sensory neurons and their projections are used to define the quality of the sensory stimulus. In the vertebrate olfactory system, spatial segregation could occur in the sensory epithelium such that neurons that express a given receptor, and therefore respond to a given odorant, may be topographically localized with the olfactory epithelium. This topographic localization would also be maintained in the projections of the sensory axons, such that neurons expressing the same receptor would project to the same set of glomeruli within the olfactory bulb (Kauer et al. 1991; Shepherd 1991; Ngai et al. 1993b). Alternatively, sensory neurons expressing a given receptor may be randomly distributed within the sensory epithelium. However, all neurons responsive to a given odorant would project to discrete glomeruli within the olfactory bulb. This second model does not require spatial control of receptor gene expression, but does require other complex recognition mechanisms to segregate distinct axonal subsets within the olfactory bulb.

In situ hybridization was therefore used to discern whether neurons expressing individual receptors are topographically segregated in the mammalian olfactory epithelium. The expression of specific odorant receptors is restricted to at least four broad zones in the olfactory epithelium of rodents. Within a given zone, however, the distribution of cells expressing a given receptor appears to be randomly distributed rather than spatially localized (Ressler et al. 1993; Vassar et al. 1993). Although these data demonstrate that specific receptor expression is restricted to one of four broad domains, perhaps the most important feature of this sort of organization is the random distribution of receptor expression within a given domain. Thus, if spatial segregation is indeed employed to encode odor quality, neurons expressing a given receptor, although randomly distributed throughout a domain, must project their axons to one or a subset of spatially defined glomeruli within the olfactory bulb.

We have therefore devised two independent experimental approaches to discern whether neurons expressing a given receptor project their axons to common glomeruli within the olfactory bulb. Experiments were designed to ask whether neurons expressing a given receptor converge on a discrete subset of glomeruli within the olfactory bulb. To define a spatial map of the projections of the olfactory neurons within the bulb, it is necessary to identify markers that distinguish the axons of neurons expressing different receptors. The specific receptors or their respective mRNAs would provide obvious markers if they were expressed in axons. mRNA in neurons is largely localized to the cell body; occasionally, specific RNAs are observed in dendrites, but mRNA is rarely found in axonal projections (for review, see Steward and Banker 1992). The mRNA encoding specific odorant receptors is abundant within the neuronal cell bodies in the sensory epithelium. Estimates from in situ hybridization analyses suggest that an olfactory sensory neuron expresses about 1000 copies of the mRNA for a single, specific receptor (data not shown). Each glomerulus in the bulb results from the convergence of axonal projections from about 3000 neurons (Meisami 1979, 1989). If a receptor mRNA molecule is infrequently found at the axon terminal and neurons expressing a given receptor indeed synapse on a single glomerulus, this convergence should permit the detection of specific receptor mRNAs in individual glomeruli by in situ hybridization.

A ^{33}P-labeled RNA probe for the mouse M50 receptor gene (which anneals with only a single receptor gene within the genome) was used in in situ hybridization on coronal sections of the olfactory bulb (Fig. 3). The M50 receptor probe reveals hybridization signals over only two discrete glomeruli, one lateral and one medial, among the 2500 glomeruli present in the bulb (Fig. 3). Importantly, the positions in each of these two glomeruli are bilaterally symmetrical: Positive glomeruli occupy the same relative position in the right and left bulb. These results provide initial evidence that sensory neurons expressing a given receptor project to one or a small number of glomeruli that are spatially defined within the olfactory bulb. A more complete topographic map was established in both the mouse and rat olfactory system by in situ hybridization with probes to several additional receptor subfamilies (Fig. 4) (Ressler et al. 1994; Vassar et al. 1994). Our data with five different rat receptor probes that hybridize to 22 genes and identify only 19 of the 3000 glomeruli strongly suggest that a significant subpopulation of axons from sensory neurons expressing a given receptor converge on one or a small number of glomeruli within the olfactory bulb. Moreover, these projections define specific glomeruli that maintain a fixed position in the brains of all animals within a species.

Visualizing an Olfactory Sensory Map

In independent experiments, we have developed a genetic approach to visualize axons from olfactory neurons as they project to the olfactory bulb (Mombaerts 1996; Mombaerts et al. 1996). We have modified the P2 olfactory receptor gene by targeted mutagenesis in the germ line of mice. The P2 locus now encodes a bicistronic mRNA that allows the translation of the P2 receptor along with tau-lacZ, a fusion of the microtubule-associated protein, tau, with β-galactosidase. In these mutant strains of mice, olfactory neurons that transcribe the P2 gene also express tau-lacZ in their axons, permitting the direct visualization of the pattern of projections in the brain.

To restrict the expression of tau-lacZ to the subpopulation of sensory neurons that express the odorant receptor P2, it is necessary to place tau-lacZ under the control of P2 regulatory sequences, such that cells expressing P2 will also express tau-lacZ. However, the

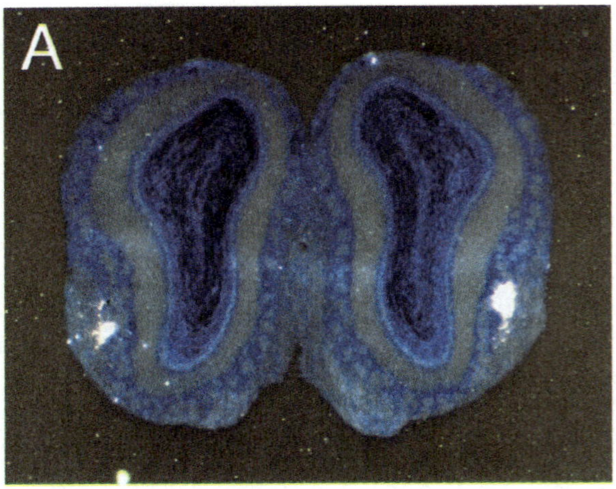

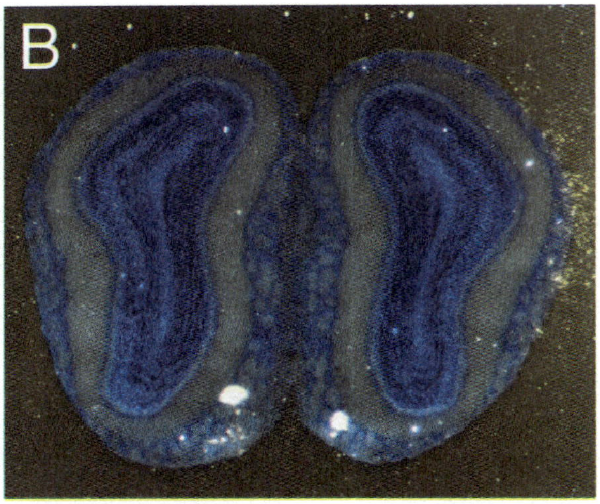

Figure 3. Localization of odorant receptor M50 RNA to discrete glomeruli within the olfactory bulb. Coronal sections of the mouse olfactory bulb were annealed with a ^{33}P-labeled M50 receptor antisense probe. The ventromedial M50 glomeruli (*B*) are ventral and posterior to the ventrolateral glomeruli (*A*).

elements regulating receptor gene expression have not yet been identified. We therefore chose to introduce tau-lacZ into the P2 locus by homologous recombination in embryonic stem (ES) cells. A gene-targeting approach in which the P2 sequence is simply replaced by tau-lacZ would eliminate P2 receptor expression from the modified allele. However, olfactory neurons express a receptor from only one of the two alleles (Chess et al. 1994). Therefore, in this targeting strategy, cells expressing the modified allele would express tau-lacZ, but not receptor. Conversely, cells expressing the P2 receptor would not express tau-lacZ. Instead, we designed a bicistronic targeting vector to assure that cells expressing a functional P2 receptor also express tau-lacZ (Fig. 5).

A genomic clone containing the P2 receptor gene was modified by the insertion of a cassette immediately 3′ of the P2 stop codon. This cassette consists of two parts: an internal ribosome entry site (IRES) from the encephalomyocarditis virus driving translation of the tau-lacZ fusion gene, followed by LTNL (loxP-tk-neo-loxP). This targeting vector was electroporated into ES cells. G418-resistant clones resulting from homologous recombination at the P2 locus were identified (Fig. 5). Targeted ES clones were then transiently transfected with a vector directing expression of Cre recombinase resulting in deletion of the tk and neo sequences, leaving only a single loxP site. Removal of the selectable markers ensures that the modified P2 locus is free of exogenous promoter elements that may affect P2 expression. These ES clones were then introduced into blastocysts to generate chimeric mice, and germ-line transmission was obtained with two clones.

In these P2-IRES-tau-lacZ mice, cells that express the P2 receptor from the modified allele should also express tau-lacZ, allowing the visualization of their axonal projections in the brain. Whole-mount analysis of mice heterozygous for the P2-IRES-tau-lacZ mutation reveals a subpopulation of sensory neurons whose dendrites, cell bodies, and axons exhibit blue color after staining with X-gal (Fig. 6). The blue axons are readily visualized as they emerge from the epithelium and pass through the cribriform plate into the olfactory bulb, where they converge on a single glomerulus on either the medial or the lateral aspect of the olfactory bulb.

Analysis of the olfactory bulb, either in whole-mount preparations or after sectioning, permits the direct visualization of the axonal projections from neurons expressing P2-IRES-tau-lacZ. The blue axons converge on a single glomerulus centrally located on the medial aspect of the bulb (Fig. 6). In the lateral half of the olfactory bulb, axons converge to a single, more dorsally and anteriorly placed glomerulus (data not shown). A similar pattern with one medial and one lateral P2 glomerulus has been observed in 37 mice. A small fraction of the blue fibers (< 5%) project to a third glomerulus in the immediate vicinity of one of the two P2 glomeruli. In 2 of 37 mice, projection to an additional glomerulus is also observed. This minor variance is also observed by in situ hybridization experiments in wild-type mice. At this level of resolution, we see no stray fibers: All axons appear to project to the two or three glomeruli we have identified. The positions of these glomeruli are relatively constant in all mice examined.

The ability to visualize neurons expressing the P2 receptor also allows us to observe the generation of a topographic map over developmental time. Neurons expressing P2-IRES-tau-lacZ can be visualized by embryonic day 13 (data not shown). Convergence of axons from P2-expressing neurons is apparent at E15, and the medial and lateral glomeruli are clearly visible at birth. Moreover, the relative positions of these glomeruli remain fixed throughout the life of the

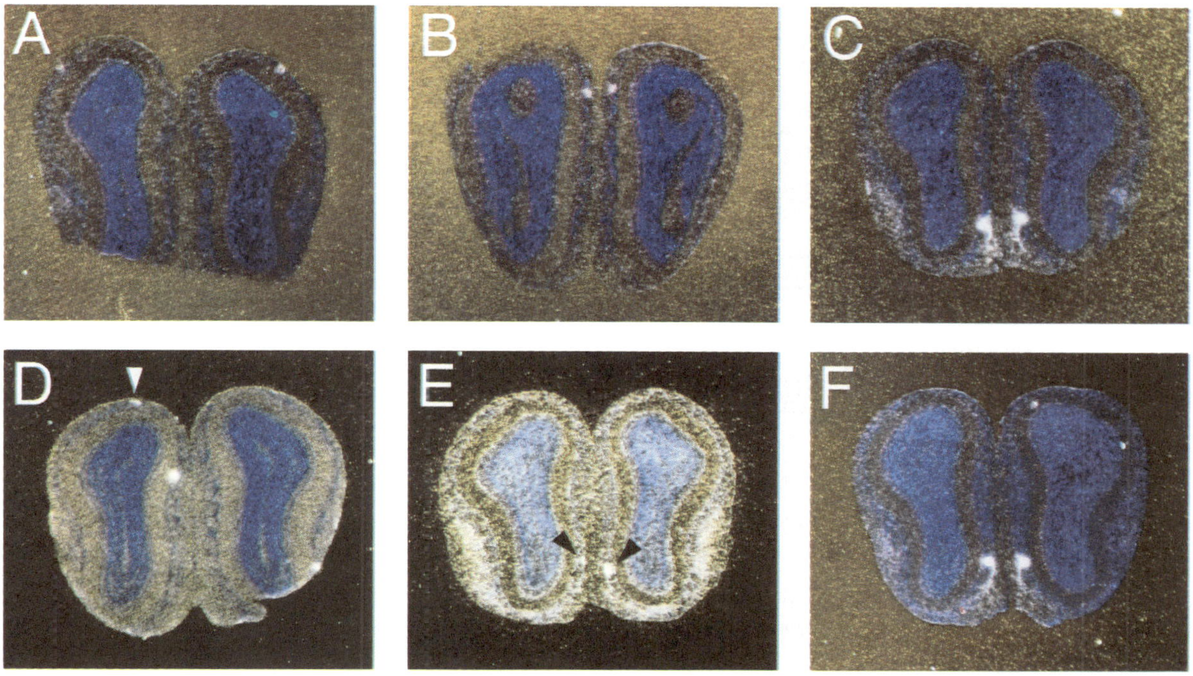

Figure 4. Positions of specific glomeruli on the mouse olfactory bulb. Examples of positive glomeruli after hybridization of the olfactory bulb with different ^{33}P-labeled mouse receptor probes. (*A*,*B*) I9. (*C*,*F*) P2 in two different animals. (*D*) M12. (*E*) P3.

organism. Control experiments demonstrate that this genetic alteration of the P2 receptor locus does not alter the pattern of expression of P2 receptor in the epithelium or the pattern of projections to the olfactory bulb (Mombaerts et al. 1996). Therefore, the pattern of P2-IRES-tau-lacZ expression accurately represents the convergence of axons from neurons expressing the P2 receptor on two topographically fixed glomeruli in the mouse olfactory bulb.

DISCUSSION

How does the vertebrate olfactory system recognize and distinguish among thousands of odors? In the main olfactory epithelium, the repertoire of odorant receptor genes consists of about 1000 genes, each encoding a distinct seven-transmembrane-domain protein. Individual sensory neurons are likely to express only 1 of 1000 receptor genes. Neurons expressing a given receptor, although randomly distributed in domains in the epithelium, project their axons to a small number of topographically fixed loci in the olfactory bulb. These observations, which derive from molecular biological and genetic experiments, are consistent with previous physiological experiments demonstrating that different odorants elicit spatially defined patterns of glomerular activity in the olfactory bulb. Thus, a two-dimensional map of receptor activation is maintained in the olfactory bulb. The quality of an olfactory stimulus would therefore be encoded by the specific combination of glomeruli activated by a given odorant.

Implications for Sensory Processing

How does the olfactory cortex decode this two-dimensional map within the bulb to allow the discrimination among a diverse array of odors? A given neuron is likely to express only 1 receptor from the repertoire of 1000 genes. Since the organism can detect far more than 1000 discrete odors, this implies that a given odorant interacts with multiple receptors, and a single receptor interacts with multiple odorous ligands. In this manner, an odorant, even one that consists of a single molecular species, will interact with a unique combination of receptors, which in turn results in the activation of specific combinations of glomeruli. The maintenance of a fixed map of glomeruli in the bulb therefore provides a mechanism to relay the information resulting from the activation of receptors in the periphery to the brain.

The ability of an odorant to activate a combination of glomeruli allows the discrimination of a diverse array of odors far exceeding the number of receptors and their associated glomeruli. Despite the diversity afforded by combinatorial activation of glomeruli, the organism is likely to be capable of discriminating only an extremely small subset of potential odors. As in other sensory systems, the olfactory system only perceives a meager image of the sensory information in the environment. This restricted array of recognizable odors is a function of the repertoire of receptors expressed by the organism as well as the nature of the glomerular combinations that are encoded in the

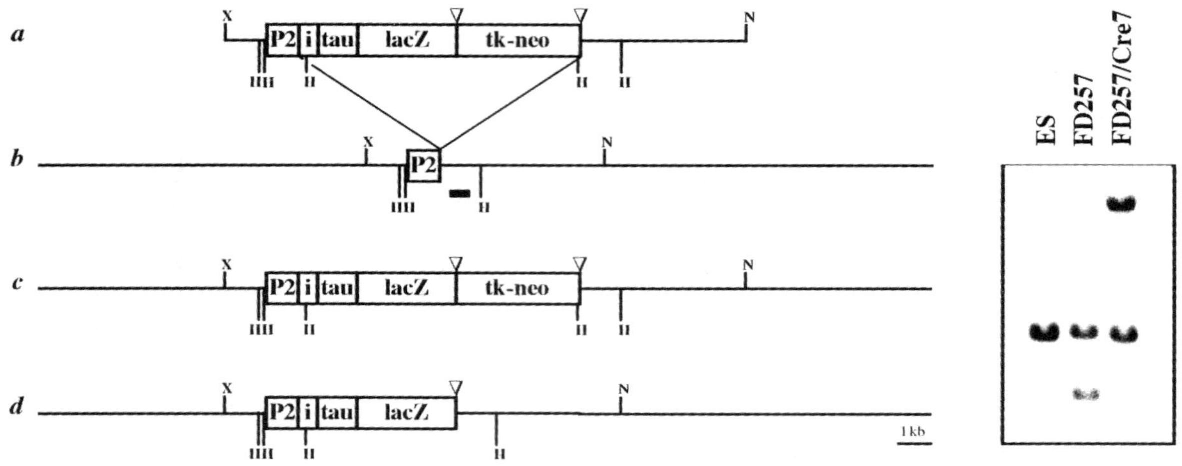

Figure 5. Targeted mutagenesis of the P2 locus. (*Left*) Schematic representation of the genetic strategy. (*Right*) Genomic Southern blot. (*a*) Targeting vector, P2-KO-13, consists of a 5′-flanking sequence, the P2 coding sequence, the IRES-tau-lacZ, and an LTNL cassette containing the tk and neo genes flanked by loxP sites. The relevant *Hin*dIII sites (*H*) are indicated, and inverted triangles indicate loxP sites. (*b*) The wild-type P2 locus. A horizontal bar below the line represents the P2 probe used to hybridize the Southern blot on the right. (*c*) The P2 locus after homologous recombination. The IRES-tau-lacZ/LTNL cassette is inserted in the genome three nucleotides downstream from the P2 stop codon. (*d*) The P2 locus after Cre-mediated site-specific recombination. (*Right*) Southern blot of genomic blot DNA from wild-type ES cells, one targeted clone, and a Cre-recombinase-treated subclone.

cortex. Those odors that are perceived from the universe of potential odorants presumably reflect selection for that subset of odorants that are biologically important for only the species. In this manner, individuals within a species maintain a repertoire of receptor genes and a combination of cortical connections that permit the detection of those odors important for its survival and reproduction.

This model of olfactory perception shares several basic features with perception in other sensory systems. The brain analyzes a visual image by interpreting the individual components of the image: form, location, movement, and color (Livingstone and Hubel 1987; Zeki and Shipp 1988). The unity of an image is accomplished by several parallel processing pathways, such that the image is initially dissected into tractable components and then reconstructed in higher visual centers of the cortex. A similar logic may be employed to discriminate olfactory stimuli. Olfactory processing initially requires that the odorant molecule is analyzed by "dissecting" its structural features, such that each of its structural elements activates a unique subset of receptors, which in turn results in the activation of a unique subset of glomeruli. The odorous stimulus is then reconstructed by the olfactory cortex, which determines which of the numerous glomeruli have been activated.

The Development of a Topographic Map in the Olfactory Bulb

The establishment of a topographic map of sensory projections may initially involve the expression of receptors by sensory cells. The choice of a given receptor would then be linked to the expression of guidance molecules, such that neurons expressing a given receptor project axons to a single glomerulus. Alternatively, it is possible that immature neurons, not yet expressing receptor, randomly project axons to any one of multiple glomeruli within the olfactory bulb. Contact with an individual gomerulus may then elicit a retrograde signal that directs the expression of specific receptor genes. In this manner, receptor gene expression would be regulated by the ultimate position of its axon terminal within the olfactory bulb. This model is unlikely, since receptor expression is observed in sensory neurons early in embryogenesis prior to the birth of mitral cells and the presence of glomeruli (Sullivan et al. 1995; Mombaerts et al. 1996). Moreover, analysis of receptor gene expression in individual neurons suggests that the choice of receptor expressed by a neuron is not regulated, but rather is stochastic (Chess et al. 1994). Thus, it is likely that neurons stochastically express one receptor gene prior to synapse formation. Neurons expressing a given receptor then form synapses with one or a small number of topographically fixed glomeruli.

How is this precise topographic map established? One attractive model combines guidance mechanisms during development with activity-dependent refinement to achieve the precision of connections between the sensory epithelium and olfactory bulb. It is possible, for example, that axons of neurons expressing a subpopulation of the receptor repertoire are restricted in their projections to broad but defined regions of the olfactory bulb. Neuronal growth cones may, for exam-

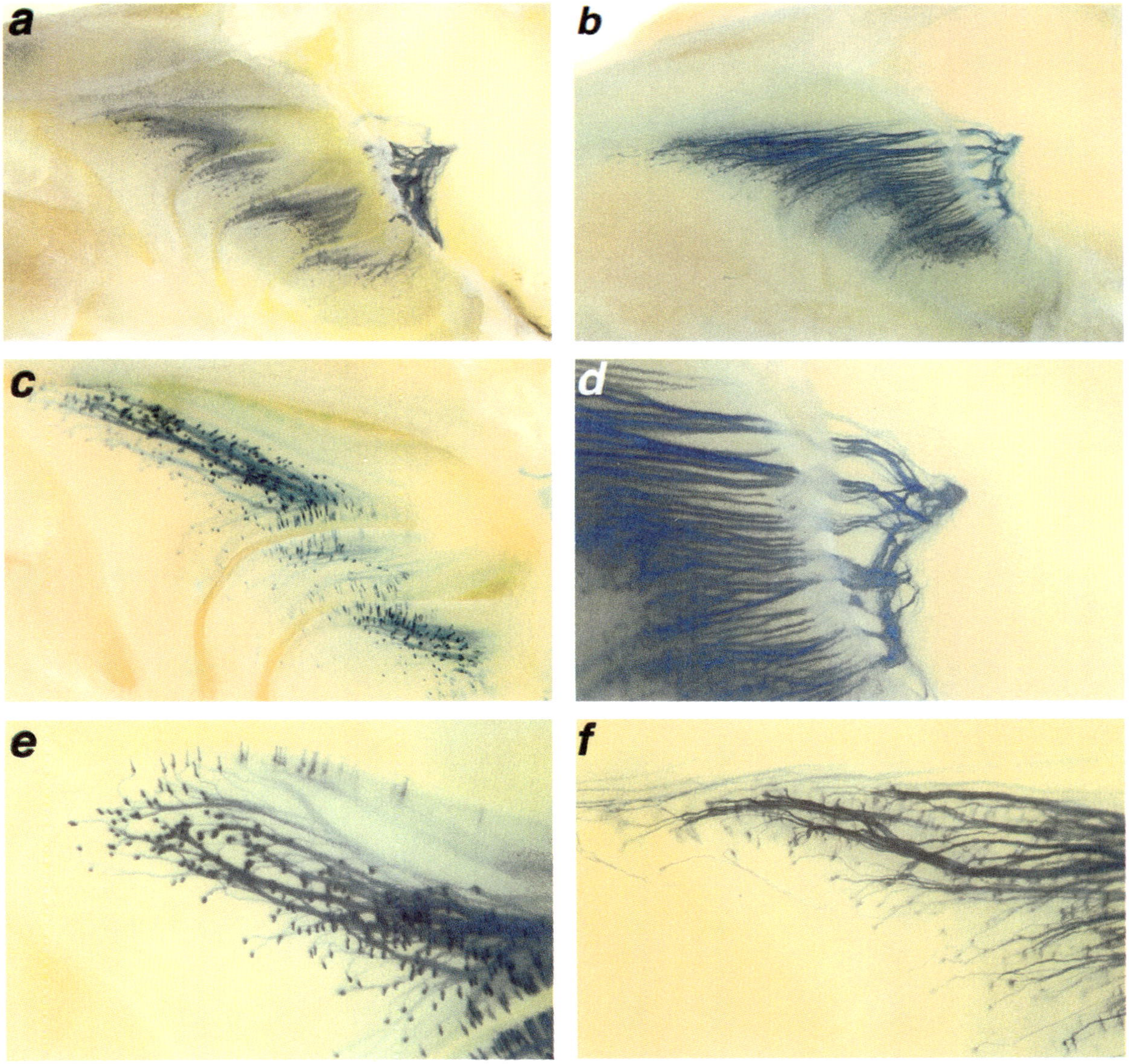

Figure 6. P2-IRES-tau-lacZ mice stained with X-Gal. (*a*) Whole-mount view from the midline of the nasal cavity. Blue neurons are distributed in a single zone in the epithelium. The axons converge on a single glomerulus on the medial aspect of the bulb. (*b*) View of the nasal septum and medial side of the bulb. (*c*) High-power view of the turbinates demonstrating neurons located in a narrow zone in the epithelium. (*d*) High-power view of neurons within the septum. (*e,f*) High-power view of the epithelium showing individual neurons with staining of the dendrite cell body and axon.

ple, be guided to their appropriate target by a gradient of recognition molecules. This guidance process could establish a coarse topographic map. Activity-dependent mechanisms, as a consequence of the synchronous firing of neurons responsive to a given odorant, could refine the pattern of synaptic connections within this restricted region of the bulb to establish a relatively precise topographic map. Such a model draws heavily on observations in the visual system indicating that retinal axons first use activity-independent mechanisms to form a coarse retinotopic map. Activity-dependent processes progressively refine this coarse map to provide a level of precision required to perceive the visual image (for review, see Constantine-Paton et al. 1990; Goodman and Shatz 1993). Alternatively, mechanisms involving multiple guidance cues that provide each glomerulus with a unique identity, coupled with multiple receptors on the different sensory neurons, may provide the precision of bulbar connections.

The nature of the putative guidance cues in the target, as well as the recognition molecules on the sensory axons, remains elusive. One particularly attractive possibility is that the odorant receptors themselves play a role in patterning the projections of olfactory sensory axons. These presynaptic receptors may be activated by guidance cues expressed by the postsynaptic mitral cells. In this manner, the odorant receptors may function in the dendrite in the recognition of odors and may exhibit a distinct function in the axon in the establishment of a topographic map that encodes odor quality in the olfactory bulb.

ACKNOWLEDGMENTS

This research was supported by the Howard Hughes Medical Institute and by grants from the National Institutes of Health (5 PO1 CA-23767, 5P-50 MH-50733, and NS-29832 [to R.A.]).

REFERENCES

Bakalyar, H.A. and R.R. Reed. 1990. Identification of a specialized adenylyl cyclase that may mediate odorant detection. *Science* **250:** 1403.

Ben-Arie, N., D. Lancet, C. Taylor, M. Khen, N. Walker, D.H. Ledbetter, R. Carrozzo, K. Patel, D. Sheer, H. Lehrach, and M.A. North. 1994. Olfactory receptor gene cluster on human chromosome 17: Possible duplication of an ancestral receptor repertoire. *Hum. Mol. Genet.* **3:** 229.

Berkley, K.J. 1985. Multiple systems diverging from the dorsal column nuclei in the cat. In *Development, organization, and processing in somatosensory pathways* (ed. M. Rowe and W.D. Willis), p. 191. A.R. Liss, New York.

Bertmar, G. 1981. Evolution of vomeronasal organs in vertebrates. *Evolution* **35:** 359.

Broadwell, R.D. 1975. Olfactory relationships of the elencephalon and diencephalon in the rabbit. I. An autoradiographic study of the efferent connections of the main and accessory olfactory bulbs. *J. Comp. Neurol.* **163:** 329.

Buck, L.B. 1996. Information coding in the vertebrate olfactory system. *Annu. Rev. Neurosci.* **19:** 517.

Buck, L. and R. Axel. 1991. A novel multigene family may encode odorant receptors: A molecular basis for odor recognition. *Cell* **65:** 175.

Chess, A., I. Simon, H. Cedar, and R. Axel. 1994. Allelic inactivation regulated olfactory receptor gene expression. *Cell* **78:** 823.

Constantine-Paton, M., H.T. Cline, and E. Debski. 1990. Patterned activity, synaptic convergence, and the NMDA receptor in developing visual pathways. *Annu. Rev. Neurosci.* **13:** 129.

Dhallan, R.S., K.W. Yau, K.A. Schrader, and R.R. Reed. 1990. Primary structure and functional expression of a cyclic nucleotide-activated channel from olfactory neurons. *Nature* **347:** 184.

Dulac, C. and R. Axel. 1995. A novel family of genes encoding putative pheromone receptors in mammals. *Cell* **83:** 195.

Dykes, R.W., D.D. Rasmusson, D. Sretavan, and N.B. Rehman. 1982. Submodality segregation and receptive-field sequences in cuneate, gracile, and external cuneate nuclei of the cat. *J. Neurophysiol.* **47:** 389.

Eisthen, H.L. 1992. Phylogeny of the vomeronasal system and of receptor cell types in the olfactory and vomeronasal epithelia of vertebrates. *Microsc. Res. Tech.* **23:** 1.

Garcia-Velasco, J. and M. Mondragon. 1991. The incidence of the vomeronasal organ in 1000 human subjects and its possible clinical significance. *J. Steroid Biochem. Mol. Biol.* **39:** 561.

Goodman, C.S. and C.J. Shatz. 1993. Developmental mechanisms that generate precise patterns of neuronal connectivity. *Cell* **72:** 77.

Halpern, M. 1987. The organization and function of the vomeronasal system. *Annu. Rev. Neurosci.* **10:** 325.

Imamura, K, N. Mataga, and K. Mori. 1992. Coding of odor molecules by mitral/tufted cells in rabbit olfactory bulb. I. Aliphatic compounds. *J. Neurophysiol.* **68:** 1986.

Jones, D.T. and R.R. Reed. 1989. G_{olf}, an olfactory neuron specific G-protein involved in odorant signal transduction. *Science* **244:** 790.

Katoh, K., H. Koshimoto, A. Tani, and K. Mori. 1993. Coding of odor molecules by mitral/tufted cells in rabbit olfactory bulb. II. Aromatic compounds. *J. Neurophysiol.* **70:** 2161.

Kauer, J.S., D.M. Senseman, and L.B. Cohen. 1987. Odor-elicited activity monitored simultaneously from 124 regions of the salamander olfactory bulb using a voltage-sensitve dye. *Brain Res.* **418:** 255.

Kauer, J.S., S.R. Neff, K.A. Hamilton, and A.R. Cinelli. 1991. The salamander olfactory pathway: Visualizing and modeling circuit activity. In *Olfaction: A model system for computational neuroscience* (ed. J.L. Davis and H. Eichenbaum), p. 43. MIT Press, Cambridge, Massachusetts.

Kevetter, G.A. and S.S. Winans. 1981. Connections of the corticomedial amygdala in the golden hamster. I. Efferents of the "vomeronasal amygdala." *J. Comp. Neurol.* **197:** 81.

Krettek, J.E. and J.L. Price. 1978. Amygdaloid projections to subcortical structures within the basal forebrain and brainstem in the rat and cat. *J. Comp. Neurol.* **178:** 225.

Lancet, D., C.A. Greer, J.S. Kauer, and G.M. Shepherd. 1982. Mapping of odor-related neuronal activity in the olfactory bulb by high resolution 2-deoxyglucose autoradiography. *Proc. Natl. Acad. Sci.* **79:** 670.

Levy, N.S. and H.A. Bakalyar. 1991. Signal transduction in olfactory neurons. *J. Steroid Biochem. Mol. Biol.* **39:** 633.

Livingstone, M.S. and D. Hubel 1987. Psychophysical evidence for separate channels for the perception of form, color, movement, and depth. *J. Neurosci.* **7:** 3416.

Meisami, E. 1979. The developing rat olfactory bulb: Prospects for a new model system in developmental neurobiology. In *Neural growth and differentiation* (ed. E. Meisami and M.A.B. Brazier), p. 528. Raven Press, New York.

———. 1989. A proposed relationship between increases in the number of olfactory receptor neurons, convergence ratio and sensitivity in the developing rat. *Dev. Brain. Res.* **46:** 9.

Mombaerts, P. 1996. Targeting olfaction. *Curr. Opin. Neurobiol.* **6:** 481.

Mombaerts, P., F. Wang, C. Dulac, S.K. Chao, A. Nemes, M. Mendelsohn, J. Edmondson, and R. Axel. 1996. Visualizing an olfactory sensory map. *Cell* (in press).

Moran, D.T., B.W. Jafek, and J.C. Rowley III. 1991. The vomeronasal (Jacobson's) organ in man: Ultrastructure and frequency of occurrence. *J. Steroid Biochem. Mol. Biol.* **39:** 545.

Mountcastle, V.B. 1957. Modality and topographic properties of single neurons of cat's somatic sensory cortex. *J. Neurophysiol.* **20:** 408.

Ngai, J., M.M. Dowling, L. Buck. R. Axel, and A. Chess. 1993a. The family of genes encoding odorant receptors in the channel catfish. *Cell* **72:** 657.

Ngai, J., A. Chess, M.M. Dowling, N. Necles, E.R. Macagno, and R. Axel. 1993b. Coding of olfactory information: Topography of odorant receptor expression in the catfish olfactory epithelium. *Cell* **72:** 667.

Parmentier, M., F. Libert, S. Schurmans, S. Schiffmann, A. Lefort, D. Eggerickx, C. Ledent, C. Moilereau, C. Gerard, J. Perret, A. Grootgoed, and G. Vassart. 1992. Expression of members of the putative olfactory receptor gene family in mammalian germ cells. *Nature* **355:** 453.

Perl, E.R., D.G. Whitlock, and J.R. Gentry. 1962. Cutaneous projection to second-order neurons of the dorsal column system. *J. Neurophysiol.* **25:** 337.

Potiquet, M. 1891. Le canal de Jacobson. *Rev. Laryngol.* **2:** 737.

Reed, R.R. 1992. Signaling pathways in odorant detection. *Neuron* **8:** 205.

Ressler, K.J., S.L. Sullivan, and L.B. Buck. 1993. A zonal organization of odorant receptor gene expression in the olfactory epithelium. *Cell* **73:** 597.

———. 1994. Information coding in the olfactory system: Evidence for a stereotyped and highly organized epitope map in the olfactory bulb. *Cell* **79:** 1245.

Sengupta, P., J.H. Chou, and C.I. Bargmann. 1996. odr-10 encodes a seven transmembrane domain olfactory receptor required for responses to the odorant diacetyl. *Cell* **84:** 899.

Scalia, F. and S.S. Winans. 1975. The differential projections of the olfactory bulb and accessory olfactory bulb in mammals. *J. Comp. Neurol.* **161:** 31.

Shepherd, G.M. 1991. Computational structure of the olfactory system. In *Olfaction: A model system for computational neuroscience* (ed. J.L. Davis and H. Eichenbaum), p. 3. MIT Press, Cambridge, Massachusetts.

———. 1994. Discrimination of molecular signals by the olfactory receptor neuron. *Neuron* **13:** 771.

Stensaas, L.J., R.M. Lavker, L. Moni-Bloch, B.I. Grossier, and D.L. Berliner. 1991. Ultrastructure of the human vomeronasal organ. *J. Steroid Biochem. Mol. Biol.* **39:** 553.

Steward, O. and G.A. Banker. 1992. Getting the message from the gene to the synapse: Sorting and intracellular transport of RNA in neurons. *Trends Neurosci.* **15:** 180.

Sullivan, S., S. Bohm, K.J. Dressler, L.F. Horowitz, and L.B. Buck. 1995. Target-dependent pattern specification in the olfactory epithelium. *Neuron* **15:** 779.

Troemel, E., J. Chou, N.D. Dwyer, H.A. Colbert, and C.I. Bargmann. 1995. Divergent seven transmembrane receptors are candidate chemosensory receptors in *C. elegans*. *Cell* **83:** 207.

Vassar, R., J. Ngai, and R. Axel. 1993. Spatial segregation of odorant receptor expression in the mammalian olfactory epithelium. *Cell* **74:** 309.

Vassar, R., S.K. Chao, R. Sitcheran, J.M. Nunez, L.B. Vosshall, and R. Axel. 1994. Topographic organization of sensory projections to the olfactory bulb. *Cell* **79:** 981.

Winans, S.S. and F. Scalia. 1970. Amygdaloid nucleus: New afferent input from the vomeronasal organ. *Science* **170:** 525.

Wysocki, C.J. 1989. Vomeronasal chemoreception: Its role in reproductive fitness and physiology. In *Neural control of reproductive function* (ed. J.H. Lakosi et al.), p. 545. A.R. Liss, New York.

Zeki, S. and S. Shipp. 1988. The functional loci of cortical connections. *Nature* **335:** 311.

Information Coding in the Mammalian Olfactory System

L.B. Buck
Howard Hughes Medical Institute, Department of Neurobiology, Harvard Medical School, Boston, Massachusetts 02115

The mammalian olfactory system is able to discriminate an immense variety of odorous molecules of differing shapes and sizes. The discriminatory capacity of the system is thought to derive from a series of information-processing steps that occur at different sites in the olfactory neural pathway (for review, see Shepherd 1988; Shipley et al. 1995; Buck 1996). These include the olfactory epithelium of the nose, where olfactory sensory neurons initially detect odorous molecules; the olfactory bulb of the brain, which receives signals from the sensory neurons; and the olfactory cortex, which receives information from the olfactory bulb and relays that information to multiple other brain regions.

Here I discuss experiments that we have done to gain insight into the molecular mechanisms and organizational strategies used by the mammalian olfactory system to transduce, encode, and process information at various levels in the olfactory pathway.

INFORMATION CODING IN THE OLFACTORY EPITHELIUM

In mammals, odorants are detected by millions of olfactory sensory neurons, which are located in a specialized olfactory neuroepithelium that lines the posterior nasal cavity. Each neuron extends cilia into the nasal lumen and projects a single axon to the olfactory bulb (Graziadei and Monti-Graziadei 1979). Electrophysiological recordings indicate that different neurons respond to different odorants, suggesting that odor discrimination derives from differential patterns of activity in the sensory neuron population (for review, see Shepherd 1994).

Odorant Receptors

In the early 1980s, olfactory cilia of fish were shown to have binding sites for amino acids that the fish smells, thus providing evidence for the existence of receptors for odorants (Rhein and Cagan 1980, 1983). Theoretically, the ability to discriminate odors could derive from the existence of a very large number of different types of odorant receptors (ORs), each specific for one or a few odorants, or, at the other extreme, from a rather small set of ORs, each capable of recognizing a variety of odorants. Each olfactory sensory neuron might express one receptor type or, alternatively, a combination of different receptors.

To investigate these questions, we first tried to identify ORs by searching for genes that might encode these molecules. In these studies, we found a large multigene family that appeared to code for G-protein-coupled ORs on rat olfactory sensory neurons (Buck and Axel 1991). Subsequent studies identified homologous families of ORs in a variety of vertebrate species (Nef et al. 1992; Parmentier et al. 1992; Ngai et al. 1993a; Barth et al. 1996; Byrd et al. 1996) and provided experimental evidence that members of this family recognize odorants (Raming et al. 1993). Current estimates indicate that mammals have as many as 1000 OR genes. Although ORs share novel sequence motifs with one another, they are extremely diverse in amino acid sequence (Buck and Axel 1991; Lancet and Ben-Arie 1993; Ngai et al. 1993a). The unprecedented size and diversity of the OR family are consistent with an ability to interact with an immense variety of structurally diverse odorants.

Odorant Receptor Gene Expression in the Olfactory Sensory Neuron

How does the olfactory system organize the information provided by 1000 different sensory receptors? To address this question, we isolated a large number of mouse OR genes and then examined the expression of these genes by in situ hybridization (Ressler et al. 1993). These studies, and others, showed that, in rodents, each OR gene is expressed in only a small percentage (on average, ~0.1%) of olfactory sensory neurons (Fig. 1) (Ressler et al. 1993; Vassar et al. 1993; Chess et al. 1994; Strotmann et al. 1994). Thus, each neuron is likely to express only one type of OR and transmit to the brain only information provided by that OR.

Spatial Zones of Odorant Receptor Gene Expression

The studies of OR gene expression also showed that neurons that express the same OR gene are dispersed over large areas of the olfactory epithelium (Nef et al. 1992; Strotmann et al. 1992, 1994; Ressler et al. 1993; Vassar et al. 1993). However, comparisons of the patterns of expression of different OR genes revealed that the olfactory epithelium is divided into at least four spatial zones, each of which expresses a different complement of OR genes (Ressler et al. 1993; Vassar et al. 1993; Strotmann et al. 1994). Neurons that express the

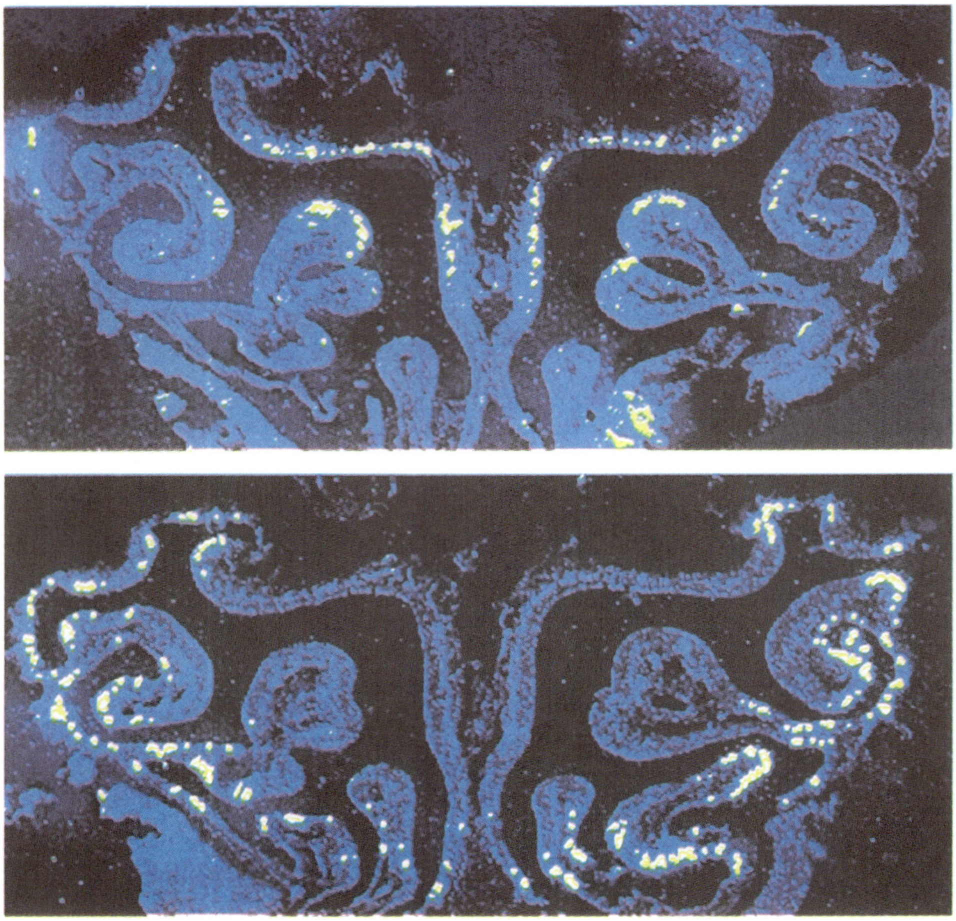

Figure 1. Spatial zones of odorant receptor gene expression. These sections through the mouse nose were hybridized to two different OR gene probes; the nasal septum is in the center with the two nasal cavities on either side. Two different OR expression zones are evident in the two sections. They are bilaterally symmetrical in the two nasal cavities. Two additional zones lie between the two shown here. (Reprinted, with permission, from Sullivan et al. 1996 [copyright Cell Press].)

same OR gene are typically confined to one zone but appear to be randomly distributed throughout that zone (Fig. 1). Each zone is thus a mosaic of neurons expressing several hundred different types of ORs.

The patterning of OR gene expression in the nose indicates that incoming sensory information is organized into four large sets prior to transmission to the brain. However, information provided by each OR is still dispersed over about 25% of the epithelial sheet. Comparisons of the OR expression zones with the results of previous anatomical studies of the olfactory epithelium/olfactory bulb axonal projection (Saucier and Astic 1986; Schwob and Gottlieb 1986; Stewart and Pedersen 1987; Schwarting and Crandall 1991; Schoenfeld et al. 1994) suggest that different zones project axons to different domains in the olfactory bulb (Ressler et al. 1993). Thus, the initial zonal organization seen in the nose is maintained in at least the first relay in the olfactory pathway. The functional significance of the zonal organization is not clear. However, one intriguing possibility is that information derived from different zones is ultimately relayed to different parts of the brain that mediate different effects of olfactory stimuli.

Odorant Receptor Gene Choice

During its development, each olfactory sensory neuron may select only one OR gene to express from among as many as 1000 candidate OR genes. The patterning of OR gene expression suggests that, when this choice is made, the neuron may be restricted to a particular zonal set of several hundred OR genes, but chooses one allele from among the members of that set by a stochastic mechanism (Ngai et al. 1993b; Ressler et al. 1993; Vassar et al. 1993; Chess et al. 1994).

Proposed models to explain this "OR gene choice" fall into two categories, "locus-dependent" and "locus-independent" (Ressler et al. 1993; Vassar et al. 1993; Chess et al. 1994). Locus-dependent models suggest that OR genes are clustered in the genome, perhaps with members of different zonal gene sets clustered at different chromosomal loci. A single gene in one cluster might be selected for expression by an immunoglobulin-like gene rearrangement to a cluster-specific expression site (Tonegawa 1983; Alt et al. 1987) or by juxtaposition of a cluster-specific enhancer with the promoter of one gene by DNA looping (Choi and Engel 1988). In locus-independent models, OR genes need not be clustered. For example, a single gene might be activated, at random, by a complex of transcriptional regulatory proteins present at limiting concentration during a brief developmental period, or, as with trypanosome VSG genes (Van der Ploeg 1991), a single OR gene might be copied into a unique, unlinked expression site.

To assess the feasibility of these models, we used interspecies mouse crosses to determine the chromosomal locations of OR genes expressed in different zones in the olfactory epithelium (Sullivan et al. 1996). Using 21 different OR genes as probes, we identified 11 different OR gene loci on 7 different mouse chromosomes. Multiple OR genes mapped to many of these loci. Thus, consistent with a previous characterization of one human OR gene locus (Ben-Arie et al. 1994), there are clusters of OR genes in the genome. Our studies also showed that genes expressed in different spatial zones can be found at the same locus and, consistent with in situ hybridization studies (Chess et al. 1994), genes expressed in the same zone are found at multiple loci.

The chromosomal organization of OR genes that we observed rules out simple locus-dependent models of OR gene choice that would rely on one or a few clusters of OR genes. One possibility is that a locus-dependent mechanism is used to select a single gene from one locus, but that this random receptor choice is preceded by a random "locus choice." On the other hand, OR gene choice might be a locus-independent event. A differential timing of replication of allelic OR loci similar to that seen with imprinted genes has been reported (Chess et al. 1994), raising the further possibility that OR gene choice involves novel mechanisms. Regardless of what mechanisms are used to initiate the expression of a single OR gene, there must be additional mechanisms to prevent the cell from subsequently activating additional OR genes. In the case of immunoglobulin heavy-chain genes, this is accomplished by a feedback mechanism that requires the expression of a functional heavy chain (Schatz et al. 1992). A similar strategy could conceivably be used to restrict the expression of OR genes to one per cell.

INFORMATION CODING IN THE OLFACTORY BULB

In the olfactory bulb, the axons of olfactory sensory neurons synapse with the dendrites of olfactory bulb neurons within bundles of neuropil, called glomeruli (for review, see Shepherd 1988; Kauer and Cinelli 1993; Scott et al. 1993; Shipley et al. 1995). In each glomerulus, information is transferred from several thousand sensory neurons to bulb relay neurons that transmit signals to the olfactory cortex. There are approximately 2000 glomeruli arrayed over the surface of each mouse bulb (Royet et al. 1988). The axon of each sensory neuron is confined to one glomerulus, as is the dendrite of each relay neuron. Numerous studies of odor-induced activity in the bulb have shown that different glomeruli (and different relay neurons) are activated by different odorants (Adrian 1950; Leveteau and MacLeod 1966; Stewart et al. 1979; Jourdan et al. 1980; Astic and Saucier 1983; Coopersmith et al. 1986; Onoda 1992; Guthrie et al. 1993; Kauer and Cinelli 1993; Sallaz and Jourdan 1993). However, these studies have also indicated that a single odorant can activate many glomeruli, and moreover, that each glomerulus can be stimulated by many odorants.

A Spatial Map of Information in the Olfactory Bulb

Theoretically, a glomerulus responsive to many odorants could receive input from different ORs specific for those different odorants or, alternatively, from a single OR that recognizes all of them. Similarly, different glomeruli that respond to the same odorant could all receive input from the same OR, or each of those glomeruli might receive input from a different OR that interacts with that odorant. To investigate these possibilities, we examined the patterns of synapses formed in the mouse olfactory bulb by sensory neurons expressing different ORs (Ressler et al. 1994). In these experiments, and similar experiments in rat (Vassar et al. 1994), the presence of OR mRNAs in sensory axons permitted a visualization of patterns of innervation in the bulb by in situ hybridization.

In these studies, each OR gene probe that was tested hybridized to a few glomeruli, indicating that the axons of neurons expressing the same OR gene converge on those glomeruli (Fig. 2). It was also found that different OR gene probes hybridize to different glomeruli; thus, the axons of neurons expressing different OR genes converge on different glomeruli. Interestingly, the percentage of glomeruli that hybridize to a given OR probe (~0.1–0.3%) approximates the percentage of OR genes that hybridize to that probe (~0.1–0.4%), suggesting that each glomerulus may receive input from only one type of OR. In the mouse, each OR probe hybridized to glomeruli located at only two sites in each bulb, one on the medial side and one on the lateral side or dorsal surface of the bulb. Surprisingly, glomeruli that hybridized to a given probe had the same positions in different animals. Thus, input from each OR is mapped onto a fixed site in the glomerular array on either side of the bulb.

These observations indicate that information is refined in the olfactory bulb into a highly organized, and spatially stereotyped, information map in which information provided by different ORs is mapped onto different glomeruli (Fig. 3). Actually, there are four

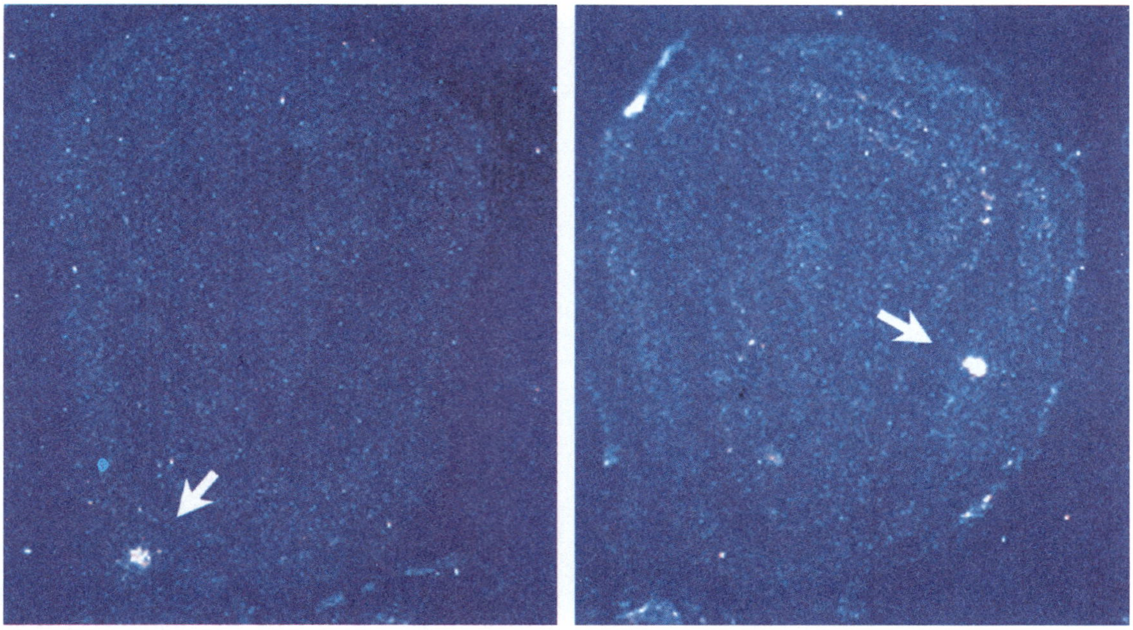

Figure 2. The axons of olfactory sensory neurons expressing the same OR gene converge to form synapses in only a few glomeruli in the olfactory bulb. A probe prepared from OR gene A16 hybridizes to a few olfactory bulb glomeruli clustered at only two sites in the mouse olfactory bulb, one on the medial side of the bulb (*left*) and the other on the lateral side (*right*). Glomeruli that hybridize to this probe have virtually identical locations in different animals. (Reprinted, with permission, from Ressler et al. 1994 [copyright Cell Press].)

such maps in each animal, one on either side of the animal's two bulbs, and the maps in the two bulbs are bilaterally symmetrical.

How the Identity of an Odorant Is Encoded

The patterning of OR inputs in the olfactory bulb suggests that a single glomerulus that responds to many odorants receives input from only one type of OR. Thus, a single OR is likely to recognize many odorants. The patterning further suggests that the many glomeruli that can be activated by a single odorant receive input from a variety of different ORs. Therefore, one odorant can be recognized by many ORs. This conclusion is, in fact, consistent with observations that a single olfactory sensory neuron can be activated by many odorants (Sicard and Holley 1984; Firestein et al. 1993) even though it probably expresses only one receptor type (see above).

These considerations suggest a model of information coding in which the identity of an odorant is encoded by a unique combination of ORs, each of which can serve as one component of the neural code for many different odorants (Fig. 4). In this model, each OR recognizes a particular structural feature, or by analogy with antibodies, an "epitope," that can be shared by different odorants, even those with very different perceived qualities. Such combinatorial coding could allow the discrimination of a virtually limitless variety of different odors. From this point of view, the information map in the bulb might be thought of as an "epitope map," in which different epitopes, or structural features of odorants, are mapped onto different glomeruli (Beets 1970; Ham and Jurs 1985; Kauer 1991; Katoh et al. 1993; Mori and Shepherd 1994; Ressler et al. 1994; Vassar et al. 1994). This idea is consistent with functional studies, which have shown that a single bulb relay neuron can be stimulated by different odorants that have only one structural feature in common (Imamura et al. 1992; Mori et al. 1992; Katoh et al. 1993).

How the Information Map in the Olfactory Bulb Is Formed

How do sensory neurons that are randomly distributed in one zone in the nose come to synapse at a few, fixed sites in the olfactory bulb? Suggestions regarding the development of the olfactory epithelium/olfactory bulb projection have evoked a variety of schemes, including targeting molecules differentially coexpressed with different ORs, the use of the OR itself as a targeting molecule, activity-dependent mechanisms, temporal asynchrony in the onset of expression of different ORs and the development of different bulb regions, and retrograde signals from synaptic partners that "tell" the neuron which OR gene to express (Brunjes and Frazier 1986; Graziadei and Monti-Graziadei 1986; Lancet 1986; Schwob 1992; Mori 1993; Farbman 1994;

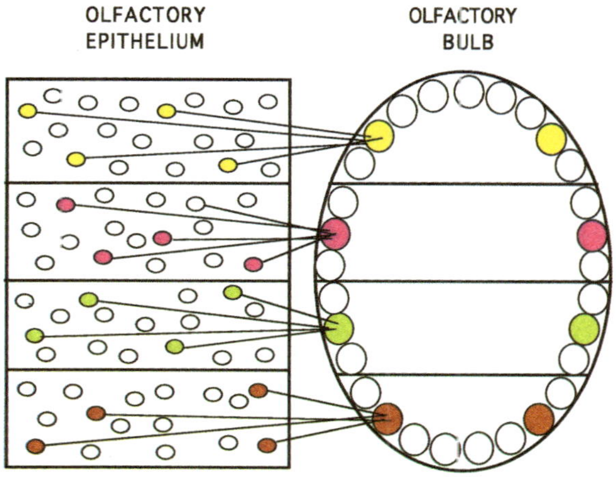

Figure 3. A schematic illustrating how information provided by different ORs is organized in the mouse olfactory epithelium and olfactory bulb. Four distinct spatial zones in the epithelium express different sets of OR genes; they also project axons to different domains in the olfactory bulb. Neurons expressing the same OR gene are dispersed throughout one zone, but their axons converge on only a few glomeruli at fixed locations in the bulb. It appears that sensory information undergoes an initial broad organization in the nose, and then is refined in the bulb into a highly organized, and spatially stereotyped, information map in which input from different ORs is mapped onto different glomeruli.

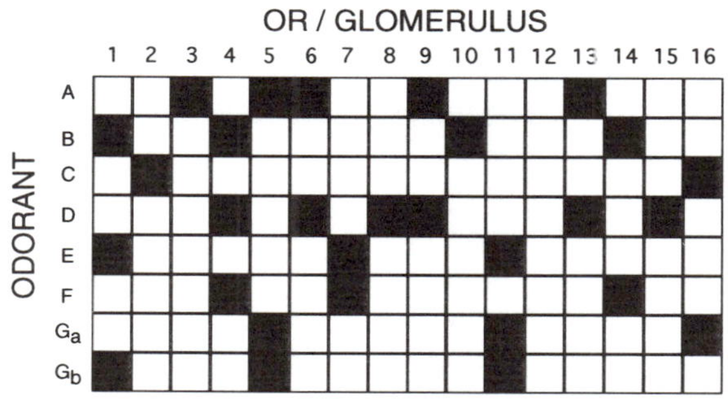

Figure 4. Combinatorial codes for odorants. The patterning of inputs to the olfactory bulb, together with functional studies of the bulb, suggests that the identity of an odorant is encoded by a combination of ORs (and the glomeruli that receive information provided by these ORs). Each OR (1–16) might serve as part of the code for many different odorants (A–G_b), thus allowing the discrimination of a vast number of odorants. In this model, different ORs can recognize different structural features, or epitopes, of the same odorant.

Lewin 1994; Ressler et al. 1994; Vassar et al. 1994; Singer et al. 1995; Sullivan et al. 1995).

To explore some of these possibilities, we examined the onset and patterning of OR gene expression during mouse development (Sullivan et al. 1995). These studies indicate that OR genes are all initially expressed at about the same time, at around embryonic day 12 (E12). This argues against the possibility that a coordination between the onset of expression of different OR genes and the development of different parts of the bulb plays a role in laying down a specific pattern of projections in the bulb.

As early as E13, the earliest time at which it is possible to discern patterns, zonal patterns of OR gene expression similar to those in the adult are present in the olfactory epithelium (Sullivan et al. 1995). Although sensory axons are visible outside the bulb at this time, they do not enter the bulb and begin to form synapses until 1–2 days later. Thus, retrograde signals provided by synaptic partners in the bulb cannot instruct sensory neurons to express specific OR genes. Further evidence for this conclusion is that embryonic *Xt^J* mutant mice, which fail to develop olfactory bulbs, also show normal patterns of OR gene expression (Sullivan et al. 1995).

One model that we find attractive would involve an initial guidance, or restriction, of the growing axon to a specific bulb domain via corresponding zone-specific and domain-specific receptors/ligands. The targeting of the axon to the correct glomerulus within that domain would then be accomplished by odor-dependent, activity-dependent mechanisms (Shatz 1990; Goodman and Shatz 1993) by which the axon would finally come to synapse at the same site as the axons of neurons that have coincident patterns of activity due to expression of the same OR. In this model, a stereotyped map might evolve from functional interrelationships among different ORs, which might, for example, favor close neighbor relationships among inputs from related ORs (Sullivan et al. 1995). The embryonic expression of olfactory sensory transduction components as early as 2–3 days prior to birth is consistent with this possibility (Sullivan et al. 1995).

INFORMATION CODING IN THE VOMERONASAL ORGAN

Many animals possess an accessory olfactory sensory structure, called the vomeronasal organ (VNO), which is thought to be specialized to detect pheromones (for review, see Keverne 1983; Halpern 1987; Wysocki and Meredith 1987). The VNO is a tubular structure at the base of the nasal septum. It is connected to the nasal cavity by a duct and is lined by a sensory epithelium that resembles the olfactory epithelium. In rodents, the VNO has been implicated in the detection of pheromones that have behavioral or neuroendocrine effects on conspecifics. Like the olfactory epithelium, which detects volatile odorants as well as some pheromones, the VNO neuroepithelium contains sensory neurons that project axons to the olfactory bulb. However, the pathways followed by sensory information that enters the olfactory system through the VNO and olfactory epithelium, the "accessory" and "main" olfactory pathways, respectively, are separate. Olfactory epithelium-derived signals ultimately reach multiple brain regions, including the frontal cortex, which is thought to mediate the conscious perception of odors. In contrast, VNO-derived signals are targeted to hypothalamic structures thought to play roles in reproduction (Krettek and Price 1978; Kevetter and Winans 1981).

Sensory Transduction Differs in VNO Neurons and Olfactory Sensory Neurons

In olfactory sensory neurons, interaction of an odorant receptor with its ligand is thought to initiate a cascade of events in which stimulation of adenylyl cyclase type III (AC III) by a Gαs-like G protein, Gαolf, leads to an increase in cAMP and the consequent opening of cyclic nucleotide-gated cation channels that are composed of two types of subunits (oCNC1 and oCNC2) (for review, see Reed 1992; Ronnett and Snyder 1992; Zufall et al. 1994; Buck 1996). Morphological and biochemical similarities between sensory neurons in the VNO and olfactory epithelium initially suggested that the two types of neurons might transduce signals by the same mechanisms. However, efforts to identify OR genes expressed in the VNO revealed that these genes are rarely expressed by VNO neurons.

We and other investigators subsequently found by in situ hybridization that VNO neurons also lack Gαolf, AC III, and oCNC1 (Dulac and Axel 1995; Berghard et al. 1996; Wu et al. 1996). Quantitative Northern blotting experiments confirmed that the inability to detect these molecules in tissue sections was not due to their simply being expressed at a lower level in VNO neurons than in olfactory sensory neurons (Berghard et al. 1996). These observations indicated that sensory transduction in the VNO differs from that in the olfactory epithelium. However, we found that the second subunit (oCNC2) of the olfactory cyclic nucleotide-gated cation channel is expressed by VNO neurons, suggesting that sensory transduction in the VNO, as in the olfactory epithelium, might involve cyclic nucleotide-gated ion channels (Berghard et al. 1996).

Sensory Transduction May Differ in Two Subsets of VNO Neurons

Although VNO neurons lack many elements of the olfactory sensory transduction cascade, they may nonetheless transduce sensory signals via a G-protein-coupled mechanism. Given the expression of a cyclic nucleotide-gated channel subunit in VNO neurons, VNO transduction may also involve the generation of cyclic nucleotides by an adenylyl or guanylyl cyclase. mRNAs encoding components of the olfactory sensory transduction cascade are highly expressed in olfactory sensory neurons, consistent with the idea that rapid sensory signaling via G-protein-coupled receptors may be facilitated by high concentrations of signaling components (Lamb and Pugh 1992). With this in mind, we used reverse transcriptase-polymerase chain reaction (RT-PCR) with degenerate primers to identify G-protein α subunits and adenylyl and guanylyl cyclases expressed in the VNO and then used in situ hybridization to determine whether any of the molecules that we had identified were highly expressed in VNO neurons (Berghard and Buck 1996).

In these experiments, we cloned a number of Gα subunits and adenylyl and guanylyl cyclases from VNO cDNA. However, we found that mRNAs encoding only three of these molecules are highly expressed in VNO neurons: Gαo, Gαi2, and adenylyl cyclase type II (AC II) (Fig. 5). Immunohistochemical studies using antibodies against Gαo and Gαi2 further showed that both molecules are enriched in the microvilli of VNO neurons, where sensory transduction is presumed to occur (antibodies against AC II have not been tested). Interestingly, Gαo and Gαi2 are highly expressed in separate subsets of VNO neurons; furthermore, the two subsets have different locations in the VNO neuroepithelium (Fig. 5). The spatial domains occupied by the two subsets are quite different from the spatial zones of OR expression in the nose; they consist of adjacent bands of cells that run parallel to the epithelial surface and extend throughout the extent of the VNO neuroepithelium. AC II is expressed by both subsets.

These findings, and similar findings regarding Gαo and Gαi2 subsets of VNO neurons from other groups (Dulac and Axel 1995; Halpern et al. 1995; Jia and Halpern 1996), suggest that spatially segregated subsets of VNO neurons may utilize different, but related, sensory transduction pathways in which G proteins and an adenylyl cyclase play major roles. The electrophysiological and biochemical effects of sensory ligands on mammalian VNO neurons have not yet been explored. Therefore, one can only speculate as to the precise roles played by these molecules. In garter snakes, where VNO neurons express both Gαo and Gαi2, a cuticle protein shed by earthworms (their prey) stimulates increases in inositol triphosphate in the VNO (Luo et al. 1994). This response is blocked by pertussis toxin, suggesting the involvement of Gαo or Gαi2 (or both). This response could conceivably be due to the stimulation of phospholipase C (PLC) by βγ subunits derived from G proteins containing either Gαo or Gαi2 (Sternweis 1994). A similar mechanism could operate in mammals.

The high expression of AC II, as well as the expression of one subunit of the olfactory cyclic nucleotide-gated channel, suggests that cAMP may also (or instead) be involved in VNO transduction in mammals. AC II can be stimulated by βγ subunits (Tang and Gilman 1991), thus suggesting a mechanism by which G proteins containing Gαo or Gαi2 could stimulate cAMP production. However, other schemes are equally plausible (Berghard and Buck 1996), and an understanding of the precise mechanisms underlying VNO

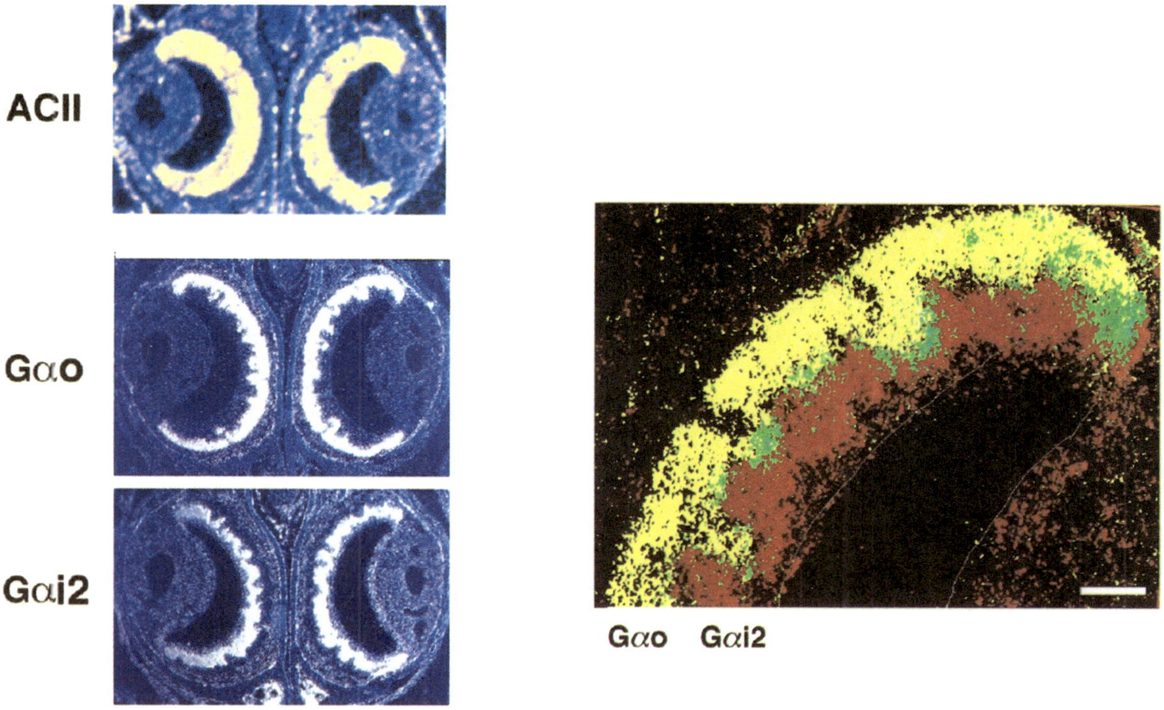

Figure 5. Sensory transduction in the vomeronasal organ. In sections through the paired VNOs of the mouse (*left*), ACII, Gαo, and Gαai2 probes all hybridize strongly to VNO neurons. In the composite on the right, it is evident that Gαo (*yellow*) and Gαi2 (*red*) mRNAs are highly expressed in separate subsets of VNO neurons that have different locations in the VNO neuroepithelium (overlap in the Gαo and Gαi2 hybridization signals is shown in green). (Reprinted, with permission, from Berghard and Buck 1996.)

sensory transduction awaits information on the effects of ligands on VNO neurons.

Why are there two subsets of neurons that differentially express Gαo and Gαi2? Do the two subsets mediate responses to different ligands, or do they mediate different responses to the same ligands? A large gene family was recently identified that codes for candidate G-protein-coupled pheromone receptors on VNO neurons (Dulac and Axel 1995). All members of this family thus far tested are expressed exclusively in the Gαi2 subset (Dulac and Axel 1995; A. Berghard and L.B. Buck, unpubl.), suggesting that the Gαo and Gαi2 subsets recognize different ligands. Interestingly, immunohistochemical studies further suggest that the two subsets form synapses in separate parts of the olfactory bulb (Shinohara et al. 1992; Jia and Halpern 1996). This raises the intriguing possibility that the separation of information provided by the Gαo and Gαi2 subsets is also maintained further along in the pathway, and that information provided by Gαo- and Gαi2-expressing VNO neurons is ultimately delivered to different regions of the hypothalamus that serve different functions.

REFERENCES

Adrian, E.D. 1950. Sensory discrimination with some recent evidence from the olfactory organ. *Br. Med. Bull.* **6:** 330.

Alt, F., T. Blackwell, and G. Yancopoulos. 1987. Development of the primary antibody repertoire. *Science* **238:** 1079.

Astic, L. and D. Saucier. 1983. Ontogenesis of the functional activity of guinea-pig olfactory bulb: Autoradiographic study with the 2-deoxyglucose method. *Dev. Brain Res.* **10:** 257.

Barth, A.L., N.J. Justice, and J. Ngai. 1996. Asynchronous onset of odorant receptor expression in the developing zebrafish olfactory system. *Neuron* **16:** 23.

Beets, M. 1970. The molecular parameters of olfactory response. *Pharmcol. Rev.* **22:** 1.

Ben-Arie, N., D. Lancet, C. Taylor, M. Khen, N. Walker, D.H. Ledbetter, R. Carrozzo, K. Patel, D. Sheer, H. Lehrach, and M.A. North. 1994. Olfactory receptor gene cluster on human chromosome 17: Possible duplication of an ancestral receptor repertoire. *Hum. Mol. Genet.* **3:** 229.

Berghard, A. and L.B. Buck. 1996. Sensory transduction in vomeronasal neurons: Evidence for Gao, Gai2, and adenylyl cyclase II as major components of a pheromone signaling cascade. *J. Neurosci.* **16:** 909.

Berghard, A., L.B. Buck, and E.R. Liman. 1996. Evidence for distinct signaling mechanisms in two mammalian olfactory sense organs. *Proc. Natl. Acad. Sci.* **93:** 2365.

Brunjes, P.C. and L.L. Frazier. 1986. Maturation and plasticity in the olfactory system of vertebrates. *Brain Res. Rev.* **11:** 1.

Buck, L.B. 1996. Information coding in the vertebrate olfactory system. *Annu. Rev. Neurosci.* **19:** 517.

Buck, L. and R. Axel. 1991. A novel multigene family may encode odorant receptors: A molecular basis for odor recognition. *Cell* **65:** 175.

Byrd, C.A., J.T. Jones, J.M. Quattro, M.E. Rogers, P.C. Brunjes, and R.G. Vogt. 1996. Ontogeny of odorant receptor gene expression in zebrafish, *Danio rerio*. *J. Neurobiol.* **29:** 445.

Chess, A., I. Simon, H. Cedar, and R. Axel. 1994. Allelic inactivation regulates olfactory receptor gene expression. *Cell* **78:** 823.

Choi, O.-R.B. and J.D. Engel. 1988. Developmental regulation of β-globin gene switching. *Cell* **55:** 17.

Coopersmith, R., S.R. Henderson, and M. Leon. 1986. Odor specificity of the enhanced neural response following early odor experience in rats. *Dev. Brain Res.* **27:** 191.

Dulac, C. and R. Axel. 1995. A novel family of genes encoding putative pheromone receptors in mammals. *Cell* **83:** 195.

Farbman, A.I. 1994. Developmental biology of olfactory sensory neurons. *Semin. Cell Biol.* **5:** 3.

Firestein, S., C. Picco, and A. Menini. 1993. The relation between stimulus and response in olfactory receptor cells of the tiger salamander. *J. Physiol.* **468:** 1.

Goodman, C.S. and C.J. Shatz. 1993. Developmental mechanisms that generate precise patterns of neuronal connectivity. *Cell* **10:** 77.

Graziadei, P.P.C. and G.A. Monti-Graziadei. 1979. Neurogenesis and neuron regeneration in the olfactory system of mammals. I. Morphological aspects of differentiation and structural organization of the olfactory sensory neurons. *J. Neurocytol.* **8:** 1.

———. 1986. Principles of organization of the vertebrate olfactory glomerulus: An hypothesis. *Neuroscience* **19:** 1025.

Guthrie, K.M., A.J. Anderson, M. Leon, and C. Gall. 1993. Odor-induced increases in c-*fos* mRNA expression reveal an anatomical "unit" for odor processing in olfactory bulb. *Proc. Natl. Acad. Sci.* **90:** 3329.

Halpern, M. 1987. The organization and function of the vomeronasal system. *Ann. Rev. Neurosci.* **10:** 325.

Halpern, M., L.S. Shapiro, and C.P. Jia. 1995. Differential localization of G proteins in the opossum vomeronasal system. *Brain Res.* **677:** 157.

Ham, C. and P. Jurs. 1985. Structure-activity studies of musk odorants using pattern recognition: Monocyclic nitrobenzenes. *Chem. Senses* **10:** 491.

Imamura, K., N. Mataga, and K. Mori. 1992. Coding of odor molecules by mitral/tufted cells in rabbit olfactory bulb. I. Aliphatic compounds. *J. Neurophysiol.* **68:** 1986.

Jia, C.P. and M. Halpern. 1996. Subclasses of vomeronasal receptor neurons: Differential expression of G proteins (G(I-α-2) and G(O-α)) and segregated projections to the accessory olfactory bulb. *Brain Res.* **719:** 117.

Jourdan, F., A. Duveau, L. Astic, and A. Holley. 1980. Spatial distribution of 2-deoxyglucose uptake in the olfactory bulb of rats stimulated with two different odors. *Brain Res.* **188:** 139.

Katoh, K., H. Koshimoto, A. Tani, and K. Mori. 1993. Coding of odor molecules by mitral/tufted cells in rabbit olfactory bulb. II. Aromatic compounds. *J. Neurophysiol.* **70:** 2161.

Kauer, J. 1991. Contributions of topography and parallel processing to odor coding in the vertebrate olfactory pathway. *Trends Neurcsci.* **14:** 79.

Kauer, J.S. and A.R. Cinelli. 1993. Are there structural and functional modules in the vertebrate olfactory bulb? *Microsc. Res. Tech.* **24:** 157.

Keverne, E.B. 1983. Pheromonal influences on endocrine regulation of reproduction. *Trends Neurosci.* **6:** 381.

Kevetter, G.A. and S.S. Winans. 1981. Connections of the corticomedial amygdala in the golden hamster. I. Efferents of the "vomeronasal amygdala." *J. Comp. Neurol.* **197:** 81.

Krettek, J.E. and J.L. Price. 1978. Amygdaloid projections to subcortical structures within the basal forebrain and brainstem in the rat and cat. *J. Comp. Neurol.* **178:** 225.

Lamb, T.D. and E.N. Pugh, Jr. 1992. G-protein cascades: Gain and kinetics. *Trends Neurosci.* **15:** 291.

Lancet, D. 1986. Vertebrate olfactory reception. *Annu. Rev. Neurosci.* **9:** 329.

Lancet, D. and N. Ben-Arie. 1993. Olfactory receptors. *Curr. Biol.* **3:** 668.

Leveteau, J. and P. MacLeod. 1966. Olfactory discrimination in the rabbit olfactory glomerulus. *Science* **153:** 175.

Lewin, B. 1994. On neuronal specificity and the molecular basis of perception. *Cell* **79:** 935.

Luo, Y., S. Lu, P. Chen, D. Wang, and M. Halpern. 1994. Identification of chemoattractant receptors and G-proteins in the vomeronasal system of garter snakes. *J. Biol. Chem.* **269:** 16867.

Mori, K. 1993. Molecular and cellular properties of mammalian primary olfactory axons. *Microsc. Res. Tech.* **24:** 131.

Mori, K. and G.M. Shepherd. 1994. Emerging principles of molecular signal processing by mitral/tufted cells in the olfactory bulb. *Semin. Cell Biol.* **13:** 771.

Mori, K., N. Mataga, and K. Imamura. 1992. Differential specificities of single mitral cells in rabbit olfactory bulb for a homologous series of fatty acid odor molecules. *J. Neurophysiol.* **67:** 786.

Nef, P., I. Hermans-Borgmeyer, H. Artieres-Pin, L. Beasley, V.E. Dionne, and S.F. Heinemann. 1992. Spatial pattern of receptor expression in the olfactory epithelium. *Proc. Natl. Acad. Sci.* **89:** 8948.

Ngai, J., M.M. Dowling, L. Buck, R. Axel, and A. Chess. 1993a. The family of genes encoding odorant receptors in the channel catfish. *Cell* **72:** 657.

Ngai, J., A. Chess, M.M. Dowling, N. Necles, E.R. Macagno, and R. Axel. 1993b. Coding of olfactory information: Topography of odorant receptor expression in the catfish epithelium. *Cell* **72:** 667.

Onoda, N. 1992. Odor-induced fos-like immunoreactivity in the rat olfactory bulb. *Neurosci. Lett.* **137:** 157.

Parmentier, M., F. Libert, F. Schurmans, S. Schiffmann, A. Lefort, D. Eggerickx, C. Ledent, C. Mollereau, C. Gerard, J. Perret, A. Grootegoid, and G. Vassart. 1992. Expression of members of the putative olfactory receptor gene family in mammalian germ cells. *Nature* **355:** 453.

Raming, K., J. Krieger, J. Strotmann, I. Boekhoff, S. Kubick, C. Baumstark, and H. Breer. 1993. Cloning and expression of odorant receptors. *Nature* **361:** 353.

Reed, R.R. 1992. Signaling pathways in odorant detection. *Neuron* **8:** 205.

Ressler, K.J., S.L. Sullivan, and L.B. Buck. 1993. A zonal organization of odorant receptor gene expression in the olfactory epithelium. *Cell* **73:** 597.

———. 1994. Information coding in the olfactory system: Evidence for a stereotyped and highly organized epitope map in the olfactory bulb. *Cell* **79:** 1245.

Rhein, L.D. and R.H. Cagan. 1980. Biochemical studies of olfaction: Isolation, characterization, and odorant binding activity of cilia from rainbow trout olfactory rosettes. *Proc. Natl. Acad. Sci.* **77:** 4412.

———. 1983. Biochemical studies of olfaction: Binding specificity of odorants to a cilia preparation from rainbow trout olfactory rosettes. *J. Neurochem.* **41:** 569.

Ronnett, G.V. and S.H. Snyder. 1992. Molecular messengers of olfaction. *Trends Neurosci.* **15:** 508.

Royet, J.P., C. Souchier, F. Jourdan, and H. Ploye. 1988. Morphometric study of the glomerular population in the mouse olfactory bulb: Numerical density and size distribution along the rostrocaudal axis. *J. Comp. Neurol.* **270:** 559.

Sallaz, M. and R. Jourdan. 1993. c-*fos* expression and 2-deoxyglucose uptake in the olfactory bulb of odour-stimulated awake rats. *NeuroReport* **4:** 55.

Saucier, D. and L. Astic. 1986. Analysis of the topographical organization of olfactory epithelium projections in the rat. *Brain Res. Bull.* **16:** 455.

Schatz, D.G., M.A. Oettinger, and M.S. Schlissel. 1992. V(D)J recombination: Molecular biology and regulation. *Annu. Rev. Immunol.* **10:** 359.

Schoenfeld, T.A., A.N. Clancy, W.B. Forbes, and F. Macrides. 1994. The spatial organization of the peripheral olfactory system of the hamster. 1. Receptor neuron projections to the main olfactory bulb. *Brain Res. Bull.* **34:** 183.

Schwarting, G.A. and J.E. Crandall. 1991. Subsets of olfactory and vomeronasal sensory epithelial cells and axons revealed by monoclonal antibodies to carbohydrate antigens. *Brain Res.* **547:** 239.

Schwob, J.E. 1992. The biochemistry of olfactory neurons: Stages of differentiation and neuronal subsets. In *Science of olfaction.* (ed. M.L. Serby and K.L. Chodor), pp. 80–125. M.I.T. Press, Cambridge, Massachusetts.

Schwob, J.E. and D.I. Gottlieb. 1986. The primary olfactory projection has two chemically distinct zones. *J. Neurosci.* **6:** 3393.

Scott, J.W., D.P. Wellis, M.J. Riggott, and N. Buonviso. 1993. Functional organization of the main olfactory bulb. *Microsc. Res. Tech.* **24:** 142.

Shatz, C.J. 1990. Impulse activity and the patterning of connections during CNS development. *Neuron* **5:** 745.

Shepherd, G.M. 1988. Neurobiology. Oxford University Press, New York.

———. 1994. Discrimination of molecular signals by the olfactory receptor neuron. *Neuron* **13:** 771.

Shinohara, H., T. Asano, and K. Kato. 1992. Differential localization of G-proteins Gi and Go in the accessory olfactory bulb of the rat. *J. Neurosci* **12:** 1275.

Shipley, M., J. McLean, and M. Ennis. 1995. Olfactory system. In *The rat nervous system* (ed. G Paxinos), p. 899. Academic Press, New York.

Sicard, G. and A. Holley. 1984. Receptor cell responses to odorants: Similarities and differences among odorants. *Brain Res.* **292:** 283.

Singer, M.S., G.M. Shepherd, and C.A. Greer. 1995. Olfactory receptors guide axons. *Nature* **376:** 19.

Sternweis, P.C. 1994. The active role of bg in signal transduction. *Curr. Opin. Cell Biol.* **6:** 198.

Stewart, W.B. and P.E. Pedersen. 1987. The spatial organization of olfactory nerve projections. *Brain Res.* **411:** 248.

Stewart, W.B., J.S. Kauer, and G.M. Shepherd. 1979. Functional organization of rat olfactory bulb, analyzed by the 2-deoxyglucose method. *J. Comp. Neurol.* **185:** 715.

Strotmann, J., I. Wanner, T. Helfrich, A. Beck, and H. Breer. 1994. Rostro-caudal patterning of receptor expressing neurones in the rat nasal cavity. *Cell Tissue Res.* **278:** 11.

Strotmann, J., I. Wanner, J. Krieger, K. Raming, and H. Breer. 1992. Expression of odorant receptors in spatially restricted subsets of chemosensory neurones. *Neuroreport* **3:** 1053.

Sullivan, S.L., M.C. Adamson, K.J. Ressler, C.A. Kozak, and L.B. Buck. 1996. The chromosomal distribution of mouse odorant receptor genes. *Proc. Natl. Acad. Sci.* **93:** 884.

Sullivan, S.L., S. Bohm, K.J. Ressler, L.F. Horowitz, and L.B. Buck. 1995. Target-independent pattern specification in the olfactory epithelium. *Neuron* **15:** 779.

Tang, W.-J. and A.G. Gilman. 1991. Type-specification regulation of adenylyl cyclase by G-protein bg subunits. *Science* **254:** 1500.

Tonegawa, S. 1983. Somatic generation of antibody diversity. *Nature* **302:** 575.

Van der Ploeg, L. 1991. Antigenic variation in African trypanosomes: Genetic recombination and transcriptional control of VSG genes. In *Gene rearrangement* (ed. B.D. Hames and D.M. Glover), p. 51. Oxford University Press, New York.

Vassar, R., J. Ngai, and R. Axel. 1993. Spatial segregation of odorant receptor expression in the mammalian olfactory epithelium. *Cell* **74:** 309.

Vassar, R., S.K. Chao, R. Sitchern, J.M. Nunez, L.B. Vosshall, and R. Axel. 1994. Topographic organization of sensory projections to the olfactory bulb. *Cell* **79:** 981.

Wu, Y.M., R. Tirindeli, and N.J.P. Ryba. 1996. Evidence for different chemosensory signal transduction pathways in olfactory and vomeronasal neurons. *Biochem. Biophys. Res. Commun.* **220:** 900.

Wysocki, C.J. and M. Meredith, Eds. 1987. The neurobiology of taste and smell. In *The vomeronasal system*, p. 125. Wiley, New York.

Zufall, F., S. Firestein, and G.M. Shepherd. 1994. Cyclic nucleotide-gated ion channels and sensory transduction in olfactory receptor cells. *Annu. Rev. Biophys. Struct.* **23:** 577.

Olfactory Recognition and Discrimination in *Caenorhabditis elegans*

J.H. Chou, E.R. Troemel, P. Sengupta,[1] H.A. Colbert, L. Tong, D.M. Tobin, K. Roayaie, J.G. Crump, N.D. Dwyer, and C.I. Bargmann

Howard Hughes Medical Institute, Programs in Developmental Biology, Neuroscience, and Genetics, Department of Anatomy, The University of California, San Francisco, California 94143-0452

An animal generates appropriate behavioral responses to a stimulus based on the intrinsic qualities of the stimulus, the context in which it appears, and the animal's previous experience. Olfactory stimuli elicit responses that are often reproducible across different individuals in a species: Many animals display characteristic behaviors in response to the smell of members of their species, food sources, or dangerous conditions. Other sensory modalities can also evoke innate responses, but in the olfactory system, odorants that elicit distinct behaviors are differentiated at the first step of sensory detection by the olfactory receptor neurons. Therefore, the neuronal circuitry responsible for different behaviors can be traced starting from the initial sensory events.

Our studies have focused on olfaction and chemosensation in the nematode *Caenorhabditis elegans*. Chemosensation is the richest mechanism *C. elegans* has for interacting with its environment, both in the number of different stimuli that are recognized and in the variety of different responses that can be elicited. Virtually all behaviors in *C. elegans* are modulated by chemical cues. Individual molecules can be attractants or repellents, or they can regulate egg-laying, feeding, or movement. In addition, pheromone cues control development of the animal and mating behavior between males and hermaphrodites. How are these chemical cues recognized and discriminated from one another? The answer to this question lies partly in the biochemical mechanisms that recognize individual odorants, and partly in the neuronal circuitry that drives particular responses.

SPECIFIC SENSORY NEURONS MEDIATE CHARACTERISTIC BEHAVIORAL RESPONSES

An adult hermaphrodite *C. elegans* has 302 neurons, whose morphology and connections have been defined through reconstruction of serial section electron micrographs (White et al. 1986). Of these, 32 neurons are anatomically defined as potential chemosensory neurons because they have endings that are associated with openings in the animal's cuticle. These neurons are divided into 14 types, where all of the neurons of one type have similar morphology and synaptic connections; there are usually two bilaterally symmetrical neurons of one type. Each neuron type has a three-letter name (e.g., AWA).

Evidence for chemosensory function has been obtained for 11 types of putative chemosensory neurons, all of which are associated with a head sensory structure called the amphid (Fig. 1). Functions are defined in experiments in which individual neurons or groups of neurons are killed using a laser microbeam, and the operated animals are tested for their responses to chemicals. For example, chemotaxis to volatile olfactory attractants depends on the AWA and AWC neurons, whereas chemotaxis to water-soluble attractants like salts depends on the ASE neurons (Bargmann and Horvitz 1991a; Bargmann et al. 1993). Importantly, the functions of individual cell types are the same from animal to animal, indicating that reproducible genetic or developmental events lead to the differentiation of distinct sensory cell types.

Some types of neurons regulate both chemotaxis and developmental responses to pheromones, suggesting that a single type of sensory neuron can generate two different patterns of activity in response to two different stimuli (Bargmann and Horvitz 1991b). The mechanisms by which this specificity is generated are not clear, but genetic results suggest that these differences may result from different patterns of neurotransmitter release. For example, pheromonal regulation of development depends on the production of a transforming growth factor (TGF-β)-related peptide by the sensory neurons (P. Ren and D. Riddle, pers. comm.), but this peptide is not essential for normal chemotaxis (Vowels and Thomas 1994).

Differential regulation of neurotransmitter release may also contribute to the ability of some neurons to sense multiple modalities. The ASH neurons are required for avoidance of chemical repellents and some repulsive mechanical stimuli (Kaplan and Horvitz 1993). The mechanosensory function of the ASH sensory neurons requires a particular glutamate receptor *(glr-1)* on the postsynaptic targets of ASH, but ASH chemosensory functions do not depend on this neurotransmitter receptor (Hart et al. 1995; Maricq et al. 1995). The difference between mechanosensation

[1]Present address: Department of Biology, Brandeis University, Waltham, Massachusetts 02254.

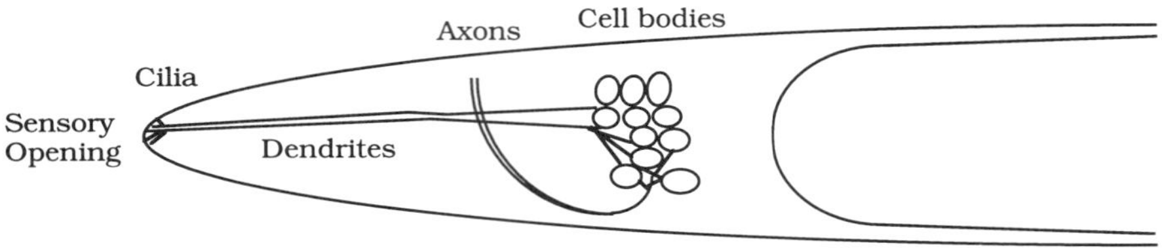

AWA	volatile chemotaxis
AWB	volatile avoidance
AWC	volatile chemotaxis
ASE	water-soluble chemotaxis, egg-laying
ADF	dauer pheromone; water-soluble chemotaxis (minor)
ASG	dauer pheromone (minor); water-soluble chemotaxis (minor)
ASH	osmotic avoidance, nose touch avoidance, volatile avoidance
ASI	dauer pheromone; water-soluble chemotaxis (minor)
ASJ	dauer pheromone (recovery)
ASK	water-soluble chemotaxis, egg laying
ADL	octanol avoidance

Figure 1. Morphology and function of the amphid chemosensory structure. All neurons are members of bilaterally symmetric pairs; only the left member of each pair is shown. Functions have been ascribed to neurons by cell killing of defined chemosensory neurons: AWA and AWC (Bargmann et al. 1993), ASE, ADF, ASG, ASI, ASK (chemotaxis) (Bargmann and Horvitz 1991a), ADF, ASG, ASI, ASJ (dauer formation) (Bargmann and Horvitz 1991b), ASH (Bargmann et al. 1990; Kaplan and Horvitz 1993; Troemel et al. 1995), ADL (Troemel et al. 1995), ASE, ASK (egg-laying) (E. Sawin, pers. comm.), AWB (E.R. Troemel and C.I. Bargmann, unpubl.).

and chemosensation could arise from a quantitative or a qualitative difference in the ASH response to the stimuli. Mechanical stimulation might generate a weak or transient ASH response and release of one transmitter (glutamate), and chemical stimulation might generate a strong or sustained ASH response and release of two transmitters. Alternatively, mechanical and chemical stimuli could activate different second-messenger cascades within ASH. One argument against the latter model is provided by analysis of *odr-3*, which encodes a G-protein α subunit that is expressed in ASH neurons and required for both their chemosensory and their mechanosensory functions (K. Roayaie et al., in prep.). Most models of G-protein function would place *odr-3* at the very first step of sensory transduction, immediately downstream from the receptors that detect chemical and mechanical stimuli. Therefore, the shared *odr-3* requirement suggests that the signaling cascades used for mechanosensation and chemosensation in the ASH neurons overlap to some degree.

Some forms of avoidance require collaboration between multiple sensory neurons. Acute avoidance of 1-octanol depends on the function of both the ASH and the ADL neurons: If either of these sensory neurons is killed, octanol avoidance is delayed or absent (Troemel et al. 1995). In contrast, acute avoidance of benzaldehyde depends on the ASH neurons but not the ADL neurons. These results suggest that ASH activation can be sufficient for avoidance under some circumstances, but that in other contexts multiple sensory neurons including ASH must act together to generate an avoidance response.

SINGLE OLFACTORY NEURONS DISCRIMINATE AMONG DIFFERENT ODORANTS

Two odorants that are recognized by a single neuron can be discriminated by the animal in behavioral assays. Uniform high levels of a single odorant block the ability of an animal to chemotax to a point source of that odorant, but the same animals respond normally to other odorants detected by the same sensory neuron (Bargmann et al. 1993). In addition, prolonged exposure to an odorant decreases the response to that odorant without decreasing responses to other odorants detected by the same cell (Colbert and Bargmann 1995). These two results could be explained by two classes of models. One neuron might have several distinct binding sites for different odorants that are regulated independently, allowing odorant discrimination by regulation of the ligand-bound receptors within a single cell. This mechanism is analogous to homologous desensitization of adrenergic receptors (Premont et al. 1995) and bacterial chemosensory receptors (Adler 1975). Alternatively, integration of information from multiple sensory neurons might contribute to discrimination between odorants, as integration of information from several types of cone cells contributes to color discrimination in the visual system. To distinguish between these two models, we analyzed animals in which only a single type of sensory neuron contributes to odorant responses. Animals doubly mutant for the *osm-3* and *odr-1* genes have defects in all amphid chemosensory neurons except the AWA olfactory neurons, whereas animals doubly mutant for

Table 1. Olfactory Discrimination in Wild-type and Mutant Animals

Odorants detected	Wild-type	*osm-3 odr-1*	*osm-3 odr-7*
Benzaldehyde	+	–	+
Butanone	+	–	+
Isoamyl alcohol	+	–	+
2,3-Pentanedione	+	(high)	+
Diacetyl	+	+	(high)
Pyrazine	+	+	–
2,4,5-Trimethyl thiazole	+	+	+
Odorants discriminated:	all distinct	diacetyl = 2,3 pd	diacetyl = 2,3 pd

In *osm-3 odr-1* mutants, the AWA neurons function; in *osm-3 odr-7* mutants, the AWC neurons function. All other amphid chemosensory neurons are structurally or functionally inactivated in the mutants. Odorants marked (high) are detected only at high concentration in the mutants, whereas wild-type animals detect the odorant at both high and low concentrations. Wild-type animals discriminate between at least seven odorant classes, *osm-3 odr-1* mutants discriminate between at least three odorant classes, and *osm-3 odr-7* mutants discriminate between at least five odorant classes.

the *osm-3* and *odr-7* genes have defects in all chemosensory neurons except the AWC olfactory neurons. Each of the double mutants *osm-3 odr-1* and *osm-3 odr-7* can be regarded as an animal with one sensory cell type, AWA or AWC, respectively. These mutant animals are still able to discriminate between at least three different odorant classes (Table 1) (J.H. Chou and C.I. Bargmann, unpubl.). Therefore, a single sensory neuron is likely to have at least three different receptor proteins or binding sites for odorants, each of which allows independent saturation and adaptation to its odorant ligand. These results are supported by molecular analysis of receptor expression and function in sensory neurons (see below).

Interestingly, some degradation of olfactory discrimination between odorants with similar structures is observed in these doubly mutant animals (J.H. Chou and C.I. Bargmann unpubl.). Wild-type animals discriminate between the odorants diacetyl (2,3-butanedione) and 2,3-pentanedione, both of which are detected by both AWA and AWC when present at very high concentrations. Both *osm-3 odr-1* animals and *osm-3 odr-7* animals detect both odorants at high concentrations, but these mutants fail to discriminate between the two odorants. These results suggest that some forms of olfactory discrimination require the function of multiple olfactory neurons.

odr-10 ENCODES A CANDIDATE RECEPTOR FOR THE ODORANT DIACETYL

Mutations in the *odr-10* gene were identified in a screen for animals that failed to chemotax to the odorant diacetyl (Sengupta et al. 1996). *odr-10* animals are about 100-fold less sensitive to diacetyl than are wild-type animals. However, their responses to all other tested odorants are normal, including responses to other odorants detected by the same sensory neurons as sense diacetyl (the AWA neurons). Thus, the AWA neurons have their normal fates in *odr-10* mutants and can function when challenged with some, but not all, of their normal odorant ligands.

odr-10 encodes a predicted protein with seven hydrophobic domains and key residues characteristic of G-protein-coupled receptors. Mammalian olfactory receptors are believed to be members of this receptor family (Buck and Axel 1991). This sequence similarity, combined with its mutant phenotype, suggests that *odr-10* might encode a receptor for the odorant diacetyl.

The expression of *odr-10* is consistent with that expected for a diacetyl receptor. A reporter gene driven by the *odr-10* promoter is expressed strongly only in the AWA neurons, the sensory neurons that respond to diacetyl (Sengupta et al. 1996). Moreover, a tagged Odr-10 protein is localized to the sensory cilia of the AWA neurons. Odorant detection and transduction are thought to be localized to olfactory cilia, which make up only about 2% of the volume of the AWA neurons, so the presence of the Odr-10 protein in the cilia argues for a sensory function.

odr-10 mutants are defective only in their response to diacetyl, suggesting that the receptor encoded by *odr-10* is highly specific for one odorant. However, if multiple receptors on the AWA neurons each detect overlapping sets of odorants, a "specific" olfactory defect could result from the loss of a more promiscuous receptor (Fig. 2). The use of an AWA-specific transcription factor, *odr-7,* allowed *odr-10* function to be explored in more detail. *odr-7* mutants lack all known AWA functions; they fail to express *odr-10* and probably other AWA receptor genes (Sengupta et al. 1994, 1996). The diacetyl responses of *odr-7* mutants can be restored by expressing *odr-10* under an *odr-7*-independent promoter (Fig. 2). However, the *odr-7* response to other AWA odorants is not rescued by *odr-10*. Thus, in both loss-of-function and gain-of-function experiments, *odr-10* affects only diacetyl responses.

odr-10 null mutants respond to high concentrations of diacetyl, indicating that worms have a second

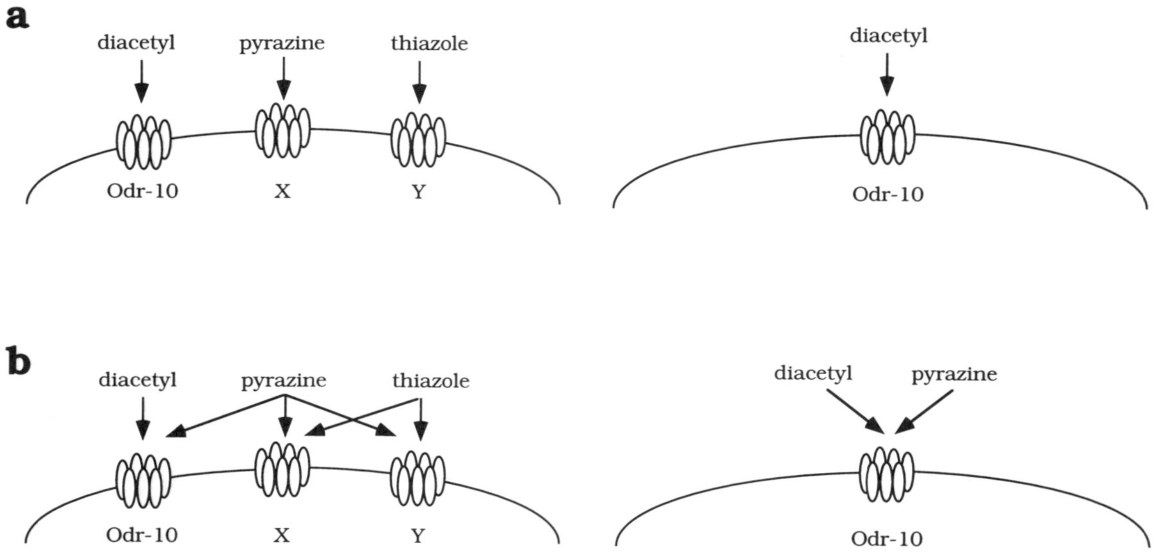

Figure 2. Analysis of *odr-10* specificity. (*Left*) An AWA neuron probably has multiple receptors, but only the *odr-10* (diacetyl) receptor is defined. Each receptor might detect a small number of odorants (*a*) or many odorants (*b*). (*Right*) Expression of only *odr-10* in an *odr-7* mutant restores only the diacetyl response, suggesting that *odr-10* is relatively diacetyl-specific (model *a*).

diacetyl receptor with approximately 100-fold lower sensitivity to the odorant. Although diacetyl is sensed mostly by the AWA olfactory neurons at low concentrations, it is sensed redundantly by both the AWA and the AWC neurons at high concentrations (P. Sengupta and C.I. Bargmann, in prep.). Cell-killing experiments in *odr-10* mutants indicate that the second, low-affinity diacetyl receptor is found in the AWC neurons. It is unlikely that the primary function of this receptor is detection of diacetyl, since the concentrations required to activate it are in excess of those that would ever be observed in nature. It is more likely that the second receptor is a receptor for a second odorant that cross-reacts with diacetyl at very high odorant concentrations. Cross-saturation experiments suggest that this receptor might have a higher affinity for 2,3-pentanedione (J.H. Chou and C.I. Bargmann, unpubl.). Other seven-transmembrane-domain receptors can also cross-react with heterologous ligands at high ligand concentrations.

MULTIPLE FAMILIES OF SEVEN-TRANSMEMBRANE-DOMAIN RECEPTORS ARE CANDIDATE *C. ELEGANS* CHEMOSENSORY RECEPTORS

The similarity between *odr-10* and G-protein-coupled receptors is consistent with data from other animals implicating similar receptors in olfaction. In vertebrates, odorants stimulate the production of cAMP via a G-protein-regulated adenylyl cyclase, whereas both G-protein-stimulated cAMP and inositol triphosphate (IP_3) pathways may participate in invertebrate olfaction. A candidate olfactory receptor gene family that includes hundreds of potential G-protein-coupled receptors has been cloned from vertebrate olfactory neurons (Buck and Axel 1991). Individual members of the vertebrate gene family are expressed in small numbers of olfactory neurons, and each olfactory neuron expresses only a few receptor genes, possibly only one (Ressler et al. 1993; Vassar et al. 1993; Chess et al. 1994). A second family of vertebrate receptor genes has been identified in the vomeronasal organ, an olfactory organ involved in species-specific behaviors (Dulac and Axel 1995). The vomeronasal receptors are unrelated to the olfactory receptors by sequence. Indeed, they show no similarity to any known G-protein-coupled receptor family and may have evolved independently of the other receptor genes.

odr-10 is not highly similar either to the vertebrate olfactory receptors or to the vomeronasal receptors. Like the vertebrate olfactory receptors, it is a classic seven-transmembrane-domain receptor, but it is unclear whether the nematode olfactory receptors and the vertebrate olfactory receptors share a common ancestor in the G-protein-coupled receptor superfamily. Database searches with *odr-10* indicate that the closest known vertebrate genes are olfactory receptors, but this similarity is slight and may represent convergent or divergent evolution.

Within *C. elegans*, *odr-10* appears to be one member of a large gene family that could encode additional olfactory receptor genes (A. Coulson et al., pers. comm.; E. Troemel et al., unpubl.). At least 80 *odr-10*-like genes have been identified within the approximately 50% of the *C. elegans* genome that has been sequenced. Any two members of the family share 20–30% amino acid identity. These genes have seven hydrophobic domains with conserved residues clustered in the second, third, sixth, and seventh transmembrane domains as well as the linker region between the fifth and sixth transmembrane domains. This pattern of conservation is characteristic of subfamilies of G-protein-coupled receptors, supporting the idea that genes in the *odr-10* family share a common G-protein-coupled function.

Several additional gene families also encode candidate chemosensory receptors in *C. elegans*. These gene families were discovered not through genetics, but through direct inspection of the *C. elegans* genomic sequence (Troemel et al. 1995)(A. Coulson et al., pers. comm.; J.H. Chou et al., unpubl.). *C. elegans* has homologs of many classic G-protein-coupled receptors, including potential serotonin receptors, metabotropic glutamate receptors, and peptide receptors. In addition, there are many *C. elegans* genes that lack primary sequence similarity with known receptors. but that contain seven hydrophobic regions and other features of G-protein-coupled receptors. These novel candidate receptor genes are called *sr* genes (for *s*even-transmembrane *r*eceptor) and have been divided into several families; within each gene family, the genes share about 30% amino acid identity. The *sra* family (at least 23 genes) and the *srb* family (at least 21 genes) are distantly related to each other by sequence, so that about 10% of residues are conserved between all *sra* and *srb* genes. The *srd* genes (at least 28 genes) are unrelated to the *sra* or *srb* genes, but are very distantly related to the *odr-10*-like genes. The *srg* genes (at least 26 genes) are unrelated to all of the other gene families, as are the *sre* genes (at least 10 genes). Within each gene family, the same regions tend to be conserved (second, third, sixth, seventh transmembrane domains, linker between fifth and sixth transmembrane domains).

Several features of the *sr* genes and *odr-10*-like genes are reminiscent of vertebrate olfactory receptor genes. Like the vertebrate genes, they are all unusually small for seven-transmembrane-domain receptors, typically 300–370 amino acids in length. The high sequence diversity within each family is also reminiscent of vertebrate olfactory receptors.

GENOMIC ORGANIZATION OF CANDIDATE RECEPTOR GENES

Mammalian olfactory receptor genes are found in large gene clusters; at least eleven different receptor gene clusters have been mapped in the mouse (Sullivan et al. 1996). Likewise, more than half of the candidate *C. elegans* receptors are also found in clusters, although these tend to be small clusters of 2–10 genes. In both *C. elegans* and mammals, the most similar receptor genes within a family are usually in the same cluster. The significance of this arrangement is unknown. In particular, the clustering of genes does not always predict a common expression pattern. Although 4 *odr-10*-like genes in one cluster all appear to be expressed in one type of olfactory neuron (see below; E. Troemel and C.I. Bargmann, unpubl.), 4 *sra* receptors from a single cluster yielded three different expression patterns, although all were predominantly within sensory neurons (Troemel et al. 1995).

One of the forces that may drive receptor clustering in *C. elegans*, but not in mammals, is the clustering of related genes in operons. In *C. elegans*, a single primary transcript can be cleaved into multiple mature transcripts that are presumably coregulated at the transcriptional level (Zorio et al. 1994). Genes within operons are invariably located within about 500 nucleotides of one another and transcribed in the same orientation. Some of the *C. elegans* candidate receptor genes are found in such configurations, but none of them has been shown directly to be transcribed in operons.

None of the mammalian olfactory or vomeronasal receptor genes has introns. In contrast, all of the known *C. elegans* receptors have multiple introns. The positions of these introns are conserved, but not invariant, between different members of a single receptor gene family (e.g., *sra* genes), but they are completely different between different receptor gene families (e.g., the *odr-10*-like genes have different intron placement than the *sra* genes).

EXPRESSION OF CANDIDATE RECEPTOR GENES

Many of the *odr-10*-like genes and *sr* genes appear to be expressed in subsets of chemosensory neurons (Troemel et al. 1995; E. Troemel and C.I. Bargmann, unpubl.). Expression was analyzed by fusing the promoter of an *odr-10*-like gene or an *sr* gene to the green fluorescent protein (GFP) marker and introducing these fusion genes to generate transgenic worms. Expression of such transgenes is usually similar to that of endogenous transcripts, but some differences have been observed, probably because the gene copy number is high, and any control sequences within the body of the gene are deleted.

Eleven of fifteen *odr-10*-like gene fusions and eleven of fourteen *sr* gene fusions (including members of the *sra, srb, srd, srg,* and *sre* families) are expressed in chemosensory neurons. Some genes are expressed only in a single type of neuron, whereas others are expressed in up to five different chemosensory cell types. These data match with the results of cell-killing experiments which indicate that some chemicals are detected by a single neuron type, whereas others are detected by several redundant types of neurons. An individual neuron can express at least four different fusion genes from three different gene families; this result is consistent with the behavioral data suggesting that there are several receptors per neuron.

The *odr-10*-like genes are expressed in multiple cell types, including cells that detect volatile or water-soluble attractants, repellents, and pheromones (E.

Troemel and C.I. Bargmann, unpubl). The *sr* genes are expressed in cells that detect water-soluble attractants, repellents, and pheromones. Interestingly, three of the *sr* genes have sex-specific patterns of expression, suggesting that they might detect mating pheromones. All three genes are expressed in putative chemosensory neurons that are associated with male mating structures, such as the spicule sensory neurons, which regulate sperm release. One of the three genes is also expressed in the ADF sensory neurons in males, but not in the same neurons in hermaphrodites. This pattern of gene expression suggests that even neurons such as ADF, which appear similar in both sexes, may actually be functionally dimorphic.

The subcellular localization of these putative receptor proteins is also consistent with a sensory function. Tagged versions of an *sra* protein, an *srd* protein, and an *srg* protein are all localized to the sensory cilia, where chemosensation takes place (Fig. 3) (L. Tong et al., unpubl.). This localization in the cilia is inconsistent with a function in axon guidance or neurotransmission and supports the notion that these genes are sensory receptors. A tagged *sre* protein is localized to the base of the cilia, and the other proteins are found along the length of the cilia.

Some of the *sr* and *odr-10*-like genes are expressed in both chemosensory neurons and interneurons, and some are expressed only in non-chemosensory neurons (Troemel et al. 1995; E. Troemel and C.I. Bargmann, unpubl.). In addition, one *odr-10*-like gene is expressed in a nonneuronal cell type (the rectal gland cells) and one *srg* gene is expressed in the gut. Unless these expression patterns are misleading, some of the *odr-10* or *sr* genes probably function in processes other than chemosensation. What might their functions be? Several of the molecules that are attractive to *C. elegans*, such as amino acids, are closely related in structure to neurotransmitters (e.g., histidine is a *C. elegans* attractant, whereas histamine is a neurotransmitter). Therefore, a receptor that detects attractants in a sensory neuron could be related to a receptor that detects a similar neurotransmitter in an interneuron.

Based on the current number of sequenced receptors in 50% of the genome, the total number of *sr* and *odr-10*-like genes in the entire genome should be about 400. The expression experiments suggest that about half of these are likely to be chemoreceptors (70% of gene fusions yielded expression patterns; of those, 75% were expressed in chemosensory neurons), suggesting that *C. elegans* uses a total of about 200 receptors to detect chemicals. This complexity is of the same order of magnitude as the mammalian candidate receptors (1000 genes) and is initially surprising, given the smaller nervous system of the nematode. Nonetheless, a diversity of receptors may be necessary for the animal's life-style. *C. elegans* probably eats many different species of bacteria associated with decaying animal and vegetable material. The by-products of bacterial metabolism vary depending on the species of bacteria and the bacteria's food source, so no single odorant or small group of odorants will necessarily predict the presence of food supplies (Zechman and Labows 1985). The known *C. elegans* attractants include typical products of bacterial fermentation (ketones, alcohols, esters), any one of which might be useful to identify food. In addition, the specificity of the *odr-10*-diacetyl interaction is quite striking; even closely related odorants are apparently not detected by *odr-10*. If this is a general property of receptor-ligand interactions under physiological conditions, the number of receptors required to detect relevant odorants may be quite large.

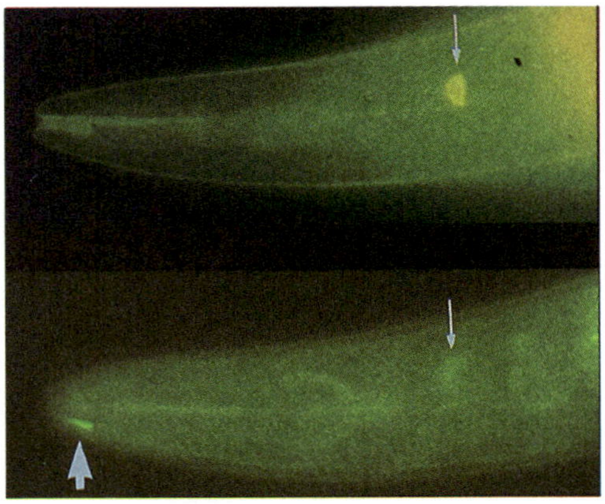

Figure 3. Protein localization of Srg-2::GFP. (*Top*) The ASK neuron visualized in an *sra-9::GFP* promoter fusion where GFP diffuses freely through the cell. The cell body fluoresces strongly (*arrow*), with weaker fluorescence in the axon and dendrite. (*Bottom*) Localization of Srg-2::GFP protein to the sensory cilia of the ASK neuron. The ASK cilium fluoresces strongly (*arrowhead*) and the cell body fluoresces weakly (*arrow*).

Taken together, the expression patterns of the receptors provide a first answer to the question of how olfactory stimuli are recognized and discriminated. We propose that a single odorant activates a small number of receptor proteins encoded by the *odr-10* and *sr* gene families, perhaps only one or two receptor types per odorant at physiological odorant concentrations. Receptors present on one group of neurons lead to the activation of chemotaxis responses, whereas receptors on other neurons preferentially activate avoidance or other responses.

REGULATION OF OLFACTORY FUNCTION BY ODORANT-SPECIFIC ADAPTATION

A *C. elegans* olfactory neuron can down-regulate one odorant response after prolonged exposure to the odorant, while maintaining its responsiveness to other odorants (Colbert and Bargmann 1995). Therefore, there must be a mechanism to regulate different receptors or signaling pathways within the sensory neurons. Genetic data suggest that the signal transduction mechanisms within the sensory neurons are largely shared by all odorants. Mutations in the G-protein α subunit encoded by the *odr-3* gene reduce all olfactory responses in the AWA and AWC neurons (K. Roayaie et al., in prep.), suggesting that all olfactory receptors within AWA or AWC might converge on common G proteins. Similarly, mutations in the channels used in olfactory transduction affect all of the olfactory responses in the cells in which they are expressed (C. Coburn et al., in prep.). If these results are taken at face value, specific adaptation of individual odorant responses probably involves regulation of the olfactory receptors. Nonetheless, the mechanisms of regulation need not be entirely receptor-specific; indeed, some heterologous adaptation can occur between different odorants (Colbert and Bargmann 1995).

Vertebrate and *Drosophila* seven-transmembrane-domain receptors are regulated by kinases of the βARK/rhodopsin kinase family and arrestins (Premont et al. 1995). The kinases phosphorylate and down-regulate only ligand-bound receptors, thereby providing a mechanism to specifically reduce the activity of only one receptor type in a cell expressing multiple receptors. A *C. elegans* βARK-related kinase is expressed in sensory neurons, but its function has not been analyzed genetically (J.G. Chou and C.I. Bargmann, unpubl.).

Genetic analysis of olfactory adaptation has led to the identification of several genes that are required for olfactory adaptation, but not for the responses of naive animals to odorants. Interestingly, these genes are also odorant-specific in their effects. The three odorants benzaldehyde, butanone, and isoamyl alcohol are detected primarily by the AWC olfactory neurons, but *adp-1* mutants are defective only in adaptation to benzaldehyde and butanone, whereas *osm-9* mutants are defective only in adaptation to butanone and isoamyl alcohol (Colbert and Bargmann 1995). These results indicate that one sensory neuron may rely on different adaptation mechanisms to regulate different odorant responses. Other observations suggest that one odorant can have multiple adaptation pathways. For example, *osm-9* null mutations cause a partial adaptation defect to butanone and isoamyl alcohol, suggesting that at least one *osm-9*-independent mechanism of adaptation persists in the mutants. Butanone adaptation appears to be blocked completely in the *adp-1 osm-9* double mutant, indicating that for this one odorant, two distinct adaptation pathways function in parallel to regulate the response.

Why should adaptation be so complex? Perhaps regulation of the receptors provides a significant route for behavioral regulation within the *C. elegans* chemosensory system. The environments in which *C. elegans* usually finds itself (compost heaps or river banks) are likely to contain many odorants; some of these odorants would be present at high uniform concentrations that could make them uninformative for finding food. An animal with many sensory neurons might regulate olfactory responses by inhibiting or potentiating all responses from a single sensory neuron, but this would not be useful in *C. elegans*, where one neuron expresses many different receptors. Distinct adaptation pathways could help prioritize odorant cues; for example, responses to odorants that are released by many species of bacteria might be slower to adapt than responses to relatively rare odorants.

Adaptation may also contribute to the discrimination of multiple stimuli by a single neuron. Behavioral studies, and analysis of the *glr-1* glutamate receptor mutant, indicate that the ASH neuron may have three distinct signaling states: off, mechanical stimuli (propagated through the *glr-1* receptor on postsynaptic targets of ASH), and chemical stimuli (*glr-1*-independent) (see above). This sensory distinction correlates with a distinction in sensory adaptation; responses to mechanical stimuli are rapidly adapting, whereas responses to chemical repellents adapt slowly, if at all. These adaptation mechanisms might create an intrinsic difference in ASH between mechanical stimuli (transient neuronal activity, glutamate released) and chemical stimuli (sustained neuronal activity, glutamate and a second transmitter released?) regardless of the temporal properties of the external stimuli. The glutamate receptor then provides a means to propagate this difference across the synapse to other neurons.

Other results are consistent with the possibility that receptor regulation could contribute not only to adaptation over time, but also to sensory discrimination. The *adp-1* adaptation mutant has the interesting property of discriminating between more classes of odorants than wild-type animals, suggesting a common pathway in olfactory discrimination and olfactory adaptation (H.A. Colbert and C.I. Bargmann, unpubl.). The contribution of different cellular and molecular components to this and other forms of behavioral regulation are currently under study.

ACKNOWLEDGMENTS

This work was supported by U.S. Public Health Service grant DC-01393, The Markey Charitable Trust, The Searle Scholars Program, and The Howard Hughes Medical Institute. C.I.B. is an assistant investigator of the Howard Hughes Medical Institute. E.R.T. and D.M.T. were supported by National Science Foundation predoctoral fellowships; P.S. was supported by a postdoctoral grant from the American Cancer Society, California division; and K.R. and J.G.C. were supported by Howard Hughes Medical Institute predoctoral fellowships.

REFERENCES

Adler, J. 1975. Chemotaxis in bacteria. *Annu. Rev. Biochem.* **44:** 341.

Bargmann, C.I. and H.R. Horvitz. 1991a. Chemosensory neurons with overlapping functions direct chemotaxis to multiple chemicals in *C. elegans*. *Neuron* **7:** 729.

———. 1991b. Control of larval development by chemosensory neurons in *Caenorhabditis elegans*. *Science* **251:** 1243.

Bargmann, C.I., E. Hartwieg, and H.R. Horvitz. 1993. Odorant-selective genes and neurons mediate olfaction in *C. elegans*. *Cell* **74:** 515.

Bargmann, C.I., J.H. Thomas, and H.R. Horvitz. 1990. Chemosensory cell function in the behavior and development of *Caenorhabditis elegans*. *Cold Spring Harbor Symp. Quant. Biol.* **55:** 529.

Buck, L. and R. Axel. 1991. A novel multigene family may encode odorant receptors: A molecular basis for odor recognition. *Cell* **65:** 175.

Chess, A., I. Simon, H. Cedar, and R. Axel. 1994. Allelic inactivation regulates olfactory receptor gene expression. *Cell* **78:** 823.

Colbert, H.A. and C.I. Bargmann. 1995. Odorant-specific adaptation pathways generate olfactory plasticity in *C. elegans*. *Neuron* **14:** 803.

Dulac, C. and R. Axel. 1995. A novel family of genes encoding putative pheromone receptors in mammals. *Cell* **83:** 195.

Hart, A., S. Sims, and J. Kaplan. 1995. Synaptic code for sensory modalities revealed by *C. elegans* GLR-1 glutamate receptor. *Nature* **378:** 82.

Kaplan, J. and H. Horvitz. 1993. A dual mechanosensory and chemosensory neuron in *Caenorhabditis elegans*. *Proc. Natl. Acad. Sci.* **90:** 2227.

Maricq, A.V., E. Peckol, M. Driscoll, and C.I. Bargmann. 1995. Mechanosensory signalling in *C. elegans* mediated by the GLR-1 glutamate receptor. *Nature* **378:** 78.

Premont, R.T., J. Inglese, and R.J. Lefkowitz. 1995. Protein kinases that phosphorylate activated G protein-coupled receptors. *FASEB J.* **9:** 175.

Ressler, K.J., S.L. Sullivan, and L.B. Buck. 1993. A zonal organization of odorant receptor gene expression in the olfactory epithelium. *Cell* **73:** 597.

Sengupta, P., J.C. Chou, and C.I. Bargmann. 1996. *odr-10* encodes a seven transmembrane domain olfactory receptor required for responses to the odorant diacetyl. *Cell* **84:** 899.

Sengupta, P., H.A. Colbert, and C.I. Bargmann. 1994. The *C. elegans* gene *odr-7* encodes an olfactory-specific member of the nuclear receptor superfamily. *Cell* **79:** 971.

Sullivan, S.L., M.C. Adamson, K.J. Ressler, C.A. Kozak, and L.B. Buck. 1996. The chromosomal distribution of mouse odorant receptor genes. *Proc. Natl. Acad. Sci.* **93:** 884.

Troemel, E.R., J.H. Chou, N.D. Dwyer, H.A. Colbert, and C.I. Bargmann. 1995. Divergent seven transmembrane receptors are candidate chemosensory receptors in *C. elegans*. *Cell* **83:** 207.

Vassar, R., J. Ngai, and R. Axel. 1993. Spatial segregation of odorant receptor expression in the mammalian olfactory epithelium. *Cell* **74:** 309.

Vowels, J. and J. Thomas. 1994. Multiple chemosensory defects in *daf-11* and *daf-21* mutants of *Caenorhabditis elegans*. *Genetics* **138:** 303.

White, J.G., E. Southgate, J.N. Thomson, and S. Brenner. 1986. The structure of the nervous system of the nematode *Caenorhabditis elegans*. *Philos. Trans. R. Soc. Lond. B* **314:** 1.

Zechman, J.M. and J.N. Labows, Jr. 1985. Volatiles of *Pseudomonas aeruginosa* and related species by automated headspace concentration-gas chromatography. *Can. J. Microbiol.* **31:** 232.

Zorio, D., N. Cheng, T. Blumenthal, and J. Spieth. 1994. Operons as a common form of chromosomal organization in *C. elegans*. *Nature* **372:** 270.

Genetic Approaches to Mammalian Olfaction

R.R. Reed
Howard Hughes Medical Institute, Department of Molecular Biology and Genetics, Johns Hopkins University School of Medicine, Baltimore, Maryland 21205

The mammalian olfactory system can sense and discriminate among a very large number of odorants. The perception of an odor is a complex process involving the initial events of odorant recognition in the nasal epithelium and neuronal processing in both the olfactory bulb and the brain (for review, see Kauer 1991; Shepherd 1994). A complete understanding of this pathway will require the identification and characterization of the molecules responsible for stimulus detection, sensory adaptation, and the patterning of neuronal connections. Considerable success has been achieved in identifying the proteins of the mammalian signaling system analogous to those components present in other sensory systems. The application of genetic, electrophysiological, and molecular analysis of olfactory function in mammals has shed light on the mechanisms that account for sensitivity and specificity in this remarkable sensory system. To address the mechanisms that contribute to the overall sensitivity and specificity of the olfactory system, we have focused our recent research efforts on two central issues. In this paper, we describe distinct genetic methods that provide insight into the fundamental processes that underlie olfaction.

A major issue in olfactory function is understanding the basis of odorant coding; that is, how the identities of individual odorants are recognized by the olfactory system. Remarkably, little is known about the nature of the ligand-receptor interactions in the olfactory system. In the half-decade since the description of putative odorant receptors by Buck and Axel (1991), there have been no compelling experiments to demonstrate that odorants specifically bind to the seven transmembrane receptors. A complete understanding of the discrimination ability of the mammalian olfactory system requires that information on the selectivity and affinity of individual odorant ligands for their cognate receptors be determined. This information should allow computer modeling studies to direct future experimentation on the overall physiology and connectivity of the olfactory system.

The second problem in olfaction is to understand the transcriptional control of olfactory neuronal development and differentiation. In large part, the special properties of the mammalian olfactory system arise from the specialized transduction components that are expressed in this tissue. In addition to a common mechanism that directs the high-level expression of all downstream components of the second-messenger signaling pathway, there must be other processes that are responsible for odorant receptor expression. The selection of a single receptor for expression from among the repertoire of more than 500 independently encoded genes is likely to derive from a hierarchical cascade of transcriptional control mechanisms. We have utilized molecular genetic methods to elucidate at least one aspect of this process.

SPECIFIC ANOSMIAS

The ability to detect olfactory stimuli is easily assessed by behavioral and physiological responses. This has provided a wealth of data documenting variations in olfactory function in species as diverse as humans, fruit flies, and worms. In humans, heritable loss of olfactory function occurs in patients with X-linked Kallman's syndrome due to mutations in an N-CAM-like protein apparently essential for neuronal migration and olfactory bulb formation. This leads to a complete general anosmia (loss of all odorant detection). Perhaps more interestingly, there are well-documented variations in the human population in an individual's ability to detect individual odorant stimuli.

Specific anosmia is defined as the failure to perceive a given odorant at ten times the mean normal threshold (Amoore 1967, 1991). At even higher concentrations, the odorant is often detected, so the specific anosmia condition is actually a variety of narrowly limited hyposmia. However, for some odorants, the variation in the human population for detection of the odorant may be as great as 8 orders of magnitude and may reflect an absolute inability to detect that compound. Up to 89 specific anosmias have been reported, with considerable redundancy among the odorants (Amoore 1991).

Human twin studies support the hypothesis that specific anosmias have a genetic basis. The thresholds for the detection of androstenone and isoamyl acetate show greater concordance in monozygotic twins, relative to dizygotic twins (Wysocki and Beauchamp 1984; Wysocki et al. 1989; Gross-Isseroff et al. 1992; Segal et al. 1992). No difference in odorant detection thresholds is observed between fraternal and identical twins among several other odorants (Hubert et al. 1980), although a high variance in phenotype may be masking the genetic basis. The specific anosmias for both *n*-butyl mercaptan and the scent of freesia flowers are inherited as autosomal recessive traits (Patterson and

Lauder 1948). The prevalence of specific anosmias varies greatly in the human population. Studies have documented that 47% of the human population displays a specific anosmia to androstenone and perhaps 3% are unable to detect isovaleric acid (see Table 1) (Wysocki and Kare 1991).

It has been suggested that specific anosmia or "smell blindness" in the olfactory system is analogous to color blindness in vision, where unequal crossing-over between the highly homologous receptors within a cluster during gametogenesis would result in the formation of new hybrid receptors and/or the deletion of receptor genes (Nathans et al. 1986a,b). In humans, the specific anosmia to pentadecalactone is inherited as a recessive genetic trait (Whissell-Buechy and Amoore 1973), consistent with mutation or loss of the receptor gene for this particular odorant.

Our understanding of the origins of specificity and sensitivity in detecting odorants requires a complete elucidation of the structure/function relationships among odorant receptors and their ligands. Toward this end, we have undertaken a functional approach to identify the receptors for particular odorant stimuli. The recently described family of putative odorant receptor proteins, with 100 genes in fish and up to 1000 genes in rodents, are structurally related to other G-protein-coupled receptors (Buck and Axel 1991; Levy et al. 1991; Ngai et al. 1993b). These proteins are expressed in the olfactory epithelium, with a single receptor subfamily expressed in only 0.1% to 0.5% of all olfactory neurons (Nef et al. 1992; Ngai et al. 1993a; Ressler et al. 1993; Kishimoto et al. 1994; Koshimoto et al. 1994; Strotmann et al. 1994). In the absence of functional expression of the odorant receptors, an indirect approach to identify genes essential for the detection of odors may prove to be a useful alternative approach.

The molecular mapping of the olfactory receptor genes has shown them to be located in clusters of 5–20 receptor genes over regions of several hundred kilobases (Ben-Arie et al. 1994; Chess et al. 1994). The linkage studies in human and in mouse indicate that they are encoded on many different chromosomes. The large number of receptors and their distribution on many autosomes suggest that targeted deletion studies which remove only a single receptor or a number of receptors might not lead to a detectable deficit in odorant detection repertoire. In particular, in the absence of a candidate ligand for a specific receptor, the identification of the odorant that normally binds to a deleted receptor would be problematic.

Specific Anosmias in Mice

There are several advantages to studying olfactory perception in nonhuman subjects. In human studies, eating, smoking, and sinus conditions have all been shown to affect the threshold level of detection of odorants (Amoore 1991). These variables can be controlled in experiments with nonhuman subjects. Studies of specific anosmia in inbred strains of mice confirm that the specific anosmias to both androstenone (H.-W. Wang et al. 1993) and isovaleric acid (Wysocki et al. 1977; Pourtier and Sicard 1989) have a genetic basis. These behaviors are better named a specific hyposmia, since the animals can detect the compound at high concentrations. Electrophysiological analysis of the olfactory epithelium from the mice with specific anosmia show that the defects are within the epithelium (H.-W. Wang et al. 1993), rather than affecting the mechanism of central processing in the brain.

Table 1. Specific Anosmias in Humans

Odorant	Percent anosmic
Androstenone	47
Isobutylaldehyde	36
1,8 Cineole	33
1-Pyrroline	16
Exaltolide	12
L-Carvone	8
Isovaleric acid	3

We have used a genetic approach to identify the origin of the specific anosmia to isovaleric acid in C57BL/6J mice. Conditioned avoidance behavior assays that test the ability of animals to detect odorants (Wysocki et al. 1977; Pourtier and Sicard 1989) have been developed and validated with electrophysiological studies (H.-W. Wang et al. 1993). Wysocki and colleagues (1977) described a behavior assay that used conditioned avoidance, where the mice that can smell the compound associate the smell with an aversive stimulus (Fig. 1). Mice avoid the test odorant when exposed to the same compound at a later time. Measurement of preference ratio (volume of odorant solution consumed/total solution consumed) as determined in this two-bottle preference assay has been shown to assess olfactory function rather than taste (Wysocki et al. 1977; Pourtier and Sicard 1989). The ability of C57BL/6J and DBA/2J mice to detect isovaleric acid differs at 10^{-5} and 10^{-6} M isovaleric acid. Specifically, DBA/2J mice detect the compound, whereas C57BL/6J mice are anosmic (Fig. 2).

The DBA/2J and C57BL/6J strains of mice detect other odorants equally well. We tested both strains of mice for their ability to detect pentadecalactone; Wysocki and colleagues had previously shown that C57BL/6J and AKR/J mice were equally capable of detecting isoamyl acetate (Wysocki et al. 1977). The inability to detect one compound while retaining the ability to detect several other unrelated odors is consistent with C57BL/6J mice having a specific anosmia to isovaleric acid, phenotypically similar to that previously described in humans.

Locus Encoding Isovaleric-acid-specific Anosmia

The olfactory defect in C57BL/6J mice was examined in F_1 progeny of a cross between C57BL/6J and

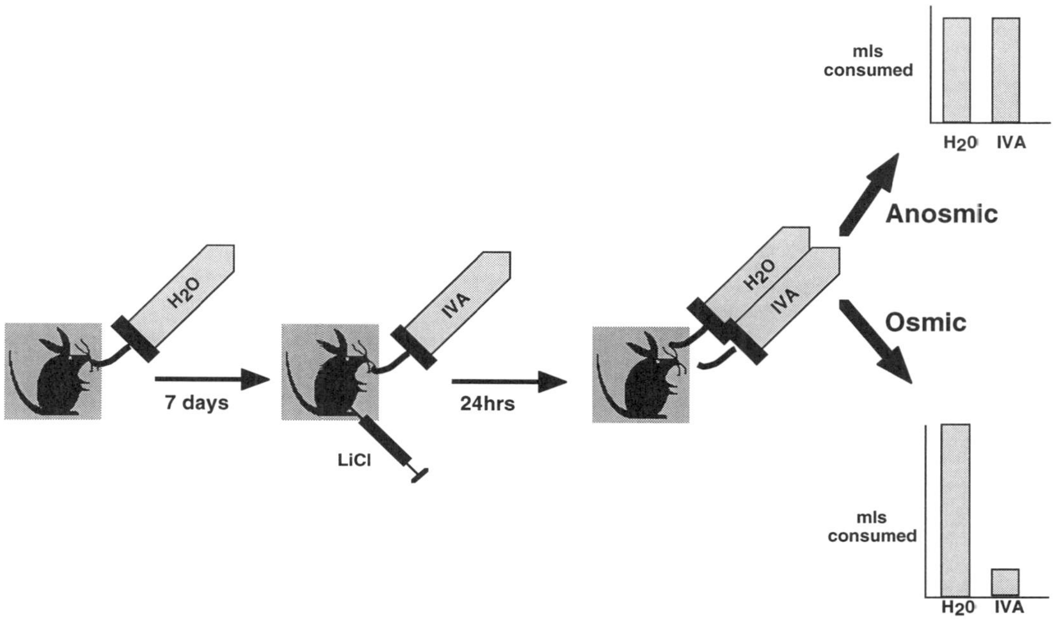

Figure 1. The conditioned aversion test for specific anosmia. Mice are given 1 hr of fluid access a day for 7 days, so that they drink readily when given liquid. On the 8th day, the mice are given access to a bottle containing isovaleric acid for 10 min. Immediately following this exposure, each mouse is injected with the LiCl solution (the aversive stimulus). Preference testing begins 24 hr after the injection. The mice are given two drinking bottles, one with and one without isovaleric acid. The amount of liquid consumed from each bottle is measured, and the ratio of isovaleric acid to total liquid consumed is defined as the preference ratio.

DBA/2J. All of the animals detected isovaleric acid at the discriminatory concentration, indicating that the specific anosmia is recessive and is consistent with the loss of a receptor or other component essential for the specific detection of isovaleric acid.

The use of recombinant inbred (RI) strains of mice, derived from systematic inbreeding from the cross of two preexisting progenitor strains (Bailey 1971), allows the efficient localization of genes important in complex traits. These strains are generated by intercrossing two strains that differ in a trait of interest and then continuing to cross their descendants for at least 20 generations. Each RI strain is homozygous at all alleles and fixes different combinations of alleles from the progenitors (here, C57BL/B6J and DBA/2J). Thus, multiple, genetically identical individuals from one strain can be phenotypically tested and compared to mice from other strains of that RI set to map markers or characteristics of interest. Two markers found on the distal region of mouse chromosome 4, *D4MIT12* and *Ckb-rs1*, had an identical strain distribution pattern as the anosmic behavior. We have named this locus on chromosome 4, *ival* (Griff and Reed 1995).

The experiments with RI strains and F_2 backcrossed individuals do not permit one to determine whether the *ival* locus is sufficient to impart the osmic phenotype. To address this question, (DBA/2J x C57BL/6J) F_1 x C57BL/6J animals were analyzed for the presence of the DBA alleles of markers flanking the *ival* locus. Congenic strains were then generated by backcrossing mice for 6 generations, while scoring for the presence of DBA markers at the *ival* locus. In these strains, more than 95% of the genome outside of the *ival* locus should derive from the C57BL/6J (anosmic) parent. Behavioral testing using the conditioned aversion assay of homozygous ($ival^+/ival^+$) animals reveals that this locus is sufficient to allow the animal to detect isovaleric acid at the test concentration (Fig. 3).

The region on chromosome 4 encoding *ival* was further refined to a segment of 0.27 cM using a large backcross and selecting from among the progeny those that had recombined in the region of interest. The recombinant mice from this screen, in combination with closely linked markers, represent valuable tools to isolate the physical DNA that carries the genes responsible for the ability of the DBA2J mice to detect isovaleric acid. Based on estimates from elsewhere in the genome, we expect that the 0.27-cM region identified on chromosome 4 represents approximately 300,000 bp of DNA. We have recently isolated cloned DNA fragments from this region and have initiated a search for the genetic differences in the osmic and anosmic strains. The ability to identify homologous genes in humans and mice will be a major focus of future work and should allow us to extend our understanding of the mouse *ival* locus to identify similar genes in human and gain insight into the mechanisms responsible for the significant diversity in odorant detection in the human population.

An interesting phenomenon associated with specific anosmias in humans and mice is the ability of appar-

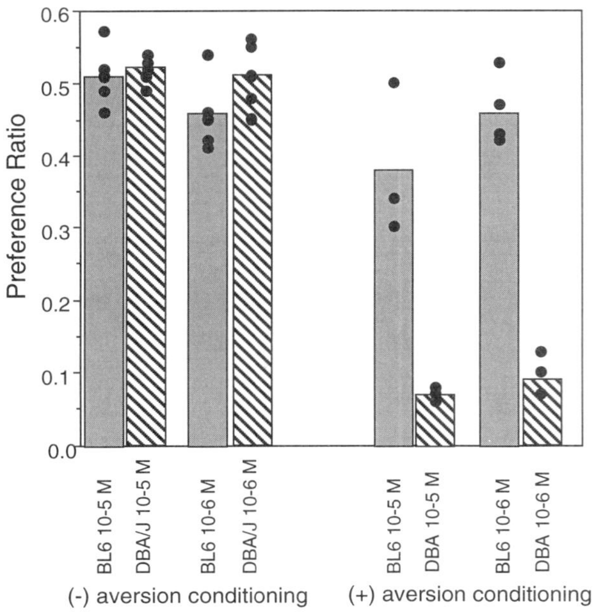

Figure 2. Strain differences in the detection of isovaleric acid. Two mouse strains (C57BL/6J and DBA/2J) known to differ in their ability to detect isovaleric acid are tested at several concentrations in the two-bottle preference test. C57BL/6J (*filled bars*) and DBA/2J (*striped bars*) mice are tested without (*left*) or with (*right*) the aversive stimulus. The preference ratio is the total amount of odorant consumed/total amount of liquid consumed. Each bar represents a minimum of 4 animals. Filled circles represent individual mice, and the bars represent the average of the points in the respective category.

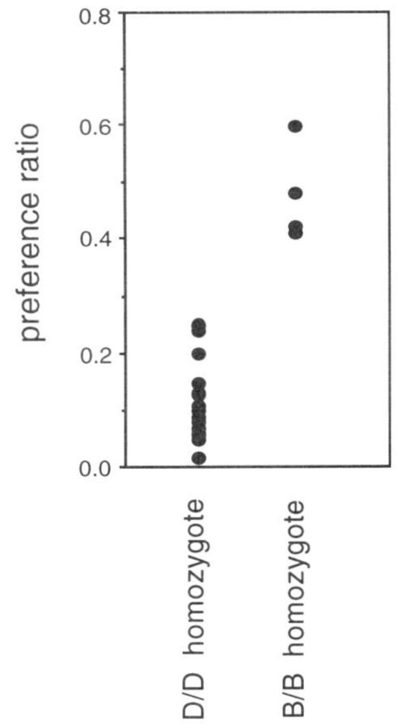

Figure 3. Analysis of specific anosmia in congenic *ival*+/+ and *ival* –/– animals. Each circle represents the data from a single animal. D refers to animals carrying the DBA/2J (osmic) genotype in the region of the *ival* locus. B indicates the animals that are C57BL/6J (anosmic) at the *ival* locus.

ently anosmic individuals to acquire long-term peripheral sensitivity to that odorant after repeated long-term exposure to high concentrations of the compound (Wysocki and Beauchamp 1984; H.-W. Wang et al. 1993). This induction does not occur in subjects that initially have sensitivity to the inducing odorant and is specific to the odorant being tested. The induction is stable, lasting at least 6 weeks in humans (Wysocki and Beauchamp 1984). Since a change in the EOG correlates with this induction, the induction results from changes within the olfactory epithelium. It has been suggested that this increase in sensitivity arises from the stimulus-induced activation of specific receptor expression. This induction could occur through an increase in cell number or level of expression in each cell. An alternative explanation, consistent with models based on the loss of receptor genes, is that long-term exposure to the stimulus leads to elevated second messengers that might positively regulate gene expression for one or more of the components of the signaling pathway. One would have to hypothesize that these changes in gene expression would occur in cells that were expressing related receptor genes and responding at subthreshold levels. These changes in expression could lead to increased sensitivity, specifically in those particular cells that expressed structurally related receptors capable of responding to the odorant.

REGULATION OF OLFACTORY GENE EXPRESSION

The expression of components of the olfactory signal transduction pathway, as well as additional proteins, is likely to establish the phenotype of the olfactory neuron. The patterned differentiation of the neuronal precursor into the terminally differentiated neuron arises from the sequential and coordinate regulation-specific gene products. The identification of the factors that regulate this process and the DNA-binding sites at which they act will provide insight into the mechanisms that contribute to olfactory sensitivity.

The developing vertebrate nervous system acquires its characteristic form and diverse cellular composition via extrinsic and intrinsic cues generated by a programmed pattern of gene expression. The replacement of olfactory neurons with an average life span of 60–90 days (Costanzo and Graziadei 1987) must be regulated in a dynamic fashion to maintain proper balance of proliferation and differentiation. The importance of extrinsically derived trophic factors and receptors (FGFs, TGF-β, and NGF-Rs) in modulating olfactory neuronal development has been described recently (Mahanthappa and Schwarting 1993; DeHamer et al.

1994; Calof 1995; Roskams et al. 1996). During olfactory receptor neuron (ORN) replacement, new neurons arise from neuroblast-like precursor cells that migrate apically through the epithelium (Mackay-Sim and Kittel 1991). The components of the odorant transduction pathway and other markers of mature ORNs are expressed as these cells achieve the differentiated state. Transcription factors are likely to play an equally important role as intrinsic regulators of neurogenesis and in expression of gene products characteristic of the differentiated olfaction neuron.

Analysis of the promoter regions of components of the odorant transduction pathway and other markers of mature olfactory neurons revealed the presence of a consensus sequence, the Olf-1 site, that bound a factor present in olfactory nuclear extracts (Kudrycki et al. 1993; M.W. Wang et al. 1993). Transgenic studies suggested that this site was important in directing olfactory-specific OMP expression in vivo (Walters et al. 1996). The factor that bound to this site, the Olf-1 protein (since renamed O/E-1), was identified using a yeast genetic selection scheme (Wang and Reed 1993), and its expression in the neuronal lineage within olfactory epithelium was confirmed by immunocytochemistry. Olf-1 encodes a novel form of helix-loop-helix (HLH) domain without the characteristic basic residues and can function as a homodimer to specifically bind the Olf-1 site and activate transcription. O/E-1 was independently identified and cloned as an early B-cell factor (EBF) that regulated the mb-1 gene (Hagman et al. 1993).

Recently, we identified two novel Olf-1/EBF-like transcription factors, named O/E-2 and O/E-3, from a mouse embryonic day-12.5 complementary DNA (cDNA) library. The biochemical characterization of these proteins reveals that O/E-1, O/E-2, and O/E-3 possess similar DNA-binding and transcriptional activation properties. Interestingly, expression of O/E-2 and O/E-3 displays a more restricted pattern than does O/E-1 among the 11 tissues examined in adult mice. In situ hybridization revealed that the three O/E genes were expressed in an identical, overlapping pattern in adult olfactory epithelium but were differentially expressed in other neuronal tissues of developing mouse embryo. These results suggest that the O/E proteins together regulate olfactory gene expression, and that they have a more general function during neuronal differentiation and maturation.

The sequences of the O/E cDNAs reveal a family of highly homologous proteins. Analysis of the predicted O/E proteins reveals >75% overall identity and >90% identity over a stretch of 370 residues suggested to be essential for dimerization and DNA binding (Hagman et al. 1995). The HLH dimerization motif of these proteins is located at the carboxyl end of this highly homologous region, and each displays a high degree of identity between helix 1 and helix 2 that was previously noted in O/E-1 and named the repeat helix-loop-helix (rHLH) motif (Wang and Reed 1993). Each of the O/E proteins has a carboxy-terminal domain that is rich in serine (>20%) and proline (>10%). This region of O/E-1 is sufficient to activate transcription when fused to a heterologous DNA-binding motif (Hagman et al. 1995).

Previous studies demonstrated that O/E-1 formed a homodimer that bound to DNA and activated transcription (Hagman et al. 1993; Wang and Reed 1993). The presence of nearly identical rHLH domains of the O/E proteins suggests that they could form heterodimers as well as homodimers. The coexpression of full-length and truncated forms of O/E-1 resulted in the formation of an additional protein-DNA complex of intermediate mobility representing a dimeric protein complex containing a full-length and a truncated O/E-1 (Wang and Reed 1993). Using truncated forms of O/E-1, O/E-2, and O/E-3, we observed protein-DNA complexes of intermediate mobility in electrophoretic mobility shift assay (EMSA) for all combinations of the family members and confirmed that all O/E proteins are able to dimerize with themselves and with other members of the O/E family. The ability of O/E-1 to activate transcription of a reporter gene, and the high degree of conservation among the O/E family members, imply that O/E-2 and O/E-3 exhibit similar *trans*-activational capacity. When HEK293 cells were cotransfected with O/E expression vectors and a reporter construct containing the luciferase gene driven by ten O/E-binding sites adjacent to an SV40 minimal promoter, an increase in luciferase activity was observed. The O/E proteins also activate transcription on native promoters, including ACIII and OMP promoters, which supports a functional role for the O/E proteins in the regulation of olfactory gene expression. These data suggest that the O/E proteins are very similar in their ability to interact with members of the O/E family and with specific DNA sequences to activate transcription.

Mice with an O/E-1 null mutation display a profound defect in their B-cell development but a morphologically normal olfactory epithelium expressing mature olfactory neuronal markers (Lin and Grosschedl 1995). We hypothesized that additional Olf-1/EBF-like proteins, analogous to the functional redundancy suggested for Engrailed and MyoD family members (Hanks et al. 1995; Wang et al. 1996), account for the absence of an olfactory phenotype in the O/E-1 knockout animals. By RNase protection assay (RPA), O/E-2 and O/E-3 are readily detectable only in olfactory tissue, and by in situ hybridization, they are expressed in a pattern identical to O/E-1 in the cells of neuronal lineage. On the basis of these observations, we propose that in the O/E-1 null mutant mice, failure to express the single O/E protein present in spleen, O/E-1, accounts for the B-cell defect, whereas the presence of O/E-2 and O/E-3 compensates for the loss of O/E-1 in olfactory epithelium.

The high-level expression of the downstream components of the signal transduction cascade appears to arise from the coordinate, direct activation of promoter regions for these genes by the O/E family of transcription factors. The differential expression of odorant receptor genes clearly requires a more complex mechanism. The characterization of odorant receptor promoter regions could identify at least some of the participants in this regulatory network. Experiments with transgenic mice carrying a region upstream of an odorant receptor reveal that 5 kb of genomic sequence is sufficient to reproduce several aspects of regulation. These properties include the zonal restriction and stochastic expression within a zone observed for the endogenous receptor (P. Qasba and R.R. Reed, in prep.).

DNA sequence analysis of transcription initiation sites in four mouse olfactory receptors reveals that each contains at least one sequence that closely matches the consensus binding site for the O/E proteins. Moreover, each of these sites can be shown by biochemical methods to bind the O/E proteins in nuclear extracts (A.G. Betz and R.R. Reed, unpubl.). Presumably, there will be additional factors that control, through positive or negative transcriptional modulation, the selection of individual receptor genes for expression. We suggest a model in which additional factors function early in neuronal development to select individual receptor genes and make them competent for expression. The subsequent activation of receptor gene expression then occurs through the action of the O/E proteins in a parallel and similar manner as the downstream components of the transduction pathway (Fig. 4).

The absence of expression of the presumed targets of O/E proteins from the basal cell layer, despite the expression of O/E proteins, suggests an additional mechanism that negatively regulates O/E *trans*-activational activity. We have identified a protein, Roaz, that inhibits the transcriptional activity of the O/E proteins by disrupting the formation of O/E homodimers. The Roaz mRNA is exclusively expressed in the neuronal precursor cells and can account for the absence of target gene expression in these cells. The Roaz protein possesses DNA-binding activity at distinct DNA sequences. The heteromultimeric complex of O/E proteins and Roaz appears to activate transcription from these distinct sites. The similar functional properties resulting from Roaz interaction with each of the O/E proteins (R.Y.L. Tsai and R.R. Reed, in prep.) suggest a common regulatory role for O/E proteins earlier in olfactory neuronal differentiation.

The expression of mature ORN markers in olfactory epithelium and of the O/E-1-regulated gene in B-cells, *mb-1*, are mutually exclusive. Similarly, the vomeronasal organ (VNO), site of pheromone perception, and the main olfactory epithelium express different mature neuronal markers (Berghard et al. 1996; Wu et al. 1996). The presence of O/E proteins in all three structures (olfactory epithelium, spleen, and VNO) suggests that their presence alone is insufficient to activate their

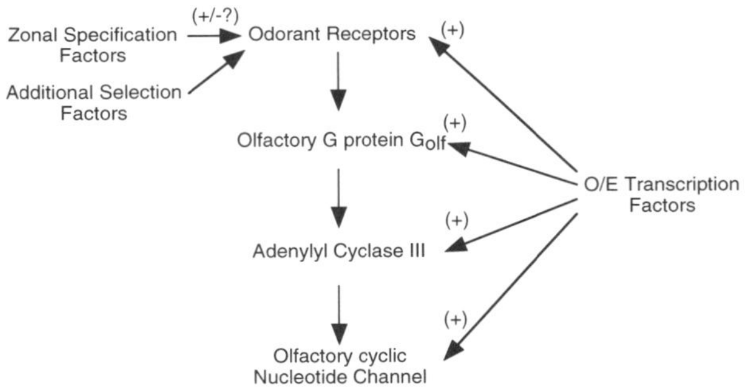

Figure 4. Schematic of the regulation of olfactory transduction components.

target genes in each tissue; additional factors in conjunction with activated O/E proteins select the repertoire of target genes and are required for high levels of tissue-specific target gene expression in vivo.

Families of related transcription factors play important roles in mammalian development, and the O/E proteins share several features with other transcription protein families. The MyoD family (MyoD, Myf-5, MRF4, and myogenin) of myogenic bHLH proteins can homodimerize and heterodimerize with other bHLH proteins and regulate the expression of target genes (Murre et al. 1989; Buckingham 1992; Molkentin et al. 1995). The MyoD proteins have been shown to be functionally redundant and display overlapping patterns of expression (Wang et al. 1996). In summary, the MyoD family of transcription factors forms a molecular circuitry that governs muscle fate determination and differentiation by activating their target genes. Similar to the MyoD family, the vertebrate bHLH proteins, MASH, NeuroD, and Neurogenin, also play a role in neural development and can induce ectopic neurogenesis when expressed in *Xenopus* embryos (Chitnis and Kintner 1996; Ma et al. 1996). Each of these genes appears to be expressed in the adult olfactory epithelium by the basal neuroblasts, the most immature cells of the neuronal lineage. The possibility that these early cells, involved in neuronal fate, induce the expression of the O/E proteins represents an attractive model that can be directly tested in the mouse olfactory system.

O/E genes are expressed in the nervous system during development and enriched in a number of structures that mediate sensory activities. Although each O/E protein could potentially perform a different task during development, our in vitro characterization suggests that they are functionally redundant, analogous to the redundancy demonstrated in MyoD and Engrailed family members (Hanks et al. 1995; Wang et al. 1996), and their physiological roles in development are determined by their temporal and spatial patterns of expression. The product of the *Caenorhabditis elegans unc-3* gene is highly homologous to the mammalian O/E proteins (B. Prasad and R. Reed, unpubl.) and is required for proper axonal connectivity

(Herman 1987) and a specific set of chemosensory functions in the nematode. By analogy, the O/E proteins may regulate the expression of factors essential for axonal pathfinding in developing neurons and in adult olfactory epithelium.

REFERENCES

Amoore, J.E. 1967. Specific anosmia: A clue to the olfactory code. *Nature* **214:** 1094.

———. 1991. Specific anosmias. In *Smell and taste in health and disease* (ed. T.V. Getchell et al.), p. 555. Raven Press, New York.

Bailey, D.W. 1971. Recombinant inbred strains. *Transplantation* **11:** 325.

Ben-Arie, N., D. Lancet, C. Taylor, M. Khen, N. Walker, D.H. Ledbetter, R. Carrozzo, K. Patel, D. Sheer, H. Lehrach, and M.A. North. 1994. Olfactory receptor gene cluster on human chromosome 17: Possible duplication of an ancestral receptor repertoire. *Hum. Mol. Genet.* **3:** 229.

Berghard, A., L.B. Buck, and E.R. Liman. 1996. Evidence for distinct signaling mechanisms in two mammalian olfactory sense organs. *Proc. Natl. Acad. Sci.* **93:** 2365.

Buck, L. and R. Axel. 1991. A novel multigene family may encode odorant receptors: A molecular basis for odor recognition. *Cell* **66:** 175.

Buckingham, M. 1992. Making muscle in mammals. *Trends Genet.* **8:** 144.

Calof, A.L. 1995. Intrinisic and extrinisic factors regulating vertebrate neurogenesis. *Curr. Opin. Neurobiol.* **5:** 19.

Chess, A., I. Simon, H. Cedar, and R. Axel. 1994. Allelic inactivation regulates olfactory receptor gene expression. *Cell* **78:** 823.

Chitnis, A. and C. Kintner. 1996. Sensitivity of proneural genes to lateral inhibition affects the pattern of primary neurons in *Xenopus* embryos. *Development* **122:** 2295.

Costanzo, R.M. and P.P.C. Graziadei. 1987. Development and plasticity of the olfactory system. In *Neurobiology of taste and smell* (ed. T.E. Finger and W.L. Silver), p. 233. Wiley, New York.

DeHamer, M.K. J.L. Guevara, K. Hannon, B.B. Olwin, and A.L. Calof. 1994. Genesis of olfactory receptor neurons in vitro: Regulation of progenitor cell divisions by fibroblast growth factors. *Neuron* **13:** 1083.

Griff, I.C. and R.R. Reed. 1995. The genetic basis for specific anosmia to isovaleric acid in the mouse. *Cell* **83:** 407.

Gross-Isseroff, R., D. Ophir, A. Bartana, H. Voet, and D. Lancet. 1992. Evidence for genetic determination in human twins of olfactory thresholds for a standard odorant. *Neurosci. Lett.* **141:** 115.

Hagman, J., C. Belanger, A. Travis, C.W. Turck, and R. Grosschedl. 1993. Cloning and functional characterization of early B-cell factor, a regulator of lymphocyte-specific gene expression. *Genes Dev.* **7:** 760.

Hagman, J., M.J. Gutch, H. Lin, and R. Grosschedl. 1995. EBF contains a novel zinc coordination motif and multiple dimerization and transcriptional activation domains. *EMBO J.* **14:** 2907.

Hanks, M., W. Wurst, L. Anson-Cartwright, A.B. Auerbach, and A.L. Joyner. 1995. Rescue of the En-1 mutant phenotype by replacement of En-1 with En-2. *Science* **269:** 679.

Herman, R.K. 1987. Mosaic analysis of two genes that affect nervous system structure in *Caenorhabditis elegans*. *Genetics* **116:** 377.

Hubert, H.B., R.R. Fabsitz, M. Feinlieb, and K.S. Brown. 1980. Olfactory sensitivity in humans: Genetic versus environmental control. *Science* **208:** 607.

Kauer, J. S. 1991. Contributions of topography and parallel processing to odor coding in the vertebrate olfactory pathway. *Trends Neurosci.* **14:** 79.

Kishimoto, J., H. Cox, E.B. Keverne, and P.C. Emson. 1994. Cellular localization of putative odorant receptor mRNAs in olfactory and chemosensory neurons: A non radioactive in situ hybridization study. *Brain Res. Mol. Brain Res.* **23:** 33.

Koshimoto, H., K. Katoh, Y. Yoshihara, Y. Nemoto, and K. Mori. 1994. Immunohistochemical demonstration of embryonic expression of an odor receptor protein and its zonal distribution in the rat olfactory epithelium. *Neurosci. Lett.* **169:** 73.

Kudrycki, K., C. Stein-Izsak, C. Behn, M. Grillo, R. Akeson, and F. Margolis. 1993. Olf-1-binding site: Characterization of an olfactory neuron-specific promoter motif. *Mol. Cell. Biol.* **13:** 3002.

Levy, N.S., H.A. Bakalyar, and R.R. Reed. 1991. Signal transduction in olfactory neurons. *J. Ster. Biochem. Mol. Biol.* **39:** 263.

Lin, H. and R. Grosschedl. 1995. Failure of B-cell differentiation in mice lacking the transcription factor EBF. *Nature* **376:** 653.

Ma, Q., C. Kintner, and D.J. Anderson. 1996. Identification of neurogenin, a vertebrate neuronal determination gene. *Cell* **87:** 43.

Mackay-Sim, A. and P. Kittel. 1991. Cell dynamics in the adult mouse olfactory epithelium: A quantitative autoradiographic study. *J. Neurosci.* **11:** 979.

Mahanthappa, N.K. and G.A. Schwarting. 1993. Peptide growth factor control of olfactory neurogenesis and neuron survival in vitro: Roles of EGF and TGF-βs. *Neuron* **10:** 293.

Molkentin, J.D., B.L. Black, J.F. Martin, and E.N. Olson. 1995. Cooperative activation of muscle gene expression by MEF2 and myogenic bHLH proteins. *Cell* **83:** 1125.

Murre, C., P.S. McCaw, H. Vaessin, M. Caudy, L.Y. Jan, Y.N. Jan, C.V. Cabrera, J.N. Buskin, S.D. Hauschka, A.B. Lassar, H. Weintraub, and D. Baltimore. 1989. Interactions between heterologous helix-loop-helix proteins generate complexes that bind specifically to a common DNA sequence. *Cell* **58:** 537.

Nathans, J., P. Thomas, and D.S. Hogness. 1986a. Molecular genetics of human color vision: The genes encoding blue, green and red pigments. *Science* **232:** 193.

Nathans, J., T.P. Piantanida, R.L. Eddy, T.B. Shows, and D.S. Hogness. 1986b. Molecular genetics of inherited variation in human color vision. *Science* **232:** 203.

Nef, P., I. Hermans-Borgmeyer, H. Artieres-Pin, L. Beasley, V.E. Dionne, and S.F. Heinemann. 1992. Spatial pattern of receptor expression in the olfactory epithelium. *Proc. Natl. Acad. Sci.* **89:** 8948.

Ngai, J., M.M. Dowling, L. Buck, R. Axel. and A. Chess. 1993a. The family of genes encoding odorant receptors in the channel catfish. *Cell* **72:** 657.

Ngai, J., A. Chess, M.M. Dowling, N. Necles, E.R. Macagno, and R. Axel. 1993b. Coding of olfactory information: Topography of odorant receptor expression in the catfish olfactory epithelium. *Cell* **72:** 667.

Patterson, P.M. and B.A. Lauder. 1948. The incidence and probable inheritance of "Smell blindness". *J. Hered.* **602:** 295.

Pourtier, L. and G. Sicard. 1989. Comparison of the sensitivity of C57BL/6J and AKR/J mice to airborne molecules of isovaleric acid and amyl acetate. *Behav. Genet.* **20:** 449.

Ressler, K.J., S.L. Sullivan, and L.B. Buck. 1993. A zonal organization of odorant receptor gene expression in the olfactory epithelium. *Cell* **73:** 597.

Roskams, A.J., M.A. Bethel, K.J. Hurt, and G.V. Ronnett. 1996. Sequential expression of Trks A, B and C in the regenerating olfactory neuroepithelium. *J. Neurosci.* **16:** 1294.

Segal, N.L., K.W. Brown, and T.D. Topolski. 1992. A twin study of odor identification and olfactory sensitivity. *Acta Genet. Med. Gemellol.* **41:** 113.

Shepherd, G.M. 1994. Discrimination of molecular signals by the olfactory receptor neuron. *Neuron* **13:** 771.

Strotmann, J., I. Wanner, T. Helfrich, A. Beck, C. Meinken, S. Kubick, and H. Breer. 1994. Olfactory neurones expressing distinct odorant receptor subtypes are spatially segregated in the nasal neuroepithelium. *Cell Tissue Res.* **276:** 429.

Walters, E., M. Grillo, G. Tarozzo, C. Stern-Izsak, J. Corbin, C. Bocchiaro, and F. Margolis. 1996. Proximal regions of the olfactory marker protein gene promoter direct olfactory neuron-specific expression in transgenic mice. *J. Neurosci. Res.* **43:** 146.

Wang, H.-W., C.J. Wysocki, and G.H. Gold. 1993. Induction of olfactory receptor sensitivity in mice. *Science* **260:** 998.

Wang, M.M. and R.R. Reed. 1993. Molecular cloning of the olfactory neuronal transcription factor Olf-1 by genetic selection in yeast. *Nature* **364:** 121.

Wang, M.M., R.Y. Tsai, K.A. Schrader, and R.R. Reed. 1993. Genes encoding components of the olfactory signal transduction cascade contain a DNA binding site that may direct neuronal expression. *Mol. Cell. Biol.* **13:** 5805.

Wang, Y., P.N. Schnegelsberg, J. Dausman, and R. Jaenisch. 1996. Functional redundancy of the muscle-specific transcription factors Myf5 and myogenin. *Nature* **379:** 823.

Whissell-Buechy, D. and J.E. Amoore. 1973. Odour-blindness to musk: Simple recessive inheritance. *Nature* **245:** 157.

Wu, Y., R. Tirindelli, and N.J. Ryba. 1996. Evidence for different chemosensory signal transduction pathways in olfactory and vomeronasal neurons. *Biochem. Biophys. Res. Commun.* **220:** 900.

Wysocki, C.J. and G.K. Beauchamp. 1984. Ability to smell androstenone is genetically determined. *Proc. Natl. Acad. Sci.* **81:** 4899.

Wysocki, C.J. and M.R. Kare. 1991. Genetics of perception and communications. *Chem. Senses* **3:** 331.

Wysocki, C.J., K.M. Dorries, and G.K. Beauchamp. 1989. Ability to perceive and androstenone can be acquired by ostensibly anosmic people. *Proc. Natl. Acad. Sci.* **86:** 7976.

Wysocki, C.J., C. Whitney, and D. Tucker. 1977. Specific anosmia in the laboratory mouse. *Behav. Genet.* **7:** 171.

Biochemical and Transgenic Analysis of Gustducin's Role in Bitter and Sweet Transduction

G.T. WONG, L. RUIZ-AVILA, D. MING, K.S. GANNON, AND R.F. MARGOLSKEE
Department of Physiology and Biophysics, The Mount Sinai School of Medicine, New York, New York 10029

Taste perception in mammals can be divided into at least four submodalities: sweet, bitter, salty, and sour. Taste transduction occurs in neuroepithelial taste receptor cells (TRCs), organized within taste buds. Salty and sour tastants (e.g., Na^+ and H^+, respectively) are thought to interact with TRC ion channels. Several lines of evidence suggest that both sweet and bitter tastes are transduced via seven transmembrane-helix receptors coupled to heterotrimeric guanine nucleotide-binding proteins (G proteins) (for review, see Kinnamon and Margolskee 1996). Gustducin is a taste-specific G protein expressed in about 40% of rat and human TRCs (McLaughlin et al. 1992; Takami et al. 1994). The α subunit of gustducin (α-gustducin) is 80% identical (90% similar) to the α subunits of rod and cone transducin. Recombinant gustducin is biochemically indistinguishable from transducin in its interactions with rhodopsin, retinal cGMP phosphodiesterase (PDE), and G-protein βγ subunits (Hoon et al. 1995). Interestingly, the α subunit of rod transducin is also expressed in TRCs, although at much lower levels than is α-gustducin (Ruiz-Avila et al. 1995).

It has been proposed that gustducin and transducin function in taste transduction in a manner similar to the way in which transducin functions in phototransduction (McLaughlin et al. 1992; Ruiz-Avila et al. 1995). This model predicts that gustducin and/or transducin couple seven transmembrane-helix taste receptors to TRC-specific PDEs to regulate intracellular cyclic nucleotides (cNMPs). To test this model, we set out to biochemically identify taste-specific proteins that might couple to gustducin or transducin and function in taste transduction (see Ruiz-Avila et al. 1995). In this regard, we partially purified a taste-specific PDE activity from bovine taste tissue that could be stimulated by transducin, transducin-derived peptides, or gustducin. We also identified a taste receptor activity that, in the presence of the bitter compound denatonium benzoate, activated transducin and gustducin but not G_i. These results suggest that gustducin/transducin couple taste receptor(s) to taste cell PDE.

We have further tested the hypothesis that gustducin mediates bitter transduction by generating α-gustducin-deficient transgenic mice and analyzing their taste responses (Wong et al. 1996). The mice are viable, healthy, and fertile, suggesting that α-gustducin is not required for normal development. As expected, behavioral tests demonstrated a difference between homozygous α-gustducin null mice and their wild-type siblings in the aversion to two bitter compounds. Surprisingly, the α-gustducin null animals also showed reduced preferences for two sweet compounds. Furthermore, the α-gustducin null mice had diminished nerve responses to both bitter and sweet compounds. These data provide clear in vivo evidence that gustducin plays a key role in both bitter and sweet taste transduction. By combining in vitro biochemical analysis of taste transduction proteins with in vivo analysis of transgenic and knockout mice, we hope to gain a clear understanding of the molecular mechanisms underlying taste transduction.

METHODS

Taste PDE. Bovine circumvallate papillae and nongustatory lingual epithelia were harvested and rapidly frozen in liquid nitrogen; subsequent purification procedures were carried out at 4°C. Tissues were homogenized in DEAE buffer (Ruiz-Avila et al. 1995) with a rotor-stator homogenizer. Centrifugation removed particulate (1500*g*) and membrane fractions (45,000*g*). The supernatant was applied to a DEAE-Sephacel column, the column was washed with DEAE buffer, and PDEs eluted with a 0–600 mM NaCl linear gradient in DEAE buffer. PDE activity was measured as described previously (Alvarez and Daniels 1992). Effector peptide was used at a final concentration of 200 μM. Results are the average ± S.E.M. of triplicate determinations and are representative of three independent tissue preparations. The 15-amino-acid-long effector interaction peptide #25 corresponding to amino acids 293–308 of rod α-transducin was synthesized and purified as described Spickofsky et al. (1994). Rod transducin was purified as described previously (Fung et al. 1981) with an additional gel filtration chromatography step through AcA 44. Aluminum-magnesium-fluoride activation of transducin was in a reaction mix of 5 mM NaF and 50 μM $AlCl_3$.

Denatonium responsive receptor. Bovine taste and non-taste membranes were prepared as described above for PDE purification. The membrane fractions were resuspended in DEAE buffer (250–500 μl) lacking protease inhibitors, then further homogenized by

10 passages through 25-gauge needles. G-protein activation by taste receptors was as described previously (Ruiz-Avila et al. 1995). Quinine sulfate, sodium saccharin, and denatonium benzoate were all purchased from Sigma (St. Louis, Missouri). Rhodopsin was used at 0.1–1 μM final concentration. The mixtures were incubated 0.5–1 hour at 30°C, then analyzed by trypsin digestion (Fung and Nash 1983; Halliday et al. 1984; Ruiz-Avila et al. 1995) or by GTPγS binding (Fawzi and Northup 1990). Intact $\alpha_{t\text{-rod}}$ and its 23-kD and 32-kD tryptic fragments were visualized using the transducin-specific antibody and the ECL system (Amersham, Arlington Heights, Illinois). Basal values without added G protein were ≤5% of the maximum value obtained upon activation. All binding experiments were performed in duplicate; the results presented are averages of at least two independent experiments. The peptides used for the inhibition experiments were derived from the carboxy-terminal region of bovine rod α-transducin (peptide G_t, aa 311–329) and from the effector interaction region of bovine G_{i-1} (peptide G_i, aa 297–315). The peptides were added to the membranes and the mixtures were preincubated on ice (10 min) prior to the addition of transducin (0.3–0.6 μM) and denatonium (5 mM). The 100% control value corresponds to 0.106 ± 0.019 pmole of GTPγS bound to G_t in the presence of taste membranes and denatonium (incubated 1 hr at 30°C) without added peptides.

Gustducin null mice. The murine α-gustducin gene was cloned from a 129/Sv mouse genomic λ library (Lambda FIX II, Stratagene, La Jolla, California) (see Wong et al. 1996). A 1.4-kb *Nde*I fragment containing sequences homologous with the 5′-most sequence of the rat α-gustducin cDNA, and an 8.5-kb *Hin*dIII fragment derived from the first intron, were subcloned into a *neo*/*tk* selection vector. Transformation of the embryonic stem (ES) cell line, W9.5 (Szabo and Mann 1994), was as described previously (Kwee et al. 1995) using *Sal*I-linearized α-gustducin targeting vector. Electroporation, selection, and expansion of G418- and FIAU-resistant ES cell colonies was as described previously (Stewart et al. 1992). ES cell and tail biopsy DNAs were prepared as described previously (Laird et al. 1991). DNA (~ 5 μg) was digested with *Xba*I, electrophoresed, electroblotted, and hybridized with a radiolabeled 0.7-kb *Bgl*II–*Xba*I α-gustducin probe (probe A). Southern analysis of genomic DNA from clonally expanded ES cell colonies indicated a homologous recombination frequency of 7%. Two independent clones with 40XY karyotypes were used to produce chimeric mice by blastocyst injection. Chimeric males were bred to C57BL/6J females. Heterozygous progeny (GUS/*gus*) containing the mutant α-gustducin allele were intercrossed. Both lines yielded homozygous α-gustducin null (*gus/gus*) pups with approximately 25% frequency. Male mice (both *gus/gus* and GUS/GUS) were about a 50/50 mix of 129/SvEmsJ and C57BL/6J backgrounds.

Immunohistochemistry. Mouse tongues were excised and then fixed (1 hr; rt) in 4% (w/v) paraformaldehyde in PBS. The fixed tissue was transferred to 20% (w/v) sucrose in PBS, and kept at 4°C until used. Frozen sections (10–12 μM) were saturated with blocking solution (3% BSA, 1% horse serum, 0.3% triton X100 in PBS) for 30 minutes at room temperature, then incubated (1 hr; rt) with a gustducin-specific antibody (GD1-KLH) elicited against a KLH-conjugated peptide (corresponding to amino acids 95–109 of the published rat α-gustducin) that had been adsorbed overnight against cow tongue muscle. After washes in PBS, the sections were incubated with anti-rabbit-IgG antibodies coupled to the fluorochrome Cy3 (Jackson Immunologicals, West Grove, Pennsylvania) and photographed on a Zeiss Axiomat microscope.

Two-bottle preference tests. Tested mice ranged in age from 8 weeks to 20 weeks. Mice were individually housed, provided with food ad libitum, and presented with distilled water in two sipper bottles for 48 hours prior to testing. During each 48-hour test period, a given concentration of tastant was provided in one sipper bottle, while the other contained distilled water. After 24 hours, volumes consumed were recorded, the bottles were refilled, and their positions were reversed (to control for positional cues that may affect preference). Tastants were presented in ascending series. Preference ratios were calculated as the fraction of tastant consumed compared to total volume consumed. ANOVAs (strain x concentration) were performed on data excluding those animals missing data at any concentration. Mean preference ratios shown in graphs and independent-groups t-tests were calculated from total collected data.

Chorda tympani nerve recording. Male mice were anesthetized with sodium pentobarbital (60 mg/kg). Surgical, taste-stimulation, and recording procedures were as described previously (Gannon and Contreras 1995). Neural signals were amplified (10,000x) and integrated using an RMS-DC converter (Hendrick and Assoc., Tallahassee, Florida) with a time constant of 0.5 seconds. Taste solutions were presented for a duration of 10 seconds followed by at least a 1-minute rinse with distilled water at a constant flow rate of 3 ml/min. Each tastant concentration was presented at least twice, and the mean response was calculated. Tastants were presented as an ascending concentration series. The mean phasic response to 0.1 M NH_4Cl was used to normalize responses (see Wong et al. 1996). Data were analyzed using Strain x Concentration ANOVAs for each tastant (presented in the text and Table 1) and independent groups t-tests (see Fig. 5 legend).

Generation of transgenic animals. 8.4 kb of the mouse α-gustducin gene immediately upstream of the transcription initiation site is sufficient to drive expression of β-galactosidase to the gustducin lineage of

Table 1. Summary of Analyses of Variance (*S*train x *C*oncentration) Performed on Behavioral and Neurophysiological Data

Response		Preference[a]		Phasic response[b]		Tonic[c]	
tastant	effect	F value	*p* value	F value	*p* value	F value	*p* value
NaCl	S	0.687	0.4171	0.060	0.8103	0.066	0.8003
	C	134.017	0.0000[d]	79.623	0.0000	202.547	0.0000
	SC	1.651	0.1871	1.850	0.1760	1.642	0.2117
HCl	S	0.416	0.5271	0.498	0.4930	0.560	0.4677
	C	118.852	0.0000	132.368	0.0000	27.505	0.0000
	SC	1.040	0.3929	1.495	0.2429	0.080	0.9238
Denatonium	S	68.614	0.0000	34.827	0.0000	15.754	0.0014
	C	45.691	0.0000	80.897	0.0000	6.478	0.0011
	SC	10.384	0.0000	7.954	0.0003	3.136	0.0353
QSO_4	S	32.204	0.0000	5.806	0.0304	7.045	0.0189
	C	15.278	0.0000	114.061	0.0000	13.504	0.0001
	SC	6.580	0.0000	5.486	0.0098	5.607	0.0090
Sucrose	S	30.534	0.0001	14.569	0.0021	21.265	0.0005
	C	21.520	0.0000	22.692	0.0000	20.775	0.0000
	SC	10.293	0.0000	16.612	0.0000	17.653	0.0000
SC45647	S	21.211	0.0002	42.066	0.0000	39.029	0.0000
	C	20.294	0.0000	45.181	0.0000	20.422	0.0000
	SC	8.707	0.0001	25.342	0.0000	23.294	0.0000

[a]Based on data shown in Fig. 4.
[b]Based on data shown in Fig. 5.
[c]Based on data not shown.
[d]*p* values < 0.00005 are presented as p=0.0000.

TRCs (G.T. Wong et al., in prep.). The $GUS_{8.4}$*gustducin* construct contained the 8.4-kb promoter (including the α-gustducin transcriptional initiation site), the rabbit βII globin intron, the complete rat α-gustducin cDNA, and the SV40 polyadenylation signal. Transgenic mice were generated by microinjection into the male pronucleus of (B6CBAF1/J x 129SvEmsJ [*gus/gus*]) zygotes (Hogan et al. 1994). Linearized $GUS_{8.4}$*gustducin* DNA was isolated away from plasmid vector sequences prior to microinjection. Seven transgenic G_0 mice were obtained from the 63 animals tested. The G_0 animals were crossed to 129SvEmsJ (*gus/gus*) animals to obtain a backcrossed first generation of all possible phenotypes: $GUS_{8.4}$*gustducin* transgenic GUS/*gus*; transgenic *gus/gus*; nontransgenic GUS/gus; nontransgenic *gus/gus*. Four lines were tested for gustducin protein expression, and one line (#28) expressing wild-type levels was chosen for the behavioral tests.

RESULTS

A Taste Phosphodiesterase Can Be Activated by Transducin

In the visual system, rod α-transducin activates PDE by binding to the regulatory (γ) subunits and inducing a conformational change that disinhibits the PDE catalytic subunits. Rarick et al. (1992) identified a portion of rod α-transducin (aa 293–314) involved in this interaction. They synthesized a 22-amino-acid-long effector interaction peptide from rod α-transducin that fully activated rod PDE. The effector interaction region of α-gustducin is very similar to that of rod α-transducin. Even though the effector interaction peptide from α-gustducin does not activate rod PDE (Spickofsky et al. 1994), recombinant gustducin protein does activate rod PDE (Hoon et al. 1995). To deter-mine if there is a PDE in taste tissue that interacts with gustducin or transducin, we isolated PDEs from bovine taste and non-taste lingual tissues, then assayed for stimulation by the activated α subunit of transducin or by the transducin-derived effector interaction peptide.

Three chromatographically distinct peaks of PDE activity were identified in both taste (Fig. 1A) and non-taste (Fig. 1B) tissues. Peak I from taste tissue showed a fivefold increase in cGMP PDE activity upon the addition of the rod transducin peptide (peptide #25) (Fig. 1C); peak I from non-taste tissue was not stimulated by the rod transducin peptide. Activated rod transducin protein stimulated taste peak I cGMP PDE activity more than tenfold, whereas non-taste peak I activity was slightly inhibited by transducin protein (see Fig. 1D). In sum, we have identified a PDE in taste tissue that is stimulated by rod transducin or the rod transducin effector interaction peptide but not by the gust-

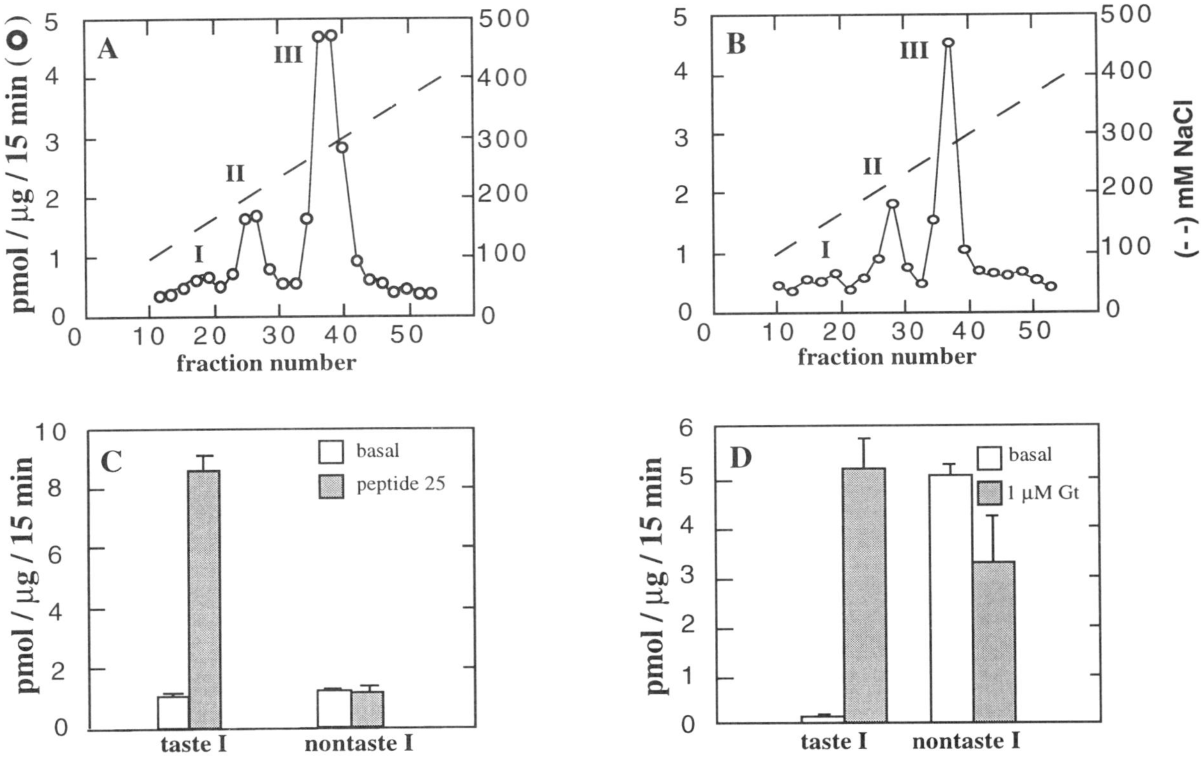

Figure 1. PDE isolated from bovine taste tissue is activated by rod transducin. Fractionation of PDE activity from (*A*) bovine fungiform papillae and (*B*) non-taste lingual tissue revealed three peaks of PDE activity in each tissue. (*C*) Assays of taste (fungiform papillae) versus non-taste peak I cGMP PDE activity: the rod transducin effector interaction peptide (*gray* bars, peptide 25) activated taste peak I but not non-taste peak I; basal activity (*open* bars) in the absence of added peptide. (*D*) Assays of taste (circumvallate papillae) versus non-taste peak I cGMP PDE activity: activated α rod transducin protein (*gray* bars 1 µM G_t) activated taste peak I but not non-taste peak I; basal activity (*open* bars) in the absence of activated $\alpha_{t\text{-rod}}$. Dashed lines indicate salt gradient.

ducin peptide. Presumably, this PDE is the taste cell target of gustducin or transducin action during taste transduction. Preliminary data (L. Ruiz-Avila and R.F. Margolskee, unpubl.) indicate that recombinant gustducin protein also activates this same taste PDE.

Reconstitution of a Taste Receptor That Activates Transducin

To seek a taste receptor that could couple to gustducin or transducin, we isolated membranes from bovine tongue tissues, reconstituted them with transducin, then assayed for transducin activation (Ruiz-Avila et al. 1995). We used trypsin sensitivity and GTPγS binding to monitor activation of transducin by rhodopsin (positive control), taste membranes, or non-taste lingual membranes in the presence of various tastants (Fig. 2). In the absence of membranes, in the presence of non-taste membranes, or in the presence of taste membranes without added tastants, there was no activation of transducin (evidenced by the 23-kD fragment derived from GDP-bound transducin) (Fig. 2B). Three different tastants (quinine, saccharin, and denatonium) were assayed for their ability to activate transducin. Only bitter denatonium activated transducin (evidenced by the 32-kD fragment derived from GTPγS-bound transducin) and only in the presence of taste membranes (Fig. 2B): Quinine and saccharin did not activate transducin, and denatonium in the absence of taste membranes likewise did not activate transducin. In the presence of taste membranes, activation of transducin could readily be detected with 100 µM denatonium (Fig. 2B). However, in the presence of non-taste membranes, even 10 mM denatonium failed to activate transducin (Fig. 2B). Presumably, a denatonium-responsive receptor present in the taste membrane extract couples to the exogenously added transducin.

To determine if this taste membrane fraction selectively couples to transducin-like G proteins, we carried out reconstitution with exogenously added G_i protein. Neither rhodopsin nor taste membranes plus denatonium activated G_i (assayed by GTPγS binding), whereas denatonium in the presence of taste membranes or activated rhodopsin alone activated transducin (~ 4-fold and ~ 10-fold, respectively) (Fig. 2C). This argues for a taste-specific receptor that couples to transducin but not to the similar G protein G_i. Similar

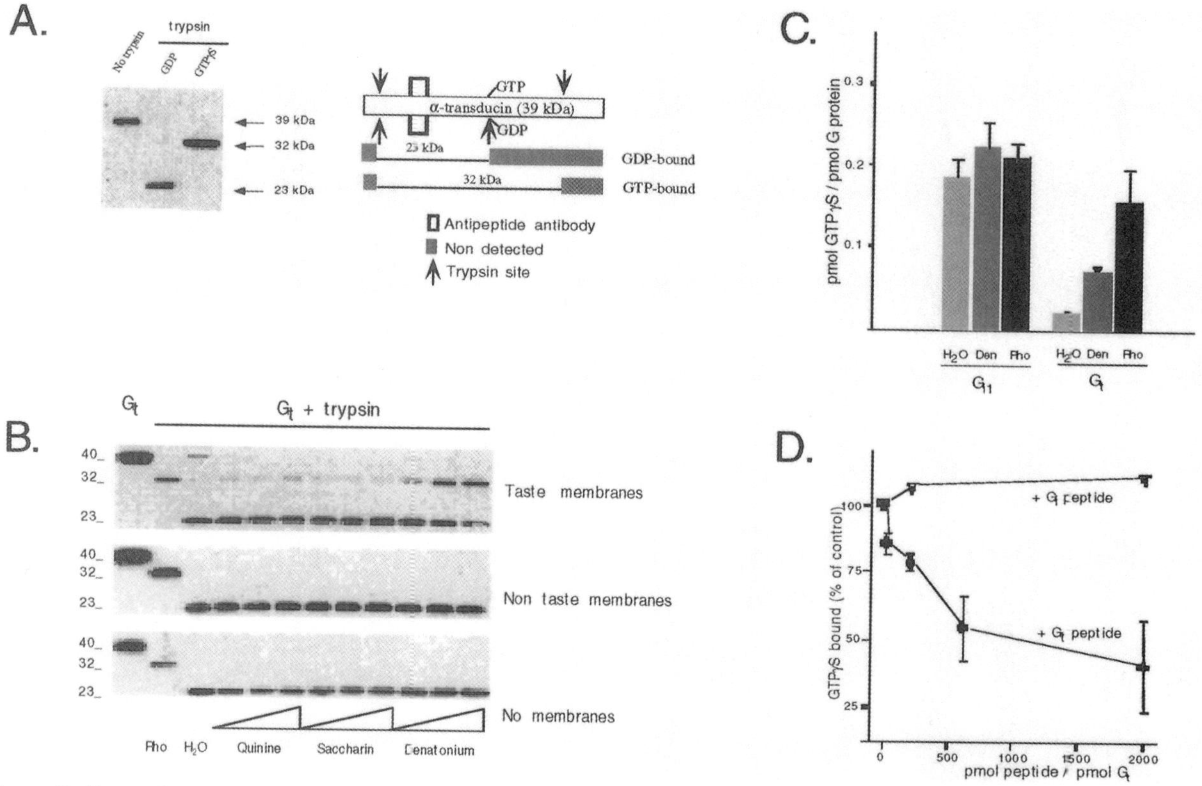

Figure 2. Reconstituted bovine taste receptor activates transducin. (*A*) (*Left* panel) Tryptic patterns distinguish GTPγS-transducin (32-kD immunoprecipitated product) from GDP-bound-transducin (23-kD fragment) from undigested transducin (~39 kD). (*Right* panel) Transducin's tryptic sites, antibody recognition site, and the location of the fragments are indicated. (*B*) Transducin was mixed with taste membranes (*top* panel), non-taste membranes (*middle* panel), or no membranes (*bottom* panel). In the presence of trypsin, rhodopsin (Rho, positive control) generated a 32-kD fragment; water (negative control) generated a 23-kD fragment. The effect of various tastants on transducin activation was assessed. Neither quinine (2.5 μM, 25 μM, 250 μM) nor saccharin (100 μM, 1 mM, 10 mM) activated transducin, whereas denatonium (100 μM, 1 mM, 10 mM) activated transducin (note the shift from 23 kD [GDP bound] to 32 kD [GTPγS bound]). (*C*) Taste receptor activated transducin but not G_i. Samples contained taste membranes and G_i or transducin; water, denatonium (Den), or rhodopsin (Rho) was added as indicated. GTPγS binding to G_i is not stimulated by either denatonium or rhodopsin. (*D*) Competitive inhibition of taste-receptor-mediated activation of transducin by a transducin peptide but not by a G_i peptide.

experiments with recombinant gustducin show that this receptor also couples to and activates gustducin (L. Ruiz-Avila and R.F. Margolskee, unpubl.).

To determine if an opsin-like receptor was involved in the taste-membrane-mediated activation of transducin, we used a peptide competition assay. A peptide derived from the carboxy-terminal region of transducin (amino acids 311–329) competitively inhibits the rhodopsin-transducin interaction (Hamm et al. 1988). This peptide blocked rhodopsin-mediated activation of transducin (data not shown) and likewise blocked taste receptor activation of transducin (Fig. 2D) or gustducin (data not shown), whereas a control peptide derived from G_i did not interfere with transducin activation (Fig. 2D). These results suggest that a seven-transmembrane taste receptor binds denatonium and activates transducin by interaction with its carboxyl terminus. However, denatonium does not nonspecifically enhance the rhodopsin-transducin interaction (data not shown).

Generation of α-Gustducin-deficient Mice

Gene replacement was used to generate a null mutation (*gus*) of the α-gustducin gene (Wong et al. 1996). The wild-type allele (GUS) of the murine α-gustducin gene was cloned, and sequences surrounding the first protein coding exon were used to create the targeting vector (Fig. 3A). Positive/negative selection was used to enrich for ES cell clones with a homologously recombined α-gustducin allele. Chimeric mice, generated from these ES cells by blastocyst injection, were backcrossed to C57BL/6J mice. Homozygous null (*gus/gus*) mice harboring the recombined α-gustducin allele, genetically (C57BL/6J x 129/SvEmsJ)F_2, were produced by intercrossing heterozygous (GUS/*gus*) animals (Fig. 3B). Heterozygous and homozygous null mice were viable, healthy, and fertile.

Taste epithelia from homozygous null mice were morphologically indistinguishable from epithelia of wild-type littermates (Fig. 3). Mice have three types of

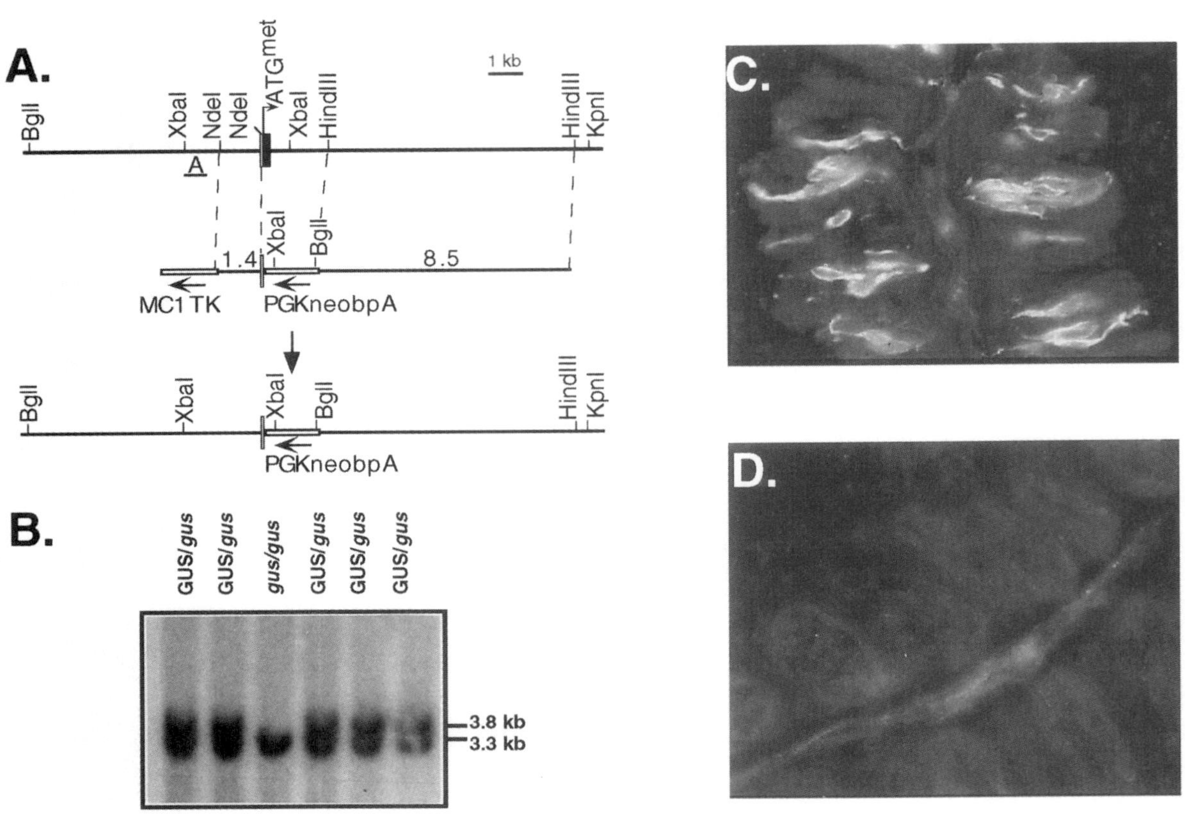

Figure 3. Generation of α-gustducin null (*gus/gus*) mice. (*A*) (*Top* line) Map of the murine α-gustducin gene showing the first exon (*open/filled* box): 5′-untranslated leader sequence (*open* box), coding region for first 18 amino acids (*filled* box), and initiation codon (ATG^{met}). The probe used to screen G418-resistant ES cell clones is indicated (line A below map). (*Middle* line) Map of the targeting vector, indicating the MC1*tk* and PGK*neo*bpA genes. The direction of transcription is indicated by the arrows. The gustducin-homologous 5′ region is a 1.4-kb *Nde*I fragment which includes the transcription initiation sequences and 30 nucleotides of untranslated leader sequence from exon 1 (*open* box). The 3′ homologous region is an 8.5-kb *Hin*dIII fragment derived from the first intron. (*Bottom* line) Map of the predicted structure of the homologously recombined gustducin allele, showing the presence of the first exon (*open* box) immediately preceding the PGK*neo* gene. (*B*) Genomic analysis of offspring from a (GUS/*gus*) x (GUS/*gus*) mating. *Xba*I-digested genomic DNA purified from tail biopsies was screened with probe A (see *A*, above). The wild-type α-gustducin restriction fragment is 3.8 kb long. The targeting event generates a novel 3.3-kb fragment that includes a portion of the first exon fused to the *neo* gene. The third lane (*gus/gus*) identifies a homozygous null (*gus/gus*) mouse. Immunofluorescence photomicrographs of frozen sections of wild-type (GUS/GUS) (*C*) and null (*gus/gus*) (*D*) mouse circumvallate papillae treated with α-gustducin-specific antibody and Cy3-conjugated secondary antibody.

taste papillae: fungiform, scattered throughout the anterior two-thirds of the tongue; foliate, in lateral grooves; and a single circumvallate, at the back of the tongue. The null mice had all three types of taste papillae, with an appropriate number of taste buds in each papilla and a normal complement of TRCs per bud. Results from immunohistochemistry on TRCs from circumvallate (Fig. 3C,D) and foliate (data not shown) papillae demonstrated that the null mice expressed no detectable α-gustducin, whereas the wild-type mice expressed high levels. Consistent results were obtained by in situ hybridization: The null mice expressed no α-gustducin mRNA in TRCs of their circumvallate, foliate, or fungiform taste papillae (Wong et al. 1996). We conclude that the targeting event resulted in a null allele of α-gustducin.

Behavioral Analysis of Taste Responses

We used 48-hour two-bottle preference tests (Harder et al. 1989) to assess the taste responses of α-gustducin null (*gus/gus*) mice versus their wild-type (GUS/GUS) siblings (Wong et al. 1996). A preference ratio was calculated for each animal at each concentration. Tastants that are primarily salty (NaCl), sour (HCl), bitter (denatonium benzoate and quinine sulfate), and sweet (sucrose and SC45647) to humans were tested.

Behavioral responses of null mice to a concentration series of NaCl were similar to those of wild-type mice ($p > 0.05$, Table 1; Fig. 4A). Similarly, no strain differences were evident in the behavioral responses to a range of HCl solutions ($p > 0.05$, Table 1; Fig. 4B). All mice were indifferent to initial (low) concentrations of NaCl or HCl and exhibited aversive responses to higher concentrations of NaCl or HCl. These data demonstrate that salty and sour behavioral responses are unaffected by the absence of α-gustducin.

In contrast, aversive responses to two bitter substances, denatonium benzoate (Fig. 4C) and quinine sulfate (Fig. 4D) (p values < 0.00005, Table 1), were diminished in the null mice compared to wild type. Wild-type mice began to avoid denatonium at the 100 μM concentration, whereas the null mice remained indifferent to denatonium at ≤ 1 mM concentrations. The null mice required about a 40-fold higher concentration of denatonium and about a 100-fold higher concentration of quinine than did their wild-type siblings to elicit comparable aversive responses. These data demonstrate that avoidance responses to these two bitter compounds are profoundly diminished in the absence of α-gustducin.

Unexpectedly, preference responses to two sweet substances, sucrose (Fig. 4E) and the high-potency guanidine sweetener SC45647 (Fig. 4F) (Tinti and Nofre 1991), were reduced in the null mice compared to their wild-type siblings (p values < 0.0001, Table 1). Wild-type mice greatly preferred sucrose at ≥ 50 mM concentrations. However, the null mice remained indifferent at concentrations below 500 mM sucrose: At this point, the null mice required about a 17-fold higher concentration of sucrose than did their wild-type siblings to elicit a similar preference response. Similar strain differences were found with SC45647 (Fig. 4F). Wild-type mice greatly preferred SC45647 at 0.1 mM and 0.5 mM concentrations, but the null mice remained indifferent at both of these concentrations. Additional testing indicated that the null mice weakly preferred 2 mM SC45647 (preference ratio = 0.71; data not shown). These data demonstrate that preference responses to these two sweet compounds are profoundly diminished in the absence of α-gustducin.

Electrophysiological Analysis of Taste Responses

The two-bottle preference test measures behavioral responses, which are dependent on all levels of signal processing from the TRC to peripheral and central nervous systems. In addition, factors outside of the taste system (e.g., post-ingestional influences) could affect preference behaviors. To determine if the behavioral deficit observed in the null mice was due to a peripheral taste defect, electrophysiological recordings were obtained from the chorda tympani branch of the facial (VII) nerve in null and wild-type control mice. The chorda tympani innervates the anterior tongue and is responsive to salty, sweet, sour, and bitter stimuli (Ninomiya and Funakoshi 1989). Summated chorda tympani responses were recorded during lingual stimulation with NaCl, HCl, quinine sulfate, denatonium benzoate, sucrose, and SC45647 (Wong et al. 1996). Examples of integrated neural responses to a subset of the tested compounds are presented (Fig. 5A,B,G). Each response was quantified by measuring two parameters: (1) the maximum amplitude of the neural response within 4 seconds of stimulus onset (phasic response) and (2) the response magnitude occurring 10 seconds after stimulus onset (tonic response). The phasic response represents the initial nerve response to tastant stimulation of TRCs. The tonic response represents the sustained nerve response to continuous tastant stimulation of TRCs.

Both phasic (Fig. 5B) and tonic responses of null mice were similar to those of wild-type mice for a concentration series of NaCl (p values > 0.05, Table 1). Similarly, no strain differences were evident in electrophysiological responses to a range of HCl solutions (p values > 0.05, Table 1; Fig. 5C). The electrophysiological results with NaCl and HCl are consistent with the behavioral results (Fig. 4) and indicate that α-gustducin null mice are unaltered in their ability to sense and respond to salty and sour stimuli. However, chorda tympani responses to bitter substances were diminished in the null mice compared to wild type. Null mice had reduced neural responses to denatonium benzoate, apparent in both phasic ($p < 0.0005$, Table 1; Fig. 5E) and tonic ($p < 0.05$, Table 1) responses. Furthermore, chorda tympani responses of null mice to quinine were significantly reduced when compared to wild type for both phasic ($p < 0.01$; Fig. 5F, Table 1) and tonic responses ($p < 0.01$, Table 1). Chorda tympani responses of null mice to both sucrose (Fig. 5H) and SC45647 (Fig. 5I) were significantly lower than those of wild type mice for both phasic (p values < 0.00005, Table 1) and tonic (p values < 0.00005, Table 1) measurements. Surprisingly, the responses of the null mice to the sweet compounds lacked a concentration response function. Responses were minimal at high concentrations (0.5 M sucrose and 10 mM SC45647) that are intensely sweet to humans. The chorda tympani recordings demonstrate that null mice possess peripheral deficits in their ability to transduce the tastes of both bitter and sweet compounds.

Rescue of the Null Phenotype by the Rat α-Gustducin Transgene

To confirm that the absence of α-gustducin is responsible for the loss of bitter and sweet responsiveness in the null (*gus/gus*) mice (Fig. 6A), we introduced into the null background the rat gustducin cDNA as a transgene under the murine gustducin promoter ($GUS_{8.4}$*gustducin*). Immunofluorescence indicated that the transgenic/null ($GUS_{8.4}$*gustducin gus/gus*) mice (Fig. 6B) expressed gustducin in a pattern indistinguishable from wild type (compare to Fig. 3C). To determine if the rat gustducin transgene was functional, we carried out two-bottle preference tests with one bitter (denatonium benzoate) and one sweet (SC45647) compound (Fig. 6C,D). We compared the behavioral responses of four types of matched lit-

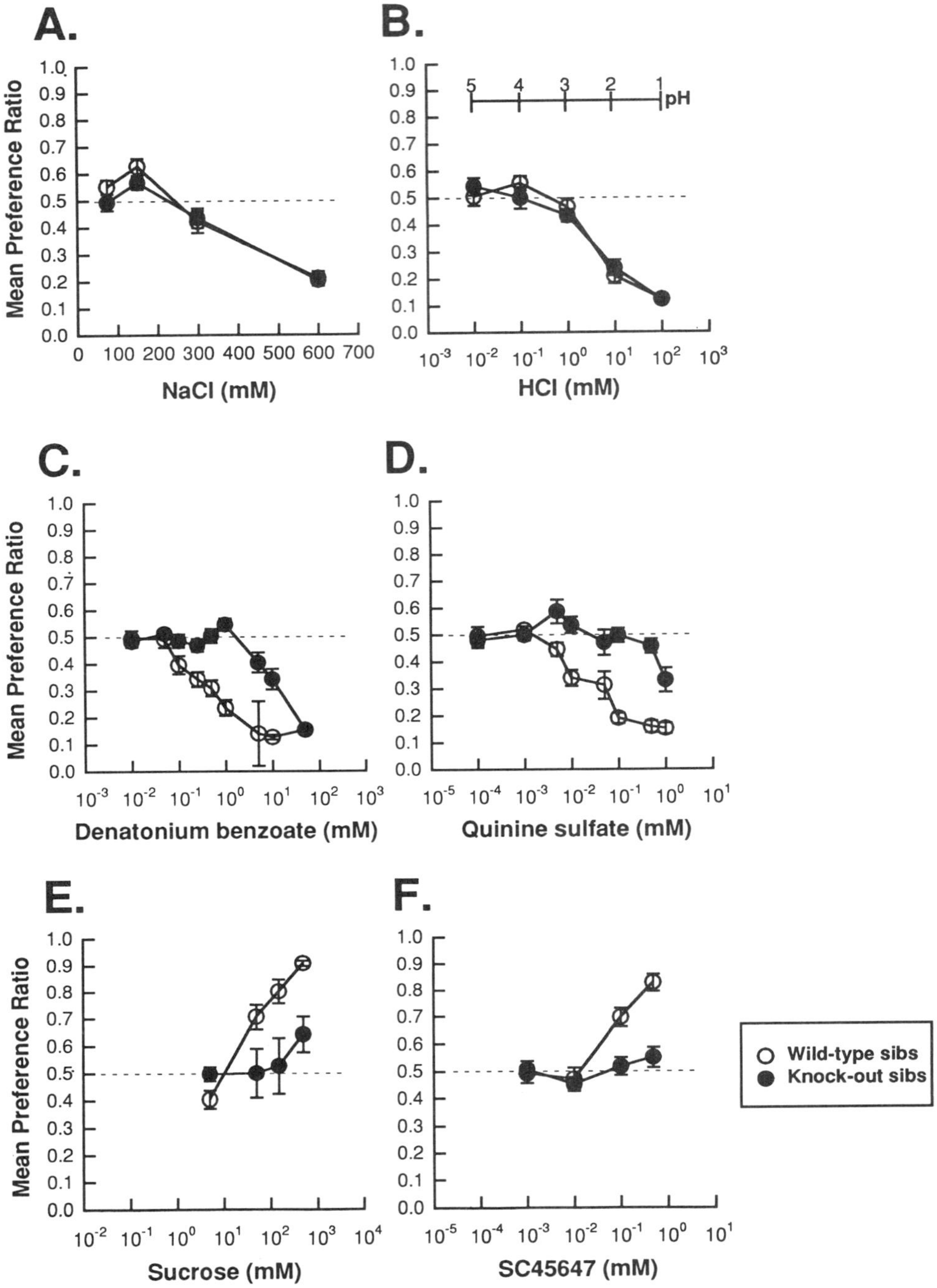

Figure 4. Mean preference ratios from 48-hr two-bottle (tastant versus distilled water) preference tests of male wild-type (GUS/GUS) (*open* circles) and null (*gus/gus*) (*filled* circles) mice. Tastant concentrations are listed in order of presentation. (*A*) Behavioral responses to NaCl (75, 150, 300, and 600 mM) of wild-type mice (n=11) and their null siblings (n=11). No significant strain or interaction effects were found (p values > 0.05, Table 1). (*B*) Behavioral responses to HCl (0.01, 0.1, 1, 10, and 100 mM; a pH range of 5.0–1.0) of wild-type mice (n=10–12) and their null siblings (n=10–12). No significant strain or interaction effects were found (p values > 0.05, Table 1). (*C*) Behavioral responses to denatonium benzoate (0.01, 0.05, 0.1, 0.25, 0.5, 1.0, 5.0, 10.0, and 50.0 mM) of wild-type mice (n=10–11) and their null siblings (n=10–11). Results of t-tests are as follows: 0.25 mM ($p < 0.01$); 0.5–10.0 mM ($p < 0.0001$). (*D*) Behavioral responses to quinine sulfate (0.1, 1.0, 5.0, 10.0, 50.0, and 100.0 μM; 0.5 and 1.0 mM) of wild-type mice (n=9–12) and their null siblings (n=10–12). Results of t-tests are as follows: 5.0 μM, 50.0 μM, and 1.0 mM ($p < 0.05$); 10.0, 100, and 500 μM ($p < 0.01$). (*E*) Behavioral responses to sucrose (5, 50, 150, and 500 mM) of wild-type mice (n=7–12) and their null siblings (n=11–12). Results of t-tests are as follows: 50–500 mM ($p < 0.001$). (*F*) Behavioral responses to SC45647 (1, 10, 100, and 500 μM) of wild-type mice (n=10–12) and their null siblings (n=10–12). Results of t-tests are as follows: 100 μM and 500 μM ($p < 0.001$).

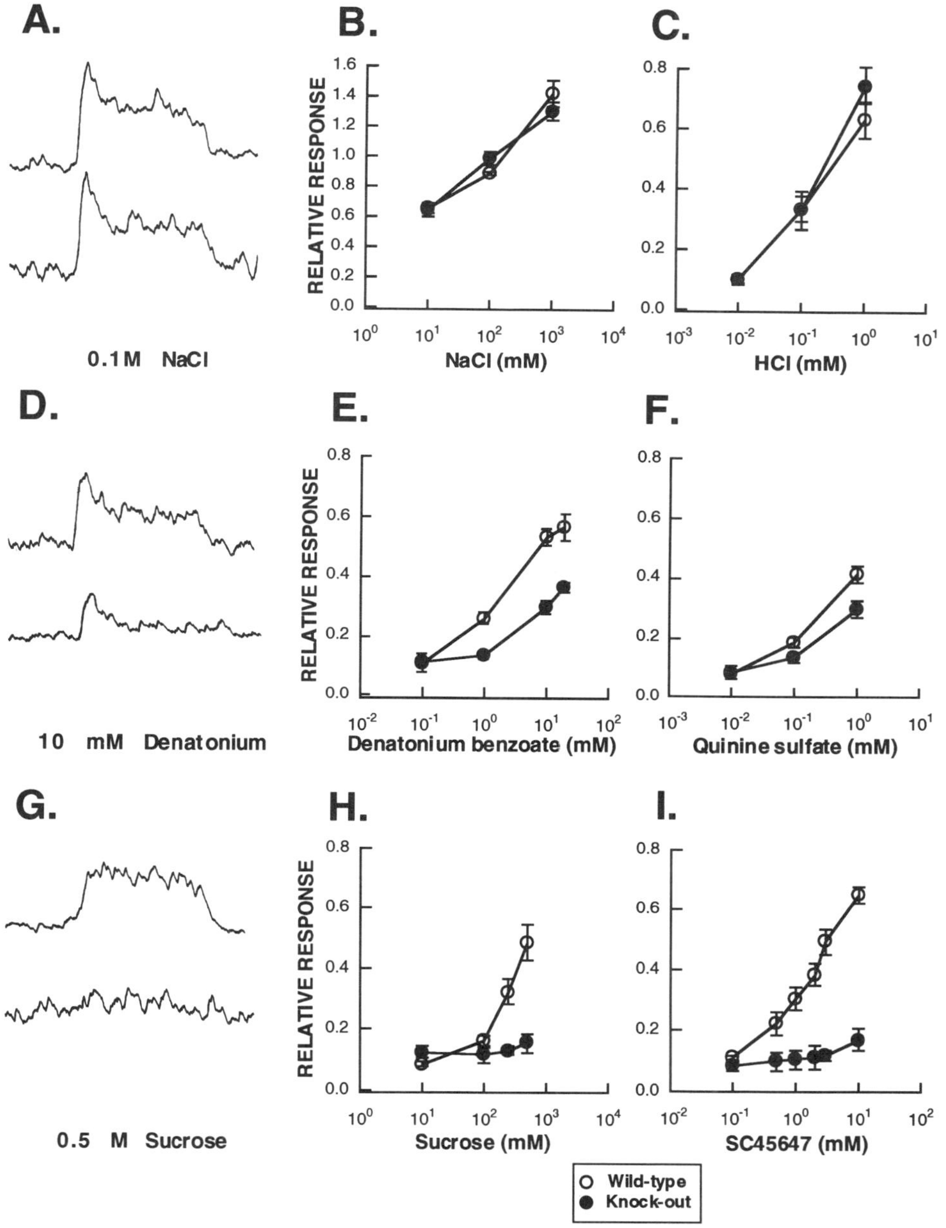

Figure 5. Chorda tympani responses to lingual application of taste stimuli for wild-type control and α-gustducin null mice. (*Left* panels) Integrated neural responses of a wild-type (*upper* trace) and a null mouse (*lower* trace) to 0.1 M NaCl (*A*), 10 mM denatonium benzoate (*D*), and 0.5 M sucrose (*G*). (*Right* panels) Chorda tympani phasic responses of null (n=6, *filled* circles) and wild-type mice (n=9–10, *open* circles) to taste compounds. Data shown represent the maximum neural response amplitude occurring within 4 sec following stimulus onset and are expressed relative to the response to 0.1 M NH_4Cl. Due to the large response of the chorda tympani to NaCl, the y-axis of panel *A* ranges from 0 to 1.4, whereas the y-axes for the other tastants range from 0 to 0.8. (*B*) Neural responses to NaCl concentrations (0.01, 0.1, and 1.0 M). No significant strain or interaction effects were present (p values > 0.05, Table 1). (*C*) Neural responses to HCl concentrations (0.01, 0.1, and 1.0 mM). No significant strain or interaction effects were present (p values > 0.05, Table 1). (*E*) Neural responses to denatonium benzoate concentrations (0.1, 1.0, 10.0, and 20.0 mM). Results of t-tests are as follows: 1.0 mM ($p < 0.001$) 10.0 mM ($p < 0.0001$), and 20 mM ($p < 0.01$). (*F*) Neural responses to quinine sulfate concentrations (0.01, 0.1, and 1.0 mM). Results of t-tests are as follows: 0.1 mM ($p < 0.05$), 1.0 mM ($p < 0.01$). (*H*) Neural responses to sucrose concentrations (0.01, 0.1, 0.25, and 0.5 M). Results of t-tests are as follows: 0.25 ($p < 0.01$), and 0.5 M ($p < 0.001$). (*I*) Neural responses to SC45647 concentrations (0.1, 0.5, 1.0, 2.0, 3.0, and 10.0 mM). Results of t-tests are as follows: 0.5 mM ($p < 0.05$); 1.0 mM ($p < 0.01$), 2.0 mM ($p < 0.001$), 3.0–10 mM ($p < 0.0001$).

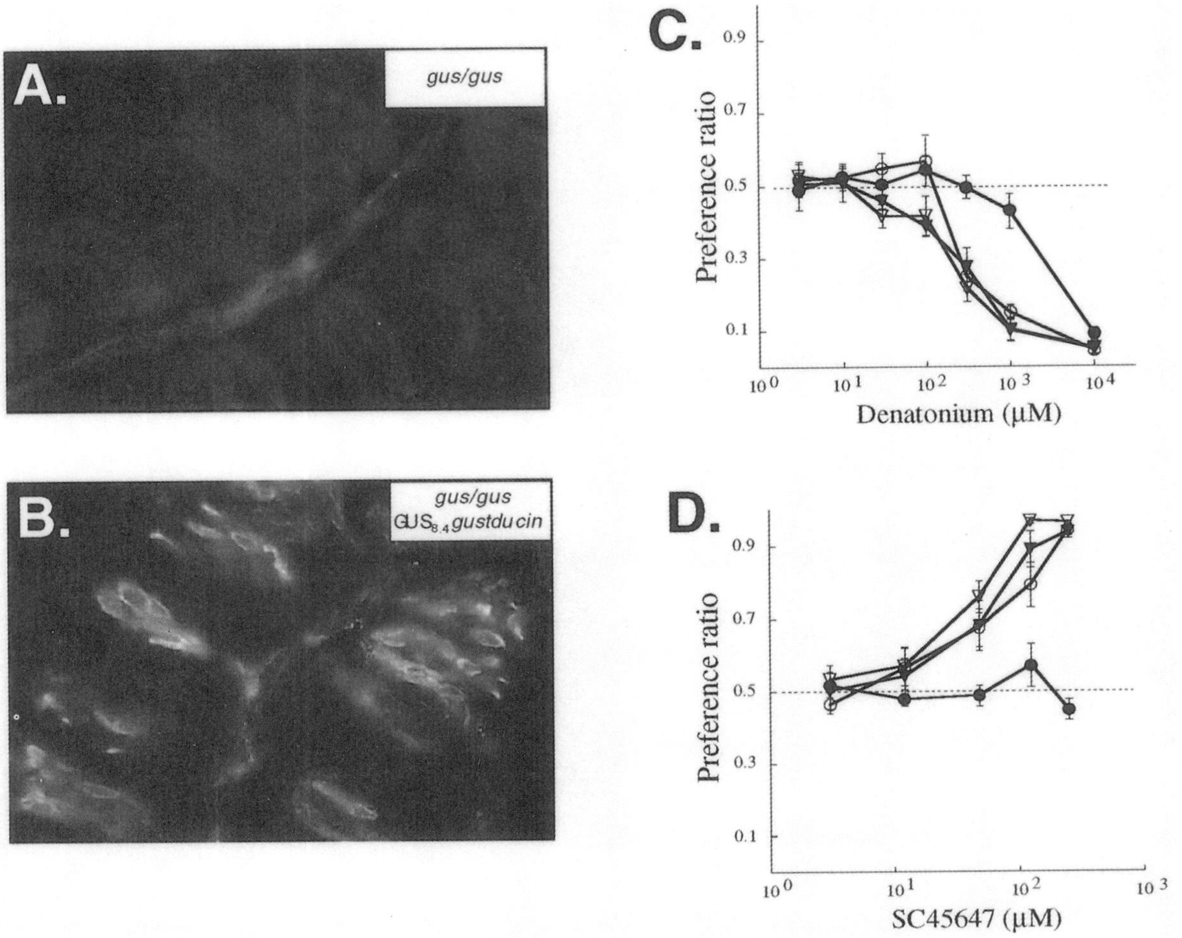

Figure 6. Rescue of taste responses of gustducin null mice by the rat gustducin cDNA. The 8.4-kb gustducin promoter ($GUS_{8.4}$) was used to drive transgenic expression of a rat gustducin cDNA to TRCs from null mice. Immunofluorescence photomicrographs of frozen sections treated with α-gustducin-specific antibody and Cy3-conjugated secondary antibody. Circumvallate papillae from nontransgenic null (*gus/gus*) (*A*) and transgenic null ($GUS_{8.4}$*gustducin gus/gus*) (*B*) mice. (*C*) Behavioral responses to denatonium benzoate of matched siblings: nontransgenic heterozygotes (GUS/*gus*: *open* circles); nontransgenic nulls (*gus/gus*: *filled* circles); transgenic nulls ($GUS_{8.4}$*gustducin gus/gus*: *filled* triangles) and transgenic heterozygotes ($GUS_{8.4}$*gustducin* GUS/*gus*: *open* triangles). (*D*) Behavioral responses to SC45647.

termates: nontransgenic GUS/*gus* ("wild-type" control); nontransgenic *gus/gus* (negative control); $GUS_{8.4}$*gustducin gus/gus* (rescued nulls); and $GUS_{8.4}$*gustducin* GUS/*gus*. Expression of the wild-type rat α-gustducin transgene in the null background restored both the bitter and sweet responses to the wild-type level, thus confirming gustducin's involvement in bitter and sweet transduction.

DISCUSSION

We have identified a taste-specific PDE that can be regulated by transducin and that we presume is normally regulated by gustducin and/or transducin. We have also identified a bitter denatonium-responsive receptor that can activate exogenously added transducin or gustducin. These results are consistent with the existence in TRCs of a photoreceptor-like cascade: receptor-gustducin/transducin-PDE. To gain further insight into the in vivo function of gustducin in taste transduction, we used a combination of molecular genetics and behavioral and electrophysiological analysis. We generated α-gustducin-deficient (null) mice and demonstrated that they were indistinguishable from their wild-type siblings in their behavioral and electrophysiological responses to NaCl and HCl. In sharp contrast, the null mice had significantly diminished behavioral and electrophysiological responses to the bitter compounds and, unexpectedly, to the sweet compounds. Introduction into null mice of the rat gustducin cDNA as a transgene under the control of the mouse gustducin promoter restored the wild-type phenotype for both bitter and sweet behavioral responses. We conclude that gustducin is a principal mediator of both bitter and sweet taste transduction, but that it is not involved in salty and sour transduction. At high tastant concentrations, the α-gustducin null mice avoid bitter and prefer sweet, suggesting that other G proteins may be involved in these taste responses (candidate G proteins expressed in TRCs include G_s, G_{i-3}, G_{14}, and rod transducin). Olfactory, tactile, and other nongustatory factors may also contribute to these behavioral responses. Interestingly, the behavioral responses of the null mice to bitter were affected more than were those to sweet, whereas the chorda tympani responses to sweet were affected more than were those to bitter. The glossopharyngeal nerve contains a larger proportion of bitter-specific fibers than does the chorda tympani (Ninomiya and Funakoshi 1989) and would therefore be expected to play a major role in behavioral responses to bitter compounds. Consistent with this idea, preliminary glossopharyngeal nerve recordings demonstrated profoundly diminished responses of the null mice to quinine sulfate and denatonium benzoate (K.S. Gannon et al., unpubl.).

Several lines of evidence implicate G proteins and their coupled receptors in the transduction of bitter and sweet tastes (for review, see Kinnamon and Margolskee 1996). Denatonium increases inositol trisphosphate levels in mouse taste tissue (Spielman et al. 1996) and leads to the release of intracellular Ca^{++} from rat TRCs (Akabas et al. 1988). Bitter transduction may involve activation of phospholipase C (PLC) by gustducin's βγ subunits and/or by an α_q-like subunit (e.g., α_{14}). Sucrose causes a GTP-dependent increase in taste-tissue cAMP, apparently by activating adenylyl cyclase (AC) (Striem et al. 1989, 1991; Naim et al. 1991). Microinjection of cAMP into TRCs (Tonosaki and Funakoshi 1988), or the addition of membrane-permeant cyclic nucleotides (Avenet and Lindemann 1987; Avenet et al. 1988), leads to inactivation of K^+ channels and TRC depolarization. Genetic ablation of α-gustducin would block the coupling of bitter- and/or sweet-responsive receptors to the regulation of certain intracellular second messengers, thereby blocking bitter/sweet TRC responses such as depolarization and neurotransmitter release. Any bitter or sweet compound that acts primarily on an α-gustducin-coupled taste receptor would be expected to have diminished behavioral and electrophysiological effects in the absence of α-gustducin. Compounds that act primarily via other G proteins, or that bypass taste receptors to act directly on intracellular targets (Naim et al. 1994), would not be expected to be affected by α-gustducin deficiency. We presume that gustducin-containing sweet-responsive and bitter-responsive cells are separate and physically distinct. Alternatively, gustducin-containing sweet- and bitter-responsive cells may utilize different downstream pathways (i.e., different second-messenger effector enzymes and different ion channels). The absence of the α subunit of gustducin may also have significant secondary effects on TRCs. Excess free βγ subunits of gustducin may act directly to activate PLC, activate or inhibit AC, or open Ca^{++} and/or K^+ channels (for review, see Neer 1995). Excess free βγ subunits may act indirectly by interfering with receptor activation of various α subunits (e.g., $G\alpha_s$, $G\alpha_{14}$) or by interfering with α-subunit activation of effector enzymes (e.g., AC, PLC). By introducing specifically mutated forms of gustducin into the null background, we will be able to study the gustducin/PDE and gustducin/receptor interactions underlying bitter and sweet transduction. Single-cell electrophysiological recordings from the gustducin lineage of TRCs from wild-type, α-gustducin null, and α-gustducin mutant mice may enable us to determine gustducin's specific roles in bitter and sweet transduction.

ACKNOWLEDGMENTS

This work was supported by National Institutes of Health grants DC-03055 (R.F.M.), DC-00142 (G.T.W.), and DC-00231 (K.S.G.), and by a grant from CIRIT BEAI-300089 (L.R.-A.). In compliance with federal regulations (42 CFR 50.604, [g], [2]) it must be noted that R.F.M. has a financial interest that might affect the design, conduct, or reporting of this federally funded research.

REFERENCES

Akabas, M.H., J. Dodd, and Q. Al-Awqati. 1988. A bitter substance induces a rise in intracellular calcium in a subpopulation of rat taste cells. *Science* **242:** 1047.

Alvarez, R. and D.V. Daniels. 1992. A separation method for the assay of adenylylcyclase, intracellular cyclic AMP, and cyclic-AMP phosphodiesterase using tritium-labeled substrates. *Anal. Biochem.* **203:** 76.

Avenet, P. and B. Lindemann. 1987. Patch-clamp study of isolated taste receptor cells of the frog. *J. Membr. Biol.* **97:** 223.

Avenet, P., F. Hofmann, and B. Lindemann. 1988. Transduction in taste receptor cells requires cAMP-dependent protein kinase. *Nature* **331:** 351.

Fawzi, A.B. and J.K. Northup. 1990. Guanine nucleotide binding characteristics of transducin: Essential role of rhodopsin for rapid exchange of guanine nucleotides. *Biochemistry* **29:** 3804.

Fung, B.K.-K. and C.R. Nash. 1983. Characterization of transducin from bovine retinal rod outer segments. II. Evidence for distinct binding sites and conformational changes revealed by limited proteolysis with trypsin. *J. Biol. Chem.* **258:** 10503.

Fung, B.K.-K., J.B. Hurley, and L. Stryer. 1981. Flow of information in the light-triggered cyclic nucleotide cascade of vision. *Proc. Natl. Acad. Sci.* **78:** 152.

Gannon, K.S. and R.J. Contreras. 1995. Sodium intake linked to amiloride-sensitive gustatory transduction in C57BL/6J and 129/J mice. *Physiol. Behav.* **57:** 231.

Halliday, K.R., P.J. Stein, N. Chernoff, G.L. Wheeler, and M.W. Bitensky. 1984. Limited trypsin proteolysis of photoreceptor GTP-binding protein. Light- and GTP-induced conformational changes. *J. Biol. Chem.* **259:** 516.

Hamm, H.E., D. Deretic, A. Arendt, P.A. Hargrave, B. Koenig, and K.P. Hofmann. 1988. Site of G protein binding to rhodopsin mapped with synthetic peptides from the alpha subunit. *Science* **241:** 832.

Harder, D.B., J.C. Maggio, and G. Whitney. 1989. Assessing

gustatory detection capabilities using preference procedures. *Chem. Senses* **14:** 547.

Hogan, B., R. Beddington, F. Costantini, and E. Lacy, eds. 1994. *Manipulating the mouse embryo.* Cold Spring Harbor Laboratory Press, Cold Spring Harbor, New York.

Hoon, M.A., J.K. Northup, R.F. Margolskee, and N.J.P. Ryba. 1995. Functional expression of the taste specific G-protein, α-gustducin. *Biochem. J.* **309:** 629.

Kinnamon, S. and R.F. Margolskee. 1996. Mechanisms of taste transduction. *Curr. Opin. Neurobiol.* **6:** 506.

Kwee, L., H.S. Baldwin, H.M. Shen, C.S. Stewart, C. Buck, C.A. Buck, and M. Labow. 1995. Defective development of the embryonic and extraembryonic circulatory systems in vascular cell adhesion molecule (VCAM-1) deficient mice. *Development* **121:** 489.

Laird, P.W., A. Zijderveld, K. Linders, M.A. Rudnicki, R. Jaenisch, and A. Berns. 1991. Simplified mammalian DNA isolation procedure. *Nucleic Acids Res.* **19:** 4293.

McLaughlin, S.K., P.J. McKinnon, and R.F. Margolskee. 1992. Gustducin is a taste-cell-specific G protein closely related to the transducins. *Nature* **357:** 563.

Naim, M., T. Ronen, B.J. Striem, M. Levenson, and U. Zehavi. 1991. Adenylate cyclase responses to sucrose stimulation in membranes of pig circumvallate taste papillae. *Comp. Biochem. Physiol.* **100B:** 455.

Naim, M., R. Seifert, B. Nurnberg, L. Grunbaum, and G. Schultz. 1994. Some taste substances are direct activators of G-proteins. *Biochem. J.* **297:** 451.

Neer, E. 1995. Heterotrimeric G proteins: Organizers of transmembrane signals. *Cell* **80:** 249.

Ninomiya, Y. and M. Funakoshi. 1989. Peripheral neural basis for behavioural discrimination between glutamate and the four basic taste substances in mice. *Comp. Biochem. Physiol.* **92A:** 371.

Rarick, H.M., N.O. Artemyev, and H.E. Hamm. 1992. A site on rod G protein alpha subunit that mediates effector activation. *Science* **256:** 1031.

Ruiz-Avila, L., S.K. McLaughlin, D. Wildman, P.J. McKinnon, A. Robichon, N. Spickofsky, R.F. Margolskee. 1995. Coupling of bitter receptor to phosphodiesterase through transducin in taste receptor cells. *Nature* **376:** 80.

Spickofsky, N., A. Robichon, W. Danho, D. Fry, B. Graves, V. Madison, and R.F. Margolskee. 1994. Biochemical analysis of the transducin phosphodiesterase interaction. *Nat. Struct. Biol.* **1:** 771.

Spielman, A.I., H. Nagai, G. Sunavala, M. Dasso, H. Breer, I. Boekhoff, T. Huque, G. Whitney, and J.G. Brand. 1996. Rapid kinetics of second messenger production in bitter taste. *Am. J. Physiol.* **270:** C926.

Stewart, C.L., P. Kaspar, L.J. Brunet, H. Bhatt, I. Gadi, F. Kontgen, and S.J. Abbondanzo. 1992. Blastocyst implantation depends on maternal expression of leukaemia inhibitory factor. *Nature* **359:** 76.

Striem, B.J., M. Naim, and B. Lindemann. 1991. Generation of cyclic AMP in taste buds of the rat circumvallate papillae in response to sucrose. *Cell. Physiol. Biochem.* **1:** 46.

Striem, B.J., U. Pace, U. Zehavi, M. Naim, and D. Lancet. 1989. Sweet tastants stimulate adenylate cyclase coupled to GTP binding protein in rat tongue membranes. *Biochem. J.* **260:** 121.

Szabo, P. and J.R. Mann. 1994. Expression and methylation of imprinted genes during in vitro differentiation of mouse parthenogenetic and androgenetic embryonic stem cell lines. *Development* **120:** 1651.

Takami, S., M.L. Getchell, S.K. McLaughlin, R.F. Margolskee, and T.V. Getchell. 1994. Human taste cells express the G protein α-gustducin and neuron-specific enolase. *Mol. Brain Res.* **22:** 193.

Tinti, J.-M. and C. Nofre. 1991. Design of sweeteners: A rational approach. In *Sweeteners: Discovery, molecular design and chemoreception* (ed. D.E. Walters et al.), p. 88. American Chemical Society, Washington, D.C.

Tonosaki, K. and M. Funakoshi. 1988. Cyclic nucleotides may mediate taste transduction. *Nature* **331:** 354.

Wong, G.T., K.S. Gannon, and R.F. Margolskee. 1996. Transduction of bitter and sweet by gustducin. *Nature* **381:** 796.

Memory, Memory Impairment, and the Medial Temporal Lobe

L.R. SQUIRE AND S.M. ZOLA
Veterans Affairs Medical Center, San Diego, and Departments of Psychiatry and Neurosciences, University of California, San Diego, La Jolla, California 92093

In the most biological sense, questions about memory are questions about synaptic plasticity, i.e., cellular and molecular questions about how individual neurons can exhibit history-dependent behavior in the short term and long term and about how neurons can behave differently as a function of their recent input. Yet, many important questions about memory are systems questions and functional questions that address a more global, neuropsychological level of analysis. Is memory one thing or many things? What brain systems are involved in memory, and what jobs do they do?

In this paper, we consider three themes that have been important in recent neuropsychological work on memory. The first theme is that memory is to some extent a separable function of the brain that is dissociable from other cognitive functions. Thus, memory can sometimes be severely impaired in the absence of other intellectual deficits. The second theme focuses on the successful development in the monkey of an animal model of human memory impairment and the identification of the brain structures in the medial temporal lobe that are important for memory. The third theme is that the role of the medial temporal lobe system is important for only one kind of memory. It is essential for conscious recollection of recently occurring facts and events (declarative memory) but not for a large collection of nondeclarative memory abilities (e.g., skills and habits, simple classic conditioning, and the phenomenon of priming).

MEMORY AS A SEPARABLE FUNCTION OF THE BRAIN

Bilateral damage to the medial temporal lobe or diencephalic midline can cause memory impairment without affecting other cognitive functions. For example, amnesiac patients with medial temporal lobe damage can obtain average or above-average IQ scores on conventional intelligence tests (e.g., the Wechsler Adult Intelligence Scale-Revised) and yet be severely impaired on conventional memory tests (e.g., the Wechsler Memory Scale-Revised). A priori, one might have supposed that the structures of the brain are so interconnected and interdependent that removal of any single structure should produce a broad band of impairment distributed across many functions. However, one important lesson of modern neuroscience is that the brain is highly differentiated and specialized, and one of the clear findings from empirical work is that brain lesions can produce highly specific cognitive deficits exquisitely related to the particular structures and connections that are damaged.

Even allowing that localized lesions can produce selective deficits, some additional explanation is needed to understand how a lesion of the medial temporal lobe can selectively impair memory. The problem is that the concept of an isolated defect in memory appears at first to conflict with the widely held view that perception, information processing, and memory are closely connected. For example, long-term memory is thought to be stored in the same cortical areas where the information to be remembered is processed and analyzed (Mishkin 1982; Squire 1987; Damasio 1989; Horel 1994; Ungerleider 1995). Accordingly, if memory is affected, one should also expect some related defect in information processing. As it turns out, the concept of an isolated memory defect can be understood without contradicting this larger principle that memory functions are closely tied to the functions of information processing and analysis.

Consider that the medial temporal lobe does in fact accomplish certain kinds of processing and analysis, with memory as the product (Teyler and Discenna 1986; Milner 1989; Alvarez and Squire 1994; McClelland et al. 1995). Specifically, the medial temporal lobe is needed at the time of learning to establish functional connections with widespread areas of neocortex, based on synaptic changes within the medial temporal lobe that occur at the time of learning. Perception and short-term memory are thought to depend on coordinated and distributed activity within neocortex and not on the medial temporal lobe.

Studies of memory-impaired patients using tests that make strong demands on perceptual operations and short-term memory have consistently found that the patients are entirely intact. For example, amnesiac patients exhibit entirely intact digit-span memory, even when the estimate of digit-span ability approaches a resolution of one decimal point (Baddeley and Warrington 1970; Cave and Squire 1992). Both control subjects and amnesiac patients with radiologically confirmed damage to the hippocampal formation were able to repeat back an average of 6.8 digits. Similarly, amnesiac patients with medial temporal lobe lesions were fully intact at identifying words flashed briefly on a computer screen, and they exhibited normal performance across a wide range of accuracies (Hamann et al. 1995). Specifically, as the experimental conditions were varied such that control subjects improved from nearly 0% correct (with a 33-msec exposure time) to about 90% correct (with a 116-msec exposure time), amnesiac patients matched the control subjects at each performance level.

Medial temporal lobe damage thus has not been shown to impair perception or short-term memory. Nevertheless, the role of the medial temporal lobe begins at the time of learning when it receives highly processed input from neocortical association areas, and it is needed at the time of learning to interact with neocortex. However, its essential role is not manifest with the lesion technique until so much time has passed after learning that performance based on prior experience must draw on long-term, recollective memory. Stated differently, its essential role is not observed until short-term memory can no longer support performance. In summary, the medial temporal lobe, like other brain structures, is involved in processing and analyzing, but the deficit that follows damage to this structure is best described as a memory deficit because the normal contribution of the structure is not essential until some time has passed after learning.

If the medial temporal lobe is to be understood as having a memory function, it should be possible to distinguish such a contribution to cognition from the contributions made by other areas of cortex. Lesion studies identify three key features of medial temporal lobe function. First, as suggested above, medial temporal lobe lesions spare short-term memory while impairing long-term memory. The deficit can be described as profound forgetfulness, and the deficit emerges most clearly after some time has elapsed beyond the moment of learning. This dissociation between perception and short-term memory, on the one hand, and long-term memory, on the other hand, is now well established in humans (Baddeley and Warrington 1970; Cave and Squire 1992), monkeys (Overman et al. 1991; Alvarez et al. 1994), and rats (Kesner and Novak 1982; Vnek et al. 1995; Vnek and Rothblat 1996). In contrast, lesions of neocortex impair performance at very short delays as well as at longer delays (Goldman-Rakic 1987; Squire 1987; Fuster 1995).

A second key feature of medial temporal lobe function is that damage to this region produces a memory impairment that is global and multimodal; i.e., memory is impaired for many kinds of material (e.g., objects, odors, or designs) and regardless of the sensory modality in which information is presented (for humans, see Milner 1968; Corkin 1984; for monkeys, Murray and Mishkin 1984; Suzuki et al. 1993; for rats, Jarrard 1993; Bunsey and Eichenbaum 1996). In contrast, the memory problems associated with neocortical lesions are domain-specific; i.e., they are specific to the kind of material that is ordinarily processed and analyzed by the damaged area (e.g., faces or words).

The third defining feature of medial temporal lobe function is that the medial temporal lobe is involved in memory for a limited period of time after learning. As time passes, memory is gradually reorganized (or consolidated), and information storage in neocortex becomes independent of the medial temporal lobe system (for review, see Squire and Alvarez 1995). The key finding is that, when a medial temporal lobe lesion is sufficiently delayed after learning, memory is not affected. Six prospective studies in experimental animals now support this conclusion; i.e., recently acquired information is impaired while more remotely acquired information is spared. This finding of temporally graded retrograde amnesia has been obtained using several different species and tasks: object discrimination learning in monkeys (Zola-Morgan and Squire 1990), context-specific fear conditioning in rats (Kim and Fanselow 1992), acquired food preference in rats (Winocur 1990), maze learning in mice (Cho et al. 1993), and trace conditioning of the eyeblink reflex in rabbits (Kim et al. 1995). In contrast, there is no evidence for temporally graded retrograde amnesia following a neocortical lesion. In another study, rats were trained beginning 0.5, 2, 4, and 6 weeks before receiving surgical lesions of entorhinal cortex or parietal cortex (Cho and Kesner 1996). Entorhinal lesions produced temporally graded retrograde amnesia, such that information acquired up to 4 weeks before surgery was impaired, but information acquired 6 weeks before surgery was intact. In contrast, parietal lesions disrupted performance to an equivalent extent regardless of the training-to-surgery interval (0.5 weeks to 6 weeks).

Recent theoretical accounts of temporally graded retrograde amnesia propose that medial temporal lobe structures direct consolidation in neocortex by gradually binding together the multiple, geographically separate cortical regions that together store memory for a whole event. Furthermore, recent experimental studies show that gradual changes in cortical connectivity can occur as the result of behavioral experience, and they give some hints as to how consolidation in neocortex might occur: Gradual morphological changes, driven by continuing input, modify the strength of connections between cortical areas (Black et al. 1990; Darian-Smith and Gilbert 1994; for review, see McClelland et al. 1995; Squire and Alvarez 1995).

In summary, medial temporal lobe lesions produce memory impairment, which occurs against a background of normal cognitive function. The brain has to some extent separated its capacity for intellectual functions and perceptual functions from its capacity to lay down in memory the records that ordinarily result from engaging in intellectual and perceptual work. Inevitably, this conclusion has been easier to reach with humans than with nonhuman animals. The possibility of speaking with amnesiac patients about their condition and the availability of many testing instruments that can be administered quickly greatly facilitate the assessment of human cognitive functions. As a result, the idea that medial temporal lobe lesions selectively impair memory now rests securely on quantitative neuropsychological data. It should also be said that one eventually arrives at the same conclusion simply by spending time with a well-circumscribed amnesiac patient and his or her family. The patient and the family describe the problem as a selective memory impairment, and the visitor readily recognizes it as such after observing the patient repeatedly in various natural settings.

In comparison, the analysis of cognitive impairment in nonhuman animals is more challenging. Indeed, a few investigators still debate whether a medial temporal lobe lesion in monkeys or a hippocampal lesion in rats really impairs memory, or whether the lesion instead impairs perception, motivation, or some other factor that affects performance (Ringo 1991; Horel 1994; Vanderwolf and Cain 1994). One cannot interview the experimental animals, and the available tests are necessarily indirect assessments of performance that sometimes require weeks or months to administer. Nevertheless, a considerable body of compelling work has been carried out with nonhuman animals. The important finding is that lesions in experimental animals, when placed in the same brain regions that are damaged in human amnesia, produce effects similar to what is observed in humans. Indeed, the impairment in rats and monkeys satisfies the three criteria outlined above for identifying memory impairment: The deficit spares short-term memory but impairs delayed (long-term) memory; the deficit is multimodal; and impairment is temporally graded for information acquired before the onset of amnesia.

During the last two decades, research in monkeys and humans has identified a system of anatomically related structures in the medial temporal lobe that is important for memory (for reviews, see Mishkin 1982; Squire and Zola-Morgan 1991; Murray 1992; Zola-Morgan and Squire 1993; Mishkin and Murray 1994). This system is schematically illustrated in Figure 1, and comprises what we here term the hippocampal region (i.e., the cell fields of the hippocampus proper, the dentate gyrus, and the subicular complex), and the cortical areas adjacent to the hippocampal region (i.e., the entorhinal, perirhinal, and parahippocampal cortices). All of these cortical areas are anatomically related to the hippocampal region (Van Hoesen and Pandya 1975a,b; Van Hoesen 1982; Insausti et al. 1987; Suzuki and Amaral 1994a,b). In particular, the perirhinal cortex and the parahippocampal cortex provide nearly two-thirds of the cortical input to the entorhinal cortex (Insausti et al. 1987; Suzuki and Amaral 1994a). The entorhinal cortex, in turn, provides the major source of cortical projections to the hippocampus and dentate gyrus (Van Hoesen 1982; Suzuki and Amaral 1994b). The hippocampal region and the entorhinal cortex, together, make up the hippocampal formation.

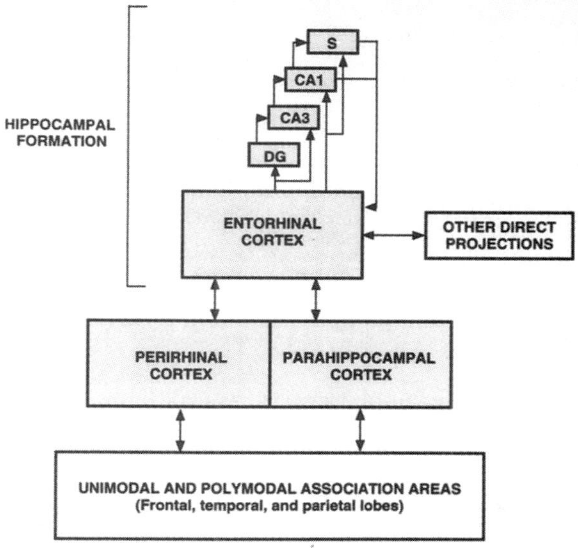

Figure 1. Schematic view of the medial temporal lobe memory system. The perirhinal and parahippocampal cortices receive projections from unimodal and polymodal areas in the frontal, temporal, and parietal lobes. In turn, the perirhinal and parahippocampal cortices account for nearly two-thirds of the cortical input to the entorhinal cortex, the primary source of cortical input to the hippocampal region (i.e., the cell fields of the hippocampus proper, the dentate gyrus, and the subicular complex). The hippocampal region together with the entorhinal cortex make up the hippocampal formation. The entorhinal cortex also receives other direct inputs from orbital frontal cortex, cingulate cortex, insular cortex, and superior temporal gyrus. All these projections are reciprocal. (Reprinted, with permission, from Squire and Zola 1996b.)

THE SEVERITY OF MEMORY IMPAIRMENT DEPENDS ON THE LOCUS AND EXTENT OF DAMAGE WITHIN THE MEDIAL TEMPORAL LOBE MEMORY SYSTEM

A large number of individual studies in monkeys have been carried out, such that performance can be compared on memory tasks for groups of monkeys with varying damage to the medial temporal lobe. Initially, these efforts began with large bilateral lesions of the medial temporal lobe that approximated the damage sustained by the well-studied amnesiac patient H.M. (Scoville and Milner 1957). This lesion involved the hippocampal formation, the amygdala, and the surrounding perirhinal and parahippocampal cortices. This lesion, and others in the same region that removed less tissue, reproduced many important features of the memory impairment in patient H.M. and other amnesiac patients (Table 1) (Squire and Zola-Morgan 1991). Note that the first three entries in the table refer to the three key features of medial temporal lobe dysfunction outlined above.

We recently took advantage of cumulated data from more than 10 years of testing involving 30 monkeys to examine the relationship between severity of memory

Table 1. Characteristics of Human Amnesia That Have Been Produced in Monkeys with Bilateral Lesions of the Medial Temporal Lobe

1.	Immediate memory is spared.
2.	Memory for events prior to the onset of amnesia can be affected in a temporally graded fashion (retrograde amnesia).
3.	Memory impairment is not limited to one sensory modality.
4.	Memory is impaired on a variety of tasks including tasks identical to those failed by amnesiac patients.
5.	Memory impairment is exacerbated by increasing the retention delay or the amount of material to be learned.
6.	Memory impairment is exacerbated by distraction.
7.	Memory impairment can be enduring.
8.	Skill-based memory is spared.

(Reprinted, with permission, from Squire and Zola-Morgan 1991 [copyright AAAS].)

impairment and extent of damage in the medial temporal lobe (Zola-Morgan et al. 1994). The memory performance in three groups of monkeys with differing extents of damage to the medial temporal lobe memory system was compared to the memory performance in 10 normal monkeys. All monkeys had completed testing on a standard memory battery (Zola-Morgan et al. 1994), and all monkeys had been tested on the tasks in the same order. Findings from a correlational analysis and a factor analysis indicated that four measures derived from the test battery were sensitive to medial temporal lobe damage, presumably because they were good measures of the kind of memory that is dependent on the medial temporal lobe (see below for a discussion of declarative memory). The four measures were: (1) the number of trials to obtain learning criterion on the trial-unique delayed nonmatching-to-sample task the first time it was administered; (2) the percent correct score averaged across the 15-second, 60-second, and 10-minute delay intervals from the delayed nonmatching-to-sample task; (3) the percent correct score averaged across all three test days for four separate object pairs from the delayed retention of object discriminations task; (4) the percent correct score averaged across the 15-second, 60-second, and 10-minute delay intervals when the delayed nonmatching-to-sample task was administered a second time, usually more than one year after surgery. The four measures from each of the 30 monkeys were converted to z scores, so that different performance measures could be considered together.

The main finding was that the severity of memory impairment depended on the locus and extent of damage within the medial temporal lobe memory system (Fig. 2). Damage limited to the hippocampal region, i.e., the cell fields of the hippocampus proper, the dentate gyrus, and the subicular complex (group H), caused significant memory impairment. More severe memory impairment occurred following H damage that also included the adjacent entorhinal and parahippocampal cortex (group H$^+$). The severity of impairment was greater still following H damage that also included all the adjacent cortical regions, i.e., the perirhinal, entorhinal, and parahippocampal cortices (group H^{++}).

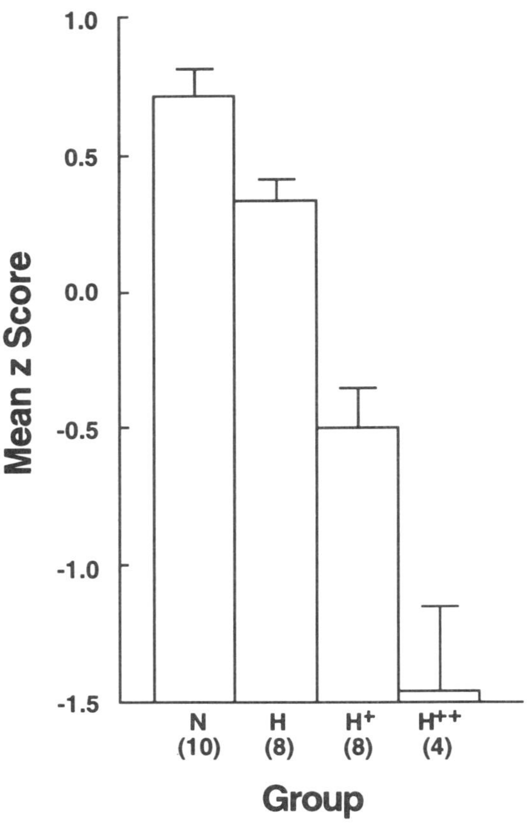

Figure 2. Mean z scores based on data from four measures of memory for 10 normal monkeys (group N), 8 monkeys with damage limited to the hippocampal region (H: the dentate gyrus, the cell fields of the hippocampus proper, and the subicular complex), 8 monkeys with damage that also included the adjacent entorhinal and parahippocampal cortices (group H$^+$), and 4 monkeys in which the H$^+$ lesion was extended forward to include the anterior entorhinal cortex and the perirhinal cortex (group H^{++}). Conversion of the data from the four behavioral measures into z scores permitted tasks that used different performance measures (e.g., trials to criterion and percent correct) to be compared with each other. As more components of the medial temporal lobe were included in the lesion, the severity of memory impairment increased. Error bars indicate standard errors of the mean. (Reprinted, with permission, from Zola-Morgan et al. 1994.)

The finding that monkeys with damage to the hippocampal region together with adjacent cortical regions (groups H$^+$ and H^{++}) exhibited more severe impairment than monkeys with damage limited to the hippocampal region (group H) emphasizes the importance for memory function of the adjacent cortical regions. Indeed, the damage to these cortical regions likely contributes substantially to the severe memory impairment produced by medial temporal lobe lesions in both monkeys and humans (Squire and Zola-Morgan 1991). Direct evidence for the importance of the cortical regions has come from studies in which circumscribed damage has been made to the perirhinal, entorhinal, or parahippocampal cortices, either separately or in combination (Moss et al. 1981; Zola-Morgan et al. 1989; Gaffan and Murray 1992; Meunier et al. 1993; Suzuki et al. 1993; Leonard et al. 1995). For example, monkeys with combined lesions of the perirhinal and parahippocampal cortices (the PRPH lesion) exhibited severely impaired performance on both a visual (Zola-Morgan et al. 1989; Suzuki et al. 1993) and tactual (Suzuki et al. 1993) version of the delayed nonmatching-to-sample task. Moreover, the monkeys with PRPH lesions continued to exhibit impaired performance when retested on the visual version of the delayed nonmatching-to-sample task approximately 2 years after surgery (Suzuki et al. 1993).

More limited lesions of the cortical regions also produce memory impairment. The clearest findings involve lesions limited to the perirhinal cortex. Several studies have now found that monkeys with bilateral lesions limited to the perirhinal cortex exhibit impaired memory (Horel et al. 1987; Meunier et al. 1993; Ramus et al. 1994). Moreover, damage to perirhinal cortex appears to produce more substantial impairment on the visual delayed nonmatching-to-sample task than damage to any other single component of the medial temporal lobe memory system (Meunier et al. 1993; Leonard et al. 1995). In addition, the memory impairment following perirhinal lesions is long-lasting (Ramus et al. 1994).

It is important to note that the relationship between severity of memory impairment and extent of damage to the medial temporal lobe cannot be attributed to a principle like mass action (Lashley 1929). That is, the severity of memory impairment exhibited by the monkeys with H^{++} lesions was not simply due to the fact that they had more damage overall than the monkeys with H^{+} lesions. When the H^{+} lesion was extended forward to include the amygdala (the $H^{+}A$ lesion), the memory impairment associated with the H^{+} lesion was not increased (Zola-Morgan et al. 1993). Thus, it is not just the extent of damage in the medial temporal lobe that is critical, but which specific structures are damaged (Zola-Morgan et al. 1994).

The finding that larger medial temporal lobe lesions produce more severe amnesia than smaller lesions, as measured by a particular group of tasks, is also compatible with the idea that structures within the medial temporal lobe could make qualitatively different contributions to memory function. For example, consider that anatomical projections from different parts of neocortex enter the medial temporal lobe memory system at different points. Thus, visual association cortex, i.e., area TE, projects more strongly to perirhinal cortex than to parahippocampal cortex, whereas parietal cortex projects to parahippocampal cortex but not to perirhinal cortex (Suzuki et al. 1993; Suzuki and Amaral 1994a). Accordingly, one might suppose that damage to perirhinal cortex could produce different effects on memory than damage to parahippocampal cortex. This idea has also been considered by other investigators. In the case of the monkey, the effects of fornix damage have been contrasted to the combined effects of perirhinal and entorhinal damage (Gaffan 1994). In the case of the rat, the function of the hippocampal region (hippocampus, dentate gyrus, subiculum, and fornix) has been proposed to be distinct from the function of the parahippocampal region (entorhinal, perirhinal, and parahippocampal cortices) (Eichenbaum et al. 1994).

MEMORY, THE HIPPOCAMPAL FORMATION, AND THE HIPPOCAMPAL REGION

It is useful to consider further the impairment in monkeys with circumscribed hippocampal damage (group H, Fig. 2). Group H consisted of monkeys from two different studies, four monkeys with ischemic damage limited to the hippocampal region (Zola-Morgan et al. 1992) and four monkeys with stereotaxic radiofrequency lesions limited to the hippocampal region (Alvarez et al. 1995). Each group exhibited significant and long-lasting memory impairment when evaluated in their respective studies using the delayed nonmatching-to-sample task. Two recent preliminary reports also described memory impairment in monkeys with lesions of the hippocampal region made by ibotenic acid (Beason-Held et al. 1993; Murray and Gaffan 1993).

The finding of impaired memory following bilateral damage limited to the hippocampal region in monkeys is consistent with findings from human amnesia. Since the report of amnesiac patient R.B. (Zola-Morgan et al. 1986), who developed memory impairment following an ischemic episode that destroyed the entire CA1 field of the hippocampus, four additional case studies of amnesia associated with damage limited to the hippocampal region (or the hippocampal region together with the entorhinal cortex) have become available (Victor and Agamanolis 1990; Rempel-Clower et al. 1996).

Three of the patients were involved in our research program at the Veterans Affairs Medical Center in San Diego, and our laboratory had the opportunity to carry out extensive postmortem analyses of the brains (Fig. 3). All three patients sustained significant memory impairment (Table 2). Detailed descriptions of the neuropsychological findings together with detailed descriptions of the neuropathological findings for each patient are described elsewhere (Rempel-Clower et al. 1996). Patient G.D., like patient R.B. (Zola-Morgan et al. 1986), had damage restricted primarily to the CA1 region of the hippocampus. Patients L.M., W.H., and an amnesiac patient reported by Victor and Agamanolis (1990) all had more extensive lesions than R.B. and G.D., involving all the cell fields of the hippocam-

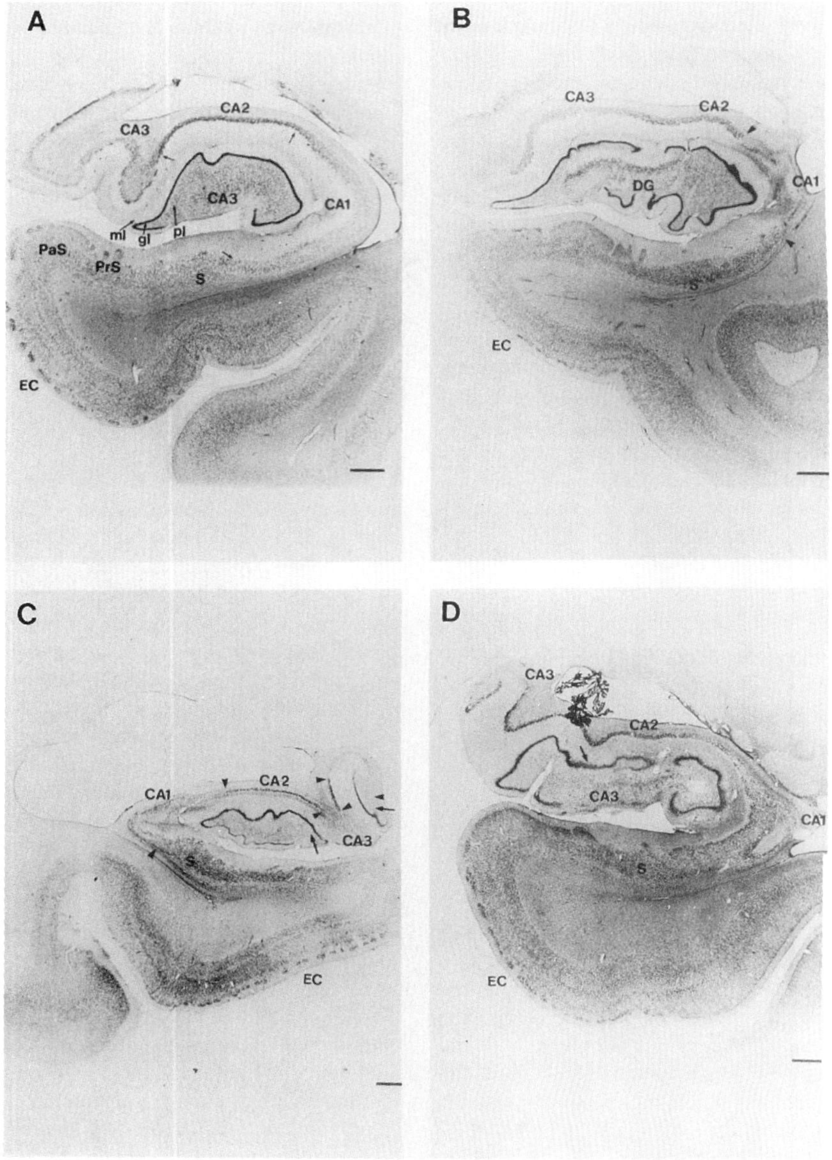

Figure 3. (*A*) Coronal section through a normal right hippocampal region stained with thionin. The hippocampus proper can be divided into three distinct fields, designated CA1, CA2, and CA3 (the CA3/CA2, CA2/CA1, and CA1/subiculum borders are indicated by arrows). The CA1 region begins where the pyramidal cell layer begins to broaden at the border of the CA2 field and extends to the subiculum (S). The CA1 field and the subiculum overlap at their border, which runs oblique to the cell fields. (*B*) Coronal section through the right hippocampal region of patient G.D. The lesion includes most of the cells in the CA1 region (marked by arrowheads). (*C*) Coronal section through patient L.M.'s left hippocampal region. Note the extensive loss of CA3 pyramidal cells and the nearly complete loss of CA1 pyramidal cells (arrowheads indicate the borders of the CA fields). There is also extensive loss of polymorphic cells in the hilus of the dentate gyrus (*arrows*). (*D*) Coronal section through W.H.'s right hippocampal region. Extensive pyramidal cell loss is evident in cell fields CA1 and CA3. Less substantial cell loss occurred in field CA2. The dentate gyrus appears very abnormal, with dispersion of the granule cells (*arrow*) and complete loss of polymorphic cells. Patchy cell loss is evident in the subiculum, and there was patchy cell loss in the entorhinal cortex as well. (CA1, CA2, CA3) Cell fields of the hippocampus; (ml) molecular layer; (gl) granular layer; (pl) polymorphic layer; (DG) dentate gyrus; (S) subiculum; (PrS) presubiculum; (PaS) parasubiculum; (EC) entorhinal cortex. For summary of findings for patients, see Table 2.

pus and the dentate gyrus. L.M. also had some cell loss in the entorhinal cortex; W.H. also had entorhinal damage as well as cell loss in the subicular complex.

The finding of impaired memory following bilateral ibotenic (fiber-sparing) damage limited to the hippocampal region has also been reported for rats for

Table 2. Summary of Neuropsychological and Neuropathological Findings from Four Patients with Bilateral Damage to the Hippocampal Formation

	Anterograde amnesia	Retrograde amnesia	Damage to the hippocampal formation
R.B.	moderate	minimal	CA1 field
G.D.	moderate	minimal (?)	CA1 field
L.M.	moderate	extensive	CA1, CA2, CA3 fields dentate gyrus entorhinal cortex
W.H.	severe	extensive	CA1, CA2, CA3 fields dentate gyrus subiculum entorhinal cortex

G.D. and R.B. had damage restricted primarily to the CA1 field of the hippocampus bilaterally. G.D. and R.B. additionally had cell loss in the region of the CA1/subiculum border. L.M., in addition to substantial cell loss in the dentate gyrus and all cell fields of the hippocampus, evidenced some loss of cells in layers II and III of entorhinal cortex. W.H. sustained more distributed damage to the hippocampal region overall than the other patients, including considerable loss of cells in the subiculum, complete loss of polymorphic cells in the dentate gyrus, and dispersion of the granule cell layer in the dentate gyrus. In addition, W.H. sustained cell loss in layers III, V, and VI of entorhinal cortex (slight cell loss also occurred in layer II of entorhinal cortex). The severity of memory impairment correlated with the extent of damage to the hippocampal formation. Thus, R.B. and G.D. had moderate anterograde amnesia and minimal retrograde amnesia. (The question mark for G.D. indicates that some uncertainty remains about the interpretation of his performance on remote memory tests.) L.M. had moderate anterograde amnesia, together with extensive, temporally graded retrograde amnesia covering at least 15 years. W.H. had severe anterograde amnesia together with extensive, temporally graded/retrograde amnesia that was probably more severe than in L.M. and involved as much as 25 years. (Reprinted, with permission, from Rempel-Clower et al. 1996.)

both spatial and nonspatial memory tasks (see Jaffard and Meunier 1993; Jarrard 1993; Bunsey and Eichenbaum 1996). Accordingly, the findings from rats, monkeys, and humans are in correspondence (Squire 1992b), and damage limited to the hippocampal region in all three species produces significant and long-lasting memory impairment. Moreover, the work in monkeys (specifically, the finding that the severity of memory impairment increases as more components of the medial temporal lobe memory system are damaged) is fully consistent with the findings from human amnesia. The moderately severe memory impairment in the patients just described, who had damage limited to the hippocampal formation, can be contrasted with the more severe memory impairment observed in the amnesiac patient H.M. and in the newly described patient E.P. Patient H.M. sustained bilateral resection of the medial temporal lobe, including the hippocampal region and adjacent cortical regions (Scoville and Milner 1957; Corkin 1984; Corkin et al. 1997). E.P. sustained similarly extensive damage to the medial temporal lobe following a viral illness (herpes simplex encephalitis) (Squire and Knowlton 1995).

Although the neuropathological findings from well-studied individual patients support the idea that the hippocampus itself is an important and essential component of the medial temporal lobe memory system, there is one possible concern. Is it possible that, in addition to the pathological changes detected within the hippocampus itself, some additional (covert) pathology occurred outside the hippocampus that did not progress to cell death and that would therefore not have been detected in a postmortem histopathological examination? This is a concern because if covert damage did occur in structures important for memory, then the undetected neuronal damage and not the hippocampal damage that was detected might account for the memory impairment.

This possibility can be addressed by evaluating the behavioral performance of monkeys who sustained a period of global ischemia. In our study, the ischemia produced identifiable bilateral damage to the CA1 field of the hippocampus and the hilar region of the dentate gyrus (Zola-Morgan et al. 1992). How did the memory performance of the ischemic animals compare to the performance of normal monkeys and monkeys with different surgical lesions (specifically, the H, H^+, and H^{++} lesions described in Fig. 2)? To make this comparison, we used the data from the lesion groups as a behavioral assay for evaluating the ischemic animals. The result, illustrated in Figure 4, is that the ischemic animals had a mild memory impairment, similar in severity to the impairment of the H group. The deficit of the ischemic group was significantly less severe than the impairment exhibited by the H^+ and H^{++} groups. Accordingly, it seems unlikely that ischemia produced significant, widespread neuropathology in areas related to memory function beyond what was detected within the CA1 and hilar regions. That is, it appears that the ischemic monkeys, and by extension patients R.B. and G.D., did not have substantial, covert neuropathology beyond the hippocampus that contributed to their memory impairment (see also Squire and Zola 1996a).

A different conclusion about the possible significance of covert pathological change was reached in an earlier study of two groups of monkeys: three with surgical lesions of the hippocampal formation and three with lesions due to posterior cerebral artery (PCA) occlusion. The PCA animals appeared to have less neuronal damage than the surgical group but a more severe memory impairment (Bachevalier and Mishkin 1989). However, the monkeys in the two groups did not have equivalent preoperative experience with the test used to assess memory, so it is unclear how to compare their memory performance (see Squire and Zola 1996a). (For additional discussion of the issue of covert damage in ischemia, see Bachevalier and Meunier 1996.)

MULTIPLE FORMS OF MEMORY

An important finding of neuropsychological studies of memory is that medial temporal lobe damage affects only one kind of memory. This finding, and others, have led to the idea that memory is not a single entity

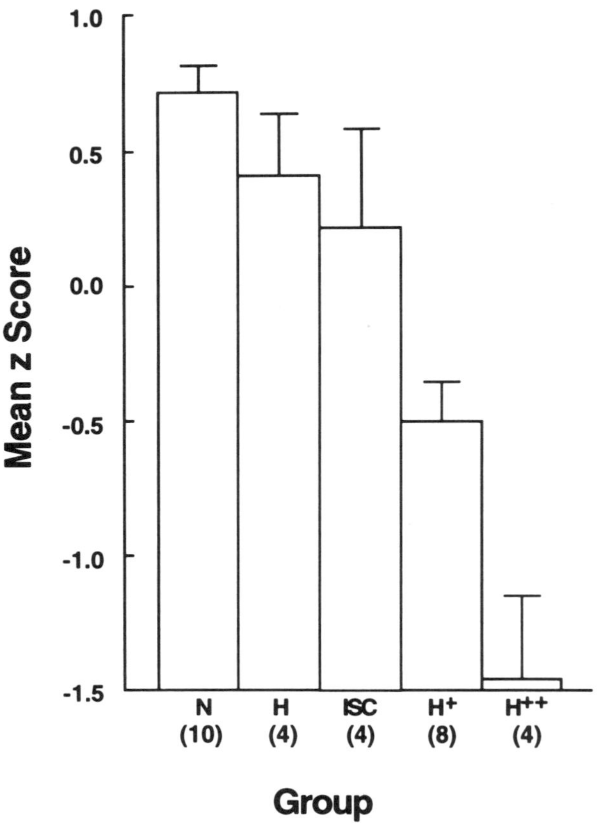

Figure 4. Same as Fig. 2, but with the two groups that comprised the H monkeys shown separately. The 4 monkeys here designated group H sustained neurosurgical lesions limited to the hippocampal region. The 4 monkeys in the ISC group sustained ischemic lesions limited to the hippocampal region. The H and the ISC groups performed similarly, and both performed better overall than the other operated groups.

but is composed of several separate systems. The kind of memory impaired in amnesia has been termed declarative or explicit memory. Nondeclarative (or implicit) memory is unaffected. (The term "procedural" has also been used to describe some kinds of nondeclarative memory, particularly skill learning). Declarative memory is typically assessed by tests of recall, recognition, or cued recall. It refers to the capacity for conscious recollections about facts and events. It is specialized for rapid, even one-trial, learning and for forming conjunctions between arbitrarily different stimuli as in paired-associate learning.

It should be emphasized that the concept of declarative memory does not derive its meaning solely from a determination of what amnesiac patients can and cannot learn. That is, the concept of declarative memory is not locked into a circularity around the performance of amnesiac patients. Studies with human and nonhuman animals have begun to develop a property list that describes the characteristics of declarative memory, independently of data from amnesia. One important idea is that declarative memory is specialized to detect variance; i.e., to detect what is different or unique about the events of a particular time and place. Nondeclarative memory is specialized for detecting invariance; i.e., for extracting from moment to moment what is common to the stimulus environment (Sherry and Schacter 1987; Squire 1992b; Knowlton et al. 1994). An additional proposal is that declarative memory is flexible and available to multiple response systems, whereas nondeclarative memory is inflexible and limited to the response systems that participated in the original learning (Cohen and Eichenbaum 1993; Cohen 1984; Squire 1994; Bunsey and Eichenbaum 1996; Reber et al. 1996).

Whereas declarative memory is a brain-systems construct, tied to the brain structures and connections damaged in amnesia, nondeclarative memory refers to a heterogeneous collection of several kinds of memory that in turn depend on distinct brain systems. Thus, classic conditioning of skeletal musculature depends on the cerebellum (Thompson and Krupa 1994), conditioning of emotional responses depends on the amygdala (LeDoux 1987; Davis 1992), and habit learning (win-stay, lose-shift responding) depends on the neostriatum (Packard et al. 1989; Salmon and Butters 1995; B.J. Knowlton et al., in prep.). Perceptual priming likely depends on changes in early-stage cortical areas involved in processing the stimuli that are primed (Fig. 5) (Squire et al. 1992; Schacter et al. 1996).

Nondeclarative memory thus refers to a variety of ways in which experience can lead to altered dispositions, preferences, and judgments without affording any conscious memory content. Performance changes as the result of experience and in this sense deserves the term memory, but performance changes without an accompanying sense that memory is being consulted. The organism simply behaves differently than it did previously. In many cases, performance changes gradually, as when one learns gradually about the causal structure of the world and acquires procedures for interacting with the world (in the case of conditioning, or skill learning, or win-stay/lose-shift habit learning). Sometimes performance can change rapidly (in the case of priming, or fear conditioning, or conditioned taste aversion). In the latter cases, the possibility of rapid change may be built into evolutionarily important systems that are specialized to process particular kinds of information.

In summary, memory is not a unitary faculty but is composed of multiple, separate systems. The medial temporal lobe memory system, which has been the primary focus of this paper, supports declarative memory. Amnesiac patients with damage to this system have an impairment of declarative memory, but they are intact at a wide variety of tasks that assess priming (Schacter et al. 1993) and skills and habits (Knowlton et al. 1994; Reber and Squire 1994), and they are able to acquire knowledge about categories when given a series of examples, as in artificial grammar learning or prototype

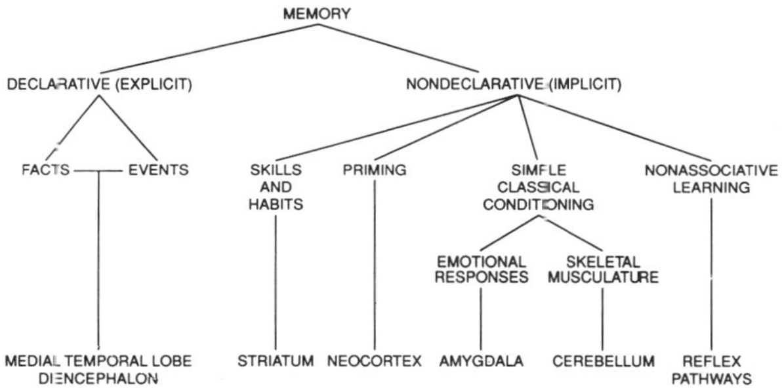

Figure 5. A taxonomy of long-term memory systems together with specific brain structures especially important for each system. (Reprinted, with permission, from Squire and Knowlton 1994.)

learning (Knowlton et al. 1992; Knowlton and Squire 1994a,b, 1996; Squire and Knowlton 1995).

SUMMARY

The cognitive and neuroanatomical work described here should be viewed as a first step in analyzing how the brain has organized its memory functions, which can open the door to more detailed neurobiological analysis. With respect to declarative memory, it should soon be possible to study representations directly in neocortex with the technique of single-cell recording, to observe directly the development of neuronal plasticity important for declarative memory, and to determine how the medial temporal lobe interacts with neocortex during learning, consolidation, and retrieval. In this regard, the paradigms developed by Miyashita and his colleagues appear to hold particular promise (Sakai and Miyashita 1991; Higuchi and Miyashita 1996). With respect to nondeclarative memory, it is now possible to identify particular brain systems that are essential for particular kinds of memory. An important next step will be to determine whether these systems are essential for the acquisition, storage, or expression of memory, and to identify exactly where the synaptic changes occur that support each kind of memory.

ACKNOWLEDGMENTS

The research summarized here was supported by the Medical Research Service of the Department of Veterans Affairs and The National Institutes of Health (grants MH-24600 and NS-19063). Some of the material in this chapter appeared in Squire and Zola (1996c) and appears here with permission.

REFERENCES

Alvarez, P. and L.R. Squire. 1994. Memory consolidation and the medial temporal lobe: A simple network model. *Proc. Natl. Acad. Sci.* **91:** 7041.

Alvarez, P., S. Zola-Morgan, and L.R. Squire. 1994. The animal model of human amnesia: Long-term memory impaired and short-term memory intact. *Proc. Natl. Acad. Sci.* **91:** 5637.

———. 1995. Damage limited to the hippocampal region produces long-lasting memory impairment in monkeys. *J. Neurosci.* **15:** 3796.

Bachevalier, J. and M. Meunier. 1996. Cerebral ischemia: Are the memory deficits associated with hippocampal cell loss? *Hippocampus* **5:** 553.

Bachevalier, J. and M. Mishkin. 1989. Mnemonic and neuropathological effects of occluding the posterior cerebral artery in *Macaca mulatta. Neuropsychologia* **27:** 83.

Baddeley, A.P. and E.K. Warrington. 1970. Amnesia and the distinction between long and short-term memory. *J. Verb. Learn. Verb. Behav.* **9:** 176.

Beason-Held, L., D.L. Rosene, and M.B. Moss. 1993. Memory deficits associated with ibotenic acid lesions of the hippocampal formation in rhesus monkeys. *Soc. Neurosci. Abstr.* **19:** 438.

Black, J.E., K.R. Isaacs, B.J. Anderson, A.A. Alcantara, and W.T. Greenough. 1990. Learning causes synaptogenesis, whereas motor activity causes angiogenesis, in cerebellar cortex of adult rats. *Proc. Natl. Acad. Sci.* **87:** 5568.

Bunsey, M. and H. Eichenbaum. 1996. Conservation of hippocampal memory function in rats and humans. *Nature* **379:** 225.

Cave, C. and L.R. Squire. 1992. Intact verbal and non-verbal short-term memory following damage to the human hippocampus. *Hippocampus* **2:** 151.

Cho, Y.H., D. Beracochea, and R. Jaffard. 1993. Extended temporal gradient for the retrograde and anterograde amnesia produced by ibotenate entorhinal cortex lesions in mice. *J. Neurosci.* **13:** 1759.

Cho, Y.H. and R.P. Kesner. 1996. Involvement of entorhinal cortex or parietal cortex in long term spatial discrimination memory in rats: Retrograde amnesia. *Behav. Neurosci.* **110:** 436.

Cohen, N.J. 1984. Preserved learning capacity in amnesia: Evidence for multiple memory systems. In *Neuropsychology of memory* (ed. L.R. Squire and N. Butters), vol. 1, p. 83. Guilford Press, New York.

Cohen, N.J. and H. Eichenbaum. 1993. *Memory, amnesia, and the hippocampal system.* MIT Press, Cambridge, Massachusetts.

Corkin, S. 1984. Lasting consequences of bilateral medial temporal lobectomy: Clinical course and experimental findings in H.M. *Semin. Neurol.* **4:** 249.

Corkin, S., D.G. Amaral, R.G. Gonzalez, K.A. Johnson, and B.T. Hyman. 1997. Medial temporal lobe lesion: Findings from MRI. *J. Neurosci.* (in press).

Damasio, A.R. 1989. Time-locked multiregional retroactivation: A systems-level proposal for the neural substrates of recall and recognition. *Cognition* **33:** 25.

Darian-Smith, C. and C.D. Gilbert. 1994. Axonal sprouting accompanies functional reorganization in adult cat striate cortex. *Nature* **354:** 152.

Davis, M. 1992. The role of the amygdala in fear-potentiated startle: Implications for animal models of anxiety. *Trends Pharmacol. Sci.* **13:** 35.

Eichenbaum, H., T. Otto, and N.J. Cohen. 1994. Two functional components of the hippocampal memory system. *Brain Behav. Sci.* **17:** 449.

Fuster, J.M. 1995. *Memory in the cerebral cortex: An empirical approach to neural networks in the human and nonhuman primate*. MIT Press, Cambridge.

Gaffan, D. 1994. Dissociated effects of perirhinal cortex ablation, fornix transection and amygdalectomy: Evidence for multiple memory systems in the primate temporal lobe. *Exp. Brain Res.* **99:** 411.

Gaffan, D. and E.A. Murray. 1992. Monkeys (*Macaca fascicularis*) with rhinal cortex ablations succeed in object discrimination learning despite 24-hr intertrial intervals and fail at matching to sample despite double sample presentations. *Behav. Neurosci.* **106:** 30.

Goldman-Rakic, P.S. 1987. Circuitry of primate prefrontal cortex and regulation of behavior by representational memory. In *Handbook of physiology* (ed. V.B. Mountcastle), vol. 5, part 1, p. 373. American Physiological Society, Bethesda, Maryland.

Hamann, S.B., L.R. Squire, and D. Schacter. 1995. Perceptual thresholds and priming in amnesia. *Neuropsychologia* **9:** 3.

Higuchi, S. and Y. Miyashita. 1996. Formation of mnemonic neuronal responses to visual paired associates in inferotemporal cortex is impaired by perirhinal and entorhinal lesions. *Proc. Natl. Acad. Sci.* **93:** 739.

Horel, J. 1994. Some comments on the special cognitive functions claimed for the hippocampus. *Cortex* **30:** 269.

Horel, J.A., D.E. Pytko-Joiner, M.L. Voytko, and K. Salsbury. 1987. The performance of visual tasks while segments of the inferotemporal cortex are suppressed by cold. *Behav. Brain Res.* **23:** 29.

Insausti, R., D.G. Amaral, and W.M. Cowan. 1987. The entorhinal cortex of the monkey: II. Cortical afferents. *J. Comp. Neurol.* **264:** 356.

Jaffard, R. and M. Meunier. 1993. Role of the hippocampal formation in learning and memory. *Hippocampus* **3:** 203.

Jarrard, L.E. 1993. On the role of the hippocampus in learning and memory in the rat. *Behav. Neural Biol.* **60:** 9.

Kesner, R.P. and J.M. Novak. 1982. Serial position curve in rats: Role of the dorsal hippocampus. *Science* **218:** 173.

Kim, J.J. and M.S. Fanselow. 1992. Modality-specific retrograde amnesia of fear. *Science* **256:** 675.

Kim, J.J., R.E. Clark, and R.F. Thompson. 1995. Hippocampectomy impairs the memory of recently, but not remotely, acquired trace eyeblink conditioned responses. *Behav. Neurosci.* **109:** 195.

Knowlton, B.J. and L.R. Squire. 1994a. The learning of categories: Parallel brain systems for item memory and category knowledge. *Science* **262:** 1747.

———. 1994b. The information acquired during artificial grammar learning. *J. Exp. Psychol. Learn. Mem. Cogn.* **20:** 79.

———. 1996. Artificial grammar learning depends on implicit acquisition of both rule-based and exemplar-based information. *J. Exp. Psychol. Learn. Mem. Cogn.* **22:** 1691.

Knowlton, B.J., S.J. Ramus, and L.R. Squire. 1992. Intact artificial grammar learning in amnesia: Dissociation of classification learning and explicit memory for specific instances. *Psychol. Sci.* **3:** 172.

Knowlton, B.J., L.R. Squire, and M. Gluck. 1994. Probabilistic classification learning in amnesia. *Learn. Mem.* **1:** 106.

Lashley, K.S. 1929. *Brain mechanisms and intelligence: A quantitative study of injuries to the brain*. Chicago University Press, Chicago, Illinois.

LeDoux, J.E. 1987. Emotion. In *Handbook of physiology* (ed. V.B. Mountcastle), vol. 5, part 1, p. 419. American Physiological Society, Bethesda, Maryland.

Leonard, B.W., D.G. Amaral, L.R. Squire, and S. Zola-Morgan. 1995. Transient memory impairment in monkeys with bilateral lesions of the entorhinal cortex. *J. Neurosci.* **15:** 5637.

McClelland, J.L., B.L. McNaughton, and R.C. O'Reilly. 1995. Why there are complementary learning systems in the hippocampus and neocortex: Insights from the successes and failures of connectionist models of learning and memory. *Psychol. Rev.* **102:** 419.

Meunier, M., J. Bachevalier, M. Mishkin, and E.A. Murray. 1993. Effects on visual recognition of combined and separate ablations of the entorhinal and perirhinal cortex in rhesus monkeys. *J. Neurosci.* **13:** 5418.

Milner, B. 1968. Disorders of memory after brain lesions in man. Preface: Material-specific and generalized memory loss. *Neuropsychologia* **6:** 175.

Milner, P. 1989. A cell assembly theory of hippocampal amnesia. *Neuropsychologia* **27:** 23.

Mishkin, M. 1982. A memory system in the monkey. *Philos. Trans. R. Soc. Lond. B Biol. Sci.* **298:** 85.

Mishkin, M. and E.A. Murray. 1994. Stimulus recognition. *Curr. Opin. Neurobiol.* **4:** 200.

Moss, M., H. Mahut, and S. Zola-Morgan. 1981. Concurrent discrimination learning of monkeys after hippocampal, entorhinal, or fornix lesions. *J. Neurosci.* **1:** 227.

Murray, E.A. 1992. Medial temporal lobe structures contributing to recognition memory: The amygdaloid complex versus the rhinal cortex. In *The amygdala: Neurobiological aspects of emotion, memory, and mental dysfunction* (ed. J.P. Aggleton), p. 453. Wiley-Liss, New York.

Murray, E.A. and D. Gaffan. 1993. Effects of lesions of rhinal cortex, hippocampus, or parahippocampal gyrus in rhesus monkeys on object and spatial reversals. *Soc. Neurosci. Abstr.* **23:** 438.

Murray, E.A. and M. Mishkin. 1984. Severe tactual as well as visual memory deficits following combined removal of the amygdala and hippocampus in monkeys. *J. Neurosci.* **4:** 2565.

Overman, W.H., G. Ormsby, and M. Mishkin. 1991. Picture recognition vs. picture discrimination learning in monkeys with medial temporal removals. *Exp. Brain Res.* **79:** 18.

Packard, M.G., R. Hirsh, and N.M. White. 1989. Differential effects of fornix and caudate nucleus lesions on two radial maze tasks: Evidence for multiple memory systems. *J. Neurosci.* **9:** 1465.

Ramus, S.J., S. Zola-Morgan, and L.R. Squire. 1994. Effects of lesions of perirhinal cortex on memory in monkeys. *Soc. Neurosci. Abstr.* **24:** 1975.

Reber, P.J. and L.R. Squire. 1994. Parallel brain systems for learning with and without awareness. *Learn. Mem.* **2:** 1.

Reber, P.J., B.J. Knowlton, and L.R. Squire. 1996. Dissociable properties of memory systems: Differences in the flexibility of declarative and nondeclarative knowledge. *Behav. Neurosci.* **110:** 861.

Rempel-Clower, N., S.M. Zola, L.R. Squire, and D.G. Amaral. 1996. Three cases of enduring memory impairment following bilateral damage limited to the hippocampal formation. *J. Neurosci.* **16:** 5233.

Ringo, J.L. 1991. Memory decays at the same rate in macaques with and without brain lesions when expressed in d' or arcsine terms (Comments). *Behav. Brain Res.* **42:** 123.

Sakai, K. and Y. Miyashita. 1991. Neural organization for the long-term memory of paired associated. *Nature* **354:** 152.

Salmon, D.P. and N. Butters. 1995. Neurobiology of skill and habit learning. *Curr. Opin. Neurobiol.* **5:** 184.

Schacter, D.L., C.-Y. Chiu, and K.N. Ochsner. 1993. Implicit memory: A selective review. *Annu. Rev. Neurosci.* **16:** 159.

Schacter, D.L., N.A. Alpert, C.R. Savage, S.L. Ranch, and M.S. Albert. 1996. Conscious recollection and the human hippocampal formation: Evidence from positron emission tomography. *Proc. Natl. Acad. Sci.* **93:** 321.

Scoville, W.B. and B. Milner. 1957. Loss of recent memory after bilateral hippocampal lesions. *J. Neurol. Neurosurg. Psychiatry* **20:** 11.

Sherry, D.F. and D.L. Schacter. 1987. The evolution of multiple memory systems. *Psychol. Rev.* **94:** 439.

Squire, L.R. 1987. *Memory and brain.* Oxford University Press, New York.

———. 1992a. Declarative and nondeclarative memory: Multiple brain systems supporting learning and memory. *J. Cog. Neurosci.* **4:** 232.

———. 1992b. Memory and the hippocampus: A synthesis from findings with rats, monkeys, and humans. *Psychol. Rev.* **99:** 195.

———. 1994. Declarative and nondeclarative memory: Multiple brain systems support learning and memory. In *Memory systems: 1994* (ed. D. Schacter and E. Tulving), p. 203. MIT Press, Cambridge, Massachusetts.

Squire, L.R. and P. Alvarez. 1995. Retrograde amnesia and memory consolidation: A neurobiological perspective. *Curr. Opin. Neurobiol.* **5:** 169.

Squire, L.R. and B.J. Knowlton. 1994. Memory, hippocampus and brain systems. In *The cognitive neurosciences* (ed. M. Gazzaniga), p. 825. MIT Press, Cambridge, Massachusetts.

———. 1995. Learning about categories in the absence of memory. *Proc. Natl. Acad. Sci.* **92:** 12470.

Squire, L.R. and S.M. Zola. 1996a. Ischemic brain damage and memory impairment: A commentary. *Hippocampus* **5:** 546.

———. 1996b. Structure and function of declarative and nondeclarative memory systems. *Proc. Natl. Acad. Sci.* (in press).

———. 1996c. Biological and psychological perspectives on memory and memory disorders. In *ARNMD Proceedings* (ed. L.R. Squire and D.L. Schechter). American Psychiatric Association, Washington, D.C. (In press.)

Squire, L.R. and S. Zola-Morgan. 1983. The neurology of memory: The case for correspondence between the findings for human and nonhuman primate. In *The physiological basis of memory* (ed. J.A. Deutsch), p. 199. Academic Press, New York.

———. 1991. The medial temporal lobe memory system. *Science* **253:** 1380.

Squire, L.R., J.G. Ojemann, F.M. Miezin, S.E. Petersen, T.O. Videen, and M.E. Raichle. 1992. Activation of the hippocampus in normal humans: A functional anatomical study of memory. *Proc. Natl. Acad. Sci.* **89:** 1837.

Suzuki, W.A. and D.G. Amaral. 1994a. Perirhinal and parahippocampal cortices of the macaque monkey: Cortical afferents. *J. Comp. Neurol.* **350:** 497.

———. 1994b. Topographic organization of the reciprocal connections between the monkey entorhinal cortex and the perirhinal and parahippocampal cortices. *J. Neurosci.* **4:** 1856.

Suzuki, W.A., S. Zola-Morgan, L.R. Squire, and D.G. Amaral. 1993. Lesions of the perirhinal and parahippocampal cortices in the monkey produce long-lasting memory impairment in the visual and tactual modalities. *J. Neurosci.* **13:** 2430.

Teyler, T.J. and P. Discenna. 1986. The hippocampal memory indexing theory. *Behav. Neurosci.* **100:** 147.

Thompson, R.F. and D.J. Krupa. 1994. Organization of memory traces in the mammalian brain. *Annu. Rev. Neurosci.* **17:** 519.

Ungerleider, L.G. 1995. Functional brain imaging studies of cortical mechanisms for memory. *Science* **270:** 769.

Vanderwolf, C.H. and D.P. Cain. 1994. The behavioral neurobiology of learning and memory: A conceptual reorientation. *Brain Res. Rev.* **19:** 264.

Van Hoesen, G. 1982. The parahippocampal gyrus: New observations regarding its cortical connections in the monkey. *Trends Neurosci.* **5:** 345.

Van Hoesen, G. and D.N. Pandya. 1975a. Some connections of the entorhinal (area 28) and perirhinal (area 35) cortices of the rhesus monkey. I. Temporal lobe afferents. *Brain Res.* **95:** 1.

———. 1975b. Some connections of the entorhinal (area 28) and perirhinal (area 35) cortices of the rhesus monkey. III. Efferent connections. *Brain Res.* **95:** 39.

Victor, M. and J. Agamanolis. 1990. Amnesia due to lesions confined to the hippocampus: A clinical-pathological study. *J. Cog. Neurosci.* **2:** 246.

Vnek, N. and L.R. Rothblat. 1996. The hippocampus and long-term object memory in the rat. *J. Neurosci.* **16:** 2780.

Vnek, N., T.C. Gleason, L.F. Kromer, and L.A. Rothblat. 1995. Entorhinal-hippocampal connections and object memory in the rat: Acquisition versus retention. *J. Neurosci.* **15:** 3193.

Winocur, G. 1990. Anterograde and retrograde amnesia in rats with dorsal hippocampal or dorsomedial thalamic lesions. *Behav. Brain Res.* **38:** 145.

Zola-Morgan, S. and L.R. Squire. 1990. The primate hippocampal formation: Evidence for a time-limited role in memory storage. *Science* **250:** 288.

———. 1993. Neuroanatomy of amnesia. *Annu. Rev. Neurosci.* **16:** 547.

Zola-Morgan, S., L.R. Squire, and D.G. Amaral. 1986. Human amnesia and the medial temporal region: Enduring memory impairment following a bilateral lesion limited to field CA1 of the hippocampus. *J. Neurosci.* **6:** 2950.

Zola-Morgan, S., L.R. Squire, and S.J. Ramus. 1994. Severity of memory impairment in monkeys as a function of locus and extent of damage within the medial temporal lobe memory system. *Hippocampus* **4:** 483.

Zola-Morgan, S., L.R. Squire, D.G. Amaral, and W.A. Suzuki. 1989. Lesions of perirhinal and parahippocampal cortex that spare the amygdala and hippocampal formation produce severe memory impairment. *J. Neurosci.* **9:** 4355.

Zola-Morgan, S., L.R. Squire, R.P. Clower, and N.L. Rempel. 1993. Damage to the perirhinal cortex but not the amygdala exacerbates memory impairment following lesions to the hippocampal formation. *J. Neurosci.* **12:** 2582.

Zola-Morgan, S., L.R. Squire, N.L. Rempel, R.P. Clower, and D.G. Amaral. 1992. Enduring memory impairment in monkeys after ischemic damage to the hippocampus. *J. Neurosci.* **9:** 4355.

Neural Mechanisms of Declarative Memory

H. EICHENBAUM,[1] J. DUSEK,[1] B. YOUNG,[2] AND M. BUNSEY[3]
[1]*Laboratory of Cognitive Neurobiology, Psychology Department, Boston University, Boston, Massachusetts 02215;* [2]*Department of Psychology, University of Otago, Dunedin, New Zealand;* [3]*Department of Psychology, Kent State University, Kent, Ohio 44242*

During the last two decades, considerable progress has been made toward understanding the brain mechanisms supporting memory representation. This success is due in great part to insights gained from studies of amnesia where memory breaks down into identifiable constituent elements that are differentially lost or spared after localized brain damage. In particular, studies of human amnesia associated with damage to the hippocampal region have shown that this part of the brain supports a capacity for declarative memory, the memory of everyday facts and events that can be brought to conscious recollection and are subject to verbal and other explicit means of expression (Cohen and Squire 1980; Cohen 1984; Corkin 1984; Squire et al. 1993). Our efforts have been directed at improving the resolution of this characterization through studies of hippocampal memory function in animals. This work is focused on key unresolved questions about the fundamental associative mechanisms, critical circuitry, and neural coding schemes that underlie declarative memory.

Characterization of human declarative memory as involving "conscious" and "explicit" recollection has been exceedingly useful for the understanding of hippocampal function in humans, but offers little direction for the development of animal models. Yet, there has been considerable progress in the study of hippocampal function in animals revealing that, as in humans, damage to the hippocampal region results in a selective impairment in some forms of memory while other memory performances are spared (for review, see Cohen and Eichenbaum 1993). Indeed, *two* kinds of dissociation have been prominent in this literature. In monkeys, several studies have shown that damage to the hippocampal region results in a selective impairment in object recognition memory, as well as in several related object memory tasks that involve rapid acquisition and extended retention (Mishkin 1982; Zola-Morgan and Squire 1985). In contrast, incremental learning of stimulus-reward associations and motor skills were completely preserved in animals with hippocampal region damage despite their deficits on object memory tasks. In rats, several dissociations have been demonstrated (see Eichenbaum 1994), the most prominent of which is that damage to the hippocampus results in impairments on spatial learning and memory versus sparing of various forms of stimulus-response and stimulus-reward association (O'Keefe and Nadel 1978; Nadel 1991). Furthermore, electrophysiological studies in rats have shown that hippocampal neurons encode spatial relations among environmental stimuli such that many hippocampal cells can be described as "place cells" that fire only when the animal is in a particular location of its environment, regardless of its orientation or ongoing behavior (O'Keefe 1976). Thus, there are strong parallels between dissociable forms of memory in animals and in humans, although the commonalities among object recognition memory and spatial memory in animals and declarative memory in humans are vague at best.

The connections between these types of memory may be further drawn by examining two general distinctions of hippocampal-dependent memory that are revealed in the studies across species and are differentially emphasized in experiments on monkeys and rats (Eichenbaum et al. 1992a, 1994). First, there is a *temporal distinction* by which the hippocampal region has been shown to be critical to very rapid acquisition of information and to persistent memory representations bridging the gap between short-term and long-term memory. Capacities for rapid acquisition and prolonged memory persistence are evident in a broad range of human memory tasks and are particularly prominent in the studies on object recognition in monkeys. Second, there is a *representational distinction* by which the hippocampal region is involved in aspects of memory organization and expression that mediate capacities for declarative memory in humans and are particularly evident in studies on spatial learning in rats. In this paper, we summarize some of our own explorations of the temporal and representational distinctions of hippocampal memory function using a rodent model system. Our data suggest that the neural mechanisms underlying these distinctions are dissociable and may be supported differentially by specific components of the hippocampal system.

MAJOR PATHWAYS OF HIPPOCAMPAL PROCESSING

Before we describe our results, we provide a brief review of the anatomy of the hippocampal system to introduce the components of the system that are the focus of the experiments described below (Fig. 1). The hippocampus is connected with other structures of the brain via two pathways, one that might be thought of

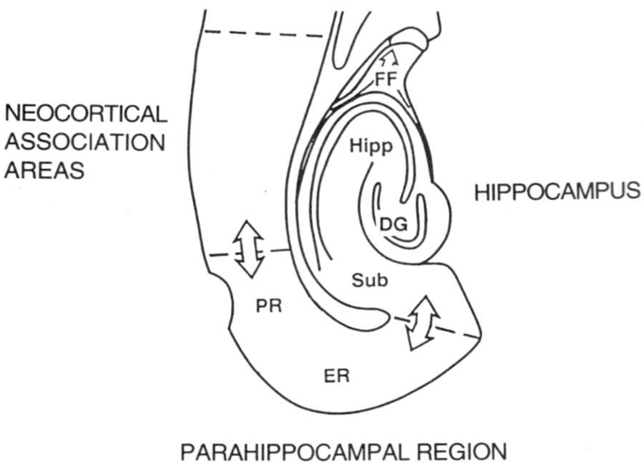

Figure 1. Simple schematic diagram of cortical-hippocampal connections illustrated on the outline of a horizontal rat brain section. (DG) Dentate gyrus; (ER) entorhinal cortex; (FF) fimbria-fornix; (Hipp) hippocampus proper; (PR) perirhinal cortex; (Sub) subiculum.

as the pathway bearing specific memory representations and the other that likely mediates modulatory and timing functions of the hippocampus. The information-bearing circuit involves the convergence of wide-ranging inputs directed from virtually every cortical association area into the parahippocampal region, a set of cortical structures including the perirhinal cortex, entorhinal cortex, and parahippocampal gyrus (Amaral and Witter 1989; Witter et al. 1989; Burwell et al. 1995). The parahippocampal region sends the major cortical inputs from intermediate layers II and III to the hippocampus proper within each of its major subfields, including the dentate gyrus, CA3, CA1, and the subiculum. Hippocampal outputs of this pathway return to deep layers of the parahippocampal region, and then this area projects heavily back to the same cortical association areas that were the origin of its inputs. Thus, the information-bearing pathway consists of two stages of bidirectional interaction: direct interactions between the cortex and parahippocampal region, and interactions between the cortex and hippocampus itself mediated via the parahippocampal region. In this paper, we present evidence that direct cortical-parahippocampal interactions are sufficient to support some memory functions independent of the hippocampus, and that the hippocampus itself mediates a distinct memory-processing function.

The pathway mediating modulatory and timing circuits of hippocampus involves bidirectional connections between subfields within the hippocampus itself and several subcortical nuclei (primarily the septal complex, mammillary bodies, and anterior thalamus) via the fornix (Fig. 1). The functions of this pathway are not the focus of the present paper. However, in some of the studies described below, we transected the fornix as one way to produce a selective dysfunction of the hippocampus, taking advantage of the fact that fornix transection disrupts subcortical connections of hippocampus while sparing bidirectional cortical-parahippocampal connections as well as the subcortical connections of the parahippocampal region, which do not pass through the fornix.

CRITICAL ROLE OF THE PARAHIPPOCAMPAL REGION IN RECOGNITION MEMORY

As introduced above, one way the temporal properties of declarative memory have been studied extensively is with a simple recognition memory test known as delayed nonmatch to sample. In the task originally designed for monkeys, animals are presented with a novel sample object and rewarded for displacing it (Gaffan 1974; Mishkin and Delacour 1975). Then, after a variable memory delay, they are presented with two objects, one identical to the sample and the other a novel object. In this choice phase, monkeys are rewarded for selecting the novel, nonmatching object (this rule is easily learned because monkeys are naturally attracted to novel objects). The delayed nonmatch-to-sample task is ideal for measuring the persistence of memory representations for single, isolated stimuli. Indeed, to the extent that memory performance can be related specifically to variations in the length of the memory delay, it would seem this task selectively assesses the temporal distinction of hippocampal memory processing.

We have described the role of components of the hippocampal system in recognition memory using two strategies, neuropsychological studies that determine the effects of damage to different hippocampal structures on performance of the delayed nonmatch-to-sample task, and electrophysiological studies that characterize the firing properties of neurons in different components of the hippocampal region of animals performing this task. In both lines of study, we exploited rats' superb olfactory learning and memory in the development of a variant of the delayed nonmatch-to-sample task, called continuous delayed nonmatch-to-sample (cDNM), which employed odor cues and involved a stimulus presentation protocol suitable for characterizing neural firing patterns to single memory stimuli as well as behavioral responses in accordance with the nonmatch memory contingency (Otto and Eichenbaum 1992a,b). On each trial, one of a large set of odors was presented with the contingency that an appropriate response to the odor was rewarded only if that odor was different from (that is, a nonmatch with) the immediately preceding odor. Rats were trained initially with a very brief interval between odor presentations. Subsequently, the interstimulus interval was manipulated to vary the retention delay, allowing an assessment of the persistence of memory as in the earlier studies on monkeys.

In an initial experiment, we compared the effects of selective ablation of the parahippocampal region versus fornix transection that selectively disrupts hippocampal function (Otto and Eichenbaum 1992a).

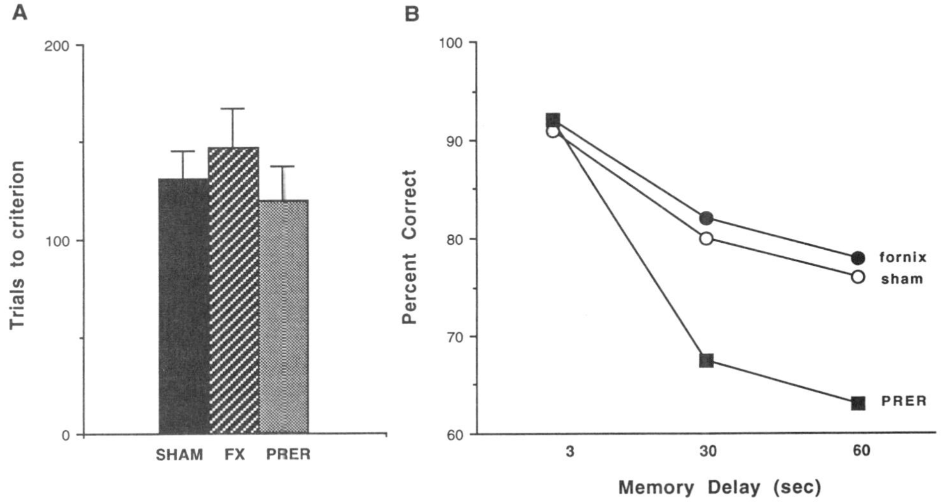

Figure 2. Performance of sham-operated rats (SHAM) and rats with transection of the fornix (FX) or lesions of the parahippocampal region (PRER) on initial acquisition of the cDNM task (*A*) and when the memory delay was increased (*B*).

Normal rats acquired the task within approximately 150 trials, and neither lesion affected the acquisition rate (Fig. 2A). In subsequent tests across memory delays, intact rats showed 90% or better retention at the shortest delay, and their memory performance gradually declined as the retention interval was increased (Fig. 2B). Rats with damage to the parahippocampal region also showed good retention at the shortest delay, but their performance declined abnormally rapidly, showing a severe deficit within 1 minute. In contrast, rats with fornix lesions performed identically with normal rats both during task acquisition and across delays, showing both intact performance at the short delay and the same gradual memory decay as normal rats. These findings indicated that neither the parahippocampal region nor the hippocampus is critical to the perception of the odor cues, nor is either component of the system necessary for acquisition of the nonmatch rule or short-term memory for odors. However, the parahippocampal region is critical to mediating a memory representation that persists beyond immediate memory in rats, as it is in monkeys. Furthermore, we may infer from these results that through its direct, reciprocal connections with the cortex, the parahippocampal region is sufficient to mediate the persistence of single-item memories independent of hippocampal processing.

In complementary electrophysiological studies, we have also examined the response properties of neurons in the parahippocampal region and in the hippocampus in rats performing the odor-guided cDNM task (Young et al. 1995). In our studies on the parahippocampal region, we examined the firing patterns of cells in these areas both during the period when rats were sampling the odor cues, in order to assess the extent to which odors were selectively encoded, and during the memory delay to determine the capacity of these areas to maintain an odor memory representation. For the latter, we focused on the trial period at the end of the memory delay, that is, immediately preceding the initiation of trials succeeding a particular odor presentation. At this time, the overt behavior of the animal is consistent (it is approaching the stimulus port), allowing us to determine if neural activity varies with the identity of the preceding odor just before the recognition judgment must be made.

We found that a substantial proportion of cells in each of the subdivisions of the parahippocampal region and subiculum encode the identity of the odor cues during the odor sampling period (Fig. 3A). Some of these cells fired selectively or differentially to odors at odor onset and ceased firing when odor sampling was concluded, much as one would expect of a sensory neuron (Fig. 4A). In addition, other cells showed striking odor-specific activity during odor sampling and then throughout the delay period, such as the example shown in Figure 4B. Indeed, substantial numbers of cells in each of the subdivisions of the parahippocampal region demonstrated selective or differential firing patterns that were apparent in our systematic analysis of firing patterns at the end of the delay period (Fig. 3B).

To assess odor memory representations in the hippocampus itself, we recorded from CA1 pyramidal neurons of rats performing the cDNM task (Otto and Eichenbaum 1992b). A large proportion of hippocampal cells was actively associated with virtually every identifiable behavioral event in the task. A substantial subset of these cells was selectively active during the odor stimulus sampling period, and the activity of some of these hippocampal cells reflected the match or nonmatch relationship critical to performance in this task (Fig. 5). In contrast to cells in the parahippocampal region, no hippocampal cells fired associated with the sampling of a particular odor or with particular combinations of odors that composed specific

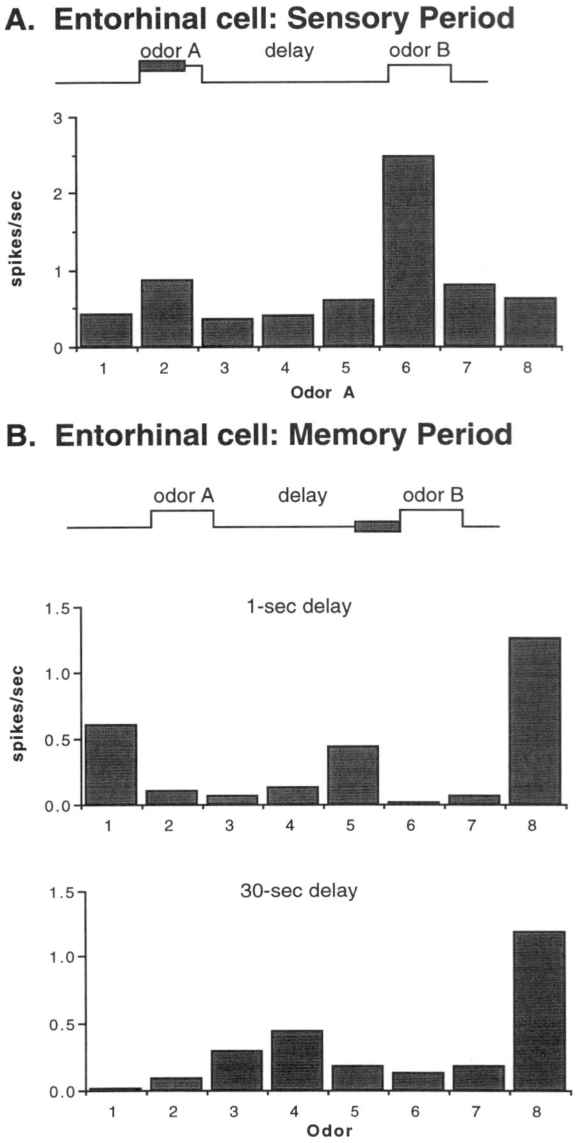

Figure 3. Neural activity in the parahippocampal region associated with delayed nonmatch-to-sample performance. Firing rates are shown for 0.5-sec periods of odor cue sampling or at the end of the memory delay associated with each of eight different odors. (A) Firing patterns of a cell that was selectively active during the odor sampling period. (*B*) Firing patterns of a cell that was differentially activated at the end of the memory delay regardless of the length of the delay.

matching comparisons. Rather, hippocampal cellular activity reflected all comparisons with the same outcome. We interpreted this finding as entirely consistent with the results of our lesion studies. It appears that the hippocampus itself is not involved in the encoding and storage of representations for specific items in this task. Instead, it appears that the hippocampus encodes abstract relations among cues, as it does in many other test situations. Thus, for example, the match/mismatch relationship reflected in the activity of hippocampal cells in animals performing the cDNM task can be viewed as analogous to the spatial relations among cues reflected in the firing patterns of hippocampal place cells when rats explore open fields (O'Keefe 1979). Indeed, across a broad range of tasks, hippocampal cells encode all manner of relations among salient stimuli as well as behavioral actions (Eichenbaum and Cohen 1988; Eichenbaum 1993, 1996; Deadwyler et al. 1995). In the cDNM task, "relational" cells in the hippocampus may mediate memory for match and nonmatch trial outcomes, even though this information contributes little directly to performance on this simple recognition task. Consistent with our data from the lesion study, the parahippocampal region, but not the hippocampus, maintains specific and persistent representations sufficient to support recognition performance.

THE HIPPOCAMPUS, MEMORY FOR STIMULUS RELATIONS, AND FLEXIBLE MEMORY EXPRESSION

The above-described findings on hippocampal neuronal firing patterns, among a substantial body of other neuropsychological and electrophysiological evidence, led us to suggest that the hippocampus is critical for mediating the organization of memories according to the relevant relationships among remembered stimuli (Eichenbaum et al. 1992a, 1994; Cohen and Eichenbaum 1993). In addition, we have proposed that such a relational representation supports the ability to express knowledge about indirectly related items in the memory organization in a variety of ways outside repetition of learning events. We have assessed the role of the hippocampus in several different memory tasks, each of which requires the animal to learn an organization of relationships among odor cues, and each of which requires the animal to use its memory representations flexibly, that is, in situations that challenge the animal to employ the learned memory organization outside repetition of the learning trials.

Three such tasks that exploit rats' superb memory capacities with odors are described here. Each experiment focused on the role of the hippocampus itself and exploited some aspect of "natural" rodent behavior in using odor memory cues. However, the tasks differed in the nature of the learned association and how it was expressed in behavior. A brief summary of our results emphasizes both the generality of associations supported by the hippocampus and its common role in mediating relational organizations and flexible memory expression.

Paired Associate Learning

One memory test that requires learning specific relationships among cues is the paired associate task. The verbal paired associate task has been exceedingly useful in understanding cognitive aspects of associative

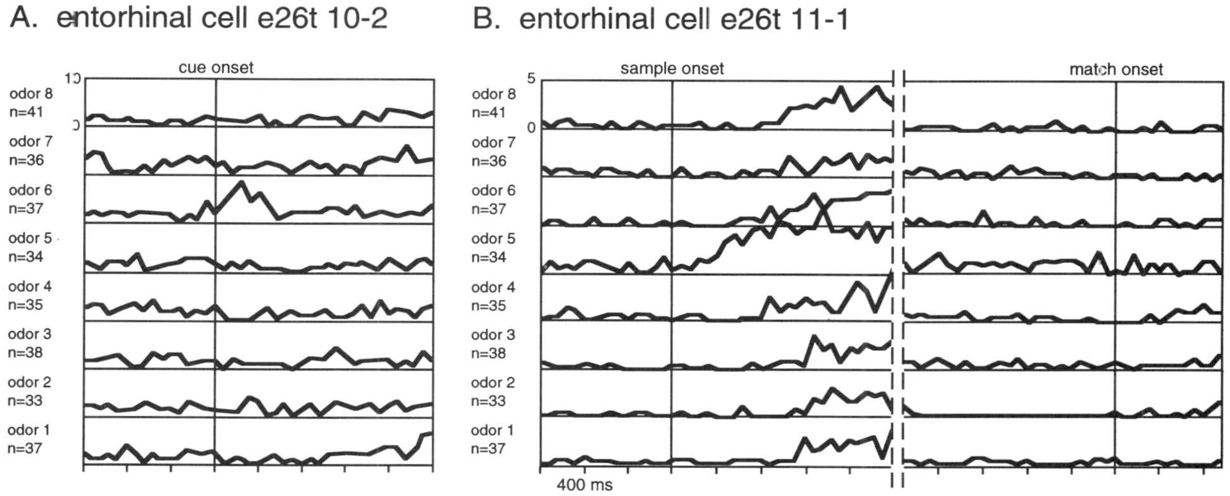

Figure 4. Neural activity in the parahippocampal region associated with delayed nonmatch-to-sample performance. (*A*) Responses of a cell during the 2 sec following the onset of different odors. (*B*) Activity of another cell during the cue sampling period and during the last 2 sec of that delay period; i.e., prior to the onset of the subsequent odor matching cue.

learning in humans and is often applied in the assessment of human amnesia. It seemed to us that a paired associate task adapted for animals was the simplest paradigm that we could exploit for neurobiological studies on the learning of new associations between distinct and neutral stimulus events. The paired associate task as typically used for humans involves presentation of a list of arbitrarily paired words followed by testing in which the subject is cued with the first item of each pair and must recall the second item. For rats, we designed an analogous task using odor stimuli and a recognition format that required subjects to distinguish in each of a series of trials the appropriate associate for a sample odor (Bunsey and Eichenbaum 1996). Exploiting rodents' natural foraging strategies that employ olfactory cues, animals were trained with stimuli that consisted of distinctive odors added to a mixture of ground rat chow and sand through which they dug to obtain buried cereal rewards. On each paired associate trial one of two sample odors initially presented was followed by two choice odors, each assigned as the "associate" of one of the samples and baited only when preceded by that sample (Fig. 6A,B). Following training on two sets of overlapping odor-odor associations, subsequent probe tests were used to characterize the extent to which learned representations supported two forms of flexible memory expression: *transitivity,* the ability to judge inferentially across stimulus pairs that share a common element; and *symmetry,* the ability to associate paired elements presented in the reverse of training order.

Intact rats learned paired associates rapidly, and hippocampal damage did not affect acquisition rate on either of the two training sets (Fig. 6C). Intact rats also showed strong transitivity across the sets with a preference of approximately 2:1 in favor of choice items directly associated with the presented sample (Fig. 6D). In contrast, rats with selective hippocampal lesions were severely impaired in that they showed no evidence of transitivity. In the symmetry test, intact rats again showed the appropriate preference of approximately 3:1 in the direction of the symmetrical association (Fig. 6E). In contrast, rats with hippocampal lesions again were severely impaired, showing no significant capacity for symmetry. These findings indicate that some form of representation that supports stimulus-stimulus learning is intact in rats with selective hippocampal damage, as previously reported for rats and monkeys with hippocampal region damage (Saunders and Weiskrantz 1989; Murray et al. 1993; Cho and Kesner 1995; Eichenbaum and Bunsey 1995), as well as for human amnesiacs (Musen and Squire 1993; Moscovitch 1994). However, this form of representation does not support the inferential expression of indirect or symmetrical associations among stimuli—such "flexibility" in representation and memory expression relies on the hippocampus itself.

Serial Order Learning

The paired associate task described above involves learning that odor elements are associated with one another, perhaps the simplest kind of relationship that can exist between remembered items. However, we and other investigators (see, e.g., McClelland et al. 1995) believe that declarative memory organizations in humans, as well as spatial memories dependent on hippocampal function in rats (O'Keefe and Nadel 1978), involve learning a systematic organization of many interrelated items. A task that was developed to examine the capacity for expression of a systematic organization is the serial order learning test. In this task, subjects

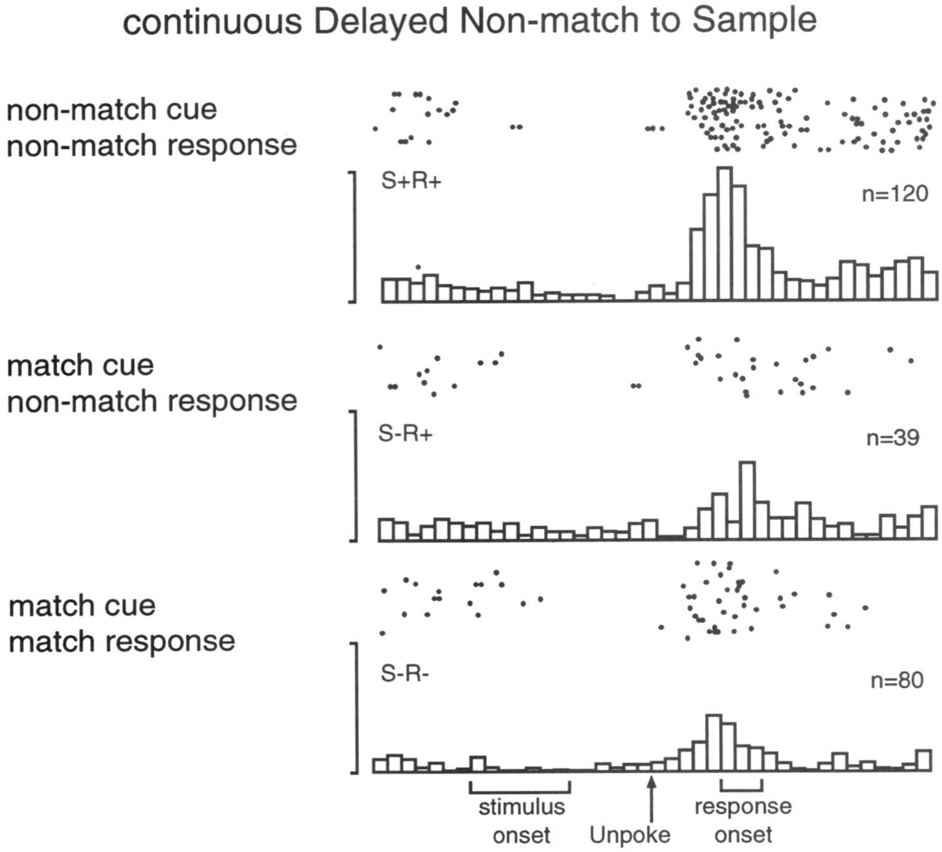

Figure 5. Neural activity in the hippocampus associated with delayed nonmatch-to-sample performance. The "unpoke" represents the instant when the rat ceases odor sampling and begins to make the discriminative response. See text for description.

learn pairwise comparisons that can be organized as a serial ordering of arbitrary stimuli. Thus, a typical training set involves comparisons A > B, then B > C, then C > D, then D > E, where rats are trained to select items to the left of the ">" over those on the right. This set of comparisons can be efficiently represented by the serial organization A > B > C > D > E. A central asset of the serial representation is that it can be expected to support novel judgments about nonadjacent items in the ordered series, in particular, the judgment B > D. Note that each stimulus (with the exception of A and E) is associated with reward on only half of the choices, so the choice of B over D cannot be made solely on the basis of differential reward history. A direct control for the capacity for such a noninferential judgment is provided in presentation of the A > E comparison, where the appropriate selection of A can be based on acquisition of a preference for this object whose selection was always followed by reward, and avoidance of object E, whose selection was never followed by reward. It has previously been determined that children acquire the capacity for serial organization, revealed by consistent transitive judgments of this type, at about age 6 (Bryant and Trabasso 1971). Several experiments have shown that chimpanzees (Gillian 1981), new world monkeys (McGonigle and Chalmers 1977), and rats (Davis 1992) can also learn this type of one-dimensional serial organization.

Using the same foraging behavior described for our paired associate task above, subjects were initially rewarded for selecting the appropriate item in adjacent premise pairs (A > B, B > C, etc.) with blocks of 10 trials for each of the pairs presented in sequence (Dusek and Eichenbaum 1996). Then the number of trials in training blocks was gradually reduced until each pair was presented only once, and finally, all the premise pairs were intermixed in the same session. In the probe testing sessions we presented the critical probe pair B > D, as well as the nontransitive probe A > E, 10 times intermixed among 180 repetitions of the premise pairs. Because rats rapidly extinguish on nonrewarded probe trials, the expected choice on each of these tests (B and A, respectively) was rewarded on these probe trials. To test whether any observed differences in performance on these probes could have been due to learning the new pairings within the 10 presentations, we included additional testing sessions where new odor pairs were presented on 10 intermingled trials with one of each pair consistently rewarded.

We found that intact rats can acquire each of the

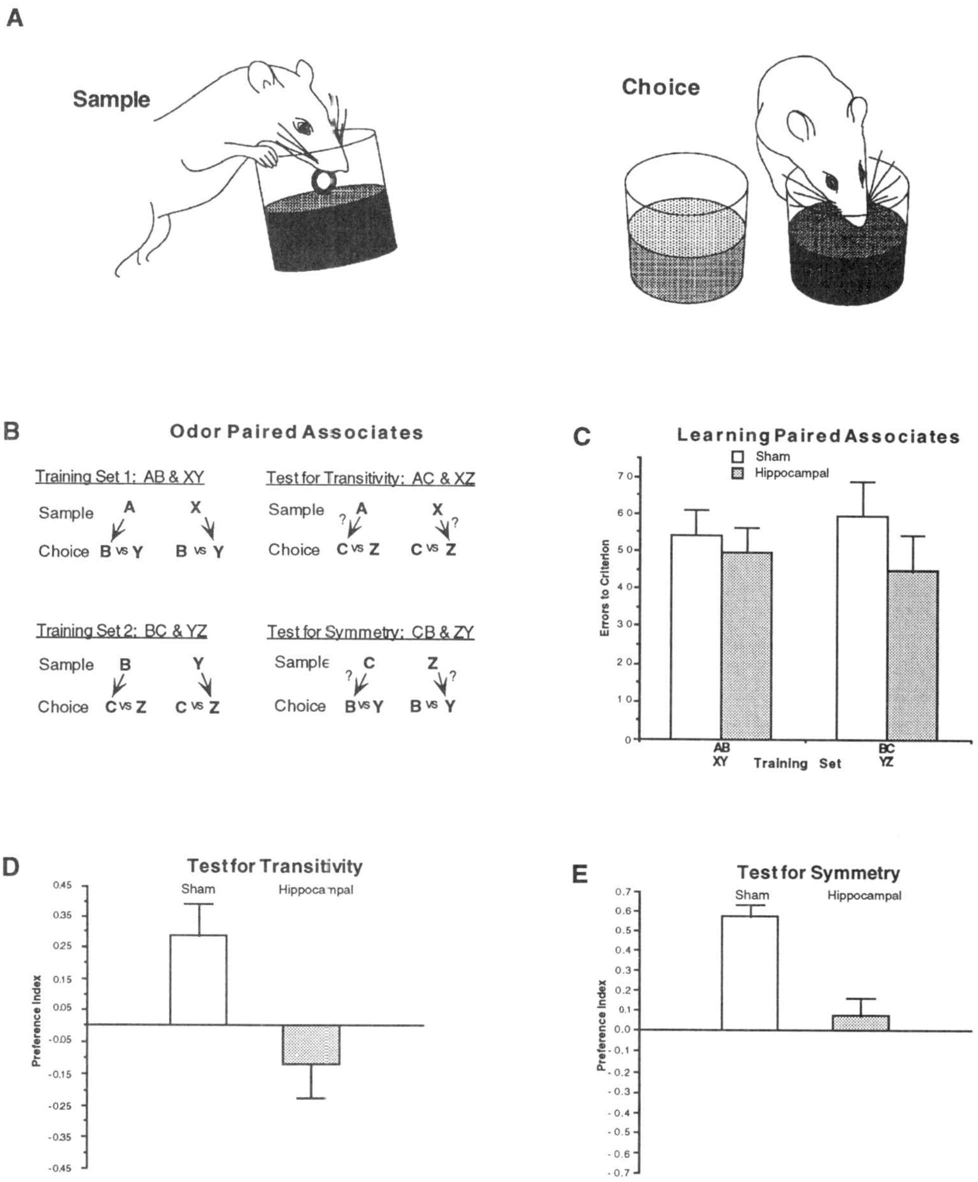

Figure 6. Inferential expression of odor-odor associations in sham-operated rats and rats with selective neurotoxic lesions of the hippocampus. (*A*) Rat and stimulus cups during sample and choice phases of the task. (*B*) Schematic diagram of paired associate training and probe testing. Letters represent odor stimulus items; arrows without question marks indicate trained pairings, whereas arrows with question marks indicate expected transitive and symmetrical choices. (*C*) Errors to criterion on acquisition of the two sets of paired associates for sham-operated and hippocampal subjects. (*D*) Preference indices on the test for transitive inference. For these probe trials, a preference score was calculated as (X–Y)/(X+Y), where X and Y were the digging times in the transitive and alternate choices, respectively. (*E*) Preference indices on the test for symmetrical expression.

premise pairs of the serial order problem, and they perform well on concurrent presentations of all of these pairings during probe testing (Fig. 7). Furthermore, normal rats made the appropriate transitive judgment between stimuli B and D about as accurately as their overall performance on the premise pairs. Rats with fornix transection or perirhinal-entorhinal cortex lesions also acquired the premise pairs at the normal rate and performed them in concurrent presentations. However, rats with either fornix transection or removal of the parahippocampal region showed no capacity for the transitive inference. They performed much worse than normal rats on the B > D transitive judgment, and their performance was not better than that expected by chance. In the control trials, intact rats and rats with fornix or perirhinal-entorhinal lesions accurately selected stimulus A over stimulus E, which could be guided by a bias for stimulus A and a bias against E. This finding indicates that the deficit in rats with fornix or parahippocampal lesions was not due merely to the

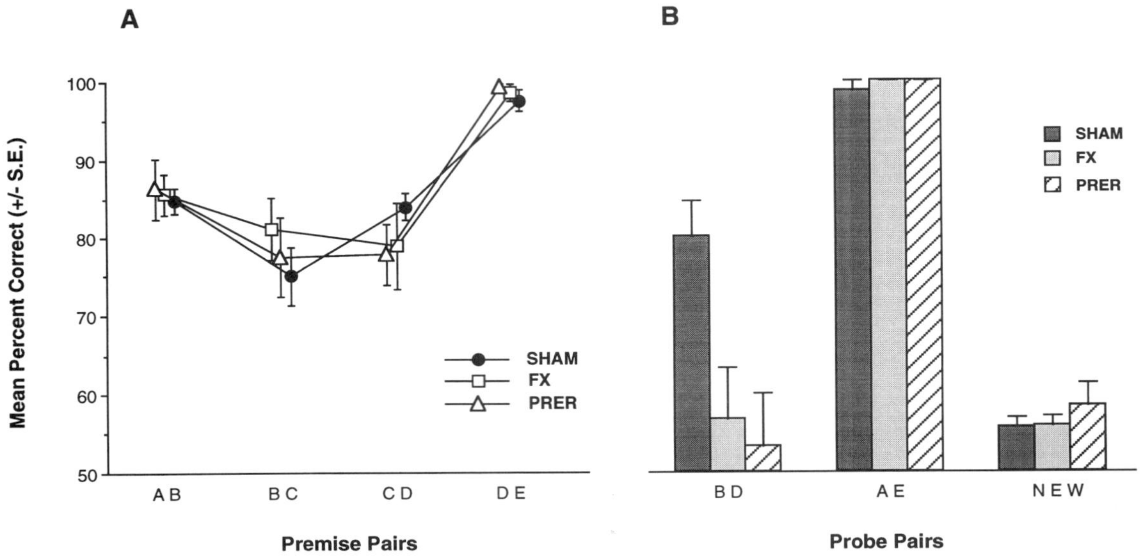

Figure 7. Transitive inference in serial ordering by sham-operated rats (SHAM) and rats with transection of the fornix (FX) or lesions of the parahippocampal region (PRER). (*A*) Performance levels after training on the premise pairs A > B, B > C, C > D, and D > E. (*B*) Performance on probe trials: BD involves the critical transitive judgment, AE can be solved by a nontransitive judgment, and columns labeled NEW reflect the extent of learning of two new odor pairings. See text for explanation.

novelty of the stimulus presentation when no transitive judgment was required. Finally, none of the groups learned the new pairs in the few intermixed trials on the novel discriminations. This pattern of results, combined with those from paired associate learning, indicates that some form of stimulus-stimulus representations can be acquired independent of the hippocampus itself, although these representations are "hyperspecific," that is, they can only be expressed within the confined context of reproduction of the learning event (Eichenbaum et al. 1992b). Only a hippocampally mediated representation can support the flexible expression of associations among items within a larger organization in various and even novel situations.

Social Learning of Odor-odor Associations

To further investigate the range of hippocampal involvement in natural forms of stimulus association, we also assessed the role of the hippocampal region in a type of social olfactory learning and memory that relies on flexible expression of an odor-odor association. The paradigm we used, called the social transmission of food preferences (Galef 1990), involves alterations in food selection patterns consequent to experience with a conspecific that has recently eaten a particular food. When an "observer" rat encounters another ("demonstrator") rat that has recently eaten a distinctively scented food, the probability that the observer will later select that same food over other foods increases. This form of social learning is interpreted within the adaptive heuristic that a food recently consumed by a conspecific is safe. In a series of studies, Galef (1990) has shown that the mechanism underlying this learning involves an association between two odors present in the observer rat's breath, the odor of the recently eaten food and an odorous constituent of rat's breath, carbon disulfide. It is of particular importance that exposing the observer to the distinctive food odor alone, or to carbon disulfide alone, has no effect on later food preference. Thus, the shift in food choice cannot be attributed to mere familiarity with the food odor. In contrast, exposure to the scented food mixed with carbon disulfide, even without the social context in which this association is usually experienced, increased later consumption of food with the same odor. The clear conclusion from these studies is that the formation of a specific stimulus-stimulus association, in the absence of any primary reinforcement, is both necessary and sufficient to influence later food selection.

Following on a previous observation that this type of learning is dependent on the hippocampal region (Winocur 1990), we investigated the role of the hippocampus itself in this task, assessing both immediate memory and delayed (24 hour) memory for social exposure to the odor of a novel food (Bunsey and Eichenbaum 1995). Normal rats showed strong memory in both tests (Fig. 8B). In contrast, rats with damage selective to the hippocampus itself showed intact short-term memory but completely forgot the association within 24 hours. These findings, similar to the pattern of sparing of immediate memory and impairment in delayed recall in human amnesiacs, indicate that the hippocampus is not required for perceptual or motivational components of learning or for the ability to express a learned food selection. However, the hip-

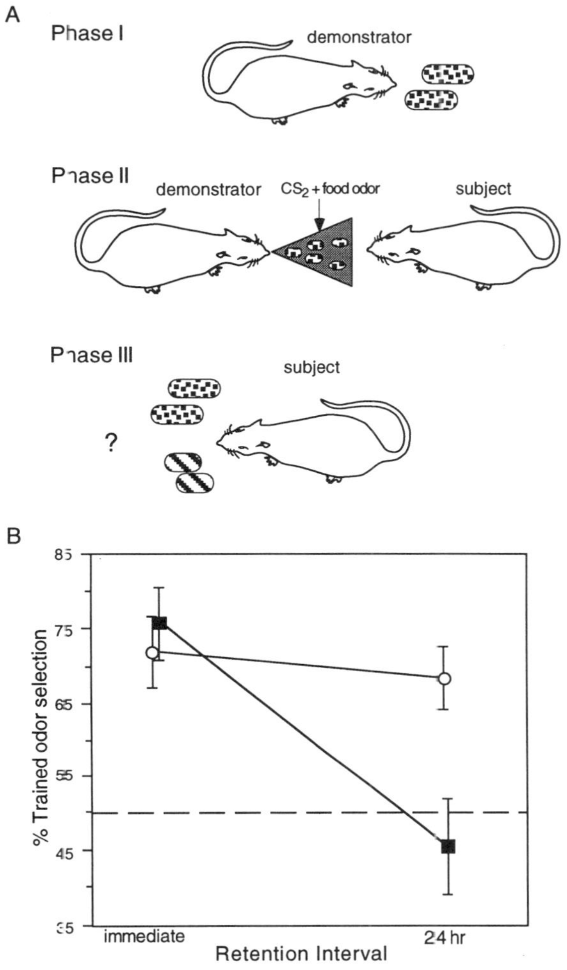

Figure 8. (*A*) Training and testing on a "naturalistic" odor-odor association. In Phase I, a "demonstrator" rat is given a distinctively scented food. Then, in Phase II, the demonstrator is presented to an experimental subject for a brief period of social interaction. In Phase III, subjects are presented with the same food or another distinctively scented food, either immediately or after a 24-hr delay. (*B*) Effects of hippocampal lesions on performance in an immediate or 24-hr delayed retention test.

pocampus itself is required for long-term expression of this natural stimulus association in guiding behavior in a test well outside the original learning situation.

CONCLUSIONS

The findings described here support the view that the contributions of the hippocampal system to declarative memory can be fractionated into distinct components. One component is the ability to form representations following a single experience and to maintain the memory for an extended period through interfering events. Complementary neuropsychological and electrophysiological evidence presented here indicates that this function can be supported by the parahippocampal region even in the absence of hippocampal processing.

With regard to the hippocampus itself, the findings presented here provide compelling evidence for a role of the hippocampus itself in relational memory representation and in flexible memory expression. This capacity should be thought of as an extension of classic views on human memory, such as William James's (1890) description of memory as involving an elaborate network of associations that can be applied across a broad range of situations, as distinct from habits that depend on rigid associative sequences. These findings are also entirely consistent with present-day characterizations of human declarative memory, such as Cohen's (Cohen and Eichenbaum 1993) description of declarative memory as "promiscuous" in its accessibility by novel routes of expression.

Taken together, the results of the studies presented here provide a preliminary picture of the processes that mediate declarative memory. It appears the parahippocampal region contributes to declarative memory by "buffering" specific representations that can be accessed and manipulated by the hippocampus. Then the hippocampus represents the critical relations among the items held by the parahippocampal region and, indeed, has access to the much larger organization of item representations in cortical association areas via the parahippocampal region. We presume the full relational memory organization comes about through multiple iterations of cortical input to the parahippocampal region and temporary storage there. This might be followed by hippocampal relational processing that adds to or restructures interconnections among parahippocampal and then cortical representations. Over extended time periods, new experiences that bear on the established organization reactivate established representations as well as add new ones, and these are processed together by this hippocampal circuit to weave the new information into the established relational network. Precisely because this network is so extensive and systematically interconnected, access to items via novel routes and in novel experiences not only is possible, but also occurs continuously as we express memories to guide almost every aspect of daily life.

ACKNOWLEDGMENTS

This work was supported by the National Institute of Mental Health, the National Institute on Aging, and the Office of Naval Research.

REFERENCES

Amaral, D.G. and M.P. Witter. 1989. The three-dimensional organization of the hippocampal formation: A review of anatomical data. *Neuroscience* **31:** 571.

Bryant, P.E. and T. Trabasso. 1971. Transitive inferences and memory in young children. *Nature* **232:** 456.

Bunsey, M. and H. Eichenbaum. 1995. Selective damage to the hippocampal region blocks long term retention of a natural and nonspatial stimulus-stimulus association. *Hippocampus* **5:** 546.

———. 1996. Conservation of hippocampal memory function in rats and humans. *Nature* **379:** 255.

Burwell, R.D., M.P. Witter, and D.G. Amaral. 1995. Perirhinal and postrhinal cortices in the rat: A review of the neuroanatomical literature and comparison with findings from the monkey brain. *Hippocampus* **5:** 390.

Cho, Y.H. and R.P. Kesner. 1995. Relational object association learning in rats with hippocampal lesions. *Behav. Brain Res.* **67:** 91.

Cohen, N.J. 1984. Preserved learning capacity in amnesia: Evidence for multiple memory systems. In *The neuropsychology of memory* (ed. N. Butters and L.R. Squire), p. 83. Guilford Press, New York.

Cohen, N.J. and H. Eichenbaum. 1993. *Memory, amnesia, and the hippocampal system.* M.I.T. Press, Cambridge, Massachusetts.

Cohen, N.J. and L.R. Squire. 1980. Preserved learning and retention of a pattern- analyzing skill in amnesia: Dissociation of knowing how and knowing that. *Science* **210:** 207.

Corkin, S. 1984. Lasting consequences of bilateral medial temporal lobectomy: Clinical course and experimental findings in H.M. *Semin. Neurol.* **4:** 249.

Davis, H. 1992. Transitive inference in rats. *J. Comp. Psychol.* **106:** 342.

Deadwyler, S.A., T. Bunn, and R. E. Hampson. 1995. Hippocampal ensemble activity during spatial delayed-non-match-to-sample performance in rats. *J. Neurosci.* **16:** 354.

Dusek, J. and H. Eichenbaum. 1996. The effects of lesions to the perirhinal and entorhinal cortices or fornix on the transitive inference task. *Soc. Neurosci. Abstr.* (in press).

Eichenbaum, H. 1993. Thinking about brain cell assemblies. *Science* **261:** 993.

———. 1994. The hippocampal system and declarative memory in humans and animals: Experimental analysis and historical origins. In *Memory systems 1994* (ed. D.L. Schacter and E. Tulving), p. 147. M.I.T. Press, Cambridge, Massachusetts.

———. 1996. Is the rodent hippocampus just for "place"? *Curr. Opin. Neurobiol.* **6:** 187.

Eichenbaum, H. and M. Bunsey. 1995. On the binding of associations in memory: Clues from studies on the role of the hippocampal region in paired-associate learning. *Curr. Dir. Psychol. Sci.* **4:** 19.

Eichenbaum, H. and N.J. Cohen. 1988. Representation in the hippocampus: What do the neurons code? *Trends Neurosci.* **11:** 244.

Eichenbaum, H., T. Otto, and N.J. Cohen. 1992a. The hippocampus—What does it do? *Behav. Neural Biol.* **57:** 2.

———. 1994. Two functional components of the hippocampal memory system. *Brain Behav. Sci.* **17:** 449.

Eichenbaum, H., N.J. Cohen, T. Otto, and C.G. Wible. 1992b. A snapshot without the album. *Brain Res. Rev.* **16:** 209.

Gaffan, D. 1974. Recognition impaired and association intact in the memory of monkeys after transection of the fornix. *J. Comp. Physiol. Psychol.* **86:** 1100.

Galef, B.G. 1990. An adaptionist perspective on social learning, social feeding, and social foraging in Norway rats. In *Contemporary issues in comparative psychology* (ed. D.A. Dewsbury), p. 55. Sinauer, Sunderland, Massachusetts.

Gillian, D.J. 1981. Reasoning in the chimpanzee. II. Transitive inference. *J. Exp. Psychol.* **7:** 150.

James, W. 1890. *The principles of psychology*. (1918 edition) Holt, New York.

McClelland, J.L., B.L. McNaughton, and R.C. O'Reilly. 1995. Why there are complementary learning systems in the hippocampus and neocortex: Insights from successes and failures of connectionist models of learning and memory. *Psychol. Rev.* **102:** 419.

McGonigle, B. and M. Chalmers. 1977. Are monkeys logical? *Nature* **267:** 694.

Mishkin, M. 1982. A memory system in the monkey. *Philos. Trans. R. Soc. Lond. Biol. Sci.* **B209:** 85.

Mishkin, M. and J. Delacour. 1975. An analysis of short-term visual memory in the monkey. *J. Exp. Psychol. Anim. Behav. Processes* **1:** 326.

Moscovitch, M. 1994. Memory and working with memory: Evaluation of a component process model comparisons with other models. In *Memory systems 1994* (ed. D.L. Schacter and E. Tulving), p. 269. M.I.T. Press, Cambridge, Massachusetts.

Murray, E.A., D. Gaffan, and M. Mishkin. 1993. Neural substrates of visual stimulus-stimulus association in rhesus monkeys. *J. Neurosci.* **13:** 4549.

Musen, G. and L.R. Squire. 1993. On the implicit learning of novel associations by amnesic patients and normal subjects. *Neuropsychologia* **7:** 119.

Nadel, L. 1991. The hippocampus and space revisited. *Hippocampus* **1:** 221.

O'Keefe, J.A. 1976. Place units in the hippocampus of the freely moving rat. *Exp. Neurol.* **51:** 78.

———. 1979. A review of hippocampal place cells. *Prog. Neurobiol.* **13:** 419.

O'Keefe, J. and L. Nadel. 1978. *The hippocampus as a cognitive map*. Oxford University Press, New York.

Otto, T. and H. Eichenbaum. 1992a. Neuronal activity in the hippocampus during delayed non-match to sample performance in rats: Evidence for hippocampal processing in recognition memory. *Hippocampus* **2:** 323.

———. 1992b. Complementary roles of orbital prefrontal cortex and the perirhinal-entorhinal cortices in an odor-guided delayed non-matching to sample task. *Behav. Neurosci.* **106:** 763.

Saunders R.C. and L. Weiskrantz. 1989. The effects of fornix transection and combined fornix transection, mammillary body lesions and hippocampal ablations on object pair association memory in the rhesus monkey. *Behav. Brain Res.* **35:** 85.

Squire, L.R., B. Knowlton, and G. Musen. 1993. The structure and organization of memory. *Annu. Rev. Psychol.* **44:** 453.

Winocur, G. 1990. Anterograde and retrograde amnesia in rats with dorsal hippocampal or dorsomedial thalamic lesions. *Behav. Brain Res.* **38:** 145.

Witter, M.P., H.J. Groenewegen, F.H. Lopes da Silva, and A.H.M. Lohman. 1989. Functional organization of the extrinsic and intrinsic circuitry of the parahippocampal region. *Prog. Neurobiol.* **33:** 161.

Young, B.J., T. Otto, G.D. Fox, and H. Eichenbaum. 1995. Neuronal activity in the parahippocampal region of rats performing a delayed non-match to sample task. *Soc. Neurosci. Abstr.* **21:** 943.

Zola-Morgan, S. and L.R. Squire. 1985. Medial temporal lesions in monkeys impair memory on a variety of tasks sensitive to human amnesia. *Behav. Neurosci.* **99:** 22.

A Return to Genetic Dissection of Memory in *Drosophila*

T. TULLY, G. BOLWIG, J. CHRISTENSEN, J. CONNOLLY, M. DELVECCHIO, J. DEZAZZO, J. DUBNAU, C. JONES, S. PINTO, M. REGULSKI, B. SVEDBERG, AND K. VELINZON
Cold Spring Harbor Laboratory, Cold Spring Harbor, New York 11724

Initial attempts to identify and characterize single-gene mutants with defective learning or memory were begun by S. Benzer and colleagues at the California Institute of Technology. Quinn et al. (1974) developed for *Drosophila* an olfactory learning task, which associated an odor cue with footshock. Dudai et al. (1976) then used this olfactory learning assay to screen mutant strains derived from an ethylmethane sulfonate (EMS) mutagenesis. D. Byers discovered that mutations of *dunce* failed to learn this task. W.G. Quinn and coworkers continued the EMS mutant screen at Princeton University, identifying the "vegetable" mutants *rutabaga*, *radish*, *turnip*, *cabbage*, and *zucchini*, each of which showed no olfactory learning, and *amnesiac*, which showed normal learning but no memory 45 minutes after training when memory retention still was appreciable in wild-type (normal) flies.

By the early 1980s, biochemical deficiencies were identified for the *dunce* and *rutabaga* mutations (Byers et al. 1981; Livingstone et al. 1984). Subsequent cloning of these genes (Chen et al. 1986; Levin et al. 1992) confirmed that both reside in enzymatic components of the cAMP second-messenger pathway (see below), which previously was shown from cell biological experiments to underlie associative learning in *Aplysia* (Kandel et al. 1987). Thus began molecular-genetic studies of learning and memory, which now extend into mammals via gene knockout techniques in mouse (Tonegawa et al. 1995; Wehner et al. 1996).

Molecular-genetic analyses of learning and memory in *Drosophila* stalled, however, for three primary reasons. First, no further biochemical abnormalities could be identified for the other learning/memory genes. Second, EMS mutageneses yielded (point) mutations that could not be identified molecularly, thereby thwarting attempts to clone the genes. Third, the behavioral assay produced only moderate olfactory learning in normal flies, which then decayed away completely within a few hours.

Each of these problems has been minimized over the last 15 years. Development of a Pavlovian assay simplified the task that flies were required to master, producing strong olfactory learning and long-lasting memory (Tully and Quinn 1985; see below). Along with systematic control of genetic backgrounds (Tully 1996), this behavioral assay now yields robust, reproducible mutant effects. Transposon-mediated mutagenesis has identified a new set of molecularly tagged learning/memory genes (Boynton and Tully 1992; Dura et al. 1993), which are more readily cloned (Bolwig et al. 1995). Reverse genetics and molecular markers have extended our understanding of the cell biological underpinnings of olfactory learning (Drain et al. 1991; Yin et al. 1994, 1995a; Connolly et al. 1996; P.-L. Han et al. 1996; S.F. Goodwin et al., in prep.). Combined with more traditional behavioral and pharmacological techniques, these molecular-genetic tools continue to support the hypothesis that memory retention is composed of functionally distinct temporal phases (Tully et al. 1990; DeZazzo and Tully 1995). Below is an update on this perspective.

PAVLOVIAN OLFACTORY LEARNING

Pavlovian olfactory learning was accomplished by designing a "teaching machine" composed of two parts: a training chamber, in which flies are trapped on an electrifiable floor and through which odors sequentially are piped on air currents, and a T-maze testing chamber, through which two odors simultaneously are piped again on air currents from the distal ends of the T-maze arms to the center choice point. An "elevator" conveniently shuttles flies from the training chamber to the choice point of the testing chamber (see Tully and Quinn 1985). During one training session, flies are exposed to (1) odor plus footshock for 60 seconds (the CS+), (2) fresh air for 45 seconds, (3) a second odor without footshock for 60 seconds (the CS–), and (4) fresh air for 45 seconds. To test for initial learning levels, the flies are transported within 90 seconds to the testing chamber via the elevator. They then are exposed to the CS+ and the CS– (without footshock in both cases) piped through opposite arms of the T-maze and are given 120 seconds to run into one arm or the other (the flies are induced to run by amenotactic responses to air current). To test for memory, flies first are transferred from the training chamber to a standard food vial for the duration of the retention interval and then are loaded into the elevator and transferred to the testing chamber as above.

Usually, octanol (OCT) and methylcyclohexanol (MCH) are used at concentrations that are aversive to the flies (Dudai 1977; Tully and Quinn 1985; Boynton and Tully 1992; Dura et al. 1993; Folkers et al. 1993; Tully et al. 1994a,b; Bolwig et al. 1995; Connolly et al. 1996). OCT and MCH concentrations are adjusted, however, so that naive flies show no preference when given a simultaneous choice between them in the T-maze. Such distributions in the T-maze are expressed as a performance index (PI), which equals 0 for a 50:50 distribution and 100 for a 100:0 distribution (see Boynton and Tully 1992). After training, typically 90–95% of flies avoid either odor as the CS+, yielding a PI ≥ 85. One complete experiment also is composed of two groups of flies: one trained with OCT as the CS+ and the other with MCH as the CS+. The two resulting distributions in the T-maze then are averaged for one experimental PI (N = 1).

These procedural and computational aspects of the Pavlovian olfactory learning assay inherently control for daily fluctuations in naive odor preference and for nonassociative changes in odor avoidance (see Tully 1984). In short, a PI can be greater than zero only if flies preferentially avoid the CS+, regardless of which odor it is. Some concern has been raised about the validity of this assay, because about 100 flies are trained and tested en masse and the PI is a population-based measure of associative learning (Holliday and Hirsch 1986; Tully 1986). Control experiments have established, however, that (1) choice behavior of individual flies in the T-maze is independent of other flies (Tempel et al. 1983; Tully and Gergen 1986) and (2) the probability of making a correct choice is similar among the individual flies (Tully et al. 1994b). Given these results, a PI computed from two reciprocal groups of 100 flies represents a valid and highly reproducible population (and genotypic) average (Tully 1996).

"Learning" cannot be observed. It is a hypothetical construct, which is presumed to underlie some changes in behavioral responses. Hence, we only can define learning by what it is not, rather than by what it is. This conceptualization becomes particularly relevant in learning studies that quantify the effects of genetic, biochemical, or anatomical lesions. Sensorimotor responses must be shown to be normal (unaffected) before conclusions can be drawn from such effects on learning per se. A potential problem arises from the fact that these lesions may affect a wide range of (behavioral) functions—due to pleiotropic effects of genes, side effects of drugs, or widespread effects of anatomical lesions on network properties. Consequently, some aspect of sensorimotor function likely will be disrupted in every lesion experiment. This realization does not necessarily represent an impasse, however, because only a subset of sensorimotor functions may be involved with any particular learning task. Hence, only "task-relevant" sensorimotor responses need be normal to assess properly the effects of lesions on learning.

For Pavlovian olfactory learning, flies must sense and react to odor cues and footshock. Thus, we have designed task-relevant assays of olfactory acuity and shock reactivity (Boynton and Tully 1992; Luo et al. 1992). For the former, naive flies are exposed to one odor versus air at the choice point of the T-maze and are given 120 seconds to distribute themselves. Different groups of (lesioned and control) flies are used to quantify these odor avoidance responses for several different concentrations of each odor used in the learning assay. To assess shock reactivity, naive flies are exposed to footshock versus no footshock in the T-maze for 120 seconds. Again, different groups of flies are used to quantify these shock avoidance responses at several different voltages. For both olfactory acuity and shock reactivity assays, a PI is calculated as for the learning assay. Thus, naive and conditioned avoidance responses to odor and shock each are quantified in an equivalent manner and in the same context (T-maze) for the same length of time (120 seconds). In this manner, effects of lesions on learning can be interpreted properly when naive responses to odor and footshock are normal but conditioned responses (to odor) are not.

BEHAVIORAL PROPERTIES OF LEARNING AND MEMORY

A primary motive for developing the Pavlovian procedure for flies was to permit systematic investigations of the phenomenology of conditioned responses (see Mackintosh 1974). Several of these behavioral properties of learning have been characterized (Table 1). Each of the experimental protocols designed to assay particular properties of learning include various temporally specific and order-dependent parameters of stimulus presentations, thereby comprising additional "subproperties" of learning. To date, flies have shown every established property (and subproperty) of learning that has been investigated. Such "homology of function" among flies and other animals predicts similar molecular mechanisms underlying simple associative learning. This perspective also presages the identification of a conserved core of genes involved with behavioral plasticity (see below).

A homology of function for memory formation also is apparent. In addition to general characteristics like longer-lasting memory with overtraining and an exponential decay of memory with time, memory formation in flies displays three important properties: (1) Spaced training produces longer-lasting memory than massed training, (2) the appearance of long-lasting memory is dependent on protein synthesis, and (3) memory becomes progressively more resistant to disruption.

Ebbinghaus (1885) first showed that repeated training sessions with a rest interval between sessions (spaced training) produced a stronger, longer-lasting

Table 1. Behavioral Properties of Learning in *Drosophila*

Acquisition	US preexposure
Extinction	Blocking
CS, US saliency	Overshadowing
Temporal specificity	Conditioned excitation
Order dependence	Conditioned inhibition

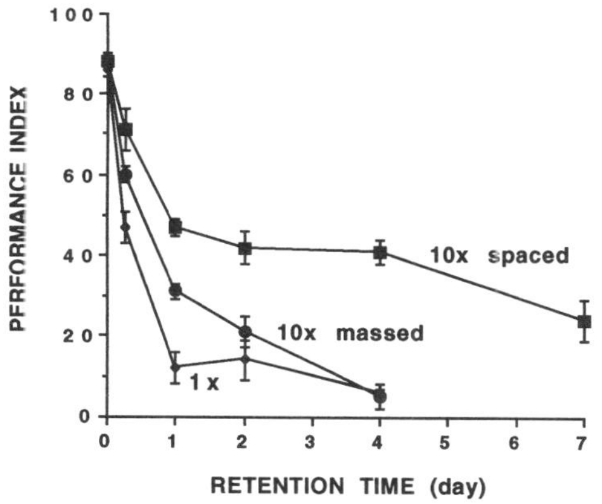

Figure 1. Memory is stronger and longer-lasting after spaced training. Memory retention was quantified in normal (wild-type) flies from 1 to 7 days after different groups of flies were subjected to one (1x), ten massed (no rest interval between each) (10x massed), or ten spaced (15-min rest between each) (10x spaced) training sessions. Massed training produced an improvement in 1-day memory, which nevertheless decayed away within 4 days. In contrast, spaced training produced a greater improvement in 1-day memory, which lasted at least 1 week. (Data from Tully et al. 1994b.)

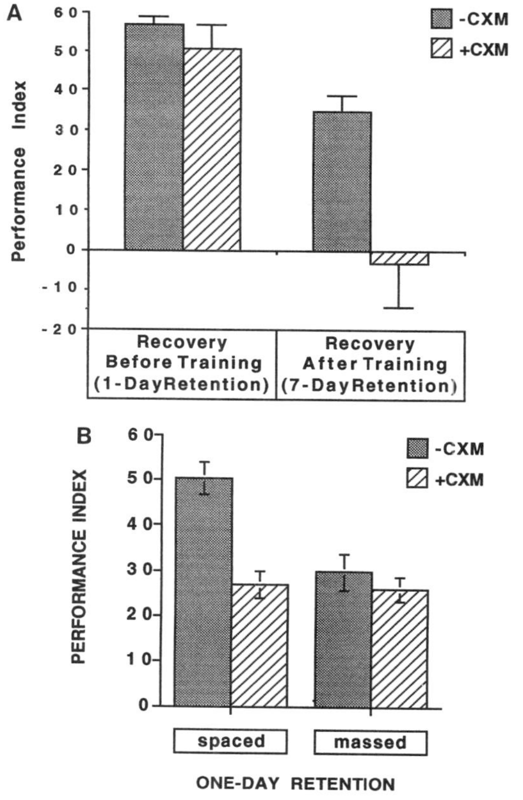

Figure 2. The storage of long-lasting memory is dependent on protein synthesis. (*A*) Normal flies were fed the protein synthesis inhibitor, cycloheximide, overnight (+CXM) or not (–CXM). One set of flies was allowed to recover from this CXM feeding for 6 days before they were subjected to spaced training. One-day memory thereafter was normal, indicating that exposure to CXM did not permanently alter the mechanisms involved with acquisition, storage, or retrieval of memory. A second set of flies was trained immediately after CXM feeding and then allowed to recover from the drug for 7 days. Seven-day memory in these flies was gone, when retrieval mechanisms were intact (see above). Thus, inhibition of protein synthesis during or shortly after training blocked the storage rather than retrieval of memory. (Data from DeZazzo and Tully 1995). (*B*) Normal flies were fed CXM (+CXM) or not (–CXM) overnight and then were subjected to either ten massed or ten spaced training sessions. One-day memory after spaced training was partially disrupted by CXM, whereas that after massed training was not. (Data from Yin et al. 1994.)

memory than the same number of training sessions delivered one right after the other (massed training). Since then, this property of memory formation has been shown for a majority of tasks in almost every species tested (Carew 1996). Flies are no exception (Fig. 1). Compared to 1-day memory after one training session, ten massed training sessions produce a moderate improvement in 1-day memory, which nevertheless does not last. In contrast, ten spaced training sessions (with a 15-minute rest interval between each) produce even better 1-day memory, which then lasts at least 7 days (Tully et al. 1994b).

Seven days is a long time for fruit flies, which normally live in the laboratory for about 8 weeks. This observation suggested that spaced training may induce a long-lasting memory qualitatively different from that produced by lesser training (one or ten-massed training sessions). To test this notion, a second property of long-lasting memory—that its appearance depends on protein synthesis—was evaluated experimentally.

In one experiment, 7-day memory was quantified in flies fed glucose laced with 35 mM cycloheximide or not (±CXM) overnight and then subjected to spaced training. One-day memory also was assayed in flies fed glucose ±CXM overnight, allowed to recover for 6 days, and then subjected to spaced training (DeZazzo and Tully 1995). Seven-day memory is abolished in flies subjected to spaced training immediately after CXM feeding. In contrast, 1-day memory is normal in flies fed CXM and then allowed to recover before spaced training (Fig. 2A). The latter result indicated that inhibition of protein synthesis produces no lasting detrimental effects on the storage or retrieval of (1-day) memory in flies which first recover from CXM feeding before spaced training. Given this result, the former result then indicated that the *storage* of (7-day) memory is blocked when protein synthesis is inhibited during or shortly after spaced training.

In a second experiment, 1-day memory was evaluated in flies that were fed solutions of glucose ±CXM overnight and then subjected immediately to massed or spaced training (Yin et al. 1995b). In this temporal context, CXM feeding had no effect on 1-day memory after massed training and only partially disrupted one-day memory after spaced training (Fig.

2B). Taken together, these data suggested that massed training produces only a CXM-insensitive memory, whereas spaced training produces a new, CXM-sensitive form of memory in addition to the CXM-insensitive memory (Tully et al. 1994b). The alternative hypothesis, of course, was that the CXM-feeding regimen produces only a partial inhibition of protein synthesis (cf. Davis and Squire 1984).

Further experiments delineated additional aspects of memory formation that are not affected by CXM feeding (Tully et al. 1994b). The most obvious results were that immediate learning and (early) memory retention within the first few hours after a single training session are normal in CXM-fed flies. A more subtle and informative result was obtained from investigations of a third property of memory formation: that it becomes more resistant to disruption with time.

This ubiquitous property of memory formation is gleaned from experiments on retrograde amnesia (McGaugh and Herz 1972; Yamada et al. 1992; Quinn and Dudai 1976). In fruit flies, such amnesia is produced by "cold-shock," which is accomplished by placing a group of flies in a glass vial and then submerging the flies in ice water for 2 minutes (Tully et al. 1990, 1994b). Within a few seconds, the flies cool down and pass out; just as quickly they recover from this treatment when they are removed to room temperature. Flies first are subjected to one training session, and then different groups are cold-shocked at different times after training (or an hour before, as a control for nonspecific effects of cold-shock). In each case, the disruptive effects of this treatment are quantified 3 hours after training. Cold-shock administered before training has no effect on 3-hour memory (Fig. 3). In contrast, such memory retention is almost completely abolished in flies cold-shocked immediately after training. With time, however, 3-hour memory becomes progressively more resistant to cold-shock. Asymptotic levels of cold-shock resistance are reached within 2 hours after training. Its maximum level nevertheless comprises only about 50% of normal levels of 3-hour memory. Importantly, the appearance of anesthesia-resistant memory in these experiments is normal in CXM-fed flies (Tully et al. 1994b).

These results suggest that "early" memory retention can be subdivided into an anesthesia-sensitive memory (ASM) and an anesthesia-resistant memory (ARM) component. Seven hours after one training session, memory retention appears to be composed mostly of ARM (Tully et al. 1994b), suggesting that ASM is induced during training but decays away quickly, whereas ARM is induced more slowly and decays away more slowly. More generally, retrograde amnesia experiments suggest a critical period for memory disruption soon after training. Interestingly, a similar critical period has been observed for the effects of protein synthesis inhibitors—which has led to the notion that resistance to disruption and dependence on protein synthesis are two different manifestations (properties)

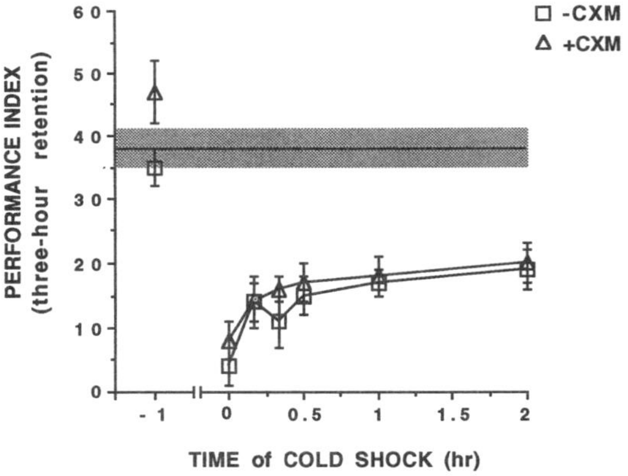

Figure 3. Early memory is composed of anesthesia-sensitive memory (ASM) and anesthesia-resistant memory (ARM). Retrograde amnesia in normal flies was assessed by measuring 3-hour retention after one training session. Different groups of flies were fed CXM (+CXM) or not (–CXM) overnight but all were exposed to 2 min of cold-shock (0°C) either 60 min before training or various times after training. Cold-shock before training had no effect on 3-hr memory. In contrast, cold-shock immediately after training severely disrupted 3-hr memory. Thereafter, 3-hr memory became progressively more resistant to cold-shock disruption, even in CXM-fed flies. The asymptotic level of this ARM nevertheless was lower than 3-hr memory retention, suggesting that such memory is composed of ARM, which is not blocked in CXM-fed flies, and an ASM. (Data from Tully et al. 1994b.)

of long-lasting memory (McGaugh 1966; Andrew 1980; Squire et al. 1980; Rosenzweig and Bennett 1984).

Behavioral experiments on fruit flies, then, have revealed two major distinctions in memory formation. First, long-lasting memory is protein synthesis-dependent, whereas learning and early memory are not. Second, early memory is composed of both an (diminishing) anesthesia-sensitive phase and an (augmenting) anesthesia-resistant phase for several hours after training. Analyses of single-gene mutants have confirmed and extended this interpretation, thereby suggesting a biological organization of memory formation along these dimensions of behavioral analysis.

BEHAVIORAL CLASSIFICATION OF SINGLE-GENE MUTANTS

Behavioral screens for mutations affecting olfactory learning or memory have identified seven genes. The *dunce* (Dudai et al. 1976), *rutabaga* (Livingstone et al. 1984), *amnesiac* (Quinn et al. 1979), *cabbage* (Booker and Quinn 1981), and *radish* (Folkers et al. 1993) genes were isolated using an instrumental olfactory learning procedure (Quinn et al. 1974), and the Pavlovian olfactory learning procedure (Tully and Quinn 1985) was used to isolate the *latheo* (Boynton and Tully 1992) and *linotte* (Dura et al. 1993) genes. Mutants for all seven of these genes show lower-than-normal learning scores in the Pavlovian task, while sensorimotor responses to odors and footshock are normal. Biochemical and molecular studies have determined that *dunce* and *rutabaga* encode a cAMP-specific phosphodiesterase and a calcium/calmodulin-dependent adenylyl cyclase, respectively (see above), revealing the involvement of the cAMP second-messenger pathway in olfactory associative learning (Fig. 4).

Four additional genes were shown to function during olfactory learning and memory by focusing on disruptions of the cAMP pathway. Learning is abolished in transgenic flies overexpressing a mutant, constitutively active α subunit of G protein (G_s; Connolly et al. 1996). Learning and memory retention are reduced in flies homozygous for mutations in *DCO* or *PKA-RI*, which encode catalytic or regulatory subunits of cAMP-dependent protein kinase (PKA), respectively (Skoulakis et al. 1993; S.F. Goodwin et al., in prep.). Similar learning/memory deficits also have been produced in transgenic flies by overexpressing a PKA catalytic subunit, a (mammalian) RII regulatory subunit, or a PKA-specific inhibitor peptide (Drain et al. 1991). Protein synthesis-dependent memory produced by spaced training is abolished specifically in transgenic flies overexpressing a repressor isoform of the cAMP-responsive transcription factor, *dCREB2* (Yin et al. 1994). (A report by Feany and Quinn [1995] that *amnesiac* encodes an AC-activating neuropeptide awaits confirmation via transgenic rescue of defective memory or in vivo demonstration of defective biochemical function in *amnesiac* mutants.)

A twelfth gene was identified from an enhancer-trap screen for preferential reporter-gene expression in adult mushroom bodies (P.-L. Han et al. 1996), an anatomical region of the brain implicated in associative learning (de Belle and Heisenberg 1994; Hammer and Menzel 1995; Connolly et al. 1996). Mutations in *14-3-3* (Swanson and Ganguly 1992), which is known to associate physically with tyrosine hydroxylase and Raf (Burbelo and Hall 1995), disrupt olfactory learning and memory retention (Skoulakis and Davis 1996). Interestingly, this enhancer-trap screen also identified additional mutations in *dunce*, *rutabaga*, and *DCO* (Nighorn et al. 1991; Han et al. 1992; Skoulakis et al. 1993).

When the memory curves for mutants of these 12 genes are compared, they appear to fall into one of five classes: acquisition (LRN) mutants, short-term memory (STM) mutants, middle-term memory (MTM) mutants, anesthesia-resistant memory (ARM) mutants (Fig. 5), and long-term memory (LTM) mutants. LRN mutants show reductions in initial learning levels, but memory decay rates thereafter appear normal. Such is the case for mutants of *DCO*, *PKA-RI*, *14-3-3*, *latheo*, and *linotte*. (G_s mutants also may be placed in this class, since associative learning is abolished completely.) STM mutants show reductions in initial learning, and memory within the first 30 minutes after training decays more rapidly than normal. Mutant *dunce* and *rutabaga* flies are examples of this class. MTM mutants show minimal effects on initial learning and on memory 7 hours after training, but memory retention between these times is lower than normal. This was first observed for *amnesiac* mutants. The definitive aspect of ARM mutants is that memory decays away entirely within 8 hours after training—a time when memory retention normally can be accounted for by an anesthesia-resistant memory. Retrograde amnesia experiments on *radish* mutants, in fact, have failed to detect any ARM (Folkers et al. 1993; Tully et al. 1994b). That the entire memory curve is lower than normal in *radish* mutants suggests that ARM may be induced during or soon after training. Finally, LTM mutants disrupt the protein synthesis-dependent

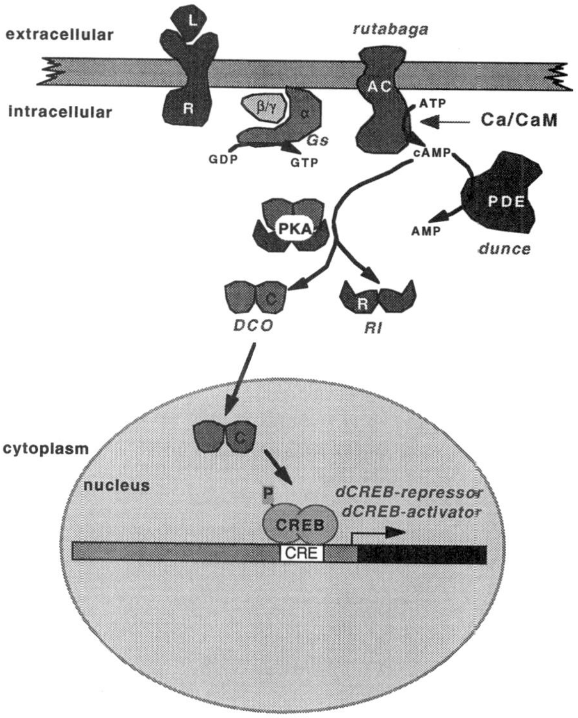

Figure 4. Genetic disruptions of cAMP signaling produce deficits in olfactory learning and memory. This cartoon depicts major steps in the cAMP second-messenger system. Learning stimulates synaptic transmission among relevant neurons. A ligand (L) binds to its receptor (R) (these components are unknown for Pavlovian olfactory learning in flies), which then stimulates adenylyl cyclase (AC) via G protein ($G_{\alpha\beta\gamma}$). AC synthesizes cAMP, which then is hydrolyzed by phosphodiesterase (PDE). Binding of cAMP to a regulatory subunit dimer (R) of cAMP-dependent protein kinase (PKA) causes its dissociation from a catalytic subunit dimer (C). Free C then translocates into the nucleus where it activates a cAMP-responsive transcription factor (CREB) via phosphorylation. CREB then regulates the expression of downstream genes presumably that lead to a synaptic growth process underlying long-term memory formation. Genetic disruptions of G protein (G_s), AC (*rutabaga*), PDE (*dunce*), PKA catalytic subunit (*DC0*), PKA regulatory subunit (*RI*), or CREB (*dCREB2b*) all affect some aspect of learning or memory (see text). (Figure designed by U. Heberlein.)

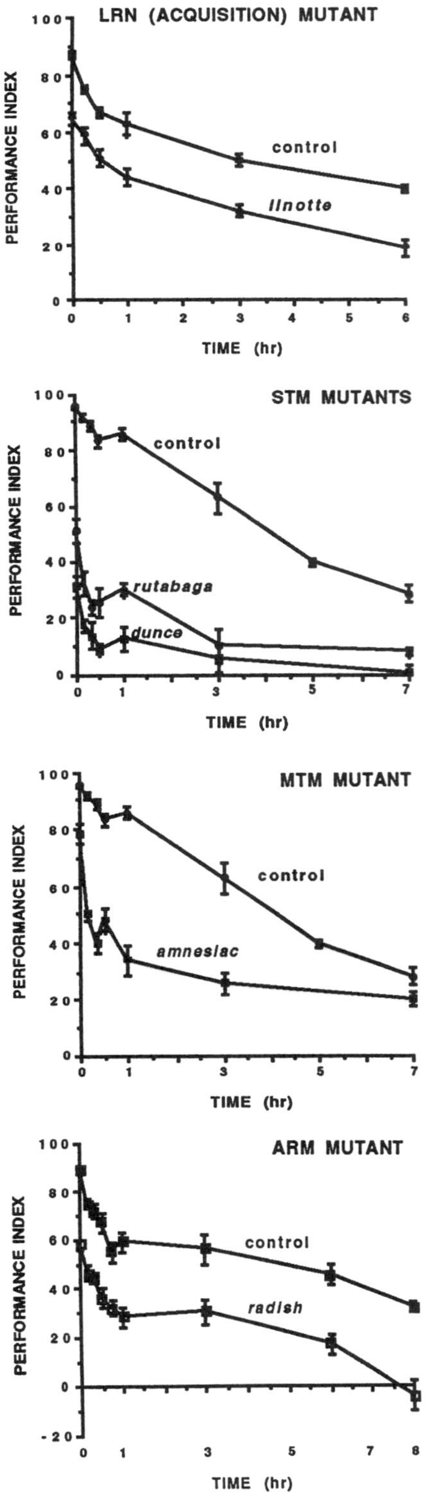

Figure 5. Single-gene mutations disrupt learning and memory in four distinct ways. *linotte* flies are typical of learning (LRN) mutants; *dunce* and *rutabaga* represent STM mutants; *amnesiac* an MTM mutant; and *radish* an ARM mutant. (Data from Dura et al. 1993; Tully and Quinn 1985; Tully et al. 1994b.) Transgenic flies expressing a repressor form of CREB (*dCREB2*) represent LTM mutants (see Fig. 7).

memory induced by spaced training. Transgenic flies overexpressing a repressor form of *dCREB2* show this effect. Consequently, memory retention after spaced training appears similar to that after massed training in *dCREB2-b* transgenic (or normal) flies (see Fig. 7).

Do these mutant defects result primarily from functional deficits in the molecular machinery underlying learning and memory per se, or rather secondarily from maldevelopment? For most of the mutants mentioned above, this issue cannot be resolved completely. The fact that task-relevant sensorimotor responses were normal in these mutants, however, argues against any gross developmental defects. Maldevelopment also seems less likely—or more anatomically restricted (and thereby informative nonetheless)—in mutants that show abnormal memory decay rates, since memory processing is largely a functional consequence of acquisition. Interpretation of LRN mutants, in particular, is problematic, since structural abnormalities in the brain simply may yield "mentally retarded" flies (see Heisenberg 1989).

Four reverse-genetic studies have tackled this "structure-function conundrum" (see Tully 1994) by using inducible transgenes in mutant flies. Bolwig et al. (1995) were able to rescue completely the learning deficit of *linotte* mutants by inducing the expression of a lio^{+} transgene 3 hours before training, clearly indicating an acute, direct role for *linotte* in olfactory associative learning (thus, its inclusion in Fig. 5). In contrast, induced expression of a dnc^{+} transgene produces only partial rescue of the *dunce* learning defect (Dauwalder and Davis 1995). This result suggests either a suboptimal level of expression of the transgene or some maldevelopment in *dunce* mutants (cf. Bellen and Kiger 1988). Drain et al. (1991) used inducible transgenes to overexpress a peptide inhibitor and catalytic or regulatory subunit of PKA. In each case, a dominant-negative effect on learning and (early) memory was observed, which certainly implies an acute role for PKA function in adults but which may not reflect a specific molecular disruption of olfactory learning because the transgene was expressed ectopically. This general critique applies similarly to experiments by Yin et al. (1994), although the dominant-negative effect of CREB repressor disrupted LTM specifically (see Fig. 7). More pertinently, induced overexpression of a CREB activator transgene enhanced LTM (Yin et al. 1995a). The combination of loss-of-function and gain-of-function effects from transgenic constructs encoding protein isoforms of opposing function strongly supports a specific functional role for CREB in long-term memory formation.

MEMORY PHASES

Once the "average effects" of these various mutants are carefully quantified (see Tully 1996), they can be combined with the effects of different training protocols (massed versus spaced training, cold-shock,

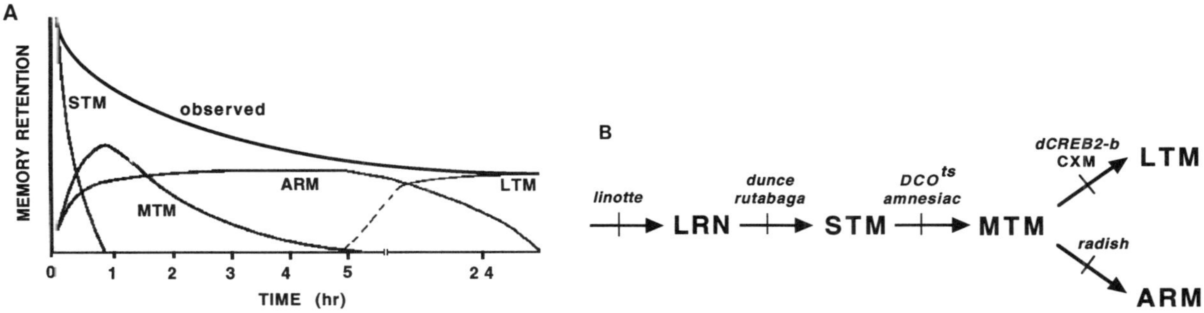

Figure 6. Memory retention derives from component memory phases and involves a genetic pathway of information flow. (*A*) Four functionally distinct memory phases underlie *observed* memory retention. STM, MTM, ARM, and LTM appear sequentially, and each has a progressively slower rate of decay. All eventually decay away completely, except for the protein synthesis-dependent LTM. (*B*) Genetic model of information flow showing where in the pathway disruptions of particular genes have their primary effects. The primary effects of (1) *linotte*, (2) *dunce* or *rutabaga*, (3) *amnesiac* or *DCO*^{ts}, (4) *radish*, and (5) *dCREB2-b* (or CXM) are on LRN, STM, MTM, ARM, or LTM, respectively. The pathway is sequential from LRN to MTM, but then it branches into two independent paths—one leading to ARM and the other leading to LTM, which coexist as parallel memories for some time. These independent paths may represent a branch in the biochemical path within a given neuron or a branch in anatomical paths of memory processing in the brain.

etc.) or different pharmacological agents (CXM, for instance) to reveal a biobehavioral organization of memory formation. By assuming (simplistically) that these various effects act additively, memory formation can be "decomposed" into four functionally distinct memory components—STM, MTM, ARM, and LTM—each with different temporal kinetics (Fig. 6A).

Here again a functional homology is apparent. Memory phases similar to STM, MTM, and LTM have been inferred from pharmacological experiments in vertebrates (McGaugh and Herz 1972; Gibbs and Ng 1977; Allweis 1991). In several studies, long-lasting "consolidated" memory was shown to have a critical period shortly after training, during which time disruptive treatments or protein synthesis inhibitors can block its formation (see Tully et al. 1994b). (More recent studies suggest two or more critical periods in some species: Rose 1995; Chew et al. 1996.) Thus, anesthesia resistance and protein synthesis dependence were considered to be different manifestations of a singular memory process. Most of these studies supported the notion that a newly acquired experience was processed sequentially through each of these memory phases, ultimately to be stored as an LTM. Disruptions of early memory phases affected subsequent ones.

GENETIC DISSECTION OF MEMORY PHASES

Behavioral analyses of single-gene mutants not only support the notion of component memory phases, but also suggest a "pathway of information flow" (Fig. 6B). Genetic disruptions of LRN, STM, or MTM secondarily affect all downstream memory phases. The memory curves of *linotte*, *dunce*, and *rutabaga* suggest this sequential effect. Direct measurements of ARM (from cold-shock experiments and as 1-day memory after massed training) and LTM (as 7-day memory after spaced training) have been made in *amnesiac* mutants, and both are reduced (T. Tully and M. DelVecchio, unpubl.), indicating a branch after MTM into independent ARM and LTM processes.

This genetic path analysis in flies has revealed three new properties of memory formation, which, given the general functional homology, likely will be discovered in other species as well. First, ARM and LTM are not different aspects of one, consolidated memory, but rather define two distinct memory phases. Second, ARM and LTM are functionally independent "parallel" memory phases that coexist for a few days after training (cf. Clark and Kandel 1993; Emptage and Carew 1993). Third, early memory (ASM) can be decomposed into separate STM and MTM components (cf. Ghirardi et al. 1995; Mauelshagen et al. 1996).

Key experiments to delineate the first two aspects revolve around behavior-genetic analysis of the single-gene mutant *radish* and *dCREB2-b* transgenic flies which overexpress a repressor form of CREB. ARM is absent in *radish* mutants (Folkers et al. 1993; Tully et al. 1994b), as is 1-day memory after massed training (Fig. 7A) (Tully et al. 1994b). One-day memory after spaced training is reduced but not abolished in *radish* mutants and is blocked completely by CXM (Fig. 7B), in contrast to the partial effect of CXM in normal flies (see Fig. 2B). Nevertheless, 2- to 7-day memory in *radish* flies remains normal (Tully et al. 1994b). The opposite effects were observed in *dCREB2-b* transgenic flies (Yin et al. 1994). Induced expression of the CREB repressor blocks the protein synthesis-dependent "extra" memory (LTM) produced by spaced training, without affecting memory after massed training (ARM; Fig. 7). When expressed in *radish dCREB2-b* "double" mutants, CREB repressor (like CXM) completely blocks 1-day memory after spaced training.

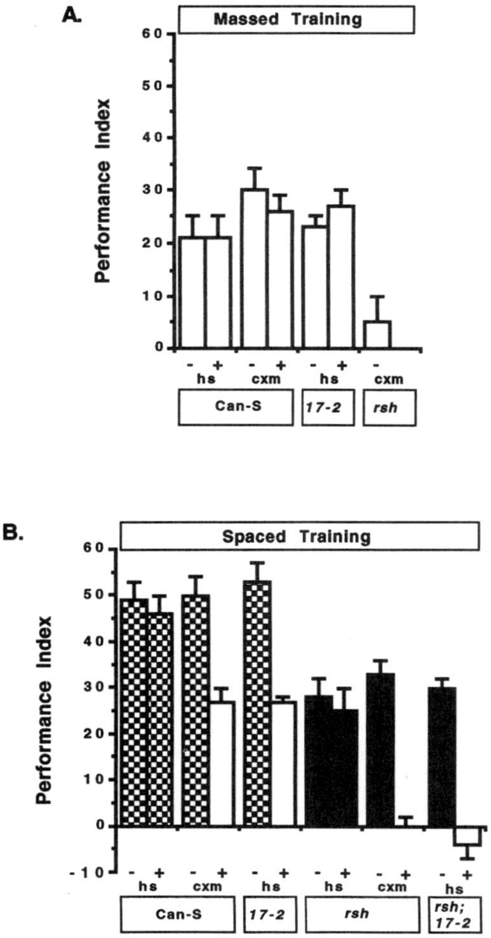

Figure 7. Genetic dissection of consolidated memory into ARM and LTM. (*A*) One-day memory after ten massed training sessions in normal (Can-S), in *dCREB2-b* flies carrying an inducible CREB repressor transgene (*17-2*), or *radish* mutants (*rsh*), which either were heat-shocked (37° C for 30 min) or not (± hs) 3 hr before training or were fed CXM overnight (± cxm) before training. One-day memory after massed training is composed only of ARM (see text). Thus, heat-shock or CXM does not affect ARM in normal flies. Heat-shock also produces no effect on ARM in *dCREB2-b* flies. The *radish* mutation disrupts ARM, however. (*B*) One-day memory after ten spaced training sessions with the same treatments (± cxm or ± hs) and in the same flies as in *A*, with the addition of *radish dCREB2-b* "double mutants" (*rsh*; *17-2*). One-day memory in normal flies is disrupted 50% by CXM but not by heat shock and also is disrupted 50% after heat-shock induction of CREB repressor protein in *dCREB2-b* transgenic flies. One-day memory after spaced training in *radish* mutants is only 50% that of normal flies and is completely disrupted (0%) in *radish* mutants fed CXM or in *radish dCREB2-b* double mutants after heat-shock induction of CREB repressor protein. Taken together, these data indicate a genetic dissection of normal memory one day after spaced training (*checkered bars*) into two underlying components: a CXM- and CREB repressor-insensitive ARM (*open bars*), and a CXM- and CREB repressor-sensitive LTM (*closed bars*). Under these conditions, ARM and LTM sum to yield normal memory. (Data from Tully et al. 1994b; Yin et al. 1994.)

These data establish the decomposition of 1-day memory into two memory components, ARM and LTM, which coexist independently 1 day after training. ARM is disrupted by *radish* but is normal in *dCREB2-b* flies, and LTM is normal in *radish* but disrupted in *dCREB2-b* flies. Importantly, ARM levels in induced *dCREB2-b* flies and LTM levels in *radish* mutants literally sum to yield normal 1-day memory after spaced training (see Fig. 7B), thereby providing an empirical demonstration of the additivity assumption that underlies the component memory model of memory formation (see above).

Behavioral experiments initially decomposed early memory into ASM and ARM (see above). Behavior-genetic analysis of *amnesiac* mutants, however, suggested that ASM might be further subdivided into MTM and STM (Tully et al. 1990). Consistent with this inference, reversal retention experiments appeared to disrupt MTM preferentially, leaving STM and ARM largely intact (Tully et al. 1990). Recently, another piece of evidence consistent with this view has been generated using a temperature-sensitive allele of *DCO*. Although PKA activity in DCO^{ts} mutants is not normal at permissive temperature, it nevertheless is further reduced at restrictive temperature to levels that produce lethal effects during development (Li et al. 1996). At permissive temperature, adult mutants show reduced levels of learning and memory that are remniscent of the effects of other *DCO* mutants (see above). At restrictive temperature, performance levels for both normal and mutant flies generally are lower, indicating a nonspecific effect of temperature on learning and or memory.

A temperature shift-specific effect of the DCO^{ts} mutation was quantified, however, by expressing mutant scores at each temperature as a "PI ratio" of their corresponding wild-type control scores. When mutant memory curves from permissive and restrictive temperatures then were compared, learning and 3-hour retention appear similar, but mutant memory between these retention intervals is reduced at restrictive temperature (Fig. 8). This observation suggested that an acute reduction of PKA activity in adult mutants disrupts MTM. Consistent with this notion, the memory curve of *amnesiac* mutants, when expressed as a PI ratio, is similar to that of DCO^{ts} mutants at restrictive temperature (Fig. 8). Thus, reversal training, the *amnesiac* mutation, and the temperature-shift-specific effects of DCO^{ts} all appear to affect MTM preferentially, leaving STM and ARM (at least somewhat) intact.

SIGNAL TRANSDUCTION AND MEMORY FORMATION

It seems amazing that six of twelve genes known to affect olfactory associative learning in flies all encode components in the cAMP second-messenger system. This certainly solidifies a central role for cAMP signal-

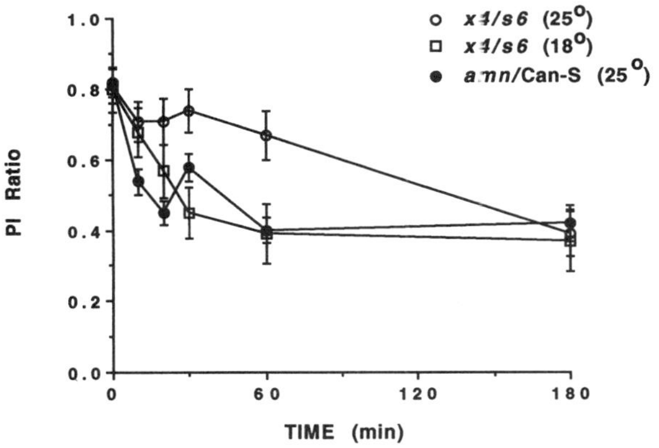

Figure 8. Genetic dissection of ASM into STM and MTM. Memory retention from 0 to 180 min after one training session was quantified in normal and in hemizygous DCO^{ts} flies (*x4/s6*) at permissive (25°) or restrictive (18°) temperature. Scores for mutant flies then were expressed as a "PI Ratio" of their corresponding control (normal) flies to reveal temperature-shift-specific effects of the DCO^{ts} mutation. Learning and 180-min retention were similar in DCO^{ts} mutants trained and tested at both temperatures. Memory retention at the intervening times was reduced at restrictive temperature, however, suggesting an acute effect of reduced PKA activity on MTM. Consistent with this notion, memory retention (expressed as a PI ratio) in *amnesiac* mutants, which show deficits in MTM (see text), is similar to that in DCO^{ts} mutants at restrictive temperature. (Data from Li et al. 1996.)

ing in behavioral plasticity and predicts that lesions of other components of this signal transduction pathway, such as the relevant neurotransmitters (cf. Tempel et al. 1984) and receptors (cf. Feng et al. 1996; K.-A. Han et al. 1996), also will affect olfactory learning.

A closer look at these gene disruptions suggests an interesting correspondence between steps in the cAMP signaling pathway (Fig. 4) and information flow from acquisition to induction of long-term memory (Fig. 6A). Disruptions of G protein, of adenylyl cyclase (AC) or phosphodiesterase (PDE), of PKA and of CREB—each at successively later steps in the cAMP pathway—produce deficits in LRN, in STM, in MTM, and in LTM, respectively. (Gene disruptions of AC, PDE, PKA, and RI also affect LRN, but nonspecific effects such as maldevelopment may be responsible [see above]. Alternatively, these proteins may play a multifunctional role in learning and memory formation.) Perhaps these discrete effects on memory formation reflect differences in the half-lives of various biochemical functions, such as cAMP synthesis or hydrolysis, phosphorylation/dephosphorylation of PKA substrates, and subcellular compartmentalization of such proteins.

The alternative observation—that six of the twelve extant genes are not known to affect the cAMP pathway—may be even more important. The known biochemical functions of some genes eventually may provide new links to the cAMP pathway. *14-3-3*, for instance, interacts with rate-limiting enzymes (tyrosine hydroxylase and tryptophan hydroxylase) in the synthesis of monoamine neurotransmitters (dopamine and octopamine, respectively), which are known to modulate AC (Hall 1992). In contrast, *linotte* encodes a novel protein, and the molecular identification of *cabbage*, *radish*, and *latheo* remain to be determined. Possibly, they will identify new biochemistries that act in concert with cAMP signaling during memory formation.

That relatively clean dissections of memory formation have emerged from analyses of *linotte* (LRN), DCO^{ts} (MTM), *radish* (ARM), and *dCREB2* (LTM) presages continued insight to the biobehavioral organization of memory formation as more genes are discovered. To this end, crude estimates suggest that 100 or more genes may be involved with olfactory learning and memory in *Drosophila*. Chances seem quite high then that new signal transduction pathways and new modulatory components of extant biochemistries will emerge from further gene discovery efforts.

BEYOND FRUIT FLIES

There is every reason to believe that many of the genes discovered in *Drosophila* will be involved with learning and memory in other species. Flies show behavioral properties of learning and memory that are common in many vertebrate and invertebrate species (Mackintosh 1974; Hawkins and Kandel 1984; Carew and Sahley 1986). This homology of behavioral function likely reflects the fact that an "elemental" form of associative learning evolved early in the animal kingdom and has been conserved. Also implied is that acquisition and memory storage are largely cellular processes, since the cellular properties of individual neurons appear similar across species. In contrast, the diversity in types of tasks that various animals are capable of learning likely reflects species differences in neuronal circuitry.

It also is apparent that this homology of function extends to the molecular machinery involved with associative learning and memory (cf. Hawkins and Kandel 1984; Bailey et al. 1996). The cAMP signaling pathway has been shown to be involved with learning in *Aplysia* (Byrne and Kandel 1996) and with long-term potentiation in vertebrate hippocampus (Bliss and Collinridge 1993; Huang et al. 1994; Weisskopf et al. 1994; Blitzer et al. 1995; Nicoll and Malenka 1995; Huang and Kandel 1996; Nguyen and Kandel 1996; Salin et al. 1996). Importantly, other signal transduction pathways have been shown to be involved in other forms of behavioral plasticity in flies (Griffith et al. 1993), as well as in associative learning in *Hermissenda* (Yamoah and Crow 1996). Minimally, this observation predicts that further gene discovery in fruit flies will implicate additional biochemistries. Maximally, it suggests that the evolutionarily conserved "core" mechanism has recruited additional molecular machinery as genome (and neuronal) complexity has increased and diversified throughout the animal kingdom.

Mention of long-term potentiation above further emphasizes the idea that the acquisition and storage of a new experience likely is a cellular phenomenon. Thus, numerous reports of experience-dependent (and developmental) synaptic plasticity probably *do* represent the neural substrates of behavioral plasticity (Stewart and Rusakov 1995; Gilbert 1996; Martin and Kandel 1996; Muller et al. 1996; Rosenzweig 1996; Wu et al. 1996). A persuasive demonstration of this lies in the observations that opposite manipulations of CREB produce opposite effects on long-term memory in flies (Yin et al. 1995a) and on the structure and function of identified synapses in mollusks (Bartsch et al. 1995).

Work in mollusks (Dash et al. 1991; Bartsch et al. 1995), flies (Yin et al. 1994, 1995a; Davis et al. 1996), and mice (Bourtchuladze et al. 1994; Impey et al. 1996; Kogan et al. 1997) supports the view that CREB is an evolutionarily conserved "molecular switch" for an activity-dependent synaptic growth process that underlies long-term memory (see Martin and Kandel 1996; Yin and Tully 1996). Two expectations emerge. First, despite the fact that different tasks in various species may involve different signal transduction pathways, they nevertheless may converge onto CREB or may participate in parallel transcription factor cascades to drive the same synaptic growth process underlying long-term memory. Second, many "downstream" genes may participate in such transcription factor-mediated cascades of gene expression. Continued identification and behavior-genetic characterization of new genes in *Drosophila* promise to help clarify and to extend our understanding of these molecular mechanisms.

ACKNOWLEDGMENTS

This work has been supported by the McKnight Foundation, the John A. Hartford Foundation, the John Merck Foundation, and National Institutes of Health grants HD-32245 and HD-33098 (to T.T.), NS-09763 (to J.D.), NS-09619 (to G.B.), HD-08087 (to J.D.), and an H. Wendt Neuroscience fellowship (to M.R.).

REFERENCES

Allweis, C. 1991. The congruity of rat and chick multiphasic memory-consolidation models. In *Neural and behavioural plasticity* (ed. R.J. Andrew), p. 370. Oxford University Press, New York.

Andrew, R.J. 1980. *The functional organization of phases of memory consolidation.* Academic Press, New York.

Bailey, C.H., D. Bartsch, and E.R. Kandel. 1996. Toward a molecular definition of long-term memory storage. *Proc. Natl. Acad. Sci.* **93:** 13445.

Bartsch, D., M. Ghirardi, P.A. Skehel, K.A. Karl, S.P. Herder, M. Chen, C.H. Bailey, and E.R. Kandel. 1995. *Aplysia* CREB2 represses long-term facilitation: Relief of repression converts transient facilitation into long-term functional and structural change. *Cell* **83:** 956.

Bellen, H.J. and J.A. Kiger. 1988. Maternal effects of general and regional specificity on embyros of *Drosophila melanogaster* caused by *dunce* and *rutabaga* mutant combinations. *Roux's Arch. Dev. Biol.* **197:** 258.

Bliss, T.V.P. and G.L. Collinridge. 1993. A synaptic model of memory: Long-term-potentiation. *Nature* **361:** 31.

Blitzer, R.D., T. Wong, R. Nouranifar, R. Iyengar, and E.M. Landau. 1995. Postsynaptic cAmp pathway gates early LTP in hippocampal CA1 region. *Neuron* **15:** 1403.

Bolwig, G.M., M. Del Vecchio, G. Hannon, and T. Tully. 1995. Molecular cloning of *linotte* in *Drosophila:* A novel gene that functions in adults during associative learning. *Neuron* **15:** 829.

Booker, R., and W.G. Quinn. 1981. Conditioning of leg position in normal and mutant *Drosophila. Proc. Natl. Acad. Sci.* **78:** 3940.

Bourtchuladze, R., B. Frenguelli, J. Blendy, D. Cioffi, G. Schutz, and A.J. Silva. 1994. Deficient long-term memory in mice with a targeted mutation of the cAMP-responsive element-binding protein. *Cell* **79:** 59.

Boynton, S., and T. Tully. 1992. *latheo*, a new gene involved in associative learning and memory in *Drosophila melanogaster* identified from P element mutagenesis. *Genetics* **131:** 655.

Burbelo, P.D. and A. Hall. 1995. Hot numbers in signal transduction. *Curr. Biol.* **5:** 95.

Byers, D., R.L. Davis, and J.A. Kiger, Jr. 1981. Defect in cyclic AMP phosphodiesterase due to the *dunce* mutation of learning in *Drosophila melanogaster. Nature* **289:** 79.

Byrne, J.H. and E.R. Kandel. 1996. Presynaptic facilitation revisited: State and time dependence. *J. Neurosci.* **16:** 425.

Carew, T.J. 1996. Molecular enhancement of memory formation. *Neuron* **16:** 5.

Carew, T.J., and C.L. Sahley. 1986. Invertebrate learning and memory: From behavior to molecules. *Annu. Rev. Neurosci.* **9:** 435.

Chen, C.-N., S. Denome, and R.L. Davis. 1986. Molecular analysis of cDNA clones and the corresponding genomic coding sequences of the *Drosophila dunce*$^+$ gene, the structural gene for cAMP phosphodiesterase. *Proc. Natl. Acad. Sci.* **83:** 9313.

Chew, S.J., D.S. Vicario, and F. Nottebohm. 1996. Quantal duration of auditory memories. *Science* **274:** 1909.

Clark, G.A. and E.R. Kandel. 1993. Induction of long-term facilitation in *Aplysia* siphon sensory neurons by local application of serotonin to remote synapses. *Proc. Natl. Acad. Sci.* **90:** 11411.

Connolly, J.B., I.J.H. Roberts, D. Armstrong, K. Kaiser, M. Forte, T. Tully, and C.J. O'Kane. 1996. Associative learning disrupted by impaired Gs signaling in *Drosophila* mushroom bodies. *Science* **274:** 2104.

Dash, P.K., K.A. Karl, M.A. Colicos, R. Prywes, and E.R. Kandel. 1991. cAMP response element-binding protein is activated by Ca^{2+}/calmodulin- as well as cAMP-dependent protein kinase. *Proc. Natl. Acad. Sci.* **88:** 5061.

Dauwalder, B. and R.L. Davis. 1995. Conditional rescue of the *dunce* learning/memory and female fertility defects with *Drosophila* or rat transgenes. *J. Neurosci.* **15:** 3490.

Davis, G.W., C.M. Schuster, and C.S. Goodman. 1996. Genetic dissection of structural and functional components of synaptic plasticity. III. CREB is necessary for presynaptic functional plasticity. *Neuron* **17:** 669.

Davis, H.P. and L.R. Squire. 1984. Protein synthesis and

memory: A review. *Psychol. Bull.* **96:** 518.

de Belle, J.S. and M. Heisenberg. 1994. Associative odor learning in *Drosophila* abolished by chemical ablation of mushroom bodies. *Science* **263:** 692.

DeZazzo, J. and T. Tully. 1995. Dissection of memory formation: From behavioral pharmacology to molecular genetics. *Trends Neurosci.* **18:** 212.

Drain, P., E. Folkers, and W.G. Quinn. 1991. cAMP-dependent protein kinase and the disruption of learning in transgenic flies. *Neuron* **6:** 71.

Dudai, Y. 1977. Properties of learning and memory in *Drosophila melanogaster. J. Comp. Physiol. A* **114:** 69.

Dudai, Y., Y.-N. Jan, D. Byers, W. Quinn, and S. Benzer. 1976. *dunce*, a mutant of *Drosophila melanogaster* deficient in learning. *Proc. Natl. Acad. Sci.* **73:** 1684.

Dura, J.M., T. Preat, and T. Tully. 1993. Identification of *linotte*, a new gene affecting learning and memory in *Drosophila melanogaster. J. Neurogenet.* **9:** 1.

Ebbinghaus, H. 1885. *Über das Gedächtnis*. Dover, New York.

Emptage, N.J. and T.J. Carew. 1993. Long-term synaptic facilitation in the absence of short-term facilitation in aplysia neurons. *Science* **262:** 253.

Feany, M.B. and W.G. Quinn. 1995. A neuropeptide gene defined by the *Drosophila* memory mutant *amnesiac*. *Science* **268:** 869.

Feng, G., F. Hannan, V. Reale, Y.Y. Hon, C.T. Kousky, P.D. Evans, and L.M. Hall. 1996. Cloning and functional characterization of a novel dopamine receptor from *Drosophila melanogaster. J. Neurosci.* **16:** 3925.

Folkers, E., P.F. Drain, and W.G. Quinn. 1993. *radish*, a *Drosophila* mutant deficient in consolidated memory. *Proc. Natl. Acad. Sci.* **90:** 8123.

Ghirardi, M., P.G. Montarolo, and E.R. Kandel. 1995. A novel intermediate stage in the transition between short- and long-term facilitation in the sensory to motor neuron synapse of *Aplysia. Neuron* **14:** 413.

Gibbs, M.E. and K.T. Ng. 1977. Psychobiology of memory: Towards a model of memory formation. *Biobehav. Rev.* **1:** 113.

Gilbert, C.D. 1996. Learning and receptive field plasticity. *Proc. Natl. Acad. Sci.* **93:** 10546.

Griffith, L.C., L.M. Verselis, K.M. Aitken, C.P. Kyriacou, W. Danho, and R.J. Greenspan. 1993. Inhibition of calcium/calmodulin dependent protein kinase in *Drosophila* disrupts plasticity. *Neuron* **10:** 501.

Hall, Z.W. 1992. *An introduction to molecular neurobiology*. Sinauer Associates, Sunderland, Massachusetts.

Hammer, M. and R. Menzel. 1995. Learning and memory in the honeybee. *J. Neurosci.* **15:** 1617.

Han, K.-A., N.S. Millar, M.S. Grotewiel, and R.L. Davis. 1996. DAMB, a novel dopamine receptor expressed specifically in *Drosophila* mushroom bodies. *Neuron* **16:** 1127.

Han, P.-L., V. Meller, and R.L. Davis. 1996. The *Drosophila* brain revisited by enhancer detection. *J. Neurobiol.* (in press).

Han, P.-L., L.R. Levin, R.R. Reed, and R.L. Davis. 1992. Preferential expression of the *Drosophila rutabaga* gene in mushroom bodies, neural centres for learning in insects. *Neuron* **9:** 619.

Hawkins, R.D. and E.R. Kandel. 1984. Is there a cell biological alphabet for learning? *Psychol. Rev.* **91:** 375.

Heisenberg, M. 1989. Genetic approach to learning and memory (mnemogenetics) in *Drosophila melanogaster*. In *Fundamentals of memory formation: Neuronal plasticity and brain function* (ed. H. Rahmann), p. 3. Gustav Fischer Verlag, New York.

Holliday, M. and J. Hirsch. 1986. A comment on the evidence for learning in diptera. *Behav. Genet.* **16:** 439.

Huang, Y.-Y. and E.R. Kandel. 1996. Modulation of both the early and the late phase of mossy fiber LTP by the activation of β-adrenergic receptors. *Neuron* **16:** 611.

Huang, Y.-Y., X.-C. Li, and E.R. Kandel. 1994. cAMP contributes to mossy fiber LTP by initiating both a covalently mediated early phase and macromolecular synthesis-dependent late phase. *Cell* **79:** 69.

Impey, S., M. Mark, E.C. Villacres, S. Poser, C. Chavkin, and D. Storm. 1996. Induction of CRE-mediated gene expression by stimuli that generate long-lasting LTP in area CA1 of the hippocampus. *Neuron* **16:** 973.

Kandel, E.R., M. Klein, B. Hochner, M. Shuster, S.A. Siegelbaum, R.D. Hawkins, D.L. Glanzman, V.F. Castellucci, and T.W. Abrams. 1987. Synaptic modulation and learning: New insights into synaptic transmission from the study of behavior. In *Synaptic function* (ed. G.M. Edelman et al.), p. 471. Wiley, New York.

Kogan, J.H., P.W. Frankland, J.A. Blendy, J. Coblentz, Z. Marowitz, G. Schütz, and A.J. Silva. 1997. Spaced training induces normal long-term memory in CREB mutant mice. *Curr. Biol.* **7:** 1.

Levin, L.R., P.-L. Han, P.M. Hwang, P.G. Feinstein, R.L. Davis, and R.R. Reed. 1992. The *Drosophila* learning and memory gene *rutabaga* encodes a Ca^{2+}/calmodulin-responsive adenylyl cylase. *Cell* **68:** 479.

Li, W., T. Tully, and D. Kalderon. 1996. Effects of a conditional *Drosophila* PKA mutant on learning and memory. *Learn. Mem.* **2:** 320.

Livingstone, M.S., P.P. Sziber, and W.G. Quinn. 1984. Loss of calcium/calmodulin responsiveness in adenylate cyclase of rutabaga, a *Drosophila* learning mutant. *Cell* **137:** 205.

Luo, L., T. Tully, and K. White. 1992. Human amyloid precursor protein ameliorates behavioral deficit of flies deleted for *Appl* gene. *Neuron* **9:** 595.

Mackintosh, N.J. 1974. *The psychology of animal learning*. Academic Press, London.

Martin, K.C. and E.R. Kandel. 1996. Cell adhesion molecules, CREB, and the formation of new synaptic connections. *Neuron* **17:** 567.

Mauelshagen, J., G.R. Parker, and T.J. Carew. 1996. Dynamics of induction and expression of long-term synaptic facilitation in *Aplysia. J. Neurosci.* **16:** 7099.

McGaugh, J.L. 1966. Time-dependent processes in memory storage. *Science* **153:** 1351.

McGaugh, J.L. and M.L. Herz. 1972. *Memory consolidation*. Albion, San Fransisco, California.

Muller, D., C. Wang, G. Skibo, N. Toni, H. Cremer, V. Calaora, G. Rougon, and J.Z. Kiss. 1996. PSA-NCAM is required for activity-induced synaptic plasticity. *Neuron* **17:** 413.

Nguyen, P.V. and E.R. Kandel. 1996. A macromolecular synthesis-dependent late phase of long-term potentiation requiring cAMP in the medial perforant pathway of rat hippocampal slices. *J. Neurosci.* **16:** 3189.

Nicoll, R.A. and R.C. Malenka. 1995. Contrasting properties of two forms of long-term potentiation in the hippocampus. *Nature* **377:** 115.

Nighorn, A., M.J. Healy, and R.L. Davis. 1991. The cyclic AMP phosphodiesterase encoded by the *Drosophila dunce* gene is concentrated in the mushroom body neuropil. *Neuron* **6:** 455.

Quinn, W.G. and Y. Dudai. 1976. Memory phases in

Drosophila. *Nature* **262:** 576.

Quinn, W.G., W.A. Harris, and S. Benzer. 1974. Conditioned behavior in *Drosophila melanogaster*. *Proc. Natl. Acad. Sci.* **71:** 707.

Quinn, W., P.P. Sziber, and R. Booker. 1979. The *Drosophila* memory mutant *amnesiac*. *Nature* **277:** 212.

Rose, S.P. 1995. Cell-adhesion molecules, glucocorticoids and long-term-memory formation. *Trends Neurosci.* **18:** 502.

Rosenzweig, M.R. 1996. Aspects of the search for neural mechanisms of memory. *Annu. Rev. Psychol.* **47:** 1.

Rosenzweig, M.R. and E.L. Bennett. 1984. Basic processes and modulatory influences in the stages of memory formation. In *Neurobiology of learning and memory* (ed. G. Lynch McGaugh et al.), p. 263. Guilford Press, New York.

Salin, P.A., R.C. Malenka, and R.A. Nicoll. 1996. Cyclic AMP mediates a presynaptic form of LTP at cerebellar parallel fiber synapses. *Neuron* **16:** 797.

Skoulakis, E.M.C. and R.L. Davis. 1996. Olfactory learning deficits in mutants for *leonardo*, a *Drosophila* gene encoding a 14-3-3 protein. *Neuron* **17:** 931.

Skoulakis, E.M.C., D. Kalderon, and R.L. Davis. 1993. Preferential expression in mushroom bodies of the catalytic subunit of protein kinase A and its role in learning and memory. *Neuron* **11:** 197.

Squire, L.R., H.P. Davis, and C.W. Spanis. 1980. Neurobiology of amnesia. *Science* **209:** 836.

Stewart, M.G. and D.A. Rusakov. 1995. Morphological changes associated with stages of memory formation in the chick following passive avoidance training. *Behav. Brain Res.* **66:** 21.

Swanson, K.D. and R. Ganguly. 1992. Characterization of a *Drosophila melanogaster* gene similar to the mammalian genes encoding the tyrosine/tryptophan hydroxylase activator and protein kinase C inhibitor proteins. *Gene* **113:** 183.

Tempel, B.L., M.S. Livingstone, and W.G. Quinn. 1984. Mutations in the dopa decarboxylase gene affect learning in *Drosophila*. *Proc. Natl. Acad. Sci.* **81:** 3577.

Tempel, B.L., N. Bonini, D.R. Dawson, and W.G. Quinn. 1983. Reward learning in normal and mutant *Drosophila*. *Proc. Natl. Acad. Sci.* **80:** 1482.

Tonegawa, S., Y. Li, R.S. Erzurumlu, S. Jhaveri, C. Chen, Y. Goda, R. Paylor, A.J. Silva, J.J. Kim, J.M. Wehner, C.F. Stevens, and A. Abelovich. 1995. The gene knockout technology for the analysis of learning and memory, and neural development. *Prog. Brain Res.* **105:** 3.

Tully, T. 1984. *Drosophila* learning: Behavior and biochemistry. *Behav. Genet.* **14:** 527.

———. 1986. Measuring learning in individual flies is not necessary to study the effects of single-gene mutations in *Drosophila*: A reply to Holliday and Hirsch. *Behav. Genet.* **16:** 449.

———. 1994. Gene disruption of learning and memory: A structure-function conundrum? *Semin. Neurosci.* **6:** 108.

———. 1996. Discovery of genes involved with learning and memory: An experimental synthesis of Hirschian and Benzerian perspectives. *Proc. Natl. Acad. Sci.* **93:** 13460.

Tully, T. and J.P. Gergen. 1986. Deletion mapping of the *Drosophila* memory mutant *amnesiac*. *J. Neurogenet.* **3:** 33.

Tully, T. and W.G. Quinn. 1985. Classical conditioning and retention in normal and mutant *Drosophila melanogaster*. *J. Comp. Physiol. A* **157:** 263.

Tully, T., V. Cambiazo, and L. Kruse. 1994a. Memory through metamorphosis in normal and mutant *Drosophila*. *J. Neurosci.* **14:** 68.

Tully, T., T. Preat, S.C. Boynton, and M. Del Vecchio. 1994b. Genetic dissection of consolidated memory in *Drosophila*. *Cell* **79:** 35.

Tully, T., S. Boynton, C. Brandes, J.-M. Dura, R. Mihalek, T. Preat, and A. Villella. 1990. Genetic dissection of memory formaton in *Drosophila melanogaster*. *Cold Spring Harbor Symp. Quant. Biol.* **55:** 203.

Wehner, J.M., B.J. Bowers, and R. Paylor. 1996. The use of null mutant mice to study complex learning and memory processes. *Behav. Genet.* **26:** 301.

Weisskopf, M.G., P.E. Castillo, R.A. Zalutsky, and R.A. Nicoll. 1994. Mediation of hippocampal mossy fiber long-term potentiation by cyclic AMP. *Science* **265:** 1878.

Wu, G.-Y., R. Malinow, and H.T. Cline. 1996. Maturation of a central glutamatergic synapse. *Science* **274:** 972.

Yamada, A., T. Sekiguchi, H. Susuki, and A. Mizukami. 1992. Behavioral analysis of internal memory states using cooling-induced retrograde amnesia in *Limax flavus*. *J. Neurosci.* **12:** 729.

Yamoah, E.N. and T. Crow. 1996. Protein kinase and G-protein regulation of Ca2+ currents in Hermissenda photoreceptors by 5-HT and GABA. *J. Neurosci* **16:** 4799.

Yin, J.C.P. and T. Tully. 1996. CREB and the formation of long-term memory. *Curr. Opin. Neurobiol.* **6:** 264.

Yin, J.C.P., M.D. Vecchio, H. Zhou, and T. Tully. 1995a. CREB as a memory modulator: Induced expression of a *dCREB2* isoform enhances long-term memory in *Drosophila*. *Cell* **81:** 107.

Yin, J.C.P., J.S. Wallach, M. Del Vecchio, E.L. Wilder, H. Zhou, W.G. Quinn, and T. Tully. 1994. Induction of a dominant-negative CREB transgene blocks long-term memory in *Drosophila*. *Cell* **79:** 49.

Yin, J.C.P., J.S. Wallach, E.L. Wilder, J. Klingensmith, D. Dang, N. Perrimon, H. Zhou, T. Tully, and W.G. Quinn. 1995b. *Drosophila* CREB/CREM homolog encodes multiple isoforms, including a cyclic AMP-dependent protein kinase-responsive transcriptional activator and antagonist. *Mol. Cell. Biol.* **15:** 5123.

CaMKII Function in the Nervous System Explored from a Genetic Perspective

M. MAYFORD, M.E. BACH, AND E. KANDEL
Center for Neurobiology and Behavior, College of Physicians & Surgeons of Columbia University and Howard Hughes Medical Institute, New York, New York 10032

Calcium functions as an important signaling molecule in nerve cells by regulating a variety of physiological as well as pathological processes. These processes include the regulation of neurotransmitter release, the induction of both short- and long-lasting forms of synaptic plasticity, and activity-induced cell death. One mechanism by which Ca^{++} signals are transduced into physiological changes in the neuron is through the activation of protein kinases. One class of serine/threonine protein kinase that is directly activated by Ca^{++} is the Ca^{++}/calmodulin-dependent protein kinase II (CaMKII) family. The regulation of CaMKII activity has been studied extensively in vitro (Hanson and Schulman 1992). The enzyme can regulate its own activity via a series of activating and inhibiting autophosphorylations. A single subunit of the holoenzyme can have at least four independent states (Fig. 1). The ability to phosphorylate itself imparts to the holoenzyme the capacity to modulate its own activity in response to the size and frequency of transient Ca^{++} signals, as well as to control the activity of other Ca^{++}-stimulated molecules through the regulation of free levels of calmodulin (Miller and Kennedy 1986; Thiel et al. 1988; Fong et al. 1989; Waldmann et al. 1990; Meyer et al. 1992).

In the basal unphosphorylated state, the purified enzyme has a low level of Ca^{++}-independent activity due to the interaction of the autoinhibitory domain with the catalytic domain (Fig. 1,i). Upon stimulation with Ca^{++}/calmodulin, the interaction of the autoinhibitory and the kinase domains is reduced, with the result that the kinase activity is increased by about 100-fold (Fig. 1,ii). The Ca^{++}-stimulated kinase is able to phosphorylate a broad range of cellular substrates, including other subunits of CaMKII itself. In fact, the CaMKII enzyme is one of its own best substrates. As a consequence of this Ca^{++}-stimulated autophosphorylation, the enzyme is converted into a form that can maintain enzymatic activity even in the absence of Ca^{++}/calmodulin binding. This self-regulation has been the subject of a great deal of study because of its potential role as a biochemical substrate of memory (Miller and Kennedy 1986; Lisman 1994). The Ca^{++}-independent state of the enzyme is produced by phosphorylation of a single threonine residue within the autoinhibitory domain of the protein. In the case of CaMKIIα, this critical residue is Thr-286 (Thiel et al. 1988; Fong et al. 1989; Waldmann et al. 1990). Autophosphorylation of CaMKII at Thr-286 has two important consequences: (1) It increases the Ca^{++}-independent activity of the enzyme and (2) it increases the affinity of the enzyme for Ca^{++}/calmodulin by three orders of magnitude (Fig. 1, iii and iv) (Meyer et al. 1992). This dramatic increase in affinity for calmodulin allows kinase molecules that are autophosphorylated at Thr-286 to trap calmodulin and thereby to regulate calmodulin availability. This second nonenzymatic mechanism is particularly intriguing because calmodulin is essential not only for the regulation of CaMKII, but also for the regulation of a large variety of other Ca^{++}-dependent processes. Thus, this mechanism serves to amplify functionally the diversity of target processes CaMKII can modulate.

The ability of the kinase to convert a transient Ca^{++} signal into a long-lasting increase in enzyme activity has led to the suggestion that the kinase can mediate the induction and maintenance of long-term potentiation (LTP) (Lisman 1994). LTP is an activity-dependent form of synaptic strengthening produced by high-frequency synaptic activation (Bliss and Collingridge 1993). The induction of LTP is known to require the activation of postsynaptic NMDA receptors and an influx of Ca^{++} into the postsynaptic dendrite. According to the simple model initially suggested by Lisman, LTP is produced at a synapse when sufficient Ca^{++} enters the postsynaptic cell to activate CaMKII. Upon activation by Ca^{++}, the CaMKII quickly converts to the Ca^{++}-independent state, which is then maintained through continuous autophosphorylation even in the absence of Ca^{++} (Fig. 1, iii and iv). The elevated CaMKII activity is thought to both produce and maintain LTP through continuous phosphorylation of substrate proteins. Candidates for possible substrate effector proteins are the postsynaptic glutamate receptors of the AMPA type. Phosphorylation of these receptors by CaMKII potentiates the flow of ionic current through the receptor channel (Tan et al. 1994).

The initial suggestion that CaMKII serves an essential role in the initiation of LTP came from studies using inhibitors of the kinase (Malenka et al. 1989; Malinow et al. 1989). However, at the concentrations used, these inhibitors did not affect CaMKII specifically (Hvalby et al. 1994). More recently, several groups have turned to genetically modified mice to study the

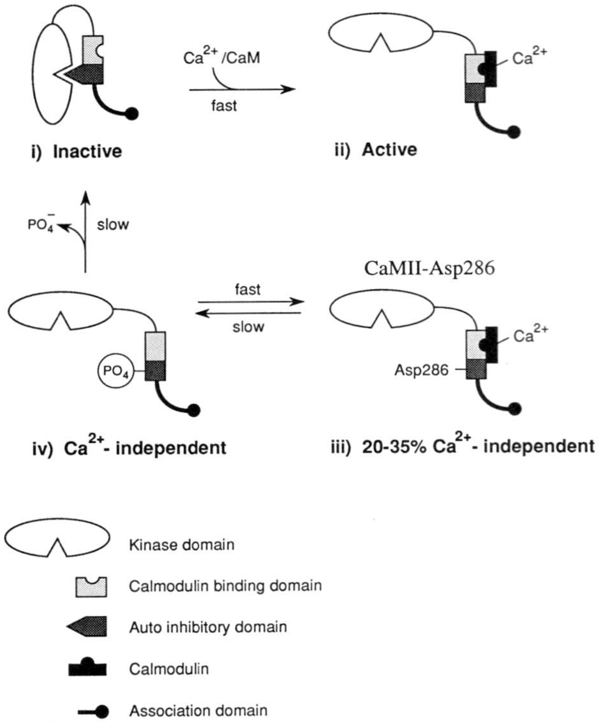

Figure 1. Regulation of CaMKII activity. Individual subunits of CaMKII can exist in at least four independent states as shown. (i) Basal unphosphorylated; (ii) unphosphorylated, but activated by bound Ca^{++}/calmodulin; (iii) autophosphorylated at Thr-286 and with Ca^{++}/calmodulin bound; and (iv) autophosphorylated at Thr-286 without bound Ca^{++}/calmodulin.

role of CaMKII in LTP and in learning and memory.

Alcino Silva, Susumu Tonegawa, and their colleagues used gene targeting to generate a mouse in which the CaMKIIα gene was inactivated (Silva et al. 1992a,b). They found a 50% reduction in the level of CaMKII activity in the hippocampus. When examined physiologically, the mice showed an almost complete loss of normal high-frequency LTP. Moreover, the animals displayed a severe deficit in hippocampal-based spatial memory tasks. These results provided genetic support for the notion that CaMKII activation is necessary for the induction of LTP. They also provided a link between CaMKII signaling, LTP, and learning.

Recently, we have attempted to test the simple Lisman model of LTP. One prediction of this model is that CaMKII activation alone is sufficient to produce LTP. To test this idea, we expressed an activated form of CaMKII in the forebrain of transgenic mice.

SWITCHING ON CAMKII IN THE MOUSE BRAIN

To test whether activation of CaMKII alone is sufficient to induce LTP, we took advantage of a mutation in the kinase that mimics autophosphorylation at Thr-286. In this mutant form of CaMKII, Thr-286 is replaced with an acidic aspartate group (CaMKII-Asp286). The mutant kinase is 20- to 30-fold more active in the absence of Ca^{++} than the wild-type enzyme (Fong et al. 1989; Waldmann et al. 1990). Using the CaMKIIα promoter to limit expression to the forebrain, we generated transgenic mice that express CaMKII-Asp286 in the hippocampus at a level of Ca^{++} independence greater than that reached during LTP. In addition, we included the entire 3′UTR of the CaMKIIα gene, which targets the mRNA to dendrites (M. Mayford and E.R. Kandel, unpubl.).

We were now in a position to ask directly: Does activating CaMKII in the hippocampus switch on LTP? If LTP were produced at many or all of the hippocampal synapses in mice expressing the CaMKII-Asp286 mutant transgene, two changes in physiology would be expected. First, an increase in the basal synaptic transmission should occur secondary to the induction of LTP. Second, the ability to induce further LTP should be occluded, since LTP is saturable. We observed neither of these two changes in the CaMKII-Asp286 mice, even though Ca^{++}-independent CaMKII activity was elevated to a level greater than that produced by LTP itself (Mayford et al. 1995). These results suggest that even though CaMKII is important for the induction of LTP, its activation alone is not sufficient to produce and maintain LTP.

LTP is commonly studied experimentally by using brief 100-Hz stimulation trains. However, lower frequency stimulation can also produce LTP. In fact, there is a direct correlation between the frequency of synaptic stimulation and the size and direction of the synaptic change produced, with high frequencies causing LTP and low frequencies causing a long-lasting synaptic depression or LTD. The CaMKII-Asp286 transgenic mice showed perfectly good LTP at 100 Hz. However, at lower frequencies it differed significantly from wild-type. When stimulated at 10, 5, and 1 Hz, wild-type mice show 29% LTP, 17% LTP, and 5% LTD, respectively. However, in the CaMKII-Asp286 transgenic mice there was a systematic shift in the response to low-frequency stimulation such that LTP was reduced and LTD was favored (Fig. 2). Thus, in the transgenic mice, stimulation at 10, 5, and 1 Hz now produced 9% LTP, 15% LTD, and 28% LTD, respectively (Fig. 2). These results give a somewhat novel view of the role of CaMKII in synaptic plasticity. They suggest that rather than being a direct effector that mediates the biochemical signal for the production of LTP, CaMKII activation is a modulator that regulates the conditions under which a synapse will undergo either LTP or LTD.

The view of CaMKII as a modulator of synaptic plasticity seems in turn to provide an explanation for two previously unrelated phenomena: the developmental loss of LTD in the adult hippocampus and the ability of high-frequency stimulation to reactivate the capacity for LTD in the adult animal. During normal

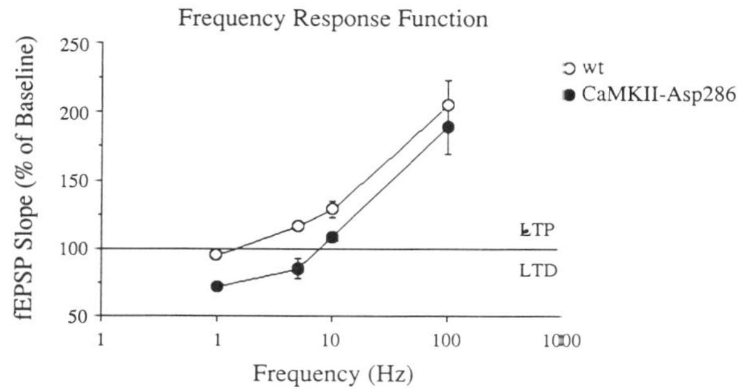

Figure 2. Shift in LTP/LTD frequency threshold. Changes in synaptic strength produced 1 hr after stimulation at 1, 5, 10, and 100 Hz in wild-type (wt) and CaMKII-Asp 286 transgenic mice. (Adapted from Mayford et al. 1995.)

development of the hippocampus there is a change in the ability to obtain LTP and LTD. In neonatal animals (5–10 days of age), LTD is readily obtained, whereas LTP is absent (Müller et al. 1989). In the juvenile hippocampus (3–4 weeks of age), both LTP and LTD can be obtained by high- and low-frequency stimulation, respectively (Dudek and Bear 1993; Mayford et al. 1995). In the adult hippocampus (>8 weeks), LTP is readily obtained by high-frequency stimulation, whereas LTD is weak or absent (Dudek and Bear, 1993; O'Dell and Kandel 1994; Mayford et al. 1995). This developmental loss in the capacity for LTD with age is accompanied by a developmental decrease in the levels of Ca^{++}-independent CaMKII activity (Molloy and Kennedy 1991; Mayford et al. 1995). Our results with the CaMKII-Asp286 transgenic mice suggest that the loss of LTD with age may be caused by the developmental decrease in Ca^{++}-independent CaMKII activity. When Ca^{++}-independent activity is maintained in the adult at the higher juvenile level by expression of the CaMKII-Asp286 transgene, the capacity for LTD is also maintained (Mayford et al. 1995).

Efficient information storage in the brain presumably requires the capacity not only for increasing, but also for decreasing, synaptic strength. How might this be achieved in the adult animal if LTD is lost? Previous studies have shown that the production of LTP at the hippocampal CA1 synapse by high-frequency stimulation causes a reactivation of the capacity for LTD in the adult animal (Fujii et al. 1991; O'Dell and Kandel 1994). This same stimulation also leads to a sustained increase in the levels of Ca^{++}-independent CaMKII activity at the synapse. Our previous study of the CaMKII-Asp286 mice showed that the genetic activation of CaMKII occludes the effect of high-frequency stimulation on LTD (Mayford et al. 1995). That is, in the CaMKII-Asp286 mice in which LTD is present in the adult animal, high-frequency stimulation does not produce a further increase in the capacity for LTD. These results suggest that the high-frequency-induced reactivation of the capacity for LTD in the adult hippocampus involves the activation of the CaMKII pathway.

To summarize, our studies of transgenic mice expressing an activated mutant form of CaMKII which mimics the effects of autophosphorylation at Thr-286 suggest a new role for the Ca^{++}-independent form of the kinase. These results suggest that the activation of CaMKII by itself does not induce LTP. Rather, CaMKII acts to regulate the frequency threshold for the production of both LTP and LTD. Moreover, our data suggest that endogenous changes in CaMKII autophosphorylation during development and following high-frequency synaptic activation similarly control this frequency threshold. Modulating the frequency threshold may be an important mechanism for regulating the absolute level of synaptic strength that can be obtained at any frequency and for providing the synapse with the forms of plasticity that are appropriate at different stages in development.

A MODEL FOR THE ROLE OF CAMKII IN REGULATING THE FREQUENCY THRESHOLD

In the CaMKII-Asp286 mice there is no alteration in the total amount of LTP produced at high frequencies but a systematic shift to favor LTD at medium-to-low frequencies. How might the expression of the CaMKII-Asp286 transgene mediate this effect? Both LTP and LTD induction require the activation of NMDA-type glutamate receptors and Ca^{++} influx into the postsynaptic dendrite. The current view is that high levels of Ca^{++} influx lead to LTP, whereas lower levels of Ca^{++} influx activate only LTD (Bear and Malenka 1994). Thus, one way for CaMKII to control the balance between LTP and LTD is by controlling the levels of free Ca^{++} or Ca^{++}/calmodulin in the postsynaptic neuron following a given frequency of stimulation.

The biochemical basis for this effect is not yet known. However, there are two possible explanations. First, the effect of CaMKII activation on the LTP/LTD frequency threshold could be due to a direct effect of the enzyme on particular substrate proteins that control Ca^{++} entry or intracellular Ca^{++} handling. For example, a direct phosphorylation of the NMDA receptor by CaMKII might reduce the influx of Ca^{++} through the receptor upon activation. In this case, stimulation in the low-frequency range would lead to a smaller intracellular Ca^{++} signal in the CaMKII-Asp286 transgenic mice and thus to a systematic shift away from LTP and in favor of LTD at those frequencies. Phosphorylation of a number of other possible substrate proteins could produce a similar effect either by directly altering the size of the Ca^{++} signal or by affecting intracellular Ca^{++}-binding proteins.

Alternatively, it is possible that it is not the enzymatic activity of the autophosphorylated form of CaMKII that is critical, but the 1000-fold increased affinity of the autophosphorylated CaMKII subunit for

Ca^{++}/calmodulin (Meyer et al. 1992). Here, the CaMKII would function as a self-regulatable Ca^{++}/calmodulin sink (Fig. 3). In this case, CaMKII enzyme activity is not necessary for the induction of either LTP or LTD. However, the amount of the autophosphorylated form of CaMKII regulates the balance between the two processes by regulating the levels of free Ca^{++}/calmodulin in the dendritic spine. The dissociation constant for calmodulin from CaMKII increases from about 0.2 second in the unphosphorylated state to about 20 seconds for CaMKII that is autophosphorylated at Thr-286 (Meyer et al. 1992). Thus, at higher levels of autophosphorylated CaMKII, the same size Ca^{++} signal would produce a smaller increase of free Ca^{++}/calmodulin, due to the sequestration of a larger fraction of the Ca^{++}/calmodulin by the high-affinity autophosphorylated form of the kinase. This in turn would lead to a systematic shift in favor of LTD at all submaximal levels of Ca^{++} influx, as would be obtained at low frequencies of stimulation. This effect of the autophosphorylated kinase should be overcome at saturating levels of Ca^{++}/calmodulin, as might be achieved by high-frequency stimulation.

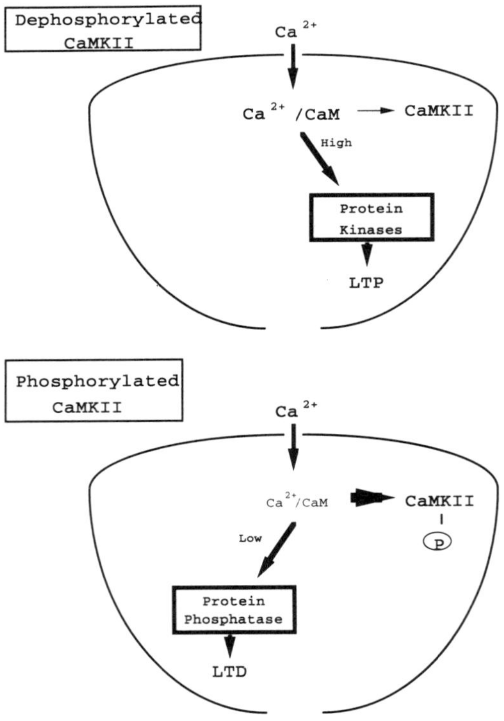

Figure 3. Calmodulin trapping model. Model depicts the effect of CaMKII autophosphorylation state on the generation of LTP or LTD for a constant amount of Ca^{++} influx. In the dephosphorylated state, CaMKII will bind relatively little Ca^{++}/calmodulin so that the free Ca^{++}/calmodulin levels will be sufficient to activate LTP. However, when autophosphorylated at Thr-286, the CaMKII will bind to and trap a large fraction of Ca^{++}/calmodulin. This will lead to a lower level of free Ca^{++}/calmodulin and the production of LTD.

A SECOND GENERATION OF GENETICALLY MODIFIED MICE: REGULATED GENE EXPRESSION

The standard approaches to genetic modification of the mouse suffer from the fact that the genetic alteration is present throughout the developmental lifetime of the animal. This makes the interpretation of a phenotype observed in adult mutant animals difficult, since it may result from a developmental defect or genetic compensation, rather than from a direct effect of the genetic change in the adult. Moreover, many molecular signaling processes are not all-or-none events, but may produce varying effects depending on the quantitative degree of pathway activation. It would thus be useful to obtain control over the timing and level of transgene expression in adult mice.

We have been influenced by the recent work by H. Bujard and his colleagues on a regulatable genetic switch (Gossen and Bujard 1992; Furth et al. 1994). Bujard has adapted for use in eukaryotic cells the tetracycline repressor system of *Escherichia coli* as outlined in Figure 4. In this system, a hybrid protein is constructed consisting of the tetracycline repressor protein of the *E. coli* Tn10 gene fused to the transcription activation domain of the herpes simplex VP16 protein. The resulting protein, called the tetracycline *trans*-activator, or tTA, gene is able to bind specifically to a sequence from the Tn10 gene called the tetracycline operator or tetO. Binding of tTA to tetO will activate transcription in eukaryotic cells of any gene that is linked to the tetO element. However, the administration of small amounts of tetracycline disrupts the binding of tTA to tetO and suppresses expression of the tetO-linked gene.

We have adapted this system to the brain to obtain forebrain-specific regulated expression of the CaMKII-Asp286 transgene. Toward this end, two lines of mice are produced. In the first mouse line, the CaMKIIα promoter is used to drive expression of the tTA gene into forebrain neurons. In the second line, the tetO promoter element is linked to the CaMKII-Asp286 gene. In this mouse line, the CaMKII-Asp286 transgene is not expressed, since there is no tTA present to activate its transcription from the tetO promoter. However, when both transgenes are introduced into the same mouse through mating, the CaMKII-Asp286 transgene is activated, but only in those forebrain neurons that express tTA. Now, administration of the tetracycline analog doxycycline to the double transgenic mice at 1 mg/ml in the drinking water will completely suppress expression of the CaMKII-Asp286 transgene to basal levels. Withdrawal of the drug will cause a reactivation of the transgene to levels seen in the untreated animal.

We have been able to reexamine the stimulation frequency threshold for the production of LTP and LTD in mice that differ from wild type in two ways: (1) the expression of the transgene is regulated and (2) the expression is restricted to the CA1 pyramidal neurons

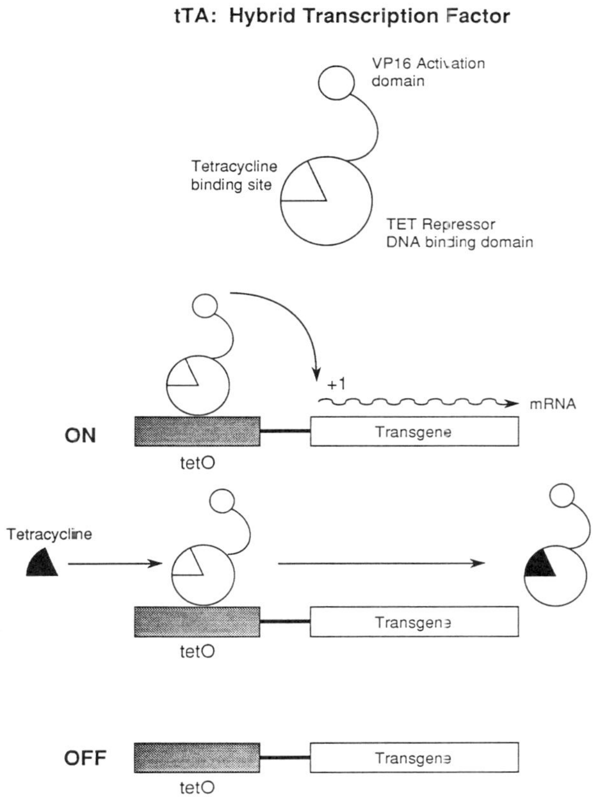

Figure 4. tTA regulation of transcription. The tTA transcription activator consisting of the Tn10 tetracycline repressor and VP16 transcription activation domains. Binding of tTA to tetO activates transcription of a linked transgene. This transcription can be suppressed by tetracycline (Gossen and Bujard 1992).

with little or no expression in the CA3 neurons. Thus, when examining the Schaffer collateral pathway in these mice, the transgene expression is limited exclusively to the postsynaptic neuron.

In these mice, we examined the response to 10-Hz stimulation and found that whereas wild-type mice show LTP, the transgenic mice show a small amount of LTD. However, when the expression of the CaMKII-Asp286 transgene is suppressed with doxycycline, the transgenic mice show LTP similar to wild-type animals. Thus, the CaMKII-Asp286 transgene functions in the postsynaptic neuron to cause the shift in the LTP/LTD frequency threshold, and this effect is due to the acute expression of the transgene rather than to an irreversible developmental defect.

We then examined a line of transgenic mouse that expressed the CaMKII-Asp286 transgene at moderate levels in the hippocampus as well as the striatum and amygdala. We tested these mice on an explicit hippocampal-based memory task, the Barnes circular maze. The animals showed a memory deficit in the Barnes circular maze that was again reversed by suppression of the transgene with doxycycline. Thus, the genetic activation of CaMKII through expression of the Ca^{++}-independent mutant CaMKII-Asp286 as a transgene can interfere with synaptic plasticity, as well as with explicit memory storage in a manner independent of its possible effects on neuronal development.

OVERALL VIEW

Recent genetic studies of CaMKII function in the nervous system have revealed a role in long-lasting forms of synaptic plasticity such as LTP and LTD. The use of a Ca^{++}-independent mutant form of CaMKII expressed as a transgene suggests that the enzyme may function not directly to produce the synaptic change, but to regulate the type of synaptic activity that will lead to either LTP or LTD. In addition, the genetic studies point to a role for CaMKII signaling in learning and memory, possibly through its effects on synaptic plasticity. A new generation of genetic methodologies is becoming available that will allow the regulation of genetic change in transgenic and knockout mice. These techniques should permit a rigorous and detailed dissection of the cellular and molecular mechanism of higher cognitive functions such as learning and memory.

REFERENCES

Bach, M.E., R.D. Hawkins, M. Osman, E.R. Kandel, and M. Mayford. 1995. Impairment of spatial but not contextual memory in CaMKII mutant mice with a selective loss of hippocampal LTP in the range of the θ frequency. *Cell* **81:** 905.

Bear, M.F. and R.C. Malenka. 1994. Synaptic plasticity: LTP and LTD. *Curr. Opin. Neurobiol.* **4:** 389.

Bliss, T.V.P. and G.L. Collingridge. 1993. A synaptic model of memory: Long-term potentiation in the hippocampus. *Nature* **361:** 31.

Dudek, S.M. and M.F. Bear. 1993. Bidirectional long-term modification of synaptic effectiveness in the adult and immature hippocampus. *J. Neurosci.* **13:** 2910.

Fong, Y.-L, W.L. Taylor, A.R. Means, and T.R. Soderling. 1989. Studies of the regulatory mechanism of Ca^{2+}/calmodulin-dependent protein kinase II: Mutation of threonine 286 to alanine and aspartate. *J. Biol. Chem.* **264:** 16759.

Fujii, S., K. Saito, H. Miyakawa, K. Ito, and H. Kato. 1991. Reversal of long-term potentiation (depotentiation) induced by tetanus stimulation of the input to CA1 neurons of guinea pig hippocampal slices. *Brain Res.* **555:** 112.

Furth, P.A., L. St. Onge, H. Böger, P. Gruss, M. Gossen, A. Kistner, H. Bujard, and L. Henninghausen. 1994. Temporal control of gene expression in transgenic mice by a tetracycline-responsive promoter. *Proc. Natl. Acad. Sci.* **91:** 9302.

Gossen, M. and H. Bujard. 1992. Tight control of gene expression in mammalian cells by tetracycline-responsive promoters. *Proc. Natl. Acad. Sci.* **89:** 5547.

Hanson, P.I. and H. Schulman. 1992. Neuronal Ca^{2+}/calmodulin-dependent protein kinases. *Annu. Rev. Biochem.* **61:** 559.

Hvalby, O., H.C. Hemmings, O. Paulsen, A.J. Czernik, A.C.

Nairn, J.M. Godfraind, V. Jensen, M. Raastad, F. Storm, and P. Andersen. 1994. Specificity of protein kinase inhibitor peptides and induction of long-term potentiation. *Proc. Natl. Acad. Sci.* **91:** 4761.

Lisman, J. 1994. The CaM kinase II hypothesis for the storage of synaptic memory. *Trends Neurosci.* **17:** 406.

Malenka, R.C., J.A. Kauer, D.J. Perkel, M.D. Mauk, P.T. Kelly, R.A. Nicoll, and M.N. Waxham. 1989. An essential role for postsynaptic calmodulin and protein kinase activity in long-term potentiation. *Nature* **340:** 554.

Malinow, R., H. Schulman, and R.W. Tsien. 1989. Inhibition of postsynaptic PKC or CaMKII blocks induction but not expression of LTP. *Science* **245:** 862.

Mayford, M., J. Wang, E.R. Kandel, and J. O'Dell. 1995. CaMKII regulates the frequency-response function of hippocampal synapses for the production of both LTD and LTP. *Cell* **81:** 891.

Meyer, T., P.I. Hanson, L. Stryer, and H. Schulman. 1992. Calmodulin trapping by calcium-calmodulin-dependent protein kinase. *Science* **256:** 1199.

Miller, S.G. and M.B. Kennedy. 1986. Regulation of brain type II Ca^{2+}/calmodulin-dependent protein kinase by autophosphorylation: A Ca^{2+}-triggered molecular switch. *Cell* **44:** 861.

Molloy, S.S. and M.B. Kennedy. 1991. Autophosphorylation of type II Ca^{2+}/calmodulin-dependent protein kinase in cultures of postnatal rat hippocampal slices. *Proc. Natl. Acad. Sci.* **88:** 4756.

Müller, D., M. Oliver, and G. Lynch. 1989. Developmental changes in synaptic properties in hippocampus of neonatal rats. *Dev. Brain Res.* **49:** 105.

O'Dell, T.J. and E.R. Kandel. 1994. Low-frequency stimulation erases LTP through an NMDA receptor-mediated activation of protein phosphatases. *Learn. Mem.* **1:** 129.

Silva, A.J., R. Paylor, J.M. Wehner, and S. Tonegawa. 1992a. Deficient hippocampal long-term potentiation in α-calcium-calmodulin kinase II mutant mice. *Science* **257:** 206.

Silva, A.J., C.F. Stevens, S. Tonegawa, and Y. Wang. 1992b. Impaired spatial learning in α-calcium-calmodulin kinase II mutant mice. *Science* **257:** 201.

Tan, S.-E., R.J. Wenthold, and T.R. Soderling. 1994. Phosphorylation of AMPA-type glutamate receptors by calcium/calmodulin-dependent protein kinase II and protein kinase C in cultured hippocampal neurons. *J. Neurosci.* **14:** 1123.

Thiel, G., A.J. Czernik, F. Gorelick, A.C. Nairn, and P. Greengard. 1988. Ca^{2+}/calmodulin-dependent protein kinase II: Identification of threonine-286 as the autophosphorylation site in the α subunit associated with the generation of Ca^{2+}-independent activity. *Proc. Natl. Acad. Sci.* **85:** 6337.

Waldmann, R., P.I. Hanson, and H. Schulman. 1990. Multifunctional Ca^{2+}/calmodulin-dependent protein kinase made Ca^{2+}/independent for functional studies. *Biochemistry* **29:** 1679.

Hippocampal CA1-region-restricted Knockout of NMDAR1 Gene Disrupts Synaptic Plasticity, Place Fields, and Spatial Learning

S. TONEGAWA,[1-5] J.Z. TSIEN,[1-5] T.J. MCHUGH,[1-5] P. HUERTA,[1-5] K.I. BLUM,[2,4,5] AND M.A. WILSON[2,4,5]
[1]*Howard Hughes Medical Institute,* [2]*Center for Learning and Memory,* [3]*Center for Cancer Research,* [4]*Department of Biology, and* [5]*Department of Brain and Cognitive Sciences, Massachusetts Institute of Technology, Cambridge, Massachusetts 02139*

It has long been hypothesized that memory storage in the mammalian brain involves modifications of the synaptic connections between neurons. In 1949, Hebb introduced an influential theory consisting of principles that neurons must exhibit for implementing associative memory. The most important principle, known as Hebb's rule, is that when the presynaptic and the postsynaptic neurons are active simultaneously, their connections become strengthened. Subsequently, a synaptic phenomenon termed long-term potentiation (LTP) was discovered in the hippocampus that fits Hebb's rule. Hippocampal LTP, and the more recently discovered long-term depression (LTD), have been subjected to excruciating molecular and cellular studies as the promising candidate mechanisms for memory storage. A large body of research has shown that various artificial protocols in vitro and in vivo can induce LTP or LTD.

The hippocampus is also well situated for its role in memory from the anatomical point of view. It is a high-level multimodal association cortex that has reciprocal connections to many other cortical regions (Amaral and Witter 1989). Numerous neurophysiological studies have revealed that humans with hippocampal lesions are severely impaired in their ability to acquire new long-term memories of people, places, and events (Scoville and Milner 1957; Zola-Morgan et al. 1986). Rodents with hippocampal lesions are impaired in a variety of spatial and order discrimination tasks (O'Keefe and Nadel 1978; Morris et al. 1982; Eichenbaum et al. 1988; Jarrard 1993).

Does the hippocampal synaptic plasticity, LTP and LTD, indeed underlie natural learning and memory? Two types of experiments have been carried out to address this central issue. Morris and his coworkers reported that an NMDA receptor antagonist delivered to the hippocampus caused spatial learning deficits similar to hippocampal lesions and prevented LTP induction (Morris et al. 1986; Morris 1989; Davis et al. 1992). Although qualified later (Bannerman et al. 1995; Saucier and Cain 1995), this work raised the possibility that NMDA-dependent plasticity would affect the natural learning of spatial information. This correlation between impairments in hippocampal synaptic plasticity and spatial learning has also been observed in several mutant mice generated by conventional gene knockout techniques (Grant et al. 1992; Silva et al. 1992a,b; Stevens et al. 1994; Chen and Tonegawa 1997). For instance, mice with a deletion in the gene encoding the α subunit of Ca^{++}/calmodulin-dependent protein kinase II (αCaMKII) displayed impaired LTP and LTD in the CA1 region of the hippocampus and a deficit in spatial learning (Silva et al. 1992a,b). Although the results of these pharmacological and genetic experiments are consistent with the notion that hippocampal synaptic plasticity underlies spatial memory, other interpretations could not be excluded because of the lack of regional (and in the case of the mutant studies, temporal) specificity of molecular blockade. It is possible that the observed behavioral defects arose from the functions of NMDA receptors or αCaMKII in processes other than the induction of hippocampal synaptic plasticity. Furthermore, even if the linkage between hippocampal synaptic plasticity and spatial memory is established, one would like to know more about how the former enables the latter.

In vivo hippocampal electrical recordings reveal that as a rodent moves freely throughout its environment, pyramidal cells in the hippocampus fire when the animal is within highly restricted regions (O'Keefe and Dostrovsky 1971). Each cell has its own region of elevated firing, termed a place field, and large numbers of hippocampal place cells will tile each environment with overlapping place fields. Information about the location of the animal is of high enough quality that the position can be well estimated by simultaneously examining the firing patterns of many hippocampal neurons (Wilson and McNaughton 1993). The relative locations of these place receptive fields change in different environments and, thus, place fields clearly must be learned anew in each environment with spatial information represented in the firing of ensembles rather than single cells. The question then is, Does hippocampal LTP (or LTD) subserve spatial memory by enabling the formation of spatial fields?

To address these questions critically, it is highly desirable to establish a method that permits post-developmental elimination of a crucial gene exclusively in a subset of hippocampal cells. Using the *Cre/loxP* recombination system derived from the phage P1, we recently produced mice in which the gene encoding NMDA receptor subunit 1, an essential component of all known forms of NMDA receptors, is knocked out exclusively in the pyramidal cells of the hippocampal CA1 region. We show that these mice lack NMDA-receptor-mediated synaptic currents and LTP specifically in the CA1 synapses and exhibit impaired spatial memory. Furthermore, we have discovered that although the CA1 pyramidal cells of these mice retain place-related activity, there is a significant decrease in the spatial specificity of individual place fields. We have also found a striking deficit in the coordinated firing of pairs of neurons tuned to similar spatial locations. These results demonstrate that NMDA-receptor-mediated synaptic plasticity is necessary for the proper representation of space in the CA1 region of the hippocampus and suggest that such representation is essential for spatial memory.

METHODS

All of the methods used in this paper are described in Tsien et al. (1996a,b) and McHugh et al. (1996).

RESULTS

Generation of CA1-restricted NMDAR1 Mutant Mice

Figure 1A illustrates the general strategy for cell-type-restricted, gene knockout technology. Using the transcriptional promoter derived from the αCaMKII gene to drive *Cre* gene expression, we recently produced a transgenic *Cre* mouse line, T29-1, with which one can accomplish *Cre/loxP*-mediated gene knockout efficiently and exclusively in the CA1 pyramidal cells of the hippocampus. This is demonstrated in Figure 1B using a *lacZ* reporter mouse in which the expression of the transgenic *lacZ* gene depends on *Cre-loxP* recombination.

To apply this cell-type-restricted gene knockout technology to the NMDAR1 gene, we constructed a targeting vector in which two *loxP* sequences were inserted into the NMDAR1 gene as shown in Figure 2A. Using this vector, mice homozygous for the *loxP*-NMDAR1-*loxP* sequences (henceforth named "floxed NR1" or "fNR1" mice) were generated through standard embryonic stem (ES) cell gene-targeting procedures (Bradley 1987; Capecchi 1989).

We crossed fNR1 mice with heterozygous *Cre* transgenic mice, T29-1, which have the capacity to mediate *Cre/loxP* recombination exclusively in the CA1 pyramidal cells (Tsien at al. 1996a). After crossing, we obtained mice carrying the *Cre* transgene and the homozygous fNR1 gene (*Cre/+, fNR1/fNR1*), that is CA1-KO mice, as well as various types of siblings (see Methods). From the latter, wild-type (wt) mice (+/+, +/+), T29-1 mice (*Cre*/+, +/+), and homozygous fNR1 mice (+/+, *fNR1/fNR1*) were used as experimental controls. The proportions of mice of the various genotypes indicated that (1) *Cre* and *fNR1* segregate as independent Mendelian loci and (2) the CA1-KO mice and the homozygous fNR1 mice are not lethal at the embryonic or perinatal stage. Indeed, these two types of mice grow and mate normally, and their overall behavior is indistinguishable from that of wt and T29-1 mice. These characteristics of the CA1-KO and the homozygous fNR1 mice are in contrast to the perinatal lethality of NMDAR1 KO mice produced by conventional gene knockout techniques (Forrest et al. 1994; Li et al. 1994). The absence of a gross behavioral phenotype suggests both that the *loxP* insertions do not interfere with normal expression of the fNR1 gene and that the NMDAR1 deletion in CA1-KO mice must be regionally restricted, as expected. Histochemical examination showed that the brains from the CA1-KO mice did not exhibit any obvious abnormalities at the macroscopic level (data not shown).

We confirmed the CA1-restricted deletion of the NMDAR1 gene in the CA1-KO mice by in situ hybridization with a probe whose sequence should be deleted at the DNA level by the *Cre/loxP* recombination. The CA1 region of the mutant mice appeared to lack NMDAR1 mRNA (Fig. 2B), whereas the level of this RNA in other brain regions (such as CA3, dentate gyrus, and neocortex) was indistinguishable from that of control mice (Fig. 2B).

Synaptic Transmission in CA1 and Dentate Gyrus

Synaptic responses of CA1 pyramidal neurons were evoked by stimulation of Schaffer collateral/commissural (Scc) afferents in acute slices. Whole-cell recordings revealed that the CA1-KO cells lacked the slow component of the excitatory postsynaptic current (EPSC) that is mediated by NMDARs (Hestrin et al. 1990a,b). Conversely, the early component of the EPSC that is mediated by AMPA receptors was intact in the mutants. Blockade of AMPA receptors with CNQX (20 μM) resulted in a complete inhibition of the EPSC in the mutant cells, whereas the control cells displayed a robust isolated NMDAR-dependent EPSC (data not shown).

We used field recordings of excitatory postsynaptic potentials (EPSPs) to further examine the synaptic properties of mutant slices. The time courses of the EPSPs measured in CA1 were similar between mutant slices (Fig. 3A, left) and control slices (not shown) when they were bathed with standard saline solution. However, addition of a solution that isolates the NMDARs resulted in the complete blockade of the EPSPs in mutant slices (n = 12, Fig. 3A, left). Conversely, the control slices showed a distinct isolated NMDA EPSP in CA1 (not shown).

A key control experiment was to examine whether functional NMDARs are present in other brain structures in the CA1-KO mice. We studied the synaptic responses of granule cells in the dentate gyrus upon

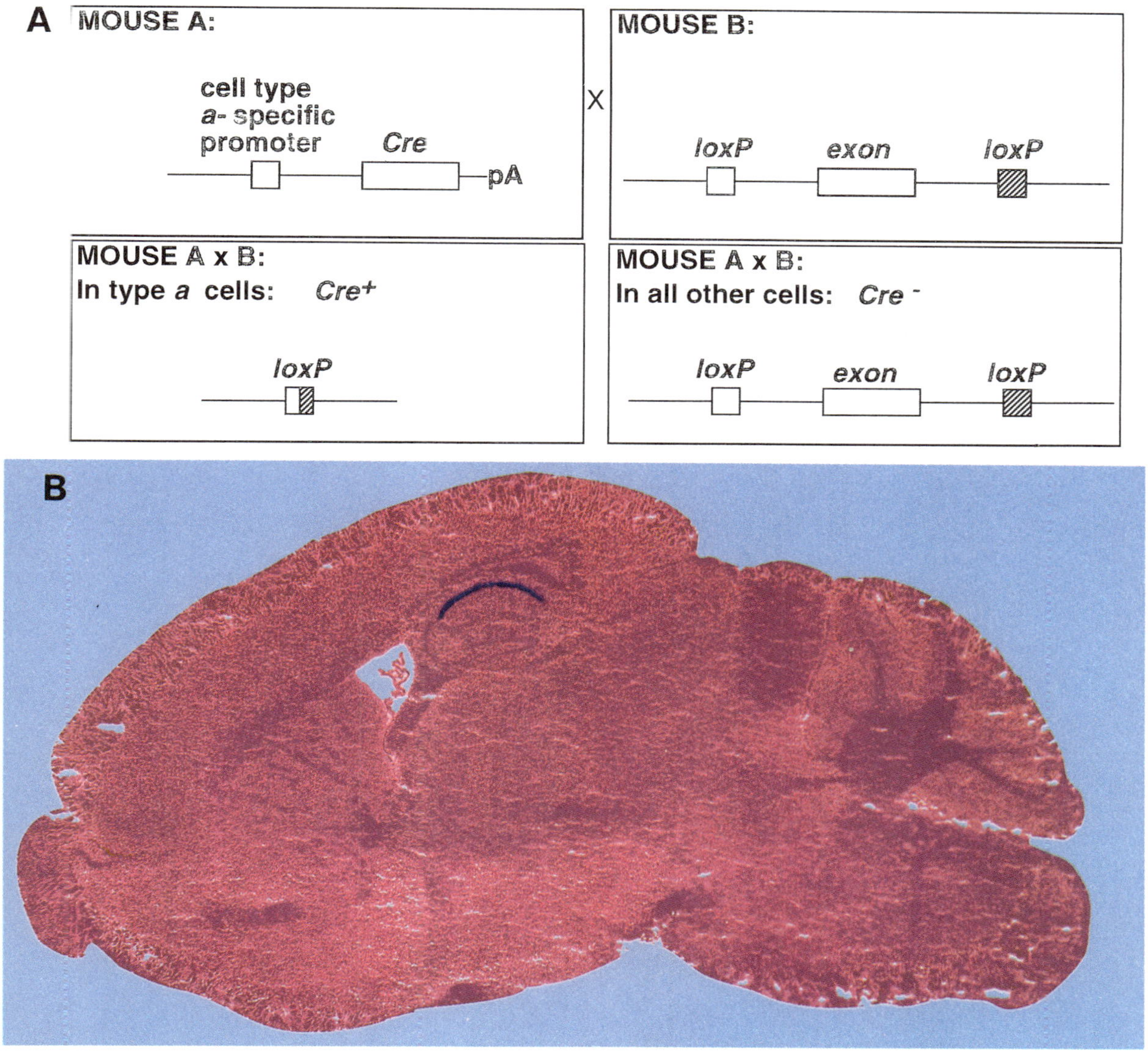

Figure 1. Strategy for cell-type-restricted gene knockout and *Cre/loxP* recombination pattern in the brain for a T29-1/*lacZ* mouse. (*A*) Strategy. *Cre* is a site-specific recombinase that mediates deletional recombination on a pair of tandemly repeated *loxP* DNA sequences. Mouse A carries the *Cre* transgene under the control of a tissue-type or cell-type-specific transcriptional promoter. Mouse B carries a pair of *loxP* sequences targeted to the gene of interest (dubbed "floxed gene") such that the mouse is homozygous with the floxed gene and the insertion itself does not interfere with the expression of the gene. This mouse can be made by the standard ES cell homologous recombination techniques. In progeny that are homozygous for the floxed gene and that carry the *Cre* transgene, the floxed gene will be deleted via *Cre/loxP* recombination but only in the tissue or cell type in which the *Cre* gene-associated promoter is active. (*B*) *Cre/loxP* pattern in T29-1/*lacZ* mouse. T 29-1 is a mouse line with a *Cre* transgene under the control of the αCaMKII promoter. This mouse was crossed to a *lacZ* reporter mouse in which β-galactosidase expression depended on *Cre/loxP* recombination. The sagittal brain section of the T29-1/*lacZ* mouse was stained with X-gal and then counterstained with eosin. Blue X-gal stain is observed only in the CA1 pyramidal cell layer of the hippocampus.

stimulation of the lateral perforant path (Hanse and Gustafsson 1992). We found that the time courses of field EPSPs in mutant slices (Fig. 3A, right) looked normal when compared with control slices (not shown). Importantly, after addition of a solution that isolates NMDARs, the mutant slices showed clear NMDA EPSPs (n =12, Fig. 3A, right) as well as the control slices (not shown). In conclusion, our electrophysiological analysis reveals that the CA1-KO mice lack functional postsynaptic NMDARs in the CA1 pyramidal cells. In contrast, postsynaptic AMPA receptors seem to operate normally in CA1. Finally, the CA1-KO mice show normal NMDAR function in the dentate gyrus.

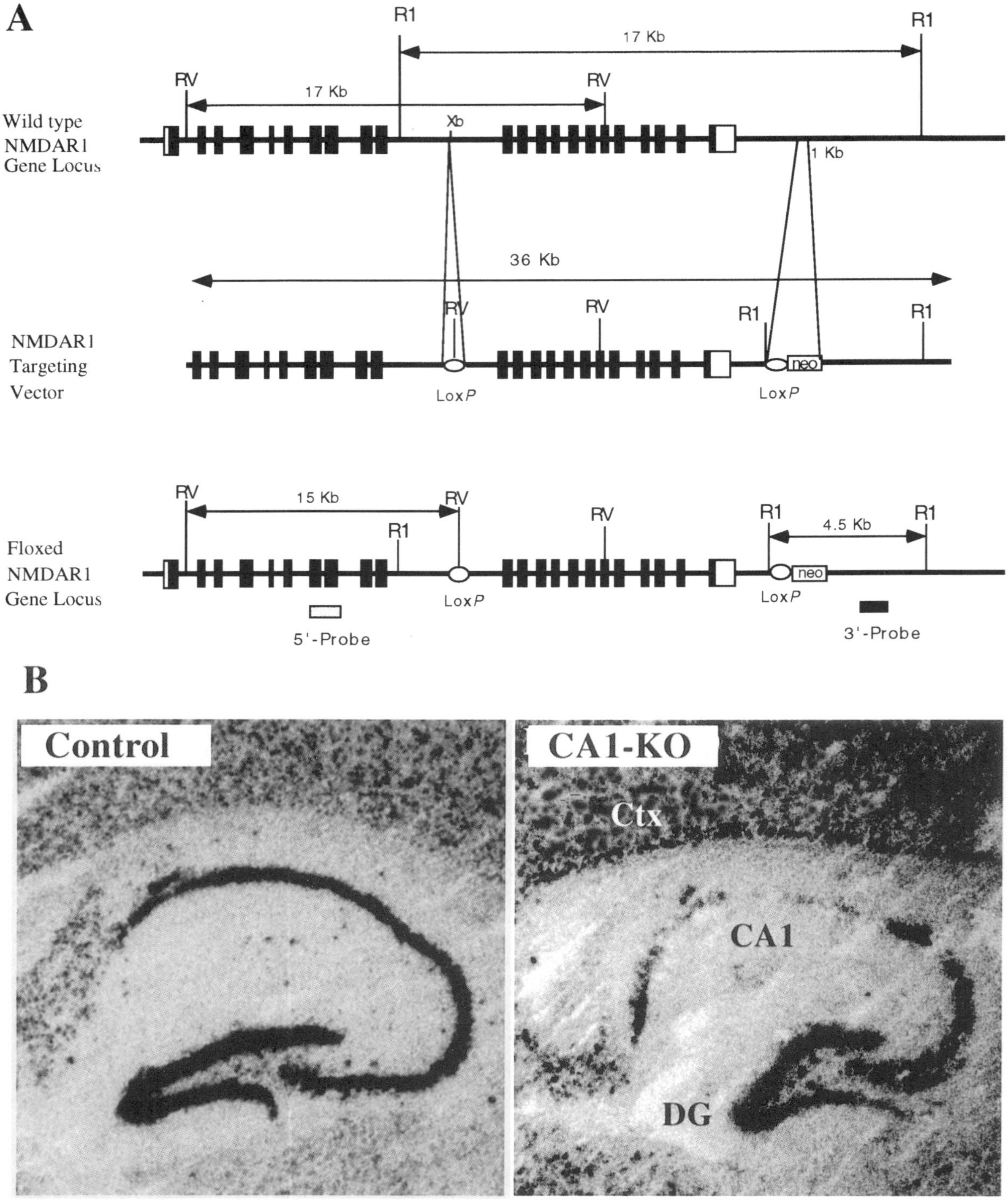

Figure 2. Strategy and demonstration of CA1-restricted deletion of the NMDAR1 gene. (*A*) The NMDAR1 locus and targeting construct. The top drawing represents the wild-type genomic region that contains the intron between exons 10 and 11 of the NMDAR1 gene. The middle drawing represents the NMDAR1 targeting vector that contains two *loxP* sequences. The lower drawing represents the floxed NMDAR1 gene. (*B*) In situ hybridization of NMDAR1 mRNA from wild-type and CA1-KO brains.

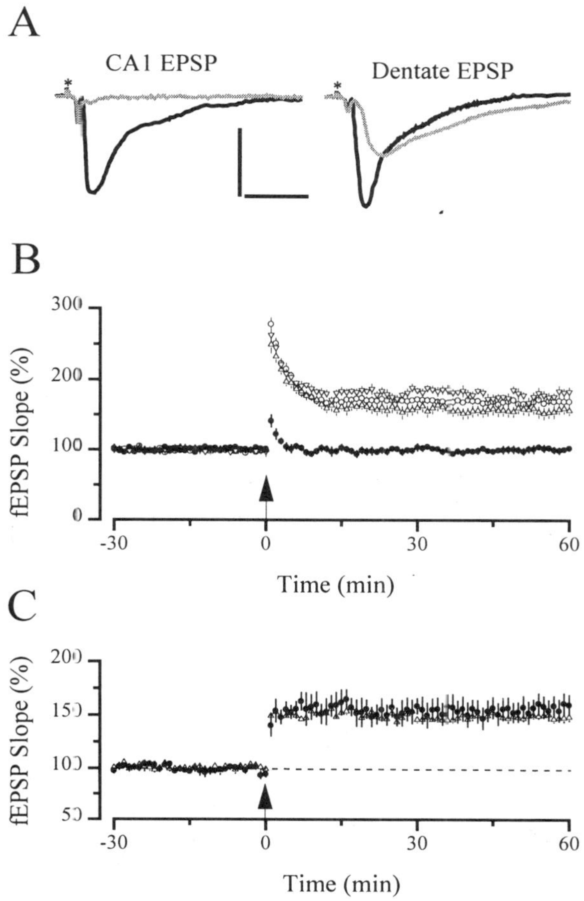

Figure 3. Field EPSPs and LTP in CA1 and dentate gyrus. (*A*) Representative traces (average of 10 responses) of field EPSPs measured in the stratum radiatum of the CA1 region (*left*) and in the stratum moleculare of the dentate gyrus (*right*) in CA1-KO slices. The black traces correspond to EPSPs measured in standard saline, and the gray traces correspond to EPSPs measured in CNQX (20 μM), 2-OH-saclofen (200 μM), glycine (1 μM) and nominally Mg^{++} free. The isolated NMDA EPSP is absent in CA1 (*left*) and clearly distinguishable in dentate (*right*). (*B*) The graph represents the mean (±S.E.M.) field EPSPs in the four groups tested for LTP induction. The CA1-KO (*filled circles*, $n = 21$) did not show LTP, whereas the control groups presented clear LTP (T29-1, *open circles*, $n = 12$; fNR1, *up triangles*, $n = 4$; wt, *inverted triangles*, $n = 5$). (*C*) The graph represents the mean (±S.E.M.) field EPSPs in the CA1-KO (*filled circles*, $n = 10$) and fNR1 (*open triangles*, $n = 6$) dentate gyrus. Significant LTP was elicited in both groups after the tetanus.

Synaptic Plasticity in CA1 and Dentate Gyrus

Application of tetanic stimulation (100 Hz for 1 sec) failed to induce LTP in the CA1-KO slices. Moreover, short-term potentiation (STP) was not detectable in the mutant slices. On average, the synaptic responses were unchanged in CA1-KO slices 45 minutes after the tetanus (100.4 ± 4.9%, $n = 21$, Fig. 3B), whereas LTP was readily obtained in control slices (T29-1, 168.5 ± 4.9 %, $n = 12$; fNR1, 156.9 ± 8.3%, $n = 4$; wt 177.7 ± 6.2%, $n = 5$; Fig. 3B).

Furthermore, we attempted to induce NMDAR-dependent LTD in CA1-KO slices by giving a low frequency train of 1 Hz for 10 minutes (Dudek and Bear 1992). This stimulation was unable to produce LTD (94.8 ± 12.6%, 45 min after train, $n = 4$; not shown). In contrast, we were able to elicit NMDAR-independent LTP in mutant slices by giving a very high frequency tetanus (four trains, each train was 250 Hz for 0.2 sec; 5 sec between trains). This paradigm induced a slowly rising synaptic increase (35.2 ± 8.4%, 60 min after tetanus, $n = 4$, $p < 0.01$, t-test; not shown), demonstrating the preservation of an NMDAR-independent LTP mechanism in the CA1 region (Grover and Teyler 1990).

Finally, we examined whether LTP could be induced in the mutant dentate gyrus. Lateral perforant path (LPP) and medial perforant path inputs onto granule cells were stimulated at 0.1 Hz (Hanse and Gustafsson 1992). Tetanic stimulation (40 shocks at 100 Hz) was able to induce LTP in either of the two inputs. On average, the LPP pathway showed a statistically significant increase in synaptic efficacy 45 minutes after the tetanus (154.6 ± 10.1%, $n = 10$, $p < 0.01$, t-test, Fig. 3C). In a few experiments, we confirmed that this LTP is NMDAR-dependent because addition of AP5 (50 μM) completely blocked its induction (99.1 ± 3.1%, $n = 3$; data not shown).

Spatial Memory

To test for spatial memory, we trained mice in a water maze to find a fixed, hidden platform by using distal cues (Morris et al. 1982; Huerta et al. 1996). We found that the CA1-KO mice were deficient in learning this task when compared to control siblings. The control mice showed a significant decrease in their latencies from block 1 to block 12. The CA1-KO mice also exhibited a significant decrease in their latencies as the training proceeded, but they never reached the level of learning displayed by the control mice.

Even though the mutant mice showed an improvement in their escape latencies, they could have been relying on nonspatial strategies to find the hidden platform. Thus, we used a "transfer" test (TT) to determine whether the mice had formed a spatial memory of the task. During this test, the platform is absent and the mice swim for 60 seconds in the pool. If the animals use a spatial strategy (i.e., they map the position of the hidden platform by using the relations among the distal visual cues around the pool), it is expected that they should spend a significantly greater amount of time than chance actively searching for the platform in the location where they were trained to find it. In contrast, if the mice use nonspatial strategies, they should spend approximately an equal amount of time in each quadrant of the pool. This could occur, for instance, if the mice learned that the platform is at a

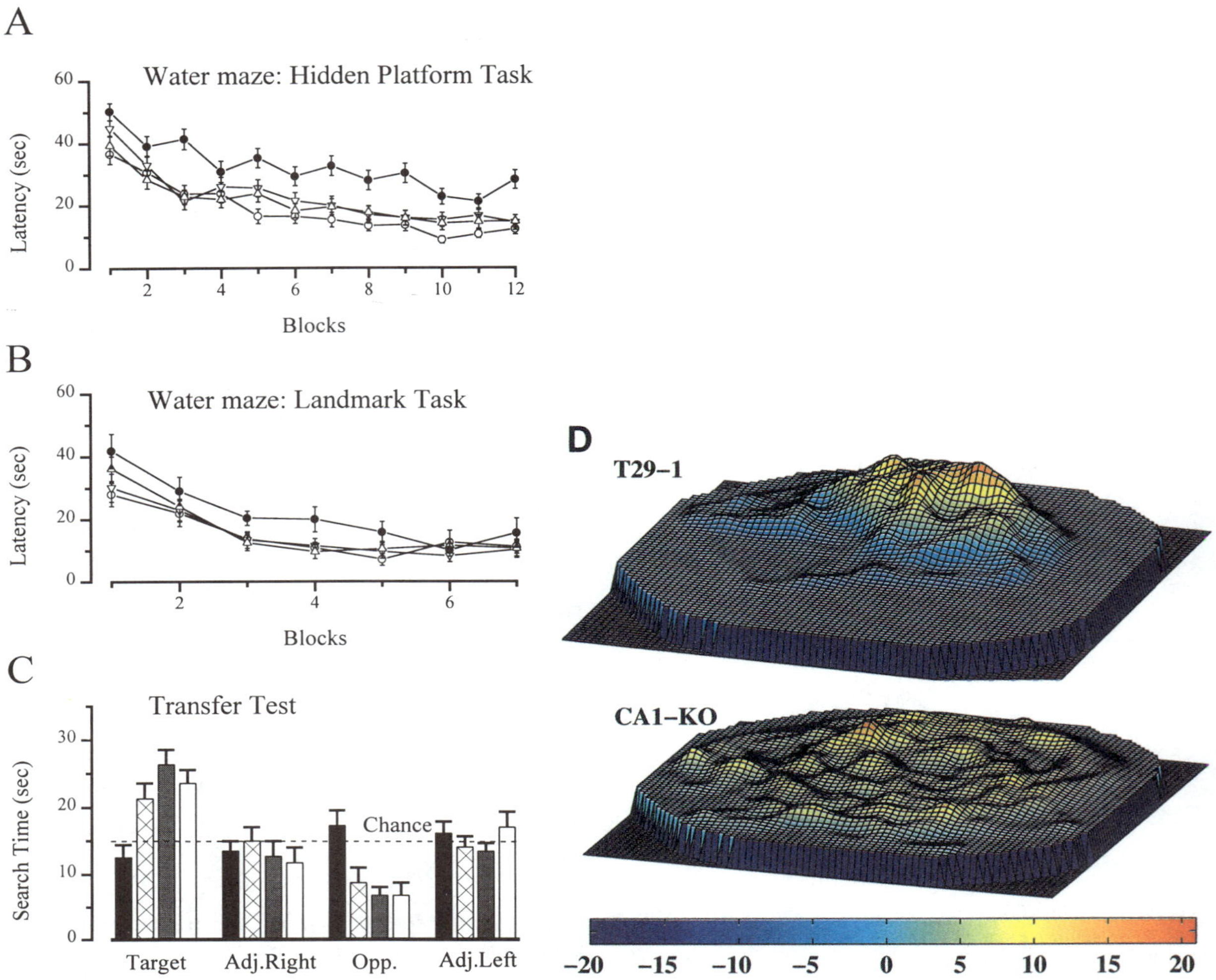

Figure 4. Morris water maze analysis. (*A*) CA1-KO mice are slower in learning the hidden platform version of the Morris water maze. The graph represents the escape latencies of mice trained to find a hidden platform in a water maze by using the distal cues surrounding it. The CA1-KO mice (*filled circles*, *n* =11) display a longer latency in every block (4 trials per day) than the control mice (T29-1, *open circles*, *n* =12; fNR1, *up triangles*, *n* = 13; wt, *inverted triangles*, *n* = 12). In addition, CA1-KO mice do not reach the optimal performance attained by the control mice, even though the mutants show some improvement. (*B*) CA1-KO mice appear normal in the performance of the landmark task in the water maze. The graph represents the escape latencies of mice trained to find a hidden platform in a water maze by using the proximal cue (a black rectangle attached to the pool wall). The CA1-KO mice (*filled circles*, *n* = 6) display a somewhat longer latency during the initial block (3 trials per day) but improved their performance to the same level as the control mice (T29-1, *open circles*, *n* = 6; fNR1, *up triangles*, *n* = 6; wt, *inverted triangles*, *n* = 6). (*C*) Transfer test. Average time (± S.E.M.) in each quadrant for the four groups (CA1-KO, *dark*; T29-1, *hatch*; fNR1, *gray*; wt, *white*). The CA1-KO mice spent equal amounts of time in every quadrant, whereas the control groups spent significantly more time than chance in the target quadrant. (*D*) Three-dimensional graphs representing the total occupancy by six T29-1 mice and six CA1-KO mice during the transfer test. The control mice focused their search in the trained location (where the platform used to be during training), whereas the mutant mice visited the whole maze area equivalently.

certain distance from the edge of the pool, a memory independent of hippocampal function. The CA1-KO mice did not show any place preference for the target quadrant. In contrast, the control groups showed a marked preference for the target quadrant (T29-1, 22.6 ± 2.7 sec; fNR1, 27.6 ± 1.5 sec; wt, 20.2 ± 2.4 sec; TT3: T29-1, 21.4 ± 2.2 sec; fNR1, 23.6 ± 1.9 sec; wt, 26.5 ± 2.2 sec; $p < 0.0001$ for all the values, paired t-test, Fig. 4C). Analysis of the navigational strategies of mice demonstrated that the control mice focused their search in the trained area and thus produced a high total occupancy peak in the position in which the platform was previously located (Fig. 4D, upper panel), whereas the mutants navigated all over the pool's area (Fig. 4D, lower panel). Finally, to ensure that our apparatus was well suited for measuring spatial memory, we tested homozygous αCaMKII knockout mice. These mice are known to be deficient in spatial memory (Silva et al.

1992b) and indeed showed, in our apparatus, the same complete deficit in spatial memory as the CA1-KO mice (data not shown).

To assess whether the impaired behavior of the mutants in the hidden platform version of the water maze was due to some sensorimotor or motivational deficit, we trained the mice in a simpler task in the water maze (Kolb et al. 1994). In this task, the animals are required to find a slightly submerged platform whose location is marked by a large proximal cue, known as the "landmark." We found that the mutant mice learned the task at a somewhat slower rate, but reached the same level of optimal performance as the control mice (Fig. 4B).

In conclusion, our behavioral analysis reveals that the CA1-KO mice display a selective and significant deficit in spatial memory, because they are unable to develop a navigational strategy in the Morris water maze. In contrast, they could perform nonspatial learning tasks that rely on simple association strategies.

Most Electrophysiological Properties of Control and Knockout Neurons In Vivo Are Indistinguishable

We employed multi-electrode recording techniques to characterize hippocampal activity in CA1-KO mice and in their littermate controls. Mice were fitted with microdrive arrays containing six independently adjustable tetrodes capable of simultaneously recording the activity of large numbers of neurons (Fig. 5). We recorded activity from 112 complex spiking cells and 13 interneurons in five control animals during 12 recording sessions, and 198 complex spiking cells and 16 interneurons in five CA1 knockout animals during 16 recording sessions. We evaluated basic spike waveform and firing characteristics of these cells and found that pyramidal cells and interneurons in CA1-KO animals are largely indistinguishable from those of the control animals. Overall firing rates of pyramidal cells were approximately 2 Hz while running and 1 Hz while resting or sleeping. Overall firing rates of inhibitory interneurons were 20–35 Hz while running and 10–15 Hz while resting or sleeping. Most neurons in control and knockout animals showed rhythmic modulation of firing rate in the theta frequency range (8–10 Hz) while the animals were running. Thus, basic neuronal firing characteristics appear normal in knockout animals during behavior. We observed no large shifts in the balance of excitation and inhibition in the CA1-KO animals, although we detected a small reduction in the firing rate of pyramidal cells. This was a weak effect, but it is consistent with the lack of an excitatory NMDA current. It is important to note that although NMDA-mediated synaptic plasticity is absent in the CA1-KO mice, two endogenous hippocampal firing patterns that have been implicated in synaptic modification, the theta modulation of hippocampal activity and the complex spiking of pyramidal cells, are intact (Larson et al. 1986; Huerta and Lisman 1993). The retention of these firing patterns is a further indication that there has been no gross alteration of hippocampal physiology.

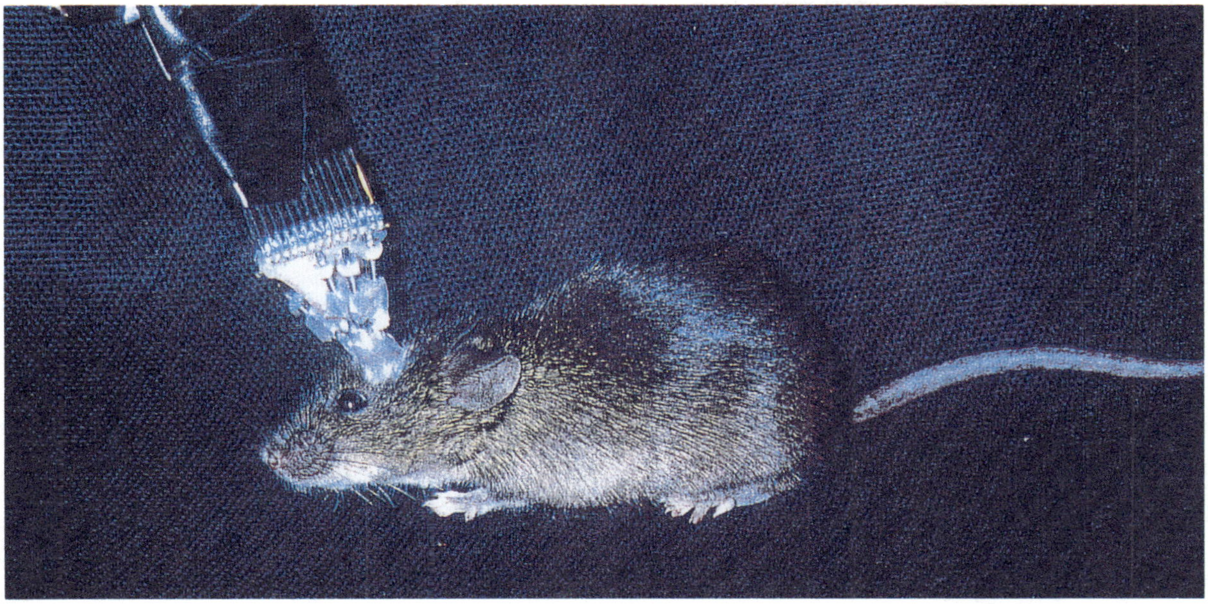

Figure 5. NMDAR1 CA1-KO mouse with implanted microdrive. A microdrive array housing six independently adjustable four-channel tetrodes was affixed to the mouse's skull directly above the hippocampus (2.0 mm L 1.8 mm P bregma coordinates), allowing large numbers of individual cells to be recorded during behavior (see Methods). All mice subjected to multiple electrode recording were littermates with CBA-C57BL/6J-129/SV background and consisted of three T29-1 mice, five CA1-KO mice, one floxed-NMDAR1 mouse, and one wild-type mouse of between 4 and 6 months of age and between 24 and 34 grams in weight.

Place Fields Are Larger in CA1-KO Animals

In our efforts to identify possible impairments of hippocampal function that could contribute to the behavioral deficit identified in CA1-KO mice, we first examined the spatial specificity of pyramidal cell activity as these animals explored an environment. We found that although pyramidal cells from CA1-KO animals fired in a place-related manner, the specificity was markedly poorer than the firing pattern of cells from control animals. Figure 6A shows representative examples of place fields recorded from control and knockout animals in three environments. Place fields recorded from control animals usually had a single salient peak. Place fields recorded from knockout animals, although sometimes individually indistinguishable from control fields, were more likely to be broad and diffuse, with multiple peaks.

We measured place field size by counting the number of pixels (pixels cover a 2-cm x 2-cm area) where average firing rates exceeded 1 spike per second. The open field environment most closely approximates the environment of a Morris water maze but has the drawback that the animal visits each pixel a few times. We therefore restricted our analysis to data from the linear and L-shaped tracks where sampling was high and uniform. Figure 6B shows the distribution of field sizes measured for both control and knockout animals. A significant difference in the means was found with control fields averaging 106 pixels and knockout fields averaging 140 pixels. The distributions also appear roughly Gaussian with similar variances; this ensures that Student's t-test will be meaningful. We find that the probability that the means are the same is less than 0.0004.

To check the possibility that this effect may arise as a consequence of the slight increase in firing rates in the knockout animals, we calculated the place field size for both high and low rate cells. The median firing rate for pyramidal cells that fired significantly while animals were running in an environment was approximately 1.6 Hz in both knockout and control animals. We divided these cells into two categories: those that fired, on average, between 1 Hz and 1.6 Hz and those that fired, on average, between 1.6 Hz and 6 Hz. Figure 6C shows that for both high and low rates, the place fields of knockout pyramidal cells are larger than those of controls.

Neuronal Ensemble Effects

It is likely that the coordinated firing of large numbers of place cells is necessary to accurately communicate the location of the animal to downstream brain regions. We took advantage of our multiple electrode array to measure the covariance coefficient (variance-normalized covariance) of firing rates averaged over 200-msec windows between pairs of cells with overlapping fields. Average covariance coefficient was computed as $< [(\Sigma_i (R_i - R_{avg})(r_i - r_{avg})] / [\sqrt{(\Sigma_i (R_i - R_{avg})^2} \sqrt{(\Sigma_i (r_i - r_{avg})^2}]>$, where $< >$ is an average over cell pairs, i is an index that runs over all included 200-msec bins in a session, and R and r refer to different cells in a pair. Figure 7A shows that pairs of knockout cells exhibit completely uncorrelated firing whereas control pairs exhibit significant correlations. As an animal moves through a region covered by several place cells, the firing of those cells is nevertheless uncorrelated over 200-msec windows. We have observed this effect for time bins ranging from milliseconds to one second. This dramatic effect in CA1-KO mice means that downstream regions cannot use these correlations to learn about place.

This point is elaborated by examining the estimate of the location of the animal conveyed simultaneously by multiple cells, i.e., the ensemble representation of location. We were able to record from as many as 29 neurons simultaneously and were thus able to estimate the position of the animal from knowledge of its fields and spike trains alone. Figure 7B shows that for small numbers of cells, the ensemble of neurons in knockout animals carries as much information about location as the ensemble in controls. For large numbers of cells, however, where place fields begin to overlap, an ensemble of CA1-KO neurons represents the location of the animal more poorly than an ensemble of control neurons. Because we always chose the best matching location, however poor the match, we may have overestimated the performance of the knockout animal ensembles. Even for ensembles with uncorrelated firing, the reconstruction improves with larger ensembles. Figure 7C shows an example of trajectory reconstruction. Ensembles of cells from the knockouts are more likely to make large errors in estimating the location of the animal. Cells that ought to fire together because they are tuned to similar locations do not robustly do so in the knockouts.

Model: Place Cells in CA1-specific NMDAR1 Knockout Mice

How can there be place fields in CA1 without NMDA receptors? We cannot rule out the possibility that other forms of plasticity are sufficient to generate place fields with poor specificity. It is also possible that a residue of fixed topologically organized input to CA1 exists. We consider both of these to be unlikely. The puzzle is this: Assuming that CA3, the major input to CA1 (Amaral and Witter 1989), has normal place fields, the random unchanging connections from CA3 to CA1 that should exist in the CA1 knockouts might be expected to destroy all place-specific responses in CA1.

To address this problem, we constructed a model (K.I. Blum and M.A. Wilson, in prep.) of the random hard-wired CA3 network connections to a single post-synaptic CA1 cell, similar in architecture to what exists in the CA1-KO animals (see Fig. 8). We used numbers

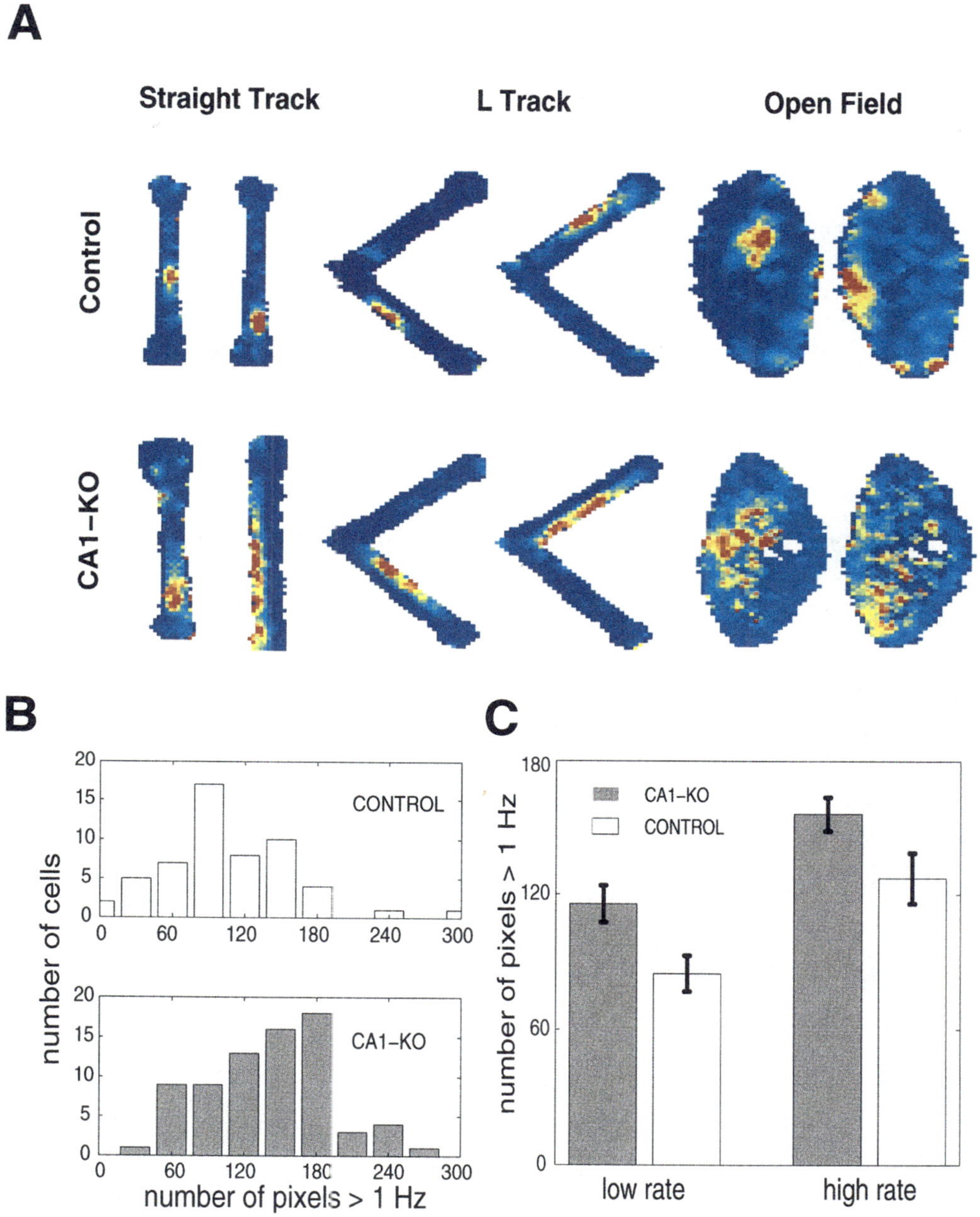

Figure 6. Place fields of NMDAR1 CA1-KO mice are significantly larger in all behavioral environments. (*A*) Rate maps of place-specific activity of two pyramidal cells from control animals and two pyramidal cells from knockout animals in each behavioral environment. The peak rate of each panel has been adjusted to reveal areas of highest activity. The field sizes of the pyramidal cells of the NMDAR1 CA1-KO animals were significantly larger in both the linear track (one-dimensional) environments and the two-dimensional open field environment. (*B*) Histogram demonstrating the distribution of CA1 pyramidal cell field sizes in control (n=55 cells) and mutant animals (n=74 cells). Pixels in which the average rate of firing exceeded 1 Hz were included when calculating field size. CA1 complex spike cells were identified on the basis of average spike width and complex spike index score (see Results). The mean field size in NMDAR1 CA1-KO animals was 140.3 pixels (~560 cm^2) and in control animals the mean size was 106.0 pixels (~420 cm^2). (*C*) Increase in place field size in NMDAR1 CA1-KO animals is not caused by a general increase in rate. The histogram shows place field size for low rate (<1.6 Hz) and high rate (>1.6 Hz) cells from both mutant and control animals. In both cases, the NMDAR1 CA1-KO animals have significantly larger fields.

of neurons and connections that match literature values for these brain regions (Amaral and Witter 1989; Paxinos 1995). We assumed that place fields are normal in CA3. Random connections generate an input to CA1 that fluctuates in a place-related manner but with an amplitude of only 5–10%. We therefore

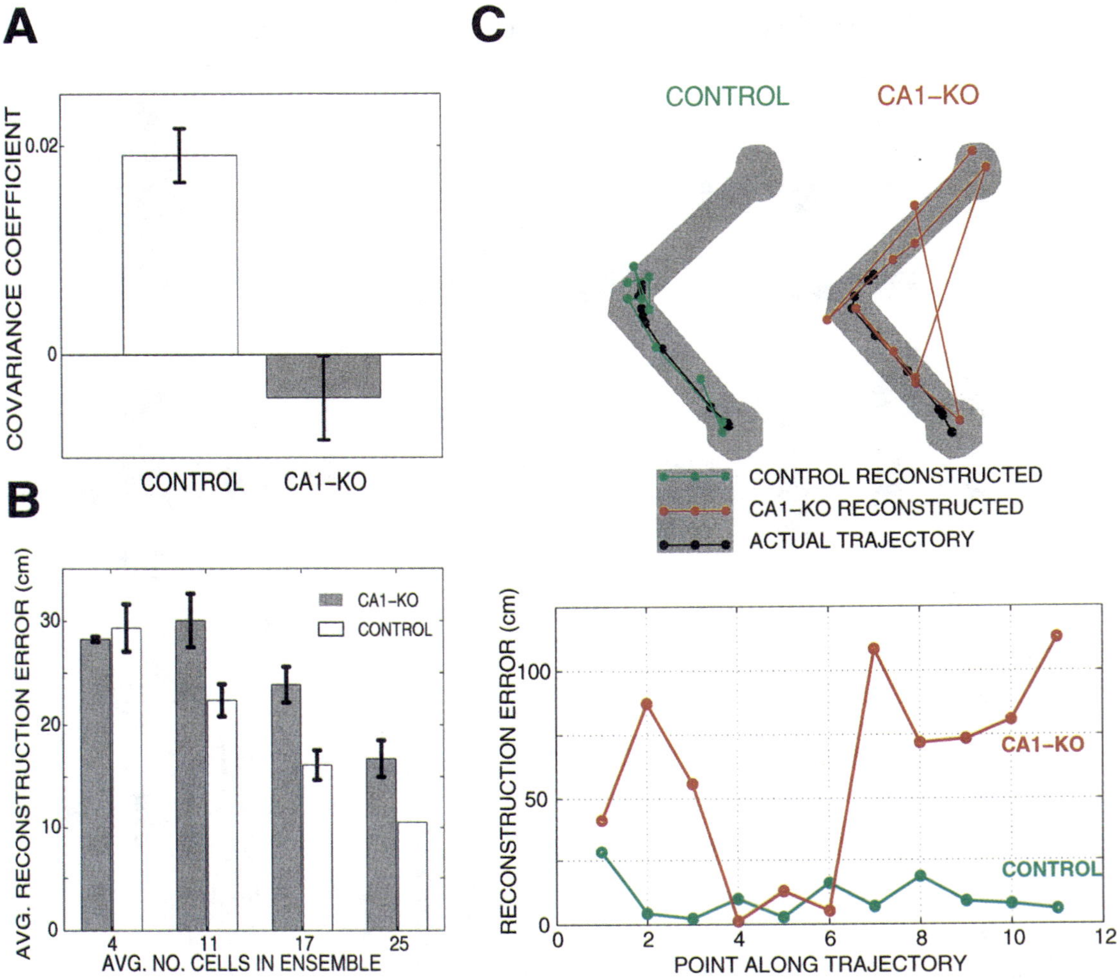

Figure 7. Ensemble coding properties of CA1 pyramidal cells in NMDAR1 CA1-KO and control mice. (*A*) The average covariance coefficient of firing rates between overlapping pairs of control and pairs of knockout pyramidal cells. Pairs of cells in knockouts fired randomly with respect to each other when their place fields overlapped. The average firing rate of each neuron was calculated for successive 200-msec bins over one 15- to 20-min RUN session. The firing rate covariance coefficient of all pairs of cells on different tetrodes with place fields that overlapped by 10 or more pixels (161 control pairs, 555 CA1-KO pairs) was calculated only when the animal was visiting common pixels. Common pixels were those where both cells fired at least one spike. Control pairs overlapped by 21.8 ± 2.2 pixels; CA1-KO pairs overlapped by 22.5 ± 3.1 pixels. Error bars represent S.E.M. for 8 control and 11 CA1-KO data sets. (*B*) Average error in path reconstruction. Trajectory reconstruction error is larger in CA1-KO mice. With few simultaneously recorded cells there was no significant difference between knockouts and controls. With large numbers of cells, the chance of overlapping fields increased, and the lack of covariance in the knockouts appeared as an increased reconstruction error compared to controls. 16 knockout and 13 control data sets were grouped by number of active place cells in that session. Reconstruction errors were averaged over the entire 15- to 20-min RUN sessions. Error bars represent S.E.M.; the number of degrees of freedom was taken to be the number of data sets, 4 on average. The same trend was observed in straight and L-shaped tracks, so the data were pooled. The position was reconstructed every 2 sec by comparing a list of the average firing rate of each cell for a 2-sec bin with a list of the average rates over the entire session and finding the position that gave the closest match. Firing rates of each cell were normalized to their peak values, and match was determined by the angle between these rate vectors. Error at each point was calculated by computing the distance between the estimated location and the average position during the 2-sec bin. (*C*) Examples of trajectory reconstruction. The upper panel illustrates trajectories reconstructed for control and CA1-KO animals for a 20-sec stretch of behavior. The ensemble firing of place cells of knockouts does not coincide with the actual location of the animal. Points indicate locations at which position estimates and measurements were made. Lines connect successive points in time. Each arm of the L-track was 75 cm long. The lower panel shows the differences between the reconstructed and actual locations for the same data. The knockouts had a highly variable reconstruction error with occasional large values. The data sets used in this figure had 19 control and 26 mutant cells. The average reconstruction errors over 15–20 min were 17 cm and 23.5 cm, respectively.

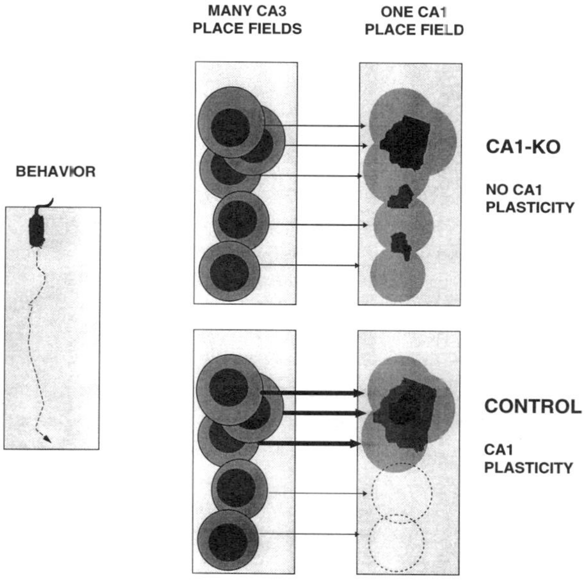

Figure 8. Schematic view of a model detailing possible role of NMDA-receptor-mediated synaptic plasticity in the refinement of place fields in CA1 pyramidal neurons. Each large rectangular panel is a copy of the environment. As the animals move around, various place cells in CA3 are activated, and these in turn drive CA1 cells to fire. In knockout animals, CA1 cells have place-related activity because some regions of space happen by chance to be densely covered by place fields, and because a sliding threshold for firing amplifies these variations. In control animals, those synapses are strengthened that connect simultaneously highly active CA3 and CA1 cells.

added another ingredient to the model: homeostatic firing rates (Turrigiano et al. 1994; Miller 1996). A firing threshold that adapts to average or peak postsynaptic activity will tend to stay in the middle range of a fluctuating response. Place-specific variations in CA1 response will thus be amplified. Without plasticity but with an adapting firing rate, we obtain location-dependent firing in CA1 cells with poor spatial specificity. Furthermore, the model suggests that without plasticity, CA1 firing may be more variable and pairs may exhibit less correlated firing.

What is gained with plasticity? We assumed that the adapting threshold for firing is also an adapting threshold for plasticity (Bienenstock et al. 1982; Kirkwood et al. 1996). We also employed a conventional "Hebbian" learning rule: If the postsynaptic response was large, all input synapses were strengthened proportionally to their contribution to the response. With these simple ingredients, the model produced a more specific place field transmitted from CA3 to CA1 compared to the model without plasticity. The model suggests that plasticity may also increase signal to noise in CA1 and raise the covariance coefficient for cell pairs.

DISCUSSION

CA1 LTP Underlies the Formation of Spatial Memory

We have generated a knockout mouse strain lacking the NMDAR1 subunit in the CA1 region of the hippocampus. These mice seem to grow normally and do not present obvious behavioral abnormalities. We have shown that the mutant mice lack NMDAR-mediated EPSCs and LTP in the CA1 region and are impaired in the hidden platform version of the Morris water maze (a measure of spatial memory), but not in nonspatial learning tasks. Previously, it was suggested that NMDA-receptor-dependent LTP underlies the acquisition of new memories in the hippocampus (for review, see Morris et al. 1991; Bliss and Collingridge 1993). Our results provide a strong support for this view and make it more specific: The NMDA-receptor-dependent LTP in the CA1 region is crucially involved in the formation of certain types of memory. We cannot exclude the possibility that the NMDA-receptor-dependent synaptic plasticity crucial for memory formation is LTD, given that the CA1-KO mice seem to lack NMDAR-dependent LTD. However, we think that this is unlikely because spatial learning is apparently intact in knockout mice deficient in protein kinase A (PKA) that lack CA1 LTD (Brandon et al. 1995).

Gene Knockout Studies Point to a Pivotal Role of CA1 Synaptic Plasticity

Previous studies examined the correlation between spatial memory and the site of hippocampal LTP (i.e., CA1, CA3, and dentate gyrus) by using a variety of conventional knockout mice (for review, see Chen and Tonegawa 1997). These studies found a correlated impairment in Sch-CA1 LTP and spatial memory (but see Conquet et al. 1994). It is important to point out that the only exceptional case, namely that of the mGluR1 mutant mice, is complicated by the fact that two groups have generated and analyzed these mutants independently and obtained opposing results (Aiba et al. 1994; Conquet et al. 1994; Chen and Tonegawa 1997). In contrast, it has been shown that impairments of mossy fiber-CA3 LTP (Huang et al. 1995) and perforant path-dentate LTP (Nosten-Bertrand et al. 1996) are not correlated with spatial memory deficit.

Our new evidence, although still correlational, is much stronger than the earlier reports because we have singled out the CA1 synapses as a site of plasticity impairment. What structural and functional features could explain this pivotal role of CA1 synapses as sites of plasticity underlying spatial memory? It is well known that the CA1 region is a crucial component of the "hippocampal formation" system that is involved in the acquisition of certain types of memory. In rodents, this system consists of several structures connected within a loop that encompasses the entorhinal cortex (EC), with inputs from higher sensory cortices;

dentate gyrus (DG), with inputs from EC; CA3, with "external" inputs from EC and DG and "internal" inputs from CA3; CA1, with inputs from CA3 and EC; and subiculum (SUB), with inputs from CA1 and outputs to EC (Lorente de Nó 1934; Amaral and Witter 1989). In view of the evidence currently available, it would seem that the minimal system required as a locus for memory acquisition would be the EC-CA3-CA1-SUB-EC loop. This is because (1) the plasticity in the EC-DG and DG-CA3 synapses seems to be dispensable (Huang et al. 1995; Nosten-Bertrand et al. 1996); (2) the direct EC-CA1 connection appears to be too weak to sustain the EC-CA1-SUB-EC loop as the locus for memory (Empson and Heinemann 1995); and (3) the evidence presented in this paper points to the special role of the CA3-CA1 synapses.

Interestingly, the plasticity of the EC-CA3 synapses has not been well studied, but our proposed scenario predicts that they are important in implementing the memory system. Most probably, both the EC-CA3 pathway and the EC-DG-CA3 pathway provide parallel inputs to the CA3 network during learning, and the CA3-CA3 synapses work as autoassociative memory devices, as it has long been proposed (Marr 1971). Thus, it is desirable to generate a CA3-region-specific knockout of the NMDA receptor to allow a direct examination of the contribution of these synapses to learning.

Loss of Place Field Specificity as a Mechanism for Behavioral Impairment

If the spatially restricted activity of a place cell was so poor that no field could be reasonably discerned, then it could be concluded that all spatial learning should be lost. Our data reflect, however, that the CA1 pyramidal cells of CA1-KO mice do retain a fairly high degree of spatially restricted activity. Although fields in CA1-KO mice are present and stable, there are significant alterations of the quality and size of individual fields. These alterations, although appearing rather small when compared to the magnitude of the behavioral deficit reported for these mice (Tsien et al. 1996b), may have significant effects on several levels. The fields observed in CA1-KO mice may convey locally unstable information due to their lack of a true salient peak or center. This ambiguity, when combined with the increased field size, may cause a significant decrease in the quality of information each cell can convey to the rest of the brain. If appropriate behavior in navigational tasks requires that specific spatial representations be recalled, and if plasticity within CA1 allows unambiguous association of refined place representations with appropriate behavioral response, then the reduced spatial specificity seen in many CA1 pyramidal cells of the knockout animals may account for the behavioral impairment found in the spatial water maze task.

Reduction in Covariance of Firing between Cells Disrupts Ensemble Coding

The observation that 30–50% of cells within the hippocampus become active within a given environment strongly indicates that rodents use ensemble representations of location rather than mapping places to individual cells. For an ensemble code to provide accurate spatial information, there must be robust covariance of the firing of cells that have overlapping spatial fields. We found that the covariance coefficient (variance-normalized covariance, see Fig. 5A) of cell pairs with overlapping place fields is approximately zero in CA1-KO animals and is significantly lower than in controls. This would radically impair the ability of the animal to use a hippocampal ensemble code as a robust indicator of spatial location. "Hebbian" learning rules operating in downstream brain regions will fail to learn anything about place from CA1 in the knockouts. We propose that this can explain the navigational deficit observed in these animals (Tsien et al. 1996b).

We have further evidence that the combination of more broadly tuned firing with decreased covariance yields a neuronal representation that may not be sufficiently robust to serve as the basis for mnemonic associations needed to perform navigational tasks such as the water maze. Impaired trajectory reconstruction in knockout animals reveals the inability of groups of neurons to coordinate their firing on a time scale relevant to tasks like the Morris water maze. Impaired trajectory reconstruction has also been seen in rats exploring a novel environment (Wilson and McNaughton 1993). We speculate that knockout animals may be unable to establish coherent representations of an environment following novel exposure.

CONCLUSION

Creation of cell-type-restricted gene knockout techniques made it possible to examine the relationship between the function of NMDA receptors, synaptic plasticity, place fields in the hippocampal CA1 region, and spatial memory. We are convinced that, for the first time, controlled changes in synaptic plasticity can be linked to electrophysiological changes that can explain a behavioral impairment. On the basis of our experiments, we propose that the uncorrelated activity of CA1 place cells during exploration causes downstream navigational learning impairments. We also suggest that cortical inputs must be associated in CA1 with CA3 inputs. This approach promises to establish the specific relationship between targeted cellular physiological mechanisms, regional neuronal function, and behavior.

ACKNOWLEDGMENTS

We thank David Gerber, Dong Feng Chen, Cindy Tom, Jason Derwin, Tamara Ochoa, and Athanassios

Siapas for assistance. We also thank Eric H. Mercer and David J. Anderson for the *lacZ* reporter mouse, Mark Mayford and Eric Kandel for the αCaMKII promoter, and Brian Sauer for the *Cre* plasmid. This work was supported by National Institutes of Health grant NS-32925 and by gifts from Shionogi Institute for Medical Science and Amgen, Inc. to S.T. P.H. was also supported by the Pew Latin American Fellows Program. This work was also supported by awards from the Seaver Institute and the Sloan Foundation to M.A.W.

REFERENCES

Aiba, A., C. Chen, K. Herrup, C. Rosenmund, C.F. Stevens, and S. Tonegawa. 1994. Reduced hippocampal long-term potentiation and context-specific deficit in associative learning in mGluR1 mutant mice. *Cell* **79:** 365.

Amaral, D.G. and M.P. Witter. 1989. The three-dimensional organization of the hippocampal formation: A review of anatomical data. *Neuroscience* **31:** 571.

Bannerman, D.M., M.A. Good, S.P. Butcher, M. Ramsay, and R.G.M. Morris. 1995. Distinct components of spatial learning revealed by prior training and NMDA receptor blockade. *Nature* **378:** 182.

Bienenstock, E.L., L.N. Cooper, and P.W. Munro. 1982. Theory for the development of neuron selectivity: Orientation specificity and binocular interaction in visual cortex. *J. Neurosci.* **2:** 32.

Bliss, T.V.P. and G.L. Collingridge. 1993. A synaptic model of memory: Long-term potentiation in the hippocampus. *Nature* **361:** 31.

Bradley, A. 1987. Production and analysis of chimeric mice. In *Teratocarcinomas and embryonic stem cells: A practical approach* (ed. E.J. Robertson), p. 113. IRL Press, Oxford, United Kingdom.

Brandon, E.P., M. Zhuo, Y. Huang, M. Qi, and K. Gerhold. 1995. Hippocampal long-term depression and depotentiation are defective in mice carrying a targeted disruption of the gene encoding the RI subunit of the cAMP-dependent protein kinase. *Proc. Natl. Acad. Sci.* **92:** 8851.

Capecchi, M.R. 1989. Altering the genome by homologous recombination. *Science* **244:** 1288.

Chen, C. and S. Tonegawa. 1997. Molecular genetic analysis of synaptic plasticity, activity-dependent neural development, learning, and memory in the mammalian brain. *Annu. Rev. Neurosci.* **20:** 157.

Conquet, F., Z.I. Bashir, C.H. Davies, H. Daniel, and F. Ferraguti. 1994. Motor deficit and impairment of synaptic plasticity in mice lacking mGluR1. *Nature* **372:** 237.

Davis, S., S.P. Butcher, and R.G.M. Morris. 1992. The NMDA receptor antagonist D-2-amino-5-phosphonopentanoate (D-AP5) impairs spatial learning and LTP *in vivo* at intracerebral concentrations comparable to those that block LTP *in vitro*. *J. Neurosci.* **12:** 21.

Dudek, S. and M. Bear. 1992. Homosynaptic long-term depression in area CA1 of hippocampus and effects of *N*-methyl-D-aspartate receptor blockade. *Proc. Natl. Acad. Sci.* **89:** 4363.

Eichenbaum, H., A. Fagan, P. Matthews, and N.J. Cohen. 1988. Hippocampal system dysfunction and odor discrimination learning in rats: Impairment or facilitation depending on representational demands. *Behav. Neurosci.* **102:** 331.

Empson, R.M. and U. Heinemann. 1995. The perforant path projection to hippocampal area CA1 in the rat hippocampal-entorhinal cortex combined slice. *J. Physiol.* **484:** 707.

Forrest, D., M. Yuzaki, H.D. Soares, L. Ng, D.C. Luk, M. Sheng, C.L. Stewart, J.I. Morgan, J.A. Connor, and T. Curran. 1994. Targeted disruption of NMDA receptor 1 gene abolishes NMDA response and results in neonatal death. *Neuron* **13:** 325.

Grant, S.G., T.J. O'Dell, K.A. Karl, P.L. Stein, P. Soriano, and E.R. Kandel. 1992. Impaired long-term potentiation, spatial learning, and hippocampal development in *fyn* mutant mice. *Science* **258:** 1903.

Grover, L.M. and T.J. Teyler. 1990. Two components of long-term potentiation induced by different patterns of afferent activation. *Nature* **347:** 477.

Hanse, E. and B. Gustafsson. 1992. Long-term potentiation and field EPSPs in the lateral and medial perforant paths in the dentate gyrus *in vitro:* A comparison. *Eur. J. Neurosci.* **4:** 1191.

Hebb, D.O. 1949. The organization of behavior. New York, NY, John Wiley.

Hestrin, S., P. Sah, and R. Nicoll. 1990a. Mechanisms generating the time course of dual component excitatory synaptic currents recorded in hippocampal slices. *Neuron* **5:** 247.

Hestrin, S., R. Nicoll, D. Perkel, and P. Sah. 1990b. Analysis of excitatory synaptic action in pyramidal cells using whole-cell recording from rat hippocampal slices. *J. Physiol.* **422:** 203.

Huang, Y., E. Kandel, L. Varshavsky, E.P. Brandon, and M. Qi. 1995. A genetic test of the effects of mutations in PKA on mossy fiber LTP and its relation to spatial and contextual learning. *Cell* **83:** 1211.

Huerta, P.T. and J.E. Lisman. 1993. Bidirectional synaptic plasticity induced by a single burst during cholinergic theta oscillation in CA1 *in vitro*. *Neuron* **15:** 1053.

Huerta, P.T., K. Scearce, S. Farris, R. Empson, and G. Prusky. 1996. Preservation of spatial learning in fyn tyrosine kinase knockout mice. *Neuroreport* **7:** 1685.

Jarrard, L.E. 1993. On the role of the hippocampus in learning and memory in the rat. *Behav. Neural Biol.* **60:** 9.

Kirkwood, A., M.G. Rioult, and M.F. Bear. 1996. Experience-dependent modification of synaptic plasticity in visual cortex. *Nature* **381:** 526.

Kolb, B., K. Buhrmann, R. McDonald, and R. Sutherland. 1994. Dissociation of the medial prefrontal, posterior parietal, and posterior temporal cortex for spatial navigation and recognition memory in the rat. *Cereb. Cortex* **4:** 664.

Larson, J., D. Wang, and G. Lynch. 1986. Patterned stimulation at the theta frequency is optimal for the induction of hippocampal long-term potentiation. *Brain Res.* **368:** 347.

Li, Y., R. Erzurumlu, C. Chen, S. Jhaveri, and S. Tonegawa. 1994. Whisker-related neuronal patterns fail to develop in the trigeminal brainstem nuclei of NMDAR1 knockout mice. *Cell* **76:** 427.

Lorente de Nó, R. 1934. Studies of the structure of the cerebral cortex: II. Continuation of the study of the ammonic system. *J. Psychol. Neurol.* **46:** 113.

Marr, D. 1971. Simple memory: A theory for archicortex. *Philos. Trans. R. Soc. Lond. B Biol. Sci.* **262:** 23.

McHugh, T.J., K.I. Blum, J.Z. Tsien, S. Tonegawa, and M.A. Wilson. 1996. Impaired hippocampal representation of space in CA1-specific NMDAR1 knockout mice. *Cell* **87:**

1339.

Miller, K.D. 1996. Synaptic economics: Competition and cooperation in synaptic plasticity. *Neuron* **17:** 371.

Morris, R.G.M. 1989. Synaptic plasticity and learning: Selective impairment of learning in rats and blockade of long-term potentiation *in vivo* by the *N*-methyl-D-aspartate receptor antagonist AP5. *J. Neurosci.* **9:** 3040.

Morris, R.G.M., S. Davis, and S.P. Butcher. 1991. Hippocampal synaptic plasticity and NMDA receptors: A role in information storage? In *Long-term potentiation. A debate of current issues* (ed. M. Baudry and J. Davis), p. 267. MIT Press, Cambridge, Massachusetts.

Morris, R.G.M., A. Anderson, G.S. Lynch, and M. Baudry. 1986. Selective impairment of learning and blockade of long-term potentiation by an *N*-methyl-D-aspartate receptor antagonist, AP5. *Nature* **319:** 774.

Morris, R.G.M., P. Garrud, J.N.P. Rowlins, and J. O'Keefe. 1982. Place navigation impaired in rats with hippocampal lesions. *Nature* **297:** 681.

Nosten-Bertrand, M., M. Errington, K. Murphy, Y. Tokugawa, E. Barboni, E. Kozlova, D. Michalovich, R.G.M. Morris, J. Silver, C. Stewart, T.V.P. Bliss, and R.J. Morris. 1996. Normal spatial learning despite regional inhibition of LTP in mice lacking Thy-1. *Nature* **379:** 826.

O'Keefe, J. and J. Dostrovsky. 1971. The hippocampus as a spatial map. Preliminary evidence from unit activity in the freely-moving rat. *Brain Res.* **34:** 171.

O'Keefe, J. and L. Nadel. 1978. *The hippocampus as a cognitive map.* Clarendon Press, Oxford, United Kingdom.

Paxinos, G., ed. 1995. *The rat nervous system*, 2nd edition. Academic Press, Boston, Massachusetts.

Rioult,M.G. and M.F. Bear. 1996. Experience-dependent modification of synaptic plasticity in visual cortex. *Nature* **381:** 526.

Saucier, D. and D.P. Cain. 1995. Spatial learning without NMDA receptor-dependent long-term potentiation. *Nature* **378:** 186.

Scoville, W.B. and B. Milner. 1957. Loss of recent memory after bilateral hippocampal lesions. *J. Neurol. Neurosurg. Psychiatry* **20:** 11.

Silva, A.J., R. Paylor, J.M. Wehner, and S. Tonegawa. 1992a. Impaired spatial learning in α-calcium calmodulin kinase II mutant mice. *Science* **257:** 206.

Silva, A.J., C.F. Stevens, S. Tonegawa, and Y. Wang. 1992b. Deficient hippocampal long-term potentiation in a-calcium-calmodulin kinase II mutant mice. *Science* **257:** 201.

Stevens, C.F., S. Tonegawa, and Y. Wang. 1994. The role of calcium-calmodulin kinase II in three forms of synaptic plasticity. *Curr. Biol.* **4:** 687.

Tsien, J.Z., P. Huerta, and S. Tonegawa. 1996a. The essential role of hippocampal CA1 NMDA receptor-dependent synaptic plasticity in spatial learning. *Cell* **87:** 1317.

Tsien, J.Z., D.F. Chen, D. Gerber, C. Tom, E. Mercer, D.J. Anderson, M. Mayford, E.R. Kandel, and S. Tonegawa. 1996b. Subregion- and cell-restricted gene knockout in mouse brain. *Cell* **87:** 1329.

Turrigiano, G.G., L.F. Abbot, and E. Marder. 1994. Activity dependent changes in the intrinsic properties of cultured neurons. *Science* **264:** 974.

Wilson, M.A. and B.L. McNaughton. 1993. Dynamics of the hippocampal ensemble code for space. *Science* **261:** 1055.

Zola-Morgan, S., L.R. Squire, and D. Amaral. 1986. Human amnesia and the medial temporal region: Enduring memory impairment following a bilateral lesion limited to field CA1 of the hippocampus. *J. Neurosci.* **6:** 2950.

Genetic Analysis of Function and Dysfunction in the Central Nervous System

A.J. Silva, N. Fedorov, J. Kogan, P. Frankland, J. Coblentz, R. Lundsten, E. Friedman, A. Smith, Y. Cho, and K.P. Giese
Cold Spring Harbor Laboratory, Cold Spring Harbor, New York 11724

The last decade has been witness to unprecedented advances in mammalian genetics. Techniques have been developed that allow the addition, deletion, or modification of any cloned gene. Recent developments also promise control over when and where mutations take place. These genetic tools have already been used successfully in the study of learning and memory. The results show that it is possible to derive mutants with informative molecular, cellular, neuroanatomical, and behavioral phenotypes. These findings have both complemented and expanded previous neuroanatomical and pharmacological studies, demonstrating that genetic techniques will be an important tool in developing explanations of learning and memory.

Genetic studies of brain function must be developed from a solid behavioral foundation, since the design and interpretation of experiments is dependent on the clarity of the behavioral concepts under analysis. Beyond careful behavioral work, these studies must also include information about the neuroanatomy and physiology of the brain regions involved, as well as a solid theoretical backbone to structure the inevitable complexity of this information. Knowledge about molecular and cellular processes is also an essential component of these studies, because it can both constrain and guide system level models.

HIPPOCAMPAL-DEPENDENT LEARNING AND MEMORY

A large number of behavioral and neuroanatomical experiments suggest that the hippocampus is a central node in the network of brain regions involved in learning and memory. Current models describe the hippocampus as a structure that quickly integrates information processed elsewhere, functioning as a comparing device that assesses and contrasts incoming signals, as well as a temporary storage buffer for this information. It seems that hippocampal lesions affect performance in many complex tasks requiring unique solutions and flexible handling of learned information (Eichenbaum and Otto 1992; Squire 1992). Our studies (Y. Cho and A.J. Silva, unpubl.) have suggested that the extensive hippocampal lesion work done with rats may apply to mice, too. For example, hippocampal lesions in mice and rats disrupt performance in the hidden (spatial), but not in the visible, platform versions of the water maze.

LTP AND LEARNING

Important connections between hippocampal physiology and behavior were derived from studies of animals exposed to a variety of compounds, such as antagonists of the *N*-methyl-D-aspartate (NMDA) receptor. When delivered to the hippocampus, these antagonists block long-term potentiation (LTP) and also appear to impair some measures of hippocampal-dependent learning (Davis et al. 1992). These findings are consistent with the idea that stable, long-lasting changes in synaptic function may be required for learning and memory. However, the involvement of this receptor in other electrophysiological functions complicates the interpretation of these studies, and recent results show that under some conditions antagonists of this receptor do not seem to block hippocampal-dependent learning (Bannerman et al. 1995; Cain et al. 1996).

Another approach to study learning and memory is to analyze directly the physiology of behaving animals. For example, electrophysiological recordings of rat hippocampal neurons during learning showed that their firing patterns are optimal for the induction of LTP in vitro (Larson and Lynch 1986; Otto et al. 1991), a finding that considerably strengthened the connection between LTP and learning. However, the physiological complexity of a working brain can obscure the relevance of any single physiological phenomenon. For example, increases in synaptic currents previously believed to be correlates of learning could actually be caused by increases in brain temperature due to active exploration (Moser et al. 1993). The many possible artifacts associated with any one technique, together with the overwhelming complexity of the problem, argue for the use of multiple approaches in the study of learning and memory.

Most of the genetic work based on hippocampal-dependent learning and memory has focused on long-lasting changes in synaptic efficacy (i.e., LTP and long-term depression or LTD). The idea behind these studies is that information can be stored in neural circuits by adjusting the synaptic weights of neurons activated by the learning experience. This concept has been implemented with surprising success by computational models with ever-increasing power and sophistication. Furthermore, structures with an acknowledged participation in learning and memory (e.g., hippocampus) are capable of LTP-like phenomena. Importantly, LTP has the very properties thought to be crucial for memory formation: associativity, specificity, reversibility, and stability.

Despite much controversy regarding the mechanisms of LTP, most researchers agree that the induction of LTP in the CA1 region involves the activation of NMDA receptors, and a consequent postsynaptic increase in calcium (for review, see Bliss and Collingridge 1993). This increase in calcium is known to activate a number of protein kinases and other enzymes (e.g., adenylate cyclase) that are thought to trigger the biochemical cascade of events that modulate synaptic strength. Interestingly, genetic deletions of the NMDA receptor ε1 subunit (Sakimura et al. 1995), α-calcium-calmodulin kinase II (αCaMKII) (Silva et al. 1992a,b), Fyn tyrosine kinase (Grant et al. 1992), protein kinase (PKCγ) (Abeliovich et al. 1993a,b), and type I adenylate cyclase (Wu et al. 1995) all affect to some extent LTP in the hippocampal CA1 region and hippocampal-dependent learning and memory. Together, the genetic studies carried out to date show that disrupting mechanisms required for LTP disrupt, in some but not in all cases (Huang et al. 1995), processes that are needed for memory formation.

Nevertheless, many problems remain unsolved: First, there is the possibility that LTP is not involved in learning or memory, but that it shares many biochemical components with the cellular mechanism(s) of learning and memory. Second, there is a fundamental philosophical problem with claiming that a single class of cellular mechanisms could be responsible for learning and memory in the hippocampus or in any other structure. Learning is a property of circuits, and it is likely to involve a variety of mechanisms. The gene-targeting studies that follow address these two issues.

αCaMKII, PHYSIOLOGY, AND LEARNING

The first gene-targeting study of LTP and learning used mice with a null mutation for αCaMKII (Silva et al. 1992a,b), a gene expressed postnatally in forebrain structures (Burgin et al. 1990). CaMKII can be in a number of activity states that depend mainly on the interaction with Ca^{++}/calmodulin (Ca/CaM) and on autophosphorylation (for review, see Hanson and Schulman 1992). The enzyme is most active when unphosphorylated and bound to Ca/CaM. The autophosphorylated enzyme traps Ca/CaM and is only partly active. These complex responses to Ca^{++} are likely to be involved in the induction of LTP, because electrophysiological studies have shown that peptides designed to simulate the inhibitory domain of the enzyme, and thus inhibit its activity, can also block the induction of LTP in the CA1 region of the hippocampus (Malenka et al. 1989; Malinow et al. 1989; but see Hvalby et al. 1994).

The studies with the αCaMKII mutants showed that in the absence of this isoform, LTP as well as LTD is severely impaired in hippocampus and neocortex (Silva et al. 1992b; Kirkwood et al. 1994; Stevens et al. 1994). A number of studies suggest that these LTP deficits are not due to gross developmental abnormalities: (1) Electron microscopic analysis in the CA1 region suggests that there are similar neuronal and synaptic numbers in these mutants, and that the size and general structure organization of postsynaptic densities is unaltered by the mutation (Comery et al. 1994). (2) Studies in the somatosensory and visual cortices demonstrated that the functional topography and general properties of these regions are normal in the mutants (Gordon et al. 1994; Glazewski et al. 1996). (3) Recent studies show that phosphatase inhibitors can rescue the LTP loss in these mutants (Tonegawa, this volume). (4) Extensive electrophysiological analysis showed that the mutants do not have a general loss of synaptic function (Silva et al. 1992b; Stevens et al. 1994).

Behavioral studies found that the αCaMKII mutant mice were severely impaired in the hippocampal-dependent version of the water maze, but that they were able to learn the visible-platform version of this task, which is known not to depend on hippocampal function (Silva et al. 1992a). Thus, the αCaMKII mutants can learn that the platform is the only escape from the pool; they have the motivation to escape the water, and the motor coordination and sensory perception required to efficiently swim to the escape platform, but they are nevertheless unable to learn the spatial relationships required to guide them to the hidden platform.

In vivo electrophysiological studies found that repetitive stimuli delivered to the amygdala cannot kindle the αCaMKII mice and that their hippocampal and amygdala circuits are hyperexcitable (Butler et al. 1995). Perhaps, the same cellular mechanisms that are required for the induction of LTP are also involved in kindling. Both phenomena involve stable and long-lasting changes in synaptic function that are severely impaired in the αCaMKII mutants. Alternatively, the deficits in LTP and kindling may represent two independent consequences of the mutation. Therefore, either of these two abnormalities could potentially impair learning in the αCaMKII homozygotes, thus confounding the original interpretation of the learning deficits.

This illustrates a common problem with studies of learning and memory: Very often the manipulations used (genetics, pharmacology, neuroanatomical lesions, etc.) have unintended effects that add unwanted variables to the experiment. This problem emphasizes the need to test important physiological explanations of behavior with multiple experimental approaches. Finding a convergence of experimental results strengthens the involvement of LTP in learning. Thus, it is important to note that the expression of a transgene encoding a constitutively active αCaMKII also affects hippocampal LTP and learning (Bach et al. 1995; Mayford et al. 1995).

PLASTICITY, DEVELOPMENT, AND LEARNING

Since calcium-dependent signaling pathways have been implicated in hippocampal neuronal plasticity, αCaMKII homozygous and heterozygous mutants were used also in studies of neocortical plasticity (Gordon et al. 1994). In wild-type mice, brief occlusion of vision in one eye during a critical period (between 20 and 50 days postnatally) reduces responses in the visual cortex to stimuli presented to the deprived eye (Gordon and Stryker 1996). These studies found that the homozygous mutants have reduced plasticity following monocular deprivation. In contrast with the homozygotes, heterozygous mutants with deficits in short-term plasticity and in learning showed normal neocortical visual plasticity. It is important to note that despite impaired plasticity, the homozygous mice have normal visual receptive fields (size and location), ocular dominance, orientation selectivity, and single-unit response strength. Thus, the deficit in plasticity is not due to deficits in either the organization, structure, or basic properties of the neocortex.

These αCaMKII mutants were also used in similar studies in the somatosensory cortex (Glazewski et al. 1996). The mammalian sensory cortex shows experience-dependent plasticity such that neurons modify their responses according to changes in sensory experience. Plasticity in adult mice can be induced by changes in the patterns of stimulation to the barrel neocortex. Unlike the visual cortex, where there is a narrow critical period for plasticity, the somatosensory cortex shows plasticity during the adult life of the animal. These plastic responses were found to be compromised in adult homozygotes (more than 3 months old) but, surprisingly, not in young homozygotes (less than 2 months old). In contrast, control animals of both age groups reveal robust plasticity. Once again, these studies showed that the general properties of the neocortex of the mutants (topography, responsiveness, etc.) were unchanged by the mutation.

Together, these results demonstrate that this kinase is required for adult neocortical plasticity and that similar mechanisms may underlie the learning and the neocortical (somatosensory and visual) plasticity deficits. Nevertheless, these results raise the possibility that the learning deficits described for the homozygous mutants may be due to changes in the plasticity of the neocortex. Current studies with tissue-specific knockouts will address this possibility.

SHORT-LIVED PLASTICITY AND LEARNING

Genetic experiments can be used to test a favorite hypothesis, such as the connection between LTP and learning. However, genetics can also uncover novel mechanisms and open new possibilities that may expand the range of mechanisms included in theories of learning and memory. An example of this is short-lived plasticity (SLP). Changes in synaptic strength lasting milliseconds, seconds, or minutes have been implicated in habituation and sensitization (for review, see Zucker 1989). Interestingly, abnormal SLP was found in the neuromuscular junction of *Drosophila* learning mutants (Zhong and Wu 1991). These results suggest that SLP, along with long-term plasticity, could have a role in learning. Modeling work has also suggested that SLP has a role in learning and in short-term memory (Little and Shaw 1975; Buonomano and Merzenich 1995). Together, these studies suggest that SLP is not simply a by-product of the complex regulation of longer-lasting changes in synaptic strength but that it may have a significant role of its own in information processing. The availability of mutants with normal LTP, but abnormal SLP, allowed the testing of this hypothesis.

Unlike the homozygotes, mice heterozygous for αCaMKII (αCaMKII$^{+/-}$) can show LTP and LTD (A.J. Silva et al., in prep.). However, studies of SLP revealed that post-tetanic potentiation (PTP) and paired-pulse facilitation (PPF) are abnormal in these mice (Silva et al. 1992b; Chapman et al. 1995). Similarly, mice lacking synapsin II (SyII$^{-/-}$) (Rosahl et al. 1995), and synapsin I/II mutants (SyI/II$^{-/-}$) (Rosahl et al. 1995; Spillane et al. 1995), have abnormal hippocampal PTP, although studies of LTP revealed no abnormalities in these mutants. Both synapsins and αCaMKII have been implicated in the modulation of presynaptic function (Greengard et al. 1993; Rosahl et al. 1993, 1995; Chapman et al. 1995). Remarkably, all these mutants show marked impairments in hippocampal-dependent learning, as measured by contextual conditioning and water maze tests. In contrast, the loss of only synapsin I (SyI$^{-/-}$) (Rosahl et al. 1993, 1995; Li et al. 1995), which affects PPF but not PTP, does not affect learning in a number of tasks and conditions used (A.J. Silva et al., in prep.). Together, these results suggest that hippocampal PTP is involved in learning.

It is noteworthy that the electrophysiological abnormalities detected in the mutant mice were specific, and that LTP in the CA1 region of the hippocampus seemed unaffected in all of these mutants. The mutation of synapsin II also is known not to affect LTP in the CA3 of the hippocampus, even though it affects PTP there (Spillane et al. 1995). Importantly, SyII$^{-/-}$, SyI/II$^{-/-}$, and αCaMKII$^{+/-}$ mutants with abnormal PTP reveal learning impairments, but the increase in PPF in SyI$^{-/-}$ mutants does not seem to affect learning. These results demonstrate that it is possible to have abnormal SLP while having normal long-term synaptic plasticity, a finding that argues against the view that SLP is just a by-product of LTP and LTD.

All four mutant lines mentioned have no general deficits in brain morphology and synaptic connectivity, they have normal life expectancies, they show normal nociception, and they are not ataxic (Silva et al. 1992b; Rosahl et al. 1993, 1995; Comery et al. 1994; Li et al. 1995). Nevertheless, some of the mutants appear to be epileptic, and this could complicate the interpretation of the learning experiments. However, $SyI^{-/-}$ and $SyII^{-/-}$ mutants show similar seizure frequencies (Rosahl et al. 1995), but only $SyII^{-/-}$ mutants have abnormal learning. Importantly, despite hippocampal hyperexcitability (Li et al. 1995; Rosahl et al. 1995), the $SyI^{-/-}$ mice showed normal learning and memory in an extensive series of tests involving both fear conditioning and the water maze. Furthermore, even though the homozygous αCaMKII did show evidence for seizures, the heterozygotes studied did not.

It is important to note that without sound theories or explanations, correlations between electrophysiology and behavior are meaningless. However, there are two neuro-network models that implicate SLP in learning (Little and Shaw 1975; Buonomano and Merzenich 1995) and provide a formal justification for how SLPs could have a critical role in learning.

The finding of abnormal PTP and learning would be less interesting, and perhaps trivial, if all abnormalities in the basic properties of synaptic transmission led to learning abnormalities. However, our results show that $SyI^{-/-}$ mutants, with abnormally enhanced PPF and with hyperexcitable synapses, nevertheless have normal learning.

These findings suggest that SLPs are involved in learning. As information flows through the hippocampus, these brief but highly dynamic changes in synaptic strength could have a role in transforming that information. This may be a consequence of the dynamic properties of SLP: This form of plasticity is highly responsive to a neuron's recent history of activation, to the architecture of circuits, and to brain-wide modulatory mechanisms (Zucker 1989). It is likely that hippocampal circuits use these properties to implement complex algorithms that process, modify, filter, and integrate information. It is important to note that the potential involvement of SLP in learning does not exclude LTP. These two mechanisms may have complementary functions, both contributing to the complex set of events that allow an animal to learn and remember.

CREB AND MEMORY

The mechanisms mentioned above are likely to be involved in early stages of memory formation (i.e., during learning). However, little is known about the molecular and cellular processes required to support memory. Previous pharmacological studies showed that the synthesis of new proteins is a pivotal requirement of long-term memory (LTM) (for reviews, see Davis and Squire 1984; Matthies 1989). A variety of inhibitors of protein and RNA synthesis have been shown to effectively block long-term, but not short-term, memory.

Experiments with *Aplysia* demonstrate that serotonin applications activate cAMP-dependent signal transduction (for review, see Byrne 1987), including the cAMP-dependent protein kinase A (PKA), which regulates the activation of transcription factors, such as cAMP-responsive element-binding protein (CREB), in the nucleus. To trigger transcription, CREB binds to a specific regulatory DNA sequence (CRE) in the promoter region of certain genes (for review, see Lee and Masson 1993). Interestingly, oligonucleotides with CRE sequences injected into *Aplysia* sensory neurons in culture selectively block long-term, but not short-term, facilitation (Dash et al. 1990). Work in *Drosophila* showed that a dominant-negative mutant form of CREB can block LTM without having a measurable effect in other memory stages (Tully et al. 1994; Yin et al. 1994). Strikingly, induction of a transgenic CREB activator can induce LTM with a single trial, whereas in control flies, the induction of LTM requires multiple spaced trials (Yin et al. 1995). Similarly, removing CREB repression, with an antibody against a natural CREB blocker, also avoids the requirement for multiple spaced serotonin applications in the induction of long-term synaptic facilitation in *Aplysia* (Bartsch et al. 1995). These results argue for a role of CREB in the induction of LTM and suggest that the requirement for spaced training during the induction of LTM is related to the levels of CREB activator (Yin et al. 1995). These results, however, do not show that all forms of memory could be facilitated by simply providing additional CREB. Instead, they illustrate the involvement of this factor in cellular processes required for memory formation.

Mice lacking the α and the δ isoform of CREB also show memory deficits. Nevertheless, the CREB mutant mice appear normal in most respects studied, suggesting that this mutation has a very specific impact on function. Remarkably, contextual conditioning is normal in CREB mice 30 minutes after training, but not at 1 or 24 hours after training (Bourtchuladze et al. 1994). Similar results were also obtained for conditioning to a sound (cued conditioning). In contrast to contextual conditioning, cued conditioning produced nearly normal fear responses in CREB mice tested 1 hour after training, but not thereafter, demonstrating that the onset of the amnesia is different for these two forms of conditioning. Training in the water maze confirmed that these mutants have deficits in specific types of learning and memory, since the CREB mice were unable to learn this task with 1 trial per day for 15 days, even though controls learn to search selectively for the hidden platform after only 10 days of similar training (Bourtchuladze et al. 1994). However, performance in the visible-platform task is unaffected by the CREB mutation. Thus, two tasks sensitive to hippocampal lesions (contextual conditioning and the spatial version of the water maze) detected a deficit in the CREB mutants.

Protein synthesis is not only essential for LTM, but is also required for late LTP (for review, see Matthies 1989). In studies of CREB mutant mice, LTP was measured in hippocampal slices of adult mice by stimulating Schaffer collaterals and recording field potentials in stratum radiatum. LTP induced by a train of 100 pulses (250-μsec pulse width) at 100 Hz was stable for at least 2 hours in controls. In contrast, LTP returned to baseline levels within 1.5 hours in CREB mutants (Bourtchuladze et al. 1994). Thus, both LTP and memory seem to be unstable in these mutants.

Previous studies found that cAMP inhibitors caused a drastic decrease in LTP between 45 and 90 minutes post-tetanus, and addition of cAMP agonists induced a potentiation within the first 90 minutes, both suggesting that a cAMP-dependent mechanism can affect LTP as early as 90 minutes after the tetanus (Frey et al. 1988, 1993). It is possible that this potentiation is protein-synthesis-dependent and that it requires CREB function. Indeed, several studies have shown clear evidence of synthesis of new proteins as early as 20–30 minutes after tetanic stimulation (Feig and Lipton 1993; Frey et al. 1993). Recently, transgenic studies with a reporter gene driven by a promoter sensitive to CREB function suggested that LTP stimuli can induce gene expression (Impey et al. 1996). Together, these results are consistent with the hypothesis that the instability of LTP and the decay of memory in the CREB mutants are dependent on the down-regulation of a protein-synthesis-dependent phase of LTP and memory. The electrophysiological studies also showed that not all other aspects of synaptic function are affected in the mutants. For example, PPF and PTP do not appear to be changed by the CREB mutation (Bourtchuladze et al. 1994).

It is noteworthy that studies in *Drosophila*, *Aplysia*, and mice—three widely divergent species—found evidence for a requirement for CREB in LTM processes. This strongly suggests that the insights about the molecular and electrophysiological mechanisms responsible for the LTM loss in CREB mutants may also be directly applicable to humans. Indeed, a dysfunction of CREB may account for the mental retardation observed in patients with Rubinstein-Taybi syndrome (Petrij et al. 1995).

It is important to stress that CREB is almost certainly not the only transcription factor modulating the induction of protein synthesis required for LTM, since CREB is known to function in association with other factors (for review, see Lee and Masson 1993). Additionally, organismal memory cannot be explained purely in terms of transcriptional regulation. Instead, the CREB mutants have been valuable in unraveling the molecular cascade of events that are required to support memory formation.

CONCLUSIONS

The history of neuroscience is full of examples that eloquently demonstrate the difficulty of connecting molecular, electrophysiological, neuroanatomical, and behavioral findings into explanations of behavior. Consequently, it may be difficult to interpret the interdisciplinary findings of the mutants, despite the many advances of transgenic technology. However, all other approaches for the integrative study of learning face similar difficulties, which simply stem from the dimensions of the problem, and not just from limitations of any one of the approaches used.

Undoubtedly, these problems will be partially overcome by the convergence of data and approaches. Each approach provides a unique window into the seemingly inscrutable complexity of cognition. New research strategies often provide opportunities both to test key hypotheses and to enrich existing theories with new questions and new emphasis. Indeed, the work presented here combined these two aspects: Not only were existing questions tested by genetics (e.g., is LTP required for learning?), but also new models and avenues of research have been and will continue to be unveiled by this approach (e.g., is short-lived plasticity involved in learning?).

The complex behavioral and electrophysiological phenotypes of these mice will probably raise more questions than they will immediately answer, since our understanding of mechanisms of behavior is so incomplete. The strength of genetics is that it often uncovers hidden processes, thus making them amenable for analysis. For example, homeotic mutations in *Drosophila* resulted in flies with duplicated thoracic or abdominal segments, etc. Indeed, the changes caused by those mutations were extremely complex. However, the study of homeotic mutants has had a widespread and profound impact on our understanding of development. Analogously, in some cases, mutations in synaptic proteins might result in grossly abnormal physiological and behavioral patterns that could nevertheless reshape our concepts of how organisms learn and remember information. Thus, the potential complexity of the mutant phenotypes is not a disadvantage of this approach, since genetic manipulations do not create complexity, but simply reveal it.

One of the most important aspects of the results obtained with gene targeting is that the mutations studied had such a specific effect on the electrophysiology and behavior of the mutant mice. This specificity is crucial for determining how changes in hippocampal physiology affect hippocampal-dependent behaviors. These complex connections between cellular biology, circuit function, and behavior will not be established with individual mutant mice, but with a collection of genetic studies confirmed with results obtained by other methodologies. This process is well under way, and the hippocampal studies described here illustrate the feasibility of using this approach to derive explanations of learning and memory. Although the focus of our studies is on hippocampal function, similar results have also been obtained for other systems, including the cerebellum (Aiba et al. 1994; Chen et al. 1995; Shibuki et al. 1996).

The beginning of a new field is marked by a period of excitement but also uncertainty, when key elements of the approach are being tested, criticisms examined, and misconceptions explained. For a new field, those who strongly oppose it with well-constructed intellectual arguments are just as important as those who enthusiastically support it. This dialectical process, which sharpens the structure and direction of the field, has already helped genetic studies of learning and memory. First, it helped to question the notion that single genes have organismal function. This concept was a useful simplification that emerged from genetic and cell biological studies with genes. Certainly, proteins can have well-defined biochemical roles, and mutations of single genes can also have exquisitely specific effects on cells and on organisms.

It is complicated to assign function to proteins beyond the exact confines of controlled biochemical reactions, however. The functional output of a protein summates, synergizes, antagonizes, and integrates with the functional outputs of millions of other proteins in a variety of interacting neurons and glial cells. These cells form networks with many millions of other neurons which finally affect the behavioral output of the animal. To ascribe meaning to the function of a single protein in behavioral terms is a difficult, if not meaningless, task. Nevertheless, the studies described here, and the many spectacular applications of genetics in biology, show that the disruption of single genes can be a powerful way to understand important biological processes underlying complex organismal phenomena such as behavior.

The current development of inducible transgenic technologies was also partially fueled by the recurrent criticism that the interpretation of genetic studies of learning and memory is confounded by possible developmental effects of the mutations. These novel techniques will allow the control of the place and the time of the mutation. Reversibility will be another important facet of some of these techniques. These advantages will lead to a new class of experiments that will go well beyond simply eliminating developmental concerns. For example, these techniques will allow investigators to specifically disrupt key cellular processes at different stages of learning and memory, and thus to test hypotheses about the biochemical mechanisms required to support different stages of memory formation.

Despite all the excitement surrounding their potential usefulness, mutant mice are simply tools. All that can be asked from a tool is specificity, flexibility, reliability, and reproducibility. The studies presented here have certainly shown that this approach can have all of those properties, which suggests that it has been a fruitful addition to the growing number of other tools that might one day allow us to understand the brain.

ACKNOWLEDGMENTS

This work was funded by grants from the Whitehall Foundation, Beckman Foundation, McKnight Foundation, Klingenstein Foundation, Merck Foundation, and the National Institutes of Health.

REFERENCES

Abeliovich, A., C. Chen, Y. Goda, A.J. Silva, C.F. Stevens, and S. Tonegawa. 1993a. Modified hippocampal long-term potentiation in PKCγ-mutant mice. *Cell* **75:** 1253.

Abeliovich, A., R. Paylor, C. Chen, J.J. Kim, J.M. Wehner, and S. Tonegawa. 1993b. PKCγ mutant mice exhibit mild deficits in spatial and contextual learning. *Cell* **75:** 1263.

Aiba, A., M. Kano, C. Chen, M.E. Stanton, G.D. Fox, K. Herrup, T.A. Zwingman, and S. Tonegawa. 1994. Deficient cerebellar long-term depression and impaired motor learning in mGluR1 mutant mice. *Cell* **79:** 377.

Bach, M.E., R.D. Hawkins, M. Osman, E.R. Kandel, and M. Mayford. 1995. Impairment of spatial but not contextual memory in CaMKII mutant mice with a selective loss of hippocampal LTP in the range of the 25 theta frequency. *Cell* **81:** 905.

Bannerman, D.M., M.A. Good, S.P. Butcher, M. Ramsay, and R.G.M. Morris. 1995. Distinct components of spatial learning revealed by prior training and NMDA receptor blockade. *Nature* **378:** 182.

Bartsch, D., M. Ghirardi, P.A. Skehel, K.A. Karl, S.P. Herder, M. Chen, C.H. Bailey, and E.R. Kandel. 1995. *Aplysia* CREB2 represses long-term facilitation: Relief of repression converts transient facilitation into long-term functional and structural change. *Cell* **83:** 979.

Bliss, T.V.P. and G.L. Collingridge. 1993. A synaptic model of memory: Long-term potentiation in the hippocampus. *Nature* **351:** 31.

Bourtchuladze, R., B. Frenguelli, J. Blendy, D. Cioffi, G. Schütz, and A.J. Silva. 1994. Deficient long-term memory in mice with a targeted disruption of the cAMP-responsive element-binding protein. *Cell* **79:** 59.

Buonomano, D.V. and M.M. Merzenich. 1995. Transformation of temporal information into a spatial code by a neural network based on realistic neuronal properties. *Science* **267:** 1028.

Burgin, K.E., M.N. Waxham, S. Rickling, S.A. Westgate, W.C. Mobley, and P.T. Kelly. 1990. In situ hybridization histochemistry of Ca^{2+}/calmodulin-dependent protein kinase in developing rat brain. *J. Neurosci.* **10:** 1788.

Butler, L.S., A.J. Silva, A. Abeliovich, Y. Watanabe, S. Tonegawa, and J.O. McNamara. 1995. Limbic epilepsy in transgenic mice carrying a Ca^{2+}/calmodulin-dependent kinase II α-subunit mutation. *Proc. Natl. Acad. Sci.* **92:** 6852.

Byrne, J.H. 1987. Cellular analysis of associative learning. *Physiol. Rev.* **67:** 329.

Cain, D.P., D. Saucier, J. Hall, E.L. Hargreaves, and F. Boon. 1996. Detailed behavioral analysis of water maze acquisition under APV or CNQX: Contribution of sensorimotor disturbances to drug-induced acquisition deficits. *Behav. Neurosci.* **110:** 86.

Chapman, P.F., B.G. Frenguelli, A. Smith, C.-M. Chen, and

A.J. Silva. 1995. The α-Ca^{2+}/calmodulin kinase II: A bidirectional modulator of presynaptic plasticity. *Neuron* **14:** 591.

Chen, C., M. Kano, A. Abeliovich, L. Chen, S. Bao, J.J. Kim, K. Hashimoto, R.F. Thompson, and S. Tonegawa. 1995. Impaired motor coordination correlates with persistent multiple climbing fiber innervation PKCψ mutant mice. *Cell* **83:** 1233.

Comery, T.A., J.A. Kleim, A. Silva, and W.T. Greenough. 1994. Hippocampal anatomy and ultrastructural morphology of α-calcium calmodulin kinase II deletion mice. *Soc. Neurosci. Abstr.* **24:** 1506.

Dash, P.K., B. Hochner, and E.R. Kandel. 1990. Injection of the cAMP-responsive element into the nucleus of *Aplysia* sensory neurons blocks long-term facilitation. *Nature* **345:** 718.

Davis, H.P. and L.R. Squire. 1984. Protein synthesis and memory. *Psychol. Bull.* **96:** 518.

Davis, S., S.P. Butcher, and R.G.M. Morris. 1992. The NMDA receptor antagonist D-2-amino-5-phosphonopentanoate (D-AP5) impairs spatial learning and LTP in vivo at intracerebral concentrations comparable to those that block LTP in vitro. *J. Neurosci.* **12:** 21.

Eichenbaum, H. and T. Otto. 1992. The hippocampus—What does it do? *Behav. Neural Biol.* **57:** 2.

Feig, S. and P. Lipton. 1993. Pairing the cholinergic agonist carbachol with patterned Schaffer collateral stimulation initiates protein synthesis in hippocampal CA1 pyramidal cell dendrites via a muscarinic, NMDA-dependent mechanism. *J. Neurosci.* **13:** 1010.

Frey, U., Y.-Y. Huang, and E.R. Kandel. 1993. Effects of cAMP stimulate a late stage of LTP in hippocampal CA1 neurons. *Science* **260:** 1661.

Frey, U., M. Krug, K.G. Reymann, and H. Matthies. 1988. Anisomycin, an inhibitor of protein synthesis, blocks late phases of LTP phenomena in the hippocampal CA1 region in vitro. *Brain Res.* **452:** 57.

Glazewski, S., C.-M. Chen, A. Silva, and K. Fox. 1996. Requirement for α-CaMKII in experience-dependent plasticity of the barrel cortex. *Science* **272:** 421.

Gordon, J.A. and M.P. Stryker. 1996. Experience-dependent plasticity of binocular responses in the primary visual cortex of the mouse. *J. Neurosci.* **10:** 3274.

Gordon, J.A., A. Silva, R. Morris, C. Stewart, J. Silver, Y. Tokugawa, and M.P. Stryker. 1994. Plasticity in mouse visual cortex: Critical period and effects of αCaMKII and Thy-1 mutations. *Soc. Neurosci. Abstr.* **24:** 465.

Grant, S.G.N., J. O'Dell, K.A. Karl, P.L. Stein, P. Soriano, and E.R. Kandel. 1992. Impaired long-term potentiation, spatial learning, and hippocampal development in *fyn* mutant mice. *Science* **258:** 1903.

Greengard, P., F. Valtorta, A.J. Czernik, and F. Benfenati. 1993. Synaptic vesicle phosphoproteins and regulation of synaptic function. *Science* **259:** 780.

Hanson, P.I. and H. Schulman. 1992. Neuronal Ca^{2+}/calmodulin-dependent protein kinases. *Annu. Rev. Biochem.* **61:** 559.

Huang, Y.Y., E.R. Kandel, L. Varshavsky, E.P. Brandon, M. Qi, R.L. Idzerda, G.S. McKnight, and R. Bourtchouladze. 1995. A genetic test of the effects of mutations in PKA on mossy fiber LTP and its relation to spatial and contextual learning. *Cell* **83:** 1211.

Hvalby, O., H.C. Hemmings, O. Paulsen, A.J. Czernik, A.C. Nairn, J.-M. Godfraind, V. Jensen, M. Raastad, J.F. Storm, P. Andersen, and P. Greengard. 1994. Specificity of protein kinase inhibitor peptides and induction of long-term potentiation. *Proc. Natl. Acad. Sci.* **91:** 4761.

Impey, S., M. Mark, E.C. Villacres, S. Poser, C. Chavkin, and D.R. Storm. 1996. Induction of CRE-mediated gene expression by stimuli that generate long-lasting LTP in area CA1 of the hippocampus. *Neuron* **16:** 973.

Kirkwood, A., A. Silva, and M.F. Bear. 1994. Reduced synaptic plasticity in visual cortex slices of a-CaM-KII knockout transgenic mice. *Soc. Neurosci. Abstr.* **24:** 1471.

Larson, J. and G. Lynch. 1986. Induction of synaptic potentiation in hippocampus by patterned stimulation involves two events. *Science* **232:** 985.

Lee, K.A. and N. Masson. 1993. Transcriptional regulation by CREB and its relatives. *Biochim. Biophys. Acta* **1174:** 221.

Li, L., L.-S. Chin, O. Shupliakov, L. Brodin, T.S. Sihra, Ø. Hvalby, V. Jensen, D. Zheng, J.O. McNamara, P. Greengard, and P. Andersen. 1995. Impairment of synaptic vesicle clustering and of synaptic transmission, and increased seizure propensity, in synapsin I-deficient mice. *Proc. Natl. Acad. Sci.* **92:** 9235.

Little, W.A. and G.L. Shaw. 1975. A statistical theory of short and long-term memory. *Behav. Biol.* **14:** 115.

Malenka, R.C., J.A. Kauer, D.J. Perkel, M.D. Mauk, P.T. Kelly, R.A. Nicoll, and M.N. Waxham. 1989. An essential role for postsynaptic calmodulin and protein kinase activity in long-term potentiation. *Nature* **340:** 554.

Malinow, R., H. Schulman, and R.W. Tsien. 1989. Inhibition of postsynaptic PKC or CaMKII blocks induction but not expression of LTP. *Science* **245:** 862.

Matthies, H. 1989. In search of cellular mechanisms of memory. *Prog. Neurobiol.* **32:** 277.

Mayford, M., J. Wang, E.R. Kandel, and T.J. O'Dell. 1995. CaMKII regulates the frequency-response function of hippocampal synapses for the production of both LTD and LTP. *Cell* **81:** 891.

Moser, E., I. Mathiesen, and P. Andersen. 1993. Association between brain temperature and dentate field potentials in exploring and swimming rats. *Science* **259:** 1324.

Otto, T., H. Eichenbaum, S.I. Wiener, and C.G. Wible. 1991. Learning-related patterns of CA1 spike trains parallel stimulation parameters optimal for inducing hippocampal long-term potentiation. *Hippocampus* **1:** 181.

Petrij, F., R.H. Giles, H.G. Dauwerse, J.J. Saris, R.C.M. Hennekam, M. Masuno, N. Tommerup, G.-J.B. van Ommen, R.H. Goodman, D.J.M. Peters, and M.H. Breuning. 1995. Rubinstein-Taybi syndrome caused by mutations in the transcriptional co-activator CBP. *Nature* **376:** 348.

Rosahl, T.W., M. Geppert, D. Spillane, J. Herz, R.E. Hammer, R.C. Malenka, and T.C. Südhof. 1993. Short-term synaptic plasticity is altered in mice lacking synapsin I. *Cell* **75:** 661.

Rosahl, T.W., D. Spillane, M. Missler, J. Herz, D.K. Selig, J.R. Wolff, R.E. Hammer, R.C. Malenka, and T.C. Südhof. 1995. Essential functions of synapsins I and II in synaptic vesicle regulation. *Nature* **375:** 488.

Sakimura, K., T. Kutsuwada, I. Ito, T. Manabe, C. Takayama, E. Kushiya, T. Yagi, S. Aizawa, Y. Inoue, H. Sugiyama, and M. Mishina. 1995. Reduced hippocampal LTP and spatial learning in mice lacking NMDA receptor ε1 subunit. *Nature* **373:** 151.

Shibuki, K., H. Gomi, L. Chen, S. Bao, J.J. Kim, H. Wakatsuki, T. Fujisaki, T. Ikeda, C. Chen, R.F. Thompson, and S. Itohara. 1996. Deficient cerebellar long-term depression, impaired eyeblink conditioning, and normal motor coordination in GFAP mutant mice. *Neuron* **16:** 587.

Silva, A.J., R. Paylor, J.M. Wehner, and S. Tonegawa. 1992a. Impaired spatial learning in alpha-calcium calmodulin kinase II mutant mice. *Science* **257:** 206.

Silva, A.J., C.F. Stevens, S. Tonegawa, and Y. Wang. 1992b. Deficient hippocampal long-term potentiation in alpha-calcium calmodulin kinase II mutant mice. *Science* **257:** 201.

Spillane, D.M., T.W. Rosahl, T.C Südhof, and R.C. Malenka. 1995. Long term potentiation in mice lacking synapsins. *Neuropharmacology* **34:** 1573.

Squire, L.R. 1992. Memory and the hippocampus; A synthesis from findings with rat, monkeys, and humans. *Psychol. Rev.* **99:** 195.

Stevens, C.F., S. Tonegawa, and Y. Wang. 1994. The role of calcium-calmodulin kinase II in three forms of synaptic plasticity. *Curr. Biol.* **4:** 687.

Tully, T., T. Preat, S.C. Boynton, and M.D. Vecchio. 1994. Genetic dissection of consolidated memory in *Drosophila. Cell* **79:** 35.

Wu, Z.-L., S.A. Thomas, E.C. Villacres, Z. Xia, M.L. Simmons, C. Chavkin, R.D. Palmiter, and D.R. Storm. 1995. Altered behavior and long-term potentiation in type I adenylyl cyclase mutant mice. *Proc. Natl. Acad. Sci.* **92:** 220.

Yin, J., M. Del Vecchio, H. Zhou, and T. Tully. 1995. CREB as a memory modulator: Induced expression of a dCREB2 activator isoform enhances long-term memory in *Drosophila. Cell* **81:** 107.

Yin, J., J.S. Wallach, M.D. Vecchio, E.L. Wilder, H. Zhou, W.G. Quinn, and T. Tully. 1994. Induction of a dominant-negative CREB transgene specifically blocks long-term memory in *Drosophila melanogaster. Cell* **79:** 49.

Zhong, Y. and C.-F. Wu. 1991. Altered synaptic plasticity in *Drosophila* memory mutants with a defective cyclic AMP cascade. *Science* **251:** 198.

Zucker, R. 1989. Short-term synaptic plasticity. *Annu. Rev. Neurosci.* **12:** 13.

Emotional Memory: A Search for Sites of Plasticity

G.J. Quirk, J.L. Armony, J.C. Repa, X.-F. Li, and J.E. LeDoux
Center for Neural Science, New York University, New York, New York 10003-6621

Traumatic experiences can leave lasting scars, in the form of emotional memories, in one's mind. Studies over the past several decades have begun to illuminate exactly how such memories are formed (Davis 1992; Kapp et al. 1992; McCabe et al. 1992; Fanselow 1994; LeDoux 1995). This work has, for the most part, involved studies of experimental animals trained using aversive conditioning procedures, especially classic fear conditioning. In fear conditioning, the subject, often a rat, is exposed to a noxious stimulus, such as footshock, in conjunction with some other stimulus (a tone, for example) that has no strong preexisting meaning. As a result of the training session, the tone acquires aversive properties and will, on next occurrence, trigger a panoply of species-typical fear (defense) responses. Such responses include freezing behavior, alterations in autonomic nervous system activity, release of stress hormones, suppression of pain reactivity, and facilitation of bodily reflexes. These responses are hard-wired into the brain's circuitry and occur in a similar fashion in a variety of species. Fear conditioning allows novel stimuli that warn of danger to call upon this tried and true response repertoire. The advantage of having a fear conditioning mechanism in the brain is that we can learn about the stimuli that predict danger and use this information to avoid situations in which we are likely to encounter dangerous things. The disadvantage is that in order for this mechanism to work, we have to carry the aversive memories around in our brains. When these memories are caused by severe trauma, any adaptive advantage they confer can be outweighed by the detrimental effects on emotional well-being. Understanding the mechanisms of fear conditioning thus offers us the opportunity to clarify how emotional memories are formed normally, as well as how devastating traumatic memories might be established.

The neural pathways involved in fear conditioning have been elucidated in considerable detail using brain lesion and tract tracing techniques (Davis 1992; Kapp et al. 1992; McCabe et al. 1992; Fanselow 1994; LeDoux 1995). These studies indicate that the amygdala plays a pivotal role. Sensory pathways transmit the learned trigger stimulus to the amygdala. Within the amygdala, specific internal connections exist, and projections from the amygdala to motor systems mediate the control of the individual defense response systems. The amygdala is thus involved in fear conditioning regardless of the sensory modality of the conditioned stimulus (CS) and independent of which motor response is used as a measure (Fig. 1A).

The mechanisms of fear conditioning are best understood for auditory conditioned stimuli (see Campeau and Davis 1995a,b; LeDoux 1995). The pathways involved are shown in Figure 1B. Following processing by brain stem regions, auditory fibers synapse at the level of the thalamus in the medial geniculate body, specifically its medial part (MGm) and adjacent posterior intralaminar nucleus (PIN). From there, the signals are transmitted directly to the amygdala and to the auditory cortex. The auditory cortex then also sends fibers to the amygdala. Thus, the amygdala receives acoustic information about an external conditioned stimulus from both the thalamus and cortex. Although either of these paths is sufficient to mediate conditioning to a single tone (for an alternative view, see Campeau and Davis 1995b; for a rebuttal, see Corodimas and LeDoux 1995), more complex stimulus analysis may require the auditory cortex and its connections with the amygdala (McCabe et al. 1992). Within the amygdala, the lateral nucleus (LA), especially the dorsal subnucleus of LA, is the main recipient of the inputs from both the auditory thalamus and auditory cortex (LeDoux et al. 1990; Turner and Herkenham 1991; Bordi and LeDoux 1992; Mascagni et al. 1993; Romanski and LeDoux 1993). Sensory information is mainly directed to the dorsal subnucleus of LA, which then projects to the more ventral parts of LA (including the ventral lateral and medial nuclei, which will be collectively referred to throughout as the ventral parts of LA), as well as to the basal, accessory basal, and central nuclei (Stefanacci et al. 1992; Pitkanen et al. 1995). The basal and accessory basal also project to the central nucleus (Savander et al. 1995). The central nucleus, in turn, is the interface with brain stem areas involved in the control of each of the various responses that are expressed in the presence of a conditioned fear stimulus (see Gray et al. 1991; Davis 1992; Kapp et al. 1992; McCabe et al. 1992; Fanselow 1994; LeDoux 1995).

Cortical inputs to the amygdala may play a role in modulating fear associations. The hippocampus has been shown to be essential for conditioning to contextual cues (Blanchard et al. 1970; Selden et al. 1991; Kim and Fanselow 1992; Phillips and LeDoux 1992), and prefrontal and sensory cortices have been implicated in the extinguishing of conditioned fear respon-

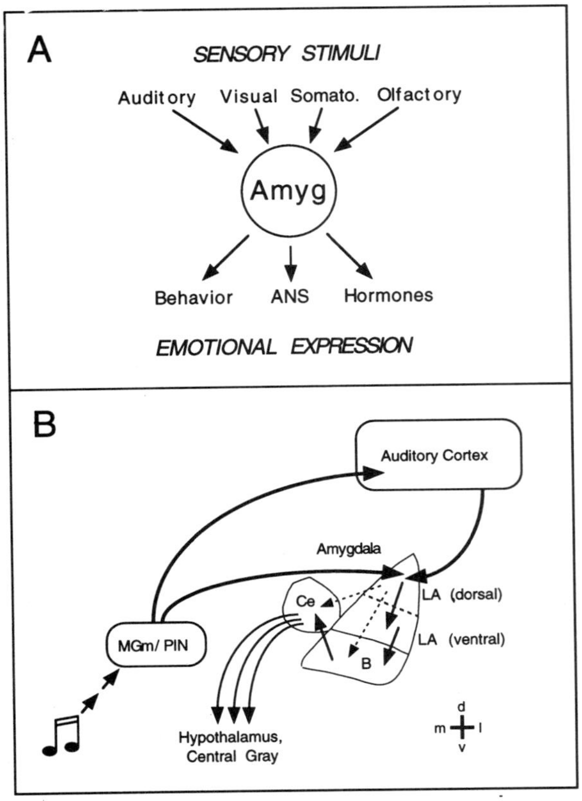

Figure 1. (*A*) The amygdala receives sensory information from all the modalities and has outputs mediating species-specific behavioral responses as well as autonomic and hormonal responses to threatening stimuli. (*B*) The detailed pathways of fear conditioning are best understood for auditory stimuli, which enter the amygdala by way of the lateral nucleus (LA). LA receives auditory information from two pathways: directly from the medial geniculate and indirectly via the auditory cortex. Intra-amygdala projections end in the central nucleus, which mediates emotional expression via efferents to the hypothalamus and midbrain. Intraamygdala circuits from the LA to the central nucleus are direct and by way of the basal and accessory basal nuclei. (MGm/PIN) Medial geniculate nucleus/posterior intralaminar nucleus of the thalamus; (LA) lateral amygdala; (B) basal nucleus of the amygdala; (Ce) central nucleus of the amygdala. Dashed lines indicate weaker projections than solid lines.

ses (LeDoux et al. 1989; Morgan and LeDoux 1995). It is likely that these structures exert their effects via projections to the amygdala.

The conditioning pathways described above have mostly been identified by assessing the effects of brain lesions on the acquisition of conditioned responses. Although the brain lesion method has clearly implicated the amygdala and its afferent and efferent systems in fear conditioning, many important questions remain unanswered. Some of these are listed below.

1. At which stage of amygdala processing is plasticity observed, and what advantages are conferred by downstream processing in the amygdala?
2. Is the amygdala really a site of plasticity during fear learning or simply a throughput for expression of conditioned responses learned elsewhere?
3. Are subcortical (thalamic) inputs sufficient for amygdala plasticity or is cortical processing a prerequisite?
4. Which aspects of the learning experience do amygdala cells encode?
5. Is the amygdala a site of extinction-resistant storage?

These questions cannot be answered with behavioral analyses of lesioned animals, but only by measuring amygdala function during learning. Single-unit recordings, especially in freely behaving animals, are well suited for this purpose. Although there have been a few such studies of the amygdala in the past, they were not designed to address, and have thus not provided answers to, the questions posed above. Recently, we have begun a systematic program of such recordings to address these questions. This paper documents our progress to date.

AT WHICH STAGE OF AMYGDALA PROCESSING IS PLASTICITY OBSERVED?

There is a long and rich tradition involving the use of unit recordings to study the plasticity or modifiability of neuronal activity as a result of some learning experience. Typically, conditioned plasticity is believed to occur if the firing rate of the cell is significantly altered after the experiment relative to before, and if the changes are specifically due to the association of the two stimuli. Previous unit studies, focused on the basal and central nuclei, have found evidence for plasticity in the amygdala (Segal 1973; Applegate et al. 1982; Pascoe and Kapp 1985; Maren et al. 1991; Muramoto et al. 1993; McEchron et al. 1995; Uwano et al. 1995). However, observing a conditioned unit response in a structure does not confirm that the structure is, in fact, a site of local changes. This was recognized long ago by Olds and colleagues (Olds et al. 1972), who proposed a strategy for identifying primary sites of plasticity. They suggested that one should search for the earliest conditioned responses (shortest latency after tone onset), which presumably would be the first possible locus of plasticity in the system. We have adopted this strategy in our work on the search for the mechanisms of plasticity within the amygdala. Specifically, we have sought to determine: (1) whether plastic changes in neural activity occur in LA (the sensory interface of the amygdala and thus the first possible site in the amygdala where such changes could occur) and (2) whether changes in LA occur at response latencies earlier than those reported for other amygdala areas.

Figure 2 reviews the auditory response latencies of neurons in LA and auditory afferent regions in the ab-

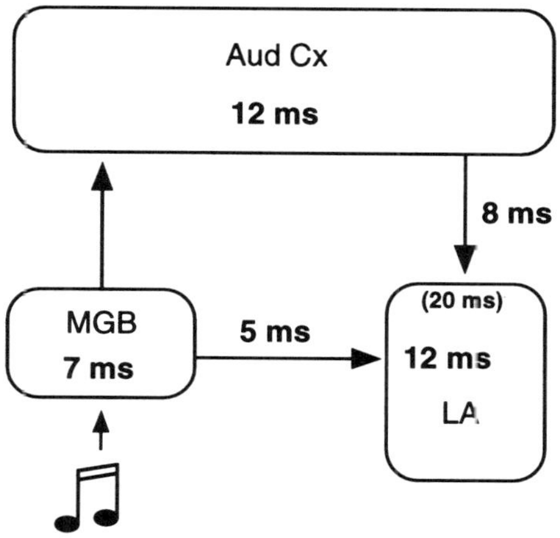

Figure 2. The minimum latencies of activation of single neurons in response to auditory stimuli (tones) are shown. Numbers next to arrows are minimum stimulation latencies between the two structures. The earliest auditory inputs activate the auditory thalamus about 7 msec after stimulus onset. These inputs are then transmitted to both the auditory cortex and LA, yielding a 12-msec response time in both structures. Given these latencies, the earliest responses in LA can only be due to thalamic input, as at least an additional 8 msec is required for cortical activation. Thalamic input to LA originates in the medial subdivision of the medial geniculate body (MGB).

sence of any prior experimentally imposed conditioning procedure. Cells in MGm/PIN fire as early as 7 msec (Bordi and LeDoux 1994), and in the LA as early as 12 msec (Bordi and LeDoux 1992; Bordi et al. 1993; Romanski et al. 1993), following tone onset. Consistent with these figures, electrical stimulation of the MGm/PIN fires neurons in the LA with a latency of 5 msec (Li et al. 1995, 1996a). Similar to the LA, cells in the auditory cortex also respond at 12 msec (Quirk et al. 1995), probably resulting from direct projections to both structures from the medial geniculate body. Stimulation of the auditory cortex region that projects to the amygdala (TE3) activates LA with a minimum latency of 8 msec (Li et al. 1996b). Thus, following tone onset, the lateral amygdala is activated directly via the thalamus at 12 msec and indirectly via the cortex with a minimum latency of 20 msec. This latency difference can be exploited to determine the path of CS processing by measuring the earliest latency of conditioned responses in LA neurons.

We implanted rats with a movable bundle of 20 microwires to record action potentials extracellularly from single LA cells (Quirk et al. 1995). Fear conditioning consisted of pairing a tone CS (5 kHz, 80 dB, 2 sec) with a footshock (0.5 mA, 0.5 sec). To control for nonassociative changes due to shock presentation, a sensitization phase consisting of unpaired tones and shocks was followed by a conditioning phase where the shocks and tones coterminated. After a 1-hour delay, 30 extinction trials (tone alone) were carried out. In all phases of the experiment, tones were separated by an average intertrial interval of 2 minutes. Figure 3 shows the waveforms of 7 simultaneously recorded LA cells before conditioning (sensitization phase) and after conditioning (extinction phase). Post-stimulus time histograms (PSTHs) show the effect of training on the tone responses of the neurons. Conditioning had different effects on the various simultaneously recorded cells. For each cell, standard scores were calculated from sensitization data and used to test for significant increases in tone response after conditioning (at the beginning of extinction). The earliest conditioned response was considered to occur in the bin that had a significantly greater number of spikes after conditioning, compared to before. The latency of the earliest conditioned responses (using bins of 10-msec duration) in the dorsal subregion of LA was below 20 msec in the majority of cells (see Fig. 4). Subdividing the bins even further showed that the majority of cells conditioned prior to 15 msec, ruling out the contribution of the cortical pathway to the earliest conditioned responses. Thus, projections from the thalamus are sufficient to generate plasticity in the dorsal part of LA. The ventral half of LA showed later conditioning (~40 msec). This is consistent with the fact that this area receives anatomical inputs from the dorsal part of LA (see Pitkanen et al. 1995; Savander et al. 1995). Because these changes in LA (dorsal and ventral parts) were observed 1 hour after conditioning, they can be thought of as reflecting long-term changes, presumably long-term changes in synaptic efficacy in the thalamo-amygdala pathway.

Previous studies have reported considerably longer conditioned response latencies in the amygdala: 30–50 msec in the central nucleus (Pascoe and Kapp 1985; Uwano et al. 1995) and 49 msec (Muramoto et al. 1993) and 70 msec (Maren et al. 1991) in the basal nucleus. Other studies (McEchron et al. 1995; Uwano et al. 1995) did not specifically measure the latency of conditioned responses. Our data suggest that plasticity observed at later stages of amygdala processing (basal, central nuclei) may depend on earlier processing in LA.

IS THE AMYGDALA REALLY A SITE OF PLASTICITY DURING FEAR LEARNING?

The observation of rapid conditioned responses in LA neurons (<15 msec) would seem to rule out a necessary role of cortical involvement in the plasticity of the earliest responses in LA but does not necessarily implicate LA as a critical site of CS–US (unconditioned stimulus) pairing. It is possible that the short-latency conditioned responses are due to plastic changes that are established first in the MGm/PIN and projected to the LA via thalamo-amygdala fibers. If so, conditioned responses in the MGm/PIN should unequivocally precede those of LA. Numerous studies dating from the early 1970s have examined units in

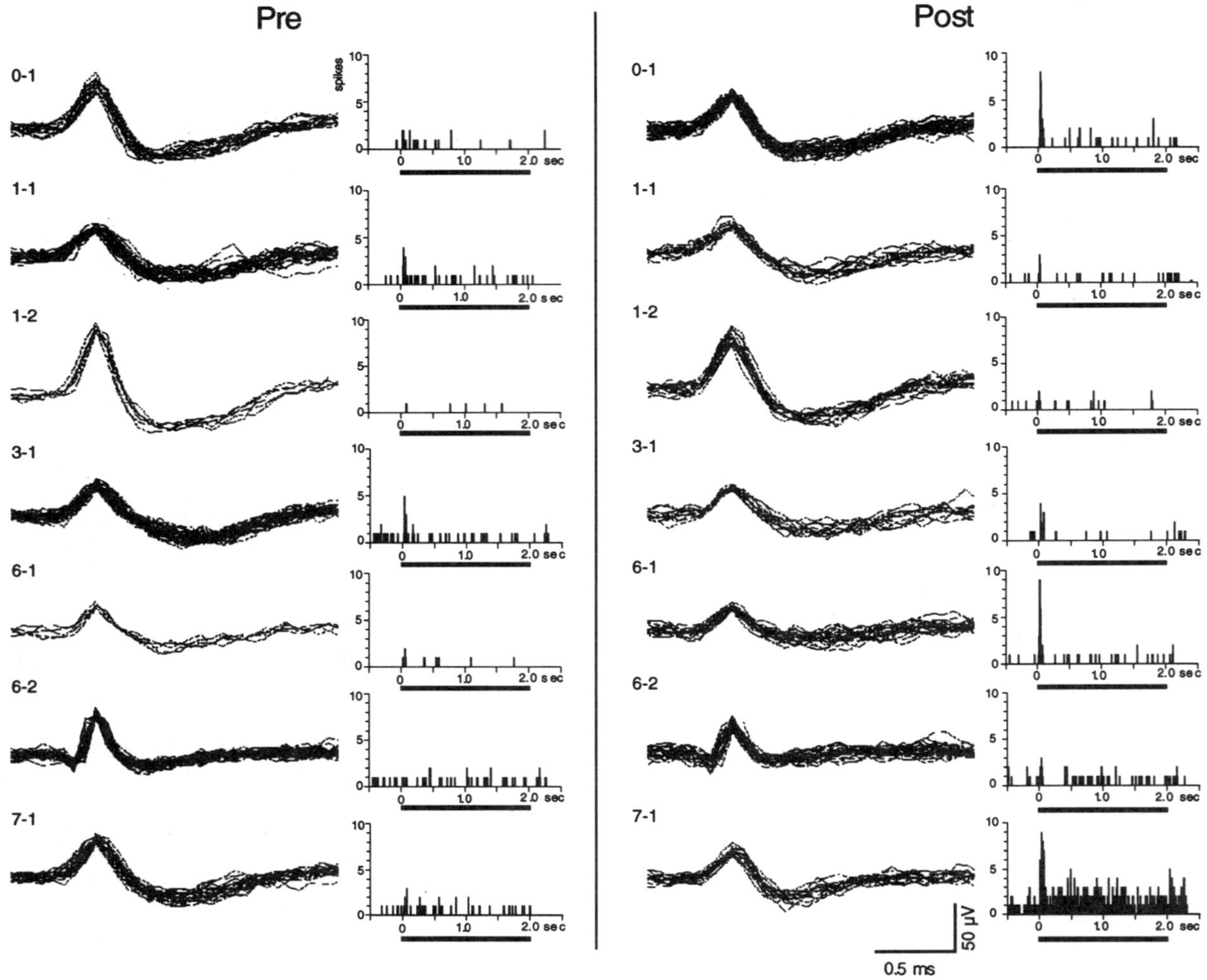

Figure 3. Waveforms and post-stimulus time histograms for 7 simultaneously recorded LA neurons are shown prior to conditioning (during sensitization trials, Pre) and after conditioning (during extinction trials, Post). The numbers in the upper left-hand corner of each waveform indicate the wire and cell number, respectively. The histograms show 10 trials with 10 msec bins, tone onset marked by a bar. Note that the waveforms were constant across training, and tone responses of several cells were increased, especially for early parts of the response.

MGm and other areas of the auditory thalamus during classic conditioning, but few have actually measured the latency of conditioned responses with fine temporal resolution. Olds et al. (1972) noted that only 2/8 MG units conditioned with a latency of less than 20 msec. A minimum conditioning latency of 20 msec was also reported by Supple and Kapp (1989) and Edeline et al. (1990). Two studies reported a range of latencies of plasticity that included values lower than 10 msec and up to 35 msec (Gabriel et al. 1976; Birt et al. 1979), but the prevalence of the short-latency responses was not indicated. Furthermore, the Gabriel study used multiunit rather than single unit recordings and tested avoidance conditioning, and the Birt et al. study involved appetitive conditioning. Given the conclusions stated above for the two single-unit studies involving fear conditioning, it seems that minimum conditioned response latencies in the MGm are around 20 msec for fear conditioning. However, due to the importance of this issue, we are currently conducting a detailed investigation of the latency of conditioned responses in the auditory thalamus (Repa et al. 1996). Thus, previous latency data do not provide much support for the hypothesis that learning-related changes in the thalamus are modifications of ascending projections from the brain stem, as the latencies tend to be fairly long. The data suggest instead that plastic changes may result from descending influences from higher centers, such as the auditory neocortex (Disterhoft and Olds 1972).

That a descending mechanism from cortex may explain MGm plasticity is also suggested by the results of a recent study that examined the effects of fear conditioning on synaptic efficacy in the ascending inputs to

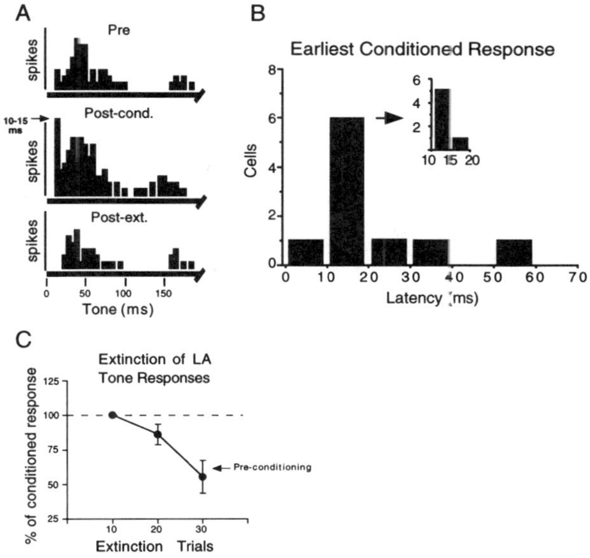

Figure 4. (*A*) Post-stimulus time histograms showing the tone response of an LA neuron at 3 points during training: before conditioning, after conditioning, and after extinction. Note the modulation of the early (10–15 msec) tone response. (*B*) Latency of the earliest conditioned response for all cells that conditioned in dorsal LA. Note that the majority of cells conditioned prior to 15 msec, which is too brief a latency for cortical auditory transmission to LA and must be due to thalamic input. (*C*) Extinction of tone responses of LA neurons ($n = 10$) to preconditioning levels following 30 extinction trials. (Adapted from Quirk et al. 1995.)

the auditory thalamus. In this study, stimulation of the inferior colliculus was used to evoke field potentials in the medial geniculate region (McEchron et al. 1996). A larger response after conditioning would suggest that conditioning increased synaptic strength in the pathway. Although significant changes were observed immediately after conditioning in several measures of synaptic efficacy, most had diminished 1 hour following conditioning. Since conditioned plasticity of single units in MGm is long-lasting (Edeline and Weinberger 1992), it is possible, as McEchron et al. (1996) suggest, that centrifugal projections from higher centers rather than ascending inputs to MGm may be responsible for sustained plasticity in the thalamus. Rather than a passive throughput for plasticity established in the thalamus, LA may be a site where stable plasticity originates. It should be noted, however, that a local plastic change is not the only explanation of early conditioned responses. Tonic influences from higher centers could also modulate short latency responses (Gabriel 1976).

LA is particularly suited as a site of associative plasticity because it receives multi-modal inputs from a wide range of cortical and thalamic areas involved in processing sensory stimuli from all modalities (Ottersen 1982; de Olmos et al. 1985; Price et al. 1987; LeDoux et al. 1990; Turner and Herkenham 1991; Amaral et al. 1992; Mascagni et al. 1993; Romanski and LeDoux 1993). In addition, amygdala units have been conditioned to visual, olfactory, and somatosensory stimuli as well as tones (Nishijo et al. 1988; Uwano et al. 1995). LA is thus the first site in the sensory processing stream leading to the amygdala where there is massive sensory convergence, encompassing all the sensory modalities. Furthermore, LA has the molecular machinery necessary for long-term synaptic plasticity, including glutamatergic terminals (LeDoux and Farb 1991), acting through NMDA and AMPA receptors (Li et al. 1995, 1996b), and exhibiting long-term potentiation (Chapman et al. 1990; Clugnet and LeDoux 1990; Rogan and LeDoux 1995). Furthermore, blockade of NMDA receptors in LA (and in the adjacent basal nucleus) prevents the acquisition of fear conditioning (Miserendino et al. 1990; Kim et al. 1991). Much remains unknown about the neural basis of conditioning in LA, but it seems clear that cells in this region are primary sites of synaptic modification during fear conditioning.

Research by McGaugh and colleagues challenges the notion that the amygdala is a site of plasticity in certain types of aversive learning (Liang et al. 1982; Parent et al. 1995). They have tested the effects of posttraining amygdala manipulations (lesions or pharmacological manipulations) on the retention of inhibitory avoidance conditioning in rats. When the lesions are made soon after training (<1 week), deficits are observed, but when the delay between training and amygdala inactivation is long (>1 week), there are no deficits. This suggests that whatever role the amygdala plays in inhibitory avoidance, it is a temporary role, and the amygdala is not a site of permanent storage in this task. In contrast, posttraining lesions of the amygdala block conditioned fear (fear potentiated startle), regardless of the training-lesion interval (Kim and Davis 1993). Therefore, the amygdala may be a permanent repository of conditioned fear memories, but this issue is not fully resolved since studies to date do not distinguish effects of amygdala lesions on long-term storage and on the ability to express conditioned fear responses. The apparent discrepancy between the effects of posttraining amygdala lesions on conditioned fear and inhibitory avoidance might reflect the different contribution of the amygdala to each. Once animals have learned an avoidance response, they no longer express emotional responses to the fearful stimulus (Solomon and Wynne 1954; Linden 1969). Whereas conditioned fear may always depend on the amygdala, inhibitory avoidance (once established) could be maintained as a habit in the so-called habit systems of the brain, striatum and neocortex (McDonald and White 1993; Petri and Mishkin 1994), rather than the amygdala. At a minimum, the amygdala is required for the initial formation of aversive associations and may be permanently required as long as the aversive stimulus cannot be safely avoided. Again, it is likely that unit recordings rather than additional lesion studies will be required to address this issue.

WHICH ASPECTS OF THE LEARNING EXPERIENCE DO AMYGDALA CELLS ENCODE?

Short-latency conditioned increases in tone responses indicate that LA neurons encode the onset of the CS. What about other components of the conditioning experience? In addition to the short-latency analysis described above, we also examined long-latency tone responses by dividing the tone into 8 bins of 250-msec duration. The histograms of Figure 5 show the number of cells that had significant tone responses (5A) and conditioned responses (5B) in each bin for dorsal LA. Prior to training, dorsal LA cells show onset and offset tone responses, as well as sustained responses. Conditioning, however, increased the tone responses at onset and offset only (Fig. 5B). Thus, it appears that dorsal LA neurons are primarily concerned with signaling the onset and offset of the CS, or changes in the state of a stimulus that has been identified as dangerous. Cells in the ventral part of LA, on the other hand, showed considerably more conditioned responses throughout the tone. Sustained conditioned responses in ventral LA might result from intra-amygdala processing (transmission from dorsal to ventral LA) or might be due to projections from cortical areas (including perirhinal, hippocampal, and prefrontal areas) to the ventral LA (Ottersen 1982; Romanski and LeDoux 1993). To more thoroughly characterize the contribution of ventral LA and other amygdala nuclei to fear conditioning, additional studies will be required.

So far we have focused on the tone response of amygdala neurons to the CS as an indicator of learning-induced plasticity. However, if circuits involving LA are altered as a function of experience, spontaneous neural activity might also be affected (Ben-Ari 1972). We made measurements of spontaneous activity of LA neurons before and after conditioning and after extended extinction training and analyzed the firing rate of individual neurons and the correlation in the time of the firing of pairs of simultaneously recorded cells (Quirk et al. 1995). The mean firing rate of LA cells did not change with training. Effects were seen, however, in the functional connections between LA cells, as evidenced in the cross-correlations of the spike trains of simultaneously recorded cell pairs. In the cross-correlation of two cells, A and B, the occurrences of spikes in cell B are binned relative to the occurrences of spikes of cell A (cell A spikes occur at t=0, by definition). The cross-correlograms of Figure 6A show examples of direct interactions between two cells. These cross-correlograms have a peak at around +3 msec, which suggests that the two cells are monosynaptically linked, A being presynaptic to B. The fact that the correlation increased with training suggests that conditioning increased the functional coupling between the cells. In Figure 6B, the coupling between the cells also increased following conditioning, but in this case the correlation was over a longer time scale. The increase in synchrony of firing over a prolonged period suggests that conditioning may have facilitated a common input to the two cells. Although preliminary, these findings can be interpreted as evidence for the formation of cell assemblies (Hebb 1949) in LA during conditioning. These modifications of synaptic function may represent a critical component of the long-term storage of information about the conditioning experience.

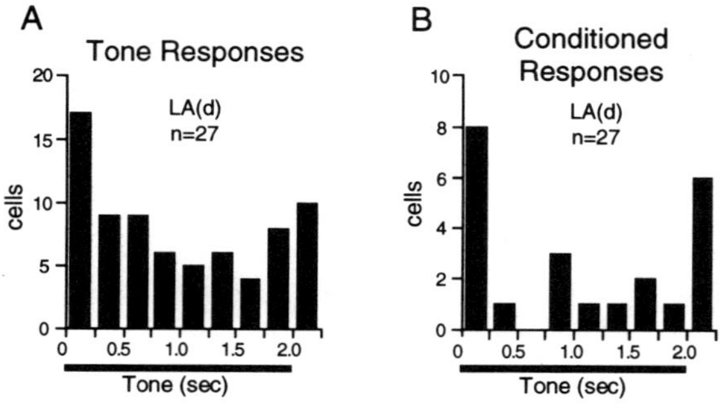

Figure 5. (*A*) Tone responses of LA neurons throughout the 2-sec tone. Note that most cells had onset responses and some showed sustained tone responses. (*B*) The majority of conditioned responses in LA cells occurred at tone onset and offset, only.

WHAT IS THE CONTRIBUTION OF THE AUDITORY CORTEX TO THE ACQUISITION AND EXPRESSION OF CONDITIONED FEAR?

The auditory cortex is not a necessary part of the circuitry underlying fear conditioning, especially when a single tone is used as a CS (DiCara et al. 1970; LeDoux et al. 1984; Romanski and LeDoux 1992), but may nevertheless contribute in important ways, especially when the CS involves more complex analysis of stimulus properties (McCabe et al. 1992). However, response properties of cells in auditory cortex are modified during conditioning, even when single tones are used as a CS (see Weinberger and Diamond 1987; Weinberger 1995). In an effort to understand how learning-induced plasticity in auditory cortex relates to the plasticity occurring in LA, we (Armony et al. 1996a; Quirk et al. 1996) have begun to record from cells in cortical area TE3, the area of auditory cortex that projects to LA (Romanski and LeDoux 1993; Mascagni et al. 1993). As previously reported (see Weinberger 1995), we observed facilitation of onset responses in auditory cortex cells by fear conditioning. The earliest latencies of conditioned increases were approximately 12 msec following tone onset. These latencies are similar to those recorded in LA and are consistent with the fact that both LA and TE3 receive a monosynaptic projection from the auditory thalamus.

In addition to cells responsive to tone onset, we ob-

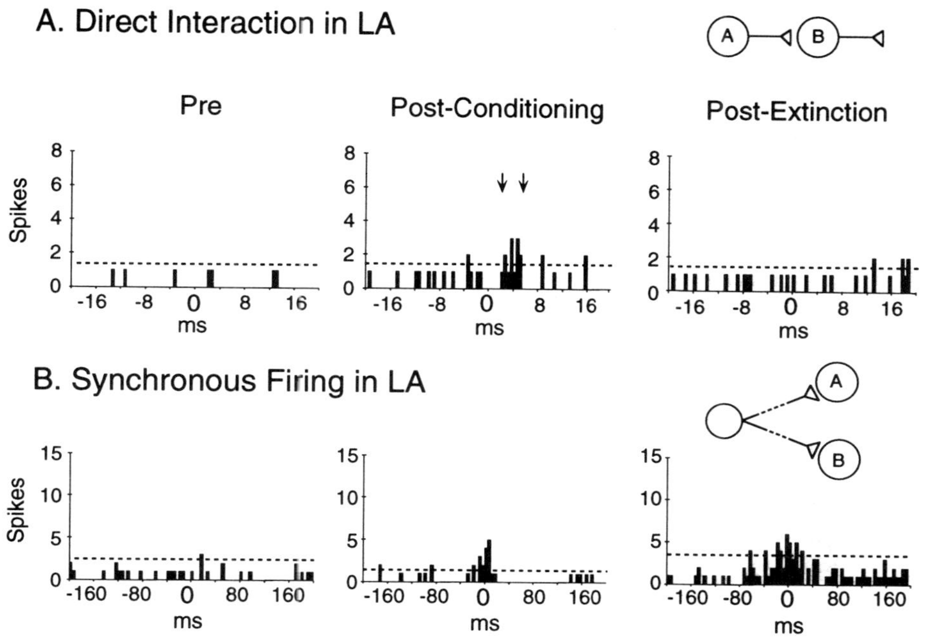

Figure 6. Cross-correlograms between simultaneously recorded neurons in LA. (*A*) Conditioning induced a significant interaction with a latency of 3 msec, suggesting facilitation of a direct interaction between LA cells. This change was reversed following 30 extinction trials. (*B*) Conditioning induced synchronous firing (peak at $t = 0$) between LA cells that persisted following 30 extinction trials, suggesting LA has access to an extinction-resistant memory trace. Dotted line indicates confidence interval of $p<0.01$. Bin width is 0.5 msec in *A* and 5.0 msec in *B*. (Adapted from Quirk et al. 1995.)

served a class of neurons in the auditory cortex not found in the LA. These cells show a conditioned response characterized by an extremely long onset latency (about 500 msec following tone onset) lasting until the time when the US would normally occur (1500 msec following tone onset). There was no US present, as these were extinction trials. The firing pattern of a typical LA cell and auditory cortex neuron are shown in Figure 7. The color plots represent a modified raster, where the firing of the cells is binned and color-coded to indicate the number of standard deviations above the mean firing rate for the entire experiment shown, across trials (red indicates 2 or more S.D. above the mean). In the LA cell, the conditioned response is confined to the start of the tone, whereas the cortical cell is an example of the late conditioned response described above.

Inputs from the auditory cortex and auditory thalamus converge onto single neurons in LA, suggesting direct interactions between the two auditory input paths to the amygdala (Li et al. 1996b). An example of such convergence is shown in Figure 8. Both of the auditory inputs to LA use glutamate as an excitatory transmitter (Li et al. 1995, 1996b). Whereas the thalamic inputs require both NMDA and AMPA receptor activation for the elicitation of action potentials from LA neurons, cortical inputs only require AMPA receptors. As cited above (Fig. 2), the minimum times of activation of LA by auditory thalamus and auditory cortex are 12 msec and 20 msec, respectively. The involvement in thalamic transmission of NMDA receptors, which have slower kinetics leading to longer effects on postsynaptic membranes (Hestrin et al. 1990), suggests that the effect of thalamic activation of LA cells is prolonged. LA cells activated by thalamic inputs could remain active until cortical inputs, driven by the same stimuli, arrive, allowing temporal summation and/or plasticity. In this way, the crude thalamic input could prime a relevant subset of LA cells to receive more specific information about the auditory stimulus from the cortex.

It is possible that the sustained response of auditory cortex cells is related to attentional processes. Such a mechanism could play a role in maintaining cortical (cognitive) vigilance to dangerous stimuli, once the amygdala has signaled the onset of the danger and initiated defense responses. Although LA does not appear to use this information directly (since LA activity does not reflect it), it is possible that the sustained cortical response is dependent on the amygdala as the trigger. We are currently examining this issue by recording from cortical cells in animals who have sustained lesions of the amygdala (Armony et al. 1996a). Several investigators have proposed contributions of the amygdala in modulating cortical attention systems (Kapp et al. 1992; Gallagher and Holland 1994; Weinberger 1995), and we are currently exploring such a contribution (Armony et al. 1996b) using a variation of a connectionist network model of the fear conditioning circuitry (Armony et al. 1995).

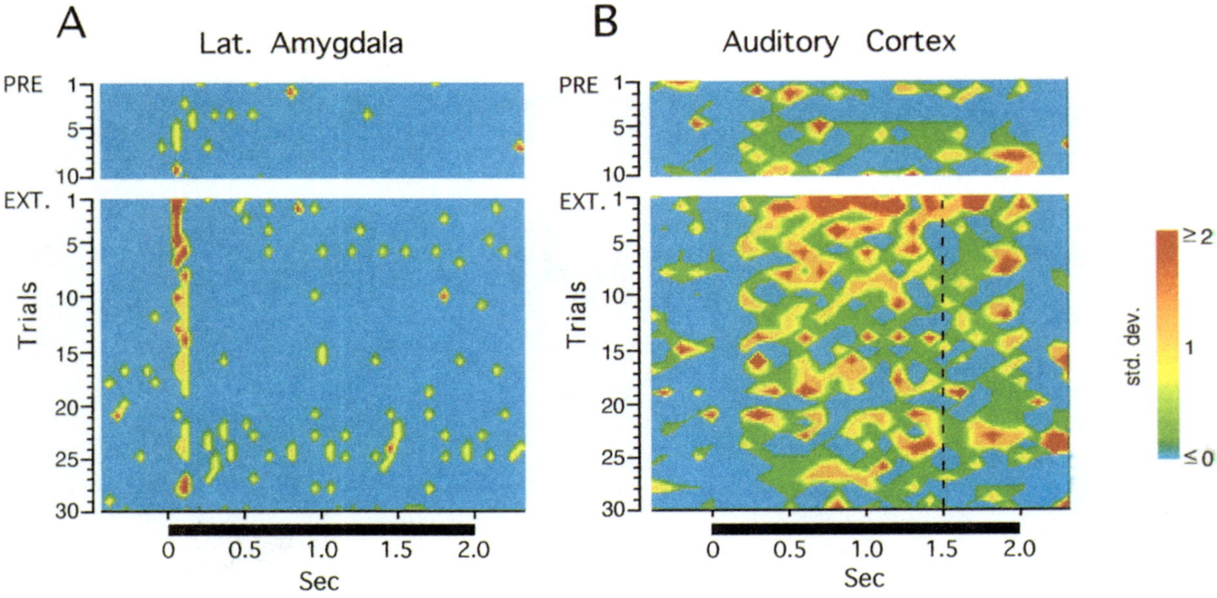

Figure 7. Color-coded firing rate plots showing the tone response of neurons across training. Firing rate bins were color coded for the number of standard deviations above the mean rate for the entire experiment. The upper part of each plot (PRE) is from the sensitization phase, where tones and shocks were unpaired. The lower part (EXT) shows the extinction trials that followed conditioning (not shown). (*A*) Typical LA cell signaling tone onset following conditioning. Note the rapid extinction. Bin width, 50 msec. (*B*) Cell from the auditory cortex showing the late onset, sustained conditioned response leading up to the time when the shock was expected, based on previous training (*dotted line*). Bin width was 100 msec.

IS THE AMYGDALA A SITE OF EXTINCTION-RESISTANT STORAGE?

Following conditioning, presentation of the CS without the US leads to extinction of the conditioned response, but behavioral experiments since the time of Pavlov (1927) have shown that extinction does not erase the memory for the CS–US association. Conditioned responses can be quickly reinstated in the extinguished animal by a number of methods, including re-presentation of the US or changing the environmental context (for review, see Bouton 1994). These observations suggest that extinction-resistant memories exist somewhere in the brain.

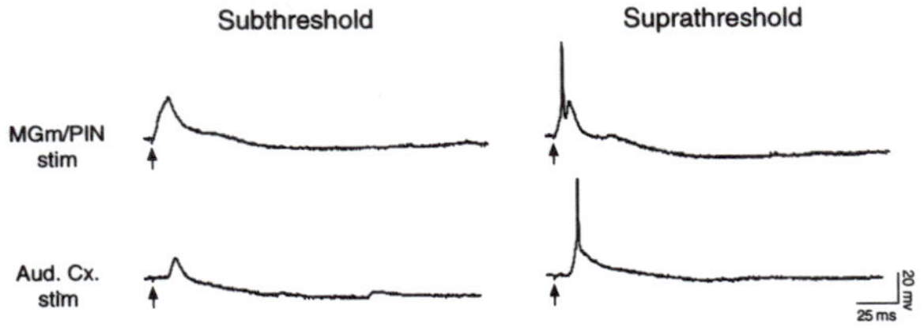

Figure 8. Intracellular recordings from an LA neuron showing convergence of thalamic (MGm/PIN) and cortical (auditory cortex) afferents. Subthreshold stimulation shows EPSPs only (*left*) while more intense stimulation produced spikes (*right*). Note the shorter latency response resulting from thalamic vs. cortical stimulation. Arrow marks stimulus onset. (Adapted from Li et al. 1996b.)

In our recordings from LA, we found that cells lost their conditioned increases in tone responses following 30 extinction trials (Quirk et al. 1995). The return of LA tone responses to their original value can be clearly seen in Figure 4C. In contrast, previous investigators have observed some persistence of conditioned responses in the amygdala following extinction trials (Ben-Ari and Le Gal La Salle 1972; Applegate et al. 1982; McEchron et al. 1995). Of course, the rate of extinction depends on a number of experimental parameters (the number of conditioning and extinction trials, the intensity of the US, etc.) that varied across studies, precluding direct comparisons. However, existing data are consistent with the possibility that conditioned responding to the CS resists extinction in the basal and central amygdala but not in LA, suggesting differences in amygdala subnuclei to extinction susceptibility.

The foregoing suggests that LA may not retain conditioned associations beyond extinction, but other findings provide evidence that it may. As described above, in addition to increasing the response of cells to the conditioned stimulus, fear conditioning results in an increase in the functional coupling of neurons in LA, as revealed by analyzing the correlation of firing between the cells. For some cell pairs, changes in correlated spontaneous activity persisted following extinction trials (Quirk et al. 1995). For example, Figure 6B shows a cross-correlogram in which the synchrony between the cell pair induced by training was still present following 30 extinction trials. It is possible that conditioning-induced changes in the circuitry within LA and/or between LA and other structures may persist through extinction and facilitate re-expression of the fear response at a later time.

CONCLUSION

Building on a wealth of lesion data implicating auditory input pathways to the amygdala in fear conditioning, we have begun to analyze the firing properties of single neurons in these pathways in an effort to further understand how fear conditioning is accomplished by the brain. Our results to date show that, following conditioning, long-term plasticity of tone responsivity is present in LA, the earliest stage of auditory processing in the amygdala. Thalamic transmission of auditory information seems to be sufficient for the initiation of this plasticity, since the conditioned changes occur at latencies that are inconsistent with cortical transmission to LA. One of the main contributions of LA appears to be to signal the onset and offset of the CS. Later stages of amygdala processing may incorporate other features of tone response plasticity. Following extinction, LA cells lose the conditioned response while nuclei downstream may maintain them. Finally, conditioning induces long-term changes in the correlational structure between LA neurons that are observable in spontaneous activity, suggesting that LA has access to a memory for the CS–US association, even following extinction trials. Whether this memory is wholly maintained by local circuits within LA or by circuits that involve other (perhaps cortical) areas remains to be determined.

These experiments suggest that the functions of the amygdala are to filter ascending sensory signals identifying potentially dangerous stimuli, initiate rapid defensive behaviors, and direct cortical attention to the stimulus. A goal of future studies will be to characterize the response properties of neurons in the various subnuclei of the amygdala, as well as in associated cortical and thalamic structures that project to the amygdala, in order to determine the sequence of events that underlie fear learning.

ACKNOWLEDGMENTS

This work was supported by U.S. Public Health Service grants MH-38774, MH-46516, and MH-00956.

REFERENCES

Amaral, D.G., J.L. Price, and A. Pitkanen. 1992. Anatomical organization of the primate amygdaloid complex. In *The amygdala* (ed. J.P. Aggleton), p. 1. Wiley-Liss, New York.

Applegate, C.D., R.C. Frysinger, B.S. Kapp, and M. Gallagher. 1982. Multiple unit activity recorded from amygdala central nucleus during Pavlovian heart rate conditioning in rabbit. *Brain Res.* **238:** 457.

Armony, J.L., G.J. Quirk, and J.E. LeDoux. 1996a. Amygdala control of cortical plasticity in fear conditioning. *Soc. Neurosci. Abstr.* **22:** (in press).

Armony, J.L., D. Servan-Schreiber, J.D. Cohen, and J.E. LeDoux. 1995. An anatomically constrained neural network model of fear conditioning. *Behav. Neurosci.* **109:** 246.

———. 1996b. Emotion and cognition interactions in the thalamo-cortico-amygdala network: Theory and model. In *Abstracts from the 3rd Annual Cognitive Neuroscience Society Meeting.*

Ben-Ari, Y. 1972. Plasticity at unitary level. I. An experimental design. *Electroencephalogr. Clin. Neurophysiol.* **32:** 655.

Ben-Ari, Y. and G. Le Gal La Salle. 1972. Plasticity at the unitary level. II. Modifications during sensory-sensory association procedures. *Electroencephalogr. Clin. Neurophysiol.* **32:** 667.

Birt, D., R. Nienhuis, and M. Olds. 1979. Separation of associative from non-associative short latency changes in medial geniculate and inferior colliculus during differential conditioning and reversal in rats. *Brain Res.* **167:** 129.

Blanchard, R.J., D.C. Blanchard, and R.A. Fial. 1970. Hippocampal lesions in rats and their effect on activity, avoidance and aggression. *J. Comp. Physiol. Psychol.* **71:** 92.

Bordi, F. and J.E. LeDoux. 1992. Sensory tuning beyond the sensory system: An initial analysis of auditory properties of neurons in the lateral amygdaloid nucleus and overlying areas of the striatum. *J. Neurosci.* **12:** 2493.

———. 1994. Response properties of single units in the areas of rat auditory thalamus that project to the amygdala. II. Cells receiving convergent auditory and somatosensory inputs and cells antidromically activated by amygdala stimulation. *Exp. Brain Res.* **98:** 275.

Bordi, F., J.E. LeDoux, M.C. Clugnet, and C. Pavlides. 1993. Single unit activity in the lateral nucleus of the amygdala and overlying areas of the striatum in freely-behaving rats: Rates, discharge patterns, and responses to acoustic stimuli. *Behav. Neurosci.* **107:** 757.

Bouton, M.E. 1994. Context, ambiguity, and classical conditioning. *Curr. Dir. Psychol. Sci.* **3:** 49.

Campeau, S. and M. Davis. 1995a. Involvement of the central nucleus and basolateral complex of the amygdala in fear conditioning measured with fear-potentiated startle in rats trained concurrently with auditory and visual conditioned stimuli. *J. Neurosci.* **15:** 2301.

———. 1995b. Involvement of subcortical and cortical afferents to the lateral nucleus of the amygdala in fear conditioning measured with fear-potentiated startle in rats trained concurrently with auditory and visual conditioned stimuli. *J. Neurosci.* **15:** 2312.

Chapman, P.F., E.W. Kairiss, C.L. Keenan, and T.H. Brown. 1990. Long-term synaptic potentiation in the amygdala. *Synapse* **6:** 271.

Clugnet, M.C. and J.E. LeDoux. 1990. Synaptic plasticity in fear conditioning circuits: Induction of LTP in the lateral nucleus of the amygdala by stimulation of the medial geniculate body. *J. Neurosci.* **10:** 2818.

Corodimas, K.P. and J.E. LeDoux. 1995. Disruptive effects of posttraining perirhinal lesions on conditioned fear: Contributions of contextual cues. *Behav. Neurosci.* **109:** 613.

Davis, M. 1992. The role of the amygdala in conditioned fear. In *The Amygdala* (ed. J.P. Aggleton), p. 255. Wiley-Liss, New York.

de Olmos, J., G. Alheid, and C. Beltramino. 1985. Amygdala. In *The rat nervous system* (ed. G. Paxinos), p. 223. Academic Press, Orlando, Florida.

DiCara, L., J.J. Braun, and B. Pappas. 1970. Classical conditioning and instrumental learning of cardiac and gastrointestinal responses following removal of neocortex in the rat. *J. Comp. Physiol. Psychol.* **73:** 208.

Disterhoft, J.F. and J. Olds. 1972. Differential development of conditioned unit changes in thalamus and cortex of rat. *J. Neurophysiol.* **35:** 665.

Edeline, J.-M., and N.M. Weinberger. 1992. Associative retuning in the thalamic source of input to the amygdala and auditory cortex: Receptive field plasticity in the medial division of the medial geniculate body. *Behav. Neurosci.* **106:** 81.

Edeline, J.-M., N. Neuenschwander-El Massioui, and G. Dutrieux. 1990. Frequency-specific changes in the auditory system during acquisition and reversal of discriminative conditioning. *Psychobiology* **18:** 382.

Fanselow, M.S. 1994. Neural organization of the defensive behavior system responsible for fear. *Psychon. Bull. Rev.* **1:** 429.

Gabriel, M. 1976. Short-latency discriminative unit response: Engram or bias? *Physiol. Psychol.* **4:** 275.

Gabriel, M, J.D. Miller, and S.E. Saltwick. 1976. Multiple-unit activity of the rabbit medial geniculate nucleus in conditioning, extinction and reversal. *Phys. Psychol.* **4:** 124.

Gallagher M. and P.C. Holland. 1994. The amygdala complex: Multiple roles in associative learning and attention. *Proc. Natl. Acad. Sci.* **91:** 11771.

Gray, J.A. 1991. Neural systems, emotion and personality. In *Neurobiology of learning, emotion and affect* (ed. J.I. Madden), p. 273. Raven Press, New York.

Hebb, D.O. 1949. *The organization of behavior.* Wiley, New York.

Hestrin, S., P. Sah, and R.A. Nicoll. 1990. Mechanisms generating the time course of dual component excitatory synaptic currents recorded in hippocampal slices. *Neuron* **5:** 247.

Kapp, B.S., P.J. Whalen, W.F. Supple, and J.P. Pascoe. 1992. Amygdaloid contributions to conditioned arousal and sensory information processing. In *The amygdala* (ed. J. P. Aggleton), p. 229. Wiley-Liss, New York.

Kim, J.J. and M.S. Fanselow. 1992. Modality-specific retrograde amnesia of fear. *Science* **256:** 675.

Kim, J.J., J.P. DeCola, J. Landeira-Fernandez, and M.S. Fanselow. 1991. *N*-methyl-D-aspartate receptor antagonist APV blocks acquisition but not expression of fear conditioning. *Behav. Neurosci.* **105:** 126.

Kim, M. and M. Davis. 1993. Lack of a temporal gradient of retrograde amnesia in rats with amygdala lesions assessed with the fear-potentiated startle paradigm. *Behav. Neurosci.* **107:** 1088.

LeDoux, J.E. 1995. Emotion: Clues from the brain. *Annu. Rev. Psychol.* **46:** 209.

LeDoux, J.E. and C.F. Farb. 1991. Neurons of the acoustic thalamus that project to the amygdala contain glutamate. *Neurosci. Lett.* **134:** 145.

LeDoux, J.E., C.F. Farb, and D.A. Ruggiero. 1990. Topographic organization of neurons in the acoustic thalamus that project to the amygdala. *J. Neurosci.* **10:** 1043.

LeDoux, J.E., L.M. Romanski, and A.E. Xagoraris. 1989. Indelibility of subcortical emotional memories. *J. Cogn. Neurosci.* **1:** 238.

LeDoux, J.E., A. Sakaguchi, and D.J. Reis. 1984. Subcortical efferent projections of the medial geniculate nucleus mediate emotional responses conditioned by acoustic stimuli. *J. Neurosci.* **4:** 683.

Li, X.F., J.L. Armony, and J.E. LeDoux. 1996a. GABAa and GABAb receptors differentially regulate synaptic transmission in the rat thalamo-amygdala pathway: An *in vivo* microiontophoretic study and a model. *Synapse* **24:** 115.

Li, X.F., R.G. Phillips, and J.E. LeDoux. 1995. NMDA and non-NMDA receptors contribute to synaptic transmission between the medial geniculate body and the lateral nucleus of the amygdala. *Exp. Brain Res.* **105:** 87.

Li, X.F., G.E. Stutzmann, and J.E. LeDoux. 1996b. Convergent but temporally separated inputs to lateral amygdala neurons from the auditory thalamus and auditory cortex use different postsynaptic receptors: *In vivo* intracellular and extracellular recordings in fear conditioning pathways. *Learn. Mem.* (in press).

Liang, K.C., J.L. McGaugh, J.L. Martinez, Jr., R.A. Jensen, B.J. Vasquez, and R.B. Messing. 1982. Post-training amygdaloid lesions impair retention of an inhibitory avoidance response. *Behav. Brain Res.* **4:** 237.

Linden, D.R. 1969. Attenuation and reestablishment of the CER by discriminated avoidance conditioning in rats. *J. Comp. Physiol. Psychol.* **69:** 573.

Maren, S., A. Porembra, and M. Gabriel. 1991. Basolateral amygdaloid multi-unit neuronal correlates of discriminative avoidance learning in rabbits. *Brain Res.* **549:** 311.

Mascagni, F., A.J. MacDonald, and J.R. Coleman. 1993. Cortico-amygdaloid and cortico-cortical projections of the rat temporal cortex: A *Phaselous vulgaris* leucoagglutinin study. *Neuroscience* **57:** 697.

McCabe, P.M., N. Schneiderman, T.W. Jarrell, C.G. Gentile, A.H. Teich, R.W. Winters, and D.R. Liskowsky. 1992. Central pathways involved in differential classical conditioning of heart rate responses. In *Learning and memory: The behavioral and biological substrates* (ed. I. Gormenzano and E. A. Wasserman), p. 321. Erlbaum, Hillsdale.

McDonald, R.J. and N.M. White. 1993. A triple dissociation of memory systems: Hippocampus, amygdala, and dorsal striatum. *Behav. Neurosci.* **107:** 3.

McEchron, M.D., P.M. McCabe, E.J. Green, M.M. Llabre, and N. Schneiderman. 1995. Simultaneous single unit recording in the medial nucleus of the medial geniculate and amygdaloid central nucleus throughout habituation, acquisition, and extinction of the rabbit's classically conditioned heart rate. *Brain Res.* **682:** 157.

McEchron, M.D., E.J. Green, R.W. Winters, T.G. Nolen, N. Schneiderman, and P.M. McCabe. 1996. Changes of synaptic efficacy in the medial geniculate nucleus as a result of auditory classical conditioning. *J. Neurosci.* **16:** 1273.

Miserendino, M.J.D., C.B. Sananes, K.R. Melia, and M. Davis. 1990. Blocking of acquisition but not expression of conditioned fear-potentiated startle by NMDA antagonists in the amygdala. *Nature* **345:** 716.

Morgan, M.A. and J.E. LeDoux. 1995. Differential contribution of dorsal and ventral medial prefrontal cortex to the acquisition and extinction of conditioned fear in rats. *Behav. Neuroscience* **109:** 681.

Muramoto, K., T. Ono, H. Nishijo, and M. Fukada. 1993. Rat amygdaloid neuron responses during auditory discrimination. *Neuroscience* **52:** 621.

Nishijo, H., T. Ono, and H. Nishino. 1988. Single neuron responses in amygdala of alert monkey during complex sensory stimulation with affective significance. *J. Neurosci.* **8:** 3570.

Olds, J., J. Disterhoft, M. Segal, C. Kornbluth, and R. Hirsch. 1972. Learning centers of rat brain mapped by measuring latencies of conditioned unit responses. *J. Neurophysiol.* **35:** 202.

Ottersen, O.P. 1982. Connections of the amygdala of the rat. IV. Corticoamygdaloid and intraamygdaloid connections as studied with axonal transport of horseradish peroxidase. *J. Comp. Neurol.* **205:** 30.

Parent, M.B., G.L. Quirarte, L. Cahill, and J.L. McGaugh. 1995. Spared retention of inhibitory avoidance learning after posttraining amygdala lesions. *Behav. Neurosci.* **109:** 803.

Pascoe, J.P. and B.S. Kapp. 1985. Electrophysiological characteristics of central nucleus neurons during Pavlovian fear conditioning in the rabbit. *Behav. Brain Res.* **16:** 117.

Pavlov, I.P. 1927. *Conditioned reflexes.* Dover, New York.

Petri, H.L. and M. Mishkin. 1994. Behaviorism, cognitivism and the neuropsychology of memory. *Am. Sci.* **82:** 30.

Phillips, R.G. and J.E. LeDoux. 1992. Differential contribution of amygdala and hippocampus to cued and contextual fear conditioning. *Behav. Neurosci.* **106:** 274.

Pitkanen, A., L. Stefanacci, C.F. Farb, C.G. Go, J.E. LeDoux, and D.G. Amaral. 1995. Intrinsic connections of the rat amygdaloid complex: Projections originating in the lateral nucleus. *J. Comp. Neurol.* **356:** 288.

Price, J.L., F.T. Russchen, and D.G. Amaral. 1987. The limbic region. II. The amygdaloid complex. In *Handbook of chemical neuroanatomy: Integrated systems of the CNS* (ed. A. Bjorklund et al.), vol. 5, p. 279. Elsevier, Amsterdam.

Quirk, G.J., J.L. Armony, and J.E. LeDoux. 1996. A comparison of lateral amygdala and auditory cortex neurons during fear conditioning. *Soc. Neurosci. Abstr.* **22:** (in press).

Quirk, G.J., J.C. Repa, and J.E. LeDoux. 1995. Fear conditioning enhances short-latency auditory responses of lateral amygdala neurons: Parallel recordings in the freely behaving rat. *Neuron* **15:** 1029.

Repa, J.C., S.J. Williamson, and J.E. LeDoux. 1996. Simultaneous recordings in the auditory thalamus and lateral amygdala: Effects of fear conditioning on spontaneous and tone evoked activity. *Soc. Neurosci. Abstr.* **22:** (in press).

Rogan, M.T. and J.E. LeDoux. 1995. LTP is accompanied by commensurate enhancement of auditory-evoked responses in a fear conditioning circuit. *Neuron* **15:** 127.

Romanski, L.M. and J.E. LeDoux. 1992. Equipotentiality of thalamo-amygdala and thalamo-cortico-amygdala projections as auditory conditioned stimulus pathways. *J. Neurosci.* **12:** 4501.

———. 1993. Information cascade from primary auditory cortex to the amygdala: Corticocortical and corticoamygdaloid projections of the temporal cortex in the rat. *Cereb. Cortex* **3:** 515.

Romanski, L.M., M.C. Clugnet, F. Bordi, and J.E. LeDoux. 1993. Somatosensory and auditory convergence in the lateral nucleus of the amygdala. *Behav. Neurosci.* **107:** 444.

Savander, V., C.G. Go, J.E. LeDoux, and A. Pitkanen. 1995. Internal connections of the rat amygdaloid complex: Projections originating in the basal nucleus. *J. Comp. Neurol.* **361:** 345.

Segal, M. 1973. Flow of conditioned responses in limbic telencephalic system of the rat. *J. Neurophysiol.* **36:** 840.

Selden, N.R.W., B.J. Everitt, L.E. Jarrard, and T.W. Robbins. 1991. Complementary roles for the amygdala and hippocampus in aversive conditioning to explicit and contextual cues. *Neuroscience* **42:** 335.

Solomon, R.L. and L.C. Wynne. 1954. Traumatic avoidance learning: The principles of anxiety conservation and partial irreversibility. *Psychol. Rev.* **61:** 353.

Stefanacci, L., C.F. Farb, A. Pitkanen, C.G. Go, J.E. LeDoux, and D.G. Amaral. 1992. Projections from the lateral nucleus to the basal nucleus of the amygdala: A light and electron microscopic PHA-L study in the rat. *J. Comp. Neurol.* **323:** 2.

Supple, W.F. and B.S. Kapp. 1989. Response characteristics of neurons in the medial component of the medial geniculate nucleus during Pavlovian differential fear conditioning in rabbits. *Behav. Neurosci.* **103:** 1276.

Turner, B. and M. Herkenham. 1991. Thalamoamygdaloid projections in the rat: A test of the amygdala's role in sensory processing. *J. Comp. Neurol.* **313:** 295.

Uwano, T., H. Nishijo, T. Ono, and R. Tamura. 1995. Neuronal responsiveness to various sensory stimuli and associative learning in the rat amygdala. *Neuroscience* **68:** 339.

Weinberger, N.M. 1995. Dynamic regulation of receptive fields and maps in the adult sensory cortex. *Annu. Rev. Neurosci.* **18:** 129.

Weinberger, N.M. and D.M. Diamond. 1987. Physiological plasticity in auditory cortex: Rapid induction by learning. *Prog. Neurobiol.* **29:** 1.

Neurobiology of Memory for Emotional Events: Converging Evidence from Infra-human and Human Studies

L. CAHILL
Center for the Neurobiology of Learning and Memory, University of California, Irvine, California 92697-3800

The experiments described here aim at understanding the neurobiological basis of the formation of long-term memory for emotional events. The primary hypothesis is that hormones released during emotionally stressful events affect memory storage processes via an interaction with the amydgala complex (AC) (see McGaugh 1989; McGaugh et al. 1995). Much of the evidence supporting this hypothesis comes from studies involving animal subjects. However, recent studies involving human subjects give the hypothesis strong new support. In this review, I first briefly summarize some of the evidence from animal research which suggests that stress hormones and the AC interact to modulate memory storage for emotionally arousing events. Next, I describe converging evidence for this view of the mechanisms of emotional memory from recent studies involving human subjects.

STRESS HORMONES AND MEMORY FOR STRESSFUL EVENTS

It is well known that endogenous stress hormones like epinephrine, norepinephrine, ACTH, and corticosterone are released during and after emotionally arousing events (Levi 1975). The fact that new memories are susceptible to modulating influences for a limited time after acquisition (McGaugh 1966) led to the hypothesis that stress hormones may modulate memory storage for emotional events in which they are released. Perhaps the first person to propose this function for endogenous stress hormones was Ralph Gerard. In discussing the evidence that memory is susceptible to post-training drug treatments (Breen and McGaugh 1961), he suggested that epinephrine may "hasten the fixation process" for a "vivid emotional experience" (Gerard 1961).

Considerable evidence from animal studies indicates that recently formed memories can be modulated by endogenous hormones (Gold and McGaugh 1975; McGaugh 1989; Bohus 1994). The mnemonic effects of epinephrine, the hormone most studied in relation to memory, are characteristic of stress hormones in general. First, the dose-response function of epinephrine on memory is an "inverted-U." Mid-range doses enhance memory, but doses higher or lower than that range do not. Second, the effect of epinephrine on memory (enhancement or impairment) depends on an interaction between endogenous levels of the hormone produced by the learning event and the exogenously administered dose (Gold and McGaugh 1975). Finally, the effects of epinephrine on memory are time-dependent: Post-training injections of the hormone influence memory only if given soon after learning occurs. The time-dependent nature of hormone effects on memory are generally interpreted as evidence that they affect memory storage (consolidation) processes (McGaugh 1989).

Although catecholamines are the stress hormones most consistently implicated in memory modulation, it is clear that many other endogenous hormones also influence memory (McGaugh 1989; Bohus 1994). Additionally, a growing body of evidence suggests that adrenomedullary and adrenocortical hormones interact to affect memory storage (Bohus 1994). For example, a recent experiment showed that suppression of the adrenocortical system (via injection of the corticosterone synthesis blocker metyrapone) blocks the enhancing effect of epinephrine on memory (Roozendaal et al. 1996).

INTERACTIONS BETWEEN STRESS HORMONES AND THE AC IN MEMORY

Through what brain regions do endogenous stress hormones affect memory? The region most consistently implicated is the AC. With very few exceptions (see, e.g., Flood et al. 1995), lesions of the AC or the stria terminalis (a primary AC pathway) block memory modulation by peripherally administered drugs and hormones. Both memory-enhancing and memory-impairing effects of peripheral agents are blocked by AC lesions (McGaugh et al. 1995; Packard et al. 1995). For example, AC lesions block memory enhancement produced by epinephrine (Cahill and McGaugh 1991), and stria terminalis lesions block amnesia caused by peripheral administration of the endogenous opiate, β-endorphin (McGaugh et al. 1986). Many other experiments involving direct pharmacological stimulation of the AC further implicate this structure in memory modulation by peripheral stress hormones (McGaugh et al. 1995; Packard et al. 1995). Thus, considerable evidence suggests that stress hormones, released during emotionally arousing events, affect memory via influences mediated by the AC.

THE ROLE OF THE AC IN MEMORY

The fact that endogenous stress hormones modulate memory via the AC appears an important clue to the role of the AC in memory. Additional clues come from experiments involving direct AC stimulation in learning situations. It has long been known that electrical stimulation of the AC can modulate—i.e., enhance or impair—memory (Gold et al. 1975). More recent experiments document that pharmacological stimulation of the AC can also modulate memory (see McGaugh et al. 1995; Packard et al. 1995). Additionally, the effects of AC stimulation on memory depend on integrity of adrenal hormones (Bennett et al. 1985; Liang et al. 1985). On the basis of such evidence, McGaugh and colleagues proposed that the AC modulates memory formation (Gold et al. 1975; McGaugh 1992) through an interaction with endogenous stress hormones. This hypothesis predicts that the AC should be more clearly involved in arousing learning situations in which training conditions induce stress hormone release.

Cahill and McGaugh (1990) directly tested the prediction that the AC is preferentially involved in memory for arousing learning situations. They found that AC-lesioned rats learned normally tasks involving relatively non-arousing stimuli (sucrose, quinine-laced water) but were impaired in learning tasks involving a highly arousing stimulus, footshock. The findings clearly do not support the widely held view that the AC is involved in the formation of stimulus-reinforcement associations (Weiskrantz 1956). Instead, the findings suggest that "the degree of arousal produced by the unconditioned stimulus...determines the level of AC involvement" in a learning situation (Cahill and McGaugh 1990). These results are consistent with the view that the AC modulates memory for emotionally arousing events.

There is evidence that the AC modulates memory processes in other brain structures. For example, lesions of the stria terminalis, a major AC pathway, block both the memory-enhancing and memory-impairing effects of direct AC stimulation (McGaugh et al. 1995). A recent experiment by Packard et al. (1994) supports this view. They studied the effects of intra-AC injection of D-amphetamine in two learning tasks—one known to require the hippocampus, the other requiring the caudate nucleus. In a circular pool, rats were trained to swim either to a hidden platform always located in the same spatial position (the hippocampus-dependent task) or to a visible platform whose location changed from trial to trial (the caudate-dependent task). Immediately after training, rats received unilateral injections of D-amphetamine into either the AC, the hippocampus, or the caudate nucleus (left side in all cases). Retention (assessed as latency to find the platform) was tested 24 hours later. D-Amphetamine injected into the hippocampus improved retention of the hippocampus-dependent (hidden platform) task relative to saline-injected controls, but had no effect on the caudate-dependent (visible platform) task. Conversely, D-amphetamine injected into the caudate improved retention of the caudate-dependent, but not hippocampus-dependent, task. However, D-amphetamine injected into the AC improved retention for both tasks. Furthermore, for both tasks, injection of a local anesthetic (lidocaine) into the AC prior to the retention test did not block the enhanced performance caused by the post-training injection of D-amphetamine into the AC. Because the AC was inactivated at the time of retention testing, the critical change underlying the improved retention must have been located *outside* the AC.

The hippocampus is a prime candidate region at which the AC may modulate memory. Considerable anatomical (Amaral et al. 1992), electrophysiological (Thomas et al. 1984; Ikegaya et al. 1994, 1995), functional anatomical (Packard et al. 1995; L. Cahill, unpubl.), and behavioral evidence (Packard et al. 1994; Maren and Fanselow 1995; B. Roozendaal and J.L. McGaugh, in prep.) strongly suggests that the hippocampus and AC interact in the formation of memory. An improved understanding of this interaction is an important goal for future animal research.

STRESS HORMONES, THE AC, AND MEMORY FOR EMOTIONAL EVENTS: EVIDENCE FROM HUMAN SUBJECT STUDIES

As indicated above, substantial evidence from animal studies indicates that memory is modulated by the interaction of stress hormones released during emotionally arousing events (in particular, catecholamines acting at β-adrenergic receptors) and the AC. New evidence from studies involving human subjects reinforces this view.

Recently, we have tested the hypothesis that enhanced long-term memory for emotional events requires activation of β-adrenergic receptors. We first established a paradigm in which a reliable effect of emotional arousal on memory could be produced (Cahill and McGaugh 1995). Subjects viewed one of two stories: a relatively neutral story (the "neutral" group) or a closely matched but more emotionally arousing story (the "arousal" group). For both stories, identical slides were presented sequentially to the subjects; however, the narration accompanying the slides differed in certain portions. The emotional story elements (concerning a boy whose feet are cut off in an accident) were introduced in the middle portion of the slide presentation (referred to as "phase 2"). The degree of emotional reaction to the story was assessed in each subject immediately after viewing the story. Memory for the stories was tested in surprise free-recall and multiple-choice tests 2 weeks later. Subjects who viewed the arousal story both experienced a significantly greater emotional reaction to the story and demonstrated significantly better memory for story elements than did subjects who viewed the neutral story, especially for the story elements associated with emotional arousal (phase 2 elements).

Next, we examined the effect of β-adrenergic impairment (via administration of the β-adrenergic blocker propranolol) on the enhancement of memory produced by emotional arousal in our paradigm (Cahill et al. 1994). Propranolol is a β1/β2 adrenergic blocker that freely crosses the blood-brain barrier and therefore acts at β-adrenergic receptors throughout the body. Subjects received either a placebo or 40 mg of propranolol 1 hour before viewing either the neutral or arousal story. Memory for the story was assessed in both recognition and free-recall tests 1 week later. Propranolol significantly impaired memory only in subjects who viewed the emotional story, primarily for the story phase in which the emotional story elements were introduced (phase 2, see Fig. 1). Because propranolol selectively affected only the emotional story, its impairing effect on memory cannot be attributed to any general effects of the drug on attention or level of sedation. In addition, because the propranolol subjects did not differ from placebo subjects in their emotional reaction to either story, the memory impairment cannot easily be attributed to reduced emotional responsiveness of the subjects to viewing the emotional story.

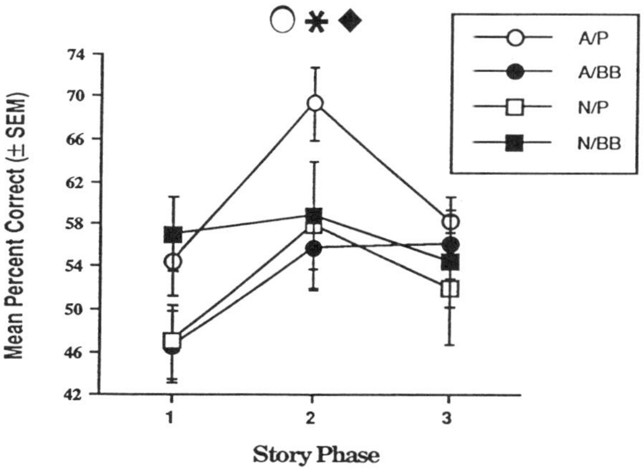

Figure 1. Performance on a multiple-choice memory test for subjects taking either a placebo or propranolol 1 hr before viewing either an emotional or neutral story. The emotional story elements were introduced into the middle phase of the emotional story (phase 2). Enhanced memory for these elements was seen only in the placebo group: Memory in the arousal story/placebo group for story phase 2 was significantly better than for either phase 1 (O, $p<.01$) or phase 3 (*, $p<.05$). No other group showed any significant differences in retention between any story phases. Propranolol blocked the enhancing effect of emotion on memory: (*filled* diamond, $p<.02$) compared to the arousal/β-blocker (A/BB) group score for story phase 2. Memory was tested 1 week after story viewing. (A/P) Arousal story/placebo. (A/BB) Arousal story/β-blocker. (N/P) Neutral story/placebo. (N/BB) Neutral story/β-blocker. (Reprinted, with permission, from Cahill et al. 1994 [copyright Macmillan].)

The findings of Cahill et al. (1994) confirm in humans the prediction of many animal studies that enhanced long-term memory for emotional (especially aversive) events depends on an activation of the β-adrenergic system. The results also help explain why most controlled tests of the effects of β-blockers on memory to date have been negative, despite persistent clinical and anecdotal reports of memory impairments associated with β-blocker treatment: Previous experiments have generally tested only short-term memory for relatively emotionally neutral stimuli.

Another recent study by Nielson and Jensen (1994) employing physically induced arousal (muscle tension) to enhance memory for written material reported that young subjects, healthy elderly subjects, and elderly hypertensive subjects taking non-β-blocker medications all showed enhanced retention performance resulting from the arousal manipulations. In contrast, elderly hypertensive subjects taking β-blocker medication showed no evidence of enhanced retention with arousal. Although this study differs from that of Cahill et al. (1994) in several key respects (e.g., very different retention intervals, chronic versus acute dosing), both studies support the general conclusion that the enhancing influence of arousal on memory depends on β-adrenergic receptor activation.

THE HUMAN AMYGDALA AND MEMORY FOR EMOTIONAL EVENTS

At least since the famous report of Scoville and Milner (1957) in which the patient H.M. was first described, a role for the AC in what is now commonly called "declarative" (or "conscious") memory in humans has been questioned. However, considerable evidence from animal studies implicates the AC in types of emotionally influenced memory that can be considered declarative, such as memory for a single training event (e.g., one-trial avoidance learning). Recent studies involving human subjects indicate that the AC plays a role in declarative memory; specifically, in long-term, declarative memory for emotionally arousing events. Evidence for a role for the human AC in declarative memory comes from two main sources: Studies of AC activity using brain-imaging techniques, and investigations of rare patients with brain damage centered on, or confined to, the AC.

Cahill et al. (1995) examined memory of a patient with bilateral, selective damage to the AC using the same paradigm shown to be sensitive to β-adrenergic blockade by Cahill et al. (1994). They found that the patient exhibited a memory deficit similar to that of healthy subjects under β-adrenergic blockade: a selective impairment of enhanced memory normally associated with emotional arousal (see Fig. 2). This finding indicates that the AC is involved in long-term, declarative memory in humans. The fact that both the β-adrenergic system (Cahill et al. 1994) and the AC (Cahill et al. 1995) are implicated in memory within a

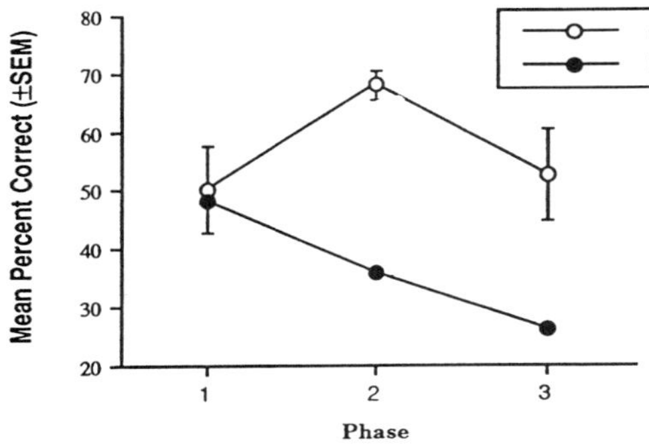

Figure 2. Retention of a short story by controls (n=6) and patient B.P., who has a selective, bilateral AC lesion. The results show performance on a multiple-choice test given 1 week after story viewing. Controls show the expected increase in memory for the phase of the story in which the emotional elements were introduced (phase 2). In contrast, B.P. showed no evidence of enhanced memory for the emotional story elements. (Reprinted, with permission, from Cahill et al. 1995 [copyright Macmillan].)

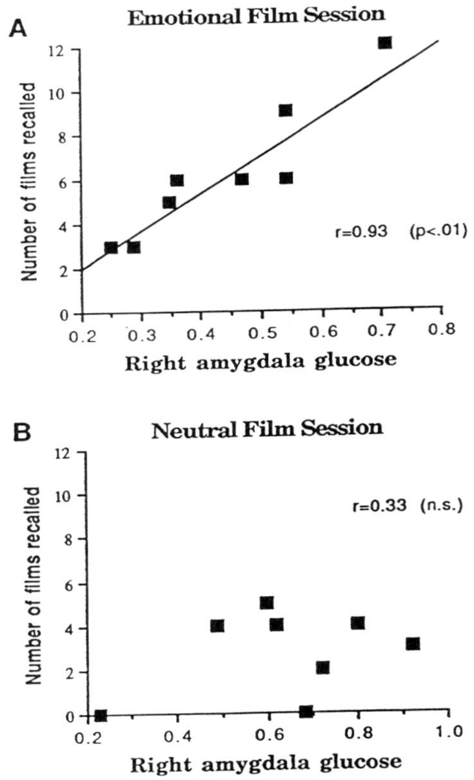

Figure 3. Scatterplots of right AC relative glucose metabolic rate versus recall of films for (A) a series of relatively emotionally arousing (E) films and (B) a series of relatively emotionally neutral (N) films. The activity of the right AC while viewing the E films was highly correlated with the number of those films recalled. Activity of the same region while subjects viewed the N films was not correlated with recall. (Reprinted, with permission, from Cahill et al. 1996.)

single experimental paradigm further argues for an interaction between the two in memory for emotional events. Other recent investigations of patients with bilateral AC lesions report generally intact cognitive functions, with the primary exception of memory for "affect-related" material (Babinsky et al. 1993; Markowitsch et al. 1994). As expected on the basis of animal studies, the AC appears not to be required for short-term declarative memory, especially of relatively non-arousing events (Bechara et al. 1995).

Only a few studies employing functional brain-imaging techniques have examined AC functions in memory in humans. Using the positron emission tomography (PET) technique, Hugdahl et al. (1995) found no evidence for AC involvement in an aversive classical conditioning procedure (a tone paired with a shock to the wrist). Other recent reports suggest that the right AC is activated during retrieval of memories for emotional events (Fink et al. 1996; Rauch et al. 1996).

Cahill et al. (1996) studied the involvement of the AC in the formation, rather than retrieval, of memory for emotional events. Subjects in this study received two PET scans: one while viewing a series of relatively emotionally neutral (N) films, a second (on a different day) while viewing a series of relatively emotionally arousing (E) films. Subjects rated their personal emotional reaction to each film immediately after viewing it. Memory for the films from both PET sessions was tested in a surprise memory test 3 weeks later. On average, subjects rated their emotional reaction to the E films as significantly greater than that to the N films. In addition, subjects remembered significantly more of the E films than the N films. The PET results showed that the activity of the right AC while viewing the emotional films was highly correlated with later recall of those films. In contrast, activity of the same region while the subjects viewed the N films was not correlated with recall (see Fig. 3). These results are consistent with the studies of AC-damaged patients: The AC is not involved with declarative memory for all events. Rather, it is selectively involved with long-term memory for emotionally arousing events. Furthermore, the results of Cahill et al. (1996) support the view that the AC is involved with the formation (as opposed to storage or retrieval) of memories for emotional events.

CONCLUSIONS

Considerable evidence from both animal and human studies now converges on the view that the AC plays a selective role in declarative memory. The AC is not involved with the formation of memory in all situations, but appears to have a selective role in memory formation for periods of emotional arousal. New findings from studies involving human subjects are consistent with those from animal investigations (McGaugh 1992) in suggesting that the AC, through an interaction with endogenous stress hormones, modulates long-term storage of declarative (conscious) memory for emotionally arousing events.

ACKNOWLEDGMENT

The author thanks James L. McGaugh for helpful comments on an earlier draft of this manuscript and for his consistent support of the research conducted by the author.

REFERENCES

Amaral, D.G., J.L. Price, A. Pitkaenen, and S.T. Carmichael. 1992. Anatomical organization of the primate amygdaloid complex. In *The amygdala* (ed. J. Aggleton), p. 1. Wiley-Liss, New York.

Babinsky, R., P. Calabrese, H.F. Durwen, H.J. Markowitsch, D. Brechtelsbauer, L. Heuser, and W. Gehlen. 1993. The possible contribution of the amygdala to memory. *Behav. Neurol.* **6:** 167.

Bechara, A., D. Tranel, H. Damasio, R. Adolphs, C. Rockland, and A.R. Damasio. 1995. Double dissociation of conditioning and declarative knowledge relative to the amygdala and hippocampus in humans. *Science* **269:** 1115.

Bennett, C., K.C. Liang, and J.L. McGaugh. 1985. Depletion of adrenal catecholamines alters the amnestic effect of amygdala stimulation. *Behav. Brain. Res.* **15:** 83.

Bohus, B. 1994. Humoral modulation of learning and memory processes: Physiological significance of brain and peripheral mechanisms. In *The memory systems of the brain* (ed. J. Delacour), p. 337. World Scientific, Singapore.

Breen, R.A. and J.L. McGaugh. 1961. Facilitation of maze learning with posttrial injections of picrotoxin. *J. Comp. Physiol. Psychol.* **54:** 498.

Cahill, L. and J.L. McGaugh. 1990. Amygdaloid complex lesions differentially affect retention of tasks using appetitive and aversive reinforcement. *Behav. Neurosci.* **104:** 532.

———. 1991. NMDA-induced lesions of the amygdaloid complex block the retention enhancing effect of post-training epinephrine. *Psychobiology* **19:** 206.

———. 1995. A novel demonstration of enhanced long-term memory associated with emotional arousal. *Conscious. Cogn.* **4:** 410.

Cahill, L., R. Babinsky, H. Markowitsch, and J.L.McGaugh. 1995. The amygdala and emotional memory. *Nature* **377:** 295.

Cahill, L., B. Prins, M. Weber, and J.L. McGaugh. 1994. β-Adrenergic activation and memory for emotional events. *Nature* **371:** 702.

Cahill, L., R.J. Haier, J. Fallon, M.T. Alkire, C. Tang, D. Keator, J. Wu, and J.L. McGaugh. 1996. Amygdala activity at encoding correlated with long-term, free recall of emotional information. *Proc. Natl. Acad. Sci.* **93:** 8016.

Fink, G., H. Markowitsch, M. Reinkemeier, T. Bruckbauer, J. Kessler, and W. Heiss. 1996. Cerebral representation of one's own past: Neural networks involved in autobiographical memory. *J. Neurosci.* **16:** 4275.

Flood, J.F., M.O. Merbaum, and J.E. Morley. 1995. The memory enhancing effects of cholecystokinin octapeptide are dependent on an intact stria terminalis. *Neurobiol. Learn. Mem.* **64:** 139.

Gerard, R.W. 1961. The fixation of experience. In *Brain mechanisms and learning* (ed. J.F. Delafresnaye), p. 21. C.C. Thomas, Springfield, Illinois.

Gold, P.E. and J.L. McGaugh. 1975. A single-trace, two-process view of memory storage processes. In *Short-term memory* (ed. D. Deutsch and J.A. Deutsch), p. 355. Academic Press, New York.

Gold, P.E., L. Hankins, R.M. Edwards, J. Chester, and J.L. McGaugh. 1975. Memory interference and facilitation with posttrial amygdala stimulation: Effect on memory varies with footshock level. *Brain Res.* **86:** 509.

Hugdahl, K., A. Berardi, W. Thompson, S. Kosslyn, R. Macy, D. Baker, N. Alpert, and J. LeDoux. 1995. Brain mechanisms in human classical conditioning: A PET blood flow study. *NeuroReport* **6:** 1723.

Ikegaya, Y., H. Saito., and K. Abe. 1994. Attenuated hippocampal long-term potentiation in basolateral amygdala-lesioned rats. *Brain Res.* **656:** 157.

———. 1995. Requirement of basolateral amygdala neuron activity for the induction of long-term potentiation in the dentate gyrus in vivo. *Brain Res.* **671:** 351.

Levi, L. (Ed.) 1975. *Emotions—Their parameters and measurement.* Raven Press, New York.

Liang, K.C., C. Bennett, and J.L. McGaugh. 1985. Peripheral epinephrine modulates the effects of posttraining amygdala stimulation on memory. *Behav. Brain Res.* **15:** 93.

Maren, S. and M. Fanselow. 1995. Synaptic plasticity in the basolateral amygdala induced by hippocampal formation stimulation *in vivo*. *J. Neurosci.* **15:** 7548.

Markowitsch, H.J., P. Calabrese, M. Wuerker, H.F. Durwen, J. Kessler, R. Babinsky, D. Brechtelsbauer, L. Heuser, and W. Gehlen. 1994. The amygdala's contribution to memory—A study on two patients with Urbach-Wiethe disease. *NeuroReport* **5:** 1349.

McGaugh, J.L. 1966. Time-dependent processes in memory storage. *Science* **153:** 1351.

———. 1989. Involvement of hormonal and neuromodulatory systems in the regulation of memory storage. *Annu. Rev. Neurosci.* **12:** 255.

———. 1992. Affect, neuromodulatory systems, and memory storage. In *The handbook of emotion and memory: Research and theory* (ed. S.-A. Christianson), p. 245. Lawrence Erlbaum, Hillsdale, New Jersey.

McGaugh, J.L., I.B. Introini-Collison, R. Juler, and I. Izquierdo. 1986. Stria terminalis lesions attenuate the effects of posttraining β-endorphin and naloxone on retention. *Behav. Neurosci.* **100:** 839.

McGaugh, J.L., L. Cahill, M.B. Parent, M.H. Mesches, K. Coleman-Mesches, and J. Salinas. 1995. Involvement of the amygdala in the regulation of memory storage. In *Plasticity in the central nervous system* (ed. J.L. McGaugh et al.), p. 17. Lawrence Erlbaum, Hillsdale, New Jersey.

Nielson, K.A. and R.A. Jensen. 1994. β-Adrenergic receptor antagonist antihypertensive medications impair arousal-induced modulation of working memory in elderly humans. *Behav. Neural. Biol.* **62:** 190.

Packard, M.G., L. Cahill, and J.L. McGaugh. 1994. Amygdala modulation of hippocampal-dependent and caudate nucleus-dependent memory processes. *Proc. Natl. Acad. Sci.* **91:** 8477.

Packard, M., C. Williams, L. Cahill, and J.L. McGaugh. 1995. The anatomy of a memory modulatory system: From periphery to brain. In *Neurobehavioral plasticity* (ed. N.E. Spear et al.), p. 149. Lawrence Erlbaum, Hillsdale, New Jersey.

Rauch, S., B. van der Kolk, R. Fisler, N. Alpert, S. Orr, C.

Savage, A. Fischman, M. Jenike, and R. Pitman. 1996. A symptom provocation study of posttraumatic stress disorder using positron emission tomography and script-driven imagery. *Arch Gen. Psychol.* **53:** 380.

Roozendaal, B., O. Carmi, and J.L. McGaugh. 1996. Adrenocortical suppression blocks the memory-enhancing effects of amphetamine and epinephrine. *Proc. Natl. Acad. Sci.* **93:** 1429.

Scoville, B. and W.B. Milner. 1957. Loss of recent memory after bilateral hippocampal lesions. *J. Neurol. Neurosurg. Psychiatry* **29:** 11.

Thomas, S.R., S.Y. Assaf, and S.D. Iverson. 1984. Amygdaloid complex modulates neurotransmission from the entorhinal cortex to the dentate gyrus of the rat. *Brain Res.* **307:** 363.

Weiskrantz, L. 1956. Behavioral changes associated with ablation of the amygdaloid complex in monkeys. *J. Comp. Physiol. Psychol.* 49: 381.

A *Drosophila* Circadian Clock

M. Rosbash, R. Allada, M. Dembinska, W.Q. Guo, M. Le, S. Marrus,
Z. Qian, J. Rutila, J. Yaglom, and H. Zeng
Howard Hughes Medical Institute, National Science Foundation Science & Technology Center for Biological Timing, Department of Biology, Brandeis University, Waltham, Massachusetts 02254

The circadian clock (pacemaker, oscillator) is considered endogenous, as opposed to driven, because rhythmic oscillations persist with near 24-hour periodicity under constant conditions. It is, however, connected with the environment because the rhythm is usually entrained or synchronized by the 24-hour light-dark cycle, the major environmental zeitgeber or time cue. The clock is also connected to downstream outputs; namely, the biochemical and behavioral fluctuations that are generally observed as rhythmic phenomena.

In metazoan organisms, several pacemaker locations are known (see King and Takahashi; Lamas et al.; both this volume). The eye (retina), the avian pineal, and the suprachiasmatic nucleus (SCN) all contain independent self-sustaining oscillators (Takahashi et al. 1989; Underwood et al. 1990; Klein et al. 1991; Tosini and Menaker 1996). The current prevailing view is that these tissue pacemakers are a collection of single-cell oscillators and that the tissue-pacemaker properties are similar to those of an individual cell. Original studies by Takahashi and colleagues indicated that individual pinealocytes keep proper circadian time with little or no intercellular contact (Robertson and Takahashi 1988). Physiological studies in individual Bulla pacemaker neurons showed that the clock is functional without cell-cell contact (Michel et al. 1993). A recent study recorded circadian rhythms of spontaneous action potentials from rat SCN cultures on fixed microelectrode arrays (Welsh et al. 1995). The results suggest that the SCN contains a large population of autonomous, single-cell oscillators; functional synaptic connections formed in culture are neither necessary for the rhythms nor sufficient to synchronize them. Perhaps melatonin participates in synchronizing the SCN neurons (Reppert et al. 1994).

The broad acceptance of an intracellular circadian pacemaker mechanism has been facilitated by three additional areas of investigation. The first is the excellent circadian biology of single-cell organisms. For example, *Neurospora* has one of the best-studied clock mechanisms (Dunlap et al. 1993). Even cyanobacteria have bona fide circadian rhythms that meet all the traditional criteria (Kondo et al. 1994). Although multiple clocks may "run" independently in cultures of the dinoflagellate *Gonyaulax* (Roenneberg and Morse 1993), there is little doubt that the basic oscillatory mechanism is intracellular. The second is the importance of macromolecular synthesis. The application of RNA and protein synthesis inhibitors indicates that the clock requires macromolecular synthesis (Raju et al. 1991; Khalsa et al. 1992; Takahashi et al. 1993), in some cases at defined times of the circadian cycle. Recent results in cyanobacteria indicate that transcription of a sizable fraction of the genome is under circadian control (Liu et al. 1995). An apparently universal and important role of macromolecular synthesis reinforces intracellular as opposed to tissue-based (i.e., systems) circadian mechanisms. The third is the molecular genetic studies in *Drosophila* and *Neurospora*, where the predominant foci have been three clock genes: *period* (*per*) and *timeless* (*tim*) in flies and *frequency* (*frq*) in *Neurospora*.

For 25 years, an impressive array of genetic evidence has been accumulating that *per* and *frq* encode bona fide components of their organisms' pacemakers. The two genes were cloned, and several mutations were identified within the coding regions. The genes were also defined by germ-line transformation and rescue of the arrhythmic null mutant phenotype. More recent results from the Young laboratory indicate that *tim* is also a member of the clock gene club (Sehgal et al. 1994; Vosshall et al. 1994; Gekakis et al. 1995; Myers et al. 1995; Sehgal et al. 1995). Molecular characterization indicates that the two clock mechanisms include the rhythmic accumulation and disappearance of the gene products; protein cycling depends on transcriptional autoregulation, which is part of the intracellular mechanism in both organisms (Hardin et al. 1990; Aronson et al. 1994; Sehgal et al. 1995; Zeng et al. 1996). In this paper, we concentrate on recent studies from our laboratory that have contributed to this *Drosophila* clock story.

THE *DROSOPHILA* CLOCK PARADIGM

The modern era began with studies that examined the spatial expression pattern of PER within *Drosophila* heads. The goal was to identify a pacemaker location, the predicted head region that governed locomotor activity rhythms. A series of papers indicated widespread PER expression (even in nonneural tissues) and pointed to a group of central brain neurons, the "lateral neurons," as the likely cen-

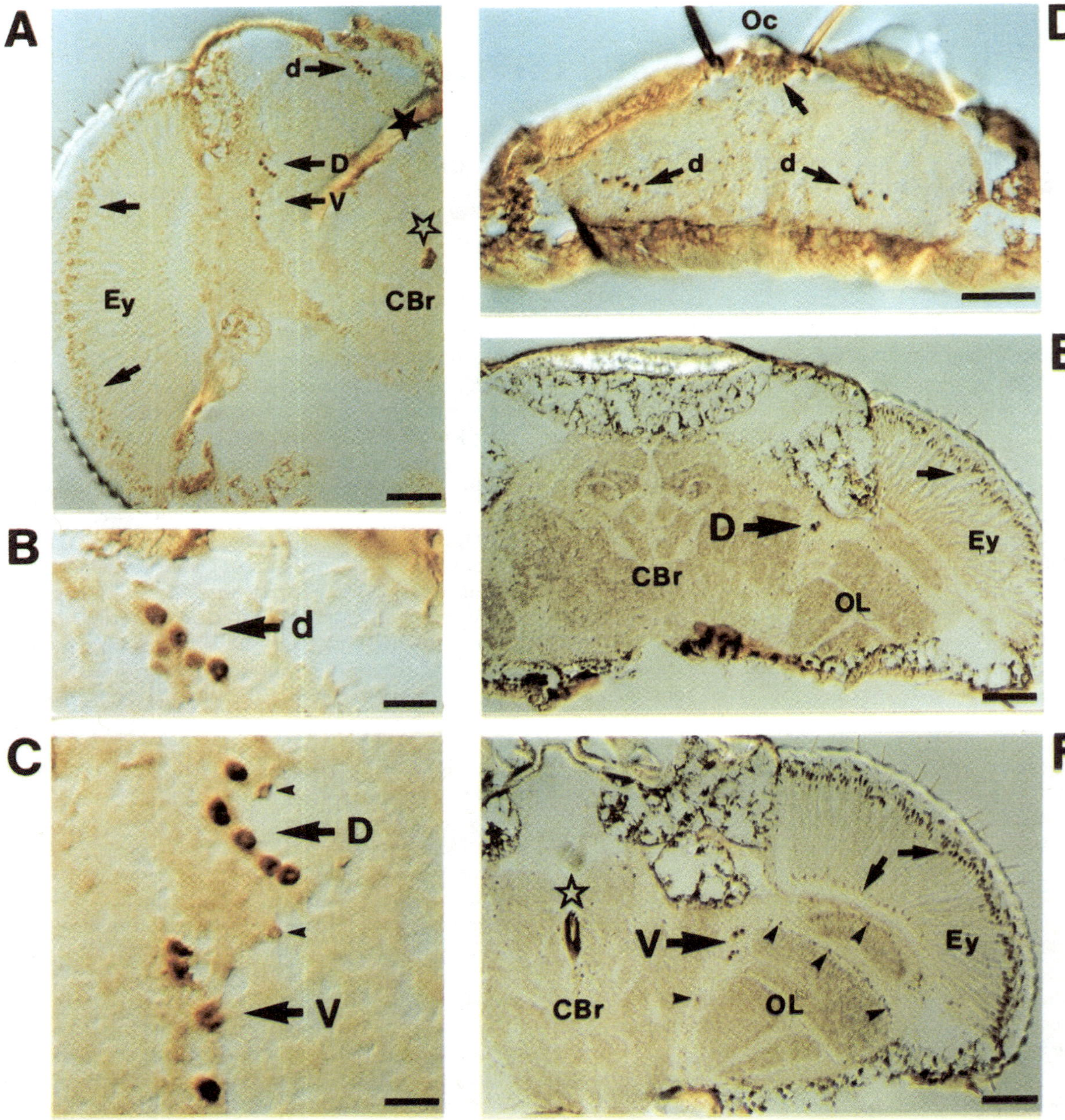

Figure 1. Distribution of *per* immunoreactivity in the brain of wild-type (Canton-S) flies, visualized using the anti-Eco*per* (*A-D*) or the anti-S antibody (*E,F*). (*A*) Distribution of *per* immunoreactivity in a frontal section of a wild-type fly. Note the occurrence of a dorsalmost cluster (d), and that of the more ventral group of dorsal (D) and ventral (V) lateral neurons. Unlabeled arrows point to photoreceptor nuclei. (*Solid star*) Piece of cuticle. Bar, 50 μm. (*B,C*) Higher-magnification views of *A* (*B*, dorsal; *C*, more ventral). (*Arrowheads*) *per*-immunoreactive cells occurring at the margins of the cells in the cortex of the central brain. Bars, 10 μm. (*D*) Horizontal section through the dorsalmost region of the head showing the *per*-immunoreactive cells in the cortex of the central brain (d). The unlabeled arrow points to the photoreceptor nuclei of the ocelli (Oc). Bar, 50 μm. (*E, F*) Sections showing *per* immunoreactivity on horizontal sections of wild-type flies (*E*, dorsal; *F*, more ventral). Note the conspicuous staining in the dorsal (*E*, labeled D) and ventral (*F*, labeled V) lateral neurons. In addition, *per*-specific labeling occurred in the nuclei of the photoreceptors of the eye (*unlabeled arrows* in *E* and *F*), at the margins of the cortex and the neuropil in the optic lobes and the central brain (*F*, *arrowheads*), and within the neuropil of the lamina (*F*, *arrowhead*). Bars, 50 μm. Other abbreviations: (CBr), central brain; (Ey) eye; (OL) optic lobes. (*Open star*) Esophagus. (Reprinted, with permission, from Ewer et al. 1992.)

tral pacemaker (Fig. 1) (Liu et al. 1988; Siwicki et al. 1988; Zerr et al. 1990; Ewer et al. 1992). Two additional approaches support the hypothesis that these are indeed pacemaker cells. First, the anatomical mutant *disco* appears to eliminate some of the key lateral neurons as well as apparent circadian rhythmicity

(Steller et al. 1987; Zerr et al. 1990; Helfrich-Forster and Homberg 1993). Second, Helfrich has shown that pigment dispersing hormone (PDH), a molecule known to be involved in insect as well as crustacean and mollusk circadian rhythms, is coexpressed with PER in a subset of these cells. One imagines that PDH is released in rhythmic fashion and is involved in communicating with the output pathway (Helfrich-Forster 1995). A recent contribution from Vosshall and Young (1995) may also be relevant. They expressed PER from a *glass* promoter, known to drive gene expression in photoreceptor cells. Surprisingly, the transgene rescued the rhythms of the arrhythmic per^{01} host animal. PER was expressed in the brain within or near the lateral neurons as well as in the eyes. Because the eyes have been shown to be irrelevant for the behavioral rescue, these results are also consistent with a subset of the lateral neurons being the location of the locomotor activity clock. Because the *glass* promoter is active in these cells, they may have some direct photoreceptor function important perhaps for light entrainment (see below).

Importantly, these early studies suggested that PER levels undergo robust circadian oscillations; the histochemical observations were subsequently confirmed by biochemical studies (Edery et al. 1994b; Zeng et al. 1994). RNA analyses accompanied the early histochemistry and showed that *per* mRNA levels also undergo robust circadian oscillations that depend on the presence of their translation products (Fig. 2) (Hardin et al. 1990). The RNA cycling was linked to rhythmic changes in *per* transcription (Hardin et al. 1992). Because missense mutations alter the periods of the RNA fluctuations, the protein fluctuations, and the rhythmic outputs in parallel, PER participates in an autoregulatory feedback loop that influences its own gene's transcription (Hardin et al. 1990). Similar results and conclusions subsequently emerged from the FRQ-*Neurospora* system (Aronson et al. 1994). Taken together, the evidence suggests that the protein fluctuations and the transcriptional feedback loop lie at the heart of the circadian oscillators.

This *Drosophila* clock model has support from four sets of experiments. First, PER was shown to be a nuclear protein at peak levels of expression (Liu et al. 1992). Second, PER contains a single motif, the PAS domain, with similarity to other proteins. The PAS motif is also present in a set of bHLH-type transcription factors and has been shown to function in vitro as a protein-protein interaction domain (Huang et al. 1993). Both of these results are consistent with the notion that PER acts rather directly to modulate transcription. Third, a construct encoding a rhodopsin promoter–*per* fusion gene was introduced into otherwise wild-type flies (Zeng et al. 1994). The high-level constitutive eye expression from the transgene stopped the clock in a tissue-specific manner; i.e., the rhythmic *per* mRNA expression in the eye was eliminated without affecting the molecular rhythms in the brain or the locomotor activity behavioral rhythms. The *per* eye RNA from the endogenous gene was pegged at trough levels, suggesting not only that the *per* feedback loop is intracellular, but also that PER acts negatively to inhibit the transcription of its own gene. Fourth, and to address the importance of the PER fluctuations in a more dynamic fashion, a heat-shock-promoter-driven *per* gene (hs-*per*) was introduced into an otherwise wild-type strain (Edery et al. 1994a). Consistent with the notion that PER is a clock component, exposure to a 1-hour 37°C heat pulse caused stable phase shifts of the flies' rhythms that were different from those experienced by wild-type flies. The magnitude and direction (advance or delay) of the phase shifts were dependent on time, i.e., on the state of the clock at the time of the heat shock. The measurements created a HS-*per* phase response curve (PRC), analogous to the more traditional light PRC that describes the temporal variation in the clock's response to a pulse of light. A comparison of the hs-*per* PRC with PER's normal fluctuations indicates that the latter are integral to the clock mechanism (Edery et al. 1994a). In circadian parlance, PER is not only a clock component but also a state variable (Tyson 1976). Using a recombinant DNA construct expressing the FRQ gene product from a strong regulated promoter, Dunlap and colleagues have drawn a similar conclusion for the *Neurospora* system (Aronson et al. 1994).

timeless AND THE PER-TIM HETERODIMER

Among the most exciting developments in the *per*-fly-rhythm business over the past 2 years has been the emergence of *timeless* as the second bona fide rhythm gene in this organism (Sehgal et al. 1994; Vosshall et al. 1994). Although the genetics is compelling and there are period-altering alleles as well as arrhythmic alleles of *tim* (Rutila et al. 1996; M.W. Young, pers. comm.), it is the interaction with the *per* system that has attracted so much well-deserved attention. In a tim^0 (arrhythmic null allele) background, there is no detectable *per* RNA cycling (Sehgal et al. 1994). *tim* RNA also undergoes cycling in a manner very similar to *per*, and the *tim* fluctuations are largely eliminated in tim^0 or per^{01} backgrounds (Sehgal et al. 1995). Therefore, there is unusual reciprocal autoregulation of the two proteins on their own transcription. The cloning of TIM was not revealing at the primary amino acid sequence level (Myers et al. 1995), but the cloning showed that PER and TIM can physically interact in vitro and in yeast (Gekakis et al. 1995), suggesting that the observed mislocalization of a *per*–β-galactosidase fusion protein in a tim^0 mutant background might reflect the absence of this physical association (Vosshall et al. 1994). Indeed, TIM was recently shown to be a stoichiometric partner of PER in fly head extracts, which offers a formal explanation for the reciprocal autoregulation: The heterodimer acts in some unknown way to regulate the transcription of both genes (Zeng et al. 1996).

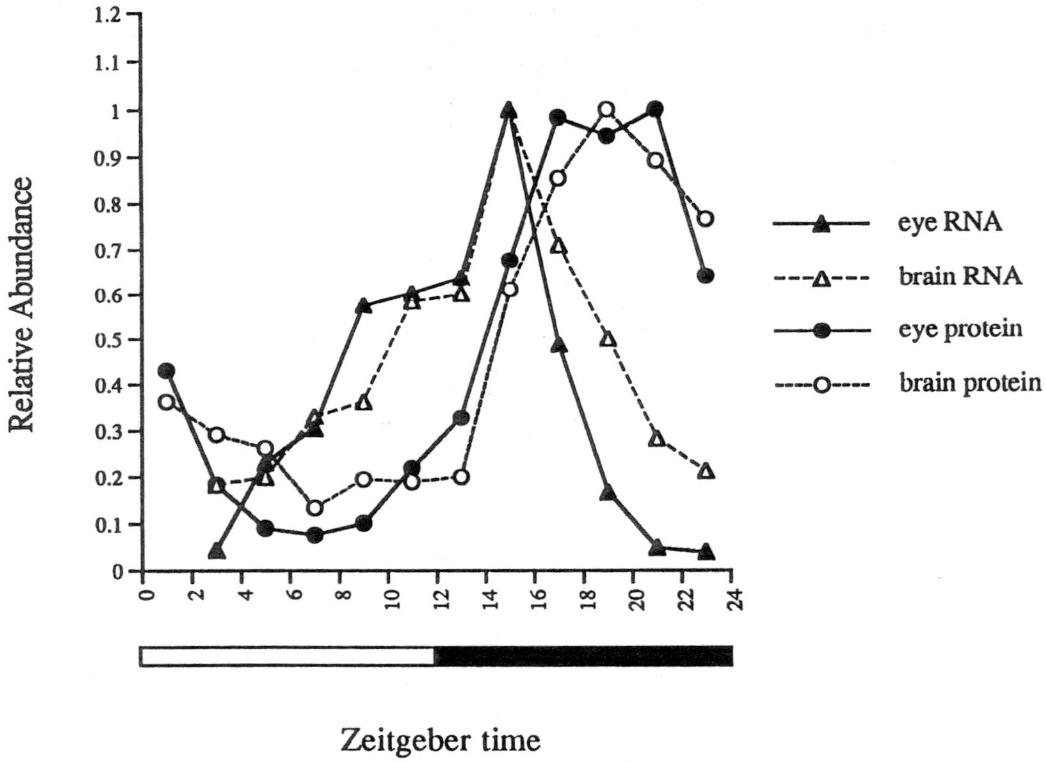

Figure 2. Quantitation of the relative abundance of *per* RNA and protein from dissected eyes (including *per*-expressing photoreceptor cells) and brains (including *per*-expressing neurons and glial cells) of wild-type flies. Although the actual peak values of both RNA and protein are about three times higher in eyes than in brains, the relative abundance is adjusted such that the maximum level in each set of data (eye or brain, RNA or protein) is 1.0. (Reprinted, with permission of Oxford University Press, from Zeng et al. 1994.)

POSTTRANSCRIPTIONAL REGULATION

There are strong indications that one or more posttranscriptional mechanisms contribute to PER and TIM cycling (Zwiebel et al. 1991). A comparison of the *per* RNA and protein curves suggests that the latter cannot be easily derived from the former without some form of posttranscriptional regulation; PER translation and/or PER degradation must be temporally regulated (Zeng et al. 1994; Dembinska et al. 1997). The same conclusions can be drawn from the *tim* RNA and protein curves (Sehgal et al. 1995; Hunter-Ensor et al. 1996; Lee et al. 1996; Zeng et al. 1996). We have some evidence to favor the notion that PER lifetime is not uniform across the circadian cycle; i.e., there is temporal regulation of protein half-life (Dembinska et al. 1997; Stanewsky et al. 1997).

A second posttranscriptional phenomenon is protein phosphorylation. The original biochemical characterization of PER cycling by Western blotting indicated that PER is subject to temporal phosphorylation (Edery et al. 1994b). It appears to be progressive, because the phosphorylation becomes more extensive during the night. Recent experiments indicate that TIM undergoes a similar phenomenon (Zeng et al. 1996). In the early morning, PER undergoes an even more extensive phosphorylation about the time when TIM disappears. PER hyperphosphorylation appears to presage PER turnover, which then takes place predominantly during the early morning hours.

A third regulatory step is the timing of nuclear entry. We recently reported that PER's nuclear localization is under temporal control: PER remains cytoplasmic throughout its accumulation phase and then undergoes nuclear entry during a narrow time window (Fig. 3) (Curtin et al. 1995). It is important to note that this temporal control of nuclear entry was visible only in the putative brain pacemaker neurons and not detected in other PER-expressing tissues, such as photoreceptor cells. The reason for this discrepancy is not clear (it may be purely technical), but it limits the general significance of the observation.

The timing of apparent nuclear entry, compared to the timing of protein accumulation, makes it unlikely that the change in subcellular localization is driven solely by the increase in protein levels (Zeng et al. 1994; Curtin et al. 1995). Consistent with the importance of posttranscriptional regulation, a *tim* null mutant inhibits nuclear localization of a PER–β-galactosidase fusion protein without affecting fusion protein levels; this suggests that the substrate for nuclear entry may be the TIM-PER heterodimer

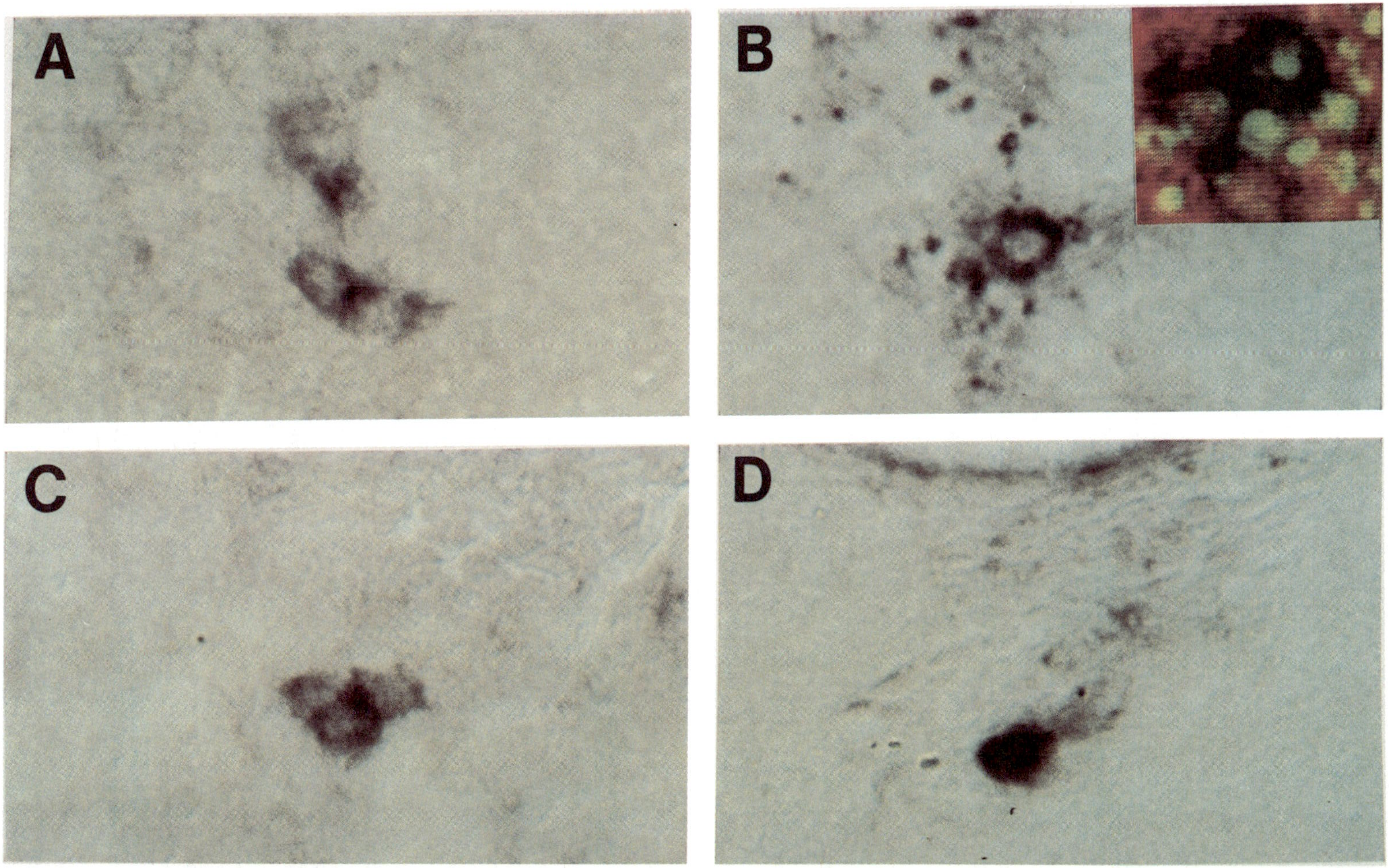

Figure 3. PER immunoreactivity in pacemaker neurons of wild-type flies at indicated times: (*A*) ZT16; (*B*) ZT17; (*C*) ZT18; (*D*) ZT19. The inset in *B* shows PER staining in black and nuclear staining with propidium iodide in yellow. Propidium iodide normally emits red fluorescence. The yellow color was computer-generated. *Note*: the neurons shown in *D* represent a subgroup of pacemaker neurons that are larger than those shown in *A–C* (Helfrich-Forster 1995). (Reprinted, with permission, from Curtin et al. 1995 [copyright Cell Press].)

(Zeng et al. 1996). This raises the fourth level of posttranscriptional regulation, PER-TIM dimerization.

It is important to emphasize that these four posttranscriptional regulatory events have not been ordered. As a consequence, we do not know which ones occur first and are necessary for which others. For example, phosphorylation could influence the PER-TIM dissociation constant or the PER lifetime. Alternatively, phosphorylation could affect the timing of nuclear entry. It is equally likely, however, that an opposite relationship obtains; for example, nuclear entry could be upstream of and lead to a change in the phosphorylation pattern or the PER-TIM dimerization constant (Lee et al. 1996).

Although the relationship of these posttranscriptional regulatory steps to transcriptional regulation is also undefined, we suspect that one or more of them are upstream of the changes in transcription. This order is attractive, because oscillatory negative feedback loops require a substantial delay between the synthesis of a factor and its inhibitory activity; otherwise the system comes to equilibrium and the fluctuations stop. For example, one can imagine that proper nuclear entry contributes to such a delay step. PER temporal phosphorylation might also be related to the gating of nuclear entry. Indeed, two groups have independently based computer models of *per* RNA and protein cycling on a possible link between phosphorylation, nuclear entry, and negative autoregulation of transcription (Goldbeter 1995; L.F. Abbott et al., unpubl.). All of these ideas are unproven and remain speculative. Moreover, it remains possible that some of the posttranscriptional regulatory steps are downstream from the transcriptional changes and caused by changes in protein levels. PER-TIM dimerization is a good candidate for a posttranscriptional event that should be sensitive to changes in transcription and protein levels.

PER-L, TIM-SL, AND PER-S

The effects of missense mutations in PER and TIM should be revealing about the order and dependency of events during the cycle. This is analogous to the classic genetic approach of cell cycle analysis (see, e.g., Hartwell and Weinert 1989). TIM missense mutants are just beginning to be uncovered and studied (see below), but the original long period and short period *per* mutations (*per*^{L} and *per*^{s}, respectively) have been available for decades (Konopka and Benzer 1971). The studies on these mutants are intriguing, but the interpretation of the results is still not entirely straightforward.

The *per*^{L} mutation lengthens the circadian period, weakens the strength of the rhythms, and abrogates temperature compensation; i.e., the period lengthens with increasing temperature. The mutation is a single amino acid change within the PER PAS domain, consistent with the notion that the mutation's direct effect is on protein-protein interactions (Baylies et al. 1987; Huang et al. 1993). Indeed, it appears to affect the PER-TIM interaction in a temperature-sensitive manner (Gekakis et al. 1995). Thus, temperature compensation may be related to temperature insensitivity of the PER-TIM heterodimer interaction (Gekakis et al. 1995; Huang et al. 1995).

Another effect of PER-L is to manifest delayed nuclear entry into circadian pacemaker neurons in lateral brain regions (Curtin et al. 1995; Lee et al. 1996). *per*^{L} is temperature-sensitive for this property, too, since nuclear entry is even further delayed at higher temperatures (Curtin et al. 1995). Yet a third molecular effect of *per*^{L} is to dampen the normally robust PER protein cycling and phosphorylation profile (Fig. 4). A similar effect is seen for TIM protein cycling and phosphorylation as well (Rutila et al. 1996). These events need to be ordered with respect to the effects on PER-TIM dimerization and on the timing of nuclear entry. Finally, all three molecular effects are not yet linked with certainty to the behavioral effects of the mutation. Because the dimerization effects are manifest in vitro and in yeast, they are probably upstream and the cause of the other molecular and behavioral phenotypes. Less likely perhaps, these dimerization effects are an independent consequence of the mutation and not critical for the other phenotypes.

Relevant to these considerations is a new *tim* mutation we have recently isolated. We screened chemically mutagenized flies for suppressors or enhancers of the *per*^{L} phenotype and isolated a new period-altering missense allele of the *timeless* gene (Rutila et al. 1996). *tim*^{SL} suppresses the *per*^{L} phenotype, as double mutant flies have a 25.5-hour period instead of the 29-hour period characteristic of the single mutant *per*^{L} strain. Preliminary experiments suggest that the single amino acid change in the *tim* coding region is indeed responsible for the behavioral phenotype: Germ-line transformation with a *tim*^{SL}-derived construct reduces the period of the *per*^{L} host strain by 3 hours (Table 1). Although control wild-type *tim* transformants are not yet available, we have never observed such a reduction in period in transformation experiments with wild-type *per*-derived DNA (Hall and Kyriacou 1990; Dushay et al. 1992).

Importantly, the *tim*^{SL} suppressor also restores proper temperature compensation to the double mutant flies, consistent with a putative posttranscriptional effect on the PER-TIM interaction. It also advances the apparent entry time of the *per*^{L} protein into pacemaker cell nuclei. *tim*^{SL} more generally manifests specific interactions with different *per* alleles. For example, it has minimal effects in an otherwise wild-type background. The identification of this first period-altering *tim* allele provides further evidence that TIM is a major component of the *Drosophila* biological clock, and the allele-specific interactions with PER provide evidence that the PER-TIM heterodimer is a unit of circadian function (Rutila et al. 1996).

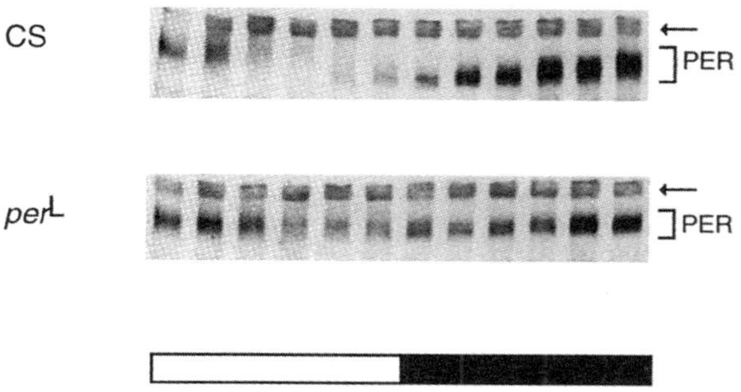

Figure 4. Western blots of PER in wild-type and per^L flies. Extracts made from CS wild-type or per^L heads (collected during LD) were run on 6% SDS gels, blotted, and probed with anti-PER antibody. Brackets indicate the differently phosphorylated forms of either PER, and the small arrows refer to a cross-reacting band. White bar is the light phase, and filled bar the dark phase of a 12-hr light:12-hr dark cycle. (Reprinted, with permission, from Rutila et al. 1996 [copyright Cell Press].)

Surprisingly, the tim^{SL} mutation fails to restore temperature insensitivity to the PER-L/TIM-SL complex in yeast, contrary to the simple expectation from the restoration of behavioral temperature compensation in the double mutant flies (Rutila et al. 1996). Although this could be some kind of in vitro (i.e., in yeast) artifact, the location of the single tim^{SL} amino acid change is outside the minimal PER-TIM interaction domain in yeast (Gekakis et al. 1995). We therefore suggest that tim^{SL} is acting as a second site (intergenic) suppressor that is affecting another important interaction rather than the formation or stability of the PER-L/TIM heterodimer. Either the PER-L/TIM yeast phenotype is unrelated to the mutant effects in the fly or, more likely perhaps, tim^{SL} is acting as a bypass suppressor of per^L. A tim^{SL} bypass suppressor could affect the interaction of TIM with another protein rather than affect the formation or stability of the heterodimer itself. tim^{SL} can only be a partial bypass suppressor, however, because per^0;tim^{SL} flies are still arrhythmic (J. Rutila, unpubl.).

Western blot results also support this bypass interpretation. The cycling profile of PER-L in a per^L background has a number of differences from what has been described for a wild-type background. However, we observed the surprising result that the PER-L profile is unaltered in the doubly mutant flies. It is as if the TIM-SL protein is "short circuiting" the protein cycling pattern by altering the time that the PER-TIM heterodimer is acting or acted upon in some downstream clock event(s) (Rutila et al. 1996).

The interaction between TIM and a kinase appears to be a reasonable candidate for the downstream clock event. TIM-SL migrates at a higher molecular weight than TIM late in the night (ZT19-23), and this difference appears to take place similarly if not identically in a per^+ genetic background. The actual phosphorylation sites for TIM are unknown, making it impossible

Table 1. Germ-line Transformation with a tim^{SL}-derived DNA Construct

Genotype	Period (τ) ± S.E.M.	% Arrhythmic	N
per^L/Y; tim^{SL}/tim^+; +/+	26.7 ± 0.2	0	16
per^L/Y; tim^0/tim^+; P(tim^{SL})/+	26.0 ± 0.1	54	26
per^L/Y; tim^0/tim^+; +/+	29.8 ± 0.3	38	29

Flies were entrained for two 12-hr light:12-hr dark cycles before being assayed for locomotor activity in constant conditions at 25°C for 5 days (Hamblen et al. 1986). Activity periods were determined by χ^2 periodogram analysis, α = 0.01 (Hamblen-Coyle et al. 1992). Periods are given in hours, plus or minus S.E.M. N = Number of individual flies tested. P(tim^{SL}) refers to the transgenic tim^{SL} cDNA gene which is driven by ~6.5 kb of *tim* genomic sequence upstream of the translation start and has 2 kb of *per* 3′ genomic sequence after the translation stop site.

to offer a detailed molecular interpretation of how the TIM-SL missense mutation affects the phosphorylation pattern. TIM-SL could accelerate TIM phosphorylation, alter the phosphorylation sites, or indirectly affect the heterodimer and make the phosphorylation of its TIM subunit more robust as well as more PER-independent (Fig. 5). Accelerated phosphorylation would presumably be related to the accelerated entrance of the heterodimer into nuclei.

The bypass hypothesis is predicated on the interpretation that the in vivo dimer is biologically active and that PER-L has a more primary effect on heterodimer dissociation, which then indirectly affects TIM phosphorylation. This model also assumes that dimer formation occurs upstream of and is necessary for phosphorylation. If, in fact, per^L has separate effects on phosphorylation and dimerization, then tim^{SL} would function as a real suppressor instead of as a bypass suppressor. In any case, the results arguably provide the best evidence for the importance of the PER-TIM heterodimer to the clock mechanism (Lee et al. 1996; Zeng et al. 1996).

In contrast to per^L, the per^S clock runs fast and is strong. Although there is no in vitro information on the direct effect of the per^s missense mutation, the in vivo experiments suggest that it too acts directly on a posttranscriptional regulatory step. Earlier experiments indicated that the protein cycle is accelerated (Zerr et al. 1990; Edery et al. 1994b), and more recent experiments also show that there is less PER and TIM in a per^s as compared to a wild-type background in constant darkness (DD) conditions (Marrus et al. 1996). (The assay in constant darkness eliminates the confounding effects of light, which have a substantial effect in LD [12:12] conditions; see below.) The low protein levels suggest that protein half-life, or perhaps phosphorylation leading in turn to more rapid turnover, may be directly affected by the mutation (Marrus et al. 1996). For example, a shorter half-life would lead to a more rapid disappearance of the PER-TIM complex in the late night/early morning.

The premature disappearance of PER-S and TIM anticipates the premature rise of *per* and *tim* RNA that

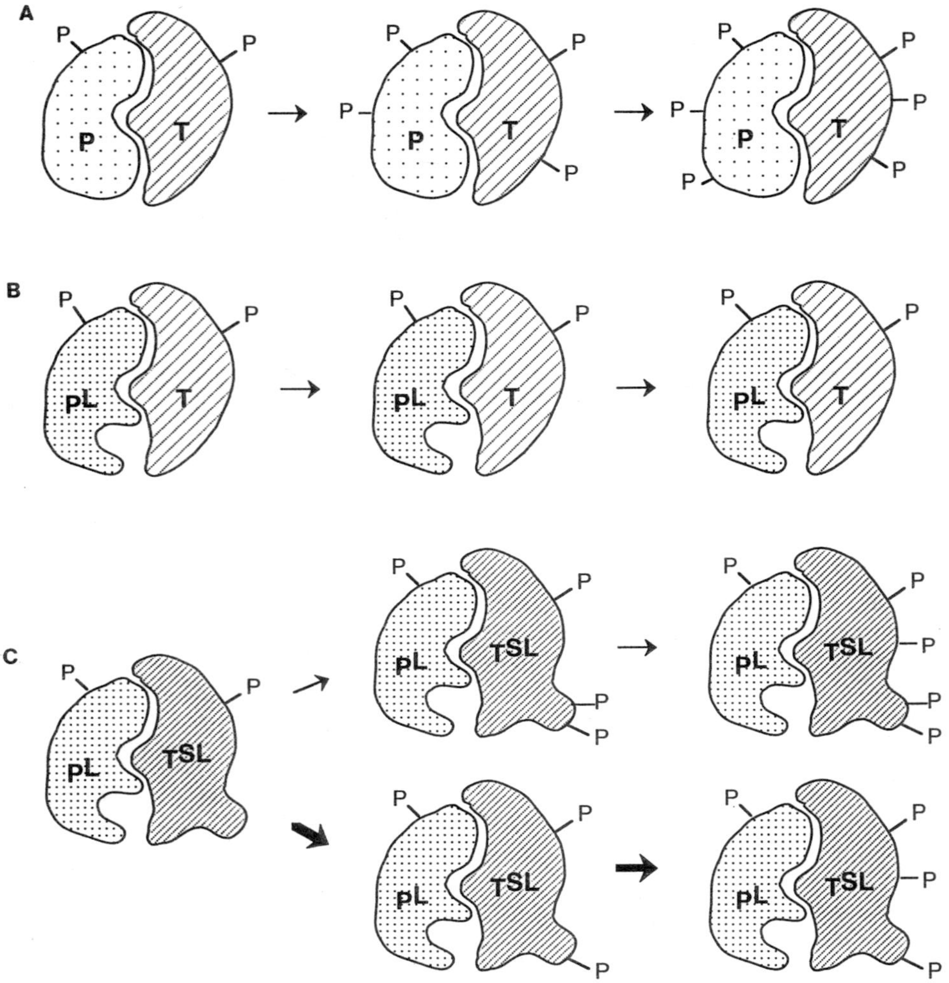

Figure 5. Bypass suppressor model for TIM-SL. (*A*) PER (**P**) and TIM (**T**) heterodimerize, and that dimer is phosphorylated (P) with time (*arrows*). (*B*) PER-L ($\mathbf{P^L}$) weakens the PER-TIM interaction, and the PER-L/TIM dimer stays relatively unphosphorylated throughout the cycle. (*C*) TIM-SL ($\mathbf{T^{SL}}$) does not alter the interaction with PER, but changes another part of TIM so that the protein could be phosphorylated more quickly (*heavy arrows*), differently (extra phosphates), or have an altered interaction with another substrate (not shown). (Reprinted, with permission, from Rutila et al. 1996 [copyright Cell Press].)

occurs in the early morning (Marrus et al. 1996). The 4- or 5-hour advance in the RNA rise occurs indistinguishably in LD or DD conditions, i.e., light in the early morning plays no detectable role in the timing (Marrus et al. 1996). This indicates that the timing of the posttranscriptional events that PER and TIM undergo during the night, phosphorylation and degradation, determine when the subsequent increase in *per* and *tim* transcription will occur several hours later; i.e., feedforward effects on the timing of the next cycle (see also below). Theoretical considerations suggest that the feedforward circuit may be simply the reversal of negative feedback (see below). However, there may be more to it; i.e., the timing of the rise in transcription may involve mechanisms distinct from those used to time the decline in transcription.

LIGHT

Similar feedforward regulation is part of the very recent and exciting *Drosophila* light story recently published in four reports from four different laboratories (Hunter-Ensor et al. 1996; Lee et al. 1996; Myers et al. 1996; Zeng et al. 1996). Our own interest in this problem began with a characterization of TIM cycling. Although it is very similar to PER cycling, careful inspection of the TIM and PER curves indicated a quantitative difference: During the late night/early morning, the decrease in TIM levels is rapid and complete in LD, and it precedes the more gradual decrease that PER undergoes (Zeng et al. 1996). This suggests that the conversion of PER from dimer to monomer, which also occurs in the late night/early morning, is caused by the disappearance of TIM. Moreover, the morning decline in TIM levels is more rapid in LD than in DD. Because there are very low *per* and *tim* mRNA levels at these cycle times, TIM disappearance is very likely due to TIM turnover, and this is probably facilitated by the lights-on event at ZT0 (Zeng et al. 1996).

Because light is the major temporal cue, we considered that it might act more generally to cause TIM degradation. To test this possibility, we exposed flies to light at different times of night and examined the levels of both TIM and PER by Western blotting. At all times, TIM levels decreased after only 1 hour, and there was little further decrease after 2 or 3 hours; indeed, the decrease was significant after only 20 minutes of light or short light pulses. In the late night, TIM disappearance was virtually complete, and this leads to a premature rise in the next day's *per* and *tim* RNA cycle; i.e., feedforward regulation similar to that shown by the per^{S} mutation (Lee et al. 1996; Zeng et al. 1996; data not shown).

These experiments do not indicate which clock component (e.g., PER, TIM, or the PER-TIM complex) is a more direct light target, but a prominent role for TIM alone is indicated by examining per^{01} flies. Although tim^{0} flies have only low levels of PER (suggesting that PER is unstable in the absence of TIM [Price et al. 1995]), TIM levels are quite high in per^{01} flies, i.e., in the absence of PER. Remarkably, there is an oscillation of TIM levels in this genetic background in LD but not in DD (Fig. 6) (Myers et al. 1996; Zeng et al. 1996). Since *tim* RNA levels do not oscillate in per^{01} flies (Sehgal et al. 1995), the light effect must be mediated by a posttranscriptional mechanism, e.g., degradation or translational inhibition. The light-induced decrease in TIM levels, evident in wild-type flies at ZT21 to ZT24 when *tim* RNA levels are extremely low (Sehgal et al. 1995; Hunter-Ensor et al. 1996; Myers et al. 1996; Zeng et al. 1996), indicates that a translational mechanism is unlikely.

In response to a light pulse, less TIM is degraded in the early evening than in the late night; in both cases, only the higher mobility (hypophosphorylated) forms of TIM persist (Zeng et al. 1996). These probably reflect newly synthesized TIM that has not yet undergone substantial phosphorylation. In addition, the lower mobility (more phosphorylated) forms of TIM, which predominate late at night, may be preferential degradation substrates. The same light protocol affects PER to a much lesser extent; its levels were not very different from what would normally be observed at these times. However, PER's phosphorylation pattern is altered after exposure to light (Lee et al. 1996; Zeng et al. 1996). Although the response of PER suggests that it is affected by light less directly than TIM, the *per* mutants are known to affect the magnitude of the light response (Saunders et al. 1994). A parsimonious explanation posits that they act by affecting the structure of the PER-TIM heterodimer, the primary clock light target (Zeng et al. 1996).

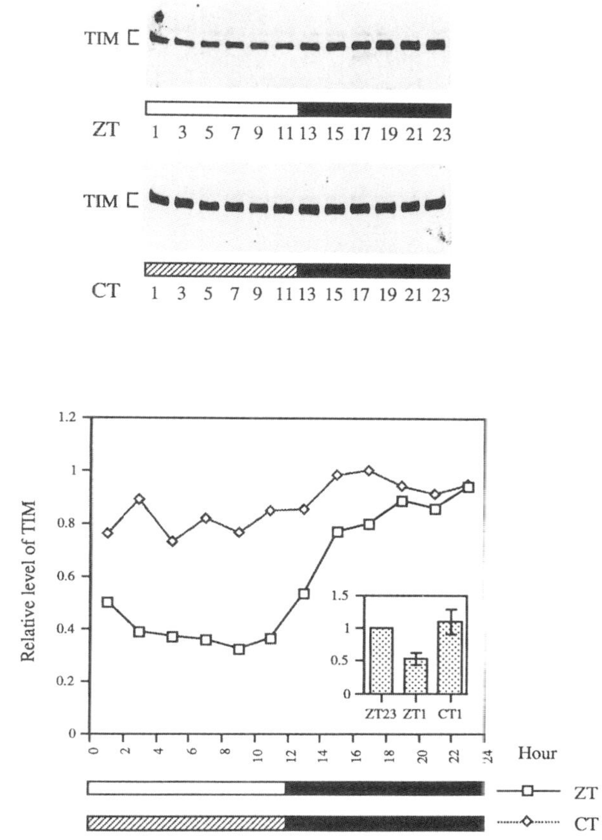

Figure 6. TIM levels in per^{01} flies in LD (ZT) and DD (CT). (*Bottom*) Quantification of the top. The inset compares TIM levels 1 hr after lights on (ZT1) with lights not on (CT1) plotted as mean ± S.E.M. (n=3). (Reprinted, with permission, from Zeng et al. 1996 [copyright Macmillan].)

A rapid light effect on the amount and state of the PER-TIM heterodimer also fits with several recent results from our laboratory on the effects of constant light (LL; Marrus et al. 1996). The most immediate and obvious effect of constant light, manifest shortly after ZT12 when the lights would normally turn off, is an inhibition of the PER and TIM phosphorylation that would normally take place in the first few hours of the night. TIM accumulation is also rapidly inhibited, as TIM levels remain almost constant in LL. PER accumulation is more modestly affected. Similar short-term effects were observed with light pulses in the early night, where there was observed a preferential disappearance of the more highly phosphorylated forms of TIM and an inhibition of PER phosphorylation (Lee et al. 1996; Zeng et al. 1996). This suggests that there is a rapid and primary posttranscriptional effect on the PER:TIM phosphorylation status, perhaps a light-mediated inhibition of the sequential phosphorylation program that normally takes place in the dark after ZT12 (Edery et al. 1994b; Lee et al. 1996; Zeng et al. 1996). However, we prefer the interpretation that the primary effect of constant light is rapid

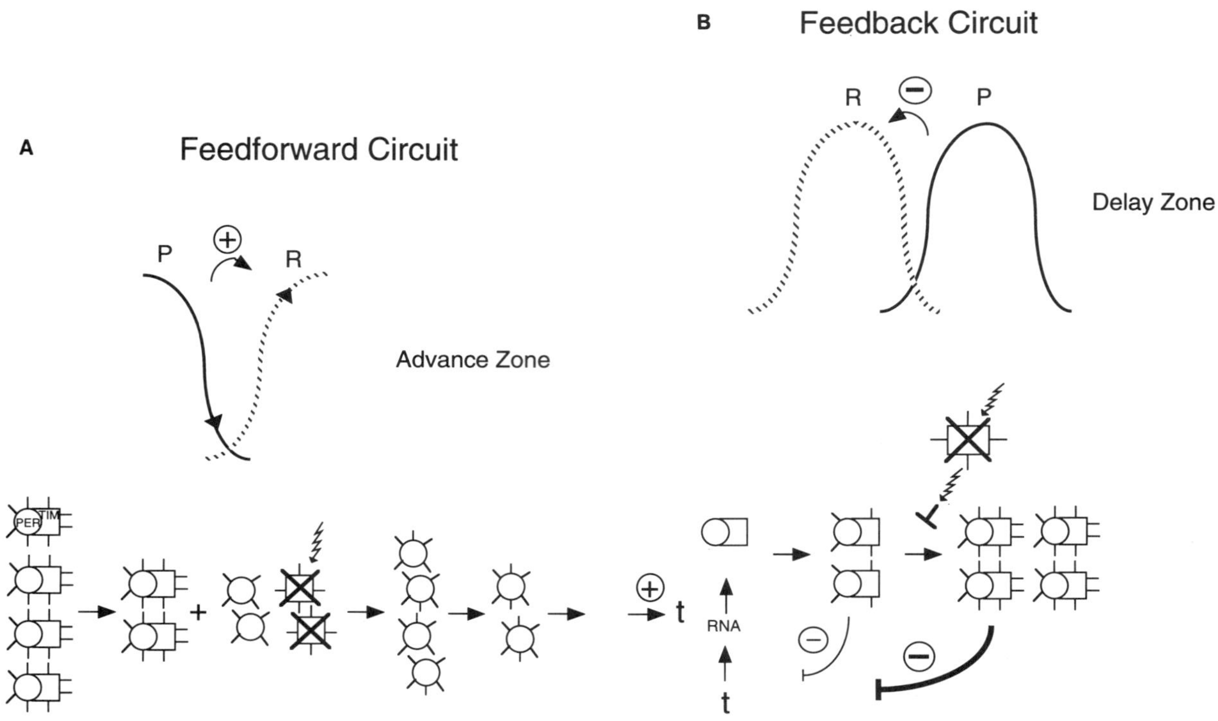

Figure 7. Feedforward (*A*) and feedback (*B*) circuits. (*A*) Disappearance of protein (P) positively affects RNA levels (R) in the advance zone. PER (*circles*)-TIM (*squares*) heterodimers are highly phosphorylated (*lines*) late in the night. When light turns on prematurely (*lightning bolt*), TIM is degraded and PER monomers become more highly phosphorylated. PER degradation then feeds forward to activate transcription and advances the cycle. (*B*) Protein negatively affects RNA in the delay zone. PER-TIM heterodimers are at low levels and less phosphorylated early in the evening. If light prematurely turns on at this time, the phosphorylation and accumulation cycles are inhibited at a posttranscription level, which slows the negative feedback of transcription and results in phase delays. For details, see Zeng et al. (1996) and Marrus et al. (1996).

destabilization (proteolysis?) of the more highly phosphorylated forms of TIM (Fig. 7) (Zeng et al. 1996). We assume that the phosphorylation inhibition is a secondary effect, because the light effect on TIM levels is even stronger in the late night when PER and TIM have already undergone their early night phosphorylation programs (Zeng et al. 1996) and because a qualitatively similar light effect on TIM levels is manifest in the absence of PER (Myers et al. 1996; Zeng et al. 1996).

Importantly, the short-term effects of constant light on PER and TIM in the early evening are accompanied and followed by extended RNA and protein profiles: The persistence of the RNA is presumably responsible for the persistence of the proteins (Marrus et al. 1996). Putting all of this together, we favor the parsimonious hypothesis that the light effects on transcription depend on a more primary effect on the PER-TIM system, revealing a negative feedback feature of the circuit. We therefore propose that PER, TIM, or the PER-TIM heterodimer is involved in the inhibition of *per* and *tim* transcription and that the posttranscriptional effects of light on the clock proteins result in delayed transcriptional inhibition, causing the delayed decline in RNA levels (Fig. 7).

The early evening (ZT12-17) is also the delay zone of the phase response curve (PRC), i.e., the region where a light pulse causes a phase delay. These light-pulse-mediated phase delays are presumably related to the delays caused by constant light. Indeed, light pulses in this time window not only delay PER-TIM accumulation and phosphorylation, but also delay the decline in RNA levels (Lee et al. 1996), consistent with the suggestion that the former causes the latter. Although it is unknown which protein species participates more directly in the negative feedback (PER, TIM, or the PER-TIM dimer), the more highly phosphorylated versions may be more potent transcriptional repressors or may lead to higher repressor concentrations. For example, PER monomers may be the direct repressor, and phosphorylation may decrease the stability of the PER-TIM dimer.

In LD conditions, *per* and *tim* RNA fails to cycle in *per*^{01} and *tim*^{0} flies (Hardin et al. 1990; Sehgal et al. 1994, 1995). Because there are also no short-term effects of light pulses on *per* transcription in a *per*^{01} null background (data not shown; Hardin et al. 1990), this further suggests that light cannot bypass the PER-TIM system and affect transcription directly. Results from the *Neurospora* circadian clock, the only other molec-

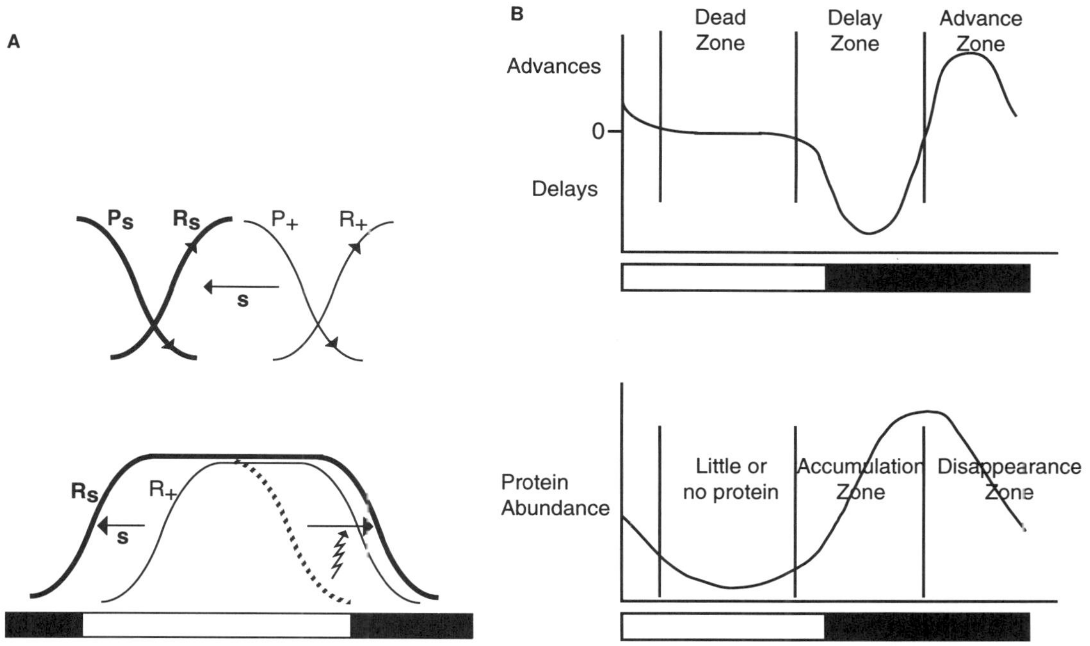

Figure 8. (*A*) Light entrainment of the per^S cycle. (*Top* panel) The early decline of per^S protein (P_S) relative to wild-type protein (P_+) leads to an early rise of per^S RNA (R_S) compared to wild-type RNA (R_+). (*Bottom* panel) The per^S RNA also falls earlier during the cycle compared to wild-type RNA in constant darkness (*dashed line* shows RNA decline). If light turns on, however, the fall of per^S RNA amount is delayed, similar to what is normally seen for wild-type RNA (R_S fall in LD shown as a *heavy line*, compared to the fall in R_+ shown as a *thin line*). (*B*) The phase response curve (PRC) and PER-TIM cycling. A PRC to light for *Drosophila* is shown in the top panel, with the phase advances indicated above 0 and the phase delays below 0. There are three zones: the dead zone, where light has little effect on the phase of activity; the delay zone, where light gives phase delays; and the advance zone, where light results in phase advances. The lower panel compares this to the pattern of PER or TIM cycling. The protein curves can also be divided into three parts, where little or no protein corresponds to the dead zone, PER and TIM accumulation corresponds to the delay zone, and the disappearance of PER and TIM corresponds to the advance zone.

ularly well characterized system, provide a different picture: Light has a potent stimulatory effect on transcription of the *frequency* gene even in the absence of FRQ gene product (Crosthwaite et al. 1995).

Constant light has an enhanced effect on the per^s genotype; namely, a reduced accumulation of PER-S relative to PER and a more pronounced inhibition of the downturn in per^s and *tim* transcription that normally occurs in the early evening (Marrus et al. 1996). This srongly supports the negative feedback hypothesis, i.e., a direct role of PER and/or TIM in transcriptional inhibition. Moreover, it explains how per^S is entrained to 24-hour cycles: The mutant advances the feedforward circuit, and light causes a counteracting inhibition of the feedback circuit (Fig. 8A). The advance is caused by a truncated protein accumulation phase and a subsequent premature per^S RNA increase. The light inhibition of the feedback circuit extends the RNA profile and, as a consequence, the protein profile, restoring them to a correct (wild-type-like) time of day, leading to 24-hour periods (Marrus et al. 1996).

More generally, the effects of light on the PER-TIM cycle explain light entrainment in the *Drosophila* system. The dark-light transition advances the cycle at ZT0 by causing TIM degradation. Light then delays the cycle until ZT12, when the light-dark transition relieves the inhibition of TIM accumulation and PER phosphorylation. The results also account for the fact that phase-shifting light pulses have three different time-dependent effects: delays in the early evening, advances late at night, and relatively little effect during much of the subjective day (Fig. 8B). (1) In the early evening, light inhibits protein accumulation, leading to phase delays. (2) Late at night, the same inhibition advances the feedforward circuit, i.e., TIM is degraded, PER monomers are released, and the next day's transcriptional cycle is advanced. (3) During much of the day (subjective day), there is little TIM and PER and therefore little or no light response. There may of course be other system components that also influence the magnitude and direction of the light response, but this scheme explains the major features of entrainment and phase resetting in *Drosophila*, suggesting that the PER-TIM heterodimer may be close to the initial light target of the circadian oscillator.

FUTURE PROSPECTS

Genetics will continue to make major contributions to the story. In the wings are several potentially exciting clock mutants (data not shown). They will probably fill some of the holes in our current *Drosophila* clock picture. These include one or more transcription factors, proteases, and kinases.

The awaited transcription factor should make a predicted connection with the PER-TIM system on the one hand and DNA on the other. The former may reveal which component (PER monomer, TIM monomer, the PER-TIM heterodimer, or an as-yet-unidentified complex) participates more directly in transcriptional inhibition. The latter may reveal which are the most direct DNA targets of the PER-TIM clock system. Although it is possible that the *per* and *tim* genes are direct targets, there is no evidence to indicate that they are not indirect targets: Circadian induction or repression of *per* and *tim* transcription may require the transcriptional induction or repression of an intermediate transcription factor. One of the newly identified *Drosophila* clock-controlled genes (CCGs) may be a transcription factor and correspond to such an intermediate (Van Gelder et al. 1995; Van Gelder and Krasnow 1996; F. Rouyer and M. Rosbash, in prep.). Alternatively, *per* and *tim* may be direct targets, and a transcription factor CCG may correspond to as-yet-undefined connections with an output pathway.

A protease or a kinase is anticipated from the light effects on TIM (Hunter-Ensor et al. 1996; Myers et al. 1996; Zeng et al. 1996) as well as the properties of different *per*–β-galactosidase fusion genes (Dembinska et al. 1997). Complex dissociation mediated by signal-dependent destabilization of one subunit is not without precedent, e.g., NF-κB/IκB (Verma et al. 1995) where IκB degradation activates NF-κB, or cyclin/cdk (Norbury and Nurse 1992; Jeffrey et al. 1995) where cyclin degradation inactivates cdk. In contrast to these examples, the biochemical mechanism of light-induced TIM degradation is completely unknown. Light might lead to the activation of a dedicated protease, or it might cause TIM modification.

A role for kinases is also indicated by the phosphorylation that PER as well as TIM undergoes. We know nothing concrete about the sites modified, the enzymes involved, or the role played by this temporally regulated phosphorylation program. As described above, phosphorylation is only one of several post-transcriptional regulatory steps experienced by the PER-TIM complex. The relevant kinase mutants or site-directed mutants at the positions of PER and TIM modification might help define the function of the phosphorylation as well as order the multiple post-transcriptional events. Mutants might also help identify which of these events contribute to the delay(s) necessary to sustain the RNA oscillations.

Defining additional clock components in the *Drosophila* system might also help resolve one of the major enigmas in the circadian field. PER, TIM, and FRQ are the only bona fide eukaryotic clock proteins. Although the identification of TIM is quite recent, the sequences of PER and FRQ have been available for years. Nonetheless, efforts in many laboratories and the explosion of sequence information from mammals have failed to reveal credible mammalian ortholog candidates. Although it is dangerous (i.e., often incorrect) to speculate from negative results, this may indicate that the core circadian clock mechanism is not conserved across vast phylogenetic distances: The circadian pacemaker may have arisen multiple times in evolution. Its similarities may therefore reflect convergent evolution and the requirement to accomplish the same tasks, e.g., entrainment to the light-dark cycle. These may be soluble in few ways and may explain the shared mechanistic features, such as a reliance on the regulation of macromolecular metabolism. Alternatively, they may reflect a common origin which is not yet apparent at the sequence level. Resolution requires the usual prescription: the identification of more clock components in a more diverse set of organisms (see King and Takahashi; Lamas et al.; both this volume). This will also lead to a much broader picture of how circadian clocks work, in the vertebrate pineal glands and suprachiasmatic nuclei as well as in *Drosophila* lateral neurons.

ACKNOWLEDGMENTS

M.R. thanks J.C. Hall for his enthusiastic and effusive introduction into the field of circadian rhythms, as well as for numerous enjoyable collaborations. M.R. also thanks all of his prior collaborators in this endeavor, the National Institutes of Health (GM-33205) and the National Science Foundation for financial support, and L.A. Monaghan for expert secretarial assistance.

REFERENCES

Aronson, B.D., K.A. Johnson, J.J. Loros, and J.C. Dunlap. 1994. Negative feedback defines a circadian clock: Autoregulation of the clock gene *frequency*. *Science* **263:** 1578.

Baylies, M.K., T.A. Bargiello, F.R. Jackson, and M.W. Young. 1987. Changes in abundance and structure of the *per* gene product can alter periodicity of the *Drosophila* clock. *Nature* **326:** 390.

Crosthwaite, S.K., J.J. Loros, and J.C. Dunlap. 1995. Light-induced resetting of a circadian clock is mediated by a rapid increase in *frequency* transcript. *Cell* **81:** 1003.

Curtin, K., Z.J. Huang, and M. Rosbash. 1995. Temporally regulated nuclear entry of the *Drosophila period* protein contributes to the circadian clock. *Neuron* **14:** 365.

Dembinska, M.E., R. Stanewsky, J.C. Hall, and M. Rosbash. 1997. Circadian cycling of a *period-lacZ* fusion protein in *Drosophila*: Evidence for an instability cycling element in PER. *J. Biol. Rhythms* (in press).

Dunlap, J.C., Q. Liu, K.A. Johnson, and J.J. Loros. 1993. Genetic and molecular dissection of the *Neurospora* clock. In *Molecular genetics of biological rhythms* (ed. M.W. Young), p. 37. Marcel Dekker, New York.

Dushay, M.S., M. Rosbash, and J.C. Hall. 1992. Mapping the *clock* rhythm mutation to the *period* locus of *Drosophila melanogaster* by germline transformation. *J. Neurogenet.* **8:** 173.

Edery, I., J.E. Rutila, and M. Rosbash. 1994a. Phase shifting of the circadian clock by induction of the *Drosophila period* protein. *Science* **263:** 237.

Edery, I., L.J. Zwiebel, M.E. Dembinska, and M. Rosbash. 1994b. Temporal phosphorylation of the *Drosophila period* protein. *Proc. Natl. Acad. Sci.* **91:** 2260.

Ewer, J., B. Frisch, M.J. Hamblen-Coyle, M. Rosbash, and J.C. Hall. 1992. Expression of the *period* clock gene within different cell types in the brain of *Drosophila* adults and mosaic analysis of these cells' influence on circadian behavioral rhythms. *J. Neurosci.* **12:** 3321.

Gekakis, N., L. Saez, A.-M. Delahaye-Brown, M.P. Myers, A. Sehgal, M.W. Young, and C.J. Weitz. 1995. Isolation of *timeless* by PER protein interactions: Defective interaction between *timeless* protein and long-period mutant PER^L. *Science* **270:** 811.

Goldbeter, A. 1995. A model for circadian oscillations in the *Drosophila period* protein (PER). *Proc. R. Soc. Lond. B Biol. Sci.* **261:** 319.

Hall, J.C. and C.P. Kyriacou. 1990. Genetics of biological rhythms in *Drosophila*. *Adv. Insect Physiol.* **22:** 221.

Hamblen, M., W.A. Zehring, C.P. Kyriacou, P. Reddy, Q. Yu, D.A. Wheeler, L.J. Zwiebel, R.J. Konopka, M. Rosbash, and J.C. Hall. 1986. Germ-line transformation involving DNA from the *period* locus in *Drosophila melanogaster*: Overlapping genomic fragments that restore circadian and ultradian rhythmicity to per^O and per^- mutants. *J. Neurogenet.* **3:** 249.

Hamblen-Coyle, M.J., D.A. Wheeler, J.E. Rutila, M. Rosbash, and J.C. Hall. 1992. Behavior of period-altered circadian rhythm mutants of *Drosophila* in light:dark cycles. *J. Insect Behav.* **5:** 417.

Hardin, P.E., J.C. Hall, and M. Rosbash. 1990. Feedback of the *Drosophila period* gene product on circadian cycling of its messenger RNA levels. *Nature* **343:** 536.

———. 1992. Circadian oscillations in *period* gene mRNA levels are transcriptionally regulated. *Proc. Natl. Acad. Sci.* **89:** 11711.

Hartwell, L.H. and T.A. Weinert. 1989. Checkpoints: Controls that ensure the order of cell cycle events. *Science* **246:** 629.

Helfrich-Forster, C. 1995. The period clock gene is expressed in central nervous system neurons which also produce a neuropeptide that reveals the projections of circadian pacemaker cells within the brain of *Drosophila melanogaster*. *Proc. Natl. Acad. Sci.* **92:** 612.

Helfrich-Forster, C. and U. Homberg. 1993. Pigment-dispersing hormone-immunoreactive neurons in the nervous system of wild-type *Drosophila melanogaster* and of several mutants with altered circadian rhythmicity. *J. Comp. Neurol.* **337:** 177.

Huang, Z.J., K. Curtin, and M. Rosbash. 1995. PER protein interactions and temperature compensation of a circadian clock in *Drosophila*. *Science* **267:** 1169.

Huang, Z.J., I. Edery, and M. Rosbash. 1993. PAS is a dimerization domain common to *Drosophila* Period and several transcription factors. *Nature* **364:** 259.

Hunter-Ensor, M., A. Ousley, and A. Sehgal. 1996. Regulation of the *Drosophila* protein *timeless* suggests a mechanism for resetting the circadian clock by light. *Cell* **84:** 677.

Jeffrey, P.D., A.A. Russo, K. Polyak, E. Gibbs, J. Hurwitz, J. Massague, and N.P. Pavletich. 1995. Mechanism of CDK activation revealed by the structure of a cyclinA-CDK2 complex. *Nature* **376:** 313.

Khalsa, S.B.S., D. Whitmore, and G.D. Block. 1992. Stopping the circadian pacemaker with inhibitors of protein synthesis. *Proc. Natl. Acad. Sci.* **89:** 10862.

Klein, D.C., R.Y. Moore, and S.M. Reppert. 1991. *Suprachiasmatic nucleus: The mind's clock.* Oxford University Press, New York.

Kondo, T., N.F. Tsinoremas, S.S. Golden, C.H. Johnson, S. Kutsuna, and M. Isjiura. 1994. Circadian clock mutants of *Cyanobacteria*. *Science* **266:** 1233.

Konopka, R.J. and S. Benzer. 1971. Clock mutants of *Drosophila melanogaster*. *Proc. Natl. Acad. Sci.* **68:** 2112.

Lee, C., V. Parikh, T. Itsukaichi, K. Bae, and I. Edery. 1996. Resetting the *Drosophila* clock by photic regulation of PER and a PER-TIM complex. *Science* **271:** 1740.

Liu, X., L. Lorenz, Q. Yu, J.C. Hall, and M. Rosbash. 1988. Spatial and temporal expression of the *period* gene in *Drosophila melanogaster*. *Genes Dev.* **2:** 228.

Liu, X., L.J. Zwiebel, D. Hinton, S. Benzer, J.C. Hall, and M. Rosbash. 1992. The *period* gene encodes a predominantly nuclear protein in adult *Drosophila*. *J. Neurosci.* **12:** 2735.

Liu, Y., N.F. Tsinoremas, C.H. Johnson, N.V. Lebedeva, S.S. Golden, M. Ishiura, and T. Kondo. 1995. Circadian orchestration of gene expression in cyanobacteria. *Genes Dev.* **9:** 1469.

Marrus, S.B., H. Zeng, and M. Rosbash. 1996. Effect of constant light and circadian entrainment of per^S flies: Evidence for light-mediated delay of the negative feedback loop in *Drosophila*. *EMBO J.* (in press).

Michel, S., M.E. Geusz, J.J. Zaritsky, and G.D. Block. 1993. Circadian rhythm in membrane conductance expressed in isolated neurons. *Science* **259:** 239.

Myers, M.P., K. Wager-Smith, A. Rothenfluh-Hilfiker, and M.W. Young. 1996. Light-induced degradation of TIMELESS and entrainment of the *Drosophila* circadian clock. *Science* **271:** 1736.

Myers, M.P., K. Wager-Smith, C.S. Wesley, M.W. Young, and A. Sehgal. 1995. Positional cloning and sequence analysis of the *Drosophila* clock gene *timeless*. *Science* **270:** 805.

Norbury, C. and P. Nurse. 1992. Animal cell cycles and their control. *Annu. Rev. Biochem.* **61:** 441.

Price, J.L., M.E. Dembinska, M.W. Young, and M. Rosbash. 1995. Suppression of PERIOD protein abundance and circadian cycling by the *Drosophila* clock mutation *timeless*. *EMBO J.* **14:** 4044.

Raju, U., K. Constantinos, M. Nuneu-Regueiro, and A. Eskin. 1991. Alteration of the phase and period of a circadian oscillator by a reversible transcription inhibitor. *Science* **253:** 673.

Reppert, S.M., D.R. Weaver, and T. Ebisawa. 1994. Cloning and characterization of a mammalian melatonin receptor that mediates reproductive and circadian responses. *Neuron* **13:** 1177.

Robertson, L.M. and J.S. Takahashi. 1988. Circadian clock in cell culture: II. In vitro photic entrainment of melatonin oscillation from dissociated chick pineal cells. *J. Neurosci.* **8:** 22.

Roenneberg, T. and D. Morse. 1993. Two circadian oscillators in one cell. *Nature* **362:** 362.

Rutila, J.E., H. Zeng, M. Le, K.D. Curtin, J.C. Hall, and M. Rosbash. 1996. The tim^{SL} mutant of the *Drosophila* rhythm gene *timeless* manifests allele-specific interactions with *period* gene mutants. *Neuron* **17:** 921.

Saunders, D.S., S.W. Gillanders, and R.D. Lewis. 1994. Light-pulse phase response curves for the locomotor activity rhythm in *Period* mutants of *Drosophila melano-*

gaster. J. Insect Physiol. **40:** 957.

Sehgal, A., J.L. Price, B. Man, and M.W. Young. 1994. Loss of circadian behavioral rhythms and *per* RNA oscillations in the *Drosophila* mutant *timeless*. *Science* **263:** 1603.

Sehgal, A., A. Rothenfluh-Hilfiker, M. Hunter-Ensor, Y. Chen, M. Myers, and M.W. Young. 1995. Circadian oscillations and autoregulation of *timeless* RNA. *Science* **270:** 808.

Siwicki, K.K., C. Eastman, G. Petersen, M. Rosbash, and J.C. Hall. 1988. Antibodies to the *period* gene product of *Drosophila* reveal diverse tissue distribution and rhythmic changes in the visual system. *Neuron* **1:** 141.

Stanewsky, R., B. Frisch, C. Brandes, M.J. Hamblen-Coyle, M. Rosbash, and J.C. Hall. 1997. Temporal and spatial expression patterns of transgenes containing increasing amounts of the *Drosophila* clock gene *period* and *lacZ* reporter: Mapping elements of the PER protein involved in circadian cycling. *J. Neurosci.* (in press).

Steller, H., K.F. Fischbach, and G.M. Rubin. 1987. *disconnected*: A locus required for neuronal pathway formation in the visual system of *Drosophila*. *Cell* **50:** 1139.

Takahashi, J.S., J.M. Kornhauser, C. Koumenis, and A. Eskin. 1993. Molecular approaches to understanding circadian oscillations. *Annu. Rev. Physiol.* **55:** 729.

Takahashi, J.S., N. Murakami, S.S. Nikaido, B.L. Pratt, and L.M. Robertson. 1989. The avian pineal, a vertebrate model system of the circadian oscillator: Cellular regulation of circadian rhythms by light, second messengers, and macromolecular synthesis. *Recent Prog. Horm. Res.* **45:** 279.

Tosini, G. and M. Menaker. 1996. Circadian rhythms in cultured mammalian retina. *Science* **272:** 419.

Tyson, J.J. 1976. Mathematical background group report. In *The molecular basis of circadian rhythms* (ed. J.W. Hastings and H.-G. Schweiger), p. 85. Abakon Verlagsgesellschaft, Berlin.

Underwood, H., R.K. Barrett, and T. Siopes. 1990. The quail's eye: A biological clock. *J. Biol. Rhythms* **5:** 257.

Van Gelder, R.N. and M.A. Krasnow. 1996. A novel circadianly expressed *Drosophila melanogaster* gene dependent on the period gene for its rhythmic expression. *EMBO J.* **15:** 1625.

Van Gelder, R.N., H. Bae, M.J. Palazzolo, and M.A. Krasnow. 1995. Extent and character of circadian gene expression in *Drosophila melanogaster*: Identification of twenty oscillating mRNAs in the fly head. *Curr. Biol.* **5:** 1424.

Verma, I.M., J.K. Stevenson, E.M. Schwarz, D. Van Antwerp, and S. Miyamoto. 1995. Rel/Nf-kB/IkB family: Intimate tales of association and dissociation. *Genes Dev.* **9:** 2723.

Vosshall, L.B. and M.W. Young. 1995. Circadian rhythms in *Drosophila* can be driven by *period* expression in a restricted group of central brain cells. *Neuron* **15:** 345.

Vosshall, L.B., J.L. Price, A. Sehgal, L. Saez, and M.W. Young. 1994. Specific block in nuclear localization of period protein by a second clock mutation, *timeless*. *Science* **263:** 1606.

Welsh, D.K., D.E. Logothetis, M. Meister, and S.M. Reppert. 1995. Individual neurons dissociated from rat suprachiasmatic nucleus express independently phased circadian firing rhythms. *Neuron* **14:** 697.

Zeng, H., P.E. Hardin, and M. Rosbash. 1994. Constitutive overexpression of the *Drosophila period* protein inhibits *period* mRNA cycling. *EMBO J.* **13:** 3590.

Zeng, H., Z. Qian, M.P. Myers, and M. Rosbash. 1996. A light-entrainment mechanism for the *Drosophila* circadian clock. *Nature* **380:** 129.

Zerr, D.M., J.C. Hall, M. Rosbash, and K.K. Siwicki. 1990. Circadian fluctuations of *period* protein immunoreactivity in the *CNS* and the visual system of *Drosophila*. *J. Neurosci.* **10:** 2749.

Zwiebel, L.J., P.E. Hardin, X. Liu, J.C. Hall, and M. Rosbash. 1991. A post-transcriptional mechanism contributes to circadian cycling of *per*-β-galactosidase fusion protein. *Proc. Natl. Acad. Sci.* **88:** 3882.

Molecular Anatomy of a Light-sensitive Circadian Pacemaker in *Drosophila*

M.W. YOUNG, K. WAGER-SMITH, L. VOSSHALL,[1] L. SAEZ, AND M.P. MYERS
National Science Foundation Science and Technology Center for Biological Timing, Howard Hughes Medical Institute, and Laboratory of Genetics, The Rockefeller University, New York, New York 10021

Adult *Drosophila* produce locomotor activity rhythms with strain-specific periods close to 24 hours. These circadian behavioral rhythms resemble mammalian sleep/wake cycles; the phase of such a rhythm can be set by environmental cycles of light and dark or temperature, but the rhythm persists under constant environmental conditions. In sustained darkness, pulses of light advance or delay the rhythm in a fashion that is dependent on the time of light administration with respect to the phase of the behavioral cycle.

The generation of circadian rhythms in *Drosophila* requires the activity of two genes, *period* (*per*, Konopka and Benzer 1971) and *timeless* (*tim*, Sehgal et al. 1994; Vosshall et al. 1994). Loss of either gene abolishes circadian rhythmicity, and missense mutation of either gene can alter period length (Konopka and Benzer 1971; Baylies et al. 1987, 1992; Yu et al. 1987; Rutila et al. 1992, 1996; Sehgal et al. 1994; A. Rothenfluh-Hilfiker and M.W. Young, unpubl.). The period length of *Drosophila*'s circadian rhythms is also sensitive to changes in the dosage of these genes. Using transgenic flies, Baylies et al. (1987) showed a uniform relationship for *per* RNA titer and period. Lowering the dose of *per* lengthened circadian rhythms. For example, a 20-fold reduction in *per* RNA was associated with a lengthening of period to 37–38 hours.

Transgenic flies expressing *per* in restricted regions of the brain have identified pacemaker cells that promote circadian behavioral rhythms (Ewer et al. 1992; Frisch et al. 1994; Vosshall and Young 1995). In these and other central brain cells, and in photoreceptor cells composing the eyes, the amounts of PER and TIM proteins fluctuate with a circadian rhythm (Siwicki et al. 1988; Edery et al. 1994; Hunter-Ensor et al. 1996; Myers et al. 1996; Zeng et al. 1996). These oscillations occur with similar phases (Siwicki et al. 1988; Edery et al. 1994; Hunter-Ensor et al. 1996; Myers et al. 1996; Zeng et al. 1996) such that peak levels of the PER and TIM proteins are observed late at night. *per* and *tim* mRNAs also accumulate with the same circadian rhythm (Hardin et al. 1990; Sehgal et al. 1995), but the phase of RNA accumulation precedes that of protein accumulation by 4–6 hours. Highest RNA levels are observed late in the day and into the early evening.

A functional interaction between these genes was originally revealed by molecular studies of *per* RNA and PER protein in *tim* mutants (Sehgal et al. 1994; Vosshall et al. 1994). Circadian cycles of *per* mRNA accumulation were eliminated by arrhythmic (null) mutations of *tim* (Sehgal et al. 1994). However, a key observation was that the product of *tim* appeared to be a posttranslational regulator of PER; null mutations of *tim* (*tim*^{0}) blocked nuclear localization of the PER protein (Vosshall et al. 1994; see below). Evidently, nuclear localization of PER is a control point in the circadian system; without *tim*'s regulation of PER's subcellular distribution, oscillations in transcription are no longer possible (Vosshall et al. 1994). In addition to blocking PER's nuclear entry, *tim* null mutations also appear to destabilize PER. Very low levels of the PER protein accumulate in the cytoplasm of *tim*^{0} flies (Vosshall et al. 1994; Price et al. 1995).

Positional cloning of *tim* (Myers et al. 1995) allowed the mechanism of this *per*/*tim* interaction to be resolved. The PER and TIM proteins are physical partners, binding to each other, in part, through PER's PAS domain (Gekakis et al. 1995; Saez and Young 1996), a protein interaction sequence supporting dimerization of several previously characterized proteins (Huang et al. 1993). The proteins bind to each other in vitro, in yeast, and in flies (Gekakis et al. 1995; Lee et al. 1996; Saez and Young 1996; Zeng et al. 1996). Moreover, this binding is highly specific, allowing efficient selection of cDNAs encoding TIM from *Drosophila* total head cDNA libraries using PER protein baits in yeast two-hybrid screens (Gekakis et al. 1995). Immunocytochemical studies have shown that TIM proteins do not translocate to nuclei in *per* null mutants. Thus, PER and TIM must both be present in a cell to afford nuclear localization of either protein (Hunter-Ensor et al. 1996; Myers et al. 1996). However, unlike PER, TIM is stable in the cytoplasm when its partner protein is missing (Myers et al. 1996).

Figure 1 presents a model for generation of circadian rhythms in *Drosophila* in which cycles of *per* and *tim* transcription are regulated by alternating cycles of nuclear localization of a PER/TIM protein complex. Our model is based on the following observa-

[1]Present address: Center for Neurobiology and Behavior, Howard Hughes Medical Institute, Columbia University, 701 W. 168th Street, New York, New York 10032.

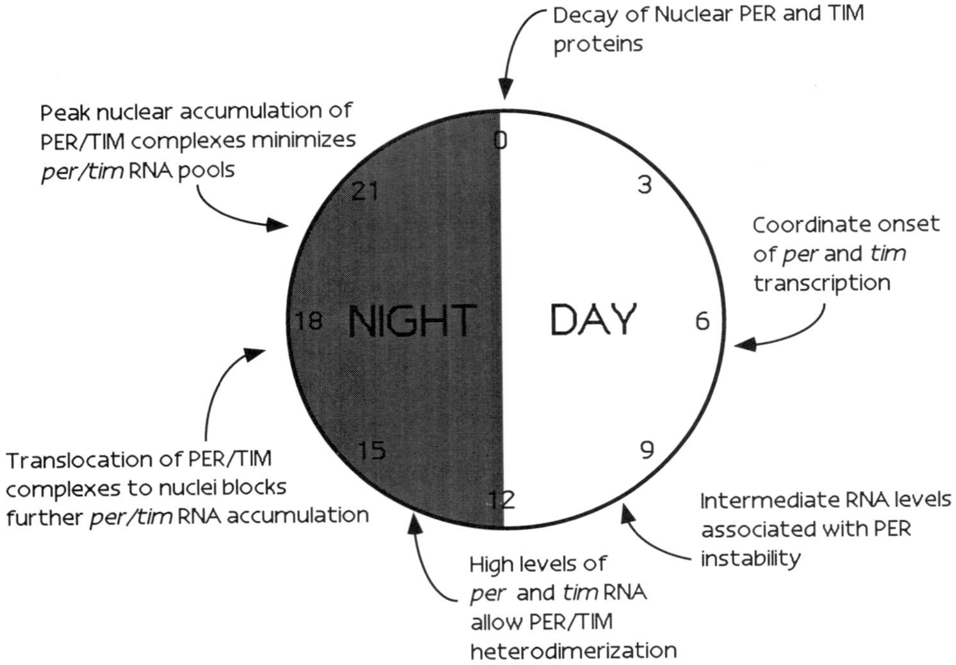

Figure 1. Physical interaction of PER and TIM produces circadian cycles in feedback regulation (see text).

tions and interpretations: (1) Several studies have suggested that, on assembly and nuclear localization, the PER/TIM complex suppresses *per* and *tim* transcription (discussed below). (2) As PER protein accumulation and nuclear localization are suppressed in *tim*^{0} mutants (Vosshall et al. 1994; Price et al. 1995), and the TIM and PER proteins bind to each other in vitro, in vivo, and in yeast, heterodimerization of the proteins is likely to be required for nuclear translocation and stabilization of PER. Because TIM accumulates in the cytoplasm of *per*^{0} mutants (Hunter-Ensor et al. 1996; Myers et al. 1996), heterodimerization is probably required for TIM nuclear localization. (3) *tim* RNA expression cycles, so PER stabilization should be restricted to only some times of day. (4) Given the instability of PER in the absence of TIM, PER proteins would accumulate in conjunction with *per* mRNA only if TIM proteins were amassed prior to *per* transcription. Because *per* and *tim* RNAs accumulate with the same phase, delays in PER accumulation and nuclear localization of PER/TIM complexes are expected, probably reflecting times of PER/TIM heterodimer formation. (5) If high levels of PER and TIM protein suppress *per* and *tim* expression, cycles in this regulation will result from separate temporal phases of *per* and *tim* RNA accumulation and PER/TIM nuclear localization. In the absence of a mechanism supporting such delays, feedback control would lead to constitutive gene and protein synthesis, albeit at intermediate levels, rather than to clock-like oscillations of RNA and protein as observed.

PER AND TIM MONOMERS ARE RETAINED IN THE CYTOPLASM

Vosshall et al. (1994) found that proteins composed of the amino-terminal half of PER (a.a. 1–636) fused to β-galactosidase translocated to brain and photoreceptor nuclei in wild-type, but not in *tim*^{0} flies. The fusion protein was expressed in the correct tissues of the head in *tim*^{0} flies but was retained in the cytoplasm (Fig. 2) (Vosshall et al. 1994). Western blots showed no effect of the *tim*^{0} mutation on the level of the fusion protein produced in these flies (Vosshall et al. 1994). In contrast, PER-β-gal fusion proteins lacking PER amino acids 95–529 were nuclear in *tim*^{0} flies (Vosshall et al. 1994). Two additional reporter genes have been constructed for analysis of expression patterns in wild-type and *tim*^{0} mutant backgrounds. The first of these reporters encoded PER amino acids 1–212 fused to β-gal and was transported to nuclei in both *tim*$^+$ and *tim*^{0} flies (data not shown). The second, a fusion protein, composed of PER 1-515 followed by β-gal, moved to nuclei in a *tim*$^+$ background but was cytoplasmic in *tim*^{0} flies (data not shown). Thus, a 303-amino-acid region (between amino acids 212 and 515, and including PAS) contains sequences promoting cytoplasmic accumulation. This segment of PER has been shown to support TIM binding in yeast and in vitro (Gekakis et al. 1995; Saez and Young 1996).

Consistent with the behavior of PER-β-gal fusion proteins in transgenic flies, cultured *Drosophila* cells (Schneider line 2, S2) show cytoplasmic accumulation

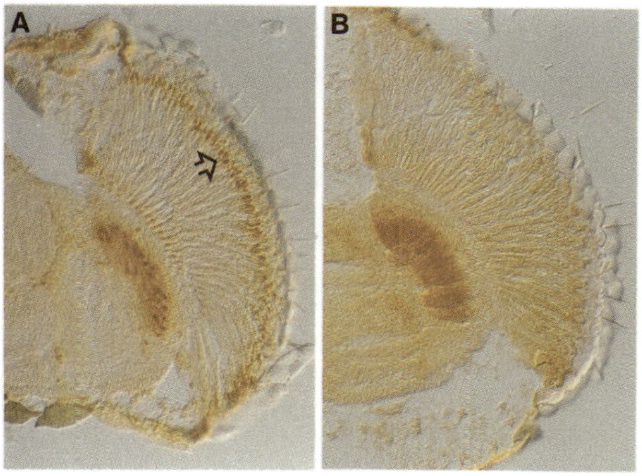

Figure 2. Nuclear localization of a PER reporter protein is blocked by the *tim*⁰ mutation. Transgenic (*A*) *tim*⁺ or (*B*) *tim*⁰ mutants that express a PER-β-galactosidase fusion protein were stained with antibody to β-gal. Open arrowhead (*A*) marks PER accumulation in nuclei of photoreceptor cells in the wild-type eye. No reactivity is observed in photoreceptor nuclei in *tim*⁰ mutants, but intense cytoplasmic staining can be seen in the elongated photoreceptor cells (*B*). PER amino acids 1–636 are present at the amino terminus of the β-gal fusion protein (for methods, see Vosshall et al. 1994).

of full-length PER proteins when transfected with *per* genomic or cDNA (Saez and Young 1996). Full-length TIM proteins, which fail to translocate to nuclei in *per*⁰ flies, also accumulate in the cytoplasm of *tim*-transfected S2 cells (Saez and Young 1996). S2 cells produce no detectable PER or TIM prior to transfection (Saez and Young 1996). When *per* and *tim* are coexpressed in S2 cells, both proteins are translocated to nuclei. This suggests that in the cultured cells and in vivo, nuclear translocation depends on physical association of the PER and TIM proteins (Saez and Young 1996). The results also show that no other clock proteins are required for nuclear localization.

Deletion studies of PER proteins expressed in S2 cells show that, as predicted from work with transgenic flies, a sequence near PAS inhibits PER nuclear accumulation (Saez and Young 1996). A sequence inhibiting TIM nuclear localization was also revealed near the TIM carboxyl terminus. Protein-binding studies indicate that PER sequences that inhibit PER nuclear translocation form a site for physical interaction with TIM. In fact, at least two binding sites on each protein mediate PER/TIM dimerization (Saez and Young 1996). Thus, formation of PER/TIM complexes is restricted to the cytoplasm by binding and localization activities carried on both proteins.

A consequence of this requirement for cytoplasmic assembly of PER/TIM heterodimers is that factors affecting rates of PER and TIM synthesis and accumulation should affect timing of nuclear localization. Aspects of PER regulation in *tim*⁰ flies may be especially important in this regard: Monomeric PER proteins appear quite unstable when restricted to the cytoplasm of brain and photoreceptor cells in *tim*⁰ flies (Vosshall et al. 1994; Price et al. 1995). This suggests that PER is unstable when not complexed with TIM. In wild-type flies, as titers of *tim* and *per* RNA and TIM protein rise, rates of nuclear translocation may become largely dependent on the half-life of monomeric PER proteins. For flies maintained in a light/dark cycle (such as the solar day), daytime levels of PER and TIM will remain low due to TIM's light sensitivity (below) and PER's dependence on TIM. After sunset, dark-dependent stabilization of TIM should be followed by TIM-dependent stabilization of PER.

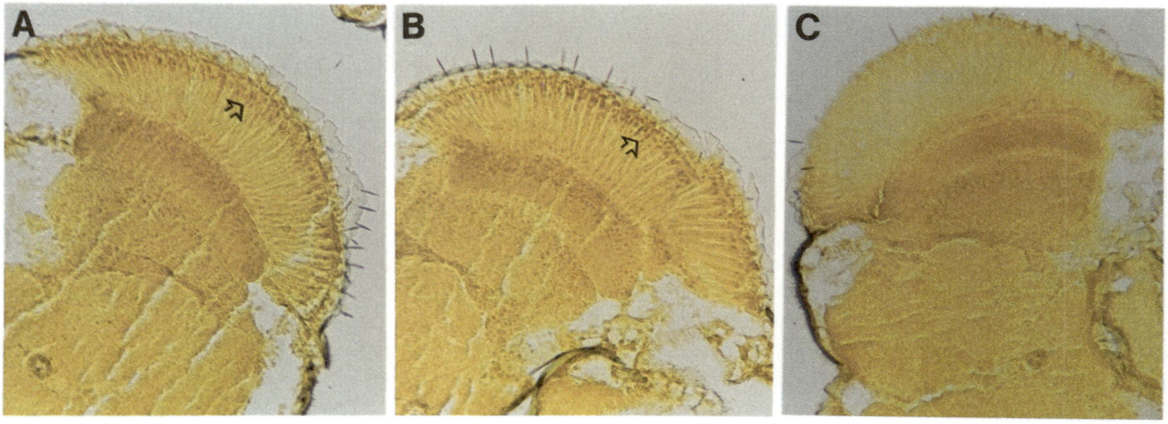

Figure 3. TIM proteins are degraded following a brief exposure to light. Immunocytochemical detection of TIM proteins in photoreceptor nuclei (*open arrowheads*) of control (non-light-pulsed) flies at CT 20.5 (*A*) and CT 22 (*B*). A 10-min light pulse (~8,000 lux) was administered to flies at CT 16. Flies were returned to constant darkness and collected for immunocytochemical detection of TIM at CT 21 (*C*). Note absence of TIM staining. The light pulse produces a phase delay in the behavioral rhythm of about 4 hr. For methods, see Myers et al. (1996).

LIGHT INDUCES RAPID LOSS OF TIM

The model presented in Figure 1 describes how a self-sustained molecular rhythm can be produced in constant darkness, but it does not provide an explanation for the rapid alignment of molecular and behavioral rhythms with the phase of environmental rhythms such as 24-hour cycles of light and dark. In wild-type flies, constant light induces arrhythmicity and low levels of PER as in *tim*^{0} mutants (Price et al. 1995). Because *tim*^{0} mutants produced indistinguishable levels of PER proteins in light/dark cycles (LD), constant darkness, and constant light, it was suggested that constant light might eliminate circadian rhythms in wild-type flies by reducing an activity dependent on *tim* (Price et al. 1995). The level of TIM protein was subsequently investigated in *per*^{0} fly heads (Myers et al. 1996; Zeng et al. 1996). TIM was expressed at fairly high levels in *per*^{0} flies reared in constant darkness, but the level of TIM was found to oscillate in *per*^{0} flies when they were exposed to light/dark cycles. Since earlier work had clearly shown that *tim* RNA levels do not oscillate in *per*^{0} mutants (Sehgal et al. 1995), the results suggested that the TIM protein is lost when flies are exposed to light.

This phenomenon was investigated more fully by exposing *per*^{0} flies to 1-hour pulses of light, followed by a recovery period in constant darkness. Western blot analysis showed that TIM levels dropped rapidly after the light treatment and began to rise within the first hour after return to darkness (Myers et al. 1996). The rapidity of this response was further indicated by measuring TIM protein amounts immediately following a 15-minute pulse of light. Substantial loss of TIM was again observed (Myers et al. 1996). As shown in Figure 3, this sensitivity to light is also readily detectable in immunocytochemical studies of TIM proteins in the eyes and brains of wild-type flies (data in Fig. 3C show response to a 10-min light pulse). The data derived from *per*^{0} mutants indicate that there exists a mechanism for the light-induced degradation of TIM protein that does not require PER, and thus, by definition, is clock-independent (Myers et al. 1996).

These and related observations (Hunter-Ensor et al. 1996; Lee et al. 1996) suggested a role for TIM in light-dependent entrainment of the *Drosophila* clock. Pulses of light given to wild-type flies during the night portion of their behavioral cycle can advance or delay the behavioral rhythm. Studies of *Drosophila melanogaster* show resetting of the locomotor activity rhythm by such light pulses within 24 hours (cf. Myers et al. 1996). It was found that light pulses in the early evening produce a delay in the phase of TIM diminution within the current cycle of the molecular rhythm, whereas light pulses delivered late at night (1–3 hr before dawn) produce a monotonic advance in the phase of TIM diminution within the current cycle of the molecular rhythm (Myers et al. 1996). Because TIM's light-dependent degradation is clock-independent (occurs in *per*^{0} flies), and the phase of the TIM protein rhythm is reset within hours of exposure to light, TIM's response to light appears to be at the core of the *Drosophila* entrainment mechanism (Myers et al. 1996; see also below).

LIGHT-DEPENDENT DEGRADATION OF TIM RESETS *per* AND *tim* MRNA RHYTHMS

What is the function of the PER/TIM complex once transported to the nucleus? Because null mutations of *per* and *tim* abolish rhythms of *per* and *tim* mRNA synthesis (Hardin et al. 1990; Sehgal et al. 1995), and constitutive expression of PER (from the rhodopsin promoter) suppresses transcriptional cycling of the endogenous gene in the adult eye (Zeng et al. 1994), it has been suggested that the PER/TIM complex may contribute to an autoregulatory loop affecting *per* and *tim* transcription (Sehgal et al. 1995; Hunter-Ensor et al. 1996; Lee et al. 1996; Myers et al. 1996; Zeng et al. 1996). One way to test this model would be to acutely perturb PER or TIM protein levels posttranscriptionally and to measure any derived effect on *per* and *tim* RNA levels. A tool for carrying out such an experiment emerged with the discovery that TIM protein is rapidly eliminated in vivo by exposure to light. Because *per* and *tim* RNA levels in the head undergo a rhythmic oscillation in flies entrained to a normal cycle of 12 hours of light and 12 hours of dark (LD 12:12), we asked how a pulse of light delivered either before the declining phase of the RNA curve, or before the rising phase, would affect subsequent RNA levels. Since TIM proteins are degraded in response to light, secondary changes in *per* and *tim* mRNA synthesis are expected following the light pulse if PER/TIM complexes regulate transcription.

Prior studies showed that *tim* RNA levels do not oscillate in *per*^{0} or *tim*^{0} flies, even when maintained in LD cycles (Sehgal et al. 1995; Hunter-Ensor et al. 1996). As predicted from those results, Figure 4 indicates no acute effect of light on either *per* or *tim* RNA levels in wild-type flies pulsed with light 2 hours after sunset (ZT14), which produces behavioral delays, or 1 hour prior to expected dawn (ZT23), which produces behavioral advances. Figure 4 does, however, show an elevation relative to control in *tim* and *per* RNA levels following times of TIM degradation. This elevation in RNA level is seen 4–5 hours after the light pulse and is therefore distinct from the timing of TIM degradation, which was previously shown to be completed within 1 hour, whether TIM loss was induced by an advancing or delaying light pulse (Myers et al. 1996). A similar elevation in *per* RNA level following exposure to light was recently reported by Lee et al. (1996). Together, the results suggest that TIM/PER complexes repress both *per* and *tim* transcription. Whether the PER/TIM complex regulates transcription by directly binding DNA or by indirect means is unknown.

Figure 4 also shows that as a consequence of the elevated *per* and *tim* RNA levels, the phases of *tim* and

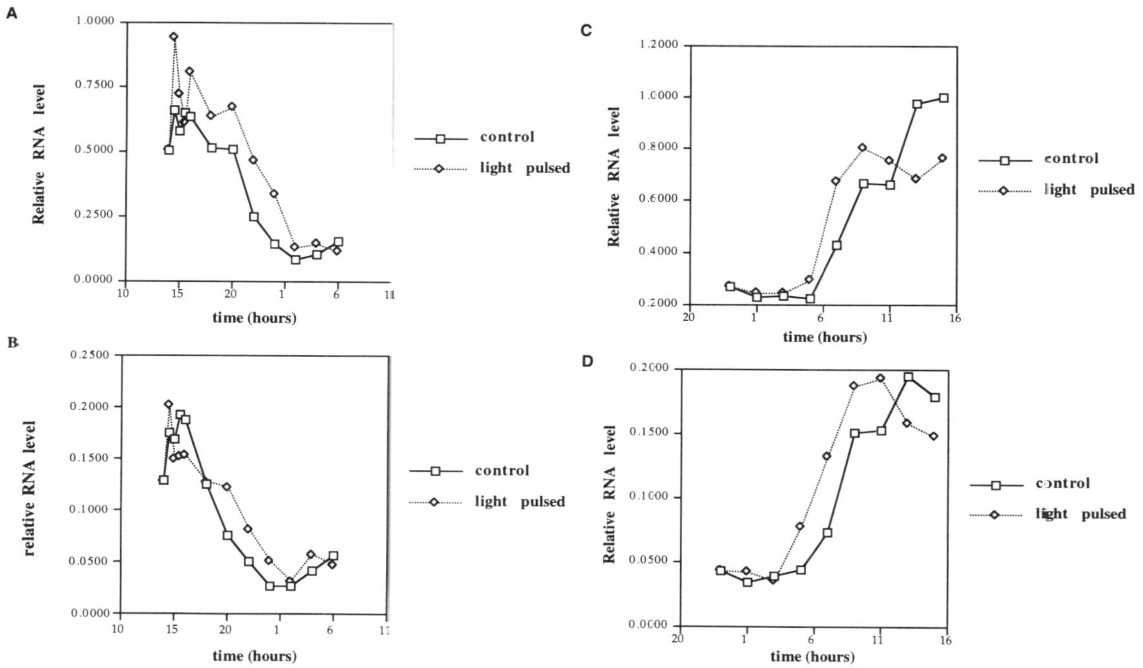

Figure 4. Light pulses lead to elevated *per* and *tim* RNA levels. Relative RNA levels for control flies (*solid line*) or flies which received a 1-hr light pulse (*dotted line*). (*A*) *tim* RNA, CT 14 light pulse. (*B*) *per* RNA, CT 14 light pulse. (*C*) *tim* RNA, CT 23 light pulse. (*D*) *per* RNA, CT 23 light pulse. Numbers on the X axis indicate circadian time (CT0= subjective lights on; CT12= subjective lights off in constant darkness). Canton S flies were entrained for several days to cycles of 12 hr light and 12 hr dark (LD 12:12). Records begin at CT 14 (*A*, *B*) or CT 23 (*C*, *D*) in the final LD cycle. At CT 12 in the last LD cycle, the lights were turned off for the remainder of the experiment. Each point is the mean of six RNase protection assays representing three separate experiments with all protection assays performed twice. RNA was derived from adult heads. *per* and *tim* values were normalized to tubulin (for methods, see Sehgal et al. 1995).

per RNA diminution are delayed by light pulses given at ZT14, and the phase of RNA accumulation is advanced by pulses supplied at ZT23. Such phase shifts are consistent with a previously suggested mechanism for the resetting of the TIM protein rhythm by light (Myers et al. 1996). For light pulses in the early evening (e.g., ZT14), rapid elimination of TIM is followed by resynthesis of the protein from an existing *tim* RNA pool that is high at that time of day (Fig. 1) (Myers et al. 1996). Because the decline in the RNA pool is delayed by extended RNA synthesis that resulted from transient loss of TIM, resynthesis of TIM protein continues with a new and delayed phase. For light pulses prior to dawn (ZT23), TIM is again rapidly degraded, but the existing *tim* RNA pool is low (Fig. 1) (Myers et al. 1996). TIM cannot be replaced in the current molecular cycle, but advanced protein synthesis occurs in the following day's cycle due to prematurely rising *tim* and *per* RNA pools (Fig. 4C,D).

Our results suggest that light-induced degradation of TIM protein causes an elevation of *per* and *tim* RNA levels. Figure 4 demonstrates that stimulation of *tim* and *per* RNA levels accompanies both advancing and delaying light pulses, and conforms to studies that indicated complete resetting of *D. melanogaster* behavioral rhythms within a single circadian cycle (cf. Myers et al. 1996). An important feature of this mechanism is that phases of PER and TIM protein synthesis appear to be coordinately reset by all light pulses. This would move both central components of the pacemaker mechanism to the new phase. The findings support a model in which PER and TIM function as negative transcriptional regulators, probably as a PER/TIM molecular complex.

ACKNOWLEDGMENTS

This work was supported by the National Science Foundation Science and Technology Center for Biological Timing and the Howard Hughes Medical Institute. M.W.Y. is an investigator in the Howard Hughes Medical Institute. L.V. was partially supported by National Research Service Awards training grant GM-07982-09.

REFERENCES

Baylies, M. K., T.A. Bargiello, F.R. Jackson, and M.W. Young. 1987. Changes in abundance of the *per* gene product can affect periodicity of the *Drosophila* clock. *Nature* **326:** 390.

Baylies, M.K., L.B. Vosshall, A. Sehgal, and M.W. Young.

1992. New short period mutations of the *Drosophila* clock gene *per*. *Neuron* **9:** 575.

Edery, I., L.J. Zwiebel, M.E. Dembinska, and M. Rosbash. 1994. Temporal phosphorylation of the *Drosophila* period protein. *Proc. Natl. Acad. Sci.* **91:** 2260.

Ewer, J., B. Frisch, M.J. Hamblen-Coyle, M. Rosbash, and J.C. Hall. 1992. Expression of the *period* clock gene within different cell types in the brain of *Drosophila* adults and mosaic analysis of these cells' influence on circadian behavioral rhythms. *J. Neurosci.* **12:** 3321.

Frisch, B., P.E. Hardin, M.J. Hamblen-Coyle, M. Rosbash, and J.C. Hall. 1994. A promoterless *period* gene mediates behavioral rhythmicity and cyclical per expression in a restricted subset of the *Drosophila* nervous system. *Neuron* **12:** 555.

Gekakis, N., L. Saez, A.-M. Delahaye-Brown, M.P. Myers, A. Sehgal, M.W. Young, and C.J. Weitz. 1995. Isolation of *timeless* by PER protein interaction: Defective interaction between *timeless* protein and long-period mutant Per^L. *Science* **270:** 811.

Hardin, P.E., J.C. Hall, and M. Rosbash. 1990. Feedback of the *Drosophila period* gene product on circadian cycling of its messenger RNA levels. *Nature* **343:** 536.

Huang, Z.J., I. Edery, and M. Rosbash. 1993. PAS is a dimerization domain common to *Drosophila* period and several transcription factors. *Nature* **364:** 259.

Hunter-Ensor, M., A. Ousley, and A. Sehgal. 1996. Regulation of *Drosophila* protein *timeless* suggests a mechanism for resetting the circadian clock by light. *Cell* **84:** 677.

Konopka, R.J. and S. Benzer. 1971. Clock mutants of *Drosophila melanogaster*. *Proc. Natl. Acad. Sci.* **68:** 2112.

Lee, C., V. Parikh, T. Itsukaichi, K. Bae, and I. Edery. 1996. Resetting the *Drosophila* clock by photic regulation of PER and PER-TIM complex. *Science* **271:** 1740.

Myers, M.P., K. Wager-Smith, A. Rothenfluh-Hilfiker, and M.W. Young. 1996. Light-induced degradation of TIMELESS and entrainment of the *Drosophila* circadian clock. *Science* **271:** 1736.

Myers, M.P., K. Wager-Smith, C.S. Wesley, M.W. Young, and A. Sehgal. 1995. Positional cloning and sequence analysis of the *Drosophila* clock gene, *timeless*. *Science* **270:** 805.

Price, J.L., M.A. Dembinska, M.W. Young, and M. Rosbash. 1995. Suppression of PERIOD protein abundance and circadian cycling by the *Drosophila* clock mutation *timeless*. *EMBO J.* **14:** 4044.

Rutila, J.E., I. Edery, J.C. Hall, and M. Rosbash. 1992. The analysis of new short-period circadian rhythm mutants suggests features of *D. melanogaster period* gene function. *J. Neurogenet.* **8:** 101.

Rutila, J.E., H. Zeng, L. Myai, K.D. Curtin, J.C. Hall, and M. Rosbash. 1996. The tim^{SL} mutant of the *Drosophila* rhythm gene *timeless* manifests allele-specific interactions with period gene mutants. *Neuron* (in press).

Saez, L. and M.W. Young. 1996. Regulated nuclear localization of the *Drosophila* clock proteins PERIOD and TIMELESS. *Neuron* (in press).

Sehgal, A., J.L. Price, B. Man, and M.W. Young. 1994. Loss of circadian behavioral rhythms and *per* RNA oscillations in the *Drosophila* mutant timeless. *Science* **263:** 1603

Sehgal, A., A. Rothenfluh-Hilfiker, M. Hunter-Ensor, Y. Chen, M.P. Myers, and M.W. Young. 1995. Rhythmic expression of *timeless:* A basis for promoting circadian cycles in *period* gene autoregulation. *Science* **270:** 808.

Siwicki, K.K., C. Eastman, G. Petersen, M. Rosbash, and J.C. Hall. 1988. Antibodies to the *period* gene product of *Drosophila* reveal diverse tissue distribution and rhythmic changes in the visual system. *Neuron* **1:** 141.

Vosshall, L.B. and M.W. Young. 1995. Circadian rhythms in *Drosophila* can be driven by *period* expression in a restricted group of central brain cells. *Neuron* **15:** 345.

Vosshall, L.B., J. Price, A. Sehgal, L. Saez, and M. Young. 1994. Block in nuclear localization of *period* protein by a second clock mutation, *timeless*. *Science* **263:** 1606.

Yu, Q., Y. Jacquier, Y. Citri, M. Hamblen, J.C. Hall, and M. Rosbash. 1987. Molecular mapping of point mutations in the *period* gene that stop or speed up biological clocks in *Drosophila melanogaster*. *Proc. Natl. Acad. Sci.* **84:** 784.

Zeng , H., P.E. Hardin, and M. Rosbash. 1994. Constitutive overexpression of the *Drosophila period* protein inhibits *period* mRNA cycling. *EMBO J.* **13:** 3590.

Zeng, H., Z. Qian, M.P. Myers, and M. Rosbash. 1996. A light-entrainment mechanism for the *Drosophila* circadian clock. *Nature* **380:** 129.

Rhythmic Transcription and Autoregulatory Loops: Nuclear *Pacemaker* CREM

M. LAMAS, E. LALLI, N.S. FOULKES, AND P. SASSONE-CORSI
Institut de Génétique et de Biologie Moléculaire et Cellulaire, Illkirch-Strasbourg, 67404 France

An important step forward in the study of transcription factors has been the discovery that many constitute final targets of specific signal transduction pathways. The two major signal transduction systems are those including cAMP and diacylglycerol (DAG) as secondary messengers (Nishizuka 1986). Each pathway is also characterized by specific protein kinases (protein kinase A [PKA] and protein kinase C [PKC], respectively) and its ultimate target DNA control element (cAMP-responsive element [CRE] and TPA-responsive element [TRE], respectively). Although initially characterized as distinct systems, accumulating evidence points toward extensive cross-talk between these two pathways (Cambier et al. 1987; Yoshimasa et al. 1987; Masquilier and Sassone-Corsi 1992).

Intracellular levels of cAMP are regulated primarily by adenylyl cyclase. This enzyme is in turn modulated by various extracellular stimuli mediated by receptors and their interaction with G proteins (McKnight et al. 1988). cAMP binds cooperatively to two sites on the regulatory subunits of PKA, releasing the active catalytic subunits (Roesler et al. 1988; Lalli and Sassone-Corsi 1994). These are translocated from cytoplasmic and Golgi complex anchoring sites and phosphorylate a number of cytoplasmic and nuclear proteins on serines in the context X-Arg-Arg-X-Ser-X. In the nucleus, PKA-mediated phosphorylation ultimately influences the transcriptional regulation of various genes through distinct, cAMP-inducible promoter-responsive sites (Ziff 1990; Lalli and Sassone-Corsi 1994).

RESULTS AND DISCUSSION

Coupling Transcription to Signal Transduction

The consensus CRE is constituted by the 8-bp palindromic sequence 5′-TGACGTCA-3′. Several genes which are regulated by a variety of endocrine stimuli contain similar sequences in their promoter regions although at different positions (Lalli and Sassone-Corsi 1994). The first CRE-binding factor to be characterized was CREB (CRE-binding protein; Hoeffler et al. 1988), but subsequently at least ten additional CRE-binding-factor cDNAs have been cloned, obtained by screening a variety of cDNA expression libraries (Hai et al. 1989; Foulkes et al. 1991). All these proteins belong to the bZip transcription factor class.

The different CRE-binding factors are able to heterodimerize with each other but only in certain combinations. A "dimerization code" exists which seems to be a property of the leucine zipper structure of each factor. Some CRE-binding factors are able to heterodimerize with Fos and Jun, and this may change the specific affinity of binding to a CRE with respect to a Fos-Jun binding site (Hai and Curran 1991). This property resides in the similarity between the CRE (TGACGTCA) and TRE (TGACTCA) sequences (Sassone-Corsi et al. 1990) and demonstrates the versatility of the transcriptional response to signal transduction.

There are both activators and repressors of cAMP-responsive transcription. Some alternatively spliced CREM isoforms act as antagonists of cAMP-induced transcription (Foulkes et al. 1991). The inducible cAMP early repressor (ICER) product deserves special mention since it is generated from an alternative promoter of the CREM gene and is responsible for its early response inducibility which is unique among CRE-binding factors (Molina et al. 1993; Stehle et al. 1993).

Activation by Phosphorylation

The characterization of the transcriptional activators CREB and CREM (Gonzalez and Montminy 1989; Foulkes et al. 1992) has helped the elucidation of the molecular mechanisms involved in transcriptional activation. These factors contain a transcriptional activation domain which is divided into two independent regions (Lalli and Sassone-Corsi 1994). The first, known as the phosphorylation box (P-box), contains several consensus phosphorylation sites for various kinases, such as PKA, PKC, p34cdc2, glycogen synthase kinase-3, and casein kinases (CK) I and II (Gonzalez and Montminy 1989; Lee et al. 1990; de Groot et al. 1993a,b). The second region flanks the P-box and is constituted by domains rich in glutamine residues (Lalli and Sassone-Corsi 1994).

Upon activation of the adenylyl cyclase pathway, a serine residue at position 133 of CREB and at position 117 of CREM is phosphorylated by PKA (Gonzalez and Montminy 1989; de Groot et al. 1993b). The major effect of phosphorylation is to convert CREB and CREM into powerful transcriptional activators. Within the P-box, Ser-133/117 is located in a region of about 50 amino acids containing an abundance of phosphorylatable serines and acidic residues which was shown to be essential for *trans*-activation by CREB and CREM (Lee et al. 1990; de Groot et al. 1993b).

Interestingly, in PC12 cells, increases in the levels of intracellular Ca^{++} caused by membrane depolarization have been shown to induce the phosphorylation of Ser-133 in CREB and a concomitant activation of c-*fos* gene expression mediated by a CRE in the promoter (Sassone-Corsi et al. 1988a,b; Sheng et al. 1990). Although Ca^{++}-dependent CamK was shown to be able to phosphorylate Ser-133 in vitro (Dash et al. 1991), the in vivo significance remains unclear, since PKA also seems to be necessary for c-*fos* induction mediated by Ca^{++} influx in PC12 cells (Ginty et al. 1991).

An important finding that reveals the complexity of the transcriptional response elicited by these factors concerns the mitogen-induced p70 S6 kinase, which phosphorylates and activates CREM (de Groot et al. 1994). This finding implicates $p70^{s6k}$, a kinase generally considered cytoplasmic, in the mitogenic response also at the nuclear level. Interestingly, since CREM and other factors of the family represent the final targets of the cAMP pathway, these results show that they may also act as effectors of converging signaling systems and possibly as mediators of pathway cross-talk (de Groot et al. 1994).

Interaction with Coactivator CBP

The two domains flanking the P-box contain about three times more glutamine residues than in the remainder of the protein in both CREB and CREM. Glutamine-rich domains have been characterized in other factors, such as AP-2 and Sp1 (Williams et al. 1988; Courey and Tjian 1989), as transcriptional activation domains. The current notion is that they constitute surfaces of the protein that can interact with other components of the transcriptional machinery. Indeed, further steps toward an understanding of the mechanism of action of the P-box have come with the identification of a 265K, 2441-amino-acid protein, CBP (CREB-binding protein), that is able to interact specifically with the phosphorylated CREB P-box domain (Chrivia et al. 1993). The CBP sequence reveals two zinc finger domains, a glutamine-rich domain at its carboxyl terminus, and a single consensus PKA recognition site. Phosphorylation of Ser-133 promotes binding to CBP and, consequently, the interaction with TFIIB, a general transcription factor involved in RNA polymerase II activity (Kwok et al. 1994). Thus, CBP may act as a link between CREB and the transcription preinitiation complex. This interaction may need some RNA polymerase II cofactors, such as TAF110. Finally, the adenoviral E1A oncoprotein-associated p300, which is thought to play a role in preventing the cell cycle G_0/G_1 transition, is structurally very closely related to CBP (Arany et al. 1995). Both CBP and p300 appear to have intrinsic activating properties that are inhibited by the E1A protein (Arany et al. 1995). Thus, it is clear that studies of the transcriptional activation domain of CRE-binding bZip factors continue to provide important insights into the function of transcription factors in general.

CREM Is an Early-response Gene

During studies of CREM expression within the neuroendocrine system, an unexpected new facet emerged: Namely, the transcription of the CREM gene is inducible by cAMP (Molina et al. 1993; Lamas and Sassone-Corsi 1996). Furthermore, the kinetics of this induction are those of an early response gene (Sassone-Corsi et al. 1988a). This important finding further reinforces the notion that CREM products play a fulcral role in the nuclear response to cAMP, since the expression of no other CRE-binding factor has been shown to be inducible to date.

The demonstration that the CREM gene is cAMP-inducible first came from the finding that adrenergic signals direct CREM transcription in the pineal gland (Stehle et al. 1993). The inducibility phenomenon was then characterized in detail in the pituitary corticotroph cell line AtT20. In unstimulated cells, the level of CREM transcript is undetectable. However, upon treatment with forskolin (or other cAMP analogs), within 30 minutes there is a rapid increase in CREM transcript levels, which peak after 2 hours and

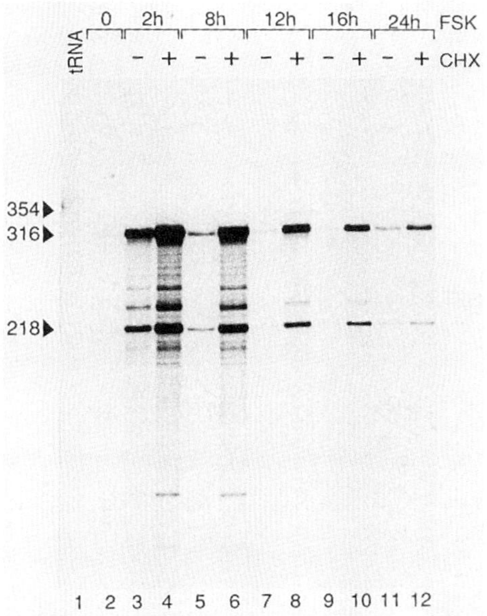

Figure 1. Superinduction of ICER expression. CREM expression in AtT20 corticotroph cells during time courses of forskolin treatment. Cells were treated with forskolin alone (FSK, lanes *3*, *5*, *7*, *9*, and *11*) or with forskolin in combination with cycloheximide (FSK/CHX, lanes *4*, *6*, *8*, *10*, and *12*) for 2, 8, 12, 16, and 24 hr. RNA from untreated AtT20 cells (lane *2*) and tRNA (lane *1*) were used as controls. The migration of the probe (p6N/1; Stehle et al. 1993) and two protected fragments corresponding to ICER transcripts is indicated.

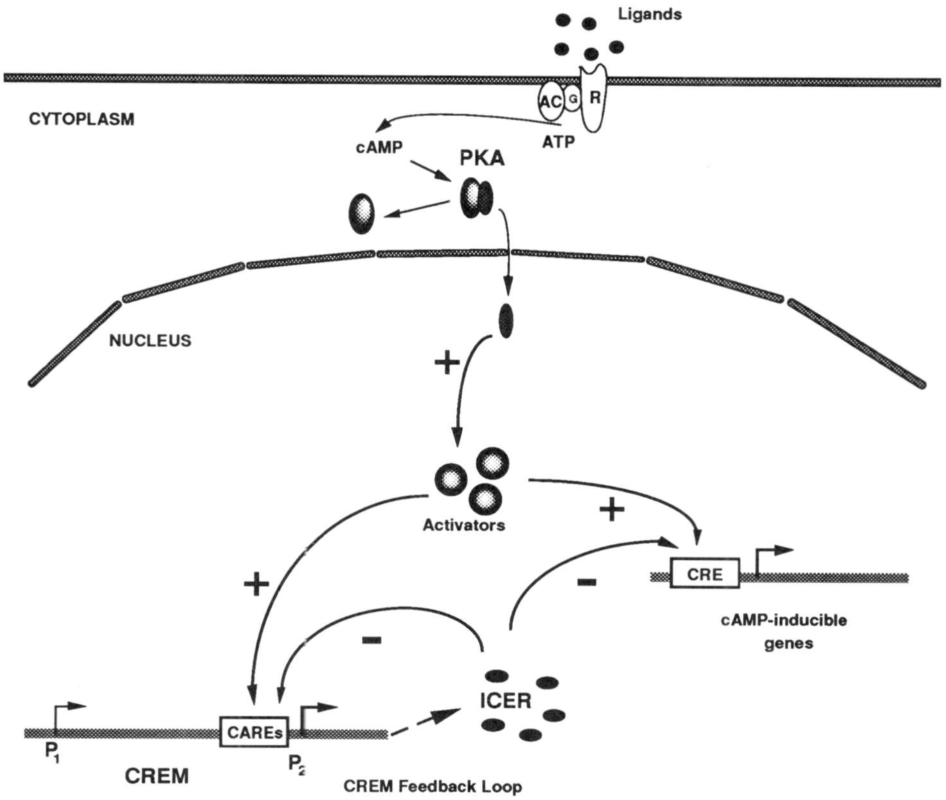

Figure 2. The cAMP signal transduction pathway and the CREM feedback loop. Schematic representation of the route whereby ligands at the cell surface interact with membrane receptors (R) and result in modulated gene expression. Ligand binding activates coupled G proteins (G) which in turn stimulates the activity of the membrane-associated adenylyl cyclase (AC). This converts ATP to cAMP, which causes the dissociation of the inactive tetrameric PKA complex into the active catalytic subunits and the regulatory subunits. Catalytic subunits migrate into the nucleus where they phosphorylate and thereby activate transcriptional activators such as CREB, CREMτ, and ATF1 (Lalli and Sassone-Corsi 1994). Attenuation of the activators may occur via a nuclear phosphatase. Activators then interact with the CRE found in the promoters of cAMP-responsive genes to activate transcription. Phosphorylated factors also activate transcription from the CREM P2 promoter via the CARE elements and ultimately lead to a rapid increase in ICER protein levels. ICER represses cAMP-induced transcription, including that from its own promoter, constituting an autoregulatory loop. The consequent fall in ICER protein levels eventually leads to a release of repression and permits a new cycle of transcriptional activation.

then progressively decline to basal levels by 5 hours (Fig. 1).

These characteristic kinetics classify CREM as an "early response gene" and thus directly implicate the cAMP pathway in the cell's early response for the first time. CREM inducibility is specific for the cAMP pathway since it is not inducible by TPA or dexamethasone treatment. The inducible CREM transcript corresponds to a truncated product, termed ICER (Molina et al. 1993; Stehle et al. 1993).

The 5′ends of the ICER clones correspond to an alternative transcription start site. The start of transcription, which identifies the P2 promoter, is within the 10-kb intron which is carboxy-terminal to the Q2 glutamine-rich domain exon. In contrast to the promoter generating all the previously characterized CREM isoforms (P1), which is GC-rich and not inducible by cAMP, the P2 promoter has a normal A-T and G-C content and is strongly inducible by cAMP. It contains two pairs of closely spaced CRE elements organized in tandem, where the separation between each pair is only three nucleotides. These features make P2 unique among cAMP-regulated promoters and are suggestive of cooperative interactions among the factors binding to these sites.

The ICER open reading frame is constituted by the carboxy-terminal segment of CREM. The predicted open reading frame encodes a small protein of 120 amino acids with a predicted molecular weight of 13.4 kD. This protein, compared with the previously described CREM isoforms, essentially consists of only the DNA-binding domain, which is constituted by the leucine zipper and basic region. The structure of ICER is suggestive of its function and makes it one of the smallest transcription factors ever described (Molina et al. 1993; Stehle et al. 1993).

The intact DNA-binding domain directs specific ICER binding to a consensus CRE element. Importantly, ICER is able to heterodimerize with the other CREM proteins and with CREB. ICER functions as a powerful repressor of cAMP-induced transcription in transfection assays using an extensive range of reporter plasmids carrying individual CRE elements or cAMP-inducible promoter fragments (Molina et al. 1993). Interestingly, ICER-mediated repression is obtained at substoichiometric concentrations, similarly to the previously described CREM antagonists (Laoide et al. 1993). ICER escapes from PKA-dependent phosphorylation and thus constitutes a new category of CRE-binding factor, for which the principal determinant of their activity is their intracellular concentration and not their degree of phosphorylation. Recent data implicate dynamic ICER expression as a more general feature of neuroendocrine systems (Lalli and Sassone-Corsi 1995; Monaco et al. 1995). Indeed, it has been shown that ICER expression is induced in the thyroid gland and in testicular Sertoli cells upon stimulation with the corresponding TSH and FSH pituitary hormones. ICER inducibility has been correlated with the phenomenon of long-term desensitization of the homologous TSH and FSH receptors (Lalli and Sassone-Corsi 1995; Monaco et al. 1995).

Mechanisms of Attenuation: Autoregulatory Loop and Refractory Period

Dephosphorylation appears to represent a key mechanism in the negative regulation of CREB activation function. It has been proposed that a mechanism to explain the attenuation of CREB activity following induction by forskolin is dephosphorylation by specific phosphatases (Hagiwara et al. 1992). After the initial burst of phosphorylation in response to cAMP, CREB is dephosphorylated in vivo by protein phosphatase-1 (PP1). However, the situation is more complex, since it has been shown that both PP1 and PP2A can dephosphorylate CREB in vitro (Nichols et al. 1992), resulting in an apparent decreased binding to low-affinity CRE sites in vitro. Therefore, the precise role of PP1 and PP2A in the dephosphorylation of CREB remains to be determined.

Upon cotreatment with cycloheximide, the kinetics of CREM gene induction by forskolin are altered in that there is a significant delay in the postinduction decrease in the transcript; elevated levels persist for as long as 12 hours (Fig. 1). This implicates a de novo synthesized factor which might down-regulate CREM transcription (Molina et al. 1993). This observation, combined with the presence of CRE elements in the P2 promoter, suggested that the transient nature of the inducibility could be due to ICER itself. Consistently, the CRE elements in the P2 promoter have been shown to bind the ICER proteins. Detailed studies have demonstrated that the ICER promoter is indeed a target for ICER negative regulation (Molina et al. 1993). Thus, there exists a negative autoregulatory mechanism controlling ICER expression (Fig. 2). The CREM feedback loop predicts the presence of a refractory inducibility period in the gene's transcription (Sassone-Corsi 1994). The refractory period (Fig. 3) is determined by the noninducibility of the gene: This phenomenon is due to the dephosphorylation of the activators by an endogenous phosphatase (Hagiwara et al. 1992) and by the increase in the intracellular levels of the dominant repressor ICER (Fig. 3) (Molina et al. 1993; M. Lamas and P. Sassone-Corsi, in prep.).

Circadian Expression of CREM

Crucial elements for the synchronization of biological rhythms in mammals are the pineal gland (Tamarkin et al. 1985) and the suprachiasmatic nucleus (SCN) (Moore 1983). Environmental lighting conditions are transduced by the pineal gland from a neuronal to an endocrine message, the rhythmic secretion of melatonin (Tamarkin et al. 1985). This hormone synthesis is controlled by the SCN, being elevated at night and low during the day (Moore 1983). The cAMP-dependent signal transduction pathway serves as a relay to stimulate melatonin synthesis. Thus, from neuronal pathways which include the retina and the SCN, the pineal gland acts as a temporal regulator for the function of the hypothalamic-pituitary-gonadal axis (Tamarkin et al. 1985).

The study of CREM expression in the rat brain indicated a specific pattern of expression (Mellström et al. 1993). Analysis of CREM expression in the pineal gland has revealed a dramatic day-night regulation, with peak during the night (Fig. 4). The CREM iso-

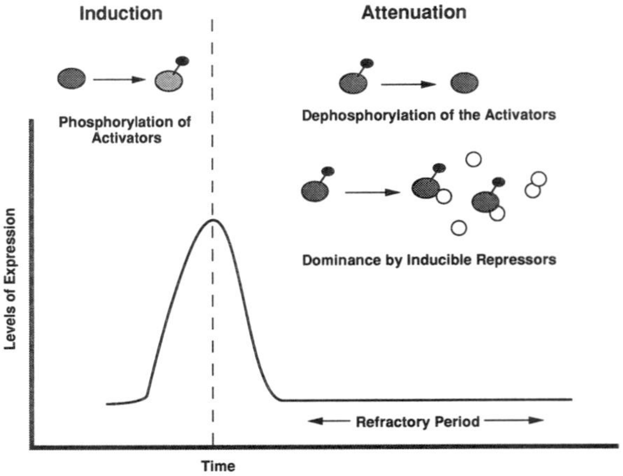

Figure 3. Kinetics of CREM inducibility. After the induction phase, due to the phosphorylation of the activators (i.e., CREB), expression is attenuated by at least two mechanisms: (1) dephosphorylation of the activators by some specific phosphatases; (2) negative autoregulation by the de novo synthesized ICER repressor on the P2 promoter (see Fig. 2) (Molina et al. 1993; Sassone-Corsi 1994).

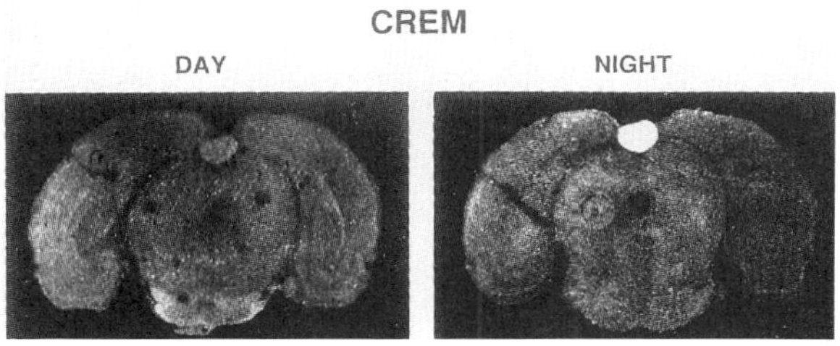

Figure 4. CREM expression is elevated at night in the pineal gland. In situ hybridization of rat brain sections with an antisense CREM-specific riboprobe. Rats maintained in 12 hr light/12 hr dark conditions (light on 07:00) were sacrificed at consecutive time points. Representative sections from 12:00 (DAY) and 02:00 (NIGHT) are shown. An intense hybridization signal is present in the pineal gland at night corresponding to ICER transcripts induced by clock-derived adrenergic signals (Stehle et al. 1993).

form in the pineal gland corresponds to ICER, the early response repressor known to be cAMP-inducible in endocrine cells (Stehle et al. 1993). The transcriptional kinetics of ICER is very characteristic. It appears likely that the autoregulatory loop shown to control ICER transient inducibility (Molina et al. 1993) would also play a role in the day-night cyclic expression in the pineal gland (Foulkes et al. 1996).

By a series of physiological experiments, the mechanism controlling this pattern of ICER expression was determined and found to require clock-distal elements. Indeed, it is known that at night, postganglionic fibers originating from the superior cervical ganglia (SCG) release norepinephrine (Axelrod 1974), which in turn regulates melatonin synthesis via β-adrenergic receptors. These analyses have shown that signals from the SCN direct the induction of CREM expression (Stehle et al. 1993). We have also shown that the only additional site of rhythmic ICER expression within the photoneuroendocrine system is the lamina intercalaris (Stehle et al. 1995). Ontogenetically, the ICER day-night switch and cAMP-inducibility mature in the pineal gland at the end of the first postnatal week. Importantly, this correlates with the onset of melatonin synthesis and the establishment of functional adrenergic innervation. At this developmental phase, we document a significant increase in PKA levels, thus suggesting that ICER inducibility reflects a complete maturation of the cAMP-dependent signaling pathway at the nuclear level (Stehle et al. 1995).

The question of possible targets for down-regulation by ICER in the gland is of particular interest. It has been proposed that a reasonable target could be the enzyme that catalyzes the rate-limiting step of melatonin synthesis (Takahashi 1994), namely, serotonin *N*-acetyl transferase or factors that regulate its activity (N.S. Foulkes et al., in prep.).

Another important finding about the role of CRE-binding factors in circadian rhythms concerns the cyclic phosphorylation of CREB in the SCN (Ginty et al. 1993). During the night, upon light stimuli which phase-shift the clock, CREB appears to be efficiently phosphorylated by an SCN-endogenous kinase at the

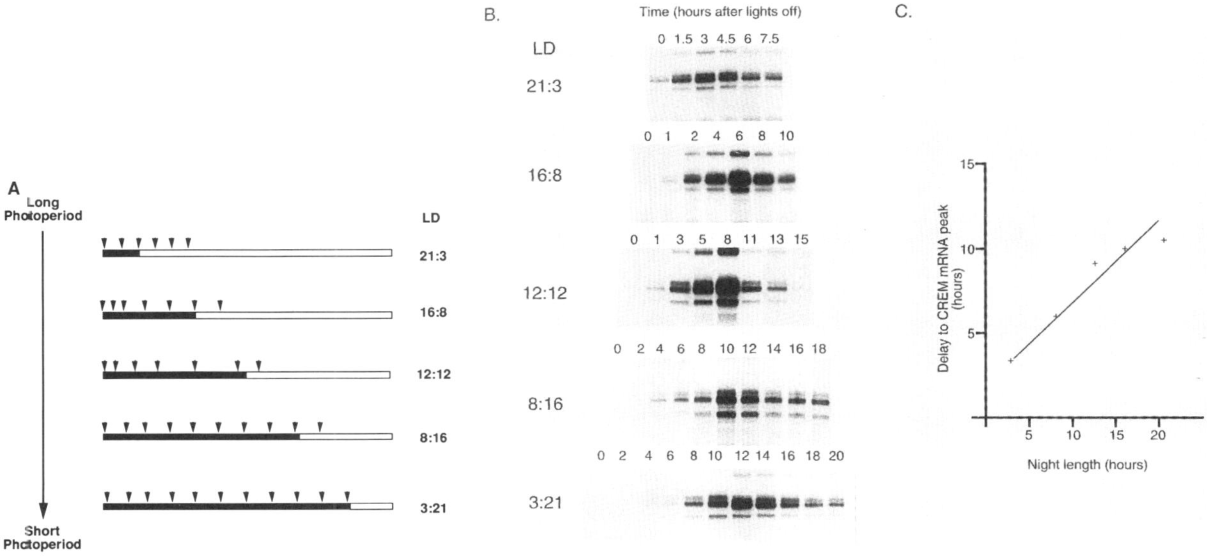

Figure 5. Changes in CREM expression in different photoperiods. (*A*) Schematic representation of different long and short photoperiod regimes. Dark bars represent night; light bars denote daytime. Arrowheads indicate the times of animal sacrifice. (*B*) RNase protection analysis of ICER mRNA levels during long and short photoperiods. ICER mRNA levels rise more rapidly under long photoperiod to reach peak values within 1.5–3 hr, whereas under short photoperiod, equivalent ICER expression is reached only after 12–14 hr. Numbers above each lane indicate the time of sacrifice (hr) following the beginning of each night. (*C*) Graphic representation of the linear relationship between the time required for the CREM gene to reach peak expression levels and the night length. (Reprinted, with permission from Foulkes et al. 1996 [copyright Macmillan].)

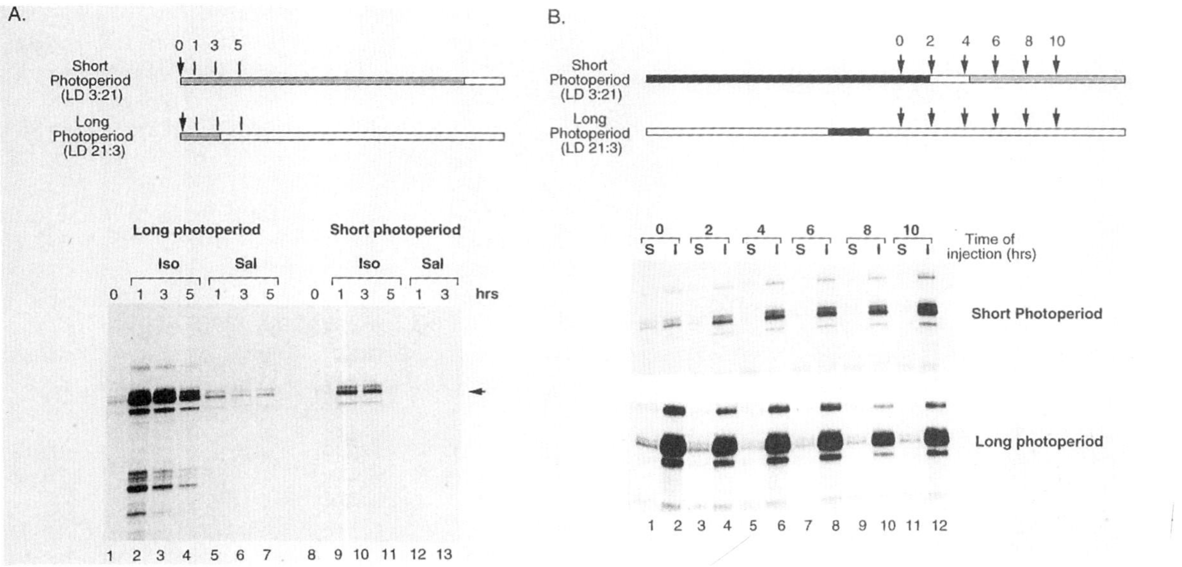

Figure 6. CREM inducibility is dependent on the photoperiod. (*A*) Differential CREM inducibility at the beginning of long or short nights. Animals were maintained under long (LD 21:3) and short (LD 3:21) photoperiods for 2 weeks prior to the analysis. During the night of treatment, rats were transferred into constant light to prevent the natural nighttime rise in ICER levels. The top panel shows the times of isoproterenol (Iso) or control saline (Sal) injections (*arrowheads*; and see bottom panel) during the period of the adapted night (*gray bars*). Vertical lines indicate the times of subsequent sacrifice of the injected animals. (*Lower panel*) RNase protection analysis of CREM expression. Induction is maximal between 1 and 3 hr during long photoperiod (lanes *1–4*), whereas inducibility is strikingly reduced under short photoperiod conditions (lanes *8–11*). (*B*) Differential CREM inducibility following long and short nights. (*Top panel*) Animals were adapted to long and short photoperiod conditions and then injected with isoproterenol (I) or saline (S) following the night at the time points indicated (*arrowheads*). Animals were sacrificed 2 hr following each injection. In the case of the short photoperiod, the course of injections starts at the end of the night (*black bar*) and overlaps with the beginning of the subsequent night, at which point the animals were transferred into constant light (indicated by a *gray bar*). (*Bottom panel*) Inducibility is maximal at all time points tested under long photoperiod (*bottom* section, lanes *1–12*). In the short photoperiod the gene is not inducible immediately at the end of the night (*top* section, lanes *1–2*), whereas it gradually gains inducibility at subsequent time points (lanes *3–12*). (Reprinted, with permission from Foulkes et al. 1996 [copyright Macmillan].)

Ser-133 residue. Phosphorylation at this site turns CREB into an activator and may be obtained by a number of kinases (Gonzalez and Montminy 1989; Lee et al. 1990; de Groot et al. 1993a,b). Although the nature of the SCN-endogenous kinase has not been established, it seems likely that it could be PKA (Ginty et al. 1993). This result would suggest a key role for this kinase or for a counteracting phosphatase in the regulation of the clock function. The target genes for the activated CREB in the SCN have yet to be established.

Changes in the Day-Night Cycle Affect CREM Transcription

It is established that night length modulates SCN adrenergic output and thereby profoundly affects the neuroendocrine response (Reiter 1991). We decided to investigate whether the pattern of ICER expression could be intimately determined by changes in the photoperiod.

We tested the effect of changing the photoperiod upon ICER expression in the pineal gland. Rats were adapted for 2 weeks in various photoperiods (LD 3:21; 6:18; 12:12; 18:6; 21:3) (Fig. 5A). With increasing photoperiod we observed a proportional increase in the speed of ICER induction at the beginning of the night (Fig. 5B,C). Under long photoperiod, ICER behaves as an early response gene, showing a peak of induction by 1.5 hours following the onset of the 3-hour night. This peak is transient, declining to basal levels within 6 hours. In striking contrast, under short photoperiods, the rate of induction is considerably slower. Peak levels occurred only 12 and 14 hours after the beginning of the 16- and 21-hour nights. From these results it is evident that the dynamics of ICER expression are versatile, since its kinetics are determined by night length.

Is CREM able to adapt to changes in photoperiod by modifying its mode of induction in response to adrenergic stimuli? Indeed, CREM is refractory to cAMP stimulation during the daytime under 12:12 conditions (Stehle et al. 1993). Rats adapted to long or short photoperiods were challenged with injections of the adrenergic agonist isoproterenol at the beginning of the night (Fig. 6). CREM is strongly inducible under

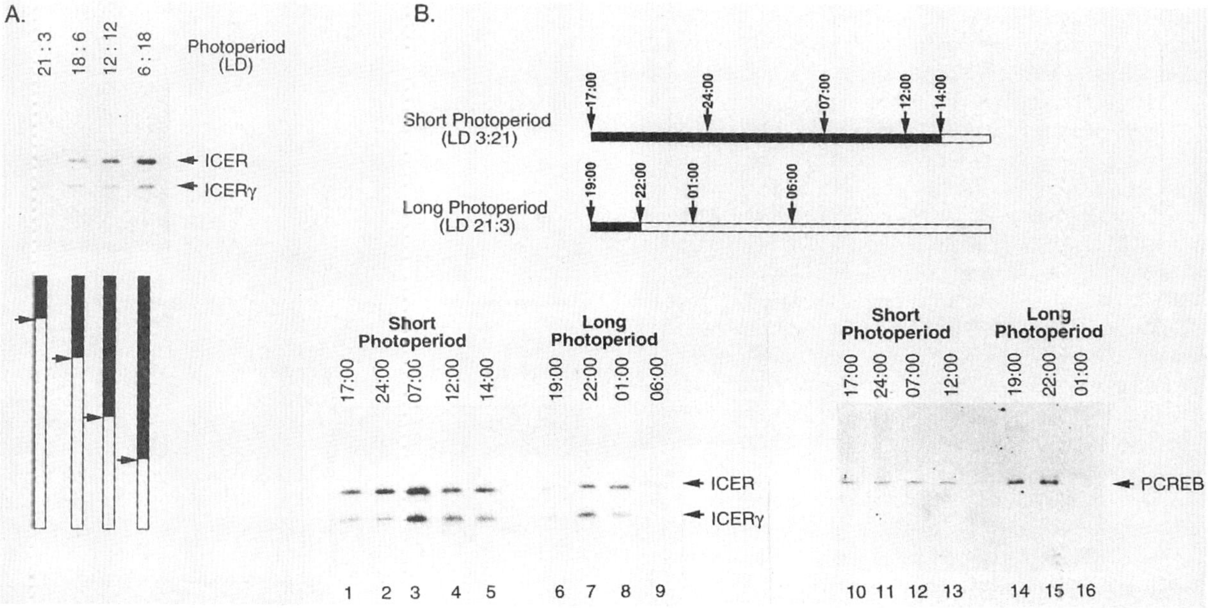

Figure 7. Contribution of CREB and ICER proteins to differential inducibility. (*A*) Rats were adapted for at least 2 weeks to various long and short photoperiods (represented below by vertical black and white bars) and then killed at the onset of the night (*arrowheads*). Pineal gland protein extracts were analyzed by Western blot using an anti-ICER antibody. Arrowheads indicate the ICER and ICERγ (Molina et al. 1993) proteins whose levels rise with increasing night length. (*B*) (*Top panel*) Rats were adapted for 2 weeks to long (LD 21:3) and short (LD 3:21) photoperiods and then sacrificed at the times indicated (*arrowheads*). (*Bottom panels*) Western blot analysis of pineal extracts using the anti-ICER antibody (lanes *1-9*) and an anti-phosphoCREB antibody (lanes *10–16*). Arrowheads indicate the ICER and ICERγ protein bands which are expressed at higher levels under short than under long photoperiod. Additional analysis confirms that the peak of ICER protein is consistently during the second half of the night. Levels of phosphorylated CREB (PCREB) are low and nonfluctuating under short photoperiod. Under long photoperiod, instead, high levels are visible for the duration of the 3-hr night. These then drop to undetectable levels from the onset of the following day. (Reprinted, with permission from Foulkes et al. 1996 [copyright Macmillan].)

long photoperiod (lanes 1–4) but only weakly inducible under short photoperiod (lanes 8–11). We then tested whether CREM inducibility at the end of the night would similarly adapt to the night length (Fig. 6B). Under long photoperiod CREM displays a high level of induction (lower panel, lanes 1–2), but the gene is refractory to isoproterenol stimulation immediately following a short photoperiod night (top panel, lanes 1–2). Thus, the CREM transcriptional response may be either supersensitive or subsensitive to the same stimulus. Interestingly, under short photoperiod, inducibility gradually increases following the night to reach a level after 10 hours comparable to that of a long photoperiod (top panel, lanes 3-12). In contrast, inducibility under long photoperiod remains elevated (lower panel, lanes 3–12). Thus, the duration of the refractory period is determined by the length of the night to which the animals are adapted. The refractory period can be considered as a memory of night length that constrains the timing of the transcriptional response at the beginning of the following night.

Molecular Mechanisms of Transcriptional Memory

We wanted to determine the role played by CREB and ICER during the CREM adaptation to changing photoperiods. Strikingly, ICER protein levels show significant differences: The overall levels are considerably higher in pineal glands from animals adapted to short photoperiods with respect to long photoperiods (Fig. 7A), consistent with the slower induction.

We then tested ICER protein levels throughout the day and night during long and short photoperiods (Fig. 7B, top panel). Consistently, at all time points we observed significantly more protein in the pineal glands under short (lanes 1–5) than under long photoperiod (lanes 6–9). Furthermore, in both photoperiods, a peak in protein occurred during the second part of the night, coincidently with ICER transcript decline. This peak has a reduced magnitude in short (compare lanes 1 and 3), compared with long, photoperiod conditions (compare lanes 6 and 7).

We assayed CREB phosphorylation using a phosphoCREB-specific antibody (PCREB; Fig. 7B, lanes 10–16) (Ginty et al. 1993). In animals adapted to short photoperiods, low, nonfluctuating levels of phosphorylated CREB were detected throughout the whole cycle (lanes 10–13). In contrast, during long photoperiods, a burst of phosphorylation accompanies the onset of the short night which persists and then subsequently drops to basal levels at the beginning of the next day (lanes 14–16). Thus, increasing phosphorylation correlates directly with more rapid CREM induction. A strict relationship exists between the changes in the kinetics of CREM expression and the status of the cAMP-responsive activators and repressors.

Transcription factors responsive to cAMP appear to play a pivotal role in long-term adaptations of neuroendocrine function (Stehle et al. 1993; Bourtchuladze et al. 1994; Huang et al. 1994; Takahashi 1994; Yin et al. 1994; Lalli and Sassone-Corsi 1995; Monaco et al. 1995). We previously documented modulation of CREM during seasonal changes in spermatogenesis (Foulkes et al. 1993). Here we demonstrate that changes in photoperiod have profound effects on ICER expression in the pineal gland. Differential inducibility of the gene supports a more general notion that the nuclear response to cAMP can be subsensitive or supersensitive (Fig. 8). This is in agreement with the original descriptions of differential sensitivity to β-adrenergic stimulation in the pineal gland (Axelrod 1974; Romero and Axelrod 1974). Importantly, our findings extend this phenomenon to mechanisms regulating gene expression in the nucleus.

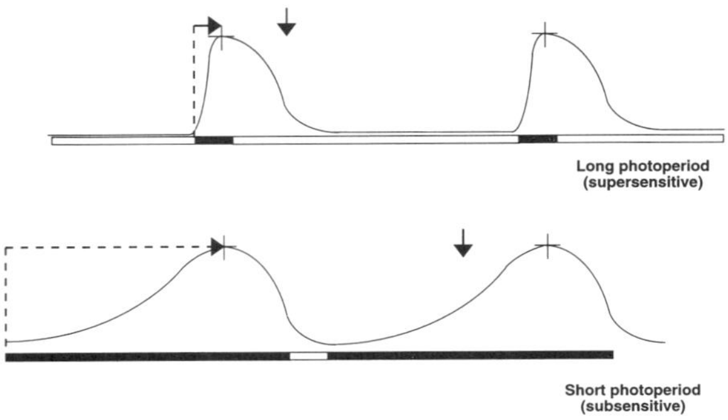

Figure 8. Schematic representation of CREM expression and inducibility following adaptation to short and long photoperiods. Although periodicity of the peak of expression is identical in both photoperiods, the kinetics of the increase are different. Thus, while rhythmicity is conserved, CREM expression increases very rapidly in a long photoperiod, whereas in a short photoperiod the increase is gradual. This is consistent with inducibility studies (see Fig. 6). The horizontal dashed arrows indicate the time required to reach the peak of expression in different photoperiods. Vertical arrows denote that the timing for maximal inducibility by cAMP following a peak of expression is different depending on the length of the night. Increasing night length dictates a slower gain in inducibility. Thereby, the CREM gene displays different modes of transcriptional regulation, being supersensitive to cAMP in the long photoperiod and subsensitive during the short photoperiod. Consequently, the length of the refractory period which precedes the subsequent induction is dependent on the nature of the previous cycle. This adaptive phenomenon represents a "memory" of transcriptional rhythmicity. (Reprinted, with permission from Foulkes et al. 1996 [copyright Macmillan].)

CONCLUSION

CREM rhythmic expression may have the characteristics of an early response gene (long photoperiod) or may have a delayed, dampened response (short photoperiod). We have shown that the length of the refractory period in CREM inducibility is determined by the photoperiod (Foulkes et al. 1996; Lamas and Sassone-Corsi 1996). Figure 8 is a schematic representation of the different kinetics of CREM expression during long and short photoperiods, displayed in combination with the subsensitive and supersensitive states of inducibility. It should be stressed that the molecular adaptation described here is likely to operate in concert with the well-documented photoperiod-dependent entrainment of the clock system (Illnerova et al. 1979). Furthermore, other photoperiod-dependent physiological changes may contribute to this phenomenon. However, the role of ICER and CREB in the adaptation to a specific state of inducibility is evident from our results (Fig. 7). Furthermore, the involvement of additional nuclear factors in this phenomenon cannot be excluded. However, the protein levels of CBP and of the regulatory and catalytic subunits of PKA do not change under different photoperiods (not shown).

In conclusion, the CREM gene has provided a remarkable example of dynamic gene regulation that enables animals to adapt to temporal changes in their environment. This adaptation involves the establishment and maintenance of different patterns of transcriptional regulation. Indeed, the CREM expression adapts to changing day-night rhythms by its experience of previous photoperiods, thus constituting a transcriptional memory.

An important aspect of our findings resides in the striking correlation between the photoperiod-dependent changes in ICER and the previously documented seasonal variations in melatonin (Illnerova et al. 1979). This further strengthens the notion that ICER may be directly involved in melatonin synthesis via the regulation of the serotonin *N*-acetyl transferase gene (Takahashi 1994; Borjigin et al. 1995; Coon et al. 1995; N.S. Foulkes et al., in prep.). The use of homologous recombination to inactivate the CREM gene products offers a powerful tool to address this question. We have generated CREM-null mice which display a phenotype including a complete block of the spermiogenesis differentiation program (Nantel et al. 1996). This result confirmed our previous observations which involved the CREM activator protein in the transcriptional regulation of postmeiotic genes (Delmas et al. 1993). We will be able to use this animal model to study the role of CREM in the regulation of melatonin synthesis and in the control of circadian rhythms.

CRE-binding proteins appear to play a central role in the physiology of the neuroendocrine system. Further studies of their molecular and functional characteristics will represent another major step forward in our understanding of hormonal regulation and metabolism.

ACKNOWLEDGMENTS

We thank all the other members of the Sassone-Corsi laboratory: E. Zazopoulos, K. Tamai, L. Penna, F. Nantel, C. Mazzucchelli, E. Heitz, and D. De Cesare. M.L. is supported by the Ministerio de Educacion y Ciencia (Spain). This work was supported by grants from Centre National de la Recherche Scientifique, Institut National de la Santé et de la Recherche Médicale, Centre Hospitalier Universitaire Régional, Fondation de la Recherche Médicale, Université Louis Pasteur, Association pour la Recherche sur le Cancer, and Rhône-Poulenc Rorer.

REFERENCES

Arany, Z., D. Newsome, E. Oldread, D.M. Livingston, and R. Eckner. 1995. A family of transcriptional adaptor proteins targeted by the E1A oncoprotein. *Nature* **374:** 81.

Axelrod, J. 1974. The pineal gland: A neurochemical transducer. *Science* **184**: 1341.

Borjigin, J., M.M. Wang, and S.H. Snyder. 1995. Diurnal variation in mRNA encoding serotonin *N*-acetyltransferase in pineal gland. *Nature* **378:** 783.

Bourtchuladze, R., B. Frenguelli, J. Blendy, D. Cioffi, G. Schutz, and A.J. Silva. 1994. Deficient long-term memory in mice with a targeted mutation of the cAMP-responsive element-binding protein. *Cell* **79:** 59.

Cambier, J.C., N.K. Newell, L.B. Justement, J.C. McGuire, K.L. Leach, and Z.Z. Chen. 1987. Ia binding ligands and cAMP stimulate nuclear translocation of PKC in β lymphocytes. *Nature* **327:** 629.

Chrivia, J.C., R.P.S. Kwok, N. Lamb, M. Haniwawa, M.R. Montminy, and R.H. Goodman. 1993. Phosphorylated CREB binds specifically to the nuclear protein CBP. *Nature* **365:** 855.

Coon, S.L., P.H. Roseboom, R. Baler, J.L. Weller, M.A.A. Namboodiri, E.V. Koonin, and D.C. Klein. 1995. Pineal serotonin *N*-acetyltransferase: Expression cloning and molecular analysis. *Science* **270:** 1681.

Courey, A.J. and R. Tjian. 1989. Analysis of Sp1 *in vivo* reveals multiple transcriptional domains, including a novel glutamine activation motif. *Cell* **55:** 887.

Dash, P.K., K.A. Karl, M.A. Colicos, R. Prywes, and E.R. Kandel. 1991. cAMP response element-binding protein is activated by Ca^{2+}/calmodulin- as well as cAMP-dependent protein kinase. *Proc. Natl. Acad. Sci.* **88:** 5061.

de Groot, R.P., L.M. Ballou, and P. Sassone-Corsi. 1994. Positive regulation of the cAMP-responsive activator CREM by the p70 S6 kinase: An alternative route to mitogen-induced gene expression. *Cell* **79:** 81.

de Groot, R.P., R. Derua, J. Goris, and P. Sassone-Corsi. 1993a. Phosphorylation and negative regulation of the transcriptional activator CREM by p34cdc2. *Mol. Endocrinol.* **7:** 1495.

de Groot, R.P., J. den Hertog, J.R. Vandenheede, J. Goris, and P. Sassone-Corsi. 1993b. Multiple and cooperative phosphorylation events regulate the CREM activator function. *EMBO J.* **12:** 3903.

Delmas, V., F. van der Hoorn, B. Mellström, B. Jégou, and P. Sassone-Corsi. 1993. Induction of CREM activator proteins in spermatids: Downstream targets and implications for haploid germ cell differentiation. *Mol. Endocrinol.* **7:** 1502.

Foulkes, N.S., E. Borrelli, and P. Sassone-Corsi. 1991. CREM gene: Use of alternative DNA binding domains generates multiple antagonists of cAMP-induced transcription. *Cell* **64:** 739.

Foulkes, N.S., G. Duval, and P. Sassone-Corsi. 1996. Adaptive inducibility of CREM as transcriptional memory of circadian rhythms. *Nature* **381:** 83.

Foulkes, N.S., B. Mellström, E. Benusiglio, and P. Sassone-Corsi. 1992. Developmental switch of CREM function during spermatogenesis: From antagonist to transcriptional activator. *Nature* **355:** 80.

Foulkes, N.S., F. Schlotter, P. Pévet, and P. Sassone-Corsi. 1993. Pituitary hormone FSH directs the CREM functional switch during spermatogenesis. *Nature* **362:** 264.

Ginty, D.D., D. Glowacka, D.S. Bader, H. Hidaka, and J.A. Wagner. 1991. Induction of immediate early genes by Ca^{2+} influx requires cAMP-dependent protein kinase in PC12 cells. *J. Biol. Chem.* **266:** 17454.

Ginty, D.D., J.M. Kornhauser, M. Thompson, H. Bading, K.E. Mayo, J.S. Takahashi, and M.E. Greenberg. 1993. Regulation of CREB phosphorylation in the suprachiasmatic nucleus by light and a circadian clock. *Science* **260:** 238.

Gonzalez, G.A. and M.R. Montminy. 1989. Cyclic AMP stimulates somatostatin gene transcription by phosphorylation of CREB at Ser 133. *Cell* **59:** 675.

Hagiwara, M., A. Alberts, P. Brindle, J. Meinkoth, J. Feramisco, T. Deng, M. Karin, S. Shenolikar, and M. Montminy. 1992. Transcriptional attenuation following cAMP induction requires PP-1-mediated dephosphorylation of CREB. *Cell* **70:** 105.

Hai, T.Y. and T. Curran. 1991. Cross-family dimerization of transcription factors Fos:Jun and ATF/CREB alters DNA binding specificity. *Proc. Natl. Acad. Sci.* **88:** 3720.

Hai, T.Y., F. Liu, W.J. Coukos, and M.R. Green. 1989. Transcription factor ATF cDNA clones: An extensive family of leucine zipper proteins able to selectively form DNA binding heterodimers. *Genes Dev.* **3:** 2083.

Hoeffler, J.P., T.E. Meyer, Y. Yun, J.L. Jameson, and J.F. Habener. 1988. Cyclic AMP-responsive DNA-binding protein: Structure based on a cloned placental cDNA. *Science* **242:** 1430.

Huang, Y.Y., X.C. Li, and E.R. Kandel. 1994. cAMP contributes to mossy fiber LTP by initiating both a covalently mediated early phase and macromolecular synthesis-dependent late phase. *Cell* **79:** 69.

Illnerova, H., J. Vanecek, L. Wetterberg, and J.J. Sääf. 1979. Effect of one minute exposure to light at night on rat pineal serotonin *N*-acetyltransferase and melatonin. *Neurochemistry* **32:** 673.

Kwok, R.P., J.R. Lundblad, J.C. Chrivia, J.P. Richards, H.P. Bachinger, R.G. Brennan, S.G.E. Roberts, M.R. Green, and R.H. Goodman. 1994. Nuclear protein CBP is a coactivator for the transcription factor CREB. *Nature* **370:** 223.

Lalli, E. and P. Sassone-Corsi. 1994. Signal transduction and gene regulation: The nuclear response to cAMP. *J. Biol. Chem.* **269:** 17359.

———. 1995. Thyroid-stimulating hormone (TSH)-directed induction of the CRME gene in the thyroid gland participates in the long-term desensitization of the TSH receptor *Proc. Natl. Acad. Sci.* **92:** 9633.

Lamas, M. and P. Sassone-Corsi. 1996. CREM and the transcriptional response to cAMP. *Curr. Opin. Endocrinol. Diabetes* **3:** (in press).

Laoide, B.M., N.S. Foulkes, F. Schlotter, and P. Sassone-

Corsi. 1993. The functional versatility of CREM is determined by its modular structure. *EMBO J.* **12:** 1179.

Lee, C.Q., Y. Yun, J.P. Hoeffler, and J.F. Habener. 1990. Cyclic-AMP-responsive transcriptional activation involves interdependent phosphorylated subdomains. *EMBO J.* **9:** 4455.

Masquilier, D. and P. Sassone-Corsi. 1992. Transcriptional cross-talk: Nuclear factors CREM and CREB bind to AP-1 sites and inhibit activation by Jun. *J. Biol. Chem.* **267:** 22460.

McKnight, S.G., C.H. Clegg, M.D. Uhler, J.C. Chrivia, G.G. Cadd, L.L. Correll, and A.D. Otten. 1988. Analysis of the cAMP-dependent protein kinase system using molecular genetic approaches. *Recent Prog. Horm. Res.* **44:** 307.

Mellström, B., J.R. Naranjo, N.S. Foulkes, M. Lafarga, and P. Sassone-Corsi. 1993. Transcriptional response to cAMP in brain: Specific distribution and induction of CREM antagonists. *Neuron* **10:** 655.

Molina, C.A., N.S. Foulkes, E. Lalli, and P. Sassone-Corsi. 1993. Inducibility and negative autoregulation of CREM: An alternative promoter directs the expression of ICER, an early response repressor. *Cell* **75:** 875.

Monaco, L., N.S. Foulkes, and P. Sassone-Corsi. 1995. Pituitary follicle-stimulating hormone (FSH) induces CREM gene expression in Sertoli cells: Involvement in long-term desensitization of the FSH receptor. *Proc. Natl. Acad. Sci.* **92:** 10673.

Moore, R.Y. 1983. Organization and function of the central nervous system circadian oscillator; the suprachiasmatic hypothalamic nucleus. *Fed. Proc.* **42:** 2783.

Nantel, F., L. Monaco, N.S. Foulkes, D. Masquilier, M. LeMeur, K. Henriksén, A. Dierich, M. Parvinen, and P. Sassone-Corsi. 1996. Spermiogenesis deficiency and germ-cell apoptosis in CREM-mutant mice. *Nature* **380:** 159.

Nichols, M., F. Weih, W. Schmid, C. DeVack, E. Kowenz-Leutz, B. Luckow, M. Boschart, and G. Schutz. 1992. Phosphorylation of CREB affects its binding to high and low affinity sites: Implications for cAMP induced gene transcription. *EMBO J.* **11:** 3337.

Nishizuka, Y. 1986. Studies and perspectives of protein kinase C. *Science* **233:** 305.

Reiter, R.J. 1991. Pineal gland. Interface between the photoperiodic environment and the endocrine system. *Trends Endocrinol. Metab.* **1:** 13.

Roesler, W.J., G.R. Vanderbark, and R.W. Hanson. 1988. Cyclic AMP and the induction of eukaryotic gene expression. *J. Biol. Chem.* **263:** 9063.

Romero, J. and J. Axelrod. 1974. Pineal β-adrenergic receptor: Diurnal variation in sensitivity. *Science* **184:** 1091.

Sassone-Corsi, P. 1994. Rhythmic transcription and autoregulatory loops: Winding up the biological clock. *Cell* **78:** 361.

Sassone-Corsi, P., W.W. Lamph, and I.M. Verma. 1988a. Regulation of proto-oncogene *fos*: A paradigm for early response genes. *Cold Spring Harbor Symp. Quant. Biol.* **53:** 749.

Sassone-Corsi, P., L.J. Ransone, and I.M. Verma. 1990. Cross-talk in signal transduction: TPA-inducible factor Jun/AP-1 activates cAMP responsive enhancer elements. *Oncogene* **5:** 427.

Sassone-Corsi, P., J. Visvader, L. Ferland, P.L. Mellon, and I.M. Verma. 1988b. Induction of proto-oncogene *fos* transcription through the adenylate cyclase pathway: Characterization of a cAMP-responsive element. *Genes Dev.* **2:** 1529.

Sheng, M., G. McFadden, and M.E. Greenberg. 1990. Membrane depolarization and calcium induce c-*fos* transcription via phosphorylation of transcription factor CREB. *Neuron* **4:** 571.

Stehle, J.H., N.S. Foulkes, P. Pévet and P. Sassone-Corsi. 1995. Developmental maturation of pineal gland function: Synchronized CREM inducibility and adrenergic stimulation. *Mol. Endocrinol.* **9:** 706.

Stehle, J.H., N.S. Foulkes, C.A. Molina, V. Simonneaux, P. Pévet, and P. Sassone-Corsi. 1993. Adrenergic signals direct rhythmic expression of transcriptional repressor CREM in the pineal gland. *Nature* **365:** 314.

Takahashi, J. 1994. ICER is nicer at night (*sir*!). *Curr. Biol.* **4:** 165.

Tamarkin, L., C.J. Baird, and O.F.X. Almeida. 1985. Melatonin: A coordinating signal for mammalian reproduction? *Science* **227:** 714.

Williams, T., A. Admon, B. Luscher, and R. Tjian. 1988. Cloning and expression of AP-2, a cell-type-specific transcription factor that activates inducible enhancer elements. *Genes Dev.* **2:** 1557.

Yin, J.C.P., J.S. Wallach, M. Del Vecchio, E.L. Wilder, H. Zhou, W.G. Quinn, and T. Tully. 1994. Induction of a dominant negative CREB transgene specifically blocks long-term memory in *Drosophila. Cell* **79:** 49.

Yoshimasa, T., D.R. Sibley, M. Bouvier, R.J. Lefkowitz, and M.G. Caron. 1987. Cross-talk between cellular signalling pathways suggested by phorbol ester adenylate cyclase phosphorylation. *Nature* **327:** 67.

Ziff, E.B. 1990. Transcription factors: A new family gathers at the cAMP response site. *Trends Genet* **6:** 69.

Forward Genetic Approaches to Circadian Clocks in Mice

D.P. KING AND J.S. TAKAHASHI
National Science Foundation Center for Biological Timing, and Department of Neurobiology and Physiology, Northwestern University, Evanston, Illinois 60208

One of the goals of neuroscience is to understand the mechanisms underlying behavior. How do genes ultimately interact with each other and with the environment to produce an organism's behavior? Properties of the mammalian circadian system have made it an ideal model in which to study the physiological mechanisms underlying behavior (Takahashi 1995). Unlike many other physiological systems, such as those regulating sleep or learning and memory, the mammalian circadian system is suprisingly simple: There is a discrete brain region, within the hypothalamus (the suprachiasmatic nuclei, SCN), responsible for the generation of circadian oscillations (Meijer and Rietveld 1989). The primary input pathway (retinohypothalamic tract) by which environmental stimuli are transmitted to the SCN is well characterized, and the behavioral end point most often studied (locomotor activity) is, in many mammals, precise, robust, and easily recorded. However, identification of genes underlying mammalian circadian rhythms has until recently been serendipitous and has not included their molecular characterization (Menaker and Takahashi 1995). In contrast, in several non-vertebrate species, genetics has provided a means to elucidate mechanisms of the circadian clock at the molecular level (Hall 1990; Dunlap 1993; Takahashi 1995). Now, with the availability of many new resources for mammalian molecular genetics, we are beginning to see the successful application of genetic analysis, as a tool of molecular discovery, to the study of mammalian circadian rhythms (Takahashi et al. 1994). This approach holds promise as a generally useful strategy by which other mammalian behaviors can be analyzed at the molecular level.

FORWARD GENETICS AND POSITIONAL CLONING

The most effective genetic tool thus far employed for the analysis of circadian rhythms has been the creation of animals with genetic mutations that affect properties of the biological clock system. Seymour Benzer (1973) articulated the strategy succinctly: "Our objectives are to discern the genetic component of a behavior, to identify it with a particular gene and then to determine the actual site at which the gene influences behavior and learn how it does so." Because the molecular elements of the circadian clock were unknown and difficult to predict, targeted mutation of genes potentially involved in this system has not been possible. Furthermore, examination of different strains of a particular species, such as *Drosophila melanogaster* (Pittendrigh 1974; Hall 1990) or *Mus musculus* (Schwartz and Zimmerman 1990; Lynch and Lynch 1992), revealed subtle differences in circadian rhythms and suggested that these differences were the result of polymorphisms at many genetic loci, making the identification of single genes underlying the behavior very difficult. However, mutagenesis followed by behavioral testing for rhythm variants has been an extremely useful method for identifying genes involved in the circadian rhythms of numerous non-vertebrate organisms. It has been especially effective in organisms for which an abundance of genetic resources is already available; this permits the cloning of the genes in question and provides the methods to analyze the function of these genes in great detail. The most successful application of this forward genetics method has been seen in mutagenesis screens involving two such "genetics-rich" organisms, *Drosophila* and *Neurospora crassa*. In *Drosophila*, two genes that are central to the circadian clock, *period* (*per*) and *timeless* (*tim*), have been identified as the result of mutagenesis screens (Konopka and Benzer 1971; Sehgal et al. 1994). Similarly, the *frequency* (*frq*) gene was identified following a mutagenesis screen in *Neurospora* (Feldman and Hoyle 1973). All of these genes have subsequently been cloned, and the mutations causing the aberrant circadian phenotypes have been identified (Baylies et al. 1987; Yu et al. 1987; McClung et al. 1989; Aronson et al. 1994a; Myers et al. 1995). The picture that is emerging from the detailed molecular genetic analysis of these three genes is one of an autoregulatory feedback loop, in which the proteins encoded by "clock" genes affect, either directly or indirectly, the rate of the clock genes' own transcription (Aronson et al. 1994b; Zeng et al. 1994; Sehgal et al. 1995). Unfortunately, despite concerted efforts from several laboratories, attempts to transfer this wealth of information regarding the clock genes of *Drosophila* and *Neurospora* to a mammalian species, in the form of a mammalian ortholog of *per*, *tim*, or *frq*, have thus far been unsuccessful.

As an alternative to the identification of mammalian orthologs of these canonical clock genes, one could instead transfer the method of forward genetics, by conducting a mutagenesis screen in the mammalian species

 0-87969-071-2/96 $5+.00

most amenable to such analysis, the laboratory mouse. In mammalian species, however, the forward genetic approach has not been used to explore the mechanisms of the circadian clock or, to our knowledge, any other behavioral phenotype. Despite this, forward genetics may be one of the few ways in which to identify genes involved in the mammalian circadian system. The cloned clock genes described above (*per*, *tim*, and *frq*) are unique and are expressed in low abundance, so it is unlikely that these genes could have been identified by other means. Parenthetically, there are two exceptions to this general "forward genetics only" rule. A single gene mutation affecting circadian rhythms in the golden hamster was identified (Ralph and Menaker 1988), but the mutation arose spontaneously (not an easily reproduced method!) and furthermore, there is not sufficient information about the hamster genome to investigate this mutation at the molecular level (Okazaki et al. 1996). The second exception involves the independent isolation of *tim* using a yeast two-hybrid screen (Gekakis et al. 1995). In this case, the previous knowledge of *per*'s involvement in the *Drosophila* circadian clock was necessary for the experiment. The use of *Drosophila per* and *tim* as "bait" has not yet been successful using mammalian expression libraries.

The general reluctance in using mutagenesis screening approaches in mice has probably been due to two limitations in mouse genetics: (1) Without an effective mutagen, such a screen would require prohibitive numbers of mice; and (2) even with a behavioral mutant isolated, identifying the gene responsible for the phenotype would be very difficult. The first of these limitations was solved several years ago by Russell et al. (1979), with the development of high-efficiency germ-line mutagenesis in mice using the alkylating agent *N*-ethyl-*N*-nitrosourea (ENU). The recent development of dense genetic maps utilizing simple sequence length polymorphisms (SSLPs) (Dietrich et al. 1992, 1996) and the availability of a number of physical mapping and cloning resources address the second limitation, making the prospects of identifying a gene, with only its phenotype as a clue, a much more feasible endeavor (Takahashi et al. 1994).

That forward genetics can be successfully applied to behavioral analysis in a mammalian system is seen with the isolation of *Clock*, a mutation affecting the circadian behavior of mice (Vitaterna et al. 1994). This semidominant mutation, which is inherited as a single gene autosomal trait, causes a lengthening of the endogenous period of mice, and in homozygous *Clock* mice, a complete loss of rhythmicity.

Mutagenesis Procedures in the Mouse

Several methods have been described for generating germ-line mutations in the mouse (Rinchik 1991). X-Irradiation and treatment with chlorambucil are efficient methods for generating large deletions in postmeiotic germ cells, with mutation rates varying from 0.00033 to 0.00127 per locus (Russell et al. 1989; Rinchik et al. 1990a,b; Cattanach et al. 1993). X-Rays can also induce small deletions in premeiotic germ cells, with a similar mutagenesis efficiency (Selby 1981). In practice, however, it has been difficult to recover sufficiently large numbers of mutant animals with these methods. Two more recently developed technologies, transgene and gene trap insertions, have the advantage of causing "tagged" mutations, but their low mutation frequencies (~0.00001 and ~0.0001 per locus per gamete, respectively) make them unsuitable for mutant screens (Rossant and Hopkins 1992). The alkylating agent ENU is best for generating point mutations, and it has a very high mutation rate, up to 0.0015 per locus per gamete (Russell et al. 1979; Hitotsumachi et al. 1985). With the development of high-efficiency germ-line ENU-mutagenesis procedures, it has become feasible to undertake large-scale mutant screens in the mouse (Rinchik 1991). An additional advantage of ENU is that, because it typically induces point mutations, one can potentially recover both gain-of-function and loss-of-function mutations.

A primary factor affecting the design of a mutagenesis screen is whether one wishes to recover mutations having dominant or recessive phenotypes. The general strategies for ENU mutagenesis screens used to identify mutations of either class are shown in Figure 1. Two aspects of a mutagen chosen for such screens are critical: the achievable mutation rate and whether the germ-line target of the mutagen is premeiotic or postmeiotic. In the case of ENU, premeiotic germ cells (spermatogonia) are the targets. Screening for mutations induced within the spermatogonia confers two advantages when compared to postmeiotic mutagenesis. Unlike postmeiotic mutagenesis, the G_1 progeny will be nonmosaic; thus, these mice can be screened directly for heterozygous mutations with dominant phenotypes. In addition, a single mutagenized male mouse can produce 100–150 progeny, each of which represents one mutagenized gamete. Achievable mutation rates are important when considering the feasibilty of mutating the majority of loci of the mouse genome. Using ENU-mutagenesis methods that can achieve a mutagenesis frequency of 0.0015 per locus per gamete (Hitotsumachi et al. 1985), one has a greater than 50% chance of recovering a mutation, on average, at any given locus, by screening about 655 gametes. To have a high probability of recovering at least one mutation for all loci, assuming Poisson statistics (3x coverage) and an average forward mutagenesis frequency described above (0.0015 per locus per gamete), one must screen about 2000 gametes. To identify mutations having dominant phenotypes, this means the direct screening of about 2000 G_1 progeny. A recessive screen, however, is more difficult, because each mutation must be rendered homozygous. To identify mutations having recessive phenotypes, a three-generation pedigree originates

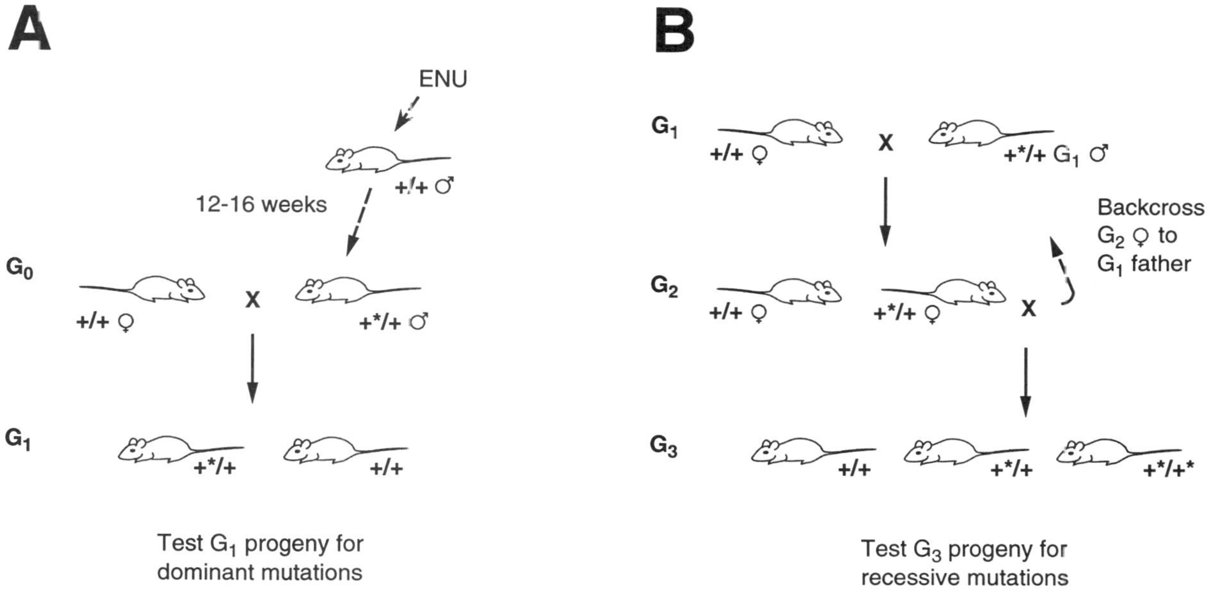

Figure 1. ENU mutagenesis screens in the mouse. (*A*) Mutagenesis screen to detect dominant (and semidominant) mutations in first generation (G_1) offspring. Male mice are injected intraperitoneally with ENU to intervene at the stage of spermatogonia. Following an ENU-induced sterile period of 12–16 weeks, these mice are bred with multiple females to produce G_1 progeny that would be heterozygous for any ENU-induced mutation (noted by an asterisk). (*B*) Mutagenesis screen to detect recessive mutations in third generation (G_3) offspring. To isolate mice homozygous for an induced mutation, a three-generation pedigree is established. G_1 male progeny are bred with wild-type females to produce second generation (G_2) progeny. G_2 female progeny are then bred with the G_1 male to produce third generation (G_3) progeny (see text for details). (Reprinted, with permission, from Takahashi et al. 1994 [copyright AAAS].)

from each G_1 male mouse. In this case, four G_2 female progeny of the G_1 male are backcrossed to the G_1 male to generate G_3 progeny, which would be homozygous for portions of the ENU-mutagenized gamete. If five G_3 progeny from each of the four G_2 females are tested, one has an 85% chance of recovering a recessive mutation (Shedlovsky et al. 1986). Thus, a recessive screen requires the analysis of about 20 times more mice than a dominant screen. For this reason, saturation mutagenesis screens for mutations having recessive phenotypes have not been done on a genome-wide scale in the mouse. However, recessive screens have been successful when applied to a specific region or locus of the mouse genome; for example, the *t* region of chromosome 17 (Shedlovsky et al. 1986) and the *Pah* (phenylalanine hydroxylase) locus (McDonald et al. 1990).

The effectiveness of ENU mutagenesis has made forward genetics feasible in the mouse. Until recently, however, mutagenesis screens with behavioral end points have not been attempted. Additional considerations are important when designing a screen with a behavioral end point. In particular, three factors are critical. First, the behavior being measured must be easily recorded, or recording it must be easily automated so that large numbers of mice can be screened, perhaps as many as 1000 or more per year. Second, the ability to determine the phenotype of individual animals will be essential for high-resolution genetic mapping experiments. Finally, if possible, performing a screen to identify mutations having dominant effects is very advantageous, because only in this case is it possible to approach genome-wide saturation mutagenesis, albeit of genes mutable to a dominant phenotype. With a mutagenesis rate of 0.0015 per locus per gamete and the ability to screen 1000 animals per year, a saturation screen for dominant mutations could be carried out in as little as 2 years.

Isolation and Characterization of the *Clock* Mutation

It was with these considerations in mind that we initiated a behavioral screen for ENU-induced mutations of the circadian system in the mouse. Circadian behavior in the mouse is precise and easily quantitated, thus it is very well suited for genetic screening. Normal C57BL/6J strain mice, which were used for this screen, exhibit a robust circadian rhythm of wheel-running activity (Pittendrigh and Daan 1976; Schwartz and Zimmerman 1990) that can be automatically recorded with an online computer system. This behavioral assay was used to screen for mice carrying mutations that cause abnormal circadian periods in constant darkness. Because most clock mutations that have been isolated in other organisms have been semidominant (Hall and Kyriacou 1990; Dunlap 1993), we chose to screen for dominant mutations using the procedure shown in Figure 1A. Analysis of about 300 progeny of ENU-treated mice revealed 1 mouse that expressed a circadian period that was more than 1 hour longer than (and six standard deviations above) the normal period of 23.7 hours (Fig. 2) (Vitaterna et al. 1994). This long-period phenotype was inherited as a single-locus, semidominant, autosomal mutation, which was designated *Clock*. Mice homozygous for the *Clock* mutation expressed extremely long circadian periods of about 28 hours for about the first 2 weeks of exposure to constant darkness, after which there was a complete loss of circadian rhythmicity (Fig. 2C).

Like many mutations in the circadian systems of other species, the *Clock* mutation has several effects on the circadian system of the mouse. In particular, two effects observed in *Clock*/+ heterozygotes are worth noting. The stability of period is decreased in *Clock*/+ mice and the amplitude of the resetting response to light pulses is increased, when compared to wild-type mice of the same strain (M. Vitaterna et al., unpublished observations). Both of these changes are consistent with the hypothesis that the circadian pacemaker of *Clock* heterozygotes cycles with a lower amplitude than that of wild-type mice.

The loss of rhythmicity in *Clock*/*Clock* mice suggested that *Clock* defines a gene essential for circadian rhythms. Recent evidence confirms and extends this conclusion (D. King et al., in prep.). We have now placed *Clock* within a radiation-induced deletion on chromosome 5, W^{-19H}, that includes the *Kit* (=*W*, *Dominant White Spotting*) locus (Lyon et al. 1984). The circadian phenotype of W^{-19H} heterozygous mice (hemizygous for the wild-type allele of *Clock*) is indistinguishable from the wild-type phenotype on a comparable strain background, suggesting that the null allele is recessive to wild type. By mating *Clock*/*Clock* mice to mice heterozygous for this deletion, we have been able to observe the phenotype of *Clock*/null animals. Of particular interest is the observation that the mean circadian period expressed by *Clock*/null animals is significantly longer than that of *Clock*/+ animals. This indicates that the wild-type allele interacts with the *Clock* mutation to ameliorate the severity of the phenotype of the *Clock* mutant allele. This is the essential feature of an antimorphic mutation (Muller 1932). That *Clock* is an antimorph, one type of dominant negative mutation, implies that the wild-type allele functions in the normal generation of circadian rhythms in the mouse. This provides strong evidence that *Clock* defines a gene central to the mammalian circadian system.

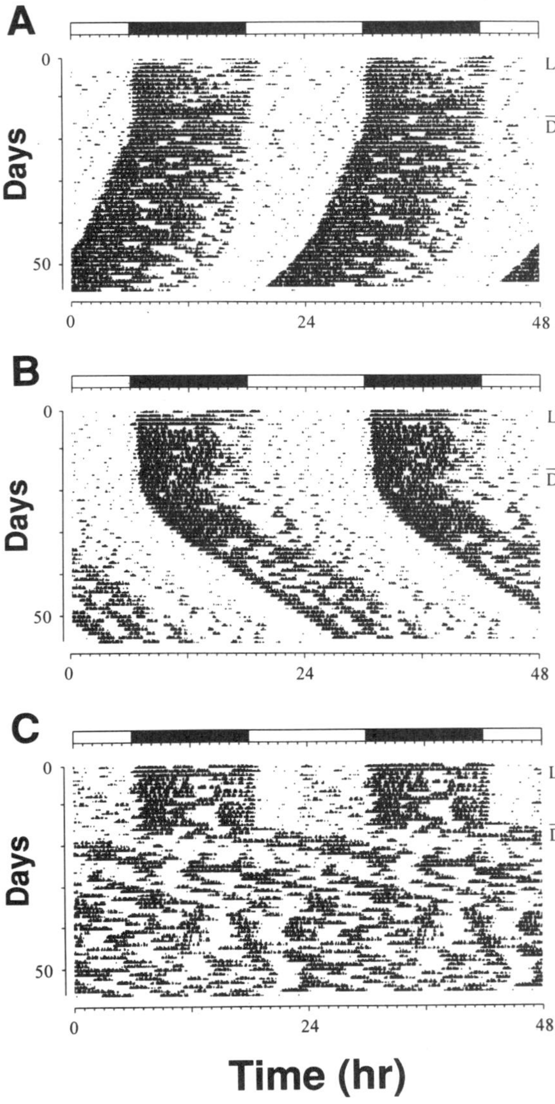

Figure 2. Circadian activity records of *Clock* mutant mice. Wheel-running activity records of three *Clock* mice on a C57BL/6J isogenic background are shown. All mice were kept on a light-dark cycle (LD 12:12) for the first 10 days of recording, then transferred to constant darkness (DD) on the day indicated by the line to the right of the record. (*A*) Activity record of a wild-type mouse. In constant darkness, this animal's activity rhythm had a period of 23.6 hr. (*B*) Activity record of a *Clock*/+ heterozygote. In DD, this animal's activity record had a rhythm of 24.8 hr. (*C*) Activity record of a *Clock*/*Clock* homozygote. This mouse had an activity rhythm period of 27.1 hr for the first 10 days in DD, which was followed by a complete loss of circadian rhythmicity. (Reprinted, with permission, from Vitaterna et al. 1994 [copyright AAAS].)

Molecular Characterization of an Induced Mutation

An effective mutagen for the mouse has been known for several years, during which time efficient screens could have been carried out to identify new mutations having effects on the behavior of mice. In fact, ENU was used in mutagenesis screens in the mouse, but the primary aim was to isolate new mutations at a known region or locus (examples include the *t* region and the *Pah* gene, mentioned above). One problem that prevented behavioral screens during this time was the lack of an effective method for identifying an unknown gene affected by the mutation. Mutagenesis screens, as a method of identifying the molecules involved in a phenotype of interest, are, of course, predicated on the belief that methods exist (or will exist) which allow for the cloning of genes affected by the mutagen. Unless, as in the case of P-element insertion in *Drosophila*, the mutagen itself allows the isolation of the affected gene, which ENU does not, identifying the gene will require positional cloning. All of the steps toward the positional cloning of a mutation in the mouse, from genetic mapping to testing of candidate genes, have benefited enormously from the development of numerous mouse molecular genetics resources. A task that once took many years can now conceivably be completed in much less time.

With the advent of dense SSLP maps, genetic mapping, the first step of any positional cloning strategy, has become a rapid process (Dietrich et al. 1992, 1994, 1996; Copeland et al. 1993). This resource allowed us to map the *Clock* mutation very rapidly in an intraspecific backcross segregating the mutation, placing it on the midportion of chromosome 5, between *D5Mit83* and *D5Mit24* (Vitaterna et al. 1994). It is important to note that it was only with the development of SSLP markers that intraspecific genetic crosses could be used on a regular basis in mapping experiments, owing to the high polymorphism rate (usually 50% or greater) that exists for these markers between strains of *M. musculus* (Dietrich et al. 1992). The SSLP map of the mouse genome includes over 6500 markers with an average interval between markers of less than 500 kb; thus, it is possible to generate a very high resolution genetic map (Dietrich et al. 1996). Without utilizing additional markers, we have been able to generate a high-resolution genetic map of the *Clock* locus (>1800 meioses), placing it within a 0.5-cM interval flanked by two SSLPs (D. King et al., in prep.).

Following the completion of a high-resolution genetic map, physical linkage of the genetic markers linked to *Clock* can be determined by long-range restriction mapping and pulsed-field gel electrophoresis, using markers converted to single-copy probes (Birren and Lai 1993). Concomitantly with the long-range mapping, large-insert genomic clones which span the critical genetic region that must contain *Clock* can be identified. In fact, much of the long-range mapping work can be done using these clones. The generation of this kind of physical map (contig) has been aided by the development of several yeast artificial chromosome (YAC) libraries of the mouse genome (Cox et al. 1993). Most of these have been pooled for high-efficiency polymerase chain reaction (PCR) screening or arrayed on high-density filters for hybridization, or both. Using one such library that is pooled for PCR screening (Kusumi et al. 1993) and SSLPs, as well as sequence tagged sites (STSs), from the region surrounding *Clock*, we have isolated more than 40 YAC clones and constructed a contig of about 4 Mb that spans the critical region (D. King et al., unpubl.). The recent development of bacterial artificial chromosome (BAC) and other large insert libraries of the mouse genome have brought new resources to physical mapping efforts (Monaco and Larin 1994). BACs, which are intermediate in size (~100–200 kb) between YACs and cosmids, have several advantages when compared to YAC clones. Although they are generally smaller than YAC clones, BACs are rarely chimeric; they are circular clones and thus much easier to manipulate, and they rarely suffer recombination or deletion damage (Shizuya et al. 1992). The transition from genetic to physical mapping has been made much easier by the ability to generate very high resolution genetic maps. In fact, marker density is sufficiently high that "walking steps" to fill in a genomic region with large clones can conceivably be avoided, at least in the case of YAC contigs. Indeed, all mapping efforts involving YAC clones may soon be eliminated, due to the planned completion of YAC contigs covering the entire extent of each of the mouse chromosomes.

With a contig covering the critical region in hand, a functional assay can be performed to identify more precisely the region that must contain *Clock*. If the number of YAC clones required to span the critical region is reasonably small and the mutation might be rescued by wild-type DNA, then an attempt can be made to express candidate YAC clones in a mutant mouse to complement the mutation or perhaps even rescue the wild-type behavior. This technical feat has been accomplished by many laboratories, with germline transmission and expression of YAC clones in the mouse either by pronuclear injection of YAC DNA with transgenic methods (Schedl et al. 1993), or by introducing YAC DNA into embryonic stem (ES) cells by lipofection and producing chimeric mice that transmitted the YAC transgene through the germ line (Strauss et al. 1993). These procedures should be easily transferred to BAC clones. In fact, if the critical region is sufficiently small, these clones would be preferable.

Once a genomic clone has been identified that either complements the *Clock* mutation or contains within it genetic markers that flank *Clock*, then efforts will be concentrated on this clone to identify transcription units and determine which gene within the clone is affected by the mutation. Several methods exist for identifying transcription units in a region of interest. Exon amplification (Church et al. 1994) and cDNA selection (Lovett 1994) of clones derived from the critical region are efficient methods of isolating expressed sequences. However, as DNA shotgun sequencing procedures become more efficient, direct sequencing of M13 subclones from the BAC clone of interest will become the most efficient way in which to identify transcription units. With candidate genes in hand, mutations can be identified using single-stranded conformational polymorphism (SSCP) (Beier 1993) or other methods, such as denaturing gradient gel electrophoresis (DGGE), chemical cleavage of mismatch (CCM) (Dianzani et al. 1993), or direct sequencing. Candidate genes may be prioritized for mutation detection based on expression patterns; we would expect, for example, that *Clock* is expressed in (at least) the brain, and in particular, the SCN. The final proof that we have identified the *Clock* gene is confirmed by expression of the gene and rescue of the mutant phenotype in transgenic mice. We are aware that it is difficult in principle to rescue a dominant mutation, but the use of hemizygous *Clock* recipients will allow us to detect wild-type *Clock* transgenes.

Recently, several resources have been developed that help to integrate the steps of positional cloning. Genetic mapping resources of high resolution (1000 meioses) and high polymorphism rates (i.e., interspecific crosses) have been generated that allow the integration and ordering of gene-based and anonymous-DNA loci. A widely used example of this kind of resource is the European Collaborative Interspecific Backcross (EUCIB), which consists of 983 backcross progeny derived from matings between *M. musculus* and *M. spretus* (Breen et al. 1994). Another resource is the growing accumulation of shotgun sequences of the 5′ and 3′ ends of hundreds of thousands of mammalian cDNA clones (Lennon et al. 1996). Although most of these sequences are from human cDNA libraries, the mouse/human sequence similarity is sufficiently high to identify mouse orthologs of human cDNAs. Candidate transcription unit sequences that have been isolated from a region of interest (in the case of *Clock*, a 0.5-cM interval in the midportion of chromosome 5) can be compared to the databases of these "expressed sequence tags" (ESTs) to determine if additional, larger, cloned sequences have already been identified. Most of the cDNAs sequenced in this way are readily available to the research community (Lennon et al. 1996). In addition, as these ESTs are mapped onto the human and mouse genomes, they will provide a rich resource of "ready-made" candidate genes. This EST mapping can be done efficiently using another recently developed resource, whole-genome radiation hybrid (RH) maps (Walter et al. 1994). An RH map of the mouse genome is now available (Schmitt et al. 1996). Loci are easily placed on RH maps by PCR and, in addition, these maps do not require the identification of intra- or interspecific polymorphisms, thus, they are ideal for integrating all loci that can be reduced to genomic DNA sequence. Some limitations to mapping 5′ cDNA sequences may be imposed by the presence of large intronic sequences between PCR primer pairs, but in most cases, the 3′ end of the cDNA clone can be placed on a RH map.

While working toward the positional cloning of the *Clock* gene, strategies can be utilized to identify additional components of the circadian system in the mouse, using *Clock* as a starting point. Two examples of such strategies are quantitative trait loci (QTL) analysis and a modifier mutagenesis screen to identify mutations affecting the expression of *Clock*. This kind of screen, which is similar in form to a dominant screen, can identify modifiers of the *Clock* mutation at unlinked loci, as well as new *Clock* alleles that might not be detected on a wild-type background. Evidence described above, indicating that the pacemaker in *Clock* heterozygotes has a reduced amplitude, suggests that a screen of this type may reveal subtle circadian mutations not detectable on a wild-type background. In addition, in light of the antimorphic behavior of the *Clock* mutation, this screen can be used to detect recessive null mutations at the *Clock* locus. Because evidence indicates that *Clock* is affected by genetic background (Vitaterna et al. 1994), it may be possible to identify multiple loci that modify the *Clock* phenotype, using a QTL strategy (Lander and Botstein 1989). The effectiveness of this strategy has been demonstrated by the identification of the *Mom-1* (*Modifier of Min-1*) locus (Dietrich et al. 1993). In this case, the expression of *Min* (*Multiple intestinal neoplasia*), itself an ENU-induced mutation (Moser et al. 1990), was dramatically affected by genetic background (Moser et al. 1992). Utilizing crosses between mouse strains with differing *Min* phenotypes, Dietrich et al. (1993) were able to identify a locus, *Mom-1*, that contributed significantly to this strain difference. Of course, once the *Clock* gene is cloned, a number of molecular approaches to find interacting proteins will become available. The independent isolation of the *tim* gene in *Drosophila*, using a yeast two-hybrid screen (Gekakis et al. 1995), provides one example of the success (and promise) of this type of approach.

SUMMARY

The study of mammalian circadian rhythms has a rich history of physiological understanding, but the molecular elements of the mammalian clock remain to be discovered. Availability of effective mutagenesis procedures and mouse molecular genetics resources sufficient for the task of positional cloning give cause for hope that the *Clock* gene, as well as other components of the mammalian circadian system, will be identified soon. The isolation of *Clock* in a deliberate mutagenesis screen provides an important proof-of-principle that forward genetics can be successfully applied toward the discovery of novel genes underlying complex behaviors in mice.

ACKNOWLEDGMENTS

The work described in this paper was supported by grants from the National Science Foundation Center for Biological Timing and the Bristol-Myers Squibb Foundation to J.S.T.

REFERENCES

Aronson, B.D., K.A. Johnson, and J.C. Dunlap. 1994a. Circadian clock locus frequency: Protein encoded by a single open reading frame defines period length and temperature compensation. *Proc. Natl. Acad. Sci.* **91:** 7683.

Aronson, B.D., K.A. Johnson, J.J. Loros, and J.C. Dunlap.

1994b. Negative feedback defining a circadian clock: Autoregulation in the clock gene *frequency*. *Science* **263:** 1578.

Baylies, M.K., T.A. Bargiello, F.R. Jackson, and M.W. Young. 1987. Changes in abundance or structure of the *per* gene product can alter periodicity of the *Drosophila* clock. *Nature* **326:** 390.

Beier, D.R. 1993. Single-strand conformation polymorphism (SSCP) analysis as a tool for genetic mapping. *Mamm. Genome* **4:** 627.

Benzer, S. 1973. Genetic dissection of behavior. *Sci. Am.* **229:** 24.

Birren, B. and E. Lai. 1993. *Pulsed field gel electrophoresis: A practical guide.* Academic Press, San Diego.

Breen, M., L. Deakin, B. Macdonald, S. Miller, R. Sibson, E. Tarttelin, P. Avner, F. Bourgade, J.L. Guenet, X. Montagutelli, C. Poirier, D. Simon, D. Tailor, M. Bishop, M. Kelly, F. Rysavy, S. Rastan, D. Norris, D. Shepherd, C. Abbott, A. Pilz, S. Hodge, I. Jackson, Y. Boyd, H. Blair, G. Malsen, J.A. Todd, P.W. Reed, J. Stoye, A. Ashworth, L McCarthy, R. Cox, L. Schalkwyk, H. Lehrach, J. Klose, U. Gangadharan, and S. Brown. 1994. Towards high resolution maps of the mouse and human genomes—A facility for ordering markers to 0.1 cM resolution. *Hum. Mol. Genet.* **3:** 621.

Cattanach, B.M., M.D. Burtenshaw, C. Rasberry, and E.P. Evans. 1993. Large deletions and other gross forms of chromosome imbalance compatible with viability and fertility in the mouse. *Nat. Genet.* **3:** 56.

Church, D.M., C.J. Stotler, J.L. Rutter, J.R. Murrell, J.A. Trofatter, and A.J. Buckler. 1994. Isolation of genes from complex sources of mammalian genomic DNA using exon amplification. *Nat. Genet.* **6:** 98.

Copeland, N.G., N.A. Jenkins, D.J. Gilbert, J.T. Eppig, L.J. Maltais, J.C. Miller, W.F. Dietrich, A. Weaver, S.E. Lincoln, R.G. Steen, L.D. Stein, J.H. Nadeau, and E.S. Lander. 1993. A genetic linkage map of the mouse: Current applications and future prospects. *Science* **262:** 57.

Cox, R.D., S. Meier-Ewert, M. Ross, Z. Larin, A.P. Monaco, and H. Lehrach. 1993. Genome mapping and cloning of mutations using yeast artificial chromosomes. *Methods Enzymol.* **225:** 637.

Dianzani, I., C. Camaschella, A. Ponzone, and R.G.H. Cotton. 1993. Dilemmas and progress in mutation detection. *Trends Genet.* **9:** 403.

Dietrich, W., H. Katz, S.E. Lincoln, H.-E. Shin, J. Friedman, N.C. Dracopoli, and E.S. Lander. 1992. A genetic map of the mouse suitable for typing intraspecific crosses. *Genetics* **131:** 423.

Dietrich, W.F., E.S. Lander, J.S. Smith, A.R. Moser, K.A. Gould, C. Luongo, N. Borenstein, and W. Dove. 1993. Genetic identification of *Mom-1*, a major modifier locus affecting *Min*-induced intestinal neoplasia in the mouse. *Cell* **75:** 631.

Dietrich, W.F., J.C. Miller, R.G. Steen, M. Merchant, D. Damron, R. Nahf, A. Gross, D.C. Joyce, M. Wessel, R.D. Dredge, A. Marquis, L.D. Stein, N. Goodman, D.C. Page, and E.S. Lander. 1994. A genetic map of the mouse with 4006 simple sequence polymorphisms. *Nat. Genet.* **7:** 220.

Dietrich, W.F., J. Miller, R. Steen, M.A. Merchant, D. Damron-Boles, Z. Husain, R. Dredge, M.J. Daly, K.A. Ingalls, T.J. O'Connor, C.A. Evans, M.M. DeAngelis, D.M. Levinson, L. Kruglyak, N. Goodman, N.G. Copeland, N.A. Jenkins, T.L. Hawkins, L. Stein, D.C. Page, and E.S. Lander. 1996. A comprehensive genetic map of the mouse genome. *Nature* **380:** 149.

Dunlap, J.C. 1993. Genetic analysis of circadian clocks. *Annu. Rev. Physiol.* **55:** 683.

Feldman, J.F. and M.N. Hoyle. 1973. Isolation of circadian clock mutants of *Neurospora crassa*. *Genetics* **75:** 605.

Gekakis, N., L. Saez, A.-M. Delahaye-Brown, M.P. Myers, A. Sehgal, M.W. Young, and C.J. Weitz. 1995. Isolation of *timeless* by PER protein interaction: Defective interaction between *timeless* protein and long-period mutant PER^{L}. *Science* **270:** 811.

Hall, J.C. 1990. Genetics of circadian rhythms. *Annu. Rev. Genet.* **24:** 659.

Hall, J.C. and C.P. Kyriacou. 1990. Genetics of biological rhythms in *Drosophila*. *Adv. Insect Physiol.* **22:** 221.

Hitotsumachi, S., D.A. Carpenter, and W.L. Russell. 1985. Dose-repetition increases the mutagenic effectiveness of *N*-ethyl-*N*-nitrosourea in mouse spermatogonia. *Proc. Natl. Acad. Sci.* **82:** 6619.

Konopka, R.J. and S. Benzer. 1971. Clock mutants of *Drosophila melanogaster*. *Proc. Natl. Acad. Sci.* **68:** 2112.

Kusumi, K., J.S. Smith, J.A. Segre, D.S. Koos, and E.S. Lander. 1993. Construction of a large-insert yeast artificial chromosome library of the mouse genome. *Mamm. Genome* **4:** 391.

Lander, E.S. and D. Botstein. 1989. Mapping Mendelian factors underlying quantitative traits using RFLP linkage maps. *Genetics* **121:** 185.

Lennon, G., C. Auffray, M. Polymeropolous, and M.B. Soares. 1996. The I.M.A.G.E. consortium: An integrated molecular analysis of genomes and their expression. *Genomics* **33:** 151.

Lovett, M. 1994. Fishing for complements: Finding genes by direct selection. *Trends Genet.* **10:** 352.

Lynch, G.R. and C.B. Lynch. 1992. Using quantitative genetic methods to understand mammalian circadian behavior and photoperiodism. In *Techniques for the genetic analysis of brain and behavior* (ed. D. Goldowitz et al.), p. 251. Elsevier, New York.

Lyon, M.F., P.H. Glenister, J.F. Loutit, E.P. Evans, and J. Peters. 1984. A presumed deletion covering the *W* and *Ph* loci of the mouse. *Genet. Res.* **44:** 161.

McClung, C.R., B.A. Fox, and J.C. Dunlap. 1989. The *Neurospora* clock gene *frequency* shares a sequence element with the *Drosophila* clock gene *period*. *Nature* **339:** 558.

McDonald, J.D., V.C. Bode, W.F. Dove, and A. Shedlovsky. 1990. Pah$^{hph\text{-}5}$: A mouse mutant deficient in phenylalanine hydroxylase. *Proc. Natl. Acad. Sci.* **87:** 1965.

Meijer, J.H. and W.J. Rietveld. 1989. Neurophysiology of the suprachiasmatic circadian pacemaker in rodents. *Physiol. Rev.* **69:** 671.

Menaker, M. and J.S. Takahashi. 1995. Genetic analysis of the circadian system of mammals: Properties and prospects. *Semin. Neurosci.* **7:** 61.

Monaco, A.P. and Z. Larin. 1994. YACs, BACs, PACs, and MACs: Artificial chromosomes as research tools. *Trends Biotechnol.* **12:** 280.

Moser, A.R., H.C. Pitot, and W.F. Dove. 1990. A dominant mutation that predisposes to multiple intestinal neoplasia in the mouse. *Science* **247:** 322.

Moser, A.R., W.F. Dove, K.A. Roth, and J.I. Gordon. 1992. The *Min* (multiple intestinal neoplasia) mutation: Its effect on gut epithelial cell differentiation and interaction with a modifier system. *J. Cell Biol.* **116:** 1517.

Muller, H.J. 1932. Further studies on the nature and causes of gene mutations. *Proc. Int. Congr. Genet.* **6:** 213.

Myers, M.P., K. Wager-Smith, C.S. Wesley, and M.W. Young. 1995. Positional cloning and sequence analysis of the *Drosophila* clock gene, *timeless*. *Science* **270:** 805.

Okazaki, Y., H. Okuizumi, T. Ohsumi, O. Nomura, S. Takada, M. Kamiya, N. Sasaki, Y. Matsuda, M. Nishimura, O. Tagaya, M. Muramatsu, and Y. Hayashizaki. 1996. A genetic linkage map of the syrian hamster and localization of cardiomyopathy locus on chromosome 9qa2.1-b1 using RLGS spot-mapping. *Nat. Genet.* **13:** 87.

Pittendrigh, C.S. 1974. Circadian oscillations in cells and the circadian organization of multicellular systems. In *The neurosciences third study program* (ed. F.C. Schmitt and F.G. Worden), p. 437. MIT Press, Cambridge.

Pittendrigh, C.S. and S. Daan. 1976. A functional analysis of circadian pacemakers in nocturnal rodents: I. The stability and lability of spontaneous frequency. *J. Comp. Physiol.* **106:** 223.

Ralph, M.R. and M. Menaker. 1988. A mutation of the circadian system in golden hamsters. *Science* **241:** 1225.

Rinchik, E.M. 1991. Chemical mutagenesis and fine-structure functional analysis of the mouse genome. *Trends Genet.* **7:** 15.

Rinchik, E.M., D.A. Carpenter, and P.B. Shelby. 1990a. A strategy for fine-structure functional analysis of a 6- to 11-centimorgan region of mouse chromosome 7 by high-efficiency mutagenesis. *Proc. Natl. Acad. Sci.* **87:** 896.

Rinchik, E.M., J.W. Bangham, P.R. Hunsicker, N.L.A. Cacheiro, B.S. Kwon, I.J. Jackson, and L.B. Russell. 1990b. Genetic and molecular analysis of chlorambucil-induced germ-line mutations in the mouse. *Proc. Natl. Acad. Sci.* **87:** 1416.

Rossant, J. and N. Hopkins. 1992. Of fin and fur: Mutational analysis of vertebrate embryonic development. *Genes Dev.* **6:** 1.

Russell, L.B., P.R. Hunsicker, N.L.A. Cacheiro, J.W. Bangham, W.L. Russell, and M.D. Shelby. 1989. Chlorambucil effectively induces deletion mutations in mouse germ cells. *Proc. Natl. Acad. Sci.* **86:** 3704.

Russell, W.L., E.M. Kelly, P.R. Hunsicker, J.W. Bangham, S.C. Maddux, and E.L. Phipps. 1979. Specific-locus test shows ethylnitrosourea to be the most potent mutagen in the mouse. *Proc. Natl. Acad. Sci.* **76:** 5818.

Schedl, A., L. Montoliu, G. Kelsey, and G. Schütz. 1993. A yeast artificial chromosome covering the tyrosinase gene confers copy number-dependent expression in transgenic mice. *Nature* **362:** 258.

Schmitt, K., J.W. Foster, R.W. Feakes, C. Knights, M.E. Davis, D.J. Spillett, and P.N. Goodfellow. 1996. Construction of a mouse whole-genome radiation hybrid panel and application to MMU11. *Genomics* **34:** 193.

Schwartz, W.J. and P. Zimmerman. 1990. Circadian timekeeping in BALB/c and C57BL/6 inbred mouse strains. *J. Neurosci.* **10:** 3685.

Sehgal, A., J.L. Price, B. Man, and M.W. Young. 1994. Loss of circadian behavioral rhythms and *per* RNA oscillations in the *Drosophila* mutant *timeless*. *Science* **263:** 1603.

Sehgal, A., A. Rothenfluh-Hilfiker, M. Hunter-Ensor, Y. Chen, M.P. Myers, and M.W. Young. 1995. Rhythmic expression of *timeless:* A basis for promoting circadian cycles in *period* gene autoregulation. *Science* **270:** 808.

Selby, P.B. 1981. Radiation genetics. In *The mouse in biomedical research* (ed. H.L. Foster et al.), p. 264. Academic Press, New York.

Shedlovsky, A., J.-L. Guenet, L.L. Johnson, and W.F. Dove. 1986. Induction of recessive lethal mutations in the *T/t-H-2* region of the mouse genome by a point mutagen. *Genet. Res.* **47:** 135.

Shizuya, H., B. Birren, U.J. Kim, V. Mancino, T. Slepak, Y. Tachiiri, and M. Simon. 1992. Cloning and stable maintenance of 300-kilobase-pair fragments of human DNA in *Escherichia coli* using an F-factor-based vector. *Proc. Natl. Acad. Sci.* **89:** 8794.

Strauss, W.M., J. Dausman, C. Beard, C. Johnson, J.B. Lawrence, and R. Jaenisch. 1993. Germ line transmission of a yeast artificial chromosome spanning the murine α_1(I) collagen locus. *Science* **259:** 1904.

Takahashi, J.S. 1995. Molecular neurobiology and genetics of circadian rhythms in mammals. *Annu. Rev. Neurosci.* **18:** 531.

Takahashi, J.S., L.H. Pinto, and M.H. Vitaterna. 1994. Forward and reverse genetic approaches to behavior in the mouse. *Science* **264:** 1724.

Vitaterna, M.H., D.P. King, A.-M. Chang, J.M. Kornhauser, P.L. Lowrey, J.D. McDonald, W.F. Dove, L.P. Pinto, F.W. Turek, and J.S. Takahashi. 1994. Mutagenesis and mapping of a mouse gene, *Clock,* essential for circadian behavior. *Science* **264:** 719.

Walter, M.A., D.J. Spillett, P. Thomas, J. Weissenbach, and P.N. Goodfellow. 1994. A method for constructing radiation hybrid maps of whole genomes. *Nat. Genet.* **7:** 22.

Yu, Q., A.C. Jacquier, Y. Citri, M. Hamblen, J.C. Hall, and M. Rosbash. 1987. Molecular mapping of point mutations in the period gene that stop or speed up biological clocks in *Drosophila melanogaster*. *Proc. Natl. Acad. Sci.* **84:** 784.

Zeng, H., P.E. Hardin, and M. Rosbash. 1994. Constitutive overexpression of the *Drosophila period* protein inhibits *period* mRNA cycling. *EMBO J.* **13:** 3590.

Confocal-microscopic Visualization of Membrane Addition during Synaptic Exocytosis at Presynaptic Active Zones of Hair Cells

A.J. HUDSPETH[1] AND N.P. ISSA[2]

[1]Howard Hughes Medical Institute and Laboratory of Sensory Neuroscience, The Rockefeller University, New York, New York 10021; [2]Medical Scientist Training Program, University of Texas Southwestern Medical Center, Dallas, Texas 75235

The vesicle hypothesis of synaptic-transmitter release (for review, see Katz 1971) was inspired by the discovery of quantal neurotransmission and the identification of synaptic vesicles. In addition to extensive physiological support, this model has been validated by several lines of morphological evidence. Rapid-freezing studies first demonstrated vesicle fusion at defined times during the release of synaptic transmitter (Heuser et al. 1979; Heuser and Reese 1981). The use of tracer molecules in the extracellular fluid (Heuser and Reese 1973), the visualization of plasmalemmal expansion and recovery (Schaeffer and Raviola 1978), and the monitoring of lipophilic fluorophores in the plasmalemma (Betz and Bewick 1992; Ryan and Smith 1995) confirmed the recycling of vesicular membrane.

Although the validity of the vesicular model of transmitter release is no longer in doubt, it only recently became possible to investigate synaptic exocytosis with a high temporal resolution. The advent of sensitive techniques for the measurement of membrane-capacitance changes (Neher and Marty 1982) has provided a means of detecting the addition of vesicular membrane at the ensemble of active zones in specialized synaptic terminals such as the retinal bipolar cell's axonal ending (von Gersdorff and Matthews 1994) and the hair cell's soma (Parsons et al. 1994).

In this paper, we demonstrate another method by which the addition of vesicular membrane to the plasmalemma may be measured with high temporal resolution. When a hair cell is stimulated, the release of neural transmitter is confined to the cell's limited number of active zones (Liberman 1980; Miller and Beck 1988; Sneary 1988; Issa and Hudspeth 1994, 1996a,b), each marked by the presence of a presynaptic dense body, clustered vesicles, and a presynaptic membrane density (Gleisner et al. 1973; Jørgensen and Flock 1973; Hama and Saito 1977; Hama 1980; Jacobs and Hudspeth 1990). Voltage-sensitive Ca^{++} channels, which are responsible for triggering synaptic-vesicle fusion, are also clustered at a presynaptic active zone (Roberts et al. 1990; Issa and Hudspeth 1994). Because a hair cell must release transmitter briskly in order to transmit information about high-frequency sounds, the rate of sustained exocytosis at each such presynaptic active zone is unusually great. It therefore stands to reason that the focal addition of vesicular membrane to the plasmalemma might be detectable by morphological techniques. By taking advantage of our ability to identify individual active zones in living hair cells (Issa and Hudspeth 1994, 1996a,b), we have been able to measure localized bulging of the plasmalemma that we believe signals the profuse fusion of synaptic vesicles.

EXPERIMENTAL PROCEDURES

Hair cells, isolated from the sacculus of the bullfrog (*Rana catesbeiana*) by exposure to protease and a solution low in divalent cations (Issa and Hudspeth 1996), were bathed in standard saline solution comprising 110 mM Na^+, 2 mM K^+, 4 mM Ca^{++}, 118 mM Cl^-, 3 mM D-glucose, and 5 mM *N*-(2-hydroxyethyl)piperazine-*N′*-(2-ethanesulfonic acid) (HEPES) at pH 7.3. Electrical recordings were made by the whole-cell, tight-seal technique. Filled with an internal solution containing 104 mM Cs^+, 2 mM Na^+, 2 mM Mg^{++}, 104 mM Cl^-, 1 mM ATP, and 5 mM HEPES at pH 7.3, the recording pipettes had resistances of 3–5 MΩ. Cytoplasmic Ca^{++} was detected by including in the internal solution 200 μM of the pentaammonium salt of the Ca^{++} indicator fluo-3 (Minta et al. 1989). To adjust the cytoplasmic Ca^{++}-buffering capacity, 1,2-*bis*(*o*-aminophenoxy)-ethane-*N,N,N′,N′*-tetraacetic acid (BAPTA; Tsien 1980) or ethylene glycol-*bis*(β-aminoethyl ether)-*N,N,N′,N′*-tetraacetic acid (EGTA) was added to the internal solution.

The electrical responses of hair cells were measured with a voltage-clamp amplifier (EPC-7, List Electronics, Darmstadt, Germany) controlled by a computer through an experimental interface (LM-900, Dagan Instruments, Minneapolis, Minnesota). Responses were filtered with an eight-pole Bessel filter whose half-power frequency was set at one quarter the sampling frequency. Linear response components were then removed by a P/6 subtraction procedure. When an experiment was performed multiple times, the result is expressed as the mean ± standard deviation for the indicated numbers of repetitions.

Confocal images were acquired with a laser-scanning microscope system (MRC-600, Bio-Rad, Hercules, California) attached to an inverted microscope (IM-35, Carl Zeiss, Jena, Germany). To produce a line-scan image, an approximately 400-nm-diameter spot of laser light was swept across a hair cell; the transect was perpendicular to the plasmalemma and intersected a presynaptic active zone (Issa and Hudspeth 1996b). After the acquisition of fluoresence-intensity data from 384 points, the scan was repeated at 2-μsec intervals. To reduce noise, line-scan images were smoothed with a 3 x 3 mask (1 : 2 : 1, 2 : 8 : 2, 1 : 2 : 1) that introduced a spread in the time domain of approximately 500 μsec. In addition to fluorescence data, the confocal microscope's computer recorded voltage-command signals that were used to synchronize confocal imaging with physiological stimulation.

RESULTS

Confocal-microscopic Measurement of Membrane Bulging

During synaptic-vesicle fusion, the surface area of a cell's membrane increases (Lim et al. 1990; Parsons et al. 1994; von Gersdorff and Matthews 1994). Because fusion occurs specifically at presynaptic active zones (Heuser et al. 1974, 1979; Heuser and Reese 1981), the plasmalemma there should be focally deformed during vigorous exocytosis.

Our ability to identify presynaptic active zones in living hair cells (Issa and Hudspeth 1994, 1996a) enabled us to visualize the addition of membrane during exocytosis. In four cells that exhibited large whole-cell Ca^{++} currents during depolarizations from –70 mV to –15 mV, the presynaptic membrane bulged away from the cell's center during Ca^{++} influx (Fig. 1A). This deformation was confined to the vicinity of the presynaptic active zone; simultaneously imaged membrane surfaces distant from an active zone did not display bulging during stimulation.

Membrane bulging in response to a large Ca^{++} current was observed only when the Ca^{++}-buffering environment permitted exocytosis (Adler et al. 1991): when a cell contained a low concentration of exogenous buffer (for example, less than 3 mM BAPTA) or a buffer with a small *on* rate for Ca^{++} binding (for example, 10 mM EGTA). During 14 depolarizations of the four cells that showed membrane movements, the Ca^{++} currents averaged 0.9 ± 0.2 nA. Even though their Ca^{++} currents averaged 1.0 ± 0.2 nA over 59 depolarizations, bulging was not observed in 12 cells loaded with 8 mM or more BAPTA. Despite a buffering environment conducive to exocytosis, the bulging phenomenon could not be detected in hair cells whose Ca^{++} currents were relatively small, averaging only 0.6 ± 0.2 nA during 110 depolarizations.

At the end of a depolarization, the plasmalemma returned to its original position within a few hundred msec (Fig. 1A). The time course of recovery was approximately exponential; for the hair cell analyzed in Figure 1, the time constant was 130 msec. Recovery from bulging was probably not caused by endocytosis, for hair cells studied by whole-cell recording lose their ability to retrieve synaptic vesicles (Parsons et al. 1994). The recovery phase was likely due to lateral flow of membrane from the site of vesicle fusion.

Estimation of the Exocytotic Rate from Membrane Bulging and Recovery

We analyzed bulging at individual presynaptic active zones on the assumption that the net local rate of change in membrane area, A_{net}, reflected the contributions of membrane addition by exocytosis and membrane clearance by lateral flow:

$$\frac{dA_{net}}{dt} = \frac{dA_{exocytosis}}{dt} + \frac{dA_{flow}}{dt} \qquad (1)$$

We estimated the rate of change in membrane area by assuming that the local membrane deformation due to exocytosis was hemispherical and that the measured displacement of the membrane represented the hemisphere's radius. In this case, the net rate of change in surface area at any time is given by

$$\frac{dA_{net}}{dt} = 4\pi r\,\frac{dr}{dt} \qquad (2)$$

in which r is the position of the membrane at a given time relative to its position before stimulation.

The rate of increase in surface area due to exocytosis is

$$\frac{dA_{exocytosis}}{dt} = A_{sv}\,\frac{dN}{dt} \qquad (3)$$

in which A_{sv} is the average surface area of an individual vesicle and dN/dt is the rate of vesicle fusion at an individual active zone.

We assumed that vesicles promptly ceased to fuse with the plasmalemma at the end of a depolarizing pulse. The change in membrane area thereafter was entirely due to lateral flow of membrane. For a hemispherical membrane deformation, the rate of membrane clearance is simply related to the rate of change in the membrane's bulge:

$$\frac{dA_{flow}}{dt} = 4\pi\left[r\frac{dr}{dt}\right]_{clearance} \qquad (4)$$

in which the bracketed term is evaluated during the recovery period following the termination of the depolarizing stimulus. Note that the numerical value of this term is negative.

Combining the equations above yields an expression for the rate of vesicle fusion at the end of the depolarizing pulse:

$$\frac{dN}{dt} = \frac{4\pi}{A_{sv}}\left\{\left[r\frac{dr}{dt}\right]_{net} - \left[r\frac{dr}{dt}\right]_{clearance}\right\} \qquad (5)$$

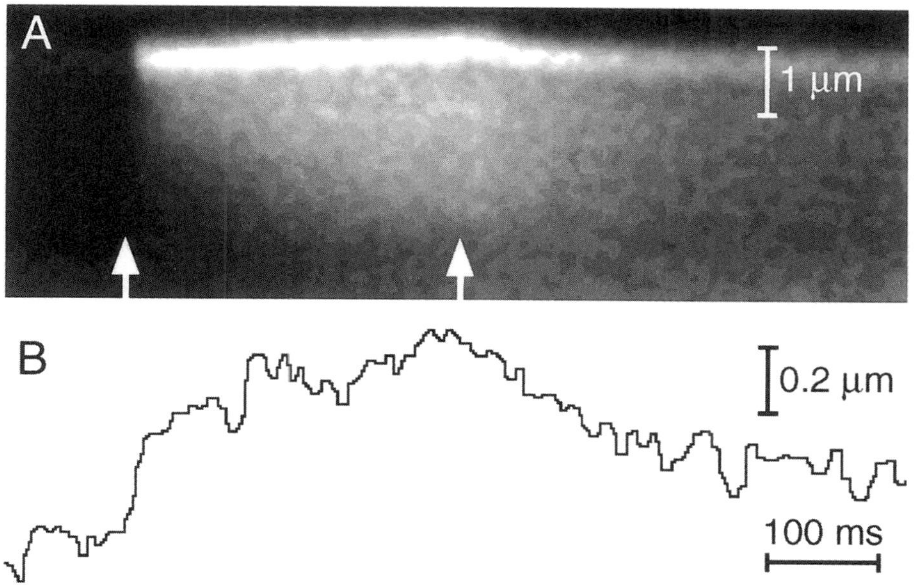

Figure 1. Deformation of the presynaptic membrane by exocytosis during a large Ca^{++} influx. (*A*) A line-scan image (Issa and Hudspeth 1994, 1996b) represents a plot of distance across a cell (*ordinate*) against time (*abscissa*); the transect of the scan intercepted a single presynaptic dense body. The brightness of individual pixels represents the fluorescence intensity of the Ca^{++} indicator fluo-3 loaded into the cell through the recording electrode. The dark horizontal strip across the image's top represents extracellular space; the lower portion of the illustration embraces the hair cell's cytoplasm. The arrows mark the onset and conclusion of a 300-msec depolarization of the membrane from –70 mV to –15 mV. Fluo-3 bound to the 450-nm-diameter presynaptic dense body just beneath the plasmalemma (Issa and Hudspeth 1996a); depolarization therefore evoked strong fluorescence from this organelle. The spread of fluorescence into the cytoplasm reflected the diffusion both of free Ca^{++} and of that bound to the indicator. Enhanced fluorescence was associated with outward bulging of the hair cell's membrane, which appears here as an upward movement of the fluorescence associated with the presynaptic dense body. Observations by differential-interference-contrast microscopy, which can be used to locate presynaptic active zones (Issa and Hudspeth 1994, 1996a), indicated that the dense body imaged here was one of a closely spaced pair of the organelles. (*B*) The bulging movement of the membrane surface was determined from the line-scan image by plotting the midpoint of the fluorescence-intensity profile at the cell's edge as a function of time. Note that, although the two panels are in temporal register, the vertical scale in *B* is exaggerated fivefold with respect to that in *A*.

in which the first term in square brackets is evaluated during electrical stimulation.

To obtain an upper bound on the rate of exocytosis, we estimated the net rate of change in membrane area from the data of Figure 1. For the 200-msec interval before the depolarizing pulse's end, the net rate of increase in membrane area was 10.5 $\mu m^2 \cdot s^{-1}$, corresponding to membrane bulging at a rate of 2.1 $\mu m \cdot s^{-1}$. The rate of membrane clearance was determined just after the pulse's termination as –18 $\mu m^2 \cdot s^{-1}$, with a rate of change in plasmalemmal position of –3.3 $\mu m \cdot s^{-1}$. The surface area of a 45-nm-diameter synaptic vesicle is about 0.005 μm^2, so the estimated rate of exocytosis was 6000 vesicles per second. Because the line scan for Figure 1 intercepted the plasmalemmal surface adjacent to two closely spaced presynaptic active zones, the exocytotic rate at each site was approximately 3000 vesicles per second.

Estimation of the Exocytotic Rate with a Steady-state Assumption

Noise in the fluorescence signals interfered with measurement of the plasmalemma's position and, thus, determination of the bulging rate. During electrical stimulation, this source of error was great enough to preclude more than approximate estimation of the rate of exocytosis. Because the signals were somewhat less noisy during the recovery phase of the response, however, less arbitrary estimation of the membrane diffusion rate was possible following depolarizations.

To estimate the rate of exocytosis without measuring the bulging rate during stimulation, we made the additional assumption that the position of the membrane at the conclusion of the depolarization was in a steady state: The rate of membrane addition due to exocytosis was balanced by the rate of membrane clearance through lateral flow. In other words, we supposed that a plot of membrane position against time (Fig. 1B) had reached a plateau by the depolarization's end. In this case, it follows that

$$\frac{dN}{dt} = -\frac{4\pi}{A_{sv}}\left[r\,\frac{dr}{dt}\right]_{clearance} \qquad (6)$$

At the conclusion of the stimulus that evoked the largest membrane deformation, the clearance rate was –18 $\mu m^2 \cdot s^{-1}$. If membrane bulging during depolarization resulted from a balance between membrane addition through exocytosis and membrane clearance by lateral flow, the rate of recovery after the Ca^{++} influx of Figure 1 implied an exocytosis of about 650 vesicles per second at a single active zone. Because of the steady-state assumption involved, this value represents a lower bound on the rate of vesicle fusion.

DISCUSSION

The present estimates of the maximal rate of exocytosis at individual presynaptic zones of hair cells are similar to that of 500 vesicles per second obtained from membrane-capacitance changes (Parsons et al. 1994). In agreement with the capacitative analysis, the relatively large presynaptic active zones of hair cells appear to mediate faster fusion of vesicles than do the smaller but more numerous active zones of retinal bipolar cells (von Gersdorff and Matthews 1994; von Gersdorff et al. 1996).

The validity of our estimates of the rate of vesicle fusion was restricted by the useful but doubtlessly simplistic assumption that the presynaptic membrane bulged hemispherically. A better appreciation of the shape of the membrane deformation due to exocytosis, and thus an improved estimate of the rate of exocytosis, might be obtained by using high-speed confocal microscopy to produce a two-dimensional image of a presynaptic active zone during vesicle fusion.

The spread of fluorescence signals beyond a cell's boundary introduced potential technical problems into our data. Because of the finite resolving power of the objective lens, the rising fluorescence intensity near the plasmalemma caused an increase in the signal attributed to the extracellular space just outside the membrane. This effect was most prominent at the onset of a pulse, when Ca^{++} rapidly entered the cell and enhanced the cytoplasmic fluorescence. Although a portion of the apparent membrane bulge could therefore have resulted from an optical artifact, not all of the movement could be attributed to this source; even the *inner* boundary of the fluorescently labeled dense body clearly receded from the cell's center.

We took two approaches to minimize the impact of the potential artifact. First, we based our estimates of the membrane's resting position not only on the images taken before stimulation, but also on those taken well after a pulse's conclusion. Because of residual cytoplasmic Ca^{++}, the latter images displayed strong fluorescence signals near the plasmalemma and thus resembled those acquired during stimulation and exocytosis. In addition, we used the midpoint in the fluorescence profile, rather than a particular intensity level, in estimating the plasmalemma's position.

The present results delineate for the first time an early step in the recycling of membrane added to the plasmalemma by vesicle fusion. During vigorous excitation of a hair cell, membrane evidently accumulates at an active zone because the rate of addition through exocytosis exceeds that of removal by lateral flow. The extent of focal plasmalemmal bulging in intact tissue is uncertain. These experiments, which involved depolarizations of hair cells more extreme than are likely to occur in situ, presumably yielded unusually high rates of exocytosis. In addition, membrane retrieval by coated vesicles, which apparently occurs immediately adjacent to active zones (Jacobs and Hudspeth 1990), was probably eliminated under our recording conditions (Parsons et al. 1994).

ACKNOWLEDGMENTS

We thank Dr. J.L. Cyr and Ms. E.A. Lumpkin for helpful comments on the manuscript. This research was supported by National Institutes of Health grant DC-00317. A.J.H. is an Investigator with the Howard Hughes Medical Institute.

REFERENCES

Adler, E.M., G.J. Augustine, S.N. Duffy, and M.P. Charlton. 1991. Alien intracellular calcium chelators attenuate neurotransmitter release at the squid giant synapse. *J. Neurosci.* **11:** 1496.

Betz, W.J. and G.S. Bewick. 1992. Optical analysis of synaptic vesicle recycling at the frog neuromuscular junction. *Science* **255:** 200.

Gleisner, L., Å. Flock, and J. Wersäll. 1973. The ultrastructure of the afferent synapse on hair cells in the frog labyrinth. *Acta Otolaryngol.* **76:** 199.

Hama, K. 1980. Fine structure of the afferent synapse and gap junctions on the sensory hair cell in the saccular macula of goldfish: A freeze-fracture study. *J. Neurocytol.* **9:** 845.

Hama, K. and K. Saito. 1977. Fine structure of the afferent synapse of the hair cells in the saccular macula of the goldfish, with special reference to the anastomosing tubules. *J. Neurocytol.* **6:** 361.

Heuser, J.E. and T.S. Reese. 1973. Evidence for recycling of synaptic vesicle membrane during transmitter release at the frog neuromuscular junction. *J. Cell Biol.* **57:** 315.

———. 1981. Structural changes after transmitter release at the frog neuromuscular junction. *J. Cell Biol.* **88:** 564.

Heuser, J.E., T.S. Reese, and D.M.D. Landis. 1974. Functional changes in frog neuromuscular junctions studied with freeze-fracture. *J. Neurocytol.* **3:** 109.

Heuser, J.E., T.S. Reese, M.J. Dennis, Y. Jan, L. Jan, and L. Evans. 1979. Synaptic vesicle exocytosis captured by quick freezing and correlated with quantal transmitter release. *J. Cell Biol.* **81:** 275.

Issa, N.P. and A.J. Hudspeth. 1994. Clustering of Ca^{2+} channels and Ca^{2+}-activated K^+ channels at fluorescently labeled presynaptic active zones of hair cells. *Proc. Natl. Acad. Sci.* **91:** 7578.

———. 1996a. Characterization of fluo-3 labeling of dense bodies at the hair cell's presynaptic active zone. *J. Neurocytol.* **25:** 257.

———. 1996b. The entry and clearance of Ca^{2+} at individual presynaptic active zones of hair cells from the bullfrog's sacculus. *Proc. Natl. Acad. Sci.* **93:** 9527.

Jacobs, R.A. and A.J. Hudspeth. 1990. Ultrastructural correlates of mechanoelectrical transduction in hair cells of the bullfrog's internal ear. *Cold Spring Harbor Symp. Quant. Biol.* **55:** 547.

Jørgensen, J.M. and Å. Flock. 1973. The ultrastructure of lateral line sense organs in the adult salamander *Ambystoma mexicanum. J. Neurocytol.* **2:** 133.

Katz, B. 1971. Quantal mechanism of neural transmitter release. *Science* **173:** 123.

Liberman, M.C. 1980. Morphological differences among radial afferent fibers in the cat cochlea: An electron-microscopic study of serial sections. *Hearing Res.* **3:** 45.

Lim, N.F., M.C. Nowycky, and R.L. Bookman. 1990. Direct measurement of exocytosis and calcium currents in single vertebrate nerve terminals. *Nature* **344:** 449.

Miller, M.R. and J. Beck. 1988. Auditory hair cell innervational patterns in lizards. *J. Comp. Neurol.* **271:** 604.

Minta, A., J.P.Y. Kao, and R.Y. Tsien. 1989. Fluorescent indicators for cytosolic calcium based on rhodamine and fluorescein chromophores. *J. Biol. Chem.* **264:** 8171.

Neher, E. and A. Marty. 1982. Discrete changes of cell membrane capacitance observed under conditions of enhanced secretion in bovine adrenal chromaffin cells. *Proc. Natl. Acad. Sci.* **79:** 6712.

Parsons, T.D., D. Lenzi, W. Almers, and W.M. Roberts. 1994. Calcium-triggered exocytosis and endocytosis in an isolated presynaptic cell: Capacitance measurements in saccular hair cells. *Neuron* **13:** 875.

Roberts, W.M., R.A. Jacobs, and A.J. Hudspeth. 1990. Colocalization of ion channels involved in frequency selectivity and synaptic transmission at presynaptic active zones of hair cells. *J. Neurosci.* **10:** 3664.

Ryan, T.A. and S.J. Smith. 1995. Vesicle pool mobilization during action potential firing at hippocampal synapses. *Neuron* **14:** 983.

Schaeffer, S.F. and E. Raviola. 1978. Membrane recycling in the cone cell endings of the turtle retina. *J. Cell Biol.* **79:** 802.

Sneary, M.G. 1988. Auditory receptor of the red-eared turtle: II. Afferent and efferent synapses and innervation patterns. *J. Comp. Neurol.* **276:** 588.

Tsien, R.Y. 1980. New calcium indicators and buffers with high selectivity against magnesium and protons: Design, synthesis, and properties of prototype structures. *Biochemistry* **19:** 2396.

von Gersdorff, H. and G. Matthews. 1994. Dynamics of synaptic vesicle fusion and membrane retrieval in synaptic terminals. *Nature* **367:** 735.

von Gersdorff, H., E. Vardi, G. Matthews, and P. Sterling. 1996. Evidence that vesicles on the synaptic ribbon of retinal bipolar neurons can be rapidly released. *Neuron* **16:** 1221.

Multiple Myosin Isozymes and Hair-cell Function

P.G. GILLESPIE,[1] T. HASSON,[2] J.A. GARCIA,[3] AND D.P. COREY[3]
[1]Departments of Physiology and Neuroscience, The Johns Hopkins University, Baltimore, Maryland 21205;
[2]Departments of Biology and Pathology, Yale University, New Haven, Connecticut 06520;
[3]Howard Hughes Medical Institute, Departments of Neurobiology and Neurology,
Massachusetts General Hospital and Harvard University, Boston, Massachusetts 02114

Transduction of auditory and vestibular stimuli is carried out by specialized sensory cells called hair cells, named for their hair-like projections of actin-based stereocilia (for review, see Hudspeth 1989; Pickles and Corey 1992; Gillespie 1995; Hackney and Furness 1995). The importance of actin filaments for hair-cell transduction and the existence of multiple actin-rich domains in hair cells suggest that myosin molecules, the only proteins known to exert force along actin filaments, carry out precise and varied tasks. Recent work has shown the myosin family to consist of a wide array of myosin classes[1]; because of the specialized requirements for actin filaments in hair cells, these cells may be ideal for investigating how a cell uses multiple myosin isozymes to carry out distinct functions.

Utilizing energy gained from hydrolysis of ATP, myosin molecules generate force by moving relative to actin filaments (Spudich 1994). Each myosin molecule contains (1) an evolutionarily conserved motor or head domain, responsible for its actin-activated ATPase activity and force production; (2) one or more regulatory domains, which bind light chains such as calmodulin; and (3) dissimilar tail structures, which presumably couple force produced by the motor domain to other cellular structures (Fig. 1). Based on motor-domain sequence similarity, 12 distinct classes of myosin genes have been identified (Mooseker and Cheney 1995; Chen et al. 1996); vertebrates express at least 7 of these classes (Hasson and Mooseker 1996). A single genome, that of the mouse, contains at least 26 myosin genes (Hasson et al. 1996). Myosin isozymes separated by enormous evolutionary distance have nearly identical ATPase mechanisms (Ostap and Pollard 1996), showing that the regulatory and tail domains fundamentally distinguish myosin molecules of different classes.

Diverse roles for myosin molecules in hair cells can be envisioned. Hair cells contain five distinct actin-rich domains: stereocilia, cuticular plate, adherens-junction network, circumferential actin belt, and lateral-wall cortical cytoskeleton. Each actin domain may employ a different complement of myosin isozymes to orchestrate its assembly and maintenance. Hair cells are motile cells, capable of diverse movement modalities that are distinguished by the region of the cell that moves, the time scales involved, and amplitudes observed. The lateral walls of cochlear outer hair cells can stretch and shrink on a time scale of microseconds, in response to membrane potential (Dallos 1992), or seconds, in response to chemical agents (Zenner 1986). Hair bundles themselves undergo evoked and spontaneous movements of a few milliseconds' duration (Crawford and Fettiplace 1985; Howard and Hudspeth 1987; Benser et al. 1996). Others investigators have reported cuticular plate tilting (Zenner et al. 1988) and kinocilium twitching (Bowen 1931). Active hair-bundle movements of about 100 nm can be elicited by manipulation of Ca^{++} entry through transduction channels (Assad et al. 1989; Assad and Corey 1992; Jaramillo and Hudspeth 1993); myosin molecules in particular are thought to mediate this latter form of cell motility. Two myosin isozymes have been shown genetically to be essential for inner-ear function (Avraham et al. 1995; Gibson et al. 1995; Weil et al. 1995); in both cases, hair cells preferentially express the unconventional myosin protein. Many myosin isozymes may be found in a single hair cell; at least six classes (I, II, V, VI, VII, and X) are expressed in a vestibular tissue, the frog's sacculus (Solc et al. 1994). Because the demonstrated significance of myosin molecules for hair cells has stimulated considerable interest in their identification and characterization, we are close to ascribing specific roles to at least some of these motors.

MYOSIN MOLECULES AND MECHANOELECTRICAL TRANSDUCTION

Hair cells are distinguished by their ability to carry out mechanoelectrical transduction with exquisite sensitivity. A hair cell detects mechanical stimuli with its hair bundle, an asymmetric cluster of actin-rich processes arising from the soma's apical surface (Fig. 2A). Hundreds of cross-linked actin filaments make up a hair bundle's 50 or so constituent stereocilia, forming rigid, membrane-enveloped rods. Because only a few dozen actin filaments enter the soma, an individual stereocilium bends at this basal insertion (Fig. 2C). Mechanical deflections cause shearing displacement between adjacent stereocilia and elicit electrical signals

[1]Myosin "superfamily" distinguishes proteins related evolutionarily by their homologous motor domains from other motor-protein superfamilies, such as the kinesins; myosin "classes" distinguishes structurally dissimilar myosins; and myosin "isozymes" distinguishes dissimilar myosin gene products, including splice variants. Many myosin isozymes may belong to a single class; e.g., the mouse genome encodes at least seven myosin-I isozymes (Hasson et al. 1996).

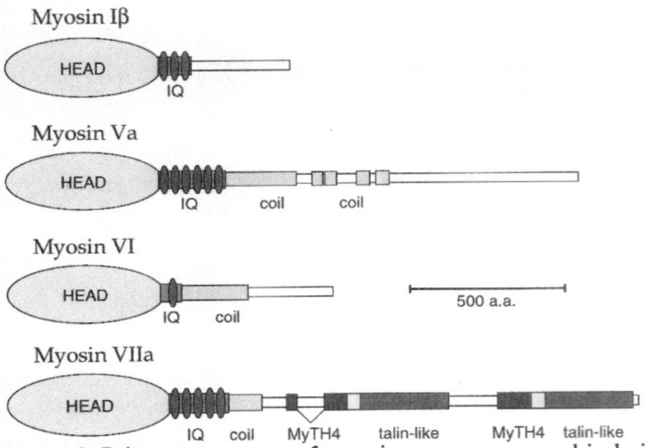

Figure 1. Primary structure of myosin genes expressed in hair cells. The conserved head domain of about 750 amino acids is shown as globular; the neck and tail segments are linear representations scaled as shown. Regulatory light chains bind to the IQ motifs in the neck region. Some myosin isozymes have predicted coiled-coil structures that would promote dimerization. Myosin VIIa has a repeated segment in the tail; each repeat contains a MyTH4 domain, similar to domains in myosins IV, X, and XII and in a plant kinesin, as well as a domain similar to the membrane-targeting region of talin and related proteins.

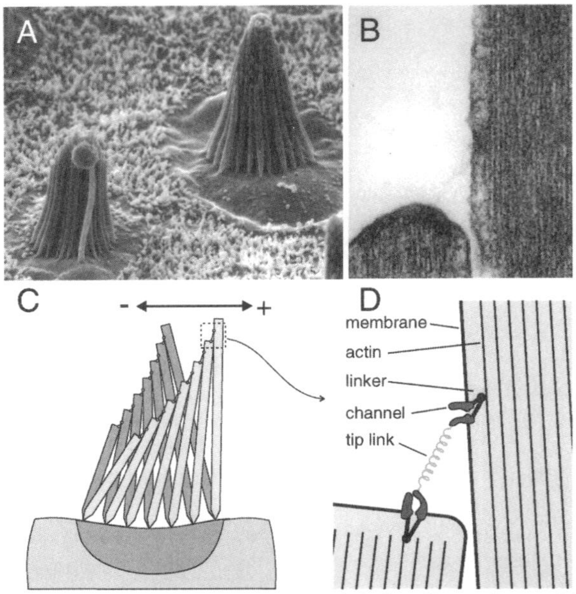

Figure 2. Morphology of vestibular hair bundles and a model for transduction. (*A*) Scanning electron micrograph of two hair bundles rising from the apical surface of the sensory epithelium of a bullfrog sacculus. (*B*) Transmission electron micrograph of a single tip link extending between two adjacent stereocilia. The actin filaments constituting the core of each stereocilium are visible, as is the osmiophilic density at each end of the tip link. (*C*) Representation of stereocilium movement upon bundle deflection. The stereocilia remain rigid and pivot at their bases, and the stereocilium tips remain in contact so that there is sliding, or shear displacement at the tips, when the bundle is deflected. (*D*) Model for the arrangement of transduction channels and tip links.

within a hair cell (Fig. 3). Deflections toward the tallest stereocilia—positive deflections—open transduction channels, whereas deflections toward shorter stereocilia—negative deflections—close them. Perpendicular deflections have no effect on channel gating. Positive deflections are thought to stretch tip links (Fig. 2B), extracellular filaments that cross-link adjacent stereocilia only along the axis of mechanical sensitivity (Pickles et al. 1984; Assad et al. 1991; Zhao et al. 1996b). Transduction channels located at the ends of a tip link (Denk et al. 1995; Lumpkin and Hudspeth 1995) would be opened by increased tip-link tension.

Each tip link is thought to bear a resting tension of ~10 pN, so that channels have an open probability at rest of ~0.1 (Corey and Hudspeth 1983a; Assad and Corey 1992; Hudspeth 1992). Resting tension ensures that inhibitory deflections, which reduce tension, also affect channel open probability. Even more importantly, resting tension ensures that transduction channels are poised at the point of optimal sensitivity on the sigmoidal displacement-response curve (Fig. 3B).

The mechanism that is responsible for setting resting tension also resets the transduction channels following a stimulus (Fig. 3). When a positive deflection is applied to a hair bundle, channels open rapidly (Corey and Hudspeth 1983b), then close within a few tens of milliseconds (Corey and Hudspeth 1983a; Eatock et al. 1987). Although inhibitory deflections close transduction channels, they reopen within a few tens of milliseconds. Because both of these phenomena restore sensitivity to small deflections, they are together referred to as adaptation; the functional assembly that carries out adaptation is called the adaptation motor (Fig. 4) (for review, see Hudspeth and Gillespie 1994). The insertional plaque, an osmiophilic structure found at the upper end of a tip link, is thought to house the adaptation motor; this structure appears to move in response to stimuli that elicit adaptation (Shepherd et al. 1992).

Myosin molecules have been touted as the probable active components of the adaptation motor (Howard and Hudspeth 1987; Hacohen et al. 1989). Hair bundles undergo a mechanical relaxation that correlates temporally with adaptation (Howard and Hudspeth 1987); by sliding down bundled polarized actin filaments within a stereocilium, a molecular motor anchoring one end of a tip link would relieve tension and allow channels to close. Because it could generate sufficient force to re-establish tension in the tip link and reopen channels, a molecular motor likewise can account for adaptation to negative deflections (Hacohen et al. 1989). By binding to calmodulin (Walker and Hudspeth 1996), Ca^{++} regulates adaptation (Eatock et al. 1987; Crawford et al. 1989, 1991; Assad et al. 1989). In a visually striking demonstration of the motor's force production, when hair cells are depolarized to prevent entry of Ca^{++}, the adaptation motor moves a

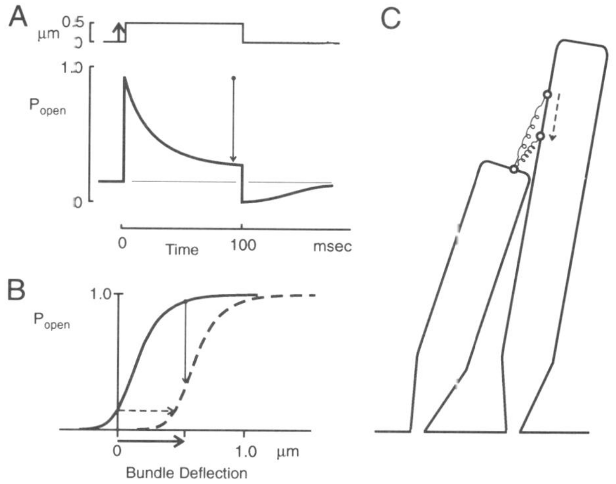

Figure 3. Electrophysiology of adaptation in bullfrog saccular hair cells. (*A*) Transduction channel open probability as a function of time. Some channels are open at rest with no bundle deflection. A deflection of 0.5 µm (*thick arrow*) opens most channels, but they spontaneously close over tens of milliseconds (*thin arrow*). (*B*) Open probability as a function of deflection (measured at the tip of the bundle). A positive 0.5-µm deflection (*thick arrow*) opens most channels; a negative 0.1-µm deflection would close the few open at rest. During adaptation to a positive deflection, the open probability declines (*thin arrow*) because the entire curve shifts to the right (*dashed arrow*), consistent with a reduction in tension on transduction channels caused by slipping of the tip-link insertion point. (*C*) Slipping of the tip-link insertion point.

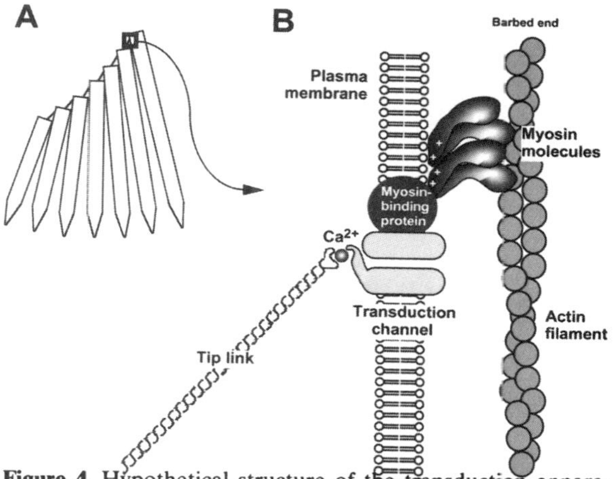

Figure 4. Hypothetical structure of the transduction apparatus, including the adaptation motor. (*A*) Diagram of hair bundle. (*B*) Detail of boxed region in *A*. Hypothetical molecular structure. Transduction channels are gated by tip-link tension (Fig. 1B). Because tip links disappear when exposed to calcium chelators such as BAPTA (Assad et al. 1991), a Ca^{++}-binding site is depicted here to mediate their interaction with a transduction channel. A cluster of myosin molecules is thought to constitute the adaptation motor; these motor molecules are organized into an "insertional plaque" by their membrane-binding properties and interaction of their tail domains. The adaptation motor couples mechanically to the remainder of the transduction apparatus through putative myosin-binding proteins that bind to exposed tail domains. All of the actin filaments in a stereocilium are arranged so that their barbed ends are at the distal tip; adaptation to positive deflections, such as illustrated in Fig. 3, requires passive movement of myosin molecules in a direction opposite to their favored direction of force generation. In contrast, when adapting to negative deflections, myosin molecules move toward the barbed end of stereociliary actin filaments; force generated by myosin molecules is transmitted to the channels' gates, restoring channel open probability to near the resting level.

hair bundle 100 nm or more (Assad et al. 1989; Assad and Corey 1992). The total force generated by an adaptation motor, as much as 30 pN, could be produced by the combined actions of several dozen myosin molecules (Jaramillo and Hudspeth 1993).

Manipulation of cellular biochemistry by introduction of compounds that perturb myosin's ATPase cycle has provided additional evidence supporting myosin's role in adaptation. Adenine nucleoside diphosphates and tight-binding phosphate analogs affect adaptation in complementary ways. As expected for agents that increase myosin's tight-binding interaction with actin, ADP analogs increase force production by adaptation motors even while inhibiting the rate of adaptation (Gillespie and Hudspeth 1993). In contrast, phosphate analogs completely eliminate motor force production, blocking adaptation to inhibitory deflections but permitting slowed adaptation to excitatory ones (Yamoah and Gillespie 1996). Both sets of results are explained well by invoking molecules that possess enzymatic and mechanical properties similar to those of skeletal-muscle myosin.

Myosin molecules constituting the adaptation motor may also participate in transduction-apparatus assembly. Following calcium-chelator eradication of tip links, mechanical transduction reappears several hours later along with newly formed tip links (Zhao et al. 1996b). At a minimum, molecular motors are essential for retensioning tip links, and perhaps also for steps involved in forming new tip links. Adaptation-motor myosin molecules may also participate in formation of the transduction apparatus during hair-bundle development (Tilney et al. 1988).

INITIAL SURVEYS AND MYOSIN II IN HAIR CELLS

The first claim for myosin's specialized presence in hair cells came from Macartney et al. (1980), who used a polyclonal antiserum produced against smooth-muscle myosin to argue that myosin was localized to hair bundles. Although later disputed as an optical (Egelman 1982) or contamination-derived (Drenckhahn et al. 1982) artifact, the original observation remains viable due to uncertainty about the antiserum's cross-reactivity with other myosin classes.

Subsequent studies using antibodies against nonmuscle myosin II have instead indicated that molecules antigenically related to myosin II do not reside in hair bundles (Drenckhahn et al. 1982, 1985; Sans et al. 1989; Slepecky and Ulfendahl 1992; Gillespie et al. 1993; Knipper et al. 1995). Nevertheless, myosin II is prominent in mammalian cochlear and vestibular hair cells, found largely in association with the circumferential actin belt that overlies the hair cell's adherens junctions or with the cuticular plate (Drenckhahn et al. 1982, 1985; Sans et al. 1989; Slepecky and Ulfendahl 1992). Although myosin II has been reported to be absent from chicken basilar-papilla hair cells (Drenckhahn et al. 1991), the authors' antisera may not have cross-reacted with myosin-II isozymes found specifically in hair cells. In the frog's sacculus, messages encoding four myosin-II isozymes are present (Solc et al. 1994); perhaps these isozymes are separately expressed by supporting and hair cells.

Other than a clearly demonstrated role in cytokinesis (De Lozanne and Spudich 1987), specific functions for nonmuscle myosin II molecules in other cell types have been difficult to ascertain. In hair cells, myosin II may permit contraction of the circumferential actin belt (Hirokawa and Tilney 1982); other myosin molecules may constrain the shape of the cuticular plate, as myosin II appears to surround the outside of this structure like a basket (Gillespie et al. 1993).

MYOSIN Iβ: THE ADAPTATION MOTOR?

As noted above, early work on the expression of myosin isozymes in hair cells was complicated by generally uncertain interclass cross-reactivity of the antibodies used. In recent years, however, development of specific monoclonal antibodies and polyclonal antisera that recognize the class-specific tail domains has enabled more conclusive localization of each myosin isozyme.

The extreme scarcity of hair bundles has also contributed to difficulties preventing conclusive identification of the motor molecule responsible for adaptation. Low bundle-protein abundance has necessitated unusual methods for isolation and detection of bundle proteins (Shepherd et al. 1989; Gillespie and Hudspeth 1991a,b; Walker et al. 1993). Photoaffinity labeling with radioactive nucleotides and vanadate trapping enables sensitive identification of myosin candidates; application of this method to purified hair bundles revealed candidate myosin molecules of 120 kD, 160 kD, and 230 kD (Gillespie et al. 1993). Of the three, the 120-kD protein best satisfies the criteria for an active myosin molecule (Gillespie et al. 1993; Yamoah and Gillespie 1996; Walker and Hudspeth 1996; A. Burlacu et al., in prep.). The 120-kD protein apparently corresponds to myosin Iβ, a myosin isozyme purified from bovine adrenal glands (Barylko et al. 1992) and cloned from several species (summarized in Mooseker and Cheney 1995). Monoclonal and polyclonal antibodies selective for myosin Iβ identify a bundle molecule of this size (Gillespie et al. 1993; T. Hasson et al., in prep.), and myosin Iβ mRNA appears to be relatively common in saccular epithelia (Solc et al. 1994).

Of the myosin molecules found in hair bundles, myosin Iβ best satisfies several criteria that have been advanced for the adaptation motor:

1. *Localization at stereociliary tips.* In hair bundles, myosin Iβ is found largely near the distal ends of the stereocilia (Fig. 5B) (Gillespie et al. 1993; T. Hasson et al., in prep.), where transduction and adaptation occur (Assad et al. 1989; Denk et al. 1995; Lumpkin and Hudspeth 1995).
2. *Sufficient bundle molecules to produce forces exerted by the adaptation motor.* The adaptation motor can exert as much as 30 pN on a single tip link (Jaramillo and Hudspeth 1993), implying that dozens of myosin molecules are clustered together. Between 100 and 200 myosin Iβ molecules are found in each stereocilium (Gillespie et al. 1993; Walker and Hudspeth 1996), consistent with a complement of several dozen in the adaptation motor and others moving through the bundle.
3. *Substantial actin-stimulated and Ca^{++}-regulated ATPase activity.* The motor molecule constituting the adaptation motor should show robust ATPase activity (Assad and Corey 1992; Hudspeth and Gillespie 1994). As judged by photoaffinity labeling, myosin Iβ behaves like an active, actin-activated ATPase (Gillespie et al. 1993; Walker and Hudspeth 1996; Yamoah and Gillespie 1996; Burlacu et al., in prep.); in contrast, the other candidate myosin molecules do not share the appropriate properties. In an in vitro assay, recombinant myosin Iβ moves actin filaments at 0.5 $\mu m \cdot s^{-1}$ (Zhu et al. 1996), similar to the maximum rate of adaptation-motor climbing of 2 $\mu m \cdot s^{-1}$ (Assad and Corey 1992). Recombinant myosin Iβ activity and motility respond to Ca^{++} (Zhu et al. 1996), as does adaptation.
4. *Small enough for dozens of molecules in an insertional plaque.* Myosin Iβ is compact compared to other candidates for the adaptation motor; because several dozen motor molecules must fit in the hair bundle's insertional plaque, a myosin isozyme with minimal tail sequence permits close packing.
5. *Mechanism for clustering.* Myosin Iβ can undergo organized self-association when tail domains bind to membranes (Reizes et al. 1994) and each other (R.A. Dumont and P.G. Gillespie, unpubl.); this tail-tail interaction also would permit ordered packing of myosin Iβ molecules into the insertional plaque.
6. *Receptors at stereociliary tips.* Recombinant myosin Iβ tail domains bind to receptors at stereociliary tips (R.A. Dumont et al., unpubl.), suggesting that

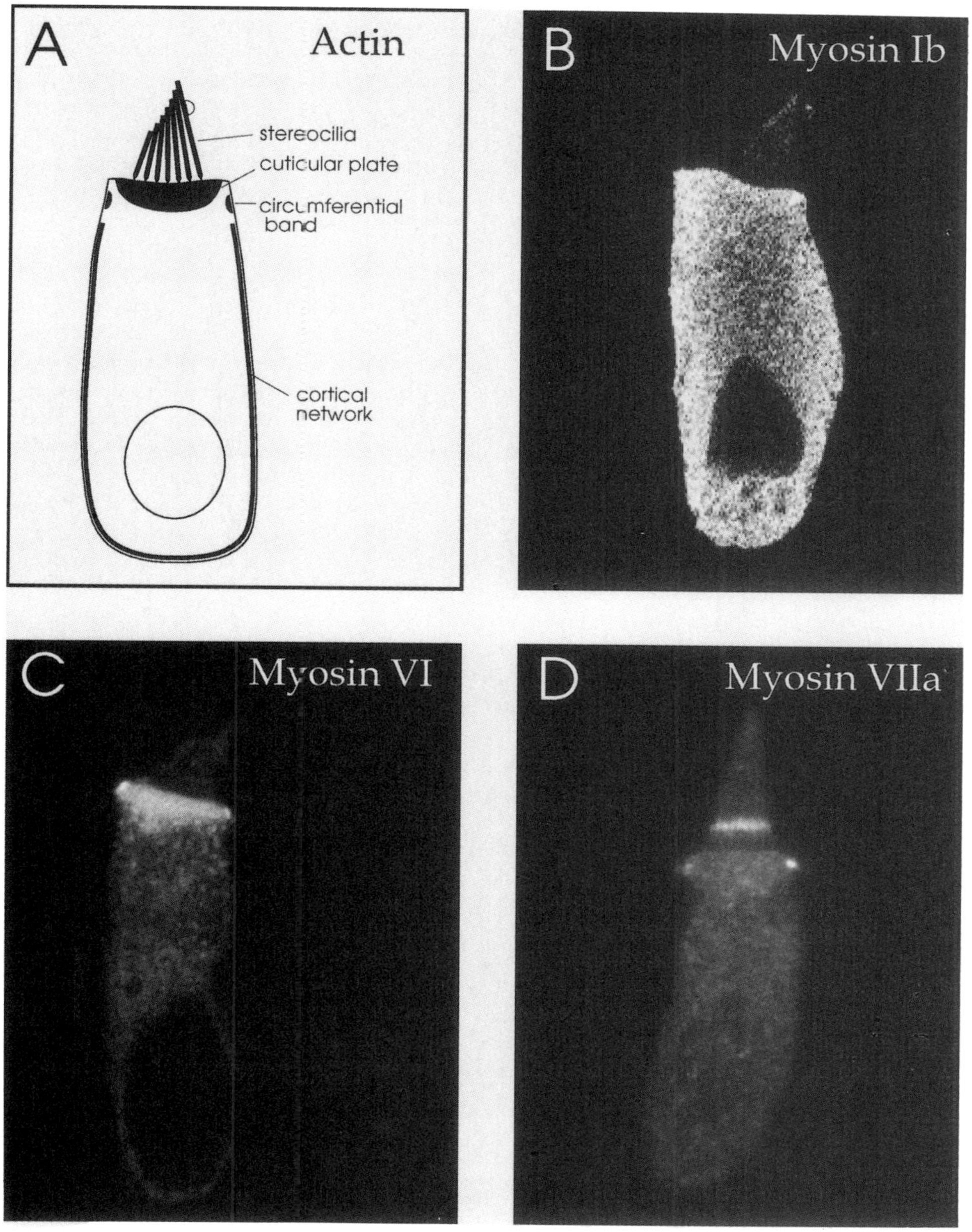

Figure 5. Localization of three myosin isozymes within hair cells. (*A*) Actin in hair cells occurs especially in stereocilia, in the cuticular plate, in a circumferential band at the apical surface, in association with the zonula adherens, and in the cortical cytoskeleton. (*B*) Myosin Iβ is distributed throughout the cell body, but is concentrated in a ring and basket around the cuticular plate. In the stereocilia, it occurs primarily in the distal one-third, but especially at the tips. (*C*) Myosin VI also occurs throughout the cell body but is bound especially to the cuticular plate and in a "pericuticular ring" between the plate and the circumferential actin band. There is a slight amount in the stereocilia. (*D*) Myosin VIIa occurs throughout the cell body and is colocalized with myosin VI in the pericuticular ring. Within the stereocilia, it occurs especially in the "ankle" zone just above the tapers, where extracellular cross-linking filaments have been observed.

myosin Iβ interacts with other components of the transduction apparatus.

Technical difficulties faced when combining difficult electrophysiological recording methods with methods that allow inhibition of single myosin isozymes have so far prevented definitive identification of the adaptation motor's active constituent as myosin Iβ. Nevertheless, compared to other isozymes, we seem closest to firmly establishing a hair-cell role for myosin Iβ as the adaptation motor.

Myosin Iβ is also found in high concentrations in a ring and a basket around the cuticular plate (Fig. 5B).

These myosin-Iβ molecules are not associated with actin filaments; perhaps they represent a pool of myosin molecules that will eventually enter the stereocilia.

Myosin Iβ may also serve to transport membrane proteins to the distal tips of stereocilia; although diffusion should readily move soluble proteins to their bundle targets, diffusion of membrane proteins in the plane of the stereociliary membrane might be too slow. Once myosin-Iβ molecules reach stereociliary tips with their membrane-protein cargo, regulatory mechanisms could disengage motor and tail domains from actin and cargo, permitting diffusion of myosin-Iβ molecules back to the soma.

MYOSIN Va: A NEURONAL MYOSIN

Myosin Va was the first vertebrate myosin isozyme cloned and sequenced that was not a myosin-I or II isozyme. A spontaneous mouse mutation called *dilute*, in which mice display diminished coat coloration, arose due to a mutation in the gene for myosin Va (Mercer et al. 1981). *dilute* is the ortholog of p190, a calmodulin-binding protein purified from chicken brain and found by molecular cloning to be an unconventional myosin (Larson et al. 1990; Espreafico et al. 1992).

Myosin Va clearly plays a significant role in the central nervous system. *dilute* mice homozygous for lethal alleles are normal until they exhibit mild ataxia at about 10 days of age and tonic-clonic seizures 1 day later; mutant mice die at about 3 weeks of age (Searle 1952). Myosin Va is abundant in the nervous system (Espreafico et al. 1992) and concentrated in neuronal growth cones (Evans et al. 1995); it may participate in actin-based motility in neuronal processes (Bearer et al. 1993). Disruption of myosin Va using chromophore-assisted laser inactivation supports a role for the protein in filopodial extension (Wang et al. 1996). At least one other myosin-V isozyme, myosin Vb, is also found in the nervous system (Zhao et al. 1996a).

Myosin Va is prominent in auditory and vestibular epithelia, but is not expressed in hair cells (T. Hasson et al., in prep.). Myosin Va is present at high levels in afferent nerve cell bodies and dendritic terminals; both bouton and calyx endings possess myosin Va. Definitive elucidation of functions carried out by myosin V isozymes in the nervous system will no doubt enlighten its role in auditory and vestibular tissues.

MYOSIN VI: A DEAFNESS GENE IN MICE

Initially identified from a degenerate-primer reverse transcriptase polymerase chain reaction (RT-PCR) screen (Bement et al. 1994) and cloned from a porcine proximal-tubule cell line (Hasson and Mooseker 1994), substantial amounts of myosin VI are found in a wide variety of tissue types. It therefore came as a surprise to discover that a spontaneous mouse deafness mutant, *Snell's waltzer*, arose from mutations in the gene encoding myosin VI (Avraham et al. 1995). Myosin VI must play a specialized and critical role in hair cells, as the *Snell's waltzer* phenotype is restricted to deafness and vestibular dysfunction.

Hair-cell epithelia transcribe myosin-VI mRNA; PCR products were also found frequently in the RT-PCR screen carried out by Solc et al. (1994), who also identified four alternatively spliced variants. Alternative splicing of myosin VI has not yet been noted in any other tissue, including mammalian cochlea.

Comparison of myosin VI's location in several auditory and vestibular tissues has permitted a comprehensive view of its location in hair cells (Fig. 5C) (Avraham et al. 1995; T. Hasson et al., in prep.). A fraction of a hair cell's myosin VI is tightly bound within the cuticular plate, the actin-rich domain that anchors a hair bundle. Although hair-cell cytoplasm is filled with freely soluble myosin VI, supporting cells lack this isozyme. Myosin VI is absent from cochlear hair bundles; although some hair bundles of the frog's sacculus possess substantial amounts of myosin VI, most do not. The concentration of bundle myosin VI appears to be greatest in small hair bundles, which are thought to arise from newly formed hair cells.

When purified frog hair bundles are examined by immunoblotting, myosin VI appears as a doublet of 145-kD and 160-kD forms (T. Hasson et al., in prep.). The larger form, which is not seen in any other tissue (Hasson and Mooseker 1994), appears in erratic amounts in bundle preparations; its variability suggests that it may reside in a hair-cell compartment that is not consistently isolated by the twist-off procedure (Gillespie and Hudspeth 1991a). Possible compartments include small bundles of newly formed hair cells, which are rich in myosin VI, or stereociliary rootlets, which apparently can contribute some cuticular-plate myosin VI to the bundle preparation.

Myosin VI's most specialized location appears to be the cuticular plate (Fig. 5C); because this isozyme is predicted to be dimeric (Fig. 1) (Hasson and Mooseker 1994), it may contribute to the actin cross-links that form this structure. Myosin VI is also prominent in terminal webs associated with microvilli of the intestine (Heintzelman et al. 1994) and kidney (Hasson and Mooseker 1994); because the terminal web plays a structural role similar to that played by the cuticular plate, myosin VI may carry out analogous functions in all of these tissues. Myosin VI is often found in association with stereocilium rootlets, suggesting that it could also cross-link these actin structures to the cuticular plate. Myosin VI's high concentration in newly formed stereocilia also implies a role in bundle formation. All three of these hypothesized roles could account for the aberrant and incomplete hair-bundle formation in *Snell's waltzer* mice (Avraham et al. 1995).

MYOSIN VIIa AND USHER SYNDROME 1β

Myosin VIIa, originally identified in the same degenerate-primer RT-PCR screen that revealed myosin VI (Bement et al. 1994), is produced from the gene responsible for the mouse deafness mutant *shaker-1* (Gibson et al. 1995). Mutations in myosin VIIa also underlie Usher syndrome type 1B, a human disease with sensorineural deafness, vestibular dysfunction, and progressive retinal degeneration (Weil et al. 1995). Association with a human deafness has led to a robust interest in myosin VIIa, and several groups have now cloned its cDNA from human tissues (Hasson et al. 1995; Chen et al. 1996; Weil et al. 1996). Several hundred families with Usher 1B have been identified; because mutations arising in the motor domain account for only a few dozen of these, many more mutations should be found in the protein's tail domain (Weil et al. 1995; Liu et al. 1996; Weston et al. 1996).

Although hair cells clearly depend on myosin VIIa, what critical function the protein mediates is unknown. Myosin VIIa extends throughout the length of a stereocilium in mammalian auditory and vestibular hair cells (Hasson et al. 1995); in frog saccular hair cells, however, myosin VIIa is concentrated in a striking band above the basal-taper region, where stereocilia narrow before inserting into the apex of the soma (Fig. 5D) (T. Hasson et al., in prep.). Because interstereociliary linkages are found at this position in frog saccular hair cells (Jacobs and Hudspeth 1990), and because similar linkages extend from base to tip of many mammalian stereocilia (Ross et al. 1987), myosin VIIa could function as the intracellular anchor of cross-links between stereocilia.

This proposed role for myosin VIIa coincides with other data. Myosin VIIa contains within its tail region a domain homologous to the membrane-associated portion of talin, a member of the protein 4.1 family; because proteins in this family serve to cross-link cytoskeleton to plasma membrane, a similar role for myosin VIIa would not be unexpected. Furthermore, in tissues such as retina (Hasson et al. 1995; El-Amraoui et al. 1996) and testis (T. Hasson, unpubl.), myosin VIIa is found in association both with actin-rich structures and with the membrane.

Because myosin VIIa is also present at stereocilium tips, it cannot be ruled out yet as the adaptation motor (T. Hasson et al., in prep.). Myosin VIIa satisfies few of the criteria posed above for the motor responsible for adaptation, however, confirming that myosin Iβ is a better candidate and that myosin VIIa's principal role may instead be to maintain hair-bundle structure.

SUMMARY AND LESSONS

The above enumeration does not conclusively summarize identities and functions of *all* hair-cell myosin isozymes. The RT-PCR screen described by Solc et al. (1994) demonstrated that other myosin isozymes, including myosin Iα and myosin X, are also found in hair-cell-containing epithelia; in addition, primer sets used may have missed other classes; for example, homologs of myosins III and Vb. Additional cataloging of myosin mRNAs from frog sacculus and other auditory and vestibular tissues will no doubt identify additional myosin isozymes expressed in hair cells.

Myosin molecules besides myosin VI and VIIa are likely to be essential for hair cells. Genes for several myosin isozymes, including those for myosins Iβ, Iγ, and VIIb, are predicted to map closely to the chromosomal locations of at least one human deafness gene (Hasson et al. 1996). Mutations in other hair-cell myosin isozymes may not manifest as human deafnesses if the isozyme in question is employed for other essential roles.

Although distribution of myosin molecules within the auditory and vestibular systems is complicated, we believe that a specific, principal role can be ascribed to each isozyme. Myosin V is not found in hair cells and likely serves the same role in afferent nerve processes that it plays elsewhere in the nervous system. Myosin Iβ probably mediates adaptation and may contribute to transport of proteins throughout stereocilia. Myosin VI appears to cross-link actin filaments within the cuticular plate and perhaps between the cuticular plate and stereociliary rootlets; mutations in myosin VI may disrupt these structures and prevent bundle formation. Myosin VIIa may actually hold stereocilia together; mutations in myosin VIIa may therefore cause stereocilia to splay apart, preventing proper assembly into a hair bundle. Myosins Iβ, VI, and VIIa are each at unusually high concentrations in bundles of the most newly formed hair cells, usually at the sensory epithelium's periphery (Gillespie et al. 1993; T. Hasson et al., in prep.); these three isozymes may therefore play additional, more specialized roles during hair-bundle development (Tilney et al. 1992). In the future, we expect that exciting results will come from experiments designed to test these predictions.

A key conclusion from hair-cell myosin localization is that these myosin molecules are not necessarily concentrated in regions of high actin density. Despite the similarity of their catalytic domains, each of the myosin isozymes found in hair cells has a distinctive subcellular localization. Furthermore, each hair-cell myosin isozyme appears in multiple specific locations. The ability of myosin molecules to bind to and translocate along actin filaments must therefore be heavily regulated; for dictating location, the affinity of myosin molecules for other proteins may be just as important as their affinity for actin. The nonhomologous tail domains of each class must contribute substantially to this differential localization. A critical goal for the field is therefore identification of hair-cell proteins that bind to myosin molecules, because their localization and abundance relative to each myosin isozyme may establish the final destination of a given myosin molecule.

Finally, we wonder why myosin molecules would be

employed in capacities that appear, at first consideration, to be entirely structural. In particular, our hypothesized roles for myosins VI and VIIa—maintaining cuticular-plate and bundle structural integrity—do not require force-producing molecules. Proteins that simply cross-link actin or connect actin to specific membrane receptors would seem to function adequately. Because the cell expends considerable energy to transcribe and translate relatively large myosin motor domains instead of smaller actin-binding structures, it seems likely that actin-activated ATPase plays a fundamental role in the behavior of these myosin isozymes. Because myosins VI and VIIa are not simply targeted to distal ends of actin filaments, but are instead found in association with specific actin-filament domains, the role of the motor activity must be relatively subtle. It seems likely that by understanding this paradox, we will understand the precise role of each myosin isozyme in the hair cell.

ACKNOWLEDGMENTS

Published and unpublished work from the authors' laboratories was supported by grants from the National Institutes of Health to P.G.G., to D.P.C., and to Mark S. Mooseker. P.G.G. is a Pew Scholar in the Biomedical Sciences; D.P.C. is an Investigator of the Howard Hughes Medical Institute.

REFERENCES

Assad, J.A. and D.P. Corey. 1992. An active motor model for adaptation by vertebrate hair cells. *J. Neurosci.* **12:** 3291.

Assad, J.A., N. Hacohen, and D.P. Corey. 1989. Voltage dependence of adaptation and active bundle movement in bullfrog saccular hair cells. *Proc. Natl. Acad. Sci.* **86:** 2918.

Assad, J.A., G.M.G. Shepherd, and D.P. Corey. 1991. Tip-link integrity and mechanical transduction in vertebrate hair cells. *Neuron* **7:** 985.

Avraham, K.B., T. Hasson, K.P. Steel, D.M. Kingsley, L.B. Russell, M.S. Mooseker, N.G. Copeland, and N.A. Jenkins. 1995. The mouse Snell's waltzer deafness gene encodes an unconventional myosin required for structural integrity of inner ear hair cells. *Nat. Genet.* **11:** 369.

Barylko, B., M.C. Wagner, O. Reizes, and J.P. Albanesi. 1992. Purification and characterization of a mammalian myosin I. *Proc. Natl. Acad. Sci.* **89:** 490.

Bearer, E.L., J. A. Degiorgis, R.A. Bodner, A.W. Kao, and T.S. Reese. 1993. Evidence for myosin motors on organelles in squid axoplasm. *Proc. Natl. Acad. Sci.* **90:** 11252.

Bement, W.M., T. Hasson, J.A. Wirth, R.E. Cheney, and M.S. Mooseker. 1994. Identification and overlapping expression of multiple unconventional myosin genes in vertebrate cell types. *Proc. Natl. Acad. Sci.* **91:** 6549.

Benser, M.E., R.E. Marquis, and A.J. Hudspeth. 1996. Rapid, active bundle movements in hair cells from the bullfrog's sacculus. *J. Neurosci.* **16:** 5629.

Bowen, R.E. 1931. Movement of the so-called hairs in the ampullar organs of fish ears. *Proc. Natl. Acad. Sci.* **17:** 192.

Chen, Z.-Y., T. Hasson, P.M. Kelley, B.J. Schwender, M.F. Schwartz, M. Ramakrishnan, W.J. Kimberling, M.S. Mooseker, and D.P. Corey. 1996. Molecular cloning and domain structure of myosin VIIa, the gene product defective in Usher Syndrome 1B. *Genomics* **36:** 440.

Corey, D.P. and A.J. Hudspeth. 1983a. Analysis of the microphonic potential of the bullfrog's sacculus. *J. Neurosci.* **3:** 942.

———. 1983b. Kinetics of the receptor current in bullfrog saccular hair cells. *J. Neurosci.* **3:** 962.

Crawford, A.C. and R. Fettiplace. 1985. The mechanical properties of ciliary bundles of turtle cochlear hair cells. *J. Physiol.* **364:** 359.

Crawford, A.C., M.G. Evans, and R. Fettiplace. 1989. Activation and adaptation of transducer currents in turtle hair cells. *J. Physiol.* **419:** 405.

———. 1991. The actions of calcium on the mechano-electrical transducer current of the turtle hair cells. *J. Physiol.* **434:** 369.

Dallos, P. 1992. The active cochlea. *J. Neurosci.* **12:** 4575.

De Lozanne, A. and J.A. Spudich. 1987. Disruption of the *Dictyostelium* myosin heavy chain by homologous recombination. *Science* **236:** 1086.

Denk, W., J.R. Holt, G.M.G. Shepherd, and D.P. Corey. 1995. Calcium imaging of single stereocilia in hair cells: Localization of transduction channels at both ends of tip links. *Neuron* **15:** 1311.

Drenckhahn, D., T. Schäfer, and M. Prinz. 1985. Actin, myosin, and associated proteins in the vertebrate auditory and vestibular organs. Immunochemical and biochemical studies. In *Auditory biochemistry* (ed. D. Drescher), p. 312. Charles C. Thomas, Springfield, Illinois.

Drenckhahn, D., K. Engel, D. Höfer, C. Merte, L. Tilney, and M. Tilney. 1991. Three different actin filament assemblies occur in every hair cell: Each contains a specific actin crosslinking protein. *J. Cell Biol.* **112:** 641.

Drenckhahn, D., J. Kellner, H.G. Mannherz, U. Gröschel-Stewart, J. Kendrick-Jones, and J. Scholey. 1982. Absence of myosin-like immunoreactivity in stereocilia of cochlear hair cells. *Nature* **300:** 531.

Eatock, R.A., D.P. Corey, and A.J. Hudspeth. 1987. Adaptation of mechanoelectrical transduction in hair cells of the bullfrog's sacculus. *J. Neurosci.* **7:** 2821.

Egelman, E. 1982. Problem of light piping in immunofluorescence studies. *Nature* **294:** 674.

El-Amraoui, A., I. Sahly, S. Picaud, J. Sahel, M. Abitol, and C. Petit. 1996. Usher IB/mouse shaker-1: The retinal phenotype discrepancy explained by the presence/absence of myosin VIIa in the photoreceptor cells. *Hum. Mol. Genet.* **5:** 1171.

Espreafico, E.M., R.E. Cheney, M. Matteoli, A.A.C. Nascimento, P.V. De Camilli, R.E. Larson, and M.S. Mooseker. 1992. Primary structure and cellular localization of chicken brain myosin-V (p190), an unconventional myosin with calmodulin light chains. *J. Cell Biol.* **119:** 1541.

Evans, L.L., J. Hammer, and P.C. Bridgeman. 1995. Subcellular localization of myosin V in nerve growth cones. *Mol. Biol. Cell* (suppl.) **6:** 145a.

Gibson, F., J. Walsh, P. Mburu, A. Varela, K.A. Brown, M. Antonio, K.W. Beisel, K.P. Steel, and S.D.M. Brown. 1995. A type VII myosin encoded by the mouse deafness gene *shaker-1*. *Nature* **374:** 62.

Gillespie, P.G. 1995. Molecular machinery of auditory and vestibular transduction. *Curr. Opin. Neurobiol.* **5:** 449.

Gillespie, P.G. and A.J. Hudspeth. 1991a. High-purity isolation of bullfrog hair bundles and subcellular and topologi-

cal localization of constituent proteins. *J. Cell Biol.* **112:** 625.
———. 1991b. Chemiluminescence detection of proteins from single cells. *Proc. Natl. Acad. Sci.* **88:** 2563.
———. 1993. Adenine nucleoside diphosphate block adaptation of mechanoelectrical transduction in hair cells. *Proc. Natl. Acad. Sci.* **90:** 2710.
Gillespie, P.G., M.C. Wagner, and A.J. Hudspeth. 1993. Identification of a 120-kD hair-bundle myosin I located near stereociliary tips. *Neuron* **11:** 581.
Hackney, C.M. and D.N. Furness. 1995. Mechanotransduction in vertebrate hair cells: Structure and function of the stereociliary bundle. *Am. J. Physiol.* **268:** C1.
Hacohen, N., J.A. Assad, W.J. Smith, and D.P. Corey. 1989. Regulation of tension on hair-cell transduction channels: Displacement and calcium dependence. *J. Neurosci.* **9:** 3988.
Hasson, T. and M.S. Mooseker. 1994. Porcine myosin-VI: Characterization of a new mammalian unconventional myosin. *J. Cell Biol.* **127:** 425.
———. 1996. Vertebrate unconventional myosins. *J. Biol. Chem.* **271:** 16431.
Hasson, T., M.B. Heintzelman, J. Santos-Sacchi, D.P. Corey, and M.S. Mooseker. 1995. Expression in cochlea and retina of myosin VIIa, the gene product defective in Usher syndrome type 1B. *Proc. Natl. Acad. Sci.* **92:** 9815.
Hasson, T., J.F. Skowron, D.J. Gilbert, K.B. Avraham, W.L. Perry, W.M. Bement, B.L. Anderson, E.H. Sherr, Z.-Y. Chen, L.A. Greene, D.C. Ward, D.P. Corey, M.S. Mooseker, N.G. Copeland, and N.A. Jenkins. 1996. Mapping of unconventional myosins in mouse and human. *Genomics* **36:** 431.
Heintzelman, M.B., T. Hasson, and M.S. Mooseker. 1994. Multiple unconventional myosin domains of the intestinal brush border cytoskeleton. *J. Cell Sci.* **107:** 3535.
Hirokawa, N. and L.G. Tilney. 1982. Interactions between actin filaments and between actin filaments and membranes in quick-frozen and deeply etched hair cells of the chick ear. *J. Cell Biol.* **95:** 249.
Howard, J. and A.J. Hudspeth. 1987. Mechanical relaxation of the hair bundle mediates adaptation in mechanoelectrical transduction by the bullfrog's saccular hair cell. *Proc. Natl. Acad. Sci.* **84:** 3064.
Hudspeth, A.J. 1989. How the ear's works work. *Nature* **341:** 397.
———. 1992. Hair-bundle mechanics and a model for mechanoelectrical transduction by hair cells. In *Sensory transduction* (ed. D.P. Corey and S.D. Roper), p. 357. Rockefeller University Press, New York.
Hudspeth, A.J. and P.G. Gillespie. 1994. Pulling springs to tune transduction: Adaptation by hair cells. *Neuron* **12:** 1.
Jacobs, R.A. and A.J. Hudspeth. 1990. Ultrastructural correlates of mechanoelectrical transduction in hair cells of the bullfrog's internal ear. *Cold Spring Harbor Symp. Quant. Biol.* **55:** 547.
Jaramillo, F. and A.J. Hudspeth. 1993. Displacement-clamp measurement of the forces exerted by gating springs in the hair bundle. *Proc. Natl. Acad. Sci.* **90:** 1330.
Knipper, M., U. Zimmermann, I. Kopschall, K. Rohbock, S. Jungling, and H.P. Zenner. 1995. Immunological identification of candidate proteins involved in regulating active shape changes of outer hair cells. *Hear. Res.* **86:** 100.
Larson, R.E., F.S. Espindola, and E.M. Espreafico. 1990. Calmodulin-binding proteins and calcium/calmodulin-regulated enzyme activities associated with brain actomyosin. *J. Neurochem.* **54:** 1288.
Liu, X.-Z., V.E. Newton, K.P. Steel, and S.D.M. Brown. 1996. Identification of a new mutation of the myosin VII head region in Usher syndrome type 1. *Hum. Mutat.* (in press).
Lumpkin, E. and A.J. Hudspeth. 1995. Detection of Ca^{2+} entry through mechanosensitive channels localizes the site of mechanoelectrical transduction in hair cells. *Proc. Natl. Acad. Sci.* **92:** 10297.
Macartney, J.C., S.D. Comis, and J.O. Pickles. 1980. Is myosin in the cochlea a basis for active motility? *Nature* **288:** 491.
Mercer, J.A., P.K. Seperack, M.C. Strobel, N.G. Copland, and N.A. Jenkins. 1991. Novel myosin heavy chain encoded by murine *dilute* coat colour locus. *Nature* **349:** 709.
Mooseker, M.S. and R.E. Cheney. 1995. Unconventional myosins. *Annu. Rev. Cell Dev. Biol.* **11:** 633.
Ostap, E.M. and T.D. Pollard. 1996. Biochemical kinetic characterization of Acanthamoeba myosin-I ATPase. *J. Cell Biol.* **132:** 1053.
Pickles, J.O. and D.P. Corey. 1992. Mechanoelectrical transduction by hair cells. *Trends Neurosci.* **15:** 254.
Pickles, J.O., S.D. Comis, and M.P. Osborne. 1984. Cross-links between stereocilia in the guinea pig organ of Corti, and their possible relation to sensory transduction. *Hear. Res.* **15:** 103.
Reizes, O., B. Barylko, C. Li, T.C. Südhof, and J.P. Albanesi. 1994. Domain structure of a mammalian myosin I. *Proc. Natl. Acad. Sci.* **91:** 6349.
Ross, M.D., T.E. Komorowski, C.M. Rogers, K.G. Pote, and K.M. Donovan. 1987. Macular suprastructure, stereociliary bonding, and kinociliary/stereociliary coupling in rat utricular maculae. *Acta Otolaryngol.* **104:** 56.
Sans, A., P. Atger, C. Cavadore, and J.C. Cavadore. 1989. Immunocytochemical localization of myosin, tropomyosin, and actin in vestibular hair cells of human fetuses and cats. *Hear. Res.* **40:** 117.
Searle, A.G. 1952. A lethal allele of *dilute* in the house mouse. *Heredity* **6:** 395.
Shepherd, G.M.G., B.A. Barres, and D.P. Corey. 1989. "Bundle-blot" purification and initial protein characterization of hair cell stereocilia. *Proc. Natl. Acad. Sci.* **86:** 4973.
Shepherd, G.M.G., J.A. Assad, M. Parakkel, B. Kachar, and D.P. Corey. 1992. Movement of the tip-link attachment is correlated with adaptation in bullfrog saccular hair cells. *J. Gen. Physiol.* **98:** 25a.
Slepecky, N.B. and M. Ulfendahl. 1992. Actin-binding and microtubule-associated proteins in the organ of Corti. *Hear. Res.* **57:** 201.
Solc, C.K., B.H. Derfler, G.M. Duyk, and D.P. Corey. 1994. Molecular cloning of myosins from bullfrog saccular macula: A candidate for the hair cell adaptation motor. *Audit. Neurosci.* **1:** 63.
Spudich, J.A. 1994. How molecular motors work. *Nature* **372:** 515.
Tilney, L.G., M.S. Tilney, and D.A. Cotanche. 1988. Actin filaments, stereocilia, and hair cells of the bird cochlea. V. How the staircase pattern of stereociliary lengths is generated. *J. Cell Biol.* **106:** 355.
Tilney, L.G., M.S. Tilney, and D.J. DeRosier. 1992. Actin filaments, stereocilia, and hair cells: How cells count and measure. *Annu. Rev. Cell Biol.* **8:** 257.
Walker, R.G. and A.J. Hudspeth. 1996. Calmodulin controls adaptation of mechanoelectrical transduction by hair cells of the bullfrog's sacculus. *Proc. Natl. Acad. Sci.* **93:** 2203.
Walker, R.G., A.J. Hudspeth, and P.G. Gillespie. 1993. Cal-

modulin and calmodulin-binding proteins in hair bundles. *Proc. Natl. Acad. Sci.* **90:** 2807.

Wang, F.-S., J.S. Wolenski, R.E. Cheney, M.S. Mooseker, and D.G. Jay. 1996. Function of myosin-V in filopodial extension of neuronal growth cones. *Science* **273:** 660.

Weil, D., G. Levy, I. Sahly, F. Levi-Acobas, S. Blanchard, A. El-Amraoui, F. Crozet, H. Philippe, M. Abitbol, and C. Petit. 1996. Human myosin VIIA responsible for the Usher 1B syndrome: A predicted membrane-associated motor protein expressed in developing sensory epithelia. *Proc. Natl. Acad. Sci.* **92:** 3232.

Weil, D., S. Blanchard, J. Kaplan, P. Guilford, F. Gibson, J. Walsh, P. Mburu, A. Varela, J. Levilliers, M.D. Weston, P.M. Kelley, W.J. Kimberling, M. Wagenaar, F. Levi-Acobas, D. Larget-Piet, A. Munnich, K.P. Steel, S.D.M. Brown, and C. Petit. 1995. Defective myosin VIIA gene responsible for Usher syndrome type 1B. *Nature* **374:** 60.

Weston, M.D., P.M. Kelley, L.D. Overbeck, D. Orten, T. Hasson, Z.-Y. Chen, D. P. Corey, M. S. Mooseker, J. Sumegi, C. Cremers, C. Moller, S. Jacobsen, S. Gorin, and W.J. Kimberling. 1996. Myosin VIIA mutation screening of 189 Usher syndrome patients. *Am. J. Hum. Genet.* (in press).

Yamoah, E.N. and P.G. Gillespie. 1996. Phosphate analogs block adaptation in hair cells by inhibiting adaptation-motor force production. *Neuron* **17:** 523.

Zenner, H.P. 1986. Motile responses in outer hair cells. *Hear. Res.* **22:** 83.

Zenner, H.P., R. Zimmermann, and A.H. Gitter. 1988. Active movements of the cuticular plate induce sensory hair motion in mammalian outer hair cells. *Hear. Res.* **34:** 233.

Zhao, L.-P., J.S. Koslovsky, J. Reinhard, M. Bähler, A.E. Witt, D.W. Provance, and J.A. Mercer. 1996a. Cloning and characterization of myr 6, an unconventional myosin of the *dilute*/myosin-V family. *Proc. Natl. Acad. Sci.* **93:** 10826.

Zhao, Y.-D., E.N. Yamoah, and P.G. Gillespie. 1996b. Regeneration of broken tip links and restoration of mechanical transduction in hair cells. *Proc. Natl. Acad. Sci.* (in press.)

Zhu, T., M. Sata, and M. Ikebe. 1996. Functional expression of mammalian myosin Iβ: Analysis of its motor activity. *Biochemistry* **35:** 513.

Molecular and Cellular Plasticity in Developing Epileptic Brain

J.L. NOEBELS, M.L. SUTHERLAND, W.K. NAHM, AND E. DIPASQUALE
Developmental Neurogenetics Laboratory, Department of Neurology, Baylor College of Medicine, Houston, Texas 77030

Epilepsy is a disorder of intermittent aberrant oscillations in cortical networks present in nearly 1% of the human population. By current estimates, 10–30% of all epilepsy is genetic, standing second only to mental retardation as the most common hereditary syndrome affecting the central nervous system. The paroxysmal cerebral excitability trait is transmitted by deleterious mutations in large numbers of genes rather than in one or a few genes; at least 120 different human Mendelian variants share epilepsy as one expression of a single gene error (McKusick 1994), whereas the remainder arise from the inheritance of multiple susceptibility loci. The genetic heterogeneity of epilepsy is clearly reflected in the diversity of the electrical seizure patterns, their variable site of origin and age of onset in the brain, and the spectrum of their sensitivity to ion channel blockers and other antiepileptic drugs. These differences are strong indicators that specific cortical synchronization defects arise from distinct alterations in the biology of neurons. Since inborn errors that produce neuronal bursting appear early in life, they pose significant risk to normal cortical development by interfering with synaptic coincidence detection and programs of activity-dependent synaptogenesis (Baumbach and Chow 1981) and often herald the onset of progressive neurodegenerative lesions. The complex interactions between defects in membrane hyperexcitability, synaptic stabilization, and altered gene expression in the developing brain make this family of neuronal membrane disorders one of the most fascinating yet elusive to understand at the molecular level.

Much as the search for oncogenes has pinpointed molecules that coordinate the transcription of interrelated sets of genes, it is reasonable to expect that the isolation and analysis of epilepsy genes will begin to define the critical molecular mechanisms that synchronize large interconnected neural networks in the brain. We would like to learn with certainty which synaptic control mechanisms regulate different types of seizure discharge; where and how the synchronization starts; why it remains focal or is allowed to spread (slowly or instantly) throughout the brain; and how the desynchronizing processes that eventually terminate each seizure are finally recruited. Some or all of the intervening steps that are illuminated by mutational analysis of epilepsies may be shared by the neural mechanisms that regulate physiological oscillations in the normal brain. A range of rhythmic frequencies, including the delta rhythms of sleep, and the theta, alpha, mu, and gamma rhythms that accompany spatial and sensorimotor information processing in the hippocampus, motor, and visual cortex remain among the most important yet least understood integrative processes in central nervous system function (Steriade et al. 1993, 1996; Freeman 1994; Lisman and Idiart 1995).

The recent identification of the first few genes for epilepsy has begun to focus attention on the challenge of dissecting the molecular pathogenesis of aberrant rhythmic activity in neural circuits whose assembly and excitability are use-dependent. Owing to the nature of their defective gene products, the solution to some epileptic phenotypes now appears to reside in the developmental dysregulation of other neural genes. Disorders of this type may prove far more difficult to analyze than, for example, the primary ion channel mutations found in hereditary disorders of muscle fiber excitability, since aberrant patterns of gene expression and firing behavior encountered in adult neurons may be either the cause or the result of seizures in the developing brain.

EPILEPSY GENES ENCODE MOLECULES OF DIVERSE FUNCTION

The genes for abnormal synchronous cortical rhythms and epilepsy are now being identified in human disease pedigrees, in spontaneous mouse mutants, and from seizure phenotypes arising in transgenic knockout and overexpression mice. Figure 1 shows the identity of genes currently associated with spontaneous seizure phenotypes.

Human Epilepsy Genes

Gene mapping studies have provided the molecular point of departure of the inherited neuronal lesion in four human epilepsy syndromes. The first, an autosomal dominant nocturnal frontal lobe epilepsy (ADNFLE), involves a point mutation in the pore region of the α4 nicotinic acetylcholinergic receptor subunit gene in one large pedigree (Steinlein et al. 1995). The effects of this mutation on the function of heteromultimeric nicotinic channels in brain have not yet been demonstrated. The second, a locus for progressive myoclonic epilepsy (EPM1) with mental deterioration was initially mapped in 12 Finnish

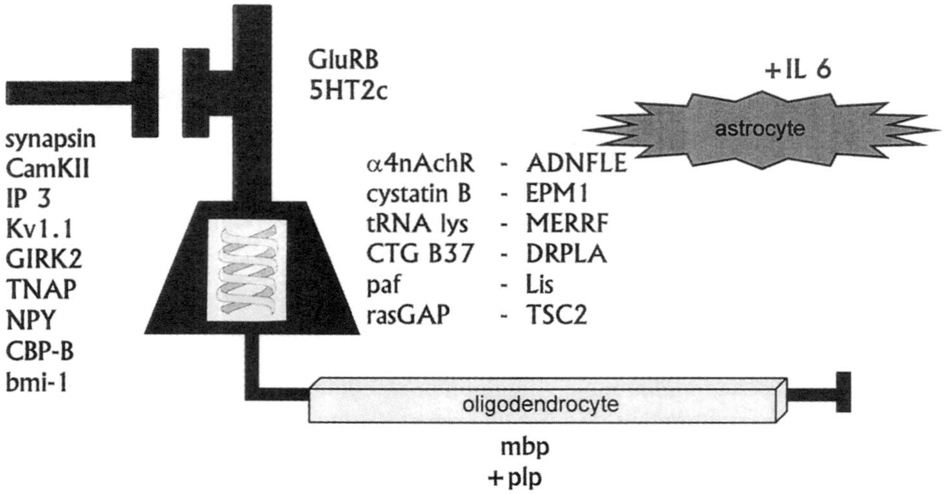

Figure 1. Genes for epilepsy in mouse and man.

families to a region on chromosome 21q22.3 and subsequently found in two affected families to contain splice-site and stop-codon mutations for the cystatin B gene. Affected individuals expressed low levels of cystatin B mRNA in lymphoblastoid cell lines (Pennacchio et al. 1996). Cystatin B is one of a family of cysteine protease inhibitors expressed ubiquitously in the brain, and the protein targets modified by the early loss of this molecule in neurons remain to be defined.

Inherited cortical malformations are associated with seizure disorders, and migration disturbances are a common neuropathological finding in human epilepsy. The gene for the Miller Dieker form of lissencephaly encodes a subunit of the heteromeric platelet-activating factor, *paf* (Hattori et al. 1994). *paf* affects neuronal growth cone morphology, suggesting that loss of this signal may favor epileptogenesis by altering synaptic strength or cortical connectivity during maturation. Malformations caused by mutations in the tuberous sclerosis gene TSC2 are the result of a defect in a rasGAP-like signaling molecule (European Consortium 1993), but the mechanism leading to aberrant cytopathology and seizures is unclear.

Epilepsy Genes in Mouse

Electrophysiological survey of mutant mice has provided an important strategy to identify candidate genes for human epilepsies, analyze the development of the epileptic circuit, and experiment with strategies to correct the molecular defect with medicine or other genes (Noebels 1979). Mutants with behavioral seizures cloned to date include *dilute-lethal* (non-muscle myosin), *shiverer* (myelin basic protein), *jimpy* (proteolipid protein), and *weaver* (GIRK2); two of the six murine genes (Fig. 2) for models of spike-wave epilepsies, *tottering* and *slow wave epilepsy* (Noebels et al. 1995) will be reported soon. Surprisingly, none of the spontaneous inherited epilepsies in man or mouse discovered so far involves direct mutations in the 35 or more genes for ion channels mediating the major form of synaptic inhibition in the brain, that is, the genes for GABA receptor-gated chloride and potassium channels, or for other voltage- and ligand-gated ion channels underlying membrane repolarization, although such mutants almost certainly exist. On the other hand, defective inhibition can be identified in epileptic mutant nervous systems. For example, the *tottering* mouse shows a latent reduction in Ca^{++}-activated K^+ currents that is revealed during synchronous network bursting (Helekar and Noebels 1991). These currents contribute a major fraction of the after-hyperpolarization observed in many central neurons and couple intracellular calcium ion levels to repetitive firing behavior. *tottering* mutants also show impaired $GABA_A$ receptor function, possibly mediated by abnormal phosphorylation patterns due to elevated protein kinase A activity (Jalilian Tehrani and Barnes 1995). The *weaver* mutation, which shows a pattern of tonic-clonic seizures in both heterozygous and homozygous mice, alters the gene for a G-protein-coupled potassium inward rectifier (Patil et al. 1995). The mutation reduces this current in cerebellar granule cells (Kofuji et al. 1996; Navarro et al. 1996; Surmeier et al. 1996); however, mutational analysis predicts different possible functional outcomes (Slesinger et al. 1996), and the actual effects of the mutation on excitable behavior must be evaluated in the CNS circuits where the epileptiform activity takes place. A recessive mutant with spike-wave seizures, *stargazer*, shows a striking increase in another inward rectifier current in deep-layer cortical neurons (Fig. 3) (DiPasquale et al. 1996). The altered current, similar to I_h, normally resists prolonged hyperpolarization from the resting membrane potential and may alter repetitive burst firing properties within thalamocortical circuits.

An unexpectedly rich source of candidate genes for epilepsy has been generated from the analysis of trans-

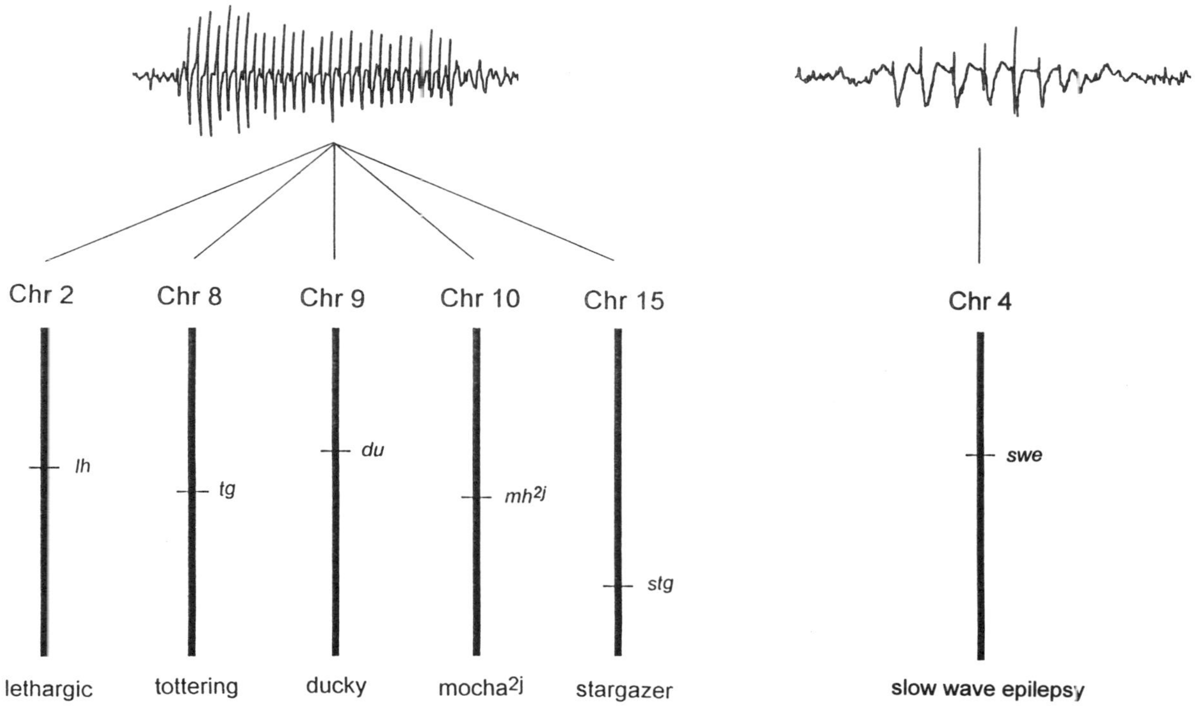

Figure 2. Genetic heterogeneity of spike-wave epilepsies. A specific frequency (6–7/sec) of intermittent thalamocortical oscillations is a common EEG phenotype shared by five single-locus mutants in the mouse. A slower pattern of 3/sec spike-wave discharge similar to that seen in children with generalized absence epilepsy is linked to the *swe* (slow wave epilepsy) locus on mouse chromosome 4.

genic mice constructed by gene targeting. The first observation was reported in the *bmi-1* proto-oncogene null mutant, where mice bearing a deletion in the widely expressed gene for a 324-amino-acid nuclear protein with zinc finger and other motifs usually found on transcriptional regulators showed seizures beginning after one month of age (van der Lugt et al. 1994). The *bmi-1* gene is believed to regulate the expression of murine homeotic genes during development. This example was followed rapidly by the recognition of tonic-clonic seizure activity in a variety of other targeted mutations, and a steadily increasing number of null mutants with epileptic phenotypes continue to emerge, including those for genes that regulate membrane excitability, signal transduction, synaptic release, neurotransmitter levels, and receptors. Transgenic modification of tyrosine kinases and growth-associated factors can also be demonstrated to modify epileptogenic potential in the brain without actually causing spontaneous seizures (for review, see Noebels 1996a).

SELECTIVE NEURONAL VULNERABILITY IN EPILEPSY GENE EXPRESSION

So far, none of the mutations implicated in human epilepsies provides direct information on how the defective gene product produces the epileptogenic lesion observed. Indeed, with few exceptions, the com-

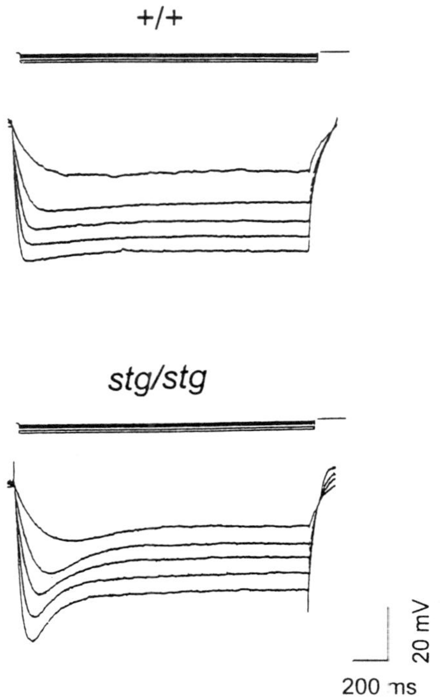

Figure 3. Inward rectifier defect in layer V cortical neurons in the spike-wave mutant mouse *stargazer*.

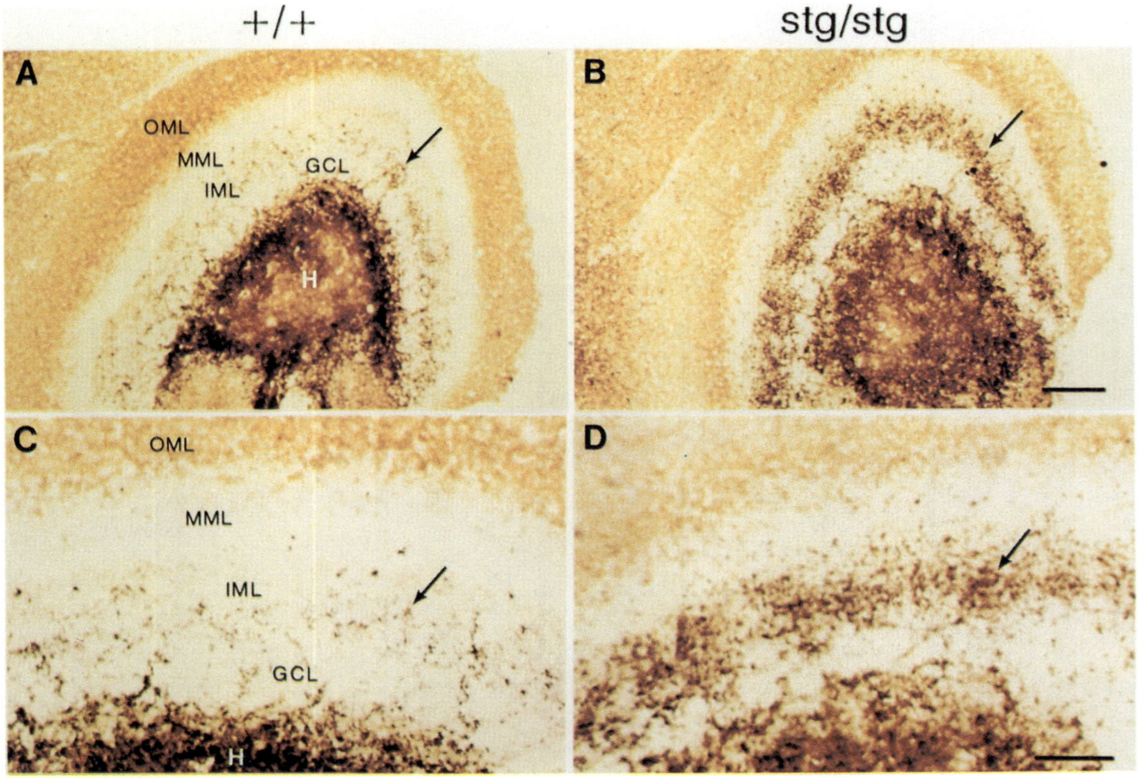

Figure 4. Altered connectivity in genetic epilepsy model. (*A*,*B*) Selenium stain selective for zinc-rich vesicles reveals laminar plexus of mossy fiber sprouting in inner molecular layer of adult stargazer dentate gyrus (*B*) compared to +/+ mouse (*A*). (*C*,*D*) Higher magnification of recurrent axon sprouting in inner molecular layer.

mon observation has been an absence of the precise spatial and temporal overlap between mutant gene expression and the population of bursting neurons that would simplify interpretation of the pathogenic process. For example, the α4 nicotinic subunit is expressed early and widely in the brain, yet seizures in ADNFLE patients arise long after infancy and are confined to the frontal lobes. Cystatin B is expressed in all neurons, yet neurological deficits in EPM1 patients are not clinically apparent until juvenile ages, and they preferentially alter neural circuits in a way that produces myoclonic seizures, suggesting a circumscribed rather than diffuse pattern of cerebral pathology.

The apparent mismatch presented by the finding of restricted cellular pathology in the presence of widespread mutant gene expression is a recurring feature in inherited neurological disease, notably in disorders featuring triplet repeat expansions. In this class of mutations, the size of the intragenic expansion can be correlated with onset and severity of the mutant phenotype, and the selective vulnerability has been hypothesized to depend on the absence of compensatory activity by other genes with overlapping function. Regardless of the nature of the mutational event, the presence of selective vulnerability and a long developmental delay before the appearance of seizures both suggest that the discovery of the mutant gene product may often have little predictive value in recognizing the remaining sequence of pathogenic steps. In these cases, the activity of other genes must be evaluated in serial developmental studies to characterize the downstream elements of the disease.

DEVELOPMENTAL PLASTICITY IN GENETIC EPILEPSY MODELS

Ongoing examination of the nervous system in epileptic mutant mice has revealed specific examples of cellular and molecular plasticity acting downstream from the gene error, some of which are known to mirror neuropathological changes in human epilepsy syndromes. These alterations fall into four general categories, and more are expected to be described at various levels of nervous system organization.

Structural Connectivity: Migration, Axon Sprouting, and Neosynaptogenesis

Epileptic nervous systems have been associated with downstream cell death, migration disturbances, and unusual lesions of axonal growth. Recent examinations of granule cells that die rather than migrate in *weaver* cerebellum reveal that the gene-linked reduction of the GIRK2 inward rectifier current is replaced by an abnormal Na^+ flux through the channel, and pharmacological blockade of this Na^+ influx restores survival and neuritic outgrowth in vitro (Kofuji et al. 1996). Another mutant phenotype of altered neurite outgrowth originally identified in human temporal epilepsy is the sprouting of recurrent collaterals from the axons (mossy fibers) of dentate granule cells. The branches leave the parent fiber in the hilar region, traverse the granule cell body layer, and emerge in the inner molecular layer of the dentate gyrus where aberrant excitatory synapses are formed on granule cell dendrites. *stargazer* epileptic mice develop this pattern of neosynaptogenesis (Fig. 4), and it has also been seen in other epileptic mutants, including *tottering* and GAP 43 overexpression mutants (Qiao and Noebels 1993; Aignier et al. 1995). Neurogenetic strategies designed to further dissect the role of growth factors in the sprouting process, as well as the impact of axon sprouting on the epilepsy phenotype, are in progress using transgenic mice as genomic reagents (Noebels 1996b).

Synaptic Signaling: Receptors, Transmitters, and "Neotransmitters"

The convulsant potential of GABA receptor antagonist synapses is well known in acute experimental epilepsy models, and reduced GABAergic signaling has been identified as a secondary mechanism of inherited epileptogenesis in the TNAP null mutant, a mouse lacking the nonspecific alkaline phosphatase enzyme required to allow membrane uptake of vitamin B6, a cofactor for GABA synthesis (Waymire et al. 1995). The *lethargic* mouse shows an increased $GABA_B$ receptor population (Lin et al. 1993), also likely to be a developmental effect of the mutant gene. The *stargazer* mutant displays a novel example of neurotransmitter-related plasticity that involves the conditional expression of a neuropeptide neurotransmitter not normally present in the cell. Immunocytochemical studies reveal the de novo appearance of neuropeptide Y (NPY) in a subcellular pattern overlapping with the releasable pool of vesicles in axons of dentate granule cells within weeks after the temporal onset of seizures (Fig. 5) (Chafetz et al. 1995). The levels of ectopic NPY vary markedly among mutants regardless of age. The interesting possibility that ectopic axonal NPY could act as a functional "neotransmitter" requires evaluation of the available NPY receptor subtypes in the postsynaptic population (Michel 1991), and the relationship to epileptogenesis must be explored further, particularly in light of the epileptic phenotype reported in NPY $^{-/-}$ null mutants (Erickson et al. 1996).

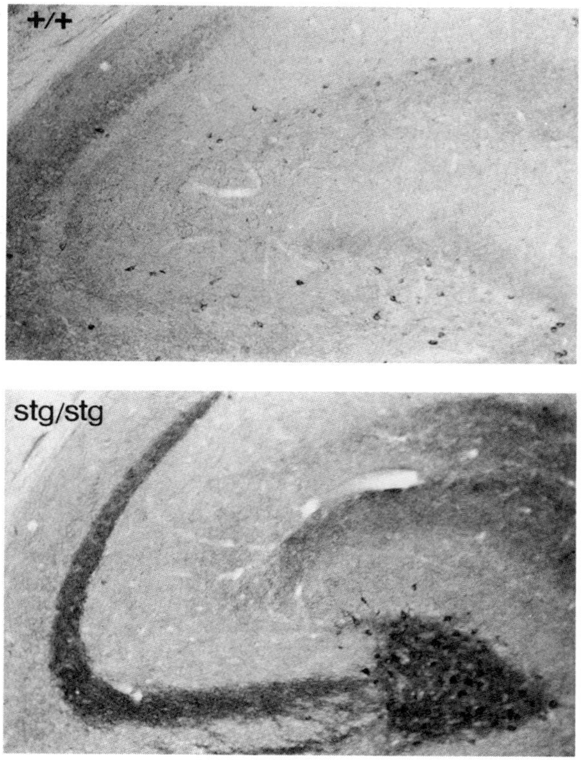

Figure 5. Molecular plasticity in genetic epilepsy model. NPY immunoreactivity reveals ectopic expression of neuropeptide Y in stargazer mossy fibers. NPY distribution overlaps with vesicle population stained in *upper* panel, suggesting NPY may be released at terminals.

Ion Channel Density and Glial Interactions

shiverer mice lack compact myelin in the CNS due to a mutation in the myelin basic protein (MBP) gene and show a neurological phenotype of early tremor and late-onset (3–5 months) seizures. Seizures are an unexpected phenotype for hypomyelinated nervous systems, and the activity of MBP, an intracellular protein expressed only in oligodendrocytes, is clearly far removed from the neuronal molecular hyperexcitability defect. Despite the glial-specific primary gene defect, hypomyelinated axons in *shiverer* brain show striking increases in the density, and alterations in the topology, of sodium (Noebels et al. 1991; Westenbroek et al. 1992) and potassium ion channels (Fig. 6) (Wang et al. 1995). Although the regulatory steps are unclear, it is reasonable to suggest that the late-onset seizures might result from a steady accumulation of axonal sodium channels to a density sufficient to support ectopic impulse generation and ephaptic interactions between corticofugal and corticopetal axons, a phenomenon that has been linked to seizures in other experimental models (Noebels and Prince 1978). Alternatively, the *shiverer* brain may be subject to synaptic reorganization favoring aberrant synchronization due to impulse-conduction abnormalities early in development.

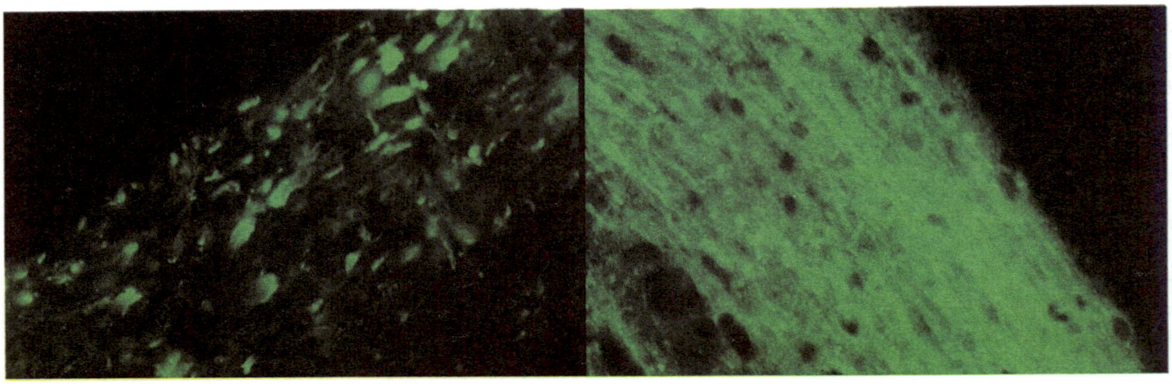

Figure 6. Fluorescence immunocytochemistry of antibody to Kv1.1 in +/+ CNS (*left*) demonstrates up-regulation and redistribution of paranodal K^+ channels in hypomyelinated axons in shiverer brain stem (*right*). Parallel changes in sodium channel population suggest a basis for ectopic excitability and seizures in hypomyelinating diseases.

Ion Channel Stoichiometry and Gene Dysregulation

A fourth level of epileptogenic neuronal plasticity has recently been uncovered following the unexpected observation of seizures in transgenic mice with over-expression of a K^+ channel construct. We used an HPRT promoter linked to a *Shaker* type aplysia aKv1.1α potassium channel containing an epitope tag, allowing us to quantitate transgene expression levels and localize the novel protein in neurons using a specific antibody (M.L. Sutherland et al., in prep.). In situ hybridization studies revealed that widespread expression of the invertebrate K^+ channel was accompanied by the appearance of immunoreactive neuronal dendrites and somas. In several brain regions, there was clear selective up- (Kv α1.4, α1.6) and down- (Kv α1.2) regulation of mRNA levels for other members of the K^+ gene subfamily, and the genes for the auxiliary β1, β2 subunits were also down-regulated (Fig. 7). The mechanisms accounting for cross-regulation remain to be explored; however, this pattern of dysregulation could result in altered subunit stoichiometry and membrane composition of the heteromultimeric proteins within this gene superfamily, with subsequent alterations of firing properties in mutant neural networks.

SUMMARY

Defined transgenic models of epilepsy in the mouse represent unique opportunities to examine interactions between synchronous synaptic activity and cellular programs of brain development. We are beginning to acquire a list of the kinds of genes favoring sudden, intermittent aberrant discharges in central neurons, and we have found that, rather than arising from a few gene superfamilies regulating membrane excitability, they are involved in many diverse functions of the cell. Whereas some primary gene defects impinge directly on membrane electrogenesis and neurotransmitter signaling at synapses, others are too far removed from these processes to clearly visualize the steps by which they promote epileptogenesis. We have tantalizing evidence that several, and probably all, epilepsy genes

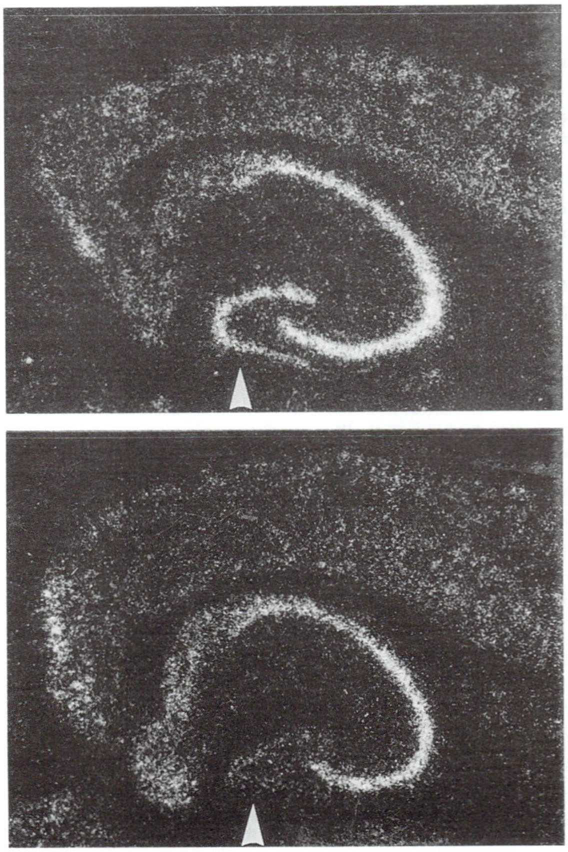

Figure 7. Developmental dysregulation of potassium channel genes in HypK transgenic mutant with aKv1.1α overexpression. Arrows show normal expression pattern of the β2 K^+ channel subunit mRNA in +/+ hippocampus (*upper* panel), and selective down-regulation restricted to the dentate granule cell layer in HypK hippocampus (*lower* panel).

entrain some degree of secondary molecular and cellular plasticity, and we can guess that these downstream rearrangements may account for the delayed onset of epileptic phenotypes in some syndromes. It is too early to tell whether these, or other induced changes, provide the basis for the reversibility of some epilepsies. The diversity of epilepsy genes and their intervening cellular phenotypes promise to provide a rich source of novel molecular targets for therapeutic discovery and will have a lot to teach us in the future about the developmental potential of neural circuits in the mammalian brain.

ACKNOWLEDGMENTS

We gratefully acknowledge the collaborative contributions of Xiaoxi Qiao, Santosh Helekar, Steve Williams, and Paul Overbeek. This work has been supported by grants from the National Institutes of Health (NINCDS NS11535 and 29702).

REFERENCES

Aignier, L., S. Arber, J.P. Kapfhammer, T. Laux, C. Schneider, F. Botteri, H.-R. Brenner, and P. Caroni. 1995. Overexpression of the neural growth-associated protein GAP-43 induces nerve sprouting in the adult nervous system of transgenic mice. *Cell* **83:** 269.

Baumbach, H.D. and K.L. Chow. 1981. Visuocortical epileptiform discharges in rabbits: Differential effects on neuronal development in the lateral geniculate nucleus and superior colliculus. *Brain Res.* **209:** 61.

Chafetz, R.S., W.K. Nahm, and J.L. Noebels. 1995. Aberrant expression of neuropeptide Y in hippocampal mossy fibers in the absence of local cell injury following the onset of spike-wave synchronization. *Mol. Brain Res.* **31:** 111.

DiPasquale, E., K. Keegan, and J.L. Noebels. 1996. Increased excitability and inward rectification in layer V cortical pyramidal neurons in the epileptic mutant mouse *stargazer*. *J. Neurophysiol.* (in press).

Erickson, J.C., K.E. Clegg, and R.D. Palmiter. 1996. Sensitivity to leptin and susceptibility to seizures of mice lacking neuropeptide Y. *Nature* **381:** 415.

European Chromosome 16 Tuberous Sclerosis Consortium. 1993. Identification and characterization of the tuberosis sclerosis gene on chromosome 16. *Cell* **75:** 1305.

Freeman, W.J. 1994. Role of chaotic dynamics in neural plasticity. *Prog. Brain Res.* **102:** 319.

Hattori, M., H. Adachi, M. Trujimoto, H. Arai, and K. Inoue. 1994. Miller Dieker lissencephaly gene encodes a subunit of brain platelet activating factor. *Nature* **370:** 216.

Helekar, S. and J.L. Noebels. 1991. Synchronous hippocampal bursting unmasks latent network excitability alterations in an epileptic gene mutation. *Proc. Nat. Acad. Sci.* **88:** 4736.

Jalilian Tehrani, M.H. and E.M. Barnes, Jr. 1995. Reduced function of γ-aminobutyric $acid_A$ receptors in tottering mouse brain: Role of cAMP-dependent protein kinase. *Epilepsy Res.* **22:** 13.

Kofuji, P., M. Hofer, K.J. Millen, J.H. Millonig, N. Davidson, H.A. Lester, and M.E. Hatten. 1996. Functional analysis of the weaver mutant GIRK2 K^+ channel and rescue of weaver granule cells. *Neuron* **16:** 941.

Lin, F., Z. Zhen Cao, and D.A. Hosford. 1993. Increased number of GabaB receptors in the lethargic (lh/lh) mouse model of absence epilepsy. *Brain Res.* **608:** 101.

Lisman, J.E. and M.A. Idiart. 1995. Storage of 7 +/− 2 short-term memories in oscillatory subcycles. *Science* **267:** 1512.

McKusick, V.A. 1994. Mendelian inheritance in man. Catalogs of human genes and genetic disorders, 11th edition. Johns Hopkins University Press, Baltimore.

Michel, M. 1991. Receptors for neuropeptide Y: Multiple subtypes and multiple second messengers. *Trends Pharmacol.* **12:** 389.

Navarro, B., M.E. Kennedy, B. Velimirovic, D. Bhat, A.S. Peterson, and D.E. Clapham. 1996. Nonselective and Gβγ-insensitive weaver K^+ channels. *Science* **272:** 1950.

Noebels, J.L. 1979. Analysis of inherited epilepsy using single locus mutations in mice. *Fed. Proc.* **38:** 2405.

———. 1996a. Targeting epilepsy genes. *Neuron* **16:** 241.

———. 1996b. Neurogenetic approaches to axon sprouting in the hippocampus. In *Neuronal regeneration, reorganization, and repair* (ed. F. Seil), p. 35. Raven Press, New York.

Noebels, J.L. and D.A. Prince. 1978. The development of focal seizures in cerebral cortex: Role of axon terminal bursting. *J. Neurophysiol.* **41:** 1267.

Noebels, J.L., C.M. Lutz, A. Fu, and W.N. Frankel. 1995. "slow-wave epilepsy", a mutant mouse with 3/sec spike-wave seizures. *Soc. Neurosci. Abstr.* **21:** 1965.

Noebels, J.L., P.K. Marcom, and M.H. Jalilian Tehrani. 1991. Sodium channel density in hypomyelinated brain increased by myelin basic protein gene deletion. *Nature* **352:** 431.

Patil, N., D.R. Cox, D. Bhat, M. Faham, R.M. Myers, and A.S. Peterson. 1995. A potassium channel mutation in weaver mice implicates membrane excitability in granule cell differentiation. *Nat. Genet.* **11:** 126.

Pennacchio, L.A., A.-E. Lehesjoki, N.E. Stone, V.L. Willour, K. Virtaneva, J. Miao, E. D'Amato, L. Ramirez, M. Faham, M. Koskiniemi, J.A. Warrington, R. Norio, A. de la Chapelle, D.R. Cox, and R.M. Myers. 1996. Mutations in the gene encoding cystatin B in progressive myoclonus epilepsy (EPM1). *Science* **271:** 1731.

Qiao, X. and J.L. Noebels. 1993. Developmental analysis of hippocampal mossy fiber outgrowth in a mutant mouse with inherited spike-wave seizures. *J. Neurosci.* **13:** 4622.

Slesinger, P.A., N. Patil, Y.J. Liao, Y.N. Jan, L.Y. Jan, and D.R. Cox. 1996. Functional effects of the mouse *weaver* mutation on G protein-gated inwardly rectifying K^+ channels. *Neuron* **16:** 321.

Steinlein, O.K., J.C. Mulley, P. Propping, R.H. Wallace, H.A. Phillips, G.R. Sutherland, I.E. Scheffer, and S.F. Berkovic. 1995. A missense mutation in the neuronal nicotinic acetylcholine receptor a4 subunit is associated with autosomal dominant nocturnal frontal lobe epilepsy. *Nat. Genet.* **11:** 201.

Steriade, M., F. Amzica, and D. Contreras. 1996. Synchronization of fast (30-40 Hz) spontaneous cortical rhythms during brain activation. *J. Neurosci.* **16:** 392.

Steriade, M., D.A. McCormick, and T.J. Sejnowski. 1993. Thalamocortical oscillations in the sleeping and aroused brain. *Science*. **262:** 679.

Surmeier, D.J., P.G. Mermelstein, and D. Goldowitz. 1996. The weaver mutation of GIRK2 results in a loss of inwardly rectifying K^+ current in cerebellar granule cells. *Proc. Natl. Acad. Sci.* **93:** 11191.

van der Lugt, N.M., J. Domen, K. Linders, M. van Roon, E. Robanus-Maandag, H. te Riele, M. van der Valk, J. Deschamps, M. Sofroniew, M. van Lohuizen, and A. Berns. 1994. Posterior transformation, neurological abnormalities, and severe hematopoietic defects in mice with a targeted deletion of the *bmi-1* proto-oncogene. *Genes Dev.* **8:** 757.

Wang, H., M.L. Allen, J.L. Noebels, and B.L. Tempel. 1995. Axonal K^+ channels are up-regulated in dysmyelinated mutants, *shiverer* and *Trembler*. *Neuron* **15:** 1337.

Waymire, K.G., J.D. Mahuren, J.M. Jaje, T.R. Guilarte, S.P. Coburn, and G.R. MacGregor. 1995. Mice lacking tissue non-specific alkaline phosphatase die from seizures due to defective metabolism of vitamin B-6. *Nat. Genet.* **11:** 45.

Westenbroek, R., J.L. Noebels, and W. Catterall. 1992. Elevated expression of type II Na^+ channels in hypomyelinated axons of *shiverer* mouse brain. *J. Neurosci.* **12:** 2259.

Glutamate Receptor Autoimmunity in Rasmussen's Encephalitis

J.O. McNamara,[1-4] M. Patel,[1] X.-P. He,[1] S. Janumpalli,[1] and K.D. Whitney[3]
Departments of [1]Medicine (Neurology), [2]Neurobiology, and [3]Pharmacology, Duke University Medical Center, Durham, North Carolina 27710, [4]Veteran's Administration Medical Center, Durham, North Carolina 27710

Almost 40 years ago, Rasmussen et al. (1958) first described the features of a chronic neurological syndrome characterized by brain dysfunction, encephalitis, and intractable epilepsy. Rasmussen's encephalitis (RE) usually starts in the first 10 years of life and, although progressive in nature, generally remains confined to one hemisphere. Although the series of 48 cases reviewed by Rasmussen and colleagues (Oguni et al. 1992) included a few patients whose neurological deterioration stabilized and one patient who partially recovered, most cases proceed inexorably from seizures and neurological deficits of limited severity to more frequent and severe seizures associated with hemiparesis, hemisensory deficits, hemianopsia, and ultimately, dementia (Rasmussen et al. 1958; Rasmussen and Andermann 1989; Oguni et al. 1992; Dulac 1996). Imaging studies of RE brains reveal progressive hemispheric atrophy (Rasmussen et al. 1958; Tampieri et al. 1991; Krauss et al. 1996), and histological analyses of brain biopsies demonstrate neuronal loss, astrogliosis, and proliferation of microglial nodules and perivascular lymphocyte infiltrates, both enriched in T cells (Rasmussen et al. 1958; Farrell et al. 1992, 1995). Numerous antiseizure drugs have been developed since the time RE was first described, but the seizures associated with this syndrome remain uncontrolled by standard pharmacotherapy. Currently, the only widely accepted and practiced therapy involves removal or functional isolation of the affected hemisphere (Oguni et al. 1992; Dulac 1996).

WHAT CAUSES RE?

It remains a matter of debate what pathophysiological processes give rise to RE. The inflammatory brain histopathology has led several researchers, including Rasmussen himself, to suggest a viral etiology (Rasmussen et al. 1958; Farrell et al. 1992; Antel and Rasmussen 1996; Dulac 1996). In a subset of RE cases, seizures have appeared at or shortly after a variety of infectious or inflammatory illnesses that were in some cases viral in nature (Rasmussen and Andermann 1989; Harvey et al. 1992; Fukuda et al. 1994). Initial studies using in situ hybridization disclosed the presence of cytomegalovirus (CMV) and Epstein-Barr virus in RE brain tissue (Walter and Renella 1989; Power et al. 1990; Farrell et al. 1992; McLachlan et al. 1993). In a more recent study (Jay et al. 1995), in situ hybridization and polymerase chain reaction (PCR) techniques uncovered the presence of CMV and herpes simplex virus 1 in some, but not all, RE tissue studied, although some controls in each study were shown to be virus-positive. Although the in situ hybridization data were not shown, the PCR data must be interpreted with caution, since even single molecules of template DNA can become amplified to produce positive viral DNA results. CMV infection in the general population is common, especially in childhood, and circulating T cells can harbor CMV DNA for an individual's lifetime (Bruggeman 1993). In one report, 80–98% of blood donors' leukocytes were positive for CMV DNA when assayed by PCR techniques (for review, see Bruggeman 1993). Positive PCR results arising from a single brain-borne affected T-cell DNA, for instance, could therefore be misinterpreted as deriving from a viral infection of the brain. Other groups have failed to find unequivocable evidence of viral infections in the brains of RE patients (Farrell et al. 1992; Atkins et al. 1995). Although multiple events, including a viral infection, might plausibly trigger the onset of RE (Farrell et al. 1992), the available evidence renders it unlikely that a persistent viral infection is the cause of RE (Antel and Rasmussen 1996; Dulac 1996).

AN AUTOIMMUNE REACTION DIRECTED AT GLUTAMATE RECEPTORS?

Recent work has shown that RE may be caused, at least in part, by an autoimmune attack directed against the glutamate receptor subunit GluR3. Glutamate receptors mediate the bulk of excitatory neurotransmission in the mammalian CNS, and the ionotropic receptors sensitive to this transmitter have been classified according to glutamate analogs by which they are activated: *N*-methyl-D-aspartate (NMDA)-, α-amino-3-hydroxy-5-methyl-4-isoxazole proprionate (AMPA)-, and kainate-preferring receptors. To date, more than 15 cDNAs encoding glutamate receptor subunits have been cloned (Seeburg 1993), and receptors composed of GluR1–4 join in heteromeric complexes to form AMPA-preferring receptors at glutamatergic synapses (Boulter et al. 1990; Keinänen et al. 1990).

The first hints of an autoimmune attack directed at GluR3 proteins emerged from an analysis of the brains of two rabbits immunized for other purposes with a *trpE* fusion protein containing a portion of the amino-terminal region of the GluR3 protein (Rogers et al. 1994). These rabbits developed an illness that included persistent seizures, while numerous rabbits immunized with fusion proteins containing other glutamate and nicotinic cholinergic receptors remained healthy. The brains from the two ill rabbits demonstrated a histopathology that, although bilateral, bore many features reminiscent of the RE inflammatory process. These observations led us to hypothesize that the rabbit syndrome stemmed from an autoimmune attack against GluR3, and that RE, too, may result from a similar autoimmune process. We showed that several patients with active RE, but not various control patients, had circulating antibodies of the IgG type directed against GluR3. When one patient was subjected to repeated plasma exchanges, seizures and cognitive functioning improved dramatically (Fig. 1). Further experimentation with plasmapheresis on additional RE patients (Andrews et al. 1996) has replicated these results. Moreover, seizure frequency and severity followed closely the serum titers of these antibodies, which tended to rise between plasma exchanges and over the course of therapy (Fig. 1), suggesting that circulating antibodies gained access to the brain and contributed to the pathogenesis of the disease.

Twyman et al. (1995) hypothesized that binding of GluR3 antibodies to their neuronal antigens might activate excitatory currents and thereby trigger the seizures seen with RE. Whole-cell patch recordings of cultured mouse cortical neurons revealed that application of either serum filtrates or IgG isolated from two *trpE*-GluR3-immunized rabbits and two RE patients evoked excitatory currents. Importantly, the excitatory currents were blocked by the glutamate receptor antagonist CNQX, as well as by preincubation of either the antibody or the serum preparation with a peptide corresponding to a region overlapping a portion of the presumed GluR3 agonist binding site (Stern-Bach et al. 1994). These results led to the interesting proposal that antibodies gaining access to the brains of RE patients may trigger seizures or other aspects of RE by acting as glutamate receptor agonists.

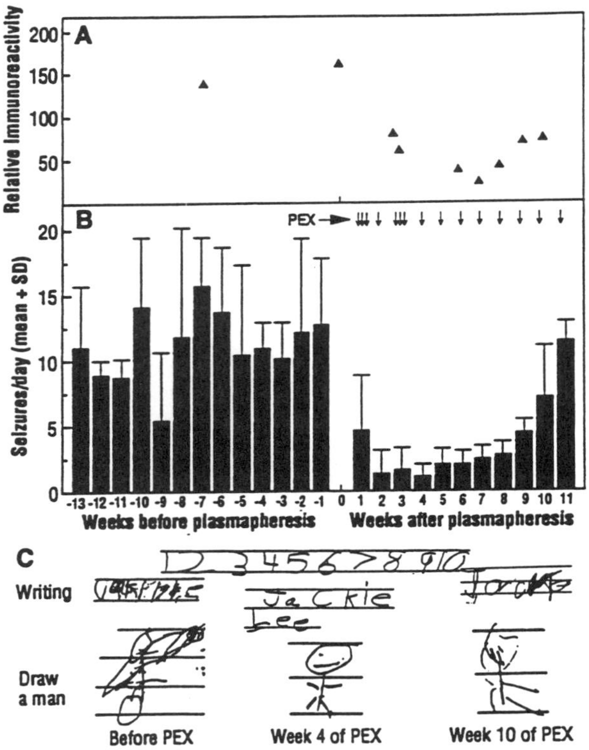

Figure 1. Correlation between seizure frequency (*B*), cognitive function (*C*), and GluR3 immunoreactivity (*A*) in one RE patient before and during 11 weeks of repeated plasma exchange (PEX), indicated by arrows in *B*. Before PEX, GluR3 antibody titers were high. She had 10–12 right-body or generalized seizures per day, mild right hemiparesis, and no spontaneous speech. She was unable to read or solve simple math problems, and her writing and drawing skills were primitive. During the first 7 weeks of PEX, GluR3 antibody titers measured immediately before each PEX decreased in temporal association with reduced seizure frequency. She spoke spontaneously in phrases and short sentences; her understanding, right hemiparesis, calculations, drawing, and writing improved remarkably. For the first time in 2 years, she resumed playing with dolls, riding a bicycle, and participating in household activities. During the last 4 weeks of PEX, GluR3 antibody titers gradually increased while cognitive skills declined. Numbers in *C* were written by the patient during week 4 of PEX therapy. Throughout the 11-week course of PEX therapy, other therapies were continued as usual.

GLUR3, AUTOIMMUNITY, AND NEURONAL DEATH

Recently, in exploring the prominent neuronal death seen in RE, we have examined whether anti-GluR3 antibodies can kill cultured cortical cells, and whether an excitotoxic mechanism is involved. We have demonstrated that serum and plasma preparations obtained from a new set of glutathione-*S*-transferase (GST)-GluR3 fusion protein-immunized rabbits can kill cultured rat cortical cells in a complement-dependent but apparently not excitotoxic manner (Patel et al. 1996). By interacting with antigen-bound antibodies and directly recognizing foreign organisms, the blood-borne complement system plays a critical role in helping the immune system fight infection. Upon interaction with the membranes of foreign organisms or recognition of antigen-bound IgG or IgM, a proteolytic cascade similar to the blood-clotting system is set in motion. The cascade culminates with the deposition of several proteins in the target cell's membrane that not only help trigger phagocytosis, but also combine to form nonselective ion channels called membrane attack complexes that can cause targeted cells to swell and lyse (Liszewski and Atkinson 1993). In agreement with these processes, plasma preparations isolated from several GluR3-immunized rabbits, but not control rabbits, kill cells, as quantified by release of lactate dehydrogenase activity into the culture supernatant. Cytotoxicity is abrogated by prior heating of the plasma samples, suggesting the involvement of heat-labile enzymes such as the complement cascade proteases. Immunocytochemical analysis of cells positive for either neuron- or glial-specific markers have indicated that a majority of neurons die at the plasma concentrations examined here (Patel et al. 1996).

Results from two experimental approaches argue against an excitotoxic mechanism for this death (Patel et al. 1996). First, toxicity is blocked by neither competitive (APV 100 μM and CNQX, 50 μM) nor noncompetitive (GYKI 52466, 50 μM, MK-801 10 μM) glutamate receptor antagonists, whereas AMPA-mediated toxicity is readily blocked by CNQX or GYKI-52466. Second, IgG alone fails to kill cells; instead, cytotoxicity is observed only upon coincubation of IgG from GluR3-immunized rabbits with non-IgG plasma components, further arguing against an excitotoxic role for the antibodies themselves. Two other observations support these results. First, the phase-contrast appearance of neurons exposed to GST-GluR3 sera is characterized by numerous bleb-like structures on their plasma membranes, which is distinct from the typical pattern of somatic swelling seen with AMPA-mediated excitotoxicity (Koh et al. 1990). Second, using electrophysiological techniques similar to those of Twyman et al. (1995), we failed to find any excitatory properties in these reagents, results which are in agreement with the apparent non-excitotoxic mechanism of cell death (Patel et al. 1996).

It is unlikely that a fruitful direct comparison can be made between the non-excitotoxic antibody preparations we have been using and the excitatory preparations of Twyman and colleagues (Twyman et al. 1995). It seems reasonable that different rabbits might generate qualitatively different immune responses to similar immunization protocols and that such differences might explain the divergent electrophysiological observations in these two reports. In fact, the observation that plasma from one of the five rabbits we immunized with GluR3 fusion proteins failed to kill cells at the doses used in our experiments, despite readily recognizing GluR3 antigen on immunoblots, supports the notion of heterogeneity among these polyclonal sera (Patel et al. 1996). Although it remains an open question, it will be interesting to determine whether excitatory antibodies can in fact kill cells by an excitotoxic mechanism.

To more directly test the involvement of complement in the cell death described here, we have incubated IgG fractions from GluR3 and control rabbit serum samples with either incomplete or complete serum complement fractions. When C1q-deficient (C1qD) serum was incubated with IgG, little cell death resulted. Cytotoxicity was enhanced by adding C1q to the mixture of C1qD and GluR3 but not control IgG (Patel et al. 1996).

In this series of experiments, we examined the cytotoxic properties of plasma and IgG obtained from five GST-GluR3- and two GST-immunized rabbits. Although the antiserum from all five GluR3-immunized rabbits detected GluR3 antigens on immunoblots, the widely ranging titers did not correlate with the degree to which the preparations killed cells in vitro. In an analysis of myasthenia gravis (MG) patient sera, Tzartos et al. (1982) demonstrated that no clear correlation existed between clinical state and anti-nicotinic receptor antibodies across patients or even within patients over the years as the disease progressed. This might imply that a small subset of antibodies, whose detection on an immunoblot would be difficult, is responsible for cytotoxicity. Perhaps the fifth GluR3 rabbit's relatively nontoxic plasma is relatively lacking in these key antibodies.

Taken together, these observations demonstrate that complement deposition triggered by anti-GluR3 antibodies promotes the cell death we have observed in vitro. Anti-GluR3 antibodies gaining access to the rabbits' brains may have promoted similar complement-mediated cell death. By analogy, the prominent cortical atrophy seen in RE patients may also be due at least in part to a complement-mediated immune attack directed against cells bearing the GluR3 antigen. Experiments are currently under way in our laboratory to demonstrate complement immunoreactivity in the brains of both RE patients and rabbits.

Complement-mediated cell death is a key means by which the immune system destroys targeted cells (Liszewski and Atkinson 1993), and some evidence suggests that complement activation may contribute to the progression of some neurological disorders, such as multiple sclerosis (MS), MG, and Alzheimer's disease (AD). Evidence for this includes immunocytochemical colocalization of complement components in the brains of MS and AD patients with sites of demyelination or senile plaque formation, respectively (for review, see Morgan 1993). Likewise, muscle endplates from MG patients demonstrate immunoreactivity for various complement cascade components (Drachman 1994). More importantly, functional decomplementation with cobra venom factor renders animals resistant to the experimentally induced animal model forms of MG and MS (for references, see Lennon et al. 1978; Linington et al. 1989, respectively).

We can hypothesize that complement activation would yield the neuronal loss, reactive gliosis, gross hemispheric atrophy, and increased seizure activity characteristic of RE via either direct deposition of complement proteins on cortical cells or more indirect mechanisms (see below). Nevertheless, in-depth analyses of the role of complement-mediated death versus, e.g., T-cell-mediated toxicity in the initiation and propagation of the rabbit RE-like syndrome must await the development of an optimal animal model.

UNANSWERED QUESTIONS

A number of interesting issues remain unresolved regarding RE. First, if as we suggest, anti-GluR3 autoantibodies play an important role in RE, how did the patients develop them? One idea, the molecular mimicry hypothesis, suggests that infection with a pathogen bearing surface epitopes similar to portions of self-antigens, in this case glutamate receptor proteins, yields antibodies that recognize both the pathogen and glutamate receptors (Oldstone 1987). In principle, these epitopes need not contain large regions of significant primary amino acid sequence identity; rather, only a few key amino acids placed in the proper spatial arrangement are required to mimic the original antigen's immunogenic site. Systematically replacing the original residues of an 11-amino-acid stretch of myelin basic protein (MBP) with alanine, Gautam et al. (1992) showed that only 5 of the original 11 residues are necessary to fully stimulate a sensitized clonal T-cell population. More importantly, experimental autoimmune encephalomyelitis (EAE), an animal model of MS, was readily induced in mice injected not only with the wild-type 11-amino-acid peptide, but also with a peptide conserving just 5 of these residues (Gautam et al. 1992). Thus, it seems plausible that a viral or bacterial pathogen with surface epitopes of even limited similarity to MBP could trigger a robust immune reaction that would produce cross-reacting antibody and/or T-cell-receptor specificities as well as the clinical features of EAE and, potentially, MS. The amino-terminal region of GluR3 bears some structural similarity to various bacterial periplasmic amino-acid-binding proteins present on the surfaces of certain *Escherichia coli* and *Salmonella* strains (Higgins et al. 1990; O'Hara et al. 1993). Perhaps RE patients experienced an infection with one of these agents that gave rise to antibodies that cross-react with GluR3 antigens.

Cross-reaction notwithstanding, for the disease process to continue according to either an excitotoxic or complement-mediated mechanism, these antibodies must locate and interact with their cognate neural antigens. Multiple mechanisms may be invoked to provide transient passage of blood-borne factors into the brain. One possibility is that focal disruption of the blood-brain barrier (BBB), perhaps following a head injury, allows circulating pathogenic antibodies to interact with GluR3 antigens (Lee 1982). In addition to promoting tissue damage, activation of complement at this point would promote further BBB disruption, chemotaxis of various cell types, and other aspects of inflammation by virtue of the chemoattractant and anaphylatoxic proteolytic fragments produced as complement is activated (Morgan 1994).

Another possibility, not mutually exclusive of the first, is that activated T cells, whose agile diapedesis is enhanced during inflammatory episodes by virtue of tumor necrosis factor-α-mediated increases in endothelial adhesion molecule expression (Merrill and Benveniste 1996; Steinman 1996), could enter the parenchyma, and upon encountering the appropriate epitope and costimulatory signals, release proinflammatory cytokines that enable other lymphocytes to cross the BBB as well (Merrill and Benveniste 1996). These events would then perpetuate the immune reaction by promoting the production of anti-GluR3 antibodies as well as the clonal expansion of subsets of T and/or B cells specific for GluR3 and perhaps other neural antigens (Yi et al. 1995; Merrill and Benveniste 1996).

Such a situation might transpire from the escape from negative selection during maturation in the thymus of small numbers of self-reactive T cells. Alternatively, T cells targeting a foreign antigen but also reacting with self may be produced during an immune process where molecular mimicry events are operative. Precedent for circulating self-reactive T cells comes from analyses of peripheral T cells isolated from normal adults, which can be stimulated by MBP and other myelin protein constituents (Steinman 1996). Likewise, GluR3-reactive T cells may persist in the circulation of at least some individuals and become activated upon interaction with cross-reacting bacterial epitopes. We are currently testing this hypothesis (see below).

Once an initial focal invasion of the brain parenchyma occurs, antibody-antigen interactions may promote seizures directly by altering neural functioning (Twyman et al. 1995) or indirectly because of the tissue damage resulting from the inflammatory process (Andrews and McNamara 1996). Moreover, inflammation can persist and even spread by virtue of the fact that the resulting seizures transiently increase BBB permeability at regions sometimes distal from the initiating focus (Nitsche and Hubauer 1986). The increased permeability would promote passage of lymphocytes, antibodies, and other serum components, leading to an inflammatory response in neighboring areas that would perpetuate cell damage, seizures, and inflammation. That a vicious cycle of this sort could propagate from a single focus may explain why most RE cases present with unihemispheric abnormalities. The unaffected hemisphere presumably remains healthy, even after hemispherectomy, because an initiating BBB disruption has not yet occurred. To more fully test these hypotheses, a unihemispheric RE animal model will have to be developed, a project now under way in our laboratory.

CONCLUDING REMARKS

Other data collected during the past 4 years have reinforced the argument that RE is caused by some sort of immune system process, perhaps autoimmune in nature. Several reports have appeared indicating that high-dose steroid, cyclophosphamide, or other immunosuppressant therapies can ameliorate the severity and frequency of seizures in at least a subset of RE cases (Walsh 1991; Chinchilla et al. 1994; Hart et al.

1994; Dulac 1996; Krauss et al. 1996). Yi et al. (1995) showed by PCR analysis of T-cell-receptor Vβ chains that the collection of T cells present in five RE patients' brains represented a small, oligoclonally expanded subset of the general peripheral lymphocyte population. Moreover, direct sequencing of the antigen-recognizing CDR3 loop region of the TCR genes from these patients revealed repeated amino acid sequence motifs that differed markedly from those deduced from peripheral T-cell TCR genes. The overrepresentation of a small number of Vβ chains and the structural similarities seen among CDR3 regions support the idea that a subset of infiltrating T cells responded to one or a few activating brain antigens as part of a larger immune reaction. What these antigens might be remains to be determined. In collaboration with Dr. Oksenberg and his colleagues, we are currently examining whether T cells collected from RE patients and healthy individuals respond to GluR3 antigens. Whether tissue damage and disease progression are primarily due to T-cell- or circulating-antibody-mediated mechanisms remains undetermined. Extensive research has shown that both mechanisms play important roles in the develoment of EAE and perhaps MS as well (Morgan 1993); in time, we may come to the same conclusions for the pathogenesis of RE.

Recently, several cases of chronic bilateral encephalitis bearing striking histopathological similarities to the typical RE pathology have been reported (Chinchilla et al. 1994). Whereas bilateral disease could be explained within the context of the model described above by postulating independent, bilateral focal BBB disruptions, we may come to recognize that what we have understood as the unitary phenomenon of RE is in fact a collection of similar diseases. The evidence reviewed above suggests that some of the symptoms of RE—or perhaps the symptoms of some forms of RE—stem from an autoimmune attack directed against the neural GluR3 antigen. Naturally, our work does not rule out other processes that may or may not act in concert with complement activation in triggering RE. Through fortuitous circumstances, we have been able to appreciate the role immune reactions against GluR3 antigens play in the rabbit and perhaps human syndromes. These experiments raise the intriguing possibility that other neurological disorders whose etiologies remain obscure are likewise caused by neural antigen autoimmunity.

ACKNOWLEDGMENTS

The work presented in this paper was supported by National Institutes of Health grant NS-17771. K.D.W. was supported by a predoctoral fellowship from the Howard Hughes Medical Institute. M.P. was supported by a grant from the Epilepsy Foundation of America.

REFERENCES

Andrews, P.I. and J.O. McNamara. 1996. Rasmussen's encephalitis: An autoimmune disorder? *Curr. Opin. Neurol.* **9:** 141.

Andrews, P.I., M.A. Dichter, S.F. Berkovic, M.R. Newton, and J.O. McNamara. 1996. Plasmapheresis in Rasmussen's encephalitis. *Neurology* **46:** 242.

Antel, J.P. and T. Rasmussen. 1996. Rasmussen's encephalitis and the new hat. *Neurology* **46:** 9.

Atkins, M.R., W. Terrell, and C.M. Hulette. 1995. Rasmussens syndrome: A study of viral etiology. *Clin. Neuropathol.* **14:** 7.

Boulter, J., M. Hollmann, A. O'Shea-Greenfield, M. Hartley, E. Deneris, C. Maron, and S. Heinemann. 1990. Molecular cloning and functional expression of glutamate receptor subunit genes. *Science* **249:** 1033.

Bruggeman, C.A. 1993. Cytomegalovirus and latency: An overview. *Virchows Arch. B Cell Pathol.* **64:** 325.

Chinchilla, D., O. Dulac, O. Robain, P. Plouin, G. Ponsot, J.F. Pinel, and D. Graber. 1994. Reappraisal of Rasmussen's syndrome with special emphasis on treatment with high doses of steroids. *J. Neurol. Neurosurg. Psychiatry* **57:** 1325.

Drachman, D.B. 1994. Myasthenia gravis. *New Engl. J. Med.* **330:** 1797.

Dulac, O. 1996. Rasmussen's syndrome. *Curr. Opin. Neurol.* **9:** 75.

Farrell, M.A., O. Droogan, D.L. Secor, V. Poukens, B. Quinn, and H.V. Vinters. 1995. Chronic encephalitis associated with epilepsy: Immunohistochemical and ultrastructural studies. *Acta Neuropathol.* **89:** 313.

Farrell, M.A., M.J. DeRosa, J.G. Curran, D. Lenard Secor, M.E. Cornford, Y.G. Comair, W.J. Peacock, W.D. Shields, and H.V. Vinters. 1992. Neuropathologic findings in cortial resections (including hemispherectomies) performed for the treatment of intractable childhood epilepsy. *Acta Neuropathol.* **83:** 246.

Fukuda, T., H. Oguni, S. Yanagaki, Y. Fuukyama, M. Kogure, H. Shimizu, and M. Oda. 1994. Chronic localized encephalitis (Rasmussen's syndrome) preceded by ipsilateral uveitis: A case report. *Epilepsia* **35:** 1328.

Gautam, A.M., C.I. Pearson, D.E. Smilek, L. Steinman, and H.O. McDevitt. 1992. A polyanine peptide with only five native myelin basic protein residues induces autoimmune encephalomyelitis. *J. Exp. Med.* **176:** 605.

Hart, Y.M., M. Cortez, F. Andermann, P. Hwang, D.R. Fish, O. Dulac, K. Silver, N. Fejerman, H. Cross, A. Sherwin, and R. Caraballo. 1994. Medical treatment of Rasmussen's syndrome (chronic encephalitis and epilepsy): Effect of high-dose steroids or immunoglobulins in 19 patients. *Neurology* **44:** 1030.

Harvey, A.S., F. Andermann, I.J. Hopkins, T. Kirkham, and S.F. Berkovic. 1992. Chronic encephalitis (Rasmussen's syndrome) and ipsilateral uveitis. *Ann. Neurol.* **32:** 826.

Higgins, C.F., S.C. Hyde, M.M. Mimmack, U. Gileadi, D.R. Gill, and M.P. Gallagher. 1990. Binding protein-dependent transport systems. *J. Bioenerg. Biomembr.* **22:** 571.

Jay, V., L.E. Becker, H. Otsubo, M. Cortez, P. Hwang, H.J. Hoffman, and M. Zielenska. 1995. Chronic encephalitis and epilepsy (Rasmussen's encephalitis): Detection of cytomegalovirus and herpes simplex virus 1 by the polymerase chain reaction and in situ hybridization. *Neurology* **45:** 108.

Keinänen, K., W. Wisedn, B. Sommer, P. Werner, A. Herb, T.A. Verdoorn, B. Sakmann, and P.H. Seeburg. 1990. A family of AMPA-selective glutamate receptors. *Science* **249:** 556.

Koh, J.-Y., M.P. Goldberg, D.M. Hartley, and D.W. Choi. 1990. Non-NMDA receptor-mediated neurotoxicity in cortical culture. *J.Neurosci.* **10:** 693.

Krauss, G.L., M.L. Campbell, K.W. Roche, R.L. Huganir, and E. Niedermeyer. 1996. Chronic steroid-responsive encephalitis without autoantibodies to glutamate receptor GluR3. *Neurology* **46:** 247.

Lee, J.C. 1982. Anatomy of the blood brain barrier under normal and pathological conditions. In *Histology and histopathology of the nervous system* (eds. W. Haymaker and R.D. Adams), p. 798. C.C. Thomas, Springfield, Illinois.

Lennon, V.A., M.E. Seybold, J.M. Lindstrom, C. Cochrane, and R. Ulevitch. 1978. Role of complement in the pathogenesis of experimental autoimmune myasthenia gravis. *J. Exp. Med.* **147:** 973.

Linington, C., B.P. Morgan, N.J. Scolding, P. Wilkins, S. Piddlesden, and D.A.S. Compston. 1989. The role of complement in the pathogenesis of experimental allergic encephalomyelitis. *Brain* **112:** 895.

Liszewski, M.K. and J.P. Atkinson. 1993. The complement system. In *Fundamental immunology,* 3rd edition (ed. W.E. Paul), p. 919. Raven Press, New York.

McLachlan, R.S., J.P. Girvin, W.T. Blume, and H.R. Reichman. 1993. Rasmussen's chronic encephalitis in adults. *Arch. Neurol.* **50:** 269.

Merrill, J.E. and E.N. Benveniste. 1996. Cytokines in inflammatory brain lesions: Helpful and harmful. *Trends Neurosci.* **19:** 331.

Morgan, B.P. 1993. Complement in diseases of the nervous system. In *Complement in health and disease,* 2nd edition (ed. K. Whaley et al.), p. 353. Kluwer, Dordrecht, The Netherlands.

———. 1994. Clinical complementology: Recent progress and future trends. *Eur. J. Clin. Invest.* **24:** 219.

Nitsche, C. and H. Hubauer. 1986. Distant blood-brain barrier opening in subfields of the rat hippocampus after intrastriatal injections of kainic acid but not ibotenic acid. *Neurosci. Lett.* **64:** 53.

Oguni, H., A. Andermann, and T.B. Rasmussen. 1992. The syndrome of chronic encephalitis and epilepsy: A study based on the MNI series of 48 cases. *Adv. Neurol.* **57:** 419.

O'Hara, P., P.O. Sheppard, H. Thogersen, D. Venezia, B.A. Haldeman, V. McGrane, K.H. Houamed, C. Thomsen, T.L. Gilbert, and E.R. Mulvhill. 1993. The ligand-binding domain in metabotropic glutamate receptors is related to bacterial periplasmic binding domains. *Neuron* **11:** 41.

Oldstone, M.B.A. 1987. Molecular mimicry and autoimmune disease. *Cell* **50:** 819.

Patel, M., X.-P. He, S. Janumpalli, K. Whitney, and J.O. McNamara. 1996. Glutamate receptor antibodies destroy cortical neurons by a complement-dependent mechanism. *Soc. Neurosci. Abstr.* **22:** 1203.

Power, C., S.D. Poland, W.T. Blume, J.P. Girvin, and G.P.A. Rice. 1990. Cytomegalovirus and Rasmussen's encephalitis. *Lancet* **336:** 1282.

Rasmussen, T. and F. Andermann. 1989. Update on the syndrome of "chronic encephalitis" and epilepsy. *Clev. Clin. J. Med.* (suppl. 2) **56:** S181.

Rasmussen, T., J. Olszewski, and D. Lloyd-Smith. 1958. Focal seizures due to chronic localized encephalitis. *Neurology* **8:** 435.

Rogers, S.W., P.I. Andrews, L.C. Gahring, T. Whisenand, K. Cauley, B. Crain, T.E. Hughes, S.F. Keinemann, and J.O. McNamara. 1994. Autoantibodies to glutamate receptor GluR3 in Rasmussen's encephalitis. *Science* **265:** 648.

Seeburg, P.S. 1993. The TINS/TIPS lecture: The molecular biology of mammalian glutamate receptor channels. *Trends Neurosci.* **16:** 359.

Steinman, L. 1996. Multiple sclerosis: A coordinated immunological attack against myelin in the central nervous system. *Cell* **85:** 299.

Stern-Bach, Y., B. Bettler, M. Hartley, P.O. Sheppard, P.J. O'Hara, and S.F. Heinemann. 1994. Agonist selectivity of glutamate receptors is specified by two domains structurally related to bacterial amino acid-binding proteins. *Neuron* **13:** 1345.

Tampieri, D., D. Melanson, and R. Ethier. 1991. Imaging of chronic encephalitis. In *Chronic encephalitis and epilepsy: Rasmussen's syndrome* (ed. A.F. Stoneham), p. 47. Butterworth-Heinemann, Boston.

Twyman, R.E., L.C. Gahring, J. Spiess, and S.W. Rogers. 1995. Glutamate receptor antibodies activate a subset of receptors and reveal an agonist binding site. *Neuron* **14:** 755.

Tzartos, S.J., M.E. Seybold, and J.M. Lindstrom. 1982. Specificities of antibodies to acetylcholine receptors in sera from myasthenia gravis patients measured by monoclonal antibodies. *Proc. Natl. Acad. Sci.* **79:** 188.

Walsh, P.J. 1991. Treatment of Rasmussen's syndrome with intravenous gammaglobulin. In *Chronic encephalitis and epilepsy: Rasmussen's syndrome* (ed. A.F. Stoneham), p. 201. Butterworth-Heinemann, Boston.

Walter, G. and R.R. Renella. 1989. Epstein-Barr virus in the brain of Rasmussen's encephalitis (Letter) *Lancet* **335:** 279.

Yi, L., A. Uccelli, K. Laxer, J.R. Oksenberg, and S.L. Hauser. 1995. Restricted T-cell repertoire in Rasmussen encephalitis brain lesions. *Neurology* (suppl. 4) **45:** A295.

Molecular and Genetic Insights into Ligand Binding and Signal Transduction at the Inhibitory Glycine Receptor

P.R. Schofield,[1] J.W. Lynch,[1] S. Rajendra,[2] K.D. Pierce,[1] C.A. Handford,[1] and P.H. Barry[2]
[1]*Garvan Institute of Medical Research, Sydney 2010, Australia;* [2]*School of Physiology and Pharmacology, University of New South Wales, Sydney 2052, Australia*

Inhibitory and excitatory synaptic neurotransmission is mediated by ligand-gated ion channel receptors (LGICs), with the neurotransmitters glycine and γ-aminobutyric acid (GABA) activating inhibitory receptors, and acetylcholine and serotonin activating excitatory receptors. However, the receptors for each of these different neurotransmitters are structurally and functionally related. In this paper, we demonstrate that the insights gained from studying the inhibitory glycine receptor (GlyR) are of relevance in understanding the mode of action of all receptors of this superfamily. In particular, we focus on the results obtained from structure/function studies using site-directed mutagenesis and on the analysis of mutations that result in inherited defects in GlyR subunits. These studies have defined receptor domains involved in ligand binding, which conform to a general model originally proposed for the nicotinic acetylcholine receptor (nAChR), and allowed the identification of a novel domain required for signal transduction.

Glycinergic inhibitory neurotransmission is essential for reflex responses, voluntary motor control, and the processing of sensory signals in the mammalian central nervous system (CNS). Inhibitory spinal cord reflex arcs include pathways for reciprocal and recurrent inhibition. In reciprocal inhibition, stretch-induced muscle contraction is accompanied by glycinergic relaxation of antagonist muscles. Recurrent inhibition provides negative feedback through the synaptic activation of Renshaw cells by the motor neuron, resulting in the inhibition of the firing of the motor neuron. The plant alkaloid, strychnine, disrupts spinal cord reflexes by potently and selectively antagonizing inhibitory neurotransmission. In the adult CNS, [^{3}H]strychnine binding occurs at high levels in the spinal cord gray matter and medulla; at lower levels in the midbrain, hypothalamus, and thalamus; and is virtually absent in the spinal cord white matter and higher brain (White et al. 1990). This accords with the distribution of endogenous glycine in the CNS and the regions in which glycine is able to elicit inhibitory synaptic activity (Kelly and Krnjevic 1969). Disruption of glycinergic inhibitory pathways, by the convulsive alkaloid strychnine or by inherited genetic disorders (Rajendra and Schofield 1995), can result in abnormal reflexes, loss of muscle control, convulsions, and death.

The primary sequences of the GlyR α (Grenningloh et al. 1987, 1990b) and β (Grenningloh et al. 1990a) subunits share considerable sequence identity with each other as well as with the subunits of the nAChR (Noda et al. 1982), GABA type A receptor ($GABA_AR$) (Schofield et al. 1987), serotonin type 3 receptor ($5HT_3R$) (Maricq et al. 1991), and the glutamate-gated chloride channel of *Caenorhabditis elegans* (GluCl) (Cully et al. 1994). Together with the GlyR, these receptors form an evolutionary superfamily of LGICs (Grenningloh et al. 1987; Schofield et al. 1987) responsible for fast excitatory (nAChR and $5HT_3R$) and inhibitory ($GABA_AR$, GluCl, and GlyR) synaptic transmission in the spinal cord and brain. LGICs comprise five subunits, arranged across the cell membrane so as to form a central, transmembrane ion channel, which for the GlyR is selective to chloride ions. Each subunit consists of a large amino-terminal extracellular domain in which ligand-binding sites reside, four transmembrane domains (M1–M4) which form the receptor channel, and a cytoplasmic domain located between M3 and M4. Ligand-binding sites of the LGICs are composed of three discontinuous extracellular domains (Devillers-Thiery et al. 1993). In the nAChR, three distinct loops form the acetylcholine binding site (Devillers-Thiery et al. 1993), and this three-loop model appears to be conserved across all LGICs, since homologous regions of the $GABA_AR$ and the GlyR also contain ligand-binding sites.

The GlyR pentamer can be formed from either α subunits alone, being composed of five α2 subunits in the neonatal GlyR (Hoch et al. 1989; Takahashi et al. 1992), or from three α and two β subunits in the adult GlyR (Fig. 1) (Langosch et al. 1988). Receptor subunit heterogeneity also exists, with four different α subunit isoforms and a single β subunit having been identified in rat, mouse, and human (Grenningloh et al. 1987, 1990a,b; Kuhse et al. 1990a,b; Akagi et al. 1991; Matzenbach et al. 1994; Handford et al. 1996). Additional α1 and α2 subunit variants arise from alternate splicing (Kuhse et al. 1990a, 1991; Akagi et al. 1991; Malosio et al. 1991). The cytoplasmic subunit, gephyrin, associates with the intracellular region of the β subunit and links the receptor complex to the cytoskeleton via attachment to tubulin (Fig. 1) (Kirsch et al. 1991; Kirsch and Betz 1995).

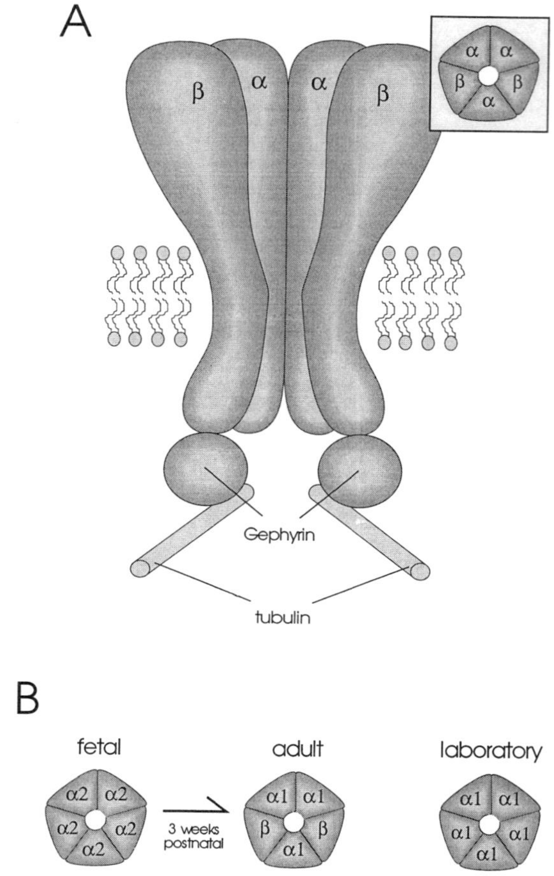

Figure 1. Model of the inhibitory GlyR. (*A*) View of the adult GlyR. The nearest α subunit has been excluded to show the ion channel. The cytosolic subunit, gephyrin, anchors the receptor to tubulin molecules of the cell cytoskeleton. (*Inset*) Top view. (*B*) The developmentally regulated switch from a fetal α2 homomeric GlyR to an adult α/β heteromeric GlyR occurs in postnatal weeks 2–3 in the rat. In recombinant expression systems, the α1 subunits can form homomeric GlyRs with functional properties similar to those observed for adult GlyRs in vivo.

To investigate the functional properties of LGICs, two recombinant expression systems have been extensively utilized. Homomeric (single-subunit-containing pentamers) GlyRs are formed by expression of α subunits in both mammalian cells (Sontheimer et al. 1989) and *Xenopus* oocytes (Schmieden et al. 1989). These receptors have properties that are almost indistinguishable from those found in native spinal cord hetero-pentameric GlyRs. Thus, the homomeric α1 GlyR, in particular, is an attractive model of an anionic LGIC, since its functional properties are similar to those of native receptors (Sontheimer et al. 1989; Grenningloh et al. 1990b), and changes in homomeric receptor complexes are more easily interpreted in mutagenesis studies due to the absence of other receptor subunits. In this manner, the α1 GlyR resembles the neuronal α7 nAChR, which is a widely regarded model of cationic LGICs (Devillers-Thiery et al. 1993). Since the GlyR is the receptor most frequently associated with the primitive brain regions of spinal cord and brain stem, this has resulted in the fact that glycine, rather than being considered as the "other" inhibitory neurotransmitter, has often been relegated to the class of the "forgotten" neurotransmitter.

The recent demonstrations that heritable mutations in the α or β subunits of the GlyR cause startle syndromes in man and mouse provide yet another important set of insights into the structure and function of the inhibitory GlyR (Rajendra and Schofield 1995). There are now more heritable mutations described in the GlyR subunits than in any other member of the LGIC superfamily. Indeed, as an allelic series of mutations have been described in the α subunits of both man and mouse, the use of genetics has now complemented the conventional structure/function studies as a powerful means by which to provide novel insights into the structure and function of the GlyR, as well as the other members of the LGIC superfamily. The GlyR can thus serve as a paradigm for molecular investigations into the structure and function of all members of the LGIC superfamily. In this paper, we review the current state of knowledge of the structure and function of the GlyR based on studies from other researchers and ourselves. In particular, these studies define the domains of the receptor and specific residues involved in the three key biological processes of ligand binding, signal transduction, and ion channel permeation.

EXPERIMENTAL PROCEDURES

Strategy. To define receptor domains and specific amino acids involved in ligand-binding and signal transduction, we have expressed recombinant human GlyR α1 subunits in the human 293 cell line (Sontheimer et al. 1989). GlyR subunits have been subjected to site-directed mutagenesis using alanine substitution to examine the role of the amino acid side chain, or by generating specific mutations as have been described in various startle disease mutations, to mimic residues found in related receptor subunits. Expressed mutated receptors have been examined by a combination of ligand-binding assays, patch-clamp electrophysiology, and immunocytochemical localization studies.

Expression of mutated GlyR α1 subunit cDNAs. The cDNA encoding the α1 subunit of the human GlyR was subcloned into the pCIS expression vector. Mutations in the cDNA were constructed using the oligonucleotide-directed PCR mutagenesis method and were confirmed by sequencing the cDNA clones. Plasmid DNA encoding wild-type or mutated α1 subunits of the human GlyR was transfected using the 3% CO_2 method into exponentially growing 293 cells. After 24 hours, the cells were washed twice with culture medium (Eagle's minimum essential medium in Hanks salts supplemented with 2 mM glutamine and 10% fetal calf serum) and refed.

Electrophysiological measurements. 48 hours after transfection, cells were patch-clamped in the whole-cell mode or outside-out excised patch configuration at a holding potential of –55 mV while continually superfused with a bath solution containing (in mM) 140 NaCl 10 glucose, 5 KCl, 2 $CaCl_2$, 2 $MgCl_2$ 10 HEPES, pH 7.4. Glycine, β-alanine, or taurine, dissolved in this solution, was rapidly applied to the chamber using a microperfusion tube system. No significant osmotic effects were observed, even at 100 mM agonist concentrations. Voltages were corrected for junction potentials using the JPCalc program. The pipette solution contained (in mM) 145 CsCl, 2 $CaCl_2$, 2 $MgCl_2$ 10 HEPES 10 EGTA, pH 7.4. Dose-response data for glycine-activated currents in individual cells were fitted using a nonlinear least squares algorithm to the Hill equation: $I/I_{max} = [G]h/(EC_{50}h + [G]h)$, where I is the magnitude of the peak current elicited by a concentration of glycine [G], I_{max} is the magnitude of the maximum peak current elicited by saturating concentrations of glycine, EC_{50} is the value of [G] required to elicit a half-maximum peak current and h is the Hill coefficient. Currents from outside-out patches were digitally stored at a sampling rate of 4 kHz and were filtered at 1 kHz before analysis using PClamp software (Axon Instruments, Foster City, California).

[^{3}H]Strychnine binding assays. 48 hours after transfection, cells were incubated with strychnine (1–50 nM; 24 5 Ci/mM, New England Nuclear) with or without 10 mM cold strychnine to determine nonspecific binding. After incubation to equilibrium at 4°C for 60 minutes, cells were collected by rapid filtration onto Whatman GF/B filter paper, and the amount of bound [^{3}H]strychnine was determined. The K_d and B_{max} for the [^{3}H]strychnine saturation isotherms and IC_{50} and K_i for glycine, β-alanine, and taurine displacement of bound [^{3}H]strychnine were estimated using the InPlot program (Graph Pad Software, San Diego, California).

RESULTS AND DISCUSSION

Ligand-binding Domains

Photoaffinity labeling studies using [^{3}H]strychnine show specific, glycine-inhibited incorporation into the α subunit (Graham et al. 1982). We therefore sought to use this antagonist to aid the dissection of the molecular pharmacology of the GlyR. Protein modification studies suggested four tyrosine residues, located at positions 128, 161, 197, and 202, which may contribute to the formation of the ligand-binding site (Marvison et al. 1986; Ruiz-Gomez et al. 1990). Mutation of either Tyr-161 or Tyr-202 to Ala resulted in the loss of

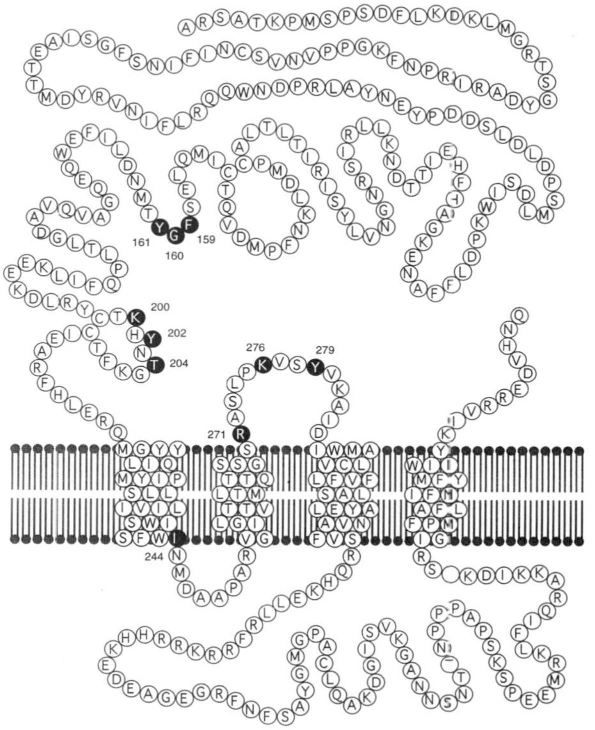

Figure 2. Model of the GlyR α1 subunit. GlyR subunits consist of a large amino-terminal extracellular region, four transmembrane regions (M1–M4), and a large intracellular loop between M3 and M4. Residues that contribute to the ligand-binding site in the amino-terminal domain of the α1 subunit are Phe-159, Gly-160, and Tyr-161, which comprise the loop-2-binding domain of the three-loop LGIC-binding site model (see text), and Lys-200, Tyr-202, and Thr-204, which comprise the loop-3-binding domain. Hyperekplexia mutations have been identified at residues Ile-244, Arg-271, Lys-276, and Tyr-279.

strychnine binding (Vandenberg et al. 1992b) and allowed Tyr-202 to be deduced as the site of photoaffinity labeling by [^{3}H]strychnine (Fig. 2). Mutation of Lys-200 also resulted in the loss of strychnine binding to the receptor (Vandenberg et al. 1992b) although relatively normal levels of glycine activation were observed (Rajendra et al. 1995b). These studies have thus identified two distinct ligand-binding sites in the extracellular region of the GlyR. These sites align with similar ligand-binding domains identified in both the nAChR and the $GABA_AR$, indicating that a conserved tertiary structure exists for all LGICs.

The presence of a ligand-binding site at Gly-160 was also inferred from the contrasting pharmacologies of the human and rat α2 subunit subtypes. GlyRs formed from the rat α2 subunit allelic variant, α2*, display markedly reduced glycine affinity and strychnine sensitivity (Kuhse et al. 1990a). The sequences of the human α2 and rat α2 differ from that of the rat α2* subunit by the presence of the nonconservative amino acid substitution occurring at position 167 (Glu in α2* and Gly in all other α subunits). The substitution

E167G in recombinant α2* GlyRs restores glycine and strychnine affinities (Kuhse et al. 1990a). Similarly, substitution of the corresponding residue in the α1 subunit, Gly-160, with Glu, results in loss of strychnine binding (Fig. 2) (Vandenberg et al. 1992b). The G160A mutation, however, does not disrupt either strychnine or glycine binding, suggesting that either the steric or charged properties of Glu are responsible for the reduced sensitivities (Vandenberg et al. 1992b). Mutation of Tyr-161 to Ala (Y161A) results in strychnine-insensitive GlyRs (Vandenberg et al. 1992b), whereas the more conservative mutation to Phe (Y161F) does not (Schmieden et al. 1993). In α1 GlyRs, transposition of Phe-159 with Tyr-161 (F159Y, Y161F) increases agonist affinity for glycine by 12-fold, but by 121- and 45-fold for β-alanine and taurine, respectively (Schmieden et al. 1993). Indeed, the F159Y, Y161F GlyR exhibits a higher affinity for β-alanine than glycine, although the strychnine affinity of the F159Y, Y161F GlyR is not altered. The F159Y, Y161F mutant GlyR is particularly significant in that the mutated GlyR is now able to be activated by GABA (Schmieden et al. 1993). Together, our findings (Vandenberg et al. 1992b) and those of Schmieden et al. (1993) indicate that the Phe-159, Gly-160, Tyr-161 triplet forms one component of the total strychnine-binding site and also determines the relative affinities of glycinergic agonists. In the context of the three-loop model, the results obtained in studying the GlyR have led to the identification of a specific sequence pattern that forms an aromatic - small - aromatic motif. Both the position and sequence of this motif are conserved in the analogous loop-2 ligand-binding sites of the $GABA_AR$ α1 and β1 subunits (Amin and Weiss 1993) and in nAChR β subunits (Schmieden et al. 1993).

The loop-3 ligand-binding region identified above is contained within the extracellular cysteine loop found only in the GlyR and GluCl (Cully et al. 1994). In the GlyR α1 subunit, this loop is formed by the disulfide bonding of Cys-198 and Cys-209 (Fig. 2). Evidence of the role of this region in ligand-binding and receptor assembly is seen from the effects of mutations to either of the Cys residues, which disrupt the disulfide bond. The C198S substitution abolishes ligand binding through disruption of receptor assembly, whereas C209S produces GlyRs unable to bind either agonists or strychnine (Rajendra et al. 1995b). Within this loop, the even-numbered residues, Lys-200, Tyr-202, and Thr-204, affect agonist and/or strychnine affinity (Fig. 2) (Vandenberg et al. 1992a,b; Rajendra et al. 1995b). This finding is consistent with a proposed β-sheet structure in which even-numbered residues are adjacent to each other. Of these three residues, Lys-200 has been demonstrated to be a determinant of strychnine binding (Vandenberg et al. 1992b) and Thr-204 has been demonstrated to be a determinant of agonist binding (Vandenberg et al. 1992a). The intervening residue, Tyr-202, is both an agonist- and antagonist-binding site. Tyr-202 has also been shown to influence receptor assembly. In α1 GlyRs, removal of the hydroxyl moiety from the aromatic ring of this residue by substitution with Phe (Y202F) produces a 480-fold reduction in glycine affinity (Rajendra et al. 1995b), but only minor reductions in taurine affinity and strychnine sensitivity (35- and 3-fold respectively). Replacement of the aromatic ring with a long-chain uncharged residue such as Leu (Y202L) produces no further decrease in glycine affinity, suggesting that glycine interacts with the hydroxyl moiety, possibly via hydrogen bonding. The Y202L substitution, however, produces taurine and strychnine insensitivity, indicating that both taurine and strychnine interact with the aromatic ring. Substitution of Tyr-202 with a short side-chain residue, such as Ala, Ser, or Thr, prevents receptor assembly. Various functions can thus be attributed to distinct structural components of the residue Tyr-202. Glycine interacts with the terminal hydroxyl group, strychnine and taurine with the aromatic ring itself, and successful receptor assembly is reliant on the size of the side chain. It is of interest to note that the β-sheet conformation of the residues Tyr-202 and Thr-204 conforms, in part, with the aromatic - small - aromatic motif (Amin and Weiss 1993; Schmieden et al. 1993) that has been shown above to form part of the glycine ligand-binding site.

Structural Model of the Agonist-binding Site

A three-loop model of agonist and antagonist binding in LGICs has been developed from studies of ligand-binding regions in the related nAChR (Devillers-Thiery et al. 1993). In this model, the binding site is composed of three discontinuous loops (loops 1–3) in the amino-terminal extracellular domain of the receptor (Kao et al. 1984; Dennis et al. 1988; Galzi et al. 1990, 1991; Cohen et al. 1991; O'Leary and White 1992). It is proposed that these distinct regions associate to form a ligand-binding structure that is conserved in the LGIC superfamily. Variations in amino acid residues would then account for the distinct pharmacologies of its different receptor types and subtypes. The extrapolation of the three-loop model to other receptors in the LGIC superfamily has been strengthened by the identification of ligand-binding residues in analogous regions in $GABA_AR$ subunits (Weiland et al. 1992; Amin and Weiss 1993). The GlyR regions identified in the studies discussed above also correspond to these loops. In the α1 subunit, Phe-159, Gly-160, Tyr-161 is in loop 2 and Lys-200, Tyr-202, Thr-204 is in loop 3 (Fig. 2). Further studies are required to investigate residues in the region corresponding to loop 1 and to confirm whether the three-loop model fully describes ligand binding in the GlyR.

The GlyR-binding site is composed of at least two discontinuous regions in the amino-terminal extracellular domain that must be in reasonable proximity to each other, since the physical dimensions of glycine are small. The site must also accommodate the strychnine molecule, which is considerably larger. Additionally, the site exhibits a marked selectivity that allows the binding of β- but not α-amino acids (Tokutomi et al. 1989; Schmieden et al. 1993). The data outlined above demonstrate that all ligand-binding-site data are consistent with the three-loop model. However, what still remains controversial is the role of each of the loops in determining ligand binding. Schmieden et al. (1992, 1993) have proposed a two-subsite ligand-binding structure for the GlyR α1 subunit, with the Gly-160 β-turn (loop 2) forming the high-affinity, agonist- and antagonist-binding subsite I, and with Ile-111 and Ala-212 contributing to the low-affinity subsite II, to which β-alanine and taurine bind. In this scheme, the Cys-198 to Cys-209 extracellular loop (loop 3) domain is able to have an interaction with the low-affinity site and, thus, would be predicted to affect taurine affinity and/or efficacy without altering that of glycine or strychnine (Schmeiden et al. 1992). This model is inconsistent with our findings that mutations in loop 3 profoundly reduce glycine sensitivity and/or confer strychnine sensitivity, without greatly affecting taurine sensitivity or efficacy (Vandenberg et al. 1992a,b; Rajendra et al. 1995b). Indeed, the reductions in glycine sensitivity in conservative mutations of residues in loop 3 are an order of magnitude greater than those produced by substitution of Gly-160, in the proposed high-affinity subsite I (Schmieden et al. 1992; Kuhse et al. 1993). Furthermore, mutations of the aromatic residues flanking Gly-160 enhance, rather than impair, the binding of glycine and glycinergic agonists and allow the binding of the α-amino acids, D- and L-alanine and D- and L-serine, and GABA (Schmieden et al. 1993). On the basis of these results, we now propose that loop 2 is important for agonist discrimination, but that agonists bind principally to residues in loop 3 (Rajendra et al. 1995b). Our model is also consistent with the description of the glycine-binding site by Tokutomi et al. (1989). Tokutomi et al. (1989) predict that mutations of residues in one domain (loop 3) would impair receptor activation, whereas mutations of residues in a second domain (loop 2) would not markedly alter agonist sensitivity but would reorder their relative affinities, as has been seen experimentally (Kuhse et al. 1990a, 1993; Schmieden et al. 1992, 1993).

Ion Permeation

The M2 transmembrane domain forms the channel in the GlyR. The sensitivity of inhibition of glycine-activated currents by cyanotriphenylborate (CTB), a recently identified noncompetitive blocker of the GlyR channel, is decreased in α1 GlyRs by mutating a residue in the M2 region (Rundström et al. 1994). The subconductance states in the GlyR are dependent on subunit composition and the sequences of the M2 domains (Bormann et al. 1993). The M2 region contains several polar residues and, in α subunits, is flanked both intracellularly and extracellularly by positively charged Arg residues (Arg-252 and Arg-271 in the α1 subunit). The M2 sequences of the various α subunits are identical, except for the residue at position 254, which is Gly in α1 and Ala in α2 and α3. The M2 sequences of β subunits differ considerably from those of α subunits. In α1 GlyRs, the Gly-254 residue in M2 is responsible for both the differences in sensitivity to CTB and the distribution of single-channel conductance states among α isoforms. Replacement with the α2/α3 homolog G254A decreases CTB channel blockade to levels seen in α2 GlyRs (Rundström et al. 1994). The G254A substitution also unmasks a high-conductance substate of 105-111 pS which is present in only α2 and α3 GlyRs (Bormann et al. 1993). α1/β GlyRs possess only three subconductance states, but conversion of the β subunit M2 sequence to the α1 sequence does not result in the conductance state distribution seen in α1 GlyRs. For this, the substitution of a proximal extracellular residue, Glu-297, with the α1 homolog, Ser, is required (Bormann et al. 1993).

Disorders of Glycinergic Neurotransmission

The blockade of inhibitory pathways by subconvulsive doses of strychnine produces an acute responsiveness to sensory stimuli, whereas acute poisoning results in severe generalized hypertonia. Inherited disorders in humans and animals also produce a characteristic exaggerated startle reflex in response to an unexpected stimulus. Recent molecular studies have demonstrated that defects in inhibitory glycinergic pathways are responsible for the pathology of a number of startle syndromes, including familial startle disease (hyperekplexia) in humans (Suhren et al. 1966), the murine mutations *spastic* (Chai 1961), *spasmodic* (Lane et al. 1987), and *oscillator* (Cook 1993), and the bovine form of myoclonus (Gundlach et al. 1988).

In response to unexpected stimuli, *spasmodic*, *oscillator*, and *spastic* homozygous mice display hypertonia, myoclonic jerks, falling, and impaired righting (Chai 1961; Lane et al. 1987; Cook 1993). The mice are phenotypically normal until 2 weeks after birth but show symptoms by 3 weeks of age. This corresponds to the time at which the fetal α2 GlyR subtype is normally replaced by the adult α1/β GlyR. *Spasmodic* is caused by a missense mutation in the extracellular amino terminus of the GlyR α1 subunit that results in the replacement of Ala-52 by Ser (Ryan et al. 1994; Saul et al. 1994). Recombinant α1 subunit homomeric GlyRs with this mutation have a 6-fold reduced glycine sensitivity but normal ligand-binding properties (Ryan et al. 1994; Saul et al. 1994). *Oscillator* is an allelic variant of *spasmodic* (Cook 1993) caused by a microdeletion that results in a frameshift mutation. This alters the α1 subunit coding sequence after the M3 domain, producing incomplete proteins that are unable to assemble into functional receptors (Buckwalter et al.

1994). This disorder is the only lethal startle syndrome identified to date.

A defect in the GlyR β-subunit gene causes the *spastic* mutation. An intronic insertion of a LINE-1 transposable element, a repetitive sequence element, causes aberrant splicing of β-subunit mRNAs, resulting in exon-skipping and the premature termination of the protein (Mulhardt et al. 1994) as well as a major reduction in the levels of normal β-subunit mRNA in the spinal cord and brain (Kingsmore et al. 1994; Mulhardt et al. 1994). Although *spastic* spinal cord GlyRs function normally, receptor numbers are dramatically reduced compared with wild-type animals (White and Heller 1982; Becker et al. 1992). Thus, the *spastic* mutation prevents the expression of normal β subunits, which are required for efficient GlyR assembly. Reduced GlyR expression in the spinal cord is characteristic of the bovine form of myoclonus (Gundlach et al. 1988), although it is not yet known if this is caused by an α- or β-subunit defect.

Suhren et al. (1966) described an autosomal dominant hereditary disease in humans which had an onset at birth, showed generalized hypertonia, and resulted in strong brain-stem reflexes and nocturnal myoclonal jerks throughout life. The exaggerated startle response was also accompanied by an uncontrolled fall during which consciousness was maintained. The disorder was termed hyperekplexia and is also known as Kok's disease, congenital stiff-baby syndrome, or familial startle disease (Suhren et al. 1966). Genetic linkage analysis of startle disease pedigrees mapped this disorder to chromosome 5q33-35 (Ryan et al. 1992), where the GlyR α1 subunit gene is located. Shiang et al. (1993) identified two mutations in the α1 subunit gene in which Arg-271 is replaced with either Leu or Gln (Fig. 2). Additional mutations have also been described in which Tyr-279 is substituted by Cys (Shiang et al. 1995) or Lys-276 is substituted by Glu (Fig. 2) (Elmslie et al. 1996). An autosomal recessive variant of the disorder results in the substitution of an Asn for Ile-244 (Fig. 2) (Rees et al. 1994). All of the hyperekplexia mutations described to date cluster within the sequences that flank the M2 domain. Examination of the effects of these hyperekplexia mutations has therefore been undertaken to probe the role of the M2-flanking domains (see below).

Channel Activation

The process by which agonist binding leads to channel gating or opening in the GlyR and other LGICs is poorly understoood. However, some clues regarding the nature of this allosteric transduction mechanism have recently emerged (O'Leary and White 1992; Schmieden et al. 1992; Aylwin and White 1994; Mihic et al. 1994). In particular, the analysis of the human startle disease mutations has led to the identification of a series of residues involved in the signal transduction or receptor activation process.

Analysis of the R271L and R271Q startle disease mutations, which remove the positively charged residue at the extracellular border of M2, result in the mutant GlyRs exhibiting a 230- to 410-fold reduced sensitivity of glycine-activated currents (Langosch et al. 1994; Rajendra et al. 1994). Glycine-binding affinity is reduced somewhat less, by only 50- to 100-fold. β-Alanine and taurine do not elicit currents from the R271L and R271Q mutant GlyRs, but surprisingly, the binding affinities of these ligands are comparable to that of wild-type α1 GlyRs (Rajendra et al. 1995a). Coapplication of either ligand with glycine inhibits glycine-activated currents in both a dose-dependent and competitive manner. This inhibition is not due to receptor desensitization, since preincubation with β-alanine or taurine does not diminish the size of glycine-activated currents. These results indicate that β-alanine and taurine binding is not impaired in these mutant GlyRs, but their ability to activate the channel is abolished. Thus, the R271L and R271Q mutations transform these wild-type GlyR agonists into competitive antagonists (Rajendra et al. 1995a).

Picrotoxin is a competitive antagonist of glycine in both α1 (Lynch et al. 1995) and α/β GlyRs (Handford et al. 1996). Glycine-activated currents at the Arg-271 mutant GlyRs are potentiated by low picrotoxin concentrations (Lynch et al. 1995). Thus, the conversion of a competitive antagonist into an allosteric enhancer, by the Arg-271 mutations, provides further compelling evidence for this residue having a major role in signal transduction (Lynch et al. 1995).

The distribution of single-channel subconductance states is also determined by Arg-271, as mutation of this positively charged residue diminishes glycine-activated whole-cell currents by up to 90% in both α1 GlyRs (Langosch et al. 1994; Rajendra et al. 1995a) and α1/β GlyRs (Langosch et al. 1994; Laube et al. 1995). This occurs by a progressive abolition of higher subconductance states (Table 1) (Langosch et al. 1994; Rajendra et al. 1995a). R271L α1 GlyRs only possess the lower four conductance states seen in wild-type α1 GlyRs, and only the lowest subconductance state (18 pS) is present in R271Q GlyRs (Table 1). The β-subunit homolog of Arg-271 is Ala, and it is possible that the lower conductance states seen in heteromeric GlyRs may be partly due to the presence of the uncharged residue at this position.

Role of M1-M2 and M2-M3 Loops in Signal Transduction

The autosomal dominant neurological disorder startle disease, or hyperekplexia, is caused by missense mutations that are located in either the M2-M3 extracellular or the M1-M2 intracellular loop regions. Expression of GlyR α1 subunits carrying the hyperekplexia mutations (K276E and Y279C) results in the expression of GlyRs that have several hundred-fold reductions in GlyR sensitivity to the agonist glycine

Table 1. Single-channel Conductance States of Human GlyRs

GlyR	Conductance state I	II	III	IV	V	VI	VII	Reference
$\alpha 1$	—	86*	64	46	30	18⁺	—	Bormann et al. (1993)
$\alpha 1$	—	88*	68	49	30	—	—	Rajendra et al. (1995b)
R271L	—	—	64*	42	27	—	—	Langosch et al. (1994)
R271L	—	—	63	47*	29	16*	—	Rajendra et al. (1995a)
R271Q	—	—	—	37⁺	25⁺	14*	—	Langosch et al. (1994)
R271Q	—	—	—	—	—	18*	—	Rajendra et al. (1995a)
$\alpha 1/\beta$	—	—	—	44*	29	20	—	Bormann et al. (1993)

All conductances are given in pS. The most frequently occurring conductance states are indicated by an asterisk, and the + denotes infrequently observed conductance states. The conductance state numbering system is based on that proposed by Bormann et al. (1993).

and transform the agonists β-alanine and taurine into competitive antagonists (J.W. Lynch et al., in prep.). The phenotype of these mutations is thus identical to that seen for the R271L and R271Q hyperekplexia mutations. The recessive startle disease mutant I244N partially disrupts signal transduction by converting the agonists β-alanine and taurine into partial agonists/partial antagonists. On the basis of these results, we suggest that each of the startle disease mutations acts in a similar manner to disrupt the ability of the receptor to convert agonist binding into channel activation (Fig. 3).

Because the various startle disease mutations are located within either the 14-amino-acid M2-M3 extracellular loop or the 9-amino-acid M1-M2 intracellular loop, they raise the possibility that these entire loop regions may form an important component of the signal transduction mechanism of this receptor. Alanine scanning mutagenesis of all 23 residues reveals that, in

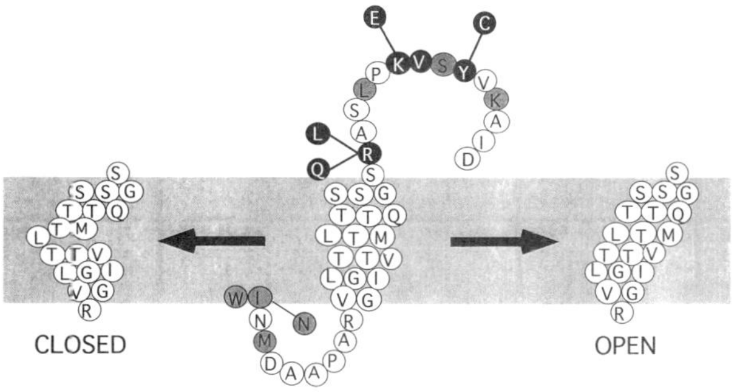

Figure 3. Model of the signal transduction domain of the GlyR channel. Representation of the putative open (extended) and closed (kinked) states of the M2 domains of the GlyR $\alpha 1$ subunit. Residues joined to the wild-type sequence by stems are hyperekplexia mutations. Residues that are shaded black show a "full" disruption phenotype, characterized by the conversion of β-alanine and taurine into competitive antagonists. Residues that are shaded gray show a "partial" disruption phenotype, characterized by the conversion of β-alanine and taurine into partial agonists/partial antagonists. The M1-M2 intracellular domain and the M2-M3 extracellular domain are postulated to act as hinges that allow the allosteric conformational change or gating of the ion channel to occur.

addition to the startle disease mutation sites, mutations at residue V277 fully disrupt, and at residues W243, I244, M246, L274, S278, and K281 partially disrupt, signal transduction (Fig. 3) (J.W. Lynch et al., in prep.). Full disruption results in the conversion of the agonists β-alanine and taurine into competitive antagonists, whereas partial disruption results in the conversion of β-alanine and taurine into partial agonists/partial antagonists. Collectively, these mutations demonstrate that a total of ten separate residues from both the extracellular and intracellular domains play a critical role in the process of signal transduction that converts ligand binding into the opening or gating of the chloride channel (Fig. 3) (J.W. Lynch et al., in prep.).

Each of the ten residues thus can be regarded as forming part of an "allosteric switch" responsible for inducing a conformational change in the receptor upon the binding of an agonist. From mutagenesis studies, it appears that the nature of this switch determines whether a particular substance will act as an agonist, potentiator, or antagonist. These residues flank the ion channel lumen formed by transmembrane domain 2, suggesting that they act as hinges, allowing the necessary conformational change required for channel gating (Fig. 3). Mutations disrupting these hinge domains affect channel gating without significantly disrupting ligand binding. These results therefore provide an unexpected molecular insight into understanding the mechanism of activation of LGICs.

Our interpretations are also consistent with several recent observations of other LGICs. Campos-Caro et al. (1996) have identified two residues in the $\alpha 7$ and $\beta 4$ subunits of the nAChR that also are involved in signal transduction. A similar interpretation may also apply to the E297S mutation (equivalent to Ser-273 in the GlyR $\alpha 1$ subunit) in the GlyR β-subunit (Bormann et al. 1993) and to the Lys to Met substitution (equivalent to Ala-272 in the GlyR $\alpha 1$ subunit) of the *Xenopus* nAChR γ and ε subunits (Murray et al. 1995), both of which result in changes to the single-channel subconductance states of the respective receptors. Finally, the mutation R316A in the $GABA_AR$ ρ subunit (homologous to Lys-276 in the GlyR $\alpha 1$ subunit) altered the allosteric coupling of the receptor through increasing the Hill coefficient of GABA activation

(Kusana et al. 1994). Collectively, these results are all supported by a theoretical analysis using an allosteric receptor model with multiple discrete conformational states (Galzi et al. 1996). Recent imaging of the nAChR by Unwin (1993, 1995) indicates that the channel region of LGICs is composed of a channel-lining kinked α helix formed by the M2 transmembrane region which is stabilized by surrounding β sheets formed by the transmembrane regions, M1, M3, and M4. It appears that agonist binding to the nAChR initiates small rotations in the subunits which realign the M2 segments, moving the kinked regions toward the side of the channel and switching the channel from a closed to an open conformation (Unwin 1995). The location of the two sets of residues in both the M1-M2 and M2-M3 loops suggests a role of these elements in the pathway that transmits this allosterically induced conformational change (Fig. 3).

PROSPECTS

The studies described in this review have provided a detailed insight into glycinergic inhibitory neurotransmission in both normal and diseased states. They have also established the GlyR as an elegant model for understanding the structure and function of the LGIC superfamily. Like the widely regarded model receptor, the neuronal α7 nAChR (Devillers-Thiery et al. 1993), the homomeric α1 GlyR is particularly amenable to mutagenesis studies due to the absence of other receptor subunits. Further unexpected insights into the function of the GlyR are provided by the growing list of mutations found to underlie various GlyR disorders. Such naturally occurring mutations have provided clues as to the manner by which agonist binding is transduced into channel opening in GlyRs. More detailed study of these mechanisms will continue to be of direct relevance to understanding receptor structure and function in all LGICs.

ACKNOWLEDGMENTS

This work was supported by the National Health and Medical Research Council of Australia.

REFERENCES

Akagi, H., K. Hirai, and F. Hishinuma. 1991. Cloning of a glycine receptor subtype expressed in rat brain and spinal cord during a specific period of neuronal development. *FEBS Lett.* **281:** 160.

Amin, J. and D.S. Weiss. 1993. $GABA_A$ receptor needs two homologous domains of the β-subunit for activation by GABA but not by pentabarbital. *Nature* **366:** 565.

Aylwin, M.L. and M.M. White. 1994. Gating properties of mutant acetylcholine receptors. *Mol. Pharmacol.* **46:** 1149.

Becker, C.-M., V. Schmieden, P. Tarroni, U. Strasser, and H. Betz. 1992. Isoform-selective deficit of glycine receptors in the mouse mutant *spastic*. *Neuron* **8:** 283.

Bormann, J., N. Rundstrom, H. Betz, and D. Langosch. 1993. Residues within the M2 determine chloride conductance of glycine receptor homo- and hetero-oligomers. *EMBO J.* **12:** 3729.

Buckwalter, M.S., S.A. Cook, M.T. Davisson, W.F. White, and S.A. Camper. 1994. A frameshift mutation in the mouse alpha 1 glycine receptor gene (Glra 1) results in progressive neurological symptoms and juvenile death. *Hum. Mol. Genet.* **3:** 2025.

Campos-Caro, A., S. Sala, J.J. Ballesta, F. Vicente-Agullo, M. Criado, and F. Sala. 1996. A single residue in the M2-M3 loop is a major determinant of coupling between binding and gating in neuronal nicotinic receptors. *Proc. Natl. Acad. Sci.* **93:** 6118.

Chai, C.K. 1961. Hereditary spasticity in mice. *J. Hered.* **52:** 241.

Cohen, J.B., S.D. Sharp, and W.S. Liu. 1991. Structure of the agonist-binding site of the nicotinic acetylcholine receptor. [^{3}H]acetylcholine mustard identifies residues in the cation-binding subsite. *J. Biol. Chem.* **266:** 23354.

Cook, S.A. 1993. *Oscillator (ot). Mouse Genome* **91:** 117.

Cully, D.F., D.K. Vassilatis, K.K. Liu, P.S. Paress, L.T.T. Van der Ploeg, J.M. Shaeffer, and J.P. Arena. 1994. Cloning of an avermectin-sensitive glutamate-gated chloride channel from *Caenorhabditis elegans*. *Nature* **371:** 707.

Dennis, M., J. Giraudat, F. Kotzyba-Hibert, M. Goeldner, C. Hirth, J.Y. Chang, C. Lazure, M. Chretien, and J.P. Changeux. 1988. Amino acids of the *Torpedo marmorata* acetylcholine receptor α subunit labelled by a photoaffinity ligand for the acetylcholine binding site. *Biochemistry* **27:** 2346.

Devillers-Thiery, A., J.L. Galzi, J.L. Eisele, S. Bertrand, D. Bertrand, and J.P. Changeux. 1993. Functional architecture of the nicotinic acetylcholine receptor: A prototype of ligand-gated ion channels. *J. Membr. Biol.* **136:** 97.

Elmslie, F.V., S.M. Hutchings, V. Spencer, A. Curtis, T. Covanis, R.M. Gardiner, and M. Rees. 1996. Analysis of GLRA1 in hereditary and sporadic hyperekplexia: A novel mutation in a family cosegragating for hyperekplexia and spastic paraparesis. *J. Med. Genet.* **33:** 435.

Galzi, J.L., S.J. Edelstein, and J.-P. Changeux. 1996. The multiple phenotypes of allosteric receptor mutants. *Proc. Natl. Acad. Sci.* **93:** 1853.

Galzi, J.-L., D. Bertrand, A. Devillers-Thiery, F. Revah, S. Bertrand, and J.-P. Changeux. 1991. Functional significance of aromatic amino acids from three peptide loops of the α7 neuronal nicotinic receptor site investigated by site-directed mutagenesis. *FEBS Lett.* **294:** 198.

Galzi, J.-L., F. Revah, D. Black, M. Goeldner, C. Hirth, and J.-P. Changeux. 1990. Identification of a novel amino acid alpha-tyrosine 93 within the cholinergic ligands-binding sites of the acetylcholine receptor by photoaffinity labeling. Additional evidence for a three-loop model of the cholinergic ligands-binding sites. *J. Biol. Chem.* **265:** 10430.

Graham, D., F. Pfeiffer, and H. Betz. 1982. Purification by affinity chromatography of the glycine receptor of rat spinal cord. *J. Biol. Chem.* **257:** 9389.

Grenningloh, G., I. Pribilla, P. Prior, G. Malthaup, K. Beyreuther, O. Taleb, and H. Betz. 1990a. Cloning and expression of the 58 kd β subunit of the inhibitory glycine receptor. *Neuron* **4:** 963.

Grenningloh, G., A. Rienitz, B. Schmitt, C. Methfessel, M. Zensen, K. Beyreuther, E. E. Gundelfinger, and H. Betz. 1987. The strychnine-binding subunit of the glycine receptor shows homology with nicotinic acetylcholine receptors. *Nature* **328:** 215.

Grenningloh, G., V. Schmeiden, P.R. Schofield, P.H. Seeburg, T. Siddique, T.K. Mohandas, C.-M. Becker, and H. Betz. 1990b. Alpha subunit variants of the human glycine receptor: Primary structures, functional expression and chromosomal localisation of the corresponding genes. *EMBO J.* **9:** 771.

Gundlach, A.L., P.S. Dodd, C.S. Grabara, W.E. Watson, G.A.R. Johnston, P.A. Harper, J.A. Dennis, and P.J. Healy. 1988. Deficit of spinal cord glycine/strychnine receptors in inherited myoclonus of Poll Hereford calves. *Science* **241:** 1807.

Handford, C.A., J.W. Lynch, E. Baker, G.C. Webb, J.C. Ford, G.R. Sutherland, and P.R. Schofield. 1996. The human glycine receptor β subunit: Primary structure, functional characterization and chromosomal localization of the human and murine genes. *Mol. Brain Res.* **35:** 211.

Hoch, W., H. Betz, and C.-M. Becker. 1989. Primary cultures of mouse spinal cord express the neonatal isoform of the inhibitory glycine receptor. *Neuron* **3:** 339.

Kao, P., A. Dwork, R. Kaldany, M. Silver, J. Wideman, S. Stein, and A. Karlin. 1984. Identification of the α-subunit half-cystine specifically labelled by an affinity reagent for the acetylcholine receptor binding site. *J. Biol. Chem.* **259:** 11662.

Kelly, J.S. and K. Krnjevic. 1969. The action of glycine on cortical neurones. *Exp. Brain Res.* **9:** 155.

Kingsmore, S.F., B. Giros, D. Suh, M. Bieniarz, M.G. Caron, and M.F. Seldin. 1994. Glycine receptor beta-subunit gene mutation in spastic mouse associated with LINE-1 element insertion. *Nat. Genet.* **7:** 136.

Kirsch, J. and H. Betz. 1995. The postsynaptic localization of the glycine receptor-associated protein gephyrin is regulated by the cytoskeleton. *J. Neurosci.* **15:** 4148.

Kirsch, J., D. Langosch, P. Prior, U.Z. Littauer, B. Schmitt, and H. Betz. 1991. The 93-kDa glycine receptor-associated protein binds to tubulin. *J. Biol. Chem.* **266:** 22242.

Kuhse, J., V. Schmieden, and H. Betz. 1990a. A single amino acid exchange alters the pharmacology of neonatal rat glycine receptor subunit. *Neuron* **5:** 867.

———. 1990b. Identification and functional expression of a novel ligand binding subunit of the inhibitory glycine receptor. *J. Biol. Chem.* **265:** 22317.

Kuhse, J., B. Laube, D. Magalei, and H. Betz. 1993. Assembly of the inhibitory glycine receptor: Identification of amino acid sequence motifs governing subunit stoichiometry. *Neuron* **11:** 1049.

Kuhse, J., A. Kuryatov, Y. Maulet, M.L. Malosio, V. Schmeiden, and H. Betz. 1991. Alternative splicing generates two isoforms of the alpha 2 subunit of the inhibitory glycine receptor. *FEBS Lett.* **283:** 73.

Kusana, T., J.B. Wang, C.E. Spivak, and G.R. Uhl. 1994. Mutagenesis of the GABA rhol receptor alters agonist affinity and channel gating. *NeuroReport* **5:** 1209.

Lane, P.W., A.L. Ganser, A.-L. Kerner, and W.F. White. 1987. *Spasmodic*, a mutation on chromosome 11 in the mouse. *J. Hered.* **78:** 353.

Langosch, D., L. Thomas, and H. Betz. 1988. Conserved quaternary structure of ligand-gated ion channels: The postsynaptic glycine receptor is a pentamer. *Proc. Natl. Acad. Sci.* **85:** 7394.

Langosch, D., B. Laube, N. Rundstrom, V. Schmieden, J. Bormann, and H. Betz. 1994. Decreased agonist affinity and chloride conductance of mutant glycine receptors associated with human hereditary hyperekplexia. *EMBO J.* **13:** 4223.

Laube, B., D. Langosch, H. Betz, and V. Schmieden. 1995b. Hyperekplexia mutations of the glycine receptor unmask the inhibitory subsite for β-amino-acids. *Neuroreport* **6:** 897.

Lynch, J.W., S. Rajendra, P.H. Barry, and P.R. Schofield. 1995. Mutations affecting the glycine receptor agonist transduction mechanism convert the competitive antagonist, picrotoxin, into an allosteric potentiator. *J. Biol. Chem.* **270:** 13799.

Malosio, M.L., G. Grenningloh, J. Kuhse, V. Schmeiden, B. Schmitt, P. Prior, and H. Betz. 1991. Alternative splicing generates two variants of the α1 subunit of the inhibitory glycine receptor. *J. Biol. Chem.* **266:** 2048.

Maricq, A.V., A.S. Peterson, A.J. Brake, R.M. Myers, and D. Julius. 1991. Primary structure and functional expression of the 5HT3 receptor, a serotonin-gated ion-channel. *Science* **254:** 432.

Marvison, J.C.G., M.G. Clavo, J. Vazques, and F. Mayor, Jr. 1986. The glycine receptor: Pharmacological studies and mathematical modelling of the allosteric interaction between the glycine- and strychnine-binding sites. *Mol. Pharmacol.* **30:** 590.

Matzenbach, B., Y. Maulet, L. Sefton, B. Courtier, P. Avner, J.-L. Guenet, and H. Betz. 1994. Structural analysis of mouse glycine receptor α subunit genes. Identification and chromosomal localization of a novel variant. *J. Biol. Chem.* **269:** 2607.

Mihic, S.J., P.J. Whiting, R.L. Klein, K.A. Wafford, and R.A. Harris. 1994. A single amino acid of the human γ-aminobutyric acid type A receptor γ2 subunit determines benzodiazepine efficacy. *J. Biol. Chem.* **52:** 32768.

Mulhardt, C., M. Fischer, P. Gass, D. Simon-Chazottes, J.-L. Guenet, J. Kuhse, H. Betz, and C.-M. Becker. 1994. The *spastic* mouse: Aberrant splicing of glycine receptor beta subunit mRNA caused by intronic insertion of L1 element. *Neuron* **13:** 1003.

Murray, N., Z. Ying-Cong, G. Mandel, P. Brehm, R. Bolinger, Q. Reuter, and R. Kullberg. 1995. A single site on the ε subunit is responsible for the change in Ach receptor channel conductance during skeletal muscle development. *Neuron* **14:** 865.

Noda, M., H. Takahashi, T. Tanabe, M. Toyosato, Y. Furutani, T. Hirose, H. Takashima, S. Inayama, T. Miyata, and S. Numa. 1982. Primary structure of α-subunit precursor of *Torpedo californica* acetylcholine receptor deduced from cDNA sequence. *Nature* **299:** 793.

O'Leary, M.E. and M.M. White. 1992. Mutational analysis of ligand-induced activation of the *Torpedo* acetylcholine receptor. *J. Biol. Chem.* **267:** 8360.

Rajendra, S. and P.R. Schofield. 1995. Molecular mechanisms of startle syndromes. *Trends Neurosci.* **18:** 80.

Rajendra, S., J.W. Lynch, K.D. Pierce, C.R. French, P.H. Barry, and P.R. Schofield. 1994. Startle disease mutations reduce the agonist sensitivity of the human inhibitory glycine receptor. *J. Biol. Chem.* **269:** 18739.

———. 1995a. Mutation of a single amino acid in the human glycine receptor transforms β-alanine and taurine from agonists into competitive antagonists. *Neuron* **14:** 169.

Rajendra, S., R.J. Vandenberg, K.D. Pierce, A.M. Cunningham, P.W. French, P.H. Barry, and P.R. Schofield. 1995b. The unique extracellular disulfide loop of the glycine receptor is a principal ligand binding element. *EMBO J.* **14:** 2987.

Rees, M.I., M. Andrew, S. Jawad, and M.J. Owen. 1994. Evidence for recessive as well as dominant forms of startle disease (hyperekplexia) caused by mutations in the α1 subunit of the inhibitory glycine receptor. *Hum. Mol. Genet.* **3:** 2175.

Ruiz-Gomez, A., E. Morato, M. Garcia-Calvo, F. Valdivieso, and F. Mayor, Jr. 1990. Location of the strychnine binding site on the 48-kilodalton subunit of the glycine receptor. *Biochemistry* **29:** 7033.

Rundström, N., V. Schmieden, H. Betz, J. Bormann, and D. Langosch. 1994. Cyanotriphenylborate: Subtype-specific blocker of glycine receptor chloride channels. *Proc. Natl. Acad. Sci.* **91:** 8950.

Ryan, S.G., S.L. Sherman, J.C. Terry, R.S. Sparkes, M.C. Torres, and R.W. Mackey. 1992. Startle disease, or hyperekplexia: Response to clonazepam and assignment of the gene (STHE) to chromosome 5q by linkage analysis. *Ann. Neurol.* **31:** 663.

Ryan, S.G., M.S. Buckwalter, J.W. Lynch, C.A. Handford, L. Segura, R. Shiang, J.J. Wasmuth, S.A. Camper, P.R. Schofield, and P. O'Connell. 1994. A missense mutation in the gene encoding the α1 subunit of the inhibitory glycine receptor in the spasmodic mouse. *Nat. Genet.* **7:** 131.

Saul, B., V. Schmieden, C. Kling, C. Mulhardt, P. Gass, J. Kuhse, and C.-M. Becker. 1994. Point mutation of glycine receptor α1 subunit in *spasmodic* mouse affects agonist responses. *FEBS Lett.* **350:** 71.

Schmieden, V., J. Kuhse, and H. Betz. 1992. Agonist pharmacology of neonatal and adult glycine receptor α subunits: Identification of amino acid residues involved in taurine activation. *EMBO J.* **11:** 2025.

———. 1993. Mutation of glycine receptor subunit creates β-alanine receptor responsive to GABA. *Science* **262:** 256.

Schmieden, V., G. Grenningloh, P.R. Schofield, and H. Betz. 1989. Functional expression in *Xenopus* oocytes of the strychnine binding 48kD subunit of the inhibitory glycine receptor. *EMBO J.* **8:** 695.

Schofield, P.R., M.G. Darlison, N. Fujita, D.R. Burt, F.A. Stephenson, H. Rodriguez, L. Rhee, J. Ramachandran, A. Reale, T. Glencorse, P.H. Seeburg, and E.A. Barnard. 1987. Sequence and functional expression of the $GABA_A$ receptor shows a ligand-gated receptor super-family. *Nature* **328:** 221.

Shiang, R., S.G. Ryan, Y.-Z. Zhu, A.F. Hahn, P. O'Connell, and J.J. Wasmuth. 1993. Mutations in the α1 subunit of the inhibitory glycine receptor cause the dominant neurologic disorder, hyperekplexia. *Nat. Genet.* **5:** 351.

Shiang, R., S.G. Ryan, Y.Z. Zhu, T.J. Fielder, R.J. Allen, A. Fryer, S. Yamashita, P. O'Connell, and J.J. Wasmuth. 1995. Mutational analysis of familial and sporadic hyperekplexia. *Ann. Neurol.* **38:** 85.

Sontheimer, H., C.-M. Becker, D.B. Pritchett, P.R. Schofield, G. Grenningloh, H. Kettenmann, H. Betz, and P.H. Seeburg. 1989. Functional chloride channels by mammalian cell expression of rat glycine receptor subunit. *Neuron* **2:** 1491.

Suhren, O., G.W. Bruyn, and J.A. Tuynman. 1966. Hyperekplexia: A hereditary startle syndrome. *J. Neurol. Sci.* **3:** 577.

Takahashi, T., A. Momiyama, K. Hirai, F. Hishinuma, and H. Akagi. 1992. Functional correlation of foetal and adult forms of glycine receptors with developmental changes in inhibitory synaptic receptor channels. *Neuron* **9:** 1155.

Tokutomi, N., M. Kaneda, and N. Akaike. 1989. What confers specificity on glycine for its receptor site? *Br. J. Pharmacol.* **97:** 353.

Unwin, N. 1993. Nicotinic acetylcholine receptor at 9Å resolution. *J. Mol. Biol.* **229:** 1101.

———. 1995. Acetylcholine receptor channel imaged in the open state. *Nature* **373:** 37.

Vandenberg, R.J., C.A. Handford, and P.R. Schofield. 1992a. Distinct agonist- and antagonist-binding sites on the glycine receptor. *Neuron* **9:** 491.

Vandenberg, R.J., C.R. French, P.H. Barry, J. Shine, and P.R. Schofield. 1992b. Antagonism of ligand-gated ion channel receptors: Two domains of the glycine receptor α subunit form the strychnine binding site. *Proc. Natl. Acad. Sci.* **89:** 1765.

Weiland, H.A., H. Luddens, and P.H. Seeburg. 1992. A single histidine in $GABA_A$ receptors is essential for benzodiazepine agonist binding. *J. Biol. Chem.* **267:** 1426.

White, W.F. and A.H. Heller. 1982. Glycine receptor alteration in the mutant mouse spastic. *Nature* **298:** 655.

White, W.F., S. O'Gorman, and A.W. Roe. 1990. Three-dimensional autoradiographic localization of quench-corrected glycine receptor specific activity in the mouse brain using ^{3}H-strychnine as the ligand. *J. Neurosci.* **10:** 795.

Nicotinic Receptors and Brain Plasticity

J.-P. Changeux, A. Bessis, J.-P. Bourgeois, P.-J. Corringer, A. Devillers-Thiery, J.-L. Eiselé, M. Kerszberg, C. Léna, N. Le Novère, M. Picciotto,[1] and M. Zoli[2]
Département des Biotechnologies, Institut Pasteur, 75724 Paris Cedex 15, France

After Langley (1906) proposed the concept of "receptive substance" to account for the pharmacological specificity of drugs on their target tissue, the chemical identity of neurotransmitter receptors remained elusive for almost two-thirds of a century. Pharmacological approaches, meanwhile, unraveled the remarkable diversity, throughout the organism and within the brain, of neurotransmitter receptors, their targets, and linked biological activity (ion channel or specialized GTP-binding protein). In retrospect, a decisive step in the understanding of receptor mechanisms was their biochemical identification as protein species, which subsequently opened the way to gene cloning techniques.

The nicotinic acetylcholine receptor became a prototype for the study of neurotransmitter receptors for several rather simple reasons: First, abundant pharmacological (H. Dale; D. Bovet) and physiological (B. Katz) data accumulated over the years on this easily accessible and rather widespread receptor. In addition, a tissue particularly rich in nicotinic synapses, the electric organ of electric fish (D. Nachmansohn), offered an exceptional source of biological material which, together with snake venom α-toxins (C.Y. Lee) (which are highly specific markers of the acetylcholine binding site), made biochemical identification possible (Changeux et al. 1970; see Changeux 1990).

The membrane protein identified and purified from electric tissue, the nicotinic acetylcholine receptor protein (nAChR), is a hetero-oligomer of about 300,000 m.w. made up of five homologous subunits with an $[\alpha 1_2 \beta 1 \gamma \delta]$ stoichiometry. Extensive biochemical studies, including reconstitution experiments, have shown that this single molecular species carries two ACh-binding sites located at the interface between subunits, a unique ion channel along its transmembrane axis of pseudo-symmetry, and all the structural elements that mediate their allosteric coupling in the course of the activation and desensitization processes (for review, see Changeux 1990; Karlin 1993; Galzi and Changeux 1995; Unwin 1995).

A fundamental outcome of the application of recombinant DNA techniques to the nAChR in the early 1980s was the demonstration of close homologies between nAChR subunit sequences from electric organ and skeletal muscle from higher vertebrates (including humans) (Numa et al. 1983) and subsequently between muscle and brain nAChRs (Boulter et al. 1986; for review, see Role and Berg 1996). These subunits together compose a multigene family (Le Novère and Changeux 1995; Ortells and Lunt 1995) that stems from a larger superfamily including $5HT_3$, $GABA_A$, and glycine receptors (Ortells and Lunt 1995) (but not the functionally related purine and glutamate receptors). To date, the sequences of ten types of neuronal nAChR subunits have been determined (for review, see Role and Berg 1996). Seven are designated as α subunits (α2–α8) and share with electric organ α1 subunit a pair of adjacent cysteines (at positions 192 and 193 in *Torpedo*; Karlin 1993), whereas the others are referred to as non-α or β subunits (β2–β4). Additional genes encoding nAChR subunits may exist, however (Role and Berg 1996). All nAChR subunits share a similar hydropathy profile, with two hydrophilic domains and four 20-amino-acid-long hydrophobic domains (M1–M4). Joint affinity labeling (with *Torpedo* nAChR) and site-directed mutagenesis experiments (primarily with α7 neuronal subunit expressed in frog oocytes, but also with *Torpedo* and muscle nAChR) have demonstrated that, in brain (as in muscle) nAChR, the large amino-terminal hydrophilic domain carries the neurotransmitter binding site, the small highly variable carboxy-terminal hydrophilic domain faces the cytoplasm where it can be phosphorylated, and the transmembrane segment M2 forms the walls of the ion channel (Bertrand and Changeux 1995; Karlin and Akabis 1996). Like electric organ and muscle nAChR, neuronal nAChRs are pentameric oligomers that undergo transitions for activation and desensitization. Yet, striking differences exist in the mode of assembly of their subunits. First, α7 and α8 subunits can form functional homopentameric ACh-gated channels after reconstitution in frog oocytes (even though they may coassemble with other subunits in situ). Additionally, multiple combinations of both α-type and β-type subunits form a wide variety of functional hetero-oligomers, with subunits of two (α2β2, α3β2, α4β2, α3β4...) or even three (α3β4α5) different types (for review, see Role and Berg 1996). These multiple combinations of nAChR subunits possess distinct pharmacological and physiological properties. Moreover, in contrast to the restricted focal localization of

Present addresses: [1]Department of Psychiatry, Yale University Medical School, Connecticut Mental Health Center, 34 Park Street, New Haven, Connecticut 06508; [2]Dipartimento di Scienze Biomediche, Sezione di Fisiologia, Universita di Modena, Via Campi 287, I-41100 Modena, Italy.

muscle nAChR at the end plate (Duclert and Changeux 1995), the distribution of neuronal nAChR subunits follows a variety of distinct patterns in the brain at the regional, cellular, and subcellular levels (Clarke 1993; Sargent 1993; Zoli et al. 1995).

The aim of this paper is to review work done primarily in our laboratory about nAChRs and brain plasticity, in particular: (1) the diversity of neuronal nAChR at the structural and functional level; (2) the regulation of nAChR gene expression in the brain in the course of development; (3) the contribution of neuronal nAChR in learning and reward processes, investigated primarily with knockout mice. Finally, possible implications of neuronal nAChR in brain dysfunction and drug abuse are mentioned.

MOLECULAR PHYLOGENY AND FUNCTIONAL DIVERSITY OF nAChR

nAChRs have a long phylogenetic history. Analysis of the sequences available (Le Novère and Changeux 1995; Ortells and Lunt 1995) shows that these nAChR subunit genes share a common origin (which might possibly derive from a prokaryotic pentameric pore-forming protein, resembling heat-labile *Escherichia coli* enterotoxin [Ortells and Lunt 1995]). Moreover, nAChR subunit sequences have been identified throughout the phylum of Bilateria, from nematodes to humans, including insects (*Drosophila*, locust). Extensive phylogenetic analysis of the nAChR gene family, performed by cladistic and phenetic methods on the gene sequences and structures, has led to a reconstruction of a putative history of the nAChR by gene duplications (Fig. 1) (Le Novère and Changeux 1995).

The reconstituted phylogenetic tree (for references, see Le Novère and Changeux 1995; Ballivet et al. 1996) shows that a nematode subunit referred to as deg3 appears to have split soon after the divergence between the serotoninergic $5HT_3$ and the ACh receptors. The next duplication involved a recently discovered α9 subunit, which, in frog oocyte reconstitution experiments, forms homo-oligomeric receptors able to respond to ACh. Yet, the α9-subunit nAChR is inhibited by α-bungarotoxin and is stimulated by both nicotine and muscarine and thus exhibits an atypical nicotinic/muscarinic pharmacology; its mRNA is detected in the nasal epithelium and in the tongue, in pars tuberalis of the adenohypophysis and in the cochlear hair cells, perhaps as a remote testimony of the ectodermal origin of nAChR in primitive metazoa. The next divergence is likely to have taken place between the vertebrate α7 and α8 subunits (together with their *Caenorhabditis* ortholog) and the remaining nAChR subunits. The α7 and α8 subunits also form homo-oligomers inhibited by α-bungarotoxin. The vertebrate muscle and neuronal high-affinity nAChR subunits comprise a large monophyletic group which, around 1000 million years ago (MYA), may have diverged from the ortholog polyphyletic set of invertebrate subunit genes. Structural gene duplications and tissue-specific promoter switches then led to muscle α1, β1, and δ/γ/ε-subunit clades and to the high-affinity neuronal subunit subfamily, which appeared at the beginning of the chordate phylum. Segregation of the ancestor gene of the β2/β4 subunits likely occurred more than 800 MYA, that for α5/β3 and the rest of the subunit genes slightly later. Finally, the duplications yielding α2 and α4, on one side, and α3 and α6, on the other side, may have taken place, respectively, more than 620 MYA and 500 MYA, anticipating the most recent β2/β4 bifurcation, a little less than 420 MYA. This last duplication coincided with the split between the teleost and the tetrapod lineages and thus accompanied an increased complexity of the brain, together with a correlative diversification of the cholinergic pathways. It is quite remarkable that no known duplication of nAChR genes took place over the course of the dramatic increase of brain complexity which characterized the recent evolution of mammals.

An outcome of these still speculative molecular phylogenetic studies is that a rather good congruence exists between the phenotypic functional properties of the nAChRs and the sequence relationships of their subunits. This is particularly striking for the ACh-binding site. Convergent affinity-labeling and site-directed mutagenesis experiments have demonstrated that the ACh-binding pocket comprises 5 loops, A, B, C, D, and E, each one identified by characteristic amino acids, and overlapping the interface between subunits (Figs. 2, 3) (Galzi and Changeux 1995). For instance, in *Torpedo* and muscle nAChR, whose subunit composition is $[\alpha1_2\beta1\gamma\delta]$, there are two binding sites per oligomer at the α-γ/ε and α–δ interfaces. The α1 subunit forms, with loops AB and C, the "principal component" of the ACh-binding site, and on the other side of the intersubunit cleft, the non-α subunits γ/ε or δ contribute to the binding pocket by loops D and E, which form the "complementary component" of the site (for references, see Corringer et al. 1995; Czajkowski and Karlin 1995). In other words, the two ACh sites are "split" between α- and non-α subunits (Figs. 2, 3).

The situation is quite different with the neuronal (and epithelial) subunits. Some of these subunits, α7, α8, and α9, are able to form homo-oligomers (at least in oocyte reconstitution experiments). As expected, each individual subunit carries all five loops (ABCDE), and the reconstituted oligomer possesses five identical acetylcholine-binding sites. Figures 1, 2, and 3 further show that the other neuronal subunits can be regrouped into two main categories, referred to as "α-type" and "non-α-type" (for references, see Sargent 1993; Role and Berg 1996), which comprise two distinct, but related, branches on the phylogenetic tree. α2, α4, and α6 possess all the characteristic amino acids of the five loops ABCDE but (for still unknown

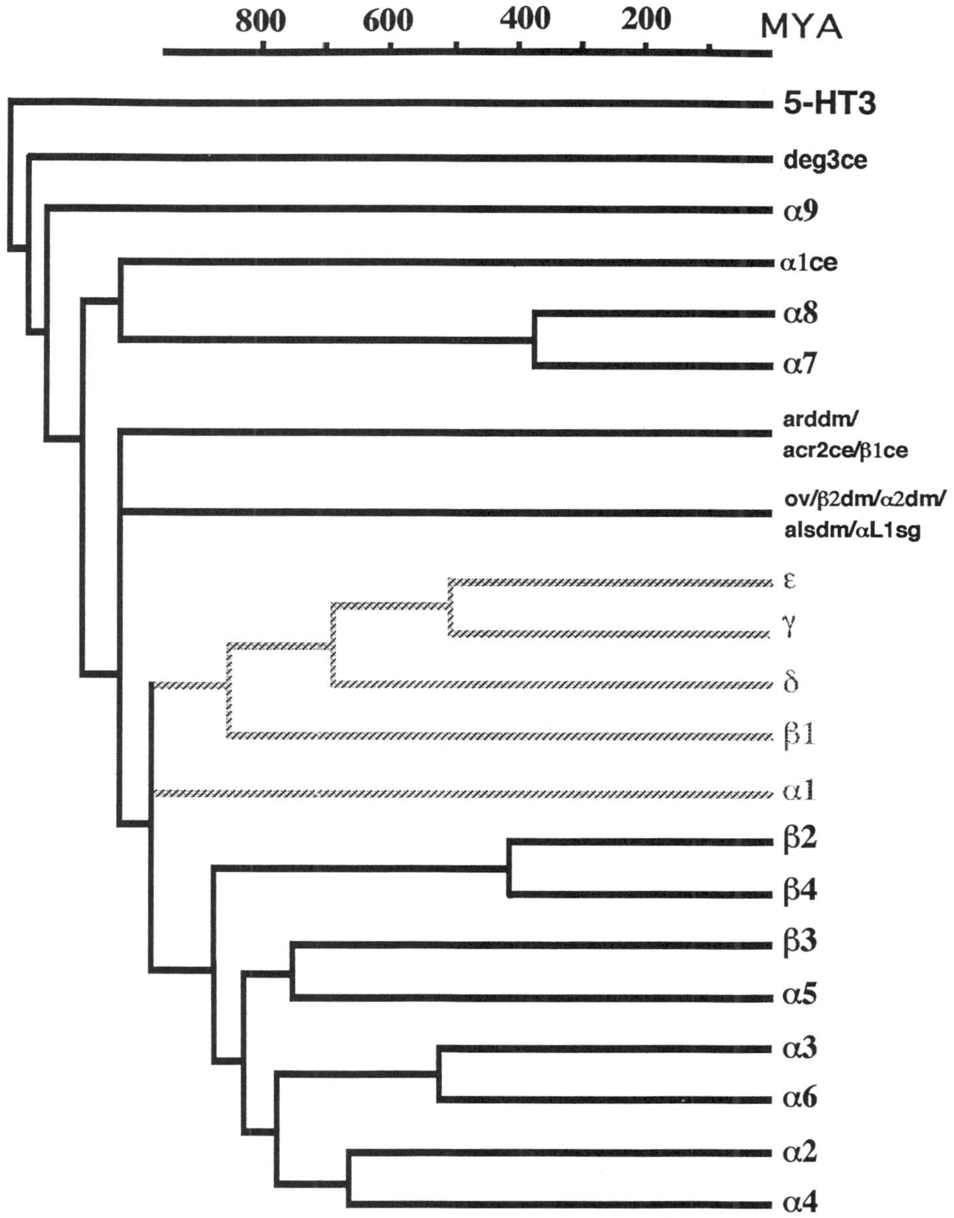

Figure 1. Evolutionary tree of nicotinic receptor subunits. The most primitive subunits (α9, α8, α7) form functional homo-oligomeric channels, as $5HT_3$ and many $GABA_A$ and glycine receptor subunits. The more recent subunits associate into hetero-oligomers with either a fixed stoichiometry (muscle) or a variable composition (neuronal) of subunits. (Modified from Le Novère and Changeux 1995.)

reasons) require hetero-oligomerization to yield functional nAChRs. Together with α3, which possesses the amino acids characteristic of loops ABC and D, but lacks loop E, they form the α-type group. The β-type group includes subunits which do *not* carry the full contingent of loops, and the so-called "α5" subunit clearly belongs to this category. All of these form hetero-oligomers $[\alpha i_2 \beta j_3]$ and thus are likely to carry only two high-affinity binding sites for ACh: As in muscle, the αi would carry the principal component of the ACh site with loop ABC, and the βi would contribute to the complementary component, with loop D and/or loop E. Yet, cross-immunoprecipitation studies and oocyte reconstitution experiments suggest that a three-partner mode of subunit association may exist for α5-containing receptors (and possibly with other subunits). This subunit does not form functional hetero-oligomers with only one α-type (α2–α4) or one β-type

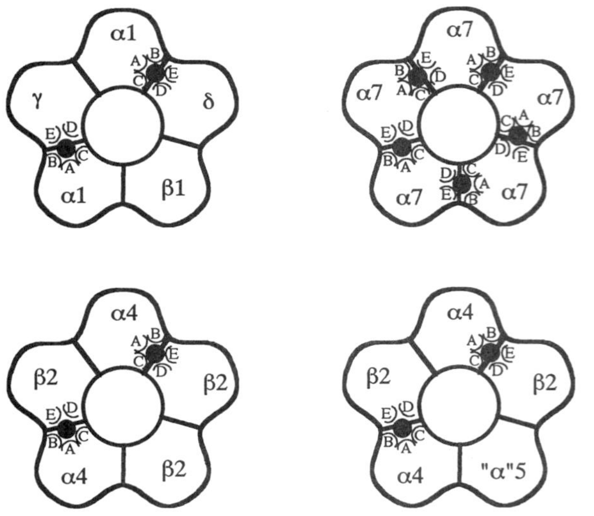

Figure 2. Plausible topological organization of the subunits and its consequences on the pharmacological diversity of the ACh-binding sites. In electric organ and muscle nAChR, the ACh nicotinic binding site comprises at least five amino acid loops subdivided into a principal component of three loops (A, B, C) from the α subunit and a complementary component of two loops (D, E) from the non-α (γ and δ) subunits. The homo-oligomeric nAChRs (α9, α8, α7) carry the five loops on the same subunit, yet on opposite faces. The combinatorial association of subunits creates sites with different binding properties within the same oligomer, and between oligomers.

(β2, β4) as a second partner; on the other hand, functionality arises when α5 associates with both α3 (or α4) *and* β2 (or β4). Under these conditions, α5 behaves like a β1-type subunit (Ramirez-Latorre et al. 1996; Wang et al. 1996). It also lacks the characteristic amino acids of loop C but possesses a full complementary component of the ACh-binding site.

A similar diversity may take place for the ion channel. Indeed, the relative permeabilities of the ion channel vary depending on the combination of subunits forming the receptors. The phylogenetically "old" α7/α8 subunits form homo-oligomers that exhibit a pCa/pNa higher than 15. Subunits α2–6 and β2–4 form a hetero-oligomeric channel with a pCa/pNa ranging between 0.5 and 2.5, whereas muscle receptors $\alpha1_2\beta1\delta\gamma/\varepsilon$ exhibit a pCa/pNa of about 0.2 (see below, "Ca^{++} Influx through nAChR in Central Neurons"; Bertrand and Changeux 1995).

These observations underline the remarkable combinatorial diversity of neuronal nAChR subunits into functional oligomers, with different pharmacological and ionic properties. A challenge of the years to come is to relate the properties of these oligomers recorded in vivo, at the level of a particular neural pathway, with a defined combination of subunits (see Role and Berg 1996), thus paving the way to a "circuit-targeted" molecular pharmacology (see below, "Subcellular Compartmentalization of Brain AChR").

nAChRs AS COMPONENTS OF "MOLECULAR SWITCHES"

An important outcome of the structural and functional studies of brain nAChRs is that, in addition to the diversity of their nicotinic ligand-binding and channel properties, they may also differ in the signal transduction processes and allosteric regulation they mediate.

Allosteric Transitions of nAChRs

As has been discussed previously (for review, see Léna and Changeux 1993; Bertrand and Changeux 1995; Edelstein et al. 1996), convergent experimental data (primarily from affinity labeling, rapid-mixing experiments with fluorescent or radioactive ligands, and site-directed mutagenesis) demonstrate that electric organ, muscle, *and* brain nAChRs may undergo similar transitions between a small number of discrete conformations with distinct binding properties and states of ion channel opening. The different conformational states are accessible in the absence of nicotinic ligands (agonists, antagonists), and allosteric effectors shift the equilibrium by cooperatively modifying the equilibrium (and kinetic) constants between the states. As a consequence, the nAChR may undergo the activation reaction (channel opening) and/or become refractory to activation (desensitization).

Recently, mutations in the M2 channel domain have been described, which support this general scheme. Indeed, a single amino acid permutation changes the elementary conductance, eliminates desensitization, increases the apparent affinity for agonists by about 100-fold, and converts competitive blocking by antagonists into a channel activation process (Révah et al. 1991; for review, see Galzi et al. 1996a). The occurrence of such highly pleiotropic effects strongly supports the view that the many functions subsumed by the nAChR molecule are "linked" by a major allosteric transition, and that a single point mutation may perturb this equilibrium.

Moreover, different subunit combinations may differentially affect both the intrinsic properties of the various ligand-binding sites and the molecular parameters of the conformational transitions they mediate. For instance, the rate of desensitization of the α3β2 oligomer is 10 times faster than that of α3β4 (Cachelin and Jaggi 1991). In addition, the diverse isomerization constants, Ls, between resting, active, and desensitized conformations, may noticeably differ from one set of wild-type (and/or mutant) subunits to another. As a consequence, the sign of the effect of nicotinic (and/or allosteric) ligands may change, for instance, from inhibitory to activatory and vice versa (for review, see Bertrand and Changeux 1995). On this basis, it was postulated that the state of the equilibrium between "activatable" and "refractory" states of the nAChR (and likely of other receptors as well) may contribute

	A	B	C	D	E	a7,8,9	α1	β1	δ	ε	γ	α2	α3	α4	α6	β3	α5	β2	β4
α789	+	+	+	+	+	+													
α1	+	+	+	–	–			+	+	+	+							*	*
β1	–	–	–	–	–		+		+	+	+							*	*
δ	–	–	–	+	+		+	+		+	+							*	*
ε	–	–	–	+	+		+	+	+		+								
γ	–	–	–	+	+		+	+	+	+								*	*
α2	+	+	+	+	+													+	+
α3	+	+	+	+	–												+	+	+
α4	+	+	+	+	+												+	+	+
α6	+	+	+	+	+														
β3	–	+	–	+	+														
α5	–	+	–	+	+								+	+				+	+
β2	+	+	–	+	–		*	*	*		*	+	+	+			+		
β4	+	+	–	+	–		*	*	*		*	+	+	+			+		

Figure 3. Combinatorial diversity of nAChR subunits in forming functional oligomers. (*Left*) Loops of the ACh-binding site. (*Right*) Association of subunits into a functional oligomer (+) in vivo, (*) in reconstituted oocyte experiments.

to the regulation of efficiency of intercellular communications mediated by the nAChR (Heidmann and Changeux 1982).

Ca^{++} Influx through nAChR in Central Neurons

Ca^{++} ions are very unequally distributed across the neuronal membrane and may exert short- and long-term regulatory effects via their entry into the nerve cell through the nAChR channel (Mulle et al. 1992b; Bertrand et al. 1993). nAChR channels from muscle and peripheral parasympathetic neurons in culture were known to permeate Ca^{++} with pCa^{++}/pNa close, respectively, to 0.1–0.3 and 1 (for references, see Dani and Mayer 1995). An important issue was thus to evaluate the magnitude of the influx of Ca^{++} through nAChRs in brain neurons under physiological conditions. This was achieved, in collaboration with H. Korn's laboratory (Mulle et al. 1992b), using freshly dissociated neurons from medial habenula using a combination of patch clamp recordings and fura 2 fluorescence measurements. The nAChR channels recorded in this semi-acute preparation display a single channel conductance of 11 pS in pure external Ca^{++} (100 mM), similar to that of NMDA receptor channels. As a consequence of nicotine activation, cytosolic calcium concentration increased to the micromolar range, and this Ca^{++} influx was much enhanced at hyperpolarized potentials (below –50 mV) where Ca^{++} influx through voltage-activated Ca^{++} channels was minimal. This contrasts with NMDA receptor channels that are blocked by Mg^{++} and produce Ca^{++} influx only at depolarized potential. A slight activation of nAChR that would not suffice to trigger a spike discharge may nevertheless allow the entry of Ca^{++} ions and subsequent activation of Ca^{++}-dependent cellular events. In other words, nAChRs in medial habenula neurons (and this is true for other nAChR types in the brain [for references, see Dani and Mayer 1995; C. Léna and J-P. Changeux, in prep.]) contribute to Ca^{++} influx, in a manner complementary to that of voltage-gated ion channels and NMDA receptors, up to intracellular levels that are sufficient to influence a variety of intracellular processes regulated by Ca^{++} (see Role and Berg 1996).

The selectivity of neuronal α7 subunit channel (with $pCa^{++}/pK^{+} < 5$) was investigated in collaboration with D. Bertrand's laboratory by site-directed mutagenesis (Bertrand et al. 1993). The primary outcome of these studies is that mutations introduced at two distinct loci within M2 almost completely abolish Ca^{++} influx, while preserving Na^{+} and K^{+} transport. One locus is the intermediate ring of negatively charged residues (E237) (Imoto et al. 1988) located at the cytoplasmic end of M2 (its substitution by alanine decreases Ca^{++}

permeability more than 1000-fold relative to Na^+). The other site comprises two adjacent rings of leucines, close to the extracellular end of M2 at positions 254 and 255. The precise contribution of E237 and L254 (or L255) to the selectivity of Ca^{++} transport is not fully understood. According to the standard view, in the wild type, these amino acids may contribute to Ca^{++} binding sites within the channel lumen. Alternatively, and in agreement with the phylogenetic investigations (Le Novère and Changeux 1995), the channel of the "oldest" nAChR subunits could be viewed as essentially nonselective for cations. The new amino acids introduced by mutation would then create barriers repelling Ca^{++} ions, while preserving Na^+/K^+ fluxes. In either case, the particular design of the M2 segment confers the high Ca^{++} permeability that characterizes brain nAChR channels.

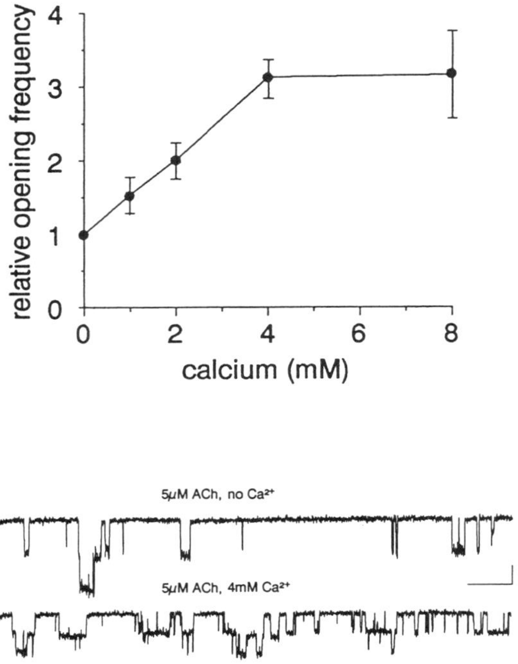

Figure 4. Potentiation by external calcium of neuronal nAChR response to ACh. External Ca^{++} increases the frequency of opening of ACh-activated elementary currents in outside-out patches. The principal Ca^{++}-binding site involved is part of the amino-terminal hydrophilic domain. (Modified from Mulle et al. 1992a.)

Allosteric Potentiation of nAChR by External Ca^{++}

External Ca^{++} ions, in addition to their permeation through the nAChR channel, exert a potent regulatory effect on nAChR response to nicotinic agonists in isolated medial habenula neurons (Mulle et al. 1992a), in chromaffin cells (Vernino et al. 1992), and in superior cervical ganglion neurons (Amador and Dani 1995). In habenular neurons, when the external Ca^{++} concentration is varied from 0 to 8 mM, the macroscopic response to ACh increases up to 3.5-fold, being maximal at low agonist concentration, an effect which is not observed with electric organ and muscle nAChR, NMDA receptors, or $5HT_3$ receptors (Fig. 4). Single-channel recordings show that potentiation by Ca^{++} ions results from an increase in opening frequency of ACh-activated channels. Moreover, among divalent cations, Ba^{++} and Sr^{++} exert a positive effect, but not Mg^{++}. In other words, Ca^{++} potentiates nAChR response upon binding to specific external regulatory sites (Mulle et al. 1992a).

The localization of these sites was analyzed in collaboration with D. Bertrand's laboratory by using functional chimeras containing the large amino-terminal hydrophilic domain of the nAChR α7 subunit joined at position V201 to the complementary carboxy-terminal portion of the $5HT_3$ receptor. Interestingly, the chimera is potentiated by Ca^{++}, as is the α7 nAChR, whereas wild-type $5HT_3$ receptor is not. The Ca^{++} regulatory site is thus located within the synaptic amino-terminal domain and not in the channel-containing moiety (Eiselé et al. 1993).

Further examination of the α7 large hydrophilic domain sequence revealed several consensus sequences for Ca^{++} binding (Galzi et al. 1996b). One of them, referred to as loop V, spans the amino acids 166–172 stretch; it exhibits significant homology with calmodulin calcium site III and with helix-loop-helix motifs referred to as EF hands from metal-binding sites with a conserved glutamate residue at position 12. Mutations of amino acids within this canonical domain alter all features of potentiation by abolishing (E172), reducing (E161, S165, Y167), or even enhancing (D163, S169) calcium effects on ionic current amplitudes, agonist affinity, and cooperativity. In addition, insertion of the [α7 161–172] domain into the Ca^{++}-insensitive $5HT_3$ receptor results in a receptor activated by 5HT and potentiated by Ca^{++}. In addition, in vitro studies with the synthetic peptide [α7 160–174] demonstrate that terbium (Tb^{+++}) binds to this sequence from which it is displaced by Ca^{++}, whereas mutation E172Q alters Ca^{++} binding to this canonical sequence. All these data support the notion that, in the intact receptor, Ca^{++} interacts with loop V to potentiate the ACh response. The data are also consistent with the assumption that Ca^{++} primarily affects the isomerization (L in the allosteric model, α/β in the sequential model) between the resting and open channel conformations of the nAChR (see above, "Allosteric Transitions of nAChRs"). Furthermore, mutations of particular residues within loop V (e.g., D163N or D163A), enhance Ca^{++} potentiation and drastically reduce apparent affinity for ACh in equilibrium binding experiments. This suggests, in agreement with data from Czajkowski and Karlin (1995) on labeling and mutagenesis of *Torpedo* nAChR, that these residues may also contribute to the ACh-binding sites at the level of loop E (Corringer et al. 1995). This regulatory Ca^{++}-binding site would therefore be in close proximity to the nicotine-binding site.

Contribution of Neuronal nAChR to a Molecular Mechanism of Synaptic Plasticity

Large variations in external Ca^{++} concentration have been noted in several brain regions during periods of high synaptic activity, and modulation of cholinergic spontaneous synaptic currents takes place in ganglionic sympathetic neurons upon rapid change of external Ca^{++} concentration (for references, see Amador and Dani 1995). These observations support the notion that nAChRs mediate efficient short-term regulation of nicotinic transmission by Ca^{++} ions, through their external Ca^{++}-binding sites and by Ca^{++} influx through their ionic channels. In addition, entry of Ca^{++} ions through nAChR channels may elicit intracellular processes such as the activation of Ca^{++}-dependent chloride and potassium channels (for references, see Role and Berg 1996) and the reduction of the response mediated by $GABA_A$ receptors (Mulle et al. 1992a,b). All these mechanisms remain to be demonstrated in physiologically recognized processes of synaptic plasticity in situ.

In addition, still from a speculative point of view, it has been suggested that nAChRs and allosteric receptors in general may serve as detectors of time coincidence (Heidmann and Changeux 1982; for references, see Changeux 1993; Edelman and Tononi 1996; Edelstein et al. 1996) and, thus, in a metaphoric sense may perform as building blocks of a "chemical Hebb synapse." Their ability to detect time coincidences would simply result from their ability (1) to recognize several convergent signals by their multiple active and allosteric binding sites and (2) to integrate their effect, within a given time window, as a result of a major, highly cooperative, allosteric transition (see above, "Allosteric Transitions of nAChRs"). Indeed, the neuronal nAChR carries on its external surface sites for binding of external Ca^{++}, for noncompetitive blockers, and for steroids (for references, see Bertrand and Changeux 1995) and, on its internal surface, phosphorylation sites. In this last instance, the kinases (and/or phosphatases) might be activated by Ca^{++} entry through the ionic channel and/or by other neurotransmitter receptors and ion channels present on the same cell (see Huganir and Greengard 1990), thereby creating molecular switches, which might even become long-lasting. A particularly important aspect of this molecular regulation is, as already mentioned (see above, "Molecular Phylogeny and Functional Diversity of nAChR"), that the physiological intervention of nAChRs in plasticity mechanisms heavily relies on their precise localization within brain circuitry. For this reason, it was of primary interest to investigate the mechanisms involved in the distribution of nAChRs within the brain.

TOPOLOGY OF nAChR SUBUNIT GENE EXPRESSION IN THE BRAIN

The three-dimensional distribution of the various nAChR subunits in the brain results from a complex cascade of transcriptional and posttranscriptional processes. In the course of motor end-plate development, two distinct molecular species of nAChR protein become expressed on the cell membrane: the embryonic, extrajunctional form and the adult, subjunctional form which, in some species, differ by the γ- versus ε-subunit contribution to the 300,000 m.w. heteropentamer (Mishina et al. 1986; for review, see Duclert and Changeux 1995). In this simple system, molecular morphogenesis reduces to a one-dimensional process of nAChR gene transcription at the level of the few specialized nuclei located under the motor nerve ending, in the middle of the multinucleated muscle fiber (for review, see Duclert and Changeux 1995). This is not the case for the nAChRs in the brain, which vary considerably in shape and connectivity, but also differ strikingly in the pattern of genes they express. Nevertheless, we have extended the strategy we adopted for the muscle nAChR to the analysis of neuronal nAChR gene expression: (1) the analysis in situ of the distribution of the nAChR subunits and mRNAs during development; (2) the identification and functional analysis of the promoter and regulatory sequences of the subunit genes; and (3) the characterization of the transcription factors and signaling mechanisms involved.

Developmental Regulation of Neuronal nAChR Genes in the Brain

Our current knowledge of the topological distribution of nAChRs in adult brain and during development relies on radiolabeled nicotinic ligand binding, immunochemistry with monoclonal and polyclonal antibodies, in situ hybridization, and local cerebral glucose utilization (for review, see Clarke 1993; Sargent 1993; Zoli et al. 1995). In a general manner, each subunit displays a distinct pattern of expression, some highly restricted (e.g., α2 in chick brain; Daubas et al. 1990), others widely distributed (e.g., β2 in rat brain; Hill et al. 1993), and many in between, often with important overlaps.

In the adult chick brain, α2-subunit mRNA detected by in situ hybridization is limited to a single small nucleus in the diencephalon: the lateral spiriform nucleus (Daubas et al. 1990). In contrast to skeletal muscle, this highly localized topology does not result from the restriction of an initially much wider distribution. The neurons that comprise the nucleus are already present at days E9 and 10; but α2 mRNA is detectable only after day E11 at which time message levels begin to increase abruptly and continue to increase until hatching. The sudden expression of α2 message at day E11 coincides with the detection by immunocytochemical methods of cholinergic projections from the semi-lunaris nucleus into the spiriform nucleus. A plausible interpretation is that the afferent axons "induce" the expression of nAChR genes. There has not yet been an actual experimental demonstration of this mechanism.

In rat brain, the developmental regulation of the more ubiquitous α3, α4, β2, β4-subunit genes differs strikingly from that of the α2 subunit in the chick (Fig. 5) (Zoli et al. 1995). Neuronal differentiation mainly occurs in a caudorostral wave between E11 (some peripheral ganglia and the first neurons of the spinal cord and rhombencephalon) and E19 (last neurons of the neocortex). The onset of nAChR subunit expression follows the same pattern. nAChR subunit mRNAs are first detected in some ganglia, the spinal cord, and the rhombencephalon at E11; in the mesencephalon at E12; in the ventral diencephalon and basal telencephalon at E13; in the dorsal diencephalon at E15; and finally in the cortical plate and subplate between E15 and E19. Therefore, the onsets of nAChR subunit mRNA expression and neuronal differentiation appear temporally related. In this respect, there are some parallels with the early expression of muscle nAChR in myoblasts and myotubes in the absence of innervation and under the control of myogenic factors (for review, see Duclert and Changeux 1995).

In most brain regions and peripheral ganglia, all four subunit mRNAs studied (α3, α4, β2, and β4) are initially detected as early as E11. Subsequently, some subunits (mostly α3 and β4 in the brain and α4 in the ganglia) are repressed in such a way that the adult pattern of expression is reached (i.e., predominance of α4-β2 in the brain and α3-β4 in the ganglia). We do not yet know the factors (first and second messengers) involved in this regulation, but, in analogy with what has been shown for the repression of nAChR expression in

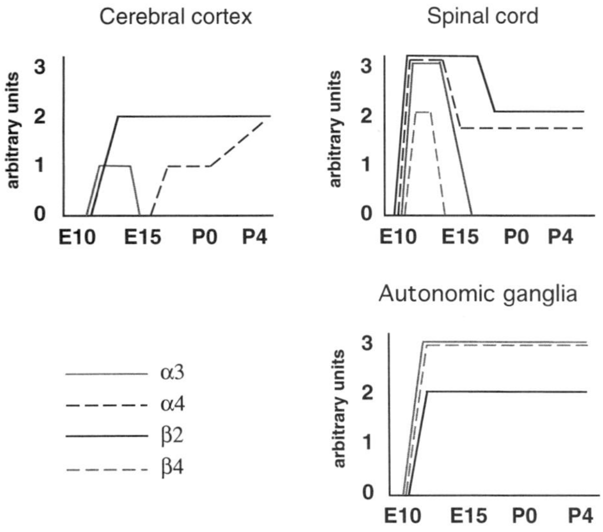

Figure 5. Compared developmental evolution of α3, α4, β2, β4 subunit mRNA levels in rat embryos in different regions of the nervous system. (Adapted from Zoli et al. 1995.)

extrajunctional nuclei of the muscle, the contribution of electrical activity and neurotrophic factors appears possible.

Expression of nAChR subunit mRNA in neocortex is interesting in several respects. α3 and β2 are first detected at E12–13 in the preplate. Subsequently, α3 mRNA disappears and β2 remains the only subunit expressed in the cortical subplate and plate until E17 (subplate) or E19 (plate), when α4 begins to be expressed. Therefore, at variance with other brain areas, α4 mRNA appearance is not temporally related to the time of the last mitosis of cortical neurons, but rather to the arrival of cholinergic innervation that penetrates into the cortical subplate and plate in the late embryonic period (Zoli et al. 1995).

We do not know if all nAChR subunit mRNAs expressed at early stages are translated into proteins. However, receptor autoradiography studies (for references, see Zoli et al. 1995) show that high-affinity nicotine binding is already detected in the rat brain at E11. In accordance with the evidence that identifies high-affinity nicotine-binding sites with α4β2-containing nAChRs (Picciotto et al. 1995), appearance of nicotine binding followed a caudorostral gradient which closely corresponds to that of the appearance of α4 subunit mRNA. It is therefore likely that the widespread and precocious expression of nAChR subunit mRNAs leads to the formation of functional nAChRs in the embryonic nervous system. This suggests that ACh, in addition to playing a role in synaptic transmission, also serves an ontogenetic function and serves as a regulatory factor for cell differentiation and/or formation of brain circuits (see Lauder 1993). For example, nAChR activation may contribute to the retraction of neurites (Pugh and Berg 1994) or to the turning of nerve growth cones (Zheng et al. 1994). In any case, a restriction of an initially widespread distribution of nAChRs and/or a selection of synapses within an initially exuberant outgrowth of connections may take place during development (see Changeux and Danchin 1976; Edelman and Tononi 1996) under the control of nAChRs.

In conclusion, each gene encoding a given nAChR subunit follows an almost unique pattern of expression throughout the central and peripheral nervous system. Consistent with this observation, the neuronal α2, α3, α4, and β2 subunit genes are found dispersed on different chromosomes (respectively, 14, 9, 2, and 3; Bessis et al. 1990), and the genes encoding α3, β5, and β4 (Boulter et al. 1990) form a tightly linked cluster of 3 genes in the rat. As illustrated in Figure 6, the localization data on human chromosomes correlates well with the mouse chromosomal localization.

The coexpression of nAChR subunit genes (α3 β4, α4 β2) at early stages of brain development (Zoli et al. 1995) mentioned above thus cannot simply be accounted for by their linkage in an operon-like structure. A detailed analysis of the promoter and regulatory sequences for each individual subunit gene is required.

	a1	a2	a3	a4	a5	a6	a7	a8	b1	b2	b3	b4	g	d	e
mouse	2	14	9	2	-	-	-	-	11	3	-	-	1	1	-
human	2	8	15	20	15	-	-	-	17	[illegible]	8	15	2	2	17

Figure 6. Chromosomic localization of nAChR subunit genes in the mouse and in human (for references, see Bessis 1993).

Functional Analysis of α2-Subunit Promoter from Chick

The very restricted localization of α2-subunit mRNA was initially demonstrated in the chick (Daubas et al. 1990). As a first step in the analysis of the regulatory mechanisms involved, transgenic mice carrying the complete structural gene encoding the α2 subunit in the chick (with 8 kb of upstream and 3 kb of downstream sequence) were constructed (Daubas et al. 1993). The gene was expressed within mouse brain in a neuron-specific manner. In situ hybridization reproducibly labeled motor cranial nuclei and mostly, but not exclusively, cholinergic areas. This indicated that some neuron-specific gene expression mechanisms are preserved between birds and mammals. Yet, important differences still exist and deserve investigation. Their understanding might shed light on evolutionarily sensitive genetic mechanisms engaged in brain morphogenesis.

A detailed analysis of the chick α2-subunit promoter and regulatory sequences was subsequently undertaken (Bessis et al. 1993). Sequence analysis of more than 7 kb of the 5′upstream region showed that the proximal 1-kb-flanking region contains a previously unidentified untranslated exon located 2.8 kb upstream of exon 1, as well as several consensus sequences for transcription factors (several AP2 sites, three Ets sites, one each of the ATF, AP4 Myc, CIIS, SCG10, NFM-binding sites, and six weakly degenerate OCT-like sites, but no TATA or CAAT boxes). Although this large putative promoter region contained many consensus sites for transcription factor binding, it was unable to drive expression of a reporter gene in any cell line tested (both neuronal and nonneuronal). We hypothesized that this was due to the presence of silencer elements within this fragment. Indeed, an 891-bp fragment was found to repress the transcription of a reporter gene (luciferase) driven by the strong heterologous promoter of the SV40 virus. Further dissection of this 5′sequence delineated an 11-bp motif (CCC CATGCAAT) repeated six times in the –130/+30 region of the gene. High-resolution mapping revealed that these six tandem repeats exert a strong silencing activity on the SV40 promoter. Paradoxically, this silencer element was able to act as a transcription activator if rather than six, four, two, or even one copy of the 11-nucleotide sequence was placed upstream of the basal promoter fragment (Bessis et al. 1993).

The remarkable behavior of this string of 11-bp motifs was further investigated, in collaboration with the laboratory of D. Lachtman (Milton et al. 1995). Three members of the Brn-3 group of the POU family, Brn3a, 3b, and 3c, are specifically expressed in the peripheral and central nervous system with each factor having a distinct expression pattern and a different effect on gene expression when they bind to Oct sequences (for references, see Milton et al. 1995). Previous work has shown that Brn3a and Brn3c *trans*-activate an artificial promoter containing one Oct consensus motif; while using the same promoter construct, Brn3b behaves as a repressor. Interestingly, in the intact α2-subunit gene promoter, Brn3b exerts the opposite effect: It acts as a very strong activator, in contrast to Brn3a and c. On the other hand, the activating effect of Brn3b is lost in derivatives containing one, two, or four copies of the Oct-like sequence. Moreover, these truncated derivatives are activated by Brn3c. Remarkably complex interactions between DNA regulatory elements and transcription factors, including strong repressors, thus contribute to the highly restricted expression of the α2-subunit promoter.

β2-Subunit Promoter Elements Involved in Neuron-specific Expression and Pattern Formation

In contrast to the extremely limited expression of the α2-subunit message, the β2-subunit mRNA is widely expressed throughout the brain (Wada et al. 1989; Hill et al. 1993); furthermore, as mentioned above (Zoli et al. 1995), the appearance of the β2-transcript occurs very early in development and its timing closely parallels that of neuronal differentiation. The mapping of the β2-subunit gene promoter was therefore undertaken with the goal of identifying the elements that underlie its ubiquitous neuronal expression (Bessis et al. 1995). Within the 1.2-kb sequence upstream of the transcription start site, several consensus DNA elements could be recognized: an Sp1 site, a cAMP-responsive element, a nuclear response element, an OCT-like motif (–522), an E-box (–118), and, within the transcribed domain, a neural restrictive silencer element (NRSE) sequence (+18 to +38). Upon transfection of an 1163-bp fragment of upstream sequence fused to a luciferase reporter gene, efficent transcriptional activation could be seen in pheochromocytoma (PC12) and neuroblastoma (SKNBe, N1E115) cell lines, but not in striatal (SVLT) or nonneuronal (3T6, 293, and HeLa) cell lines. As had been seen with the α2-subunit promoter, deletion analysis of the 1163-bp β2 promoter revealed several silencing elements: one present in the distal 5′-end region and another more proximally (between –862 and –283 bp). Both elements contribute to the neuron-specific expression of the β2-subunit gene, although in a different manner. Another important silencing NRSE is located, as mentioned, at the 3′end of the promoter between +18 and +38. A point mutation in the NRSE in the context of the 1163-

bp promoter results in a more than 100-fold increase in transcriptional activity in fibroblasts, but only a 3.2-fold increase in neuroblastomas. This strongly argues in favor of a contribution of the NRSE to the neuron-specific expression of the β2-subunit gene, primarily via repression of its transcription in nonneuronal cells. In contrast, a powerful activating element is present within the –245- to –95-bp fragment, which includes an Sp1 element and an E-box. These two elements have been shown to contribute to nAChR α1-subunit gene expression in muscle (for references, see Duclert and Changeux 1995). Consistent with these observations, point mutation of the E-box in the 1163-bp promoter context results in a 40% reduction in transcriptional activity in neuronal cell lines, demonstrating that this element behaves as an enhancer, possibly in cooperation with the neighboring Sp1-binding sites (see Bessereau et al. 1993). The HLH transcription factors involved in nerve cells are likely to differ from the myogenic proteins in muscle, however.

Two lines of transgenic mice were constructed with the 1163-bp promoter sequence linked to a β-galactosidase reporter gene. Histological examination of β-galactosidase activity in these mice showed that the β-galactosidase transgene was expressed in neurons, and that both the endogenous β2-subunit mRNA and the transgene driven by the β2 promoter had a similar pattern of expression during the development of the early embryonic nervous system. At later stages of development, most of the β2-subunit-expressing neurons in ganglia were labeled by the β2-promoter-driven expression of β-galactosidase. However, in the brain, only a subset of β2-positive regions expressed the transgene, and there was considerable variability in the expression pattern from one strain to the other. (At E13, labeling was prominent in the peripheral nervous system but also in the brain stem and in the forebrain. After E17, positive neurons were found in several basal telencephalic nuclei and in the caudate putamen. Positive clusters were also identified in reticular thalamic and many hypothalamic nuclei and in the brain stem motor nuclei of cranial nerves. Labeling persisted during postnatal development but only in limited loci in the brain.)

Recent experiments (A. Bessis, unpubl.) on transgenic mice constructed with the 1163-bp promoter carrying a point mutation in the NRSE sequence have shown that this element strikingly affects the expression of the β2 gene. At approximately day E13, β-galactosidase staining disappears from the posterior and peripheral nervous system but becomes intense in the anterior part of the brain. In other words, a switch in reporter gene expression takes place along the antero-posterior axis of the nervous system. This is a preliminary but striking piece of evidence demonstrating a contribution of defined promoter elements and transcription factors to the formation of topologically defined patterns of nAChR gene expression in the brain.

Remarks on Pattern Formation of nAChR Transcripts in the Brain

The molecular mechanisms that account for pattern formation in the brain are orders of magnitude more complex than those involved in compartmentalized expression of nAChR genes at the motor end plate. The experimental data obtained thus far on end-plate restriction of the nAChR in skeletal muscle are consistent with cybernetic models that propose autoregulation of transcription factor biosynthesis and competition among promoter elements for limiting concentrations of transcription factors as mechanisms for compartmentalization of expression (Kerszberg and Changeux 1993). The extension of the model to embryonic morphogenesis (Kerszberg and Changeux 1994) proposes that a shallow morphogenetic gradient can result in sharp boundaries as a consequence of the formation of heterodimers between two types of transcription factors: (1) a morphogen M which forms the gradient and (2) a "vernier" molecule V transcribed in the embryo. In this model, the various hetero- and homo-oligomers of M and V exert distinct activating/inhibitory effects on the responsive element of the V promoter in a manner very reminiscent of the interaction of transcription factors with silencer/enhancer elements in the α2 and β2 promoters. Quantitative simulation of the program demonstrates, depending on the parameters, either a sharp transcriptional boundary of the V gene, or a stationary or even a moving stripe. Mutations affecting the binding and/or the sign of given combinations of transcription factors are anticipated to alter the pattern of gene expression. This is found experimentally with many developmental genes in *Drosophila*. One possibility is that the above-mentioned NRSE and the REST factor that interacts with this element and which, incidentally, exhibits sequence homologies with the *Drosophila* Krüppel gene product, are parts of such a mechanism. This remains to be demonstrated, however. In any case, the model underlines the importance of combinatorial mechanisms between protein units in the activity of oligomeric transcription factors, which are also allosteric proteins.

In the course of end-plate morphogenesis, coexisting peptides, including trophic or growth factors and electrical activity, play important roles in the regulation of nAChR gene transcription (for review, see Duclert and Changeux 1995). As mentioned, similar processes may contribute to the regulation of nAChR gene expression in the brain. However, nAChR may also mediate plasticity phenomena via, for instance, Ca^{++} entry (see Sargent 1993; Galzi and Changeux 1995). nAChR activation stimulates transcription of the immediate-early gene c-*fos* in neuroblastoma cells and increases mRNA levels for brain-derived growth factor and nerve growth factor (NGF) in the hippocampus (for review, see Galzi and Changeux 1995). Such interplay between ACh and growth factors and their receptors may influence the development of cortical connectivity and its activity-dependent plasticity in barrel fields (Umbriaco et al. 1994) or in visual cortex (Singer 1985; Griesbeck et al.; Riddle et al.; both this volume). Ultimately, as with muscle nAChR, these regulatory processes will be analyzed at the promoter level. In any case, tools and ideas are in hand to undertake a reasonable analysis of the development of nAChR gene patterns of expression in the brain (see also Matter et al. 1995).

SUBCELLULAR COMPARTMENTALIZATION OF BRAIN nAChR

In adult skeletal muscle, one molecular species of nAChR protein is expressed at a single locus: the endplate postsynaptic membrane. In the brain, the situation is much more complex, since each nerve cell may express different combinations of nAChR subunits in distinct areas of the cell membrane (for review, see Duclert and Changeux 1995). Complex transcriptional mechanisms, followed by elaborate posttranscriptional processes, are necessary to establish the right combination of nAChR subunits at the right place in the nerve cell. As a first step in understanding these complex properties, the subcellular compartmentalization of nAChR has been investigated using electrophysiological techniques (Fig. 7) (Mulle et al. 1991, 1992a,b; Léna et al. 1993; C. Léna and J.-P. Changeux, in prep.).

The Somatodendritic Compartment

Many neurons in the brain generate fast inward currents upon application of nicotinic agonists to the somatodendritic membrane (in particular, cells from substantia nigra pars compacta, ventral tegmental area, medial habenula, interpeduncular nucleus [IPN], retinal ganglion, and hippocampus) (for review, see Clarke 1993; Role and Berg 1996). Medial habenula neurons are a particularly convenient system for studying these currents since, as mentioned, single channels can be recorded using patch-clamp techniques, either from freshly dissociated neurons of juvenile rats (Mulle and Changeux 1990; Mulle et al. 1991, 1992a,b) or from thin slices from the adult brain (Connolly et al. 1995; Picciotto et al. 1995). In the ventral region of the medial habenula, neurons express mRNAs encoding the α3, α4, α7, β2, β3, and β4 subunits. At least two populations of single-channel amplitudes of approximately 41 and 51 pS can be recorded from these cells whose relative proportions differ on distinct patches of the cell surface (Connolly et al. 1995). The pharmacology of the dominant single channels recorded (Mulle and Changeux 1990; Mulle et al. 1991) and of the whole-cell response (Connolly et al. 1995; Picciotto et al. 1995) reveals an equal, or higher, potency of nicotine over cytisine (nicotine > cytisine > ACh > DMPP), a block by hexamethonium and dihydro-β-erythroidine, but an insensitivity to α- and neuronal bungarotoxin. This profile differs from that of neurons from thalamus, which mostly express α4 and β2-subunit mRNAs and which give whole-cell responses with a rank order of potency of nicotine > DMPP > cytisine. No response to nicotine could be found in thalamic neurons in mice lacking the β2 subunit, using patch-clamp recording from thin brain slices, demonstrating the dominant contribution of the β2-subunit to the nicotinic response in these cells. On the other hand, in habenular neurons, the cytisine to nicotine ratio did not significantly change as a consequence of the β2 mutation, a finding consistent with a greater contribution of the β4-containing receptor to nicotinic physiology in these cells (Picciotto et al. 1995).

Neurons from the medial habenula project to the IPN via the fasciculus retroflexus. Since patch-clamp recording can be performed on IPNs both after acute isolation and in thin slices, one can compare the physiology and pharmacology of nAChRs located at both pre- and postsynaptic sites within the same system. The data show that the rank order of efficacy for agonists of presynaptic nAChRs (nicotine > cytisine > ACh > DMPP) is different from that seen for the soma of postsynaptic IPNs (cytisine > ACh > nicotine > DMPP) (Mulle et al. 1991). In other words, the physiological properties, and probably the subunit composition of pre- and postsynaptic nAChRs, may differ within a given synaptic connection. Moreover, although the recording techniques were not the same, evidence exists for pharmacological differences (IC_{50} values for antagonists) between somatic and axonal nAChRs within the same habenular neuron. Different nAChR species not only coexist within a given nerve cell, but may also segregate into different compartments (somatodendritic and axonal) on the neuronal surface.

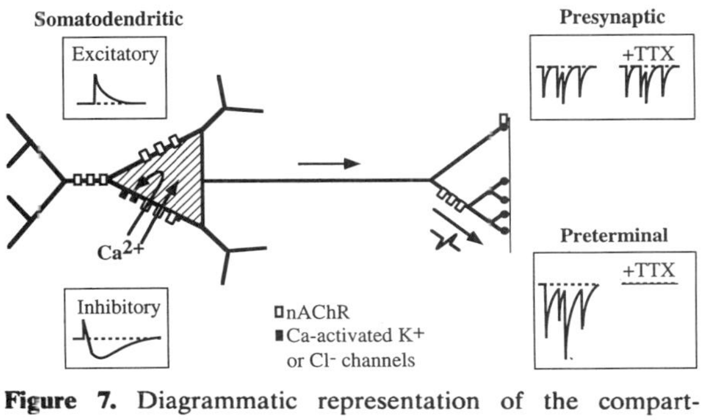

Figure 7. Diagrammatic representation of the compartmentalization of nAChRs in the nerve cell, revealed by electrophysiological techniques. (*Inset*) Responses to ACh or nicotine recorded in the somatodendritic, presynaptic, or preterminal compartments.

The "Preterminal" Axonal Compartment

The presence of nAChRs on axons has been demonstrated by a combination of nicotinic ligand-binding experiments and lesion experiments in vivo, as well as by a number of studies on nicotinic stimulation of neurotransmitter release in synaptosomes or brain slices in vitro. Whole-cell recordings (Léna et al. 1993) in thin slices and on acutely isolated IPNs that have retained synaptic contacts attached to their cell body (as evidenced by synaptophysin immunoreactivity and spontaneous GABA and glutamate release) confirm that nicotine dramatically increases the frequency of large GABAergic currents in these cells. Yet, rather unexpectedly, the Na^+ spike-blocker tetrodotoxin (TTX) was found to inhibit this effect. Because the specificity of TTX is strictly limited to Na^+ channels, these channels must intervene between the nAChR and the GABA release site. The location of these nAChRs thus differs from the "terminal" receptors described in synaptosomal preparations which are insensitive to TTX (Wonnacott et al. 1995). The term "preterminal" (Léna et al. 1993) was coined to specify the distribution of these nAChRs on the axon. The observation has been confirmed and the term adopted by other groups working with different systems (McMahon et al. 1994a,b; McGehee and Role 1996). The role of these preterminal nAChRs on terminal axon branches still remains elusive. One possibility is that they are the target of as-yet-unidentified cholinergic terminals; another is that they exert a "global" control of neurotransmitter release by a general depolarization of the afferent axons due to ACh released in a paracrine manner (Agnati et al. 1995).

nAChR on Axon Terminals

As mentioned above, TTX does not affect nicotine-enhanced neurotransmitter release in synaptosomes, and the nAChRs involved are thus authentic terminal nAChRs (McMahon et al. 1994a; McGehee et al. 1995; C. Léna and J.-P. Changeux, in prep.). The direct action of nAChRs on axon terminals was recorded using the patch-clamp technique on thin slices of the ventrobasal complex and dorsolateral geniculate nucleus from mouse sensory thalamus (C. Léna and J.-P. Changeux, in prep.). In these preparations, nicotinic agonists enhance the frequency of miniature GABA currents and decrease the failure rate of evoked inhibitory synaptic currents. Both effects disappear in β2-subunit knockout mice, indicating that the β2 subunit is a necessary component of the nAChR implicated (most likely together with the α4-subunit whose mRNA is particularly abundant in thalamic neurons). The nicotine-enhanced release disappears at low external Ca^{++} concentrations but persists when Ca^{++} is replaced by Sr^{++} or Ba^{++}, but not Mg^{++}. This Ca^{++} dependence of nAChR-enhanced neurotransmitter release might result either from the direct entry of Ca^{++} ions through the nAChR channel or, indirectly, from the activation of voltage-dependent Ca^{++} channels by the depolarization of the nerve ending membrane. Interestingly, the two situations may actually occur but in different systems. In the ventrobasal nucleus, cadmium ions (Cd^{++}), which efficiently block high-threshold voltage-sensitive Ca^{++} channels, block nAChR-mediated presynaptic facilitation. On the other hand, in the dorsolateral geniculate nucleus, Cd^{++} does not show this effect, and nicotine enhances Ca^{++}-dependent GABA release apparently without depolarizing the nerve terminal, supporting the view that Ca^{++} influx through the nAChR channel might directly contribute to nicotine facilitation of synaptic, here inhibitory, transmission.

Nicotinic versus Muscarinic Regulation of Synaptic Efficiency in Cortical Networks

The prefrontal area of the neocortex plays a key role in higher cognitive functions, which also require the integrity of cortical cholinergic systems (see below, "Nicotine Receptors in Learning and Reward"). This system was therefore selected to investigate the contribution of nAChRs at the network level. In a first approach (Vidal and Changeux 1989), extracellular recordings of field potentials and unit discharges taken from the prelimbic area of the prefrontal cortex revealed excitatory effects of nicotine that were blocked by neuronal bungarotoxin and thus possibly involved α3β2–α4β2 nAChRs. In subsequent experiments (Vidal and Changeux 1993), intracellular recordings were made from pyramidal cells located predominantly in layer II/III (where nicotine binding sites are concentrated [for review, see Clarke 1993]). Iontophoretic applications of nicotine near the recording site increased the amplitude of the postsynaptic potentials evoked by stimulation of the superficial cortical layers (14% of the cells). In contrast, muscarinic agonists decreased the amplitude of the postsynaptic response. In all instances, the early postsynaptic potentials were blocked by a specific inhibitor of non-NMDA glutamate receptors (CNQX), but not by APV, a selective blocker of NMDA glutamate receptors. Thus, presynaptic nAChRs may, in the neocortex, potentiate excitatory glutamatergic synapses, in addition to the above-mentioned facilitation of GABAergic synapses, a finding recently confirmed and extended in different systems (for review, see McGehee and Role 1996).

In conclusion, even though the evidence is still fragmentary, a compartmentalized expression of nAChR proteins takes place in central neurons at the level of the somatodendritic, preterminal, and terminal domains of the cell membrane. The posttranscriptional mechanisms necessary for this targeting remain to be identified (see Hill et al. 1993; Sargent 1993). Moreover, the available information on the relative topology of presynaptic cholinergic nerve endings and postsynaptic nAChR distribution at the subcellular level is still fragmentary. However, a contribution of diffuse, paracrine release of ACh (Agnati et al. 1995), together with more classic synaptic transmission, appears plausible. In any case, the abundance of nAChR in presynaptic compartments supports the notion that, at least at this level, nAChRs play a dominant role in the modulation of both excitatory *and* inhibitory transmission. It thus appears timely to investigate the modulatory role of nAChR in plasticity processes in the brain; in particular, those related to learning and memory.

NICOTINIC RECEPTORS IN LEARNING AND REWARD

The cellular and molecular mechanisms underlying learning and memory have been extensively investigated in simple organisms like *Aplysia* and *Drosophila*, or in simplified systems from vertebrate brain like the hippocampus (see Mayford et al.; Tonegawa; both this volume). It has been overwhelmingly difficult, however, to relate the observations made at these elementary levels with the actual behavior of the organism and its cognitive functions (for discussion, see Changeux 1993). This is why it appeared to us to be necessary to elaborate models that were already consistent with experimental observations of neural systems before embarking on further experimental investigations on the role of the nAChR in learning. The aim of these models will be to create a context for the elementary mechanisms under study and to establish a causal link between a particular network organization and the behavioral process under study (see Dehaene and Changeux 1989; Edelman and Tononi 1996; Montague et al. 1996).

Models of Learning with Reward: Role of Allosteric Receptors

Storage of learning and memory traces does not take place in a passive, nonselective, manner like a "blind" imprinting process. Quite to the contrary, mechanisms of evaluation by externally and/or internally represented reinforcement (or reward processes) efficiently contribute to the selection of the stored (or rejected) representations (see Barto et al. 1983). In a first attempt to elaborate formal models of learning by selection through external reward, together with S. Dehaene, we have focused our attention on delayed-response tasks. These tasks were initially designed to test for the acquisition of cognitive patterns—or rules of behavior—and they selectively engage the prefrontal cortex (Dehaene and Changeux 1989). The approach was subsequently extended to the related Wisconsin card-sorting task (Dehaene and Changeux 1991). In the simple case of the delayed-response tasks, the subject is first presented with a cue object, followed

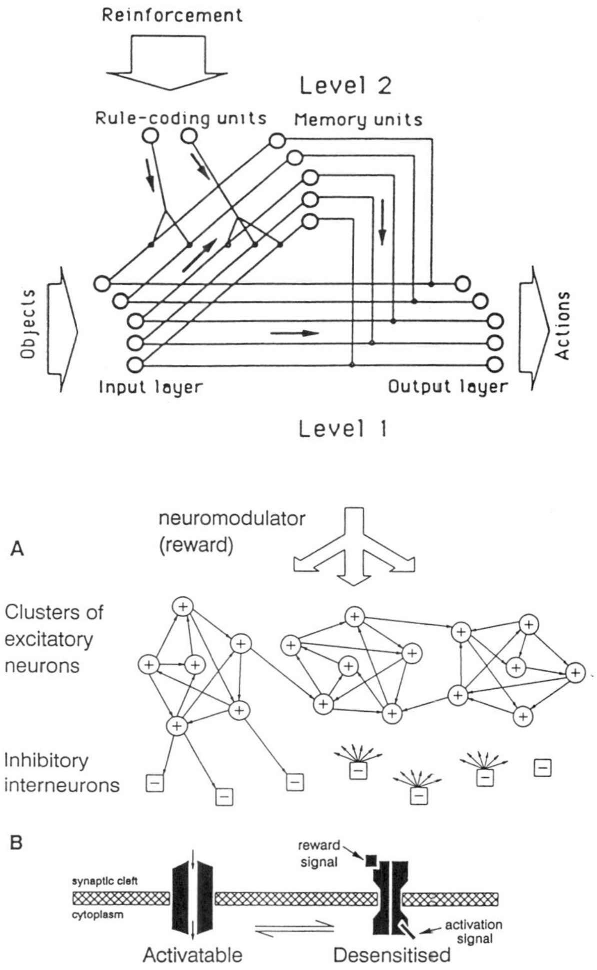

Figure 8. Model of formal neural architecture passing delayed-response tasks. The figure illustrates two main features of the model: (1) Two distinct hierarchical levels of organization occur: the higher one carries clusters coding for high-order rules of behavior (according here to position or color), and selection occurs when time coincidence takes place between positive reward and activity in the cluster. (2) The mechanism postulated for the stabilization of the selected cluster is a regulation of synaptic efficacy by the reward substance, which here behaves as effector of an allosteric receptor. (Modified from Dehaene and Changeux 1989, 1991.)

by a delay period of variable duration. Then, two objects are presented simultaneously at two separate locations and the subject has to choose one of them according to a rule, either on the basis of its *position* (task A *not* B) or of its *identity* to the cue (task matching to sample [MTS]). The *reward* given during the learning period specifies the rule that the organism subsequently follows during the test. In all these instances, formal neural architectures were built which, under conditions of computer simulation, successfully perform these tasks (Fig. 8). Common features relevant to an eventual contribution of allosteric receptors and "molecular switches" (see above, "Molecular Phylogeny and Functional Diversity of nAChR") and, more specifically, nAChRs to these network architectures include the following: (1) The formal organism comprises, at least and in a very schematic manner, two hierarchically nested levels of organization: a low, sensori-motor, routine level consisting of neurons with modifiable synaptic weights, and a higher, cognitive, supervisory level containing neural units coding for the rules or programs of behavior. (2) The rule-coding units are implemented as clusters of densely interconnected excitatory neurons, with two (or more in more complex models [Dehaene and Changeux 1991]) discrete, internally generated and self-sustained states of activity; the clusters are linked by lateral inhibitory connections in such a way that when one rule-coding unit is spontaneously active, the others are in the low-activity or silent state. (3) In the course of learning, the layer of rule-coding units plays the role of a "generator of diversity"; that is, the activity of each particular cluster spontaneously changes and alternates at random with time, in such a way that the organism is able to test successively one (or the other) of the dimension rules upon its environment. A search by trial and error takes place until (4) a positive reward is delivered from the external environment when the formal organism produces a motor output congruent with the rule to be learned; the particular cluster active at this precise moment is selected; (5) allosteric receptors regulate the efficiency of synapses at the postsynaptic level without or with (Hebb rule) timing relationships between pre- and postsynaptic activity; (6) positive and/or negative rewards are implemented as the externally driven (or even internally elicited in the case of auto-evaluation loops [Dehaene and Changeux 1991]) global release of a "reward signal," such as norepinephine, dopamine, acetylcholine, or a coexisting messenger, directly or indirectly, behaving as effectors of allosteric receptors; (7) in the currently active cluster, the reward substance stabilizes the ongoing activity by changing the synaptic efficacies, in a Hebbian manner, of the active cluster, thereby increasing the chances of selecting the same output again in subsequent trials. Negative reward, on the other hand, destabilizes current activity at the synaptic level, thereby resetting the system to a random trial-and-error mode (Dehaene and Changeux 1989, 1991; see also Edelman and Tononi 1996; Montague et al. 1996).

According to these views, allosteric receptors would play a critical role as molecular switches in the selective storage of traces in neurons by mediating, in a "bottom-up" fashion, the effect of reward on spontaneous pre-representations taking place at the cognitive level. Many other molecular devices may also contribute to synaptic switches, for instance, at the level of neurotransmitter release mechanisms (for references, see Changeux 1993). Neurotransmitters are excellent candidates for these switches, however, as their allosteric properties are well established, particularly for the nAChR (Léna and Changeux 1993; Bertrand and Changeux 1995; Edelstein et al. 1996). They may legitimately serve as short- (and even long-) term regulators of synaptic efficacy and, in particular, they may play the role of coincidence detectors (together with many other regulatory proteins in the cell). Their eventual contribution in established learning tasks was therefore experimentally tested.

nAChR in the Prefrontal Cortex: Differential Role in Delayed Response Tasks

A rich body of pharmacological and behavioral observations demonstrate the importance of cholinergic nuclei and pathways in memory, and, more specifically, in working memory and attentional processes that rely on the integration of the prefrontal cortex and are deeply affected in Alzheimer's patients (for review, see Vidal 1994). Moreover, nicotine selectively improves memory and attention (for review, see Levin 1992) and nicotine-binding sites significantly decrease (compared to muscarinic receptor sites) in the neocortex of Alzheimer patients' brains (Nordberg and Windblad 1986; for review, see Vidal 1994). To evaluate the contribution of nAChR to these functions (but also to test the theoretical models presented above), the effect of the nicotinic antagonists neuronal bungarotoxin and dihydro-β-erythroidine was assayed in collaboration with C. Thinus Blanc's laboratory, on the performance of a delayed matching-to-sample (MTS) task (Granon et al. 1995). A less difficult task, the non-matching-to-sample (NMTS) task, was used as a control as it depends on the natural tendency of the rat to spontaneously alternate, on a second run, to the branch it *did not* visit the first time. As anticipated, lesions of the prefrontal cortex selectively impaired the performance of the MTS task and caused perseverations while preserving the performance on the NMTS task (Granon et al. 1994). Interestingly, injections of neuronal bungarotoxin into the prelimbic area of the prefrontal cortex produced a significant decrease in working memory performance in the MTS, but not in the NMTS, task. In contrast, an inhibitor of the muscarinic receptor, scopolamine, impaired working memory in both tasks. These findings seem consonant with the above-mentioned ("Nicotinic versus Muscarinic Regulation of Synaptic Efficiency") nAChR-mediated enhancement of glutamate release in the prefrontal cortex, whereas muscarinic receptors exert the opposite effect (Vidal and Changeux 1993). In conclusion, consistent with the theoretical models presented above (although the models are still far from proven), nAChRs in the prefrontal cortex appear to maintain performance in delayed-response tasks requiring effortful processing for response selection, and the muscarinic system appears to be involved in more general working memory processes (Granon et al. 1995).

Avoidance Learning in β2-Subunit Mutant Mice

A rather efficient method to test for the involvement of a particular neuronal subunit in behavior, particularly in learning, is to disrupt the gene encoding this subunit. This was achieved for the β2 subunit, in collaboration with the laboratories of P. Brûlet and E. Merlo Pich (Picciotto et al. 1995). The homozygous mutant mice ($\beta2^{-/-}$) are viable, mate normally, and do not show any obvious physical and behavioral deficits. The overall brain size and morphology are normal. β2-Subunit immunoreactivity and mRNA were undetectable in total brain homogenates and in situ. The most evident biochemical modification was a complete loss of high-affinity [^{3}H]nicotine binding measured both in extracts and by in situ autoradiography. The β2 subunit containing nAChR thus comprises the high-affinity binding sites for [^{3}H]nicotine, most likely together with the α4 subunit (whose distribution closely parallels that of the β2 subunit) (see above, "Molecular Phylogeny and Functional Diversity of nAChR") (see Zoli et al. 1995). As mentioned, the electrophysiological response to nicotine of the neurons from the anterior thalamus (which express very high levels of β2- and α4-subunit mRNA) completely disappears in the mutant, whereas that of the medial habenula, which is pharmacologically distinct, largely persists.

Spatial orientation learning evaluated by the Morris water maze (with visible or hidden platform) did not show significant impairment. On the other hand, the $\beta2^{-/-}$ mice tested for the retention of an avoidance task showed marked differences compared to their nonmutant siblings. The test utilized in a standard manner for pharmacological assay of nicotine sensitivity consists in the measurement of the delay taken by a mouse placed in a well-lit compartment to enter an adjacent dark chamber. In the sample run, the mouse is delivered an electric shock upon entry into the dark chamber, and vehicle or nicotine is immediately injected into the mouse. After 24 hours, retention of the electric shock memory was assessed by measuring the delay to enter the dark chamber. Nicotine (0.01 mg/kg) consistently aided retention in wild-type animals but was completely ineffective in $\beta2^{-/-}$ mice. The effect of low nicotine concentration upon passive avoidance learning is thus mediated by a β2 subunit containing nAChR (Picciotto et al. 1995).

Moreover, preliminary observations support the view that slight modification of the learning behavior of the $\beta2^{-/-}$ mice takes place in the absence of nicotine: The mice spontaneously display longer retention latencies, as if they were able to perform better than their nonmutant littermates (Picciotto et al. 1995). This would mean that β2-subunit-containing nAChR mediates endogenous effects of ACh in the brain under defined behavioral conditions. At this stage, the response of the mutant mice in delayed matching to sample tasks has not been studied. Compensatory effects and/or reorganization of the nAChR-containing pathways may also take place in the course of development. All these aspects need further investigation.

nAChR in Reward and Addiction

Because the mice spontaneously fear light, the application of the electric shock when the animal enters the dark compartment may be viewed as a "negative reward." It is therefore tempting to propose that (as suggested in the theoretical section of this chapter) ACh, among several other neurotransmitters, is a "reward substance" contributing to the complex networks involved in reinforcement. Moreover, it has long been hypothesized and debated that such positive reinforcing properties were at the origin of nicotine addiction (Stolerman et al. 1995),

The mesolimbic dopaminergic system, and particularly its projection to the nucleus accumbens, has been identified as the critical shared substrate of the reinforcing effect of drugs of abuse (cocaine, amphetamine, morphine). These drugs are thus thought to cause addiction because they produce plastic changes (both within and outside the mesolimbic-accumbens circuits) that subsequently alter the state of activity of neurons that regulate motivated behavior and emotion (Hyman 1996; Koob 1996). The *shell* of the nucleus accumbens (ventromedial part) is thought to contribute to the integration and expression of emotions via its projection to the amygdala, lateral hypothalamus, and central gray matter. On the other hand, the *core* would contribute to somatomotor functions (for review, see Pontieri et al. 1996). Pontieri et al. (1996) have recently shown that nicotine, at concentrations that maintain self-administration, enhances extracellular dopamine release (estimated by microdialysis) in the shell of the nucleus accumbens, but *not* in the core. This fact tallies well with the notion that modulation of dopamine release is a major neurochemical effect of nicotine administration (see Dani and Heidmann 1996). Nicotine also stimulates local glucose utilization in a manner qualitatively similar to that of strongly addictive drugs (Pontieri et al. 1996). Interestingly, preliminary results (Biomed EEC Activity Report 1995; M. Picciotto et al., unpubl.) indicate that, in anesthetized $\beta2^{-/-}$ mice, dopamine release in striatum is no longer stimulated by nicotine. This supports the notion that β2-subunit-containing high-affinity nAChRs contribute to this effect.

In situ binding and hybridization studies reveal labeling for a number of nAChR α and β subunits in catecholaminergic nuclei. These include β2-subunit mRNA and high-affinity nicotine binding and mRNA, but also α6 and β3 mRNAs, which are very abundant in these aminergic neurons (Le Novère et al. 1996). It is thus proposed, as a working hypothesis, that [α6β2β3] nAChRs are likely candidates for the mediation of nicotine-enhanced stimulation of catecholamine release (Le Novère et al. 1996). In addition, the present results suggest that different nAChR isoforms may be present in subsets of dopaminergic neurons and/or at different subcellular compartments (somatodendritic, preterminal, and terminal) within them.

The site(s) that accounts for the plastic changes responsible for tolerance and addiction remains to be identified (see Dani and Heinemann 1996). Possible mechanisms include: (1) properties of the nAChR molecule itself, such as short- and long-term desensitization (see above, "Molecular Phylogeny and Functional Diversity of nAChR") and (2) posttranscriptional increase of nAChR protein without change of nAChR mRNA (Marks et al. 1992). Other possibilities, alternatively and/or in addition, are interactions between nAChR and dopamine receptors (Zoli et al. 1993; Li et al. 1995). For instance, a single subcutaneous administration of nicotine causes a significant increase of the binding of a selective dopamine D2 receptor antagonist to striatal membranes (Li et al. 1995), but no change in the level of D2 receptor mRNA was detected in the caudate-putamen or in the substantia nigra (Biomed EEC Activity Report 1995). To further test for possible nAChR-D2 receptor interaction, the levels of dopamine D2-receptor-binding sites and mRNA were investigated in nAChR $\beta2^{-/-}$ subunit mutants (M. Zoli et al., unpubl.), whereas nAChR subunit mRNA and nicotine binding were investigated in D2-receptor null mutants (Baik et al. 1995). Interestingly, none of the dopamine receptor parameters tested significantly varied in the $\beta2^{-/-}$ mutants. In contrast, preliminary investigations carried out with E. Borrelli's laboratory reveal that nAChR subunit mRNA levels increase in the D2-receptor knockout mice (M.M. Arroyo-Jimenez, unpubl.). In addition to molecular mechanisms engaging the nAChR protein itself, interactions between the nAChR and dopaminergic receptors may thus play a crucial role. This eventuality, of course, deserves additional investigations.

In conclusion, strong evidence exists for a contribution of defined species of nAChR in reward and in addiction to nicotine. Promising avenues thus open for the elucidation of molecular and cellular mechanisms involved in this socially important health problem.

CONCLUSION: nAChR IN BRAIN FUNCTIONS AND DYSFUNCTIONS

The cholinergic system in the brain contributes to a wide variety of functions, which include attentional processes and various forms of learning and memory. Lesions of cholinergic nuclei, pharmacological modifications of cholinergic systems, spontaneous alterations of cholinergic pathways during aging, intracerebral transplantations of fetal tissue, and implantation of genetically modified cells that produce acetylcholine (Winkler et al. 1995 and references therein) demonstrate the essential role of acetylcholine in cognitive behavior (see above, "nAChR in Reward and Addiction").

The data presently available on the contribution of nAChR to intercellular signaling by acetylcholine in the brain differ strikingly from those of other neurotransmitters, such as glutamate or GABA. In particular, (1) cholinergic cell bodies are restricted to a few nuclei located mainly in the basal telencephalon and dorsal pons, but their axon terminals are spread throughout the brain in a rather diffuse manner; (2) no consistent match exists between the known distribution of nAChRs in the brain and that of cholinergic terminals; and (3) preterminal nAChRs occur along axons. All these observations support the notion that ACh may be liberated following a paracrine neuromodulatory mode (Agnati et al. 1995; Role and Berg 1996). On the other hand, authentic anatomical synapses with axonal terminals immunolabeled by anticholine acetyltransferase antibodies and typical postsynaptic densities have been recognized at the electron microscopic level (Umbriaco et al. 1994) in defined brain areas, suggesting that, in fact, the classic "wiring" and the "volume" transmission modes may coexist in the brain, possibly at different loci. Moreover, muscarinic receptors are also known to regulate synaptic transmission, in some instances with a sign opposite to that of nAChR (see above, "Nicotine versus Muscarinic Regulation of Synaptic Efficiency in Cortical Networks"). Still, the relative distribution of muscarinic (metabotropic) versus nicotinic (ionotropic) receptors, in particular, at the level of synapses, has not yet been established, as in the case of glutamate receptors (Lujan et al. 1996).

nAChRs, like ligand-gated ion channels in general, are allosteric membrane proteins, but with distinct properties. In particular, they carry several categories of topographically distinct sites for diverse categories of ligands and undergo multiple conformational transitions for intercellular communications, but also higher-order regulations that might control synaptic efficiency and possibly serve as coincidence detector in a "chemical Hebb synapse" (see above, "Allosteric Transitions of nAChRs").

As reviewed above ("nAChRs as Components of 'Molecular Switches' "), Ca^{++} ions may play crucial roles in the molecular switches mediated by nAChR by two distinct mechanisms: (1) the allosteric potentiation of the ionic response to ACh and (2) the influx of Ca^{++} ions through activated nAChR channels (under conditions different from those of NMDA receptor channels and/or voltage-sensitive Ca^{++} channels). Entry of Ca^{++} ions may elicit activation of other ionic channels and ligand-gated channels (for instance, $GABA_A$ receptors) present in the cell membrane, thereby modifying both the excitability of the neuron and its ability to "integrate" synaptic and/or paracrine signal. Moreover, the intervention of phosphorylation/dephosphorylation reactions may prolong these short-term processes.

The multiple combinations of subunits forming nAChR oligomers in the brain may differ by their pharmacological sensitivity, channel open time, and allosteric properties. Their precise distribution at strategic "nodal points" of the signaling networks is therefore expected to play a decisive role in their contribution to brain plasticity. This distribution is determined by the long-term biosynthesis and/or turnover of nAChR, within the three-dimensional organization of the brain, and within the different compartments of each individual nerve cell.

Future work along these lines requires an analysis of the developmental regulation of patterns of nAChR gene transcription at the promoter and transcription factor level, but also of the posttranscriptional phenomena engaged in intracellular assembly, maturation, transport, and targeting of the nAChR oligomers to defined compartments of the neuronal surface. Opposite regulations of α3 and α4 subunit mRNA levels in the cortex during development recall the γ/ε-subunit switch in muscle; but is this a valid analogy? Possible roles of electrical activity and trophic or growth factors (in particular NGF) in these regulations deserve investigation. The same (or different) regulatory signals may also intervene, together with ACh, in the course of synaptogenesis and play important roles in the epigenetic selection of synapses such as barrel formation of the somatosensory cortex (Juliano et al. 1991) and ocular dominance columns in the visual cortex (Singer 1985; Maffei and Galli-Resta 1990; Griesbeck et al; Riddle et al.; both this volume). Spontaneous electrical activity of the developing networks has long been suggested to participate in these epigenetic processes (see Changeux and Danchin 1976; Singer 1985; Stryker, this volume). It is interesting to note, in this respect, that spontaneous electrical activity invades the retina early in development (Maffei and Galli-Resta 1990) and requires nicotinic transmission (Feller et al. 1996).

The molecular biology of brain nAChR has opened many new avenues in the understanding of the neurobiology of cognitive processes. In this respect, the attempt to model formal, although neurally plausible, networks passing cognitive tasks (like the delayed-response tasks) has at least the virtue to demonstrate that understanding the role of neurotransmitter receptors in learning requires, first, a knowledge of their intrinsic functional properties. However, it also requires the description of their precise localization within a rather complex, albeit defined, architecture that includes several levels of organization, multiple sets of interconnected "groups" of neurons, and accessibility to reward mechanisms.

Finally, in recent years, several compelling observations have underlined that alterations of nAChR structure and distribution may plausibly underlie major brain dysfunctions in humans. In aged persons and Alzheimer's patients, a differential loss of neuronal nAChR takes place, and nicotine improves their performance in cognitive learning tasks (see above, "Nicotine Receptors in Learning and Reward"). In addition, a missense mutation in nAChR α4 subunit has been recently found associated with autosomal dominant nocturnal frontal lobe epilepsy; moreover, the mutation is located at the precise amino acid position (Steinlein et al. 1995) whose labeling by chlorpromazine resulted in the first recognition that transmembrane segment M2 is a component of the ion channel (Giraudat et al. 1986; Hucho et al. 1986). These are a few of many recent examples. Studies on the contribution of nAChR to brain dysfunctions have started. Their scientific future appears most promising.

ACKNOWLEDGMENTS

This work was supported by research grants from the Association Française contre les Myopathies, Collège de France, the Centre National de la Recherche Scientifique, the Institut National de la Santé et de la Recherche Médicale, the Direction des Recherches Etudes et Techniques, Human Frontiers, and EEC Biotech and Biomed.

REFERENCES

Agnati, L.F., M. Zoli, I. Strömberg, and K. Fuxe. 1995. Intercellular communication in the brain: Wiring versus volume transmission. *Neuroscience* **69:** 711.

Amador, M. and J. Dani. 1995. Mechanisms for modulation of nicotinic acetylcholine receptors that can influence synaptic transmission. *J. Neurosci.* **15:** 4525.

Baik, J., R. Picetti, A. Saiardi, G. Thiriet, A. Dierich, A. Depaulis, M. Le Meur, and X.E. Borrelli. 1995. Parkinsonian-like locomotor impairment in mice lacking dopamine D2 receptors. *Nature* **377:** 424.

Ballivet, M., C. Alliod, S. Bertrand, and D. Bertrand. 1996. Nicotinic acetylcholine receptors in the nematode *Caenorhabditis elegans*. *J. Mol. Biol.* **258:** 261.

Barto, A.G., R.S. Sutton, and C.W. Anderson. 1983. Neuron like adaptive elements that can solve difficult learning and control problems. *IEEE Trans. Syst. Man.Cybern.* **13:** 834.

Bertrand, D. and J.P. Changeux. 1995. Nicotinic receptor: An allosteric protein specialized for intercellular communication. *Semin. Neurosci.* **7:** 75.

Bertrand, D., J.L. Galzi, A. Devillers-Thiéry, S. Bertrand, and J.P. Changeux. 1993. Mutations at two distinct sites within the channel domain M2 alter calcium permeability of neuronal alpha7 nicotinic receptor. *Proc. Natl. Acad. Sci.* **90:** 6971.

Bessereau, J.L., D. Mendelzon, C. Le Poupon, M. Fiszman, J.P. Changeux, and J. Piette. 1993. Muscle specific expression of the acetylcholine receptor α subunit gene requires both positive and negative interaction between myogenic factors Sp1 and GBF factors. *EMBO J.* **12:** 443.

Bessis, A. 1993. "Régulation de l'expression des gènes des sous-unités des récepteurs nicotiniques de l'acétylcholine dans le système nerveux." Ph.D. thesis, Université Paris.

Bessis, A., N. Savatier, A. Devillers-Thiéry, S. Béjamin, and J.P. Changeux. 1993. Negative regulatory elements upstream of a novel exon of the neuronal nicotinic acetylcholine receptor alpha2 subunit gene. *Nucleic Acids Res.* **21:** 2185.

Bessis, A., D. Simon-Chazottes, A. Devillers-Thiéry, J.L.

Guénet, and J.P. Changeux. 1990. Chromosomal localization of the mouse genes coding for α-2, 3, 4 and β-2 subunits of neuronal nicotinic acetylcholine receptor. *FEBS Lett.* **264:** 48.

Bessis, A., A.M. Salmon, M. Zoli, N. Le Novère, M. Picciotto, and J.P. Changeux. 1995. Promoter elements confering neuron specific expression of the beta-2-subunit of the neuronal nicotinic acetylcholine receptor studied in vitro and in transgenic mice. *Neuroscience* **69:** 807.

Biomed EEC Activity Report. 1995. Neuronal acetylcholine nicotinic receptors in the brain: Interactions with dopaminergic receptors. Cee, Brussels.

Boulter, J., K. Evans, D. Goldman, G. Martin, D. Treco, S. Heinemann, and J. Patrick. 1986. Isolation of a cDNA clone coding for a possible neural nicotinic acetylcholine receptor alpha-subunit. *Nature* **319:** 368.

Boulter, J., A. O'Shea-Greenfield, R.M. Duvoisin, J.G. Connolly, E. Wada, A. Jensen, P.D. Gardner, M. Ballivet, E.S. Deneris, D. McKinnon, S. Heinemann, and J. Patrick. 1990. Alpha 3, alpha 5, and beta 4: Three members of the rat neuronal nicotinic acetylcholine receptor-related gene family form a gene cluster. *J. Biol. Chem.* **265:** 4472.

Cachelin, A.B. and R. Jaggi. 1991. Beta subunits determine the time course of desensitization in rat alpha 3 neuronal nicotinic acetylcholine receptors. *Pflügers Arch.* **419:** 579.

Changeux, J.P. 1990. Functional architecture and dynamics of the nicotinic acetylcholine receptor: An allosteric ligand-gated ion channel. *Fidia Res. Found. Neurosci. Award Lect.* **4:** 21.

———. 1993. A critical view of neuronal models of learning and memory. In *Memory concepts: Basic and clinical aspects* (ed. P.O. Andersen et al.), p. 413. Elsevier Science, New York.

Changeux, J.P. and A. Danchin. 1976. Selective stabilization of developing synapses as a mechanism for the specification of neuronal networks. *Nature* **264:** 705.

Changeux, J.P., M. Kasai, and C.Y. Lee. 1970. The use of a snake venom toxin to characterize the cholinergic receptor protein. *Proc. Natl. Acad. Sci.* **67:** 1241.

Clarke, P.B.S. 1993. Nicotinic receptors in mammalian brain: Localization and relation to cholinergic function. *Prog. Brain Res.***98:** 77.

Connolly, J.G., A.J. Gibb, and D. Colquhoun. 1995. Heterogeneity of neuronal nicotinic acetylcholine receptors in thin slices of rat medial habenula. *J. Physiol.* **484:** 87.

Corringer, P.J., J.L. Galzi, J.L. Eiselé, S. Bertrand, J.P. Changeux, and D. Bertrand. 1995. Identification of a new component of the agonist binding site of the nicotinic alpha 7 homooligomeric receptor. *J. Biol. Chem.* **270:** 11749.

Czajkowski, C. and A. Karlin. 1995. Structure of the nicotinic receptor acetylcholine-binding site. *J. Biol. Chem.* **270:** 3160.

Dani, J.A. and S. Heinemann. 1996. Molecular and cellular aspects of nicotine abuse. *Neuron* **16:** 905.

Dani, J.A. and M. Mayer. 1995. Structure and function of glutamate and nicotinic acetylcholine receptors. *Curr. Opin. Neurobiol.* **5:** 310.

Daubas, P., A. Devillers-Thiéry, B. Geoffroy, S. Martinez, A. Bessis, and J.P. Changeux. 1990. Differential expression of the neuronal acetylcholine receptor α-2 subunit gene during chick brain development as detected by *in situ* hybridization and cDNA amplification. *Neuron* **5:** 49.

Daubas, P., A.M. Salmon, M. Zoli, B. Geoffroy, A. Devillers-Thiéry, A. Bessis, F. Médevielle, and J.P. Changeux. 1993. Chicken neuronal acetylcholine receptor alpha 2 subunit gene exhibits neuron-specific expression in the brain and spinal cord of transgenic mice. *Proc. Natl. Acad. Sci.* **90:** 2237.

Dehaene, S. and J.P. Changeux. 1989. A simple model of prefrontal cortex function in delayed-response tasks. *J. Cogn. Neurosci.* **1:** 244.

———. 1991. The Wisconsin card sorting test: Theoretical analysis and simulation of a reasoning task in a model neuronal network. *Cereb. Cortex* **1:** 62.

Duclert, A. and J.P. Changeux. 1995. Acetylcholine receptor gene expression at the developing neuromuscular junction. *Physiol. Rev.* **75:** 339.

Edelman, G. and G. Tononi. 1996. Selection and development: The brain as a complex system. In *Behavioral, neurobiological and psychosocial perspectives* (ed. T.G.D. Magnusson et al.), p. 107. Cambridge University Press.

Edelstein, S., O. Schaad, E. Henry, D. Bertrand, and J.P. Changeux. 1996. A kinetic mechanism for nicotinic acetylcholine receptors based on multiple allosteric transitions. *Biol. Cybern.* (in press).

Eiselé, J.L., S. Bertrand, J.L. Galzi, A. Devillers-Thiéry, J.P. Changeux, and D. Bertrand. 1993. Chimaeric nicotinic-serotonergic receptor combines distinct ligand binding and channel specificities. *Nature* **366:** 479.

Feller, M.B., D.P. Wellis, D. Stellwagen, F.S. Werblin, and C.J. Shatz. 1996. Requirement for cholinergic synaptic transmission in the propagation of spontaneous retinal waves. *Science* **272:** 1182.

Galzi, J.L. and J.P. Changeux. 1995. Neuronal nicotinic receptors: Molecular organization and regulations. *Neuropharmacology* **34:** 563.

Galzi, J.L., S.J. Edelstein, and J.P. Changeux. 1996a. The multiple phenotypes of allosteric receptor mutants. *Proc. Natl. Acad. Sci.* **93:** 1853.

Galzi, J.L., S. Bertrand, P.J. Corringer, J.P. Changeux, and D. Bertrand. 1996b. Identification of calcium binding sites which regulate potentiation of a neuronal nicotinic acetylcholine receptor. *EMBO J.* (in press).

Giraudat, J., M. Dennis, T. Heidmann, J.Y. Chang, and J.P. Changeux. 1986. Structure of the high affinity site for noncompetitive blockers of the acetylcholine receptor: Serine-262 of the delta subunit is labeled by [3H]-chlorpromazine. *Proc. Natl. Acad. Sci.* **83:** 2719.

Granon, S., B. Poucet, C. Thinus-Blanc, J.P. Changeux, and C. Vidal. 1995. Nicotinic and muscarinic receptors in the rat prefrontal cortex: Differential roles in working memory, response selection, and effortful processing. *Psychopharmacology* **119:** 139.

Granon, S., C. Vidal, C. Thinus-Blanc, J.P. Changeux, and B. Poucet. 1994. Working memory, response selection and effortful processing in rats with medial, prefrontal lesions. *Behav. Neurosci.* **108:** 883.

Heidmann, T. and J.P. Changeux. 1982. Un modèle moléculaire de régulation d'efficacité d'une synapse chimique au niveau postsynaptique. *C.R. Acad. Sci.* **295:** 665.

Hill, J.A., M. Zoli, J.P. Bourgeois, and J.P. Changeux. 1993. Immunocytochemical localization of a neuronal nicotinic receptor: The beta2 subunit. *J. Neurosci.* **13:** 1551.

Hucho, F., W. Oberthür, and F. Lottspeich. 1986. The ion channel of the nicotinic acetylcholine receptor is formed by the homologous helices M2 of the receptor subunits. *FEBS Lett.* **205:** 137.

Huganir, R.L. and P. Greengard. 1990. Regulation of neurotransmitter receptor desensibilization by protein phosphorylation. *Neuron* **5:** 555.

Hyman, S. 1996. Addiction to cocaine and amphetamine. *Neuron* **16:** 901.

Imoto, K., C. Busch, B. Sackmann, M. Mishina, T. Konno, J. Nakai, H. Bujo, Y. Mori, K. Fukuda, and S. Numa. 1988. Rings of negatively charged amino acids determine the acetylcholine receptor channel conductance. *Nature* **335:** 645.

Juliano, S.L., W. Ma, and D. Eslin. 1991. Cholinergic depletion prevents expansion of topographic maps in somatosensory cortex. *Proc. Natl. Acad. Sci.* **88:** 780.

Karlin, A. 1993. Structure of nicotinic acetylcholine receptors. *Curr. Opin. Neurobiol.* **3:** 299.

Karlin, A. and M. Akabas. 1996. Toward a structural basis for the function of the nicotinic acetylcholine receptors and their cousins. *Neuron* **15:** 1231.

Kerszberg, M. and J.P. Changeux. 1993. A model for motor endplate morphogenesis: Diffusible morphogens, transmembrane signalling and compartmentalized gene expression. *Neural Computation* **5:** 341.

———. 1994. A model for reading morphogenetic gradients: Autocatalysis and competition at the gene level. *Proc. Natl. Acad. Sci.* **91:** 5823.

Koob, G. 1996. Drug addiction: The yin and yang of hedonic homeostasis. *Neuron* **16:** 893.

Langley, J.N. 1906. On nerve endings and special excitable substances in cells. *Proc. R. Soc.* **78:** 170.

Lauder, J.M. 1993. Neurotransmitters as growth regulatory signals: Role of receptors and second messengers. *Trends Neurosci.* **16:** 233.

Léna, C. and J.P. Changeux. 1993. Allosteric modulations of the nicotinic acetylcholine receptor. *Trends Neurosci.* **16:** 181.

———. 1996. Role of Ca^{2+} ions in nicotinic facilitation of GABA release in mouse thalamus. *J. Neurosci.* **17:** (in press).

Léna, C., J.P. Changeux, and C. Mulle. 1993. Evidence for "Preterminal" nicotinic receptors on GABAergic axons in the rat interpeduncular nucleus. *J. Neurosci.* **13:** 2680.

Le Novère, N. and J.P. Changeux. 1995. Molecular evolution of the nicotinic acetylcholine receptor: An example of multigene family in excitable cells. *J. Mol. Evol.* **40:** 155.

Le Novère, N., M. Zoli, and J.P. Changeux. 1996. Neuronal nicotinic receptor alpha-6 subunit mRNA is selectively concentrated in catecholaminergic nuclei of the rat brain. *Eur. J. Neurosci.* (in press).

Levin, E.D. 1992. Nicotinic systems and cognitive function. *Psychopharmacology* **108:** 417.

Li, X.M., M. Zoli, U.B. Finnman, L. Novère, J.P. Changeux, and K. Fuxe. 1995. A single (–)-nicotine injection causes change with a time delay in the affinity of striatal D2 receptors for antagonist, but not for agonist, nor in the D2 receptor mRNA levels in the rat substantia nigra. *Brain Res.* **679:** 157.

Lujan, R., Z. Nusser, J.D.B. Roberts, R. Shigemoto, and P. Somogyi. 1996. Perisynaptic location of metabotropic glutamate receptors mGluR1 and MGluR5 on dendrites and dendritic spines in the rat hippocampus. *Eur. J. Neurosci.* **8:** 1488.

Maffei, L. and L. Galli-Resta. 1990. Correlation in the discharges of neighboring rat retinal ganglion cells during prenatal life. *Proc. Natl. Acad. Sci.* **87:** 2861.

Marks, M.J., J.R. Pauly, S.D. Gross, E.S. Deneris, I. Hermans-Borgmeyer, S.F. Heinemann, and A.C. Collins. 1992. Nicotine binding and nicotinic receptor subunit RNA after chronic nicotine treatment. *J. Neurosci.* **12:** 2765.

Matter, J.M., L. Matter-Sadzinski, and M. Ballivet. 1995. Activity of the beta-3 nicotinic receptor promoter is a marker of neuron fate determination during retina development. *J. Neurosci.* **15:** 5919.

McGehee, D.S. and L. Role. 1996. Presynaptic ionotropic receptors. *Curr. Opin. Neurobiol.* **6:** 342.

McGehee, D.S., M. Heath, S. Gelber, P. Devay, and L.W. Role. 1995. Nicotine enhancement of fast excitatory synaptic transmission in CNS by presynaptic receptors. *Science* **269:** 1692.

McMahon, L.L., K.W. Yoon, and V.A. Chiappinelli. 1994a. Nicotinic receptor activation facilitates GABAergic neurotransmission in the avian lateral spiriform nucleus. *Neuroscience* **59:** 689.

———. 1994b. Electrophysiological evidence for presynaptic nicotinic receptors in the avian ventral lateral geniculate nucleus. *J. Neurophysiol.* **71:** 826.

Milton, N., A. Bessis, J.P. Changeux, and D.S. Latchman. 1995. The neuronal nicotinic acetylcholine receptor alpha 2 subunit gene promoter is activated by the Brn-3b POU family transcription factor and not by Brn-3a or Brn-3c. *J. Biol. Chem.* **270:** 15143.

Mishina, M., T. Takai, K. Imoto, M. Noda, T. Takahashi, S. Numa, C. Methfessel, and B. Sakmann. 1986. Molecular distinction between fetal and adult forms of muscle acetylcholine receptor. *Nature* **321:** 406.

Montague, P.R., P. Dayan, and T.J. Sejnowski. 1996. A framework for mesencephalic dopamine systems based on predictive Hebbian learning. *J. Neurosci.* **16:** 1936.

Mulle, C. and J.P. Changeux. 1990. A novel type of nicotinic receptor in the rat central nervous system characterized by patch-clamp techniques. *J. Neurosci.* **10:** 169.

Mulle, C., C. Léna, and J.P. Changeux. 1992a. Potentiation of nicotinic receptor response by external calcium in rat central neurons. *Neuron* **8:** 937.

Mulle, C., D. Choquet, H. Korn, and J.P. Changeux. 1992b. Calcium influx through nicotinic receptor in rat central neurons: Its relevance to cellular regulation. *Neuron* **8:** 135.

Mulle, C., C. Vidal, P. Benoit, and J.P. Changeux. 1991. Existence of different subtypes of nicotinic acetylcholine receptors in the rat habenulo interpeduncular system. *J. Neurosci.* **11:** 2588.

Nordberg, A. and B. Winblad. 1986. Reduced number of 3H-nicotine and 3H-acetylcholine binding sites in the frontal cortex of Alzheimer brains. *Neurosci. Lett.* **72:** 307.

Numa, S., M. Noda, H. Takahashi, T. Tanabe, M. Toyosato, Y. Furutani, and S. Kikyotani. 1983. Molecular structure of the nicotinic acetylcholine receptor. *Cold Spring Harbor Symp. Quant. Biol.* **48:** 57.

Ortells, M. and G. Lunt. 1995. Evolutionary history of the ligand-gated ion channel superfamily of receptors. *Trends Neurosci.* **18:** 121.

Picciotto, M., M. Zoli, C. Léna, A. Bessis, Y. Lallemand, N. Le Novère, P. Vincent, E. Merlo Pich, P. Brûlet, and J.P. Changeux. 1995. Abnormal avoidance learning in mice lacking functional high-affinity nicotine receptor in the brain. *Nature* **374:** 65.

Pontieri, F.E., G. Tanda, F. Orzi, and G. Di Chiara. 1996. Effects of nicotine on the nucleus accumbens and similarity to those of addictive drugs. *Nature* **382:** 255.

Pugh, P.C. and D.K. Berg. 1994. Neuronal acetylcholine receptors that bind alpha-bungarotoxin mediate neurite retraction in a calcium-dependent manner. *J. Neurosci.* **14:** 889.

Ramirez-Latorre, J., C.R. Yu, X. Qu, F. Perin, A. Karlin, and L. Role. 1996. Functional contributions of alpha 5 subunit to neuronal acetylcholine receptor channels. *Nature* **380:** 347.

Révah, F., D. Bertrand, J.L. Galzi, A. Devillers-Thiéry, C. Mulle, N. Hussy, S. Bertrand, M. Ballivet, and J.P. Changeux. 1991. Mutations in the channel domain alter desensitization of a neuronal nicotinic receptor. *Nature* **353:** 846.

Role, L. and D. Berg. 1996. Nicotinic receptors in the development and modulation of CNS synapses. *Neuron* **16:** 1077.

Sargent, P.B. 1993. The diversity of neuronal nicotinic acetylcholine receptors. *Annu. Rev. Neurosci.* **16:** 403.

Singer, W. 1985. Activity-dependent self-organization of synaptic connections as a substrate of learning. In *Dahlem Workshop: Neural molecular basis of learning* (ed. J.P. Changeux and M. Konishi), p. 301. Wiley, Chichester, United Kingdom.

Steinlein, O., J. Mulley, P. Propping, R. Wallace, H. Philipps, G. Sutherland, I. Scheffer, and S. Berkovic. 1995. A missense mutation in the neuronal nicotinic acetylcholine receptor alpha 4 subunit is associated with autosomal dominant nocturnal frontal lobe epilepsy. *Nat. Genet.* **11:** 201.

Stolerman, I.P., N.R. Mirza, and M. Shoaib. 1995. Nicotine psychopharmacology: Addiction, cognition, and neuroadaptation. *Med. Res. Rev.* **15:** 47.

Umbriaco, D., K.C. Watkins, L. Descarries, C. Cozzari, and B.K. Hartman. 1994. Ultrastructural and morphometric features of the acetylcholine innervation in adult rat parietal cortex: An electron microscopic study in serial sections. *J. Comp. Neurol.* **348:** 351.

Unwin, N. 1995. Acetylcholine receptor channel imaged in the open state. *Nature* **373:** 37.

Vernino, M.A., C.W. Luetje, J. Patrick, and J.A. Dani. 1992. Calcium modulation and high calcium permeability of nicotinic acetylcholine receptors. *Neuron* **8:** 127.

Vidal, C. 1994. Nicotinic potentiation of glutamatergic synapses in the prefrontal cortex: New insight into the analysis of the role of nicotinic receptors in cognitive functions. *Drug Dev. Res.* **31:** 120.

Vidal, C. and J.P. Changeux. 1989. Pharmacological profile of nicotinic acetylcholine receptors in the rat prefrontal cortex: An electrophysiological study in a slice preparation. *Neuroscience* **29:** 261.

———. 1993. Nicotinic and muscarinic modulations of excitatory synaptic transmission in the rat prefrontal cortex in vitro. *Neuroscience* **56:** 23.

Wada, E., K. Wada, J. Boulter, E. Deneris, S. Heinemann, J. Patrick, and L.W. Swanson. 1989. Distribution of alpha2, alpha3, alpha4, and beta2 neuronal nicotinic receptor subunit mRNAs in the central nervous system: A hybridization histochemical study in the rat. *J. Comp. Neurol.* **284:** 314.

Wang, F., V. Gerzanich, G.B. Wells, R. Anand, X. Peng, K. Keyser, and J. Lindstrom. 1996. Assembly of human neuronal nicotinic receptor $\alpha5$ subunits with $\alpha3$, $\beta2$ and $\beta4$ subunits. *J. Biol. Chem.* **271:** 17656.

Wegner, M., D.W. Drolet, and M.G. Rosenfeld. 1993. POU-domain proteins: Structure and function of developmental regulators. *Curr. Opin. Cell Biol.* **5:** 488.

Winkler, J., S.T. Suhr, F.H. Gage, L.J. Thai, and L.J. Fisher. 1995. Essential role of neocortical acetylcholine in spatial memory. *Nature* **375:** 484.

Wonnacott, S., G. Wilkie, L. Soliakov, and P. Whiteaker. 1995. Presynaptic nicotinic autoreceptors and heteroreceptors in the CNS. *Adv. Pharmacol. Sci.* **2:** 87.

Zheng, J.Q., M. Felder, J.A. Connor, and M.-M. Poo. 1994. Turning of nerve growth cones induced by neurotransmitters. *Nature* **368:** 140.

Zoli, M., N. Le Novère, J. Hill, and J.P. Changeux. 1995. Developmental regulation of nicotinic receptor subunit mRNAs in the rat central and peripheral nervous system. *J. Neurosci.* **15:** 1912.

Zoli, M., L.F. Agnati, P. Hedlund, X.M. Li, S. Ferré, and K. Fuxe. 1993. Receptor-receptor interactions as an integrative mechanism in nerve cells. *Mol. Neurobiol.* **7:** 293.

The Nicotinic Acetylcholine Receptor at the Neuromuscular Junction: Assembly and Tyrosine Phosphorylation

Z.-Z. WANG, C. FUHRER, S. SHTROM,[1] J.E. SUGIYAMA, M.J. FERNS,[2] AND Z.W. HALL

National Institutes of Mental Health, National Institutes of Health, Bethesda, Maryland 20892; [1]Department of Physiology, University of California at San Francisco, San Francisco, California 94143

Rapid signaling at chemical synapses in the nervous system is mediated by a family of ligand-gated ion channels that are concentrated in the postsynaptic membrane beneath the nerve terminal. At each synapse, the neurotransmitter released by presynaptic activation binds one or more specific receptors in the postsynaptic membrane and causes the ion channels to open; the resulting current across the postsynaptic membrane is responsible for the synaptic potential. Although particular synapses use different neurotransmitters, the ion channels that act as receptors for these transmitters have similar structures and a similar disposition in the postsynaptic membrane (Unwin 1993). All are constructed of five highly homologous transmembrane subunits that surround a central aqueous pore through the membrane that serves as the ion channel. A characteristic feature of these receptors is their localization and concentration beneath the nerve terminal, where they form part of a specialized postsynaptic structure (Hall and Sanes 1993). Although the molecular structure of a wide variety of subunits of neurotransmitter receptors is known, relatively little is known about how the subunits are assembled to form oligomers of defined composition, and how they are modified during the formation of the postsynaptic membrane.

The nicotinic acetylcholine receptor (AChR) at the adult neuromuscular junction is formed of four subunits in the molecular ratio, $\alpha_2\beta\gamma\delta$ (Karlin and Akabas 1995). Each of the subunits has a characteristic transmembrane topology in which a long amino-terminal extracellular domain is followed by three transmembrane domains, an intracellular cytoplasmic loop, a fourth transmembrane domain, and a short carboxy-terminal tail (Karlin 1993). The AChR has two acetylcholine (ACh) binding sites that are associated with each of the α subunits and are thought to lie at or near the interface of the α subunits and the γ or δ subunits, respectively (Karlin and Akabas 1995).

The AChR subunits are synthesized as separate polypeptide chains and are assembled in the endoplasmic reticulum (ER) following signal sequence cleavage, core glycosylation, and folding. The intact AChR is then transported to the Golgi apparatus, where fatty acid acylation and complex carbohydrate modification take place, and finally, it becomes incorporated into the surface membrane. The entire process is remarkably slow: Folding of the α subunit, which is required for α-bungarotoxin binding, takes approximately 15 minutes; assembly takes approximately 30 minutes; and the appearance of surface AChRs takes approximately 90 minutes (Merlie and Smith 1986).

At the mature synapse, the AChR is concentrated in the postsynaptic membrane in an almost crystalline array (Fertuck and Salpeter 1976), where it is associated with a specialized postsynaptic apparatus (Hall and Sanes 1993). Although many components of this apparatus have been identified (Froehner 1993), the functions of all of the components and the mechanism that ultimately leads to the aggregation of AChRs is incompletely understood. In cultured muscle cells, AChRs are diffusely distributed on the cell surface, but aggregate upon coculture with nerves, or with the addition of agrin, a neurally derived factor (McMahan 1990). Our experiments focus on two aspects of the AChR: the mechanism by which the subunits fold and assemble to form the intact AChR; and tyrosine phosphorylation of the AChR, a modification that is most likely involved in its redistribution during synapse formation.

RESULTS

AChR Assembly

We and other investigators have previously established that the mature AChR is assembled in the ER by a defined pathway in which the first step is the formation of the two heterodimers, αδ and αγ (Fig. 1A) (Blount et al. 1990; Gu et al. 1991; Saedi et al. 1991). Each of these heterodimers has a high-affinity ligand-binding site that corresponds to one of the two ACh-binding sites in the fully assembled AChR (Blount and Merlie 1989; Karlin and Akabas 1995). On the basis of results from dominant-negative experiments using chimeric subunits, we postulated that recognition between the αδ and αγ subunits and the initial steps of heterodimer assembly are mediated by

[2]Present address: Montreal General Hospital Research Institute, 1650 Cedar Avenue, Montreal, Quebec, Canada H3G 1A4.

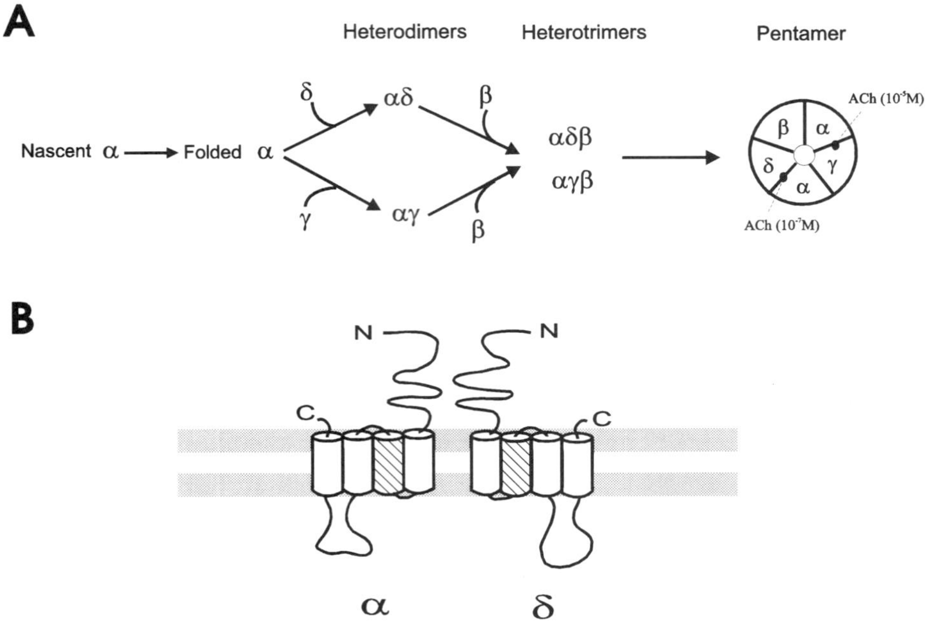

Figure 1. (*A*) Pathway of AChR assembly and formation of the two ligand-binding sites at the αδ and αγ interfaces. The folded α subunit first interacts with δ and γ subunits to form heterodimers. The addition of the β subunit creates a heterotrimer and, ultimately, the final pentameric structure containing a pore and two ligand-binding sites. (*B*) Schematic of α and δ subunits within the membrane. αδ and αγ heterodimer formation requires recognition and interaction between the amino-terminal luminal domains of the subunits. The shaded transmembrane region represents the pore-forming domain for each subunit.

the amino-terminal domains of the subunits within the ER lumen (Fig. 1B) (Yu and Hall 1991, 1994a; Verrall and Hall 1992). Recent experiments by Kreienkamp et al. (1995) have narrowed the region of the γ subunit that is critical for the specificity of assembly to amino acids 21–131 in the amino-terminal domain.

Initially, we attempted to study the folding and association of the α and δ subunits by expressing truncated amino-terminal domains of these subunits separately in bacteria (S. Hardy and Z. Hall, unpubl.). The bacterially expressed subunits were solubilized by extraction under denaturing conditions, followed by slow renaturation and oxidation. However, we were unable to achieve either correct folding, as measured by binding of α-bungarotoxin to the α subunit, or association between the amino-terminal domains, as measured by coimmunoprecipitation. To gain a better understanding of AChR folding and assembly, we have thus developed two expression systems that allow us to manipulate the maturation process: in vitro translation of subunits and transient transfection of heterologous cells.

The α Subunit Folds and Forms a Heterodimer in an In Vitro Translation System

To investigate the requirements for folding of the α subunit, we expressed it in a conventional in vitro translation system, using mRNA encoding the α subunit, a rabbit reticulocyte lysate, and dog pancreas microsomes (Shtrom and Hall 1996). Under suitable redox conditions, approximately 15% of the α subunit folded correctly. Folding of the subunit occurred with a lag time of approximately 15 minutes (Fig. 2A,B), consistent with that observed in vivo, and yielded a stable, monomeric product. When expressed with the δ subunit, a heterodimer containing a high-affinity ligand-binding site was formed. Although folding of the α subunit required glycosylation, inhibitors of the oligosaccharide-trimming reactions did not have an effect on α subunit folding or assembly (summarized in Table 1). This latter observation suggests that chaperones, such as calnexin, which have been shown to assist in the folding of viral glycoproteins by binding to trimmed oligosaccharides, may not be required for α subunit folding. Indeed, immunoprecipitation experiments showed that although the unfolded α subunit binds resident ER proteins such as BiP, calnexin, and protein disulfide isomerase, these complexes are stable, not transient, and are thus unlikely to play a role in α subunit folding (S. Shtrom and Z. Hall, unpubl.).

The Amino-terminal Domain of the α Subunit Folds In Vivo, but Must Be Tethered to the ER Membrane to Associate with the δ Subunit

When expressed in COS cells in the absence of other subunits, the α subunit folds, acquires α-bungarotoxin-binding capability, and remains in the ER,

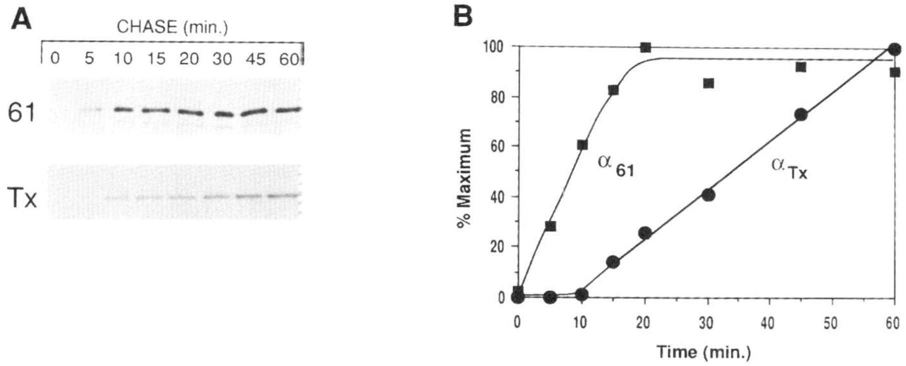

Figure 2. The newly synthesized α subunit folds with a delay. (*A*) Kinetics of α subunit synthesis and α-bungarotoxin (Tx) binding. The α subunit was synthesized in vitro in the presence of [^{35}S]methionine for 10 min (pulse) and with excess unlabeled methionine for various times thereafter (chase). At the times indicated during the chase period, aliquots from the translation reaction were analyzed via immunoprecipitation with MAb61 (61) and toxin-binding (Tx). The upper band precipitated with MAb61 corresponds to the mature, glycosylated subunit, and the lower band corresponds to the unglycosylated subunit with the signal sequence removed. The fluorograms showing MAb61 immunoprecipitation and BTX-binding were exposed for different lengths of time. (*B*) Quantitation of the fluorograms shown in *A*. Results were quantitated using a phosphorimager. (Data reproduced, with permission, from Shtrom and Hall 1996.)

but does not bind ligands such as ACh. However, when coexpressed with the δ subunit, it forms a heterodimer with a high-affinity ligand-binding site (Blount and Merlie 1989; Blount et al. 1990; Gu et al. 1991; Saedi et al. 1991). To determine the minimal domain of the α subunit required for folding and heterodimer assembly, we constructed a series of truncated amino-terminal α subunit fragments (diagrammed in Fig. 3): α211, containing the entire amino-terminal, luminal domain; α216, extending partially into the first transmembrane domain; and αM1, containing the entire first transmembrane region of the α subunit (Wang et al. 1996a). Each of these folded to acquire toxin-binding activity (Fig. 3), but α207, lacking the last four amino acids of the amino-terminal, luminal domain, did not. Thus, the entire luminal amino terminus is required for proper folding. We found, however, that only αM1 was capable of forming a heterodimer with the δ subunit (Fig. 3). On the basis of these results, we tested whether the first transmembrane domain of the α subunit contained information required for association with the δ subunit. We constructed and assayed chimeras in which α211 was fused to the transmembrane domain of the vesicular stomatitis virus (VSV) G protein or to the lymphocyte surface protein, CD8 (Fig. 3). Both chimeras folded, were retained in the ER, and formed heterodimers containing high-affinity ligand-binding sites (Wang et al. 1996b). These chimeric ligand-binding characteristics were identical to those of wild-type α-δ heterodimers.

Table 1. Folding of the α Subunit in an In Vitro Translation System

10–15% of α subunit folds to bind α-bungarotoxin
Folded subunit is monomeric and assumes native conformation based on affinity for α-bungarotoxin and cholinergic ligands
Folding requires an oxidizing environment and glycosylation
Folding does not requires oligosaccharide trimming
Conformationally mature α subunit associates specifically with the δ subunit to form a ligand-binding site
The unfolded α subunit forms long-lived complexes with BiP, calnexin, and protein disulfide isomerase

Data from Shtrom and Hall (1996).

We next examined the inability of α211 to form a heterodimer. We found that unlike αM1 or the chimeric α subunits which can form heterodimers, α211 was secreted into the medium. To determine if retention in the ER would enable α211 to form a heterodimer, we treated cells expressing α211 with brefeldin A, a drug that prevents transport from the ER to the Golgi (Klausner et al. 1992). Even under these conditions, α211 was unable to form a heterodimer with the δ subunit (Fig. 4). We then tested whether tethering of α211 to the membrane via a glycolipid anchor would enable it to form a heterodimer. We expressed a chimeric protein (α211-HPAP) by fusing α211 to the carboxy-terminal domain of human placental alkaline phosphatase (HPAP), which contains a glycosylphosphatidylinositol (GPI) attachment and cleavage site (Lin et al. 1990). Cleavage of the GPI anchor by treatment of cells with phosphatidylinositol-specific phospholipase C (PI-PLC) released toxin-binding activity to the medium, demonstrating that the chimeric protein folded correctly. Although it was rapidly transported to the cell surface, α211-HPAP did not form a heterodimer when coexpressed with the δ subunit (Wang et al. 1996b). When transport to the Golgi was blocked by brefeldin A, however, heterodimer formation did occur, with the formation of a high-affinity ligand-binding site (Fig. 4). Thus, these results imply that attachment to the membrane and retention in the ER are necessary for heterodimer formation between the α and δ subunits.

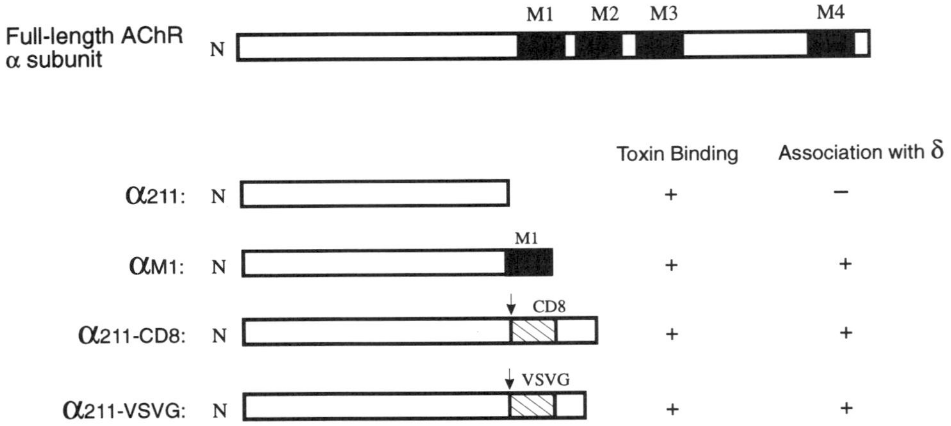

Figure 3. Schematic illustration of truncated and chimeric amino-terminal constructs of the AChR α subunit and their ability to fold and form a heterodimer with the δ subunit. Schematic illustrations of the full-length mouse AChR α subunit protein, truncated proteins encoded by α211 and αM1 cDNA, and fusion proteins encoded by a set of chimeric α subunit cDNA are shown. Hydrophobic transmembrane domains are marked by black boxes; those of the CD8 and VSV G chimeric constructs are marked by shaded boxes. Sequences derived from CD8 and VSV G are as follows: CD8, DIYIWAPLAGTCGVLLLSLVITLYCNHRN-RRRVCKCPRPVVKSGDKPSLSARYV; VSV G, SSIASFFFIIGLIIGLFLVLRVGIHLCIKLKTKKRQITDIEMNRLGK. The truncated and chimeric α subunits were assayed for their abilty to bind α-bungarotoxin and for their ability to associate with the δ subunit, as measured by the formation of a high-affinity ligand-binding site. All were able to bind toxin (+), and only α 211, which does not have a transmembrane domain, is unable to associate with the δ subunit (−). (Data from Wang et al. 1996b.)

AChR Clustering

In developing muscle fibers and in cultured myotubes, newly synthesized AChRs are diffusely distributed on the surface. When motor neurons contact the fibers, AChRs become clustered at the site of contact, along with other components of the postsynaptic apparatus (Hall and Sanes 1993). The action of the nerve in organizing and localizing the postsynaptic specializations is mediated by agrin, a proteoglycan that is synthesized and secreted by motor nerves and that becomes incorporated into the synaptic basal lamina (McMahan. 1990; Reist et al. 1992; Gautam et al. 1996). Neurons express a specific isoform of agrin, generated by alternative RNA splicing, that is much more active in clustering AChRs than isoforms found in muscle or other tissues (Ferns et al. 1992, 1993; Ruegg et al. 1992). Neural-derived agrin appears to exert its effects via a receptor tyrosine kinase, recently identified as MuSK, which then activates the AChR clustering machinery (DeChiara et al. 1996; Glass et al. 1996).

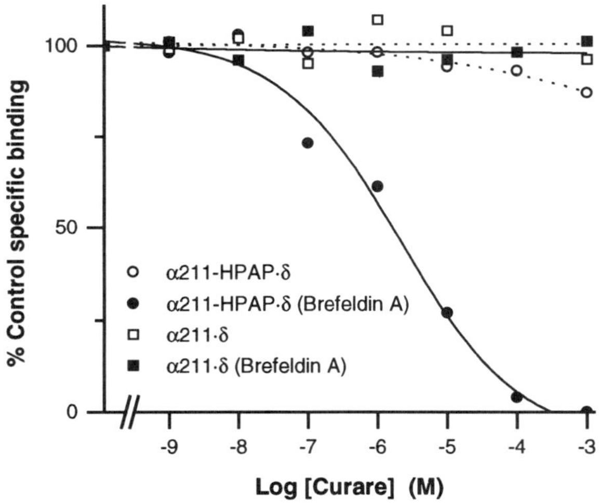

Figure 4. GPI-tethered, but not soluble, α211 assembles with the δ subunit to form a high-affinity ligand-binding site. COS cells were transfected with α211 plus δ (*squares*) or α211-HPAP plus δ (*circles*) and incubated in control growth medium (*open* symbols) or in growth medium containing 5 mg/ml brefeldin A (*filled* symbols) at 37°C for 6 hr. They were then lysed with 60 mM β-D-octylglucoside. Inhibition of ^{125}I-labeled α-bungarotoxin binding by dTC was determined as described by Blount and Merlie (1989). (Data reprinted, with permission, from Wang et al. 1996b. [copyright Rockefeller University Press])

AChRs in Mammalian Muscle are Tyrosine-phosphorylated Prior to Agrin-induced Clustering

Although the molecular mechanism by which agrin induces AChR clustering is unknown, several lines of evidence suggest that tyrosine phosphorylation is part of the signaling pathway (Qu et al. 1990; Wallace et al. 1991; Qu and Huganir 1994; Gillespie et al. 1996; Glass et al. 1996). Thus, we have examined the relationship between tyrosine phosphorylation and clustering of AChRs in mammalian muscle cells. We treated C2 myotube cultures with a biologically active, soluble form of neural agrin referred to as C-$Ag_{12,4,8}$ (Ferns et al. 1993), isolated the AChR, separated the proteins by SDS-PAGE, and immunoblotted with a phosphotyrosine antibody, 4G10. Our results showed that agrin in-

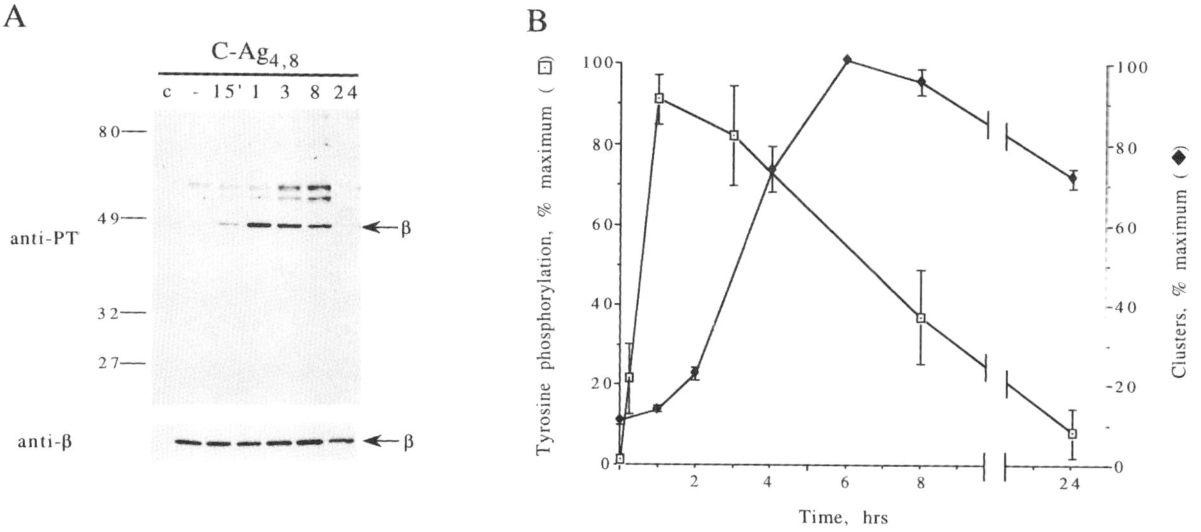

Figure 5. Time course of agrin-induced AChR phosphorylation. Agrin induces a transient tyrosine phosphorylation of the AChR. (*A*) C2 myotubes were treated with agrin for times from 15 min to 24 hr, and the AChR was purified and immunoblotted with a phosphotyrosine antibody. Agrin induces a rapid, but transient, tyrosine phosphorylation of a 49-kD band that corresponds to the β subunit. Reprobing with an anti-β-subunit antibody also confirmed that equal amounts of AChR are present in each lane. (*B*) Time course of β subunit phosphorylation compared to that of AChR clustering. Agrin-induced phosphorylation of the β subunit is rapid and peaks (1–2 hr) prior to the first formation of AChR clusters (2–4 hr). Phosphorylation is then progressively lost as the number of AChR clusters increases. (Data reproduced, with permission, from Ferns et al. 1996 [copyright Rockefeller University Press].)

duced rapid, transient tyrosine phosphorylation of the AChR β subunit (Ferns et al. 1996). Phosphorylation was detected within 15 minutes after agrin addition, peaked at approximately 1–2 hours, and steadily declined to slightly above basal levels over the next 24 hours (Fig. 5). In contrast, AChR clustering occurred more slowly, with the first clusters detected at about 2–4 hours and rising to a peak at 6 hours after agrin addition. Tyrosine phosphorylation of other receptor subunits was not detected in this system.

Agrin-induced phosphorylation of the β subunit correlated well with AChR clustering under several conditions. The dose-response curves for AChR clustering and tyrosine phosphorylation were almost identical, with activity in the picomolar range. In addition, the soluble muscle isoform of agrin, which is biologically inactive at concentrations as high as 100 nM, was likewise inactive in stimulating tyrosine phosphorylation of the AChR. Finally, genetic variants of the C2 muscle cell line that fail to respond to agrin by clustering AChRs also failed to respond when tyrosine phosphorylation of the AChR was measured (Ferns et al. 1996).

We further examined the relationship between tyrosine phosphorylation and clustering of the AChR by using tyrosine kinase inhibitors. Pretreatment of C2 myotube cultures with either 0.5 mM herbimycin A, a specific tyrosine kinase inhibitor, or 5 nM staurosporine, a more general inhibitor of protein kinases, completely blocked the induction of AChR clusters by agrin. In neither case was the overall level of AChRs affected. After removal of the inhibitors, the myotubes again became responsive to agrin. Surprisingly, we found that treatment with herbimycin or staurosporine could also cause preformed clusters to become dispersed (Ferns et al. 1996). These results suggest that tyrosine phosphorylation is required for both the formation and stability of AChR clusters and that β subunit phosphorylation may be a precursor step in the process.

Src Family Kinases Interact with the AChR

Because of the possibility that tyrosine phosphorylation of the β subunit is involved in agrin-induced AChR clustering, we wanted to identify kinases that associate with and phosphorylate the β subunit of the AChR. Src-family kinases associate with the AChR in *Torpedo* electric organ (Swope and Huganir 1993, 1994); thus, we were interested in whether they play a role in tyrosine phosphorylation of mammalian AChR. We found by immunoblotting that src, fyn, and yes (all members of the src family) are expressed in C2 myotubes (Fuhrer and Hall 1996). We then constructed glutathione-*S*-transferase (GST) fusion proteins containing all or part of the AChR β cytoplasmic loop (Fig. 6, left). Immobilized fusion proteins were incubated with C2 extracts, and bound proteins were analyzed by immunoblotting with antibodies specific for each of the src-family kinases, src, fyn, and yes, or with src-CT, an antibody that recognizes a highly conserved sequence near the end of all three kinases. None of the fusion proteins bound fyn or yes, but all of those containing the exon-9 region, which encodes the

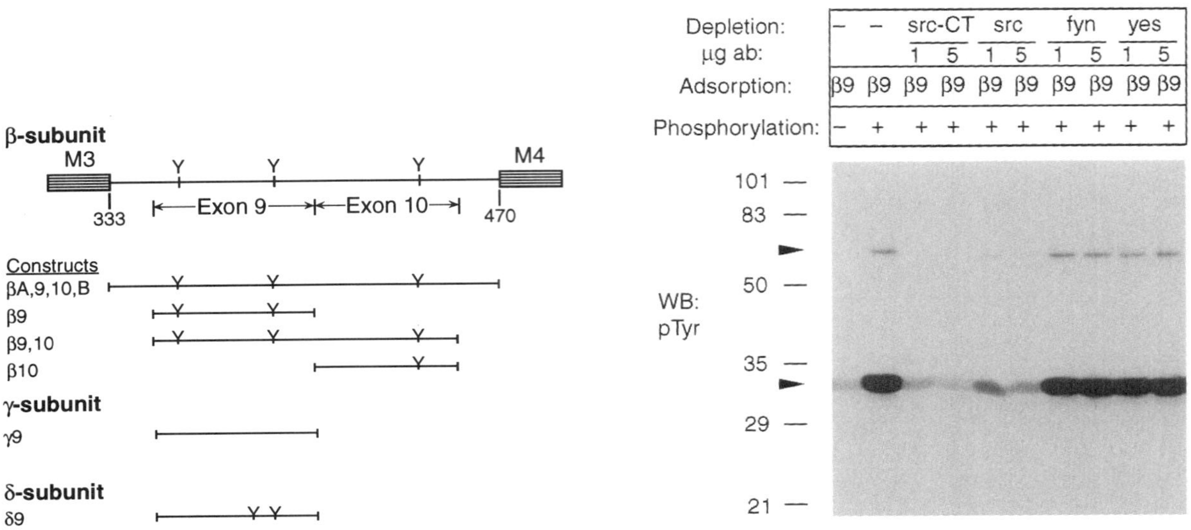

Figure 6. Construction of GST fusion proteins containing part of the AChR cytoplasmic loop and their phosphorylation by src-related kinases. (*Left*) GST fusion constructs were made with various cytoplasmic loop regions between the M3 and M4 transmembrane domains of the β, γ, and δ subunits. Tyrosine residues are noted with Y. (*Right*) Phosphorylation of β exon 9 by bound src was analyzed by adsorbing C2 lysates to immobilized fusion proteins, incubating without (–) or with (+) ATP under phosphorylating conditions, followed by SDS-PAGE and immunoblotting with a phosphotyrosine antibody. Only fusion proteins containing β exon 9 were phosphorylated; this phosphorylation was abolished by immunodepleting C2 lysates with src-specific antibodies, but not with fyn or yes antibodies. (Data reproduced, with permission, from Fuhrer and Hall 1996.)

amino-terminal half of the β cytoplasmic loop, bound src (Fuhrer and Hall 1996). This domain contains two tyrosines, one of which is conserved among species and is phosphorylated in AChRs isolated from *Torpedo*. Binding of src was specific for the β subunit, as corresponding parts of the γ or δ subunits did not bind any of the src-family kinases.

To determine if bound src is able to phosphorylate the β cytoplasmic region, complexes of β exon-9 fusion protein and bound src were incubated under conditions required for kinase activity, and the samples were analyzed by phosphotyrosine immunoblotting (Fuhrer and Hall 1996). Two tyrosine-phosphorylated proteins were detected, one of 60 kD that presumably represents src kinase, and another of 34 kD that corresponds to the β subunit fusion protein (Fig. 6, right). Again, only fusion proteins containing the β exon-9 region were phosphorylated. We then used immunodepletion experiments to determine the proportion of phosphorylating activity in C2 extracts corresponding to src. Adsorption of the C2 extracts with antibodies specific for src virtually abolished phosphorylation (Fig. 6, right). However, adsorption with fyn or yes antibodies had no effect. These experiments thus demonstrate that src specifically binds and phosphorylates the amino-terminal half of the β subunit cytoplasmic loop. We next investigated the association of src with the AChR β subunit in vivo and found that both src and fyn bound to endogenous AChRs isolated from C2 extracts (Fig. 7). When the blot was reprobed with phosphotyrosine antibodies, we observed two phosphorylated bands, corresponding to the β subunit and src. Thus, we have envisioned the following model for tyrosine phosphorylation of the AChR: src associates with the AChR, which becomes tyrosine-phosphorylated on its β subunit, allowing the SH2 domain of fyn to bind the AChR complex (Fig. 8).

DISCUSSION

To better understand neurotransmitter receptor structure and function, we have examined the molecular basis of AChR assembly and modification during development. We examined the factors critical for subunit maturation and assembly in a simple in vitro translation system and found that the α subunit folded into its native conformation and specifically associated with the δ subunit, forming a heterodimer with a high-affinity ligand-binding site. Acquisition of the folded conformation occurred with a delay and required an oxidizing potential at the time of initiation of subunit synthesis. These data support the hypothesis that disulfide-bond formation may be the rate-limiting step in conformational maturation of the α subunit (Merlie and Lindstrom 1983) and suggest that folding may take place cotranslationally.

N-linked core glycosylation and oligosaccharide trimming are among the earliest processing steps in the ER and have been demonstrated to promote glycoprotein stability, solubility, and folding (Helenius 1994; Fiedler and Simons 1995). Some molecular chaperones, such as calnexin and calreticulin, preferentially associate with partially trimmed glycoproteins (Hebert et al. 1995; Peterson et al. 1995). Our data showed that cor-

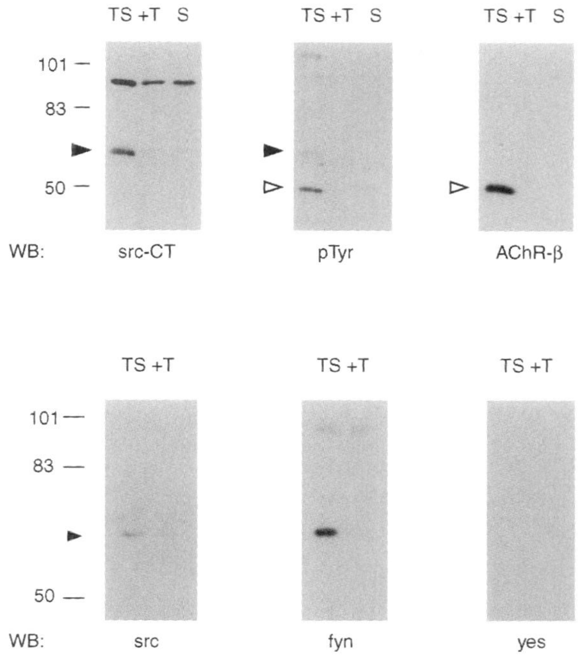

Figure 7. AChRs from C2 myotubes interact with the src-family kinases, src and fyn. AChRs were isolated from C2s by incubating lysates at 4°C for 2 hr with α-bungarotoxin Sepharose in the absence (TS) or presence (+T) of 10 mM free toxin or Sepharose only (S). Co-isolated src-related kinase(s) was identified by immunoblotting with a general src-CT antibody (*upper* panel). Src-related kinases are indicated by solid arrowheads. The nonspecific, 90-kD src-CT-reactive band was observed in both control and experimental samples. The samples were reprobed with a phosphotyrosine antibody (*upper middle*) and MAb124 (*upper right*), which recognizes the AChR β subunit (*open arrowhead*) to show that the AChR is specifically isolated and that the β subunit is tyrosine-phosphorylated. Isolated AChR-containing lysates were probed with anti-src, fyn, and yes antisera (*lower* panel) to show that src and fyn specifically associate with the AChR in C2 myotubes. (Data reprinted, with permission, from Fuhrer and Hall 1996.)

rect folding of the α subunit required N-linked core glycosylation but not oligosaccharide trimming, suggesting that calnexin and calreticulin are probably not essential for conformational maturation of the α subunit. Indeed, we found that calnexin and other chaperones such as BiP and protein disulfide isomerase only associate with the α subunit after most of the population has acquired the folded conformation and, thus, do not appear to play a role in subunit maturation (S. Shtrom and Z. Hall, unpubl.).

We have gained further insight into the minimal subunit domains required for folding and assembly by analyzing the properties of truncated amino-terminal α subunit fragments in COS cells. Using α-bungarotoxin binding as an assay for folding, we observed that the entire extracellular, amino-terminal domain through residue 211 (α211) folds efficiently, whereas fragments lacking the last 4 residues of this extracellular domain (α207) do not fold correctly. An α subunit fragment containing sequence through the first membrane-spanning segment (αM1) is sufficient to associate and form a high-affinity ligand-binding site with the δ subunit.

We also found that the first transmembrane domain of the α subunit does not contain specific information for subunit association, as α211 can efficiently form a heterodimer with the δ subunit when attached to transmembrane domains from unrelated proteins. Thus, the membrane-spanning regions of the α subunit do not contribute specificity to the assembly process but act to anchor the subunit within the membrane. In fact, an amino-terminal fragment attached to the membrane by a GPI anchor is able to associate with the δ subunit, forming a high-affinity ligand-binding site. However, the anchored peptide must be retained in the ER for a sufficient amount of time for assembly to occur. Thus, the specificity for α-δ subunit binding must be contained within the amino-terminal domain; attachment to the membrane appears to be necessary only to facilitate the assembly process.

Our work on how the AChR becomes modified in response to nerve-derived signals suggests that in mammalian muscle, both the formation and maintenance of AChR clusters are dependent on tyrosine phosphorylation. Moreover, agrin-induced clustering of the AChR appears to be linked to the tyrosine phosphorylation of the AChR itself. Agrin induces a rapid and transient phosphorylation of the AChR β subunit that occurs prior to the development of clusters; thus, it may serve as an early precursor step in the clustering mechanism. One candidate for the kinase that phosphorylates the β subunit is src. We have shown that the tyrosine kinase, src, constitutively binds and phosphorylates the amino-terminal half of the β cytoplasmic loop. This src-mediated phosphorylation probably occurs on Tyr-390: It is found within a phosphorylation consensus site (Songyang et al. 1995) and corresponds to the phosphorylated tyrosine in the *Torpedo* subunit (Wagner et al. 1991; Gillespie et al. 1996). The unique amino-terminal domain of src may be involved in its binding to the β subunit, as this region of src-related kinases mediates interactions with non-kinase transmembrane proteins (for review, see Kefalas et al. 1995). Fyn, a src-related kinase, also specifically interacts with tyrosine-phosphorylated AChRs, similar to the *Torpedo* AChR, which associates with fyn and fyk (Swope and Huganir 1993, 1994).

Our findings, together with similar observations in chick muscle (Wallace et al. 1991; Wallace 1994, 1995), suggest a model for AChR clustering in which agrin acts through the MuSK receptor tyrosine kinase, leading to phosphorylation of the AChR and other postsynaptic proteins. AChR-associated src-related kinases could be involved in agrin-induced AChR phosphorylation and in subsequent signaling steps, similar to the interleukin-2 and lymphocyte signaling pathways

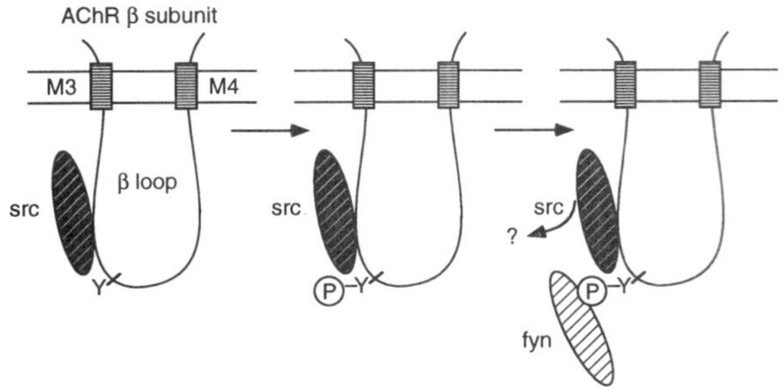

Figure 8. Model for the association of src and fyn with the AChR in C2 myotubes. Sequential interactions of src and fyn with the intracellular loop of the AChR β subunit are shown. For simplicity, the domain structure of the kinases and their membrane attachment due to myristoylation have been neglected.

(Taniguchi 1995; Weiss and Littman 1994). AChRs may first be phosphorylated by src on Tyr-390 of the β subunit, then interact with the SH2 domain of fyn via the phosphotyrosine (Swope and Huganir 1994). Src may remain bound to the β subunit to yield a fyn-src-AChR complex, or it may dissociate from the AChR prior to its association with fyn (Fig. 8). Tyrosine phosphorylation of the AChR may then regulate its interactions with proteins such as rapsyn, syntrophin, or the 87-kD protein (Hall and Sanes 1993) that could immobilize the AChR and link it to the cytoskeleton, thus resulting in its aggregation. Consistent with this model, rapsyn has been shown to aggregate the AChR when they are coexpressed in nonmuscle cells (Froehner et al. 1990; Phillips et al. 1991). Although we have found that rapsyn-associated aggregation of the AChR is not dependent on β subunit phosphorylation (Yu and Hall 1994b), this may not accurately reflect the regulated clustering that occurs in developing muscle. Experiments in muscle cells will be needed to confirm whether β subunit phosphorylation is required for agrin-induced clustering of the AChR. Further elucidation of the signaling pathways and protein-protein interactions involved in AChR clustering will determine whether src and fyn are involved in the orchestration of these events.

ACKNOWLEDGMENTS

We are grateful to Dr. Stephen Hardy for helpful advice on the construction and expression of GST fusion proteins and to Dr. Robin Taylor for critical reading of the manuscript. This work was initially supported by grants from the National Institutes of Health and the Muscular Dystrophy Association, and then intramurally by the National Institute for Mental Health. C.F. was supported by postdoctoral fellowships from the Swiss National Science Foundation, the Ciba-Geigy Jubilaeumsstiftung, and the Human Frontier Science Program.

REFERENCES

Blount, P. and J.P. Merlie. 1989. Molecular basis of the two nonequivalent ligand binding sites of the muscle nicotinic acetylcholine receptor. *Neuron* **3:** 349.

Blount, P., M.S. McHardy, and J.P. Merlie. 1990. Assembly intermediates of the mouse muscle nicotinic acetylcholine receptor in stably transfected fibroblasts. *J. Cell Biol.* **111:** 2601.

DeChiara, T.M., D.C. Bowen, D.M. Valenzuela, M.V. Simmons, W.T. Poieymirou, S. Thomas, E. Kinetz, D.L. Compton, E. Rojas, J.S. Park, C. Smith, P.S. DiStefano, D.J. Glass, S.J. Burden, and G.D. Yancopoulos. 1996. The receptor tyrosine kinase MuSK is required for neuromuscular junction formation in vivo. *Cell* **85:** 501.

Ferns, M., M. Deiner, and Z. Hall. 1996. Agrin-induced acetylcholine receptor clustering in mammalian muscle requires tyrosine phosphorylation. *J. Cell Biol.* **132:** 927.

Ferns, M.J., J.T. Campanelli, W. Hoch, R.H. Scheller, and Z. Hall. 1993. The ability of agrin to cluster AChRs depends on alternative splicing and on cell surface proteoglycans. *Neuron* **11:** 491.

Ferns, M., W. Hoch, J.T. Campanelli, F. Rupp, Z.W. Hall, and R.H. Scheller. 1992. RNA splicing regulates agrin-mediated acetylcholine receptor clustering activity on cultured myotubes. *Neuron* **8:** 1079.

Fertuck, H.C. and M.M. Salpeter. 1976. Quantitation of junctional and extrajunctional acetylcholine receptors by electron microscope autoradiography after ^{125}I-α-bungarotoxin binding at mouse neuromuscular junctions. *J. Cell Biol.* **69:** 144.

Fiedler, K. and K. Simons. 1995. The role of N-glycans in the secretory pathway. *Cell* **81:** 309.

Froehner, S.C. 1993. Regulation of ion channel distribution at synapses. *Annu. Rev. Neurosci.***16:** 347.

Froehner, S.C., C.W. Luetje, P.B. Scotland, and J. Patrick. 1990. The postsynaptic 43K protein clusters muscle nicotinic acetylcholine receptors in *Xenopus* oocytes. *Neuron* **5:** 403.

Fuhrer, C. and Z.W. Hall. 1996. Functional interaction of *src* family kinases with the acetylcholine receptor in C2 myotubes. *J. Biol. Chem.* (in press).

Gautam, M., P.G. Noakes, L. Moscoso, F. Rupp, R.H. Scheller, J.P. Merlie, and J.R. Sanes. 1996. Defective neuromuscular synaptogenesis in agrin-deficient mice. *Cell* **85:** 525.

Gillespie, S.K.H., S. Balasubramanian, E.T. Fung, and R.L. Huganir. 1996. Rapsyn clusters and activates the synapse-specific receptor kinase MuSK. *Neuron* **16:** 953.

Glass, D.J., D.C. Bowen, T.N. Stitt, C. Radziejewski, J. Bruno, T.E. Ryan, D.R. Gies, S. Shah, K. Mattsson, S.J. Burden, P.S. DiStefano, D.M. Valenzuela, T.M. DeChiara, and G.D. Yancopoulos. 1996. Agrin acts via a MuSK receptor complex. *Cell* **85:** 513.

Gu, Y., J.R. Forsayeth, S. Verrall, X.-M. Yu, and Z.W. Hall. 1991. Assembly of the mammalian acetylcholine receptor in transfected COS cells. *J. Cell Biol.* **114:** 799.

Hall, Z.W. and J.R. Sanes. 1993. Synaptic structure and development: The neuromuscular junction. *Neuron* (suppl.) **10:** 99.

Hebert, D.N., B. Foellmer, and A. Helenius. 1995. Glucose trimming and reglucosylation determine glycoprotein association with calnexin in the endoplasmic reticulum. *Cell* **81:** 425.

Helenius, A. 1994. How N-linked oligosaccharides affect

glycoprotein folding in the endoplasmic reticulum. *Mol. Biol. Cell* **5:** 253.

Karlin, A. 1993. Structure of nicotinic acetylcholine receptors. *Curr. Opin. Neurobiol.* **3:** 299.

Karlin, A. and M.H. Akabas. 1995. Toward a structural basis for the function of nicotinic acetylcholine receptor and their cousins. *Neuron* **15:** 1231.

Kefalas, P., T.R.P. Brown, and P.M. Brickell. 1995. Signalling by the p60c-src family of protein-tyrosine kinases. *Int. J. Biochem. Cell Biol.* **27:** 551.

Klausner, R.D., J.G. Donaldson, and J. Lippincott-Schwartz. 1992. Brefeldin A: Insights into the control of membrane traffic and organelle structure. *J. Cell Biol.* **116:** 1071.

Kreienkamp, H.-J., R.K. Maeda, S.M. Sine, and P. Taylor. 1995. Intersubunit contacts governing assembly of the mammalian nicotinic acetylcholine receptor. *Neuron* **14:** 635.

Lin, A., B. Devaux, A. Green, C. Sagerstrom, J. Elliott, and M. Davis. 1990. Expression of T cell antigen receptor heterodimers in a lipid-linked form. *Science* **249:** 677.

McMahan, U.J. 1990. The agrin hypothesis. *Cold Spring Harbor Symp. Quant. Biol.* **50:** 407.

Merlie, J.P. and J. Lindstrom. 1983. Assembly *in vivo* of mouse muscle acetylcholine receptor: Identification of an α subunit species that may be an assembly intermediate. *Cell* **34:** 747.

Merlie, J.P. and M.M. Smith. 1986. Synthesis and assembly of acetylcholine receptor, a multisubunit membrane glycoprotein. *J. Membr. Biol.* **91:** 1.

Peterson, J.R., A. Ora, P.N. Van, and A. Helenius. 1995. Transient, lectin-like association of calreticulin with folding intermediates of cellular and viral glycoproteins. *Mol. Biol. Cell* **6:** 1173.

Phillips, W.P., C. Kopta, P. Blount, P.D. Gardner, J.H. Steinbach, and J.P. Merlie. 1991. ACh receptor-rich membrane domains organized in fibroblasts by recombinant 43-kilodalton protein. *Science* **251:** 568.

Qu, Z. and R.L. Huganir. 1994. Comparison of innervation and agrin-induced tyrosine phosphorylation of the nicotinic acetylcholine receptor. *J. Neurosci.* **14:** 6834.

Qu, Z., E. Moritz, and R.L. Huganir. 1990. Regulation of tyrosine phosphorylation of the nicotinic acetylcholine receptor at the rat neuromuscular junction. *Neuron* **2:** 367.

Reist, N.E., M.J. Werle, and U.J. McMahan. 1992. Agrin released by motor neurons induces the aggregation of AChRs at neuromuscular junctions. *Neuron* **8:** 865.

Ruegg, M.A., K.W.K. Tsim, S.E. Horton, S. Kroger, G. Escher, E.M. Gensch, and U.J. McMahan. 1992. The agrin gene codes for a family of basal lamina proteins that differ in function and distribution. *Neuron* **8:** 691.

Saedi, M.S., W.G. Conroy, and J. Lindstrom. 1991. Assembly of *Torpedo* acetylcholine receptors in *Xenopus* oocytes. *J. Cell Biol.* **112:** 1007.

Shtrom, S.S. and Z.W. Hall. 1996. The α subunit of the acetylcholine receptor folds to bind α-bungarotoxin in an *in vitro* translation system. *J. Biol. Chem.* (in press).

Songyang, Z., K.L. Carraway III, M.J. Eck, S.C. Harrison, R.A. Feldman, M. Mohammadi, J. Schlessinger, S.R. Hubbard, D.P. Smith, C. Eng, M.J. Lorenzo, B.A.J. Ponder, B.J. Mayer, and L.C. Cantley. 1995. Catalytic specificity of protein-tyrosine kinases is critical for selective signalling. *Nature* **373:** 536.

Swope, S.L. and R.L. Huganir. 1993. Molecular cloning of two abundant protein tyrosine kinases in *Torpedo* electric organ that associate with the acetylcholine receptor. *J. Biol. Chem.* **268:** 25152.

———. 1994. Binding of nicotinic acetylcholine receptor to SH2 domains of fyn and fyk protein tyrosine kinases. *J. Biol. Chem.* **269:** 29817.

Taniguchi, T. 1995. Cytokine signaling through nonreceptor protein tyrosine kinases. *Science* **268:** 251.

Unwin, N. 1993. Neurotransmitter action: Opening of ligand-gated ion channels. *Cell* (suppl.) **72:** 31.

Verrall, S. and Z.W. Hall. 1992. The N-terminal domains of acetylcholine receptor subunits contain recognition signals for the initial steps of receptor assembly. *Neuron* **68:** 23.

Wagner, K., K. Edson, L. Heginbotham, M. Post, R.L. Huganir, and A.J. Czernik. 1991. Determination of the tyrosine phosphorylation sites of the nicotinic acetylcholine receptor. *J. Biol. Chem.* **266:** 23784.

Wallace, B.G. 1994. Staurosporine inhibits agrin-induced acetylcholine receptor phosphorylation and aggregation. *J. Cell Biol.* **125:** 661.

———. 1995. Regulation of the interaction of nicotinic acetylcholine receptors with the cytoskeleton by agrin-activated protein tyrosine kinase. *J. Cell Biol.* **128:** 1121.

Wallace, B.G., Z. Qu, and R.L. Huganir. 1991. Agrin induces phosphorylation of the nicotinic acetylcholine receptor. *Neuron* **6:** 869.

Wang, Z.-Z., S.F. Hardy, and Z.W. Hall. 1996a. Assembly of the nicotinic acetylcholine recptor: The first transmembrane domains of truncated α and δ subunits are required for heterodimer formation *in vivo*. *J. Biol. Chem.* (in press).

________. 1996b. Membranne tethering enables an extracellular domain of the acetylcholine receptor alpha subunit to form a heterodimeric ligand-binding site. *J. Cell Biol.* (in press).

Weiss, A. and D.R. Littman. 1994. Signal transduction by lymphocyte antigen receptors. *Cell* **76:** 263.

Yu, X.-M. and Z.W. Hall. 1991. Extracellular domains mediate subunit interactions of the muscle acetylcholine receptor. *Nature* **352:** 64.

———. 1994a. Amino- and carboxyl-terminal domains specify the identity of the δ subunit in assembly of the mouse nicotinic acetylcholine receptor. *Mol. Pharmacol.* **46:** 964.

———. 1994b. The role of the cytoplasmic domains of individual subunits of the acetylcholine receptor in 43 kDa protein-induced clustering in COS cells. *J. Neurosci.* **14:** 785.

The GluR2 Hypothesis: Ca^{++}-permeable AMPA Receptors in Delayed Neurodegeneration

M.V.L. BENNETT,[1] D.E. PELLEGRINI-GIAMPIETRO,[2] J.A. GORTER,[1,4] E. ARONICA,[1] J.A. CONNOR,[3,5] AND R.S. ZUKIN[1]

[1]*Department of Neuroscience, Albert Einstein College of Medicine, Bronx, New York 10461;* [2]*Dipartimento di Farmacologia Preclinica e Clinica "Mario Aiazzi Mancini," Università di Firenze, 50134 Firenze, Italy;* [3]*Roche Institute of Molecular Biology, Nutley, New Jersey 07110;* [4]*University of Amsterdam, Dept. Experimentele Dierkunde, 1098 SM Amsterdam, The Netherlands;* [5]*The Lovelace Institute, Albuquerque, New Mexico 87108*

Excessive activation of glutamate receptors is thought to contribute to neurodegeneration following a wide range of neurological insults, including ischemia, trauma, hypoglycemia, and epileptic seizures. Diseases such as Alzheimer's and Huntington's may also involve overstimulation of glutamate receptors. A major cytotoxic mechanism is increased Ca^{++} influx through NMDA receptors and voltage-activated Ca^{++} channels, and under conditions of metabolic stress, reduced Ca^{++} extrusion and sequestration. Until recently, non-NMDA receptors were thought to be Ca^{++}-impermeable, but it is now well established that AMPA receptors lacking the GluR2 subunit are Ca^{++}-permeable and provide an additional potential source of Ca^{++} overload (for references, see below). High levels of cytosolic Ca^{++} are known to induce cell degeneration by activation of proteases and endonucleases (for reviews, see Rothman and Olney 1986; Choi 1988, 1992; Sheardown et al. 1990). In cultured neurons, sufficiently high Ca^{++} levels induce necrosis, but lower levels can also induce apoptosis (Takei and Endo 1994; Choi 1995).

In this paper, we describe two different paradigms in which neurological insult is followed by delayed neurodegeneration in hippocampal structures; we present evidence that decreased expression of GluR2 subunits leads to increased Ca^{++} influx through AMPA receptors, which initiates the degenerative process. Following transient global ischemia, neurons in the hippocampus appear to recover fully in minutes to a few hours, but by 48–72 hours, most neurons in the CA1 die with characteristics of apoptosis (Bredesen 1995; Nitatori et al. 1995). This delayed neurodegeneration is of clinical importance, not only in people resuscitated from heart attacks, but also in patients undergoing cardiac surgery in whom neurological complications are frequent sequelae (Brillman 1993; Swain 1993; Roach et al. 1996). In animals, postischemic treatment with blockers of AMPA receptors can be neuroprotective when applied surprisingly long (16–24 hours) after the insult (Buchan et al. 1993; Sheardown et al. 1993; Pulsinelli 1995), and pharmacological agents of this class may have clinical application. Delayed neurodegeneration is also seen in rats after kainate-induced status epilepticus, which shows many similarities to temporal lobe epilepsy in humans (Nadler 1981; Ben Ari 1985). Following status epilepticus, it is CA3 rather than CA1 neurons that degenerate. In each condition, however, the vulnerable neurons exhibit a delayed decrease in GluR2 expression that is predicted to result in increased Ca^{++} permeability of AMPA receptors.

THE GluR2 HYPOTHESIS OF DELAYED NEURODEGENERATION

AMPA receptor subunits are encoded by four genes of the glutamate receptor family (Keinänen et al. 1990; Nakanishi 1992; Hollmann and Heinemann 1994; Dani and Mayer 1995; Seeburg 1995). These subunits, termed GluR1–GluR4 (GluR-A–GluR-D by the Seeburg group [1995]), assemble into heteromers as well as homomers. Although all the genes for GluR1–4 have Q at a critical site in the second transmembrane domain (TM2), GluR2 mRNA in cortex and hippocampus is almost entirely edited to R at this site (Burnashev et al. 1992; however, editing is less complete in human substantia nigra and corpus striatum, [Nutt and Kamboj 1994]). The effect of the editing is that the receptors are Ca^{++}-impermeable if they have edited GluR2 subunits (although homomeric edited GluR2 receptors pass little current), and they are Ca^{++}-permeable if they lack edited GluR2 subunits (Hollmann et al. 1991; Hume et al. 1991; Jonas et al. 1994). "GluR2-less" receptors in cells are also characterized by inward rectification, which is due to fast channel block by intracellular spermine (or a similar molecule) (Bowie and Mayer 1995; Donevan and Rogawski 1995; Koh et al. 1995). AMPA receptors of most neurons are Ca^{++}-impermeable and electrically linear. The subunit stoichiometry is unclear, but immunoprecipitation studies indicate that GluR1/GluR2 and GluR2/GluR3 receptors comprise the majority in the hippocampus (Wenthold et al. 1996). Some types of neurons, however, do have Ca^{++} -permeable AMPA receptors (see, e.g., Bochet et al. 1994; Isa et al. 1995; Koh et al. 1995), and in different types of neurons the level of GluR2 expression correlates with Ca^{++} impermeability (Geiger et al. 1995).

The GluR2 hypothesis states that a decrease in

GluR2 expression leads to increased formation of Ca^{++}-permeable AMPA receptors and that the resulting increase in Ca^{++} influx in response to (endogenous) glutamate causes or contributes to delayed neurodegeneration. (In the strong form of the hypothesis, GluR2 down-regulation is sufficient to cause the degeneration; in weaker forms, GluR2 down-regulation is necessary or contributory but not sufficient.) Because some neurons normally express only GluR2-less, Ca^{++}-permeable AMPA receptors, the GluR2 hypothesis is not applicable to all cells, although at least some GluR2-less cells are more susceptible to glutamate excitotoxicity (Brorson et al. 1992). Their survival may result from interesting differences in, e.g., Ca^{++} buffering or level of parvalbumin (Bering et al. 1995), faster desensitization (Geiger et al. 1995; Lambolez et al. 1996), or from simply fewer receptors or glutamatergic inputs. Evidence that delayed neurodegeneration following global ischemia is caused (at least in part) by reduction in GluR2 receptor expression includes in situ hybridization and immunocytochemistry to demonstrate reduction in receptor mRNA and protein, intracellular recording and Ca^{++} imaging to measure increased AMPA receptor-mediated Ca^{++} influx, and neuroprotection by antagonists of non-NMDA receptors (data and references below). Although basal levels of cytosolic free Ca^{++} are unchanged in cells surviving sufficiently to permit microelectrode measurements, activation of AMPA receptors causes greater rises in intracellular Ca^{++} than in controls, suggesting increased Ca^{++} influx. Moreover, selective blockers suggest increased expression of GluR2-less, Ca^{++}-permeable receptors (Tsubokawa et al. 1995; see Herlitze et al. 1993). Evidence that the GluR2 hypothesis explains neurodegeneration following kainate-induced status epilepticus is to date limited to in situ hybridization and immunocytochemistry showing reduction in GluR2 mRNA and protein.

There is evidence that delayed cell death following both global ischemia and status epilepticus is apoptotic (MacManus et al. 1995; Nitatori et al. 1995; Honkanieme et al. 1996; Morrison et al. 1996), and the GluR2 hypothesis can now be extended beyond its original formulation (Pellegrini-Giampietro et al. 1992; Friedman et al. 1994) to state that the increased Ca^{++} influx through GluR2-less receptors triggers apoptosis or programmed cell death.

OUR DATA

Global Ischemia

Rat. Altered GluR expression following transient global ischemia and preceding neurodegeneration was first observed in the rat (Pellegrini-Giampietro et al. 1992; see also Pollard et al. 1993; Heurteaux et al. 1995). Following 10-minute ischemia, hippocampal neurons are histologically quite normal at 24 hours, but by 48–72 hours, most CA1 pyramidal cells have degenerated (Kirino 1982). In contrast, CA3 and dentate gyrus show very little degeneration. In control brain, in situ hybridization showed that GluR1, GluR2, and GluR3 mRNAs were expressed at high levels in the pyramidal cell layer of CA1 and CA3 and the granule cell layer of the dentate gyrus (Boulter et al. 1990; Keinänen et al. 1990; Pellegrini-Giampietro et al. 1991). At 24 hours postischemia, GluR2 mRNA was markedly depressed in the vulnerable hippocampal CA1, to about 30% of control, but was less changed in CA3 and dentate gyrus (Fig. 1) (Pellegrini-Giampietro et al. 1992). GluR3 mRNA was also depressed in CA1 to about 50% of control, but GluR1 was maintained at 80% or more. Emulsion-dipped sections showed that the changes in mRNA expression in CA1 pyramidal neurons were more or less uniform from cell to cell. More recently, we obtained data that GluR2 protein was reduced in postischemic CA1 pyramidal neurons prior to degeneration (Pulsinelli et al. 1995). On the basis of the in situ hybridization data alone it was plausible that the observed decrease in GluR2 mRNA led to an increase in Ca^{++}-permeable AMPA receptors and that the resulting increased Ca^{++} influx in response to endogenous glutamate contributed to the neurodegeneration. Although there is a sharp rise in glutamate during the ischemic episode, its level rapidly returns to normal upon reperfusion (Torp et al. 1993), and neurons recover their resting potential and excitability; thus, the ischemic rise in glutamate cannot be directly responsible for the delayed neurodegeneration.

The initial indication that activation of AMPA receptors contributes to postischemic delayed neurodegeneration came from studies of neuroprotection with systemically administered blockers of glutamate receptors. 2,3-Dihydroxy-6-nitro-7-sulfamoyl-benzo(f) quinoxaline (NBQX), an AMPA and kainate receptor antagonist, was neuroprotective, when given on reperfusion or even 8–16 hours after an ischemic insult (Pulsinelli et al. 1993; Pulsinelli 1995). Moreover, NBQX did not prevent the postischemic reduction in GluR2 expression in the rat; GluR2 mRNA was still decreased when NBQX was given immediately after the ischemic episode (Pellegrini-Giampietro et al. 1994). Although the pharmacodynamics of NBQX have not been published, it is not very soluble and may precipitate when injected into the peritoneal cavity, from where it may gradually enter the circulation for days (Buchan et al. 1993). (There are as yet no data on how long treatment with a short-lasting AMPA blocker must be maintained to prevent degeneration, or whether short-lasting glutamate antagonists are neuroprotective when given at the time of the ischemic episode.) MK-801, in contrast, was not neuroprotective in this paradigm (Pulsinelli et al. 1993; comparable data were obtained from the gerbil, see below). Thus, protection by blockers of non-NMDA receptors indicates that activation of these receptors is necessary, and possibly sufficient, for the delayed neurodegeneration. We will return to

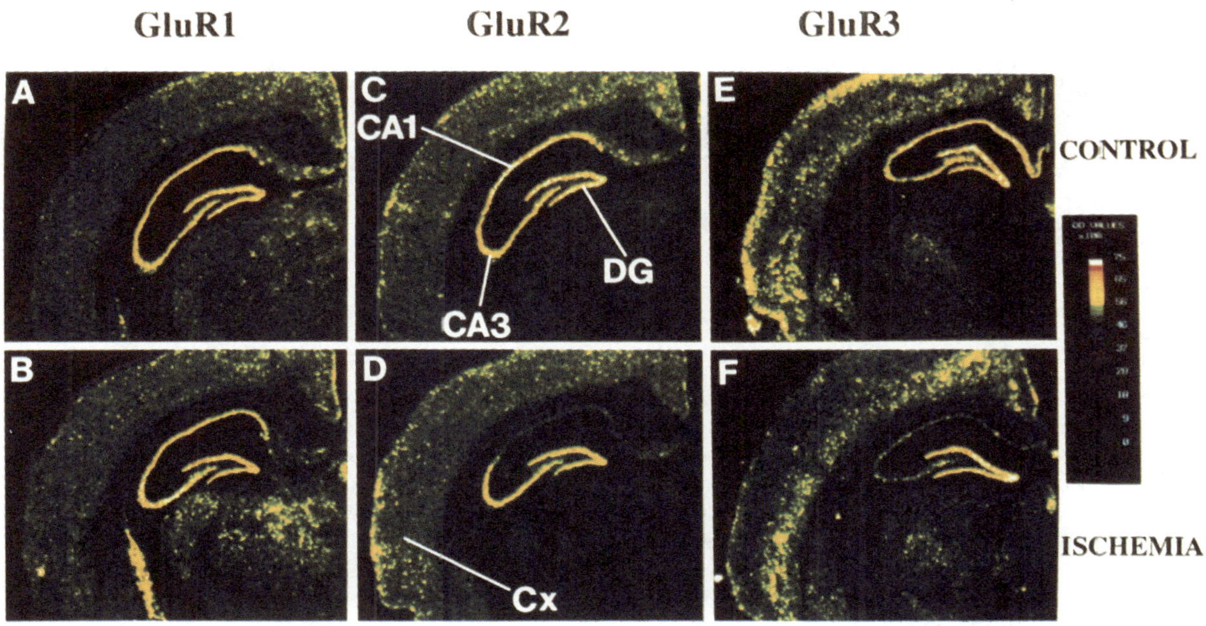

Figure 1. Specific reduction in GluR2 mRNA in CA1 after global ischemia in rat. In situ hybridization labeling of GluR1, GluR2, and GluR3 mRNAs in coronal sections of control and 24-hr postischemic brain at the level of the hippocampus. (*Upper row*) Control. (*Lower row*) 24 hr postischemia. (*A,B*) GluR1 was little changed postischemia. (*C,D*) GluR2 was markedly decreased in CA1 postischemia. (*E,F*) GluR3 was somewhat reduced in CA1 and CA3 postischemia. (DG) Dentate gyrus; (Cx) neocortex. (Reprinted, with permission, from Pellegrini-Giampietro et al. 1992.)

the question of whether activation of GluR2-less, Ca^{++}-permeable receptors is necessary for the neurodegeneration.

We obtained preliminary data with fura-2 imaging of cytoplasmic free Ca^{++} in rat CA1 neurons (Gorter et al. 1995 and unpubl.). At 24 hours postischemia, which is prior to obvious neurodegeneration, basal Ca^{++} levels were unchanged. AMPA receptor-mediated rises in Ca^{++} were similar in control and postischemic animals, but the variability was too great to conclude that Ca^{++} permeability was or was not altered. We did see that rises in Ca^{++} evoked by depolarization were similar in postischemic and control neurons but that postischemic neurons recovered the resting Ca^{++} level more slowly. This difference may reflect that the postischemic neurons had reduced Ca^{++} handling ability or that their mechanisms were normal but had been overloaded by increased Ca^{++} influx that occurred prior to our depolarizing them.

Gerbil. We also carried out molecular and physiological studies of delayed neurodegeneration following global ischemia in the gerbil. Because of differences in the circulatory system, ischemia can be produced by two-vessel occlusion, but the result is selective and delayed neurodegeneration in hippocampal CA1 as in the rat, although the time course is somewhat slower (Kirino 1982). Patterns of glutamate receptor expression were examined in control and postischemic animals by in situ hybridization with RNA probes to GluR1, GluR2, and NR1 mRNAs. In unoperated or sham-operated control gerbils, as in the rat, all three transcripts were expressed at high levels in the pyramidal cell layer of CA1 and CA3 and the granule cell layer of the dentate gyrus (Fig. 2).

Global ischemia caused a decrease of GluR2 mRNA in the CA1 pyramidal cell layer (Fig. 2) but not in the CA3 region or dentate gyrus. GluR2 mRNA in CA1 progressively decreased to 85 ± 2% of the control level at 24 hours, to 48 ± 6% at 48 hours, and to 17 ± 10% at 72 hours (Figs. 2, 3). GluR1 and NR1 mRNAs showed no change at 24 hours, a slight decrease at 48 hours (13 ± 5% and 7 ± 5%, respectively), and a substantial decrease at 72 hours (55 ± 4% and 46 ± 3%, respectively; Fig. 3). The ratio of GluR2 to GluR1 mRNAs, a possible predictor of Ca^{++} impermeability of AMPA receptors, progressively decreased at 48 hours and 72 hours. CA1 showed no obvious loss of neurons at 72 hours, and in emulsion-dipped sections, receptor labeling of pyramidal cells was reduced uniformly. In the CA3 pyramidal cell layer and dentate gyrus, none of the mRNAs was significantly altered following ischemia. By 1 week postischemia, all CA1 pyramidal neurons had died, in confirmation of earlier studies (data not shown; see Kirino 1982).

To determine whether basal levels of cytosolic free Ca^{++} and Ca^{++} levels after AMPA stimulation are affected by the altered expression of GluR2, we studied individual CA1 neurons in hippocampal slices from control and postischemic gerbils. Intracellular recording and optical Ca^{++} measurements were carried out at 48 hours and 72 hours after induction of ischemia and

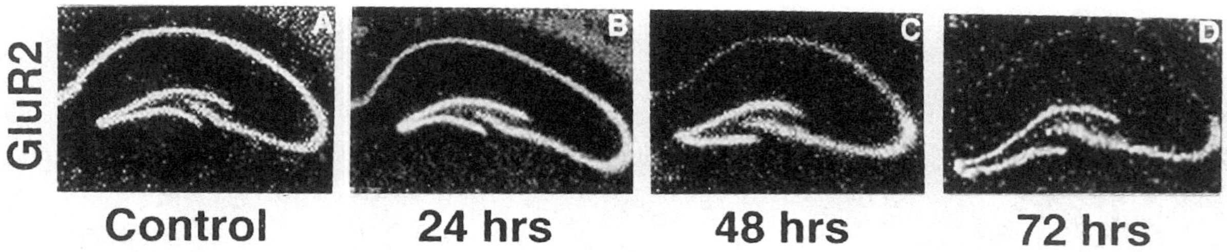

Figure 2. Reduction in GluR2 mRNA in CA1 after global ischemia in the gerbil. In situ hybridization labeling of GluR2 mRNA in coronal sections of hippocampus of control, 24-hr, 48-hr, and 72-hr postischemic brain. GluR2 labeling progressively declined in CA1, but was little changed in CA3 and dentate gyrus.

in sham-operated and unoperated control animals. In control animals, about 80% of the cells were "healthy" in that they generated action potentials in response to depolarizing currents and could be held hyperpolarized by small hyperpolarizing currents. Other, presumably damaged, cells remained depolarized under similar circumstances and were not included in the study. At 48 hours postischemia, the fraction of successful penetrations was similar to that in controls. At 72 hours postischemia, more than half of the cells slowly depolarized despite application of hyperpolarizing current; the decrease in successful penetrations may reflect the onset of degeneration.

Impaled neurons were filled with fura-2 by passing hyperpolarizing currents, and with Cs^+ by passing depolarizing currents, and the membrane potential was clamped at −80 mV. In addition, slices were bathed in solution containing DL-2-amino-5-phosphonovaleric acid (APV, 100 μM) and MK-801 (20 μM) to block Ca^{++} influx through NMDA receptors, nimodipine (10 μM) and Cd^{++} (100 μM), to block voltage-dependent Ca^{++} channels, and tetrodotoxin (3 μM) to block action

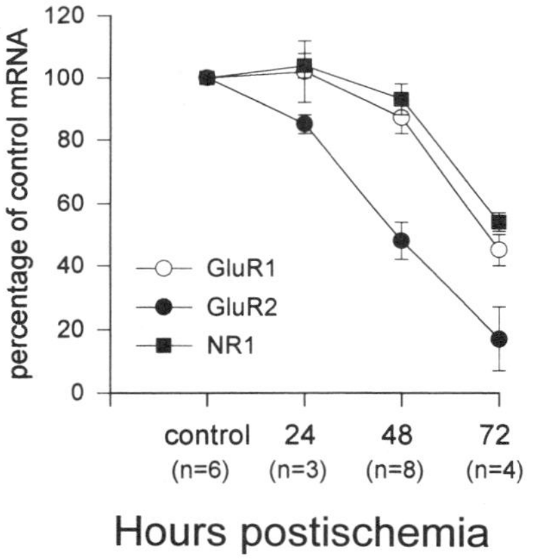

Figure 3. Time course of decreases of glutamate receptor mRNAs in CA1 after global ischemia in gerbil. Density of labeling of glutamate receptor mRNAs in CA1 of gerbil hippocampus following 5-min transient global ischemia is plotted as percent ± S.E.M. of control. GluR2 mRNA decreased more rapidly than did those of GluR1 and the NMDA receptor subunit, NR1. Numbers of animals are indicated.

potentials and synaptic glutamate release by other neurons. Ca^{++} concentrations were determined by ratio imaging of fura-2 fluorescence at 360 nm and 380 nm excitation. Healthy CA1 neurons, selected by the above criteria, exhibited low basal cytoplasmic Ca^{++} levels that did not differ significantly in control and in 48-hour and 72-hour postischemic slices (50–100 nM, Figs. 4, 5A).

After measurement of basal Ca^{++} concentrations, the slices were bathed for 30 seconds in the solution with Ca^{++} and Na^+ channel blockers with added AMPA (30 μM) to activate the receptors and cyclothiazide (10–30 μM) to prevent desensitization (Partin et al. 1995). This treatment caused the cells to generate a slowly rising inward current. Under these conditions, AMPA evoked a mean peak inward current that did not differ significantly among neurons in control, 48-hour, and 72-hour postischemic groups (Fig. 6B). The solution was then replaced with the original blocker solution with the addition of 20 μM 6-cyano-7-nitroquinoxaline-2,3-dione (CNQX) to block the AMPA receptors, and the clamping current was returned to the original level. Finally, the slices were bathed in physiological saline without blockers, when they recovered the ability to generate action potentials (although the responses were prolonged because of the injected Cs^+). Only those cells that demonstrated a Ca^{++} signal in response to depolarization at the end of the experiment were included in the study. Slices were exposed to a single sequence of solutions.

The AMPA-induced current was associated with a rise in Ca^{++} in six out of nine CA1 neurons 72 hours postischemia; there was a small rise in two of ten neurons 48 hours postischemia, and little change in Ca^{++} in control neurons (Figs. 4, 5A, 6). AMPA-induced rises in Ca^{++} paralleled the rather slow rise and fall of inward current (Fig. 4); more rapid application of AMPA would be required to measure a lag associated with accumulation or extrusion of Ca^{++}. As expected, the rises in Ca^{++} were greater for larger currents. In the 72-hour postischemic neurons, AMPA increased Ca^{++} in both somata and proximal dendrites (from a mean of ~ 70 nM to a mean of ~ 260 nM in the somata; Figs. 5, 6A,B). Ca^{++} rises in apical dendrites were always smaller and, in some cases, were un-

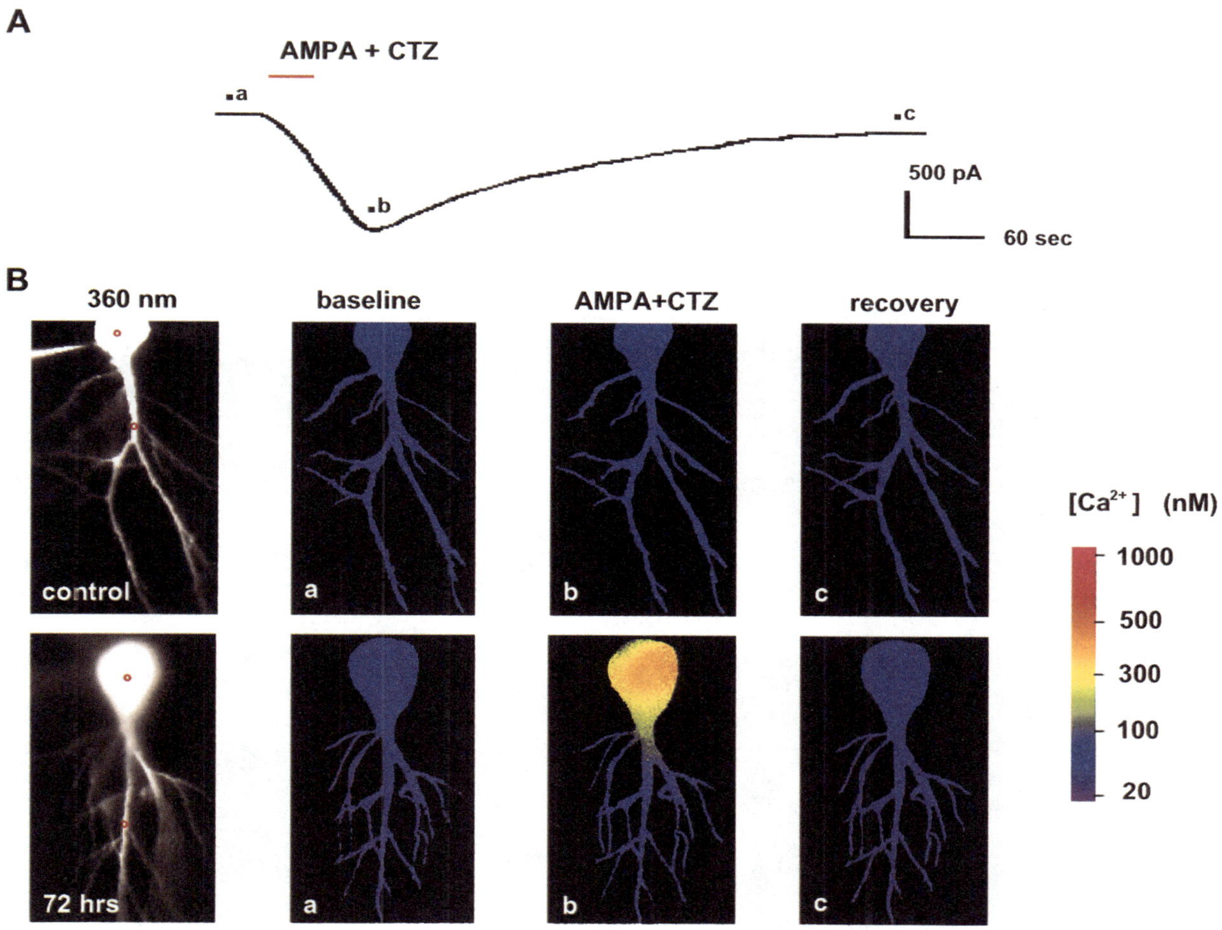

Figure 4. Ca^{++} influx induced by AMPA plus cyclothiazide (CTZ) is greater in postischemic than control CA1 neurons in gerbil. (*A*) Current recorded from a 72-hr postischemic neuron in response to 30 μM AMPA with 10 μM CTZ bath applied for 30 sec (*red bar*). Current of the control cell in *B* in response to 30 μM AMPA with 30 μM CTZ was of similar amplitude. (*B*) 360-nm excitation images taken prior to AMPA application (*left column*) and ratio images taken before, during, and after AMPA action at the times indicated on the current trace in *A*. (*Upper row*) Control. (*Lower row*) 72 hr postischemia. Red circles in the fluorescence images show typical sites of Ca^{++} measurement in somata and dendrites for data included in Figs. 5 and 6. AMPA caused little change in Ca^{++} in the control neuron but a large transient increase in the soma of the postischemic neuron and a small increase in its proximal dendrites.

detectable. The lack of Ca^{++} increases in apical dendrites is surprising, since many excitatory synapses are located in this region of the neuron. Possible explanations include earlier insertion of Ca^{++}-permeable receptors near the soma and more effective Ca^{++} buffering in the dendrites.

Since postischemic neurons may lose their excitability rather quickly after they have begun to accumulate Ca^{++}, our sample of neurons, which were selected for their ability to maintain a resting potential, may include neurons that were relatively delayed in the onset of neurodegenerative changes. Rises in Ca^{++} might have been greater in cells that were too weakened to withstand the experimental protocol for Ca^{++} measurement.

Excitatory postsynaptic potentials (EPSPs) and excitatory postsynaptic currents (EPSCs) from CA1 neurons were altered in the postischemic gerbil (Tsubokawa et al. 1994, 1995). The CNQX-sensitive, non-NMDA component of both spontaneous and evoked EPSCs was prolonged compared to control, consistent with reduction in desensitization. However, the prolongation appeared to require Ca^{++} influx, since it was reversed by lowering extracellular Ca^{++} or injecting the Ca^{++} buffer, BAPTA. Joro spider toxin and a synthetic analog, 1-naphthyl acetyl spermine, blocked a large fraction of the CNQX-sensitive current. These blockers preferentially act on GluR2-less, Ca^{++}-permeable receptors (Blaschke et al. 1993). These data indicate that there is an increase in Ca^{++}-permeable AMPA receptors in postischemic neurons and that another change, prolongation of the EPSCs, may contribute to the degeneration.

Since AMPA receptors rapidly desensitize upon glutamate stimulation, ambient interstitial glutamate is unlikely to contribute to excitoxicity through activation

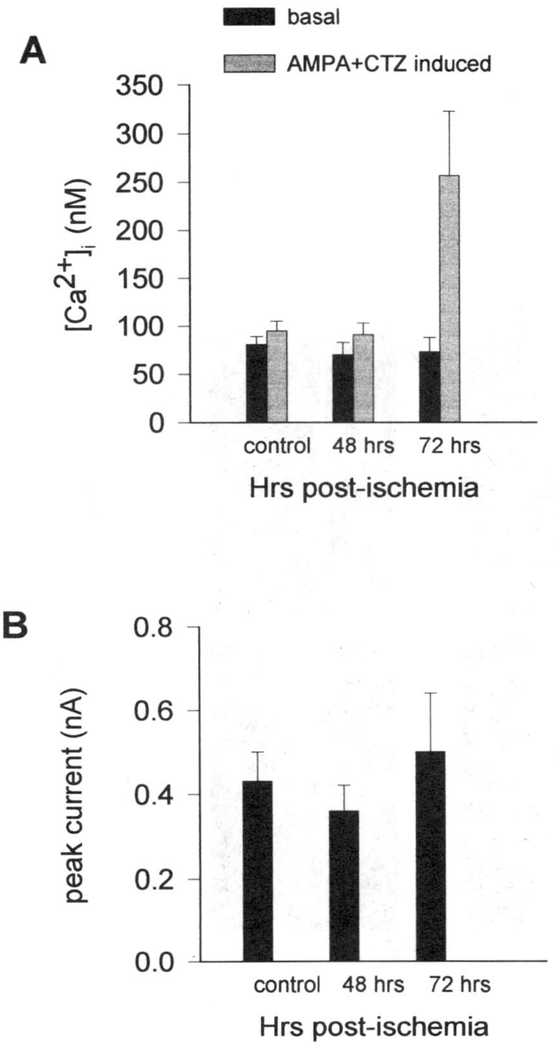

Figure 5. Mean basal levels of Ca^{++} were unchanged postischemia, but AMPA-induced levels were increased, although amplitudes of AMPA-induced currents were not. (*A*) Basal somatic Ca^{++} levels and somatic Ca^{++} levels induced by AMPA with CTZ in control and postischemic (48 hr and 72 hr) CA1 neurons. AMPA with CTZ induced a slight rise in Ca^{++} in control and at 48 hr postischemia. AMPA induced a large increase in Ca^{++} at 72 hr postischemia (p<0.01 compared to control and to 48 hr postischemia, Student's t test). (*B*) The peak AMPA-induced currents did not differ significantly among control and postischemic neurons.

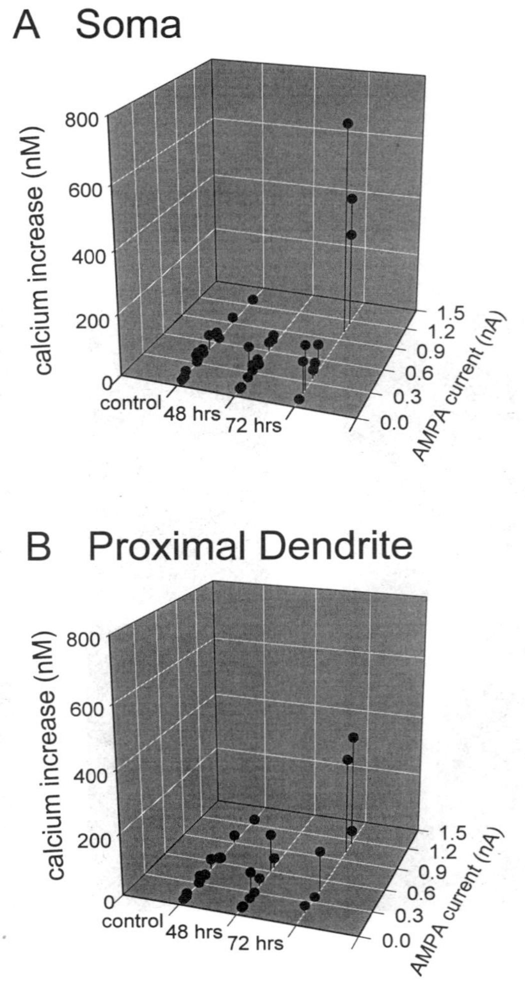

Figure 6. AMPA-induced currents and rises in Ca^{++} in individual control and postischemic neurons. (*A*) Somatic levels. (*B*) Levels in proximal dendrites. Peak current amplitudes and calcium changes induced by AMPA with CTZ are indicated in control neurons and neurons at 48 hr and 72 hr postischemia. Rises in Ca^{++} were greater at 72 hr postischemia than in controls and at 42 hr postischemia.

of either their Ca^{++}-permeable or -impermeable forms. However, synaptic release that generates EPSPs would presumably be sufficiently phasic that AMPA receptors would recover from desensitization between release events. The importance of non-NMDA receptor activation is demonstrated by the observation that delayed treatment with NBQX is neuroprotective in the gerbil as well as the rat (Buchan et al. 1993; Sheardown et al. 1993). It remains to be determined whether a specific blocker of GluR2-less, Ca^{++}-permeable (or Ca^{++}-impermeable) AMPA receptors is also neuroprotective. Since small neurons in the hippocampus that have Ca^{++}-permeable AMPA receptors may be inhibitory (Isa et al. 1995), specific block of these receptors might have excitatory as well as blocking actions.

Given the likelihood that rises in Ca^{++} are a mediator of neurotoxicity, it is surprising that NMDA antagonists are not neuroprotective in global ischemia. This negative finding suggests that there is little activation of NMDA receptors during delayed neurodegeneration. NMDA antagonists are neuroprotective in focal ischemia (Pulsinelli et al. 1993), where degree of damage is correlated with the number of episodes of spreading depression emanating from the lesion (Mies et al. 1993; Takano et al. 1996); since NMDA antagonists block spreading depression, their mode of action may be via this mechanism rather than simple block of

Ca^{++} influx through NMDA receptors (Hossmann 1994). NBQX is neuroprotective in the penumbra of focal ischemia as well (Xue et al. 1994; Graham et al. 1996), but changes in GluR2 expression have not been examined.

Mechanisms of altered gene expression. The molecular mechanisms by which global ischemia alters GluR2 expression are as yet unknown. Other postischemic changes in CA1 have been described, including elevations and decreases in mRNAs and/or proteins including transcription factors (Nowak et al. 1993; Kamme et al. 1995), enzymes (Kindy et al. 1994), stress proteins (Aoki et al. 1993; Nowak et al. 1993), and neurotrophic factors (Takeda et al. 1993; Kokaia et al. 1994). It is likely that one or more of these proteins play a role in subsequent down-regulation of GluR2 expression. Since some mRNAs and proteins are up-regulated in CA1, the decreases in GluR2 mRNA and protein are not simply a result of a loss of transcriptional or translational capability and appear to result from a regulatory, if maladaptive, change. Treatment with agonists of adenosine A1 receptors and activators of K_{ATP} channels is neuroprotective when given just prior to ischemia and blocks the down-regulation of GluR2 (Heurteaux et al. 1995). Aurintricarboxylic acid, which blocks endonucleases, among other enzymes, is neuroprotective when given intraventricularly at the time of ischemia and blocks the down-regulation of GluR2 (E.M. Aronica et al., unpubl.). Another neuroprotective treatment, block of ornithine decarboxylase (Kindy et al. 1994), has not been examined with respect to action on GluR2 expression or AMPA-induced currents. The rise in c-fos expression following global ischemia can be reduced by pretreatment with c-fos antisense oligonucleotide (Liu et al. 1994), but effects on other genes including GluR2 have not been reported. It is likely that the regulatory mechanism responsible for reduced expression of GluR2 is active in other, physiological processes, such as development (Pellegrini-Giampietro et al. 1991).

Status Epilepticus

In adult rat, kainate-induced status epilepticus leads to delayed neurodegeneration in a specific hippocampal region; however, in this paradigm it is the pyramidal cells in CA3 rather than CA1 that degenerate (Nadler 1981; Ben Ari 1985). In situ hybridization and immunocytochemistry suggest that a reduction in GluR2 expression leads to the neurodegeneration associated with status epilepticus, as it appears to do following global ischemia. At 12 hours and 24 hours following induction of status, when there is little cell loss, GluR2 and GluR3 mRNAs were reduced in the vulnerable CA3, and GluR1 and NR1 mRNAs were unchanged (Fig. 7) (Friedman et al. 1994; see also Pollard et al. 1993). The change in GluR2 mRNA would be expected to lead to increased formation of GluR2-less,

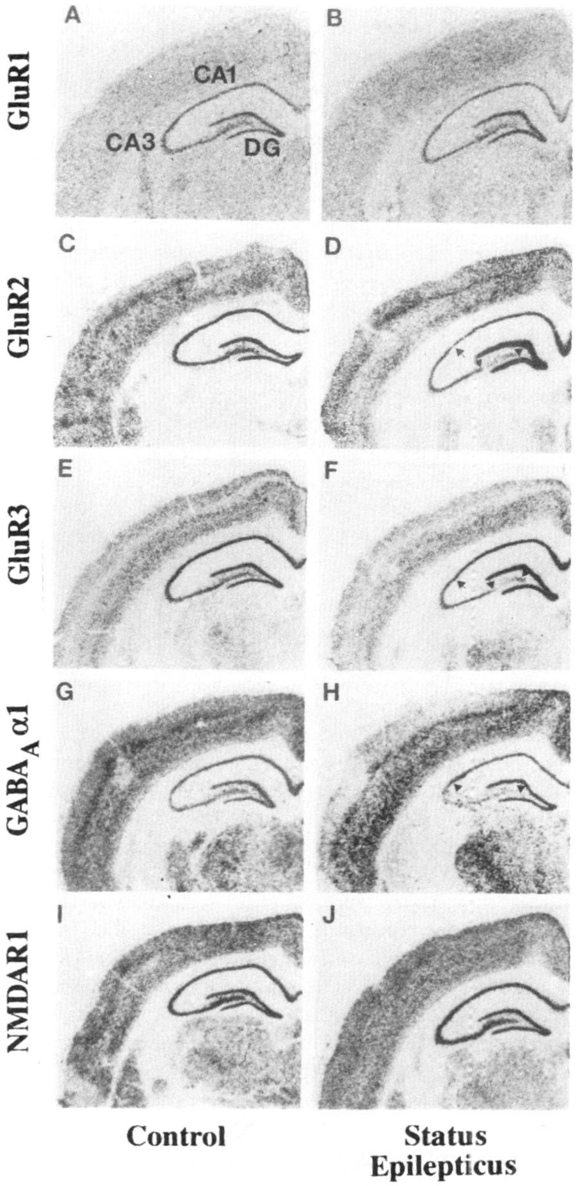

Figure 7. In situ hybridization labeling of GluR1, GluR2, GluR3, GABA$_A$α1, and NR1 mRNAs in coronal sections of control and 24-hr post-status epilepticus rat brain at the level of the hippocampus. (*Left column*) Control. (*Right column*) 24-hr post-status epilepticus. All probes labeled the pyramidal cell layer of CA1 and CA3 and the granule cell layer of dentate gyrus. (*A,B*) Status epilepticus had little effect on GluR1 mRNA. (*C,D*) Following status epilepticus, GluR2 mRNA was reduced in the CA3 region, particularly between the blades of the dentate. (*E,F*) Following status epilepticus, GluR3 mRNA was reduced to a similar degree as GluR2 mRNA. (*G,H*) Following status epilepticus, GABA$_A$α1 mRNA was reduced throughout CA3. (*I,J*) Status epilepticus had little effect on NR1 mRNA. (Reprinted, with permission, from Friedman et al. 1994.)

Ca^{++}-permeable AMPA receptors. In the resistant CA1, none of these transcripts was altered, whereas in the resistant dentate gyrus, GluR2 and GluR3 mRNAs were increased and GluR1 mRNA was unchanged. Moreover, immunoreactivity determined with a GluR2 antibody was decreased in the vulnerable CA3 but not in CA1 or dentate gyrus (L.K. Friedman et al., in prep.). Expression of GABAα1 subunit mRNA was also reduced in CA3 but not CA1 or dentate gyrus, possibly leading to reduced inhibition of CA3 neurons which could enhance excitotoxicity.

In rat pups, kainate induces status epilepticus, but without the accompanying neurodegeneration in hippocampal CA3 (Albala et al. 1984). In young animals, postnatal days 5 and 14, GluR2 expression is *not* reduced in CA3 following the induction of status epilepticus (L.K. Friedman et al., in prep.). These findings further implicate Ca^{++}-permeable, GluR2-less AMPA receptors in the neurodegeneration associated with status epilepticus. We have not yet determined whether AMPA receptor antagonists are neuroprotective following status epilepticus, although it was reported that NMDA antagonists do not protect CA3 (Clifford et al. 1990).

DISCUSSION

The previous section reviews molecular and physiological changes leading to delayed neurodegeneration in the hippocampus as a result of global ischemia and kainate-induced status epilepticus. Similar reductions in GluR2 mRNA and protein expression were triggered by an ischemic insult and by status epilepticus, but these changes were in different structures, i.e., CA1 and CA3, respectively. In postischemic gerbils, there were functional changes in the affected neurons consistent with the predicted change in subunit composition and suggesting increased AMPA-induced Ca^{++} influx. The time course of changes in receptor expression and function were appropriate for mediation of the delayed neurodegeneration by increased Ca^{++} influx through GluR2-less, Ca^{++}-permeable AMPA receptors. Neuroprotection by antagonists at non-NMDA receptors supports this mechanism. There remains the possibility that GluR5-6 and KA1-2 receptors are also changed, and depending on the degree of editing, these receptors can be Ca^{++}-permeable or -impermeable (Kohler et al. 1993; Paschen and Djuricic 1994; Ruano et al. 1995). Although GluR5 and GluR6 are expressed in hippocampus, they appear to make little contribution to synaptic currents in adult animals (Lerma et al. 1997). In our experiments, the rises in Ca^{++} evoked by AMPA plus CTZ could only have been due to activation of AMPA receptors.

The existence of neurons with AMPA receptors that are entirely GluR2-less and Ca^{++}-permeable has been clearly demonstrated (Geiger et al. 1995). These cells either lack much glutamatergic input or have mechanisms for dealing with the resulting Ca^{++} influx. Of greater concern for the GluR2 hypothesis are mice with the GluR2 gene disrupted by homologous recombination (Jia et al. 1996). Development in the GluR2 (–/–) animals is grossly normal, and neurons survive that die in the wild-type adult when their GluR2 expression is down-regulated. To "save" the GluR2 hypothesis, we predict that during development there is regulation of AMPA receptors and/or of the cells' response to Ca^{++}. Since GluR2 expression is lower in the postnatal period, it is less surprising that GluR2 (–/–) mice go through development more or less normally. In transgenic mice in which GluR2 editing was prevented by altering an intron essential for the process, hemizygotes (from one mosaic sire) had Ca^{++}-permeable AMPA receptors, developed seizures, and succumbed by 3 weeks of age with cell loss in the hippocampus (Brusa et al. 1995). In these animals, unedited GluR2 may have contributed to the formation of Ca^{++}-permeable receptors, leading to a greater number than in the GluR2 (–/–) mice. The pathology of the editing-deficient mouse makes another possibility of greater interest; formation of Ca^{++}-permeable AMPA receptors would be increased if Q to R editing of GluR2 RNA were reduced. We know of no reports of changed editing following neurological insult.

Important questions remain unanswered: (1) What are the early changes following ischemia or status epilepticus that lead to down-regulation of GluR2? As noted above, some neuroprotective interventions at early stages prevent reduction in expression of GluR2 mRNA (and also prevent certain other changes in gene expression). Further understanding of the cascade may allow somewhat later, but still effective, intervention. (2) How are the changes in mRNA level evoked, through a decrease in transcription or an increase in degradation? (3) Is decrease in GluR2 expression alone sufficient to cause neurodegeneration or are one or more of the many other changes necessary? Use of antisense oligonucleotides to GluR2 may allow more specific down-regulation of GluR2. (4) What is the mechanism by which EPSCs are prolonged postischemia, and is this change necessary for the neurodegeneration? (5) Does GluR2 expression return to normal in protected neurons, and if so when? For how long must AMPA antagonists be present to achieve neuroprotection? Since neurons survive in the GluR2 (–/–) animal, recovery of GluR2 expression is not a foregone conclusion. (6) NBQX, which blocks kainate as well as AMPA receptors, is neuroprotective, but would a specific blocker of GluR2-less receptors be more or less effective? (7) Are AMPA antagonists neuroprotective after status epilepticus? (8) Given that the delayed neurodegeneration is apoptotic, is the hypothesized Ca^{++} influx through GluR2-less receptors adequate to initiate this process, or is it dependent on other changes produced by the earlier insult? Protein synthesis inhibitors are neuroprotective in global ischemia (Goto et al. 1990; Du et al. 1996) and can be effective as late as 16 hours after the insult, but it is unclear whether they would be protective after the formation of GluR2-less receptors. Expression of immediate-early genes following global ischemia shows an early peak and a later one after 12–36 hours (Kamme et al. 1995). The late peak could represent the onset of expression of pro-apoptotic genes in response to Ca^{++} influx through GluR2-less receptors. The lack of delayed neurodegeneration following status epilepticus in the p53 knockout mouse (Morrison et al. 1996), although supporting the importance of apoptosis, does not indicate the time at which the p53 protein acts or when it is synthesized.

The GluR2 hypothesis suggests several levels at which neuroprotection could be obtained. Inhibition of transcription or protein synthesis may prevent downregulation of GluR2 and formation of GluR2-less receptors. Blocking AMPA receptors neuroprotects, presumably by blocking increased Ca^{++} influx. Block of apoptosis at transcriptional and translational levels may also be effective. Finally, block of the action of apoptotic enzymes or oxidative activity could prevent the end stages leading to cell death.

The GluR2 hypothesis may also be relevant to the delayed neurodegeneration following transient or permanent *focal* ischemia. The GluR2 mechanism may also be operative, although GluR2 expression has not been examined in these paradigms. In the penumbra, where cells have the possibility of surviving, both NMDA and AMPA antagonists are neuroprotective (Graham et al. 1996), but the action of NMDA may be in reducing the number of episodes of spreading depression (Hossman 1994). When delayed neurodegeneration occurs, it shows characteristics of apoptosis (Linnik et al. 1995; Charriaut-Marlangue et al. 1996; Du et al. 1996).

The findings discussed here have implications for human disease. It should prove advantageous for victims of cardiac arrest and stroke that the therapeutic window stays open for a long time. However, action at earlier stages of the gene expression cascade could be more effective. Also potentially important is the possibility of preoperative, in addition to postoperative, treatment of patients who undergo cardiac surgery, a patient group numbering in the hundreds of thousands (Brillman 1993; Swain 1993; Roach et al. 1996). For these patients, blockers of an earlier step in the process would be more practical than it would for the person at risk of a heart attack. Disruption of normal brain function might be acceptable for short periods while gene expression recovered, but prolonged prophylactic treatment with AMPA blockers or other neuroprotectants is a less likely prospect.

Neurodegeneration is a frequent long-term consequence of epilepsy in humans, and neurologists are concerned with neuroprotective treatment as well as antiseizure medication. Problems include knowing which kind of seizure merits which kind of neuroprotective treatment and finding drugs with few enough side effects to justify their use. The animal data suggest that the neurologist may well consider neuroprotection immediately after the first seizure.

SUMMARY

Increased glutamate-receptor-mediated Ca^{++} influx is considered an important factor underlying delayed neurodegeneration following ischemia or seizures. Until recently, the NMDA receptor was the only glutamate receptor known to be Ca^{++}-permeable. It is now well established that glutamate receptors of the AMPA type, encoded by a gene family designated GluR1–GluR4, exist in both Ca^{++}-permeable and Ca^{++}-impermeable forms, depending on their subunit composition and degree of RNA editing. Recombinant channels assembled without GluR2 are permeable to Ca^{++}; channels assembled with (edited) GluR2 are Ca^{++}-impermeable. AMPA receptors in most adult neurons are hetero-oligomers containing GluR2 subunits, but some neurons have GluR2-less, Ca^{++}-permeable receptors. The "GluR2 hypothesis" predicts that a relative reduction in the expression of GluR2 results in enhanced Ca^{++} influx through newly synthesized AMPA receptors, thereby increasing neurotoxicity of endogenous glutamate. Recent observations indicate reduction in GluR2 expression and predict formation of Ca^{++}-permeable AMPA receptors following global ischemia and kainate-induced status epilepticus; these changes are likely to be a major factor contributing to the delayed neurodegeneration that follows these pathological events. The delayed neurodegeneration appears to be primarily apoptotic. Thus, there are at least three strategies for neuroprotection: block of formation of GluR2-less receptors, which may be possible at several levels; block of the GluR2-less receptors themselves; and block of the subsequent apoptosis.

ACKNOWLEDGMENTS

This work was supported by grants from the National Institutes of Health: NS-20752 (R.S.Z.), NS-31282 (R.S.Z.), and NS-07512 (M.V.L.B); from the Aaron Diamond Foundation (E.A.); and from the Human Frontiers Science Project Organization (J.G.). M.V.L.B. is the Sylvia and Robert S. Olnick Professor of Neuroscience.

REFERENCES

Albala, B.J., S.L. Moshe, and R. Okada. 1984. Kainic-acid-induced seizures: A developmental study. *Brain Res.* **315:** 39.

Aoki, M., K. Abe, J. Kawagoe, S. Nakamura, and K. Kogure. 1993. Acceleration of HSP70 and HSC70 heat shock gene expression following transient ischemia in the preconditioned gerbil hippocampus. *J. Cereb. Blood Flow Metab.* **13:** 781.

Ben Ari, Y. 1985. Limbic seizure and brain damage produced

by kainic acid: Mechanisms and relevance to human temporal lobe epilepsy. *Neuroscience* **14:** 375.

Bering, R., N.H. Diemer, A. Draguhn, and F.F. Johansen. 1995. Co-localization of somatostatin mRNA and parvalbumin in the dorsal rat hippocampus after cerebral ischemia. *Hippocampus* **5:** 341.

Blaschke, M., B.U. Keller, R. Rivosecch, M. Hollmann, S. Heinemann, and A. Konnerth. 1993. A single amino acid determines the subunit-specific spider toxin block of α-amino-3-hydroxy-5-methylisoxazole-4-propionate/kainate receptor channels. *Proc. Natl. Acad Sci.* **90:** 6528.

Bochet, P., E. Audinat, B. Lambolez, F. Crepel, J. Rossier, M. Iino, K. Tsuzuki, and S. Ozawa. 1994. Subunit composition at the single-cell level explains functional properties of a glutamate-gated channel. *Neuron* **12:** 383.

Boulter, J., M. Hollmann, A. O'Shea-Greenfield, M. Hartley, E. Deneris, C. Maron, and S. Heinemann. 1990. Molecular cloning and functional expression of glutamate receptor subunit genes. *Science* **249:** 1033.

Bowie, D. and M. Mayer. 1995. Inward rectification of both AMPA and kainate subtype glutamate receptors generated by polyamine-mediated ion channel block. *Neuron* **15:** 415.

Bredesen, D.E. 1995. Neural apoptosis. *Ann. Neurol.* **38:** 839.

Brillman, J. 1993. Central nervous system complications in coronary artery bypass graft surgery. *Neurocardiology* **11:** 475.

Brorson, J.R., D. Bleakman, P.S. Chard, and R.J. Miller. 1992. Calcium directly permeates kainate/α-amino-3-hydroxy-5-methyl-4-isoxazolepropionic acid receptors in cultured cerebellar Purkinje neurons. *Mol. Pharmacol.* **41:** 603.

Brusa, R., F. Zimmermann, D.S. Koh, D. Feldmeyer, P. Gass, P.H. Seeburg, and R. Sprengel. 1995. Early-onset epilepsy and postnatal lethality associated with an editing-deficient GluR-B allele in mice. *Science* **270:** 1677.

Buchan, A.M., H. Lesiuk, K.A. Barnes, H. Li, Z.-G. Huang, K.E. Smith, and D. Xue. 1993. AMPA antagonists: Do they hold more promise for clinical stroke trials than NMDA antagonists? *Stroke* (suppl. 12) **24:** I148.

Burnashev, N., H. Monyer, P.H. Seeburg, and B. Sakmann. 1992. Divalent ion permeability of AMPA receptor channels is dominated by the edited form of a single subunit. *Neuron* **8:** 189.

Charriaut-Marlangue, C., I. Margaill, A. Represa, T. Popovici, M. Plotkine, and Y. Ben-Ari. 1996. Apoptosis and necrosis after reversible focal ischemia: An in situ DNA fragmentation analysis. *J. Cereb. Blood Flow Metab.* **16:** 186.

Choi, D.W. 1988. Calcium-mediated neurotoxicity: Relationship to specific channel types and role in ischemic damage. *Trends Neurosci.* **11:** 465.

———. 1992. Excitotoxic cell death. *J. Neurobiol.* **23:** 1261.

———. 1995. Calcium: Still center-stage in hypoxic-ischemic neuronal death. *Trends Neurosci.* **18:** 58.

Clifford, D.B., J.W. Olney, A.M. Benz, T.A. Fuller, and C.F. Zorumski. 1990. Ketamine, phencyclidine, and MK-801 protect against kainic acid-induced seizure-related brain damage. *Epilepsia* **31:** 382.

Dani, J.A. and M.L. Mayer. 1995. Structure and function of glutamate and nicotinic acetylcholine receptors. *Curr. Opin. Neurobiol.* **5:** 310.

Donevan, S.D. and M.A. Rogawski. 1995. Intracellular polyamines mediate inward rectification of Ca^{2+}-permeable α-amino-3-hydroxy-5-methyl-4-isoxazole-propionic acid receptors. *Proc. Natl. Acad. Sci.* **92:** 9298.

Du, C., R. Hu, C.A. Csernansky, C.Y. Hsu, and D.W. Choi. 1996. Very delayed infarction after mild focal cerebral ischemia: A role for apoptosis? *J. Cereb. Blood Flow Metab.* **16:** 195.

Friedman, L.K., D.E. Pellegrini-Giampietro, E.F. Sperber, M.V.L. Bennett, S.L. Moshé, and R.S. Zukin. 1994. Kainate-induced status epilepticus alters glutamate and $GABA_A$ receptor gene expression in adult rat hippocampus: An in situ hybridization study. *J. Neurosci.* **14:** 2697.

Geiger, J.R.P., T. Melcher, D.S. Koh, B. Sakmann, P.H. Seeburg, P. Jonas, and H. Monyer. 1995. Relative abundance of subunit mRNAs determines gating and Ca^{2+} permeability of AMPA receptors in principal neurons and interneurons in rat CNS. *Neuron* **15:** 193.

Gorter, J.A., J.J. Petrozzino, D. Rosenbaum, S. Rybak, W.A. Pulsinelli, T. Nowak, M.V.L. Bennett, R.S. Zukin, and J.A. Connor. 1995. Resting and kainate-induced Ca^{2+} levels measured by fura-2 imaging of individual CA1 neurons after global ischemia in the rat. *Soc. Neurosci. Abstr.* **21:** 1342.

Goto, K., A. Ishige, K. Sekiguchi, S. Iizuka, A. Sugimoto, M. Yuzurihara, M. Aburada, E. Hosoya, and K. Kogure. 1990. Effects of cycloheximide on delayed neuronal death in rat hippocampus. *Brain Res.* **534:** 299.

Graham, S.H., J. Chen, J.Q. Lan, and R.P. Simon. 1996. A dose-response study of neuroprotection using the AMPA antagonist NBQX in rat focal cerebral ischemia. *J. Pharmacol. Exp. Ther.* **276:** 1.

Herlitze, S., M. Raditsch, J.P. Ruppersberg, W. Jahn, H. Monyer, R. Schoepfer, and V. Witzemann. 1993. Argiotoxin detects molecular differences in AMPA receptor channels. *Neuron* **10:** 1131.

Heurteaux, C., I. Lauritzen, C. Widmann, and M. Lazdunski. 1995. Essential role of adenosine, adenosine A1 receptors, and ATP-sensitive K^+ channels in cerebral ischemic preconditioning. *Proc. Natl. Acad. Sci.* **92:** 4666.

Hollmann, M. and S. Heinemann. 1994. Cloned glutamate receptors. *Annu. Rev. Neurosci.* **17:** 31.

Hollmann, M., M. Hartley, and S. Heinemann. 1991. Ca^{2+} permeability of KA-AMPA-gated glutamate receptor channels depends on subunit composition. *Science* **252:** 851.

Honkanieme, J., S.M. Massa, M. Breckinridge, and F.R. Sharp. 1996. Global ischemia induces apoptosis-associated genes in hippocampus. *Mol. Brain Res.* **42:** 79.

Hossmann, K.A. 1994. Glutamate-mediated injury in focal cerebral ischemia: The excitotoxin hypothesis revised. *Brain Pathol.* **4:** 23.

Hume, R., R. Dingledine, and S. Heinemann. 1991. Identification of a site in glutamate receptor subunits that controls calcium permeability. *Science* **253:** 1028.

Isa, T., M. Iino, S. Itazawa, and S. Ozawa. 1995. Spermine mediates inward rectification of Ca(2+)-permeable AMPA receptor channels. *Neuroreport* **6:** 2045.

Jia, Z., N. Agopyan, P. Miu, A. Xiong, J. Henderson, R. Gerlai, F.A. Taverna, A. Velumian, J. MacDonald, P. Carlen, W. Abramow-Newerly, and J. Roder. 1996. Enhanced LTP in mice deficient in the AMPA receptor GluR2. *Neuron* **17:** 945.

Jonas, P., C. Racca, B. Sakmann, P.H. Seeburg, and H. Monyer. 1994. Differences in Ca^{2+}-permeability of AMPA-type glutamate receptor channels in neocortical neurons caused by differential GluR-B subunit expression. *Neuron* **12:** 1281.

Kamme, F., K. Campbell, and T. Wieloch. 1995. Biphasic expression of the *fos* and *jun* families of transcription factors following transient forebrain ischaemia in the rat. Effect of hypothermia. *Eur. J. Neurosci.* **7:** 2007.

Keinänen, K., W. Wisden, B. Sommer, P. Werner, A. Herb, T.A. Verdoorn, B. Sakmann, and P.H. Seeburg. 1990. A family of AMPA-selective glutamate receptors. *Science* **249:** 556.

Kindy, M.S., Y. Hu, and R.J. Dempsey. 1994. Blockade of ornithine decarboxylase enzyme protects against ischemic brain damage. *J. Cereb. Blood Flow Metab.* **14:** 1040.

Kirino, T. 1982. Delayed neuronal death in the gerbil hippocampus following ischemia. *Brain Res.* **239:** 57.

Koh, D.-S., N. Burnashev, and P. Jonas. 1995. Block of native Ca^{2+}-permeable AMPA receptors in rat brain by intracellular polyamines generates double rectification. *J. Physiol.* **486:** 305.

Kohler, M., N. Burnashev, B. Sakmann, and P.H. Seeburg. 1993. Determinants of Ca^{2+} permeability in both TM1 and TM2 of high affinity kainate receptor channels: Diversity by RNA editing. *Neuron* **10:** 491.

Kokaia, Z., M. Metsis, M. Kokaia, J. Bengzon, E. Elmer, M.L. Smith, T. Timmusk, B.K. Siesjo, H. Persson, and O. Lindvall. 1994. Brain insults in rats induce increased expression of the BDNF gene through differential use of multiple promoters. *Eur. J. Neurosci.* **6:** 587.

Lambolez B., N. Ropert, D. Perrais, J. Rossier, and S. Hestrin. 1996. Correlation between kinetics and RNA splicing of α-amino-3-hydroxy-5-methylisoxazole-4-propionic acid receptors in neocortical neurons. *Proc. Natl. Acad. Sci.* **93:** 1797.

Lerma, J., M. Morales, M.A. Vicente, and O. Herreras. 1997. Glutamate receptors of the kainate type and synaptic transmission. *Trends Neurosci.* **20:** 9.

Linnik, M.D., J.A. Miller, J. Sprinkle-Cavallo, P.J. Mason, F.Y. Thompson, L.R. Montgomery, and K.K. Schroeder. 1995. Apoptotic DNA fragmentation in the rat cerebral cortex induced by permanent middle cerebral artery occlusion. *Mol. Brain Res.* **32:** 116.

Liu, P.K., A. Salminen, Y.Y. He, M.H. Jiang. J.J. Xue, J.S. Liu, and C.Y. Hsu. 1994. Suppression of ischemia-induced *fos* expression and AP-1 activity by an antisense oligodeoxynucleotide to c-*fos* mRNA. *Ann. Neurol.* **36:** 566.

MacManus, J.P., I.E. Hill, E. Preston, I. Rasquinha, T. Walker, and A.M. Buchan. 1995. Differences in DNA fragmentation following transient cerebral or decapitation ischemia in rats. *J. Cereb. Blood Flow Metab.* **15:** 728.

Mies, G., T. Lijima, and K.A. Hossmann. 1993. Correlation between peri-infarct DC shifts and ischaemic neuronal damage in rat. *Neuroreport* **4:** 709.

Morrison, R.S., H.J. Wenzel, Y. Kinoshita, C.A. Robbins, L.A. Donehower, and P.A. Schwartzkroin. 1996. Loss of the p53 tumor suppressor gene protects neurons from kainate-induced cell death. *J. Neurosci.* **16:** 337.

Nadler, J.V. 1981. Kainic acid as a tool for the study of temporal lobe epilepsy. *Life Sci.* **29:** 2031.

Nakanishi, S. 1992. Molecular diversity of glutamate receptors and implications for brain function. *Science* **258:** 597.

Nitatori, T., N. Sato, S. Waguri, Y. Karasawa, H. Araki, K. Shibanai, E. Kominami, and Y. Uchiyama. 1995. Delayed neuronal death in the CA1 pyramidal cell layer of the gerbil hippocampus following transient ischemia is apoptosis. *J. Neurosci.* **15:** 1001.

Nowak, T.S., Jr., O.C. Osborne, and S. Suga. 1993. Stress protein and proto-oncogene expression as indicators of neuronal pathophysiology after ischemia. *Prog. Brain Res.* **96:** 195.

Nutt, S.L. and R.K. Kamboj. 1994. Differential RNA editing efficiency of AMPA receptor subunit GluR-2 in human brain. *Neuroreport* **5:** 1679.

Partin, K.M., D. Bowie, and M.L. Mayer. 1995. Structural determinants of allosteric regulation in alternatively spliced AMPA receptors. *Neuron* **14:** 833.

Paschen, W. and B. Djuricic. 1994. Extent of RNA editing of glutamate receptor subunit GluR5 in different brain regions of the rat. *Cell. Mol. Neurobiol.* **1:** 259.

Pellegrini-Giampietro, D.E., M.V.L. Bennett, and R.S. Zukin. 1991. Differential expression of three glutamate receptor genes in developing rat brain. *Proc. Natl. Acad. Sci.* **88:** 4157.

Pellegrini-Giampietro, D.E., W.A. Pulsinelli, and R.S. Zukin. 1994. NMDA and non-NMDA receptor gene expression following global ischemia in rats: Effect of NMDA and non-NMDA receptor antagonists. *J. Neurochem.* **62:** 1067.

Pellegrini-Giampietro, D. E., R.S. Zukin, M.V.L. Bennett, S. Cho, and W.A. Pulsinelli. 1992. Switch in glutamate receptor subunit gene expression in CA1 subfield of hippocampus following global ischemia in rats. *Proc. Natl. Acad. Sci.* **89:** 10499.

Pollard, H., A. Héron, J. Moreau, Y. Ben-Ari, and M. Khrestchatisky. 1993. Alterations of the GluR-B AMPA receptor subunit flip/flop expression in kainate-induced epilepsy and ischemia. *Neuroscience* **57:** 545.

Pulsinelli, W.A. 1995. The therapeutic window in ischemic brain injury. *Curr. Opin. Neurol.* **8:** 3.

Pulsinelli, W., A. Sarokin, and A. Buchan. 1993. Antagonism of the NMDA and non-NMDA receptors in global versus focal brain ischemia. *Prog. Brain Res.* **96:** 125.

Pulsinelli, W.A., L.K. Friedman, T. Nowak, D. Pellegrini, J.M. Morrison, and R.S. Zukin. 1995. GluR2 receptor protein expression is reduced in hippocampal CA1 after global ischemia. *Soc. Neurosci. Abstr.* **21:** 837.

Roach, B.W., M. Kanchuger, C.T. Mora Mangano, M. Newman, N. Nussmeier, R. Wolman, A. Aggarwal, K. Marschall, S.H. Graham, C. Ley, G. Ozanne, and D.T. Mangano. 1996. Adverse cerebral outcomes after coronary bypass surgery. *New Engl. J. Med.* **335:** 1857.

Rothman, S.M. and J.W. Olney. 1986. Glutamate and the pathophysiology of hypoxic–ischemic brain damage. *Ann. Neurol.* **19:** 105.

Ruano, D., B. Lambolez, J. Rossier, A.V. Paternain, and J. Lerma. 1995. Kainate receptor subunits expressed in single cultured hippocampal neurons: Molecular and functional variants by RNA editing. *Neuron* **14:** 1009.

Seeburg, P.H. 1995. The TINS/TIPS lecture. The molecular biology of mammalian glutamate receptor channels. *Trends Neurosci.* **16:** 359.

Sheardown, M.J., P.D. Suzdak, and L. Nordholm. 1993. AMPA, but not NMDA, receptor antagonism is neuroprotective in gerbil global ischaemia, even when delayed 24 h. *Eur. J. Pharmacol.* **236:** 347.

Sheardown, M.J., E.O. Nielsen, A.J. Hansen, P. Jacobsen, and T. Honore. 1990. 2,3-Dihydroxy-6-nitro-7-sulfamoyl-benzo(F)quinoxaline: A neuroprotectant for cerebral ischemia. *Science* **247:** 571.

Swain, J.A. 1993. Cardiac surgery and the brain. *New Engl. J Med.* **329:** 1119.

Takano, K., L.L. Latour, J.E. Formato, R.A. Carano, K.G. Helmer, Y. Hasegawa, C.H. Sotak, and M. Fisher. 1996. The role of spreading depression in focal ischemia evaluated by diffusion mapping. *Ann. Neurol.* **39:** 308.

Takeda, A., H. Onodera, A. Sugimoto, K. Kogure, M. Obinata, and S. Shibahara. 1993. Coordinated expression of messenger RNAs for nerve growth factor, brain-derived neurotrophic factor and neurotrophin-3 in the rat hippocampus following transient forebrain ischemia. *Neuroscience* **55:** 23.

Takei, N. and Y. Endo. 1994. Ca^{2+} ionophore-induced apoptosis on cultured embryonic rat cortical neurons. *Brain Res.* **652:** 65.

Torp, R., B. Arvin, E. Le Peillet, A.G. Chapman, O.P. Ottersen, and B.S. Meldrum. 1993. Effect of ischaemia and reperfusion on the extra- and intracellular distribution of glutamate, glutamine, aspartate and GABA in the rat hippocampus, with a note on the effect of the sodium channel blocker BW1003C87. *Exp. Brain Res.* **96:** 365.

Tsubokawa, H., K. Oguro, T. Masuzawa, and N. Kawai. 1994. Ca^{2+}-dependent non-NMDA receptor-mediated synaptic currents in ischemic CA1 hippocampal neurons. *J. Neurophysiol.* **71:** 1190.

Tsubokawa, H., K. Oguro, T. Masuzawa, T. Nakaima, and N. Kawai. 1995. Effects of a spider toxin and its analogue on glutamate-activated currents in the hippocampal CA1 neuron after ischemia. *J. Neurophysiol.* **74:** 218.

Wenthold, R.J., R.S. Petralia, J. Blahos II, and A.S. Niedzielski. 1996. Evidence for multiple AMPA receptor complexes in hippocampal CA1/CA2 neurons. *J. Neurosci.* **16:** 1982.

Xue, D., Z.G. Huang, K. Barnes, H.J. Lesiuk, K.E. Smith, and A.M. Buchan. 1994. Delayed treatment with AMPA, but not NMDA, antagonists reduces neocortical infarction. *J. Cereb. Blood Flow Metab.* **14:** 251.

Zinc Neurotoxicity May Contribute to Selective Neuronal Death following Transient Global Cerebral Ischemia

D.W. CHOI

Center for the Study of Nervous System Injury and Department of Neurology, Washington University School of Medicine, St. Louis, Missouri 63110

The transition metal Zn^{++} plays an essential role in biology. There are about 2.5 grams of Zn^{++} in a human; among the trace elements, Zn^{++} is present in tissues at concentrations second only to iron. Zn^{++} binds readily to the thiol and imidazole moieties of various proteins and modifies the function of many metalloenzymes such as carbonic anhydrase. In addition, many DNA-binding proteins that regulate eukaryotic gene function contain a Zn^{++}-binding sequence, the "zinc finger." Dietary deprivation of Zn^{++} is lethal in mice; dietary deficiency in man has been associated with abnormalities in widespread processes, including growth, sexual maturation, and wound healing.

Zn^{++} also plays an important role in nervous system function. Growing evidence suggests that Zn^{++} serves as a widespread mediator of central neural signaling (Frederickson 1989; Smart et al. 1994). Large amounts of chelatable Zn^{++} are present throughout the brain, especially in the neuropil of the hippocampus and neocortex, substantially localized to a subpopulation of synaptic vesicles within excitatory boutons. Neuronal firing likely produces a calcium-dependent release of endogenous Zn^{++}; with intense activity, concentrations of several hundred micromolar may be achieved in synaptic clefts (Assaf and Chung 1984). Following release, Zn^{++} is probably actively reaccumulated back into presynaptic terminals.

By these features of presence, release, and uptake removal, free Zn^{++} has the potential to serve as a central signaling substance. Zn^{++} can modify the function of sodium, potassium, and calcium channels, as well as certain γ-aminobutyric acid receptors ($GABA_A$). Perhaps most importantly, given the strong association between Zn^{++} and excitatory synapses, Zn^{++} strongly attenuates activation of the *N*-methyl-D-aspartate (NMDA) subclass of glutamate receptors (Peters et al. 1987; Westbrook and Mayer 1987). The co-release of Zn^{++} with glutamate therefore likely reduces the activation of NMDA receptor-gated channels relative to AMPA/kainate receptor-gated channels. Single-channel study with native cortical neuronal NMDA receptors has suggested two mechanisms of Zn^{++} block: one independent of membrane voltage and thus presumably reflecting a binding site outside the membrane field, and the other a voltage-dependent, fast channel block (Christine and Choi 1990). Since NMDA channels have special properties, including high calcium permeability and voltage-dependent blockade by magnesium, this reduction could dynamically regulate the nature of excitatory neurotransmission, as well as reduce NMDA receptor-mediated toxicity (Koh and Choi 1988).

Although the ability of Zn^{++} to attenuate NMDA receptor overactivation may be beneficial under conditions of brain ischemia, intense release of Zn may itself induce lethal neuronal injury (Choi et al. 1988). This toxicity is probably initiated by toxic Zn^{++} entry through glutamate receptor- or voltage-gated Ca^{++} channels (Weiss et al. 1993; Koh and Choi 1994). A pathogenic role for Zn^{++} has been suggested in ischemic or epileptic brain damage, based on the observation that presynaptic Zn^{++} translocates into selectively vulnerable hippocampal hilar neurons degenerating after transient forebrain ischemia (Tonder et al. 1990), or into limbic or cortical neurons degenerating after brain seizures induced by kainate or perforant path stimulation (Sloviter 1985; Frederickson et al. 1988).

DOES ZN^{++} TRANSLOCATION MEDIATE SELECTIVE NEURONAL DEATH AFTER GLOBAL ISCHEMIA?

We set out recently to answer three questions (Koh et al. 1996): Does Zn^{++} influx into selectively vulnerable hippocampal neurons precede the neurodegeneration induced by transient ischemic insults? Will chelation of extracellular Zn^{++}, sufficient to prevent Zn^{++} influx, reduce this neuronal death? Finally, can Zn^{++} influx be implicated in the selective vulnerability of brain neurons outside the hippocampus?

Staining of Long Evans rat brains with the Zn^{++}-specific fluorescent dye, *N*-(6-methoxy-8-quinolyl)-*para*-toluenesulfonamide (TSQ) (Frederickson et al. 1992) revealed dense fluorescence in the mossy fiber axon terminals of dentate granule neurons in the hilus and the CA3 regions of the hippocampus, as well as in the stratum radiatum and stratum oriens of CA1. Neuronal or glial cell bodies did not exhibit Zn^{++} fluorescence, appearing as dark holes in the fluorescent neuropil. Twenty-four hours after a 10-minute period of forebrain ischemia, Zn^{++} fluorescence in presynaptic fibers was reduced, and new fluorescence appeared in certain hilar neuronal cell bodies. Subsequent acid fuchsin staining on the same section revealed a near one-to-one correlation between this apparent translocation of Zn^{++} fluorescence and degenerative changes. Seventy-two hours after ischemia, Zn^{++} fluorescence in presynaptic fibers had returned to normal, but selectively degenerating CA1 pyramidal neurons also displayed Zn^{++} fluorescence. These Zn^{++} translocations were detectable prior to gross neurodegenerative changes, e.g., 30 minutes after ischemia in hilar neurons or 24 hours after ischemia in CA1.

Confirming that TSQ fluorescence in the degenerating neurons reflected increased intracellular Zn^{++}, exposure to the specific cell-permeable Zn^{++} chelator, dithizone, abolished this fluorescence. Arguing against the possibility that Zn^{++} accumulation was a nonspecific accompaniment of cell death (e.g., due to release of protein-bound Zn^{++} into the cytosol), TSQ fluorescence was prominent in cultured cortical neurons degenerating after exposure to Zn^{++} plus α-amino-3-hydroxy-5-methyl-4-isoxazolepropionic acid (AMPA), but not after the neuronal deaths induced by NMDA, ionomycin, Fe^{+++}, or staurosporine.

To block the influx of extracellular Zn^{++} into postsynaptic neurons, we turned to the cell-membrane-impermeant chelator, disodium ethylenediaminetetraacetate (EDTA), saturated with equimolar Ca^{++} (CaEDTA). EDTA has higher affinity for Ca^{++} than Mg^{++}, but a much higher affinity for Zn^{++} than either Ca^{++} or Mg^{++}. Thus, CaEDTA will bind extracellular Zn^{++} without reducing extracellular Ca^{++} or significantly reducing extracellular Mg^{++}. In addition, since EDTA is membrane-impermeant, it is unlikely to disturb intracellular Zn^{++} homeostasis or the function of Zn^{++} metalloenzymes.

Addition of 1 mM CaEDTA, but not 1 mM ZnEDTA, to the bathing medium blocked the death of cultured cortical neurons induced by 15-minute exposure to 1 mM Zn^{++} alone, or the synergistic combination of 300 mM Zn^{++} and 5 mM AMPA. CaEDTA did not reduce the Ca^{++}-overload excitotoxicity induced by exposure to NMDA, kainate, or AMPA in vitro, or hippocampal neuronal death induced by NMDA injection in vivo; furthermore, it did not reduce the neurotoxicity of Fe^{++} or Cu^{++}, probably because it did not interfere with the participation of these ions in Fenton chemistry.

Injection of CaEDTA, but not ZnEDTA, into the lateral ventricles 30 minutes prior to transient forebrain ischemia markedly reduced Zn^{++} influx into hilar or CA1 pyramidal neurons, and their degeneration 72 hours later. Similar interference with Zn^{++} translocation and neuroprotective effects were also seen in several other brain regions, including thalamic reticular nucleus, amygdala, neocortex, and striatum.

QUESTIONS FOR THE FUTURE

The possibility that selective neuronal death in several brain regions following transient brain ischemia may be mediated substantially by the toxic transsynaptic movement of Zn^{++} from presynaptic terminals into postsynaptic neurons raises several broad themes for future study. Three in particular seem pressing:

1. First is the issue of possible practical application. Even before the mechanisms underlying ischemic Zn^{++} toxicity are completely sorted out, could extracellular chelation strategies be utilized therapeutically in victims of cardiac arrest? Certainly it would be more attractive if a membrane-permeable chelating agent could be found, capable of attenuating ischemic Zn^{++} toxicity without producing intolerable disturbances in normal neuronal function. However, perhaps administration of a membrane-impermeant chelator such as CaEDTA by lumbar or cisternal puncture could be contemplated in patients facing a certain grave neurological prognosis after a slow resuscitation.
2. Given recent suggestions that selective neuronal death, at least in hippocampal CA1, occurs by apoptosis (Goto et al. 1990; Shigeno et al. 1990; Héron et al. 1993; MacManus et al. 1993; Okamoto et al. 1993; Nitatori et al. 1995), can Zn^{++} toxicity induce apoptosis? Intense exposure to Zn^{++} produces marked neuronal swelling suggestive of necrosis (Choi et al. 1988), but preliminary experiments suggest that low levels of Zn^{++} exposure can trigger neuronal cell death sensitive to inhibition by either cycloheximide or the interleukin-1β-converting enzyme, ZVAD-FMK (D. Lobner et al., unpubl.).
3. What factors determine whether neurons receive a toxic Zn^{++} insult after global ischemia? Ischemic Zn^{++} toxicity cannot simply reflect the presence of Zn^{++}-containing inputs, because then hippocampal CA3 neurons would be the most vulnerable to this damage. Indeed, not all neurons are equally vulnerable to Zn^{++}-induced death; for example, cortical GABAergic neurons exhibit heightened vulnerability to Zn^{++}-induced death (J. Weiss, pers. comm.), probably because their expression of Ca^{++}-permeable AMPA/kainate receptors (Yin et al. 1994) provides a powerful route of Zn^{++} entry. Do all voltage-gated Ca^{++} channels participate equally in Zn^{++} toxicity, or do certain classes of Ca^{++} channels play a predominant role (and can these then be considered "Zn^{++} channels")? Other factors such as the availability of transporters capable of restoring Zn^{++} homeostasis (Palmiter and Findley 1995), or the state of intracellular targets sensitive to Zn^{++} activation, may also weigh in. Delineation of these factors may permit the development of novel strategies for the therapeutic interdiction of Zn^{++} toxicity after global ischemic insults.

ACKNOWLEDGMENTS

This work was supported by National Institutes of Health grant NS-32636.

REFERENCES

Assaf, S.Y. and S.H. Chung. 1984. Release of endogenous Zn^{++} from brain tissue during activity. *Nature* **308:** 734.

Choi, D.W., M. Yokoyama, and J. Koh. 1988. Zinc neurotoxicity in cortical cell culture. *Neuroscience* **24:** 67.

Christine, C.W. and D.W. Choi. 1990. Effect of zinc on NMDA receptor-mediated channel currents in cortical neurons. *J. Neurosci.* **10:** 108.

Frederickson, C.J.. 1989. Neurobiology of zinc and zinc-containing neurons. *Int. Rev. Neurobiol.* **131:** 145.

Frederickson, C.J., B.A. Rampy, S. Reamy-Rampy, and G.A. Howell. 1992. Distribution of histochemically reactive zinc in the forebrain of the rat. *J. Chem. Neuroanat.* **5:** 521.

Frederickson, C.J., M.D. Hernandez, S.A. Goik, J.D. Morton, and J.F. McGinty. 1988. Loss of zinc staining from hippocampal mossy fibers during kainic acid induced seizures: A histofluorescence study. *Brain Res.* **446:** 383.

Goto, K., A. Ishige, K. Sekiguchi, S. Iizuka, A. Sugimoto, M. Yuzurihara, M. Aburada, E. Hosoya, and K. Kogure. 1990. Effects of cycloheximide on delayed neuronal death in rat hippocampus. *Brain Res.* **534:** 299.

Héron, A., H. Pollard, F. Dessi, J. Moreau, F. Lasbennes, Y. Ben-Ari, and C. Charriaut-Marlangue. 1993. Regional variability in DNA fragmentation after global ischemia evidenced by combined histological and gel electrophoresis observations in the rat brain. *J. Neurochem.* **61:** 1973.

Koh, J.Y. and D.W. Choi. 1988. Zinc alters excitatory amino acid neurotoxicity on cortical neurons. *J. Neurosci.* **8:** 2164.

———. 1994. Zinc toxicity on cultured cortical neurons: Involvement on *N*-methyl-δ-aspartate receptors. *Neuroscience* **60:** 1049.

Koh, J.Y., S.W. Suh, B.J. Gwag, Y.Y. He, C.Y. Hsu, and D.W. Choi. 1996. The role of zinc in selective neuronal death after transient global cerebral ischemia. *Science* **272:** 1013.

MacManus, J.P., A.M. Buchan, I.E. Hill, I. Rasquinha, and E. Preston. 1993. Global ischemia can cause DNA fragmentation indicative of apoptosis in rat brain. *Neurosci. Lett.* **164:** 89.

Nitatori, T., N. Sato, S. Waguri, Y. Karasawa, H. Araki, K. Shibanai, E. Kominami, and Y. Uchiyama. 1995. Delayed neuronal death in the CA1 pyramidal cell layer of the gerbil hippocampus following transient ischemia is apoptosis. *J. Neurosci.* **15:** 1001.

Okamoto, M., M. Matsumoto, T. Ohtsuki, A. Taguchi, K. Mikoshiba, T. Yanagihara, and T. Kamada. 1993. Internucleosomal DNA cleavage involved in ischemia-induced neuronal death. *Biochem. Biophys. Res. Commun.* **196:** 1356.

Palmiter, R.D. and S.D. Findley. 1995. Cloning and functional characterization of a mammalian zinc transporter that confers resistance to zinc. *EMBO J.* **14:** 639.

Peters, S., J. Koh, and D.W. Choi. 1987. Zinc selectively blocks the action of *N*-methyl-δ-aspartate on cortical neurons. *Science* **236:** 589.

Shigeno, T., Y. Yamasaki, G. Kato, K. Kusaka, T. Mima, K. Takakura, D.I. Graham, and S. Furukawa. 1990. Reduction of delayed neuronal death by inhibition of protein synthesis. *Neurosci. Lett.* **120:** 117.

Sloviter, R.S.. 1985. A selective loss of hippocampal mossy fiber Timm stain accompanies granule cell seizure activity induced by perforant path stimulation. *Brain Res.* **330:** 150.

Smart, T.G., X. Xie, and B.J. Krishek. 1994. Modulation of inhibitory and excitatory amino acid receptor ion channels by zinc. *Prog. Neurobiol.* **42:** 393.

Tonder, N., F.F. Johansen, C.J. Frederickson, J. Zimmer, and N.H. Diemer. 1990. Possible role of zinc in the selective degeneration of dentate hilar neurons after cerebral ischemia in the adult rat. *Neurosci. Lett.* **109:** 247.

Weiss, J.H., D.M. Hartley, J.Y. Koh, and D.W. Choi. 1993. AMPA receptor activation potentiates zinc neurotoxicity. *Neuron* **10:** 43.

Westbrook, G.L. and M.L. Mayer. 1987. Micromolar concentrations of Zn^{++} antagonize NMDA and GABA responses of hippocampal neurons. *Nature* **328:** 640.

Yin, H.Z., D.M. Turetsky, D.W. Choi, and J.H. Weiss. 1994. Cortical neurons with Ca^{2+} permeable AMPA/kainate channels display distinct receptor immunoreactivity and are GABAergic. *Neurobiol. Dis.* **1:** 43.

A Signaling Endosome Hypothesis to Explain NGF Actions: Potential Implications for Neurodegeneration

E.C. BEATTIE,[1,5] J. ZHOU,[2,5] M.L. GRIMES,[4] N.W. BUNNETT,[1] C.L. HOWE,[3] AND W.C. MOBLEY[2,3]

[1]*Department of Physiology,* [2]*Department of Neurology, and* [3]*The Neuroscience Program, University of California, San Francisco, California 94143;* [4]*Department of Biochemistry, Massey University, Palmerston North, New Zealand*

Nerve growth factor (NGF), a polypeptide neurotrophic factor of the neurotrophin (NT) gene family, acts to enhance the survival and differentiation of specific populations of neurons in the central (CNS) and peripheral (PNS) nervous systems (Levi-Montalcini 1987; Yuen and Mobley 1995). NGF acts by binding to both high- and low-affinity receptors. Its receptors are $p75^{NGFR}$ and TrkA. $p75^{NGFR}$ is a receptor for all the neurotrophins, exhibiting binding affinities in the nanomolar range (i.e., low-affinity binding) (Meakin and Shooter 1992; Bothwell 1995). The role that $p75^{NGFR}$ plays in NGF signaling is not well defined; however, in addition to a direct signaling function (Bothwell 1996; Carter et al. 1996; Taglialatela et al. 1996), $p75^{NGFR}$ has been shown to modulate NGF binding and activation of TrkA (Meakin and Shooter 1992; Davies et al. 1993; Barker and Shooter 1994; Hantzopoulos et al. 1994; Mahadeo et al. 1994; Verdi et al. 1994; Bothwell 1995). TrkA is a receptor tyrosine kinase (Kaplan et al. 1991; Klein et al. 1991; Meakin and Shooter 1991). Although the exact composition of high-affinity receptors is controversial (Hempstead et al. 1991; Meakin and Shooter 1992; Mahadeo et al. 1994; Bothwell 1995), TrkA alone has been shown to create both high- and low-affinity NGF-binding sites (Jing et al. 1992). It is also the receptor responsible for the slowly dissociating component of NGF binding that characterizes high-affinity receptors (Meakin et al. 1992). NGF binding causes TrkA dimerization with resulting activation of its kinase domain (Kaplan et al. 1991; Klein et al. 1991; Meakin and Shooter 1991; Jing et al. 1992). Autophosphorylation of certain tyrosine residues in the intracellular domain of the receptor creates sites for binding and activation of signaling intermediates which continue the signal transduction cascade (Stephens et al. 1994). Phospholipase C-γ (PLC-γ), SHC (an adapter protein containing sequences to the Src domain 2), and phosphatidylinositol 3 kinase are known intermediaries in this cascade (Stephens et al. 1994). The significance of TrkA activation for NGF signaling has been tested in vitro and in vivo. In cultured cells, TrkA activation induces many of the typical neuronal responses to NGF (Loeb and Greene 1993). TrkA also plays an important role in NGF signaling in vivo. Animals in which the gene for TrkA was disrupted showed marked abnormalities in the development of NGF-responsive neurons in the CNS and PNS (Smeyne et al. 1994).

In earlier studies, we defined NGF-responsive CNS neurons by localizing TrkA gene expression and by demonstrating that all *TrkA*-expressing populations responded to NGF with hypertrophy of the cell body (Holtzman et al. 1992, 1995). Significantly, some of these populations do not express $p75^{NGFR}$. These data suggest that in these neurons TrkA is able to transduce the NGF signal. To further characterize NGF actions, we examined gene expression in the NGF-responsive cholinergic neurons of the basal forebrain (BFCN) and caudate-putamen (CPCN). Consistent with findings in earlier studies (Johnston et al. 1987; Fusco et al. 1989; Higgins et al. 1989), NGF treatment induced an increase in mRNA for choline acetyltransferase (ChAT) in both populations (Holtzman et al. 1992). Remarkably, *TrkA* expression was also increased by NGF. Intracerebroventricular infusion of NGF into adult rats for 2 weeks led to approximately a 60% increase in TrkA mRNA in both BFCNs and CPCNs (Holtzman et al. 1992). These data show that NGF signaling is positively linked to expression of *TrkA*. Such a relationship also appears to exist under physiological conditions. Studies in developing animals show that *TrkA* expression in BFCNs parallels that for *NGF* expression in the hippocampus and neocortex, the target fields of BFCN axons, and that *TrkA* expression is suppressed by infusion of specific NGF antibodies (Li et al. 1995). It is often the case that ligands negatively regulate their receptors (Collins et al. 1992). Thus, the NGF effect on *TrkA* was surprising and unexplained.

To pursue further the mechanism and significance of NGF actions on *TrkA* expression, we carried out studies in PC12 cells, a neuron-like cell line that has been used extensively to characterize NGF signaling (Tischler and Greene 1975; Stephens et al. 1994; Zhou et al. 1995). Our findings demonstrate that NGF has widespread effects on TrkA, regulating activation, trafficking, degradation, and synthesis. How these actions are integrated was suggested by noting distinct phases in the NGF response: an early phase characterized by down-regulation of TrkA and a later phase that featured enhanced *TrkA* expression. Dramatic down-regulation of surface TrkA within minutes of NGF treatment, with subsequent degradation of TrkA,

[5]These authors contributed equally to the work.

raised the possibility that NGF induces internalization of activated TrkA receptors and targets them to lysosomes. We gathered evidence to show that this is the case. Our findings suggest that it is through the formation and retrograde transport of activated TrkA-containing signaling endosomes that NGF released in the target of responsive neurons acts to regulate gene expression to support survival, differentiation, and maintenance. NGF-induced increases in *TrkA* expression may serve to replace receptors degraded after carrying the retrograde signal. Certain aspects of these studies have been reported previously (Zhou et al. 1995; Grimes et al. 1996).

MATERIALS AND METHODS

Materials

Bis(sulfosuccinimidyl)suberate (BS^3), disuccinimidyl suberate (DSS), and NHS-SS-biotin were obtained from Pierce (Rockford, Illinois). Normal goat serum and Vectashield mounting medium were from Vector Laboratories, Inc. (Burlingame, California). Except as noted herein, or as indicated (M.L. Grimes et al., in prep.), Sigma (St. Louis, Missouri) was the source of all other reagents and chemicals. NGF was prepared as described previously (Mobley et al. 1986) and was labeled with ^{125}I (Amersham, Arlington Heights, Illinois) using lactoperoxidase, as modified from Vale and Shooter (Vale and Shooter 1985; M.L. Grimes et al., in prep.). 1088 is a rabbit antibody against the carboxyl terminus of human TrkA. It was purified using protein A–Sepharose (Pierce) and has been characterized previously (Zhou et al. 1995). Sc11 is another rabbit antibody to the carboxyl terminus of human TrkA (Santa Cruz Biotechnology, Santa Cruz, California). RTA is a rabbit antibody against the extracellular domain of rat TrkA (Clary et al. 1994; Lucidi-Phillipi et al. 1996). X22 is a mouse monoclonal antibody to the clathrin heavy chain (Brodsky 1985). AP.6 is a mouse monoclonal antibody to the α-adaptin 100-kD subunits (Chin et al. 1989). GM10 is a mouse monoclonal antibody that stains lysosomes (Grimaldi et al. 1987; Grady et al. 1995). The antibody to PLC-γ1 was a mixed monoclonal antibody; 4G10 is a mouse monoclonal antibody to phosphorylated tyrosine; the antibody to SHC is a rabbit polyclonal antibody (all from Upstate Biotechnology Inc., Lake Placid, New York). ^{125}I-labeled goat anti-mouse was prepared using $Na^{125}I$ (Amersham), iodobeads (Pierce), and goat-anti-mouse (Pierce) according to the manufacturer's instructions, and desalted on a PD-10 column (Pharmacia Biotech, Inc., Piscataway, New Jersey).

Methods

Cell culture procedures for biochemical examinations. PC12 cells were maintained in Dulbecco's modified Eagle's (DME H-21) medium supplemented with 10% heat-inactivated horse serum, 5% fetal calf serum, 100 units/ml penicillin, and 100 μg/ml streptomycin. PC12 cells not treated with NGF are also referred to as "naive" cells. PC12 cells were "primed" by incubating with mouse NGF (50 ng/ml = 1.9 nM) for at least 1 week (Zhou et al. 1995). For binding and surface cross-linking experiments, culture plates (Falcon) were precoated with rat tail collagen (Collaborative Biomedical, Bedford, Massachusetts). Immediately before each experiment on primed cells, the cells were washed three times with NGF-free, fresh tissue culture medium for 2 hours at 37°C.

RNA isolation and Northern blot analysis. The procedures used were essentially those described previously (Holtzman et al. 1992). PC12 cells grown to 30% confluence were treated with mouse NGF (50 ng/ml) at 37°C for the times indicated. Cells were harvested and total RNA was prepared using guanidinium isothiocyanate extraction. For Northern blots, 20 μg of total RNA was electrophoresed on 1% agarose-formaldehyde gels and blotted to Genescreen (Dupont, Boston, Massachusetts). Blots were probed with ^{32}P-labeled cDNAs for rat *trkA*, rat $p75^{NGFR}$, or 18S rRNA. After washing at high stringency, blots were exposed to X-ray films and quantitated as described previously (Zhou et al. 1995).

Immunoprecipitation and Western blotting of whole-cell lysates. Immunoprecipitation and Western blotting were performed as described previously (Zhou et al. 1995). PC12 cells were lysed at 4°C in lysis buffer #1 (20 mM Tris HCl, pH 8.0, 150 mM NaCl, 1% NP-40, 10% glycerol, 1 mM sodium orthovanadate, and a cocktail of protease inhibitors (1 mM phenylmethylsulfonyl fluoride 10 mg/ml benzamidine, 1 mg/ml *o*-phenanthroline, 0.1 mg/ml each of pepstatin, chymostatin, leupeptin, and aprotinin). Lysates (1 ml) were immunoprecipitated while rocking overnight at 4°C with antibodies to TrkA (1088) (10 mg), PLC-γ1 (5 mg), or $p75^{NGFR}$ (7 mg) (REX), and immunoprecipitates were collected and processed according to the method of Zhou et al. (1995). After boiling for 5 minutes in 50 μl of 2x SDS-PAGE sample buffer (2% SDS, 10% glycerol, 0.1 M DTT, 125 mM Tris, pH 6.95, 0.1% bromophenol blue), they were subjected to 7.5% SDS-PAGE and transferred to nitrocellulose. For examining TrkA, blots probed with 1088 or RTA were incubated with 1 μCi ^{125}I-labeled protein A (Amersham). For measuring phosphotyrosine, blots were incubated with 4G10, then washed and incubated with goat anti-mouse IgG antibodies (Boehringer Mannheim Corporation, Indianapolis, Indiana) prior to using ^{125}I-labeled protein A or the ECL chemiluminescence system (Amersham) for detection. All blots were exposed to X-ray film, and band intensities were quantified on a densitometer (LKB Ultroscan, Gaithersberg, Maryland) (Zhou et al. 1995).

NGF binding and cross-linking to surface receptors. PC12 cells were maintained as indicated. Naive and primed cells were seeded in six-well collagen-coated plates at a density of 5 x 10^5 cells per well 2 days before assay. Naive cells and primed cells (washed free of NGF for 2 hours at 37°C with culture medium) were washed with binding buffer at 4°C for 10 minutes and then incubated in binding buffer containing ^{125}I-labeled NGF at either 100 pM or 2 nM for 2 hours at 4°C. To measure binding to slowly dissociating receptors, cells were washed in NGF-free binding buffer at 4°C for 1 hour. For internalization studies, cells bound to NGF at steady state were incubated at 37°C for various time periods and chilled to 4°C. Internalized NGF was then measured, as indicated previously (Zhou et al. 1995). To measure down-regulation of surface gp140^{TrkA}, cells (10^7/15-cm dish), plated 2 days before the experiment, were washed and then incubated with ^{125}I-labeled NGF, as above. They were then warmed to 37°C for 1 hour, and chilled (4°C) before cross-linking. To measure cross-linking to slowly dissociating receptors, cells were washed in ligand-free binding buffer at 4°C for 1 hour prior to cross-linking.

To cross-link NGF to gp140^{TrkA}, BS^3 was added to a final concentration of 0.8 mM in binding buffer. Samples were incubated at 4°C for 30 minutes, washed, and lysed in lysis buffer, as above. ^{125}I-labeled NGF/gp140^{TrkA} complexes were immunoprecipitated with 1088. The immunoprecipitates were boiled in the SDS-PAGE sample buffer for 5 minutes and subjected to SDS-PAGE using a gradient resolving gel (5.0% acrylamide with 0.1% bisacrylamide to 12.0% acrylamide with 0.5% bisacrylamide). Gels were fixed in 20% methanol with 10% isopropanol and 10% acetic acid, dried, and exposed to X-ray film or to a phosphorimager screen. Quantitation was via a Molecular Dynamics PhosphorImager (Molecular Dynamics, Sunnyvale, California).

Cell surface biotinylation. Cells were incubated with or without NGF (1 nM) for 30 minutes at 4°C in PBS with 1 mg/ml glucose, and NHS-SS-biotin (0.5 mg/ml) was then added. The mixture was incubated with gentle rocking for 90 minutes at 4°C. Cells were pelleted (1000 rpm for 5 min) and then washed 3 times in cold PBS containing 1 mM lysine. Samples were then processed as indicated previously (M.L. Grimes et al., in prep.) producing three equal aliquots. Aliquot #1 was held at 4°C. Aliquot #2 was treated at 4°C with 50 mM reduced glutathione in 50 mM Tris, pH 8.6, 100 mM NaCl 1 mg/ml glucose, and 1 mg/ml BSA for 30 minutes. This treatment was repeated twice. Aliquot #3 was warmed to 37°C for either 10 or 20 minutes to allow endocytosis, and then treated with glutathione as above. All aliquots were then incubated 1 hour on ice in 0.2 ml lysis buffer #2 (20 mM Tris, pH 8.0, 150 mM NaCl, 1% NP-40, 1 mM EDTA) containing 1% BSA and 1 mg/ml iodoacetamide. The lysates were centrifuged 10 minutes at 10,000*g*. SDS (final concentration 0.5%) was added to the supernatant, and the lysates were boiled for 5 minutes. Lysis buffer #2 (0.8 ml) was then added, and TrkA was immunoprecipitated with 1088 (12 μg). Each lysate was divided into two parts. The first was used to detect the amount of biotinylated TrkA. Proteins were separated on nonreducing 7.5% SDS-PAGE, transferred to nitrocellulose (Hoefer Pharmacia Biotech Inc., San Francisco, California), and blotted with ^{125}I-labeled streptavidin (Amersham). Biotinylated TrkA was quantified by PhosphorImager (Molecular Dynamics, Sunnyvale, California). The second part was used to quantitate TrkA protein. It was submitted to 7.5% SDS-PAGE in a reducing environment, transferred to nitrocellulose, and blotted with 1088 (1:500). The signal was developed using ^{125}I-protein A (Amersham) and quantified using the PhosphorImager. The signal for biotinylated TrkA was normalized to the amount of TrkA protein. The TrkA available for internalization was calculated as follows: aliquot #1 – aliquot #2. TrkA internalized during warming was not susceptible to reduction with glutathione. The amount of TrkA internalized was calculated: aliquot #3 – aliquot #2. The percentage of TrkA internalized was calculated as follows: aliquot #3 – aliquot #2) (aliquot #1 – aliquot #2) x 100.

Immunostaining and confocal microscopy. Cells were plated on 8-well chamber slides (Nunc Inc., Naperville, Illinois) that had been coated with Matrigel (Collaborative Biomedical Products) using a 1:200 dilution in PBS (Ca^{++}- and Mg^{++}-free) overnight at 4°C. Wells were washed 3 times with cold PBS. PC12 cells were plated in DME H-21 medium with 10% horse serum and 5% fetal calf serum 1–2 days before experiments. After aspirating the medium, NGF (2 nM) was added to cells for 30 seconds, 2 minutes, or 60 minutes in 300 μl of DME H-21 containing 0.5 mg/ml bovine serum albumin, 10 mM HEPES at 37°C. This medium, without NGF, was added to controls.

Cells were fixed on ice with 1% paraformaldehyde in PBS for 15 minutes. Cells were permeabilized in PSS (PBS with 10% normal goat serum and saponin [1 mg/ml]) at room temperature for 30 minutes, changing the solution every 10 minutes. Primary antibodies were diluted in PSS (sc11 at 1 μg/ml; X22 at 3.1 μg/ml; GM10 at 1:6000; AP.6 at 8 μg/ml) and incubated with cells overnight at 4°C. After three 10-minute washes with PSS, secondary antibodies diluted in PSS (FITC-conjugated goat-anti-rabbit IgG at 1:100; Texas Red-conjugated goat-anti-mouse immunoglobulins 1:200; both from Cappel Research Products, Durham, North Carolina) were applied for 45 minutes at room temperature. After 3 washes in PBS, coverslips were mounted using Vectashield mounting solution. No staining was evident when primary antibodies were excluded. For Sc11, preliminary incubation (overnight, 4°C) with the peptide immunogen (10 μg/ml) eliminated staining.

Cells were observed with an MRC 1000 Laser Scanning Confocal Microscope (Biorad Laboratories, Inc.,

Hercules, California) equipped with a krypton/argon laser and attached to a Zeiss Axiovert microscope. A Zeiss Neofluor x 100 oil-immersion objective with a numerical aperture of 1.3 (∞0.17) was used, and images were collected using an aperture of 3–4 mm and a zoom of 2–3. Typically, 10–20 optical sections were taken at 0.5-μm intervals through the cells. The resolution of the confocal microscope in the X-Y axis was 170–200 nm, and in the Z axis was 230–400 nm. Images of 768 x 520 pixels were obtained. Images were processed using Adobe Photoshop 3.0 (Adobe Systems Inc., Mountain View, California) and printed using a Techtronix Printer. In experiments in which markers were colocalized, colocalization was confirmed by examining individual organelles at higher magnification. In addition, we ensured that colocalization was eliminated by merging overlaying, but noncoincident, sections. The images shown correspond to optical sections through cells at mid-height.

To count TrkA-positive vesicles or TrkA/clathrin colocalizations near the surface of cells, images of individual optical sections were examined. The edge of the cell was defined as the outermost limit of staining for the clathrin heavy chain, and this was marked with a line. A second line was drawn 0.5 μm interior to the first, and all bright, punctate TrkA-positive vesicles between the lines were counted. The number of these vesicles was then recorded per cell or was divided by the perimeter of the surface of the cell to yield a value for the number per micron of cell perimeter.

Cell fractionation. In some experiments, cells were first incubated with or without NGF (1 nM) in binding buffer at 4°C for 1 hour. They were then either washed briefly in binding buffer, or not washed, and warmed in binding buffer for 10 min at 37°C. In other experiments, NGF was added to cells at 37°C. Cells were then chilled (4°C) and washed in PBS with 1 mM EDTA and 1 mM EGTA, and then in a cytoplasm-like buffer (buffer B) (38 mM each of the potassium salts of aspartic, gluconic, and glutamic acids; 20 mM MOPS; 5 mM reduced glutathione; 10 mM potassium bicarbonate; 0.5 mM magnesium carbonate; 1 mM EGTA; 1 mM EDTA; pH adjusted to 7.1 at 37°C with potassium hydroxide). Cells were resuspended in 0.5 ml buffer B containing proteinase inhibitors (as for lysis buffer #1). Sodium orthovanadate (1 mM) was included to inhibit phosphatase activity for the experiments shown in Figures 11 and 12. To permeabilize cells, we used a ball homogenizer obtained from the European Molecular Biology Laboratory (Heidelberg, Germany) and tungsten carbide grade 25 balls obtained from Industrial Tectonics, Inc. (Ann Arbor, Michigan). The cell suspension was passed through the homogenizer (8.020 mm cylinder with an 8.0186 mm ball). Greater than 98% of the cells stained with trypan blue after this procedure. By centrifuging at 1000*g* for 10 minutes, cell ghosts (P1) were pelleted, thus separating them from the cytosol and the released vesicles. The 1000*g* supernatant was centrifuged at 8000*g* for 35 minutes in a TiSW50.1 rotor. The pellet (P2) contained large organelles. The supernatant (S2) was layered over a 0.4-ml pad of 10% sucrose in buffer B (with inclusions, as above) and centrifuged at 100,000*g* for 1 hour to produce the pellet, P3. S3 was the cytosol.

To determine whether fragments of plasma membrane contaminated released intracellular organelles, we biotinylated cell-surface proteins and determined whether amyloid precursor protein (APP), a relatively abundant protein (Haass et al. 1992), was detected in P2 and P3. PC12 cells were harvested and cell-surface proteins were biotinylated, as indicated above, for 20 minutes at 4°C. Cells were washed 3 times with 1 mM lysine in PBS and then permeabilized and fractionated. P1, P2, and P3 were lysed in lysis buffer #2 and immunoprecipitated with α-C7, an antibody to the carboxyl terminus of APP (Podlisny et al. 1991). Immunoprecipitates were submitted to 7.5% SDS-PAGE and blotted. ^{125}I-labeled streptavidin was used to probe the blots, and the Phosphorimager was used for detection. To quantify ^{125}I-labeled NGF in intracellular organelles, fractions were assayed for ^{125}I-labeled NGF. In some experiments, acid-washing (Bernd and Greene 1984) was used to measure surface-bound ^{125}I-labeled NGF.

NGF cross-linking to intracellular TrkA. Cells incubated with ^{125}I-labeled NGF (1 nM) in binding buffer for 1 hour at 4°C were washed and then warmed for 10 minutes at 37°C prior to permeabilization, as above. Unlabeled NGF (1 mM) was added to control for nonspecific binding and cross-linking. DSS (2 mM) was added to the permeabilized cells and released membranes and the mixture was incubated while rotating for 30 minutes (4°C). The reaction was quenched with lysine (10 mM) for 10 minutes. P1, P2, and P3 were then prepared, as above. P1 was solubilized by extracting in 1% NP-40 in buffer B for 1 hour (4°C). After centrifuging at 1000*g* (10 min), SDS was added to bring the final concentration to 0.5%. P2 and P3 were resuspended in H_2O with 0.5% SDS. S3 was brought to the same SDS concentration. All samples were boiled for 5 minutes, chilled (4°C), and then brought to a volume of 1 ml and a final concentration of 0.1% SDS by diluting with immunoprecipitation (IP) buffer (20 mM HEPES, pH 7.4, 0.15 M NaCl, 1% NP-40, 0.5% DOC, 1 mM EDTA). To this was added 1088 (17 μg/ml). After incubating at 4°C overnight 1/10 volume of 20% protein A–Sepharose beads (Pierce) was added for 1 hour, with rotation. The beads were washed twice with IP buffer and once with water before resuspending in 7 M urea SDS-PAGE sample buffer with 20 mM DTT. Samples were heated to 65°C for 10 minutes and run on a 5–12% SDS-PAGE. Dried gels were exposed to XAR film for 1–3 weeks.

Immunoprecipitation and blotting of cellular fractions. PC12 cells incubated without NGF, or with NGF

(2 nm), at 37°C were chilled (4°C), mechanically permeabilized, and fractionated as above. Immunoprecipitation of cell fractions was performed by dissolving P1, P2, P3, or S3 in 1 ml of lysis buffer #1. To this was added 12 µg of 1088, or 5 µg of anti-SHC. The mixture was incubated overnight at 4°C and 1/10 volume of protein A or protein-A/G Sepharose beads was added for 2 hours at 4°C. Sepharose beads were washed 3 times in lysis buffer #1 and once with water, then treated with 50 µl of 7 M urea SDS-PAGE sample buffer (125 mM Tris, pH 6.95, 7 M urea, 2% SDS, 1 mM EDTA, 0.1% Bromphenol Blue) with 100 mM DTT and heated (55°C, 15–30 min). Samples were loaded on 7.5% SDS-PAGE. After transferring to nitrocellulose, blots were probed with antiphosphotyrosine (4G10), RTA, or anti-PLC-γ1. Immune complexes were detected with horseradish peroxidase-conjugated anti-mouse IgG or anti-rabbit IgG and chemiluminescence (Amersham).

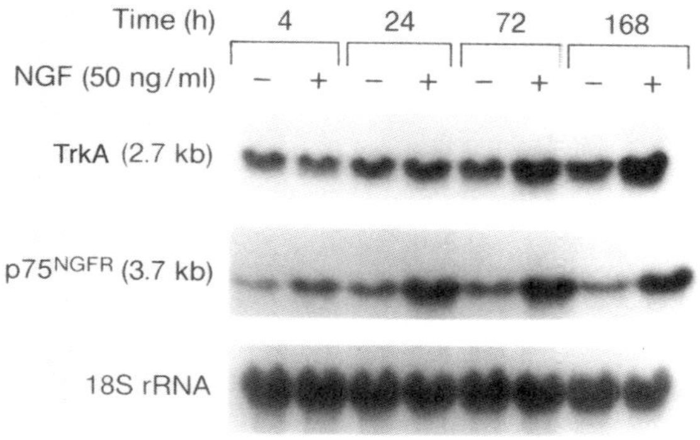

Figure 1. NGF induces gene expression for *Trk*A and $p75^{NGFR}$ in PC12 cells. PC12 cells were treated with NGF (50 ng/ml = 1.9 nM) for 4 hr, 24 hr, 72 hr, and 168 hr. Cells were harvested and total RNA from untreated (–) or NGF-treated (+) cells was prepared and analyzed on Northern blot; 20 µg was loaded in each lane. Blots were hybridized with rat *TrkA* cDNA or rat $p75^{NGFR}$ cDNA. The 18S rRNA probe was used to control for RNA loading. (Reprinted, with permission, from Zhou et al. 1995.)

RESULTS

NGF Increased TrkA mRNA in PC12 Cells

In vivo studies showed that NGF infusion into the CNS induced an increase in TrkA mRNA levels in forebrain cholinergic neurons of both developing and adult rats (Holtzman et al. 1992; Li et al. 1995). Earlier studies documenting NGF-induced increases in TrkA mRNA in PC12 cells (Holtzman et al. 1992; Meakin et al. 1992) encouraged use of these cells to examine further NGF regulation of *TrkA*. Northern blotting was used to examine total RNA isolated from naive (i.e., untreated) PC12 cells and from PC12 cells treated with NGF (50 ng/ml = 1.9 nM) for 4 hours, 24 hours, 3 days, 7 days, or 14 days. TrkA mRNA was decreased about 40% (n = 4) at 4 hours following NGF addition (Fig. 1). It was increased to 1.5-fold (n = 4) the untreated level at 2 days and reached a maximum (3.7-fold, n = 4) at day 7 (Fig. 1), remaining at this level for up to 14 days (data not shown). NGF is also known to increase $p75^{NGFR}$ expression in PC12 cells (Miller et al. 1991; Meakin et al. 1992). A different time course was seen for NGF effects on $p75^{NGFR}$ mRNA. It was increased to 2.0-fold (n = 4) the untreated level by 8 hours (data not shown), 3.4-fold (n = 4) at 24 hours, and remained at about this level through 7 days (Fig. 1). For both genes, the effect of NGF was transient. After NGF removal, mRNA levels for TrkA and $p75^{NGFR}$ fell to control levels within 48 hours (data not shown).

TrkA Protein Levels: Distinct Early and Late Responses to NGF

To ask whether the NGF-induced increase in *TrkA* expression would result in increased protein levels, we measured TrkA protein following NGF addition. The time points chosen (5 minutes, 30 minutes, 60 minutes, 2 days, and 7 days) allowed us to evaluate both immediate and long-term NGF effects. TrkA proteins were immunoprecipitated from cell lysates using 1088, an antibody directed at the carboxyl terminus of human TrkA (Zhou et al. 1995). Immunoprecipitates were submitted to SDS-PAGE and analyzed after immunoblotting with 1088. Proteins of 140 kD and 110 kD were detected. The former corresponds to the mature form of the receptor (Martin-Zanca et al. 1989; Kaplan et al. 1991; Klein et al. 1991; Meakin and Shooter 1991) and will be referred to herein as $gp140^{TrkA}$. The 110-kD species is a precursor (Martin-Zanca et al. 1989) and is referred to as $gp110^{TrkA}$. Figure 2 shows that NGF markedly influenced the levels of both $gp140^{TrkA}$ and $gp110^{TrkA}$ and that the early response was distinct from that which occurred after prolonged treatment. Soon after NGF addition, there was a marked decrease in $gp140^{TrkA}$. Although there was little change at 5 minutes, $gp140^{TrkA}$ was decreased at 30 minutes, and by 60 minutes the level was only 33% of that present in untreated cells (Fig. 2). The persistence of $gp110^{TrkA}$ at levels equal to those in untreated cells suggested that increased degradation of $gp140^{TrkA}$, and not a decrease in synthesis, was responsible.

With prolonged NGF treatment there were increases in both $gp110^{TrkA}$ and $gp140^{TrkA}$ (Fig. 2). On a per-cell basis, $gp110^{TrkA}$ was increased to 3.4-fold (n = 2) at 2 days, and at day 7 it was increased to 6.7-fold (n = 5). At day 2 of treatment, $gp140^{TrkA}$ was increased slightly relative to the level at 60 minutes. At day 7, it was increased to 3.0-fold (n = 5) that present in untreated cells. Although the increase in $gp140^{TrkA}$ was less pronounced than for $gp110^{TrkA}$, it was marked. One suggestion for the relatively smaller increase in $gp140^{TrkA}$ is that with continued NGF treatment, $gp140^{TrkA}$ continued to be targeted for degradation.

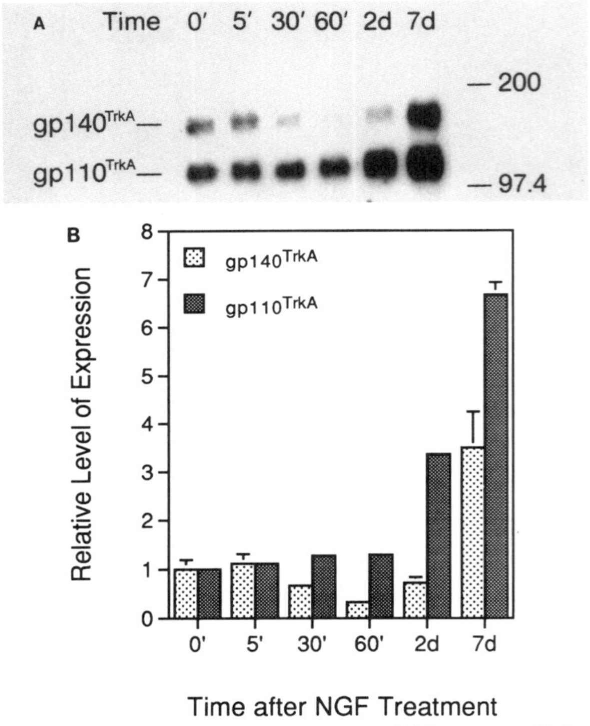

Figure 2. NGF regulates the level of gp140^{TrkA} and gp110^{TrkA}. (*A*) TrkA proteins were immunoprecipitated with 1088 from lysates of untreated PC12 cells (0′) or cells treated with NGF for 5 min, 30 min, 60 min, 2 days, and 7 days. Immunoprecipitates were analyzed on SDS-PAGE and immunoblotted with 1088. An equal number of cells was used for each lane. (*B*) gp140^{TrkA} and gp110^{TrkA} bands were quantitated by densitometry. The level of expression relative to untreated cells is plotted ($n = 2$ for each point). (Reprinted, with permission, from Zhou et al. 1995.)

Total protein increased in NGF-treated cells by 28% at 2 days and 60% at 7 days. Therefore, whether expressed on a per-cell or per-milligram of protein basis, TrkA protein increased with prolonged NGF treatment. Increased TrkA protein levels were correlated temporally with increased mRNA levels, suggesting that the increase in TrkA mRNA was responsible for the increase in TrkA protein. The same may be true of NGF effects on p75^{NGFR}; the increase in mRNA at day 7 (Fig. 1) was associated with a p75^{NGFR} protein level that was 2.4-fold ($n = 3$) that in untreated cells.

Increased gp140^{TrkA} Resulted in Increased NGF Binding and Signaling

The biphasic response of gp140^{TrkA} levels to NGF treatment suggested that NGF induces both the degradation and the synthesis of its receptors. We reasoned that both may mark important aspects of NGF signaling. To explore the significance of increased gp140^{TrkA}, we asked whether NGF treatment resulted in increased gp140^{TrkA} receptors at the cell surface. This possibility was suggested by earlier studies on PC12 cells showing that NGF produced an increase in both high-affinity and low-affinity binding (Bernd and Greene 1984). We investigated ^{125}I-labeled NGF binding to naive (i.e., untreated) and primed (i.e., NGF-treated for 7 days) cells, carrying out these experiments at 4°C to inhibit membrane traffic and endocytosis. Two NGF concentrations were used. At 100 pM NGF, one is below the ED_{50} for the neurite outgrowth response (ED_{50} ~ 400 pM), and at a level that is subsaturating for high-affinity receptors (K_D ~ 400 pM) (Bernd and Greene 1984). At 2 nM, NGF occupies most of these receptors and produces maximal neurite outgrowth. We found that ^{125}I-labeled NGF binding was increased on primed cells, when expressed on a per-cell basis. Relative to naive cells, binding to primed cells was increased to 1.8 (± 0.2)-fold (S.E.M.) ($n = 6$) at 100 pM and 1.6 (± 0.1)-fold ($n = 3$) at 2 nM. NGF bound to gp140^{TrkA} receptors dissociates slowly (Meakin et al. 1992). At 2 nM, the ^{125}I-labeled NGF bound to slowly dissociating surface receptors on primed cells was increased 1.6 (± 0.1)-fold ($n = 3$); there was a corresponding increase in fast-dissociating binding (i.e., binding to low-affinity receptors) to 1.5 (± 0.1)-fold on these cells. ^{125}I-labeled NGF internalization is known to be mediated by gp140^{TrkA} (Jing et al. 1992; Loeb and Greene 1993). After a 60-minute treatment, ^{125}I-labeled NGF internalization in primed cells was 1.8 (± 0.1)-fold ($n = 3$) that in naive cells. To show directly whether increased TrkA receptors contributed to increased NGF binding, we performed cross-linking studies. Naive and primed cells were incubated with ^{125}I-labeled NGF at 4°C for 2 hours, and then a membrane-impermeant cross-linking reagent was added. Following immunoprecipitation with 1088, the immunoprecipitates were analyzed by SDS-PAGE. For primed cells, ^{125}I-labeled NGF cross-linked to gp140^{TrkA} was increased 44% ($n = 2$) at 100 pM (Fig. 3) and 100% at 2 nM ($n = 2$). There was a comparable increase in ^{125}I-labeled NGF cross-linking to gp140^{TrkA} in slowly dissociating receptors on primed cells (data not shown). These data are evidence that increased gene expression for TrkA results in an increase in the number of cell-surface gp140^{TrkA} receptors on individual PC12 cells.

The increase in gp140^{TrkA} receptors suggested there may be increased NGF signaling in primed cells. NGF binding to gp140^{TrkA} induces receptor dimerization and autophosphorylation (Jing et al. 1992; Kaplan and Stephens 1994; Stephens et al. 1994). A pronounced increase in tyrosine-phosphorylated gp140^{TrkA} is registered within minutes of NGF treatment (Stephens et al. 1994). To ask whether NGF signaling was increased in primed cells, we examined tyrosine phosphorylation of gp140^{TrkA} in naive cells and in primed cells washed free of NGF for 2 hours before assay. After treatment for 5, 30, or 120 minutes at 37°C, cell lysates were immunoprecipitated with 1088 and probed with an antiphosphotyrosine antibody (4G10). As shown in Figure 4, a relatively high level of tyrosine phos-

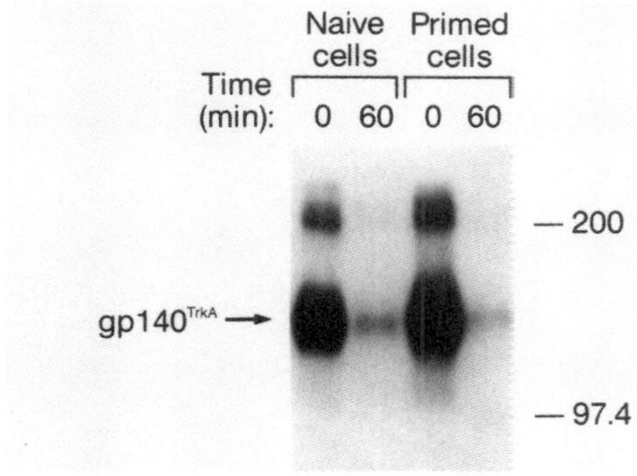

Figure 3. Cross-linking of ^{125}I-labeled NGF to surface gp140^{TrkA} in PC 12 cells. PC12 cells, naive or NGF-primed, were incubated with 100 pM ^{125}I-labeled NGF at 4°C for 2 hr and then warmed to 37°C for 0 or 60 min. Cells were then chilled and cross-linking was carried out as described in Materials and Methods. Cells were lysed and lysates were immunoprecipitated with 1088. The resulting immunoprecipitates were analyzed by SDS-PAGE. The gel was dried and exposed to X-ray film. After 60 min at 37°C, the amount of gp140^{TrkA} cross-linked to ^{125}I-labeled NGF dropped to the same level in naive and primed cells. There is also a band at 200 kD; a band of similar molecular mass has been seen in prior studies (Hartman et al. 1992). In this band, NGF specifically cross-linked to TrkA appears to be present in a higher-order complex. Each lane represents protein from an equal number of cells. The experiment was done twice with the same results. (Reprinted, with permission, from Zhou et al. 1995.)

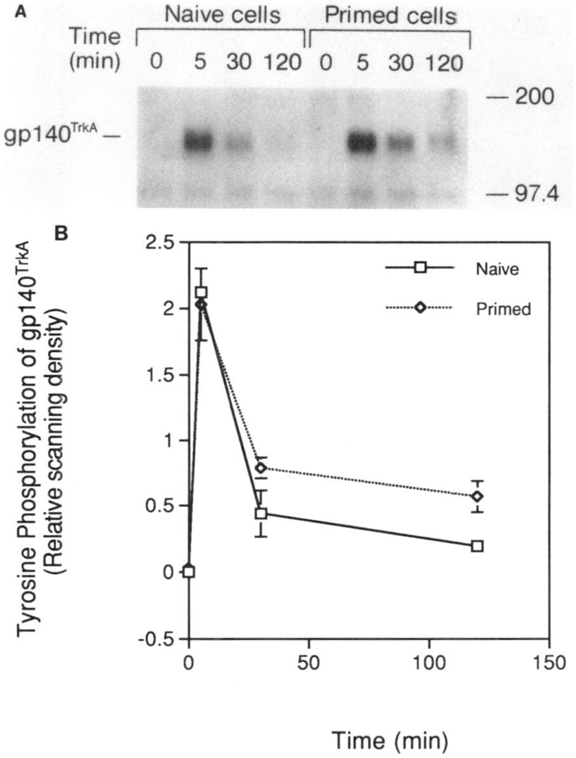

Figure 4. NGF-mediated tyrosine phosphorylation of TrkA was increased in primed cells. (*A*) Naive and primed PC12 cells were untreated (0) or treated with NGF (50 ng/ml) for 5 min, 30 min, or 120 min. Cell lysates were immunoprecipitated with 1088, subjected to SDS-PAGE, immunoblotted and the blots probed with anti-phosphotyrosine antibody (4G10). Lanes contain protein from an equal number of cells. (*B*) Tyrosine-phosphorylated TrkA was quantitated by densitometry. The data are corrected for the increase in protein that results from NGF priming. (Reprinted, with permission, from Zhou et al. 1995.)

phorylated gp140^{TrkA} was present at 5 minutes in both naive and primed cells. Tyrosine-phosphorylated gp140^{TrkA} decreased thereafter in both naive and primed cells, and the decreases followed a similar time course. However, the level of tyrosine-phosphorylated gp140^{TrkA} was greater in primed cells at each time point tested. As noted above, primed cells contain more protein. To normalize for this, the results were expressed per milligram of protein (Fig. 4B). The ratio of the signal in primed to that in naive cells was 0.9-fold (n = 3) at 5 minutes, 1.8-fold (n = 3) at 30 minutes, and 2.9-fold (n = 3) at 2 hours.

PLC-γ1 is a target of NGF-induced tyrosine phosphorylation and activation (Kim et al. 1991; Ohmichi et al. 1991; Vetter et al. 1991; Stephens et al. 1994). We investigated the level of tyrosine phosphorylation of PLC-γ1 in naive and primed PC12 cells. Tyrosine phosphorylation of PLC-γ1 was demonstrable at 5 minutes and was sustained at lower levels through 7 days of NGF treatment (Fig. 5, first five lanes). In primed cells washed free of NGF, tyrosine-phosphorylated PLC-γ1 was barely detected (Fig. 5, lane 6). When primed cells were then reexposed to NGF for 5 minutes, the level of tyrosine phosphorylation of PLC-γ1 was 1.7-fold (n = 3) that in naive cells on a per-milligram-of-protein basis (Fig. 5, lane 7). An increased ratio was also present at later time points. The data for tyrosine phosphorylation of gp140^{TrkA} and PLC-γ1 are evidence for a modest increase in NGF signaling through gp140^{TrkA} in primed cells.

NGF Induced Endocytosis of gp140^{TrkA}

Quite distinct from the increase in gp140^{TrkA} seen after prolonged NGF treatment, the early response to NGF was characterized by a rather dramatic decrease in gp140^{TrkA} (Fig. 2). Given that gp110^{TrkA} was not affected, this finding was most consistent with an NGF-mediated increase in the degradation of gp140^{TrkA} receptors. There are relatively few data for NGF effects on the cellular disposition of gp140^{TrkA}. However, ligand-mediated cell-surface down-regulation of other receptor tyrosine kinases is linked to lysosomal degradation of these receptors (Beguinot et al. 1984; Stoscheck and Carpenter 1984; Sorkin and Waters 1993), and in earlier studies it was shown that NGF treatment induced down-regulation of surface

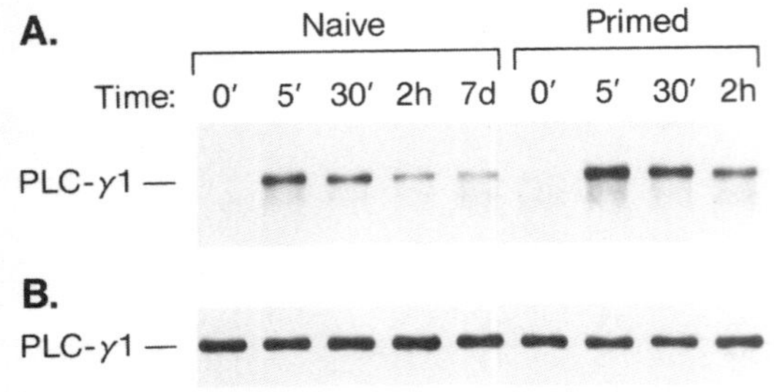

Figure 5. NGF-mediated tyrosine phosphorylation of PLC-γ1 was increased in primed cells. Naive and primed PC12 cells were untreated (0′) or treated with NGF (50 ng/ml) for 5 min, 30 min, 2 hr, or 7 days. Cells were lysed, and equal amounts of protein were immunoprecipitated with anti-PLC-γ1 antibody. Immunoprecipitated proteins were analyzed on SDS-PAGE and probed first with anti-phosphotyrosine antibody (*A*) and then with anti-PLC-γ1 antibody (*B*). (Reprinted, with permission, from Zhou et al. 1995.)

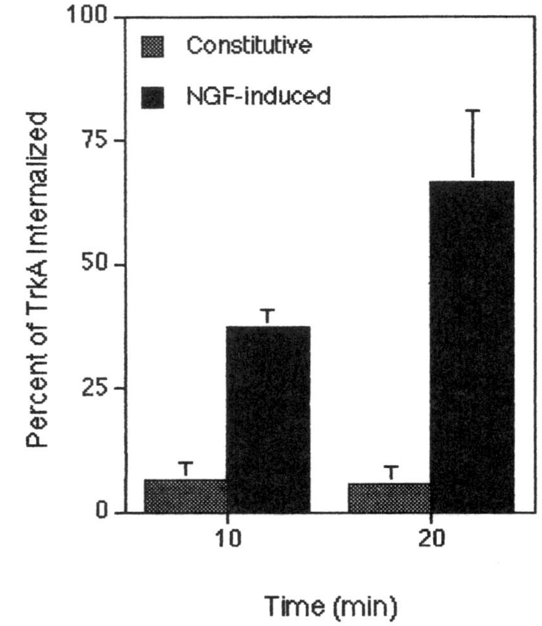

Figure 6. Constitutive and NGF-induced TrkA internalization. Experiments were performed as described in Materials and Methods, and the percent internalization of TrkA was computed as described. Values are mean (± S.E.M) from three separate experiments at 10 min and two at 20 min. There was a low level of constitutive internalization. NGF markedly increased TrkA internalization.

$gp140^{TrkA}$ in PC12 cells (Hosang and Shooter 1987). To ask if trafficking of $gp140^{TrkA}$ is similar to that of other receptor tyrosine kinases, we attempted first to confirm that NGF decreased surface $gp140^{TrkA}$. For these experiments, ^{125}I-labeled NGF (100 pM) was bound to its receptors on PC12 cells at 4°C to inhibit membrane traffic. In the continued presence of ^{125}I-labeled NGF, the cells were then either warmed to 37°C for 60 minutes or kept at 4°C. ^{125}I-labeled NGF was then cross-linked to $gp140^{TrkA}$ at 4°C, and TrkA immunoprecipitates were analyzed by SDS-PAGE. There was a marked decrease in cross-linking to $gp140^{TrkA}$ under these conditions; indeed, in naive cells only 16% of the amount detected in cells held at 4°C was present after warming (Fig. 3). Surface $gp140^{TrkA}$ was also down-regulated in primed cells.

To show that NGF-mediated down-regulation of surface TrkA was due to enhanced endocytosis of these receptors, we used surface biotinylation (Schmid and Carter 1990) to examine trafficking of $gp140^{TrkA}$. Cells were incubated either in the presence of NGF (1 nM) or in its absence at 4°C. NHS-SS-biotin was used to biotinylate surface proteins. After removing unreacted NHS-SS-biotin, cells were warmed to 37°C for 10 minutes to allow endocytosis, or not warmed. After chilling (4°C) the samples, glutathione was added to release biotin only on cell-surface proteins (Schmid and Carter 1990). TrkA immunoprecipitates were submitted to SDS-PAGE and blotting; ^{125}I-labeled streptavidin was used to detect biotinylated TrkA. Endocytosed $gp140^{TrkA}$ molecules would be expected to retain their biotin; the extent of $gp140^{TrkA}$ biotinylation was therefore taken as a measure of $gp140^{TrkA}$ endocytosis. Figure 6 shows the results of these studies. Whether or not cells were treated with NGF, endocytosis of $gp140^{TrkA}$ was increased by warming. In the absence of NGF, 6% of surface $gp140^{TrkA}$ was internalized after 10 minutes. This finding points to constitutive endocytosis of TrkA receptors. Remarkably, after 10 minutes warming with NGF, approximately 37% of TrkA was internalized. More than 66% of labeled TrkA was internalized after 20 minutes warming with NGF (Fig. 6). Thus, NGF induced extensive, rapid endocytosis of cell-surface $gp140^{TrkA}$.

Evidence that Endocytosis of $gp140^{TrkA}$ Creates a Signaling Endosome

Endocytosis of activated receptor tyrosine kinases targets these receptors to lysosomes where degradation prevents the possibility of further signaling (Beguinot et al. 1984; van der Geer et al. 1994). Some have suggested that activated receptors in endosomes could have a role in signaling (Baass et al. 1995), but the physiological significance of such signaling is uncertain. We entertained the intriguing possibility that via endocytosis of activated $gp140^{TrkA}$ receptors, NGF signaling could be communicated from axon tips to neuronal cell bodies. This arrangement was suggested by noting that NGF is a target-derived factor. For many NGF-responsive neurons, the target field of innervation provides the principal source of NGF (Longo et al. 1993). Thus, NGF is available to bind and activate its receptors on distal axons. Prior studies have made clear the importance of signaling through receptors on axons (Campenot 1977), but they did not elucidate how this signaling is communicated down the

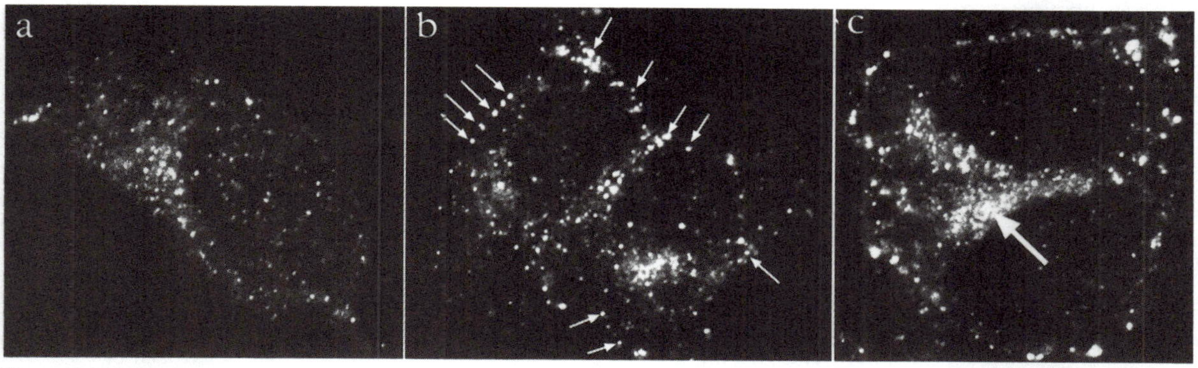

Figure 7. NGF changed the distribution of TrkA immunostaining in PC12 cells. Cells were exposed to media at 37°C without NGF (*a*), or with NGF (2 nM) for 2 min (*b*) or 60 min (*c*). A Trk-specific antibody, sc11, was used to examine the distribution of TrkA. Most TrkA staining was intracellular. With NGF treatment there was an increase in bright punctate staining near the plasma membrane (e.g., *small arrows* in *b*). Note the marked increase with NGF treatment of TrkA staining in the juxtanuclear region at 60 min (*large arrow* in *c*).

axon to the cell body. Evidence that NGF induced rapid, robust endocytosis of gp140^{TrkA} suggested that retrograde transport of activated gp140^{TrkA} receptors in endocytic vesicles could serve as the signal.

TrkA was present in endocytic vesicles. The signaling endosome hypothesis predicts that activated gp140^{TrkA} would be present in endocytic vesicles. To test this we used immunofluorescence and confocal mi-

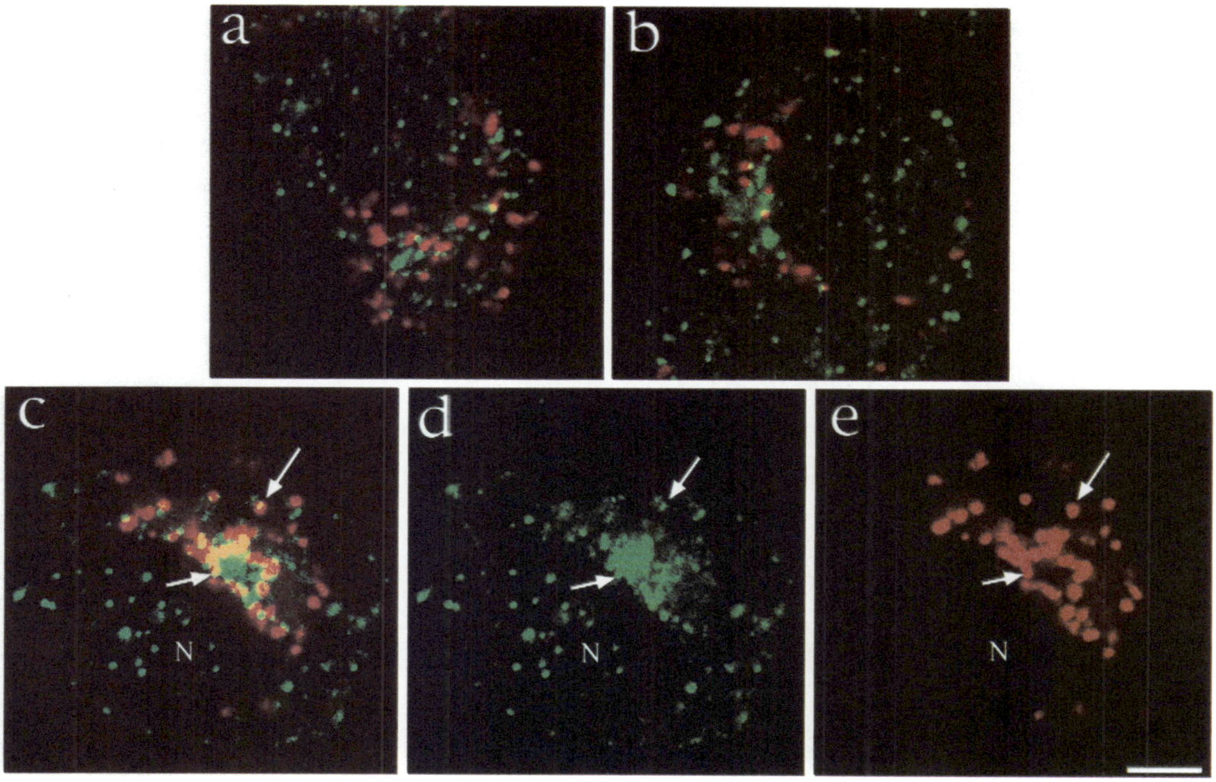

Figure 8. TrkA staining was colocalized with a lysosomal marker after 60 min of NGF treatment. Cells were exposed to media at 37°C without NGF (*a*), or with NGF (2 nM) for 2 min (*b*) or 60 min (*c, d,* and *e*). A Trk-specific antibody, sc11, was used to examine the distribution of TrkA. TrkA immunoreactivity was detected using an FITC-conjugated goat anti-rabbit IgG. GM-10 was used to visualize lysosomal staining. GM-10 immunoreactivity was detected with a Texas-Red-bound goat anti-mouse IgG. Panels *a, b,* and *c* show the labeling patterns for both markers. The immunostaining patterns after 60 min NGF treatment for TrkA (*d*) and GM10 (*e*) are also shown. N denotes the nucleus. The bar in panel *e* is 4 μM.

croscopy to localize TrkA proteins. PC12 cells were incubated with or without NGF (2 nM) at 37°C. Cells were then fixed, permeabilized, and incubated with sc11, an antibody to the carboxyl terminus of human TrkA. Fluoresceinated goat anti-rabbit IgG was used to detect antibody binding. In cells not exposed to NGF, TrkA staining was predominantly intracellular (Fig. 7a). Some immunoreactivity was found near the

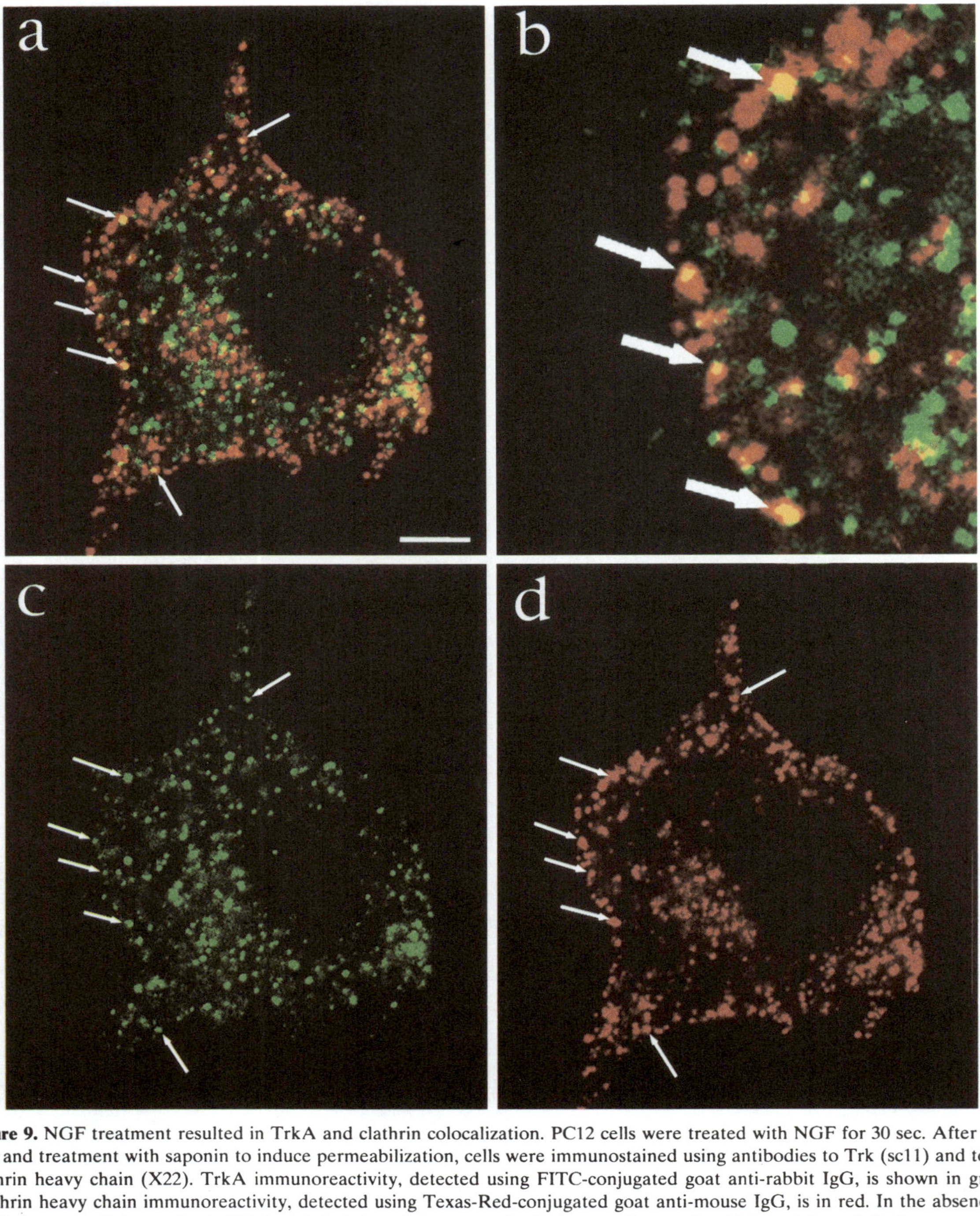

Figure 9. NGF treatment resulted in TrkA and clathrin colocalization. PC12 cells were treated with NGF for 30 sec. After fixation and treatment with saponin to induce permeabilization, cells were immunostained using antibodies to Trk (sc11) and to the clathrin heavy chain (X22). TrkA immunoreactivity, detected using FITC-conjugated goat anti-rabbit IgG, is shown in green. Clathrin heavy chain immunoreactivity, detected using Texas-Red-conjugated goat anti-mouse IgG, is in red. In the absence of NGF, there was little overlap in TrkA and clathrin staining except in the juxtanuclear region (data not shown). In the presence of NGF, TrkA (*c*) and clathrin (*d*) staining were widely distributed in the cytosol; some staining was seen for both near the plasma membrane. Panel *a* shows colocalization of TrkA and clathrin staining near the plasma membrane (*arrows*) (yellow denotes colocalization). The organelles showing colocalization had the same distribution and size as those seen with increased frequency following NGF treatment (Fig. 7). Panel *b* shows a 3-fold magnification of panel *a* to provide a better view of the colocalizations on the left side of the cell. Bar in panel *a* is 6 μm. (Modified, with permission, from Grimes et al. 1996.)

nucleus; most was present as small punctate accumulations distributed throughout the cytoplasm. With NGF treatment there was within minutes the appearance of many densely stained punctate structures, most of which were present near the cell surface (Fig. 7b). The number of bright punctate organelles located within 0.5 μm of the cell surface was quantified. After 30-second treatment, the number increased approximately 3-fold from 0.08 (± 0.01) puncta/μm of cell perimeter in untreated cells (n = 12) to 0.21 (± 0.02) puncta/μm in NGF-treated cells (n = 12) (student's t-test, $p < 0.05$). At later times (Fig. 7c), TrkA staining was most prominent in the perinuclear region. To examine the possibility that this perinuclear staining was due to the presence of TrkA in lysosomes, we looked at the subcellular localization of immunostaining for TrkA and the lysosomal marker, GM10. In the absence of NGF, there was little colocalization (Fig. 8a). The same was true after brief NGF treatment (Fig. 8b). However, after NGF treatment for 60 minutes, TrkA present in the perinuclear region was colocalized, in part, with GM10 (Fig. 8c). The presence of TrkA immunostaining in lysosomes at 60 minutes, and the observations on gp140^{TrkA} cited above, suggest that endocytosed TrkA was destined for degradation.

To characterize further the immunostained puncta seen near the plasma membrane with NGF treatment, we attempted to colocalize TrkA with markers of the clathrin-coated pit endocytic pathway. Cells incubated with or without NGF at 37°C for 30 seconds were chilled and fixed. Clathrin was visualized with antibodies to the clathrin heavy chain (X22) and to α-adaptin (AP.6). Without NGF treatment there was a small amount of TrkA and clathrin colocalization near the nucleus (data not shown). This was probably due to the presence of these proteins in the biosynthetic pathway. Only rarely were TrkA and clathrin colocalized in puncta near the cell surface. In the presence of NGF, however, TrkA and clathrin could be colocalized in many more puncta near the cell surface. The result shown in Figure 9 demonstrates a particularly marked example. The number of organelles in which TrkA and clathrin were colocalized within 0.5 mM of the plasma membrane was quantified. In cells not treated with NGF there was a range of 0 to 2 puncta/cell with a mean of 0.68 (± 0.10) (n = 40 cells). With NGF the range was 1 to 18 puncta per cell, and the mean increased nearly 5-fold to 3.25 (± 0.56) (n = 31 cells) (student's t-test, $p<0.001$). TrkA was also colocalized with α-adaptin in NGF-treated cells (data not shown). These data are evidence that TrkA is found in endocytic vesicles produced via the clathrin-coated pit pathway.

NGF was bound to gp140^{TrkA} in endocytic vesicles. TrkA expression confers on cells the ability to internalize NGF (Jing et al. 1992). To characterize further the endocytic organelles that contain TrkA, we examined those that could be labeled with ^{125}I-labeled NGF. After incubating PC12 cells with ^{125}I-labeled NGF (1 nM) for 1 hour at 4°C, we washed them briefly to enrich for binding to slowly dissociating receptors (Zhou et al. 1995) and to minimize fluid-phase endocytosis of free ligand. Cells were then warmed for 10 minutes and chilled (4°C). To prepare intracellular organelles, we took advantage of the fact that mechanically permeabilized cells release untethered organelles (Grimes and Kelly 1992a,b). A Balch homogenizer (Balch and Rothman 1985; Martin and Walent 1989) was used to permeabilize cells, and released membranes were then harvested. Cytosol and released organelles were separated from the cell ghosts (P1) by centrifugation at 1000g (10 minutes). Differential centrifugation was used to separate large vesicle-containing fractions (P2) and small vesicle-containing fractions (P3) from cytosol (S3) (see Methods). Using these methods, we showed that endocytic vesicles could be isolated free of plasma membrane. In one series of experiments, cells incubated with ^{125}I-labeled NGF at 4°C were washed, and the cross-linker BS^3 was added prior to permeabilization and fractionation. Under these conditions, we did not detect a cross-linked NGF/gp140^{TrkA} complex in either P2 or P3. In a second series, we asked whether surface amyloid precursor protein (APP) could be detected in P2 or P3. Cells were incubated with NHS-SS-biotin at 4°C to biotinylate surface APP; they were then permeabilized and fractionated. The amount of surface-labeled APP detected in P2 was 2.9% (n = 2), of that in P1; the corresponding value for P3 was 0.6% (n = 2), and for S3 it was 0.1% (n = 2). Thus, the intracellular organelles that emerged from permeabilized cells were virtually free of plasma membrane. We quantified the amount of internalized ^{125}I-labeled NGF that was recovered in membrane fractions: 6.9% (± 0.6; n = 9) of total cell-associated ^{125}I-labeled NGF was recovered in P2 and 3.1% (± 0.4; n = 9) was present in P3. Using acid washing, we found that 49.8% (± 4.9%, n = 3) of the total bound ^{125}I-labeled NGF was on the cell surface under these conditions. Therefore, P2 and P3 together contained about one-fifth of total intracellular ^{125}I-labeled NGF. These studies showed that the fractionation scheme allowed us to recover a substantial fraction of intracellular organelles that contained internalized NGF, and that ^{125}I-labeled NGF was present in both the large and small vesicle-containing fractions.

To ask whether gp140^{TrkA} was bound to NGF in intracellular organelles, PC12 cells were incubated with ^{125}I-labeled NGF (1 nM) at 4°C, washed, warmed 10 minutes as above, then chilled. Following permeabilization, DSS, a membrane-permeable cross-linking reagent, was added to the cell suspension prior to fractionation. gp140^{TrkA} was immunoprecipitated from lysates prior to SDS-PAGE. A radiolabeled band that migrated at the position expected for a complex containing ^{125}I-labeled NGF cross-linked to TrkA was seen in P1, P2, and P3 but not in the cytosol (S3) (Fig. 10). These data are evidence that gp140^{TrkA} and NGF

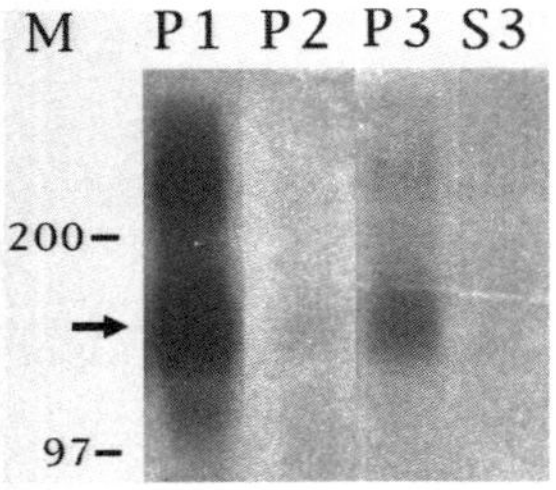

Figure 10. TrkA was cross-linked to NGF in intracellular organelles. Cells were incubated with ^{125}I-labeled NGF (1 nM), washed, warmed 10 min (37°C), chilled (4°C), and then permeabilized and fractionated. The membrane-permeable cross-linking reagent DSS was added before fractionation. One-fifth of the cell ghost membranes (P1), the entire 8000*g* pellet (P2), the entire 100,000*g* pellet (P3), and one-tenth of the 100,000*g* supernatant (S3) were immunoprecipitated with 1088 and analyzed by SDS-PAGE and autoradiography. The arrow marks the 150-kD cross-linked complex containing TrkA and ^{125}I-labeled NGF in P1, P2, and P3. The more slowly migrating complex may correspond to that seen in Fig. 3. There was no cross-linking when the experiment was carried out in the presence of unlabeled NGF (1 μM). The amount of ^{125}I-labeled NGF cross-linked to TrkA was quantified by Phosphorimager.

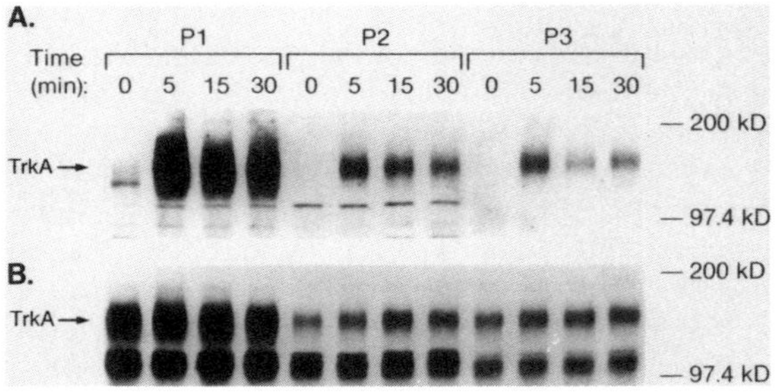

Figure 11. TrkA and tyrosine-phosphorylated TrkA were detected in intracellular organelles. PC12 cells were incubated without NGF (0) or with NGF (2 nM) for 5, 15, or 30 min at 37°C. Cells were then chilled (4°C), permeabilized, and fractionated. Using 1088, TrkA was immunoprecipitated from 1/3 of P1, or from the entire P2 or P3 fractions. (*A*) A Western blot of immunoprecipitates probed with antiphosphotyrosine antibody (4G10) followed by HRP-conjugated anti-mouse IgG. Chemiluminescence was used for detection. (*B*) The blot in *A* was stripped and probed with RTA followed by HRP-conjugated anti-rabbit IgG. Chemiluminescence was used for detection. In P1, there was a modest (9%) but significant decrease at 5 min in gp140^{TrkA} ($p<0.04$); although gp140^{TrkA} was increased at 5 min in P2 and P3 in the experiment shown, the increases varied across experiments and the changes were not significant.

were present together in the same compartments after internalization, and that NGF remained bound to gp140^{TrkA} after endocytosis.

Endocytic vesicles contained activated gp140^{TrkA}. To determine whether organelles derived from endocytosis contained activated TrkA, cells were cultured at 37°C in the absence of NGF, or with NGF (2 nM) for 5, 15, or 30 minutes. They were then chilled and submitted to permeabilization and fractionation, as above. TrkA present in lysates was immunoprecipitated and submitted to SDS-PAGE and blotting. Both gp140^{TrkA} and gp110^{TrkA} were detected in P1, P2, and P3 (Fig. 11, panel B). Neither was detected in S3 (data not shown). The presence of gp110^{TrkA} suggests that the endoplasmic reticulum, or vesicles derived from it, emerge upon permeabilization. Regulated and constitutive secretory vesicles also emerge from permeabilized cells (Grimes and Kelly 1992a,b). Newly synthesized TrkA should be present in these. Since receptors in the biosynthetic pathway have no direct access to NGF, it can be assumed that they have not been activated. The presence of phosphotyrosine on TrkA is a measure of its activation (Stephens et al. 1994). Thus, tyrosine-phosphorylated TrkA should comprise plasma membrane and internalized TrkA. Activated TrkA was detected by blotting TrkA immunoprecipitates with an anti-phosphotyrosine antibody. Fractions prepared from cells not exposed to NGF contained very little tyrosine-phosphorylated TrkA (Fig. 11A). In the NGF-treated cells, there was a marked increase in tyrosine-phosphorylated TrkA in P1, P2 and P3. Only gp140^{TrkA} was tyrosine-phosphorylated. The amount of tyrosine-phosphorylated gp140^{TrkA} was greatest at 5 minutes in all three fractions. Although the amount decreased at later time points, it was present through 30 minutes. These data are evidence that activated gp140^{TrkA} is present in endocytic vesicles following NGF treatment.

Another measure of TrkA activation, one that contributes to TrkA signaling leading to differentiation, is binding and tyrosine phosphorylation of SHC (Stephens et al. 1994). To ask whether SHC was bound to internalized TrkA receptors, we examined immunoprecipitates from cells that were incubated without NGF, or with NGF (2 nM), for 5 or 15 minutes at 37°C prior to chilling (4°C). After permeabilization, cells were fractionated. Lysates from P2, P3, and S3 were immunoprecipitated with antibodies to SHC. SHC immunoprecipitates were submitted to SDS-PAGE, and blotted proteins were probed with antibodies to phosphotyrosine (Fig. 12, panel A), TrkA (panel B), or SHC (panel C). As reported previously (Stephens et al. 1994), three SHC proteins were detected in PC12 cell immunoprecipitates: p68SHC, p53SHC, and p48SHC. Although the amount of each was greatest in S3, each SHC protein was also present in P2 and P3. With NGF treatment there was no apparent increase in SHC in P2 or P3, but two changes were evident. First, all three SHC species were more heavily tyrosine-phosphorylated (panel A); the change was most apparent in P2 and P3. Second, NGF treatment induced a shift in the electrophoretic mobility of p68SHC, a finding consistent with earlier studies (Stephens et al. 1994). Importantly, gp140^{TrkA} was

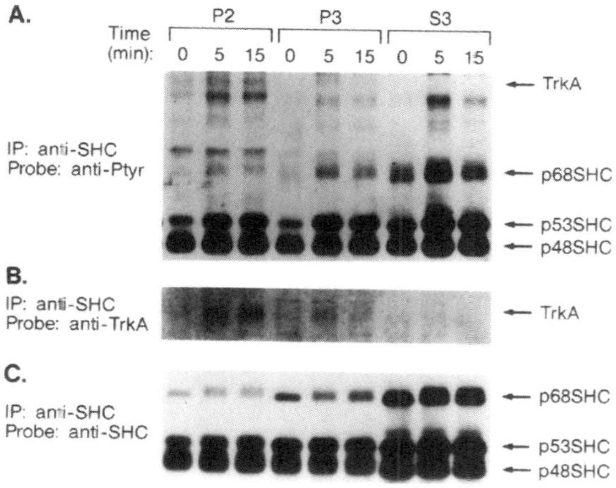

Figure 12. SHC was bound to TrkA in intracellular organelles. PC12 cells were incubated without NGF (0) or with NGF (2 nM) for 5 or 15 min at 37°C. Cells were chilled (4°C), permeabilized, and fractionated. P2, P3, and S3 were lysed and immunoprecipitated with anti-SHC antibodies. Immunoprecipitates were Western blotted with antiphosphotyrosine antibody (4G10) (*A*), then stripped and reprobed with anti-TrkA (RTA) (*B*), and finally, with anti-SHC (*C*). Chemiluminescence was used for detection. NGF increased the amount of tyrosine-phosphorylated SHC and its association with gp140^{TrkA} in P2 and P3. NGF treatment also increased the amount of a tyrosine-phosphorylated band that migrated slightly faster than gp140^{TrkA}. Unlike gp140^{TrkA}, it was also present in S3; its identity is unknown.

present in the SHC immunoprecipitates of NGF-treated cells. Panel A shows a tyrosine-phosphorylated band in the P2 and P3 fractions at the position for TrkA; the amount was increased by NGF treatment and was greatest at 5 minutes. That this band is gp140^{TrkA} is indicated by immunostaining for TrkA in panel B. Here again, the amount of gp140^{TrkA} was increased with NGF treatment. These data show that activated gp140^{TrkA} in intracellular organelles is associated with tyrosine-phosphorylated SHC. In other studies, we discovered that activated PLC-γ1 is also associated with tyrosine-phosphorylated gp140^{TrkA} in the P2 and P3 fractions (Grimes et al. 1996). These findings are strong evidence for the ability of activated gp140^{TrkA} in endocytic vesicles to signal.

DISCUSSION

NGF acts to evoke the responses required for maintenance of neuronal viability and enhanced neuronal differentiation. Defining the biochemical and cellular events that characterize these responses is an important objective. The discovery that TrkA is a receptor tyrosine kinase for NGF (Kaplan et al. 1991; Klein et al. 1991; Meakin and Shooter 1991) and that it has an essential role in NGF signaling (Loeb and Greene 1993) has greatly facilitated these studies. We discovered that NGF regulated TrkA in PC12 cells in distinct early and late phases. Within minutes of NGF treatment there was activation of TrkA and marked changes in TrkA trafficking, with resulting down-regulation of surface and cellular TrkA. After prolonged NGF treatment there was increased *TrkA* expression, and this was associated with a modest enhancement of NGF signaling. To understand how these responses are integrated in vivo, we entertained the hypothesis that endocytosis of activated TrkA at axon tips provides a means for retrogradely transporting the NGF signal to cell bodies, where it influences gene expression prior to its degradation in lysosomes. In testing this hypothesis, we discovered in PC12 cells that: (1) NGF induced rapid internalization of TrkA; (2) NGF and TrkA were both found in intracellular vesicles; (3) NGF was bound to TrkA in these vesicles; (4) TrkA receptors in vesicles were activated, as assessed by tyrosine-phosphorylation and association with activated SHC and PLC-γ1; and (5) TrkA receptors were targeted to lysosomes in NGF-treated cells. Our findings raise the possibility that it is through the creation of signaling endosomes containing activated TrkA that NGF signals retrogradely to regulate neuronal survival and differentiation. Since continuous NGF signaling may be required to maintain the trophic effect (Zhou et al. 1995), NGF induction of *TrkA* expression may be necessary for replacing degraded receptors. Thus, NGF may increase *TrkA* expression to both maintain and enhance signaling through this receptor.

In earlier work, it was apparent that NGF induces expression of TrkA (Holtzman et al. 1992; Meakin et al. 1992). To explore the biological significance of this finding, we examined NGF signaling in PC12 cells. We discovered that after prolonged NGF exposure there was an increase in gene expression for both gp140^{TrkA} and p75^{NGFR}. Increased receptor gene expression was correlated with increased receptor binding. In cross-linking studies, NGF induction of *TrkA* expression was shown to result in increased cell-surface gp140^{TrkA} receptors. Interestingly, the increase in NGF binding to gp140^{TrkA} was smaller than the increase in gp140^{TrkA} protein. When expressed on a per-cell basis, a greater than 200% increase in total gp140^{TrkA} protein was associated with only a 60% increase in NGF binding to slowly dissociating receptors and a 100% increase in cross-linking to gp140^{TrkA} at the cell surface. When these data are expressed on a per-milligram of protein basis, gp140^{TrkA} was nearly doubled, while there was little, if any, increase in binding. These observations suggest that the number of surface gp140^{TrkA} receptors is not simply a function of the total protein level. Although further studies are required, our data suggest that trafficking of gp140^{TrkA} is complex, even in the absence of NGF. For example, we noted that much immunostaining for TrkA was intracellular, pointing to possible controls on exocytosis. There was also constitutive endocytosis of gp140^{TrkA}. Regulation of the extent to which newly synthesized receptors are inserted at the cell surface and on the recycling of receptors to the plasma membrane could have an important influence on the number of surface receptors. Our data raise the possibility that the number of cell-surface TrkA receptors is regulated at several levels.

There was enhanced NGF signaling in primed cells, as evidenced by increased tyrosine phosphorylation of $gp140^{TrkA}$ and PLC-γ. These experiments link increased *TrkA* expression to increased signaling and suggest that the increase in $gp140^{TrkA}$ played a role. Of note, the difference in signaling between primed and naive cells was greatest 2 hours after NGF addition, at which time it more closely approximated the increase in total cellular $gp140^{TrkA}$ than the increase in receptor binding. It is tempting to speculate that increased signaling in primed cells was due, in part, to increased trafficking of $gp140^{TrkA}$ to the plasma membrane. If so, NGF may have influenced its own signaling through increasing the number of receptors as well as through enhancing their movement to the plasma membrane. It will be important to more carefully examine TrkA trafficking in primed cells and to show whether there is a link between increased $gp140^{TrkA}$ and increased NGF signaling in vivo. It is known that early exposure to exogenous NGF enhances the response to later treatment (Johnston et al. 1987), but it is not known that increased signaling through TrkA is responsible.

Whereas up-regulation of $gp140^{TrkA}$ marked the response to prolonged NGF treatment, a very different response was seen within the first 60 minutes, during which time there was a marked decrease in $gp140^{TrkA}$. Two studies gave direct evidence that NGF treatment targeted $gp140^{TrkA}$ for degradation. First, NGF was shown to down-regulate $gp140^{TrkA}$ surface receptors through enhanced endocytosis. This was apparent in both biochemical and confocal microscopy studies. In the latter, the increase in TrkA-positive puncta near the cell surface and the increase in colocalization of TrkA and clathrin were consistent with increased TrkA endocytosis. Second, NGF treatment increased colocalization of TrkA with a lysosomal marker, suggesting that $gp140^{TrkA}$ in endocytic vesicles was delivered to lysosomes. Surface down-regulation targets other receptor tyrosine kinases to lysosomes and is believed to serve an important role in signal up-regulation (van der Geer et al. 1994). For example, in the case of the receptor for the epidermal growth factor (EGF), EGF addition results in a pronounced and rapid decrease in surface receptors and accelerated receptor degradation (Beguinot et al. 1984, Stoscheck and Carpenter 1984; Murthy et al. 1986). In the case of EGF and EGFR, it has been presumed that endocytosis of receptors serves simply to turn off the signal. However, some have suggested that since EGFR is still activated following endocytosis, these receptors could have a role in intracellular signaling (Baass et al. 1995). Most TrkA signaling in vivo is likely to be initiated by NGF in contact with receptors on axons (Longo et al. 1993); we were intrigued by the possibility that, if these receptors continue to signal after endocytosis, trafficking them retrogradely would provide a means to convey the NGF signal to the cell body. In studies to address this hypothesis, we examined organelles and found continued NGF binding to $gp140^{TrkA}$. Moreover, we detected tyrosine-phosphorylated TrkA in intracellular organelles following NGF treatment. In studies similar to those reported here, we showed that NGF markedly increased the specific activity of tyrosine-phosphorylated TrkA in intracellular organelles (Grimes et al. 1996). Finally, we discovered that internalized activated TrkA formed complexes with tyrosine-phosphorylated SHC and with activated PLC-γ1 (Grimes et al. 1996). Taken together, our data suggest strongly that endocytosis of activated TrkA receptors has two consequences for NGF signaling. One is the creation of a signaling endosome. The second is the eventual degradation of this signal in lysosomes.

NGF is critical for the normal survival and differentiation of several populations of PNS and CNS neurons (Levi-Montalcini 1987; Longo et al. 1993; Crowley et al. 1994; Li et al. 1995). Since NGF gene expression is localized to target tissues (Longo et al. 1993), a mechanism must exist to carry the NGF signal retrogradely from the processes of neurons to their cell bodies. Earlier studies characterizing retrograde NGF signaling showed that, although NGF and the signaling process were similar with respect to both the time course for transport and the requirement for microtubules (Hendry et al. 1974a,b; Paravicini et al. 1975; Hendry and Bonyhady 1980), NGF itself was not the signal (Heumann et al. 1984). Internalized, activated TrkA is an attractive candidate for the NGF retrograde signal. Recently, Ehlers et al. (1995) showed that NGF infusion into the rat foot-pad, the target of sciatic nerve sensory neurons, induced an increased accumulation of tyrosine-phosphorylated TrkA distal to a ligature on the sciatic nerve. Their experiments showed that target-derived NGF regulates retrograde transport of TrkA. However, they did not examine the mechanism by which NGF accomplishes this effect or demonstrate its significance for NGF signaling. The studies reported herein suggest that the increased retrograde transport of activated TrkA seen in their studies followed induction of rapid, extensive endocytosis of these receptors in the distal processes of DRG neurons.

Current evidence suggests that activated TrkA in axonal endosomes would be protected from degradation. Studies on the endosomal-lysosomal pathway in neurons (Parton et al. 1992; Hollenbeck 1993; Parton and Dotti 1993; Nixon and Cataldo 1995) indicate that late endosomes and lysosomes are located predominantly in the cell body and proximal dendrites. Indeed, there was no evidence for these organelles in the axons or presynaptic terminals of cultured hippocampal neurons (Parton et al. 1992). Recent evidence shows that only a few acidified organelles can be found in distal axons (Overly et al. 1995). There are few observations that address directly axonal transit of endocytosed NGF and TrkA. As just indicated, TrkA retrogradely transported in the sciatic nerve was apparently intact (Ehlers et al. 1995). In earlier studies, retrogradely transported NGF was also shown to be intact (Claude et al. 1982), and, using electron microscopy (EM), an NGF-HRP conjugate was not found in degradative organelles in axons (Schwab 1977). Indeed, it is possible that NGF would remain bound to gp140^{TrkA} during axonal transport since, even at a pH characteristic of acidified endocytic organelles in axons (pH 5.5) (Overly et al. 1995), most NGF remains bound to gp140^{TrkA} (J. Zhou et al., unpubl.). These data combine to suggest that NGF, and the TrkA receptors endocytosed in response to NGF binding, would resist degradation during retrograde transport.

Our observations support the hypothesis that through endocytosis of activated TrkA, NGF creates signaling endosomes that convey its retrograde signal and that, following delivery to the cell body, activated receptors are degraded. It is reasonable to suggest that because there is degradation of activated TrkA receptors, NGF induction of *TrkA* gene expression is required for NGF signaling to continue. How it is that retrograde TrkA signaling is linked to new TrkA synthesis is uncertain, but a direct effect of TrkA signaling on *TrkA* gene expression is possible. This arrangement creates some interesting consequences, as well as problems. One consequence would be that the levels of TrkA receptors are buffered. For example, although increased NGF levels would result in a rapid increase in endocytosis and degradation, the resulting increase in TrkA synthesis would act over a longer interval to blunt the decrease. Thus, the trophic state of NGF-responsive neurons would be driven by NGF levels in the postsynaptic target without major changes in the number of cell-surface TrkA receptors. This situation would ensure that even with marked increases or decreases in NGF levels, responsive neurons would be able to continue to respond to NGF in their target. However, this same arrangement predisposes to potentially serious problems if there is uncoupling of degradation and synthesis. For example, one can envision a situation in which there is degradation of activated receptors without the benefit of enhanced receptor synthesis. In this case, there would be a progressive decrease in the number of NGF receptors and NGF signaling would fail, possibly with neuronal atrophy and death as consequences. It is interesting to consider disease states in which NGF-responsive neurons are affected. BFCNs are known to atrophy and die in Alzheimer's disease (AD), and their loss may contribute to cognitive decline (Coyle 1983). One aspect of AD neuropathology, highlighted by the studies of Nixon and colleagues (Cataldo et al. 1996), is a marked increase in the number of late endosomes and lysosomes in AD neurons. Cataldo et al. (1996) recently reported that pyramidal neurons of the cortex and hippocampus of the AD brain showed a 2- to 8-fold increase in the number of such structures. Lysosomal structures have also been shown to be increased in the axons and dendrites of AD patients. In early EM studies, Suzuki and Terry (1967) showed a marked increase in dense bodies in dystrophic neurites in the AD cortex. These dense bodies were acid phosphatase-positive, signifying their lysosomal character (Suzuki and Terry 1967). These observations may have relevance to NGF signaling. If endocytic vesicles containing activated TrkA are trafficked to lysosomes in BFCN axons, rather than to their cell bodies, the NGF signal would be destroyed prematurely. There are data to suggest this scenario. Whereas NGF levels in the cortex and hippocampus of AD patients are increased 2-fold relative to normal, the NGF level in the basal forebrain is only one-half normal (Scott et al. 1995). These data suggest a failure of NGF retrograde transport. Indeed, Mufson et al. (1995) have used immunocytochemical studies to suggest that less NGF is present in individual BFCNs in the AD brain. Although a number of alternatives can be envisioned to explain these results, the most attractive possibility is that retrograde transport of NGF and of activated TrkA are decreased in AD. Studies to test these ideas in animal models will help to define whether activation of the endosomal-lysosomal system can interrupt retrograde NGF signaling and, if so, what significance this has for the death of BFCNs in AD.

ACKNOWLEDGMENTS

The authors thank Drs. Steven Morris and Frances Brodsky for helpful discussions and antibodies, and Dianne Esson for secretarial assistance. We acknowledge the support of the Adler Foundation (J.Z.), National Institutes of Health grant T32 NS-07219 (E.B.), and a Howard Hughes Medical Institute predoctoral fellowship (C.L.H.). M.L.G. was supported by the National Alliance for Research on Schizophrenia and Depression (NARSAD), Whitehall Foundation, Cancer Society of New Zealand, Lottery Health and Science, National Child Health Research Foundation, and the Palmerston North Medical Research Foundation. W.C.M. acknowledges support from the March of Dimes (FY-95-0625), the McGowan Charitable Trust, and the National Institutes of Health (NS-24054, AG10672, and AG08938-10).

REFERENCES

Baass, P.C., G.M. Di Guglielmo, F. Authier, B.I. Posner, and J.J.M. Bergeron. 1995. Compartmentalized signal transduction by receptor tyrosine kinases. *Trends Cell Biol.* **5:** 465.

Balch, W.E. and J.E. Rothman. 1985. Characterization of protein transport between successive compartments of the Golgi apparatus: Asymmetric properties of donor and acceptor activities in a cell-free system. *Arch. Biochem. Biophys.* **240:** 413.

Barker, P.A. and E.M. Shooter. 1994. Disruption of NGF binding to the low affinity neurotrophin receptor p75LNTR reduces NGF binding to trkA on PC12 cells. *Neuron* **13:** 203.

Beguinot, L., R.M. Lyall, M.C. Willingham, and I. Pastan. 1984. Down-regulation of the epidermal growth factor receptor in KB cells is due to receptor internalization and subsequent degradation in lysosomes. *Proc. Natl. Acad. Sci.* **81:** 2384.

Bernd, P. and L.A. Greene. 1984. Association of ^{125}I-nerve growth factor with PC12 pheochromocytoma cells: Evidence for internalization via high-affinity receptors only and for long-term regulation by nerve growth factor of both high- and low-affinity receptors. *J. Biol. Chem.* **259:** 15509.

Bothwell, M. 1995. Functional interactions of neurotrophins and neurotrophin receptors. *Annu. Rev. Neurosci.* **18:** 223.

———. 1996. p75NTR: A receptor after all. *Science* **272:** 506.

Brodsky, F.M. 1985. Clathrin structure characterized with monoclonal antibodies. I. Analysis of multiple antigenic sites. *J. Cell Biol.* **101:** 2047.

Campenot, R.B. 1977. Local control of neurite development by nerve growth factor. *Proc. Natl. Acad. Sci.* **74:** 4516.

Carter, B.D., C. Kaltschmidt, B. Kaltschmidt, N. Offenhäuser, R. Böhm-Matthaei, P.A. Baeuerle, and Y.-A. Barde. 1996. Selective activation of NF-κB by nerve growth factor through the neurotrophin receptor p75. *Science* **272:** 542.

Cataldo, A.M., D.J. Hamilton, J.L. Barnett, P.A. Paskevich, and R.A. Nixon. 1996. Properties of the endosomal-lysosomal system in the human central nervous system: Disturbances mark most neurons in populations at risk to degenerate in Alzheimer's disease. *J. Neurosci.* **16:** 186.

Chin, D.J., R.M. Straubinger, S. Acton, I. Nathke, and F.M. Brodsky. 1989. 100-kDa polypeptides in peripheral clathrin-coated vesicles are required for receptor-mediated endocytosis. *Proc. Natl. Acad. Sci.* **86:** 9289.

Clary, D.O., G. Weskamp, L.R. Austin, and L.F. Reichardt. 1994. TrkA cross-linking mimics neuronal responses to nerve growth factor. *Mol. Biol. Cell* **5:** 549.

Claude, P., E. Hawrot, D.A. Dunis, and R.B. Campenot. 1982. Binding, internalization, and retrograde transport of ^{125}I nerve growth factor in cultured rat sympathetic neurons. *J. Neurosci.* **2:** 431.

Collins, S., M.G. Caron, and R.J. Lefkowitz. 1992. From ligand binding to gene expression: New insights into the regulation of G-protein-coupled receptors. *Trends Biochem Sci.* **17:** 37.

Coyle, J.T., D.L. Price, and M.R. DeLong. 1983. Alzheimer's disease: A disorder of cortical cholinergic innervation. *Science* **219:** 1184.

Crowley, C., S.D. Spencer, M.C. Nishimura, K.S. Chen, M.S. Pitts-Meek, M.P. Armanini, L.H. Ling, S.B. McMahon, D.L. Shelton, A.D. Levinson, and H.S. Phillips. 1994. Mice lacking nerve growth factor display perinatal loss of sensory and sympathetic neurons yet develop basal forebrain cholinergic neurons. *Cell* **76:** 1001.

Davies, A.M., K.-F. Lee, and R. Jaenisch. 1993. p75-deficient trigeminal sensory neurons have an altered response to NGF but not to other neurotrophins. *Neuron* **11:** 565.

Ehlers, M.D., D.R. Kaplan, D.L. Price, and V.E. Koliatsos. 1995. NGF-stimulated retrograde transport of TrkA in the mammalian nervous system. *J. Cell Biol.* **130:** 149.

Fusco, M., B. Olderfeld-Nowak, G. Vantini, N. Schiavo, M. Gradkowska, M. Zaremba, and A. Leon. 1989. Nerve growth factor affects uninjured, adult rat septohippocampal cholinergic neurons. *Neuroscience* **33:** 47.

Grady, E.F., A.M. Garland, P.D. Gamp, M. Lovett, D.G. Payan, and N.W. Bunnett. 1995. Delineation of the endocytic pathway of substance P and its seven-transmembrane domain NK1 receptor. *Mol. Biol. Cell* **6:** 509.

Grimaldi, K.A., J.C. Hutton, and K. Siddle. 1987. Production and characterization of monoclonal antibodies to insulin secretory granule membranes. *Biochem. J.* **245:** 557.

Grimes, M.L. and R.B. Kelly. 1992a. Sorting of chromogranin B into immature secretory granules in pheochromocytoma (PC12) cells. *Ann. N.Y. Acad. Sci.* **674:** 38.

———. 1992b. Intermediates in the constitutive and regulated secretory pathways released in vitro from semi-intact cells. *J. Cell Biol.* **117:** 539.

Grimes, M.L., J. Zhou, E.C. Beattie, E.C. Yuen, D.E. Hall, J.S. Valletta, K.S. Topp, J.H. LaVail, N.W. Bunnett, and W.C. Mobley. 1996. Endocytosis of activated TrkA: Evidence that nerve growth factor induces formation of signaling endosomes. *J. Neurosci.* **16:** 7950.

Haass, C., E.H. Koo, A. Mellon, A.Y. Hung, and D.J. Selkoe. 1992. Targeting of cell-surface β-amyloid precursor protein to lysosomes: Alternative processing into amyloid-bearing fragments. *Nature* **357:** 500.

Hantzopoulos, P.A., C. Suri, D.J. Glass, M.P. Goldfarb, and G.D. Yancopoulos. 1994. The low affinity NGF receptor, p75, can collaborate with each of the Trks to potentiate functional responses to the neurotrophins. *Neuron* **13:** 187.

Hartman, D.S., M. McCormack, R. Schubenel, and C. Hertel. 1992. Multiple trkA proteins in PC12 cells bind NGF with a slow association rate. *J. Biol. Chem.* **267:** 24516.

Hempstead, B.L., D. Martin-Zanca, D.R. Kaplan, L.F. Parada, and M.V. Chao. 1991. High-affinity NGF binding requires coexpression of the *trk* proto-oncogene and the low-affinity NGF receptor. *Nature* **350:** 678.

Hendry, I. and R. Bonyhady. 1980. Retrogradely transported nerve growth factor increases ornithine decarboxylase activity in rat superior cervical ganglia. *Brain Res.* **200:** 39.

Hendry, I.A., R. Stach, and K. Herrup. 1974a. Characteristics of the retrograde axonal transport system for nerve growth factor in the sympathetic nervous system. *Brain Res.* **82:** 117.

Hendry, I.A., K. Stockel, H. Thoenen, and L.L. Iversen. 1974b. The retrograde axonal transport of nerve growth factor. *Brain Res.* **68:** 103.

Heumann, R., M. Schwab, R. Merkl, and H. Thoenen. 1984. Nerve growth factor-mediated induction of choline acetyltransferase in PC12 cells: Evaluation of the site of action of nerve growth factor and the involvement of lysosomal degradation products of nerve growth factor. *J. Neurosci.* **4:** 3039.

Higgins, G.A., S. Koh, K.S. Chen, and F.H. Gage. 1989. NGF induction of NGF receptor gene expression and cholinergic neuronal hypertrophy within the basal forebrain of the adult rat. *Neuron* **3:** 247.

Hollenbeck, P.J. 1993. Products of endocytosis and autophagy are retrieved from axons by regulated retrograde organelle transport. *J. Cell Biol.* **121:** 305.

Holtzman, D.M., J. Kilbridge, Y. Li, E.T. Cunningham, N.J. Lenn, D.O. Clary, L.F. Reichardt, and W.C. Mobley. 1995. *TrkA* expression in the CNS: Evidence for the existence of several novel NGF-responsive CNS neurons. *J. Neurosci.* **15:** 1567.

Holtzman, D.M., Y. Li, L.F. Parada, S. Kinsman, C.K. Chen, J.S. Valletta, J. Zhou, J. Long, and W.C. Mobley. 1992. p140trk mRNA marks NGF-responsive forebrain neurons: Evidence that *trk* gene expression is induced by NGF.

Neuron **9:** 465.

Hosang, M. and E.M. Shooter. 1987. The internalization of nerve growth factor by high-affinity receptors on pheochromocytoma PC12 cells. *EMBO J.* **6:** 1197.

Jing, S., P. Tapley, and M. Barbacid. 1992. Nerve growth factor mediates signal transduction through trk homodimer receptors. *Neuron* **9:** 1067.

Johnston, M.V., J.L. Rutkowski, B.H. Wainer, J.B. Long, and W.C. Mobley. 1987. NGF effects on developing forebrain cholinergic neurons are regionally specific. *Neurochem. Res.* **12:** 985.

Kaplan, D.R. and R.M. Stephens. 1994. Neurotrophin signal transduction by the Trk receptor. *J. Neurobiol.* **25:** 1404.

Kaplan, D.R., B.L. Hempstead, D. Martin-Zanca, M.V. Chao, and L.F. Parada. 1991. The trk proto-oncogene product: A signal transducing receptor for nerve growth factor. *Science* **252:** 554.

Kim, U.H., D.J. Fink, H.S. Kim, D.J. Park, M.L. Contreras, G. Guroff, and S.G. Rhee. 1991. Nerve growth factor stimulates phosphorylation of phospholipase C-γ in PC12 cells. *J. Biol. Chem.* **266:** 1359.

Klein, R., S.Q. Jing, V. Nanduri, E. O'Rourke, and M. Barbacid. 1991. The *trk* proto-oncogene encodes a receptor for nerve growth factor. *Cell* **65:** 189.

Levi-Montalcini, R. 1987. The nerve growth factor 35 years later. *Science* **237:** 1154.

Li, Y., D.M. Holtzman, L.F. Kromer, D.R. Kaplan, J. Chua-Couzens, D.O. Clary, B. Knusel, and W.C. Mobley. 1995. Regulation of TrkA and ChAT expression in developing rat basal forebrain: Evidence that both exogenous and endogenous NGF regulate differentiation of cholinergic neurons. *J. Neurosci.* **15:** 2888.

Loeb, D.M. and L.A. Greene. 1993. Transfection with *trk* restores "slow" NGF binding, efficient NGF uptake, and multiple NGF responses to NGF-nonresponsive PC12 cell mutants. *J. Neurosci.* **13:** 2919.

Longo, F.M., D.M. Holtzman, M.L. Grimes, and W.C. Mobley. 1993. Nerve growth factor: Actions in the peripheral and central nervous systems. In *Neurotrophic factors* (ed. J. Fallon and S. Loughlin), p. 209. Academic Press, New York.

Lucidi-Phillipi, C.A., D.O. Clary, L.F. Reichardt, and F.H. Gage. 1996. TrkA activation is sufficient to rescue axotomized cholinergic neurons. *Neuron* **16:** 653.

Mahadeo, D., L. Kaplan, M.V. Chao, and B.L. Hempstead. 1994. High affinity nerve growth factor binding displays a faster rate of association than p140^{trk} binding. *J. Biol. Chem.* **269:** 6884.

Martin, T.F. and J.H. Walent. 1989. A new method for cell permeabilization reveals a cytosolic protein requirement for Ca^{2+}-activated secretion in GH3 pituitary cells. *J. Biol. Chem.* **264:** 10299.

Martin-Zanca, D., R. Oskam, G. Mitra, T. Copeland, and M. Barbacid. 1989. Molecular and biochemical characterization of the human *trk* proto-oncogene. *Mol. Cell. Biol.* **9:** 24.

Meakin, S.O. and E.M. Shooter. 1991. Tyrosine kinase activity coupled to the high-affinity nerve growth factor-receptor complex. *Proc. Natl. Acad. Sci.* **88:** 5862.

———. 1992. The nerve growth factor family of receptors. *Trends Neurosci.* **15:** 323.

Meakin, S.O., U. Suter, C.C. Drinkwater, A.A. Welcher, and E.M. Shooter. 1992. The rat trk protooncogene product exhibits properties characteristic of the slow nerve growth factor receptor. *Proc. Natl. Acad. Sci.* **89:** 2374.

Miller, T., T.C. Mathew, and J.G. Toma. 1991. Regulation of nerve growth factor receptor gene expression by nerve growth factor in the developing peripheral nervous system. *J. Cell Biol.* **112:** 303.

Mobley, W.C., J.L. Rutkowski, G.I. Tennekoon, J. Gemski, K. Buchanan, and M.V. Johnston. 1986. Nerve growth factor increases choline acetyltransferase activity in developing basal forebrain neurons. *Mol. Brain Res.* **387:** 53.

Mufson, E.J., J.M. Conner, and J.H. Kordower. 1995. Nerve growth factor in Alzheimer's disease: Defective retrograde transport to nucleus basalis. *NeuroReport* **6:** 1063.

Murthy, U., M. Basu, A. Sen-Majumdar, and M. Das. 1986. Perinuclear location and recycling of epidermal growth factor receptor kinase: Immunofluorescent visualization using antibodies directed to kinase and extracellular domains. *J. Cell Biol.* **103:** 333.

Nixon, R.A., and A.M. Cataldo. 1995. The endosomal-lysosomal system of neurons: New roles. *Trends Neurosci.* **18:** 489.

Ohmichi, M., S.J. Decker, L. Pang, and A.R. Saltiel. 1991. Nerve growth factor binds to the 140 kd *trk* proto-oncogene product and stimulates its association with the *src* homology domain of phospholipase C γ1. *Biochem. Biophys. Res. Commun.* **179:** 217.

Overly, C.C., K.-D. Lee, E. Berthiaume, and P.J Hollenbeck. 1995. Quantitative measurement of intraorganelle pH in the endosomal-lysosomal pathway in neurons by using ratiometric imaging with pyranine. *Proc. Natl. Acad. Sci.* **92:** 3156.

Paravicini, U., K. Stoeckel, and H. Thoenen. 1975. Biological importance of retrograde axonal transport of nerve growth factor in adrenergic neurons. *Brain Res.* **84:** 279.

Parton, R.G. and C.G. Dotti. 1993. Cell biology of neuronal endocytosis. *J. Neurosci. Res.* **36:** 1.

Parton, R.G., K. Simons, and C.G. Dotti. 1992 Axonal and dendritic endocytic pathways in cultured neurons. *J. Cell Biol.* **119:** 123.

Podlisny, M.B., D.R. Tolan, and D.J. Selkoe. 1991. Homology of the amyloid beta protein precursor in monkey and human supports a primate model for beta amyloidosis in Alzheimer's disease. *Am. J. Pathol.* **138:** 1423.

Schmid, S.L. and L.L. Carter. 1990. ATP is required for receptor-mediated endocytosis in intact cells. *J. Cell Biol.* **111:** 2307.

Schwab, M.E. 1977. Ultrastructural localization of a nerve growth factor-horseradish peroxidase (NGF-HRP) coupling product after retrograde axonal transport in adrenergic neurons. *Brain Res.* **130:** 190.

Scott, S.A., E.J. Mufson, J.A. Weingartner, K.A. Skau, and K.A. Crutcher. 1995. Nerve growth factor in Alzheimer's disease: Increased levels throughout the brain coupled with declines in nucleus basalis. *J. Neurosci.* **15:** 6213.

Smeyne, R.J., R. Klein, A. Schnapp, L.K. Long, S. Bryant, A. Lewin, S.A. Lira, and M. Barbacid. 1994. Severe sensory and sympathetic neuropathies in mice carrying a disrupted Trk/NGF receptor gene. *Nature* **368:** 246.

Sorkin, A. and C.M. Waters. 1993. Endocytosis of growth factor receptors. *BioEssays* **15:** 375.

Stephens, R.M., D.M. Loeb, T.D. Copeland, T. Pawson, L.A. Greene, and D.R. Kaplan. 1994. Trk receptors use redundant signal transduction pathways involving SHC and PLC-γ1 to mediate NGF responses. *Neuron* **12:** 691.

Stoscheck, C.M. and G. Carpenter. 1984. Down regulation of epidermal growth factor receptors: Direct demonstration of receptor degradation in human fibroblasts. *J. Cell Biol.*

98: 1048.

Suzuki, K. and R.D. Terry. 1967. Fine structural localization of acid phosphatase in senile plaques in Alzheimer's presenile dementia. *Acta Neuropathol.* **8:** 276.

Taglialatela, G., C.J. Hibbert, L.A. Hutton, K. Werrbach-Perez, and J.R. Perez-Polo. 1996. Suppression of $p140^{trkA}$ does not abolish nerve growth factor-mediated rescue of serum-free PC12 cells. *J. Neurochem.* **66:** 1826.

Tischler, A.S. and L.A. Greene. 1975. Nerve growth factor-induced process formation by cultured rat pheochromocytoma cells. *Nature* **258:** 341.

Vale, R.D. and E.M. Shooter. 1985. Assaying binding of nerve growth factor to cell surface receptors. *Methods Enzymol.* **109:** 21.

van der Geer, P., T. Hunter, and R.A. Lindberg. 1994. Receptor protein-tyrosine kinases and their signal transduction pathways. *Annu. Rev. Cell Biol.* **10:** 251.

Verdi, J.M., S.J. Birren, C.F. Ibanez, H. Persson, D.R. Kaplan, M. Benedetti, M.V. Chao, and D.J. Anderson. 1994. $p75^{LNGFR}$ regulates trk signal transduction and NGF-induced neuronal differentiation in MAH cells. *Neuron* **12:** 733.

Vetter, M.L., D. Martin-Zanca, L.F. Parada, J.M. Bishop, and D.R. Kaplan. 1991. Nerve growth factor rapidly stimulates tyrosine phosphorylation of phospholipase C-γ 1 by a kinase activity associated with the product of the *trk* protooncogene. *Proc. Natl. Acad. Sci.* **88:** 5650.

Yuen, E.C. and W.C. Mobley. 1995. Therapeutic applications of neurotrophic factors in disorders of motor neurons and peripheral nerves. *Mol. Med. Today* **1:** 278.

Zhou, J., J.S. Valletta, M.L. Grimes, and W.C. Mobley. 1995. Multiple levels for regulation of TrkA in PC12 cells by nerve growth factor. *J. Neurochem.* **65:** 1146.

Neurotrophins and Their p75 Receptor

B.D. Carter,[1] G. Dechant,[2] J.M. Frade,[2] C. Kaltschmidt,[3] and Y.-A. Barde[2]
[1]*Department of Cell Biology and Anatomy, Cornell University Medical College, New York, New York 10021;* [2]*Department of Neurobiochemistry, Max-Planck-Institute for Psychiatry, 82152 Martinsried, Germany;* [3]*Institute for Biochemistry, University of Freiburg, 79104 Freiburg, Germany*

The neurotrophins are a family of structurally related proteins best known for their trophic actions on neural cells. Four neurotrophin genes have been identified in mouse and human, all coding for secretory proteins with many characteristics in common, including biosynthesis as precursor proteins, a characteristic spacing between their six cysteine residues, unusually basic isoelectric points, and the formation of noncovalently bound dimers (for a recent review, see Lewin and Barde 1996). It is becoming apparent that the neurotrophins have functions beyond preventing programmed cell death during development. These include in particular a role as effectors of morphological changes observed during synaptic plasticity, in both the developing and adult central nervous system (Thoenen 1995).

Following the discovery of nerve growth factor (NGF) (Levi-Montalcini and Hamburger 1953; Cohen 1960), which preceded by far the isolation of other neurotrophins, binding studies with radiolabeled NGF suggested the presence of two different receptors on responsive cells: one with high affinity and slow kinetics of association/dissociation and one with low affinity and fast kinetics (Sutter et al. 1979). The gene encoding the low-affinity NGF receptor, now referred to as $p75^{NTR}$, was the first to be cloned, but the sequence of its cytoplasmic domain did not indicate that it could have any catalytic activity (Johnson et al. 1986; Radeke et al. 1987), nor was this receptor sufficient to account for the survival effects of NGF. Following the identification of brain-derived neurotrophic factor (BDNF) and neurotrophin 3 (NT-3), these neurotrophins were also shown to bind to $p75^{NTR}$ with affinities similar to that of NGF (about 10^{-9} M), but with slower kinetics (Rodríguez-Tébar et al. 1990, 1992).

Subsequent to the characterization of $p75^{NTR}$, it was realized that the proto-oncogene *trk* (tropomyosin-related kinase) had an expression pattern in the developing peripheral nervous system, suggesting that it may be the long-sought receptor preventing cell death during development after activation by NGF (Martin-Zanca et al. 1990). Indeed, soon after, it was demonstrated that this receptor binds NGF, resulting in the activation of its intrinsic tyrosine kinase (Kaplan et al. 1991a,b; Klein et al. 1991). Kinetic experiments demonstrated that this second NGF receptor was part of the high-affinity NGF receptor on neurons (see below). It is now recognized that in mammals, there are three distinct, but strongly related, tyrosine kinase receptors, *trk*A, *trk*B, and *trk*C, each expressed in distinct parts of the nervous system and in several isoforms, and each selectively binding the neurotrophins (for review, see Barbacid 1994). Ligand binding triggers receptor dimerization, autophosphorylation, and activation of well-characterized signal transduction pathways, including phosphatidylinositol 3 kinase, phospholipase C, and the Ras/MAP kinase cascade (for review, see Kaplan and Stephens 1994).

A variety of experiments have demonstrated that the *trk*s are the primary mediators of the trophic and differentiating effects of neurotrophins. Most convincing is the tight correlation between the nature and the extent of neuronal losses after deletion of either a *trk* receptor or its corresponding neurotrophin gene (for review, see Barbacid 1994; Snider 1994).

Although the role of the *trk* receptors has continued to be thoroughly investigated and much has been revealed, the function of the other neurotrophin receptor, $p75^{NTR}$, has been more difficult to appreciate due to its lack of intrinsic catalytic activity and its coexpression with catalytic *trk* receptors in many cells. However, recent studies indicate that $p75^{NTR}$ has an independent signaling function.

METHODS

Cell culture. Mouse L-cells expressing recombinant rat $p75^{NTR}$ (PCNA cells) were grown in DMEM containing 10% heat-inactivated fetal calf serum in 5% CO_2. For binding and cross-linking experiments, the cells were removed from the dishes by gentle treatment with 0.01% trypsin (Worthington) for 10 minutes at 37°C. The reaction was stopped by the addition of 10% fetal calf serum (Life Sciences). The cells were centrifuged (200*g*, 5 min) and resuspended in ice-cold Ca^{++}/Mg^{++}-free Krebs-Ringer HEPES buffer containing 5 mg/ml BSA (Sigma) and 0.1 mg/ml horse heart cytochrome *c* (Serva, binding buffer).

Iodination of neurotrophins. NGF, NT-3, and BDNF were iodinated using lactoperoxidase ^{125}I (Amersham IMS30) as described previously (Rohrer and Barde 1982; Rodríguez-Tébar et al. 1992). The specific radioactivity was 125–175 cpm/pg neurotrophin with 85–95% incorporation. Radiolabeled material was used within 1 week.

Cross-linking experiments. Cross-linking experiments were performed at 37°C with 5 x 10^5 PCNA cells/ml in binding buffer. After incubation for 60 minutes with 5 x 10^{-10} M radioligand, 1 mM cross-linking reagent, *bis*(sulfosuccinimidyl)suberate (BS^3, Pierce), was added for 30 minutes, and the reaction was quenched by the addition of 40 mM Tris/HCl (pH 8.0). The cells were separated from free ligand by centrifugation, and the pellets were washed once in ice-cold Krebs-Ringer-HEPES buffer containing protease inhibitors (1 mM aprotinin, 10 mM leupeptin, 1 mM PMSF) and lysed by boiling in Laemmli gel loading solution. Equal amounts of the lysates were then analyzed by 7.5% SDS-PAGE. The dried gels were exposed for 2 days to 6 weeks to autoradiographic film (Kodak X-omat AR).

RESULTS AND DISCUSSION

Structural Aspects of $p75^{NTR}$

$P75^{NTR}$ was the first member to be isolated of a family of structurally related cytokine receptors, some having a clear biological function. These include TNF receptors type I and II (TNFRI and TNFRII), the Fas antigen (also referred to as Apo-1 or CD95), OX40, CD40, CD30, CD27, and the lymphotoxin β receptor. These receptors are characterized by an extracellular domain containing 3 or 4 repeated cysteine clusters, and most have been shown to bind their ligands as multimeric structures. Neurotrophin binding to $p75^{NTR}$ has been suggested to occur through receptor dimers, as is the case for the *trk*s. Grob et al. (1985) have reported that $p75^{NTR}$ exists, in part, as a disulfide-linked dimer when immunoprecipitated and resolved with nonreducing polyacrylamide gel electrophoresis (PAGE). The monomer was found constitutively phosphorylated on serine and threonine residues, whereas the dimer showed much less phosphorylation, suggesting that this may be a means of regulating the association. The physiological significance of $p75^{NTR}$ dimerization is not clear.

In contrast to the extracellular domains, the sequences of the intracellular domains of the family members are not obviously related and lack any catalytic domain that could provide clues as to their mechanisms of action. The only clear intracellular homology is a short segment of similarity in Fas and TNFRI. This region has been called the "death domain," as these two receptors have clearly been shown to induce apoptosis in a variety of cell types (Brakebusch et al. 1992; Itoh and Nagata 1993; Tartaglia et al. 1993). Recently, careful alignment analysis has revealed weakly homologous regions in other family members, including $p75^{NTR}$, as well as in other nonreceptor proteins (Feinstein et al. 1995). In addition, structural analysis using the solved crystal structure of the TNF receptor type I (TNFRI) as a model has suggested that $p75^{NTR}$ contains a domain that is structurally conserved with the death domain of Fas and TNFRI (Chapman and Kuntz 1995). Current findings suggest that the function of this domain is to act as a protein-protein coupling region (discussed below).

Analysis of the intracellular sequence of $p75^{NTR}$ has also drawn attention to the juxta-membrane domain, which is 95% conserved between chick and human. It undergoes palmitoylation (Barker and Shooter 1994), suggesting that its proximity to the membrane might be important. Interestingly, this region has been shown to be crucial for $p75^{NTR}$-mediated activation of the hydrolysis of the membrane lipid, sphingomyelin, to produce ceramide (Dobrowsky et al. 1995; see also below).

Modulation of Neurotrophin Binding to *trk* Receptors

Expression of either $p75^{NTR}$ or any of the *trk*s in fibroblast cell lines does not result in the formation of large numbers of high-affinity binding sites like those observed with dissociated neurons. These observations led to the suggestion that the two receptors somehow collaborate to form a high-affinity site (for recent review, see Chao and Hempstead 1995). Indeed, coexpression studies have demonstrated a need for expression of both receptors, typically with a molar excess of $p75^{NTR}$ relative to *trk*A, in order to produce high-affinity NGF-binding sites (Hempstead et al. 1991; Battleman et al. 1993). However, high levels of expression of a given *trk* receptor do lead to the formation of a minority of high-affinity sites, in addition to large numbers of low-affinity binding sites (see Klein et al. 1991; Lamballe et al. 1991; Jing et al. 1992). These sites have been proposed to result from the formation of *trk* dimers (Jing et al. 1992), which might be facilitated by $p75^{NTR}$ coexpression. Experiments in which NGF binding to $p75^{NTR}$ was blocked using antibodies to either $p75^{NTR}$ or BDNF (which binds to $p75^{NTR}$, but not to trkA) have indicated a decrease in the number of high-affinity sites, using both PC12 cells and sensory neurons (Weskamp and Reichardt 1991; Barker and Shooter 1994). Biological responses were still observed but required higher NGF concentrations. Similar results were obtained using a mutant NGF unable to bind $p75^{NTR}$: When used to culture rat sympathetic neurons, normal neurite outgrowth and survival were observed, but higher concentrations of the mutant were required than for wild-type NGF (Ibáñez et al. 1992). These data support the two-receptor model and indicate that *trk*A is the primary mediator of NGF-induced neurite outgrowth and survival.

The direct demonstration of a physical association between the *trk*s and $p75^{NTR}$ has been exceedingly difficult, and there is only one report indicating coimmunoprecipitation of $p75^{NTR}$ and *trk*A (Huber and

Chao 1995). Perhaps the most convincing evidence for interaction between both receptors in biological membranes comes from measurements of fluorescence recovery after photobleaching: *trk*A seems to substantially restrict the lateral mobility of $p75^{NTR}$, an action requiring the intracellular domain of $p75^{NTR}$ and a functional *trk* kinase (Wolf et al. 1995). In this context, it is interesting to note that recent sequence analysis of membrane proteins associated with postsynaptic-density (PSD) proteins has identified a consensus sequence also present in $p75^{NTR}$ (Kornau et al. 1995).

Signal Transduction by $p75^{NTR}$

Recent evidence indicates that $p75^{NTR}$ can activate an intracellular signal cascade. In particular, neurotrophin binding to $p75^{NTR}$ in T9 glioma cells has been shown to activate a sphingomyelinase activity, resulting in the production of the lipid second messenger ceramide (Dobrowsky et al. 1994, 1995). Ceramide forms the backbone of sphingolipids found in abundance in the nervous system, and ligands such as TNF, interferon, and interleukin-1 have been shown to increase its production. In addition, elevated intracellular concentrations of ceramide have been shown to regulate cell growth, to cause programmed cell death, and to influence gene transcription (for review, see Chao 1995; Hannun and Obeid 1995). In particular, addition of C2-ceramide to a variety of cells has been shown to induce DNA fragmentation (Yang et al. 1993; Jarvis et al. 1994). In insect cells, expression of the *Drosophila* protein REAPER was shown to result in ceramide production and programmed cell death. Both effects were blocked by a specific inhibitor of the apoptosis-inducing protease interleukin-1-converting enzyme (ICE), suggesting that activation of the protease is upstream of ceramide production (Pronk et al. 1996; White et al 1996).

The downstream effectors of ceramide action remain to be identified but may include stress-activated MAP kinases, such as the jun-kinases (JNKs) and p38 (Verheij et al. 1996). These kinases are activated by inflammatory cytokines and various stressful stimuli (for review, see Cano and Mahadevan 1995) and have been implicated in regulating apoptosis. For example, upon NGF withdrawal, PC12 cells undergoing programmed cell death were found to have active JNK and p38 MAP kinases. Interfering with this pathway by use of a dominant negative MAP kinase kinase reduced the number of apoptotic cells (Xia et al. 1995). In line with this, recent work indicates that the activation of $p75^{NTR}$ by NGF activates jun kinase and initiates programmed cell death in cultured oligodendrocytes (P. Casaccia-Bonnefil et al., in prep.).

In addition to acting in the hydrolysis of sphingomyelin and the induction of programmed cell death, cytokines such as TNF also activate the transcription factor NF-κB. Both pathways might be related, as the addition of C2-ceramide is capable of activating NF-κB in several systems (Schutze et al. 1992; Dbaibo et al. 1993; Yang et al. 1993; Carter et al. 1996). In addition, TNF-induced binding of the TNFRI interactor TRADD seems to trigger both cell death and NF-κB activation (Hsu et al. 1995). The possibility that NGF binding to $p75^{NTR}$ can activate NF-κB was tested with Schwann cells, which express $p75^{NTR}$ but not *trk*A. The addition of NGF to rat Schwann cells (but not to Schwann cells isolated from $p75^{NTR}$ –/– mice) resulted in the activation of NF-κB, as measured either by the translocation of NF-κB using immunocytochemistry or by DNA binding in gel shift assays. Interestingly, neither BDNF nor NT-3 could activate NF-κB. These neurotrophins bind to $p75^{NTR}$ with affinities similar to that of NGF, but the kinetics of binding differ, with BDNF having a slower off rate than NGF by at least one order of magnitude. Furthermore, the binding of both BDNF and NT-3, but not NGF, shows a significant degree of positive cooperativity (Rodríguez-Tébar et al. 1990, 1992; see also Bothwell 1995). Timm et al. (1994) found differences in the circular dichroism spectra of extracellular $p75^{NTR}$ when mixed with each of the neurotrophins, suggesting different conformational changes accompanying binding.

To further investigate differences in the way the various neurotrophins interact with $p75^{NTR}$, cross-linking experiments were performed using radiolabeled neurotrophins and fibroblasts constitutively expressing $p75^{NTR}$ (PCNA cells). Suspensions of PCNA cells were incubated with 5×10^{-10} M radioiodinated NGF, BDNF, or NT-3 at 37°C. The receptor-ligand complexes were cross-linked using the bifunctional cross-linking agent BS^3 and visualized by autoradiography following separation on polyacrylamide gels. With NGF, three bands with apparent molecular masses of 80, 160, and 180 kD were observed, whereas for BDNF as well as for NT-3, bands with 82, 90, and 170 kD were identified (Fig. 1). This direct comparison of complexes formed between $p75^{NTR}$ and three neurotrophins indicates that NGF-$p75^{NTR}$ complexes are different from the complexes formed between $p75^{NTR}$ and either BDNF or NT-3. The variability in the apparent size of the $p75^{NTR}$-neurotrophin complexes must involve the extracellular portion of $p75^{NTR}$, since the hydrophilic cross-linking agent BS^3 does not penetrate the cells. BS^3 also contains a spacer of 11.4 Å and potentially links moieties over considerable distances. This agent is therefore useful to detect not only short-range ligand-receptor interactions, but also to "freeze" different conformational changes in the structure of the $p75^{NTR}$ receptor, which appears to be the most likely explanation for the observed difference in the sizes of the ligand-receptor complexes. Such conformational changes might also influence the aggregation of p75 receptors on the cell surface as is indicated by the variability of the high-molecular-weight receptor isoforms on our gels, which most likely represent oligomeric $p75^{NTR}$ molecules. The results of the cross-linking experiments are thus consistent with the hy-

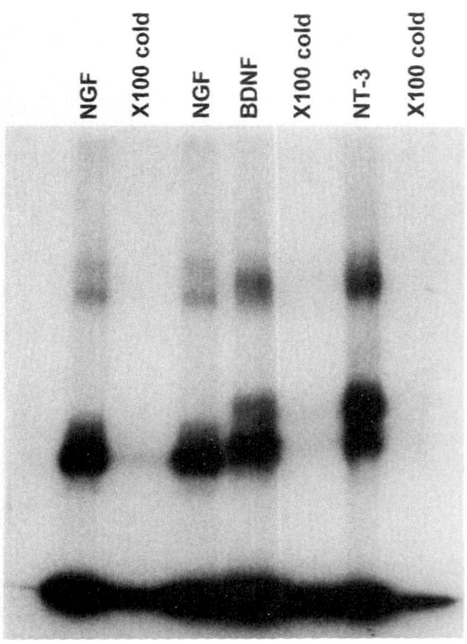

Figure 1. $p75^{NTR}$ -ligand complexes on PCNA cells. Radiolabeled NGF, BDNF, or NT-3 was cross-linked to rat $p75^{NTR}$ in the presence (100x cold) or absence of unlabeled neurotrophin using the suberate cross-linker BS^3. The receptor complexes were analyzed by 7.5% PAGE and autoradiography.

pothesis that the NGF-specific activation of NF-κB is a result of NGF-induced conformational changes of $p75^{NTR}$ different from those induced by BDNF or NT-3.

Isolation of a Neurotrophin Receptor Interacting Factor

Like other members of this gene family, $p75^{NTR}$ is likely to associate with cytoplasmic proteins to produce a signal. To understand the mechanisms of $p75^{NTR}$ signal transduction, we used the yeast two-hybrid system to identify proteins associated with the cytoplasmic domain. A similar approach has been successfully used with a number of receptors in the $p75^{NTR}$ family and has begun to elucidate a complex signaling network (Fig. 2). The group of Goeddel et al. isolated TRADD, a protein associated with TNFRI, or p55 (Hsu et al. 1995), and TRAF1 and 2 associated with TNFRII (Rothe et al. 1995b). TRAF3 (also referred to as CD40-binding protein, CRAF, or LAP1) was found to associate with the CD40 receptor (Hu et al. 1994; Cheng et al. 1995) and the Epstein-Barr virus transforming protein LMP1 (Mosialos et al. 1995). Similarly, the Fas antigen was shown to interact with novel proteins, FADD (Chinnaiyan et al. 1995), also called MORT1 (Boldin et al. 1995), and RIP (Stanger et al. 1995). Most of these interactors were found to interact with the death domain of their corresponding receptor and have been suggested to be involved in cell death signaling or activation of NF-κB. TRADD appears to be a branch point transducing a death signal to FADD or activating NF-κB via TRAF2 (Hsu et al. 1996).

Recently, a novel protein associated with FADD was isolated and referred to as MACH (Boldin et al. 1996) or FLICE (Muzio et al. 1996). This protein comes in several splice variants, some of which include a domain homologous to the ICE family of cell death-inducing proteases. Furthermore, this domain was shown to act as a protease, and overexpression induced cell death, which could be blocked by inhibitors of ICE protease (Boldin et al. 1996; Muzio et al. 1996).

TRAF2 can directly associate with CD40 or TNFRII, and its ring-finger domain was shown to be crucial for NF-κB activation (Rothe et al. 1995a). In contrast, TRAF3 was observed to attenuate TRAF2 activation of NF-κB (Rothe et al. 1995a). RIP has also been shown to activate NF-κB and to induce cell death in HeLa and 293 cells (Hsu et al. 1996). Thus Fas, TNFRI and II, and CD40 all associate with proteins regulating NF-κB, and all are known to regulate cell survival, suggesting that although the cell death pathway may be distinct (Hsu et al. 1995, 1996), it is likely that there is an interaction between regulation of apoptosis and NF-κB activation.

Using the intracellular domain of $p75^{NTR}$, we isolated a novel cDNA encoding a zinc finger protein from a human fetal brain library that we termed NRIF, for neurotrophin receptor interacting factor. This clone was used to isolate a full-length mouse clone, and recombinant protein generated from either the human or the mouse cDNA was able to bind to full-length $p75^{NTR}$ in cell lysates. The message for this clone was found to be widely distributed, as is $p75^{NTR}$ (Ernfors et al. 1988). The encoded protein is predicted to be composed of an amino terminus with little identity between human and mouse, five potential zinc fingers of the C2/H2 type with a Kruppel sequence in between, a conserved sequence with some similarities to a zinc finger, and a potential nuclear localization signal at the carboxyl terminus. The interaction between $p75^{NTR}$ and NRIF was mapped to the amino, non-zinc-finger region of NRIF and both the juxta-membrane and the death domain of $p75^{NTR}$. Interestingly, the structure of NRIF resembles that of the TRAFs, in particular, TRAF3. Although NRIF lacks the ring-finger domain seen in TRAF3, it also contains five zinc fingers resembling a DNA-binding domain, as does TRAF3. At present, it is unclear if the association of NRIF with p75 is influenced by ligand binding and if it is involved in NF-κB activation.

Physiological Function

To better understand the biological role of $p75^{NTR}$, Lee and coworkers generated mutant mice lacking exon 3 of the $p75^{NTR}$ gene (Lee et al. 1992). This exon codes for three of the four cysteine-rich repeats. Sensory deficits were observed, but the mice are viable and able to reproduce. In vitro analyses indicated that

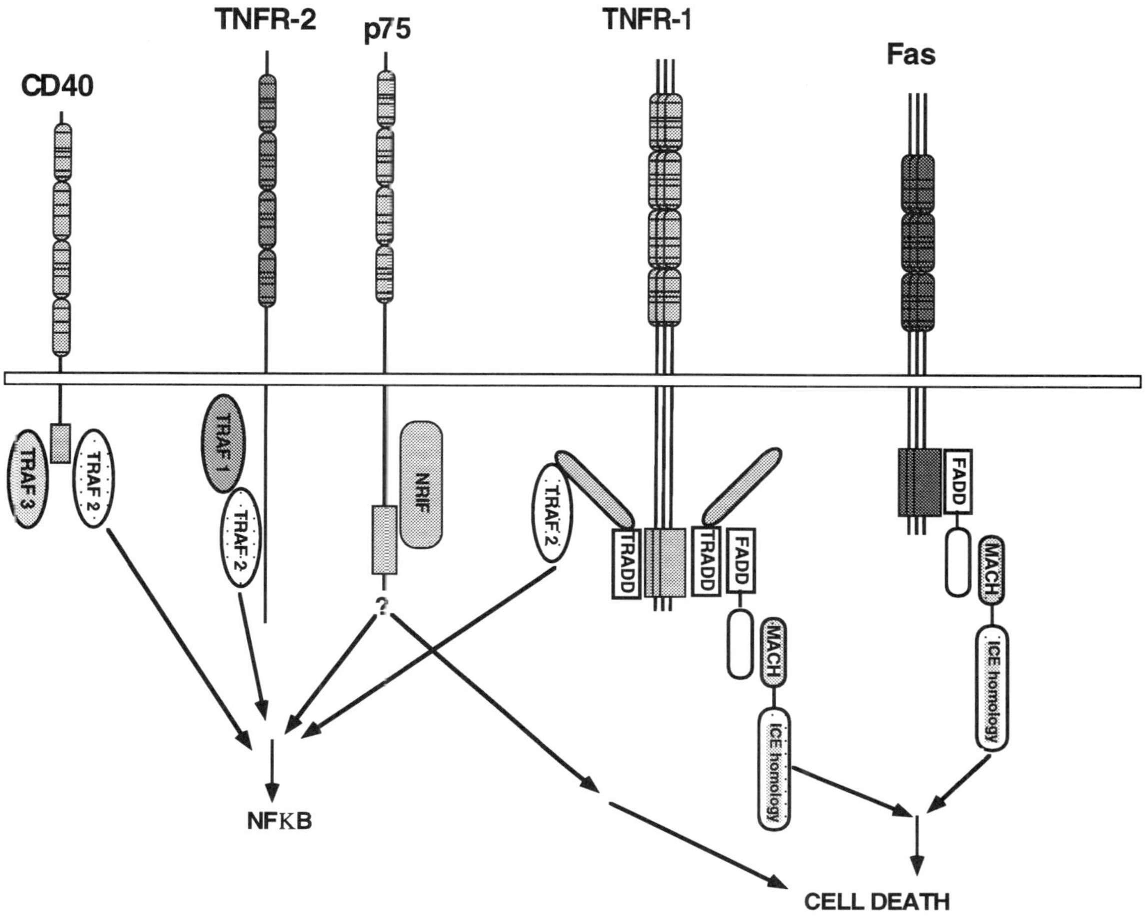

Figure 2. Schematic representation of the p75^{NTR} family of receptors and the receptor-proximal signaling components. The death domains are indicated by boxes.

both sensory and sympathetic neurons isolated from these mice require higher concentrations of NGF to survive than wild-type neurons (Davies et al. 1993; Lee et al. 1994). No differences were observed with BDNF or NT-3. Thus, these results support the notion that p75^{NTR} collaborates with trkA to form a high-affinity NGF-binding site (see above). Further analysis of these mice is needed to better understand the biological role of p75^{NTR}.

A series of in vitro findings indicate that the activation of p75^{NTR} by NGF regulates the expression of the cell adhesion molecule L1, first observed in PC12 cells (McGuire et al. 1978) and subsequently in cultured Schwann cells, which, unlike PC12 cells, do not express *trk*A (Seilheimer and Schachner 1987). A recent report indicates that NGF induction of L1 is also observed in the PC12 nnr5 mutant (expressing very low levels of *trk*A), as well as in PC12 cells treated with the *trk*A antagonist K252a (Itoh et al. 1995). Interestingly, activation of NF-κB is known to result in increased expression of a variety of adhesion molecules (Baeuerle and Henkel 1994), suggesting a mechanism by which L1 is induced. The regulation of adhesion molecules was suggested as a possible basis for the observation that NGF induces the migration of Schwann cells on denervated sciatic nerve via binding to p75^{NTR} (Anton et al. 1996). Finally, p75^{NTR} was recently shown to play a role in cholinergic neuron sprouting following fimbria-fornix lesion (Lucidi-Phillipi et al. 1996). It is conceivable that the up-regulation of molecules such as L1 plays a role in fiber outgrowth. In this regard, it is interesting to consider the observations of Maffei and coworkers, who found that addition of exogenous NGF prevents the effects of monocular deprivation, a means of testing neural plasticity in the visual cortex (Berardi et al. 1994). Furthermore, addition of monoclonal antibodies to NGF during monocular deprivation resulted in a prolonging of the critical period, possibly delaying synapse consolidation (Domenici et al. 1994). Such effects of NGF may be mediated by p75^{NTR} regulation of adhesion molecules, since there is no detectable *trk*A in these regions of the visual cortex.

p75^{NTR} and Cell Death

Using transfected cells, Bredesen and colleagues have suggested that p75^{NTR} mediates cell death in the absence of ligand and is blocked by the binding of NGF (Rabizadeh et al. 1993). In addition, postnatal rat dorsal root ganglion cells treated with antisense oligonucleotides to p75^{NTR} survive longer than controls in the absence of NGF, suggesting the presence of p75^{NTR} is responsible for their apoptosis (Barrett and Bartlett 1994). How generally applicable these observations are remains unclear, as a variety of cells, including Schwann cells, express p75^{NTR} and seem to be able to survive in vitro. In fact, it has recently been observed that NGF induces cell death of mature oligodendrocytes in vitro (P. Casaccia-Bonnefil et al., in prep.).

In vivo, following section of the facial nerve in newborn rats, the application of BDNF increased the number of surviving motor neurons. In contrast, the addition of NGF reduced the population more than 50% relative to the nerve without any addition (Sendtner et al. 1992). Interestingly, motor neurons are known to dramatically up-regulate p75^{NTR} after lesion (Raivich and Kreutzberg 1987; Yan and Johnson 1988; Ernfors et al. 1989). Similar observations were made in the isthmo-optic nuclei of chick. Naturally occurring neuronal death of these neurons can be decreased by BDNF, but increased by NGF (Von Bartheld et al. 1994). The death-promoting effects of NGF could result from the reduction of endogenous BDNF binding to p75^{NTR}, which may decrease functional responsiveness to low concentrations of BDNF via *trk*B. Alternatively, it might result from the direct activation of p75^{NTR} by NGF. Very recent in vivo data indicate that early in the development of the chick retina, neutralization of endogenous NGF considerably reduces normally occurring cell death. Although NGF and p75^{NTR} are expressed in the retina at these early developmental stages, *trk*A is not (Frade et al. 1996). It thus appears that in some systems, p75^{NTR} does actually mediate cell death, but that this is a ligand (NGF)-mediated process.

Neurotrophins and Evolution

Until recently, no evidence had been found for neurotrophin-related proteins in any invertebrates. Unlike other growth factors such as hedgehog or the wingless/int (wnts), conservation of primary structure seems to have been minimal. However, the recent elucidation of the crystal structure of the horseshoe crab protein coagulogen has shed new light on the evolution of neurotrophin-like structures (A. Bergner et al., pers. comm.). This lymph-clotting protein has a characteristic neurotrophin fold, as first identified following the crystallization of NGF (McDonald et al. 1991). Coagulogen is unrelated to the neurotrophins in primary structure, with the exception of the spacing of its cysteine residues, suggesting that they might form a "cystine-knot," as predicted by McDonald and Hendrickson (1993). In *Drosophila*, two putative ligands, Spätzle and Trunk, also show an arrangement of their cysteine residues indicating that they may form a cystine knot (Morisato and Anderson 1994; Casanova et al. 1995). Spätzle is thought to activate the receptor Toll, known to be essential for the establishment of dorso-ventral polarity in the *Drosophila* egg (for review, see St Johnston and Nüsslein-Volhard 1992). Toll activates the NF-κB-like protein Dorsal, which is regulated by Cactus, the equivalent of IkB. Trunk is likely to be a ligand for the receptor tyrosine kinase receptor Torso, whose activation is known to be necessary for the establishment of the maternal polarity system Terminal. It is thus intriguing to note that in *Drosophila* two gene products may display a neurotrophin fold (although the three-dimensional structure remains to be established), and like the neurotrophins, use two different receptor systems, one leading to activation of an NF-κB-like molecule and the other to the activation of a receptor tyrosine kinase. Controlling cell fate by diffusible ligands, be that polarity of the *Drosophila* egg or survival of neurons in vertebrates, seems to involve related receptor systems and ligands.

ACKNOWLEDGMENTS

We are grateful to Drs. Moses Chao and Patrizia Casaccia-Bonnefil for sharing unpublished data.

REFERENCES

Anton, E.S., G. Weskamp, L.F. Reichardt, and W.D. Matthew. 1996. Nerve growth factor and its low affinity receptor promote Schwann cell migration. *Proc. Natl. Acad. Sci.* **91:** 2795.

Baeuerle, P.A. and T. Henkel. 1994. Function and activation of NF-κB in the immune system. *Annu. Rev. Immunol.* **12:** 141.

Barbacid, M. 1994. The *trk* family of neurotrophin receptors. *J. Neurobiol.* **25:** 1386.

Barker, P.A. and E.M. Shooter. 1994. Disruption of NGF binding to the low affinity neurotrophin receptor p75^{LNTR} reduces NGF binding to TrkA on PC12 cells. *Neuron* **13:** 203.

Barrett, G.L. and P.F. Bartlett. 1994. The p75 nerve growth factor receptor mediates survival or death depending on the stage of sensory neuron development. *Proc. Natl. Acad. Sci.* **91:** 6501.

Battleman, D.S., A.I. Geller, and M.V. Chao. 1993. HSV-1 vector-mediated gene transfer of the human nerve growth factor receptor p75^{hNGFR} defines high-affinity NGF binding. *J. Neurosci.* **13:** 941.

Berardi, N., A. Cellerino, L. Domenici, M. Fagiolini, T. Pizzorusso, A. Cattaneo, and L. Maffei. 1994. Monoclonal antibodies to nerve growth factor affect the postnatal development of the visual system. *Proc. Natl. Acad. Sci.* **91:** 684.

Boldin M. P., T. M. Goncharov, Y. V. Goltsev, and D. Wallach. 1996. Involvement of MACH, a novel MORT1/

FADD-interacting protease, in Fas/APO-1- and TNF receptor-induced cell death. *Cell* **85**: 803.

Boldin, M.P., E.E. Varfolomeev, Z. Pancer, I.L. Mett, J.H. Camonis, and D. Wallach. 1995. A novel protein that interacts with the death domain of Fas/APO1 contains a sequence motif related to the death domain. *J. Biol. Chem.* **270:** 7795.

Bothwell, M. 1995. Functional interactions of neurotrophins and neurotrophin receptors. *Annu. Rev. Neurosci.* **18:** 223.

Brakebusch, C., Y. Nophar, O. Kemper, H. Engelmann, and D. Wallach. 1992. Cytoplasmic truncation of the p55 tumour necrosis factor (TNF) receptor abolishes signalling, but not induced shedding of the receptor. *EMBO J.* **11:** 943.

Cano, E. and L.C. Mahadevan. 1995. Parallel signal processing among mammalian MAPKs. *Trends Biochem. Sci.* **20:** 117.

Carter, B.D., C. Kaltschmidt, B. Kaltschmidt, N. Offenhäuser, R. Böhm-Matthaei, P.A. Baeuerle, and Y.A. Barde. 1996. Selective activation of NF-κB by nerve growth factor through the neurotrophin receptor p75. *Science* **272:** 542.

Casanova, J., M. Furriols, C.A. McCormick, and G. Struhl. 1995. Similarities between trunk and spatzle, putative extracellular ligands specifying body pattern in *Drosophila*. *Genes Dev.* **9:** 2539.

Chao, M.V. 1995. Ceramide: A potential second messenger in the nervous system. *Mol. Cell. Neurosci.* **6:** 91.

Chao, M.V. and B.L. Hempstead. 1995. p75 and Trk: A two-receptor system. *Trends Neurosci.* **18:** 321.

Chapman, B.S. and I.D. Kuntz. 1995. Modeled structure of the 75-kDa neurotrophin receptor. *Protein Sci.* **4:** 1696.

Cheng, G., A.M. Cleary, Z. Ye, D.I. Hong, S. Lederman, and D. Baltimore. 1995. Involvement of CRAF1, a relative of TRAF, in CD40 signaling. *Science* **267:** 1494.

Chinnaiyan, A.M., K. O'Rourke, M. Tewari, and V.M. Dixit. 1995. FADD, a novel death domain-containing protein, interacts with the death domain of Fas and initiates apoptosis. *Cell* **81:** 505.

Cohen, S. 1960. Purification of a nerve-growth promoting protein from the mouse salivary gland and its neuro-cytotoxic antiserum. 1960. *Proc. Natl. Acad. Sci.* **46**: 302.

Davies, A.M., K.-F. Lee, and R. Jaenisch. 1993. p75-deficient trigeminal sensory neurons have an altered response to NGF but not to other neurotrophins. *Neuron* **11:** 565.

Dbaibo, G.S., L.M. Obeid, and Y.A. Hannun. 1993. Tumor necrosis factor-α (TNF-α) signal transduction through ceramide. Dissociation of growth inhibitory effects of TNF-α from activation of nuclear factor-κB. *J. Biol. Chem.* **268:** 17762.

Dobrowsky, R.T., G.M. Jenkins, and Y.A. Hannun. 1995. Neurotrophins induce sphingomyelin hydrolysis—Modulation by co-expression of $p75^{NTR}$ with Trk receptors. *J. Biol. Chem.* **270:** 22135.

Dobrowsky, R.T., M.H. Werner, A.M. Castellino, M.V. Chao, and Y.A. Hannun. 1994. Activation of the sphingomyelin cycle through the low-affinity neurotrophin receptor. *Science* **265:** 1596.

Domenici, L., A. Cellerino, N. Berardi, A. Cattaneo, and L. Maffei. 1994. Antibodies to nerve growth factor (NGF) prolong the sensitive period for monocular deprivation in the rat. *NeuroReport* **5:** 2041.

Ernfors, P., A. Henschen, L. Olson, and H. Persson. 1989. Expression of nerve growth factor receptor mRNA is developmentally regulated and increased after axotomy in rat spinal cord motoneurons. *Neuron* **2:** 1605.

Ernfors, P., F. Hallböök, T. Ebendal, E.M. Shooter, M.J. Radeke, T.P. Misko, and H. Persson. 1988. Developmental and regional expression of β-nerve growth factor receptor mRNA in the chick and rat. *Neuron* **1:** 983.

Feinstein, E., A. Kimchi, D. Wallach, M. Boldin, and E. Varfolomeev. 1995. The death domain: A module shared by proteins with diverse cellular functions (Letter). *Trends Biochem. Sci.* **20:** 342.

Frade, J.M., A. Rodríguez-Tébar, and Y.-A. Barde. 1996. Induction of cell death by endogenous nerve growth factor through its p75 receptor. *Nature* (in press).

Grob, P.M., A.H. Ross, H. Koprowski, and M. Bothwell. 1985. Characterization of the human melanoma nerve growth factor receptor. *J. Biol. Chem.* **260:** 8044.

Hannun, Y.A. and L.M. Obeid. 1995. Ceramide: An intracellular signal for apoptosis. *Trends Biochem. Sci.* **20:** 73.

Hempstead, B.L., D. Martin-Zanca, D.R. Kaplan, L.F. Parada, and M.V. Chao. 1991. High-affinity NGF binding requires coexpression of the trk proto-oncogene and the low-affinity NGF receptor. *Nature* **350:** 678.

Hsu, H., J. Xiong, and D.V. Goeddel. 1995. The TNF receptor 1-associated protein TRADD signals cell death and NF-κB activation. *Cell* **81:** 495.

Hsu, H.L., H.B. Shu, M.G. Pan, and D.V. Goeddel. 1996. TRADD-TRAF2 and TRADD-FADD interactions define two distinct TNF receptor 1 signal transduction pathways. *Cell* **84:** 299.

Hu, H.M., K. O'Rourke, M.S. Boguski, and V.M. Dixit. 1994. A novel RING finger protein interacts with the cytoplasmic domain of CD40. *J. Biol. Chem.* **269:** 30069.

Huber, L.J. and M.V. Chao. 1995. A potential interaction of p75 and *trkA* NGF receptors revealed by affinity crosslinking and immunoprecipitation. *J. Neurosci. Res.* **40:** 557.

Ibáñez, C.F., T. Ebendal, G. Barbany, J. Murray-Rust, T.L. Blundell, and H. Persson. 1992. Disruption of the low affinity receptor-binding site in NGF allows neuronal survival and differentiation by binding to *trk* gene product. *Cell* **69:** 329.

Itoh, K., R. Brackenbury, and R.A. Akeson. 1995. Induction of L1 mRNA in PC12 cells by NGF is modulated by cell-cell contact and does not require the high-affinity NGF receptor. *J. Neurosci.* **15:** 2504.

Itoh, N. and S. Nagata. 1993. A novel protein domain required for apoptosis. Mutational analysis of human Fas antigen. *J. Biol. Chem.* **268:** 10932.

Jarvis, W.D., F.A. Fornari, Jr., J.L. Browning, D.A. Gewirtz, R.N. Kolesnick, and S. Grant. 1994. Attenuation of ceramide-induced apoptosis by diglyceride in human myeloid leukemia cells. *J. Biol. Chem.* **269:** 31685.

Jing, S., P. Tapley, and M. Barbacid. 1992. Nerve growth factor mediates signal transduction through *trk* homodimer receptors. *Neuron* **9:** 1067.

Johnson, D., A. Lanahan, C.R. Buck, A. Sehgal, C. Morgan, E. Mercer, M. Bothwell, and M. Chao. 1986. Expression and structure of the human NGF receptor. *Cell* **47:** 545.

Kaplan, D.R. and R.M. Stephens. 1994. Neurotrophin signal transduction by the trk receptor. *J. Neurobiol.* **25:** 1404.

Kaplan, D.R., D. Martin-Zanca, and L.F. Parada. 1991a. Tyrosine phosphorylation and tyrosine kinase activity of the *trk* proto-oncogene product induced by NGF. *Nature* **350:** 158.

Kaplan, D.R., B.L. Hempstead, D. Martin-Zanca, M.V. Chao, and L.F. Parada. 1991b. The *trk* proto-oncogene product:

A signal transducing receptor for nerve growth factor. *Science* **252:** 554.

Klein, R., S. Jing, V. Nanduri, E. O'Rourke, and M. Barbacid. 1991. The *trk* proto-oncogene encodes a receptor for nerve growth factor. *Cell* **65:** 189.

Kornau, H.C., L.T. Schenker, M.B. Kennedy, and P.H. Seeburg. 1995. Domain interaction between NMDA receptor subunits and the postsynaptic density protein PSD-95. *Science* **269:** 1737.

Lamballe, F., R. Klein, and M. Barbacid. 1991. *trk*C, a new member of the *trk* family of tyrosine protein kinases, is a receptor for neurotrophin-3. *Cell* **66:** 967.

Lee, K.-F., A.M. Davies, and R. Jaenisch. 1994. p75-deficient embryonic dorsal root sensory and neonatal sympathetic neurons display a decreased sensitivity to NGF. *Development* **120:** 1027.

Lee, K.-F., E. Li, L.J. Huber, S.C. Landis, A.H. Sharpe, M.V. Chao, and R. Jaenisch. 1992. Targeted mutation of the p75 low affinity NGF receptor gene leads to deficits in the peripheral sensory nervous system. *Cell* **69:** 737.

Levi-Montalcini, R. and V. Hamburger. 1953. A diffusible agent of mouse sarcoma producing hyperplasia of sympathetic ganglia and hyperneurotization of viscera in the chick embryo. *J. Exp. Zool.* **123**: 233.

Lewin, G.R. and Y.-A. Barde. 1996. Physiology of the neurotrophins. *Annu. Rev. Neurosci.* **78:** 289.

Lucidi-Phillipi, C.A., D.O. Clary, L.F. Reichardt, and F.H. Gage. 1995. TrkA activation is sufficient to rescue axotomized cholinergic neurons. *Neuron* **16:** 653.

Martin-Zanca, D., M. Barbacid, and L.F. Parada. 1990. Expression of the *trk* proto-oncogene is restricted to the sensory cranial and spinal ganglia of neural crest origin in mouse development. *Genes Dev.* **4:** 683.

McDonald, N.Q. and W.A. Hendrickson. 1993. A structural superfamily of growth factors containing a cystine knot motif. *Cell* **73:** 421.

McDonald, N.Q., R. Lapatto, J. Murray-Rust, J. Gunning, A. Wlodawer, and T.L. Blundell. 1991. New protein fold revealed by a 2.3-Å resolution crystal structure of nerve growth factor. *Nature* **354:** 411.

McGuire, J.C., L.A. Greene, and A.V. Furano. 1978. NGF stimulates incorporation of fucose or glucosamine into an external glycoprotein in cultured rat PC12 pheochromocytoma cells. *Cell* **15:** 357.

Morisato, D. and K.V. Anderson. 1994. The spatzle gene encodes a component of the extracellular signaling pathway establishing the dorsal-ventral pattern of the *Drosophila* embryo. *Cell* **76:** 677.

Mosialos, G., M. Birkenbach, R. Yalamanchili, T. VanArsdale, C. Ware, and E. Kieff. 1995. The Epstein-Barr virus transforming protein LMP1 engages signaling proteins for the tumor necrosis factor receptor family. *Cell* **80:** 389.

Muzio, M., A.M. Chinnaiyan, F.C. Kischkel, K. O'Rourke, A. Shevchenko, J. Ni, C. Scaffidi, J.D. Bretz, M. Zhang, R. Gentz, M. Mann, P.H. Krammer, M.E. Peter, and V.M. Dixit. 1996. FLICE, a novel FADD homologous ICE/CED-3—like protease, is recruited to the CD95 (Fas/Apo-1) death-inducing signaling complex. *Cell* **85:** 817.

Pronk, G.J., K. Ramer, P. Amiri, and L.T. Williams. 1996. Requirement of an ICE-like protease for induction of apoptosis and ceramide generation by REAPER. *Science* **271:** 808.

Rabizadeh, S., J. Oh, L. Zhong, J. Yang, C.M. Bitler, L.L. Butcher, and D.E. Bredesen. 1993. Induction of apoptosis by the low-affinity NGF receptor. *Science* **261:** 345.

Radeke, M.J., T.P. Misko, C. Hsu, L.A. Herzenberg, and E.M. Shooter. 1987. Gene transfer and molecular cloning of the rat nerve growth factor receptor: A new class of receptors. *Nature* **325:** 593.

Raivich, G. and G.W. Kreutzberg. 1987. Expression of growth factor receptors in injured nervous tissue. I. Axotomy leads to a shift in the cellular distribution of specific beta-nerve growth factor binding in the injured and regenerating PNS. *J. Neurocytol.* **16:** 689.

Rodríguez-Tébar, A., G. Dechant, and Y.-A. Barde. 1990. Binding of brain-derived neurotrophic factor to the nerve growth factor receptor. *Neuron* **4:** 487.

Rodríguez-Tébar, A., G. Dechant, R. Götz, and Y.-A. Barde. 1992. Binding of neurotrophin-3 to its neuronal receptors and interactions with nerve growth factor and brain-derived neurotrophic factor. *EMBO J.* **11:** 917.

Rohrer, H. and Y.-A. Barde. 1982. Presence and disappearance of nerve growth factor receptors on sensory neurons in culture. *Dev. Biol.* **89:** 309.

Rothe, M., V. Sarma, V.W. Dixit, and D.V. Goeddel. 1995a. TRAF2-mediated activation of NF-κB by TNF receptor 2 and CD40. *Science* **269:** 1424.

Rothe, M., M.G. Pan, W.J. Henzel, T.M. Ayres, and D.V. Goeddel. 1995b. The TNFR2-TRAF signaling complex contains two novel proteins related to baculoviral-inhibitor of apoptosis proteins. *Cell* **83:** 1243.

Schutze, S., K. Potthoff, T. Machleidt, D. Berkovic, K. Wiegmann, and M. Kronke. 1992. TNF activates NF-κB by phosphatidylcholine-specific phospholipase C-induced "acidic" sphingomyelin breakdown. *Cell* **71:** 765.

Seilheimer, B. and M. Schachner. 1987. Regulation of neural cell adhesion molecule expression on cultured mouse Schwann cells by nerve growth factor. *EMBO J.* **6:** 1611.

Sendtner, M., B. Holtmann, R. Kolbeck, H. Thoenen, and Y.-A. Barde. 1992. Brain-derived neurotrophic factor prevents the death of motoneurons in newborn rats after nerve section. *Nature* **360:** 757.

Snider, W.D. 1994. Functions of the neurotrophins during nervous system development: What the knockouts are teaching us. *Cell* **77:** 627.

St Johnston, D. and C. Nüsslein-Volhard. 1992. The origin of pattern and polarity in the *Drosophila* embryo. *Cell* **68:** 201.

Stanger, B.Z., P. Leder, T.-H. Lee, E. Kim, and B. Seed. 1995. RIP: A novel protein containing a death domain that interacts with Fas/APO-1 (CD95) in yeast and causes cell death. *Cell* **81:** 513.

Sutter, A., R.J. Riopelle, R.M. Harris-Warrick, and E.M. Shooter. 1979. Nerve growth factor receptors: Characterization of two distinct classes of binding sites on chick embryo sensory ganglia cells. *J. Biol. Chem.* **254:** 5972.

Tartaglia, L.A., T.M. Ayres, G.H.W. Wong, and D.V. Goeddel. 1993. A novel domain within the 55 kd TNF receptor signals cell death. *Cell* **74:** 845.

Thoenen, H. 1995. Neurotrophins and neuronal plasticity. *Science* **270:** 593.

Timm, D.E., P.L. De Haseth, and K.E. Neet. 1994. Comparative equilibrium denaturation studies of the neurotrophins: Nerve growth factor, brain-derived neurotrophic factor, neurotrophin 3, and neurotrophin 4/5. *Biochemistry* **33:** 4667.

Verheij, M., R. Bose, X.H. Lin, B. Yao, W.D. Jarvis, S. Grant, M.J. Birrer, E. Szabo, L.I. Zon, J.M. Kyriakis, A.

Haimovitz-Friedman, Z. Fuks, and R.N. Kolesnick. 1996. Requirement for ceramide-initiated SAPK/JNK signalling in stress-induced apoptosis. *Nature* **380:** 75.

Von Bartheld, C.S., Y. Kinoshita, D. Prevette, Q.-W. Yin, R.W. Oppenheim, and M. Bothwell. 1994. Positive and negative effects of neurotrophins on the isthmo-optic nucleus in chick embryos. *Neuron* **12:** 639.

Weskamp, G. and L.F. Reichardt. 1991. Evidence that biological activity of NGF is mediated through a novel subclass of high affinity receptors. *Neuron* **6:** 649.

White, K., E. Tahaoglu, and H. Steller. 1996. Cell killing by the *Drosophila* gene reaper. *Science* **271:** 805.

Wolf, D.E., C.A. McKinnon, M.-C. Daou, R.M. Stephens, D.R. Kaplan, and A.H. Ross. 1995. Interaction with TrkA immobilizes gp75 in the high affinity nerve growth factor receptor complex. *J. Biol. Chem.* **270:** 2133.

Xia, Z., M. Dickens, J. Raingeaud, R.J. Davis, and M.E. Greenberg. 1995. Opposing effects of ERK and JNK-p38 MAP kinases on apoptosis. *Science* **270:** 1326.

Yan, Q. and E.M. Johnson, Jr. 1988. An immunohistochemical study of the nerve growth factor receptor in developing rats. *J. Neurosci.* **8:** 3481.

Yang, Z., M. Costanzo, D.W. Golde, and R.N. Kolesnick. 1993. Tumor necrosis factor activation of the sphingomyelin pathway signals nuclear factor κB translocation in intact HL-60 cells. *J. Biol. Chem.* **268:** 20520.

Nitric Oxide, Cell Multiplication, and Cell Survival

N. Peunova,[1] B. Kuzin,[1,2] I. Roberts,[3] C. O'Kane,[3] and G. Enikolopov[1]
[1]Cold Spring Harbor Laboratory, Cold Spring Harbor, New York 11724; [2]Koltzov Institute of Developmental Biology, Russian Academy of Sciences, Moscow, Russia; [3]Department of Genetics, University of Cambridge, United Kingdom

Arrest of cell division is crucial for cells to enter a program of terminal differentiation. In the developing organ or a differentiating tissue, growth arrest defines roughly the size of the cellular population that is further committed to become a domain of differentiated cells. Eventually, the balance between the number of cell divisions and the extent of subsequent programmed cell death determines the final size of a domain, a tissue, or an organ (for review, see Bryant and Simpson 1984; Raff 1992, 1996). Mitogenesis, cytostasis, and survival of neuronal cells can be induced and maintained by the same or by different growth or trophic factors. The signaling pathways that coordinate proliferation, growth arrest, and survival of cells and groups of cells in developing organisms are not known, but they probably involve as yet undetermined inter- and intra-cellular second messenger molecules.

Nitric oxide (NO) is a diffusible multifunctional transcellular messenger that has been implicated in numerous physiological functions in mammals, ranging from contraction of muscles and dilation of blood vessels to immune response and potentiation of synaptic transmission (for review, see Bredt and Snyder 1994a; Nathan and Xie 1994; Garthwaite and Boulton 1995). NO is a highly reactive molecule that can spread from its original source and act on adjacent cells within a restricted volume, displaying properties similar to both paracrine and autocrine effectors. NO is produced from arginine by nitric oxide synthase (NOS). Three chromosomal NOS genes have been cloned from mammalian cells (for review, see Knowles and Moncada 1994; Wang and Marsden 1995). These loci give rise to numerous NOS isoforms, which differ in their tissue distribution, dependence on calcium, and mechanism of activation.

Besides its short-term physiological effects, NO can directly affect cell division and cell survival. Depending on the biochemical milieu, NO can act in some systems as a hazardous agent, inducing mutagenesis, cytotoxicity, and apoptosis. However, in other systems, NO can act as a delicate antiproliferative instrument, inducing temporary cytostasis, which is reversed if the concentration of NO decreases. These antiproliferative properties of NO may contribute to the cellular decision-making processes that control cessation of division, entry to a differentiation program, suppression or induction of programmed cell death, etc.

Here, we consider our recent studies to understand the role of NO in development. We present evidence that NO has a dual role during neuronal cell differentiation—at first it acts as an antiproliferative agent, inducing growth arrest in dividing cells, and later, when the growth arrest is firmly established and the cells have undergone differentiation, it helps to suppress programmed cell death, thus mediating the survival effects of growth factors. Moreover, we have found that the antiproliferative features of NO enable it to control cell number during the development of an intact animal. Our results suggest that NO can play a broader role as a general regulator of cell proliferation and cell survival during organism development and morphogenesis.

NO INITIATES A SWITCH FROM PROLIFERATION TO CYTOSTASIS DURING DIFFERENTIATION OF NEURONAL CELLS

When naive PC12 cells are exposed to nerve growth factor (NGF), they show few signs of neuronal differentiation within the first 3–4 days. However, after 5–6 days, the cells stop dividing, enter a cytostatic state, and develop a differentiated phenotype: They change the pattern of expressed genes, start to express a variety of differentiation markers, and, as a most visible trait, they send out processes, building a dense network of extended and branched neurites (Greene and Tishler 1976; Greene et al. 1987). Thus, the response of PC12 cells to NGF involves a proliferative phase that is followed by growth arrest and differentiation. The switch from proliferation to cytostasis is critical for the cells to establish a differentiated phenotype after exposure to NGF. If cells cannot establish growth arrest, as happens in mutant PC12-U2 cells, they cannot acquire a differentiated phenotype and instead continue to proliferate (Burstein and Greene 1982). We have found that production of NO is crucial for the NGF-induced neuronal differentiation of PC12 cells (Peunova and Enikolopov 1995). Our experiments suggest that the cytostatic effect of NGF is mediated by NO and that induction of NOS is an important step in the commitment of neuronal precursors during differentiation.

NGF Treatment Induces NOS Activity

When untreated PC12 cells were tested for NOS by the NADPH-diaphorase cytochemical reaction, which reflects total NOS activity, no staining was observed.

After the cells were treated with NGF, however, they gradually started to acquire an intense NADPH-dependent blue color after diaphorase staining, indicating that NOS accumulates in PC12 cells in response to NGF treatment. This increase in diaphorase staining was specific for NGF and did not appear after addition of fetal calf serum or epidermal growth factor (EGF). However, staining was increased after addition of the fibroblast growth factor (bFGF), which, like NGF, induces neuronal differentiation in PC12 cells. Importantly, the NGF-treated cells that were first to undergo initial morphological changes characteristic of the differentiated phenotype were also the first to show bright staining. This suggests that elevation of NOS activity precedes development of the differentiated phenotype. Induction of NOS was confirmed using in vitro assays of NOS activity, immunocytochemistry, reverse-transcriptase polymerase chain reaction (RT-PCR), and RNase protection assays of NOS transcripts. The results of these assays indicate that during the early stages of NGF action, a substantial part of the total NOS activity is due to the induction of the Ca^{++}-independent *NOS2* gene and that the neuronal NOS1 form is activated much later, following the establishment of the growth arrest (see also Hirsch et al. 1993).

NO Can Act as an Antimitogenic Agent in PC12 Cells

NO can inhibit DNA synthesis in several cell types (Garg and Hassid 1989; Lepoivre et al. 1990; Kwon et al. 1991; Hogan et al. 1992). It acts as an antimitogenic agent in PC12 cells as well. Several NO donors, sodium nitroprusside (SNP), *S*-nitroso-*N*-acetylpenicillamine (SNAP), and *S*-nitroso-*N*-penicillamine (SNOP), suppressed DNA synthesis in a concentration-dependent manner (albeit with different potencies), indicating that NO is an active inhibitor of DNA replication in PC12 cells. This inhibition, which resulted in a decrease in cell division, was not due to cytotoxicity, since the cells resumed proliferation once the source of NO was removed. NO-mediated inhibition of DNA synthesis overcomes the increase of DNA synthesis induced by serum, NGF, EGF, bFGF, insulin-like growth factor, and various growth factors in combination with NOS inhibitors (see below).

The results of the fluorescence-activated cell sorting (FACS) analysis showed that NO induces specific changes in the cell-cycle phase distribution of PC12 cells. After treatment with NO donors, cells tended to accumulate specifically in G_2 phase, and the proportion of cells in S phase decreased. Remarkably, within a specific range of concentrations of NO donors, the proportion of PC12 cells in G_2 and S phases was similar to levels reached after prolonged treatment with NGF (Buchkovich and Ziff 1994; Peunova and Enikolopov 1995). These results with externally added NO donors suggest that NO molecules produced intracellularly during the course of NGF action could play a similar role in promoting NGF-induced cytostasis.

Inhibition of NOS Activity Prevents Cytostatic Action of NGF

After several days of NGF treatment, the proliferation of PC12 cells ceases and differentiation occurs. If NO produced by the NGF-induced NOS in PC12 cells can indeed act as a crucial antiproliferative factor, then inhibition of the enzyme should uncouple the proliferative and cytostatic components of NGF action and prolong the proliferative phase while suppressing the cytostatic effect of NGF. NOS inhibitors *N*-nitro-L-arginine methyl ester (L-NAME), *N*-monomethyl-L-arginine (L-NMMA), and 2-ethyl-2-thiopseudourea (ETU) indeed reversed the cytostatic action of NGF when applied together with the growth factor, and forced the cells to continue to proliferate instead of ceasing to divide after several days of NGF treatment. In the absence of NGF, similar concentrations of inhibitors did not have a detectable effect on PC12 cell growth; in particular, they did not accelerate cell proliferation. Addition of NOS inhibitors also did not hinder one of the most important early features of NGF action on neuronal cells—rapid induction of a set of immediate early genes (IEGs). Induction of IEGs is believed to trigger further steps in a cascade of gene activity, ultimately leading to the development of the differentiated phenotype. We tested a panel of IEGs (c-*fos*, c-*jun*, *fra-1*, *egr-1*, *nur77*, and others) by RNase protection and found that addition of the NOS inhibitor L-NAME did not affect either their basal level of expression or their induction by NGF. This proves that the NOS inhibitors do not merely prevent the initial steps of NGF action (such as binding to the receptors, activation of the receptors, induction of the MAP kinase signaling pathway) and, in addition, suggests that the NOS-dependent stage(s) occurs later in the development of the differentiated phenotype.

The most visible consequence of NGF action on PC12 cells is neurite outgrowth, and this was also affected by NOS inhibition. Under normal conditions, almost every cell gradually extends neurites in response to NGF, but when PC12 cells were treated with a combination of NGF and NOS inhibitor, the number of cells with neurites decreased dramatically, in accordance with the observation that most of the cells continued to divide and did not enter the differentiated state. In summary, our data show that inhibition of NOS reverses the NGF-dependent growth arrest, indicating that NO mediates the antiproliferative action of NGF in neuronal cells.

NOS Action Is Dependent on Cell Proliferation

To determine whether in the course of response to NGF there is a critical phase during which the cells are particularly susceptible to NOS action, PC12 cells were treated with NOS inhibitor L-NAME before or after the addition of NGF. L-NAME was able to reverse the cytostatic action of NGF only when applied before NGF addition or within 2–3 days of NGF treatment;

after that the inhibitor had no effect. Note that this time is shorter than the time needed for full manifestation of cytostasis and development of the neuronal phenotype. This suggests that the critical time window for NO action is within the first days of NGF addition, after which NOS may relegate its antiproliferative functions to the other, perhaps more general, systems of growth arrest.

To test if the crucial phase of NOS action in NGF-treated cells is cell-cycle specific, we uncoupled the mitogenic and differentiating phases of NGF action by suppressing proliferation of PC12 cells. Cells were brought to G_0 by growth on a medium with low (0.5%) serum and then transferred either to low-serum medium again or to high (15%)-serum medium and treated with combinations of NGF and L-NAME. When the cells were transferred to the low-serum medium (which does not permit cells to cycle), the NOS inhibitor could not prevent neurite outgrowth even at very high concentrations (10 mM). In contrast, when starved cells were transferred to the high-serum medium, where they could resume proliferation, the same concentrations of L-NAME were quite effective at suppressing the neurite outgrowth. This implies that if growth arrest is established by means other than NO production, then NO-mediated induction of cytostasis is not evoked and NOS inhibitors do not affect the action of NGF. Taken together, these results argue that the critical period of NOS action is dependent on the cell cycle progression and that it probably occurs in a different phase of the cycle from the decision to enter the differentiation program.

Mutant Cells' Capacity to Differentiate Can Be Rescued by NO

Mutant PC12-U2 cells retain the early steps of the response to NGF but have lost the capacity to execute the later steps (Burstein and Greene 1982). They do not stop dividing after NGF treatment and, as a consequence, they do not develop the fully differentiated phenotype; in particular, they do not send out processes. To investigate whether this defect is connected to NO production, we tested whether the phenotype could be overcome by the addition of NO. Although neither NGF nor NO alone had any effect on the phenotype of U2 cells, in combination these treatments restored the differentiated neuronal phenotype. The mutant cells stopped dividing and grew extensive branched neurites, similar to wild-type PC12 cells. Thus, it was possible to rescue the defect in mutant cells and to restore the complete differentiation program by complementing NGF action with NO.

To confirm further the involvement of NOS in the differentiation of mutant U2 cells, the induction of NOS by NGF in these cells was examined by immunofluorescence and by RT-PCR analysis. Inducible NOS (NOS2) was expressed at much lower (almost tenfold) levels in U2 cells than in the wild-type PC12 cells after 4 days of NGF treatment. However, the levels of neuronal NOS (NOS1) in U2 cells were indistinguishable from those in PC12 cells. Together, these data demonstrate that the NGF-treated U2 cells are defective in NGF-dependent NOS2 induction and that this defect can be rescued by the external application of NO. Importantly, the *NOS2* gene is expressed in U2 cells, although at low levels, and it can be induced by means other than NGF. This suggests that the defect in U2 cells resides in the signaling regulatory pathway rather than in the gene for NOS2 itself.

In summary, we present evidence for a causative role for NO action in NGF-induced growth arrest in PC12 cells. Our experiments argue that NO, produced by the NGF-induced NOS, serves as a switch between the proliferative and cytostatic phases of NGF action in neuronal cells and that NOS activation is necessary for the further development of the differentiated phenotype. Our results suggest a role for *NOS* as a growth arrest gene in the commitment cascade during NGF-mediated differentiation of neuronal cells.

NO MEDIATES SURVIVAL OF FULLY DIFFERENTIATED NEURONAL CELLS

Differentiated neuronal cells become dependent on growth factors for survival. NGF is a survival factor for sympathetic neurons and for PC12 cells, and when NGF-differentiated PC12 cells are deprived of growth factors, they undergo apoptosis. Our studies indicate that during the early stages of NGF action, NO initiates growth arrest. Here we present evidence that during the later stages of NGF action, in fully differentiated PC12 cells, NO has an additional role as a mediator of the survival functions of NGF.

Fully Differentiated PC12 Cells Become Dependent on NO

When growth factors are removed from NGF-differentiated PC12 cells, these cells undergo programmed cell death by apoptosis. This process can be blocked by reapplying NGF. Since NGF-induced NO production remains very high during the late stages of NGF action, after growth arrest has been already established, we examined whether part of the NGF action as a survival agent could be supported by NO. We have found that NO, like growth factors, can inhibit apoptosis of differentiated PC12 cells after NGF withdrawal. When NO-releasing compounds were added to fully differentiated cells before or immediately after withdrawal of NGF, cell death was markedly reduced, demonstrating that NO can partially substitute for NGF in preventing apoptosis. This suggests that endogenously produced NO, like that produced by NO donors, could contribute to cell survival. It may mediate some of the survival functions of NGF and may be necessary for the suppression of cell death. Indeed, inhibition of NOS in fully differentiated cells led to massive death by apoptosis, as documented by several criteria (changes in morphology, acridine orange and DAPI staining, TUNEL assay, and FACS analysis). Importantly, no apoptosis was observed when a similar treatment was applied to naive PC12 cells or to cells that had been treated with NGF for 2–4 days and hence had not yet established growth arrest and had not differentiated (also see above). Similarly, inhibition of NOS did not impair the survival of mutant U2 cells, which retain the early steps of the response to NGF but have lost the capacity to differentiate. Together, the results with differentiated, naive, and mutant cells indicate that fully differentiated PC12 cells, in parallel with increased dependence on NGF, develop a dependence on NO production for their survival, such that inhibition of NOS activity leads to cell death, and addition of NO can suppress cell death.

NO Activates Anti-apoptotic Machinery

A possible explanation of the role of NO in preventing apoptosis may involve its antiproliferative properties. NO may prevent cells from traversing the cell cycle, thereby keeping them from reaching a critical point where mitogenic signals contradict the established cytostatic condition of the cells, prompting them to undergo apoptosis (Evan et al. 1992; Ferrari and Greene 1994). In addition, inhibition of apoptosis by NO may involve direct activation of an anti-apoptotic program by NO; for example, by changing the levels of expression of proteins that prevent or promote apoptosis. We tested whether treatment of PC12 cells with NO changes the expression of the Bcl-2 family of proteins (Bcl-2, Bcl-x_L, Bcl-x_S, Bax, Bad, Bak, Bag-1) involved in regulating programmed cell death (for review, see Steller 1995; White 1996; see also Boise et al. 1993; Oltvai et al. 1993; Yang et al. 1995) and how these changes relate to those induced by NGF. Prolonged treatment of PC12 cells with NGF leads to an increase in the level of Bcl-x_L, a product that, like Bcl-2, can prevent apoptosis in many cell types. At the same time, the amount of Bax, a protein that counters the ability of Bcl-2 and Bcl-x_L to repress apoptosis, decreased with a similar time course. In contrast, the levels of these proteins are unchanged in the mutant U2 cells after NGF treatment, indicating that changes in the expression of apoptosis-related genes are connected to withdrawal from the cell cycle and differentiation, and not just to prolonged NGF treatment. Thus, NGF-induced differentiation of PC12 cells changes the expression of genes involved in the cell death program in favor of products that prevent apoptosis. This may lead to a switch of the cell program toward prevention of cell death, in line with the known role of NGF as a survival factor.

To determine whether NO can mediate part of the effect of NGF on the apoptosis machinery, we subjected PC12 cells to sustained treatment with NO donors. The changes in expression of a panel of apoptosis-related proteins were very similar to the changes evoked by NGF treatment. When the same donors were added to U2 cells (NGF-treated and untreated), the changes observed were identical to those seen in wild-type PC12 cells; most importantly, the levels of Bcl-x_L were increased, whereas the levels of Bax were decreased. Thus, like NGF, NO is able to induce an anti-apoptotic program directly, and this ability of NO may contribute to the survival functions of NGF.

Our results indicate that action of NO is critical in both the early and late phases of NGF-driven neuronal differentiation, i.e., before and after induction of growth arrest. To examine the contribution of different NOS isoforms in these two phases of differentiation, we followed the expression of various NOS genes by Western blot analysis and by RT-PCR. We found that differentiation of PC12 cells is accompanied by a switch from expression of the inducible form (NOS2) soon after addition of NGF (before growth arrest is established), to the neuronal form of NOS (NOS1), which reaches the maximal levels after the growth arrest is established and, perhaps, is more directly associated with the survival functions.

Dual Role of NO in Neuronal Cells

Our results argue that there is a dual role for NO during NGF-driven differentiation of neuronal cells (Fig.1). NO acts as an initiator of growth arrest during the early stages of NGF action and as a mediator of the survival effects of growth factor during the later stages. In the proliferative phase of NGF action, the NOS gene(s) is induced as a delayed response to the growth factor stimulation. This produces enough NO to inhibit DNA synthesis and, probably, to activate further checkpoints, thereby blocking further progression of the cell cycle, completing the proliferative phase of NGF action, and switching the cells to the cytostatic phase. Thus, NO acts here as a permissive factor for the remaining program of differentiation traits (such as neurite outgrowth), which can only occur after cell division has ceased; in addition, NO probably induces some of the later differentiation markers directly by promoting gene activity (Peunova and Enikolopov 1993).

Later, once growth arrest is established and the cells become fully differentiated and dependent on growth factors, NO also mediates the cells' survival both by enforcing the growth arrest of differentiated cells and by activating an anti-apoptotic program. Perhaps the switch from expression of the calcium-independent form of NOS to the calcium-dependent form underlies the dual role for NOS as a trigger of cytostasis in undifferentiated cells and as an inhibitor of apoptosis in differentiated cells. Given the unconventional properties of NO, it is possible that NO diffuses from the cell that produces it to promote cessation of growth in adjacent cells and that this phenomenon contributes

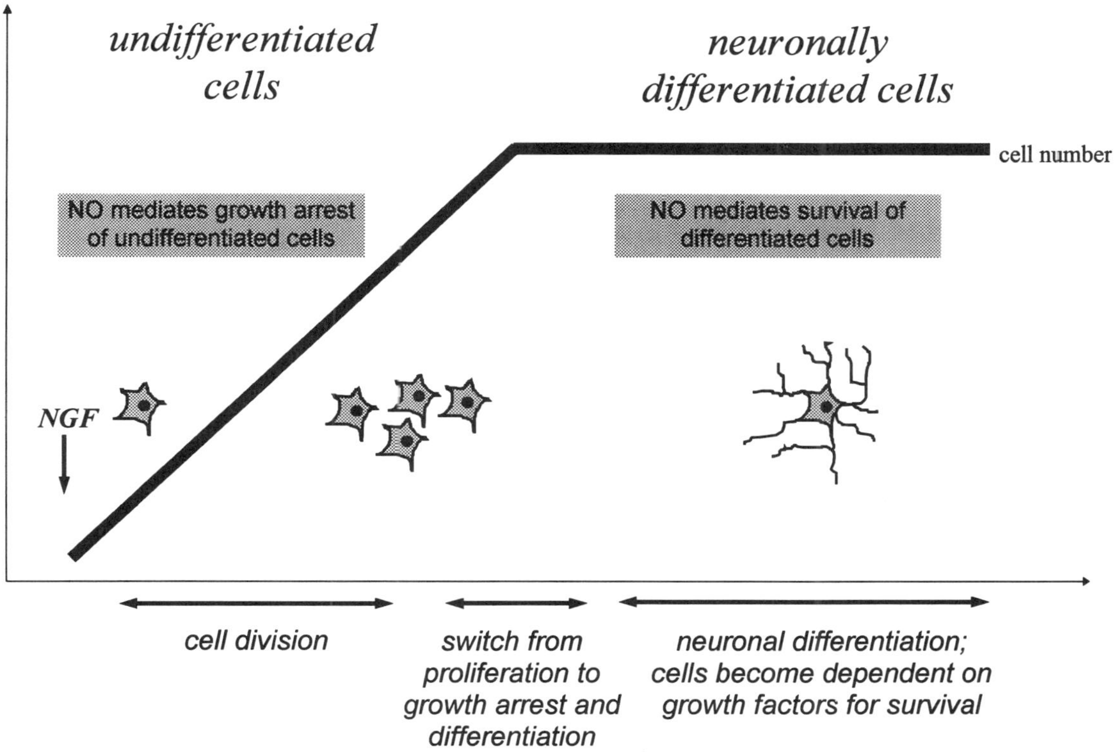

Figure 1. Schematic summary of NGF action and NOS functions. The model relates NGF-induced NOS activity to proliferation, differentiation, and survival of PC12 cells. In the early stages of the NGF action, in dividing undifferentiated cells, NO mediates transition to the cytostatic phase and neuronal differentiation. At the later stages, in fully differentiated cells, NO mediates part of the survival functions of NGF and prevents cells from programmed cell death both by enforcing the growth arrest and by activating an anti-apoptotic program.

to the synchronization of development and/or survival of a domain of neuronal precursors.

In the brain, NO production is associated with the death of neurons by necrosis and apoptosis after an ischemic stroke and, perhaps, neurodegenerative diseases (Choi 1993; Bredt and Snyder 1994a; Gross and Wolin 1995). Paradoxically, NOS-positive neurons in the brain are remarkably resistant to damage, and most of them are spared after exposure to strong insults and diseases that kill other cells (Ferrante et al. 1985, 1987; Koh et al. 1986; Koh and Choi 1988a,b; Uemura et al. 1990; Hyman et al. 1992; Mufson and Brandabur 1994). Our results suggest that preexposure to sustained NO production may be responsible for the increased resistance of NOS-positive neurons to damage. Although apoptosis can be initiated by numerous different stimuli, both the control mechanisms and the execution mechanisms of programmed cell death are remarkably uniform for different settings and appear to involve a relatively limited set of genes. The ability of NO to induce an anti-apoptotic program and prevent programmed cell death after withdrawal of a growth factor may reflect its physiological function in the brain during disease. We propose that the unusual resistance of NOS-positive neurons in the brain is related both to the role of NO in maintaining growth arrest and to its ability to fortify the cellular anti-apoptotic defense, which may later protect the cells from insults.

NO REGULATES CELL PROLIFERATION DURING *DROSOPHILA* DEVELOPMENT

Our experiments with cultured cells suggested that the antiproliferative activity of NO is crucial for the transition from proliferation to differentiation during neuronal differentiation. To investigate whether NO has a similar role during normal development of organisms, we have used *Drosophila* as a model organism. During *Drosophila* development, the structure, size, and shape of most of the organs of the adult fly are determined in the imaginal structures of the larvae (Cohen 1993; Fristrom and Fristrom 1993). Disc cells divide rapidly throughout larval development and cease proliferating at the end of the third instar period (Fig. 2). In leg, wing, and haltere discs, progression through the cell cycle stops in G_2 phase 3–4 hours before puparium formation. It resumes 15–18 hours later and then stops again in a defined spatial pattern after 12–14 hours (Fain and Stevens 1982; Graves and Schubiger 1982; Schubiger and Palka 1987). Although most of the dividing cells in the late larvae and in the

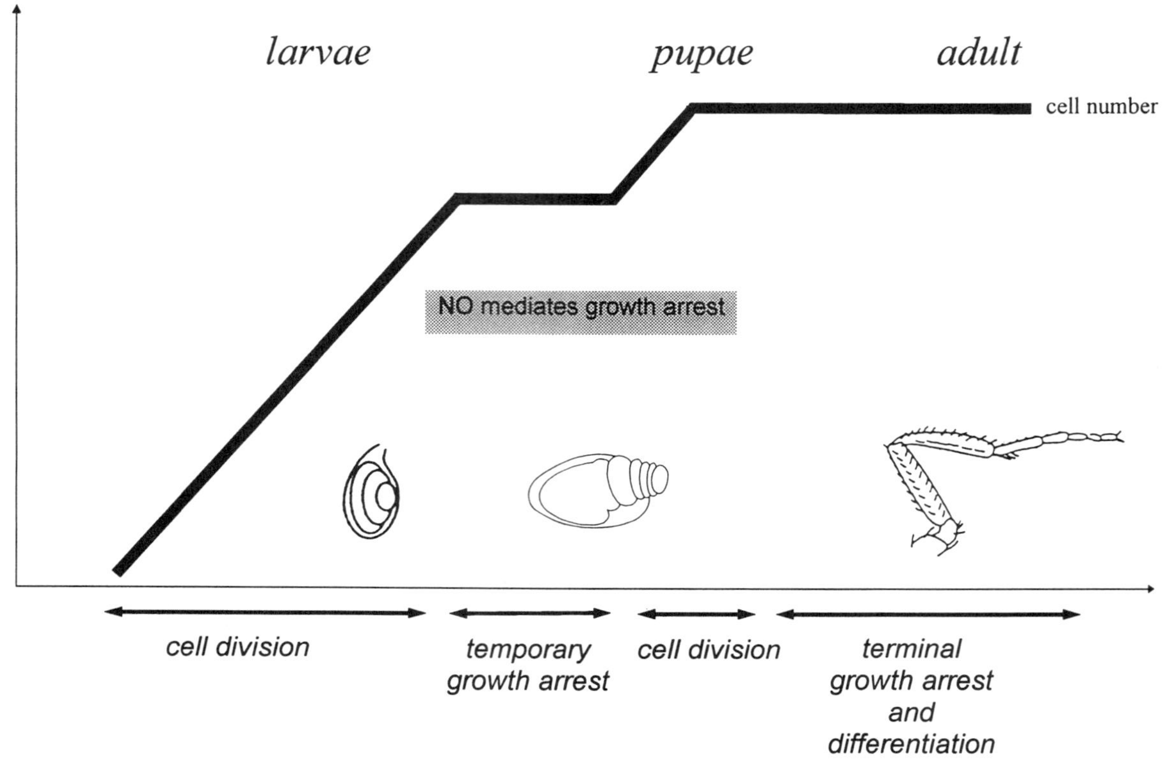

Figure 2. Schematic summary of cell proliferation in imaginal discs and organ development in *Drosophila.* Antiproliferative properties of NO mediate part of the temporary and, perhaps, terminal growth arrest during development of imaginal discs, and thus control the balance between cell proliferation and cell differentiation.

early pupae are already committed to their adult fate, they do not develop a fully differentiated phenotype until growth arrest is firmly established. Thus, cell proliferation is temporally separated from cell differentiation, which takes place later during metamorphosis. We tested whether NO is involved in the signaling pathways that control coordinated temporary growth arrest in larvae and pupae and subsequent terminal growth arrest in pupae and adults. We have found that NO acts as an antiproliferative agent during *Drosophila* development and controls the switch from cell proliferation to cell differentiation. Our data suggest that NO controls cell number and thus the size of anatomical structures in an intact animal. We propose that induction of NOS is a crucial step in *Drosophila* development and that NO may be a general regulator of cell proliferation and differentiation during organism development and morphogenesis.

NOS Is Expressed in Imaginal Discs during Larval Development

When imaginal discs of the third instar and early pupae were examined for the NADPH-diaphorase activity of NOS, staining was observed in all imaginal discs, imaginal rings, histoblasts, and the brain of the larvae, beginning in the third instar. Staining became more intense as development proceeded, indicating accumulation of the NOS activity. In late third-instar larvae and early pupae, a highly specific and reproducible pattern of very intense staining was evident. Later in development, when the discs began to evert in the prepupae, diaphorase staining of the forming structures became less intense and a distinct characteristic staining pattern of individual segments became evident. Diaphorase staining further decreased in a specific spatial pattern during early pupal development. Thus, there is a gradual and specific accumulation of NOS in those developing imaginal structures, which undergo radical changes during metamorphosis before giving rise to adult organs. This staining reaches its highest levels at the time when progression through the cell cycle slows down.

Inhibition of NOS Results in Hypertrophy of Leg Segments

The strong antiproliferative properties of NO and the specific pattern of diaphorase staining seen in mature imaginal discs imply that NO may act as a growth arrest agent in these structures and be capable of inhibiting DNA synthesis and supporting temporary cytostasis during the switch to metamorphosis. If NO indeed acts as an antiproliferative agent during the late stages of larval development, then inhibition of NOS might result in excessive growth of organs and tissues, whereas ectopic overexpression of the NOS gene might have the opposite effect.

To test this hypothesis, we inhibited NOS activity by injecting various NOS inhibitors in the developing larvae at the end of the third instar, several hours before metamorphosis. The resulting adults exhibited dramatic enlargements of many structures: legs, wings, genital structures, tergites, and sternites, etc. The changes most often affected and were most profound in the legs of the adults, where the diameter of certain segments increased 3- to 4-fold. The number of bristles and the number of rows of bristles were also increased, confirming that hyperproliferation of the cells had occurred. The leg segments most strongly affected were those (first and second tarsal segments, tibia, and femur) whose primordia had the highest levels of NOS at the larval and prepupal stages. Identical changes were observed when structurally unrelated inhibitors of NOS were used, indicating that the observed effect resulted specifically from blocking NOS activity. To test whether changing the NO levels directly affects DNA synthesis in the imaginal discs, we labeled the nuclei with 5-bromo-deoxyuridine (BrdU) after inhibition of NOS activity. There were significantly more BrdU-labeled cells in the imaginal discs of flies in which NOS activity was blocked than in those of control flies. Thus, inhibition of NOS at the late stages of larval development results in excessive cell proliferation and increased size of the structures of the body of the adult fly.

Ectopic Expression of a Mouse NOS Transgene Results in Reduced Size of Leg Segments

The ability of NO to inhibit DNA synthesis and cell proliferation suggests that overexpression of NOS in developing larvae may lead to diminished cell proliferation in the imaginal discs and to a reduction in the size of organs of the adult fly. To increase NO production, we induced expression of *NOS* transgene in transformed larvae carrying the mouse *NOS2* cDNA gene under the control of the heat-shock promoter. NOS2 is a calcium-independent form of NOS that is capable of efficient constitutive NO production. Transgenic larvae were heat shocked within 1 hour after puparıation to induce ectopic expression of NOS before the final cell divisions take place. This resulted, among other changes, in a reduction in the size of the limbs of the fly. The distal segments of the legs were affected most frequently and to the greatest degree. In extreme cases, the whole tarsus was shortened 1.5- to 2-fold and several segments were fused together with poorly defined boundaries. The most terminal structures of the appendage remained intact in these defective legs, suggesting that the observed reduction in size was due to incomplete growth of the developing appendage, rather than to complete loss of its distal structures. The number of bristles in a row on the affected segments also decreased, although the number of rows did not change. The segments of the adult leg most often affected by the overexpression of NOS (third, fourth, and fifth tarsal segments) were those that were not affected by the NOS inhibitors and whose precursors exhibited particularly low levels of diaphorase staining in the early prepupal stages. In contrast to experiments with inhibition of NOS, when imaginal discs were labeled with BrdU after induction of ectopic NOS expression, there were markedly fewer labeled cells in imaginal discs from induced NOS-transformed flies than in uninduced controls. Thus, ectopic expression of NOS at the late stages of larval development results in a decrease in cell proliferation and a reduction in the size of the structures of the body of the adult fly.

Inhibition of Apoptosis Unmasks Excessive Proliferation

For some *Drosophila* structures, for instance, the eye, we consistently detected an increase in the number of cells in S-phase in the imaginal disc after inhibition of NOS, but the resulting adult organ usually appeared normal. We tested the possibility that the apparently normal eye phenotype occurred as a result of programmed cell death, which counteracts excessive cell proliferation induced by NOS inhibition and restores the normal number of cells in the eye during metamorphosis. To suppress programmed cell death, we used GMR-P35 flies in which apoptosis in the developing eye is largely prevented by expression of recombinant baculovirus p35 protein (Hay et al. 1994).

When NOS was inhibited in GMR-P35 larvae, the eyes of the adult flies showed numerous changes, reflecting the surplus proliferation of various cell types in the developing eye. The most dramatic of these changes was in the number of ommatidia in the adult eye, which increased from the nearly invariant complement of 750 in wild-type flies and untreated GMR-P35 flies to nearly 820 after NOS inhibition in GMR-P35 flies. In addition, different types of accessory cells in the ommatidia proliferated after NOS inhibition to levels higher than those achieved by blocking apoptosis by p35 (Hay et al. 1994). For instance, the number of secondary and tertiary pigment cells was increased from 12 per sample area in normal eyes to more than 35 in GMR-P35 flies after inhibition of NOS. This number exceeds the maximal number of pigment cells saved from programmed cell death in untreated GMR-P35 flies (~25 per sample area) and suggests that extra pigment cells arise as a result of excessive cell proliferation caused by inhibition of NOS combined with suppression of cell death caused by p35. Furthermore, the number of bristles was increased in some areas of the eye in GMR-P35 flies after NOS inhibition, up to four to five per ommatidium, instead of the three seen in normal flies and untreated GMR-P35 flies. Similarly, the number of cone cells was increased from four in normal and in untreated GMR-P35 ommatidia to five and six in many ommatidia of GMR-P35 flies after NOS inhibition. Thus, prevention of apoptosis in the developing *Drosophila* eyes revealed excessive proliferation of various cell types after NOS inhibition, which was otherwise masked by programmed cell death in the larvae and pupae.

Together, our experiments with *Drosophila* have demonstrated that inhibition of NOS in larvae leads to enlargement of organs in adults and, conversely, that ectopic expression of NOS in larvae leads to a reduction in the size of organs in adults. In addition, the distribution of affected segments in the adult leg corresponds to the distribution of NOS in the larvae, and the changes in segment size can be directly correlated to changes in DNA synthesis in imaginal discs after manipulations of NOS activity. The increased cell proliferation that occurs in response to NOS inhibition is masked in some structures by apoptosis, and it can be revealed by suppressing programmed cell death. Taken together, these results indicate that NO acts as an antiproliferative agent to control cell proliferation during *Drosophila* development (Fig. 2).

NO AND DEVELOPMENT

This study provides support for the hypothesis that NO acts as an antiproliferative agent during cell differentiation and organism development and controls the cell number in an intact developing organism. It suggests a novel role for NO as a regulator of the balance between cell proliferation and cell differentiation during development. How general is the phenomenon of NO-mediated growth arrest in organism development? NOS expression can be induced to high levels in a large number of tissues and cell types by appropriate stimulation (Bredt and Snyder 1994a; Forstermann et al. 1995). In most cases, the pattern of NOS distribution in a developing organism differs strongly from the distribution in the adult organism. Furthermore, transient elevation of NOS expression in a given tissue often coincides with the cessation of division of committed precursor cells. For instance, in the brain, a strong elevation of NOS activity in the developing cerebral cortical plate and hippocampus at days 15–19 of embryonic development correlates with the time course of cessation of precursor cell proliferation, tight growth arrest, and cell differentiation; notably, NOS activity goes down after the proliferation of committed neuronal precursors is completed (Bredt and Snyder 1994b; Blottner et al. 1995). NOS levels are also transiently increased in developing lungs, bones, blood vessels, nervous system, and other tissues and organs (Blottner et al. 1995; Collin-Osdoby et al. 1995; Cramer et al. 1995; Shaul 1995; Wetts et al. 1995). Elsewhere, NOS activity is greatly elevated in regenerating tissues when cessation of cell division is crucial for prevention of unregulated growth (Roscams et al. 1994; Blottner et al. 1995; Decker and Obolenskaya 1995; Hortelano et al. 1995). In all these cases, a transient elevation of NOS activity might trigger a transition from proliferation to growth arrest and differentiation, thus contributing to the proper morphogenesis of the tissue and the organ.

We propose that production of NO is required during embryonic development and during tissue regeneration in the adult organism for the proper control of cell proliferation. The antiproliferative properties of NO may be particularly important in situations in which terminal differentiation of committed cells is temporally separated from cell proliferation and is strictly dependent on cessation of cell division. Given the multiplicity of the NOS isoforms, their overlapping tissue distribution, and the possibility that NO can be transferred within the organism by hemoglobin (Jia et al. 1996), it is conceivable that any group of cells in the embryo and fetus can be exposed to NO action.

NO is easily diffusible, and it may therefore exert its antiproliferative properties not only in the cell that produces it, but in the adjacent cells as well. Thus, it is possible that NO can contribute to the coordinated development of a group of neighboring cells committed to form a particular structure and thus may participate in tissue and organ morphogenesis. An efficient source of readily diffusible transcellular messengers, such as NO, may induce synchronized changes in the adjacent cells within a limited volume of a tissue. Moreover, several adjacent cells producing easily diffusible antiproliferative molecules may share the total pool of these molecules, produced by the neighbors as well as by themselves. If a particular threshold level of a signal is needed to initiate a signaling chain that eventually leads to growth arrest, then the cells in this group could stop dividing when a certain number of cells and, therefore, a certain local concentration of messenger molecules is reached. This way, by organizing groups of cells in functional clusters, NO may instruct the developing structures to terminate their growth when they attain the appropriate size and shape, at the same time coordinating their growth with the growth of the adjacent tissues.

ACKNOWLEDGMENTS

We are grateful to the members of the Enikolopov laboratory for advice and support. We are indebted to Santosh John for expert assistance with the experiments. We thank Gerald Rubin and Bruce Hay for their gift of GMR-p35 flies, and Charles Lowenstein and Solomon Snyder for the NOS2 gene. We thank Michael Regulski and Tim Tully for sharing their results on the *Drosophila* NOS gene. This work was supported by a National Institutes of Health grant, an American Cancer Society grant, and a Klingenstein Foundation grant to G.E.; by funding from the Human Frontiers Science Program and the Biotechnology and Biological Sciences Research Council to C.O'K.; by a National Science Foundation grant to N.P., and by a grant from the Russian Foundation for Basic Research (RFFI) to B.K.

REFERENCES

Blottner, D., Z. Grozdanovic, and R. Gossrau. 1995. Histochemistry of nitric oxide synthase in the nervous system. *Histochem. J.* **27:** 785.

Boise, L.H., M. Gonzalez-Garcia, C.E. Postema, L. Ding, T. Lindsten, L.A. Turka, X. Mao, G. Nunez, and C.B. Thompson. 1993. bcl-x, a bcl-2-related gene that functions as a dominant regulator of apoptotic cell death. *Cell* **74:** 597.

Bredt, D.S. and S.H. Snyder. 1994a. Nitric oxide: A physiologic messenger molecule. *Annu. Rev. Biochem.* **63:** 175.

———. 1994b. Transient nitric oxide synthase neurons in embryonic cerebral cortical plate, sensory ganglia, and olfactory epithelium. *Neuron* **13:** 301.

Bryant, P.J. and P. Simpson. 1984. Intrinsic and extrinsic control of growth in developing organs. *Q. Rev. Biol.* **59:** 387.

Buchkovich, K.J. and E.B. Ziff. 1994. Nerve growth factor regulates the expression and activity of p33cdk2 and p34cdc2 kinases in PC12 pheochromocytoma cells. *Mol. Biol. Cell* **5:** 1225.

Burstein, D.E. and L.A. Greene. 1982. Nerve growth factor has both mitogenic and antimitogenic activity. *Dev. Biol.* **94:** 477.

Choi, D.W. 1993. Nitric oxide: Foe or friend to the injured brain? *Proc. Natl. Acad. Sci.* **90:** 9741.

Cohen, S.M. 1993. Imaginal disc development. In *The Development of* Drosophila melanogaster (ed. M. Bate and A. Martinez Arias), p. 747. Cold Spring Harbor Laboratory Press, Cold Spring Harbor, New York.

Collin-Osdoby, P., G.A. Nickols, and P. Osdoby. 1995. Bone cell function, regulation, and communication: A role for nitric oxide. *J. Cell. Biochem.* **57:** 399.

Cramer, K.S., C.I. Moore, and M. Sur. 1995. Transient expression of NADPH-diaphorase in the lateral geniculate nucleus of the ferret during early postnatal development. *J. Comp. Neurol.* **353:** 306.

Decker, K.F. and M.Y. Obolenskaya. 1995. Cytokines, nitric oxide synthesis and liver regeneration. *J. Gastroenterol. Hepatol.* **1:** S12.

Evan, G.I., A.H. Wyllie, C.S. Gilbert, T.D. Littlewood, H. Land, M. Brooks, C.M. Waters, L.Z. Penn, and D.C. Hancock. 1992. Induction of apoptosis in fibroblasts by c-myc protein. *Cell* **69:** 119.

Fain, M.J. and B. Stevens. 1982. Alterations in the cell cycle of *Drosophila* imaginal disc cells precede metamorphosis. *Dev. Biol.* **92:** 247.

Ferrante, R.J., N.W. Kowall, M.F. Beal, J.B Martin, E.D. Bird, and E.P. Richardson, Jr. 1987. Morphologic and histochemical characteristics of a spared subset of striatal neurons in Huntington's disease. *J. Neuropathol. Exp. Neurol.* **46:** 12.

Ferrante, R.J., N.W. Kowall, M.F. Beal, E.P. Richardson, Jr., E.D. Bird, and J.B. Martin. 1985. Selective sparing of a class of striatal neurons in Huntington's disease. *Science* **230:** 561.

Ferrari, G. and L.A. Greene. 1994. Proliferative inhibition by dominant-negative Ras rescues naive and neuronally differentiated PC12 cells from apoptotic death. *EMBO J.* **13:** 5922.

Forstermann, U., H. Kleinert, I. Gath, P. Schwarz, E.I. Closs, and N.J. Dun. 1995. Expression and expressional control of nitric oxide synthases in various cell types. *Adv. Pharmacol.* **34:** 171.

Fristrom, D. and J.W. Fristrom. 1993. The metamorphic development of the adult epidermis. In *The Development of* Drosophila melanogaster (ed. M. Bate and A. Martinez Arias), p. 843. Cold Spring Harbor Laboratory Press, Cold Spring Harbor, New York.

Garg, U.C. and A. Hassid. 1989. Nitric oxide-generating vasodilators and 8-bromo-cyclic guanosine monophosphate inhibit mitogenesis and proliferation of cultured rat vascular smooth muscle cells. *J. Clin. Invest.* **83:** 1774.

Garthwaite, J. and C.L. Boulton. 1995. Nitric oxide signaling in the central nervous system. *Annu. Rev. Physiol.* **57:** 683.

Graves, B.J. and G. Schubiger. 1982. Cell cycle changes during growth and differentiation of imaginal leg discs in *Drosophila melanogaster. Dev. Biol.* **93:** 104.

Greene, L.A. and A.S. Tischler. 1976. Establishment of a noradrenergic clonal line of rat adrenal pheochromocytoma cells which respond to nerve growth factor. *Proc. Natl. Acad. Sci.* **73:** 2424.

Greene, L.A., J.M. Aletta, A. Rukenstein, and S.H. Green. 1987. PC12 pheochromocytoma cells: Culture, nerve growth factor treatment, and experimental exploitation. *Methods Enzymol.* **147:** 207.

Gross, S.S. and M.S. Wolin. 1995. Nitric oxide: Pathophysiological mechanisms. *Annu. Rev. Physiol.* **57:** 737.

Hay, B.A., T. Wolff, and G.M. Rubin. 1994. Expression of baculovirus P35 prevents cell death in *Drosophila. Development* **120:** 2121.

Hirsch, D.B., J.P. Steiner, T.M. Dawson, A. Mammen, E. Hayek, and S.H. Snyder. 1993. Neurotransmitter release regulated by nitric oxide in PC12 cells and brain synaptosomes. *Curr. Biol.* **3:** 749.

Hogan, M., A. Cerami, and R. Bucala. 1992. Advanced glycosylation endproducts block the antiproliferative effect of nitric oxide. Role in the vascular and renal complications of diabetes mellitus. *J. Clin. Invest.* **90:** 1110.

Hortelano, S., B. Dewez, A.M. Genaro, M.J. Diaz-Guerra, and L. Bosca. 1995. Nitric oxide is released in regenerating liver after partial hepatectomy. *Hepatology* **21:** 776.

Hyman, B.T., K. Marzloff, J.J. Wenniger, T.M. Dawson, D.S. Bredt, and S.H. Snyder. 1992. Relative sparing of nitric oxide synthase-containing neurons in the hippocampal formation in Alzheimer's disease. *Ann. Neurol.* **32:** 818.

Jia, L., C. Bonaventura, J. Bonaventura, and J.S. Stamler. 1996. S-nitrosohaemoglobin: A dynamic activity of blood involved in vascular control. *Nature* **380:** 221.

Knowles, R.G. and S. Moncada. 1994. Nitric oxide synthases in mammals. *Biochem. J.* **298:** 249.

Koh, J.Y. and D.W. Choi. 1988a. Cultured striatal neurons containing NADPH-diaphorase or acetylcholinesterase are selectively resistant to injury by NMDA receptor agonists. *Brain Res.* **446:** 374.

———. 1988b. Vulnerability of cultured cortical neurons to damage by excitotoxins: Differential susceptibility of neurons containing NADPH-diaphorase. *J. Neurosci.* **8:** 2153.

Koh, J.Y., S. Peters, and D.W. Choi. 1986. Neurons containing NADPH-diaphorase are selectively resistant to quinolinate toxicity. *Science* **234:** 73.

Kwon, S.K., D.J. Stuehr, and C.F. Nathan. 1991. Inhibition of tumor cell ribonucleotide reductase by macrophage-derived nitric oxide. *J. Exp. Med.* **174:** 761.

Lepoivre, M., B. Chenais, A. Yapo, G. Lemaire, L.

Thelander, and J.P. Tenu. 1990. Alterations of ribonucleotide reductase activity following induction of the nitrite-generating pathway in adenocarcinoma cells. *J. Biol. Chem.* **265:** 14143.

Mufson, E.J. and M.M. Brandabur. 1994. Sparing of NADPH-diaphorase striatal neurons in Parkinson's and Alzheimer's diseases. *NeuroReport* **5:** 705.

Nathan, C. and Q.-W. Xie. 1994. Nitric oxide synthases: Roles, tolls and controls. *Cell* **78:** 915.

Oltvai, Z.N., C.L. Milliman, and S.J. Korsmeyer. 1993. Bcl-2 heterodimerizes in vivo with a conserved homolog, Bax, that accelerates programmed cell death. *Cell* **74:** 609.

Peunova, N. and G. Enikolopov. 1993. Amplification of calcium-induced gene transcription by nitric oxide in neuronal cells. *Nature* **364:** 450.

———. 1995. Nitric oxide triggers a switch to growth arrest during differentiation of neuronal cells. *Nature* **375:** 68.

Raff, M.C. 1992. Social control on cell survival and cell death. *Nature* **356:** 397.

———. 1996. Size control: The regulation of cell number in animal development. *Cell* **86:** 327.

Roskams, A.J., D.S. Bredt, T.M. Dawson, and G.V. Ronnett. 1994. Nitric oxide mediates the formation of synaptic connections in developing and regenerating olfactory receptor neurons. *Neuron* **13:** 289.

Schubiger, M. and J. Palka. 1987. Changing spatial patterns of DNA replication in the developing wing of *Drosophila. Dev. Biol.* **123:** 145.

Shaul, P.W. 1995. Nitric oxide in the developing lung. *Adv. Pediatr.* **42:** 367.

Steller, H. 1995. Mechanisms and genes of cellular suicide. *Science* **267:** 1445.

Uemura, Y., N.W. Kowall, and M.F. Beal. 1990. Selective sparing of NADPH-diaphorase-somatostatin-neuropeptide Y neurons in ischemic gerbil striatum. *Ann. Neurol.* **27:** 620.

Wang, Y. and P.A. Marsden. 1995. Nitric oxide synthases: Gene structure and regulation. *Adv. Pharmacol.* **34:** 71.

Wetts, R., P.E. Phelps, and J.E. Vaughn. 1995. Transient and continuous expression of NADPH diaphorase in different neuronal populations of developing rat spinal cord. *Dev. Dyn.* **202:** 215.

White, E. 1996. Life, death, and the pursuit of apoptosis. *Genes Dev.* **10:** 1.

Yang, E., J. Zha, J. Jockel, L.H. Boise, C.B. Thompson, and S.J. Korsmeyer. 1995. Bad, a heterodimeric partner for Bcl-XL and Bcl-2, displaces Bax and promotes cell death. *Cell* **80:** 285.

The Role of Neuregulin (ARIA) at the Neuromuscular Junction

K.M. Rosen, A.W. Sandrock, Jr., A.D.J. Goodearl, J.A. Loeb, and G.D. Fischbach
Department of Neurobiology, Harvard Medical School, Boston, Massachusetts 02115

AChR SYNTHESIS AT EMBRYONIC AND MATURE ENDPLATES

*A*cetylcholine *r*eceptor *i*nducing *a*ctivity (ARIA) is a protein purified from acid extracts of adult chicken brains that can stimulate the synthesis of acetylcholine receptors (AChRs) in cultured embryonic chick myotubes (Jessell et al. 1979; Buc-Caron et al. 1983; Usdin and Fischbach 1986; Falls et al. 1990, 1993). The purification was undertaken with the assumption that one or more ARIAs were synthesized in motor neurons, transported to the motor nerve terminals, and then released into the synaptic cleft where they would exert their effects on the postsynaptic partner, skeletal muscle. From the beginning, it was assumed that ARIA-induced AChR synthesis contributed to the accumulation of AChRs at developing neuromuscular junctions (NMJ) as well as the maintenance of the high AChR density that is found at mature endplates.[1] The effect seen on synthesis would complement the effects of agrin and related molecules that act to immobilize AChRs in the lipid bilayer and restrict their lateral diffusion. In this view, the high postsynaptic AChR density is due to the trapping of newly synthesized AChRs inserted in the immediate vicinity of the postsynaptic membrane.

The purification of ARIA to homogeneity and the determination of the predicted amino acid sequence from a cloned cDNA have provided powerful new tools that were needed to test several aspects of this model. What follows is a review of the results of recent experimentation in our laboratory aimed at understanding ARIA's role in synapse formation. (For more systematic reviews of the relevant literature, see Hall and Sanes 1993; Ben-Baruch and Yarden 1994; Grinnell 1995; Fischbach and Rosen 1996; Lemke 1996.)

METHODS

Chick muscle bioassays. The preparation of chicken pectoral muscle cultures for bioassay was performed as described previously (Falls et al. 1993). For bioassay, cultures were prepared in 96-well plates. Myotubes were treated for 24 hours with specified samples in quadruplicate, and this was followed by a block of preexisting surface receptors with an excess (100 nM) of cold α-bungarotoxin (BTX). After washing out unbound toxin, fresh medium containing ^{125}I-labeled α-BTX was added and the cells were incubated for 5 hours. After washing, cells were extracted in 1 M sodium hydroxide and 0.5 mg/ml sodium deoxycholate, and the extract was counted in a γ counter (Packard Instruments). Values are represented as the experimental sample value minus the value of an untreated control.

Compound muscle action potential (CMAP) measurements. Mice were placed under general anesthesia and a pair of monopolar needle electrodes were inserted at Erb's point to supramaximally stimulate the brachial plexus. CMAPs were recorded from the flexor muscles of the ipsilateral forelimb with an indwelling monopolar needle electrode. The motor nerves were stimulated with alternating 3-Hz and 30-Hz trains of 10 current pulses delivered at 1-minute intervals. D-Tubocurarine was administered in doses of 2.5, 5, 10, 20, 40, and 80 μmol/kg at 10-minute intervals through an intraperitoneal catheter.

^{125}I-labeled α-BTX binding to hemidiaphragms. Diaphragms were removed from 6 wild-type (+/+) and 6 heterozygote (+/–) mice and incubated in Puck's saline containing 2 nM ^{125}I-labeled α-BTX for 2 hours at room temperature. After rinsing, the diaphragms were divided midsagittally. Endplate-rich strips were cut from each right hemidiaphragm and counted in a γ counter. Specific binding was calculated by subtracting the values obtained for binding to a right hemidiaphragm strip, isolated from BALB/c mice, that had been similarly treated but in the presence of an excess of unlabeled BTX.

A FAMILY OF PROTEINS

Analysis of sequences, derived either from tryptic peptides isolated from brain-purified material or from the entire predicted protein sequence deduced from the cloned cDNA, identifies ARIA as one member of a group of proteins that activate transmembrane receptor tyrosine kinases of the epidermal growth factor receptor (EGF-R) family. These related receptors have been called HER (*h*uman *E*GF-*R*), *neu* (*neu*roblastoma), or erbB (*e*rythro*b*lastosis *B*), depending on the

[1] The latter may seem surprising considering the relatively slow rate of AChR turnover at mature endplates, but when one considers the enormous increase in receptor number as the endplate matures, and if one assumes that degradation is a first-order process, the need for maintaining a high rate of synthesis at mature junctions is evident.

tissue and the species from which they were isolated. Given the variation in the receptor names, it has also happened that the ligands for this receptor family bear differing names, including the human heregulins (HRGs) (Holmes et al. 1992) and the rat neu differentiation factors (NDFs) (Wen et al. 1992). Another member of the family is glial growth factor (GGF), which was purified (Goodearl et al. 1993) and cloned (Marchionni et al. 1993) on the basis of its ability to stimulate the proliferation of Schwann cells in culture. After years of effort, all of these related ligands were cloned within a few months of one another. There are a substantial number of structural isoforms of these ligands that all appear to be generated through alternative splicing of transcription products from a single gene. With an abundance of names that nearly rivals the number of currently known isoforms, there is a need for a simplifying nomenclature. The name "neuregulin" has been suggested, and we use it to refer to all the proteins generated from this gene.[2]

The original chick cDNA (called λ12) predicted a protein (proARIA-1) with several distinct structural domains (diagrammed in Fig. 1). This protein is substantially larger than the species purified from adult brain. A stretch of hydrophobic amino acids near the middle of the sequence presumably spans the membrane, so the protein appears to be synthesized as a transmembrane precursor. The brain-purified material likely represents the soluble, extracellular portion of the precursor. This is supported by the finding that all five of the tryptic peptides that were isolated and sequenced are found within the predicted extracellular domain (Falls et al. 1993). Although ARIA is present in medium conditioned by certain neurons, the precursor does not predict an obvious amino-terminal signal sequence. An immunoglobulin-like fold is found beginning approximately 50 residues from the amino terminus, and this is followed by a serine- and threonine-rich segment that contains several sites for both O- and N-linked sugars. Immediately after this "spacer" segment is an EGF-like domain, characterized by the presence of six conserved cysteines within a span of approximately 40 residues. The EGF-like domain is a site of extensive variation in the isoforms characterized to date (see Ben-Baruch and Yarden 1994; Fischbach and Rosen 1997). Following the EGF-like domain is the transmembrane segment and then the largest portion of the precursor, the cytoplasmic domain, another site of alternative splicing.

THE IMPORTANCE OF ARIA AT THE NMJ

First, ARIA is a potent activator of AChR synthesis. The ability of purified recombinant ARIA (λ12) ex-

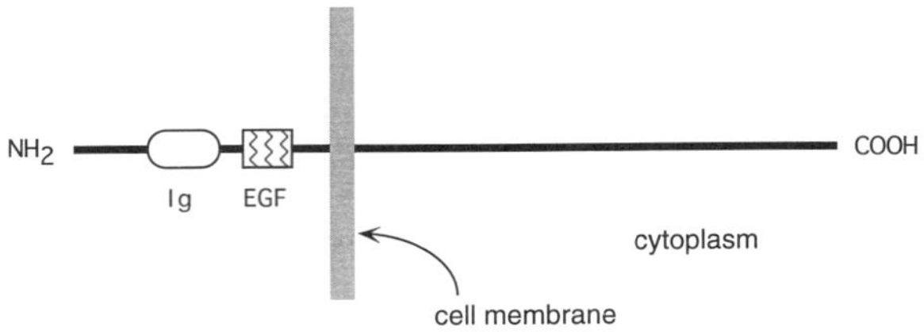

Figure 1. Schematic representation of the 67-kD proARIA-1 precursor. Ig and EGF refer to the location of the immunoglobulin-like and EGF-like domains found in the extracellular portion of the protein. Amino and carboxyl termini are indicated.

pressed in yeast (*Pichia pastoris*) to induce the synthesis and insertion of new AChRs into the sarcolemma is evident at concentrations of 1–5 pM, and the effect is half-maximal at 25–50 pM. This is comparable to the potency of the neurotrophins acting on their respective receptors. In the chick, the major effect of ARIA is on the synthesis of the AChR α subunit mRNA (Harris et al. 1988), whereas in mammals, the most profound effect is on the developmentally regulated ε subunit (Martinou et al. 1991; Chu et al. 1995).

A variety of isoforms of the EGF-like domain have been expressed in isolation in *Escherichia coli*. Alterations in sequence due to alternative splicing following the fifth cysteine of the EGF-like domain identify two classes of EGF-like domains named α and β. When properly folded, β isoforms (see below) stimulate AChR synthesis with the same potency and efficacy as the entire extracellular domain. In our experiments, α isoforms are about 1000-fold less potent and may not be full agonists (Fig. 2). Few or no α isoforms have been found in the nervous system; it seems that their expression and function may be limited to cells and tissues of mesenchymal lineages.

Second, the neuregulin gene is expressed beginning early in development in motor neurons. In situ hybridization identifies a clear signal in motor neurons on embryonic day (E) 4–5 in the chick, a time when motor axons first invade the peripheral muscle masses (Goodearl et al. 1995). In the rat, silver grains are concentrated over the ventral horn of the spinal cord on E15 (Chen et al. 1994; Corfas et al. 1995), the time when the first NMJs are forming in this species.

Third, the ARIA protein can be detected at motor endplates. Our first studies of chick junctions with an antiserum (HM22) raised against the amino-terminal 27 amino acids showed staining that corresponded precisely with rhodamine-labeled α-bungarotoxin on E18 (Goodearl et al. 1995). Although no staining of the NMJ was evident prior to E16 with this antiserum, ARIA-like immunoreactivity has been detected in chick motor neurons and motor axons as early as E5 with affinity-purified antibodies (HM 183) from a rabbit immunized with the entire recombinant proARIA molecule. It is likely that the affinity of HM22 is not high enough to detect the antigen until it is con-

[2]Neuregulin implies that all members of the family are present in the nervous system or that they act only on neurons or glia. This is certainly not the case. Some isoforms are restricted to mesenchymal tissue and have little or no effect on neural cells.

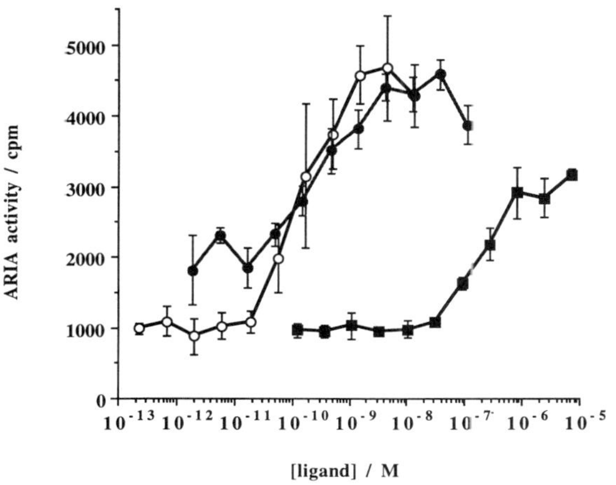

Figure 2. Comparison of dose response curves for receptor-inducing activity of three different forms of neuregulin. ^{125}I-labeled α-BTX binding is listed on the Y-axis. Molar concentration of ligand is listed on the X-axis. (*Open circles*) Extracellular domain of proARIA expressed in yeast. (*Closed circles*) β1 EGF-like domain expressed in *E. coli*. (*Closed squares*) α2 EGF-like domain expressed in *E. coli*.

centrated in the synaptic cleft or, alternatively, another isoform may be present at that time, although nuclease protection experiments show that, the proARIA-1 isoform is being produced in spinal cord at the earliest examined developmental times. Complementary immunohistochemical studies performed in the rat have shown ARIA to be localized at the adult NMJ, and its levels decrease dramatically, but not completely, after denervation (Jo et al. 1995; Moscoso et al. 1995; Sandrock et al. 1995).

ARIA is retained on a heparin column (Falls et al. 1993), so it is not surprising that it is concentrated in the matrix of the synaptic cleft—adding to an already large number of proteins that have found a home in this narrow crevice. In immuno-electron microscopy studies with gold particles or with horseradish peroxidase (HRP) as the reporter, it is evident that ARIA is in the cleft (Goodearl et al. 1995; for description of an activity in the synaptic cleft of the NMJ that can stimulate AChR synthesis, see Goldman et al. 1991; Brenner et al. 1992; Jo and Burden 1992). ARIA-like immunoreactivity extends beyond the zone of nerve/muscle contact at the earliest junctions, but it does seem to be confined to the region of contact between the muscle fiber and the overlying Schwann cell. This is interesting because of the dual role of neuregulin as an AChR-inducing activity and as a GGF. The effect of neuregulin on terminal Schwann cells remains to be fully determined, but recent studies have indicated that it may serve to regulate survival of Schwann cells during early postnatal development in the rat (Trachtenberg and Thompson 1996).

Since it appears that the ability of neuregulins to bind to and activate erbB receptors resides in the EGF-like domain, the other domains are likely involved in roles relating to regulation of processing of the precursors or to the localization of the released ligands. The immunoglobulin-like (Ig) domain is responsible for ARIA binding to heparin and is probably essential for binding to the extracellular matrix of the NMJ (Loeb and Fischbach 1995). There are abundant precedents in the literature for the involvement of Ig domains in cell/matrix interactions (see Vaughn and Bjorkman 1996). Limited proteolysis that preserves AChR-inducing activity (presumably as the 6-kD EGF-like domain) but degrades the rest of the molecule can release AChR-inducing activity from the surface of intact neuronal cells (Loeb and Fischbach 1995). Moreover, AChR-inducing activity can be released into the medium by the addition of heparin. Earlier studies of an axonal-associated Schwann cell mitogen, which in retrospect is likely a neuregulin, also showed that the mitogen was not covalently attached to the cell surface and could be released by high salt treatment (Ratner et al. 1985, 1988).

Interestingly, not all neuregulins contain an Ig fold. cDNAs have been characterized from chicken (Kuo et al. 1994), human (Ho et al. 1995), and rat (D. Wen, pers. comm.) that instead of an Ig fold, use a novel 222-amino-acid amino-terminal region that contains a hydrophobic 34-amino-acid segment, 8 of which are cysteines. Transfection experiments in our laboratory have indicated that the addition of heparin has no apparent effect on the Ig$^-$ isoforms, and these isoforms are capable of stimulating AChR synthesis in our chick skeletal muscle bioassay. The importance of the Ig$^-$ isoforms at the NMJ remains unclear, although motor neurons may express higher levels of Ig$^-$ isoforms than Ig$^+$ isoforms at specific times during development (Kuo et al. 1994; Corfas et al. 1995; Ho et al. 1995). However, it is important to remember that the efficacy of any given isoform is likely to be influenced most by its local concentration and interactions, rather than simply by its total abundance. We await the availability of additional tools with which to characterize these two classes of isoforms more fully.

Fourth, the receptors for ARIA are present at the NMJ. Immunohistochemical and molecular biological studies have indicated that of these various receptors, erbB2 and erbB3 are the most abundant in skeletal muscle, whereas lower but clearly detectable levels of erbB4 are found (Altiok et al. 1995; Jo et al. 1995; Moscoso et al. 1995; Zhu et al. 1995). This result may be taken to indicate that erbB4 is either not important or that it is the most important component of the postsynaptic complex. It may be that the least abundant protein is limiting in establishing the postsynaptic response. The issue is significant because the intracellular phosphorylation cascades triggered by the various erbB homo- and heterodimers are almost certainly different from one another. They probably do not, therefore, regulate AChR genes (or other synapse-specific genes) in exactly the same way.

Fifth, ARIA increases the number of voltage-gated sodium channels. Over the same time course in which

ARIA increases AChRs in cultures of chick skeletal muscle, there is an increase in voltage-gated sodium channels (Corfas and Fischbach 1993). Sodium channels are present at a high density in the lower third of the postjunctional folds (Flucher and Daniels 1989; Boudier et al. 1992). The high density lowers the threshold for activation of muscle action potentials. The fact that ARIA/neuregulin elevates the levels of two channels that directly increase the safety factor for neuromuscular transmission provides further support for the relevance of these proteins in vivo.

Sixth, and most importantly, mice in which one allele of the neuregulin gene has been inactivated are myasthenic. This is the most crucial piece of evidence for the necessity of ARIA/neuregulin at the motor endplate (Sandrock et al.1997). Two types of ligand knockout have been reported. In one, the common EGF-like domain sequence has been disrupted (Meyer and Birchmeier 1995). This type of alteration should lead to the abrogation of expression of all neuregulin isoforms. In the other class, the Ig domain sequence was targeted (Kramer et al. 1996). The presumption is that this type of inactivation would yield a gene that only produced Ig^- isoforms. In both types of knockouts, homozygous animals die on approximately E10. Death is most likely due to cardiac defects: Hearts are enlarged and thin, and the muscular invaginations of the ventricular wall, called trabeculae, which help propel the blood through the embryonic heart, are diminished or absent. Endocardial cushions are thin and incomplete. In retrospect, death by heart failure is not surprising, because the neuregulin gene is expressed in the endocardium and in the endothelium of the great vessels (Corfas et al. 1995; Meyer and Birchmeier 1995). The cardiac defect merits further study at the level of membrane function and myocyte precursor maturation, but the important point here is that homozygous animals die before the time at which motor axons contact target muscle cells and NMJ formation can be assayed. We turned, therefore, to heterozygous Ig domain knockout animals ($Ig^{+/-}$)[3] to obtain evidence for ARIA action at motor endplates.

Heterozygous knockout animals appear to both move about their cages normally and reproduce without difficulty. However, they are much more susceptible to the effects of low doses of curare. CMAPs, recorded with indwelling EMG electrodes, do not run down (i.e., fade) when evoked at rates between 3 Hz and 30 Hz. When challenged with incremental doses of curare, CMAP amplitude decrements are seen at a lower dose in heterozygotes than in controls (Fig. 3). Presumably, the evoked endplate potential is reduced at all endplates, and at some, it has dropped below the threshold for action potential generation. The "dropout" of individual fibers is reflected in the fade of the population spike. Assuming that transmitter release is unchanged in the heterozygotes, this implies a postsynaptic deficit, some combination of decreased AChR density and/or Na^+ channel density.

Intracellular microelectrode recordings and measurements of ^{125}I-labeled α-BTX binding indicate that the postsynaptic AChR density is indeed decreased. The amplitude of miniature endplate potentials (mepps), recorded in an isolated diaphragm preparation, is reduced by approximately 30% in heterozygotes as compared to controls, and the number of BTX binding sites in endplate-rich zones of the diaphragm is decreased by a comparable amount (Table 1).

The mean stimulus-evoked epp amplitude was not reduced like the spontaneously occurring mepps. Statistical analyses of series of evoked epps showed that the mean quantum content of the epp was increased at heterozygote endplates. Presynaptic changes (an increase in transmitter release per impulse) compensate, in part, for the deficit in postsynaptic AChR density. The same compensation has been observed in human myasthenia gravis (Plomp et al. 1995) and in experimental myasthenia produced by chronic AChR blockade (Plomp et al. 1992). The compensation, however, does not mask the myasthenia, because during brief tetani the amplitude of successive epps declines more rapidly in heterozygotes than in controls—as expected from terminals with an augmented release per impulse.

In addition to the neuregulin gene, the genes encoding the receptors erbB2 (Lee et al. 1995) and erbB4 (Gassman et al. 1995) have been insertionally inactivated through homologous recombination. Both types of knockouts result in homozygous animals that also die on E10 with the same cardiac defect as the neuregulin knockouts. It will be interesting to examine neuromuscular transmission in the receptor knockouts as well as animals derived from neuregulin (+/–)/erbB2 or erbB4 (+/–) crosses.

In light of the evidence described above, we conclude that neuregulins play an important role at the developing and mature NMJ. There may be additional factors that regulate endplate AChR synthesis, but ARIA, or a closely related neuregulin isoform (i.e., an Ig-containing form), is an important one. Our data suggest that neuregulins are present in limiting amounts at the NMJ. A presumed reduction of mRNA and protein by only a factor of 2 (making the simplest assumptions about gene expression and mRNA translation) is sufficient to decrease AChR levels despite the persistence of powerful aggregating forces at the junction. In this regard, neuregulins resemble the neurotrophins. Heterozygote knockout animals for either neurotrophin genes or their *trk* receptors exhibit significant defects in neurotrophin-dependent tissues and cells (for review, see Snider 1994).

Our findings also suggest that there are very few "spare" receptors in the adult postsynaptic membrane.

[3]Genotyped animals were generously provided by R. Kramer and L. Theill of AMGEN, Inc.

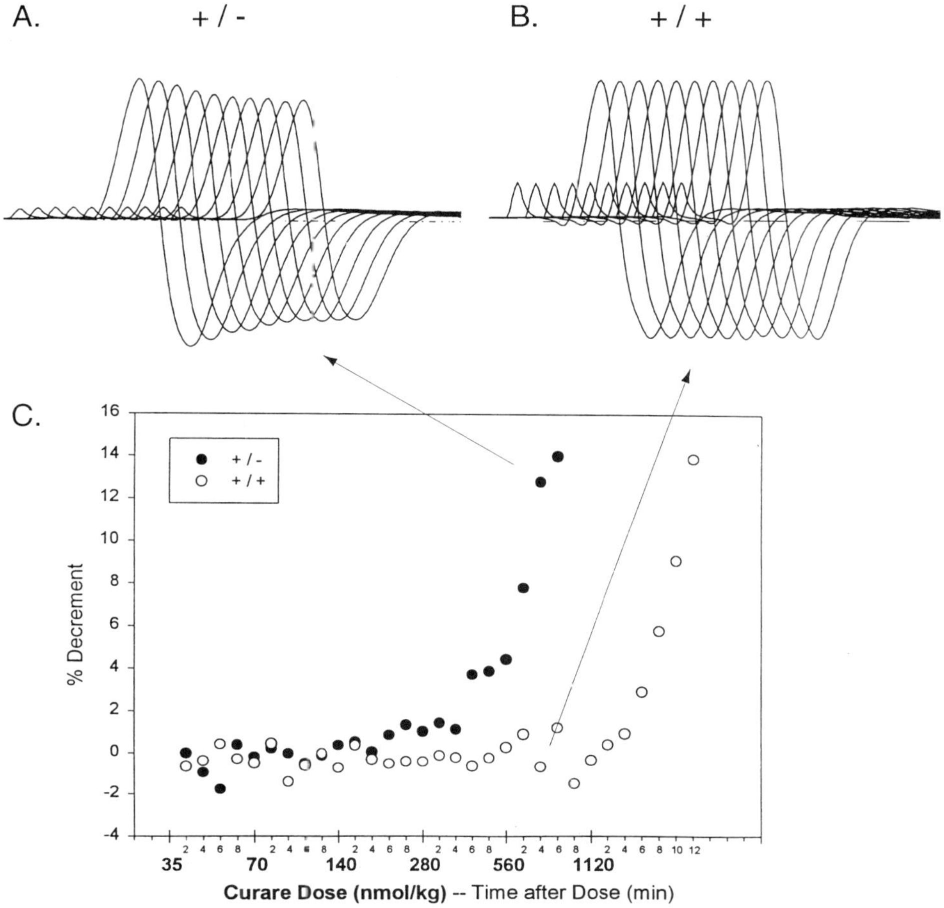

Figure 3. Measurement of CMAP amplitude in a wild-type (+/+) and a heterozygous (+/–) littermate pair during incremental curare injections. (*a*) CMAPs recorded from the heterozygote animal 4 min after the 40-μmol/kg injection of D-tubocurarine. (*b*) CMAPs recorded from the wild-type animal at the same time and dose point. (*c*) The magnitude of the decrement (as percentage decrease of the 6th CMAP compared to the 2nd CMAP) of each 3-Hz train plotted against D-tubocurarine dose (shown in bold on X-axis) and the time after each dose. In wild-type mice, no significant CMAP decrement was evident until 6 min after the 80 μmol/kg dose, whereas CMAP decrements began at ~6 min after the 280 nmol/kg dose in the heterozygote.

The decline in mepp amplitude is most consistent with the notion that each quantum of transmitter saturates the AChRs within its sphere of influence as dictated by buffered diffusion and the action of acetylcholinesterase. AChR synthesis at a high rate is, therefore, important for the maintenance of normal neuromuscular transmission in adults and presumably in developing animals as well.

FUTURE DIRECTIONS

One area of investigation is how total neuregulin levels are regulated, as well as the processing of both cell-surface and "soluble" neuregulin in various cell types. Considering the continued requirement for AChR synthesis at mature as well as developing endplates, this is an important issue. The neuregulin gene is transcriptionally active in spinal motor neurons even before their axons invade their targets in the periphery (Falls et al. 1993; Marchionni et al. 1993; Chen et al. 1994; Meyer and Birchmeier 1994; Corfas et al. 1995; Goodearl et al. 1995). Recent experiments in our laboratory indicate that muscle-derived neurotrophins, as well as glial-derived neurotrophic factor (GDNF), may influence the expression of the neuregulin gene in cultured spinal cord neurons (J.A. Loeb and G.D. Fischbach, in prep.). Once synthesized, the neuregulins are presumably transported via a vesicular pathway to the motor nerve terminal. The extracellular domain is likely cleaved by a cell-surface-associated protease. Recent studies have indicated that the processing of transmembrane forms of neuregulin can be increased by the addition of phorbol esters via a protein-kinase-C-dependent mechanism (Burgess et al. 1995). Regula-

Table 1. Specific ^{125}I-labeled α-BTX Binding to Endplate-rich Zones of Wild-type (+/+) and Heterozygote (+/–) Mouse Hemidiaphragm

+/+	–/–
12,462 ± 949 cpm $n = 6$	8,756 ± 765 cpm $n = 6$

tion of the protease responsible for the cleavage, whether emanating from the motor neuron or the postsynaptic muscle cell, may be a key point of regulation of neuregulin action, a situation similar, perhaps, to the processing of the amyloid precursor protein (APP).

Neuregulins may be evident on the surface of the axon along its length. These molecules may well be serving to signal not only to muscle, but also to Schwann cells, as studies of purified recombinant GGF-II have clearly indicated an important role for this isoform in Schwann cell regulation in developing muscle tissue (Trachtenberg and Thompson 1996). Consistent with this role is the immunocytochemical identification of this particular isoform along intramuscular axons utilizing an isoform-specific antiserum (Jo et al. 1995).

The extensive conservation of sequence in the cytoplasmic domain of the transmembrane isoforms of neuregulin between species strongly argues for an important function for this portion of the molecule. Alterations between different splice forms change the occurrence of consensus phosphorylation sites as well as other sequences. These changes likely lead to alterations in neuregulin processing. An additional possibility deserving of investigation is whether transmembrane neuregulins may act themselves as receptors for "retrograde" signaling molecules.

Chick ARIA was purified from extracts of brain. In situ hybridization analyses by many groups have shown that the neuregulin gene is widely expressed in the central nervous system (see above). Our own studies have indicated that every identifiable cholinergic neuron in the brain expresses the neuregulin gene (Corfas et al. 1995). However, the gene is expressed in many noncholinergic cells as well, including cerebellar granule cell neurons and the reticular nucleus of the thalamus. It is attractive to think that neuregulins may regulate ion channels in the CNS as well as in the periphery. The neuregulin gene is also expressed in germinal zones of the developing brain, and several laboratories have suggested a role for these ligands in precursor cell proliferation or differentiation in both neuronal and glial precursors (Shah et al. 1994; Vartanian et al. 1994; Verdi et al. 1996).

The finding that neuregulin knockout mice die during early embryonic development with cardiac malformations makes it extremely important to understand the role(s) that these molecules play during development of the heart. Several attractive possibilities include (1) regulation of cardiomyocyte proliferation, (2) modulation of the rate of differentiation of cells of the myo- and/or endocardium, and (3) regulation of sodium channels, and perhaps other channels, leading to alterations in the electrical behavior of cardiomyocytes. The regulation of sodium channels is particularly interesting, since we have found that ARIA regulates sodium channel number in skeletal muscle. As mentioned above, ARIA's most prominent effect on mammalian skeletal muscle AChR subunit genes is seen with the developmentally regulated ε subunit. This subunit replaces the embryonic γ subunit during development in a nerve-dependent manner (for review, see Hall and Sanes 1993). An analogous alteration in subunit specification is seen with the mammalian skeletal muscle sodium channel, where a developmentally regulated switch occurs, with the embryonic tetrodotoxin (TTX)-insensitive channel (SkM2) being replaced by the postnatal TTX-sensitive channel (SkM1) (Kallen et al. 1990). Interestingly, the SkM2 channel of embryonic skeletal muscle is the same as the channel that is expressed in cardiac muscle.

It is clear that neuregulins and their receptors are likely to play key roles in a number of different cellular contexts. Studies of carcinogenesis, glial cell proliferation/differentiation, and synapse formation have all implicated members of this complex ligand-receptor family. Continued investigation of these molecules will not only help to better understand the functions already attributed to them, but also will undoubtedly reveal more.

REFERENCES

Altiok, N., J.L. Bessereau, and J.P. Changeux. 1995. ErbB3 and ErbB2/neu mediate the effect of heregulin on acetylcholine receptor gene expression in muscle: Differential expression at the endplate. *EMBO J.* **14:** 4258.

Ben-Baruch, N. and Y. Yarden. 1994. Neu differentiation factors: A family of alternatively spliced neuronal and mesenchymal factors. *Proc. Soc. Exp. Biol. Med.* **206:** 221.

Boudier, J., T. Le Treut, and E. Jover. 1992. Autoradiographic localization of voltage-dependent sodium channels on the mouse neuromuscular junction using ^{125}I-alpha scorpion toxin. II. Sodium channel distribution on postsynaptic membranes. *J. Neurosci.* **12:** 454.

Brenner, H.R., A. Herczeg, and C.R. Slater. 1992. Synapse-specific expression of acetylcholine receptor genes and their products at original synaptic sites in rat soleus muscle fibers regenerating in the absence of innervation. *Development* **116:** 41.

Buc-Caron, M.H., P. Nystrom, and G.D. Fischbach. 1983. Induction of acetylcholine receptor synthesis and aggregation: Partial purification of low-molecular-weight activity. *Dev. Biol.* **95:** 378.

Burgess, T.L., S.L. Ross, Y. Quian, D. Brankow, and S. Hu. 1995. Biosynthetic processing of neu differentiation factor. *J. Biol. Chem.* **270:** 19188.

Chen, M.S., O. Bermingham-McDonogh, F.T. Danehy, C. Nolan, S.S. Scherer, J. Lucas, D. Gwynne, and M.A. Marchionni. 1994. Expression of multiple neuregulin transcripts in postnatal rat brains. *J. Comp. Neurol.* **349:** 389.

Chu, G.C., L.M. Moscoso, M.X. Sliwkowski, and J.P. Merlie. 1995. Regulation of the acetylcholine receptor ε subunit gene by recombinant ARIA: An in vitro model for transynaptic gene regulation. *Neuron* **14:** 329.

Corfas, G. and G.D. Fischbach. 1993. The number of Na^+ channels in cultured chick muscle is increased by ARIA, an acetylcholine receptor-inducing activity. *J. Neurosci.* **13:** 2118.

Corfas, G., K.M. Rosen, H. Aratake, R. Krauss, and G.D. Fischbach. 1995. Differential expression of ARIA isoforms in the rat brain. *Neuron* **14:** 103.

Falls, D.L., K.M. Rosen, G. Corfas, W.S. Lane, and G.D. Fischbach. 1993. ARIA, a protein that stimulates acetylcholine receptor synthesis, is a member of the neu ligand family. *Cell* **72:** 801.

Falls, D.L., D.A. Harris, F.A. Johnson, M.M. Morgan, G. Corfas, and G.D. Fischbach. 1990. M_r 42,000 ARIA: A protein that may regulate the accumulation of acetylcholine receptors at developing chick neuromuscular junctions. *Cold Spring Harbor Symp. Quant. Biol.* **55:** 397.

Fischbach, G.D. and K.M. Rosen. 1997. ARIA: A neuromuscular junction neuregulin. *Annu. Rev. Neurosci.* **20:** 429.

Flucher, B.E. and M.P. Daniels. 1989. Distribution of Na^+ channels and ankyrin in neuromuscular junctions is complementary to that of acetylcholine receptors and the 43 kd protein. *Neuron* **3:** 163.

Gassman, M., F. Casagranda, D. Orioli, H. Simon, C. Lai, R. Klein, and G. Lemke. 1995. Aberrant neural and cardiac development in mice lacking the erbB4 neuregulin receptor. *Nature* **378:** 390.

Goldman, D., B.M. Carlson, and J. Staple. 1991. Induction of adult-type nicotinic acetylcholine receptor gene expression in noninnervated regenerating muscle *Neuron* **7:** 649.

Goodearl, A.D.J., A.G. Yee, A.W. Sandrock, Jr., G. Corfas, and G.D. Fischbach. 1995. ARIA is concentrated in the synaptic basal lamina of the developing chick neuromuscular junction. *J. Cell Biol.* **130:** 1423.

Goodearl, A.D.J., J.B. Davis, K. Mistry, L. Minghetti, M. Otsu, M.D. Waterfield, and P. Stroobant. 1993. Purification of multiple forms of glial growth factor. *J. Biol. Chem.* **268:** 18905.

Grinnell, A.D. 1995. Dynamics of nerve-muscle interaction in developing and mature neuromuscular junctions. *Physiol. Rev.* **75:** 789.

Hall, Z.W. and J.R. Sanes. 1993. Synaptic structure and development: The neuromuscular junction. *Cell* **72:** 99.

Harris, D.A., D.L. Falls, R.M. Dill-Devor, and G.D. Fischbach. 1988. Acetylcholine receptor-inducing factor from chicken brain increases the level of the mRNA encoding the receptor α subunit. *Proc. Natl. Acad. Sci.* **85:** 1983.

Ho, W., M.P. Armanini, A. Nuijens, H.S. Phillips, and P.L. Osheroff. 1995. Sensory and motor neuron derived factor. *J. Biol. Chem.* **270:** 14523.

Holmes, W.E., M.X. Sliwkowski, R.W. Akita, W.J. Henzel, J. Lee, J.W. Park, D. Yansura, N. Abadi, H. Raab, G.D. Lewis, H.M. Shepard, W.-J. Kuang, W.I. Wood, D.V. Goeddel, and R.L. Vandlen. 1992. Identification of heregulin, a specific activator of p185 erbB2. *Science* **256:** 1205.

Jessell, T.M., R.E. Siegel, and G.D. Fischbach. 1979. Induction of acetylcholine receptors on cultured skeletal muscle by a factor extracted from brain and spinal cord. *Proc. Natl. Acad. Sci.* **76:** 5397.

Jo, S.A. and S.J. Burden. 1992. Synaptic basal lamina contains a signal for synapse-specific transcription. *Development* **115:** 673.

Jo, S.A., X. Zhu, M.A. Marchionni, and S.J. Burden. 1995. Neuregulins are concentrated at nerve-muscle synapses and activate ACh-receptor gene expression. *Nature* **373:** 158.

Kallen, R.G., Z. Sheng, J. Yang, L. Chen, R.B. Rogart, and R.L. Barchi. 1990. Primary structure and expression of a sodium channel characteristic of denervated and immature rat skeletal muscle. *Neuron* **4:** 233.

Kramer, R., N. Bucay, D.J. Kane, L.E. Martin, J.E. Tarpley, and L.E. Theill. 1996. Neuregulins with an Ig-like domain are essential for mouse myocardial and neuronal development. *Proc. Natl. Acad. Sci.* **93:** 4833.

Kuo, Y., X. Yang, and L. Role. 1994. Isolation and characterization of chick and human nARIA, a novel member of the erbB2/HER ligand family which lacks the immunoglobulin domain. *Soc. Neurosci. Abstr.* **20:** 452.18.

Lee, K., H. Simon, H. Chen, B. Bates, M. Hung, and C. Hauler. 1995. Requirement for neuregulin receptor erbB2 in neural and cardiac development. *Nature* **378:** 394.

Lemke, G. 1996. Neuregulins in development. *Mol. Cell. Neurosci.* **7:** 247.

Loeb, J.A. and G.D. Fischbach. 1995. ARIA can be released from extracellular matrix through cleavage of a heparin-binding domain. *J. Cell Biol.* **130:** 127.

Marchionni, M.A., A.D.J. Goodearl, M. Chen, O. Bermingham-McDonogh, C. Kirk, M. Hendricks, F. Danehy, D. Misumi, J. Sudhalter, K. Kobayashi, D. Wroblewski, C. Lynch, M. Baldassare, I. Hiles, J.B. Davis, J.J. Hsuan, N.F. Totty, M. Otsu, R.N. McBurney, M.D. Waterfield, P. Stroobant, and D. Gwynne. 1993. Glial growth factors are alternatively spliced erbB2 ligands expressed in the nervous system. *Nature* **362:** 312.

Martinou, J.C., D.L. Falls, G.D. Fischbach, and J.P. Merlie. 1991. Acetylcholine receptor-inducing activity stimulates expression of the ε-subunit gene of the muscle acetylcholine receptor. *Proc. Natl. Acad. Sci.* **88:** 7669.

Meyer, D. and C. Birchmeier. 1994. Distinct isoforms of neuregulin are expressed in mesenchymal and neuronal cells during mouse development. *Proc. Natl. Acad. Sci.* **91:** 1064.

———. 1995. Multiple essential functions of neuregulin in development. *Nature* **378:** 386.

Moscoso, L.M., G.C. Chu, M. Gautam, P.G. Noakes, J.P.X. Merlie, and J.R. Sanes. 1995. Synapse associated expression of an acetylcholine receptor-inducing protein, ARIA/heregulin, and its putative receptors. erbB2 and erbB3, in developing mammalian muscle. *Dev. Biol.* **172:** 158.

Plomp, J.J., G.T. Van Kempen, and P.C. Molenaar. 1992. Adaptation of quantal content to decreased postsynaptic sensitivity at single endplates in alpha-bungarotoxin-treated rats. *J. Physiol.* **458:** 487.

Plomp, J.J., G.T. Van Kempen, M.B. De Baets, Y.M. Graus, J.B. Kuks, and P.C. Molenaar. 1995. Acetylcholine release in myasthenia gravis: Regulation at single end-plate level. *Ann. Neurol.* **37:** 627.

Ratner, N., R.P. Bunge, and L. Glaser. 1985. A neuronal cell surface heparan sulfate proteoglycan is required for dorsal root ganglion neuron stimulation of Schwann cell proliferation. *J. Cell Biol.* **101:** 744.

Ratner, N., D. Hong, M.A. Lieberman, R.P. Bunge, and L. Glaser. 1988. The neuronal cell-surface molecule mitogenic for Schwann cells is a heparin-binding protein. *Proc. Natl. Acad. Sci.* **85:** 6992.

Sandrock, A.W., Jr., A.D. Goodearl, Q.W. Yin, D. Chang, and G.D. Fischbach. 1995. ARIA is concentrated in nerve terminals at neuromuscular junctions and at other synapses. *J. Neurosci.* **15:** 6124.

Sandrock, A.W., Jr., S.E. Dryer, K.M. Rosen, S.N. Gozani, R. Kramer, L.E. Theill, and G.D. Fischbach. 1997. Maintenance of acetylcholine receptor number by neuregulins at the neuromuscular junction *in vivo*. *Science* (in press).

Shah, N.M., M.A. Marchionni, I. Isaacs, P. Stroobant, and D.J. Anderson. 1994. Glial growth factor restricts mammalian neural crest stem cells to a glial fate. *Cell* **77:** 349.

Snider, W.D. 1994. Functions of the neurotrophins during nervous system development: What the knockouts are teaching us. *Neuron* **77:** 627.

Trachtenberg, J.T. and W.J. Thompson. 1996. Schwann cell apoptosis at developing neuromuscular junctions is regulated by glial growth factor. *Nature* **379:** 174.

Usdin, T.B. and G.D. Fischbach. 1986. Purification and characterization of a polypeptide from chick brain that promotes the accumulation of acetylcholine receptors in chick myotubes. *J. Cell Biol.* **103:** 493.

Vartanian, T., G. Corfas, Y. Li, G.D. Fischbach, and K. Stefansson. 1994. A role for the acetylcholine receptor-inducing protein ARIA in oligodendrocyte development. *Proc. Natl. Acad. Sci.* **91:** 11626.

Vaughn, D.E. and P.J. Bjorkman. 1996. The (greek) key to structures of neural adhesion molecules. *Neuron* **16:** 261.

Verdi, J.M., A.K. Groves, I. Farinas, K. Jones, M.A. Marchionni, L.F. Reichardt, and D.J. Anderson. 1996. A reciprocal cell-cell interaction mediated by NT-3 and neuregulins controls the early survival and development of sympathetic neuroblasts. *Neuron* **16:** 515.

Wen, D., E. Peles, R. Cupples, S.V. Suggs, S.S. Bacus, Y. Luo, G. Trail, S. Hu, S.M. Silbiger, R. Ben Levy, R.A. Koski, H.S. Lu, and Y. Yarden. 1992. Neu differentiation factor: A transmembrane glycoprotein containing an EGF domain and an immunoglobulin homology unit. *Cell* **69:** 559.

Zhu, X.J., C. Lai, S. Thomas, and S.J. Burden. 1995. Neuregulin receptors, erbB3 and erbB4, are localized at neuromuscular synapses. *EMBO J.* **14:** 5842.

The Receptor Tyrosine Kinase MuSK Is Required for Neuromuscular Junction Formation and Is a Functional Receptor for Agrin

D.J. Glass, T.M. DeChiara, T.N. Stitt, P.S. DiStefano, D.M. Valenzuela, and G.D. Yancopoulos
Regeneron Pharmaceuticals, Inc., Tarrytown, New York 10591

Intercellular communication is often mediated by receptors on the surface of one cell, which recognize and are activated by specific protein ligands released by other cells. Members of one class of cell-surface receptors, known as receptor tyrosine kinases (RTKs), are characterized by having a cytoplasmic domain containing intrinsic tyrosine kinase activity (Schlessinger and Ullrich 1992). This kinase activity is regulated by the binding of a cognate ligand to the extracellular portion of the receptor. The few RTKs known to be expressed in cell-type-specific fashions have been shown to play roles critical for the growth and differentiation of those cell types. For example, members of the neural-specific trk family of RTKs, which recognize the neurotrophin family of growth factors (Barbacid 1993; Glass and Yancopoulos 1993), are required for the survival and development of discrete neuronal subpopulations (Snider 1994).

We described a receptor-like tyrosine kinase that appears to be restricted to skeletal muscle in its expression, and named it MuSK for muscle-specific kinase (Valenzuela et al. 1995). The mouse MuSK ortholog has been termed Nsk2 (Ganju et al. 1995), and a potential MuSK ortholog has been cloned from the *Torpedo* ray (Jennings et al. 1993).

MuSK protein is detectable in proliferating myoblasts but is dramatically up-regulated as myoblasts exit the cell cycle and fuse to form multinucleated myotubes (Valenzuela et al. 1995). In vivo, innervation by motor axons shortly follows myoblast fusion (Hall and Sanes 1993). Functional innervation depends on the formation of a highly specialized synaptic connection, termed the neuromuscular junction (NMJ), between the incoming motor nerve and the muscle fiber (Hall and Sanes 1993).

The NMJ can be understood as having three distinct components: the presynaptic nerve terminal, where acetylcholine is packaged into synaptic vesicles, and whose end-process is marked by a polarized arrangement of synaptic vesicles and active zones; the postsynaptic motor endplate on the surface of the muscle, a small patch comprising less than 2% of the total surface area of the muscle surface, which is characterized by a dense clustering of particular proteins, some of which may receive nerve-derived signals, as AChRs are known to do, whereas others may be involved in creating the molecular scaffold for this postsynaptic specialization; and a biochemically distinct protein layer called the "basal lamina," which lies between the nerve terminal and the motor endplate. This basal lamina is distinguished from the adjacent extracellular matrix by the accumulation of a number of proteins, such as acetylcholinesterase and s-laminin; as noted below, the synaptic basal lamina also serves as a reservoir for signaling molecules exchanged between nerve and muscle.

As muscle matures, MuSK becomes highly localized to the motor endplate (Valenzuela et al. 1995). Thus, MuSK is strategically positioned to recognize and mediate a nerve-derived ligand and, in turn, to relay a key signal to muscle. It has long been known that important signals are exchanged across the NMJ (Nitkin et al. 1987; Hall and Sanes 1993; Bowe and Fallon 1995; Burden et al. 1995; Sanes 1995). These signals include the chemical transmitter, acetylcholine, which is released from vesicles in the nerve terminal, recognized by acetylcholine receptors (AChRs) on the muscle, and ultimately results in electrical activation and contraction of the muscle. Muscle also provides neurotrophic factors that support survival of motor neurons (DeChiara et al. 1995), and the nerve may in turn provide myotrophic factors that maintain muscle mass (Helgren et al. 1994). Reciprocal signaling interactions are also critical for both the formation and the maintenance of the NMJ itself. Such signals regulate recognition of nerve-to-muscle contact, arrest the growth of the incoming nerve ending, and induce formation of the highly specialized nerve terminal.

Signals produced by the nerve induce postsynaptic clusters by at least two mechanisms. First, these signals can induce redistribution of preexisting molecules that are initially expressed throughout the myofiber, and second, they can induce localized transcription of specific genes only by subsynaptic nuclei underlying the NMJ. The realization that empty sheaths of the synaptic basal lamina could induce formation of both nerve terminal specializations and motor endplates suggested that key signaling molecules might be embedded in the extracellular matrix (Sanes et al. 1978; Burden et al. 1979; McMahan and Slater 1984; Kuffler 1986).

One nerve-derived factor, embedded in the synaptic basal lamina, is a protein termed agrin, which was discovered for its ability to cause the clustering of preexisting AChRs on the surface of cultured myotubes (Godfrey et al. 1984; McMahan 1990; Rupp et al. 1991; Tsim et al. 1992). Agrin has subsequently been shown to co-cluster a number of synaptic components along with AChRs on the surface of cultured myotubes (Wallace 1989). Agrin is a 200-kD protein that can be subdivided into a number of distinct domains. The amino-terminal half contains nine follistatin-like repeats that are homologous to Kazal-type protease inhibitor domains, and the carboxy-terminal half contains four epidermal growth factor (EGF)-like repeats and three regions homologous to the G domains of laminin (Rupp et al. 1991; Tsim et al. 1992). The clustering activity of agrin has been mapped to the carboxy-terminal region; whereas the full-length form of agrin interacts tightly with the extracellular matrix, the carboxy-terminal region can be made in soluble form, and is referred to as "c-agrin" (Ruegg et al. 1992; Tsim et al. 1992; Ferns et al. 1993; Hoch et al. 1994).

A number of different forms of agrin have been discovered, encoded by alternatively spliced transcripts (Ferns et al. 1992; Ruegg et al. 1992; Tsim et al. 1992; Hoch et al. 1993). The carboxy-terminal region of agrin can contain variable insertions at two critical sites, referred to as the Y and Z sites, that can affect the clustering ability of the agrin (Ferns et al. 1992, 1993; Ruegg et al. 1992; Hoch et al. 1994); differential splicing results in transcripts encoding agrins with different combinations of these insertions. Importantly, expression of these different agrin forms is restricted to either muscle or nerve (Ruegg et al. 1992; Hoch et al. 1993). A neuronal-specific insertion at the Z position is absolutely required for the clustering ability of soluble c-agrin, and agrins with an 8-amino-acid insertion at this position are at least 10,000-fold more active than agrins lacking an insert at this position (Ruegg et al. 1992; Ferns et al. 1993). Muscle-derived agrins lack the insertion at the Z position, and thus are not potent clustering agents. A 4-amino-acid insertion at the Y position causes a modest additional increase in the activity of agrins having an insertion at the Z position, and the Y insertion also seems to be involved in the binding of agrin to heparin and proteoglycans (Ferns et al. 1993; Hoch et al. 1994).

A variety of data are consistent with the notion that the in vitro clustering actions of agrin reflect an in vivo role for agrin in the formation of the NMJ (McMahan 1990). Most important among these are the findings that the highly active forms of agrin are exclusively made by neurons and are deposited in the synaptic basal lamina (Ruegg et al. 1992; Hoch et al. 1993), and that antibodies to agrin block nerve-induced clustering of AChRs on cultured myotubes (Reist et al. 1992). Agrin induces intracellular tyrosine phosphorylations, including that of the β-subunit of the AChR, and inhibitors of tyrosine phosphorylation block agrin-mediated clustering (Wallace et al. 1991; Qu and Huganir 1994; Wallace 1994, 1995; Ferns et al. 1996). Intriguing recent findings have revealed that agrin can directly bind to an extrinsic peripheral membrane protein, known as α-dystroglycan, via its laminin-like domains (Bowe et al. 1994; Campanelli et al. 1994; Gee et al. 1994; Sugiyama et al. 1994). α-Dystroglycan is part of a protein complex, herein referred to as the dystroglycan complex, that seems to provide crucial anchoring between the extracellular basal lamina and the underlying cytoskeleton (Fallon and Hall 1994). Extrasynaptically, the dystroglycan complex binds laminin in the extracellular matrix and associates with the actin scaffold via a spectrin-like protein known as α dystrophin, whereas at the synapse, agrin can substitute for laminin and utrophin replaces dystrophin (Fallon and Hall 1994). In addition, the dystroglycan complex is apparently coupled to AChRs by a 43-kD cytoplasmic protein known as rapsyn (Noakes et al. 1993; Apel et al. 1995).

Despite the findings that agrin can bind directly to α-dystroglycan, and that the dystroglycan complex is coupled to AChRs via rapsyn, the role of α-dystroglycan as an agrin receptor remains unclear (Sealock and Froehner 1994). Dystroglycan could be a required component of the functional agrin receptor that is responsible for initiating the signaling response, and it might even be directly involved in activating signaling pathways. However, an agrin mutant has been recently reported that maintains the ability to cluster AChRs without binding to dystroglycan (Gesemann et al. 1996), suggesting that agrin induces clustering via another cell-surface receptor. Here we review recent findings (DeChiara et al. 1996; Glass et al. 1996) demonstrating that agrin acts via a MuSK receptor complex to induce all aspects of NMJ formation.

THE ROLE OF MUSK IN VIVO

MuSK Gene Disruption Results in Perinatal Lethality due to Lack of NMJ Formation

To determine the role of MuSK during skeletal muscle development, we generated mice homozygous for a deletion of an exon encoding the catalytic region of the MuSK tyrosine kinase domain, since such a mutation would abolish MuSK's ability to mediate signals (DeChiara et al. 1996). All the $MuSK^{-/-}$ mice died shortly after birth. Not a single mouse homozygous for the mutation survived the perinatal period. Although normal in their gross anatomy and body weight at birth, the $MuSK^{-/-}$ pups were apparently different in several striking ways from their littermate controls (DeChiara et al. 1996). First, they showed no spontaneous movement and did not respond to a mild tail or leg pinch. Only a strong tail pinch was able to elicit a weak uncoordinated movement. Second, the $MuSK^{-/-}$ pups were cyanotic at birth and appeared not to breathe; histological examination revealed that the lung alveoli of $MuSK^{-/-}$ pups were not expanded, indicating that the pups had never taken a breath.

Neuronal Differentiation and Termination

Given the synaptic localization of MuSK (Valenzuela et al. 1995), we reasoned that the mutant animals' immobility and inability to breathe could be a result of aberrant neuromuscular synapse formation. To determine whether synapse formation is aberrant in MuSK$^{-/-}$ mutant mice, we stained whole mounts of diaphragm muscle with probes that allowed us to assess presynaptic (e.g., synaptophysin antibodies) and postsynaptic (e.g., bungarotoxin to label AChRs) differentiation. In diaphragm from normal animals, nerve processes are restricted to the central region of the muscle, where they terminate shortly after branching from the innervating phrenic nerve. In MuSK$^{-/-}$ mutant mice, synaptophysin-stained nerve processes are not restricted to the central region of diaphragm muscle, and instead are found throughout the muscle. Indeed, synaptophysin-stained nerve processes are nearly as abundant at the ends of the muscle as in the central region (DeChiara et al. 1996). Moreover, the shape of synaptophysin-stained processes in MuSK$^{-/-}$ mutant mice resembles that of preterminal axons rather than that of nerve terminals, and highly arborized nerve terminals are absent in MuSK$^{-/-}$ mice, indicating that MuSK is required for at least some aspects of presynaptic differentiation. Since MuSK is expressed in skeletal muscle and not in motor neurons (Valenzuela et al. 1995), it is likely that the exuberant growth of motor axons and the absence of nerve terminal arborization is due to a lack of MuSK function in muscle and a consequent loss of appropriate retrograde signals that normally prevent continued axon growth and also induce presynaptic differentiation (see Discussion).

AChR clusters, which are found in postsynaptic membrane patches underlying synaptophysin-stained nerve terminals in normal muscle, are absent from MuSK$^{-/-}$ mutant muscle (DeChiara et al. 1996). The absence of AChR clusters in MuSK$^{-/-}$ mutant muscle is not due to a lack of AChR expression, since quantitation using ^{125}I-labeled α-bungarotoxin reveals more—albeit diffusely distributed—AChRs in MuSK$^{-/-}$ mutant muscle as compared to normal muscle, and similar numbers of AChRs in cultured MuSK$^{-/-}$ and control myotubes (Glass et al. 1996). Thus, MuSK is required to cluster but not to express AChRs.

The absence of differentiated nerve terminals and AChR clusters in MuSK$^{-/-}$ mutant mice is consistent with the notion that these mice die at birth due to severe abnormalities in both presynaptic and postsynaptic aspects of NMJ formation, and that MuSK is essential for normal formation of neuromuscular synapses in vivo (DeChiara et al. 1996).

In addition to the AChRs, approximately one dozen proteins are known to be concentrated in the postsynaptic membrane of neuromuscular synapses, or locally deposited in the overlying synaptic basal lamina, and serve as markers of appropriate postsynaptic differentiation (Hall and Sanes 1993; Bowe and Fallon 1995). We examined the distributions of several of these markers to further characterize the extent of postsynaptic deficits in MuSK$^{-/-}$ mice. Although clusters of AChE, ErbB4, utrophin, and rapsyn are all precisely juxtaposed with nerve terminals in sections of muscle from control and MuSK$^{+/-}$ pups, these proteins were concentrated neither at sites stained with antibodies to synaptic vesicle proteins nor anywhere else in muscle from MuSK$^{-/-}$ mutant pups (DeChiara et al. 1996). These results indicate that MuSK was required for every marker of presynaptic, postsynaptic, and basal lamina organization studied.

MuSK$^{-/-}$ Mutant Mice Lack Synapse-specific AChR Gene Expression

In addition to the characteristic localization of proteins presynaptically, postsynaptically, and in the basal lamina, the NMJ junction is notable in that the nuclei underlying the motor endplate (referred to as synaptic nuclei) express a unique set of transcripts. To learn whether MuSK is indeed required for induction of this synapse-specific expression, we used in situ hybridization to determine the expression pattern of transcripts encoding the α and δ subunits of the AChR. In control mice, these transcripts are concentrated near myofiber nuclei that are situated near synaptic sites, which appear as a band in the central region of the muscle. In contrast, transcripts encoding both the α and δ subunits are distributed uniformly throughout the myofibers of MuSK$^{-/-}$ mice (DeChiara et al. 1996). Thus, MuSK is required for onset of transcription, and these results suggest that an inability to selectively express AChR genes in synaptic nuclei is responsible, at least in part, for the lack of AChR clustering in muscle from MuSK$^{-/-}$ mice (DeChiara et al. 1996).

THE ROLE OF AGRIN IN MUSK-MEDIATED SIGNALING

Agrin Fails to Induce AChR Clustering in Myotubes Lacking MuSK

The localization of MuSK to the NMJ, together with the absence of NMJs in mice lacking MuSK (MuSK$^{-/-}$ mice), inspired us to ask whether MuSK is required for responsivity to agrin. Myoblasts isolated from newborn MuSK$^{-/-}$ mice or from control pups were equally able to fuse and form long, twitching myotubes in culture. Together with the observation that skeletal muscle appears rather normal in MuSK$^{-/-}$ mice, these findings indicate that MuSK is not critical for early muscle development and myoblast fusion. On the other hand, MuSK appeared to be absolutely required for AChR clustering in vitro, in response to agrin (Glass et al. 1996). After stimulation with the most active form of c-agrin (c-agrin4,8), AChR clusters were evident only in the myotubes from control mice, and not in myotubes from MuSK$^{-/-}$ mice.

Agrin Induces Prominent and Rapid Tyrosine Phosphorylation of MuSK

The inability of agrin to induce AChR clustering in myotubes from MuSK$^{-/-}$ mice demonstrated that MuSK is required for agrin responsiveness and is consistent with the possibility that MuSK serves as the functional agrin receptor. However, since clustering occurs over a period of hours, these results are also consistent with the possibility that MuSK acts much farther downstream in the agrin signaling pathway. To begin to distinguish between these possibilities, we took advantage of the fact that RTKs become rapidly autophosphorylated on tyrosine upon challenge with their cognate ligand. We decided to assay four of the known forms of soluble agrin, which exhibit differing AChR clustering activities (Ferns et al. 1992, 1993; Ruegg et al. 1992; Hoch et al. 1994), for their ability to induce phosphorylation of the MuSK receptor. Phosphorylation was assessed on the endogenous MuSK receptor that is highly expressed in myotube cultures, obtained by differentiating either the C2C12 mouse myoblast cell line (Valenzuela et al. 1995) or primary rat myoblasts. Strikingly, soluble agrins containing the 8-amino-acid insert at position Z (c-agrin4,8 and c-agrin0,8), which are the forms capable of inducing AChR clustering, were also the forms that induced prominent tyrosine phosphorylation of MuSK (Glass et al. 1996). The agrin most active in clustering (c-agrin4,8) was also most active in inducing MuSK phosphorylation. In contrast, the soluble agrins lacking the 8-amino-acid insert (c-agrin4,0 and c-agrin0,0), which cannot induce AChR clustering, also could not induce MuSK phosphorylation.

The activation of a RTK by its cognate ligand typically tends to occur rapidly, and we could demonstrate that agrin induces tyrosine phosphorylation of MuSK with kinetics similar to those seen for well-characterized RTK/ligand systems; induction was detectable by 1 minute, peaked within the first 5 minutes, and remained elevated for over an hour (Glass et al. 1996). The tyrosine phosphorylation of MuSK also occurred using agrin at concentrations similar to those noted for other ligands that act on RTKs (Ip et al. 1993), with phosphorylation detectable using 1 nM agrin (Glass et al. 1996).

The requirement of MuSK for agrin responsiveness, the ability of agrin to induce rapid and prominent MuSK phosphorylation, the specificity of agrin for MuSK as compared to other factors tested, and the precise correlation of agrin forms active in AChR clustering assays and in MuSK phosphorylation assays together continued to support the notion that MuSK serves as the functional agrin receptor.

Agrin Does Not Directly Bind to an Isolated MuSK Ectodomain

If MuSK is indeed the functional agrin receptor, we would have expected to be able to demonstrate binding of agrin to MuSK. In an attempt to demonstrate such binding, we first constructed an expression construct encoding a fusion protein between the ectodomain of rat MuSK and the Fc portion of human immunoglobulin G1 (designated MuSK-Fc). Similar receptor-Fc fusions have previously been used to characterize binding between RTKs and their ligands (see, e.g., Davis et al. 1994; Stitt et al. 1995). We tried to demonstrate binding of MuSK and agrin ex vivo through a variety of methods, including simply by attempting to use MuSK-Fc to detect agrin immobilized onto nitrocellulose. In contrast to our control experiments, in which immobilized brain-derived neurotrophic factor (BDNF) was easily detected by an Fc fusion of its cognate receptor (TrkB-Fc), and in which immobilized agrin was easily detected by the agrin-specific monoclonal antibody, immobilized agrin could not be detected by MuSK-Fc (Glass et al. 1996). All other methods undertaken to get direct binding of MuSK-Fc to agrin ex vivo were similarly unsuccessful (Glass et al. 1996).

The negative binding results showed that the isolated MuSK receptor was not sufficient to bind agrin. Thus, despite much functional data indicating that agrin acts via MuSK, the possibility was raised that MuSK may not directly serve as a receptor for agrin. Alternatively, MuSK may require additional components or modifications to bind and respond to agrin.

Agrin Activates MuSK in a Cell-context-dependent Fashion

Seeing the results described above, we considered the possibility that the agrin-MuSK interaction required additional components. We reasoned that if an accessory component was required, it might be specifically expressed only on cells normally responding to agrin. Thus, we ectopically expressed full-length cDNAs encoding rat, human, and chicken MuSK in fibroblasts and assayed whether these MuSK receptors could be inducibly phosphorylated by agrin. When expressed in fibroblasts or undifferentiated myoblasts, the three transfected species of MuSK could not be phosphorylated in response to agrin (Glass et al. 1996).

When transfected myoblasts were differentiated into myotubes, however, the introduced MuSK receptors were as effectively activated by agrin as was the endogenous mouse MuSK (Glass et al. 1996). Both introduced and endogenous MuSK had identical profiles of responsivity to the various forms of agrins, with activations mediated only by forms having the 8-amino-acid insert at the Z position. Thus, our cDNAs encode MuSK proteins that are perfectly competent to undergo agrin-induced phosphorylation, but they can only be activated by agrin in the context of a differentiated myotube, consistent with the notion that agrin activation of MuSK requires a myotube-specific accessory component that is not expressed in fibroblasts or undifferentiated myoblasts.

A Receptor Complex Can Be Demonstrated between Agrin, MuSK, and a Myotube-associated Specificity Component

Altogether, the data indicate that agrin requires MuSK to mediate clustering and that agrin activates MuSK very rapidly, but that agrin does not directly bind to a purified MuSK ectodomain and can only activate MuSK in the context of a myotube. These findings are consistent with the possibility that MuSK is a requisite part of an agrin receptor complex, but that although MuSK provides a key signaling function for this complex, it requires another component(s) to bind to agrin. Similar types of receptor complexes have been described for other ligands. Perhaps some of the best-characterized examples include the receptor complexes for ciliary neurotrophic factor (CNTF) and its cytokine relatives (Davis et al. 1993; Stahl and Yancopoulos 1993). In order to interact with its two signal transducing β receptor components, gp130 and LIFRβ, CNTF must first bind to its α receptor component, known as CNTFRα. CNTFRα serves no signaling role, and is in fact linked to the surface via a glycosylphosphatidylinositol linkage and thus has no cytoplasmic domain. The receptor complex for CNTF is built in step-wise fashion: CNTF first binds to CNTFRα; this initial complex can then bind to and recruit a single β component; finally, a complete complex forms that involves β component dimerization, which is required for signal initiation. In the final complex, CNTF seems to make contacts with all three receptor components, and can be directly cross-linked to all three components (Stahl and Yancopoulos 1993). Interestingly, receptor complexes for CNTF can be built in solution using just the soluble ecto-domains of the various components. Furthermore, if just one of the receptor components is linked to the surface, a receptor complex can be built around it using soluble versions of the other components, but only in a CNTF-dependent fashion.

To confirm that MuSK directly interacts with agrin as part of its receptor complex, we next demonstrated that radiolabeled agrin could be cross-linked to MuSK receptors on the surface of myotubes. Immunoprecipitations using a MuSK-specific antibody, from lysates of myotubes chemically cross-linked to radiolabeled recombinant human agrin, contained complexes corresponding in size to agrin/MuSK complexes. These agrin/MuSK complexes were not seen in the presence of excess unlabeled agrin, or if a peptide was used to block MuSK precipitation.

Since agrin appears to bind MuSK directly in a receptor complex, we reasoned that we might be able to manipulate this complex in much the same way the CNTF receptor complex can be manipulated. To confirm the possibility that myotubes specifically express an accessory component(s) required for agrin to bind MuSK, we decided to test whether we could specifically build a receptor complex on the surface of myotubes, but not on other cells, using agrin together with a soluble version of the MuSK receptor to complex to the putative accessory component(s) on the surface of myotubes. Confirming this possibility, we found that soluble MuSK-Fc can be directly cross-linked to radiolabeled agrin, but only in the presence of membranes from differentiated myotubes, and not with membranes from fibroblasts (T.N. Stitt et al., unpubl.). These data demonstrate that complexes can form between agrin and MuSK, but only in the presence of a myotube-associated specificity component(s), which we call MASC. Potential ternary complexes were identified that might contain agrin, MuSK, and MASC.

DISCUSSION

Whereas early skeletal muscle development apparently proceeds rather normally in MuSK$^{-/-}$ mice, every aspect of NMJ formation that we examined is absent in these mice (DeChiara et al. 1996). Branches of the main intramuscular nerve do not establish normal contacts with the muscle, do not form correctly positioned or specialized nerve terminals, and are apparently not given appropriate signals to stop their wandering aimlessly across the muscle. Furthermore, we found no evidence of postsynaptic differentiation, since muscle-derived proteins that are normally localized to the synaptic basal lamina or the postsynaptic membrane are instead uniformly distributed in MuSK$^{-/-}$ myofibers. The defects in NMJ formation are sufficient to account for the perinatal lethality of the MuSK$^{-/-}$ mice resulting from their inability to breathe, and for their immobility.

Because of the absence of NMJs in mice lacking the MuSK RTK, we proceeded to test the possibility that agrin acts via the MuSK receptor and demonstrated that MuSK indeed serves as a required signaling component of a complex receptor that specifically responds to the neural forms of agrin (Glass et al. 1996). Together, our findings indicate that agrin, acting via the MuSK receptor, is required for all aspects of NMJ formation.

The defects in NMJ formation in mice lacking MuSK are more profound than might have been predicted, based on the in vitro actions of agrin, for mice lacking a functional agrin receptor. The previously described in vitro actions of agrin are largely limited to its organizing effects on postsynaptic differentiation (McMahan 1990; Hall and Sanes 1993; Bowe and Fallon 1995). The aberrant behavior of the preterminal axons and the lack of synapse-specific transcription represent deficits that would not necessarily have been expected to occur in mice in which agrin-mediated signaling pathways had been disrupted. However, recent generation of mice lacking agrin reveals NMJ defects that are indeed as profound as those described here for mice lacking MuSK (Gautam et al. 1996), consistent with the idea that MuSK is a required component of the functional receptor for agrin. Since MuSK is located only on the postsynaptic side of the NMJ (Valenzuela et al. 1995), it seems likely that the aberrant be-

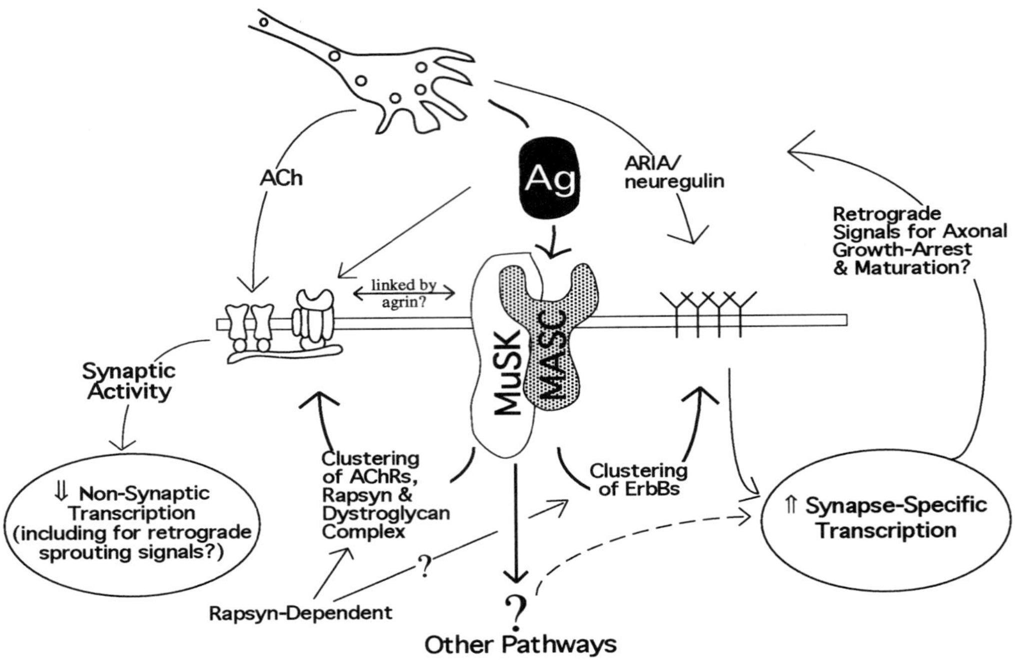

Figure 1. Schematic representation of role played by the agrin/MuSK/MASC signaling system. MuSK appears to activate signaling cascades that are responsible for all aspects of NMJ formation, including postsynaptic organizations, synapse-specific-transcription, and presynaptic growth and differentiation (perhaps by regulating the elaboration of retrograde signals, or simply by promoting synaptic activity that down-regulates production of sprouting factors). MuSK is diagrammed as being recruited after agrin binds MASC, since agrin does not bind directly to MuSK ex vivo. MuSK activates at least two independent pathways, one that is rapsyn-dependent and leads to AChR and dystroglycan clustering, and one that appears to be rapsyn-independent and results in synapse-specific transcription. In the model depicted, synapse-specific transcription is presumed to involve clustering of erbB receptors. However, it has recently been shown that synapse-specific transcription occurs in rapsyn-deficient mice although they lack clustered erbB3 receptors (Moscoso et al. 1995), indicating that synapse-specific expression does not require clustering of erbB3 in particular; it may still involve clustering of other erbB receptors (e.g., erbB4), or alternatively, it may depend on erbB-independent pathways. (Modified, with permission, from DeChiara et al. 1996 [copyright Cell Press].)

havior of the presynaptic terminals in MuSK$^{-/-}$ mutant mice is due to indirect actions of the agrin/MuSK signaling system (Fig. 1). Thus, we favor the idea that agrin released from the nerve terminal causes the postsynaptic muscle cell, via MuSK activation, to reciprocally release a recognition signal back to the nerve (Fig. 1) to indicate that a functional contact has occurred. In response to this muscle-derived recognition signal, the nerve stops growing and undergoes presynaptic differentiation; the ability of basal lamina sheaths to induce presynaptic differentiation in the absence of the underlying muscle suggests that muscle-derived signals may be embedded in synaptic basal lamina, like agrin and neuregulin (Sanes et al. 1978). Alternatively, we cannot eliminate the possibility that excessive neuronal growth in MuSK$^{-/-}$ mutant mice is caused by persistent production of a muscle-derived sprouting factor that is normally down-regulated following functional innervation (Brown et al. 1981), or by the absence of appropriate synaptic activity (Balice-Gordon and Lichtman 1994). It should be noted that despite the defects displayed by nerve branches, the main intramuscular nerves appear to be properly positioned within the muscle in MuSK$^{-/-}$ mice, indicating that guidance mechanisms which bring motor axons to muscle remain intact and operate independently of the agrin/MuSK signaling system.

As with the deficits in presynaptic differentiation, it seems likely that the lack of synapse-specific transcription in MuSK$^{-/-}$ mice also results from an indirect mechanism (Fig. 1). That is, although AChR genes are expressed uniformly in muscle fibers from MuSK$^{-/-}$ mice, we do not favor the idea that MuSK is the receptor for the extracellular signal that activates synapse-specific transcription. At present, the best candidate for such a signal is neuregulin, acting via the ErbB3 and/or ErbB4 receptors localized in the postsynaptic membrane (Altiok et al. 1995; Moscoso et al. 1995; Zhu et al. 1995). Thus, it seems likely that the loss of synapse-specific transcription is another indirect by-product of the fact that disruption of agrin/MuSK signaling blocks normal synaptic differentiation, resulting in an inability of the muscle cell to cluster ErbB receptors and possibly an inability of mutant nerve terminals to provide neuregulin.

Despite our findings, the role of dystroglycan as an agrin receptor remains unclear. The comparison of MuSK$^{-/-}$ and agrin$^{-/-}$ mutant mice, together with the signaling data for MuSK, indicate that MuSK is the critical receptor component that initiates agrin-mediated signaling pathways. Recent evidence demonstrates that a 27-kD protein fragment of agrin is sufficient to induce AChR clustering and yet does not bind dystroglycan at all (Gesemann et al. 1996), casts doubt on any functional role for dystroglycan in agrin-mediated phosphorylation or clustering.

The essential role of MuSK at the NMJ raises the possibility that MuSK or related RTKs are playing similar roles in other synapses, particularly since low levels of MuSK mRNA are detectable in the central nervous system (Valenzuela et al. 1995; and data not shown). Agrin, as well as binding sites for agrin, has been detected in the central nervous system (Bowe and Fallon 1995), suggesting that analysis of synapses in the central nervous systems of $MuSK^{-/-}$ mice is warranted. In this regard, a pair of receptors known as the RORs (Masiakowski and Carroll 1992), which are expressed during early development of the central nervous system and whose closest relative is MuSK, should probably also be evaluated for roles in synapse formation. In any case, the complex types of spatial organizing events initiated by MuSK have not previously been noted in response to other RTKs, which have instead been largely characterized for their ability to mediate responses to growth factors that elicit mitogenic, survival, or differentiative actions (Schlessinger and Ullrich 1992). It remains possible that, in addition to its organizing role at the NMJ, the agrin/MuSK system is also involved in more classic growth-factor-like responses.

MuSK Is a Requisite Subunit of the Agrin Receptor Complex but Requires a Myotube-associated Specificity Component

Our data have indicated that MuSK is a requisite subunit of a multicomponent receptor complex used by agrin and that it requires a myotube-specific accessory component(s) to bind and mediate responses to agrin. There are many other examples of ligands that use multicomponent receptor complexes (Stahl and Yancopoulos 1993). Most cytokines, as noted above for CNTF and its relatives, use such receptor complexes. In these receptor complexes, there are often components whose primary role is to bind ligand, whereas other subunits can both bind and signal. In the case of RTKs, there are also examples of multicomponent receptors. For example, fibroblast growth factors (FGFs) need to bind heparin, usually presented on surface proteoglycans, in order to bind and activate their RTK subunits (Goldfarb 1990). The trk family of RTKs, which bind to nerve growth factor (NGF) and the related neurotrophins, present a less well-understood example of RTKs which may interact with an accessory component known as p75 (Barbacid 1993). In the case of ARIA/neuregulin, receptor complexes can include two different members of the ErbB family (Burden et al. 1995). Most recently, and most analagous to MuSK/MASC, it has been shown that binding and activation of the ret RTK by glial cell-line-derived neurotrophic factor (GDNF) requires an accessory component termed GDNFRα (Jing et al. 1996; Treanor et al. 1996). In all these examples of multicomponent receptor complexes, signal initiation seems to depend on ligand-mediated dimerization of signal-transducing subunits that are included within the receptor complex; this dimerization can involve either homodimerization of identical subunits or heterodimerization of related subunits.

Before considering potential candidates for the other component(s) of the agrin receptor complex, it is worth remembering that the signaling function of MuSK appears quite unusual as compared to other RTKs. Whereas most RTKs are thought to mediate growth or survival responses, or quite simple differentiative events, MuSK seems instead to mediate a very complicated organizing function. The structure of the NMJ has already been shown to depend on complex molecular scaffolds that anchor components in place by linking them to the extracellular matrix as well as to the cytoskeleton. Since they combine to initiate formation of the entire postsynaptic macrostructure, and also are contained within it, it seems likely that both agrin and MuSK have many interactions with molecules at the NMJ, for both structural and signaling purposes. One can imagine that MuSK interacts with proteins that serve to link it to the molecular scaffold at the junction, both extracellularly and intracellularly; it may bind to other proteins that are direct substrates for its kinase activity or that act merely as couplers of MuSK to its substrates. Thus, the myotube-specific accessory component(s) required for agrin to bind and activate MuSK may be difficult to distinguish from other (perhaps more abundant) molecules interacting with agrin and MuSK that serve other functions; even the accessory component(s) itself may be multifunctional, and not only serve to help bind agrin, but to couple this ligand/receptor system to other proteins as well.

There are clues concerning the possible identity of accessory receptor components for agrin. Recent data implicate a synapse-specific carbohydrate in agrin responses (Martin and Sanes 1995); enzymatic removal of this carbohydrate blocks agrin responsiveness, whereas lectin-mediated clustering of proteins with this carbohydrate, or enzymatic unmasking of more of this carbohydrate, potentiate or even mimic agrin. These data could be reconciled with the concept of a MuSK receptor complex if such a carbohydrate marked and was required for agrin recognition by the MuSK accessory component. Alternatively, it could be that such a carbohydrate is required on MuSK itself. Along these lines, it should be pointed out that a myotube-specific modification of MuSK, whether it involves carbohydrate or other modifications, may allow MuSK to directly bind agrin, and thus raises the possibility that modified MuSK itself might correspond to the myotube-specific "accessory" component; in this case, soluble recombinant MuSK would presumably be able to dimerize with the correctly modified MuSK—via agrin—on the myotube surface. A related scenario might involve the expression of a MuSK relative in myotubes, and the need for heterodimerization between MuSK and this relative—as can occur with the ErbBs—to create a functional agrin receptor. Finally, since agrin forms lacking the ability to bind heparin are still active, it seems unlikely that binding to a proteoglycan at the "Y" site would be critical for linking agrin to its accessory component.

Mechanism by Which MuSK Activation Triggers Postsynaptic Organization

Previous studies had implicated tyrosine phosphorylation in the agrin response (Wallace et al. 1991; Wallace 1994, 1995; Qu and Huganir 1994; Ferns et al. 1996). The finding that the critical signaling component of the agrin receptor complex is a RTK validates the notion that specific agrin-induced tyrosine phosphorylations initiate organization and formation of the NMJ. The only well-characterized agrin-induced tyrosine phosphorylation, other than that of MuSK, is of the AChR β component (Wallace et al. 1991; Qu and Huganir 1994; Ferns et al. 1996). As would be expected, although phosphorylation of AChRβ is relatively rapid and begins by 15 minutes after agrin addition, it trails MuSK phosphorylation. It is unknown whether AChRβ phosphorylation is required for, or contributes to, AChR clustering, or whether it is a direct substrate of MuSK. The critical MuSK-mediated phosphorylations may well involve proteins that are clustered or directly involved in building the molecular scaffold that maintains the postsynaptic specialization. It is easy to imagine that direct phosphorylation of key proteins may trigger complexes or aggregations to form; for example, AChRβ phosphorylation may trigger its association and co-aggregation with rapsyn or other coupling proteins. Since MuSK appears to be much less abundant than many of the proteins that are clustered, it would presumably act catalytically on such structural targets. Alternatively, MuSK-mediated phosphorylations may not directly trigger clustering events, but rather, MuSK may activate downstream enzymes or signaling pathways that in turn trigger clustering. These possibilities emphasize the need to identify direct substrates and signaling pathways activated by MuSK.

MuSK Signaling in Other Contexts: In the Adult, Atrophies and Dystrophies?

The complex type of organizational role played by MuSK at the NMJ distinguishes it from other growth factors that use RTKs. However, this unusual role does not preclude MuSK from having more traditional growth-factor-like effects. Exploration of the signaling pathways activated by MuSK will certainly help address whether MuSK uses unique signaling pathways or instead shares pathways with other RTKs. When it was realized that the trk family of RTKs served as the receptors for NGF and its relatives, it was thought that the trks might prove to have unusual substrates because they mediated neuronal survival and differentiation responses, as opposed to the conventional type of proliferative responses that had previously been attributed to RTKs. It turns out, instead, that the trks activate much the same substrates as mitogenic RTKs, but that these activations are ultimately interpreted much differently within the context of a postmitotic neuron (Glass and Yancopoulos 1993). In fact, ectopic expression of the trks in proliferation-competent cells, such as fibroblasts, allows them to mediate conventional mitogenic responses indistinguishable from those of FGFs or EGFs (Glass et al. 1991). Thus, it will be important to determine whether the unusual actions of MuSK are a consequence of unique signaling capabilities, or simply of its unique site of expression.

Current studies of agrin and MuSK have almost completely focused on their roles during formation of the NMJ. In the entirely different context of an adult muscle, MuSK is dramatically up-regulated in situations where the muscle is at risk for atrophy, including during forced immobilization (Valenzuela et al. 1995). It will certainly be of interest to determine what kinds of actions MuSK mediates in the context of an adult muscle, whether these are more along the trophic types more usual for a RTK, and whether these actions would be of benefit during muscle atrophy or other muscle diseases. Along these lines, it is worth noting that MuSK, via agrin, now appears to be linked to the dystroglycan complex. Mutations in at least three of the components of this complex (dystrophin, emerin, and adhalin) account for different types of muscular dystrophies (Campbell 1995). The mechanism by which problems in the dystroglycan complex lead to progressive muscle wasting are poorly understood, and efforts to understand this mechanism are primarily focused on problems with sarcolemmal stability. The association of a RTK with the dystroglycan complex would certainly raise the possibility that signaling defects play an important contributory role in dystrophies.

ACKNOWLEDGMENTS

We thank Drs. L.S. Schleifer and P. Roy Vagelos, along with the rest of the Regeneron community, for their consistent support. This manuscript was largely the result of combining and expanding on two recently published papers by DeChiara et al. (1996) and Glass et al. (1996), and the figure represents a modified version of the figure contained therein.

REFERENCES

Altiok, N., J.L. Bessereau, and J.P. Changeux. 1995. ErbB3 and ErbB2/neu mediate the effect of heregulin on acetylcholine receptor gene expression in muscle: Differential expression at the endplate. *EMBO J.* **14:** 4258.

Apel, E.D., S.L. Roberds, K.P. Campbell, and J.P. Merlie. 1995. Rapsyn may function as a link between the acetylcholine receptor and the agrin-binding dystrophin-associated glycoprotein complex. *Neuron* **15:** 115.

Balice-Gordon, R.J. and J.W. Lichtman. 1994. Long-term synapse loss induced by focal blockade of postsynaptic receptors. *Nature* **372:** 519.

Barbacid, M. 1993. Nerve growth factor: A tale of two receptors. *Oncogene* **8:** 2033.

Bowe, M.A. and J.R. Fallon. 1995. The role of agrin in synapse formation. *Annu. Rev. Neurosci.* **18:** 443.

Bowe, M.A., K.A. Deyst, J.D. Leszyk, and J.R. Fallon. 1994. Identification and purification of an agrin receptor from *Torpedo* postsynaptic membranes: A heteromeric complex related to dystroglycans. *Neuron* **12:** 1173.

Brown, M.C., R.L. Holland, and W.G. Hopkins. 1981. Motor nerve sprouting. *Annu. Rev. Neurosci.* **4:** 17.

Burden, S.J., P.B. Sargent, and U.J. McMahan. 1979. Acetylcholine receptors in regenerating muscle accumulate at original synaptic sites in the absence of the nerve. *J. Cell Biol.* **82:** 412.

Burden, S.J., S.A. Jo, J. Tang, X. Zhu, J.E. Yeadon, and A.M. Simon. 1995. Polarity in skeletal muscle cells is induced by innervation. *Dev. Biol.* **6:** 59.

Campanelli, J.T., S.L. Roberds, K.P. Campbell, and R.H. Scheller. 1994. A role for dystrophin-associated glycoproteins and utrophin in agrin-induced AChR clustering. *Cell* **77:** 673.

Campbell, K.P. 1995. Three muscular dystrophies: Loss of cytoskeleton-extracellular matrix linkage. *Cell* **80:** 675.

Davis, S., T.H. Aldrich, N. Stahl, T. Taga, T. Kishimoto, N.Y. Ip, and G.D. Yancopoulos. 1993. LIFRb and gp130 as heterodimerizing signal transducers of the tripartite CNTF receptor. *Science* **260:** 1805.

Davis, S., N.W. Gale, T.H. Aldrich, P.C. Maisonpierre, V. Lhotak, T. Pawson, M. Goldfarb, and G.D. Yancopoulos. 1994. Ligands for the EPH-related receptor tyrosine kinases that require membrane attachment or clustering for activity. *Science* **266:** 816.

DeChiara, T.M., R. Vejsada, W.T. Poueymirou, A. Acheson, C. Suri, J.C. Conover, B. Friedman, J. McClain, L. Pan, N. Stahl, N.Y. Ip, A. Kato, and G.D. Yancopoulos. 1995. Mice lacking the CNTF receptor, unlike mice lacking CNTF, exhibit profound motor neuron deficits at birth. *Cell* **83:** 313.

DeChiara, T.M., D.C. Bowen, D.M. Valenzuela, M.V. Simmons, W.T. Pouemirou, S. Thomas, E. Kinetz, D.L. Compton, E. Rojas, J.S. Park, C. Smith, P.S. DiStefano, D.J. Glass, S.J. Burden, and G.D. Yancopoulos. 1996. The receptor tyrosine kinase, MuSK, is required for all aspects of neuromuscular junction formation in vivo. *Cell* **85:** 501.

Fallon, J.R. and Z.W. Hall. 1994. Building synapses: Agrin and dystroglycan stick together. *Trends Neurosci.* **17:** 469.

Ferns, M., M. Deiner, and Z. Hall. 1996. Agrin-induced acetylcholine receptor clustering in mammalian muscle requires tyrosine phosphorylation. *J. Cell Biol.* **132:** 937.

Ferns, M., J.T. Campanelli, W. Hoch, R.H. Scheller, and Z.W. Hall. 1993. The ability of agrin to cluster AChRs depends on alternative splicing and on cell surface proteoglycans. *Neuron* **11:** 491.

Ferns, M., W. Hoch, J.T. Campanelli, F. Rupp, Z.W. Hall, and R.H. Scheller. 1992. RNA splicing regulates agrin-mediated acetylcholine receptor clustering activity on cultured myotubes. *Neuron* **8:** 1079.

Ganju, P., E. Walls, J. Brennan, and A.D. Reith. 1995. Cloning and developmental expression of NsK2, a novel receptor tyrosine kinase implicated in skeletal myogenesis. *Oncogene* **11:** 281.

Gautam, M., P.G. Noakes, L. Moscoso, F. Rupp, R.H. Scheller, J.P. Merlie, and J.R. Sanes. 1996. Defective neuromuscular synaptogenesis in agrin-deficient mutant mice. *Cell* **85:** 525.

Gee, S.H., F. Montanaro, M.H. Lindenbaum, and S. Carbonetto. 1994. Dystroglycan-alpha, a dystrophin-associated glycoprotein, is a functional agrin receptor. *Cell* **77:** 675.

Gesemann, M., V. Cavalli, A.J. Denzer, A. Brancaccio, B. Schumacher, and M.A. Ruegg. 1996. Alternative splicing of agrin alters its binding to heparin, dystroglycan, and the putative agrin receptor. *Neuron* **16:** 755.

Glass, D.J. and G.D. Yancopoulos. 1993. The neurotrophins and their receptors. *Trends Cell Biol.* **3:** 262.

Glass, D.J., S.H. Nye, P. Hantzopoulos, M.J. Macchi, S.P. Squinto, M. Goldfarb, and G.D. Yancopoulos. 1991. TrkB mediates BDNF/NT-3-dependent survival and proliferation in fibroblasts lacking the low affinity NGF receptor. *Cell* **66:** 405.

Glass, D.J., D.C. Bowen, C. Radziejewski, J. Bruno, T.N. Stitt, T.E. Ryan, D.R. Gies, K. Mattsson, S. Shah, S.J. Burden, D.M. Valenzuela, T.M. DeChiara, and G.D. Yancopoulos. 1996. Agrin acts via a MuSK receptor complex. *Cell* **85:** 513.

Godfrey, E.W., R.M. Nitkin, B.G. Wallace, L.L. Rubin, and U.J. McMahan. 1984. Components of *Torpedo* electric organ and muscle that cause aggregation of acetylcholine receptors on cultured muscle cells. *J. Cell. Biol.* **99:** 615.

Goldfarb, M. 1990. The fibroblast growth factor family. *Cell Growth Differ.* **1:** 439

Hall, Z.W. and J.R. Sanes. 1993. Synaptic structure and development: The neuromuscular junction. *Cell* (suppl.) **72:** 99.

Helgren, M.E., S.P. Squinto, H.L. Davis, D.J. Parry, T.G. Boulton, C.S. Heck, Y. Zhu, G.D. Yancopoulos, R.M. Lindsay, and P.S. DiStefano. 1994. Trophic effects of ciliary neurotrophic factor on denervated skeletal muscle. *Cell* **76:** 493.

Hoch, W., J.T. Campanelli, S. Harrison, and R.H. Scheller. 1994. Structural domains of agrin required for clustering of nicotinic acetylcholine receptors. *EMBO J.* **13:** 2814.

Hoch, W., M. Ferns, J.T. Campanelli, Z.W. Hall, and R.H. Scheller. 1993. Developmental regulation of highly active alternatively spliced forms of agrin. *Neuron* **11:** 479.

Ip, N.Y., T.N. Stitt, P. Tapley, R. Klein, D.J. Glass, J. Fandl, L.A. Greene, M. Barbacid, and G.D. Yancopoulos. 1993. Similarities and differences in the way neurotrophins interact with the Trks in neuronal and nonneuronal cells. *Neuron* **10:** 137.

Jennings, C.G., S.M. Dyer, and S.J. Burden. 1993. Muscle-specific trk-related receptor with a kringle domain defines a distinct class of receptor tyrosine kinases. *Proc. Natl. Acad. Sci.* **90:** 2895.

Jing, S., D. Wen, Y. Yu, P. Holst, Y. Luo, M. Fang, R. Tamir, L. Antonio, Z. Hu, R. Cupples, J.-C. Louis, S. Hu, B.W. Altrock, and G.M. Fox. 1996. GDNF-induced activation of the Ret protein tyrosine kinase is mediated by GDNR-α, a novel receptor for GDNF. *Cell* **85:** 1113.

Kuffler, D.P. 1986. Accurate reinnervation of motor end plates after disruption of sheath cells and muscle fibers. *J. Comp. Neurol.* **250:** 228.

Martin, P.T. and J.R. Sanes. 1995. Role for a synapse-specific carbohydrate in agrin-induced clustering of acetylcholine receptors. *Neuron* **14:** 743.

Masiakowski, P. and R.D. Carroll. 1992. A novel family of cell surface receptors with tyrosine kinase-like domain. *J. Biol. Chem.* **267:** 26181.

McMahan, U.J. 1990. The agrin hypothesis. *Cold Spring Harbor Symp. Quant. Biol.* **55:** 407.

McMahan, U.J. and C.R. Slater. 1984. The influence of basal lamina on the accumulation of acetylcholine receptors at synaptic sites in regenerating muscles. *J. Cell. Biol.* **98:** 1453.

Moscoso, L.M., G.C. Chu, M. Gautam, P.G. Noakes, J.P. Merlie, and J.R. Sanes. 1995. Synapse-associated expression of an acetylcholine receptor-inducing protein, ARIA/heregulin, and its putative receptors, ErbB2 and ErbB3, in developing mammalian muscle. *Dev. Biol.* **172:** 158.

Nitkin, R.M., M.A. Smith, C. Magill, J.R. Fallon, Y.M.-Y. Yao, B.G. Wallace, and U.J. McMahan. 1987. Identification of agrin, a synaptic organizing protein from *Torpedo* electric organ. *J. Cell. Biol.* **105:** 2471.

Noakes, P.G., W.D. Phillips, T.A. Hanley, J.R. Sanes, and J.P. Merlie. 1993. 43K protein and acetylcholine receptors colocalize during the initial stages of neuromuscular synapse formation in vivo. *Dev. Biol.* **155:** 275.

Qu, Z. and R.L. Huganir. 1994. Comparison of innervation and agrin-induced tyrosine phosphorylation of the nicotinic acetylcholine receptor. *J. Neurosci.* **14:** 6834.

Reist, N.E., M.J. Werle, and U.J. McMahan. 1992. Agrin released by motor neurons induces the aggregation of acetylcholine receptors at neuromuscular junctions. *Neuron* **8:** 865.

Ruegg, M.A., K.W.K. Tsim, S.E. Horton, S. Kroger, G. Escher, E.M. Gensch, and U.J. McMahan. 1992. The agrin gene encodes for a family of basal lamina proteins that differ in function and distribution. *Neuron* **8:** 691.

Rupp, F., D.G. Payan, C. Magill-Solc, D.M. Cowan, and R.H. Scheller. 1991. Structure and expression of a rat agrin. *Neuron* **6:** 811.

Sanes, J.R. 1995. The synaptic cleft of the neuromuscular junction. *Dev. Biol.* **6:** 163.

Sanes, J.R., L.M. Marshall, and U.J. McMahan. 1978. Reinnervation of muscle fiber basal lamina after removal of myofibers. Differentiation of regenerating axons at original synaptic sites. *J. Cell. Biol.* **78:** 176.

Schlessinger, J. and A. Ullrich. 1992. Growth factor signaling by receptor tyrosine kinases. *Neuron* **9:** 383.

Sealock, R. and S.C. Froehner. 1994. Dystrophin-associated proteins and synapse formation: Is alpha-dystroglycan the agrin receptor? *Cell* **77:** 617.

Snider, W.D. 1994. Functions of the neurotrophins during nervous system development: What the knockouts are teaching us. *Cell* **77:** 627.

Stahl, N. and G.D. Yancopoulos. 1993. The alphas, betas and kinases of cytokine receptor complexes. *Cell* **74:** 587.

Stitt, T.N., G. Conn, M. Gore, C. Lai, J. Bruno, C. Radziejewski, K. Mattson, J. Fisher, D.R. Gies, P.F. Jones, P. Masiakowski, T.E. Ryan, N.J. Tobkes, D.H. Chen, P.S. DiStefano, G.L. Long, C. Basilico, M.P. Goldfarb, G. Lemke, D.J. Glass, and G.D. Yancopoulos. 1995. The anticoagulation factor protein S and its relative, Gas6, are ligands for the Tyro3/Axl family of receptor tyrosine kinases. *Cell* **80:** 661.

Sugiyama, J., D.C. Bowen, and Z.W. Hall. 1994. Dystroglycan binds nerve and muscle agrin. *Neuron* **13:** 103.

Treanor, J.J.S., L. Goodman, F. de Sauvage, D.M. Stone, K.T. Poulsen, C.D. Beck, C. Gray, M.P. Armanini, R.A. Pollock, F. Hefti, H.S. Phillips, A. Goddard, M.W. Moore, A. Buh-Bello, A.M. Davies, N. Asai, M. Takahashi, R. Vandlen, C.E. Henderson, and A. Rosenthal. 1996. Characterization of a multicomponent receptor for GDNF. *Nature* **382:** 80.

Tsim, K.W., M.A. Ruegg, G. Escher, S. Kroger, and U.J. McMahan. 1992. cDNA that encodes active agrin. *Neuron* **8:** 677.

Valenzuela, D.M., T.N. Stitt, P.S. DiStefano, E. Rojas, K. Mattsson, D.L. Compton, L. Nunez, J.S. Park, J.L. Stark, D.R. Gies, S. Thomas, M.M. Le Beau, A.A. Fernald, N.G. Copeland, N.A. Jenkins, S.J. Burden, D.J. Glass, and G.D. Yancopoulos. 1995. Receptor tyrosine kinase specific for the skeltal muscle lineage: Expression in embryonic muscle, at the neuromuscular junction, and after injury. *Neuron* **15:** 573.

Wallace, B.G. 1989. Agrin-induced specializations contain cytoplasmic, membrane, and extracellular matrix-associated components of the postsynaptic apparatus. *J. Neurosci.* **9:** 1294.

———. 1994. Staurosporine inhibits agrin-induced acetylcholine receptor phosphorylation and aggregation. *J. Cell. Biol.* **125:** 661.

———. 1995. Regulation of the interaction of nicotinic acetylcholine receptors with the cytoskeleton by agrin-activated protein tyrosine kinase. *J. Cell Biol.* **128:** 1121.

Wallace, B.G., Z. Qu, and R.L. Huganir. 1991. Agrin induces phosphorylation of the nicotinic acetylcholine receptor. *Neuron* **6:** 869.

Zhu, X., C. Lai, S. Thomas, and S.J. Burden. 1995. Neuregulin receptors, erbB3 and erbB4, are localized at neuromuscular synapses. *EMBO J.* **14:** 5842.

GDNF Is Required for Kidney Development and Enteric Innervation

J.G. PICHEL,[1] L. SHEN,[1] H.Z. SHENG,[1] A.-C. GRANHOLM,[2] J. DRAGO,[3]
A. GRINBERG,[1] E.J. LEE,[1] S.P. HUANG,[1] M. SAARMA,[4] B.J. HOFFER,[2]
H. SARIOLA,[4,5] AND H. WESTPHAL[1]

[1]Laboratory of Mammalian Genes and Development, National Institutes of Health, Bethesda, Maryland 20892; [2]Departments of Pharmacology and Basic Dental Science, University of Colorado Health Sciences Center, Denver, Colorado 80262; [3]Department of Anatomy, Monash University, Clayton, 3168 Victoria, Australia; [4]Programs of Molecular Neurobiology and Developmental Biology, Institute of Biotechnology, Biocentre 1, University of Helsinki, FIN-00014 Helsinki, Finland; [5]Laboratory of Pediatric Pathology, Childrens Hospital, University of Helsinki, FIN-00380 Helsinki, Finland

Glial cell line-derived neurotrophic factor (GDNF) was first isolated as a survival and differentiation factor for midbrain dopaminergic neurons (Lin et al. 1993). Its neurotrophic activity has been documented in vitro and in vivo on a range of different neuronal subpopulations including midbrain dopaminergic (DA) neurons (Hoffer et al. 1994; Beck et al. 1995; Clarkson et al. 1995; Kearns and Gash 1995; Sauer et al. 1995; Tomac et al. 1995a,b; Hou et al. 1996), cranial nerve and spinal motor neurons (Henderson et al. 1994; Zurn et al. 1994; Bowenkamp et al. 1995; Kreiglstein et al. 1995; Li et al. 1995; Oppenheim et al. 1995; Yan et al. 1995; Gouin et al. 1996; Yamamoto et al. 1996), sympathetic, ciliary, and sensory neurons (Buj-Bello et al. 1995; Ebendal et al. 1995; Trupp et al. 1995), brain stem noradrenergic neurons (Arenas et al. 1995), and cerebellar Purkinje neurons (Mount et al. 1995). On the basis of these findings, GDNF is considered to be a potential protective and reparative agent for treating neurodegenerative disorders involving central dopaminergic and noradrenergic neurons, including Parkinson's, Alzheimer's, and Huntington diseases (Lin et al. 1993; Strömberg et al. 1993; Drago et al. 1994; Poulsen et al. 1994; Arenas et al. 1995; Beck et al. 1995; Bowenkamp et al. 1995; Hudson et al. 1995; Lindner et al. 1995; Opackkajuffry et al. 1995; Sauer et al. 1995; Tomac et al. 1995a,b; Gash et al. 1996; Hou et al. 1996), and motor neuron diseases such as spinal muscular atrophy and amyotrophic lateral sclerosis (Henderson et al. 1994; Zurn et al. 1994; Li et al. 1995; Oppenheim et al. 1995).

GDNF is a distantly related member of the transforming growth factor-β (TGF-β) superfamily with which it shares seven conserved cysteine residues. It is posttranscriptionally processed from a precursor polypeptide and secreted as a disulfide-bonded N-glycosylated homodimer (Lin et al. 1993, 1994). TGF-β factors are known to mediate inductive interactions during development (Hogan et al. 1994; Kingsley 1994; Wall and Hogan 1994), and some also show potent neurotrophic effects (Poulsen et al. 1994; Kreiglstein et al. 1995). Two distinct GDNF transcripts have been detected in almost every region of the rat newborn brain and developing embryo by reverse transcription-polymerase chain reaction (RT-PCR) (Schaar et al. 1993; Springer et al. 1994, 1995; Suter-Crazzolara and Unsicker 1994; Choi-Lundberg and Bohn 1995; Cristina et al. 1995) or ribonuclease protection assay (Arenas et al. 1995; Trupp et al. 1995). By oligonucleotide hybridization, low levels of GDNF expression have been detected in many fields of the perinatal rat brain that do not receive dopaminergic innervation (Strömberg et al. 1993). mRNA in situ hybridization revealed GDNF transcripts in the anterior neuroectoderm during early stages of mouse development (Hellmich et al. 1996). During organogenesis the main areas of GDNF expression include, in addition to the brain (Strömberg et al. 1993; Poulsen et al. 1994), many tissues undergoing epithelial-mesenchymal interactions (notably the metanephric kidney), and also the gastrointestinal tract, suggesting possible functions during organogenesis, innervation, or both (Suter-Crazzolara and Unsicker 1994; Choi-Lundberg and Bohn 1995; Trupp et al. 1995; Hellmich et al. 1996; Suvanto et al. 1996).

Although the therapeutic potential of GDNF as a neurotrophic molecule is being assessed, its in vivo role remains to be elucidated. Toward this goal, we have used targeted mutagenesis of the GDNF locus to generate mice that lack GDNF expression. The resulting mutant phenotype indicates that GDNF is required for effective branching of the ureter during early kidney development and for innervation of the gastrointestinal tract.

EXPERIMENTAL PROCEDURES

Targeting the murine GDNF locus. The targeting construct, containing 1.6 kb of 5′flank (*Bam*HI-*Xba*I fragment) and 4.0 kb of 3′sequence (*Nco*I-*Nco*I fragment), obtained from a mouse 129/Sv-derived GDNF genomic sequence and subcloned in pPNT (Tybulewicz et al. 1991), was linearized with *Not*I and transfected into J1 (Li et al. 1992) or R1 (Nagy et al. 1993) embryonic stem (ES) cell lines by electroporation. After selection with G418 and gancyclovir (Love et al. 1992), 180 independent clones (98 from J1 and 82 from R1-derived ES cells) were screened by Southern analysis using *Eco*RV digestion and 3′*probe*. Three J1-derived (J47, J67, and J84) and 4 R1-derived (R10, R13, R29, and R52) clones yielded the expected restriction fragments. When analyzed for homologous recombination at the 5′flank, using either *Eco*RV or *Eco*RI enzymes with 5′*probe*, all clones except J67 proved to contain the expected GDNF mutant allele. Chimeric mice were produced either by blastocyst injection (Li et al. 1992) or by morula aggregation (Nagy et al. 1993) of CD1 or C57BL/6 recipient strains to obtain germ-line transmission of the targeted allele. Embryos or newborns derived from the intercross of heterozygotes were genotyped by Southern blot or PCR. The wild-type GDNF allele was detected by PCR using the p1 5′ oligonucleotide (5′-CCAGAGAATTCCAGAGGGA AAGGTC) and the p2 3′ oligonucleotide (5′-CAG ATACATCCACACCGTTTAGCGG) that generate a 338-bp fragment corresponding to exon 3 of the GDNF gene. The targeted GDNF allele was identified by the p3 3′ primer (5′-GATCCCCTCAGAAGAACTCGT) and the p4 5′ primer (5′-CTGTGCTCGACGTTGTC ACTG) within the *PGK-neo* cassette that amplify 567 bp. PCR conditions were: 5 minutes at 94°C; 33 cycles of 30 seconds at 94°C, 55 seconds at 66°C, and 1 minute at 72°C; followed by 10 minutes at 72°C.

Embryo dissections and histological analysis. Newborns or fetuses at different developmental stages were collected in saline phosphate buffer (PBS) and tails or yolk sacs were removed for DNA analysis by Southern blot or PCR. For histology and in situ hybridization, the specimens were fixed either in buffered 10% formalin or 4% paraformaldehyde for 12–24 hours and then transferred to 70% ethanol. After genotyping, the samples were placed in successive ethanol and xylene baths and finally embedded in Paraplast Plus (Oxford). Specimens were sectioned in a microtome (5-μm sections) and for histological analysis stained with hematoxylin and eosin. Urogenital systems and digestive tubes were dissected out and cleaned of adjacent tissues.

In situ hybridization. Transverse sections of paraffin-embedded embryos were hybridized to a ^{33}P-labeled antisense riboprobe corresponding to the carboxy-terminal 107 amino acids of the predicted mature GDNF peptide, according to published procedures (Robinson et al. 1991). Sections were stained with Hoechst solution and simultaneously viewed in dark field and ultraviolet illumination for photography.

Kidney explant cultures. Urogenital specimens, consisting of mesonephros, Wolffian duct, ureteric bud, and metanephric mesenchyme, were dissected from embryonic day 11.5 (E11.5) embryos. They were cultured on a 1.0-μm Nucleopore filter (Costar) for 72 hours in chemically defined Improved MEM Zinc Option medium (Richter's Modification) (GIBCO) supplemented with 50 μg/ml transferrin (Sigma), fixed in cold methanol, and whole-mount immunostained as described previously (Sariola et al. 1988). The primary antibody was a mouse monoclonal anti-mouse cytokeratin-18 (Virtanen et al. 1985) and the secondary antibody was a donkey FITC-labeled anti-mouse IgG (Jackson Immunoresearch). For the effects on restoration of GDNF function, Affi-Gel blue agarose beads, 100–200 mesh (Bio-Rad), saturated in recombinant GDNF at 100 ng/μl or in 1% BSA (control not shown) (Vainio et al. 1993), were placed on top of or next to the metanephric mesenchyme and incubated and analyzed as described above.

Immunohistological analysis. Intestines from GDNF$^{+/-}$ and GDNF$^{-/-}$ and normal newborn mice were immersion fixed in 4% paraformaldehyde in PBS overnight and stored in 30% sucrose in PBS. After embedding in O.C.T. medium (Miles Inc.), 10-μm cryostat coronal sections were collected and mounted on glass slides. Immunostaining was performed as described elsewhere (Harlow and Lane 1988) using antibodies directed against ChAT (Boehringer-Mannheim). FITC-conjugated anti-rat IgG (Dako Corporation) was used as secondary antibody.

RESULTS

Mice Lacking GDNF Show Renal Agenesis and Digestive System Abnormalities

We generated a nonfunctional allele of the GDNF gene by replacing part of the third exon that encodes the mature GDNF molecule (Lin et al. 1993; Hellmich et al. 1996) with a cassette that expresses the selectable marker neomycin phosphotransferase (*neo*) (Fig. 1A). After introducing the construct into the ES cell lines J1 (Li et al. 1992) and R1 (Nagy and Rossant 1993), six clones, J47, J84, R10, R13, R29, and R52, were identified as homologous recombinants with the predicted mutant allele (called GDNF^{-}; Fig. 1B). When clone J47 was injected into CD1 mouse blastocysts, and clones R10, R13, and R29 were injected into, or aggregated with, C57BL/6 embryos, all produced chimeric mice that transmitted the mutation to their progeny.

Heterozygous offspring were viable and fertile whereas mice homozygous for the mutant allele (GDNF$^{-/-}$) (Fig. 1C,D), although born with the expected Mendelian frequency, died within 12–24 hours after birth. Dissection revealed that their kidneys were either absent or rudimentary. Some GDNF$^{-/-}$ mutant mice contained blind-ending ureters with no renal tissue, and others displayed a complete absence of ureter and kidney (renal agenesis), either unilateral or

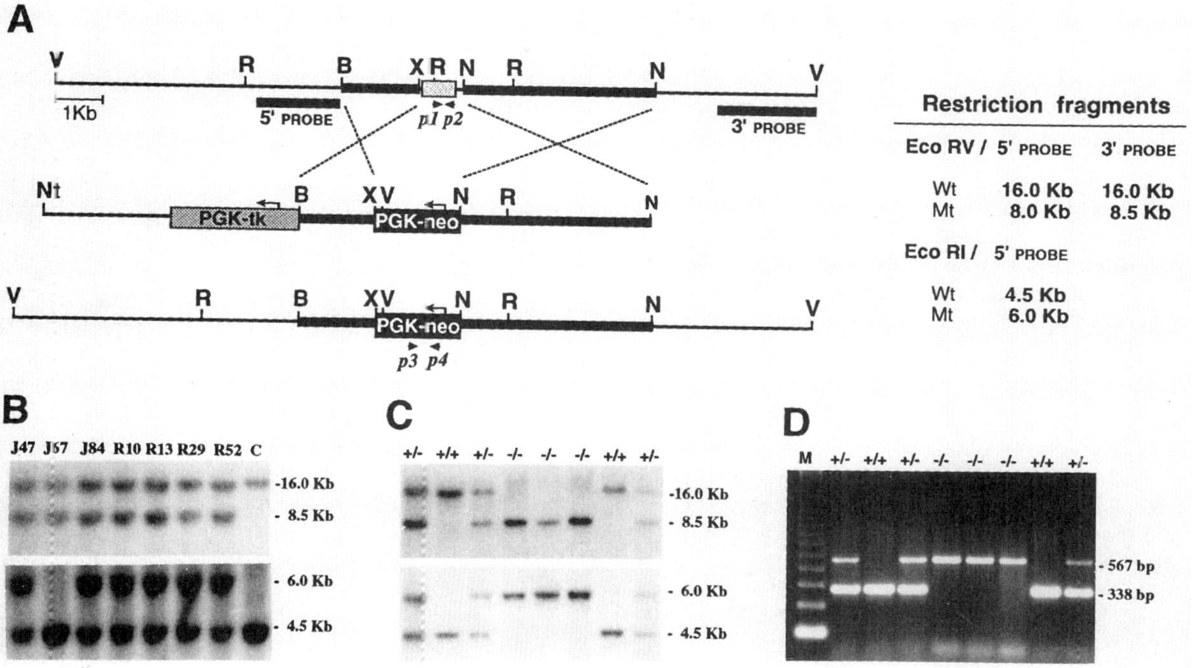

Figure 1. Generation of GDNF mutant mice. (*A*) Schematic representation of the GDNF locus (*upper*), GDNF targeting vector (*middle*), expected mutant allele after the homologous recombination event (*bottom*), and restriction fragment lengths using the 5′ or 3′ probes (*right table*). Successful gene replacement results in the deletion of just under 1 kb of GDNF genomic sequence, including all exon-3-derived coding sequences (*hatched box*) that encode the predicted GDNF mature peptide (amino acids 52 to the carboxyl terminus) (Lin et al. 1993; Hellmich et al. 1996). In its place, a 1.6-kb PGK-neo selection cassette (Tybulewicz et al. 1991) is inserted in opposite transcriptional orientation. Restriction enzyme sites: (V) *Eco*RV; (R) *Eco*RI; (B) *Bam*HI; (X) *Xba*I; (N) *Nco*I; (Nt) *Not*I. Symbols p1, p2, p3, and p4 indicate PCR primers. (Wt) Wild type; (Mt) mutant. (*B*) Southern blot analysis of targeted (J47, J67, J84, R10, R13, R29, R52) and parental (*C*) ES cell clones. Wild-type and mutant alleles show bands of 16.0 and 8.5 kb, respectively, when *Eco*RV-digested DNA is probed with the 3′-flanking probe (*upper panel*). If a 5′-flanking probe is used, the *Eco*RV digestion yields 16.0-kb and 8.0-kb fragments (not shown), whereas *Eco*RI enzyme yields bands of 4.5 kb (wild type) and 6.0 kb (mutant) (*lower panel*). Note that clone J67 shows the expected 3′, but not 5′ homologous recombination. (*C*) Southern blot analysis of progeny from a GDNF$^{+/-}$ heterozygous intercross showing the three possible genotypes: normal (+/+), lanes *2* and *7*; heterozygous mutant (+/–), lanes *1*, *3*, and *8*; and homozygous mutant (–/–), lanes *4*, *5*, and *6*. Restriction enzymes and probes were the same as used in *B*. (*D*) Routine PCR assay used to genotype the GDNF locus. The 567-bp amplification product is generated from the mutant allele (*neo* primers p3 and p4), whereas the 338-bp product (primers p1 and p2 within the 1.0-kb deleted segment) corresponds to the wild-type allele. DNA samples and distribution in lanes shown in *D* are the same as in *C*. (M) Molecular marker 123-bp ladder (GIBCO/BRL).

bilateral (Figs. 2C and 3B). The timing of death and the lack of functional renal tissue pointed to renal failure as the more likely cause of death. Surprisingly, heterozygous GDNF$^{+/-}$ animals also showed renal abnormalities (Figs. 2B and 4B). When analyzed macroscopically, 35% (*n* = 89) of the adult heterozygotes between 3 and 5 months of age presented a wide spectrum of renal abnormalities: small kidneys with abnormal shape and/or cortical cysts or rough surface (23%), unilateral kidney agenesis or severe dysgenesis (8%), or kidneys seriously affected bilaterally (4%) (Table 1). Animals presenting the last phenotype mentioned develop a prominent renal disease that jeopardizes their life around 4 months of age. Histological analysis of kidneys from these animals revealed papillary hypoplasia, segmental cortical dysplasia, and glomerular sclerosis (data not shown). In addition, one heterozygous embryo was found with bilateral renal agenesis. This variability in phenotype may be due, at least in part, to differences in the genetic background of the parent mouse strains used in our study. Adrenal glands, gonads, and the rest of the urogenital system components appear macroscopically normal. The second consistent abnormality found in GDNF$^{-/-}$ mutant newborn pups was the presence of milk in the esophagus and often reduced progression of milk into the stomach and to the intestine, suggesting a defect in gastrointestinal peristalsis (Fig. 2F,H).

These two major abnormalities correlate with the pattern of GDNF gene expression during development. Among the tissues that show the highest expression of GDNF mRNA are the embryonic metanephros and the gastrointestinal tract (Fig. 3A) (Trupp et al. 1995; Hellmich et al. 1996; Suvanto et al. 1996), suggesting that the mutation affected the development of these tissues. Indeed, GDNF$^{-/-}$ mice lack any discernible accumulation of GDNF transcripts (Fig. 3B), strongly supporting the notion that the observed phenotypes are due to a lack of GDNF function.

Abnormal Metanephric Development in GDNF Mutant Mice Is the Result of Reduced Ureteric Bud Formation and Branching

Metanephric kidney development is critically dependent on reciprocal inductive interactions between the ureteric bud, an outgrowth of the Wolffian duct, and the adjacent metanephric mesenchyme (for review, see Saxén 1987). The mesenchymal cells induce the ureteric bud to grow and branch repeatedly, forming the renal collecting system (Grobstein 1953, 1955), and the ureteric bud induces the mesenchyme to condense into epithelial structures that differentiate into the glomeruli and proximal and distal tubules of the nephron (Grobstein 1955; Saxén 1987; Ekblom 1989). GDNF is highly expressed in the metanephric mesenchyme, in those cells that are induced to differentiate around the tip of the ureteric bud. Expression is downregulated by the epithelial differentiation of secretory nephrons (Fig. 3A) (Hellmich et al. 1996; Suvanto et al. 1996). Histological analysis of GDNF$^{-/-}$ embryos between E11.5 and E14.5 revealed that metanephric development is halted when the ureter bud is absent, even though morphologically distinct metanephric mesenchyme is present (Fig. 4C). In some GDNF$^{-/-}$ embryos, ureter buds were present and had penetrated deeply into the mesenchyme, but the number of collecting ducts, nephric condensates, and secretory nephrons was markedly reduced (not shown). Both defects, although less pronounced, were also seen in some of the heterozygous GDNF$^{+/-}$ embryos (Fig. 4B). The observed phenotypes correspond well with the process of kidney formation; without primary bud formation, renal agenesis follows. If the ureteric bud forms, but its branching is reduced or delayed, renal dysplasia results. Thus, it is reasonable to postulate that GDNF acts as a ureteric bud-forming and branching factor.

To establish a direct link between GDNF action and ureteric branching, and to provide an explanation for reduced branching in heterozygous mutants, we performed quantitative analysis of the branching pattern in explants dissected from E11.5 embryos. The growth and branching defects of the ureteric bud postulated by histological analysis were recapitulated when explanted urogenital tissues were allowed to differentiate ex vivo for 72 hours. We observed a significant reduction in the growing arborization of the renal collecting system in the heterozygotes (Fig. 4E) and a delayed or total absence of ureteric branching in the GDNF$^{-/-}$ mutants (Fig. 4F), when compared to the control explants (Fig. 4D). The pronounced differences in ureteric branching among the GDNF$^{+/+}$, GDNF$^{+/-}$, and GDNF$^{-/-}$ samples were statistically significant (Fig. 5). Quantitative data obtained from this study support the notion that GDNF is involved in inductive interactions responsible for the formation and branching of the ureteric bud, and that normal renal development may be compromised in mice with a single copy of the wild-type GDNF allele.

To examine whether GDNF was able to rescue the defects in mutant kidneys, we incubated explanted urogenital tissue in the presence of recombinant GDNF, either embedded in agarose beads or added to the media. In the presence of GDNF-soaked beads, in vitro branching of the GDNF$^{-/-}$ ureters was significantly restored (Figs. 4I and 5). Ectopic supernumerary primary ureteric buds (Fig. 4G) and aberrant induction of ureteric buds along the Wolffian duct were occasionally observed in the control GDNF$^{+/+}$ samples. Several growth factors have been implicated in the process of ureteric branching in vitro, including TGF-β1 and hepatocyte growth factor/scatter factor (HGF/SF) (Rogers et al. 1993; Cantley et al. 1994; Woolf et al. 1995). Both of these factors are expressed in the condensing mesenchyme around the time and place at which ureteric branching takes place (Lehnert and Akhurst 1988; Sonnenberg et al. 1993). In our restoration assay, we found no significant effect of either HGF/SF or TGF-β1 on branching in GDNF$^{-/-}$ explants (data not shown). Consistent with these results, neither TGF-β1 nor HGF/SF null mutant mice show obvious defects in kidney organogenesis (Dickson et al. 1955; Schmidt et al. 1995; Uehara et al. 1995). We conclude from these results that the enhanced branching effect

Figure 2. Analysis of urogenital system and digestive tube defects in GDNF newborn mutant mice. (*A–C*) Whole mounts of dissected urogenital systems of the three genotypes showing some of the phenotypes observed. (*A*) Urogenital system from a normal newborn male mouse. (*B*) Right renal agenesis in a heterozygous GDNF$^{+/-}$ female; the affected side reveals a blind-ending ureter without renal tissue at the tip (*arrow*). (*C*) Renal agenesis or severe dysgenesis observed in a GDNF$^{-/-}$ homozygous mutant male. A rudimentary kidney with its ipsilateral ureter is present; the contralateral side shows neither kidney nor ureter. Different combinations of agenesis/dysgenesis are observed in mice with this genotype. (*D–F*) Dissected digestive tubes from each genotype. (*D,E*) Wild-type and heterozygous samples, respectively, showing no macroscopic difference between them. (*F*) Digestive tract from a mutant GDNF$^{-/-}$ animal presenting presence of milk in the esophagus. Some mutant pups did not show this feature, having instead an extremely enlarged stomach and a constricted pylorus sphincter (*arrowheads*). (*G,H*) Cross-sections of colon stained with hematoxylin and eosin. Note larger size of colon and food contents in normal mice (*G*), compared to the mutant (*H*). (ad) Adrenal gland; (b) bladder; (d) duodenum; (e) epididymis; (es) esophagus; (k) kidney; (li) large intestine; (o) ovary; (s) stomach; (si) small intestine; (t) testes; (u) ureter; (ur) urethra; (ut) uterus. Bars: *A–F*, 1 mm; *G* and *H*, 100 μm.

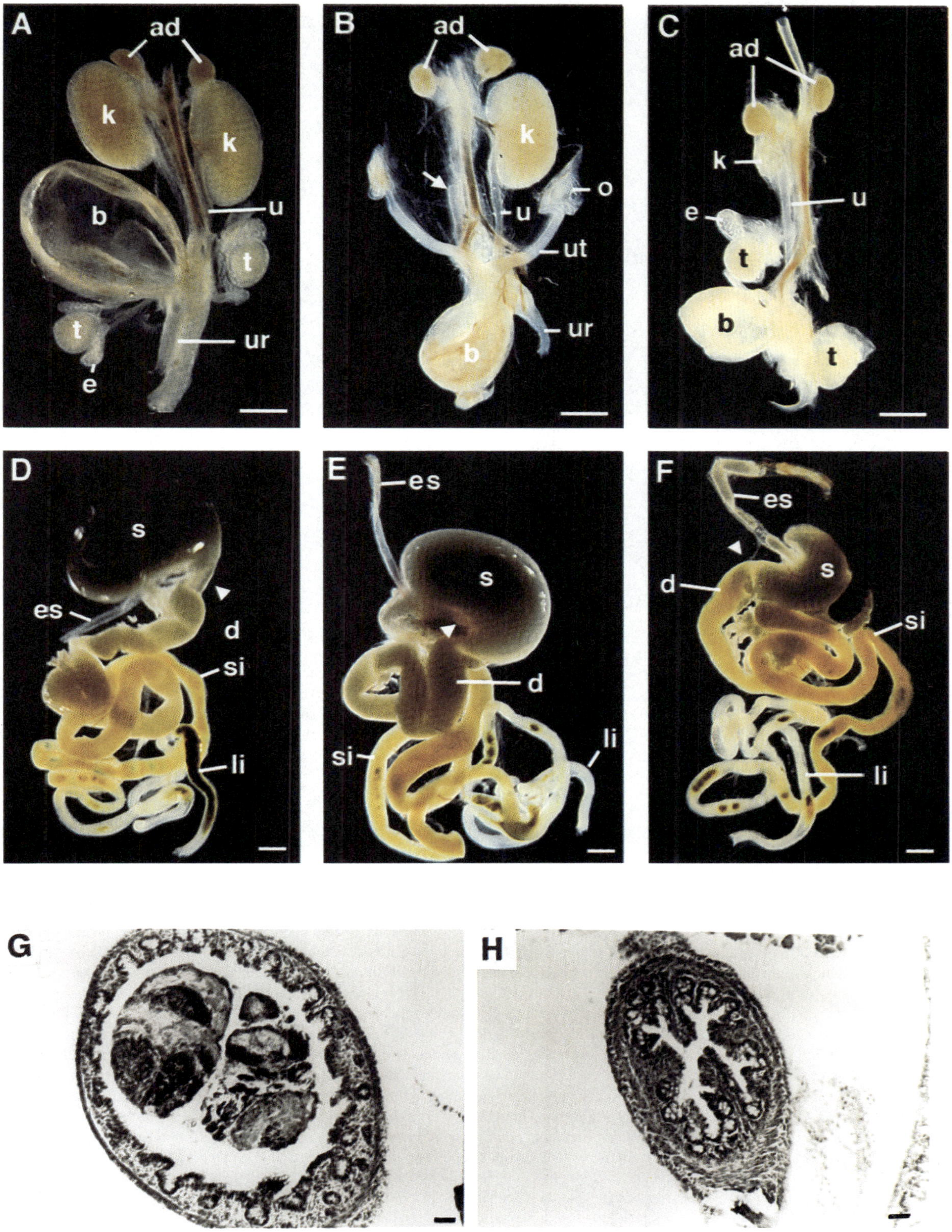

Figure 2. (*See facing page for legend.*)

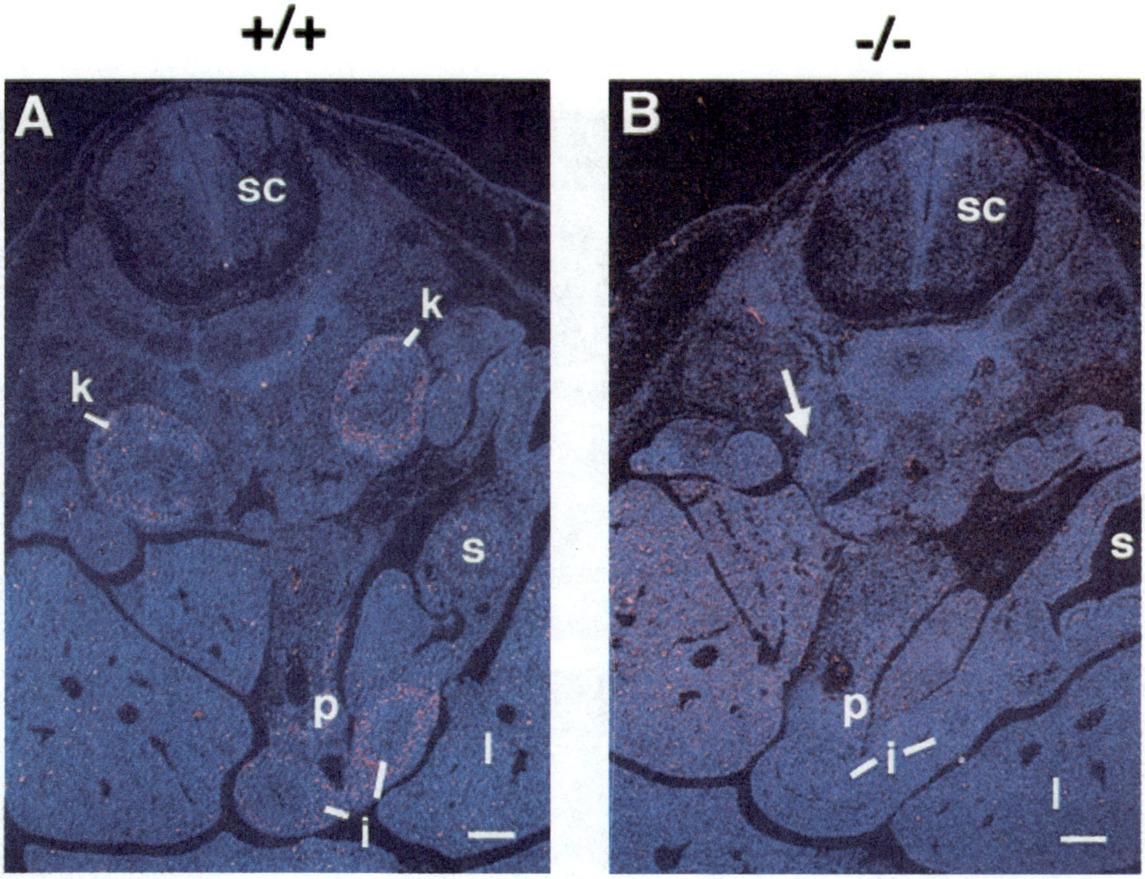

Figure 3. GDNF expression during morphogenesis of the metanephric kidney and intestinal tract of normal and mutant embryos. In situ hybridization with a ^{33}P mRNA probe was used to detect GDNF mRNA in a transverse section through the abdominal cavity of E13.5 embryos. (*A*) Transverse section of a normal $GDNF^{+/+}$ (+/+) fetus showing GDNF expression restricted to the cortical mesenchyme of the metanephric kidney (k) and the outer smooth muscle layer of the intestine (i) and stomach (s). GDNF transcripts are also seen in the pancreatic primordium (p). (*B*) Corresponding section of a mutant $GDNF^{-/-}$ (–/–) embryo lacking any detectable expression of the GDNF gene in the remnant metanephric mesenchyme (*arrow*) or the digestive tract. The ureteric buds are completely absent in this specimen, yet the metanephric mesenchyme is clearly discernible. (i) Intestine; (k) kidney; (l) liver; (p) pancreas primordium; (s) stomach; (sc) spinal cord. Bars, 200 μm.

Figure 4. Comparative analysis of the metanephros of $GDNF^{+/+}$, $GDNF^{+/-}$, and $GDNF^{-/-}$ embryos showing a ureter branching defect in the $GDNF^{+/-}$ and $GDNF^{-/-}$ genotypes and recovery using GDNF-embedded beads in ex vivo kidney cultures. (*A–C*) Hematoxylin and eosin stained transverse sections of the developing metanephros at E13.5. (*A*) Section of a normal ($GDNF^{+/+}$) kidney at the level of ureter (u) entry in the kidney; several branches of collecting ducts (cd) with condensing mesenchyme (cm) or s-shaped bodies are clearly observed. In the heterozygous $GDNF^{+/-}$ mutant kidney (*B*), the ureter enters the kidney inducing condensation (cm) and epithelization (c) of mesenchyme, but there is reduced branching (collecting ducts are not observed in the field shown). The expansion of calyx-like spaces (*asterisk*) appears more enlarged along the entering ureter. The metanephric mesenchyme (m) of the homozygous $GDNF^{-/-}$ mutant embryo (*C*) was not induced to condense due to the absence of the ureteric bud and remains histologically undifferentiated. (*D–E*) Branching defect in mutant kidney explanted at E11.5, incubated in vitro for 3 days and stained with anti-cytokeratin 18 antibodies. The number of branches of the ureter is highly reduced in the heterozygous $GDNF^{+/-}$ animal (*D*) compared with the normal phenotype (*E*). In *F*, a $GDNF^{-/-}$ mutant sample shows the Wolffian duct with complete absence of ureter budding. In this case, the tip of the Wolffian duct (*arrowhead*) has not connected with the cloaca (cl). (*G–I*) Recombinant GDNF action on ureteric branching in kidney explants. Addition of GDNF containing agarose beads (*dotted circles*) next to the explanted metanephric mesenchymes increases the branching of the Wolffian duct and ureteric bud. *G* is an example of supernumerary ureteric budding in a normal kidney explant, showing two ureters (u) that have budded from the Wolffian duct and branched toward the bead. The branching toward the GDNF source is also seen in the heterozygous (*H*) and even in the "rescued" homozygous $GDNF^{-/-}$ specimens (*I*). Note that progression of tubular structures (and progression of branching) is interrupted by the presence of the GDNF beads, resulting in a thickening of the epithelium. (c) Comma-shaped body; (cd) collecting duct; (cl) cloaca; (cm) condensing mesenchyme; (m) metanephric mesenchyme; (s) s-shaped body; (u) ureter; (wd) Wolffian duct. Bars: *A–C*, 50 μm; *D–F*, 100 μm; *G–I*, 50 μm.

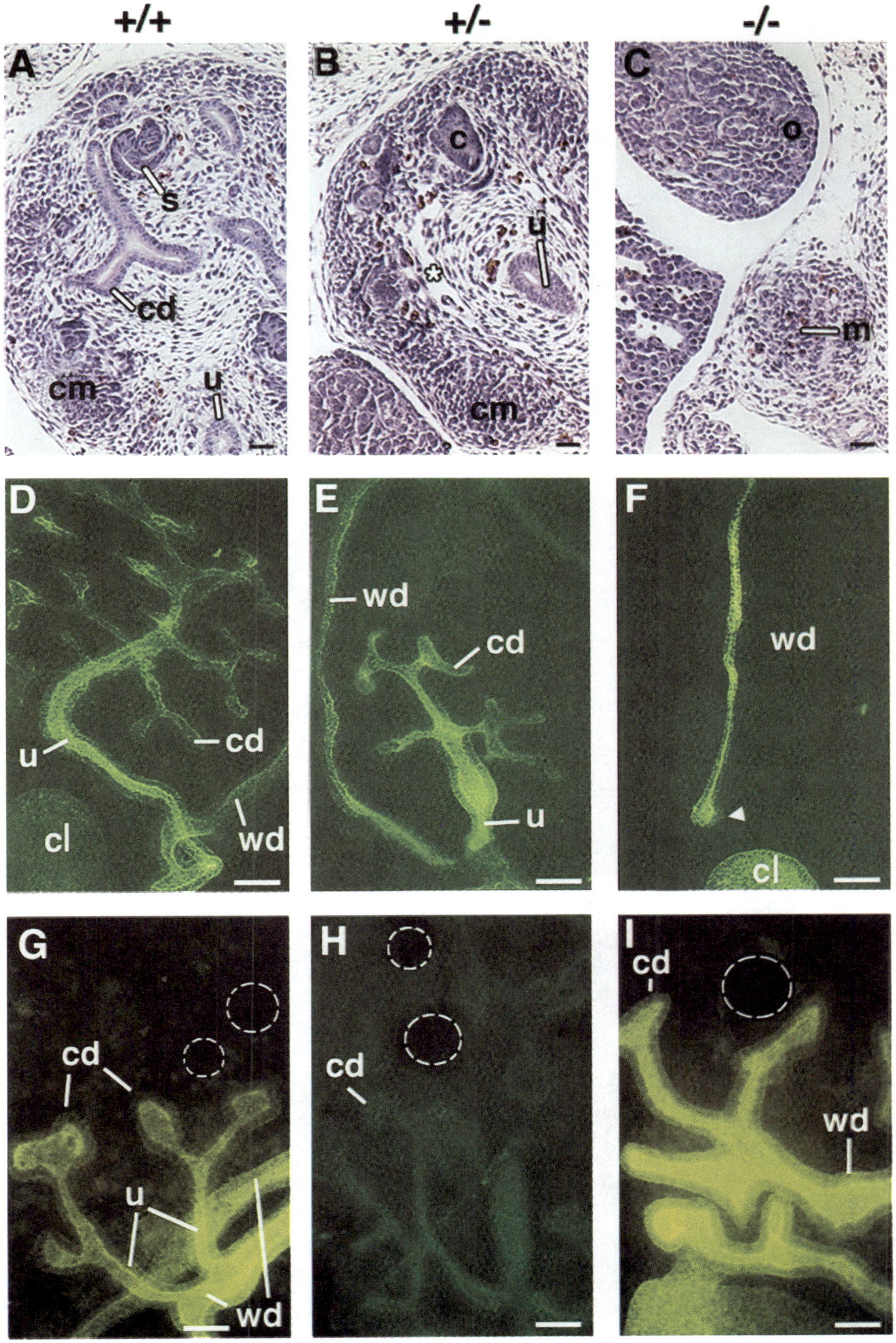

Figure 4. (*See facing page for legend.*)

Table 1. Kidney Phenotypes in Adult GDNF$^{+/-}$ Heterozygous Mutants

		Abnormal		
	Normal	small, abnormal shape and/or presence of cysts	unilateral kidney agenesis	bilateral dysplasia (sick animal)
Females	34	12	5	1
Males	24	8	2	3
Total	58	20	7	4

Phenotype is described as observed microscopically after gross dissection of 3- and 5-month-old adult animals. No significant abnormalities were found in nonmutant animals.

on mutant explants was specific for supplemented GDNF. When GDNF was added directly to the media (100 ng/ml), its action was less effective (not shown), suggesting that GDNF diffusion from the beads more closely resembles the in vivo situation. Through explant culture analysis, we demonstrated that ureteric formation and branching is a specific primary function of GDNF. Taken together, our results clearly show that GDNF is a mesenchyme-derived factor, acting in a dose-dependent manner on the growth or arborization of the ureteric bud during early stages of kidney morphogenesis.

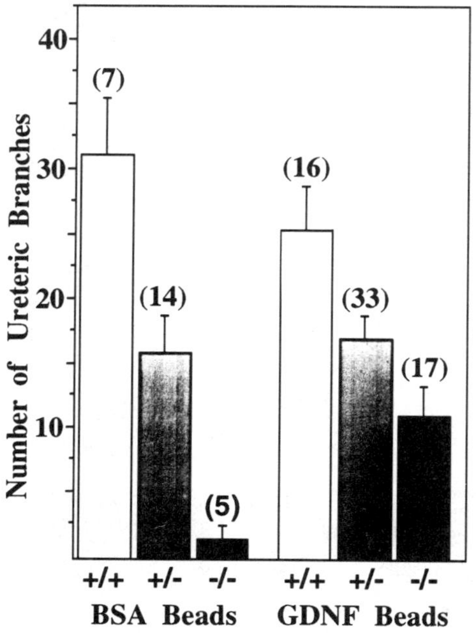

Figure 5. Quantitative assessment of ureteric branching mediated by recombinant GDNF. Shown are numbers of collecting duct tips observed in GDNF$^{+/+}$ (+/+), GDNF$^{+/-}$ (+/–), and GDNF$^{-/-}$ (–/–) urogenital specimens treated in culture in the presence of GDNF beads (100 ng/μl) or control BSA beads (1%). Values are means ± S.E.M. The difference in the number of branching tips between (+/+), (+/–), and (–/–) is statistically significant when using control BSA beads ($p<0.01$, Student t-test). Administration of GDNF in agarose beads significantly restores ureteric branching in homozygous GDNF$^{-/-}$ samples (GDNF Beads –/–) as compared to control BSA soaked beads (BSA Beads –/–) ($p<0.05$, paired t-test). Addition of GDNF to the medium was less effective. Numbers in parentheses indicate the sample size for each experimental condition.

GDNF$^{-/-}$ Mutant Mice Manifest Defective Enteric Innervation

The second phenotypic observation, an apparent defect in peristalsis in GDNF$^{-/-}$ mutant mice, raised the possibility that enteric innervation might be affected by GDNF. GDNF transcripts have been detected at high levels in the outer mesenchymal layer throughout the length of the developing gastrointestinal tract (Fig. 3A) (Hellmich et al. 1996; Suvanto et al. 1996), known to be innervated by the neural crest-derived enteric nervous system (ENS) (Yntenna and Hammond 1954; Le Douarin and Teillet 1973). Histological analysis of E18 embryos revealed that the neurons of the myenteric plexus, readily apparent in normal embryos, were absent from the intestine of mutant GDNF$^{-/-}$ (Fig. 6A,B). These observations were confirmed by immunofluorescence studies using antibodies against the neural markers choline acetyltransferase (ChAT) and neurofilament (NF). A large number of enteric parasympathetic cholinergic ganglion cells were found distributed throughout the intestine of the control GDNF$^{+/+}$ mice (Fig. 6C) or heterozygous GDNF$^{+/-}$ mutant embryos (not shown). In contrast, the GDNF$^{-/-}$ mutants were virtually devoid of these neurons (Fig. 6D). Their absence was confirmed by scoring for NF-positive neurons (data not shown). The results demonstrated that the absence of the cholinergic marker ChAT was due to lack of neurons, rather than down-regulation of ChAT expression. These data indicate a second major role for GDNF as a factor required for the proper innervation of the digestive tract. Whether GDNF is acting directly on multipotent neural crest-derived stem cells of the enteric neurons, or only on their survival after differentiation, remains to be defined.

GDNF$^{-/-}$ Mutants Do Not Reveal Major Defects in a Number of Central Nervous Tissues

On the basis of the reported neurotrophic action of GDNF, notably in dopaminergic and cholinergic neuron populations, we examined several brain areas

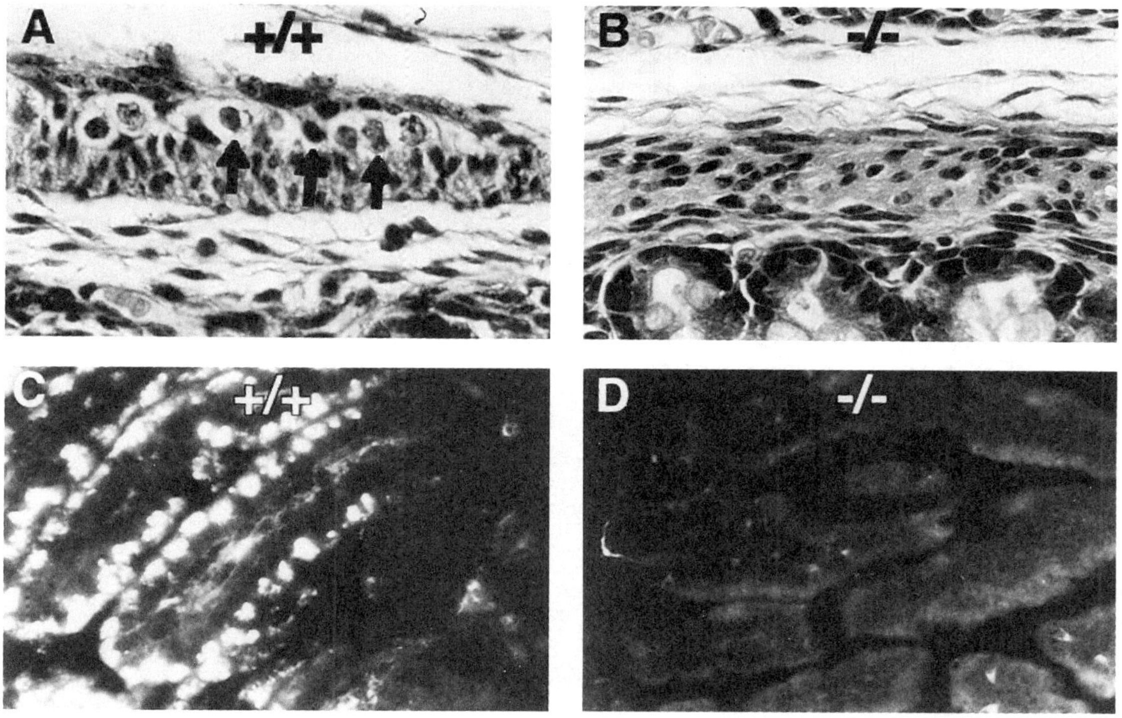

Figure 6. Histological and immunocytochemical analysis of normal and GDNF$^{-/-}$ mutant gastrointestinal tracts. (*A–D*) Sections through the gastrointestinal tract of GDNF$^{+/-}$ (*A,C*) and homozygous GDNF$^{-/-}$ mutant mice (*B,D*). (*A,B*) Hematoxylin and eosin staining of E18 embryos. The arrows in *A* point to neurons of the myenteric plexus that are identified by their large size, clear cytoplasm, and prominent nuclei. These cells are absent in *B*. Arrows point to their expected position. (*C,D*) Density and localization of enteric ganglia using antibodies directed against ChAT. Many ChAT-positive neurons are present in the intestinal wall of normal mice. None are seen in the GDNF$^{-/-}$ animals. Similar results were observed when anti-neurofilament antibodies were used, and no significant differences were observed between GDNF$^{+/+}$ and GDNF$^{+/-}$ animals (not shown). Bars: *A,B*, 25 μm; *C,D*, 32 μm.

in the GDNF mutants. Our preliminary analysis failed to reveal overt differences in either distribution, density, or tyrosine hydroxylase staining properties between substantia nigra dopamine neurons in newborn GDNF$^{-/-}$ mutant mice and the GDNF$^{+/+}$ controls. The same was true for brain stem facial motor nuclei and cortical cholinergic neurons evaluated by ChAT immunostaining. Thus, no marked developmental disturbances of these neurons could be found. Possibly, GDNF-like molecules can compensate for the lack of GDNF function in the mutant brain. Since our mutant mice die shortly after birth, we are unable to assess a possible role of GDNF in the maintenance of these neurons after birth.

GDNF is expressed in multiple areas of the developing nervous system and shows neurotrophic activity in the adult CNS (see introduction). Thus, an extensive histochemical and physiological survey of central and peripheral nervous systems in a number of inbred strains of GDNF$^{-/-}$ mutant mice will be required to precisely define the full range of nervous system abnormalities elicited by the absence of GDNF.

DISCUSSION

GDNF is well known as a potent survival factor of a variety of neural tissues, and especially of dopaminergic and motor neurons. However, the renal agenesis and hypoplasia observed in the metanephric kidney of the GDNF null mutants, and the severe depletion of enteric innervation, imply that GDNF has major effects on embryonic fields that lie outside the central nervous system.

The restoration of kidney morphogenesis by GDNF and the morphogenetic response of ureter bud branching toward GDNF-soaked beads are strong indications that GDNF controls ureteric branching and thereby a fundamental step in kidney development (Saxén 1987; Bard et al. 1994). Potential receptors for the GDNF ligand that are expressed at the time of induction at the tip of the ureteric bud (Bard et al. 1994) include the receptor tyrosine kinase molecules encoded by proto-oncogenes c-*met* (Sonnenberg et al. 1993), c-*ros* (Sonnenberg et al. 1991; Tessarollo et al. 1992), and c-*ret* (Pachnis et al. 1993). Although c-*met* has been implicated in metanephric development (Tsarfaty et al. 1994; Woolf et al. 1995), mice lacking its ligand, HGF/SF, show no defects in kidney organogenesis (Schmidt et al. 1995; Uehara et al. 1995). In contrast, direct interactions between the GDNF ligand and the c-Ret receptor are likely, based on the following observations: (1) GDNF is expressed in close vicinity of the budding ureter but not in the mesenchymal compartment (Pachnis et al. 1993); (2) as in $GDNF^{-/-}$ mutant mice, renal agenesis is observed in *c-ret*$^{-/-}$ mutants (Schuchardt et al. 1994); (3) recent studies have identified Ret as a functional GDNF receptor (for review, see Massagué 1996); (4) our preliminary results show that *c-ret* mRNA expression is down-regulated in the remnants of $GDNF^{-/-}$ ureteric buds, suggesting that maintenance of *c-ret* expression may be dependent on GDNF.

No kidney defects have been observed in heterozygous *c-ret*$^{+/-}$ mutants, yet we see a spectrum of phenotypes indicative of defective kidney development in heterozygous $GDNF^{+/-}$ mutant mice (Table 1). Conversely, we did not observe gross defects in the superior cervical ganglia of our GDNF mutant mice (data not shown), an area severely affected in *c-ret* null mutant mice (Durbec et al. 1996). These discrepancies suggest that intercellular signaling during development of these embryonic fields may not depend solely on GDNF/c-Ret interaction.

The absence of enteric neurons in $GDNF^{-/-}$ mutant mice indicates that GDNF is also necessary for the innervation of the digestive tract. Again, the lack of enteric innervation closely resembles the phenotype of *c-ret* null mutants (Schuchardt et al. 1994; Durbec et al. 1996), supporting once more the GDNF/c-Ret interaction. Future studies will determine whether GDNF is acting directly on the proliferation and specification of multipotent crest-derived cells in the gut (Gershon et al. 1993; Saffrey and Burnstock 1994), perhaps via secretion from nonneuroblastic mesenchyme (Kapur et al. 1993; Rothman et al. 1993). It also remains to be established whether development of the enteric glia is affected in $GDNF^{-/-}$ mutants (Gershon and Rothman 1991).

Some human genetic disorders, notably Hirschsprung disease (HSCR) with megacolon formation, are characterized by anomalies of enteric innervation. HSCR is caused and diagnosed as either a total loss or a segmental absence of the intrinsic enteric ganglia in the myenteric and submucosal plexi of the gastrointestinal tract. Mutations in the human RET locus that lead to intestinal aganglionosis are consistent with a genetic linkage of this locus to a familial form of HSCR (Edery et al. 1994; Romeo et al. 1994; Angrist 1995; Attie 1995; Pasini et al. 1996). On the basis of the loss of intrinsic enteric neurons in homozygous $GDNF^{-/-}$ mice, we suggest that HSCR patients should also be screened for mutations in the GDNF gene. In addition, renal dysplasias observed in mice heterozygous for the GDNF mutation are reminiscent of analogous human disorders. In man, renal dysplasias represent a spectrum of defects in renal differentiation that have not yet been linked to specific gene defects. Microdissection surveys have suggested a perturbance of ureter branching as the cause of the observed defects (Osathanondh and Potter 1966). The same cause most likely underlies the renal agenesis that we observe in $GDNF^{-/-}$ mice. This correlation should promote a thorough search for GDNF defects in patients.

In summary, in vivo characterization of the GDNF mutant phenotype and ex vivo explant culture of mutant tissues indicate that GDNF has essential roles in ureteric budding and branching, and in the innervation of the gastrointestinal tract. Similarities between GDNF and *c-ret* null phenotypes provide genetic evidence for possible Ret/GDNF receptor/ligand interactions. It is possible that the GDNF locus is implicated in human disorders in which target fields of this factor are affected.

Note Added in Proof

Results similar to those reported here have recently been reported by several laboratories (for review, see Massagué 1996).

ACKNOWLEDGMENTS

J.D. is a Basser Fellow of the Royal Australasian College of Physicians supported by the National Health and Medical Research Council of Australia. M.S. and H.S. were supported by a grant from the Academy of Finland. We thank D.F. Porter and D. Feltner for comments on drafts of this manuscript. B.J.H. thanks Nisha Srivastava and Justin Mott for assistance with histological evaluation of the nervous tissues, and acknowledges grant support from the National Institutes of Health.

REFERENCES

Angrist, M. 1995. Mutation analysis of the ret receptor tyrosine kinase in Hirschsprung's disease. *Hum. Mol. Genet.* **4:** 821.

Arenas, E., M. Trupp, P. Åkerud, and C. Ibáñez. 1995. GDNF prevents degeneration and promotes the phenotype of brain noradrenergic neurons in vivo. *Neuron* **15:** 1465.

Attie, T. 1995. Diversity of ret proto-oncogene mutations in familial and sporadic Hirschprung disease. *Hum. Mol. Genet.* **4:** 1381.

Bard, J.B.L., J.E. McConnell, and J.A. Davies. 1994. Towards a genetic basis for kidney development. *Mech. Dev.* **48:** 3.

Beck, K.D., J. Valverde, T. Alexl, K. Poulsen, B. Motaff, R.A. Vandlen, A. Rosenthal, and F. Heftl. 1995. Mesencephalic dopaminergic neurons protected by GDNF from axotony-induced degeneration in the adult brain. *Nature* **373:** 339.

Bowenkamp, K.E., A.F. Hoffan, G.A. Gerhardt, M.A. Henry, P.T. Biddle, B.J. Hoffer, and A.-C. E. Granholm. 1995. Glial cell line-derived neurotrophic factor supports survival of injured midbrain dopaminergic neurons. *J. Comp. Neurol.* **355:** 479.

Buj-Bello, A., V.L. Buchman, A. Horton, A. Rosenthal, and A.M. Davies. 1995. GDNF is an age-specific survival factor for sensory and autonomic neurons. *Neuron* **15:** 821.

Cantley, L.G, E.J. Barros, M. Gandhi, M. Rauchman, and S.K. Nigam. 1994. Regulation of mitogenesis, motogenesis, and tubulogenesis by hepatocyte growth factor in renal collecting duct cells. *Am. J. Physiol.* **267:** F271.

Choi-Lundberg, D.L. and M.C. Bohn. 1995. Ontogeny and distribution of glial cell line-derived neurotrophic factor (GDNF) mRNA in rat. *Dev. Brain Res.* **85:** 80.

Clarkson, E.D., W.M. Zawada, and C.R. Freed. 1995. GDNF reduces apoptosis in dopaminergic neurons in vitro. *NeuroReport* **7:** 145.

Cristina, N., C. Chatellard-Causse, M. Manier, and C. Feuerstein. 1995. GDNF: Existence of a second transcript in the brain. *Mol. Brain Res.* **32:** 354.

Dickson, M.C., J.S. Martin, F.M. Cousins, A.B. Kulkarni, S. Karlsson, and R.J. Akhurst. 1955. Defective haematopoiesis and vasculogenesis in transforming growth factor-β1 knock out. *Development* **121:** 1845.

Drago, J., T.J. Kilpatrick, S.A. Koblar, and P.S. Talman. 1994. Growth factors: Potential therapeutic applications in neurology. *J. Neurol. Neurosur. Psychiatry* **57:** 1445.

Durbec, P.L., L.B. Larsson-Blomberg, A. Schuchardt, F. Costantini, and V. Pachnis. 1996. Common origin and developmental dependence on c-*ret* of subsets of enteric and sympathetic neuroblasts. *Development* **122:** 349.

Ebendal, T., A. Tomac, B.J. Hoffer, and L. Olson. 1995. Glial cell line-derived neurotrophic factor stimulates fiber formation and survival in cultured neurons from peripheral autonomic ganglia. *J. Neurosci. Res.* **40:** 276.

Edery, P., S. Lyonnet, L.M. Mulligan, A. Pelet, E. Dow, L. Abel, S. Hoider, C. Nihoul-Fékété, B.A.J. Ponder, and A. Munnich. 1994. Mutations of the RET proto-oncogene in Hirschsprung's disease. *Nature* **367:** 378.

Ekblom, P. 1989. Developmental regulated conversion of mesenchyme to epithelium. *FASEB J.* **3:** 2141.

Gash, D.M., Z. Zhang, A. Ovadia, W.A. Cass, A. Yi, L. Simmerman, D. Russel, D. Martin, P.A. Lapchak, F. Collins, B.J. Hoffer, and G.A. Gerhardt. 1996. Functional recovery in Parkinsonian monkeys treated with GDNF. *Nature* **380:** 252.

Gershon, M.D. and T.P. Rothman. 1991. Enteric glia. *Glia* **4:** 195.

Gershon, M.D., A. Chalazonitis, and T.P. Rothman. 1993. From neural crest to bowel: Development of the enteric nervous system. *J. Neurobiol.* **24:** 199.

Gouin, A., E. Bloch-Gallego, H. Tanaka, A. Rosenthal, and C.E. Henderson. 1996. Transforming growth factor-beta 3, glial cell line-derived neurotrophic factor and fibroblast growth factor-2, act in different manners to promote motoneuron survival in vivo. *J. Neurosci. Res.* **15:** 454.

Grobstein, C. 1953. Inductive epithelio-mesenchymal interaction in cultured organ rudiments of the mouse. *Science* **118:** 52.

———. 1955. Inductive interactions in the development of the mouse metanephros. *J. Exp. Zool.* **130:** 319.

Harlow, E. and D. Lane. 1988. *Antibodies: A laboratory manual*, 1st edition. Cold Spring Harbor Laboratory, Cold Spring Harbor, New York.

Hellmich, H.L., L. Kos, E.S. Cho, K.A. Mahon, and A. Zimmer. 1996. Embryonic expression of glial cell-line derived neurotrophic factor (GDNF) suggests multiple developmental roles in neural differentiation and epithelial-mesenchymal interactions. *Mech. Dev.* **54:** 95.

Henderson, C.E., H.S. Phillips, R.A. Pollock, A.M. Davies, C. Lemeulle, M. Armanini, L.C. Simpson, B. Moffet, R.A. Vandlen, V.E. Koliatsos, and A. Rosenthal. 1994. GDNF: A potent survival factor for motoneurons present in peripheral nerve and muscle. *Science* **266:** 1062.

Hoffer, B.J., A. Hoffman, K. Bowenkamp, P. Huettl, J. Hudson, D. Martin, L.-F. H. Lin, and G.A. Gerhardt. 1994. Glial cell line-derived neurotrophic factor reverses toxin-induced injury to midbrain dopaminergic neurons in vivo. *Neurosci. Lett.* **182:** 107.

Hogan, B.L.M., M. Blessing, G.E. Winnier, N. Suzuki, and C.M. Jones. 1994. Growth factors in development: The role of TGF-β related polypeptide signalling molecules in embryogenesis. *Dev. Suppl.* **1994:** 53.

Hou, J.-G. G., L.-F. H. Lin, and C. Mytilineou. 1996. Glial cell line-derived neurotrophic factor exerts neurotrophic effects on dopaminergic neurons in vitro and promotes their survival and regrowth after damage by 1-methyl-4-phenylpyridinium. *J. Neurochem.* **66:** 74.

Hudson, J., A.-C. Granholm, G.A. Gerhardt, M.A. Henry, A. Hoffman, P. Biddle, N.S. Leela, L. Mackerlova, J.D. Lile, F. Collins, and B.J. Hoffer. 1995. Glial cell line-derived neurotrophic factor augments midbrain dopaminergic circuits *in vivo. Brain Res. Bull.* **36:** 425.

Kapur, R.P., C. Yost, and R.D. Palmiter. 1993. Aggregation chimera demonstrate that the primary defect responsible for a ganglionic megacolon in lethal spotted mice is not neuroblast autonomous. *Development* **117:** 993.

Kearns, C.M. and D.M. Gash. 1995. GDNF protects nigral dopamine neurons against 6-hydroxydopamine *in vivo. Brain Res.* **672:** 104.

Kingsley, D.M. 1994. The TGF-β superfamily: New members, new receptors and new genetic tests of function in different organisms. *Genes Dev.* **8:** 133.

Kreiglstein, K., C. Suter-Crazzolara, W.H. Fisher, and K. Unsicker. 1995. TGF-β superfamily members promote survival of dopaminergic neurons and protect them against MPP^+ toxicity. *EMBO J.* **14:** 736.

Le Douarin, N.M. and M.-A. Teillet. 1973. The migration of neural crest cells to the wall of the digestive tract in avian embryo. *J. Embryol. Exp. Morphol.* **30:** 31.

Lehnert, S.A. and R.J. Akhurst. 1988. Embryonic expression pattern of TGF beta type-1 RNA suggests both paracrine and autocrine mechanism of action. *Development* **104:** 263.

Li, E., T.H. Bestor, and R. Jaenisch. 1992. Targeted mutation of the DNA methyltransferase gene results in embryonic lethality. *Cell* **69:** 915.

Li, L., W. Wu, L.-F. H. Lin, M. Lei, R.W. Oppenheim, and L.J. Houenou. 1995. Rescue of adult mouse motoneurons from injury-induced cell death by glial cell line-derived neurotrophic factor. *Proc. Natl. Acad. Sci.* **92:** 9771.

Lin, L.-F.H., T.J. Zhang, F. Collins, and L.G. Armes. 1994. Purification and initial characterization of rat B49 glial cell line-derived neurotrophic factor. *J. Neurochem.* **63:** 758.

Lin, L.-F.H., D.H. Doherty, J.D. Lile, S. Bektesh, and F. Collins. 1993. GDNF: A glial cell line-derived neurotrophic factor for midbrain dopaminergic neurons. *Science* **260:** 1130.

Lindner, M.D., S.R. Winn, E.E. Baetge, J.P. Hammang, F.T. Gentile, E. Doherty, P.E. McDermott, B. Frydel, M.D. Ullman, T. Schallert, and D.F. Emerich. 1995. Implantation of encapsulated catecholamine and GDNF-producing cells in rats with unilateral dopamine depletions and parkinsonian symptoms. *Exp. Neurol.* **132:** 62.

Love, P.E., M. Tremblay, and H. Westphal. 1992. Targeting of the T-cell receptor zeta-chain gene in embryonic stem cells: Strategies for generating multiple mutations in a single gene. *Proc. Natl. Acad. Sci.* **89:** 9929.

Massagué, J. 1996. Crossing receptor boundaries. *Nature* **382:** 29.

Mount, H.T.J., D.O. Dean, J. Alberch, C.F. Dreyfus, and I.B. Black. 1995. Glial cell line-derived neurotrophic factor promotes the survival and morphologic differentiation of Purkinje cells. *Proc. Natl. Acad. Sci.* **92:** 9092.

Nagy, A. and J. Rossant. 1993. Production of completely ES cell-derived fetuses. In *Gene targeting: A practical approach* (ed. A. Joyner), p. 147. IRL Press, Oxford.

Nagy, A., J. Rossant, R. Nagy, W. Abramow-Newerly, and J.C. Roder. 1993. Derivation of completely cell culture-derived mice from early-passage embryonic stem cells. *Proc. Natl. Acad. Sci.* **90:** 8424.

Opackkajuffry, J., S. Ashworth, S.P. Hume, D. Martin, D.J. Brooks, and S.B. Blunt. 1995. GDNF protects against 6-OHDA nigrostriatal lesion. In vivo study with microdialysis and PET. *NeuroReport* **7:** 348.

Oppenheim, R.W., L.J. Houenou, J.E. Johnson, L.-F.H. Lin, L. Li, A.C. Lo, A.L. Newsome, D.M. Prevette, and S. Wang. 1995. Developing motor neurons rescued from programmed and axotomy-induced cell death by GDNF. *Nature* **373:** 344.

Osathanondh, V. and E.L. Potter. 1966. Development of human kidney as shown by microdissection. IV. Development of tubular portions of nephrons. *Arch. Pathol.* **82:** 391.

Pachnis, V., B. Mankoo, and F. Costantini. 1993. Expression of the c-*ret* proto-oncogene during mouse embryogenesis. *Development* **119:** 1005.

Pasini, B., I. Ceccherini, and G. Romeo. 1996. RET mutations in human disease. *Trends Genet.* **12:** 138.

Poulsen, K.T., M.P. Armanini, R.D. Klein, M.A. Hynes, H.S. Philips, and A. Rosenthal. 1994. TGFβ2 and TGFβ3 are potent survival factors for midbrain dopaminergic neurons. *Neuron* **13:** 1245.

Robinson, G.W., S. Wray, and K.A. Mahon. 1991. Spatially restricted expression of a member of a new family of murine Distal-less homeobox genes in the developing forebrain. *New Biol.* **3:** 1183.

Rogers, S.A., G. Ryan, A.F. Purchio, and M.R. Hammerman. 1993. Metanephric transforming growth factor β1 regulates nephrogenesis in vitro. *Am. J. Physiol.* **264:** F996.

Romeo, G., P. Ronchetto, Y. Luo, V. Barone, M. Seri, I. Ceccherini, B. Pasini, R. Bocciardi, M. Lerone, H. Kääriäinen, and G. Martucciello. 1994. Point mutations affecting the tyrosine kinase domain of the RET proto-oncogene in Hirschsprung's disease. *Nature* **367:** 377.

Rothman, T.P., D. Goldowitz, and M.D. Gershon. 1993. Inhibition of migration of neural crest-derived cells by the abnormal mesenchyme of the presumptive aganglionic bowel of *ls/ls* mice: Analysis with aggregation and interspecies chimeras. *Dev. Biol.* **159:** 559.

Saffrey, M.J. and G. Burnstock. 1994. Growth factors and the development and plasticity of the enteric nervous system. *J. Auton. Nerv. Syst.* **49:** 183.

Sariola, H., K. Holm, and S. Henke-Fahle. 1988. Early innervation of the metanephric kidney. *Development* **104:** 589.

Sauer, H., C. Rosenblad, and A. Björklund. 1995. Glial cell line-derived neurotrophic factor but not transforming growth factor β3 prevents delayed degeneration of nigral dopaminergic neurons following striatal 6-hydroxydopamine lesion. *Proc. Natl. Acad. Sci.* **92:** 8935.

Saxén, L. 1987. *Organogenesis of the kidney*. Cambridge University Press, United Kingdom.

Schaar, D.G., B-A. Sieber, C.F. Dreyfus, and I.B. Black. 1993. Regional and cell-specific expression of GDNF in rat brain. *Exp. Neurol.* **124:** 368.

Schmidt, C., F. Bladt, S. Goedecke, V. Brinkmann, W. Zschische, M. Sharpe, E. Gherardi, and C. Birchmeier. 1995. Scatter factor/hepatocyte growth factor is essential for liver development. *Nature* **373:** 699.

Schuchardt, A., V. D'Agati, L. Larsson-Blomberg, F. Costantini, and V. Pachnis. 1994. Defects in the kidney and enteric nervous system of mice lacking the tyrosine kinase receptor Ret. *Nature* **367:** 380.

Sonnenberg, E., D. Meyer, K.M. Weidner, and C. Birchmeier. 1993. Scatter factor/hepatocyte growth factor and its receptor, the c-*met* tyrosine kinase, can mediate a signal exchange between mesenchyme and epithelia during mouse development. *J. Cell Biol.* **123:** 223.

Sonnenberg, E., A. Gödecke, B. Walter, F. Bladt, and C. Birchmeier. 1991. Transient and locally restricted expression of the *ros1* protooncogene during mouse development. *EMBO J.* **10:** 3693.

Springer, J.E., X. Mu, L.W. Bergmann, and J.Q. Trojanowski. 1994. Expression of GDNF mRNA in rat and human nervous tissue. *Exp. Neurol.* **127:** 167.

Springer, J.E., J.L. Seeburger, J. He, A. Gabrea, E.P. Blankenhorn, and L.W. Bergman. 1995. cDNA sequence and differential mRNA regulation of two forms of glial cell line-derived neurotrophic factor in Schwann cells and rat skeletal muscle. *Exp. Neurol.* **131:** 47.

Strömberg, I., L. Björklund, M. Johansson, A. Tomac, F. Collins, L. Olson, B. Hoffer, and C. Humpel. 1993. Glial cell line-derived neurotrophic factor is expressed in the developing but not adult striatum and stimulates developing dopamine neurons *in vivo*. *Exp. Neurol.* **124:** 401.

Suter-Crazzolara, C. and K. Unsicker. 1994. GDNF is expressed in two forms in many tissues outside the CNS. *NeuroReport* **5:** 2486.

Suvanto, P., J.O. Hiltunen, U. Arumäe, M. Moshnyakov, H. Sariola, K. Sainio, and M. Saarma. 1996. Localization of glial cell line-derived neurotrophic factor (GDNF) mRNA in embryonic rat by *in situ* hybridization. *Eur. J. Neurosci.* **8:** 816.

Tessarollo, L., L. Nagarajan, and L.F. Parada. 1992. c-*ros:* The vertebrate homolog of the sevenless tyrosine kinase receptor is tightly regulated during organogenesis in the mouse embryonic development. *Development* **115:** 11.

Tomac, A., E. Lindqvist, L.-F. H. Lin, S.O. Ögren, D. Young, B.J. Hoffer, and L. Olson. 1995a. Protection and repair of the nigrostriatal dopaminergic system by GDNF *in vivo*. *Nature* **373:** 335.

Tomac, A., J. Widenfalk, L.-F. H. Lin, T. Kohno, T. Ebendal, B.J. Hoffer, and L. Olson. 1995b. Retrograde axonal transport of glial cell line-derived neurotrophic factor in the adult nigrostriatal system suggests a trophic role in the adult. *Proc. Natl. Acad. Sci.* **92:** 8274.

Trupp, M., M. Rydén, H. Jörnvall, H. Funakoshi, T. Timmusk, E. Arenas, and C. Ibáñez. 1995. Peripheral expression and biological activities of GDNF, a new neurotrophic factor for avian and mammalian peripheral neurons. *J. Cell Biol.* **130:** 137.

Tsarfaty, I., S. Rong, J.H. Resau, S. Rulong, P.P. da Silva, and G.F. Vande Woude. 1994. The Met proto-oncogene mesenchymal to epithelial cell conversion. *Science* **263:** 98.

Tybulewicz, V.L.J., C.E. Crawford, P.K. Jackson, R.T. Bronson, and R.C. Mulligan. 1991. Neonatal lethality and lymphopenia in mice with a homozygous disruption of the c-*abl* proto-oncogene. *Cell* **65:** 1153.

Uehara, Y., O. Minowa, C. Mori, K. Schiota, J. Kuno, T. Noda, and N. Kitamura. 1995. Placental defect and embryonic lethality in mice lacking hepatocyte growth factor/scatter factor. *Nature* **373:** 702.

Vainio, S., I. Karavanova, A. Jowett, and I. Thesleff. 1993. Identification of BMP-4 as a signal mediating secondary induction between epithelial and mesenchymal tissues during early tooth development. *Cell* **75:** 45.

Virtanen, I., M. Miettinen, V.-P. Letho, A.-L. Kariniemi, and R. Paasivuo. 1985. Diagnostic applications of monoclonal antibodies to intermediate filaments. *Ann. Rev. N.Y. Acad. Sci.* **455:** 635.

Wall, N.A. and B.L.M. Hogan. 1994. TGF-β related genes in development. *Curr. Opin. Genet. Dev.* **4:** 517.

Woolf, A.S., M. Kolatsi-Joannou, P. Hardman, E. Andermarcher, C. Moorby, L.G. Fine, P.S. Jat, M.D. Noble, and E. Gherardi. 1995. Roles of hepatocyte growth factor/scatter factor and the Met receptor in the early development of the metanephros. *J. Cell Biol.* **128:** 171.

Yamamoto, M., G. Sobue, K. Yamamoto, S. Terao, and T. Mitsuma. 1996. Expression of glial-cell line-derived growth-factor messenger-RNA in the spinal cord and muscle in amyotrophic-lateral-sclerosis. *Neurosci. Lett.* **204:** 117.

Yan, Q., C. Matheson, and O.T. Lopez. 1995. *In vivo* neurotrophic effects of GDNF on neonatal and adult facial motor neurons. *Nature* **373:** 341.

Yntenna, C.L. and W.S. Hammond. 1954. The origin of intrinsic ganglia of trunk viscera from vagal neural crest in the chick embryo. *J. Comp. Neurol.* **101:** 515.

Zurn, A.D., E.E. Baetge, J.P. Hammang, S.A. Tan, and P. Aebischer. 1994. Glial cell line-derived neurotrophic factor (GDNF), a new neurotrophic factor for motoneurones. *NeuroReport* **6:** 113.

Neuregulins as Potential Drugs for Neurological Disorders

M.A. MARCHIONNI,[1] C.J. KIRK,[1] I.J. ISAACS,[1] C.J. HOBAN,[1] N.K. MAHANTHAPPA,[1] E.S. ANTON,[2] C. CHEN,[1] F. WASON,[1] D. LAWSON,[1] F.P.T. HAMERS,[3] P.D. CANOLL,[4] R. REYNOLDS,[5] B. CANNELLA,[6] D. MEUN,[1] W.F. HOLT,[1] W.D. MATTHEW,[2] L.-E. CHEN,[7] W.H. GISPEN,[3] C.S. RAINE,[6] J.L. SALZER,[4] AND D.I. GWYNNE[1]

[1]Cambridge NeuroScience, Inc., Cambridge, Massachusetts 01239; [2]Department of Neurobiology, Duke University Medical Center, Durham, North Carolina 27710; [3]Division of Molecular Neurobiology, University of Utrecht, 3584 CH Utrecht, The Netherlands; [4]Department of Cell Biology, New York University Medical School, New York, New York 10016; [5]Department of Anatomy, Charing Cross and Westminster College, London W68RF, United Kingdom; [6]Department of Pathology (Neuropathology), Albert Einstein Medical College, Bronx, New York 10461; [7]Department of Surgery, Duke University Medical Center, Durham, North Carolina 27710

Neurological disorders affect the principal functions of neural cells. Imbalances in electrical or metabolic activity, or aberrant regulation of cellular survival, proliferation, and differentiation can result in a variety of neurological deficits. Many lines of evidence drawn from developmental biology, genetics, and pharmacology support the concept that signaling via peptide growth factors and receptor tyrosine kinases regulates numerous essential neural cell functions. Thus, neurotrophic growth factors have potential to become drugs for treatment of neurological disorders. Indeed, several growth factors currently are being evaluated in clinical trials for amyotrophic lateral sclerosis, peripheral neuropathies, and multiple sclerosis (Hefti 1994).

One growth factor signaling system receiving growing attention is that involving the neuregulins and the neuregulin receptors erbB2, erbB3, and erbB4 (for review, see Caraway and Burden 1995; Lemke 1996). As growth factors, neuregulins have deep roots in neurobiology. The discovery and purification of soluble Schwann cell mitogens (glial growth factor, [GGF]; Raff et al. 1978; Brockes et al. 1980; Lemke and Brockes 1984; Goodearl et al. 1993) led to the identification of GGF coding sequences (Marchionni et al. 1993). Interest in neuronal signals involved in neuromuscular transmission spurred the identification of the acetylcholine receptor-inducing activity (ARIA; Jessell et al. 1979; Falls et al. 1993). Sequencing of these and other neuregulins, which were discovered as specific activators of the orphan receptor tyrosine kinase erbB2 (e.g., neu differentiation factor [NDF], Peles et al. 1992; Wen et al. 1992; heregulins, Holmes et al. 1992) revealed that these various signaling proteins all are products of a single neuregulin gene. The name neuregulin, which refers to the entire group of these gene products, reflects signaling through *neu* and related receptors and points to a significant involvement of these molecules in regulating neural development and function.

The neuregulins belong to the epidermal growth factor (EGF) superfamily and exhibit a great variety of membrane-attached and secreted isoforms generated by alternative splicing and usage of three distinct promoters (Fig. 1). This diversity of isoforms may support multiple modes of delivering these peptide growth factors to target cells, such as paracrine, juxtacrine, endocrine, and autocrine modes of signaling. To what extent such diversity in form implies diversity in function is an area of active investigation.

Neuregulins mediate their biological activities through members of the EGF receptor family. These include the products of the erbB2, erbB3, and erbB4 genes (Schechter et al. 1984; Kraus et al. 1989; Plowman et al. 1993). Based on the bulk of available biochemical evidence: erbB2 cannot bind neuregulins with high affinity without aid of a co-receptor; erbB3 binds effectively, but cannot transduce a signal; and only erbB4 is capable of both binding and signaling. Hence, erbB2 and erbB3 are thought to collaborate as a heterodimer, whereas at least in some contexts, erbB4 can function independently. Disruptions of the neuregulin gene (Meyer and Birchmeier 1995), erbB2 (Lee et al. 1995), and erbB4 (Gassmann et al. 1995) have shed additional light on the molecular interactions of this signaling system, and indicate that all three genes are essential for development of both the heart and the hind brain (for reviews, see Carraway and Burden 1995; Marchionni 1995).

Neuregulins are expressed by both peripheral and central neurons (Marchionni et al. 1993; Chen et al. 1994; Meyer and Birchmeier 1994; Corfas et al. 1995) and are involved in numerous interactions between neurons and glia. Neuregulin signaling promotes survival and proliferation of peripheral and central glial cells and their progenitors (Marchionni et al. 1993; Pinkas-Kramarski et al. 1994; Vartanian et al. 1994; Dong et al. 1995; Levi et al. 1995; Morissey et al. 1995; Rutkowski et al. 1995; Canoll et al. 1996; Cheng and Mudge 1996; Grinspan et al. 1996; Trachtenburg and

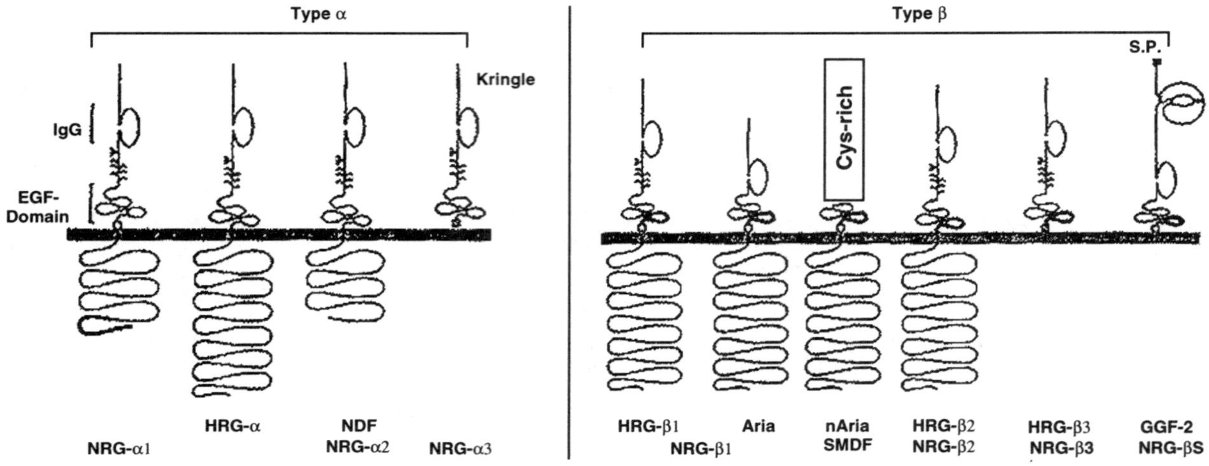

Figure 1. Schematic representation of the neuregulins. Common structural elements include an immunoglobulin fold and one EGF-like domain. The diversity of forms is generated by several molecular mechanisms: (1) Alternate promoter usage leads to at least three mutually exclusive amino termini—one containing a signal peptide and a potential kringle domain, a second with a hydrophilic sequence, and a third that has eight closely spaced cysteine residues (Ho et al. 1995). (2) At least three distinct carboxyl termini are used, which are derived from unique stop codons, 3′-untranslated sequences, and polyadenylation sites. (3) Alternative splicing generates forms that either contain or lack a linker sequence rich in serines and threonines that separate the Ig domain and the EGF-like domain, and produces two alternative EGF-like folds (α and β), which differ in the third cysteine loop. Several alternative cleavage sites adjacent to the transmembrane segment also are encoded by different DNA sequences. (Adapted from Peles and Yarden 1993.)

Thompson 1996) and restricts multipotential neural crest stem cells to a glial cell fate (Shah et al. 1994). One or more of these biological activities presumably account for the absence of erbB3-expressing Schwann cells along outgrowing peripheral axons in neuregulin-deficient mice (Meyer and Birchmeier 1995). Recently, neuregulins have been shown to stimulate the expression of soluble neurotrophic activities in nonneuronal cells of embryonic sympathetic ganglia (Verdi et al. 1996) and in Schwann cells cultured from neonatal sciatic nerve (Mahanthappa et al. 1996). Thus, it seems that neuregulins also participate in a trophic support loop between neurons and glia, which may have a significant role in neural development and function. For some CNS neurons, such as retinal ganglion cells, neuregulins may act directly, possibly via an autocrine signaling mechanism, to promote neuronal survival (Bermingham-McDonogh et al. 1996).

The involvement of neuregulins in regulating cellular differentiation has been studied in a variety of contexts, particularly in nerve/muscle interactions. The localized expression of ion channel genes, such as those encoding acetylcholine receptors and voltage-gated sodium channels, at the neuromuscular junction is induced by neuregulins (Corfas et al. 1993; Falls et al. 1993; Chu et al. 1995; Jo et al. 1995). In peripheral nerve, the expression of the myelination program appears to be regulated by signals present on the axon surface (see, e.g., Jessen and Mirsky 1991), and some recent studies suggest that neuregulins may be involved there as well. Whether neuregulins act to promote or to repress this important aspect of Schwann cell differentiation has not yet been resolved. Although neuregulin (NDFβ) can activate the transcription factor krox-20 (Murphy et al. 1996), which is required for expression of late myelin proteins (Topilko et al. 1994), it seems that detectable myelin protein zero (P0) expression in cultured Schwann cells can be shut off following treatment with neuregulin (Cheng and Mudge 1996). Finally, neuregulins also influence cellular morphogenesis of both oligodendrocytes (Vartanian et al. 1994; Canoll et al. 1996) and retinal ganglion cells (Bermingham-McDonogh et al. 1996).

We have used both in vitro and in vivo approaches to further characterize the neural activities of a secreted form of neuregulin, recombinant human glial growth factor 2 (rhGGF2). The studies have focused on both peripheral and central systems, and here we summarize recent results which indicate that neuregulin/rhGGF2 may have clinical utility in the treatment of certain neurological disorders.

EXPERIMENTAL PROCEDURES

rhGGF2, which corresponds to the structure designated GGF2 (or NRG-βS) in Figure 1, was produced in a stably transformed CHO cell line, was purified by several column chromatography steps, and was judged to be more than 98% pure by the criteria of SDS-PAGE and reverse-phase high-performance liquid chromatography (HPLC).

RESULTS

Neuregulin[1] Promotes Multiple Schwann Cell Functions

Schwann cells have important roles in the development, maintenance, and repair of peripheral nerves. In addition to proliferation, Schwann cell activities that are necessary to support peripheral nerve repair include migration, synthesis of neurotrophic factors, and the ensheathment and myelination of axons. Data from in vitro studies presented here show not only that rhGGF2 is a Schwann cell mitogen, but also that it stimulates migration and elicits the production of soluble neurotrophic activity from Schwann cells that support peripheral neuron survival and outgrowth.

Regeneration of transected peripheral nerves provides a tractable approach to model recovery from neural injuries or disease, and entubulation is a common method of bridging experimentally created peripheral nerve gaps in vivo. By suturing the proximal and distal nerve stumps of a transected nerve to opposite ends of a biocompatible (e.g., polyethylene) tube, nerve regeneration can be facilitated. In this context, the therapeutic value of various agents to this process can be evaluated by filling the tube with the agent of interest. In an effort to develop an in vitro model of this paradigm, a "tube culture" system was developed in which a portion of a peripheral ganglion (superior cervical ganglion, [SCG]) is placed at one end of a polyethylene tube filled with medium containing various concentrations of rhGGF2 in a three-dimensional (type I collagen) matrix. The ganglion serves to mimic an entubulated proximal nerve stump, and the tube provides an environment in which cellular outgrowth is physically restricted to a geometry relevant to nerve regeneration in vivo.

Schwann cells and neurites were analyzed in this culture system in varying concentrations of rhGGF2. In low doses of rhGGF2 (submaximal for stimulation of proliferation), Schwann cells were identified (by S100 staining) at greater distances from the explant after 5–10 days in culture as compared to control cultures (Fig. 2A,B). Additional studies on peripheral nerve cryosections and Schwann cell cultures on poly-D-lysine-coated plastic dishes with rhGGF2 immobilized on heparin beads support the interpretation that neuregulin/rhGGF2 stimulated migration of Schwann cells at doses that were submaximal for stimulating proliferation (Mahanthappa et al. 1996).

Neurite outgrowth also increased in the presence of rhGGF2 in the collagen tube culture system. The number of neurites (stained with anti-tubulin βIII) counted at various distances from the ganglion (on day 10) is shown in Figure 2C. It is unlikely that the effects of rhGGF2 on neurite outgrowth are direct. rhGGF2 neither promoted SCG neuron survival when administered without nerve growth factor (NGF), nor shifted NGF dose-responsiveness, and there was no obvious effect of rhGGF2 on neurite outgrowth (Mahanthappa et al. 1996). Instead, as shown in Figure 2D, rhGGF2 induced the production of neurotrophic activity by Schwann cells. This induced activity, which increased with dose of rhGGF2, stimulated the survival of isolated SCG neurons. Because of the absence of an observable effect of rhGGF2 on neurite outgrowth of purified SCG neurons, we suggest that the neuritic outgrowth observed in the SCG explant cultures derives from neurotrophic activity induced in Schwann cells present in the explant (see Fig. 2C).

These results demonstrate that neuregulins can affect the recovery of peripheral nerve from damage in several ways: by increasing the number of Schwann cells at the injury site acting through stimulation of migration and proliferation, and by providing trophic support for neurons indirectly through Schwann cells. Since Schwann cells are known to secrete many neurotrophic factors, this approach may hold a significant advantage over the use of any single neurotrophic factor that directly targets a selective subset of peripheral neurons.

Neuregulin Promotes Recovery from Peripheral Nerve Injury

A sciatic nerve transection model was selected as the initial paradigm to examine the effects of rhGGF2 in recovery from nerve damage. A 10-mm gap, bridged by a nerve guide tube, was used as a standard assay, and rhGGF2 was delivered in a slow-release formulation from a membrane sliver positioned in the center of the guide tube. The resulting regenerated nerve completely surrounded the rhGGF2-impregnated membrane under these conditions. rhGGF2-containing membrane slivers induced a statistically significant increase (>2.6-fold) in the number of myelinated axons over control membrane slivers (Fig. 3).

A complicating factor in the interpretation of these results was that the presence of the membrane slivers appeared to inhibit the capacity of the system to reach the maximum potential number of myelinated axons. The presence of control slivers (lacking rhGGF2) inhibited myelinated axon formation by more than 50%, versus saline-filled tube controls. rhGGF2, however, overcame this inhibitory effect. Numbers of myelinated axons in the tubes containing rhGGF2-treated membranes were approximately equivalent to saline-filled tube controls. Thus, it appears that rhGGF2 has the potential to promote peripheral nerve regeneration if an appropriate delivery system (material, geometry, etc.) can be designed and implemented.

A second model of peripheral nerve injury that was used to evaluate rhGGF2 was sciatic nerve crush in

---

[1]Neuregulin as used here refers to the bioactive entity associated with all forms of neuregulin gene products that contain the β type of EGF-like fold. From this perspective, neuregulin can be viewed as a growth factor that is a composite of the known isoforms. In reference to the work described here, we consider rhGGF2 as the prototype neuregulin (for further discussion of this issue, see Lemke 1996).

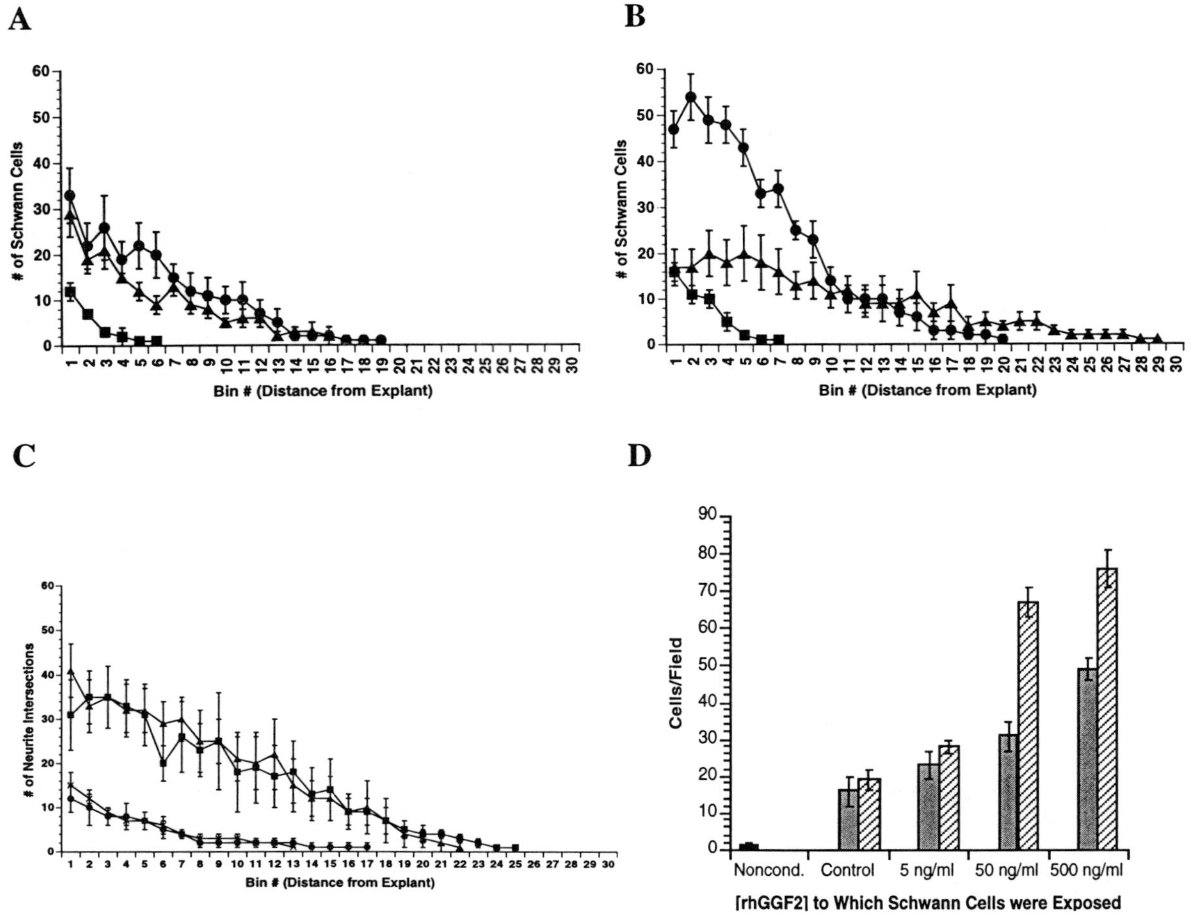

Figure 2. Neuregulins promote multiple Schwann cell functions. Superior cervical ganglia were positioned in one end of collagen-filled tubes containing either control media (*A*) or media containing 5 ng/ml rhGGF2 (*B*). The two panels quantify Schwann cell number (mean ± S.E.M., $n = 6$–7) and distance (1 bin = 50 µm) traveled from the explant at 2, 5, and 10 days (*boxes*, *circles*, *triangles*, respectively). (*C*) Effect of 0, 5, 10, and 500 ng/ml rhGGF2 (*boxes*, *circles*, *triangles*, *diamonds*, respectively) on the number (mean ± S.E.M., $n = 6$–7) of neurites crossing at various distances from the explant (on day 10). (*D*) Schwann cells (initial plating densities: 1×10^5 cells, *shaded bars*; 5×10^5 cells, *cross-hatched bars*) were cultured in rhGGF2 at various concentrations and media conditioned for 5 days were collected from the cultures, then used to culture SCG neurons in a 2-day survival assay (mean ± S.E.M., $n = 10$). (Adapted, with permission, from Mahanthappa et al. 1996.)

adult rats (Chen et al. 1993). In the model, a 100*g* force was applied over a 5-mm segment of exposed sciatic nerve for 2 hours to crush the nerve. Animals were administered either rhGGF2 or vehicle via subcutaneous injection on 5 consecutive days, beginning 1 day prior to nerve crush, and recovery of motor function was monitored until 48 days post-injury. Quantitative assessment of functional recovery from the nerve crush was performed twice per week using a walking track analysis. The parameters from the walking track that were recorded (from the injured and the uninjured limbs) were footprint length, and the distances between the first and fifth, and the second and fourth, pairs of toes. A sciatic functional index (SFI), which was derived from the measurements and normalized to a 100 point scale, was used to compare the motor function of rhGGF2-treated and placebo groups. The conditions of nerve crush were controlled precisely (Chen et al. 1993) and produced a highly reproducible motor deficit. From the day of injury until day 7, both groups were impaired to the maximum extent (as obtained with the 100*g* x 2-hr crush) and showed no signs of improvement. Signs of improvement were evident by day 10: The rhGGF2-treated group had recovered nearly 30% of normal motor function compared to 10% recovery for the placebo group. Over the ensuing 2–3 weeks, both groups continued to improve toward normal levels of motor function, with the rhGGF2-treated group advancing roughly 4–6 days ahead of the pace of the placebo group. Thus, subcutaneously administered rhGGF2 accelerated the rate of regeneration following peripheral nerve injury.

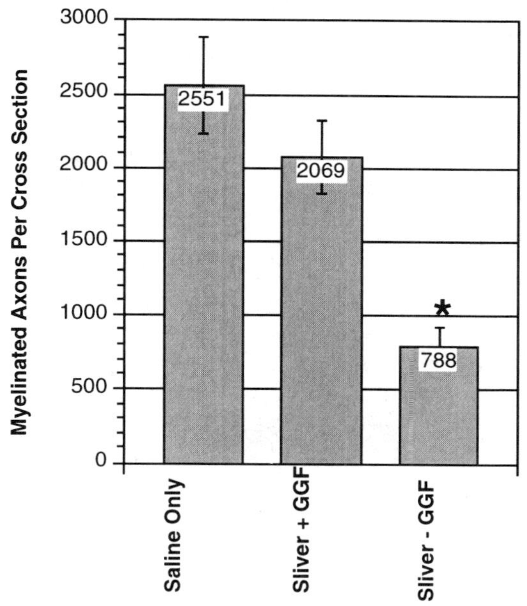

Figure 3. Evaluation of neuregulin in a rat model of sciatic nerve transection. The number of regenerated myelinated axons (thin sections stained with toluidine blue) at the midpoint of a polyethylene tube (10 mm nerve gap), at 4 weeks post-injury.

Neuregulin Prevents Drug-induced Peripheral Neuropathy in Rats

Several cancer chemotherapies induce peripheral neuropathies. For example, sensory neuropathy occurs in patients undergoing prolonged cancer chemotherapy with cisplatin and becomes a barrier to continued treatment. Hence, therapeutic agents that might slow or prevent the development of such drug-induced neuropathy would be of benefit to cancer patients. Thus, rhGGF2 was tested in a rat model of cisplatin-induced neuropathy (Gerritsen Van der Hoop et al. 1988). A 10-week study was done on four groups of young age-matched rats (n = 12), where one group was untreated and three groups received cisplatin (twice per week for 10 weeks at 1 mg per intraperitoneal injection) to induce neuropathy plus various doses of rhGGF2. The dosing regimen for rhGGF2 was three times per week (for 10 weeks) via subcutaneous injection at 0, 0.1, and 0.3 mg/kg. To assess the extent of neurological deficits from cisplatin and the protection afforded with rhGGF2 treatment, sensory nerve conduction velocities (SNCV) were measured at weeks 0, 4, 6, 8, and 10. The untreated control group showed a continuous increase in SNCV from 45 m/sec to 60 m/sec, as expected for thriving young animals over the 10-week time course. The effects of cisplatin were evident at week 6 as the SNCV leveled off at 55 m/sec, then became much more pronounced over the following 4 weeks, as the SNCV slowed to roughly 50 m/sec. Treatment with rhGGF2 showed a dose-dependent protection from cisplatin-induced neuropathy, and at 0.3 mg/kg the growth factor was completely protective. At this dosing level no differences were observed in the SNCV measurements between rhGGF2-treated and untreated control (without cisplatin) groups.

The pleiotrophic effects of rhGGF2 on Schwann cells in culture described above, and the results of tests in animal models of peripheral neuropathy and nerve injury, suggest that neuregulin might be efficacious in a variety of neurological disorders of the peripheral nervous system. As a first step toward exploring the potential of neuregulins in CNS disorders, we have focused our attention on oligodendrocytes and models of demyelinating disease.

Neuregulin Is a Potent Mitogen for Cells of the Oligodendrocyte Lineage

We have investigated the effects of rhGGF2 on the proliferation, survival, and differentiation of oligodendrocyte progenitors, which were established in culture from neonatal rat cortex as described previously (Louis et al. 1992). A highly purified population of O-2A progenitor cells depleted of neurons and astrocytes was expanded in media supplemented with B104 conditioned media (CM). These cells had a bipolar morphology and remained highly proliferative, and more than 95% of the cells expressed markers of O-2A progenitors, vimentin and A2B5, but not the markers of more mature cells in the lineage, such as O4, O1, or GFAP. When switched to a defined medium plus 0.5% serum (DM^+), the cells rapidly acquired a multipolar morphology and began to express the O4 antigen as an early sign of differentiation. After several days, the cells developed a complex network of processes and began to express the O1 antigen, which is characteristic of mature oligodendrocytes. By 3 days in DM^+, essentially all cells were $O4^+$ and more than 50% were $O1^+$. This process of differentiation coincided with reduced proliferation: The initial labeling index of O-2A progenitor cells grown in B104 conditioned media was greater than 50% after a 4-hour pulse of BrdU, but decreased to less than 5% when cells were grown in DM^+ for 3 days.

To characterize the effects of rhGGF2, cells grown in DM^+ for 3 days were treated with 200 ng/ml of rhGGF2 for 16 hours, the last 4 hours in the presence of BrdU. Cells were then fixed and stained for O4, O1, and BrdU. The results, shown in Figure 4, demonstrate that all cells remained $O4^+$ (panel B), but most rhGGF2-treated cells had a less complex morphology than control cells (panel A), with fewer and flatter processes suggestive of a less mature phenotype. In addition, significantly few $O1^+$ cells were present after rhGGF2 treatment compared to controls (panels C and D). There was a substantial increase in the number of BrdU-positive nuclei in the treated compared to the control cells (panels E and F). The labeling index was determined separately for $O4^+$ and $O1^+$ cells (Fig. 4G),

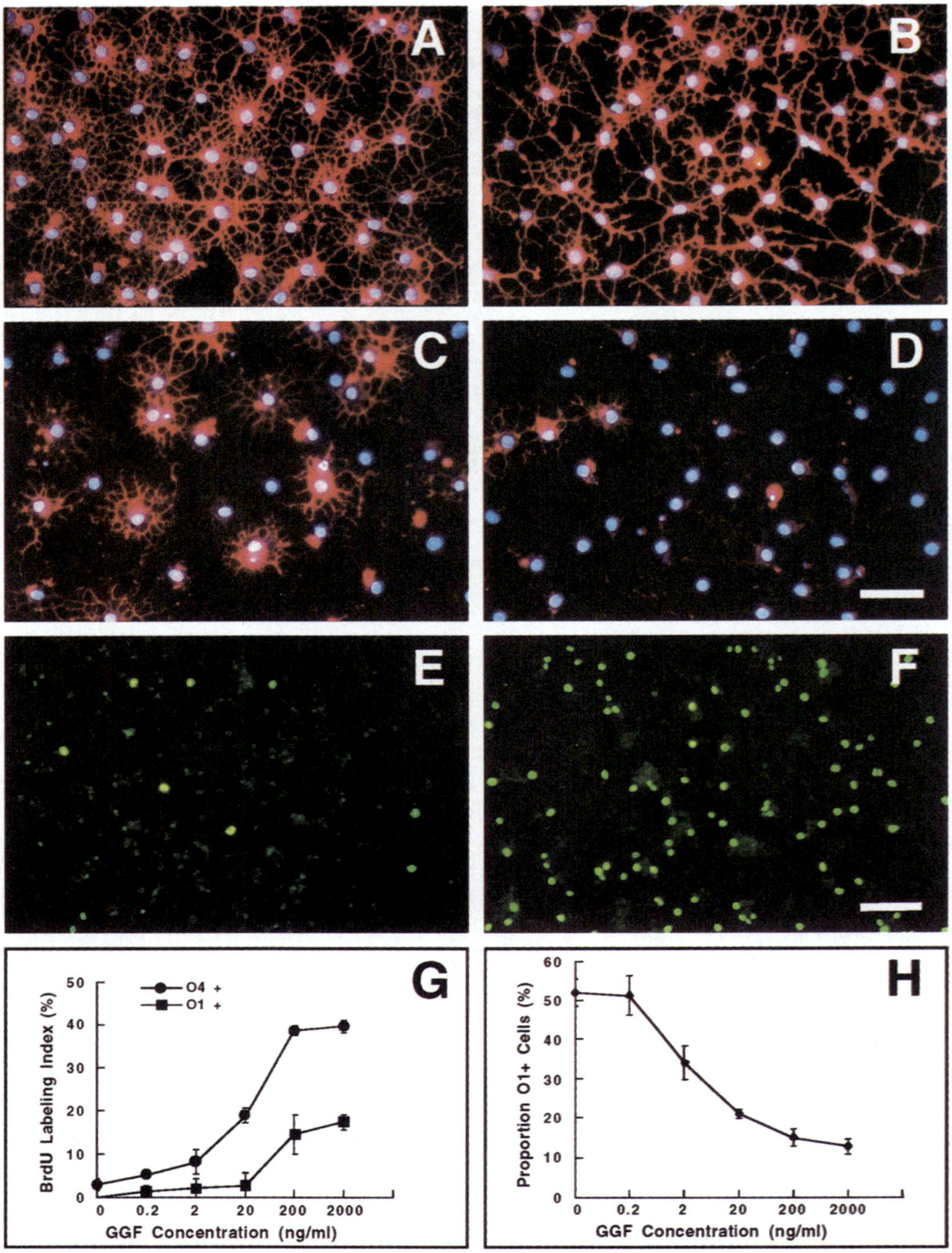

Figure 4. Pleiotropic effects of rhGGF2 on cells in the oligodendrocyte lineage. (*A–E*). Effects of rhGGF2 on cells of the oligodendrocyte lineage. Cells were allowed to differentiate in DM⁺ for 3 days; cultures were then fed with DM⁺ without (*A, C, E*) or with (*B, D, F*) 200 ng/ml of rhGGF2 for 16 hr. In each case, BrdU was added during the last 4 hr. Cultures were fixed and stained for O4 (*A, B*), O1 (*C, D*), or BrdU (*E, F*) and counterstained with Hoechst dye to identify all cells in the field (*A–D*). Separate fields from a single experiment that are representative of the staining pattern of each antibody are shown. Bars, 50 μm (*A–D*); 100 μm (*E, F*). (*G*) $O4^+$/O1- progenitors and $O1^+$ oligodendrocytes exhibit different mitogenic responses to rhGGF2. The labeling index was determined for $O4^+$ and $O1^+$ cells after adding different concentrations of rhGGF2 for 16 hr.; BrdU was added for the last 4 hr. Each point represents the mean ± S.E.M. from two independent experiments. (*H*) Loss of O1 expression with increasing concentrations of rhGGF2. The percentage of $O1^+$ cells was determined from cultures that were treated with increasing concentrations of rhGGF2 (described in *G*). Each point represents the mean ± the S.E.M. from 2 independent experiments. (Reprinted, with permission, from Canoll et al. 1996 [copyright Cell Press].)

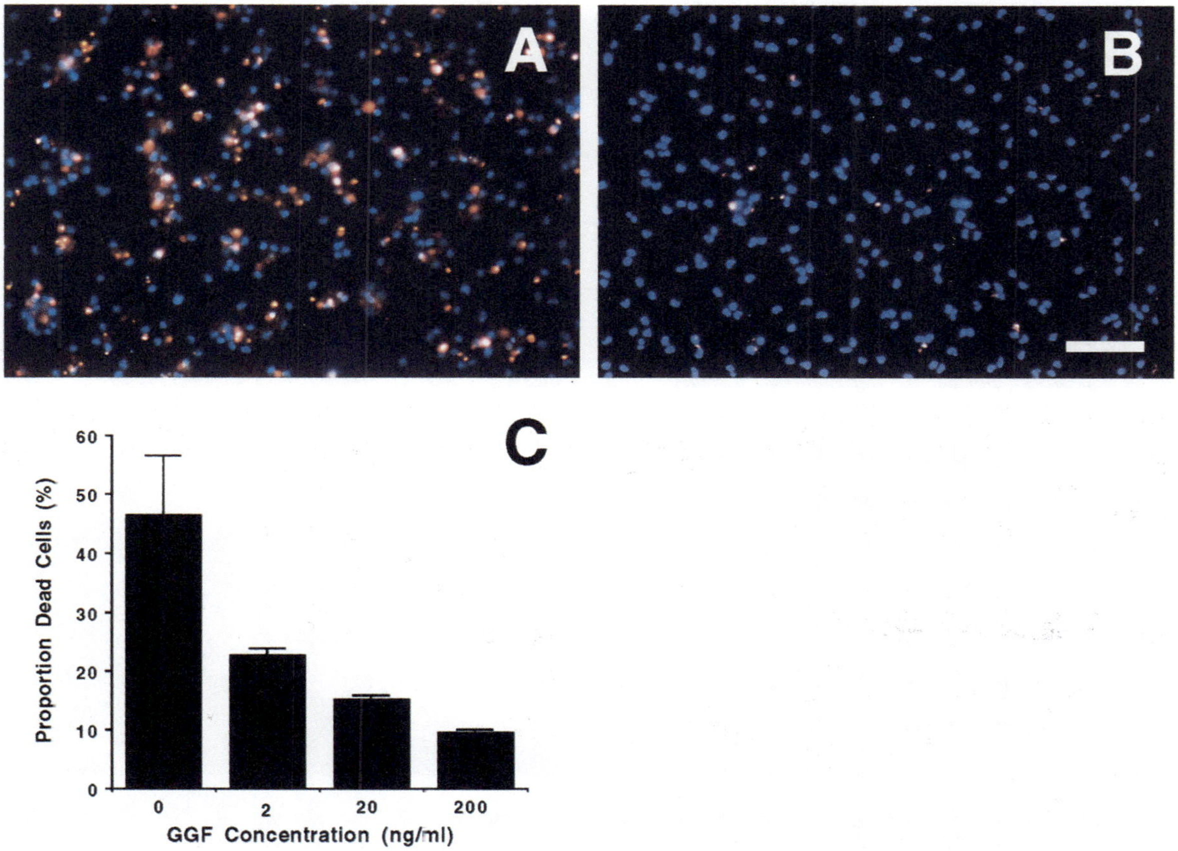

Figure 5. rhGGF2 promotes the survival of oligodendrocyte progenitors. (*A*, *B*) rhGGF2 maintains cell survival after serum withdrawal. $O4^+$ cells (3 days in DM^+) were switched to DMEM without any serum for 12 hr without (*A*) or with (*B*) 200 ng/ml of rhGGF2. Dead cells are stained with a red nuclear stain; all other nuclei are stained blue. Representative fields are shown. Bar 100 μm. (*C*) Dose response of survival effects. The percentages of dead cells after switching cells to DMEM without any serum for 12 hr in the presence of increasing concentrations of rhGGF2 are shown. Each bar represents the mean ± S.E.M. of duplicate wells from three independent experiments. (Reprinted, with permission from Canoll et al. 1996 [copyright Cell Press].)

which shows that rhGGF2 was a potent mitogen for $O4^+$ cells. This effect was paralleled by the loss of O1 expression (Fig. 4H).

Neuregulin Promotes Oligodendrocyte Progenitor Survival

Survival of oligodendrocyte progenitors in vitro is dependent on the presence of a number of growth factors or low concentrations of serum (see, e.g., Barres et al. 1992). To examine directly whether rhGGF2 had survival effects for oligodendrocyte progenitors, cells were grown in DM^+ for 3 days, then switched to a serum-free defined medium containing varying concentrations of rhGGF2 for an additional 12 or 24 hours to analyze cell death (Fig. 5). In the absence of rhGGF2, approximately 50% of the cells were dead at 12 hours (Fig. 5A). In contrast, at 200 ng/ml of rhGGF2, only about 10% of the cells were dead (Fig. 5B). The survival effects of rhGGF2 on $O4^+$ cells were dose-dependent with a half-maximal response of approximately 2 ng/ml (Fig. 5C).

Neuregulin Maintains Progenitor Cell Proliferation and Inhibits Differentiation

To study the effects of neuregulin on oligodendrocyte differentiation, cells were treated for 3 days with rhGGF2 and analyzed for their expression of oligodendrocyte markers. O-2A progenitors treated this way progressed to the $O4^+/O1^-$ stage but were inhibited from differentiating to the $O4^+/O1^+$ stage. For example, after 3 days of rhGGF2, essentially all cells were $O4^+$ and had a multipolar morphology (Fig. 6A, B), but less than 10% of the cells were $O1^+$ or had acquired the complex morphology characteristic of mature oligodendrocytes (Fig. 6C,D). This inhibition of differentiation reversed following withdrawal of rhGGF2; 3 days after rhGGF2 withdrawal, more than 50% of the cells became $O1^+$. Thus, treatment with high doses of rhGGF2 reversibly blocks oligodendrocyte differentiation at the $O4^+/O1^-$ stage.

We next examined whether rhGGF2 similarly inhibited differentiation of O-2A cells into type 2 astrocytes. Cells were switched to media containing 20% fetal bovine serum (FBS) with or without 200

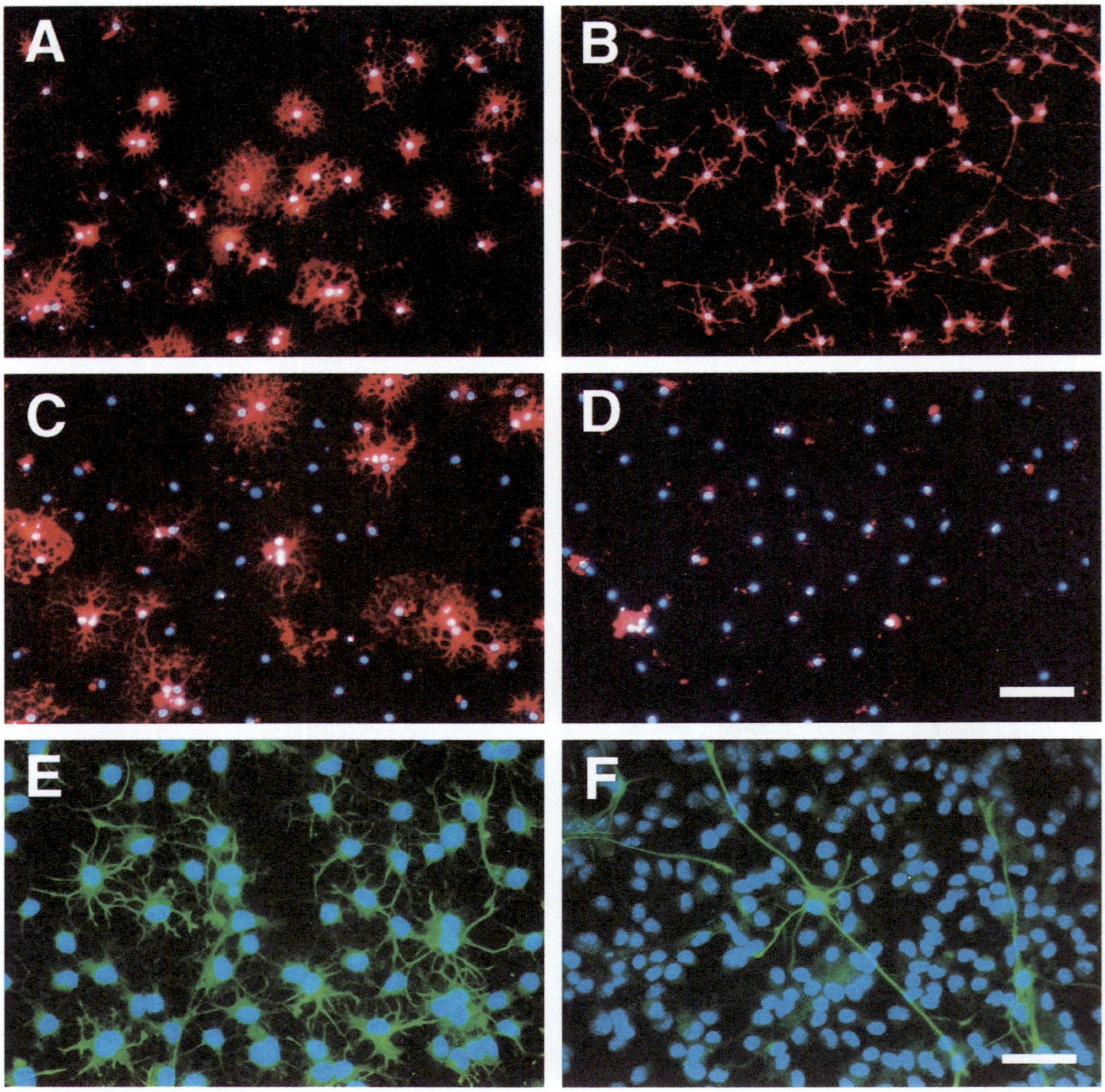

Figure 6. rhGGF2 inhibits the differentiation of O-2A cells into oligodendrocytes or astrocytes. Cells were grown in DM⁺ (*A–D*) or in 20% FBS (*E, F*) without (*A, C, E*) or with (*B, D, F*) 200 ng/ml of rhGGF2 for 3 days. Cultures were fixed and stained for O4 (*A, B*), for O1 (*C, D*), or for GFAP (*E, F*). O4 and O1 staining were visualized with a rhodamine-conjugated secondary antibody, GFAP with a fluorescein-conjugated secondary antibody; in each case nuclei were counterstained blue. Bars, 100 μm (*A–D*); 25 μm (*E, F*). (Reprinted, with permission, from Canoll et al. 1996 [copyright Cell Press].)

ng/ml of rhGGF2. Similar to its effects on oligodendrocyte differentiation, treatment with rhGGF2 inhibited differentiation down the astrocyte lineage. When grown in 20% FBS with rhGGF2, fewer cells expressed detectable levels of glial fibrillary acid protein (GFAP) than controls. Cells that did express GFAP had a unique morphology, characterized by a few highly extended, $GFAP^+$ processes (Fig. 6E,F). Cells grown in 20% FBS with rhGGF2 also continued to proliferate at high levels. After 3 days in 20% FBS with rhGGF2, for example, the labeling index was 19.7% ± 2.5% after a 4-hour BrdU pulse compared to 5.5% ± 1.4% in control cultures.

Neuregulins Are Neuronal Signals That Activate ErbB Receptors on Cells of the Oligodendrocyte Lineage

Previous studies have demonstrated that cortical neurons release mitogenic factors for O-2A progenitor cells that are distinct from basic fibroblast growth factor (bFGF) or platelet-derived growth factor (PDGF) (Hardy and Reynolds 1993). Using blocking antibodies to rhGGF2, we determined that cortical neuron-conditioned medium also contains one or more forms of neuregulin (data not shown).

To determine which of the neuregulin receptors were expressed by cells in the oligodendrocyte lineage, lysates were prepared from O-2A cells grown in B104 CM, from type 2 astrocyte-enriched cultures grown in 20% FBS, and from cells that increasingly differentiated into $O4^+/O1^+$ oligodendrocytes, which were grown in DM^+ for 1–4 days. Lysates were fractionated by SDS-PAGE and immunoblotted with a panel of receptor-specific antibodies. As controls, lysates were prepared and analyzed from rat Schwann cells and from newborn rat cerebrum. Results, shown in Figure 7A, demonstrate that with the exception of Schwann cells, which are known to express only erbB2 and erbB3 proteins (Levi et al. 1995), all three receptors were expressed in each cell type and in the brain. Of note, erbB3 is a prominent neuregulin receptor protein in Schwann cells and in cells of the oligodendrocyte lineage. In contrast, erbB4 appears to predominate in the neonatal brain. This is likely a reflection of high levels of expression by neurons in several regions of the developing brain (Lai and Lemke 1991). Of particular interest, as cells progress along the oligodendrocyte lineage, there is a decrease in erbB4 and an increase in erbB2 expression; in some experiments this transition was even more pronounced than is shown here. Because these cultures, even those maintained in DM^+ for 4 days, contain a mixture of $O1^-$ and $O1^+$ cells, the expression of erbB4 may be even further reduced in the $O1^+$ cells. Additional studies to address this point are in progress.

We next analyzed which subunits became tyrosine phosphorylated following rhGGF2 treatment. rhGGF2 was briefly added to cultures of Schwann cells, O-2A progenitors (in B104 CM), $O4^+$ cells (3 days in DM^+), and type 2 astrocyte-enriched cultures (3 days in 20% FBS). Lysates were prepared, fractionated by SDS-PAGE, blotted, and probed with an anti-phosphotyrosine antibody. In each case, rhGGF2 treatment resulted in increased phosphorylation of a protein band of ~185 kD, with the $O4^+$ cells showing the most robust response (Fig. 7B). In some experiments, a protein of similar size is constitutively phosphorylated at lower levels in the O-2A and $O4^+$ cells. To determine which of the erbB receptors were phosphorylated following rhGGF2 treatment, tyrosine-phosphorylated proteins were immunoprecipitated and analyzed by immunoblotting with antibodies specific for each of the receptor proteins (Fig. 7C). As a control, total lysate from the O-2A cells also was analyzed. In each case, phosphorylated erbB3 is quite prominent. Phosphorylated forms of erbB2 and erbB4 were only readily detected in the case of the $O4^+$ cells but were also present in the type 2 astrocytes with higher sample loading (data not shown).

In summary, the studies described above on oligodendrocyte progenitors have shown that neuregulins are neuronal signals that promote proliferation and survival and inhibit the differentiation of cells in the oligodendrocyte lineage. Since oligodendrocytes are the myelin-producing cells of the CNS, we have begun to investigate whether rhGGF2 might show efficacy in animal models of central demyelinating disorders. Of course, as with any potential protein therapeutic, delivery to the CNS via traditional parenteral routes of administration may prove difficult. In the instance of multiple sclerosis, however, breakdown in the blood/brain barrier during periods of lesion activity might provide a passageway to reach sites of demyelination.

Neuregulin Prevents Clinical Disability in Animal Models of Multiple Sclerosis

Potential approaches to therapy for multiple sclerosis (MS) patients include medicines that prevent/reduce the inflammatory response or drugs that prevent cell loss and promote the repair of damage from demyelination and glial scarring. Based on our current understanding of the biological activities of neuregulins (see above), the possibilities for neuregulin-mediated therapy for MS might include: (1) promoting survival of differentiated oligodendrocytes to prevent myelin breakdown and/or enhance remyelination; (2) promoting proliferation, differentiation, and/or migration of adult 0-2A progenitors to allow repopulation of oligodendrocytes at a lesion site (an analogous approach applies to the potential for dedifferentiation of mature oligodendrocytes, which are then recruited to lesion sites); and (3) expansion of oligodendrocytes (or Schwann cells) in culture for transplantation.

We have begun testing rhGGF2 in an animal model of MS, experimental autoimmune encephalomyelitis (EAE). Specifically, we utilized a passive T-cell transfer acute EAE model in SJL/J mice (Mokhtarian et al. 1984) to evaluate different dosing regimens for rhGGF2. Mice were injected with T cells reactive to myelin basic protein on day 0, then were given daily injections of either vehicle or a specified dose of rhGGF2 delivered by intravenous (i.v.) or subcutaneous (s.c.) routes of administration. Each day the mice were scored for signs of clinical disability (clinical index) by an observer who was blinded to the treatment regimen. Vehicle-treated EAE mice are compared to EAE mice that were given daily injections (from days 0–10) of rhGGF2 at 1 or 2 mg/kg i.v., or 2 mg/kg s.c. (Fig. 8). At 2 mg/kg rhGGF2 i.v. dosing, the average clinical index over the duration of the study was significantly reduced compared to the vehicle-treated group. The subcutaneous route of administration was extremely effective at this same dose: The animals did not show any signs of illness until 14 days post-transfer (4 days after

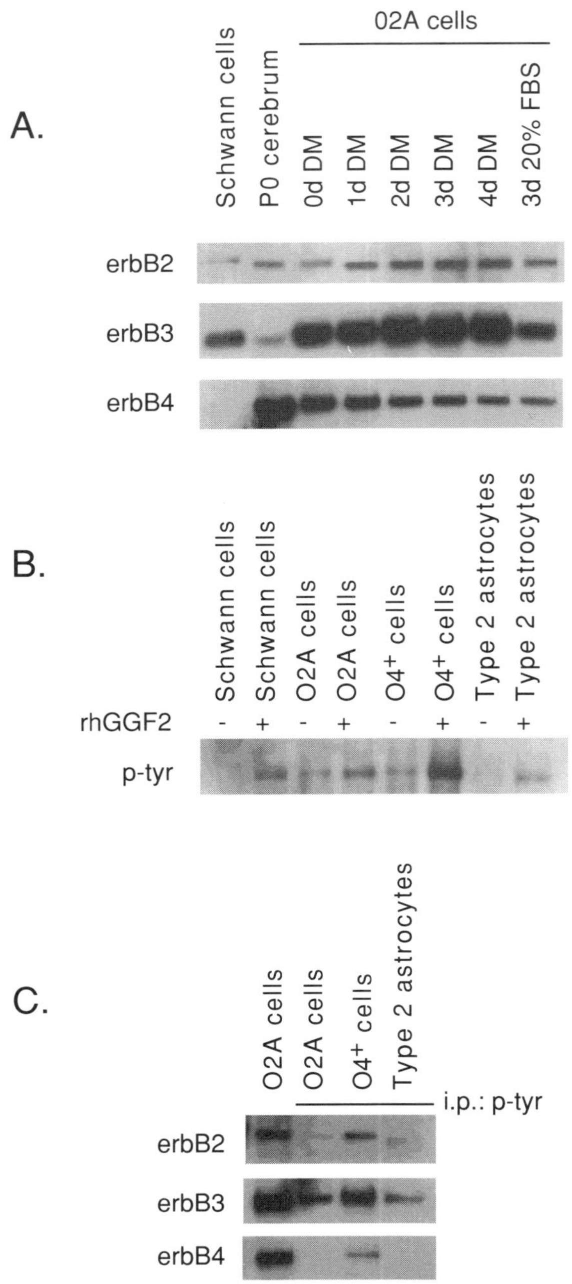

Figure 7. Expression of neuregulin receptor proteins by cells in the oligodendrocyte lineage. (*A*) Expression of erbB receptors by cells in the oligodendrocyte lineage. Detergent lysates were prepared from rat Schwann cells, from P0 cerebrum, and from O-2A cells grown in B104 CM, grown in DM^+ for 1–4 days, or grown in 20% FBS for 3 days. Samples were fractionated by SDS-PAGE, blotted and stained with antibodies specific for erbB2, erbB3, and erbB4. (*B*) rhGGF2 induces phosphorylation of p185. Schwann cells, O-2A cells grown in B104 CM, $O4^+$ cells grown in DM^+ for 3 days, and type 2 astrocyte-enriched cultures grown in 20% FBS for 3 days were treated with DM^+ without (– lanes) or with (+ lanes) 200 ng/ml of rhGGF2 for 2.5 min and then lysed in detergent. Detergent lysates were subjected to SDS-PAGE, transferred onto nitrocellulose, and immunoblotted with an anti-phosphotyrosine antibody. (*C*) rhGGF2 induces phosphorylation of erbB receptors. O-2A cells grown in B104 CM, $O4^+$ cells grown in DM^+ for 3 days, and type 2 astrocyte-enriched cultures grown in 20% FBS for 3 days were treated with 200 ng/ml of rhGGF2 for 2.5 min and lysed. Tyrosine-phosphorylated proteins were immunoprecipitated, separated by SDS-PAGE, blotted, and probed with erbB receptor-specific antibodies. A detergent lysate from untreated O-2A cells was run in the first lane as a control for antibody reactivity. (Reprinted, with permission, from Canoll et al. 1996 [copyright Cell Press].)

dosing was stopped). The reduction in mean clinical index of rhGGF2-treated EAE mice as compared to controls shows that parenterally delivered rhGGF2 produced a beneficial effect on the occurrence and/or course of the acute model. Of central importance to MS patients is whether this growth factor can affect the course of the disease once it is established. Therefore, we are currently testing rhGGF2 in the chronic phases of this animal model of MS. Whether these beneficial effects are mediated through trophic activities on oligodendrocytes, or involve the immune system directly (or both), also are significant questions to be addressed.

DISCUSSION

Neuregulins as Glial Growth Factors

The GGFs were discovered as a result of an effort to identify sources of Schwann cell mitogenic activities (Raff et al. 1978). Subsequent work has shown that these proteins are involved in a much wider spectrum

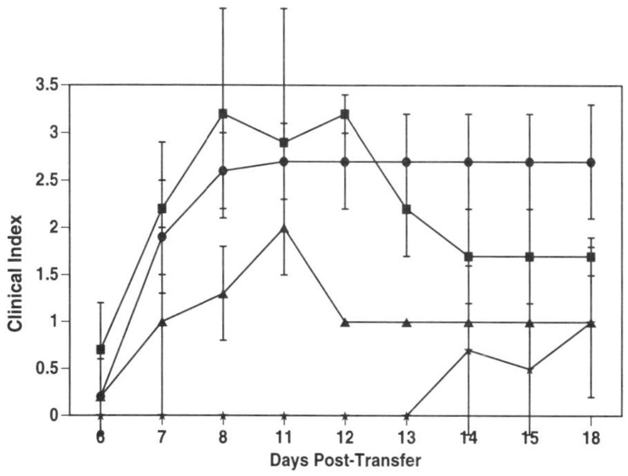

Figure 8. Neuregulin prevents clinical disability in experimental autoimmune encephalomyelitis, an animal model of multiple sclerosis. Four groups of SJL/J mice were injected in the tail vein on day 0 with myelin basic protein-reactive T lymphocytes to induce EAE. The animals were randomized, then dosing with rhGGF2 or vehicle followed a daily regimen, which also began on day 0. The dosing groups were 0, 1, and 2 mg/kg i.v. and 2 mg/kg s.c. (*squares, circles, triangles, stars,* respectively). The mice were scored on a semi-quantitative scale of disability, the clinical index, where 0 = normal, no disability; 1 = floppy tail; 2 = mild weakness of hind limbs; 3 = moderate weakness of hind limbs or forelimbs; 4 = plegia of both hind limbs and forelimbs; 5 = dead. All of the mice appeared normal until day 6. Shown is the mean ± S.E.M. ($n = 6$) of the clinical index of each of the four groups beginning on day 6 through day 18 post-T-cell transfer.

of neurobiology. With the availability of recombinant neuregulins, it has been possible to demonstrate that additional PNS and CNS glia and their progenitor cells express functional neuregulin receptors and are responsive to neuregulins both in vitro and in vivo. The range of trophic activities attributed to neuregulins also has expanded considerably. For example, neuregulins promote the survival of both embryonic precursors and neonatal Schwann cells in vitro (Dong et al. 1995; Cheng and Mudge 1996) and in vivo following nerve injury (Grinspan et al. 1996; Trachtenburg and Thompson 1996). Here we have shown that neuregulins stimulated oligodendrocyte progenitor proliferation and prevented these cells from dying following serum withdrawal (see also Canoll et al. 1996).

Much of the nervous system develops through migration of various cellular derivatives of the neuroepithelium, including the neural crest cells. Cell migration also is essential for successful recovery from nerve injury. In an in vitro model of peripheral nerve repair, low doses of rhGGF2 enhanced Schwann cell migration (see Fig. 2), which suggests that neuregulins might aid in the mobilization of Schwann cells to sites of injury, and thus promote nerve repair. Increasing the number of autologous Schwann cells seeded into a semipermeable guide tube enhanced regeneration of a transected sciatic nerve (Guenard et al. 1992). Therefore, a growth factor such as neuregulin, which can promote Schwann cell survival, proliferation, and migration, could effectively recruit endogenous Schwann cells from areas adjacent to the site of injury and thereby promote nerve regeneration. In two distinct nerve injury models—nerve transection and nerve crush—administration of rhGGF2 promoted nerve repair. We conclude that neuregulins could be of clinical benefit in traumatic nerve injuries.

Milder forms of nerve crush, for example, entrapment of the sciatic nerve, have been used to model compression neuropathies, such as carpel tunnel syndrome (O'Brien et al. 1984). The beneficial effects that we have noted in the more traumatic model of nerve crush (above) suggest that treatment with neuregulin could be of benefit in nerve compression and in other chronic peripheral neuropathies. That rhGGF2 prevented the cisplatin-induced decline in sensory nerve conduction velocity in a rat model (above) supports this point of view.

Neuregulins as Indirect Neurotrophins

Peripheral nerves are made up of both motor axons and sensory fibers of various calibers and impulse-conduction characteristics. All peripheral neurons are dependent for their survival on neurotrophic factors provided by targets and by support cells, such as Schwann cells. The distinct patterns of neurotrophin dependence are dictated largely by the segregation of trk receptor expression. In general, neurons that express trkA are supported by NGF; trkB-expressing neurons are dependent on brain-derived neurotrophic factor (BDNF) or NT4/5; and trkC-expressing neurons are supported by NT3 (for review, see Barbacid 1994). As a consequence of the specificity of these survival requirements, no single neurotrophin can be expected to directly rescue all of the various peripheral neurons that are afflicted in neurological diseases and injury.

Schwann cells not only produce myelin, but also represent a major source of trophic support for peripheral neurons. Schwann cells are known to express all of the neurotrophins as well as ciliary neurotrophic factor (CNTF), leukocyte inhibitory factor (LIF), and glial-cell-line-derived neurotrophic factor (GDNF), and produce increased quantities of these factors in response to injury (Funakoshi et al. 1993; Bunge 1994). By increasing Schwann cell number and/or by inducing the expression of multiple growth factors produced by Schwann cells, an array of neurotrophic activities can be elicited to support all of the various peripheral fiber types.

Several lines of evidence support the concept that neuregulins can act as indirect neurotrophins via induction of neurotrophin synthesis and secretion. First, the expression of NT3 was up-regulated 40-fold in non-neuronal, glial-like cells of embryonic sympathetic ganglia treated with rhGGF2. In addition, in cocultures of these nonneuronal cells and sympathetic neuroblasts, blocking antibodies to rhGGF2 diminished the neuronal signaling that induced NT3 expression (Verdi et al. 1996). Thus, neuregulin and NT3 act together to create a trophic support loop in developing sympathetic ganglia. Second, conditioned media from Schwann cells treated with rhGGF2 contained soluble neurotrophic activities that promoted survival of sympathetic neurons (see Fig. 2D). This rhGGF2-induced activity is likely to account for the extensive neurite outgrowth that was seen in SCG ganglion explant tube cultures (Fig. 2C). Since NGF is known to have both of these activities on neonatal SCG neurons, and Schwann cells express this neurotrophin, NGF is a candidate for rhGGF2-induced neurotrophic activity. Further studies will be directed at identifying which specific factor(s) is expressed in Schwann cells in response to neuregulin.

Neuregulins as Potential Drugs for Neurological Disorders

Common features of many neurological disorders include the loss of neural cells, and tissue wasting resulting from inflammatory, infectious, or neoplastic processes. Chronic neurodegenerative diseases (e.g., amyotrophic lateral sclerosls, Alzheimer's, and Parkinson's diseases) and autoimmune diseases (e.g., MS and myasthenia gravis) result in neurological deficits, as do adult-onset diabetes, cancer chemotherapy, AIDS, and various inherited peripheral neuropathies. By promoting neural growth and function, growth factors might be expected to slow the progression or reverse the course of these diseases. In animal models of neural injury, peripheral neuropathy, or neurodegeneration, several neurotrophic factors have been shown to exert beneficial effects. For example, BDNF, CNTF, and GDNF each have rescued motor neurons from death following root avulsion and can sustain the expression of choline acetyltransferase activity following axotomy (see, e.g., Li et al. 1994; Henderson et al. 1994; Lindsay 1996). BDNF effectively delayed motor neuron death in the *wobbler* mouse (Ikeda et al. 1995). Both NGF and NT3 have been evaluated in models of peripheral neuropathy with positive results (Apfel and Kessler 1996). Insulin-like growth factor I (IGF-I) has been tested in a wide range of models (Vaught et al. 1996). As a result of the encouraging results obtained in preclinical studies, several of these growth factors now have advanced into clinical trials. Since neuregulins have pleiotrophic actions in the nervous system, they also have potential as drugs for treatment of a variety of neurological disorders.

We have demonstrated beneficial effects of rhGGF2 treatment in models of neural injury, peripheral neuropathy, and MS. Continued evaluation of this growth factor in additional models of neurological disorders accompanied by further progress in understanding the basic neurobiology of neuregulins and neuregulin receptors will help to advance rhGGF2 toward eventual clinical trials. Before clinical trials can commence, however, several additional hurdles need to be cleared. Perhaps the two most critical areas to be dealt with relate to the process of developing a consistent and economical method of production and to defining the therapeutic window for dosing. Because rhGGF2 is the only neuregulin known to be efficiently secreted when produced in mammalian cells (Marchionni et al. 1993), the production process should be relatively straightforward. To begin to define the therapeutic window for dosing, one must take into account both the efficacy and safety profiles obtained in animal studies along with pharmacokinetic data. In this latter regard, the plasma half-life for rhGGF2 has been measured in hours (Katragadda et al. 1995). This property of rhGGF2 should make systemic administration of this neuregulin a viable option for drug delivery.

ACKNOWLEDGMENTS

We thank Michael Jarpe, Frank Danehy, Debra Bedell-Hogan, and Colleen Nolan for purification and analysis of rhGGF2; Beth Happel, Ruth Toms, and Nancy Ratner for characterization of neuregulin antisera; Kristen Cronin and Judith Sudhalter for Schwann cell culture; Olivia Bermingham-McDonogh and Stanley Goldin for many interesting discussions; Debbie Giampa for aid in preparation of the manuscript; Mario Pita for art work; and David J. Anderson, Jeremy Brockes, and Tom Jessell for critique. Finally, we are grateful to Robert McBurney for his steadfast support and encouragement.

REFERENCES

Apfel, S.C. and J.A. Kessler. 1996. Neurotrophic factors in the treatment of peripheral neuropathy. *CIBA Found. Symp.* **196:** 98.

Barbacid, M. 1994. The trk family of neurotrophin receptors. *J. Neurobiol.* **25:** 386.

Barres, B.A., I.K. Hart, H.S.R. Coles, J.F. Burne, J.T. Voyvodic, W.D. Richardson, and M.C. Raff. 1992. Cell death and control of cell survival in the oligodendrocyte lineage. *Cell* **70:** 31.

Bermingham-McDonogh, O., K.L. McCabe, and T.A. Reh. 1996. Effects of GGF/neuregulins on neuronal survival and neurite outgrowth correlate with erbB2/neu expression in developing rat retina. *Development* **122:** 1427.

Brockes, J.P., G.E. Lemke, and D.R. Balzer, Jr. 1980. Purification and preliminary characterization of a glial growth factor from the bovine pituitary. *J. Biol. Chem.* **255:** 8374.

Bunge, R.P. 1994. The role of the Schwann cell in trophic support and regeneration. *J. Neurol.* **241:** 19.

Canoll, P.D., J.M. Musacchio, R. Hardy, R. Reynolds, M.A. Marchionni, and J.L. Salzer. 1996. GGF/neuregulin is a neuronal signal that promotes the proliferation and survival and inhibits the differentiation of oligodendrocyte progenitors. *Neuron* **17:** 229.

Carraway, K.L. and S.J. Burden. 1995. Neuregulins and their

receptors. *Curr. Opin. Neurobiol.* **5:** 606.

Chen, L.E., A.V. Seaber, and J.R. Urbaniak. 1993. The influence of magnitude and duration of crush load on functional recovery of the peripheral nerve. *J. Reconstruct. Microsurg.* **9:** 299.

Chen, M.S., O. Bermingham-McDonogh, F. Danehy, Jr., C. Nolan, S.S. Scherer, J. Lucas, D. Gwynne, and M.A. Marchionni. 1994. Expression of multiple neuregulin transcripts in postnatal rat brains. *J. Comp. Neurol.* **349:** 389.

Cheng, L. and A.W. Mudge. 1996. Cultured Schwann cells constitutively express the myelin protein P0. *Neuron* **16:** 309.

Chu, G.C., L.M. Moscoso, M.X. Sliwkowski, and J.P. Merlie. 1995. Regulation of the acetylcholine receptor epsilon subunit gene by recombinant ARIA: An in vitro model for transynaptic gene regulation. *Neuron* **14:** 329.

Corfas, G., D.L. Falls, and G.D. Fischbach. 1993. ARIA, a protein that stimulates acetylcholine receptor synthesis, also induces tyrosine phosphorylation of a 185-kDa muscle transmembrane protein. *Proc. Natl. Acad. Sci.* **90:** 1624.

Corfas, G., K.M. Rosen, H. Aratake, R. Krauss, and G.D. Fischbach. 1995. Differential expression of ARIA isoforms in the rat brain. *Neuron* **14:** 103.

Dong, Z., A. Brennan, N. Liu, Y. Yarden, G. Lefkowitz, R. Mirsky, and K.R. Jessen. 1995. Neu differentiation factor is a neuron-glia signal and regulates survival, proliferation, and maturation of rat Schwann cell precursors. *Neuron* **15:** 585

Falls, D.L., K.M. Rosen, G. Corfas, W.S. Lane, and G.D. Fischbach. 1993. ARIA, a protein that stimulates acetylcholine receptor synthesis, is a member of the *neu* ligand family. *Cell* **72:** 801.

Funakoshi, H., J. Frisen, G. Barbany, T. Timmusk, O. Zachrisson, V.M.K. Verge, and H. Persson. 1993. Differential expression of mRNAs for neurotrophins and their receptors after axotomy of the sciatic nerve. *J. Cell Biol.* **123:** 455.

Gassmann, M., F. Casagranda, D. Orioli, H. Simon, C. Lai, R. Klein, and G. Lemke. 1995. Aberrant neural and cardiac development in mice lacking the ErbB4 neuregulin receptor. *Nature* **378:** 390.

Gerritsen Van der Hoop, R., P. De Koning, E. Boven, J.P. Neijt, F.G.I. Jennekens, and W.H. Gispen. 1988. Efficacy of the neuropeptide ORG.2766 in the prevention and treatment of cisplatin-induced neurotoxicity in rats. *Eur. J. Cancer Clin. Oncol.* **24:** 637.

Goodearl, A.D., J.B. Davis, K. Mistry, L. Minghetti, M. Otsu, M.D. Waterfield, and P. Stroobant. 1993. Purification of multiple forms of glial growth factor. *J. Biol. Chem.* **268:** 18095.

Grinspan, J. B., M.A. Marchionni, M. Reeves, M. Coulaloglou, and S.S. Scherer 1996. Axonal interactions regulate Schwann cell apoptosis in developing peripheral nerve: Neuregulin receptors and the role of neuregulins. *J. Neurosci.* (in press).

Guenard, V., N. Kleitman, T.K. Morrissey, R.P. Bunge, and P. Aebischer. 1992. Syngeneic Schwann cells derived from adult nerves seeded in semipermeable guidance channels enhance peripheral nerve regeneration. *J Neurosci.* **12:** 3310.

Hardy R. and R. Reynolds 1993. Rat cerebral cortical neurons in primary culture release a mitogen specific for early (G_{D3}^+/$O4^-$) oligodendroglial progenitors. *J. Neurosci. Res.* **34:** 589.

Hefti, F. 1994. Neurotrophic factor therapy for nervous system degenerative diseases. *J. Neurobiol.* **25:** 1418.

Henderson, C.E., H.S. Phillips, R.A. Pollock, A.M. Davies, C. Lemeulle, M. Armanini, L.C. Simpson, B. Moffet, R.A. Vandlen, V.E. Koliatsos, and A. Rosenthal. 1994. GDNF: A potent survival factor for motoneurons present in peripheral nerve and muscle. *Science* **266:** 1062.

Ho, W.H., M.P. Armanini, A. Nuijens, H.S. Phillips, and P.L. Osheroff. 1995. Sensory and motor neuron-derived factor: A novel heregulin variant highly expressed in sensory and motor neurons. *J. Biol. Chem.* **270:** 14523.

Holmes, W.E., M.X. Sliwkowski, R.W. Akita, W.J. Henzel, J. Lee, J.W. Park, D. Yansura, N. Abadi, H. Raab, G.D. Lewis, H.M. Shepard, W.J. Kuang, W.I. Wood, D.V. Goeddel, and R.L. Vandlen. 1992. Identification of heregulin, a specific activator of $p185^{erbB2}$. *Science* **256:** 1205.

Ikeda, K., B. Klinkosz, T. Greene, J.M. Cedarbaum, V. Wong, R.M. Lindsay, and H. Mitsumoto. 1995. Effects of brain-derived neurotrophic factor on motor dysfunction in wobbler motor neuron disease. *Ann. Neurol.* **37:** 505.

Jessell, T.M., R.E. Siegel, and G.D. Fischbach. 1979. Induction of acetylcholine receptors on cultured skeletal muscle by a factor extracted from brain and spinal cord. *Proc. Natl. Acad. Sci.* **76:** 5397.

Jessen, K.R. and R. Mirsky. 1991. Schwann cell precursors and their development. *Glia* **4:** 185.

Jo, S.A., X. Zhu, M.A. Marchionni, and S.J. Burden. 1995. Neuregulins are concentrated at nerve-muscle synapses and activate ACh receptor gene expression. *Nature* **373:** 158.

Katragadda, S., O. Bermingham-McDonogh, K. Cronin, D.I. Gwynne, and C. Kirk. 1995. Pharmacokinetics and distribution of ^{125}I-rhGGF2. *Soc. Neurosci. Abstr.* **21:** 314.

Kraus, M.H., W. Issing, T. Miki, N.C. Popescu, and S.A. Aaronson. 1989. Isolation and characterization of ERBB3, a third member of the ERBB/epidermal growth factor receptor family: Evidence for overexpression in a subset of human mammary tumors. *Proc. Natl. Acad. Sci.* **86:** 9193.

Lai, C. and G. Lemke 1991. An extended family of protein-tyrosine kinase genes differentially expressed in the vertebrate nervous system. *Neuron* **6:** 691.

Lee, K.F., H. Simon, H. Chen, B. Bates, M.C. Hung, and C. Hauser. 1995. Requirement for neuregulin receptor erbB2 in neural and cardiac development. *Nature* **378:** 394.

Lemke, G. 1996. Neuregulins in development. *Mol. Cell. Neurosci.* **7:** 247.

Lemke, G.E. and J.P. Brockes. 1984. Identification and purification of glial growth factor. *J. Neurosci.* **4:** 75.

Levi, A.D.O., R.P. Bunge, J.A. Lofgren, L. Meima, F. Hefti, K. Nikolics, and M.X. Sliwkowski 1995. The influence of heregulins on human Schwann cell proliferation. *J. Neurosci.* **14:** 1329.

Li, L., R.W. Oppenheim, M. Lei, and L.J. Houenou. 1994. Neurotrophic agents prevent motoneuron death following sciatic nerve section in the neonatal mouse. *J. Neurobiol.* **25:** 759.

Lindsay, R.M. 1996. Therapeutic potential of the neurotrophins and neurotrophin-CNTF combinations in peripheral neuropathies and motor neuron diseases. *CIBA Found. Symp.* **196:** 39.

Louis, J.C., E. Magal, D. Muir, M. Manthorpe, and S. Varon. 1992. CG-4, a new bipotential glial cell line from rat brain, is capable of differentiating in vitro into either mature oligodendrocytes or type-2 astrocytes. *J. Neurosci. Res.* **31:** 193.

Mahanthappa, N.K., E.S. Anton, and W.D. Mathew. 1996. Glial growth factor 2, a soluble neuregulin, directly increases Schwann cell motility and indirectly promotes neurite outgrowth. *J. Neurosci.* **16:** 4673.

Marchionni, M.A. 1995. Cell-cell signalling: *neu* tack on neuregulin. *Nature* **378:** 334.

Marchionni, M.A., A.D. Goodearl, M.S. Chen, O. Bermingham-McDonogh, C. Kirk, M. Hendricks, F. Danehy, D. Misumi, J. Sudhalter, K. Kobayashi, D. Wroblewski, C. Lynch, M. Baldassare, I. Hiles, J.B. Davis, J. Hsuan, J.J. Totty, M. Otsu, R.N. McBurney, M.D. Waterfield, P. Stroobant, and D. Gwynne. 1993. Glial growth factors are alternatively spliced erbB2 ligands expressed in the nervous system. *Nature* **362:** 312.

Meyer, D. and C. Birchmeier. 1994. Distinct isoforms of neuregulin are expressed in mesenchymal and neuronal cells during mouse development. *Proc. Natl. Acad. Sci.* **91:** 1064.

———. 1995. Multiple essential functions of neuregulin in development. *Nature* **378:** 386.

Mokhtarian, F., D.E. McFarlin, and C.S. Raine. 1984. Adoptive transfer of myelin basic protein-sensitized T cells produces chronic relapsing demyelinating disease in mice. *Nature* **309:** 356.

Morrissey, T.K., A.D.O. Levi, A. Nuijens, M.X. Sliwkowski, and R.P. Bunge 1995. Axon-induced mitogenesis of human Schwann cells involves heregulin and p185^{erbB2}. *Proc. Natl. Acad. Sci.* **92:** 1431.

Murphy, P., P. Topilko, S. Schneider-Maunoury, T. Seitanidou, A. Baron-Van Evercooren, and P. Charnay. 1996. The regulation of Krox-20 expression reveals important steps in the control of peripheral glial cell development. *Development* (in press).

O'Brien, J.P., S.E. McKinnon, A.R. MacLean, A.R. Hudson, A.L. Dellon, and D.A. Hunter. 1984. A model of chronic nerve compression in the rat. *Ann. Plastic Surg.* **19:** 430.

Peles, E. and Y. Yarden. 1993. Neu and its ligands: From an oncogene to neural factors. *BioEssays* **15:** 815.

Peles, E., S.S. Bacus, R.A. Koski, H.S. Lu, D. Wen, S.G. Ogden, R.B. Levy, and Y. Yarden. 1992. Isolation of the neu/HER-2 stimulatory ligand: A 44 kd glycoprotein that induces differentiation of mammary tumor cells. *Cells* **69:** 205.

Pinkas-Kramarski, R., R. Eilam, O. Spiegler, S. Lavi, N. Liu, D. Chang, D. Wen, M. Schwartz, and Y. Yarden. 1994. Brain neurons and glial cells express Neu differentiation factor/heregulin: A survival factor for astrocytes. *Proc. Natl. Acad. Sci.* **91:** 9387.

Plowman, G.D., J.M. Culouscou, G.S. Whitney, J.M. Green, G.W. Carlton, L. Foy, M.G. Neubauer, and M. Shoyab. 1993. Ligand-specific activation of HER4/p180erbB4, a fourth member of the epidermal growth factor receptor family. *Proc. Natl. Acad. Sci.* **90:** 1746.

Raff, M.C., E. Abney, J.P. Brockes, and A. Hornby-Smith. 1978. Schwann cell growth factors. *Cell* **15:** 813.

Rutkowski, J.L., C.J. Kirk, M.A. Lerner, and G.I. Tennekoon. 1995. Purification and expansion of human Schwann cells *in vitro*. *Nat. Med.* **1:** 80.

Schechter, A.L., D.F. Stern, L. Vaiyanathan, S.J. Decker, J.A. Drebin, M.I. Grenne, and R.A. Weinberg. 1984. The *neu* oncogene: An erbB-related gene encoding a 185,000-M_r tumour antigen. *Nature* **312:** 513.

Shah, N.M., M.A. Marchionni, I. Isaacs, P. Stroobant, and D.J. Anderson. 1994. Glial growth factor restricts mammalian neural crest stem cells to a glial fate. *Cell* **77:** 349.

Topilko, P., S. Schneider-Maunoury, G. Levi, A. Baron-Van Evercooren, A.B.Y. Chennoufi, T. Seitanidou, C. Babinet, and P. Charnay. 1994. Krox-20 controls myelination in the peripheral nervous system. *Nature* **371:** 796.

Trachtenberg, J.T. and W.J. Thompson. 1996. Schwann cell apoptosis at developing neuromuscular junctions is regulated by glial growth factor. *Nature* **379:** 174.

Vartanian, T., G. Corfas, Y. Li, G. Fischbach, and K. Stefansson. 1994. A role for the acetylcholine receptor-inducing protein ARIA in oligodendrocyte development. *Proc. Natl. Acad. Sci.* **91:** 11626.

Vaught, J.L., P.C. Contreras, M.A. Glicksman, and N.T. Neff. 1996. Potential utility of rhIGF-1 in neuromuscular and/or degenerative disease. *CIBA Found. Symp.* **196:** 18.

Verdi, J.M., A.K. Groves, I. Farinas, K. Jones, M.A. Marchionni, L.F. Reichardt, and D.J. Anderson. 1996. A reciprocal cell-cell interaction mediated by neurotrophin-3 and neuregulins controls the early survival and development of sympathetic neuroblasts. *Neuron* **16:** 515.

Wen, D., E. Peles, R. Cupples, S.V. Suggs, S.S. Bacus, Y. Luo, G. Trail, S. Hu, S.M.Silbiger, R.B. Levy, R.A. Koski, H.S. Lu, and Y. Yarden. 1992. Neu differentiation factor: A transmembrane glycoprotein containing an EGF domain and an immunoglobulin homology unit. *Cell* **69:** 559.

Molecular Biology and Genetics of Prion Diseases

S.B. PRUSINER
Departments of Neurology and of Biochemistry and Biophysics, University of California, San Francisco, California 94143-0518

Prions cause a group of human and animal neurodegenerative diseases which are now classified together because their etiology and pathogenesis involve modification of the prion protein (PrP) (Prusiner 1991). Prion diseases are manifest as infectious, genetic, and sporadic disorders. These diseases can be transmitted among mammals by the infectious particle designated "prion" (Prusiner 1982). Despite intensive searches over the past three decades, no nucleic acid has been found within prions (Alper et al. 1966, 1967; Hunter 1972; Riesner et al. 1992), yet a modified isoform of the host-encoded PrP designated PrP^{Sc} is essential for infectivity (Prusiner 1991; Büeler et al. 1993; Prusiner et al. 1983, 1993a,b). In fact, considerable experimental data argue that prions are composed exclusively of PrP^{Sc}. Earlier terms used to describe the prion diseases include transmissible encephalopathies, spongiform encephalopathies, and slow virus diseases (Sigurdsson 1954; Gajdusek 1977, 1985). The human prion disorders include kuru, Creutzfeldt-Jakob disease (CJD), Gerstmann-Sträussler-Scheinker syndrome, (GSS), and fatal familial insomnia (FFI).

Studies of the prion diseases have taken on new significance with the recent report of ten cases of atypical CJD in three teenagers and seven young adults (Bateman et al. 1995; Britton et al. 1995; Will et al. 1996). All of these cases have been reported from Great Britain, where more than 160,000 cattle have died of bovine spongiform encephalopathy (BSE), or mad cow disease, as it is often called (Wells and Wilesmith 1995). It seems possible that bovine prions have been passed to humans through the consumption of tainted beef products. How many cases of atypical CJD caused by bovine prions will occur in the years ahead is unknown. Whatever happens, the need for more knowledge about the biology of prions and the pathogenesis of prion diseases would seem to be substantial.

The experimental transmissions of CJD and kuru from humans to apes ushered in an exciting period of neurological research which focused first on kuru—a disease of epidemic proportions centered in the Fore region of the New Guinea highlands (Gajdusek and Zigas 1957)—and subsequently on CJD and GSS disease (Gibbs et al. 1968; Masters et al. 1981a). Upon transmission of kuru to apes in 1966, the possibility that kuru was transmitted among the New Guinea natives by ritualistic cannibalism was no longer remote (Gajdusek et al. 1966). Such transmission studies were stimulated by the insightful suggestion of Hadlow that the neuropathology of kuru resembled scrapie, and thus that the disease might be transmissible after intracerebral inoculation of brain extracts into apes following a prolonged incubation time (Hadlow 1959).

Scrapie of sheep and goats possesses an equally fascinating history. For many years, British scientists had argued about whether natural scrapie was a genetic or an infectious disease (Parry 1983). Scrapie, like kuru and CJD, caused death of the host without any sign of an immune response to a "foreign infectious agent." Debate about scrapie was heightened in 1966, when Tikvah Alper and colleagues reported the extraordinary resistance of the scrapie agent to inactivation by ionizing and UV irradiation (Alper et al. 1966, 1967). Speculation about the composition of the scrapie agent increased over the following decade.

ORIGIN OF THE PRION CONCEPT

Once an effective protocol was developed for preparation of partially purified fractions of scrapie agent from hamster brain, investigators could demonstrate that procedures modifying or hydrolyzing proteins diminish scrapie infectivity (Prusiner et al. 1981; Prusiner 1982). At the same time, tests done in search of a scrapie-specific nucleic acid could not demonstrate any dependence of infectivity on a polynucleotide (Prusiner 1982), in agreement with earlier studies reporting the extreme resistance of infectivity to UV irradiation at 254 nm (Alper et al. 1967). On the basis of these findings, the term "prion" was introduced to distinguish the *pro*teinaceous *in*fectious particles that cause scrapie, CJD, GSS, and kuru from both viroids and viruses (Prusiner 1982). It now seems likely that the scrapie agent may be composed only of a protein that adopts an abnormal conformation (Pan et al. 1993; Stahl et al. 1993; Kocisko et al. 1994; Kaneko et al. 1995).

PRION PROTEINS

After it was established that scrapie prion infectivity in partially purified fractions depended on protein (Prusiner et al. 1981), the search for a scrapie-specific protein intensified. Although the insolubility of scrapie infectivity made purification problematic, we took advantage of this property, along with its relative resistance to degradation by proteases, to extend the degree of purification. In subcellular fractions from Syrian hamster (SHa) brain enriched for scrapie infectivity, a protease-resistant prion protein (PrP) of 27 kD to 30 kD, designated PrP 27-30, was identified that was absent from controls (Bolton et al. 1982; Prusiner et al. 1982; McKinley et al. 1983). Radioiodination of partially purified fractions revealed a protein unique to preparations from scrapie-infected brains (Bolton et al. 1982; Prusiner et al. 1982). This protein was later named prion protein (PrP) with an apparent M_r of 27-30 kD or, more succinctly, PrP 27-30 (McKinley et al. 1983). The existence of this protein was rapidly confirmed (Diringer et al. 1983).

Purification of PrP 27-30 to homogeneity allowed determination of its amino-terminal amino acid sequence (Prusiner et al. 1984). This permitted the synthesis of an isocoding mixture of oligonucleotides that was subsequently used to identify PrP cDNA clones (Chesebro et al. 1985; Oesch et al. 1985; Basler et al. 1986; Locht et al. 1986). It was found that PrP is encoded by a chromosomal gene and not by a nucleic acid within the infectious scrapie prion particle (Oesch et al. 1985; Basler et al. 1986). Levels of PrP mRNA remain unchanged throughout the course of scrapie infection—an observation that led to the identification of the normal PrP gene product, a protein of 33 kD to 35 kD, designated PrP^C (Oesch et al. 1985; Basler et al. 1986). PrP^C is protease-sensitive, whereas PrP 27-30 is the protease-resistant core of a 33- to 35-kD disease-specific protein, designated PrP^{Sc} (Oesch et al. 1985; Meyer et al. 1986). At the same time, it was found that the brains of normal and scrapie-infected hamsters express similar levels of PrP mRNA and a protease-sensitive prion protein designated PrP^C (Oesch et al. 1985). PrP^C or a subset of PrP molecules is the substrate for PrP^{Sc}.

The discovery of PrP 27-30 in fractions enriched for scrapie infectivity was accompanied by the identification of rod-shaped amyloid particles (Prusiner et al. 1982, 1983). Solubilization of PrP 27-30 into liposomes with retention of infectivity (Gabizon et al. 1987) demonstrated that large PrP polymers are not required for infectivity, and also permitted the immunoaffinity copurification of PrP^{Sc} and infectivity (Gabizon et al. 1988; Gabizon and Prusiner 1990). Of note, the amyloid plaques in prion diseases contain PrP, as determined by immunoreactivity and amino acid sequencing (Bendheim et al. 1984; DeArmond et al. 1985; Kitamoto et al. 1986; Roberts et al. 1988; Tagliavini et al. 1991).

PrP Gene Structure, Organization, and Expression

The entire open reading frame (ORF) of all known mammalian and avian PrP genes resides within a single exon (Basler et al. 1986; Westaway et al. 1987; Hsiao et al. 1989b; Gabriel et al. 1992), which eliminates the possibility that PrP^{Sc} arises from alternative RNA splicing (Basler et al. 1986; Westaway et al. 1987, 1991). The two exons of the SHa PrP gene are separated by a 10-kb intron: Exon 1 encodes a portion of the 5′-untranslated leader sequence, and exon 2 encodes the ORF and 3′-untranslated region (Basler et al. 1986). The mouse (Mo) and sheep PrP genes contain three exons, with exon 3 analogous to exon 2 of the hamster (Westaway et al. 1991, 1994a,b). The promoters of both the SHa and MoPrP genes contain multiple copies of GC-rich repeats and are devoid of TATA boxes. These GC nonamers represent a motif that may function as a canonical binding site for the transcription factor Sp1 (McKnight and Tjian 1986). Although PrP mRNA is constitutively expressed in the brains of adult animals (Chesebro et al. 1985; Oesch et al. 1985), it is highly regulated during development. In the septum, levels of PrP mRNA and choline acetyltransferase increase in parallel during development (Mobley et al. 1988). In other brain regions, PrP gene expression occurs at an earlier age. In situ hybridization studies show that the highest levels of PrP mRNA occur in neurons (Kretzschmar et al. 1986a). It was shown that there are less than 0.002 PrP gene sequences per ID_{50} unit in purified prion fractions, indicating that a gene encoding PrP^{Sc} is not a component of the infectious prion particle (Oesch et al. 1985). This is a major feature that distinguishes prions from viruses, including those retroviruses that carry cellular oncogenes, and from satellite viruses that derive their coat proteins from other viruses previously infecting plant cells. Purified fractions enriched for prion infectivity were analyzed for a scrapie-specific nucleic acid, but no such nucleic acid was found (Meyer et al. 1991). If such a molecule exists, then its size is 80 nucleotides or less (Kellings et al. 1992; Riesner et al. 1992).

Cell Biology of PrP^{Sc} Formation

In scrapie-infected cells, PrP^C molecules destined to become PrP^{Sc} exit to the cell surface prior to conversion into PrP^{Sc} (Stahl et al. 1987; Caughey and Raymond 1991; Borchelt et al. 1992; Taraboulos et al. 1992a). Like other GPI-anchored proteins, PrP^C appears to re-enter the cell through a cholesterol/glycosphingolipid-rich subcellular compartment (DIGs) (Taraboulos et al. 1995) which may be caveolae or early endosomes (Fig. 1) (Keller et al. 1992; Anderson 1993). Within this cholesterol-rich, nonacidic compartment, GPI-anchored PrP^C can be either converted into PrP^{Sc} or partially degraded (Taraboulos et al. 1995). PrP^{Sc} is trimmed at the amino terminus in an acidic compartment in scrapie-infected cultured cells to form PrP 27-30 (Caughey et al. 1991a; Taraboulos et al. 1992a). In contrast, amino-terminal trimming of PrP^{Sc} is minimal in brain, where little PrP 27-30 is found (McKinley et al. 1991).

Recent studies have shown that redirecting PrP^C to clathrin-coated pits by creating chimeric PrP molecules with four different carboxy-terminal targeting domains prevented the formation of PrP^{Sc} (Taraboulos et al.

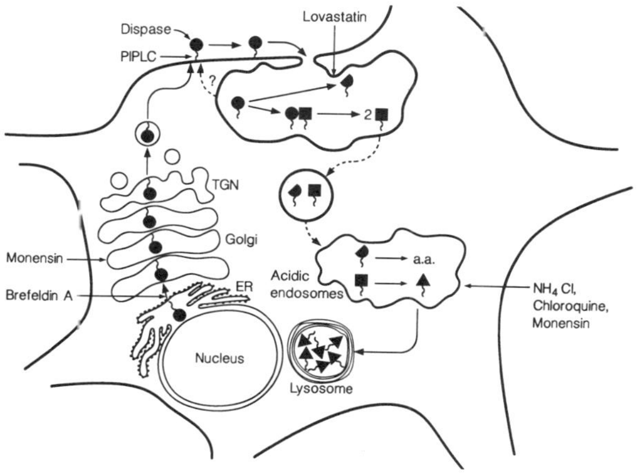

Figure 1. Pathways of prion protein synthesis and degradation in cultured cells. PrP^{Sc} is denoted by squares; PrP^{C} by circles. Prior to becoming protease-resistant, the PrP^{Sc} precursor transits through the plasma membrane and is sensitive to dispase or PIPLC added to the medium. PrP^{Sc} formation probably occurs in a compartment accessible from the plasma membrane, such as caveolae or early endosomes, both of which are nonacidic compartments. The synthesis of nascent PrP^{Sc} seems to require the interaction of PrP^{C} with existing PrP^{Sc}. In cultured cells, but not brain, the amino terminus of PrP^{Sc} is trimmed to form PrP 27-30; PrP^{Sc} then accumulates primarily in secondary lysosomes. The inhibition of PrP^{Sc} synthesis by brefeldin A demonstrates that the endoplasmic reticulum (ER)-Golgi is not competent for its synthesis and that transport of PrP down the secretory pathway is required for the formation of PrP^{Sc}.

1995; K. Kaneko et al., in prep.). To determine if these carboxy-terminal transmembrane segments prevented PrP^{C} from refolding into PrP^{Sc} by altering the structure of the polypeptide, we fused the 28-amino-acid carboxyl termini from the Qa protein (Waneck et al. 1988). Two carboxy-terminal Qa segments differing by a single residue direct the transmembrane protein (Qa[−]) to clathrin-coated pits or the GPI form (Qa[+]) to DIGs. The DIG-targeted PrP^{C} was converted into PrP^{Sc}, but the transmembrane PrP^{C} was not. Our findings argue that the formation of PrP^{Sc} occurs within a specific subcellular compartment and, as such, it is likely to involve auxiliary macromolecules that are found within the DIG microdomains.

STRUCTURES OF PrP ISOFORMS

In a search for a posttranslational chemical modification that might explain the differences in the properties of these two PrP isoforms, PrP^{Sc} was analyzed by mass spectrometry and gas phase sequencing. The amino acid sequence was the same as that deduced from the translated ORF of the PrP gene, and no modifications that might differentiate PrP^{C} from PrP^{Sc} were found (Stahl et al. 1993). These findings forced consideration of the possibility that conformation distinguishes the two PrP isoforms.

Molecular Modeling of PrP Isoforms

By comparing the amino acid sequences of 11 mammalian and 1 avian prion proteins, structural analyses using a neuronal network algorithm (Kneller et al. 1990; Presnell et al. 1993) predicted four α-helical regions (Fig. 2) (Gasset et al. 1992; Huang et al. 1994). Interestingly, the four putative α-helical domains of PrP (Gasset et al. 1992) showed both strong helix preference in the α/α class prediction and strong β-sheet preference in the β/β class prediction. These results are consistent with the hypothesis that one or more of these domains undergo conformational changes from α helices to β sheets during the formation of PrP^{Sc} (Huang et al. 1996).

Spectroscopy of PrP Isoforms

PrP^{C} and PrP^{Sc} were purified using nondenaturing procedures (Turk et al. 1988; Pan et al. 1993). Fourier transform infrared (FTIR) spectroscopy and circular dichroism (CD) demonstrated that PrP^{C} has a high α-helix content (42%) and no β-sheet content (3%) (Fig. 3) (Pan et al. 1993). In contrast, the β-sheet content of PrP^{Sc} was 43% and the α-helix 30% as measured by FTIR (Pan et al. 1993) and CD spectroscopy (Safar et al. 1993a). As determined in earlier studies, amino-terminally truncated PrP^{Sc} derived by limited proteolysis and designated PrP 27-30 has an even higher β-sheet content (54%) and a lower α-helix content (21%) (Caughey et al. 1991b; Gasset et al. 1993; Safar et al. 1993b). Denaturation of PrP 27-30 under conditions that reduced scrapie infectivity resulted in a concomitant diminution of β-sheet content (Gasset et al. 1993; Safar et al. 1993b). Since PrP^{Sc} seems to be the only component of the "infectious" prion particle, it is likely that a conformational transition is the fundamental event in the propagation of prions.

We and other workers have suggested that the conversion of PrP^{C} into PrP^{Sc} may proceed through a metastable or partially unfolded intermediate designated PrP* (Jarrett and Lansbury 1993; Cohen et al. 1994). Intermediates in the refolding of PrP 27-30 from a denatured state have been identified by fluorescence and CD spectroscopy (Safar et al. 1994). How PrP^{C} unfolds and refolds into PrP^{Sc} is unknown, but the profound change in protein structure that occurs during this process is likely to be associated with a large activation barrier (Cohen et al. 1994). Whether a catalyst such as a molecular chaperone mediates this process is unknown. Some features of PrP^{Sc} formation seem to mimic an enzymatic reaction: (1) PrP^{C} is the substrate and PrP^{Sc} is the product; (2) the reaction rate depends on the concentration of substrate, PrP^{C}, which is manifest inversely with respect to the incubation time; (3) PrP^{Sc} is an allosteric effector that regulates the conversion of PrP^{C} into PrP^{Sc}; and (4) pseudo substrates such as heterotypic PrP^{C} molecules can slow the conversion through competition. Besides being the

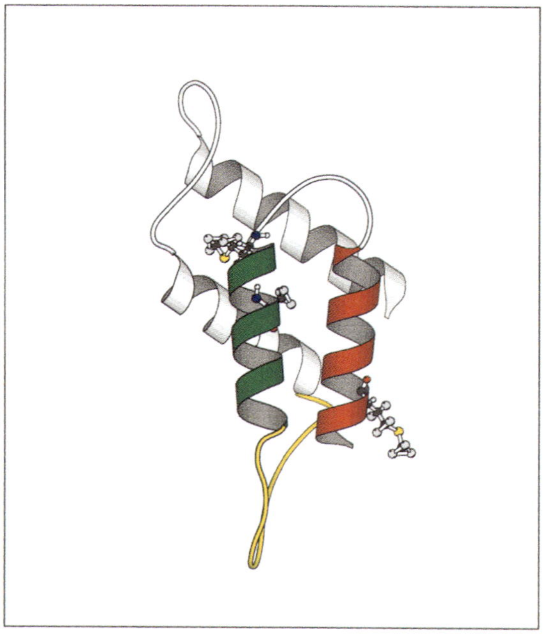

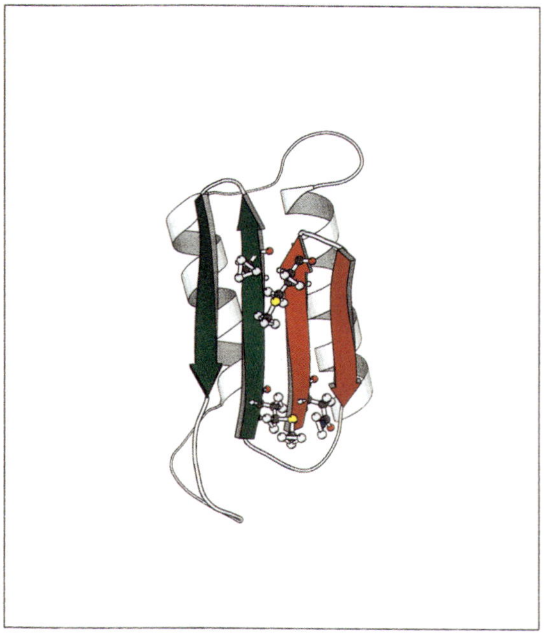

Figure 2. Plausible models for the tertiary structures of PrP^{Sc} and PrP^{C}. (*Left*) Proposed three-dimensional structure of PrP^{C} (Huang et al. 1994). Helix 1 is shown in red, and helix 2 in green. We believe that helices 1 and 2 are converted into β-sheet structure during the formation of PrP^{Sc} (*left*). The H_2-H_3 loop corresponding to the S_{2b}-H_3 loop in PrP^{Sc} is shown in yellow. Four residues (Asn-108, Met-112, Met-129, and Ala-133) are implicated in the species barrier as noted above and they are shown in the ball and stick model. (*Right*) Proposed three-dimensional structure of PrP^{Sc}. This structure was chosen from the six penultimate models of PrP^{Sc} (Fig. 1) because it appeared to correlate best with genetic data on residues involved in species barrier. It contains a 4-strand mixed β sheet with two α helices packed against one face of the sheet. Strands 1a and 1b (in red) correspond to the helix 1 in PrP^{C}, whereas strands 2a and 2b (in green) correspond to the helix 2 (*right*). Helices 3 and 4 in this model remain unchanged from the PrP^{C} model (*right*) (Huang et al. 1994). Four residues (Asn-108, Met-112, Met-129, and Ala-133) implicated in the species barrier (Schätzl et al. 1995) are shown in the ball and stick model. They cluster on the solvent-accessible surface of the β sheet which might provide a plausible interface for the PrP^{Sc}-PrP^{C} interaction. The S_{2b}-H_3 loop connecting the β sheet and helix 3 is implicated in the species barrier and is shown in yellow. This conformationally flexible loop could come into contact with PrP^{C} during the formation of the PrP^{Sc}-PrP^{C} complex. Therefore, the specific molecular recognition during prion replication might involve both the β sheet as the primary binding site and the S_{2b}-H_3 loop as an additional site for interaction. (Adapted from Huang et al. 1996.)

product of the conversion reaction and acting as a ligand, it has been suggested that PrP^{Sc} functions as a chaperone-like protein in mediating the conversion (Liautard 1993). Although unlikely, this additional role has not been ruled out by the available data. Changes in the inducibility of heat shock proteins (Hsp), some of which function as molecular chaperones, as well as their subcellular distribution, have been found in scrapie-infected cells (Kenward et al. 1994; Tatzelt et al. 1995). Whether the Hsps function as chaperones in the conversion of PrP^{C} into PrP^{Sc} or whether Hsps accumulate in response to PrP^{Sc}, which is perceived as a misfolded protein, remains to be determined.

Experiments with immunoprecipitated [^{35}S]Met-labeled $SHaPrP^{C}$ and a more than 50-fold excess of purified $SHaPrP^{Sc}$ have been interpreted as showing that PrP^{C} becomes protease-resistant under these conditions (Kocisko et al. 1994). To date, there is no evidence that the properties of PrP^{C} bound to PrP^{Sc} have been changed into those of PrP^{Sc}. Only reisolation of PrP^{C} after disruption of the PrP^{C}/PrP^{Sc} complexes will allow determination as to whether the properties of these PrP^{C} molecules have been altered. Our attempts to disrupt such PrP^{C}/PrP^{Sc} complexes formed in the presence of excess PrP^{Sc} have been unsuccessful using nondenaturing procedures (Kaneko et al. 1995). Using a similar protocol, we have shown that synthetic peptides can induce protease resistance in PrP^{C} but the resulting PrP^{C}/peptide complexes have not caused disease after injection into experimental animals (Kaneko et al. 1995).

TRANSGENETICS AND GENE TARGETING

Species Barrier

To test the hypothesis that differences in PrP gene sequences might be responsible for the species barrier, Tg mice expressing SHaPrP were constructed (Scott et al. 1989; Prusiner et al. 1990). The PrP genes of Syrian hamsters and mice encode proteins differing at 16 positions. Inoculation of Tg(SHaPrP) mice with SHa prions

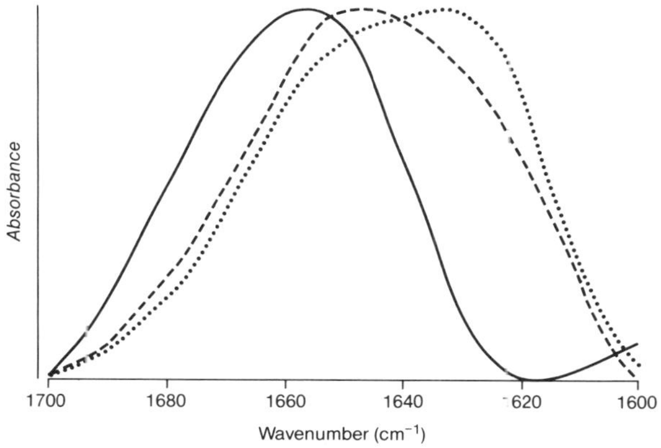

Figure 3. FTIR spectroscopy of prion proteins. The amide I′ band (1700-1600 cm^{-1}) of transmission FTIR spectra of PrP^{C} (*solid line*), PrP^{Sc} (*dashed line*), and PrP 27-30 (*dotted line*). These proteins were suspended in a buffer in D_2O containing 0.15 M NaCl/10 mM sodium phosphate, pD 7.5 (uncorrected)/0.12% ZW. The spectra are scaled independently to be full scale on the ordinate axis (absorbance). (Reprinted, with permission, from Pan et al. 1993.)

demonstrated abrogation of the species barrier, resulting in abbreviated incubation times due to a nonstochastic process (Scott et al. 1989; Prusiner et al. 1990). The length of the incubation time after inoculation with SHa prions was inversely proportional to the level of SHaPrP^{C} in the brains of Tg(SHaPrP) mice (Prusiner et al. 1990). Bioassays of brain extracts from clinically ill Tg(SHaPrP) mice inoculated with Mo prions revealed that only Mo prions, but no SHa prions, were produced. Conversely, inoculation of Tg(SHaPrP) mice with SHa prions led to the synthesis of only SHa prions.

Modeling GSS

The codon 102 point mutation found in GSS patients was introduced into the MoPrP gene, and Tg(MoPrP-P101L)H mice were created expressing high (H) levels of the mutant transgene product. Five lines of Tg(MoPrP-P101L)H mice developed CNS degeneration indistinguishable from experimental murine scrapie with neuropathology consisting of widespread spongiform morphology and astrocytic gliosis (Hsiao et al. 1990) and PrP amyloid plaques (Hsiao et al. 1994). Brain extracts prepared from spontaneously ill Tg(MoPrP-P101L)H mice transmitted CNS degeneration to about 40% of Tg196 mice and some SHa (Hsiao et al. 1994). The Tg196 mice express low levels of the mutant transgene product MoPrP^{C} (P101L) but do not develop spontaneous disease. Much higher rates of transmission of prions from ill Tg(MoPrP-P101L)H mice to Tg196/Prnp$^{0/0}$ mice have been found (Telling et al. 1996). These studies, as well as transmission of prions from patients who died of GSS to apes and monkeys (Masters et al. 1981a; Brown et al. 1994), non-Tg mice (Tateishi et al. 1996), and Tg(MHu2M-P102L) mice (Telling et al. 1995), argue persuasively that prions are devoid of nucleic acid.

PrP-Deficient Mice

Ablation of the PrP gene (Prnp$^{0/0}$) in mice did not affect the development of these animals (Büeler et al. 1992; Manson et al. 1994b), but one study of Prnp$^{0/0}$ mice reports loss of Purkinje cells in the cerebellum after 70 weeks of age (Sakaguchi et al. 1996). In fact, they are healthy at almost 2 years of age. Prnp$^{0/0}$ mice are resistant to prions and do not propagate scrapie infectivity (Fig. 4) (Prusiner et al. 1993b; Manson et al. 1994a; Sakaguchi et al. 1995). One group of investigators described a low level of prion infectivity in Prnp$^{0/0}$ mice in an initial report (Büeler et al. 1993), but that was attributed to contamination of pooled samples in a subsequent communication where the absence of infectivity in individual brains was reported (Sailer et al. 1994).

Hippocampal slices from Prnp$^{0/0}$ mice have been reported to show abnormalities in GABA-mediated synaptic transmission and diminished long-term potentiation (LTP) (Collinge et al. 1994; Manson et al. 1995; Whittington et al. 1995). However, our attempts to reproduce these findings were unsuccessful (Lledo et al. 1996).

Transmission of Human Prions to Transgenic Mice

Because our initial transgenetic studies had shown that the "species barrier" between mice and SHa for the transmission of prions can be abrogated by expression of a SHaPrP transgene in mice (Scott et al. 1989), Tg mice expressing HuPrP were constructed. These Tg(HuPrP)FVB mice inoculated with Hu prions failed to develop CNS dysfunction more frequently than non-Tg controls (Telling et al. 1994). Faced with this apparent dichotomy, we constructed mice expressing a chimeric Hu/Mo PrP transgene designated MHu2M. Earlier studies had shown that chimeric SHa/Mo PrP transgenes supported the transmission of either Mo or SHa prions (Scott et al. 1992, 1993). HuPrP differs from Mo PrP at 28 of 254 positions (Kretzschmar et al. 1986b), and chimeric Hu/MoPrP differs at nine residues. We found that mice expressing the MHu2M transgene are susceptible to human prions and exhibit abbreviated incubation times (Telling et al. 1994).

When Tg(HuPrP) mice were crossed with Prnp$^{0/0}$ mice, they were rendered susceptible to Hu prions, unexpectedly. These findings suggested that Tg(HuPrP) FVB mice were resistant to Hu prions because MoPrP^{C} inhibited the conversion of HuPrP^{C} into PrP^{Sc}; once MoPrP^{C} was removed by gene ablation, the inhibition was abolished (Telling et al. 1995). Earlier studies argued that PrP^{C} forms a complex with PrP^{Sc} during the formation of nascent PrP^{Sc} (Prusiner et al. 1990), but these findings suggested that PrP^{C} also

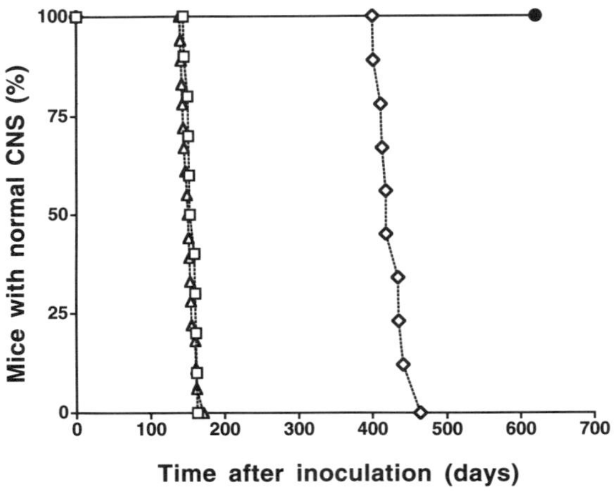

Figure 4. Incubation times in PrP gene ablated $Prnp^{0/+}$ and $Prnp^{0/0}$ mice as well as wt $Prnp^{+/+}$ and CD-1 mice inoculated with RML mouse prions. The RML prions were heated and irradiated at 254 nm prior to intracerebral inoculation into CD-1 Swiss mice (*open triangles*), $Prnp^{+/+}$ mice (*open squares*), $Prnp^{0/+}$ mice (*open diamonds*), or $Prnp^{0/0}$ mice (*filled circle*).

binds to another macromolecule during the conversion process. We provisionally designated this second macromolecule as "protein X." Like the binding of PrP^C to PrP^{Sc}, which is most efficient when the two isoforms have the same sequence (Prusiner et al. 1990), the binding of PrP^C to protein X seems to exhibit the highest affinity when these two proteins are from the same species. Whether protein X is a chaperone that is involved in catalyzing the conformational changes that feature in the formation of PrP^{Sc} (Pan et al. 1993) remains to be established.

Binding Sites on PrP^C

Based largely on the foregoing studies with chimeric transgenes, we surmise that H1 and H2 comprise the region of PrP^C that binds to PrP^{Sc} during the formation of nascent PrP^{Sc}. This conclusion is supported by correlations between species-specific amino acid substitutions and transmission studies across species (Lowenstein et al. 1990; Schätzl et al. 1995).

Molecular modeling studies suggest that PrP^C is a four-helix-bundle protein: The four putative helices are designated H1, H2, H3, and H4 (Huang et al. 1994). A comparison of amino acid substitutions among species in and adjacent to H3 and H4 suggests that the binding of PrP^C to protein X may occur through interactions at the carboxy-terminal end of H4. Such a model can explain why chimeric $MHu2MPrP^C$, but not $HuPrP^C$, is converted into PrP^{Sc} in the presence of $MoPrP^C$, and why $HuPrP^C$ is converted into PrP^{Sc} in the absence of $MoPrP^C$. The proposed model is also consistent with the observation that the Hu and MHu2M prions exhibit similar incubation times in Tg(MHu2M) mice (Telling et al. 1995). Further support is derived from studies on the transmission of prions from inherited prion diseases to mice expressing chimeric PrP transgenes. Tg(MHu2M) mice were resistant to Hu prions from a patient with GSS who carried the P102L mutation but susceptible to prions from patients with familial CJD who harbor the E200K mutation; however, Tg (MHu2M-P101L) mice were susceptible to GSS prions. These findings demonstrate that a single amino acid mismatch at codon 102 near H1 prolongs the incubation time, whereas a mismatch at codon 200 in the loop between H3 and H4 does not.

The residue 129 lies at the amino terminus of H2; this polymorphic residue is either M or V in humans. Prions from a patient homozygous for M129 produced an incubation time of about 170 days in Tg(HuPrP-M129) $440/Prnp^{0/0}$ mice expressing HuPrP encoding M129 on the null background; the same inocula gave much longer incubation times in Tg(HuPrP-V129)$152/Prnp^{0/0}$ mice expressing HuPrP with a V at codon 129 (Telling et al. 1995). Molecular modeling studies predict that residue 129 lies at the amino terminus of H2 within the putative PrP^C/PrP^{Sc} interface. These findings demonstrate that a single amino acid mismatch at codon 129, like codon 102 in the region of helices one and two, prolongs the incubation time, in contrast to a mismatch at codon 200.

Binding of PrP^C to PrP^{Sc} and Synthetic PrP Peptides

Once studies of mice expressing SHaPrP transgenes indicated that PrP^C and PrP^{Sc} form a complex during the formation of nascent PrP^{Sc} (Prusiner et al. 1990), we attempted to demonstrate PrP^{Sc} formation through such complexes by mixing purified fractions containing equimolar amounts of the two isoforms (Raeber et al. 1992). Unable to demonstrate conversion of PrP^C into PrP^{Sc} in these mixtures, we pursued the interactions of synthetic PrP peptides, since we had found that such peptides corresponding to regions of putative secondary structure display conformational pluralism (Gasset et al. 1992; Nguyen et al. 1995a). In contrast to our earlier findings, other investigators were able to demonstrate an interaction between PrP^{Sc} and PrP^C by mixing a 50-fold excess of PrP^{Sc} with labeled PrP^C (Kocisko et al. 1994).

Having found that large, synthetic PrP peptides encompassing the first two putative α-helical regions mimic more of the structural features displayed by the two PrP isoforms than smaller peptides (Nguyen et al. 1995b; Zhang et al. 1995), we asked if such peptides could alter the properties of PrP^C. Up to 70% of the PrP^C was complexed when a peptide of 56 amino acids corresponding to PrP residues 90–145 was used (Kaneko et al. 1995). Unexpectedly, the peptide in a β-sheet conformation did not bind PrP^C whereas the random coil did. The PrP^C/peptide complex was resistant to proteolytic digestion, displayed a high β-sheet content, and sedimented at 100,000*g* for 1 hour. Ultrastructure of the complexes was that of fibrous aggregates. Addition of 2% Sarkosyl disrupted the complex and rendered PrP^{C} sensitive to protease digestion. Complex formation could be prevented by including an α-PrP monoclonal antibody in the PrP^{C}/peptide mixture. When the pathological A117V mutation was substituted in the peptide, the concentration of peptide required for complex formation could be reduced by a factor of approximately 10. Our findings, in concert with transgenetic investigations, argue PrP^{C} interacts with PrP^{Sc} through a domain that contains the first two putative α helices.

Although other investigators have reported the in vitro formation of PrP^{Sc} by mixing a large excess of PrP^{Sc} with ^{35}S-labeled PrP^{C}, their conclusions assume that protease-resistant PrP^{C} is equivalent to PrP^{Sc} (Kocisko et al. 1994). Interestingly, the binding of PrP^{C} to PrP^{Sc} was found to be dependent on the same residues (Kocisko et al. 1995) that render Tg(MH2M) mice susceptible to SHa prions (Scott et al. 1993), and it seems to be strain-dependent (Bessen et al. 1995). Although we were able to confirm the binding of PrP^{C} to PrP^{Sc} in the presence of a large excess of PrP^{Sc}, we were unable to reproduce the renaturation of PrP^{Sc} from GdnHCl as judged by a restoration of protease resistance (Kaneko et al. 1995).

Attempts to separate ^{35}S-labeled PrP^{C} from PrP^{Sc} under conditions where scrapie infectivity is preserved were unsuccessful using a variety of detergents, α-PrP monoclonal antibodies, detergent-lipid-protein complexes (DLPCs), and synthetic peptides. Until such conditions are identified, we cannot determine whether PrP^{C} has been converted into PrP^{Sc} or is only tightly bound. The experiments with PrP peptides which bind to PrP^{C} and render it protease-resistant argue that the latter possibility is more likely to be correct, since Sarkosyl disrupted the PrP^{C}/peptide complex and made PrP^{C} sensitive to protease. Since the PrP peptides used in our studies have not exhibited prion infectivity, it will be possible to determine if the PrP^{C}/peptide complexes that mimic many of the features of PrP^{Sc} are capable of transmitting prion disease in inoculated animals.

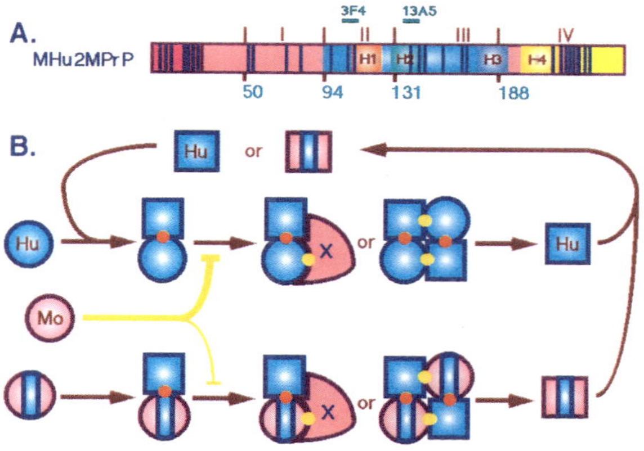

Figure 5. The chimeric Hu/Mo PrP transgene and a model for the formation of PrP^{Sc}. (*A*) Schematic representation of the ORF of the PrP gene showing the 28 differences between the Hu and Mo PrP (*vertical blue lines*). The ORF of HuPrP encoded a protein of 253 amino acids, and that of MoPrP of 254 residues. The four putative α-helical regions of PrP^{C} are designated H1 (*red*), H2 (*green*), H3 (*light blue*), and H4 (*yellow*). In segments II and III, a DNA fragment from the HuPrP gene (*cyan rectangle*) was substituted for MoPrP (*mauve rectangle*). The signal peptide at the amino terminus is denoted by the purple rectangle. The signaling sequence at the carboxyl terminus which is removed upon GPI anchor addition is denoted by the yellow rectangle. (*B*) Possible model for the formation of PrP^{Sc}. PrP^{C} is represented by circles and PrP^{Sc} by squares. HuPrP is cyan and MoPrP is mauve. The site for binding of PrP^{Sc} to PrP^{C} is denoted by the orange disk and the site for binding of PrP^{C} to protein X by the yellow disk. When present, MoPrP^{C} inhibits the formation of HuPrP^{Sc} more than it inhibits the production of MHu2MPrP^{Sc} as denoted by the yellow effector lines. An alternative model for the formation of PrP^{Sc} is shown where protein X is PrP^{Sc}. If this is the case, then the yellow disk designates the binding of the carboxy-terminal domain of PrP^{C} to PrP^{Sc}. Although a tetrameric intermediate is shown, a dimeric intermediate is also possible where the same molecule of PrP^{Sc} binds a molecule of PrP^{C} at two sites.

Monomers or Dimers?

Whether PrP^{C} and PrP^{Sc} exist as monomers, dimers, or oligomers is unknown. Molecular modeling studies suggest that PrP^{C} may form dimers through a solvent-accessible hydrophobic surface of H1 (Huang et al. 1994). The dimerization of PrP^{C} provides an explanation for the results of genetic studies using (PrP-A x PrP-B)F_1 mice inoculated with 22A prions (Dickinson and Meikle 1971; Carlson et al. 1994). These F_1 mice exhibit incubation periods exceeding those of both parents. Ionizing radiation inactivation studies suggest a target size of 55 kD for the infectious prion particle, suggesting that PrP^{Sc} is also a dimer (Alper et al. 1966; Bellinger-Kawahara et al. 1988). It remains to be established whether the PrP^{C}/PrP^{Sc} complex is a heterodimeric or heterotetrameric structure (Fig. 5B).

On the Binding of PrP^{C} to Protein X

Although MoPrP and HuPrP differ at 28 residues, only nine or fewer amino acids between codons 96 and 167 feature in the species barrier for the transmission of Hu prions into mice, as demonstrated by the susceptibility of Tg(MHu2M) mice to Hu prions (Telling et al. 1994). Breaching the species barrier by substitution of residues in H1 and H2 is analogous to the results of studies with chimeric SHa/Mo PrP transgenes, as noted above. That Tg(HuPrP) mice crossed with gene-targeted mice in which the MoPrP gene has been disrupted (Prnp$^{0/0}$) rendered the mice susceptible to Hu prions, which in combination with the susceptibility of Tg(MHu2M)/FVB mice to Hu prions argues that MoPrP^{C} inhibits the conversion of HuPrP^{C} but not

MHu2MPrP^C into PrP^{Sc} (Telling et al. 1995). Perhaps the most conservative explanation for these findings is the existence of a macromolecule other than PrP^{Sc} that binds PrP^C.

If Mo protein X has a higher affinity for MoPrP^C than it does for HuPrP^C, then MoPrP^C would inhibit the conversion of HuPrP^C into HuPrP^{Sc}. When MoPrP^C expression was eliminated by gene targeting, HuPrP^C was converted into HuPrP^{Sc} in murine cells expressing protein X. If the binding site of PrP^C to protein X occurs through the amino- or carboxy-terminal region of PrP^C, then chimeric PrP molecules such as MHu2M would be likely to compete effectively with MoPrP^C for binding to protein X. The experimental data argue that this is the case (Table 1).

Since truncation of the amino terminus of PrP in cultured cells still permitted the formation of PrP^{Sc}-like molecules based on their acquisition of protease resistance (Rogers et al. 1993), it seems more likely that the site at which PrP^C binds to protein X is at the carboxy-terminal end of PrP^C. A comparison of amino acid substitutions in and adjacent to H3 and H4 shows sufficient variation between Hu and Mo, as well as between SHa and Mo, to account for the results of studies with chimeric transgenes. These sequence comparisons suggest that the binding of PrP^C to protein X occurs through interactions at the carboxy-terminal end of H4 (Fig. 5A). PrP residue 215 is a reasonable candidate for participation in the binding of PrP^C to protein X. In HuPrP, this residue is an I, whereas in MoPrP it is a V, and in SHaPrP a T. The side chain of residue 215 is predicted to lie on the external surface of the fourth putative helix (H4). In addition to residue 215, amino acids at positions 219 and 220 may participate in the binding of PrP^C to protein X. It seems unlikely that residues at 228 or 230 are involved in the binding to protein X, since they are adjacent to the GPI anchor, which is attached to an S residue at 231. The proposed model can explain why chimeric MHu2MPrP^C but not HuPrP^C is converted into PrP^{Sc} in the presence of MoPrP^C, and why HuPrP^C is converted into PrP^{Sc} in the absence of MoPrP^C. This model is also consistent with the observation that Hu and MHu2M prions exhibit similar incubation times in Tg(MHu2M) mice if the concentration of protein X is not rate-limiting.

Table 1. Transmission of Hu Prions to Tg(MHu2MPrP) Mice

Inoculum[a]	Incubation time mean days ± S.E.M. (n/n_0)
(A) Tg(MHu2M)FVB mice inoculated with sporadic or infectious CJD	
sCJD(RG)	238 ± 3 (8/8)[b]
sCJD(EC)	218 ± 5 (7/7)[b]
iCJD(364)	232 ± 3 (9/9)[b]
iCJD(364)[c]	231 ± 6 (9/9)
sCJD(MA)	222 ± 1 (4/4)
(B) Tg(MHu2M)Prnp$^{0/0}$ mice inoculated with sporadic or infectious CJD	
sCJD(RC)	207 ± 4 (8/10)
sCJD(RG)	191 ± 3 (10/10)
iCJD(364)	192 ± 6 (8/8)
iCJD(364)[c]	211 ± 5 (8/9)
sCJD(MA)	180 ± 5 (8/8)
sCJD(RO)	217 ± 2 (9/9)
(C) Tg(MHu2M)Prnp$^{0/0}$ mice inoculated with inherited GSS or CJD	
GSS(JJ,P102L)	>310 (0/10)
fCJD(LJ1,E200K)	170 ± 2 (10/10)
fCJD(CA,E200K)	180 ± 9 (9/9)
fCJD(FH,E200K)	>290 (0/7)

[a]All samples were 10% (w/v) brain homogenates (unless otherwise noted) that were diluted 1:10 prior to inoculation. sCJD is sporadic CJD, iCJD is iatrogenic CJD, GSS is Gerstmann-Sträussler-Scheinker disease with the codon 102 mutation, and fCJD is familial CJD with the codon 200 mutation. Patient's initials referring to inocula in B are given in parentheses. If the PrP gene of the patient carried a mutation, then the mutation is noted after the patient's initials.

[b]Transmissions previously reported (Telling et al. 1994).

[c]This is a second inoculum prepared from a different brain region of iatrogenic CJD patient 364.

Does PrP^{Sc} Bind Protein X?

The transmission of Hu and MHu2M prions into Tg(MHu2M)/FVB mice yielded similar incubation times. This finding argues that the differences in the Hu or Mo sequences of PrP^{Sc} at the amino and carboxyl termini have little effect on the transmission of prions to Tg(MHu2M) mice (Tables 1 and 2). Conversely, the region of PrP containing H1 and H2 clearly governs prion transmission to Tg(MHu2M)/Prnp$^{0/0}$ mice: Inoculation of Hu or MHu2M prions produced disease, but Mo prions did not.

Although the lack of binding of PrP^{Sc} to protein X is what we expect for the product of an "enzyme-substrate" reaction, this situation can be construed as an argument favoring the hypothesis that PrP^{Sc} is protein X. If PrP^{Sc} binds to both sites on PrP^C, then the infrequent transmission of Hu prions to Tg(HuPrP)/FVB mice suggests that HuPrP^{Sc} has a higher affinity at the carboxy-terminal binding site for MoPrP^C than for HuPrP^C. This conclusion contrasts with the observation that homotypic interactions between PrP^C and PrP^{Sc} have produced the shortest incubation times when the same amino acid sequence is shared by the two PrP isoforms.

Although most cases of Hu prion disease are not readily transmitted to Tg(HuPrP)/FVB, an exception has been noted (Telling et al. 1994). Undoubtedly other such cases will be found, since it has been reported that a group of GSS cases harboring the P102L mutation transmit CNS degeneration to non-Tg mice in less than 400 days, whereas a second group of cases with the same genotype do not (Tateishi and Kitamoto 1995). One explanation for these cases of prion disease which are unusual with respect to their transmission characteristics is that they represent dif-

Table 2. Serial Transmission of Chimeric Hu/Mo Prions in Tg(MHu2M) Mice

Recipient mouse line	Inoculum[a]	Incubation times mean days ± S.E.M. (n/n_0) illness	death
(A) Chimeric prions produced in Tg(MHu2M) mice inoculated with CJD prions			
Tg(MHu2M)5378/FVB	MHu2M(sCJD)[b]	220 ± 3 (7/7)[c]	226 ± 1(5)
Non-Tg5378/FVB	MHu2M(sCJD)[b]	>400	
Tg(MHu2M)5378/FVB	MHu2M(sCJD)[d]	226 ± 3 (9/9)	228 ± 1(6)
Non-Tg5378/FVB	MHu2M(sCJD)[d]	>400	
Tg(MHu2M)5378/$Prnp^{0/0}$	MHu2M(sCJD)[b]	189 ± 4 (8/8)	192 ± 1(4)
Tg(MHu2M)5378/$Prnp^{0/0}$	MHu2M(sCJD)[d]	183 ± 5 (7/7)	190 ± 3(4)
(B) Mouse prions produced in Tg(MHu2M) or non-Tg mice inoculated with RML prions			
Tg(MHu2M)5378/FVB	Mo(RML)	178 ± 3 (19/19)	203 ± 2(14)[e]
NonTg5378/FVB	Mo(RML)	127 ± 2 (18/18)	156 ± 2(5)
Tg(MHu2M)5378/FVB	MHu2M(RML)[f]	185 ± 1 (7/7)	211 ± 1(3)
Tg(MHu2M)5378/FVB	MHu2M(RML)[g]	189 ± 2 (7/7)	211 ± 9(3)
Non-Tg5378/FVB	MHu2M(RML)[g]	134 ± 3 (5/5)	n.d.
Tg(MHu2M)5378/$Prnp^{0/0}$	Mo(RML)	>400	
Tg(MHu2M)5378/$Prnp^{0/0}$	MHu2M(RML)[f]	>360	
Tg(MHu2M)5378/$Prnp^{0/0}$	MHu2M(RML)[g]	>360	

[a]Notations in parentheses indicate inoculum used in initial passage in Tg(MHu2M) mice.
[b]Mice were inoculated with chimeric prions generated in the brain of a Tg(MHu2M)5378/FVB mouse that had been inoculated with a brain homogenate prepared from patient EC who died of sporadic CJD.
[c]Number of mice developing CNS illness divided by the number inoculated is given in parentheses.
[d]Mice were inoculated with chimeric prions generated in the brain of a second Tg(MHu2M)5378/FVB mouse that had been inoculated with a brain homogenate prepared from patient EC who died of sporadic CJD.
[e]Data from Telling et al. (1994).
[f]Mice were inoculated with Mo prions generated in the brain of a Tg(MHu2M)5378/FVB mouse that had been inoculated with RML Mo prions.
[g]Mice were inoculated with Mo prions generated in the brain of a second Tg(MHu2M)5378/FVB mouse that had been inoculated with RML Mo prions.

ferent strains of prions. Upon the binding of PrP^{Sc} to PrP^{C}, the resulting conformation of PrP^{C} allows it to bind protein X.

No Evidence That Amyloid Formation Features in PrP^{Sc} Synthesis

Some investigators have suggested that scrapie agent multiplication proceeds through a crystallization process involving PrP amyloid formation (Gajdusek 1988, 1990; Gajdusek and Gibbs 1990; Jarrett and Lansbury 1993). Although the high β-sheet content of PrP^{Sc} is clearly a hallmark distinguishing it from PrP^{C} (Pan et al. 1993; Safar et al. 1993a), there is no evidence that PrP^{Sc} forms paracrystalline arrays as is the case for amyloids, which also have a high β-sheet content (Glenner 1980; Glenner et al. 1974). Purified infectious prions isolated from scrapie-infected SHa brains with a cocktail of protease inhibitors contain only PrP^{Sc} which exists as amorphous aggregates; only if PrP^{Sc} molecules are exposed to detergents and limited proteolysis do they then polymerize into prion rods exhibiting the ultrastructural and tinctorial features of amyloid (Fig. 6) (McKinley et al. 1991; Pan et al. 1993). Furthermore, dispersion of prion rods into detergent-lipid-protein complexes results in a 10- to 100-fold increase in scrapie titer, and no rods could be identified in these fractions by electron microscopy (Gabizon et al. 1987). Consistent with these findings is the absence or rarity of amyloid plaques in many prion diseases, as well as the inability to identify any amyloid-like polymers in cultured cells chronically synthesizing prions (Prusiner et al. 1990; McKinley et al. 1991).

Although prion replication seems to be "seeded" by PrP^{Sc}, it can also be initiated by specific mutations, the specificity of which was dramatically demonstrated recently when the change from a glutamate-to-a lysine at codon 200 produced PrP^{CJD} and CJD in humans (Gabizon et al. 1993), and the same glutamate-to-lysine mutation at codon 219 is a common polymorphism occurring in about 6% of the Japanese population (Kitamoto and Tateishi 1994).

The discovery of two binding sites on PrP^{C}, one of which interacts with homotypic PrP^{Sc} and the other with protein X, argues for a high degree of specificity in the prion replication process. Whereas $SHaPrP^{C}$ or a chimeric $SHa/MoPrP^{C}$ can be converted into the corresponding PrP^{Sc} molecules in Tg mice inoculated with SHa prions (Prusiner et al. 1990; Scott et al. 1993), the situation with Hu prions is different (Telling et al. 1994, 1995). As described above, Tg(HuPrP)/FVB mice rarely produce $HuPrP^{Sc}$ after inoculation with Hu prions, but after Tg(HuPrP) mice are crossed onto the null $Prnp^{0/0}$ background, they are rendered susceptible to Hu prions. Furthermore, Tg(MHu2M)/FVB mice expressing a chimeric $Hu/MoPrP^{C}$ readily produce chimeric PrP^{Sc} after inoculation with Hu prions (Tell-

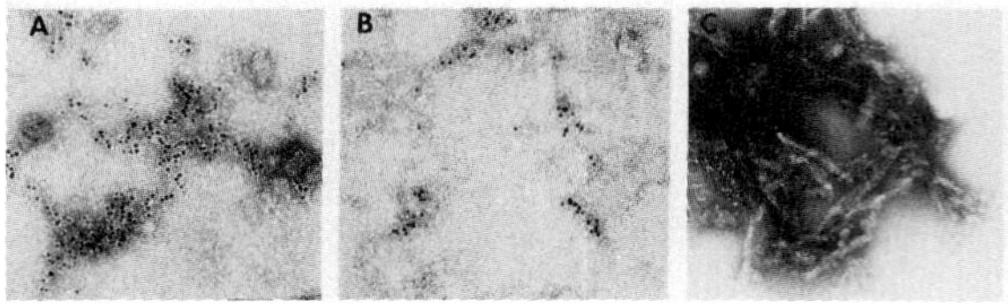

Figure 6. Electron micrographs of negatively stained and immunogold-labeled prion proteins: (*A*) PrP^C and (*B*) PrP^{Sc}. (*C*) Prion rods composed of PrP 27-30 were negatively stained with uranyl acetate. Bar, 100 nm. (Reprinted, with permission, from Pan et al. 1993.)

ing et al. 1994). These results argue persuasively for two different species-specific binding sites on PrP^C in the propagation of prion infectivity.

It is difficult to reconcile the foregoing data with the conjecture that crystallization is the mechanism by which prions replicate. A crystallization phenomenon producing multidimensional macroscopic ordered arrays implies a high degree of at least two-dimensional, and more commonly three-dimensional, organization in aggregates of PrP^{Sc}. It seems more likely that a complex process involving chaperones or similar molecules is responsible for transforming PrP^C into PrP^{Sc}.

PRION DIVERSITY

For many years, studies of experimental scrapie were performed exclusively with sheep and goats. The disease was first transmitted by intraocular inoculation (Cuillé and Chelle 1939) and later by intracerebral, oral, subcutaneous, intramuscular, and intravenous injections of brain extracts from sheep developing scrapie. Incubation periods of 1–3 years were common, and often many of the inoculated animals failed to develop disease (Dickinson and Stamp 1969; Hadlow et al. 1980, 1982). Different breeds of sheep exhibited markedly different susceptibilities to scrapie prions inoculated subcutaneously, suggesting that the genetic background might influence host permissiveness (Gordon 1966).

The diversity of scrapie prions was first appreciated in goats inoculated with "hyper" and "drowsy" isolates (Pattison and Millson 1961). There is good evidence for multiple "strains" or distinct isolates of prions, as defined by specific incubation times, distribution of vacuolar lesions, and patterns of PrP^{Sc} accumulation (Dickinson et al. 1968; Fraser and Dickinson 1973; Bruce et al. 1989; Hecker et al. 1992). The lengths of the incubation times have been used to distinguish prion strains inoculated into sheep, goats, mice, and hamsters. Dickinson and his colleagues developed a system for "strain typing" by which mice with genetically determined short and long incubation times were used in combination with the F_1 cross (Dickinson et al. 1968, 1984; Dickinson and Meikle 1971). For example, C57BL mice exhibited short incubation times of about 150 days when inoculated with either the Me7 or Chandler isolates; VM mice inoculated with these same isolates had prolonged incubation times of about 300 days.

Scrapie Incubation Times

The identification of a widely available mouse strain with long incubation times accelerated studies of prion strains (Kingsbury et al. 1983; Carp et al. 1987). Once molecular clones of the PrP gene were available, we were able to demonstrate genetic linkage between the mouse PrP (*Prnp*) and a gene modulating incubation times (*Prn-i*) (Carlson et al. 1986). Subsequently, other investigators have confirmed the genetic linkage, and one group has shown that the scrapie incubation time gene *Sinc* is also linked to PrP (Hunter et al. 1987; Race et al. 1990). Much evidence now argues that the *Prnp*, *Prn-i*, and *Sinc* genes are congruent; the term *Sinc* is no longer used (Ziegler 1993). The PrP sequences of NZW mice with short and long scrapie incubation times, respectively, differ at codons 108 (L→F) and 189 (T→V) (Westaway et al. 1987).

The discovery that incubation times are controlled by the relative dosage of $Prnp^a$ and $Prnp^b$ alleles (Carlson et al. 1994) was foreshadowed by studies of Tg(SHaPrP) mice in which the length of the incubation time after inoculation with SHa prions was inversely proportional to the transgene product, $SHaPrP^C$ (Prusiner et al. 1990). The PrP gene dose determines not only the length of the incubation time, but also the passage history of the inoculum, particularly in $Prnp^b$ mice (Carlson et al. 1994). The PrP^{Sc} allotype in the inoculum produced the shortest incubation times when it was the same as that of PrP^C in the host (Carlson et al. 1989). The term "allotype" is used to describe allelic variants of PrP. The effect of the allotype barrier was small when measured in $Prnp^{a/a}$ mice but was clearly demonstrable in $Prnp^{b/b}$ mice. Previous passage of prions in $Prnp^b$ mice shortened the incubation time by about 40% when assayed in $Prnp^b$ mice, compared to those inoculated with prions passaged in $Prnp^a$ mice (Carlson et al. 1989).

Patterns of PrP^{Sc} Deposition

In addition to measurements of the length of the incubation time, profiles of spongiform degeneration have also been used to characterize different prion strains (Fraser and Dickinson 1973; Fraser 1979). With the development of a new procedure for in situ detection of PrP^{Sc}, designated histoblotting (Taraboulos et al. 1992b), it became possible to localize and quantify PrP^{Sc} as well as to determine whether or not strains produce different, reproducible patterns of PrP^{Sc} accumulation (Hecker et al. 1992; DeArmond et al. 1993). Histoblotting overcame two obstacles that plagued PrP^{Sc} detection in brain by standard immunohistochemical techniques: the presence of PrP^C and weak antigenicity of PrP^{Sc} (DeArmond et al. 1987).

Comparisons of PrP^{Sc} accumulation on histoblots with histological sections showed that PrP^{Sc} deposition preceded vacuolation and only those regions with PrP^{Sc} underwent degeneration (Hecker et al. 1992). Microdissection of individual brain regions confirmed the conclusions of the histoblot studies: Those regions with high levels of PrP 27-30 had intense vacuolation (Casaccia-Bonnefil et al. 1993). Thus, we concluded that the deposition of PrP^{Sc} is responsible for the neuropathological changes found in the prion diseases.

Although studies with both mice and Syrian hamsters established that each isolate has a specific signature as defined by a specific pattern of PrP^{Sc} accumulation in the brain (Hecker et al. 1992; DeArmond et al. 1993; Carlson et al. 1994), comparisons must be done on an isogenic background (Scott et al. 1993; Hsiao et al. 1994). Variations in the patterns of PrP^{Sc} accumulation were found to be equally as great as those seen between two strains when a single strain is inoculated in mice expressing different PrP genes. On the basis of the initial studies which were performed in animals of a single genotype, we suggested that PrP^{Sc} synthesis occurs in specific populations of cells for a given distinct prion isolate.

Are Prion Strains Different PrP^{Sc} Conformers?

Explaining the problem of multiple distinct prion isolates might be accommodated by multiple PrP^{Sc} conformers that act as templates for the folding of de novo synthesized PrP^{Sc} molecules during prion "replication." Although the proposal for multiple PrP^{Sc} conformers is rather unorthodox, we already know that PrP can assume at least two profoundly different conformations: PrP^{C} and PrP^{Sc} (Pan et al. 1993). Of note, two different isolates from mink dying of transmissible mink encephalopathy exhibit different sensitivities of PrP^{Sc} to proteolytic digestion, supporting the suggestion that isolate-specific information might be carried by PrP^{Sc} (Marsh et al. 1991; Bessen and Marsh 1992a,b). How many conformations PrP^{Sc} can assume is unknown. The molecular weight of a PrP^{Sc} homodimer is consistent with the ionizing radiation target size of 55,000 ± 9000 daltons as determined for infectious prion particles independent of their polymeric form (Bellinger-Kawahara et al. 1988). If prions are oligomers of PrP^{Sc}, which seems likely, then this offers another level of complexity, which in turn generates additional diversity.

INHERITED PRION DISEASES

The recognition that about 10% of cases are familial led to the suspicion that genetics plays a role in this disease (Kirschbaum 1924; Meggendorfer 1930; Stender 1930; Davison and Rabiner 1940; Jacob et al. 1950; Friede and DeJong 1964; Rosenthal et al. 1976; Masters et al. 1979, 1981a,b). As in sheep scrapie, the relative contributions of genetic and infectious etiologies in the human prion diseases remained puzzling. The discovery of the PrP gene and its linkage to scrapie incubation times in mice (Carlson et al. 1986) raised the possibility that mutation might feature in the hereditary human prion diseases. A proline (P)→leucine (L) mutation at codon 102 was shown to be linked genetically to development of GSS with a LOD score exceeding 3 (Fig. 7) (Hsiao et al. 1989b). This mutation may be caused by the deamination of a methylated CpG in a germ-line PrP gene resulting in the substitution of a thymine (T) for cytosine (C). This mutation has been found in ten different families in nine different countries, including the original GSS family (Doh-ura et al. 1989; Goldgaber et al. 1989; Kretzschmar et al. 1991, 1992).

An insert of 144 bp containing six octarepeats at codon 53 was described in patients with CJD from four families residing in southern England (Owen et al. 1989; Collinge et al. 1992; Poulter et al. 1992). Genealogical investigations have shown that all four families are related, arguing for a single founder born more than two centuries ago. The LOD score for this extended pedigree exceeds 11. Studies from several laboratories have demonstrated that two, four, five, six, seven, eight, or nine octarepeats in addition to the normal five are found in individuals with inherited CJD (Collinge et al. 1989, 1990; Owen et al. 1989, 1990; Goldfarb et al. 1991a; Brown 1993), whereas deletion of one octarepeat has been identified without the neurological disease (Laplanche et al. 1990; Vnencak-Jones and Phillips 1992; Palmer et al. 1993).

The unusually high incidence of CJD among Israeli Jews of Libyan origin was thought to be due to the consumption of lightly cooked sheep brain or eyeballs (Herzberg et al. 1974; Kahana et al. 1974, 1991; Alter and Kahana 1976; Neugut et al. 1979; Zilber et al. 1991). Recent studies have shown that some Libyan and Tunisian Jews in families with CJD have a PrP gene point mutation at codon 200 resulting in a Glu→Lys substitution (Goldfarb et al. 1990b; Gabizon et al. 1991; Hsiao et al. 1991b). The E200K mutation has also been found in Slovaks originating from Orava in North Central Czechoslovakia (Goldfarb et al. 1990b), in a cluster of familial cases in Chile (Goldfarb et al. 1991c), and in a large German family living in the United States (Bertoni et al. 1992). If carriers with the codon 200 mutation live long enough, they eventually develop prion disease (Chapman et al. 1994; Spudich et al. 1995).

Many families with CJD have been found to have a point mutation at codon 178 resulting in an Asp→Asn substitution (Fink et al. 1991; Goldfarb et al. 1991a, 1992a; Haltia et al. 1991; Brown et al. 1992;). FFI which presents with insomnia is also associated with the D178N mutation (Lugaresi et al. 1986; Medori et al. 1992). The neuropathology in these patients with FFI is restricted to selected nuclei of the thalamus. It is unclear whether all patients with the D178N mutation or only a subset present with sleep disturbances. It ap-

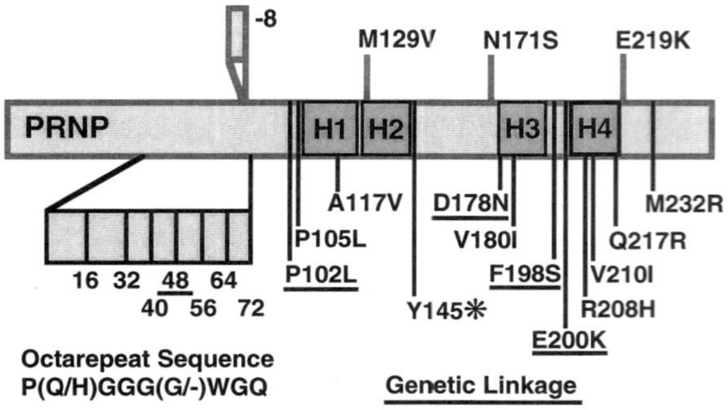

Figure 7. Human prion protein gene (*PRNP*). The ORF is denoted by the large gray rectangle. Human PRNP wild-type coding polymorphisms are shown above the rectangle, and mutations that segregate with the inherited prion diseases are depicted below. The wild-type human PrP gene contains five octarepeats (P[Q/H]GGG[G/-]WGQ) from codons 51 to 91 (Kretzschmar et al. 1986b). Deletion of a single octarepeat at codon 81 or 82 is not associated with prion disease (Laplanche et al. 1990; Puckett et al. 1991; Vnencak-Jones and Phillips 1992); whether this deletion alters the phenotypic characteristics of a prion disease is unknown. There are common polymorphisms at codons 117 (Ala→Ala) and 129 (Met→Val); homozygosity for Met or Val at codon 129 appears to increase susceptibility to sporadic CJD (Palmer et al. 1991). Additional polymorphisms have been found at codons 171 (Asn→Ser) and 219 (Glu→Lys) (Fink et al. 1994; Kitamoto and Tateishi 1994). Octarepeat inserts of 16, 32, 40, 48, 56, 64, and 72 amino acids at codons 67, 75, or 83 are designated by the small rectangle below the ORF. These inserts segregate with familial CJD, and genetic linkage has been demonstrated where sufficient specimens from family members are available (Collinge et al. 1989, 1990; Crow et al. 1990; Goldfarb et al. 1990d, 1991b; Owen et al. 1989, 1990; Palmer et al. 1993). Point mutations are designated by the wild-type amino acid preceding the codon number and the mutant residue following: e.g., P102L. These point mutations segregate with the inherited prion diseases and significant genetic linkage (underlined mutations) has been demonstrated where sufficient specimens from family members are available. Mutations at codons 102 (Pro→Leu), 117 (Ala→Val), 198 (Phe→Ser), and 217 (Gln→Arg) are found in patients with GSS (Dohura et al. 1989; Goldfarb et al. 1990b,c,d; Goldgaber et al. 1989; Hsiao et al. 1989a,b, 1991a; Hsiao and Prusiner 1990; Tateishi et al. 1990). Point mutations at codons 178 (Asp→Asn), 200 (Glu→Lys), 208 (Arg→His), and 210 (Val→Ile) are found in patients with familial CJD (Gabizon et al. 1991; Goldfarb et al. 1990a, 1991a; Hsiao et al. 1991b; Ripoll et al. 1993; Mastrianni et al. 1995). Point mutations at codons 198 (Phe→Ser) and 217 (Gln→Arg) are found in patients with GSS who have PrP amyloid plaques and neurofibrillary tangles (Dlouhy et al. 1992; Hsiao et al. 1992). Additional point mutations at codons 145 (Tyr→Stop), 105 (Pro→Leu), 180 (Val→Ile), and 232 (Met→Arg) have been recently reported (Kitamoto et al. 1993a,b). Single-letter code for amino acids is as follows: A, Ala; D, Asp; E, Glu; F, Phe; I, Ile; K, Lys; L, Leu; M, Met; N, Asn; P, Pro; Q, Gln; R, Arg; S, Ser; T, Thr; V, Val; and Y, Tyr.

pears that the allele with the D178N mutation encodes an M at position 129 in FFI, whereas a V is encoded at position 129 in familial CJD (Goldfarb et al. 1992b). The discovery that FFI is an inherited prion disease clearly widens the clinical spectrum of these disorders and raises the possibility that many other degenerative diseases of unknown etiology may be caused by prions (Johnson 1992; Medori et al. 1992). The codon 178 mutation has been linked to the development of prion disease with a LOD score exceeding 5 (Petersen et al. 1992).

BOVINE SPONGIFORM ENCEPHALOPATHY

Beginning in 1986, an epidemic of a previously unknown prion disease named BSE or "mad cow" disease appeared in cattle in Great Britain (Wells et al. 1987), in which protease-resistant PrP was found in brains of ill cattle (Hope et al. 1988; Prusiner et al. 1993c). It has been proposed that BSE represents a massive common source epidemic which has caused more than 160,000 cases (Wells and Wilesmith 1995). Dairy cows were routinely fed meat and bone meal prepared by rendering the offal of sheep and cattle as a nutritional supplement. Since 1988, the practice of using dietary protein supplements for domestic animals derived from rendered sheep or cattle offal has been banned. Recent statistics argue that the epidemic is now under control as a result of the 1988 food ban (Fig. 8).

Brain extracts from BSE cattle have transmitted disease to mice, cattle, sheep, and pigs after intracerebral inoculation (Fraser et al. 1988; Dawson et al. 1990a,b; Bruce et al. 1993). Transmissions to mice and sheep suggest that cattle preferentially propagate a single "strain" of prions (Bruce et al. 1994). Of particular significance is the transmission of BSE to the marmoset after intracerebral inoculation (Baker et al. 1993). Recent cases of atypical CJD in three teenagers and seven young adults in the United Kingdom raise the possibility of transmission of BSE to humans (Bateman et al. 1995; Britton et al. 1995; Will et al. 1996).

Our experience with Tg(HuPrP)FVB mice expressing both Hu and $MoPrP^{C}$ (Telling et al. 1994, 1995) contrasts with that reported for a case of iatrogenic CJD. When Tg(HuPrP)FVB mice were inoculated with Hu prions from this iatrogenic case of CJD, the mice developed CNS dysfunction about 300 days later (Collinge et al. 1995). When this same inoculum was injected into Tg(HuPrP)$Prnp^{0/0}$ mice, the incubation was reduced to about 200 days, which is similar to those reported by us for other Hu prions (Telling et al. 1995). On the basis of the susceptibility of Tg(HuPrP)$Prnp^{0/0}$ mice to Hu prions from this iatrogenic CJD case and the resistance of these mice to bovine prions from cattle dying of BSE, the authors concluded that BSE prions are unlikely to be pathogenic for humans (Collinge et al. 1995). This conclusion seems contrary to recent reports describing more than ten cases of atypical CJD in teenagers and young adults who are thought to have become ill after

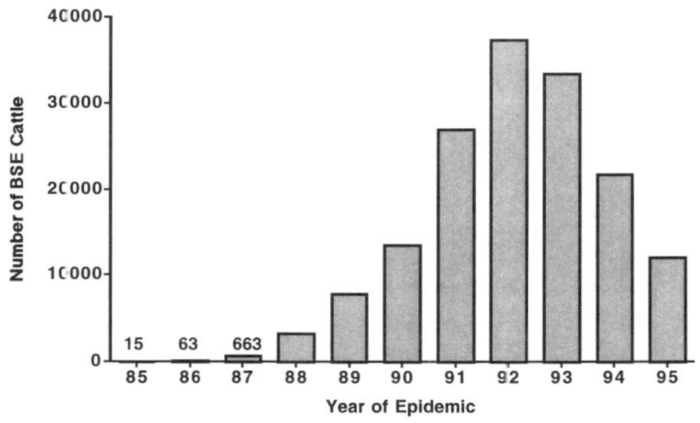

Figure 8. BSE epidemic in Great Britain. Number of annual cases of BSE in cattle is plotted for the past decade. Data were compiled by Dr. John Wilesmith from the Central Veterinary Laboratory at Weybridge, England.

consuming tainted beef in Great Britain, as well as possibly in France and Switzerland (Bateman et al. 1995; Britton et al. 1995; Will et al. 1996).

It is notable that bovine PrP is more homologous with HuPrP than is sheep PrP in the region between codons 96 and 167, which feature in the species barrier in the transmission of Hu prions into mice, as demonstrated by the susceptibility of Tg(MHu2M) mice to Hu prions (Telling et al. 1994, 1995). Whether the differences in the amino acid sequence between bovine and sheep PrP in this central domain are responsible for the apparent differential susceptibility of humans to bovine and sheep prions remains to be established. Epidemiological studies over nearly three decades have failed to establish convincing evidence for transmission of sheep prions to humans (Malmgren et al. 1979; Brown et al. 1987; Harries-Jones et al. 1988; Cousens et al. 1990). It is notable that the high incidence of CJD among Libyan Jews was initially attributed to the consumption of lightly cooked sheep brain (Kahana et al. 1974); however, subsequent studies showed that this geographic cluster of CJD is due to a mutation at codon 200 of the PrP gene (Goldfarb et al. 1990a; Hsiao et al. 1991b; Gabizon et al. 1993).

CONCLUSION

Prions Are Not Viruses

The study of prions has taken several unexpected directions over the past decade. The discovery that prion diseases in humans are uniquely both genetic and infectious has greatly strengthened and extended the prion concept. To date, 19 different mutations in the human PrP gene, all resulting in nonconservative substitutions, have been found to either be linked genetically to or segregate with the inherited prion diseases. Yet, the transmissible prion particle is composed largely, if not entirely, of an abnormal isoform of the prion protein designated PrP^{Sc} (Prusiner 1991). These findings argue that prion diseases should be considered pseudoinfections, since the particles transmitting disease appear to be devoid of a foreign nucleic acid and thus differ from all known microorganisms as well as viruses and viroids. Because much information, especially about scrapie of rodents, has been derived using experimental protocols adapted from virology, we continue to use terms such as infection, incubation period, transmissibility, and endpoint titration in studies of prion diseases.

Common Neurodegenerative Diseases

The knowledge accrued from the study of prion diseases may provide an effective strategy for defining the etiologies and dissecting the molecular pathogenesis of the more common neurodegenerative disorders such as Alzheimer's disease, Parkinson's disease, and amyotrophic lateral sclerosis (ALS). Advances in the molecular genetics of Alzheimer's disease and ALS suggest that, like the prion diseases, an important subset is caused by mutations that result in nonconservative amino acid substitutions in proteins expressed in the CNS (Levy et al. 1990; Van Broeckhoven et al. 1990, 1992; Goate et al. 1991; Mullan et al. 1992; Schellenberg et al. 1992; St. George-Hyslop et al. 1992; Corder et al. 1993; Rosen et al. 1993; Saunders et al. 1993a,b; Levy-Lahad et al. 1995a,b; Rogaev et al. 1995; Sherrington et al. 1995). Since people at risk for inherited prion diseases can now be identified decades before neurological dysfunction is evident, the development of an effective therapy is imperative.

Future Studies

Tg mice expressing foreign or mutant PrP genes now permit virtually all facets of prion diseases to be studied and have created a framework for future investigations. Furthermore, the structure and organization of the PrP gene suggest that PrP^{Sc} is derived from PrP^{C} or a precursor by a posttranslational process. Studies with scrapie-infected cultured cells have provided much evidence that the conversion of PrP^{C} to PrP^{Sc} is a posttranslational process that probably occurs within a subcellular compartment bounded by cholesterol-rich membranes. The molecular mechanism of PrP^{Sc} formation remains to be elucidated, but chemical and physical studies have shown that the conformations of PrP^{C} and PrP^{Sc} are profoundly different.

The study of prion biology and diseases is a new and emerging area of biomedical investigation. Whereas prion biology has its roots in virology, neurology, and neuropathology, its relationships to the disciplines of molecular and cell biology, as well as protein chemistry, have become evident only recently. Certainly, it is likely that learning how prions multiply and cause disease will open up new vistas in biochemistry and genetics.

ACKNOWLEDGMENTS

I thank M. Baldwin, D. Borchelt, G. Carlson, F.E. Cohen, C. Cooper, S.J. DeArmond, R. Fletterick, M. Gasset, R. Gabizon, D. Groth, R. Koehler, L. Hood, K. Hsiao, Z. Huang, V. Lingappa, K.-M. Pan, D. Riesner, M. Scott, A. Serban, N. Stahl, A. Taraboulos, G. Telling, M. Torchia, and D. Westaway for their help in these studies. This work is supported by grants from the National Institutes of Health (NS-14069, AG-08967, AG-02132, NS-22786, and AG-10770) and the American Health Assistance Foundation, as well as by gifts from the Sherman Fairchild Foundation and Bernard Osher Foundation.

REFERENCES

Alper, T., D.A. Haig, and M.C. Clarke. 1966. The exceptionally small size of the scrapie agent. *Biochem. Biophys. Res. Commun.* **22:** 278.

Alper, T., W.A. Cramp, D.A. Haig, and M.C. Clarke. 1967. Does the agent of scrapie replicate without nucleic acid? *Nature* **214:** 764.

Alter, M. and E. Kahana. 1976. Creutzfeldt-Jakob disease among Libyan Jews in Israel. *Science* **192:** 428.

Anderson, R.G.W. 1993. Caveolae: Where incoming and outgoing messengers meet. *Proc. Natl. Acad. Sci.* **90:** 10909.

Baker, H.F., R.M. Ridley, and G.A.H. Wells. 1993. Experimental transmission of BSE and scrapie to the common marmoset. *Vet. Rec.* **132:** 403.

Basler, K., B. Oesch, M. Scott, D. Westaway, M. Wälchli, D.F. Groth, M.P. McKinley, S.B. Prusiner, and C. Weissmann. 1986. Scrapie and cellular PrP isoforms are encoded by the same chromosomal gene. *Cell* **46:** 417.

Bateman, D., D. Hilton, S. Love, M. Zeidler, J. Beck, and J. Collinge. 1995. Sporadic Creutzfeldt-Jakob disease in a 18-year-old in the UK (Letter). *Lancet* **346:** 1155.

Bellinger-Kawahara, C.G., E. Kempner, D.F. Groth, R. Gabizon, and S.B. Prusiner. 1988. Scrapie prion liposomes and rods exhibit target sizes of 55,000 Da. *Virology* **164:** 537.

Bendheim, P.E., R.A. Barry, S.J. DeArmond, D.P. Stites, and S.B. Prusiner. 1984. Antibodies to a scrapie prion protein. *Nature* **310:** 418.

Bertoni, J.M., P. Brown, L. Goldfarb, D. Gajdusek, and N.E. Omaha. 1992. Familial Creutzfeldt-Jakob disease with the PRNP codon 200^{lys} mutation and supranuclear palsy but without myoclonus or periodic EEG complexes. *Neurology* (suppl. 3) **42:** 350. (Abstr.)

Bessen, R.A. and R.F. Marsh. 1992a. Biochemical and physical properties of the prion protein from two strains of the transmissible mink encephalopathy agent. *J. Virol.* **66:** 2096.

———. 1992b. Identification of two biologically distinct strains of transmissible mink encephalopathy in hamsters. *J. Gen. Virol.* **73:** 329.

Bessen, R.A., D.A. Kocisko, G.J. Raymond, S. Nandan, P.T. Lansbury, and B. Caughey. 1995. Non-genetic propagation of strain-specific properties of scrapie prion protein. *Nature* **375:** 698.

Bolton, D.C., M.P. McKinley, and S.B. Prusiner. 1982. Identification of a protein that purifies with the scrapie prion. *Science* **218:** 1309.

Borchelt, D.R., A. Taraboulos, and S.B. Prusiner. 1992. Evidence for synthesis of scrapie prion proteins in the endocytic pathway. *J. Biol. Chem.* **267:** 16188.

Britton, T.C., S. Al-Sarraj, C. Shaw, T. Campbell, and J. Collinge. 1995. Sporadic Creutzfeldt-Jakob disease in a 16-year-old in the UK (Letter). *Lancet* **346:** 1155.

Brown, P. 1993. Infectious cerebral amyloidosis: Clinical spectrum, risks and remedies. In *Developments in biological standardization* (ed. F. Brown), p. 91. Karger, Basel.

Brown, P., F. Cathala, R.F. Raubertas, D.C. Gajdusek, and P. Castaigne. 1987. The epidemiology of Creutzfeldt-Jakob disease: Conclusion of 15-year investigation in France and review of the world literature. *Neurology* **37:** 895.

Brown, P., C.J. Gibbs, Jr., P. Rodgers-Johnson, D.M. Asher, M.P. Sulima, A. Bacote, L.G. Goldfarb, and D.C. Gajdusek. 1994. Human spongiform encephalopathy: The National Institutes of Health series of 300 cases of experimentally transmitted disease. *Ann. Neurol.* **35:** 513.

Brown, P., L.G. Goldfarb, J. Kovanen, M. Haltia, F. Cathala, M. Sulima, C.J. Gibbs, Jr., and D.C. Gajdusek. 1992. Phenotypic characteristics of familial Creutzfeldt-Jakob disease associated with the codon 178^{Asn} *PRNP* mutation. *Ann. Neurol.* **31:** 282.

Bruce, M.E., P.A. McBride, and C.F. Farquhar. 1989. Precise targeting of the pathology of the sialoglycoprotein, PrP, and vacuolar degeneration in mouse scrapie. *Neurosci. Lett.* **102:** 1.

Bruce, M., A. Chree, I. McConnell, J. Foster, and H. Fraser. 1993. Transmissions of BSE, scrapie and related diseases to mice. In *Proceedings of the 9th International Congress of Virology,* Glasgow, Scotland, p. 93.

Bruce, M., A. Chree, I. McConnell, J. Foster, G. Pearson, and H. Fraser. 1994. Transmission of bovine spongiform encephalopathy and scrapie to mice: Strain variation and the species barrier. *Philos. Trans. R. Soc. Lond. B Biol. Sci.* **343:** 405.

Büeler, H., A. Aguzzi, A. Sailer, R.-A. Greiner, P. Autenried, M. Aguet, and C. Weissmann. 1993. Mice devoid of PrP are resistant to scrapie. *Cell* **73:** 1339.

Büeler, H., M. Fischer, Y. Lang, H. Bluethmann, H.-P. Lipp, S.J. DeArmond, S.B. Prusiner, M. Aguet, and C. Weissmann. 1992. Normal development and behaviour of mice lacking the neuronal cell-surface PrP protein. *Nature* **356:** 577.

Carlson, G.A., D. Westaway, S.J. DeArmond, M. Peterson-Torchia, and S.B. Prusiner. 1989. Primary structure of prion protein may modify scrapie isolate properties. *Proc. Natl. Acad. Sci.* **86:** 7475.

Carlson, G.A., D.T. Kingsbury, P.A. Goodman, S. Coleman, S.T. Marshall, S.J. DeArmond, D. Westaway, and S.B. Prusiner. 1986. Linkage of prion protein and scrapie incubation time genes. *Cell* **46:** 503.

Carlson, G.A., C. Ebeling, S.-L. Yang, G. Telling, M. Torchia, D. Groth, D. Westaway, S.J. DeArmond, and S.B. Prusiner. 1994. Prion isolate specified allotypic interactions between the cellular and scrapie prion proteins in congenic and transgenic mice. *Proc. Natl. Acad. Sci.* **91:** 5690.

Carp, R.I., R.C. Moretz, M. Natelli, and A.G. Dickinson. 1987. Genetic control of scrapie: Incubation period and plaque formation in mice. *J. Gen. Virol.* **68:** 401.

Casaccia-Bonnefil, P., R.J. Kascsak, R. Fersko, S. Callahan, and R.I. Carp. 1993. Brain regional distribution of prion protein PrP27-30 in mice stereotaxically microinjected with different strains of scrapie. *J. Infect. Dis.* **167:** 7.

Caughey, B. and G.J. Raymond. 1991. The scrapie-associated

form of PrP is made from a cell surface precursor that is both protease- and phospholipase-sensitive. *J. Biol. Chem.* **266:** 18217.

Caughey, B., G.J. Raymond, D. Ernst, and R.E. Race. 1991a. N-terminal truncation of the scrapie-associated form of PrP by lysosomal protease(s): Implications regarding the site of conversion of PrP to the protease-resistant state. *J. Virol.* **65:** 6597.

Caughey, B.W., A. Dong, K.S. Bhat, D. Ernst, S.F. Hayes, and W.S. Caughey. 1991b. Secondary structure analysis of the scrapie-associated protein PrP 27-30 in water by infrared spectroscopy. *Biochemistry* **30:** 7672.

Chapman, J., J. Ben-Israel, Y. Goldhammer, and A.D. Korczyn. 1994. The risk of developing Creutzfeldt-Jakob disease in subjects with the *PRNP* gene codon 200 point mutation. *Neurology* **44:** 1683.

Chesebro, B., R. Race, K. Wehrly, J. Nishio, M. Bloom, D. Lechner, S. Bergstrom, K. Robbins, L. Mayer, J.M. Keith, C. Garon, and A. Haase. 1985. Identification of scrapie prion protein-specific mRNA in scrapie-infected and uninfected brain. *Nature* **315:** 331.

Cohen, F.E., K.-M. Pan, Z. Huang, M. Baldwin, R.J. Fletterick, and S.B. Prusiner. 1994. Structural clues to prion replication. *Science* **264:** 530.

Collinge, J., M.A. Whittington, K.C. Sidle, C.J. Smith, M.S. Palmer, A.R. Clarke, and J.G.R. Jefferys. 1994. Prion protein is necessary for normal synaptic function. *Nature* **370:** 295.

Collinge, J., A.E. Harding, F. Owen, M. Poulter, R. Lofthouse, A.M. Boughey, T. Shah, and T.J. Crow. 1989. Diagnosis of Gerstmann-Sträussler syndrome in familial dementia with prion protein gene analysis. *Lancet* **II:** 15.

Collinge, J., F. Owen, H. Poulter, M. Leach, T. Crow, M. Rosser, J. Hardy, H. Mullan, I. Janota, and P. Lantos. 1990. Prion dementia without characteristic pathology. *Lancet* **336:** 7.

Collinge, J., M.S. Palmer, K.C. Sidle, A.F. Hill, I. Gowland, J. Meads, E. Asante, R. Bradley, L.J. Doey, and P.L. Lantos. 1995. Unaltered susceptibility to BSE in transgenic mice expressing human prion protein. *Nature* **378:** 779.

Collinge, J., J. Brown, J. Hardy, M. Mullan, M.N. Rossor, H. Baker, T.J. Crow, R. Lofthouse, M. Poulter, R. Ridley, F. Owen, C. Bennett, G. Dunn, A.E. Harding, N. Quinn, B. Doshi, G.W. Roberts, M. Honavar, I. Janota, and P.L. Lantos. 1992. Inherited prion disease with 144 base pair gene insertion. 2. Clinical and pathological features. *Brain* **115:** 687.

Corder, E.H., A.M. Saunders, W.J. Strittmatter, D.E.Schmechel, P.C. Gaskell, G.W. Small, A.D. Roses, J.L. Haines, and M.A. Pericak-Vance. 1993. Gene dose of apolipoprotein E type 4 allele and the risk of Alzheimer's disease in late onset families. *Science* **261:** 921.

Cousens, S.N., R. Harries-Jones, R. Knight, R.G. Will, P.G. Smith, and W.B. Matthews. 1990. Geographical distribution of cases of Creutzfeldt-Jakob disease in England and Wales 1970–1984. *J. Neurol. Neurosurg. Psychiatry* **53:** 459.

Crow, T.J., J. Collinge, R.M. Ridley, H.F. Baker, R. Lofthouse, F. Owen, and A.E. Harding. 1990. Mutations in the prion gene in human transmissible dementia. In *Abstracts from Seminar on Molecular Approaches to Research in Spongiform Encephalopathies in Man.* Medical Research Council, London.

Cuillé, J. and P.L. Chelle. 1939. Experimental transmission of trembling to the goat. *C.R. Seances Acad. Sci.* **208:** 1058.

Davison, C. and A.M. Rabiner. 1940. Spastic pseudosclerosis (disseminated encephalomyelopathy; corticopal-lidospinal degeneration). Familial and nonfamilial incidence (a clinico-pathologic study). *Arch. Neurol. Psychiatry* **44:** 578.

Dawson, M., G.A.H. Wells, and B.N.J. Parker. 1990a. Preliminary evidence of the experimental transmissibility of bovine spongiform encephalopathy to cattle. *Vet. Rec.* **126:** 112.

Dawson, M., G.A.H. Wells, B.N.J. Parker, and A.C. Scott. 1990b. Primary parenteral transmission of bovine spongiform encephalopathy to the pig. *Vet. Rec.* **127:** 338.

DeArmond, S.J., M.P. McKinley, R.A. Barry, M.B. Braunfeld, J.R. McColloch, and S.B. Prusiner. 1985. Identification of prion amyloid filaments in scrapie-infected brain. *Cell* **41:** 221.

DeArmond, S.J., W.C. Mobley, D.L. DeMott, R.A. Barry, J.H. Beckstead, and S.B. Prusiner. 1987. Changes in the localization of brain prion proteins during scrapie infection. *Neurology* **37:** 1271.

DeArmond, S.J., S.-L. Yang, A. Lee, R. Bowler, A. Taraboulos, D. Groth, and S.B. Prusiner. 1993. Three scrapie prion isolates exhibit different accumulation patterns of the prion protein scrapie isoform. *Proc. Natl. Acad. Sci.* **90:** 6449.

Dickinson, A.G. and J.T. Stamp. 1969. Experimental scrapie in Cheviot and Suffolk sheep. *J. Comp. Pathol.* **79:** 23.

Dickinson, A.G. and V.M.H. Meikle. 1971. Host-genotype and agent effects in scrapie incubation: Change in allelic interaction with different strains of agent. *Mol. Gen. Genet.* **112:** 73.

Dickinson, A.G., V.M.H. Meikle, and H. Fraser. 1968. Identification of a gene which controls the incubation period of some strains of scrapie agent in mice. *J. Comp. Pathol.* **78:** 293.

Dickinson, A.G., M.E. Bruce, G.W. Outram, and R.H. Kimberlin. 1984. Scrapie strain differences: The implications of stability and mutation. In *Proceedings of workshop on slow transmissible diseases* (ed. J. Tateishi), p. 105. Japanese Ministry of Health and Welfare, Tokyo.

Diringer, H., H. Gelderblom, H. Hilmert, M. Ozel, C. Edelbluth, and R.H. Kimberlin. 1983. Scrapie infectivity, fibrils and low molecular weight protein. *Nature* **306:** 476.

Dlouhy, S.R., K. Hsiao, M.R. Farlow, T. Foroud, P.M. Conneally, P. Johnson, S.B. Prusiner, M.E. Hodes, and B. Ghetti. 1992. Linkage of the Indiana kindred of Gerstmann-Sträussler-Scheinker disease to the prion protein gene. *Nat. Genet.* **1:** 64.

Doh-ura, K., J. Tateishi, H. Sasaki, T. Kitamoto, and Y. Sakaki. 1989. Pro→Leu change at position 102 of prion protein is the most common but not the sole mutation related to Gerstmann-Sträussler syndrome. *Biochem. Biophys. Res. Commun.* **163:** 974.

Fink, J.K., M.L. Peacock, J.T. Warren, A.D. Roses, and S.B. Prusiner. 1994. Detecting prion protein gene-mutations by denaturing gradient gel-electrophoresis. *Hum. Mutat.* **4:** 42.

Fink, J.K., J.T. Warren, Jr., I. Drury, D. Murman, and B.A. Peacock. 1991. Allele-specific sequencing confirms novel prion gene polymorphism in Creutzfeldt-Jakob disease. *Neurology* **41:** 1647.

Fraser, H. 1979. Neuropathology of scrapie: The precision of the lesions and their diversity. In *Slow transmissible diseases of the nervous system* (ed. S. B. Prusiner and W. J. Hadlow), vol. 1, p. 387. Academic Press, New York.

Fraser, H. and A.G. Dickinson. 1973. Scrapie in mice. Agent-strain differences in the distribution and intensity of grey matter vacuolation. *J. Comp. Pathol.* **83:** 29.

Fraser, H., I. McConnell, G.A.H. Wells, and M. Dawson. 1988. Transmission of bovine spongiform encephalopathy to mice. *Vet. Rec.* **123:** 472.

Friede, R.L. and R.N. DeJong. 1964. Neuronal enzymatic failure in Creutzfeldt-Jakob disease. A familial study. *Arch. Neurol.* **10:** 181.

Gabizon, R. and S.B. Prusiner. 1990. Prion liposomes. *Biochem. J.* **266:** 1.

Gabizon, R., M.P. McKinley, and S.B. Prusiner. 1987. Purified prion proteins and scrapie infectivity copartition into liposomes. *Proc. Natl. Acad. Sci.* **84:** 4017.

Gabizon, R., M.P. McKinley, D.F. Groth, and S.B. Prusiner. 1988. Immunoaffinity purification and neutralization of scrapie prion infectivity. *Proc. Natl. Acad. Sci.* **85:** 6617.

Gabizon, R., H. Rosenmann, Z. Meiner, I. Kahana, E. Kahana, Y. Shugart, J. Ott, and S.B. Prusiner. 1993. Mutation and polymorphism of the prion protein gene in Libyan Jews with Creutzfeldt-Jakob disease. *Am. J. Hum. Genet.* **33:** 828.

Gabizon, R., Z. Meiner, C. Cass, E. Kahana, I. Kahana, D. Avrahami, O. Abramsky, G. Scarlato, S.B. Prusiner, and K.K. Hsiao. 1991. Prion protein gene mutation in Libyan Jews with Creutzfeldt-Jakob disease. *Neurology* **41:** 160.

Gabriel, J.-M., B. Oesch, H. Kretzschmar, M. Scott, and S.B. Prusiner. 1992. Molecular cloning of a candidate chicken prion protein. *Proc. Natl. Acad. Sci.* **89:** 9097.

Gajdusek, D.C. 1977. Unconventional viruses and the origin and disappearance of kuru. *Science* **197:** 943.

———. 1985. Subacute spongiform virus encephalopathies caused by unconventional viruses. In *Subviral pathogens of plants and animals: Viroids and prions* (ed. K. Maramorosch and J.J. McKelvey, Jr.), p. 483. Academic Press, Orlando, Florida.

———. 1988. Transmissible and non-transmissible amyloidoses: Autocatalytic post-translational conversion of host precursor proteins to β-pleated sheet configurations. *J. Neuroimmunol.* **20:** 95.

———. 1990. Subacute spongiform encephalopathies: Transmissible cerebral amyloidoses caused by unconventional viruses. In *Virology*, 2nd edition (ed. B.N. Fields et al.), p. 2289. Raven Press, New York.

Gajdusek, D.C. and C.J. Gibbs, Jr. 1990. Brain amyloidoses-precursor proteins and the amyloids of transmissible and nontransmissible dementias: Scrapie-kuru-CJD viruses as infectious polypeptides or amyloid-enhancing vector. In *Biomedical advances in aging* (ed. A. Goldstein), p. 3. Plenum Press, New York.

Gajdusek, D.C. and V. Zigas. 1957. Degenerative disease of the central nervous system in New Guinea—The endemic occurrence of "kuru" in the native population. *N. Engl. J. Med.* **257:** 974.

Gajdusek, D.C., C.J. Gibbs, Jr., and M. Alpers. 1966. Experimental transmission of a kuru-like syndrome to chimpanzees. *Nature* **209:** 794.

Gasset, M., M.A. Baldwin, R.J. Fletterick, and S.B. Prusiner. 1993. Perturbation of the secondary structure of the scrapie prion protein under conditions associated with changes in infectivity. *Proc. Natl. Acad. Sci.* **90:** 1.

Gasset, M., M.A. Baldwin, D. Lloyd, J.-M. Gabriel, D.M. Holtzman, F. Cohen, R. Fletterick, and S.B. Prusiner. 1992. Predicted α-helical regions of the prion protein when synthesized as peptides form amyloid. *Proc. Natl. Acad. Sci.* **89:** 10940.

Gibbs, C.J., Jr., D.C. Gajdusek, D.M. Asher, M.P. Alpers, E. Beck, P.M. Daniel, and W.B. Matthews. 1968. Creutzfeldt-Jakob disease (spongiform encephalopathy): Transmission to the chimpanzee. *Science* **161:** 388.

Glenner, G.G. 1980. Amyloid deposits and amyloidosis. *N. Engl. J. Med.* **302:** 1283.

Glenner, G.G., E.D. Eanes, H.A. Bladen, R.P. Linke, and J.D. Termine. 1974. Beta-pleated sheet fibrils—A comparison of native amyloid with synthetic protein fibrils. *J. Histochem. Cytochem.* **22:** 1141.

Goate, A., M.-C. Chartier-Harlin, M. Mullan, J. Brown, F. Crawford, L. Fidani, L. Giuffra, A. Haynes, N. Irving, L. James, R. Mant, P. Newton, K. Rooke, P. Roques, C. Talbot, M. Pericak-Vance, A. Roses, R. Williamson, M. Rossor, M. Owen, and J. Hardy. 1991. Segregation of a missense mutation in the amyloid precursor protein gene with familial Alzheimer's disease. *Nature* **349:** 704.

Goldfarb, L., A. Korczyn, P. Brown, J. Chapman, and D.C. Gajdusek. 1990a. Mutation in codon 200 of scrapie amyloid precursor gene linked to Creutzfeldt-Jakob disease in Sephardic Jews of Libyan and non-Libyan origin. *Lancet* **336:** 637.

Goldfarb, L.G., E. Mitrova, P. Brown, B.H. Toh, and D.C. Gajdusek. 1990b. Mutation in codon 200 of scrapie amyloid protein gene in two clusters of Creutzfeldt-Jakob disease in Slovakia. *Lancet* **336:** 514.

Goldfarb, L., P. Brown, D. Goldgaber, R. Garruto, R. Yanaghiara, D. Asher, and D.C. Gajdusek. 1990c. Identical mutation in unrelated patients with Creutzfeldt-Jakob disease. *Lancet* **336:** 174.

Goldfarb, L.G., M. Haltia, P. Brown, A. Nieto, J. Kovanen, W.R. McCombie, S. Trapp, and D.C. Gajdusek. 1991a. New mutation in scrapie amyloid precursor gene (at codon 178) in Finnish Creutzfeldt-Jakob kindred. *Lancet* **337:** 425.

Goldfarb, L.G., P. Brown, D. Goldgaber, D.M. Asher, R. Rubenstein, W.T. Brown, P. Piccardo, R.J. Kascsak, J.W. Boellaard, and D.C. Gajdusek. 1990d. Creutzfeldt-Jakob disease and kuru patients lack a mutation consistently found in the Gerstmann-Sträussler-Scheinker syndrome. *Exp. Neurol.* **108:** 247.

Goldfarb, L.G., P. Brown, W. R. McCombie, D. Goldgaber, G.D. Swergold, P.R. Wills, L. Cervenakova, H. Baron, C.J.J. Gibbs, and D.C. Gajdusek. 1991b. Transmissible familial Creutzfeldt-Jakob disease associated with five, seven, and eight extra octapeptide coding repeats in the *PRNP* gene. *Proc. Natl. Acad. Sci.* **88:** 10926.

Goldfarb, L.G., P. Brown, E. Mitrova, L. Cervenakova, L. Goldin, A.D. Korczyn, J. Chapman, S. Galvez, L. Cartier, R. Rubenstein, and D.C. Gajdusek. 1991c. Creutzfeldt-Jacob disease associated with the PRNP codon 200^{Lys} mutation: An analysis of 45 families. *Eur. J. Epidemiol.* **7:** 477.

Goldfarb, L.G., P. Brown, M. Haltia, F. Cathala, W. R. McCombie, J. Kovanen, L. Cervenakova, L. Goldin, A. Nieto, M. S. Godec, D.M. Asher, and D.C. Gajdusek. 1992a. Creutzfeldt-Jakob disease cosegregates with the codon 178^{Asn} *PRNP* mutation in families of European origin. *Ann. Neurol.* **31:** 274.

Goldfarb, L.G., R.B. Petersen, M. Tabaton, P. Brown, A.C. LeBlanc, P. Montagna, P. Cortelli, J. Julien, C. Vital, W.W. Pendelbury, M. Haltia, P.R. Wills, J.J. Hauw, P.E. McKeever, L. Monari, B. Schrank, G.D. Swergold, L. Autilio-Gambetti, D.C. Gajdusek, E. Lugaresi, and P. Gambetti. 1992b. Fatal familial insomnia and familial Creutzfeldt-Jakob disease: Disease phenotype determined by a DNA polymorphism. *Science* **258:** 806.

Goldgaber, D., L.G. Goldfarb, P. Brown, D.M. Asher, W.T. Brown, S. Lin, J.W. Teener, S.M. Feinstone, R. Rubenstein, R.J. Kascsak, J.W. Boellaard, and D.C. Gajdusek. 1989. Mutations in familial Creutzfeldt-Jakob disease and Gerstmann-Sträussler-Scheinker's syndrome. *Exp. Neurol.* **106:** 204.

Gordon, W.S. 1966. Variation in susceptibility of sheep to scrapie and genetic implications. In *Report of Scrapie Seminar*, (ARS 91-53), p. 53. U.S. Department of Agriculture, Washington, D.C.

Hadlow, W.J. 1959. Scrapie and kuru. *Lancet* **II:** 289.

Hadlow, W.J., R.C. Kennedy, and R.E. Race. 1982. Natural infection of Suffolk sheep with scrapie virus. *J. Infect. Dis.* **146:** 657.

Hadlow, W.J., R.C. Kennedy, R.E. Race, and C.M. Eklund. 1980. Virologic and neurohistologic findings in dairy goats affected with natural scrapie. *Vet. Pathol.* **17:** 187.

Haltia, M., J. Kovanen, L.G. Goldfarb, P. Brown, and D.C. Gajdusek. 1991. Familial Creutzfeldt-Jakob disease in Finland: Epidemiological, clinical, pathological and molecular genetic studies. *Eur. J. Epidemiol.* **7:** 494.

Harries-Jones, R., R. Knight, R.G. Will, S. Cousens, P.G. Smith, and W.B. Matthews. 1988. Creutzfeldt-Jakob disease in England and Wales, 1980–1984: A case-control study of potential risk factors. *J. Neurol. Neurosurg. Psychiatry* **51:** 1113.

Hecker, R., A. Taraboulos, M. Scott, K.-M. Pan, M. Torchia, K. Jendroska, S.J. DeArmond, and S.B. Prusiner. 1992. Replication of distinct prion isolates is region specific in brains of transgenic mice and hamsters. *Genes Dev.* **6:** 1213.

Herzberg, L., B. N. Herzberg, C.J. Gibbs, Jr., W. Sullivan, H. Amyx, and D.C. Gajdusek. 1974. Creutzfeldt-Jakob disease: Hypothesis for high incidence in Libyan Jews in Israel. *Science* **186:** 848.

Hope, J., L.J.D. Reekie, N. Hunter, G. Multhaup, K. Beyreuther, H. White, A.C. Scott, M.J. Stack, M. Dawson, and G.A.H. Wells. 1988. Fibrils from brains of cows with new cattle disease contain scrapie-associated protein. *Nature* **336:** 390.

Hsiao, K. and S.B. Prusiner. 1990. Inherited human prion diseases. *Neurology* **40:** 1820.

Hsiao, K.K., K. Doh-ura, T. Kitamoto, J. Tateishi, and S.B. Prusiner. 1989a. A prion protein amino acid substitution in ataxic Gerstmann-Sträussler syndrome. *Ann. Neurol.* **26:** 137.

Hsiao, K.K., M. Scott, D. Foster, D.F. Groth, S.J. DeArmond, and S.B. Prusiner. 1990. Spontaneous neurodegeneration in transgenic mice with mutant prion protein. *Science* **250:** 1587.

Hsiao, K.K., C. Cass, G.D. Schellenberg, T. Bird, E. Devine-Gage, H. Wisniewski, and S.B. Prusiner. 1991a. A prion protein variant in a family with the telencephalic form of Gerstmann-Sträussler-Scheinker syndrome. *Neurology* **41:** 681.

Hsiao, K., H.F. Baker, T.J. Crow, M. Poulter, F. Owen, J.D. Terwilliger, D. Westaway, J. Ott, and S. B.Prusiner. 1989b. Linkage of a prion protein missense variant to Gerstmann-Sträussler syndrome. *Nature* **338:** 342.

Hsiao, K., S. Dlouhy, M.R. Farlow, C. Cass, M. Da Costa, M. Conneally, M.E. Hodes, B. Ghetti, and S.B. Prusiner. 1992. Mutant prion proteins in Gerstmann-Sträussler-Scheinker disease with neurofibrillary tangles. *Nat. Genet.* **1:** 68.

Hsiao, K.K., D. Groth, M. Scott, S.-L. Yang, H. Serban, D. Rapp, D. Foster, M. Torchia, S.J. DeArmond, and S.B. Prusiner. 1994. Serial transmission in rodents of neurodegeneration from transgenic mice expressing mutant prion protein. *Proc. Natl. Acad. Sci.* **91:** 9126.

Hsiao, K., Z. Meiner, E. Kahana, C. Cass, I. Kahana, D. Avrahami, G. Scarlato, O. Abramsky, S.B. Prusiner, and R. Gabizon. 1991b. Mutation of the prion protein in Libyan Jews with Creutzfeldt-Jakob disease. *N. Engl. J. Med.* **324:** 1091.

Huang, Z., S.B. Prusiner, and F.E. Cohen. 1996. Scrapie prions: A three-dimensional model of an infectious fragment. *Folding Design* **1:** 13.

Huang, Z., J.-M. Gabriel, M.A. Baldwin, R.J. Fletterick, S.B. Prusiner, and F.E. Cohen. 1994. Proposed three-dimensional structure for the cellular prion protein. *Proc. Natl. Acad. Sci.* **91:** 7139.

Hunter, G.D. 1972. Scrapie: A prototype slow infection. *J. Infect. Dis.* **125:** 427.

Hunter, N., J. Hope, I. McConnell, and A.G. Dickinson. 1987. Linkage of the scrapie-associated fibril protein (PrP) gene and Sinc using congenic mice and restriction fragment length polymorphism analysis. *J. Gen. Virol.* **68:** 2711.

Jacob, H., W. Pyrkosch, and H. Strube. 1950. Die erbliche Form der Creutzfeldt-Jakobschen Krankheit. *Arch. Psychiatry Z. Neurol.* **184:** 653.

Jarrett, J.T. and P.T. Lansbury, Jr. 1993. Seeding "one-dimensional crystallization" of amyloid: A pathogenic mechanism in Alzheimer's disease and scrapie? *Cell* **73:** 1055.

Johnson, R.T. 1992. Prion disease. *N. Engl. J. Med.* **326:** 486.

Kahana, E., N. Zilber, and M. Abraham. 1991. Do Creutzfeldt-Jakob disease patients of Jewish Libyan origin have unique clinical features? *Neurology* **41:** 1390.

Kahana, E., A. Milton, J. Braham, and D. Sofer. 1974. Creutzfeldt-Jakob disease: Focus among Libyan Jews in Israel. *Science* **183:** 90.

Kaneko, K., D. Peretz, K.-M. Pan, T. Blochberger, R. Gabizon, O.H. Griffith, F.E. Cohen, M.A. Baldwin, and S.B. Prusiner. 1995. Prion protein (PrP) synthetic peptides induce cellular PrP to acquire properties of the scrapie isoform. *Proc. Natl. Acad. Sci.* **32:** 11160.

Keller, G.A., M.W. Siegel, and I.W. Caras. 1992. Endocytosis of glycophospholipid-anchored and transmembrane forms of CD4 by different endocytic pathways. *EMBO J.* **11:** 863.

Kellings, K., N. Meyer, C. Mirenda, S.B. Prusiner, and D. Riesner. 1992. Further analysis of nucleic acids in purified scrapie prion preparations by improved return refocussing gel electrophoresis (RRGE). *J. Gen. Virol.* **73:** 1025.

Kenward, N., J. Hope, M. Landon, and R.J. Mayer. 1994. Expression of polyubiquitin and heat-shock protein 70 genes increases in the later stages of disease progression in scrapie-infected mouse brain. *J. Neurochem.* **62:** 1870.

Kingsbury, D.T., K.C. Kasper, D.P. Stites, J.D. Watson, R.N. Hogan, and S.B. Prusiner. 1983. Genetic control of scrapie and Creutzfeldt-Jakob disease in mice. *J. Immunol.* **131:** 491.

Kirschbaum, W.R. 1924. Zwei eigenartige Erkrankungen des Zentralnervensystems nach Art der spastischen Pseudosklerose (Jakob). *Z. Gesamte Neurol. Psychiatr.* **92:** 175.

Kitamoto, T. and J. Tateishi. 1994. Human prion diseases with variant prion protein. *Philos. Trans. R. Soc. Lond. B Biol. Sci.* **343:** 391.

Kitamoto, T., R. Iizuka, and J. Tateishi. 1993a. An amber mutation of prion protein in Gerstmann-Sträussler syndrome with mutant PrP plaques. *Biochem. Biophys.*

Res. Commun. **192:** 525.

Kitamoto, T., M. Ohta, K. Doh-ura, S. Hitoshi, Y. Terao, and J. Tateishi. 1993b. Novel missense variants of prion protein in Creutzfeldt-Jakob disease or Gerstmann-Sträussler syndrome. *Biochem. Biophys. Res. Commun.* **191:** 709.

Kitamoto, T., J. Tateishi, I. Tashima, I. Takeshita, R.A. Barry, S.J. DeArmond, and S.B. Prusiner. 1986. Amyloid plaques in Creutzfeldt-Jakob disease stain with prion protein antibodies. *Ann. Neurol.* **20:** 204.

Kneller, D.G., F.E. Cohen, and R. Langridge. 1990. Improvement in protein secondary structure prediction by an enhanced neural network. *J. Mol. Biol.* **214:** 171.

Kocisko, D.A., S.A. Priola, G.J. Raymond, B. Chesebro, P.T. Lansbury, Jr., and B. Caughey. 1995. Species specificity in the cell-free conversion of prion protein to protease-resistant forms: A model for the scrapie species barrier. *Proc. Natl. Acad. Sci.* **92:** 3923.

Kocisko, D.A., J.H. Come, S.A. Priola, B. Chesebro, G.J. Raymond, P.T. Lansbury, Jr., and B. Caughey. 1994. Cell-free formation of protease-resistant prion protein. *Nature* **370:** 471.

Kretzschmar, H.A., S.B. Prusiner, L.E. Stowring, and S.J. DeArmond. 1986a. Scrapie prion proteins are synthesized in neurons. *Am. J. Pathol.* **122:** 1-5.

Kretzschmar, H.A., P. Kufer, G. Riethmüller, S.J. DeArmond, S.B. Prusiner, and D. Schiffer. 1992. Prion protein mutation at codon 102 in an Italian family with Gerstmann-SträusslerScheinker syndrome. *Neurology* **42:** 809.

Kretzschmar, H.A., L.E. Stowring, D. Westaway, W.H. Stubblebine, S.B. Prusiner, and S.J. DeArmond. 1986b. Molecular cloning of a human prion protein cDNA. *DNA* **5:** 315.

Kretzschmar, H.A., G. Honold, F. Seitelberger, M. Feucht, P. Wessely, P. Mehraein, and H. Budka. 1991. Prion protein mutation in family first reported by Gerstmann, Straussler, and Scheinker. *Lancet* **337:** 1160.

Laplanche, J.-L., J. Chatelain, J.-M. Launay, C. Gazengel, and M. Vidaud. 1990. Deletion in prion protein gene in a Moroccan family. *Nucleic Acids Res.* **18:** 6745.

Levy, E., M.D. Carman, I.J. Fernandez-Madrid, M.D. Power, I. Lieberburg, S.G. van Duinen, G.T.A.M. Bots, W. Luyendijk, and B. Frangione. 1990. Mutation of the Alzheimer's disease amyloid gene in hereditary cerebral hemorrhage, Dutch type. *Science* **248:** 1124.

Levy-Lahad, E., E.M. Wijsman, E. Nemens, L. Anderson, K.A.B. Goddard, J.L. Weber, T.D. Bird, and G.D. Schellenberg. 1995a. A familial Alzheimer's disease locus on chromosome 1. *Science* **269:** 970-973.

Levy-Lahad, E., W. Wasco, P. Poorkaj, D.M. Romano, J. Oshima, W.H. Pettingell, C. Yu, P.D. Jondro, S.D. Schmidt, K. Wang, A.C. Crowley, Y.-H. Fu, S.Y. Guenette, D. Galas, E. Nemens, E.M. Wijsman, T.D. Bird, G.D. Schellenberg, and R.E. Tanzi. 1995b. Candidate gene for the chromosome 1 familial Alzheimer's disease locus. *Science* **269:** 973.

Liautard, J.-P. 1993. Prions and molecular chaperones. *Arch. Virol.* (suppl.) **7:** 227.

Lledo, P.-M., P. Tremblay, S.J. DeArmond, S.B. Prusiner, and R.A. Nicoll. 1996. Mice deficient for prion protein exhibit normal neuronal excitability and synaptic transmission in the hippocampus. *Proc. Natl. Acad. Sci.* **93:** 2403.

Locht, C., B. Chesebro, R. Race, and J.M. Keith. 1986. Molecular cloning and complete sequence of prion protein cDNA from mouse brain infected with the scrapie agent. *Proc. Natl. Acad. Sci.* **83:** 6372.

Lowenstein, D.H., D.A. Butler, D. Westaway, M.P. McKinley, S.J. DeArmond, and S.B. Prusiner. 1990. Three hamster species with different scrapie incubation times and neuropathological features encode distinct prion proteins. *Mol. Cell. Biol.* **10:** 1153.

Lugaresi, E., R. Medori, P. Montagna, A. Baruzzi, P. Cortelli, A. Lugaresi, P. Tinuper, M. Zucconi, and P. Gambetti. 1986. Fatal familial insomnia and dysautonomia with selective degeneration of thalamic nuclei. *N. Engl. J. Med.* **315:** 997.

Malmgren, R., L. Kurland, B. Mokri, and J. Kurtzke. 1979. The epidemiology of Creutzfeldt-Jakob disease. In *Slow transmissible diseases of the nervous system* (ed. S.B. Prusiner and W. J. Hadlow), vol. 1, p. 93. Academic Press, New York.

Manson, J.C., A.R. Clarke, P.A. McBride, I. McConnell, and J. Hope. 1994a. PrP gene dosage determines the timing but not the final intensity or distribution of lesions in scrapie pathology. *Neurodegeneration* **3:** 331.

Manson, J.C., A.R. Clarke, M.L. Hooper, L. Aitchison, I. McConnell, and J. Hope. 1994b. 129/Ola mice carrying a null mutation in PrP that abolishes mRNA production are developmentally normal. *Mol. Neurobiol.* **8:** 121.

Manson, J.C., J. Hope, A.R. Clarke, A. Johnston, C. Black, and N. MacLeod. 1995. PrP gene dosage and long term potentiation (Letter). *Neurodegeneration* **4:** 113.

Marsh, R.F., R.A. Bessen, S. Lehmann, and G.R. Hartsough. 1991. Epidemiological and experimental studies on a new incident of transmissible mink encephalopathy. *J. Gen. Virol.* **72:** 589.

Masters, C.L., D.C. Gajdusek, and C.J. Gibbs, Jr. 1981a. Creutzfeldt-Jakob disease virus isolations from the Gerstmann-Sträussler syndrome. *Brain* **104:** 559.

———. 1981b. The familial occurrence of Creutzfeldt-Jakob disease and Alzheimer's disease. *Brain* **104:** 535.

Masters, C.L., D.C. Gajdusek, C.J. Gibbs, Jr., C. Bernouilli, and D.M. Asher. 1979. Familial Creutzfeldt-Jakob disease and other familial dementias: An inquiry into possible models of virus-induced familial diseases. In *Slow transmissible diseases of the nervous system*, (ed. S.B. Prusiner and W.J. Hadlow), vol. 1, p. 143. Academic Press, New York.

Mastrianni, J.A., C. Iannicola, R. Myers, and S.B. Prusiner. 1995. Identification of a new mutation of the prion protein gene at codon 208 in a patient with Creutzfeldt-Jakob disease. *Neurology* (suppl.) **45:** 201. (Abstr.)

McKinley, M.P., D.C. Bolton, and S.B. Prusiner. 1983. A protease-resistant protein is a structural component of the scrapie prion. *Cell* **35:** 57.

McKinley, M.P., R. Meyer, L. Kenaga, F. Rahbar, R. Cotter, A. Serban, and S.B. Prusiner. 1991. Scrapie prion rod formation *in vitro* requires both detergent extraction and limited proteolysis. *J. Virol.* **65:** 1440.

McKnight, S. and R. Tjian. 1986. Transcriptional selectivity of viral genes in mammalian cells. *Cell* **46:** 795.

Medori, R., P. Montagna, H.J. Tritschler, A. LeBlanc, P. Cortelli, P. Tinuper, E. Lugaresi, and P. Gambetti. 1992. Fatal familial insomnia: A second kindred with mutation of prion protein gene at codon 178. *Neurology* **42:** 669.

Meggendorfer, F. 1930. Klinische und genealogische Beobachtungen bei einem Fall von spastischer Pseudosklerose Jakobs. *Z. Gesamte Neurol. Psychiatr.* **128:** 337.

Meyer, N., V. Rosenbaum, B. Schmidt, K. Gilles, C. Mirenda,

D. Groth, S.B. Prusiner, and D. Riesner. 1991. Search for a putative scrapie genome in purified prion fractions reveals a paucity of nucleic acids. *J. Gen. Virol.* **72:** 37.

Meyer, R.K., M.P. McKinley, K.A. Bowman, M.B. Braunfeld, R.A. Barry, and S.B. Prusiner. 1986. Separation and properties of cellular and scrapie prion proteins. *Proc. Natl. Acad. Sci.* **83:** 2310.

Mobley, W.C., R.L. Neve, S.B. Prusiner, and M.P. McKinley. 1988. Nerve growth factor increases mRNA levels for the prion protein and the beta-amyloid protein precursor in developing hamster brain. *Proc. Natl. Acad. Sci.* **85:** 9811.

Mullan, M., H. Houlden, M. Windelspecht, L. Fidani, C. Lombardi, P. Diaz, M. Rossor, R. Crook, J. Hardy, K. Duff, and F. Crawford. 1992. A locus for familial early-onset Alzheimer's disease on the long arm of chromosome 14, proximal to the α1-antichymotrypsin gene. *Nat. Genet.* **2:** 340.

Neugut, R.H., A.I. Neugut, E. Kahana, Z. Stein, and M. Alter. 1979. Creutzfeldt-Jakob disease: Familial clustering among Libyan-born Israelis. *Neurology* **29:** 225.

Nguyen, J., M.A. Baldwin, F.E. Cohen, and S.B. Prusiner. 1995a. Prion protein peptides induce α-helix to β-sheet conformational transitions. *Biochemistry* **34:** 4186.

Nguyen, J.T., H. Inouye, M.A. Baldwin, R.J. Fletterick, F.E. Cohen, S.B. Prusiner, and D.A. Kirschner. 1995b. X-ray diffraction of scrapie prion rods and PrP peptides. *J. Mol. Biol.* **252:** 412.

Oesch, B., D. Westaway, M. Wälchli, M.P. McKinley, S.B.H. Kent, R. Aebersold, R.A. Barry, P. Tempst, D.B. Teplow, L.E. Hood, S.B. Prusiner, and C. Weissmann. 1985. A cellular gene encodes scrapie PrP 27-30 protein. *Cell* **40:** 735.

Owen, F., M. Poulter, J. Collinge, M. Leach, R. Lofthouse, T.J. Crow, and A.E. Harding. 1992. A dementing illness associated with a novel insertion in the prion protein gene. *Mol. Brain Res.* **13:** 155.

Owen, F., M. Poulter, T. Shah, J. Collinge, R. Lofthouse, H. Baker, R. Ridley, J. McVey, and T. Crow. 1990. An in-frame insertion in the prion protein gene in familial Creutzfeldt-Jakob disease. *Mol. Brain Res.* **7:** 273.

Owen, F., M. Poulter, R. Lofthouse, J. Collinge, T.J. Crow, D. Risby, H.F. Baker, R.M. Ridley, K. Hsiao, and S.B. Prusiner. 1989. Insertion in prion protein gene in familial Creutzfeldt-Jakob disease. *Lancet* **I:** 51.

Palmer, M.S., A.J. Dryden, J.T. Hughes, and J. Collinge. 1991. Homozygous prion protein genotype predisposes to sporadic Creutzfeldt-Jakob disease. *Nature* **352:** 340.

Palmer, M.S., S.P. Mahal, T.A. Campbell, A.F. Hill, K.C.L. Sidle, J.-L. Laplanche, and J. Collinge. 1993. Deletions in the prion protein gene are not associated with CJD. *Hum. Mol. Genet.* **2:** 541.

Pan, K.-M., M. Baldwin, J. Nguyen, M. Gasset, A. Serban, D. Groth, I. Mehlhorn, Z. Huang, R.J. Fletterick, F.E. Cohen, and S.B. Prusiner. 1993. Conversion of α-helices into β-sheets features in the formation of the scrapie prion proteins. *Proc. Natl. Acad. Sci.* **90:** 10962.

Parry, H.B. 1983. Recorded occurrences of scrapie from 1750. In *Scrapie disease in sheep* (ed. D.R. Oppenheimer), p. 31–59. Academic Press, New York.

Pattison, I.H. and G.C. Millson. 1961. Scrapie produced experimentally in goats with special reference to the clinical syndrome. *J. Comp. Pathol.* **71:** 101.

Petersen, R.B., M. Tabaton, L. Berg, B. Schrank, R.M. Torack, S. Leal, J. Julien, C. Vital, B. Deleplanque, W.W. Pendlebury, D. Drachman, T.W. Smith, J.J. Martin, M. Oda, P. Montagna, J. Ott, L. Autilio-Gambetti, E. Lugaresi, and P. Gambetti. 1992. Analysis of the prion protein gene in thalamic dementia. *Neurology* **42:** 1859.

Poulter, M., H.F. Baker, C.D. Frith, M. Leach, R. Lofthouse, R.M. Ridley, T. Shah, F. Owen, J. Collinge, G. Brown, J. Hardy, M.J. Mullan, A.E. Harding, C. Bennett, R. Doshi, and T.J. Crow. 1992. Inherited prion disease with 144 base pair gene insertion. 1. Genealogical and molecular studies. *Brain* **115:** 675.

Presnell, S.R., B.I. Cohen, and F.E. Cohen. 1993. MacMatch: A tool for pattern-based protein secondary structure prediction. *CABIOS* **9:** 373.

Prusiner, S.B. 1982. Novel proteinaceous infectious particles cause scrapie. *Science* **216:** 136.

———. 1991. Molecular biology of prion diseases. *Science* **252:** 1515.

Prusiner, S.B., D.F. Groth, D.C. Bolton, S.B. Kent, and L.E. Hood. 1984. Purification and structural studies of a major scrapie prion protein. *Cell* **38:** 127.

Prusiner, S.B., D. Groth, A. Serban, N. Stahl, and R. Gabizon. 1993a. Attempts to restore scrapie prion infectivity after exposure to protein denaturants. *Proc. Natl. Acad. Sci.* **90:** 2793.

Prusiner, S.B., D.C. Bolton, D.F. Groth, K.A. Bowman, S.P. Cochran, and M.P. McKinley. 1982. Further purification and characterization of scrapie prions. *Biochemistry* **21:** 6942.

Prusiner, S.B., M.P. McKinley, K.A. Bowman, D.C. Bolton, P.E. Bendheim, D.F. Groth, and G.G. Glenner. 1983. Scrapie prions aggregate to form amyloid-like birefringent rods. *Cell* **35:** 349.

Prusiner, S.B., M.P. McKinley, D.F. Groth, K.A. Bowman, N.I. Mock, S.P. Cochran, and F.R. Masiarz. 1981. Scrapie agent contains a hydrophobic protein. *Proc. Natl. Acad. Sci.* **78:** 6675-6679.

Prusiner, S.B., D. Groth, A. Serban, R. Koehler, D. Foster, M. Torchia, D. Burton, S.-L. Yang, and S.J. DeArmond. 1993b. Ablation of the prion protein (PrP) gene in mice prevents scrapie and facilitates production of anti-PrP antibodies. *Proc. Natl. Acad. Sci.* **90:** 10608.

Prusiner, S.B., M. Fuzi, M. Scott, D. Serban, H. Serban, A. Taraboulos, J.-M. Gabriel, G. Wells, J. Wilesmith, R. Bradley, S.J. DeArmond, and K. Kristensson. 1993c. Immunologic and molecular biological studies of prion proteins in bovine spongiform encephalopathy. *J. Infect. Dis.* **167:** 602.

Prusiner, S.B., M. Scott, D. Foster, K.-M. Pan, D. Groth, C. Mirenda, M. Torchia, S.-L. Yang, D. Serban, G.A. Carlson, P.C. Hoppe, D. Westaway, and S.J. DeArmond. 1990. Transgenetic studies implicate interactions between homologous PrP isoforms in scrapie prion replication. *Cell* **63:** 673.

Puckett, C., P. Concannon, C. Casey, and L. Hood. 1991. Genomic structure of the human prion protein gene. *Am. J. Hum. Genet.* **49:** 320.

Race, R.E., K. Graham, D. Ernst, B. Caughey, and B. Chesebro. 1990. Analysis of linkage between scrapie incubation period and the prion protein gene in mice. *J. Gen. Virol.* **71:** 493.

Raeber, A.J., D.R. Borchelt, M. Scott, and S.B. Prusiner. 1992. Attempts to convert the cellular prion protein into the scrapie isoform in cell-free systems. *J. Virol.* **66:** 6155.

Riesner, D., K. Kellings, N. Meyer, C. Mirenda, and S.B. Prusiner. 1992. Nucleic acids and scrapie prions. In *Prion diseases of humans and animals* (ed. S.B. Prusiner et al.), p. 341. Ellis Horwood, London.

Ripoll, L., J.-L. Laplanche, M. Salzmann, A. Jouvet, B. Planques, M. Dussaucy, J. Chatelain, P. Beaudry, and J.-M. Launay. 1993. A new point mutation in the prion protein gene at codon 210 in Creutzfeldt-Jakob disease. *Neurology* **43:** 1934.

Roberts, G.W., R. Lofthouse, D. Allsop, M. Landon, M. Kidd, S.B. Prusiner, and T.J. Crow. 1988. CNS amyloid proteins in neurodegenerative diseases. *Neurology* **38:** 1534.

Rogaev, E.I., R. Sherrington, E.A. Rogaeva, G. Levesque, M. Ikeda, Y. Liang, H. Chi, C. Lin, K. Holman, T. Tsuda, L. Mar, S. Sorbi, B. Nacmias, S. Piacentini, L. Amaducci, I. Chumakov, D. Cohen, L. Lannfelt, P.E. Fraser, J.M. Rommens, and P.H. St. George-Hyslop. 1995. Familial Alzheimer's disease in kindreds with missense mutations in a gene on chromosome 1 related to the Alzheimer's disease type 3 gene. *Nature* **376:** 775.

Rogers, M., F. Yehiely, M. Scott, and S.B. Prusiner. 1993. Conversion of truncated and elongated prion proteins into the scrapie isoform in cultured cells. *Proc. Natl. Acad. Sci.* **90:** 3182.

Rosen, D.R., T. Siddique, D. Patterson, D.A. Figiewicz, P. Sapp, A. Hentati, D. Donaldson, J. Goto, J.P. O'Regan, H.X. Deng, Z. Rahmani, A. Krizus, D. McKenna-Yasek, A. Cayabyab, S.M. Gaston, R. Berger, R. E. Tanzi, J.J. Halperin, B. Herzfeldt, R. Van den Bergh, W.-Y. Hung, T. Bird, G. Deng, D.W. Mulder, C. Smyth, N.G. Laing, E. Soriano, M.A. Pericak-Vance, J. Haines, G.A. Rouleau, J.S. Gusella, H.R. Horvitz, and R.H. Brown, Jr. 1993. Mutations in Cu/Zn superoxide dismutase gene are associated with familial amyotrophic lateral slerosis. *Nature* **362:** 59.

Rosenthal, N.P., J. Keesey, B. Crandall, and W.J. Brown. 1976. Familial neurological disease associated with spongiform encephalopathy. *Arch. Neurol.* **33:** 252.

Safar, J., P.P. Roller, D.C. Gajdusek, and C.J. Gibbs, Jr. 1993a. Conformational transitions, dissociation, and unfolding of scrapie amyloid (prion) protein. *J. Biol. Chem.* **268:** 20276.

———. 1993b. Thermal-stability and conformational transitions of scrapie amyloid (prion) protein correlate with infectivity. *Protein Sci.* **2:** 2206.

———. 1994. Scrapie amyloid (prion) protein has the conformational characteristics of an aggregated molten globule folding intermediate. *Biochemistry* **33:** 8375.

Sailer, A., H. Büeler, M. Fischer, A. Aguzzi, and C. Weissmann. 1994. No propagation of prions in mice devoid of PrP. *Cell* **77:** 967.

Sakaguchi, S., S. Katamine, K. Shigematsu, A. Nakatani, R. Moriuchi, N. Nishida, K. Kurokawa, R. Nakaoke, H. Sato, K. Jishage, J. Kuno, T. Noda, and T. Miyamoto. 1995. Accumulation of proteinase K-resistant prion protein (PrP) is restricted by the expression level of normal PrP in mice inoculated with a mouse-adapted strain of the Creutzfeldt-Jakob disease agent. *J. Virol.* **69:** 7586.

Sakaguchi, S., S. Katamine, N. Nishida, R. Moriuchi, K. Shigematsu, T. Sugimoto, A. Nakatani, Y. Kataoka, T. Houtani, S. Shirabe, H. Okada, S. Hasegawa, T. Miyamoto, and T. Noda. 1996. Loss of cerebellar Purkinje cells in aged mice homozygous for a disrupted PrP gene. *Nature* **380:** 528.

Saunders, A.M., W.J. Strittmatter, D. Schmechel, P.H. St. George-Hyslop, M.A. Pericak-Vance, S.H. Joo, B.L. Rosi, J.F. Gusella, D.R. Crapper-MacLachlan, M.J. Alberts, C. Hulette, B. Crain, D. Goldgaber, and A.D. Roses. 1993a. Association of apolipoprotein E allele ε4 with late-onset familial and sporadic Alzheimer's disease. *Neurology* **43:** 1467.

Saunders, A.M., K. Schmader, J.C.S. Breitner, M.D. Benson, W.T. Brown, L. Goldfarb, D. Goldgaber, M.G. Manwaring, M.H. Szymanski, N. McCown, K.C. Dole, D.E. Schmechel, W.J. Strittmatter, M.A. Pericak-Vance, and A.D. Roses. 1993b. Apolipoprotein E ε4 allele distributions in late-onset Alzheimer's disease and in other amyloid-forming diseases. *Lancet* **342:** 710.

Schätzl, H.M., M. Da Costa, L. Taylor, F.E. Cohen, and S.B. Prusiner. 1995. Prion protein gene variation among primates. *J. Mol. Biol.* **245:** 362.

Schellenberg, G.D., T.D. Bird, E.M. Wijsman, H.T. Orr, L. Anderson, E. Nemens, J.A. White, L. Bonnycastle, J.L. Weber, M.E. Alonso, H. Potter, L.L. Heston, and G.M. Martin. 1992. Genetic linkage evidence for a familial Alzheimer's disease locus on chromosome 14. *Science* **258:** 668.

Scott, M.R., R. Köhler, D.Foster, and S.B. Prusiner. 1992. Chimeric prion protein expression in cultured cells and transgenic mice. *Protein Sci.* **1:** 986-997.

Scott, M., D. Groth, D. Foster, M. Torchia, S.-L. Yang, S.J. DeArmond, and S.B. Prusiner. 1993. Propagation of prions with artificial properties in transgenic mice expressing chimeric PrP genes. *Cell* **73:** 979.

Scott, M., D. Foster, C. Mirenda, D. Serban, F. Coufal, M. Wälchli, M. Torchia, D. Groth, G. Carlson, S.J. DeArmond, D. Westaway, and S.B. Prusiner. 1989. Transgenic mice expressing hamster prion protein produce species-specific scrapie infectivity and amyloid plaques. *Cell* **59:** 847.

Sherrington, R., E.I. Rogaev, Y. Liang, E.A. Rogaeva, G. Levesque, M. Ikeda, H. Chi, C. Lin, G. Li, K. Holman, T. Tsuda, L. Mar, J.-F. Foncin, A.C. Bruni, M.P. Montesi, S. Sorbi, I. Rainero, L. Pinessi, L. Nee, I. Chumakov, D. Pollen, A. Brookes, P. Sanseau, R.J. Polinsky, W. Wasco, H. A.R. Da Silva, J.L. Haines, M.A. Pericak-Vance, R.E. Tanzi, A.D. Roses, P.E. Fraser, J.M. Rommens, and P.H. St. George-Hyslop. 1995. Cloning of a gene bearing missense mutations in early-onset familial Alzheimer's disease. *Nature* **375:** 754.

Sigurdsson, B. 1954. Rida, a chronic encephalitis of sheep with general remarks on infections which develop slowly and some of their special characteristics. *Br. Vet. J.* **110:** 341.

Spudich, S., J.A. Mastrianni, M. Wrensch, R. Gabizon, Z. Meiner, I. Kahana, H. Rosenmann, E. Kahana, and S.B. Prusiner. 1995. Complete penetrance of Creutzfeldt-Jakob disease in Libyan Jews carrying the E200K mutation in the prion protein gene. *Mol. Med.* **1:** 607.

Stahl, N., D.R. Borchelt, K. Hsiao, and S.B. Prusiner. 1987. Scrapie prion protein contains a phosphatidylinositol glycolipid. *Cell* **51:** 229.

Stahl, N., M.A. Baldwin, D.B. Teplow, L. Hood, B.W. Gibson, A.L. Burlingame, and S.B. Prusiner. 1993. Structural analysis of the scrapie prion protein using mass spectrometry and amino acid sequencing. *Biochemistry* **32:** 1991.

Stender, A. 1930. Weitere Beiträge zum Kapitel "Spastische Pseudosklerose Jakobs." *Z. Neurol. Psychiat.* **128:** 528.

St. George-Hyslop, P., J. Haines, E. Rogaev, M. Mortilla, G. Vaula, M. Pericak-Vance, J.-F. Foncin, M. Montesi, A. Bruni, S. Sorbi, I. Rainero, L. Pinessi, D. Pollen, R. Polinsky, L. Nee, J. Kennedy, F. Macciardi, E. Rogaeva, Y. Liang, N. Alexandrova, W. Lukiw, K. Schlumpf, R. Tanzi, T. Tsuda, L. Farrer, J.-M. Cantu, R. Duara, L.

Amaducci, L. Bergamini, J. Gusella, A. Roses, and D.C. McLachlan. 1992. Genetic evidence for a novel familial Alzheimer's disease locus on chromosome 14. *Nat. Genet.* **2:** 330.

Tagliavini, F., F. Prelli, J. Ghisto, O. Bugiani, D. Serban, S.B. Prusiner, M.R. Farlow, B. Ghetti, and B. Frangione. 1991. Amyloid protein of Gerstmann-Sträussler-Scheinker disease (Indiana kindred) is an 11-kd fragment of prion protein with an N-terminal glycine at codon 58. *EMBO J.* **10:** 513.

Taraboulos, A., A.J. Raeber, D.R. Borchelt, D. Serban, and S.B. Prusiner. 1992a. Synthesis and trafficking of prion proteins in cultured cells. *Mol. Biol. Cell* **3:** 851.

Taraboulos, A., K. Jendroska, D. Serban, S.-L. Yang, S.J. DeArmond, and S.B. Prusiner. 1992b. Regional mapping of prion proteins in brains. *Proc. Natl. Acad. Sci.* **89:** 7620.

Taraboulos, A., M. Scott, A. Semenov, D. Avrahami, L. Laszlo, and S.B. Prusiner. 1995. Cholesterol depletion and modification of COOH-terminal targeting sequence of the prion protein inhibit formation of the scrapie isoform. *J. Cell Biol.* **129:** 121.

Tateishi, J. and T. Kitamoto. 1995. Inherited prion diseases and transmission to rodents. *Brain Pathol.* **5:** 53.

Tateishi, J., T. Kitamoto, M.Z. Hoque, and H. Furukawa. 1996. Experimental transmission of Creutzfeldt-Jakob disease and related diseases to rodents. *Neurology* **46:** 532.

Tateishi, J., T. Kitamoto, K. Doh-ura, Y. Sakaki, G. Steinmetz, C. Tranchant, J.M. Warter, and N. Heldt. 1990. Immunochemical, molecular genetic, and transmission studies on a case of Gerstmann-Sträussler-Scheinker syndrome. *Neurology* **40:** 1578.

Tatzelt, J., J. Zuo, R. Voellmy, M. Scott, U. Hartl, S.B. Prusiner, and W.J. Welch. 1995. Scrapie prions selectively modify the stress response in neuroblastoma cells. *Proc. Natl. Acad. Sci.* **92:** 2944.

Telling, G.C., T. Haga, M. Torchia, P. Tremblay, S.J. DeArmond, and S.B. Prusiner. 1996. Interactions between wild-type and mutant prion proteins modulate neurodegeneration in transgenic mice. *Genes Dev.* **10:** 1736.

Telling, G.C., M. Scott, J. Mastrianni, R. Gabizon, M. Torchia, F.E. Cohen, S.J. DeArmond, and S.B. Prusiner. 1995. Prion propagation in mice expressing human and chimeric PrP transgenes implicates the interaction of cellular PrP with another protein. *Cell* **83:** 79.

Telling, G.C., M. Scott, K.K. Hsiao, D. Foster, S.-L. Yang, M. Torchia, K.C.L. Sidle, J. Collinge, S.J. DeArmond, and S.B. Prusiner. 1994. Transmission of Creutzfeldt-Jakob disease from humans to transgenic mice expressing chimeric human-mouse prion protein. *Proc. Natl. Acad. Sci.* **91:** 9936.

Turk, E., D.B. Teplow, L.E. Hood, and S.B. Prusiner. 1988. Purification and properties of the cellular and scrapie hamster prion proteins. *Eur. J. Biochem.* **176:** 21.

Van Broeckhoven, C., H. Backhovens, M. Cruts, G. De Winter, M. Bruyland, P. Cras, and J.-J. Martin. 1992. Mapping of a gene predisposing to early-onset Alzheimer's disease to chromosome 14q24.3. *Nat. Genet.* **2:** 335.

Van Broeckhoven, C., J. Haan, E. Bakker, J.A. Hardy, W. Van Hul, A. Wehnert, M. Vegter-Van der Vlis, and R.A. Roos. 1990. Amyloid β protein precursor gene and hereditary cerebral hemorrhage with amyloidosis (Dutch). *Science* **248:** 1120.

Vnencak-Jones, C.L. and J.A. Phillips. 1992. Identification of heterogeneous PrP gene deletions in controls by detection of allele-specific heteroduplexes (DASH). *Am. J. Hum. Genet.* **50:** 871.

Waneck, G.L., M.E. Stein, and R.A. Flavell. 1988. Conversion of a PI-anchored protein to an integral membrane protein by a single amino acid mutation. *Science* **241:** 697.

Wells, G.A.H. and J.W. Wilesmith. 1995. The neuropathology and epidemiology of bovine spongiform encephalopathy. *Brain Pathol.* **5:** 91.

Wells, G.A.H., A.C. Scott, C.T. Johnson, R.F. Gunning, R.D. Hancock, M.Jeffrey, M. Dawson, and R. Bradley. 1987. A novel progressive spongiform encephalopathy in cattle. *Vet. Rec.* **121:** 419.

Westaway, D., C. Cooper, S. Turner, M. Da Costa, G.A. Carlson, and S.B. Prusiner. 1994a. Structure and polymorphism of the mouse prion protein gene. *Proc. Natl. Acad. Sci.* **91:** 6418.

Westaway, D., P.A. Goodman, C.A. Mirenda, M.P. McKinley, G.A. Carlson, and S.B. Prusiner. 1987. Distinct prion proteins in short and long scrapie incubation period mice. *Cell* **51:** 651.

Westaway, D., V. Zuliani, C.M. Cooper, M. Da Costa, S. Neuman, A.L. Jenny, L. Detwiler, and S.B. Prusiner. 1994b. Homozygosity for prion protein alleles encoding glutamine-171 renders sheep susceptible to natural scrapie. *Genes Dev.* **8:** 959.

Westaway, D., C.A. Mirenda, D. Foster, Y. Zebarjadian, M. Scott, M. Torchia, S.-L. Yang, H. Serban, S.J. DeArmond, C. Ebeling, S.B. Prusiner, and G.A. Carlson. 1991. Paradoxical shortening of scrapie incubation times by expression of prion protein transgenes derived from long incubation period mice. *Neuron* **7:** 59.

Whittington, M.A., K.C.L. Sidle, I. Gowland, J. Meads, A.F. Hill, M.S. Palmer, J.G.R. Jefferys, and J. Collinge. 1995. Rescue of neurophysiological phenotype seen in PrP null mice by transgene encoding human prion protein. *Nat. Genet.* **9:** 197.

Will, R.G., J.W. Ironside, M. Zeidler, S.N. Cousens, K. Estibeiro, A. Alperovitch, S. Poser, M. Pocchiari, A. Hofman, and P.G. Smith. 1996. A new variant of Creutzfeldt-Jakob disease in the UK. *Lancet* **347:** 921.

Zhang, H., K. Kaneko, J.T. Nguyen, T.L. Livshits, M.A. Baldwin, F.E. Cohen, T.L. James, and S.B. Prusiner. 1995. Conformational transitions in peptides containing two putative α-helices of the prion protein. *J. Mol. Biol.* **250:** 514.

Ziegler, D.R. 1993. *Genetic Maps—Locus maps of complex genomes*, 6th edition (ed. S. J. O'Brien), pp. 4.42–4.45. Cold Spring Harbor Laboratory Press, Cold Spring Harbor, New York.

Zilber, N., E. Kahana, and M.P.H. Abraham. 1991. The Libyan Creutzfeldt-Jakob disease focus in Israel: An epidemiologic evaluation. *Neurology* **41:** 1385.

Prion Protein Structure and Scrapie Replication: Theoretical, Spectroscopic, and Genetic Investigations

P. Bamborough,[1] H. Wille,[2] G.C. Telling,[2] F. Yehiely,[2]
S.B. Prusiner,[2,3] and F.E. Cohen[1,3,4]
Departments of [1]Pharmaceutical Chemistry, [2]Neurology, [3]Biochemistry, and [4]Medicine, University of California, San Francisco, California 94143-0450

The mechanism by which prions reproduce without the aid of nucleic acids remains unprecedented. In this paper we discuss the results of several years of experimental and theoretical investigation into the genetic and molecular properties of prions. Here we discuss the unusual properties of the prion protein (PrP) sequence, structural studies of prion peptide fragments, attempts to replicate prions in vitro, evidence for the involvement of additional host-specific factors in prion disease, and the kinetics of prion replication in vivo.

Substantial evidence has accumulated that scrapie-like diseases cannot be caused by a virus. Infectivity is resistant to UV radiation and other processes destructive to nucleic acids (for review, see Prusiner 1994). Although some reports (e.g., Narang 1992) have claimed to find the involvement of nucleotides, these results have not been repeated. Such reports are also inconsistent with thorough attempts to locate nucleic acids in extensively purified scrapie fractions (Kellings et al. 1992), suggesting that any nucleotide present can be no larger than 80 nucleotides. As early as the 1960s it had been recognized that the resistance of the scrapie agent to ionizing radiation was consistent with an extremely small agent (Alper et al. 1967). This result, together with additional biochemical data, led to the current picture, which involves a novel type of pathogen (dubbed a prion, or proteinaceous infectious particle; Prusiner et al. 1982) composed of PrP. PrP is frequently found in abnormal deposits in the brains of animals with scrapie-like diseases. In the laboratory, purified preparations of PrP are infectious when injected intracerebrally into rodents. The discovery that a human gene linked to inherited neurodegenerative diseases encodes the same sequence as that of the infectious protein was highly suggestive of a nonviral cause, but perhaps the most overwhelming evidence is the immunity to infection of mice in which the gene encoding this protein has been ablated (Prusiner et al. 1993a). In addition, mice engineered to produce a prion protein differing from the wild type by a single amino acid substitution corresponding to that known to cause human Gerstmann-Sträussler-Scheinker disease (GSS) also fall spontaneously ill (Hsiao et al. 1990) with neurodegeneration similar to that seen in the human disease.

TWO FORMS OF PRP

PrP is encoded by a single chromosomal gene and exists in two forms. One is the normal, cellular isoform PrP^{C}, which is attached to the outer cell membrane by a GPI anchor (Stahl et al. 1987) and is relatively soluble. The other, PrP^{Sc}, is an abnormal form found in plaques in diseased brain and also intracellularly in neuroblastoma cells permanently infected with scrapie (Taraboulos et al. 1990). PrP^{Sc} is highly insoluble in nonionic detergents and is also distinguished from PrP^{C} by partial resistance to proteinase K, which fails to digest a 27- to 30-kD core. This fragment, PrP 27-30, has been sequenced and found to possess a ragged amino terminus (Prusiner et al. 1984), starting approximately at PrP codon 90.

PrP^{Sc} can also be induced to form amyloid-like rods in vitro, suggestive of β-sheet structure, but only upon limited proteolysis in the presence of detergent (McKinley et al. 1991). The β content of PrP^{Sc} is confirmed by spectroscopy, which shows that the secondary structure of PrP^{C} is substantially different from that of PrP^{Sc}. The Fourier transform infrared (FTIR) spectrum of PrP^{C} purified from hamster brain shows an amide I′ band characteristic of a protein with a high α-helical content (Pan et al. 1993). Deconvolution of the spectrum gave an estimate of around 42%/3% helix/sheet content, with the remainder made up of turn and coil. Circular dichroism (CD) spectroscopy supported this result. These values contrast with about 30%/43% helix/sheet content for PrP^{Sc} purified from scrapie-infected hamster brain, and 21%/54% for PrP 27-30. This is in rough agreement with values obtained elsewhere by CD spectroscopy (Safar et al. 1993) showing 20%/34% helix/sheet content in liposomes for PrP^{Sc} and 0%/43% helix/sheet content for PrP 27-30. Because no covalent modifications have been found that distinguish PrP^{C} from PrP^{Sc} (Stahl et al. 1993), it has been proposed that prion infection is a disease propagated by changes in protein conformation (Cohen et al. 1994).

THE SEQUENCE OF PRP

The human Prnp gene contains a single open reading frame encoding a protein of 253 amino acids

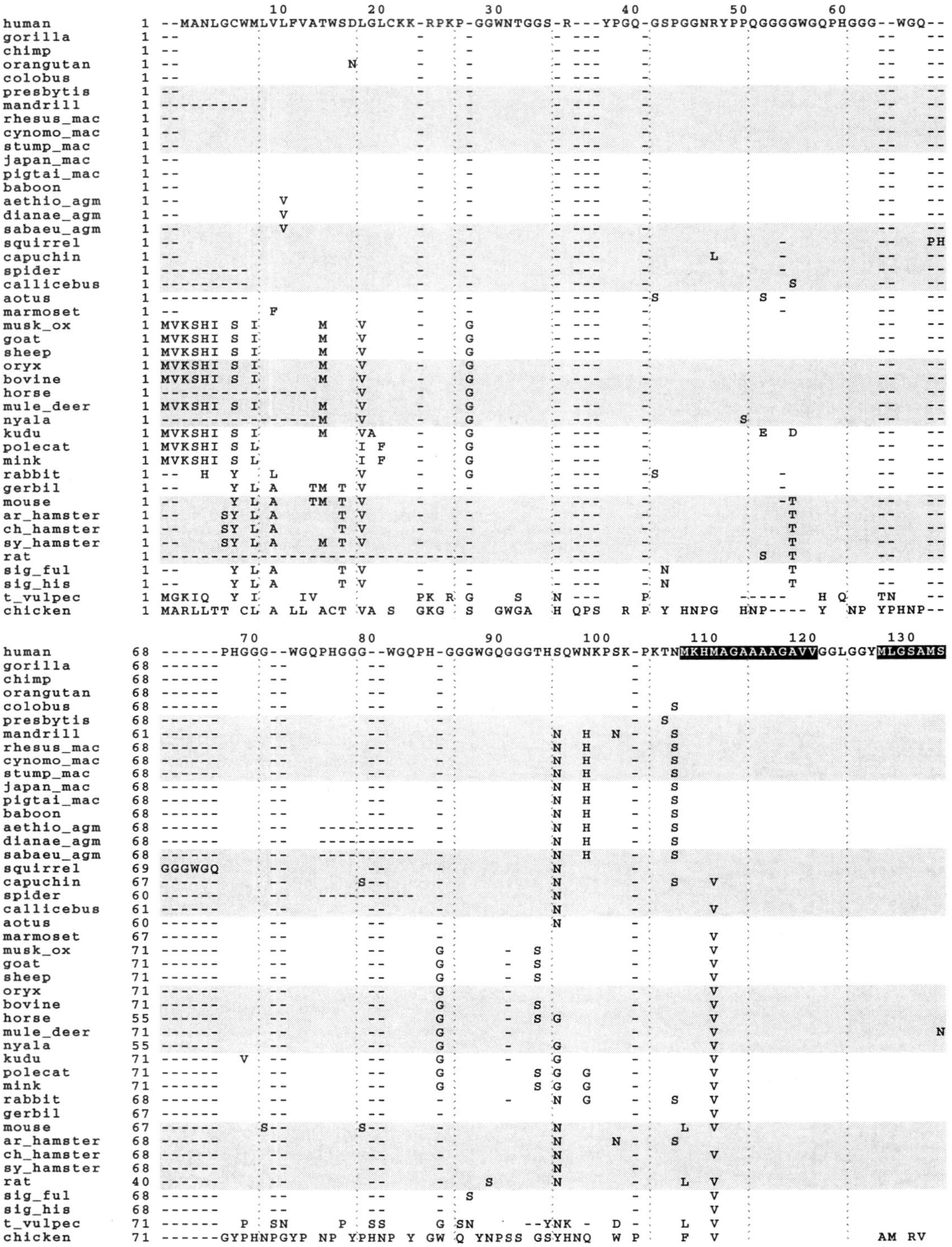

Figure 1. Alignment of 44 PrP sequences. Only the positions that differ from human are shown. The amino-terminal signal sequence and carboxy-terminal sequence that marks for the GPI anchor are lost during processing. The four predicted α helices H1–H4 are indicated above the sequences. The sequences are human (Doh-ura et al. 1989; Goldfarb et al. 1990, 1991; Hsiao et al. 1989, 1992; Kretzschmar et al. 1986; Liao et al. 1986; Medori et al. 1992; Palmer and Collinge 1993; Tagliavini et al. 1991), gorilla (Schätzl et al. 1995), chimpanzee (Schätzl et al. 1995), orangutan (Schätzl et al. 1995), colobus monkey (Schätzl et al. 1995), presbytis monkey (Schätzl et al. 1995), mandrill (Schätzl et al. 1995), rhesus macaque (Schätzl et al. 1995), cynomolgus monkey (Schätzl et al. 1995), stumptail macaque (Schätzl et al. 1995), pigtail macaque (Schätzl et al. 1995), baboon (Schätzl et al. 1995), African green monkeys (*Aethiops, Dianae, Sabaeus*) (Schätzl et al. 1995), squirrel monkey (Schätzl et al. 1995), capuchin monkey

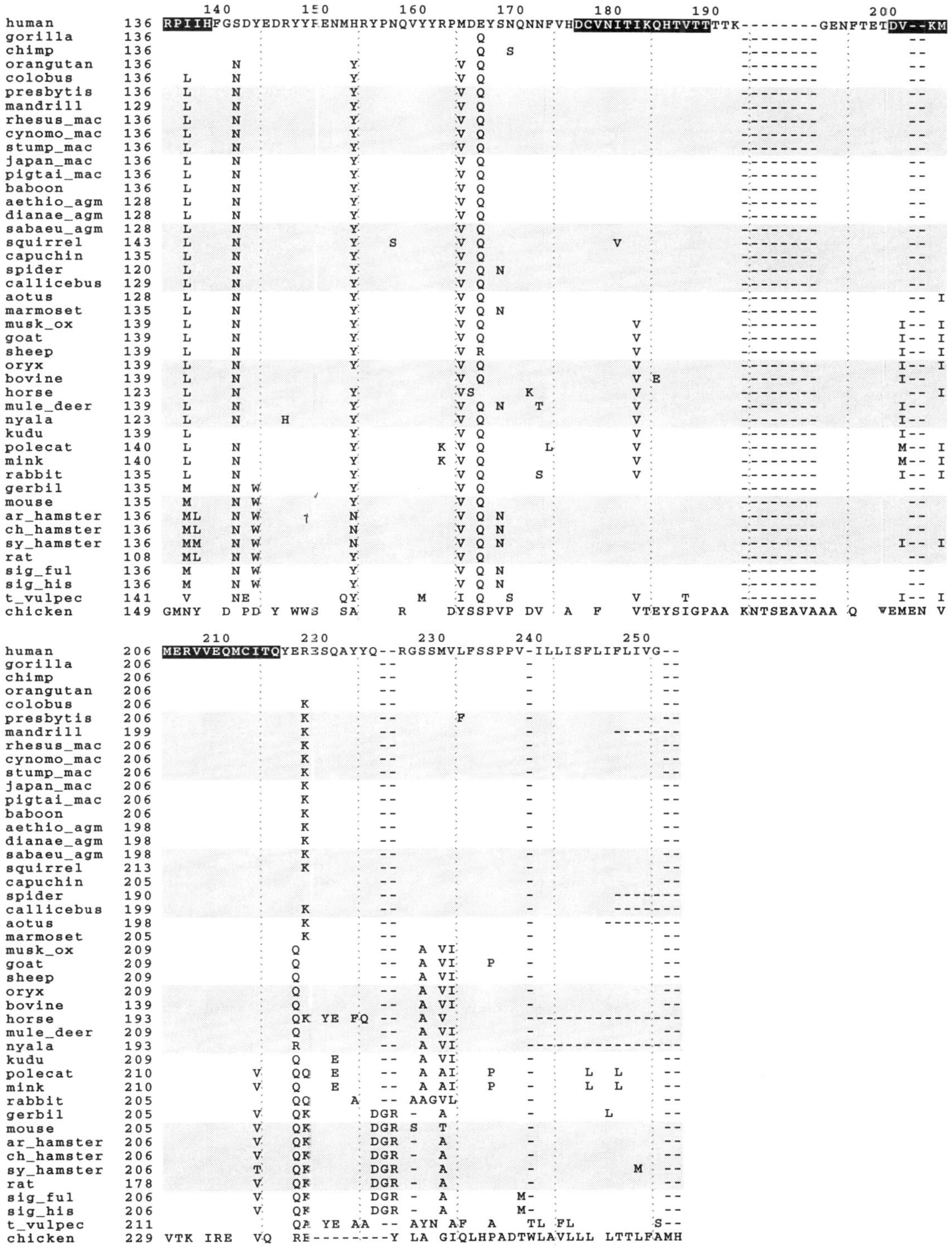

(Schätzl et al. 1995), spider monkey (Schätzl et al. 1995), callicebus monkey (Schätzl et al. 1995), aotus monkey (Schätzl et al. 1995), marmoset (Schätzl et al. 1995), musk-ox (H.M. Schätzl, unpubl.), goat (Martin et al. 1993a), sheep (Goldmann et al. 1990), oryx (Poidinger et al. 1993), bovine (Yoshimoto et al. 1992), horse (H.M. Schätzl, unpubl.), mule deer (Cervenakova et al. 1995), nyala (H.M. Schätzl, unpubl.), kudu (Martin et al. 1993b), polecat (Bartz et al. 1994), mink (Kretzschmar et al. 1992), rabbit (H.M. Schätzl, unpubl.), gerbil (H.M. Schätzl, unpubl.), mouse (Westaway et al. 1987), hamster (Armenian [Lowenstein et al. 1990], Chinese [Lowenstein et al. 1990], Syrian [Basler et al. 1986; Oesch et al. 1985; Rogers et al. 1990; Stahl et al. 1987, 1990; Turk et al. 1988]), rat (Liao et al. 1987), cotton rats (*Sigmodon fulviventur* and *hispidus*) (S.B. Prusiner, unpubl.), marsupial (*Trichosurus vulpecular*) (Windl et al. 1995), and chicken (Falls et al. 1990; Gabriel et al. 1992; Harris et al. 1991).

(Kretzschmar et al. 1986; Liao et al. 1986). This protein is posttranslationally processed to remove a 22-amino-acid amino-terminal signal peptide. A further 23 carboxy-terminal residues are also removed during the addition of a glycophosphatidyl inositol chain, capable of anchoring the protein to the cell membrane (Stahl et al. 1987). Also contributing to the mass of the protein are two asparagine side chains linked to large oligosaccharides, with multiple structures that have been shown to be complex and diverse (Endo et al. 1989). Although many species variants of PrP have been sequenced (Schätzl et al. 1995), most have been of primates, and only the chicken sequence is greatly different from the human. This makes it difficult to draw conclusions about the functional importance of many of the individual residues in the protein, because the short evolutionary distance between sequences means that many residues are conserved. The alignment of the 44 determined PrP sequences is shown in Figure 1. The degree of conservation between mammalian sequences is striking, and suggestive of the retention of some important function through evolution. However, mice with an ablated PrP gene ($PrP^{0/0}$) appeared to be normal (Büeler et al. 1992). Although $PrP^{0/0}$ mice were reported to show altered synaptic behavior (Collinge et al. 1994; Whittington et al. 1995), these results have since been questioned (Herms et al. 1995; Lledo et al. 1996). It has been reported that $PrP^{0/0}$ mice develop progressive ataxia at about 70 weeks of age and are deficient in Purkinje cells (Sakaguchi et al. 1996).

The carboxy-terminal 120 amino acids contain two conserved disulfide-bonded cysteines and a sequence that marks the addition of the GPI anchor. With the exception of the chicken sequence, amino acid conservation is fairly high. The amino-terminal amino acids contain some very unusual features, which are discussed below.

AMINO-TERMINAL SEQUENCE REPEATS

The amino-terminal domain of mammalian PrP contains five copies of a P(H/Q)GGG(G)WGQ octarepeat sequence, occasionally more, as in the case of one sequenced bovine allele that has six copies. These repeats are remarkably conserved between species, implying a functionally important role. The chicken sequence is notably different in this area and contains a different repeat, PGYP(H/Q)N. Although insertions of extra repeats have been found in patients with familial disease (Collinge et al. 1989), naturally occurring deletions of single octarepeats do not appear to cause disease, and deletion of all these repeats does not prevent PrP from undergoing the PrP^{C} to PrP^{Sc} transition (Rogers et al. 1993).

CONSERVED ALA-GLY REGION

The other region of notable conservation is in the sequence following the carboxyl terminus of the last octarepeat. This is the unusual glycine- and alanine-rich region, from A113 to Y128. From an evolutionary standpoint, it is striking to see such conservation as illustrated in Figure 2A in such a nondescript sequence, containing as it does only small, borderline-hydrophobic residues. Although no differences between species have yet been found in this part of the sequence, a single point mutation at residue 117 of A to V is linked to GSS (Hsiao et al. 1991). Several other point mutants in the same region also moderate the incubation times and phenotype of disease, as described later. Although the degree of conservation suggests a functional or structural importance, this region also appears to be of great importance to prion interconversion.

Other sequences exist in the database with similarities to this part of PrP, but it is difficult to assess their importance. Many of them are in sequences with long stretches of alanine and glycine that do not resemble proteins with compositions typical of the globular proteins of the structural databank and probably carry out a structural role for which a repetitive composition is required. A search through the SWISSPROT database reveals 1943 examples of eightfold stretches of sequence containing only alanine and glycine, out of 52,205 sequences (many sequences contain more than one such region). There are 4696 examples of runs of eight residues containing six or more alanines. Looking for similarities to the longer PrP sequence AGAAAAGAVVGGLGG, the database contains 5111 examples of 15-mers containing 12 or more alanines or glycines. Such stretches of sequence are clearly not uncommon, but are rarely as well conserved as in PrP. It is interesting to speculate about why such a sequence, containing so many side chains with no chemical functionality, or even with very high hydrophobicity, should apparently be subject to strong evolutionary constraints. The sequence gives the appearance of having been selected for its properties of flexibility and, perhaps, for the ability to undergo conformational change.

Similarity has previously been noted to part of the spider dragline silk protein sequence (Xu and Lewis 1990) that appears to be important because of its ability to form alanine-rich β-sheet aggregates (Simmons et al. 1996). This is consistent with the aggregation of PrP^{Sc} in β-rich structures. However, the silk sequence contains many such alanine-rich repeats, and therefore the pairings between strands are likely to be mostly intramolecular. This contrasts with PrP, in which only one alanine-rich section exists, and so intermolecular strand pairings are likely to play a greater part. One of the silk repeating units is shown in Figure 3A. FTIR spectroscopy showed that spider silk is predominantly antiparallel β-sheet, but that helical structure is induced by tension (Dong et al. 1991), an interesting parallel to the prion protein's conformational plasticity (Pan et al. 1993). The composition of the alanine/glycine-rich region has led to the suggestion

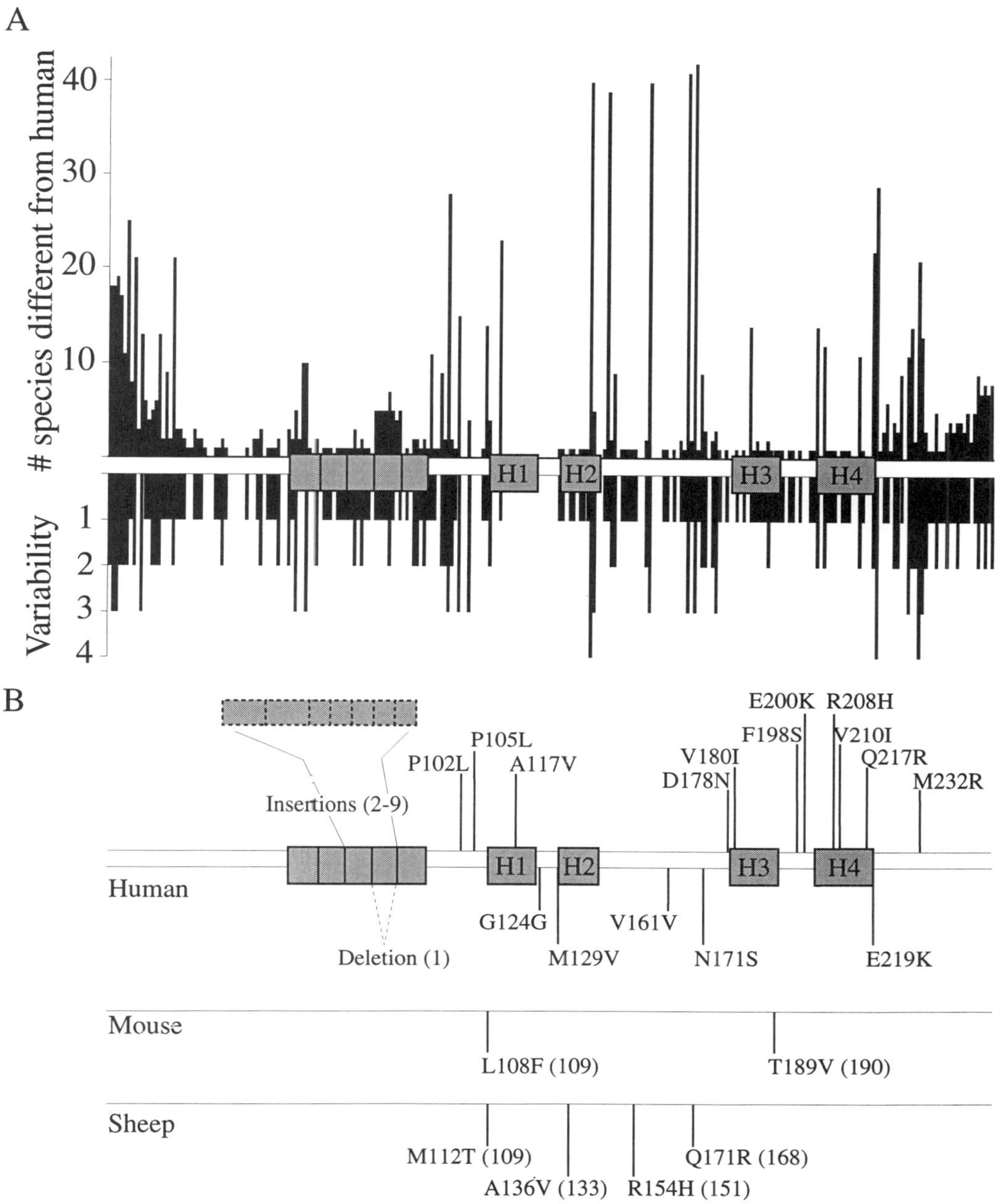

Figure 2. Natural variations in PrP. (*A*) Species variations. The x-axis represents the human PrP sequence, with the five octarepeats and H1–H4 as shown. Vertical bars above the axis indicate the number of species from Fig. 1 that differ from the human sequence at each position. Below the axis, the length of the bars indicates the number of alternative amino acids at each position in the alignment. (*B*) Mutations causing inherited human prion disease and polymorphisms in human, mouse, and sheep. Above the line of the human sequence are mutations that cause prion disease. Below the lines are polymorphisms, some, but not all, of which are known to influence the onset and phenotype of disease.

that the prion protein may share some features with viral envelope proteins, which are also known to undergo substantial structural change (Callebaut et al. 1994).

Another of the more noteworthy sequence matches is the skeletal muscle ryanodine receptor (Zorzato et al. 1990), which, although around 5000 amino acids in length, has a sequence with similarity to PrP residues 113–126 (shown in Fig. 3B). This part of the ryanodine receptor is a putative membrane-spanning region involved in a calcium channel. Interestingly, although PrP^C is normally anchored on the extracellular side of the membrane, it has been reported that under certain conditions in a cell-free system, a proportion can be

A

```
SHa PrP   111   HMAGAAAAGAVVGGLGGYML
                  | ||| ||   |||||
Fibroin   217   AAAAAAAGGAGQGGLGGQGA
```

B

```
SHa PrP   111   HMAGAAAAGAVVGGLGGYML
                  |||| |||   | ||
RynR     4335   TRAGAAGAGAAAGALGLLWG
```

Figure 3. Sequences with similarity to the alanine/glycine-rich conserved region of PrP. (*A*) One of the repeating regions of orb spider dragline silk fibroin. (*B*) A short, transmembrane region of skeletal muscle ryanodine receptor.

made in an inserted form that spans the endoplasmic reticulum membrane (Lopez et al. 1990; De Fea et al. 1994). The alanine-rich sequence is implicated in this insertion. It has not yet been shown that such a transmembrane form can be found in the plasma membrane or in the cholesterol-rich compartments thought to be the site of scrapie replication (Taraboulos et al. 1995), but it is feasible that transient or partial membrane insertion could play a part in either prion infection or the normal function of PrP. A recent study found that PrP containing six extra octarepeats, a mouse homolog of a form of PrP found in familial Creutzfeldt-Jakob disease (CJD), shows an abnormal mode of membrane association in cultured cells (Lehmann and Harris 1995).

It may also be of interest that this Ala/Gly-rich sequence is palindromic. The structure that would be adopted by a "retro-protein" (a protein whose sequence has been reversed in order) is not a new issue and has been discussed recently (Olszewski et al. 1996). If a protein chain is superimposed upon its retrosequence, running in the opposite direction, the main chains can be made to lie on top of one another, although the backbone hydrogen-bonding properties are altered. If the sequence is palindromic, the side chains occupy similar positions, but their spatial orientations are reversed in chirality, so the divergence increases with longer side chains. Such an unusual sequence as AGAAAAGA, however, is not only palindromic, but also contains short side chains only, so the structural difference between side chains in the forward and backward directions would be small. It is not known whether this feature is significant to aggregation or even to PrP^{C} to PrP^{Sc} conversion, or if it is merely coincidental.

STRUCTURAL PREDICTIONS AND DISEASE-CAUSING POINT MUTATIONS

Secondary structure prediction was used to analyze the multiple alignment of prion sequences (Gasset et al. 1992). The best of these methods assigns each residue to a state of helix, sheet, or coil with an accuracy of about 70%, and therefore the results should be treated with caution. Most methods predicted one or more stretches of sheet sequence, although the precise boundaries suggested by different algorithms did not agree with each other. However, as mentioned above, CD and IR spectra of PrP^{C} are consistent with a structure containing little or no β character. With a choice between only helix and coil, a better prediction can be made. A neural network trained on protein structures with only these two states (Kneller et al. 1990) was applied to the PrP sequence. The resulting prediction was of four helical regions, shown in Figures 1 and 2A, labeled H1 to H4. Of these, the carboxy-terminal helix was the most strongly predicted.

In support of this prediction is the apparent preference for residues that cause or modify the course of human disease to lie mainly within or close to these postulated helices. These have been summarized before (Hsiao et al. 1994) and are shown in Figure 2B. In particular, the mutation P102L is linked to the development of GSS and also to prion disease in transgenic mice carrying the same mutation (Hsiao et al. 1990). Substitutions at E200K and D178N are associated with familial CJD, whereas other mutations at positions 102, 105, 117, 145, 178, 180, 198, 200, 210, 217, and possibly 232 are also linked to inherited prion disease. One patient with prion disease has been found with a Prnp gene marked with a stop codon at position 145 (Kitamoto et al. 1993). Insertions of variable numbers of octarepeats are also associated with hereditary disease, although deletions of single repeats appear not to be (Laplanche et al. 1990). The effects of these point mutations can be explained by the hypothesis that they act to destabilize the tertiary structure of PrP^{C} and lower the barrier to conversion to PrP^{Sc}, which in turn gives rise to spontaneous disease. In addition, a site of polymorphism at codon 129 appears to alter the course of the disease in patients also possessing the D178N mutation (Goldfarb et al. 1992).

THREE-DIMENSIONAL MODELING

Using the predicted helices as a starting point, three-dimensional models were constructed (Huang et al. 1994). Sites favored for forming contact points between helices were identified, and a combinatorial algorithm (Cohen et al. 1979) was used to pair up sites on adjacent helices in an approach similar to that used earlier with some success to predict the structure of interleukin-4 (Curtis et al. 1991). This generated 300,000 test structures with different topologies that were screened to find the most reasonable possibilities. This method presupposes that the helix predictions are accurate and that the sequence 109–218 forms a globular domain. These assumptions need to be verified experimentally. The two carboxy-terminal helices are more amphipathic than the first two and are predicted to pack side-by-side, linked by a hairpin turn. They are connected at the "open" end by a disulfide bridge, making a fairly rigid structure. These helices are probably fairly stable, but would still require other amino-terminal residues to pack against them to complete the folding of the domain. Several residues linked to inherited prion disease are found buried in the center of this model (Huang et al. 1994), which is consistent with the idea that mutation of these sites would destabilize the PrP^{C} fold.

The disulfide bond between cysteine residues 179 and 214 is known to be intact in PrP^{Sc}, and so the block of amino acids between this cross-link is likely to retain the same structure as in PrP^{C}. The helix-to-sheet transition therefore probably occurs in the region between the amino terminus of PrP 27-30 and the amino terminus of the predicted helix 3, within amino acids 90–178. Models were also constructed of possible PrP^{Sc} structures, assuming that two of the PrP^{C} predicted helices are converted into four strands instead (Huang et al. 1996). The most sensible model is that in which H1 and H2 are transformed. Each helix was broken into two strands, since a strand of a given length contains about half the number of amino acids as does a comparable helix. The ends of the strands were placed at predicted strand-breaking residues where possible. A similar combinatorial approach was applied as was used to model PrP^{C}. Four residues thought to be involved in the species barrier (N108, M112, M129, A133) are close together on the surface of this model, perhaps indicating a surface for interaction with PrP^{C} (Huang et al. 1996).

PROTEIN-PROTEIN INTERACTIONS AND THE SPECIES BARRIER

Genetic evidence is suggestive of a rate-limiting, physical interaction between PrP^{C} and PrP^{Sc} during the conversion process. The species barrier, in which prions from another species have longer incubation times or do not transmit at all, is suggestive of this. In addition, mice in which the PrP gene has been ablated do not support prion infection (Prusiner et al. 1993a). Furthermore, it has been shown that mice normally resistant to hamster PrP^{Sc} become susceptible when a transgene expressing hamster PrP is introduced (Scott et al. 1989). In addition, in transgenic mice expressing both mouse (Mo) and hamster PrP^{C}, infectious prions select the most compatible PrP^{C}. Thus, inoculation with Mo prions led to neurological features and the production of prions characteristic of scrapie in mice (Prusiner et al. 1990). Conversely, inoculation with hamster prions led to the production of hamster prions. An inverse relationship between the steady-state PrP^{C} levels and the incubation time was also noted.

Additional support for PrP^{C}/PrP^{Sc} interaction comes from the different reactions of mice with subtly different PrP to different prion strains. Two different allotypes of the Prnp gene, a and b, differ at only two codons: positions 108 (Leu or Phe) and 189 (Thr or Val) (Fig. 2B) (Westaway et al. 1987). Even these conservative differences lead to altered susceptibility to different prion strains. For example, homozygous $Prnp^{b/b}$ mice are susceptible to prions from the 87V strain, but heterozygous $Prnp^{a/b}$ mice are not. The ability of strains of prions to retain differences in infectivity and disease phenotype from the original source of the prion, and in some way to remember this information despite multiple passages of the prion through different species, is likely to involve structural templating. Stable strains seem to display different structures in the scrapie isoform.

Comparison of sequences is of special importance because of the observed phenomenon of the species barrier to prion infection. Even within primates, there is considerable variation in the susceptibility of one species to prions from another (Fig. 2A) (Schätzl et al. 1995). As noted, this is believed to be because conversion requires compatibility in a physical association between PrP^{Sc} and PrP^{C}. Naturally, not all residues differing between PrP of two species take part in this PrP^{C}/PrP^{Sc} interaction. Codons 108 and 189 are obviously implicated in PrP^{C}/PrP^{Sc} interaction because of the differences between the two mouse allotypes. Species differences between the human and bovine PrP sequences are especially relevant. A comparison with the sheep sequence that may have been the source of the bovine spongiform encepthalopathy (BSE) outbreak in the United Kingdom is also interesting, since sheep scrapie prions are the most likely cause of the epidemic in cattle but do not cause infection in humans. Seven substitutions, all between codons 98 and 208, distinguish sheep from cattle PrP, as discussed previously (Prusiner et al. 1993b). There are four positions in which the human and bovine sequences are identical (Fig. 1), yet the ovine is different at positions 95 (Hu/Bo=Thr, Ov=Ser), 143 (Hu/Bo=Ser, Ov=Asn), 155 (Hu/Bo=His, Ov=Tyr), and 205 (Hu/Bo=Met, Ov=Ile). There are nine positions in which the ovine and bovine are identical and differ from the human. It is difficult to extrapolate from this to make predictions about the species barrier in this case, because all the residues taking part in the PrP^{C}/PrP^{Sc} structural interface have not yet been determined.

Aside from interaction with PrP^{Sc}, there is considerable genetic evidence for the interaction of PrP^{C} with an additional host-dependent factor (Telling et al. 1995). Transgenic mice expressing human (Hu) PrP are immune to infection with human prions but become susceptible when the endogenous MoPrP is ablated. In contrast, transgenic mice expressing the Hu-Mo chimeric protein MHu2M do support infection by Hu prions. Our interpretation of these observations is that the HuPrP sequence is incapable of competing effectively with background $MoPrP^{C}$ for a host-dependent factor that is required for replication. Infection can only proceed if MoPrP is ablated, in which case this unknown factor can interact with the next-best target, $HuPrP^{C}$. The MHu2M chimera, unlike HuPrP, can compete with MoPrP for this other component. Similar conclusions can be drawn from results with genetic prion diseases. Although mice expressing MoPrP with the GSS P102L mutation develop spontaneous disease (Hsiao et al. 1994), mice expressing the human GSS protein with endogenous MoPrP do not. The Hu-Mo chimera with the GSS mutation does lead to spontaneous disease (Telling et al. 1995).

This chimera was constructed by replacing the central part of the mouse sequence with the human equivalent (Mo residues 96–167, Fig. 1). Because MHu2M-PrP^{C} can compete effectively with MoPrP, the site of interaction with the unknown factor must include some of the residues which distinguish the human sequence from the mouse that are located in the mouse region of MHu2M (before 96 or after 167). The amino terminus up to residue 88 is dispensable for prion interaction (Rogers et al. 1993), and so the species barrier due to the alternative host-specific factor includes residues in the range 89–96 or 168–231 (mouse numbering). In the 89–96 range, only codon 96 differs, but more substantial differences are found in the 168–231 range.

It is assumed, although not explicitly proven, that the host-specific factor responsible for this is a protein, temporarily dubbed "protein X" until its identity can be determined. It interacts with PrP^{C} and may have a chaperone-like function, facilitating the folding of PrP into a more stable conformation, PrP^{Sc}. Alternatively, it may act to localize PrP^{C} to the correct subcellular environment for interaction with PrP^{Sc}. Such speculation will only be proved or disproved when protein X has been identified. Several proteins have been found that bind to PrP, but whether these are related to development of scrapie is not known. Using the yeast two-hybrid system, PrP was found to bind to Bcl-2, a protein that regulates cell death (Kurschner and Morgan 1995). Several other potential PrP-binding proteins have also been cloned and are under investigation (F. Yehiely et al., in prep.).

STRUCTURAL STUDIES OF PRP PEPTIDES

Structural studies of PrP are problematic. Obtaining sufficient quantities of PrP^{C} to carry out structural characterization is difficult but may be alleviated by the recent successful expression of recombinant PrP peptides (Mehlhorn et al. 1996). On the other hand, PrP^{C} is at least soluble in detergents, unlike PrP^{Sc}, which is very difficult to study outside the solid state. For these reasons, most structural studies to date have involved short, synthetic PrP peptides. Secondary structure prediction, as mentioned, postulated the existence of four helices between positions 109 and 218, designated H1–H4. Many disease-causing mutations seem to lie in or around these regions. The study of peptides of these regions, in particular the conserved alanine- and glycine-rich sequence within H1, has been of special interest.

Peptides corresponding to the four predicted helices H1–H4 of the Syrian hamster (SHa) sequence were synthesized, and their properties were investigated (Gasset et al. 1992). Of these, only H2 was readily soluble, and H1 was especially insoluble. Examination using attenuated total reflection FTIR spectroscopy showed that the H1 peptide had an amide I′ band characteristic of a strongly hydrogen-bonded, low-frequency (LF) β-pleated sheet. H3 and H4 also contained LF-β sheet, with a significant amount of turn structure in the case of H3. H2, on the other hand, gave a different spectrum indicative of multiple structures, including helix, sheet, and turn. There was also evidence from hydrogen-deuterium exchange that H1 was involved in intermolecular interactions. Electron microscopy showed that H1 formed clusters of fibrils when deposited from a suspension in 20 mM HEPES, which were similar in appearance to the infectious rods of PrP 27–30 isolated from hamster brain by sucrose gradient ultracentrifugation. The effect of solvent on the H1 peptide was also investigated. LF-β structure was found to be maximized by the incorporation of H1 into phospholipids. Additional peptides overlapping with H1 and H2 were also synthesized. Both 113–127 and 113–120 possessed LF-β structure. Another peptide, 121–136, gave mixed spectra similar to H2.

Other peptides in the 90–145 range have also been studied. This region was chosen because scrapie infectivity is retained by PrP 27–30, a PrP^{Sc} fragment with an amino-terminal truncation at around residue 90, and also because of the observation that a position 145 stop codon mutation has been found in a patient with disease (Kitamoto et al. 1993). IR and CD spectroscopy has shown that in aqueous solution, 90–145, 109–141, 104–122, and 129–141 adopt random coil structures (Zhang et al. 1995). In hexafluoroisopropanol or detergents, the spectra become consistent with α-helical conformations. A hydrophobic environment was found to stabilize helical structure. This was investigated further by using nuclear magnetic resonance-derived chemical shifts to assign the secondary structure of peptides 109–122, 109–141, and 90–145 in SDS micelles. Residues 113–122 exhibited helical structure, whereas residues 128–139 showed sporadic α-helical chemical shifts consistent with a transient helix.

Peptides 90–145 and 109–141 were monitored over time by FTIR spectroscopy (Zhang et al. 1995). β-Structure formed gradually over a period of up to a month in aqueous NaCl solution. The rate of formation in acetonitrile was greatly increased, but decreased in the absence of salt, suggesting that physiological salt concentrations are necessary for β-structure formation. As stated below, although peptide 90–145 could induce β conformation in full-length PrP^{C} when in random coil conformation itself, after the peptide had been allowed to form β structure it could not induce any conformational change in PrP^{C}.

X-ray diffraction was also used to examine PrP 27–30, SHa 90–145, H1, and 113–120 (Nguyen et al. 1995b). PrP 27–30 dried from sucrose had an intersheet distance of about 8.82 Å, and a hydrogen-bond distance of 4.72 Å. This compares well with values from

SHa 90–145 of 9.15 Å for an intersheet distance and a split reflection at 4.72 Å/4.82 Å. The intersheet distance was much reduced in the H1 and 113–120 peptides, suggesting that in these peptides, the small side chains in the alanine- and glycine-rich region form the interior of the sandwich.

ATTEMPTS TO MIMIC CONVERSION IN VIVO

A peptide, 104H1, containing H1 with an amino-terminal extension to residue 104, has different properties from H1 in aqueous solution, with more stable helical or coil conformation (Nguyen et al. 1995a). In acetonitrile, a small fraction was converted to β structure. The effects of mixing this peptide with H1 alone were investigated. When H1 was added, a significant fraction of 104H1(50% at a H1:104H1 ratio of 1:10) was converted to a β conformation as monitored by FTIR spectroscopy (Nguyen et al. 1995a). CD spectroscopy was also used to follow the conversion of SHa 104H1 by SHa H1. Interestingly, Mo H1 (differing by two residues from SHa H1) was less able to induce β conformation in SHa 104H1. This may be relevant to the in vivo species barrier. FTIR spectroscopy was also used to follow SHa H1 peptides labeled with ^{13}C at the carbonyl carbon of Ala-116 during mixing with 104H1. A shift in the $^{13}C{=}O$ vibration was observed, indicating recruitment of 104H1 into a common β-sheet with labeled H1.

Peptide SHa 90–145, when incubated with SHa PrP^{C}, was found to induce protease resistance, but only when in 5000-fold excess (Kaneko et al. 1995). The most efficient peptide found was SHa90-145(A117V), containing the GSS mutation. The complex formed had decreased solubility compared to PrP^{C} and showed an increase in β conformation by FTIR spectroscopy, although the extent to which this was due to conformational change in the peptide or in the PrP^{C} is not clear. Interestingly, SHa90-145 only induced protease resistance when in the random coil form, but not in the β-sheet form. Mo90–145 was incapable of inducing protease resistance in SHa PrP^{C} even at 5000-fold excess.

Mixing undenatured hamster PrP^{Sc} in 50-fold excess with ^{35}S-labeled SHa PrP^{C} produces some protease-resistant labeled PrP^{C}, as reported by Kocisko et al. (1994). However, it has not yet been possible to demonstrate that this protease-resistant form of PrP^{C} derived from in vitro conversion efforts is equivalent to PrP^{Sc}. It remains possible, especially in view of the ability of peptides to render PrP^{C} protease-resistant simply by binding, that the full-length proteins are tightly bound, but that true conversion has not taken place. Even with this caveat in mind, the observation that $SHaPrP^{Sc}$ could bind to $SHaPrP^{C}$ and protect it from proteolytic digestion, but not to $MoPrP^{C}$, demonstrates species specificity in this interaction (Kocisko et al. 1995), reinforcing the idea that direct, complementary PrP^{C}/PrP^{Sc} interaction is part of the conversion process. If it emerges that the ability of PrP^{Sc} to induce protease resistance in vitro is related to infectivity in vivo, use of $HuPrP^{C}$ with bovine PrP^{Sc} may be a useful indicator of the susceptibility of humans to BSE. Intriguingly, distinct strains of PrP^{Sc} that yield different products when treated with protease are reported to have passed on these properties to the PrP^{C} with which they interact in this cell-free system (Bessen et al. 1995). This reinforces the proposal that scrapie strains result from different interactions between the two isoforms.

In summary, several of these model systems show sequence selectivity in their interactions, supporting the idea that simple molecular interactions between PrP^{C} and PrP^{Sc} are at least part of the source of the species barrier to infection. It should be noted, however, that combinations of H1, H2, H3, and H4 peptides have so far failed to show infectivity, and so they must be regarded as model systems that do not fully mimic the conversion into infectious PrP^{Sc}.

MODELS FOR PRP^{Sc} FORMATION

Clearly, the situation in vivo is much more complex than any simple kinetic model, seemingly involving an interaction in a specialized microenvironment within the cell (Taraboulos et al. 1995) between proteins whose concentrations depend on many factors. Nevertheless, two models suggest ways that proteins can induce structural conversion at the molecular level. This in no way contradicts the widely held view that a unique sequence folds to a unique protein structure under a particular set of conditions (Anfinsen 1973), because the environments and quaternary structures in which PrP^{C} and PrP^{Sc} are found are not necessarily the same.

Any plausible replication mechanisms must be able to reproduce the observed exponential growth of infectious titer seen in the early phase of the infectious form of the disease (Oesch et al. 1985). The long incubation time is probably a consequence of this exponential growth, beginning with a small amount of PrP^{Sc}, when little effect is seen. It also explains the surprising uniformity of the time to onset of disease, which may be assumed to happen when a certain PrP^{Sc} level is reached; according to the observed growth of infectivity, the amount of PrP^{Sc} increases by about 20% each day. A model must also require species compatibility in a physical interaction between PrP^{C} and PrP^{Sc}.

One mechanism proposes a nucleated polymerization model (Come et al. 1993; Jarrett and Lansbury 1993; Lansbury et al. 1995) in which prion deposition is the driving force. The initial stage is the slow, reversible formation of a nucleating multimer. Once formed, this seed acts in a manner analogous to crystallization, permitting additional PrP monomers to add to the lengthening polymer. Intermolecular interactions stabilize an abnormal conformation that is always present as

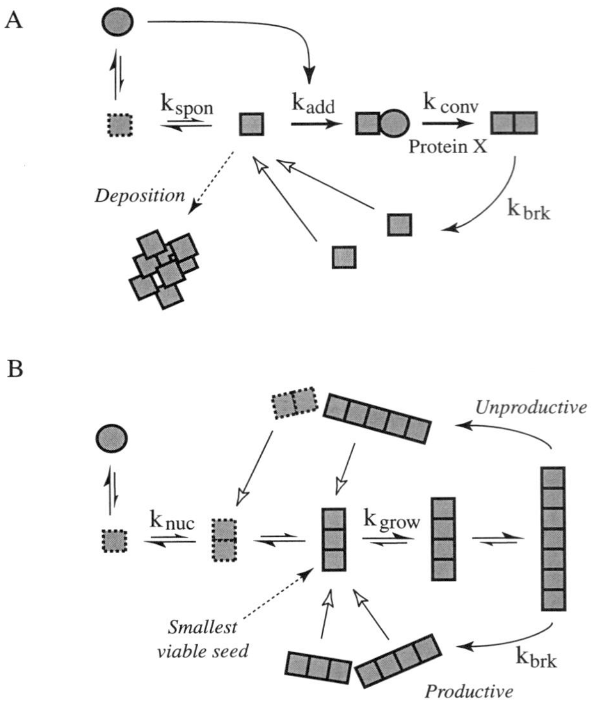

Figure 4. Schematic representations of the essential steps in (*A*) the nucleated polymerization model and (*B*) the catalytic model for prion replication. Circles represent PrP^C, and broken boxes represent stages intermediate between PrP^C and PrP^{Sc} that are not themselves infectious. The first step in inherited disease is either (*A*) nucleation, or (*B*) stochastic formation of monomeric or dimeric PrP^{Sc}. This is followed by a second order (*A*) polymer growth or (*B*) association involving PrP^C and PrP^{Sc} accompanied by conformational change. The final stage in either model is either (*A*) fragmentation of the polymer or (*B*) the breakdown of the associated intermediate, to produce two new infectious units. In *B* a slow deposition of aggregated PrP^{Sc} is not essential for prion propagation.

a minor component. To permit exponential growth in the number of nuclei, we will assume that polymers must occasionally break apart to generate new seeds. This is illustrated in Figure 4B. In favor of the nucleated polymerization model is its ability to explain prion strains as representing alternative packing arrangements within the seed particles. These would allow monomers to associate with different rates, depending on quaternary organization effects. It is also precedented, for example, in the gelation of deoxyhemoglobin (Hofrichter et al. 1974).

We have investigated the nucleated polymerization model by computer simulation, first considering the infectious disease case. We attempted to fit the model to the observed exponential increase in the number of infectious units in mice over the first 40 days of infection (Oesch et al. 1985). Estimates were made to the best of our current knowledge for the initial concentration of nuclei or infectious units per gram of brain (Ni), and for the concentration [C] of monomeric PrP^C, which was assumed to be constant throughout the simulation. These estimates assumed that the concentrations are the same in the microenvironment in which interaction occurs as the bulk values for brain, but this is unimportant, since the rate constants scale to account for inaccuracies. Another value chosen at the outset was the number of molecules of PrP contained within the multimer aggregates (Nm): The ratio of this to the number of polymers (Nm/Ni) gives an estimate of the mean size of each polymer. No assumptions were made about the statistical distribution of sizes.

Two steps were considered. The first is an addition to the polymer, a second-order process whose rate is given by

$$R_1 = k_1 \, Ni \, [C] \qquad (1)$$

The second step is the first-order fragmentation of the polymer. For this, it was assumed that each of the Nm molecules contained within polymers has an equal chance of fragmentation. However, according to this model, only particles of a minimum size S are infectious themselves, and so for Ni infectious multimers 2(S.Ni) possible fragmentation gives rise to no new productive seeds. The rate of this step is therefore given by

$$R_2 = k_2 \, \{Nm - 2(S.Ni)\} \qquad (2)$$

The rate of nucleation in animals without a mutated gene is negligible, as shown by the extremely rare incidence of spontaneous disease. Therefore, this step was not implemented in the analysis.

For the two steps of addition to the nucleus and the subsequent fragmentation, initial rate constants were chosen at random. These were then optimized using a Simplex minimization to produce the best root-mean-square fit to experimental growth kinetics (Oesch et al. 1985). Simulation of the scheme does, as expected, lead to an exponential increase in infectivity. Rate constants could be found that allowed the simulation to fit the observed growth kinetics curve over a wide range of starting conditions (data not shown).

The effects of varying the starting conditions were examined. The rate constants were optimized to reproduce experimental kinetics with a given number and average size of starting seeds. The simulation was then carried out with the same rate constants, but varying the initial number of infectious units, the average size of each infectious particle, and the minimum size for an infectious seed. It was found that the average particle size returns rapidly to an equilibrium value that is determined solely by the rate constants and is independent of starting conditions. In addition, because of the exponential increase in infectivity, even large changes in the initial multimer concentration have little effect on the time taken to generate a certain critical number of infectious units. This suggests that initial differences in the numbers of infectious units at the start would not greatly influence the incubation time in experimental disease, supported by the homogeneity of incubation times in vivo.

An alternative mechanism for replication (Cohen et al. 1994) proposes a catalytic process in which PrP^{Sc} monomers or dimers are capable of binding to PrP^{C}, or to PrP^{*}, a partially unfolded intermediate state. Once bound, the activation barrier for conversion is lowered, and a new monomer or dimer of PrP^{Sc} can be formed. This is then released as an additional infectious particle. This scheme is shown in Figure 4B. The main difference between this and nucleated polymerization is that, according to this theory, the PrP deposits found in some prion diseases are a by-product of an increasing concentration of insoluble PrP^{Sc}, rather than being the rate-limiting step. Deposition into insoluble plaques would certainly assist the overall process by mass action.

Kinetically, the nucleated polymerization model is identical to the catalytic model for the infectious disease simulation. Both models include a second-order association between PrP* and PrP^{Sc}, followed by a first-order dissociation to yield two infectious units. At the limit of the polymerization model, where the minimum seed size is only one molecule, the two models converge. There are, however, obvious physical differences in the intermediates used to propagate infection, one of which is that the catalytic scheme allows only one PrP^{C} monomer or dimer to bind to an infectious unit at a time, whereas the polymerization scheme proceeds by adding several monomers sequentially before the formation of a new infectious seed. This would lead to one detectable difference: A system with catalytic kinetics should become saturated with a large excess of PrP^{C}, whereas a polymerization scheme would not. Because the data we have is entirely from experiments carried out with a large excess of PrP^{Sc}, this cannot yet be used to distinguish the models.

Another difference would only become apparent in spontaneous or genetic disease. Normally, spontaneous prion generation is a rare event, as the 1 in 10^6 incidence of sporadic CJD shows. Therefore, even if any new prions are generated in this way during infectious prion disease, the numbers would be negligible compared to the many replicated from those introduced by infection. Such spontaneous generation is, however, important in the onset of genetic disease We are still gathering information about the time to onset of spontaneous disease in mice that express a mutant prion protein. The presence of wild-type PrP is a complicating factor, but transgenic mice that express the GSS mutant PrP-P101L on a null background allow investigation without interference from endogenous MoPrP. Recent data show that these mice expressing one copy of the transgene become ill with scrapie at 146 ± 2 days, whereas mice homozygous for the transgene array show symptoms at 85 ± 2 days roughly half the time (Telling et al. 1996). If the local PrP concentration available for conversion to PrP^{Sc} is proportional to the gene dose, this is indicative of first-order kinetics with respect to PrP^{C}. If the rate-determining step of spontaneous prion formation is really the formation of a multimolecular nucleus, higher-order dependence on the gene dose of PrP would be expected; for instance, the aggregation of deoxyhemoglobin shows a 30th-order concentration dependence (Hofrichter et al. 1974). Interestingly, the heterozygous mice with the longer incubation time seem to have more amyloid plaques, suggesting that the correlation between PrP^{Sc} deposition and death is not perfect. This result relies on only one line of mice and two data points, but experiments are under way with mice that will express 8, 16, and 32 times the quantity of mutant PrP. This should give revealing insights into the kinetics of the rate-determining step of the infectious form of the disease in vivo.

Other biochemical and biophysical data argue against the nucleated polymerization model. First, a variety of prion preparations showed resistance to ionizing radiation consistent with a particle size upper limit of 55 kD (a dimer of the polypeptide). The kinetics of inactivation was inconsistent with a model in which scrapie resistance to irradiation is due to aggregation (Bellinger-Kawahara et al. 1988); rather, it was indicative of the ability of a dimer to be infectious. Second, not all prion diseases show the presence of amyloid plaques. Although amorphous aggregates of PrP^{Sc} can be purified from scrapie-infected hamster brain, only when PrP^{Sc} is exposed to detergents and proteolysis does the protease-resistant core PrP 27–30 polymerize into rods. Amyloid-like polymers have also not been observed in scrapie-infected ScN2a cell cultures. The relevance of kinetic studies of peptide aggregation (Come et al. 1993) to scrapie in vivo is therefore questionable. Although aggregation undoubtedly occurs as the rate-limiting step in peptide aggregation studies, the evidence is against this being an indispensable part of the prion replication process. Third, infectivity increases by one or two orders of magnitude when prion rods are dispersed into detergents; this clearly frees additional infectious units, whether they are monomers or multimers. However, in this situation, no rods can be identified by electron microscopy (Gabizon et al. 1987), suggesting that if polymeric nuclei are essential for propagation, then the minimum size cannot be large. In contrast, electron microscopy was able to identify aggregated chains of deoxyhemoglobin in sickle cell anemia (Murayama 1966).

In summary, a catalytic model is consistent with the available physical data about the minimum size of an infectious prion. Although prion aggregates are undoubtedly infectious as well, a model in which an infectious unit need be no bigger than a monomer or dimer is compatible with the ionizing radiation experimental results and requires neither the formation of aggregates, which are sometimes not observed, nor the growth of rods, which are not observable by electron microscopy. In addition, it predicts first-order behavior upon varying PrP^C gene copy numbers in null background mice, which is what we observe in the admittedly sparse data available to date.

We note, however, that the differences between the two models are not so large. Both agree that in infectious disease, molecular recognition is a critical step. Some aggregation (whether into a dimer or a higher polymer) is required for either model, but the main difference is the question over whether multimeric aggregation is a prerequisite for prion propagation or a by-product of increasing concentration of the product of this conversion.

Attempts to reproduce prion conversion in vitro have also led to interesting results and promise to yield more information about the sequence requirements of species specificity in conversion. Considerable spectroscopic and theoretical evidence suggests that the region of conformational difference between PrP^C and PrP^{Sc} is in or around the H1 region of the sequence. Additional structural investigation with longer sequences is under way and should provide useful insights into the nature of the cellular prion protein. Structural studies should also assist in the interpretation of the positions of residues involved in the interaction between the different isoforms and, hence, help to explain the species barrier to infection. Finally, the apparent role in vivo of additional components, such as protein X, remains to be explained.

ACKNOWLEDGMENTS

This work was supported by grants from the International Human Frontier Science Program and the National Institutes of Health.

REFERENCES

Alper, T., W.A. Cramp, D.A. Haig, and M.C. Clarke. 1967. Does the agent of scrapie replicate without nucleic acid? *Nature* **214:** 764.

Anfinsen, C.B. 1973. Principles that govern the folding of protein chains. *Science* **181:** 223.

Bartz, J.C., D.I. McKenzie, R.A. Bessen, R.F. Marsh, and J.M. Aiken. 1994. Transmissible mink encephalopathy species barrier effect between ferret and mink: PrP gene and protein analysis. *J. Gen. Virol.* **75:** 2947.

Basler, K., B. Oesch, M. Scott, D. Westaway, M. Wälchli, D.F. Groth, M.P. McKinley, S.B. Prusiner, and C. Weissmann. 1986. Scrapie and cellular PrP isoforms are encoded by the same chromosomal gene. *Cell* **46:** 417.

Bellinger-Kawahara, C.G., E. Kempner, D.F. Groth, R. Gabizon, and S.B. Prusiner. 1988. Scrapie prion liposomes and rods exhibit target sizes of 55,000 Da. *Virology* **164:** 537.

Bessen, R.A., D.A. Kocisko, G.J. Raymond, S. Nandan, P.T. Lansbury, and B. Caughey. 1995. Non-genetic propagation of strain-specific properties of scrapie prion protein. *Nature* **375:** 698.

Büeler, H., M. Fischer, Y. Lang, H. Bluethmann, H.-P. Lipp, S.J. DeArmond, S.B. Prusiner, M. Aguet, and C. Weissmann. 1992. Normal development and behaviour of mice lacking the neuronal cell-surface PrP protein. *Nature* **356:** 577.

Callebaut, I., A. Tasso, R. Brasseur, A. Burny, D. Portetelle, and J.P. Mornon. 1994. Common prevalence of alanine and glycine in mobile reactive centre loops of serpins and viral fusion peptides: Do prions possess a fusion peptide? *J. Comput. Aided Mol. Des.* **8:** 175.

Cervenakova, L., D.C. Guiroy, P. Brown, E. Williams, J. Nagle, E.K. Lau, L.G. Goldfarb, J.C. Gibbs, and D.C. Gajdusek. 1995. Mule deer PrP gene sequence. EMBL Acc. no. P47852.

Cohen, F.E., T.J. Richmond, and F.M. Richards. 1979. Protein folding: Evaluation of some simple rules for the assembly of helices into tertiary structures with myoglobin as an example. *J. Mol. Biol.* **132:** 275.

Cohen, F.E., K.-M. Pan, Z. Huang, M. Baldwin, R.J. Fletterick, and S.B. Prusiner. 1994. Structural clues to prion replication. *Science* **264:** 530.

Collinge, J., M.A. Whittington, K.C. Sidle, C.J. Smith, M.S. Palmer, A.R. Clarke, and J.G.R. Jefferys. 1994. Prion protein is necessary for normal synaptic function. *Nature* **370:** 295.

Collinge, J., A.E. Harding, F. Owen, M. Poulter, R. Lofthouse, A.M. Boughey, T. Shah, and T.J. Crow. 1989. Diagnosis of Gerstmann-Sträussler syndrome in familial dementia with prion protein gene analysis. *Lancet* **2:** 15.

Come, J.H., P.E. Fraser, and P.T. Lansbury, Jr. 1993. A kinetic model for amyloid formation in the prion diseases: Importance of seeding. *Proc. Natl. Acad. Sci.* **90:** 5959.

Curtis, B.M., S.R. Presnell, S. Srinivasan, H. Sassenfeld, R. Klinke, E. Jeffrey, D.Cosman, C.J. March, and F.E. Cohen. 1991. Experimental and theoretic studies of the 3-dimensional structure of human interleukin-4. *Proteins* **11:** 111.

De Fea, K.A., D.H. Nakahara, M.C. Calayag, C.S. Yost, L.F. Mirels, S.B. Prusiner, and V.R. Lingappa. 1994. Determinants of carboxyl-terminal domain translocation during prion protein biogenesis. *J. Biol. Chem.* **269:** 16810.

Doh-ura, K., J. Tateishi, H. Sasaki, T. Kitamoto, and Y. Sakaki. 1989. Pro→Leu change at position 102 of prion protein is the most common but not the sole mutation related to Gerstmann-Sträussler syndrome. *Biochem. Biophys. Res. Commun.* **163:** 974.

Dong, Z., R.V. Lewis, and C.R. Middaugh. 1991. Molecular mechanism of spider silk elasticity. *Arch. Biochem. Biophys.* **284:** 53.

Endo, T., D. Groth, S.B. Prusiner, and A. Kobata. 1989. Diversity of oligosaccharide structures linked to asparagines of the scrapie prion protein. *Biochemistry* **28:** 8380.

Falls, D.L., D.A. Harris, F.A. Johnson, M.M. Morgan, G. Corfas, and G.D. Fischbach. 1990. 42 kD ARIA: A protein that may regulate the accumulation of acetylcholine receptors at developing chick neuromuscular junctions. *Cold Spring Harbor Symposium Quant. Biol.* **55:** 397.

Gabizon, R., M.P. McKinley, and S.B. Prusiner. 1987. Purified prion proteins and scrapie infectivity copartition into liposomes. *Proc. Natl. Acad. Sci.* **84:** 4017.

Gabriel, J.-M., B. Oesch, H. Kretzschmar, M. Scott, and S.B. Prusiner. 1992. Molecular cloning of a candidate chicken prion protein. *Proc. Natl. Acad. Sci.* **89:** 9097.

Gasset, M., M.A. Baldwin, D. Lloyd, J.-M. Gabriel, D.M. Holtzman, F. Cohen, R. Fletterick, and S.B. Prusiner. 1992. Predicted α-helical regions of the prion protein when synthesized as peptides form amyloid. *Proc. Natl. Acad. Sci.* **89:** 10940.

Goldfarb, L.G., E. Mitrova, P. Brown, B.H. Toh, and D.C. Gajdusek. 1990. Mutation in codon 200 of scrapie amyloid protein gene in two clusters of Creutzfeldt-Jakob disease in Slovakia. *Lancet* **336:** 514.

Goldfarb, L.G., M. Haltia, P. Brown, A. Nieto, J. Kovanen, W.R. McCombie, S. Trapp, and D.C. Gajdusek. 1991. New mutation in scrapie amyloid precursor gene (at codon 178) in Finnish Creutzfeldt-Jakob kindred. *Lancet* **337:** 425.

Goldfarb, L.G., R.B. Petersen, M. Tabaton, P. Brown, A.C. LeBlanc, P. Montagna, P. Cortelli, J. Julien, C. Vital, W.W. Pendelbury, M. Haltia, P.R. Wills, J.J. Hauw, P.E. McKeever, L. Monari, B. Schrank, G.D. Swergold, L. Autilio-Gambetti, D.C. Gajdusek, E. Lugaresi, and P. Gambetti. 1992. Fatal familial insomnia and familial Creutzfeldt-Jakob disease: Disease phenotype determined by a DNA polymorphism. *Science* **258:** 806.

Goldmann, W., N. Hunter, J.D. Foster, J.M. Salbaum, K. Beyreuther, and J. Hope. 1990. Two alleles of a neural protein gene linked to scrapie in sheep. *Proc. Natl. Acad. Sci.* **87:** 2476.

Harris, D.A., D.L. Falls, F.A. Johnson, and G.D. Fischbach. 1991. A prion-like protein from chicken brain copurifies with an acetylcholine receptor-inducing activity. *Proc. Natl. Acad. Sci.* **88:** 7664.

Herms, J.W., H.A. Kretzschmar, S. Titz, and B.U. Keller. 1995. Patch-clamp analysis of synaptic transmission to cerebellar purkinje cells of prion protein knockout mice. *Eur. J. Neurosci.* **7:** 2508.

Hofrichter, J., P.D. Ross, and W.A. Eaton. 1974. Kinetics and mechanism of deoxyhemoglobin S gelation: A new approach to understanding sickle cell disease. *Proc. Natl. Acad. Sci.* **71:** 4804.

Hsiao, K.K., M. Scott, D. Foster, D.F. Groth, S.J. DeArmond, and S.B. Prusiner. 1990. Spontaneous neurodegeneration in transgenic mice with mutant prion protein. *Science* **250:** 1587.

Hsiao, K.K., C. Cass, G.D. Schellenberg, T. Bird, E. Devine-Gage, H. Wisniewski, and S.B. Prusiner. 1991. A prion protein variant in a family with the telencephalic form of Gerstmann-Sträussler-Scheinker syndrome. *Neurology* **41:** 681.

Hsiao, K., H.F. Baker, T.J. Crow, M. Poulter, F. Owen, J.D. Terwilliger, D. Westaway, J. Ott, and S.B. Prusiner. 1989. Linkage of a prion protein missense variant to Gerstmann-Sträussler syndrome. *Nature* **338:** 342.

Hsiao, K., S. Dlouhy, M.R. Farlow, C. Cass, M. Da Costa, M. Conneally, M.E. Hodes, B. Ghetti, and S.B. Prusiner. 1992. Mutant prion proteins in Gerstmann-Sträussler-Scheinker disease with neurofibrillary tangles. *Nat. Genet.* **1:** 68.

Hsiao, K.K., D. Groth, M. Scott, S.-L. Yang, H. Serban, D. Rapp, D. Foster, M. Torchia, S.J. DeArmond, and S.B. Prusiner. 1994. Serial transmission in rodents of neurodegeneration from transgenic mice expressing mutant prion protein. *Proc. Natl. Acad. Sci.* **91:** 9126.

Huang, Z., S.B. Prusiner, and F.E. Cohen. 1996. Scrapie prions: A three-dimensional model of an infectious fragment. *Folding Design* **1:** 13.

Huang, Z., J.-M. Gabriel, M.A. Baldwin, R.J. Fletterick, S.B. Prusiner, and F.E. Cohen. 1994. Proposed three-dimensional structure for the cellular prion protein. *Proc. Natl. Acad. Sci.* **91:** 7139.

Jarrett, J.T. and P.T. Lansbury, Jr. 1993. Seeding "one-dimensional crystallization" of amyloid: A pathogenic mechanism in Alzheimer's disease and scrapie? *Cell* **73:** 1055.

Kaneko, K., D. Peretz, K.-M. Pan, T. Blochberger, R. Gabizon, O.H. Griffith, F.E. Cohen, M.A. Baldwin, and S.B. Prusiner. 1995. Prion protein (PrP) synthetic peptides induce cellular PrP to acquire properties of the scrapie isoform. *Proc. Natl. Acad. Sci.* **32:** 11160.

Kellings, K., N. Meyer, C. Mirenda, S.B. Prusiner, and D. Riesner. 1992. Further analysis of nucleic acids in purified scrapie prion preparations by improved return refocussing gel electrophoresis (RRGE). *J. Gen. Virol.* **73:** 1025.

Kitamoto, T., R. Iizuka, and J. Tateishi. 1993. An amber mutation of prion protein in Gerstmann-Sträussler syndrome with mutant PrP plaques. *Biochem. Biophys. Res. Commun.* **192:** 525.

Kneller, D.G., F.E. Cohen, and R. Langridge. 1990. Improvement in protein secondary structure prediction by an enhanced neural network. *J. Mol. Biol.* **214:** 171.

Kocisko, D.A., S. A. Priola, G.J. Raymond, B. Chesebro, P.T. Lansbury, Jr., and B. Caughey. 1995. Species specificity in the cell-free conversion of prion protein to protease-resistant forms: A model for the scrapie species barrier. *Proc. Natl. Acad. Sci.* **92:** 3923.

Kocisko, D.A., J.H. Come, S.A. Priola, B. Chesebro, G.J. Raymond, P.T. Lansbury, Jr., and B. Caughey. 1994. Cell-free formation of protease-resistant prion protein. *Nature* **370:** 471.

Kretzschmar, H.A., M. Neumann, G. Riethmüller, and S.B. Prusiner. 1992. Molecular cloning of a mink prion protein gene. *J. Gen. Virol.* **73:** 2757.

Kretzschmar, H.A., L.E. Stowring, D. Westaway, W.H. Stubblebine, S.B. Prusiner, and S.J. DeArmond. 1986. Molecular cloning of a human prion protein cDNA. *DNA* **5:** 315.

Kurschner, C. and J.I. Morgan. 1995. The cellular prion protein (PrP) selectively binds to Bcl-2 in the yeast two-hybrid system. *Mol. Brain Res.* **30:** 165.

Lansbury, P.T., P.R. Costa, J.M. Griffiths, E.J. Simon, M. Auger, K.J. Halverson, D.A. Kocisko, Z.S. Hendsch, T.T. Ashburn, R.G.S. Spencer, B. Tidor, and R.G. Griffin. 1995. Structural model for the B-amyloid fibril based on interstrand alignment of an antiparallel-sheet comprising a C-terminal peptide. *Nat. Struct. Biol.* **2:** 990.

Laplanche, J.-L., J. Chatelain, J.-M. Launay, C. Gazengel, and M. Vidaud. 1990. Deletion in prion protein gene in a Moroccan family. *Nucleic Acids Res.* **18:** 6745.

Lehmann, S. and D.A. Harris. 1995. A mutant prion protein displays aberrant membrane association when expressed in cultured cells. *J. Biol. Chem.* **270:** 24589.

Liao, Y.-C., R.V. Lebo, G.A. Clawson, and E. A. Smuckler. 1986. Human prion protein cDNA: Molecular cloning, chromosomal mapping, and biological implication. *Science* **233:** 364.

Liao, Y.-C., Z. Tokes, E. Lim, A. Lackey, C.H. Woo, J.D. Button, and G.A. Clawson. 1987. Cloning of rat "prion-related protein"' cDNA. *Lab. Invest.* **57:** 370.

Lledo, P.-M., P. Tremblay, S.J. DeArmond, S.B. Prusiner, and R.A. Nicoll. 1996. Mice deficient for prion protein exhibit normal neuronal excitability and synaptic transmission in the hippocampus. *Proc. Natl. Acad. Sci.* **93:** 2403.

Lopez, C.D., C.S. Yost, S.B. Prusiner, R.M. Myers, and V.R. Lingappa. 1990. Unusual topogenic sequence directs prion protein biogenesis. *Science* **248:** 226.

Lowenstein, D.H., D.A. Butler, D. Westaway, M.P. McKinley, S.J. DeArmond, and S.B. Prusiner. 1990. Three hamster species with different scrapie incubation times and neuropathological features encode distinct prion proteins. *Mol. Cell. Biol.* **10:** 1153.

Martin, T.C., S.L. Hughes, K.J. Hughes, and M. Dawson. 1993a. Goat PrP gene sequence. EMBL Acc. no. X74758.

———. 1993b. Kudu PrP gene sequence. EMBL Acc. no. X74771.

McKinley, M.P., R. Meyer, L. Kenaga, F. Rahbar, R. Cotter, A. Serban, and S.B. Prusiner. 1991. Scrapie prion rod formation *in vitro* requires both detergent extraction and limited proteolysis. *J. Virol.* **65:** 1440.

Medori, R., P. Montagna, H.J. Tritschler, A. LeBlanc, P. Cortelli, P. Tinuper, E. Lugaresi, and P. Gambetti. 1992. Fatal familial insomnia: A second kindred with mutation of prion protein gene at codon 178. *Neurology* **42:** 669.

Mehlhorn, I., D. Groth, J. Stöckel, B. Moffat, D. Reilly, D. Yansura, W.S. Willett, M. Baldwin, R. Fletterick, F.E. Cohen, R. Vandlen, D. Henner, and S.B. Prusiner. 1996. High-level expression and characterization of a purified 142-residue polypeptide of the prion protein. *Biochemistry* **35:** 5528.

Murayama, M. 1966. Molecular mechanism of red cell "sickling." *Science* **153:** 145.

Narang, H.K. 1992. Scrapie-associated tubulofilamentous particles in human Creutzfeldt-Jakob disease. *Res. Virol.* **143:** 387.

Nguyen, J., M.A. Baldwin, F.E. Cohen, and S.B. Prusiner. 1995a. Prion protein peptides induce α-helix to β-sheet conformational transitions. *Biochemistry* **34:** 4186.

Nguyen, J.T., H. Inouye, M.A. Baldwin, R.J. Fletterick, F.E. Cohen, S.B. Prusiner, and D.A. Kirschner. 1995b. X-ray diffraction of scrapie prion rods and PrP peptides. *J. Mol. Biol.* **252:** 412.

Oesch, B., D. Westaway, M. Wälchli, M.P. McKinley, S.B.H. Kent, R. Aebersold, R.A. Barry, P. Tempst, D.B. Teplow, L.E. Hood, S.B. Prusiner, and C. Weissmann. 1985. A cellular gene encodes scrapie PrP 27-30 protein. *Cell* **40:** 735.

Olszewski, K.A., A. Kolinski, and J. Skolnick. 1996. Does a backwardly read protein sequence have a unique native state? *Protein Eng.* **9:** 5.

Palmer, M.S. and J. Collinge. 1993. Mutations and polymorphisms in the prion protein gene. *Hum. Mutat.* **2:** 168.

Pan, K.-M., M. Baldwin, J. Nguyen, M. Gasset, A. Serban, D. Groth, I. Mehlhorn, Z. Huang, R.J. Fletterick, F.E. Cohen, and S.B. Prusiner. 1993. Conversion of α-helices into β-sheets features in the formation of the scrapie prion proteins. *Proc. Natl. Acad. Sci.* **90:** 10962.

Poidinger, M., J. Kirkwood, and W. Almond. 1993. Sequence analysis of the PrP protein from two species of antelope susceptible to transmissible spongiform encephalopathy. *Arch. Virol.* **131:** 193.

Prusiner, S.B. 1994. Molecular biology and genetics of prion diseases. *Philos. Trans. R. Soc. Lond. B* **343:** 447.

Prusiner, S.B., D.F. Groth, D.C. Bolton, S.B. Kent, and L.E. Hood. 1984. Purification and structural studies of a major scrapie prion protein. *Cell* **38:** 127.

Prusiner, S.B., D.C. Bolton, D.F. Groth, K.A. Bowman, S.P. Cochran, and M.P. McKinley. 1982. Further purification and characterization of scrapie prions. *Biochemistry* **21:** 6942.

Prusiner, S.B., D. Groth, A. Serban, R. Koehler, D. Foster, M. Torchia, D. Burton, S.-L. Yang, and S.J. DeArmond. 1993a. Ablation of the prion protein (PrP) gene in mice prevents scrapie and facilitates production of anti-PrP antibodies. *Proc. Natl. Acad. Sci.* **90:** 10608.

Prusiner, S.B., M. Fuzi, M. Scott, D. Serban, H. Serban, A. Taraboulos, J.-M. Gabriel, G. Wells, J. Wilesmith, R. Bradley, S.J. DeArmond, and K. Kristensson. 1993b. Immunologic and molecular biological studies of prion proteins in bovine spongiform encephalopathy. *J. Infect. Dis.* **167:** 602.

Prusiner, S.B., M. Scott, D. Foster, K.-M. Pan, D. Groth, C. Mirenda, M. Torchia, S.-L. Yang, D. Serban, G.A. Carlson, P.C. Hoppe, D. Westaway, and S.J. DeArmond. 1990. Transgenetic studies implicate interactions between homologous PrP isoforms in scrapie prion replication. *Cell* **63:** 673.

Rogers, M., A. Taraboulos, M. Scott, D. Groth, and S.B. Prusiner. 1990. Intracellular accumulation of the cellular prion protein after mutagenesis of its Asn-linked glycosylation sites. *Glycobiology* **1:** 101.

Rogers, M., F. Yehiely, M. Scott, and S.B. Prusiner. 1993. Conversion of truncated and elongated prion proteins into the scrapie isoform in cultured cells. *Proc. Natl. Acad. Sci.* **90:** 3182.

Safar, J., P.P. Roller, D.C. Gajdusek, and C.J. Gibbs, Jr. 1993. Conformational transitions, dissociation, and unfolding of scrapie amyloid (prion) protein. *J. Biol. Chem.* **268:** 20276.

Sakaguchi, S., S. Katamine, N. Nishida, R. Moriuchi, K. Shigematsu, T. Sugimoto, A. Nakatani, Y. Kataoka, T. Houtani, S. Shirabe, H. Okada, S. Hasegawa, T. Miyamoto, and T. Noda. 1996. Loss of cerebellar Purkinje cells in aged mice homozygous for a disrupted PrP gene. *Nature* **380:** 528.

Schätzl, H.M., M. Da Costa, L. Taylor, F.E. Cohen, and S.B. Prusiner. 1995. Prion protein gene variation among primates. *J. Mol. Biol.* **245:** 362.

Scott, M., D. Foster, C. Mirenda, D. Serban, F. Coufal, M. Wälchli, M. Torchia, D. Groth, G. Carlson, S.J. DeArmond, D. Westaway, and S.B. Prusiner. 1989. Transgenic mice expressing hamster prion protein produce species-specific scrapie infectivity and amyloid plaques. *Cell* **59:** 847.

Simmons, A.H., C.A. Michal, and L.W. Jelinski. 1996. Molecular orientation and two-component nature of the crystalline fraction of spider dragline silk. *Science* **271:** 84.

Stahl, N., M.A. Baldwin, D.B. Teplow, L. Hood, B.W. Gibson, A.L. Burlingame, and S.B. Prusiner. 1993. Structural analysis of the scrapie prion protein using mass spectrometry and amino acid sequencing. *Biochemistry* **32:** 1991.

Stahl, N., D.R. Borchelt, and S.B. Prusiner. 1990. Differential release of cellular and scrapie prion proteins from cellular membranes by phosphatidylinositol-specific phospholipase C. *Biochemistry* **29:** 5405.

Stahl, N., D.R. Borchelt, K. Hsiao, and S.B. Prusiner. 1987. Scrapie prion protein contains a phosphatidylinositol glycolipid. *Cell* **51:** 229.

Tagliavini, F., F. Prelli, J. Ghisto, O. Bugiani, D. Serban, S.B. Prusiner, M.R. Farlow, B. Ghetti, and B. Frangione. 1991. Amyloid protein of Gerstmann-Sträussler-Scheinker disease (Indiana kindred) is an 11-kd fragment of prion protein with an N-terminal glycine at codon 58. *EMBO J.* **10:** 513.

Taraboulos, A., D. Serban, and S.B. Prusiner. 1990. Scrapie prion proteins accumulate in the cytoplasm of persistently infected cultured cells. *J. Cell Biol.* **110:** 2117.

Taraboulos, A., M. Scott, A. Semenov, D. Avrahami, L. Laszlo, and S.B. Prusiner. 1995. Cholesterol depletion and modification of COOH-terminal targeting sequence of the prion protein inhibit formation of the scrapie isoform. *J. Cell Biol.* **129:** 121.

Telling, G.C., M. Scott, J. Mastrianni, R. Gabizon, M. Torchia, F.E. Cohen, S.J. DeArmond, and S.B. Prusiner. 1995. Prion propagation in mice expressing human and chimeric PrP transgenes implicates the interaction of cellular PrP with another protein. *Cell* **83:** 79.

Telling, G.T., T. Haga, M. Torchia, P. Tremblay, S.J. DeArmond, and S.B. Prusiner. 1996. Interactions between wild-type and mutant prion proteins modulate neurodegeneration in transgenic mice. *Genes Dev.* **10:** 1736.

Turk, E., D.B. Teplow, L.E. Hood, and S.B. Prusiner. 1988. Purification and properties of the cellular and scrapie hamster prion proteins. *Eur. J. Biochem.* **176:** 21.

Westaway, D., P.A. Goodman, C.A. Mirenda, M.P. McKinley, G.A. Carlson, and S.B. Prusiner. 1987. Distinct prion proteins in short and long scrapie incubation period mice. *Cell* **51:** 651.

Whittington, M.A., K.C.L. Sidle, I. Gowland, J. Meads, A.F. Hill, M.S. Palmer, J.G.R. Jefferys, and J. Collinge. 1995. Rescue of neurophysiological phenotype seen in PrP null mice by transgene encoding human prion protein. *Nat. Genet.* **9:** 197.

Windl, O., M. Dempster, P. Estibeiro, and R. Lathe. 1995. A candidate marsupial *PrP* gene reveals 2 domains conserved in mammalian PrP proteins. *Gene* **159:** 181.

Xu, M. and R.V. Lewis. 1990. Structure of a protein superfiber: Spider dragline silk. *Proc. Natl. Acad. Sci.* **87:** 7120.

Yoshimoto, J., T. Iinuma, N. Ishiguro, M. Horiuchi, M. Imamura, and M. Shinagawa. 1992. Comparative sequence analysis and expression of bovine PrP gene in mouse L-929 cells. *Virus Genes* **6:** 343.

Zhang, H., K. Kaneko, J.T. Nguyen, T.L. Livshits, M.A. Baldwin, F.E. Cohen, T.L. James, and S.B. Prusiner. 1995. Conformational transitions in peptides containing two putative α-helices of the prion protein. *J. Mol. Biol.* **250:** 514.

Zorzato, F., K. Fujii, K. Otsu, M. Phillips, N.M. Green, F.A. Lai, G. Meissner, and D.H. Maclennan. 1990. Molecular cloning of cDNA encoding human and rabbit forms of the Ca^{2+} release channel (ryanodine receptor) of skeletal muscle sarcoplasmic reticulum. *J. Biol. Chem.* **265:** 2244.

The Role of PrP in Pathogenesis of Experimental Scrapie

C. WEISSMANN,[1] M. FISCHER,[1] A. RAEBER,[1] H. BÜELER,[1] A. SAILER,[1,2] D. SHMERLING,[1] T. RÜLICKE,[3] S. BRANDNER,[4] AND A. AGUZZI[4]

[1]*Institut für Molekularbiologie der Universität Zürich, Hönggerberg, 8093 Zürich,* [3]*Biologisches Zentrallabor and* [4]*Institut für Neuropathologie, Universitätsspital Zürich, 8091 Zürich, Switzerland*

It was recognized early on that the agent responsible for transmissible spongiform encephalopathies such as scrapie in sheep or kuru, Creutzfeldt-Jakob disease (CJD), Gerstmann-Sträussler-Scheinker disease (GSS), and fatal familial insomnia (FFI) in man had quite extraordinary properties, such as unusually long incubation periods (measured in months to years) and uncommon resistance to high temperature, formaldehyde treatment, and UV irradiation. The agent has been designated as "prion" (see glossary, Table 1) to distinguish it from conventional pathogens such as bacteria and viruses (Prusiner 1982).

In recent years, a new form of prion disease emerged in Great Britain and to a lesser extent in other European countries, namely, bovine spongiform encephalopathy (BSE) or mad cow disease, which has been attributed to the consumption by cattle of feed supplements derived from scrapie-contaminated sheep and later from cattle offal (Wilesmith et al. 1992). It is, however, quite possible that BSE originated as a sporadic case in cattle and was then spread by contaminated cattle offal. Because there has recently been a cumulation in Great Britain of CJD-like disease with novel neuropathological features in humans below the age of 35 (Will et al. 1996), there is reason to believe that BSE may have been transmitted to man via the consumption of BSE-contaminated bovine offal.

Human prion diseases have a low incidence, around $1{:}10^6$ per year. Most frequently they arise spontaneously in the population at large without any apparent cause, so-called sporadic or idiopathic forms; more rarely they are familial, tightly linked to certain mutations of the *Prnp* gene or acquired by transplantation, injection, and possibly ingestion of contaminated products; in all cases the disease can usually be experimentally transmitted to mice by intracerebral inoculation.

Although incubation times are measured in years or decades, once the disease becomes clinically evident, progression to death may take as little as a few months. In man, the first symptoms are usually loss of memory or motor disturbances, leading to dementia and death. The pathological changes in the brain vary in location and intensity; characteristically, extensive vacuolation, neuronal cell death, and gliosis, singly or in combination, are evident. Accumulation of PrP^{Sc} is the major pathognomonic feature; formation of amyloid plaques

Table 1. Glossary of Terms

Prion: Agent of transmissible spongiform encephalopathy (TSE), with unconventional properties. The term does not have structural implications other than that a protein is an essential component.

"Protein only" hypothesis: Maintains that the prion is devoid of informational nucleic acid and consists of protein (or glycoprotein) as essential pathogenic component. Genetic evidence strongly suggests that the protein is an abnormal form of PrP (PrP^* or perhaps specifically PrP^{Sc}). The association with other "non-informational" molecules (e.g., lipids or glycosamino glycans) is not excluded.

PrP^C or PrP-sen: This is the naturally occurring form of the mature *Prnp* gene product. It is glycosylated and anchored to the plasma membrane by a GPI residue. Its presence in a given cell type is necessary, but not sufficient, for the replication of the prion. It is poor in β-sheet structure.

PrP^{Sc} or PrP-res: An "abnormal" form of the mature *Prnp* gene product found in tissue of TSE sufferers, operationally defined as being partly resistant to proteinase K digestion under defined reaction conditions. It is believed to differ from PrP^C only (or mainly) conformationally and is rich in β-sheet structure. Within the framework of the protein-only hypothesis, it is often considered to be the transmissible agent or prion (however, see PrP^*).

PrP^*: Within the framework of the protein-only hypothesis, PrP^* is defined as the form of PrP constituting the essential (or only) component of the prion. It may, but need not, be identical with PrP^{Sc}. This concept was introduced (Weissmann 1991) because the ratio of infectivity to PrP^{Sc} is 1:100,000 or less, and the determination of chemical or physical characteristics of purified infectious preparations consisting mainly of PrP^{Sc} does not necessarily reflect the characteristics of the infectious component.

Virino hypothesis: Maintains that the TSE agent (prion) consists of an agent-specific nucleic acid enveloped in or associated with a host protein, perhaps PrP^{Sc}. Such a nucleic acid has not been identified in highly purified preparations of infectious agent.

"Unconventional virus" hypothesis: Maintains that the TSE agent is a virus with unusual properties. The requirement for PrP in the host to allow replication and pathogenesis is explained by assuming that PrP forms part or all of a receptor for the virus. As was mentioned above, no nucleic acid specific for TSEs has been isolated.

These definitions describe our terminology, which is not agreed on by convention and is not necessarily used by others.

[2]Present address: Salk Institute, La Jolla, California 92037.

consisting mainly of PrP^{Sc} is a typical, although not invariable, finding. Neither classic inflammatory nor immunological responses are apparent.

HYPOTHESES ABOUT THE NATURE OF THE SCRAPIE AGENT

The unusual properties of the scrapie agent early on gave rise to speculations that it might be devoid of nucleic acid (Alper et al. 1967). Currently, the most widely accepted proposal is the *"protein-only" hypothesis*, first outlined in general terms by Griffith (1967) and enunciated in its updated and detailed form by Prusiner (Prusiner 1989, 1993). The *virino hypothesis* holds that the infectious agent consists of a scrapie-specific nucleic acid genome and host-derived PrP^{Sc}, which is recruited as some sort of coat (Dickinson and Outram 1988). Finally, some still believe that the scrapie agent is a *conventional virus* with unusual properties. However, no evidence for the scrapie-specific nucleic acid postulated by the virus or virino theories has been found (Kellings et al. 1993).

The protein-only hypothesis proposes that the prion contains no nucleic acid and is identical with PrP^{Sc}, a modified form of PrP^{C} (Prusiner 1989). PrP^{C} is a normal host protein (Chesebro et al. 1985; Oesch et al. 1985; Basler et al. 1986) found predominantly on the outer surface of neurons (Fig. 1). PrP^{Sc} is defined as a form of PrP^{C} that readily forms protease-resistant aggregates after treatment with detergents (Oesch et al. 1985; McKinley et al. 1991). Prusiner proposed that PrP^{Sc}, when introduced into a normal cell, causes the conversion of PrP^{C} or its precursor into PrP^{Sc} (Figs. 1–3). The exact nature of the conversion is unknown, but it is currently ascribed to conformational modifica-

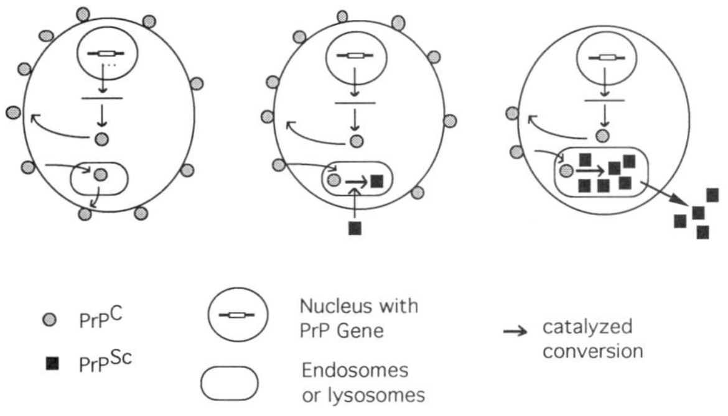

Figure 1. Models for the propagation of the prion. (*a*) In the normal cell, PrP^{C} is synthesized, transported to the cell surface, and recycled. (*b*) The "protein only" model assumes that the prion is identical with PrP^{Sc}. Exogenous prions cause the conversion of the normal cellular protein PrP^{C} into PrP^{Sc}, either at the cell surface or after internalization. (*c*) PrP^{Sc} accumulates intracellularly in late endosomes or lysosomes, and the cell surface is depleted of PrP^{C}. PrP^{Sc} is also released into the extracellular space.

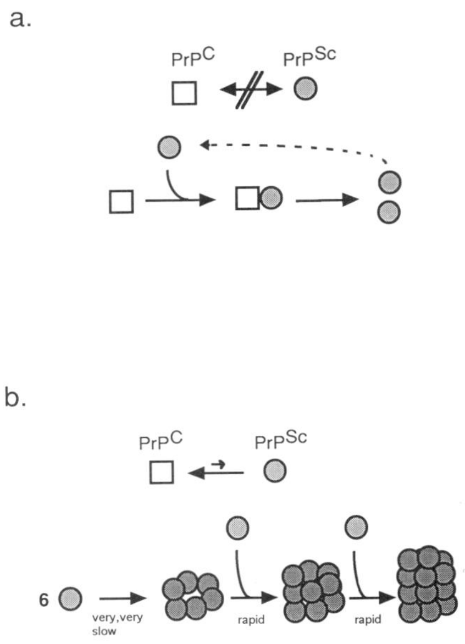

Figure 2. Models for the conformational conversion of PrP^{C} to PrP^{Sc}. (*a*) The "refolding" model. The conformational change is kinetically controlled: A high-activation-energy barrier prevents spontaneous conversion at detectable rates. As a result of an interaction with exogenously introduced PrP^{Sc}, PrP^{C} undergoes an induced conformational change to form PrP^{Sc}. This reaction may involve extensive unfolding and refolding of the protein to explain the postulated high-energy barrier and could be dependent on an enzyme or chaperone. The process leads to an exponential conversion cascade. In the case of certain mutations in PrP^{C}, spontaneous conversion to PrP^{Sc} may occur as a rare event, explaining why familial CJD or GSS arises spontaneously, albeit late in life. Sporadic CJD may come about when an extremely rare event (occurring in one among a million individuals per year) leads to spontaneous conversion of PrP^{C} to PrP^{Sc} and gives rise to a conversion cascade (Prusiner 1989; Prusiner et al. 1990). (*b*) The "seeding" model. The conformational change is thermodynamically controlled: The conformational change between PrP^{C} and PrP^{Sc} or a PrP^{Sc}-like molecule is reversible. PrP^{Sc} is only stabilized when it adds onto a crystal-like seed or aggregate of PrP^{Sc}. Seed formation is extremely slow; once a seed is present, monomer addition can ensue at a rapid rate (Brown et al. 1991; Jarrett and Lansbury 1993).

tion (Cohen et al. 1994); it has been determined that the β-sheet content of PrP^{Sc} is high, whereas that of PrP^{C} is low (Caughey et al. 1991b; Pan et al. 1993). The three-dimensional structure of a 121–231 fragment of recombinant PrP produced in *Escherichia coli* has recently been reported (Fig. 4). No chemical differences have so far been found between PrP^{C} and PrP^{Sc} (Stahl et al. 1993). However, because the ratio of infectious units to PrP^{Sc} molecules is only about 1:100,000 (Bolton et al. 1991), the structure of the PrP molecule actually associated with infectivity cannot be definitively inferred. For this reason, and because specific infectivity can vary considerably, the PrP species responsible for infectivity is presently better designated as PrP* (Weissmann 1991); it may or may

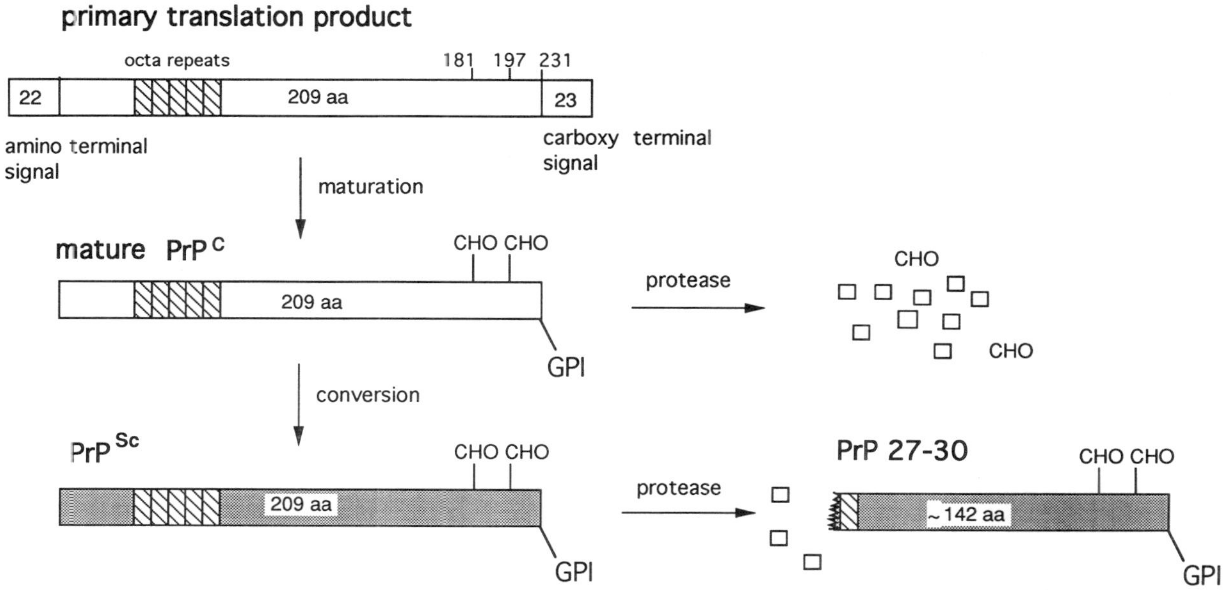

Figure 3. Biosynthesis of PrP^C and PrP^{Sc}. Maturation of the PrP precursor protein involves cleavage of the signal sequence, removal of 23 carboxy-terminal amino acids, attachment of a GPI anchor at Ser-231, and glycosylation (CHO) at Asn-181 and Asn-197. Mature PrP^C is anchored at the outer surface of the plasma membrane and is sensitive to proteinase K. Conversion of PrP^C to PrP^{Sc} occurs after exposure of the host to scrapie prions. PrP^{Sc} is partially resistant to proteinase K and yields PrP27-30 after digestion; the amino terminus is frayed and ranges from residues 73 to 90. "Octa repeats" are repeats of almost identical sequences of 8 amino acids.

not be identical with PrP^{Sc}, the major species that has been characterized chemically and physicochemically. If it is identical, the low specific activity could be due to a low efficiency of infection or to the infectious unit's being an aggregate of a large number of PrP^{Sc} molecules. The conclusion that some form of PrP is the essential, perhaps only, constituent of the infectious agent is based on biochemical and genetic evidence, as outlined below.

BIOSYNTHESIS OF PrP^C AND PrP^{Sc}

The entire PrP coding sequence is contained within one exon of the singular *Prnp* gene (Basler et al. 1986). As shown in Figure 3, an amino-terminal signal sequence of 22 amino acids is cleaved off the primary translation product, glycosylation occurs at two Asn residues, and 23 carboxy-terminal amino acids are replaced by a glycosyl phosphatidylinositol (GPI) residue that is attached to Ser-231 (Stahl et al. 1992). Mature PrP^C is anchored to the outer surface of the plasma membrane (Stahl et al. 1987) and undergoes endocytosis (Caughey et al. 1991a; Borchelt et al. 1992) and recycling (Shyng et al. 1993). The highest levels of PrP^C are found in brain, but substantial amounts are also found in heart and skeletal muscle and lesser levels in most other organs, except for liver and pancreas (Bendheim et al. 1992).

No nonallelic *Prnp*-related genes have been identified, no differences between PrP^C and PrP^{Sc} have been revealed by protein sequencing, and the amino acid sequences of both agree with that deduced from cloned genomic and cDNA (Basler et al. 1986; Hope et al. 1986; Stahl et al. 1993). Pulse-chase experiments in scrapie-infected neuroblastoma cells suggest that PrP^C is converted to PrP^{Sc} either at the cell surface or following endocytosis (Caughey and Raymond 1991). In brain, PrP^{Sc} accumulates to a level up to 100 times higher than that of PrP^C; however, PrP mRNA levels are the same in normal and scrapie-infected tissue.

PHYSICAL LINKAGE OF PrP^{Sc} AND PRIONS

Purification of scrapie infectivity led to preparations containing PrP^{Sc} as major protein component (Prusiner et al. 1982). Conversely, immunoaffinity purification of scrapie-infected hamster brain extracts using antibodies against PrP (there are currently no antibodies discriminating between PrP^C and PrP^{Sc}) led to enrichment of infectivity (Gabizon et al. 1988). These experiments show that the infectious agent is physically associated with PrP^{Sc} or a molecule antigenically related to it (PrP*) but do not preclude its association with other components. It has, however, been shown that highly purified prion preparations contain less than one molecule of nucleic acid larger than about 100 nucleotides (Kellings et al. 1992).

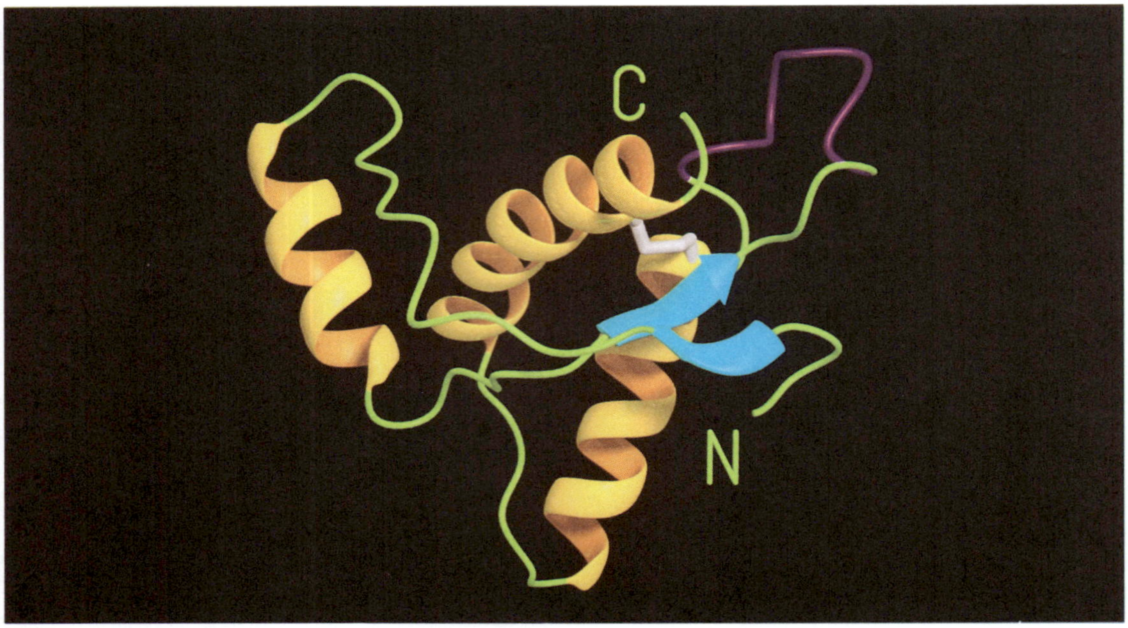

Figure 4. Ribbon diagram of the structure of recombinant mouse PrP domain 121–231. The three helices are yellow, the antiparallel two-stranded sheet is cyan. The connecting loops are displayed in green if their structure is well defined and in magenta otherwise. The disulfide bond between Cys-179 and Cys-214 is shown in white. The amino-terminal segment of residues 121–124 and the carboxy-terminal segment 220–231 are disordered and not displayed. (Reprinted, with permission, from Riek et al. 1996 [copyright Macmillan].)

GENETIC EVIDENCE LINKING THE PrP GENE WITH PRION DISEASE

Prions are transmitted from one species to another much less efficiently, if at all, than within the same species and only after prolonged incubation times. In the case of prion transmission from hamsters to mice, this so-called species barrier was overcome by introducing hamster *Prnp* transgenes into recipient wild-type mice (Scott et al. 1989; Prusiner et al. 1990). Importantly, the properties of the prions produced in these transgenic mice corresponded to the prion species used for inoculation (Prusiner et al. 1990); that is, infection with hamster prions led to production of hamster prions, but infection with mouse prions gave rise to mouse prions. Within the framework of the protein-only hypothesis, this means that hamster PrP^{C}, but not murine PrP^{C} (which differs from the former by 10 amino acids), is a suitable substrate for conversion to hamster PrP^{Sc} by hamster prions and vice versa.

Most, if not all, familial forms of human spongiform encephalopathies are linked to one of a number of mutations in the PrP gene (Hsiao et al. 1990); for review, see (Baker and Ridley 1992; Goldfarb et al. 1994). Prusiner (1989, 1991) proposed that the mutations lead to spontaneous conversion of PrP^{C} into PrP^{Sc} with a frequency sufficient to allow expression of the disease within the lifetime of the individual. Sporadic CJD could be attributed to rare instances of spontaneous conversion of PrP^{C} into PrP^{Sc} or rare somatic mutations in the *Prnp* gene. In both cases, the initial conversion is thought to be followed by autocatalytic propagation. Hsiao et al. (1990) showed that mice overexpressing a murine PrP transgene with a mutation corresponding to the human GSS mutation Pro-102→Leu spontaneously contract a lethal scrapie-like disease. The brains of these animals contain low levels of infectious prions that can be detected in indicator mice expressing the same mutant transgene, but at lower levels which do not lead to spontaneous disease (Hsiao et al. 1994).

RESISTANCE TO SCRAPIE OF MICE DEVOID OF PrP^{C}

The protein-only hypothesis predicts that mice devoid of PrP^{C} should be resistant to scrapie and fail to propagate the infectious agent. To generate mice devoid of PrP, we disrupted one *Prnp* allele of murine embryonic stem (ES) cells by homologous recombination with a recombinant DNA fragment in which two-thirds of the 254-codon open reading frame were replaced by extraneous DNA. The ES cells were introduced into blastocysts, from which chimeric mice were generated. Appropriate breeding gave rise to offspring homozygous for the disrupted *Prnp* gene ($Prnp^{0/0}$). PrP was undetectable in $Prnp^{0/0}$ brains and present at about half the normal level in the brains of heterozygous ($Prnp^{0/+}$) mice (Büeler et al. 1992). No abnormalities were noted in $Prnp^{0/0}$ mice at the macroscopic, microscopic, or behavioral levels (Büeler et al.

1992) other than the possibility of a disturbance of the circadian activity rhythm (Tobler et al. 1996). The suggestion that there may be a synaptic deficiency in *Prnp*$^{0/0}$ mice (Collinge et al. 1994; Whittington et al. 1995) has not been confirmed (Lledo et al. 1996). The claim that aged mice (with a mixed genetic background) develop ataxia and suffer a loss of Purkinje cells (Sakaguchi et al. 1996) as a consequence of PrP gene disruption is not consistent with previous investigations on independently generated *Prnp*$^{0/0}$ mouse lines (Büeler et al. 1992; Manson et al. 1994). Because the phenotype might be due to the removal of part of the large intron, or to undefined, mixed genetic background of the knockout mice (Gerlai 1996), it is necessary to show that complementation with a PrP transgene restores the normal phenotype.

When challenged with mouse prions, mice devoid of PrP were completely protected against scrapie disease (Fig. 5a). Prions were not propagated in brains of *Prnp*$^{0/0}$ mice at detectable levels, whereas in scrapie-inoculated *Prnp*$^{+/+}$ animals, infectious agent was absent up to 2 weeks post inoculation (p.i.) but was present at 8 weeks and increased to about 8.6 log LD_{50} units/ml by 20 weeks p.i. (Table 2) (Büeler et al. 1993; Sailer et al. 1994). Borderline infectivity in brains of some few of the inoculated knockout mice (Büeler et al. 1993; Sailer et al. 1994; Sakaguchi et al. 1995) is attributed to residual inoculum. As opposed to brain, spleen of *Prnp*$^{+/+}$ animals contained infectivity at the earliest time point tested, namely 2 days p.i., and increased thereafter to a level of about 7 log LD_{50} units/ml. In contrast, spleen of knockout animals showed only a low prion level at 4 days p.i., which thereafter became undetectable, suggesting that prions are initially transported from the intracerebral injection site to the spleen, where they are soon degraded. It had previously not been clear whether infectivity in spleen of wild-type animals, particularly at early times, was due to transport from the site of inoculation or whether it was synthesized in the spleen itself. The fact that in spleen of wild-type animals the prion titer is high at 2 weeks, when no infectivity can be detected in the brain, coupled with the fact that in knockout animals inoculum-derived infectivity has become undetectable by that time, strongly suggests that in wild-type animals prions are in fact synthesized in the spleen. It is, incidentally, quite puzzling that following intracerebral injection prion synthesis occurs so early in spleen and only after a long delay in brain.

Interestingly, even heterozygous *Prnp*$^{0/+}$ mice were partially protected, inasmuch as they showed prolonged incubation times of about 290 days as compared to about 180 days in the case of the wild-type controls. Moreover, the disease progressed much more slowly in *Prnp*$^{0/+}$ mice than in *Prnp*$^{+/+}$ mice, the interval between first symptoms and death being about 13 days in the case of *Prnp*$^{+/+}$ mice and 150 or more days in *Prnp*$^{0/+}$ mice (Fig. 6) (Büeler et al. 1994) These and other findings (see below; Prusiner et al. 1990) show

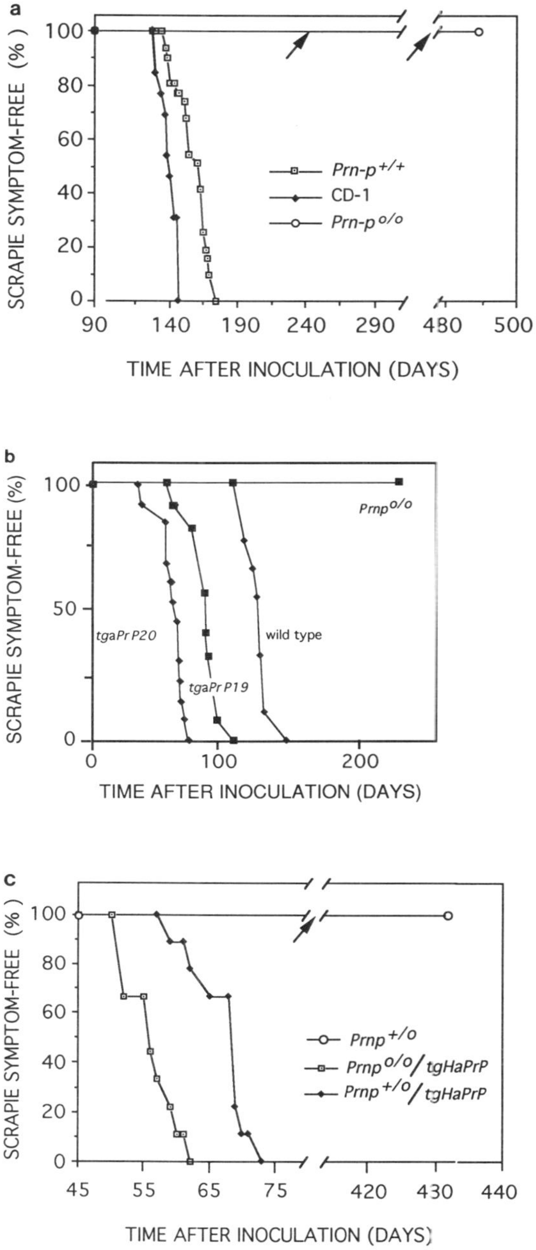

Figure 5. Scrapie resistance of mice with disrupted PrP genes. (*a*) *Prnp*$^{0/0}$ mice remain symptom-free after inoculation with mouse scrapie prions. *Prnp*$^{+/+}$ littermates or wild-type CD-1 mice show scrapie symptoms at the times indicated. (*Arrows*) Five mice were killed at various times; none had scrapie symptoms. (Modified from Büeler et al. 1993). (*b*) *Prnp*$^{0/0}$ mice were rendered transgenic for *Prnp* genes. *tga19*/+ mice had 3–4 times the normal PrP^C level; *tga20*/+ mice had 6–7 times the normal level. (Modified from Fischer et al. 1996.) (*c*) *Prnp*$^{0/0}$ and *Prnp*$^{0/+}$ mice with hamster PrP transgenes at different times after inoculation with hamster scrapie prions. Groups of 9–11 mice of each genotype were inoculated with the Sc237 isolate of hamster prions. (*Arrow*) One animal died spontaneously without scrapie symptoms and one was killed because of a tumor. (Modified, with permission, from Büeler et al. 1993 [copyright Cell Press].)

Table 2. Prion Titers in Brain and Spleen of $Prnp^{+/+}$ and $Prnp^{0/0}$ Mice

Time after inoculation	Log LD_{50} units/ml			
	brain		spleen	
	$Prnp^{+/+}$	$Prnp^{0/0}$	$Prnp^{+/+}$	$Prnp^{0/0}$
4 days	<1.5	2.0	5.7 ± 0.9	2.3
2 weeks	<1.5	<1.5	6.2 ± 0.8	<1.5
8 weeks	5.4	<1.5	6.9 ± 1.0	<1.5
12 weeks	6.8	<1.5	5.9 ± 0.6	<1.5
20 weeks	8.6	<1.5	6.9 ± 0.6	<1.5
23/25 weeks	8.1 ± 0.8	<1.5	n.d.	<1.5

Mice with the genotypes indicated were inoculated intracerebrally with mouse prions. Titers were determined by end-point titration on homogenates of pooled organs from 4 mice after heating for 20 min at 80°C. (n.d.) Not determined. Data from Büeler et al. (1993).

that susceptibility to scrapie is a function of PrP^C levels in the host. It is evident that mice can carry high levels of scrapie infectivity and PrP^{Sc} in their brains without showing clinical disease; the same might well be true for humans and other animals.

When a modified phenotype is observed following a targeted mutation or gene disruption, it is important to show that the original phenotype—in this case, susceptibility to scrapie—can be recovered by restoring wild-type function. We therefore introduced murine *Prnp* transgenes into $Prnp^{0/0}$ mice and obtained several lines with varying expression levels of PrP^C. As shown in Figure 5b, knockout mice expressing *Prnp* transgenes became susceptible to mouse prions; in fact, the higher the PrP^C content of the brain, the shorter the incubation times (Fischer et al. 1996). Even more interestingly, introduction of multiple hamster *Prnp* transgenes into $Prnp^{0/0}$ mice rendered them very susceptible to hamster-derived prions (56 days incubation time) (Fig. 5c), but much less so to mouse-derived prions (303 days incubation time) (Büeler et al. 1993), demonstrating the requirement for a homotypic relationship between incoming prion and resident PrP protein for optimal prion propagation and development of pathology, as foreshadowed by the results of Prusiner et al. (1990) described above.

MECHANISM OF PATHOGENESIS

The mechanism of pathogenesis, i.e., the events leading to vacuolization and neuronal death, are not yet well understood. Because neurons (and astrocytes) may be depleted of PrP^C, it has been speculated that this may be the cause of cell damage (Collinge et al. 1994). The fact that PrP knockout animals show no scrapie-like symptoms and appear quite healthy would argue against this hypothesis, unless one postulates that chronic deprivation of PrP allows the recruitment of compensatory mechanisms whereas acute depletion, as may occur in scrapie, does not. Alternatively, exposure to PrP^{Sc} may lead to toxic effects. Brandner et al. (1996) introduced PrP-overproducing neuroectodermal grafts into brains of knockout mice; contralateral inoculation with scrapie prions led to pronounced scrapie pathology in the graft but not in the surrounding tissue. Moreover, PrP^{Sc} was released by the infected graft, transported to distant sites, presumably by diffusion within the extracellular space (Jeffrey et al. 1994), and deposited in the form of granules without causing any apparent damage to surrounding cells. It would seem that damage is only caused to cells expressing PrP^C, perhaps because this leads to infection and intracellular processes, including accumulation of PrP^{Sc}. Interestingly, PrP-derived peptides cause toxic damage to PrP^C-expressing cortical cell cultures, but not to $PrP^{0/0}$ cultures (Brown et al. 1994, 1996).

REVERSE GENETICS OF THE PrP GENE

The demonstration that disruption of the PrP gene confers resistance to scrapie, and reintroduction of a PrP-encoding transgene restores susceptibility to the disease, opens up the possibility of practicing reverse genetics on PrP, that is, introducing deletions or mutations into the *Prnp* gene and determining the capacity of the modified gene to confer susceptibility to scrapie to a PrP knockout mouse.

As mentioned above, protease treatment of prion preparations cleaves off about 60 amino-terminal residues of PrP^{Sc} (Hope et al. 1988) but does not abrogate infectivity (McKinley et al. 1983). We introduced into PrP knockout mice transgenes encoding wild-type PrP or PrP lacking 16 or 49 amino-proximal amino acids which are protease-susceptible in PrP^{Sc}. Inoculation with prions led to fatal disease (Fig. 7), prion propagation, and accumulation of PrP^{Sc} in mice expressing both wild-type and truncated PrPs (Fischer et al. 1996). Within the framework of the protein-only hypothesis, this means that the amino-proximal segment of PrP^C, which contains 3.5 of its 5 octa repeats, is required neither for its susceptibility to conversion into the pathogenic, infectious form of PrP nor for the generation of PrP^{Sc}.

CONVERSION OF PrP^C TO PrP^{Sc}

Conversion of PrP^C to PrP^{Sc} in scrapie-infected cells is a late posttranslational process, occurring after PrP^C has reached its normal extracellular location (Borchelt et al. 1990; Caughey and Raymond 1991). Spontaneous conversion of PrP^C is obviously (and luckily) an extremely rare event. Why is this so, and how does scrapie infection promote conversion? The "refolding model" (Fig. 2a) proposes that conversion requires unfolding PrP^C to some extent and refolding it under the influence of a PrP^{Sc} molecule (Prusiner 1991), a process that would have to overcome a high activation energy barrier and might require a chaperone and an energy source. The "nucleation model" (Fig. 2b) proposes that PrP^C is in equilibrium with PrP^{Sc} (or a precursor thereof) and that PrP^{Sc} is only stabilized when it adds onto a crystal-like seed or aggregate of PrP^{Sc}. If formation of a stable aggregate requires a minimum of n PrP^{Sc} molecules, then the spontaneous formation of such aggregates would proceed at a rate proportional to the (n–1) power of the monomer concentration

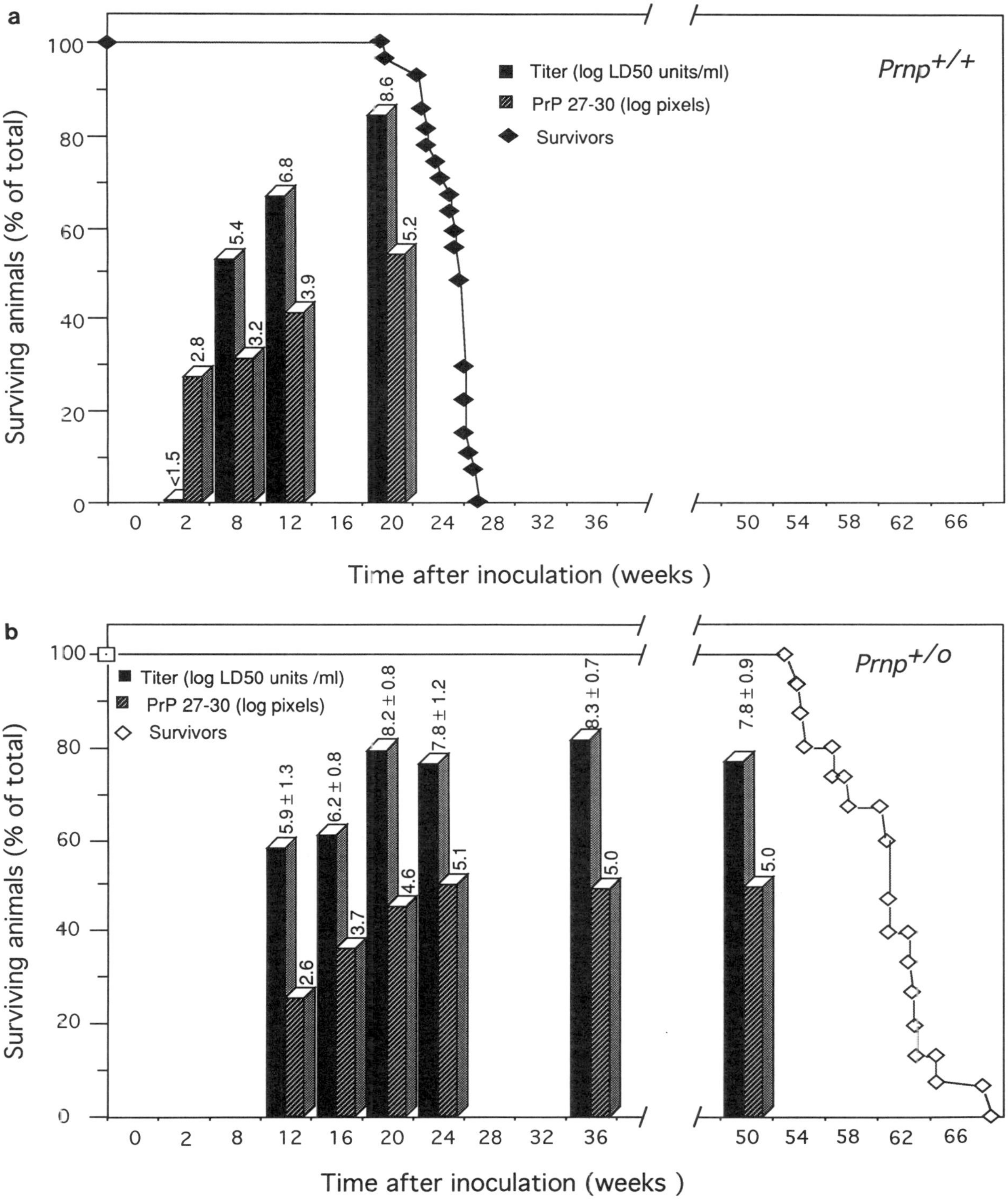

Figure 6. Survival, prion titers, and PrP^{Sc} in brains of (*a*) wild type and (*b*) $Prnp^{0/+}$ mice at various times after inoculation with mouse prions. (Reprinted, with permission, from Büeler et al. 1994.)

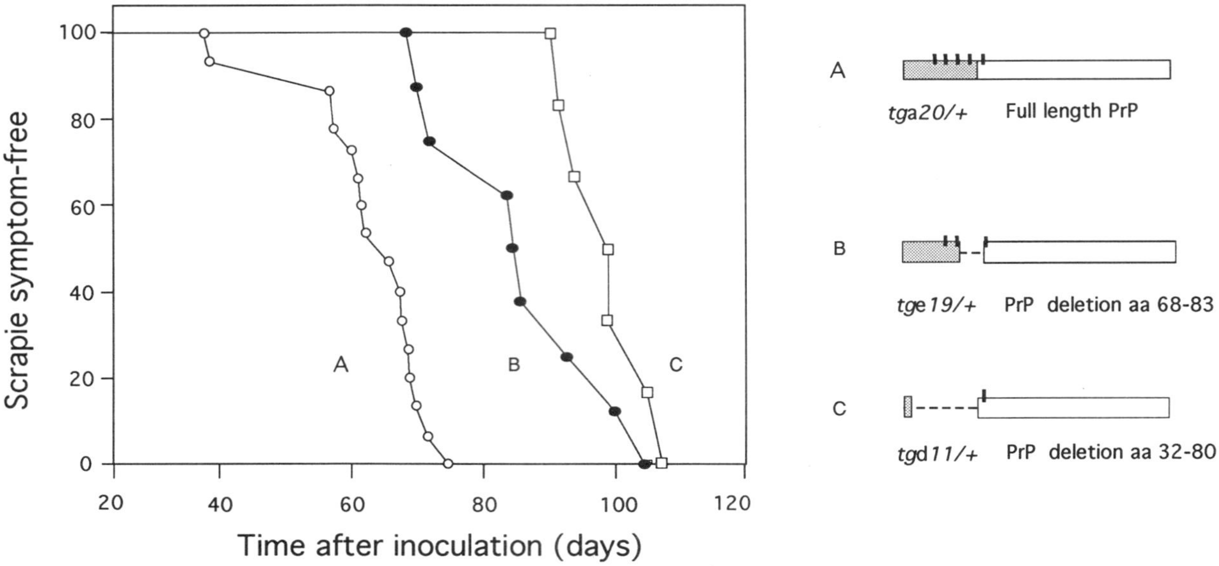

Figure 7. Susceptibility to scrapie of *Prnp* knockout mice carrying *Prnp* transgenes with amino-proximal deletions. *Prnp* transgenes with the structures indicated in the right half of the panel were introduced into $Prnp^{0/0}$ mice. *tga20/+* (*A*, wild-type), *tge19/+* (*B*, a deletion removing 2 octa repeats), and *tgd11/+* (*C*, a deletion removing 3.5 octa repeats and additional amino-proximal sequences) expressed PrP at levels 6–7, 3–4, and 6 times, respectively, those of wild-type. Mice were inoculated intracerebrally with mouse prions. Data from Fischer et al. (1996).

(Hofrichter et al. 1974), which might explain why spontaneous disease is so rare. Once a seed is present, monomer addition can ensue at a rapid rate (Gajdusek 1988; Brown et al. 1991; Jarrett and Lansbury 1993). Trapping of PrP by an essentially irreversible aggregation reaction would drive the bulk conversion process. The proposed process is akin to the assembly of, for example, (protease-sensitive) flagellin to (protease-resistant) flagellar filaments (Aizawa et al. 1990). Interestingly, the same flagellin molecule can assemble into two types of flagella, depending on the provenance of the seed (Asakura et al. 1966), thereby providing an analogy for conformationally determined prion strain specificity (see below).

Whatever the nature of the conversion process, an important experimental advance (Kocisko et al. 1994) has been the demonstration that incubation of ^{35}S-labeled biosynthetic hamster PrP^C with about 50-fold excess of PrP^{Sc} from scrapie-infected hamster brain resulted in the conversion of some labeled protein into the partly proteinase-K-resistant state characteristic for hamster PrP^{Sc}. To achieve this conversion, ^{35}S-labeled PrP^C and PrP^{Sc} were partly denatured with 3 M guanidinium chloride prior to incubation in a lower, critical concentration of the denaturant. Because of the denaturation step, the experiment is compatible with both the "refolding" and the "nucleation" models. The large amount of infectious agent associated with the PrP^{Sc} added, the modest extent of conversion, and the imprecision of the infectivity assay have so far precluded attempts to search for an increase in infectivity. The specificity of the reaction was documented by showing that murine PrP^C was converted by murine PrP^{Sc} but not by hamster PrP^{Sc}, as would be expected from the species barrier for in vivo transmission from hamster to mouse; however, in the converse reaction, conversion was observed, perhaps reflecting the less stringent barrier from mouse to hamster (Kocisco et al. 1995).

PRION STRAINS

Dickinson and his colleagues (Dickinson and Meikle 1969; Bruce et al. 1992) showed that many distinct strains of scrapie prions can be derived from sheep isolates. These strains differ by their incubation times in various inbred mouse lines and by the lesion patterns they occasion in the affected brains. Interestingly, different strains can be propagated in one inbred mouse strain (homozygous with regard to its PrP gene) (Bruce et al. 1992). Within the framework of the protein-only hypothesis, this is at first blush puzzling, because it means that one and the same polypeptide chain is able to mediate different strain phenotypes. At least two explanations can be considered in this connection. The *conformational hypothesis* postulates that each strain is associated with a different conformation of PrP^{Sc} (or PrP*) and that each of these can convert the PrP^C of its host into a likeness of itself. Bessen et al. (1995) took advantage of the finding that two hamster-adapted scrapie strains, HY and DY, give rise to PrP^{Sc} molecules that are cleaved to products of different length by proteinase K (Bessen and Marsh 1992). In the in vitro system described above, ^{35}S-labeled hamster PrP^C incubated with DY PrP^{Sc} gave a radioactive proteolytic product shorter by about 1 kD than that obtained after incubation with HY PrP^{Sc}, the same difference exhibited by the protease-resistant moieties of natural PrP^{Sc} molecules of the two strains. These remarkable results, if extended to show that conversion also results in generation of infectivity, would definitively confirm the protein-only model, allow structural characterization of the prion, and solve the strain problem.

The *targeting hypothesis* (Hecker et al. 1992; Weissmann et al. 1993; K.H. Meyer, pers. comm.) proposes that PrP^{Sc} carries a modification, for example, carbohydrate residues, which varies from strain to strain and which targets it to a particular subset of cells. These cells would impart the same modification to the newly formed PrP^{Sc} molecules. Different strains would thus be targeted to different subsets of cells and retain their specific modification. This hypothesis is supported by the observation that different hamster prion strains (Hecker et al. 1992) or mouse prion strains (Manson et al. 1992) give rise to different patterns of PrP^{Sc} deposition in the brain.

IMPLICATIONS AND OUTLOOK

Although each individual piece of evidence described above could be explained in several ways, the conjunction of data strongly supports the proposal that the prion is composed partly or entirely of a PrP-derived molecule (PrP* or PrP^{Sc}) and that protein-encoding nucleic acid is not an essential component. Probably the closest one could come to irrefutable proof for the protein-only hypothesis would be the demonstration that biosynthetic, pure PrP^{C} can be converted not only into a protease-resistant form, but to infectious scrapie agent under defined conditions in vitro.

Because mice with disrupted *Prnp* genes are viable and resistant to prion disease, it should also be possible to breed sheep or cattle that are resistant to this disease; knockout methodology is in principle available for sheep (Campbell et al. 1996) but not yet for cattle. Although it is hardly practical to consider complete replacement of conventional herds by PrP knockout counterparts, herds of BSE-resistant cattle would be useful as a source for products required for pharmaceutical purposes. Moreover, the fact that $Prnp^{0/+}$ heterozygous mice show prolonged scrapie incubation times argues that an as-yet-conjectural drug leading to moderate reduction of PrP^{C} synthesis or one retarding the conversion of PrP^{C} to PrP^{Sc} (Demaimay et al. 1994) might substantially mitigate disease progression in incipient cases of human spongiform encephalopathies.

Finally, one may raise the question whether prion-like agents cause other diseases or appear in nonvertebrate organisms. Although several human diseases accompanied by amyloid formation are known, none of them has been reproducibly transmitted. Interestingly, two yeast phenotypes are ascribed to "heritable protein conversion," namely, the [URE3] and the [psi+] systems (Chernoff et al. 1995; Masison and Wickner 1995), opening new perspectives for the elucidation of this phenomenon.

SUMMARY

The prion, the transmissible agent that causes spongiform encephalopathies such as scrapie, BSE, and CJD, is believed to be devoid of nucleic acid and identical with PrP^{Sc}, a modified form of the normal host protein PrP^{C} that is encoded by the single-copy gene *Prnp*. The protein-only hypothesis proposes that PrP^{Sc}, when introduced into a normal host, causes the conversion of PrP^{C} into PrP^{Sc}; it therefore predicts that an animal devoid of PrP^{C} should be resistant to prion diseases. We generated homozygous $Prnp^{0/0}$ ("PrP knockout") mice and showed that, after inoculation with prions, they remained free of scrapie for at least 2 years, whereas wild-type controls all died within 6 months. There was no propagation of prions in the $Prnp^{0/0}$ animals. Surprisingly, heterozygous $Prnp^{0/+}$ mice, which express PrP^{C} at about half the normal level, also showed enhanced resistance to scrapie disease despite high levels of infectious agent and PrP^{Sc} in the brain early on. After introduction of murine PrP transgenes, $Prnp^{0/0}$ mice became highly susceptible to mouse but not to hamster prions, and the insertion of Syrian hamster PrP transgenes rendered them susceptible to hamster and, to a much lesser extent, to mouse prions. These complementation experiments paved the way for the application of reverse genetics. We have prepared animals transgenic for genes encoding PrP with amino-terminal deletions of various lengths and have found that PrP lacking 49 amino-proximal amino acids, which comprise four of the five octa repeats of PrP, is still biologically active.

ACKNOWLEDGMENTS

This study was supported by the Erziehungsdirektion of the Kanton of Zürich; by grants from the Schweizerischer Nationalfonds to A.A. and C.W., from the European Union to A.A., from the Human Frontier Science Program to C.W.; and by a postdoctoral fellowship of the Ernst Hadorn Foundation to S.B.

REFERENCES

Aizawa, S.-I., F. Vonderviszt, R. Ishima, and K. Akasaka 1990. Termini of Salmonella flagellin are disordered and become organized upon polymerization into flagellar filament. *J. Mol. Biol.* **211:** 673.

Alper, T., W.A. Cramp, D.A. Haig, and M.C. Clarke. 1967. Does the agent of scrapie replicate without nucleic acid? *Nature* **214:** 764.

Asakura, S., G. Eguchi, and T. Iino. 1966. *Salmonella* flagella: In vitro reconstruction and over-all shapes of flagellar filaments. *J. Mol. Biol.* **16:** 302.

Baker, H.F. and R.M. Ridley. 1992. The genetics and transmissibility of human spongiform encephalopathy. *Neurodegeneration* **1:** 3.

Basler, K., B. Oesch, M. Scott, D. Westaway, M. Wälchli, D.F. Groth, M.P. McKinley, S.B. Prusiner, and C. Weissmann. 1986. Scrapie and cellular PrP isoforms are encoded by the same chromosomal gene. *Cell* **46:** 417.

Bendheim, P.E., H.R. Brown, R.D. Rudelli, L.J. Scala, N.L. Goller, G.Y. Wen, R.J. Kascsak, N.R. Cashman, and D.C. Bolton. 1992. Nearly ubiquitous tissue distribution of the scrapie agent precursor protein. *Neurology* **42:** 149.

Bessen, R.A. and R.F. Marsh. 1992. Biochemical and physical properties of the prion protein from two strains of the transmissible mink encephalopathy agent. *J. Virol.* **66:** 2096.

Bessen, R.A., D.A. Kocisko, G.J. Raymond, S. Nandan, P.T. Lansbury, and B. Caughey. 1995. Non-genetic propagation of strain-specific properties of scrapie prion protein. *Nature* **375:** 698.

Bolton, D.C., R.D. Rudelli, J.R. Currie, and P.E. Bendheim. 1991. Copurification of Sp33-37 and scrapie agent from hamster brain prior to detectable histopathology and clinical disease. *J. Gen. Virol.* **72:** 2905.

Borchelt, D.R., A. Taraboulos, and S.B. Prusiner. 1992. Evidence for synthesis of scrapie prion proteins in the endocytic pathway. *J. Biol. Chem.* **267:** 16188.

Borchelt, D.R., M. Scott, A. Taraboulos, N. Stahl, and S.B. Prusiner. 1990. Scrapie and cellular prion proteins differ in their kinetics of synthesis and topology in cultured cells. *J. Cell Biol.* **110:** 743.

Brandner, S., S. Isenmann, A. Raeber, M. Fischer, A. Sailer, Y. Kobayashi, S. Marino, C. Weissmann, and A. Aguzzi. 1996. Normal host prion protein necessary for scrapie-induced neurotoxicity. *Nature* **379:** 339.

Brown, D.R., J. Herms, and H.A. Kretzschmar. 1994. Mouse cortical cells lacking cellular PrP survive in culture with a neurotoxic PrP fragment. *NeuroReport* **5:** 2057.

Brown, D.R., B. Schmidt, and H.A. Kretzschmar. 1996. Role of microglia and host prion protein in neurotoxicity of a prion protein fragment. *Nature* **380:** 345.

Brown, P., L.G. Goldfarb, and D.C. Gajdusek. 1991. The new biology of spongiform encephalopathy: Infectious amyloidoses with a genetic twist. *Lancet* **337:** 1019.

Bruce, M.E., H. Fraser, P.A. McBride, J.R. Scott, and A.G. Dickinson. 1992. The basis of strain variation in scrapie. In *Prion diseases of humans and animals* (ed. S.B. Prusiner et al.), p. 487. Ellis Horwood, New York.

Büeler, H., A. Aguzzi, A. Sailer, R.A. Greiner, P. Autenried, M. Aguet, and C. Weissmann. 1993. Mice devoid of PrP are resistant to scrapie. *Cell* **73:** 1339.

Büeler, H., M. Fischer, Y. Lang, H. Bluethmann, H.P. Lipp, S.J. DeArmond, S.B. Prusiner, M. Aguet, and C. Weissmann. 1992. Normal development and behaviour of mice lacking the neuronal cell-surface PrP protein. *Nature* **356:** 577.

Büeler, H., A. Raeber, A. Sailer, M. Fischer, A. Aguzzi, and C. Weissmann. 1994. High prion and PrPSc levels but delayed onset of disease in scrapie-inoculated mice heterozygous for a disrupted PrP gene. *Mol. Med.* **1:** 19.

Campbell, K.H., J. McWhir, W.A. Ritchie, and I. Wilmut. 1996. Sheep cloned by nuclear transfer from a cultured cell line. *Nature* **380:** 64.

Caughey, B. and G.J. Raymond. 1991. The scrapie-associated form of PrP is made from a cell surface precursor that is both protease-sensitive and phospholipase-sensitive. *J. Biol. Chem.* **266:** 18217.

Caughey, B., G.J. Raymond, D. Ernst, and R.E. Race. 1991a. N-terminal truncation of the scrapie-associated form of PrP by lysosomal protease(s): Implications regarding the site of conversion of PrP to the protease-resistant state. *J. Virol.* **65:** 6597.

Caughey, B.W., A. Dong, K.S. Bhat, D. Ernst, S.F. Hayes, and W.S. Caughey. 1991b. Secondary structure analysis of the scrapie-associated protein PrP 27-30 in water by infrared spectroscopy. *Biochemistry* **30:** 7672.

Chernoff, Y.O., S.L. Lindquist, B. Ono, S.G. Inge-Vechtomov, and S.W. Liebman. 1995. Role of the chaperone protein Hsp104 in propagation of the yeast prion-like factor [psi+]. *Science* **268:** 880.

Chesebro, B., R. Race, K. Wehrly, J. Nishio, M. Bloom, D. Lechner, S. Bergstrom, K. Robbins, L. Mayer, J.M. Keith, C. Garon, and A. Haase. 1985. Identification of scrapie prion protein-specific messenger RNA in scrapie-infected and uninfected brain. *Nature* **315:** 331.

Cohen, F.E., K.M. Pan, Z. Huang, M. Baldwin, R.J. Fletterick, and S.B. Prusiner. 1994. Structural clues to prion replication (see comments). *Science* **264:** 530.

Collinge, J., M.A. Whittington, K.C.L. Sidle, C.J. Smith, M.S. Palmer, A.R. Clarke, and J.G.R. Jefferys. 1994. Prion protein is necessary for normal synaptic function. *Nature* **370:** 295.

Demaimay, R., K. Adjou, C. Lasmezas, F. Lazarini, K. Cherifi, M. Seman, J.P. Deslys, and D. Dormont. 1994. Pharmacological studies of a new derivative of amphotericin B, MS-8209, in mouse and hamster scrapie. *J. Gen. Virol.* **75:** 2499.

Dickinson, A.G. and V.M. Meikle. 1969. A comparison of some biological characteristics of the mouse-passaged scrapie agents, 22A and ME7. *Genet. Res.* **13:** 213.

Dickinson, A.G. and G.W. Outram. 1988. Genetic aspects of unconventional virus infections: the basis of the virino hypothesis. *Ciba Found. Symp.* **135:** 63.

Fischer, M., T. Rülicke, A. Raeber, A. Sailer, M. Moser, B. Oesch, S. Brandner, A. Aguzzi, and C. Weissmann. 1996. Prion protein (PrP) with amino-proximal deletions restoring susceptibility of PrP knockout mice to scrapie. *EMBO J.* **15:** 1255.

Gabizon, R., M.P. McKinley, D. Groth, and S.B. Prusiner. 1988. Immunoaffinity purification and neutralization of scrapie prion infectivity. *Proc. Natl. Acad. Sci.* **85:** 6617.

Gajdusek, D.C. 1988. Transmissible and non-transmissible amyloidoses: Autocatalytic post-translational conversion of host precursor proteins to β-pleated configurations. *J. Neuroimmunology* **20:** 95.

Gerlai, R. 1996. Gene-targeting studies of mammalian behaviour: Is it the mutation or the background genotype? *Trends Neurosci.* **19:** 177.

Goldfarb, L.G., P. Brown, L. Cervenakova, and D.C. Gajdusek. 1994. Genetic analysis of Creutzfeldt-Jakob disease and related disorders. *Philos. Trans. R. Soc. Lond. B Biol. Sci.* **343:** 379.

Griffith, J.S. 1967. Self-replication and scrapie. *Nature* **215:** 1043.

Hecker, R., A. Taraboulos, M. Scott, K.M. Pan, S.L. Yang, M. Torchia, K. Jendroska, S.J. DeArmond, and S.B. Prusiner. 1992. Replication of distinct scrapie prion isolates is region specific in brains of transgenic mice and hamsters. *Genes Dev.* **6:** 1213.

Hofrichter, J., P.D. Ross, and W.A. Eaton. 1974. Kinetics and mechanism of deoxyhemoglobin S gelation: A new approach to understanding sickle cell disease. *Proc. Natl. Acad. Sci.* **71:** 4864.

Hope, J., G. Multhaup, L.J. Reekie, R.H. Kimberlin, and K. Beyreuther. 1988. Molecular pathology of scrapie-associated fibril protein (PrP) in mouse brain affected by the ME7 strain of scrapie. *Eur. J. Biochem.* **172:** 271.

Hope, J., L.J. Morton, C.F. Farquhar, G. Multhaup, K. Beyreuther, and R.H. Kimberlin. 1986. The major polypeptide of scrapie-associated fibrils (SAF) has the same size, charge distribution and N-terminal protein sequence as predicted for the normal brain protein (PrP). *EMBO J.* **5:** 2591.

Hsiao, K.K., M. Scott, D. Foster, D.F. Groth, S.J. DeArmond, and S.B. Prusiner. 1990. Spontaneous neurodegeneration in transgenic mice with mutant prion protein. *Science* **250:** 1587.

Hsiao, K.K., D. Groth, M. Scott, S.L. Yang, H. Serban, D. Rapp, D. Foster, M. Torchia, S.J. Dearmond, and S.B. Prusiner. 1994. Serial transmission in rodents of neurodegeneration from transgenic mice expressing mutant prion protein. *Proc. Natl. Acad. Sci.* **91:** 9126.

Jarrett, J.T. and P.J. Lansbury. 1993. Seeding "one-dimensional crystallization" of amyloid: A pathogenic mechanism in Alzheimer's disease and scrapie? *Cell* **73:** 1055.

Jeffrey, M., C.M. Goodsir, M.E. Bruce, P.A. McBride, N. Fowler, and J.R. Scott. 1994. Murine scrapie-infected neurons in vivo release excess prion protein into the extracellular space. *Neurosci. Lett.* **174:** 39.

Kellings, K., N. Meyer, C. Mirenda, S.B. Prusiner, and D. Riesner. 1992. Further analysis of nucleic acids in purified scrapie prion preparations by improved return refocusing gel electrophoresis. *J. Gen. Virol.* **73:** 1025.

———. 1993. Analysis of nucleic acids in purified scrapie prion preparations. *Arch. Virol.* (suppl.) **7:** 215.

Kocisco, D.A., S.A. Priola, G.J. Raymond, B. Chesebro, P.T. Lansbury, Jr., and B. Caughey. 1995. Species specificity in the cell-free conversion of prion protein to protease-resistant forms: A model for the scrapie species barrier. *Proc. Natl. Acad. Sci.* **92:** 3923.

Kocisko, D.A., J.H. Come, S.A. Priola, B. Chesebro, G.J. Raymond, P.T. Lansbury, and B. Caughey. 1994. Cell-free formation of protease-resistant prion protein. *Nature* **370:** 471.

Lledo, P.-M., P. Tremblay, S.J. DeArmond, S.B. Prusiner, and R.A. Nicoll. 1996. Mice deficient for prion protein exhibit normal neuronal excitability and synaptic transmission in the hippocampus. *Proc. Natl. Acad. Sci.* **93:** 2403.

Manson, J., P. McBride, and J. Hope. 1992. Expression of the PrP gene in the brain of sinc congenic mice and its relationship to the development of scrapie. *Neurodegeneration* **1:** 45.

Manson, J.C., A.R. Clarke, M.L. Hooper, L. Aitchison, I. McConnell, and J. Hope. 1994. 129/Ola mice carrying a null mutation in PrP that abolishes mRNA production are developmentally normal. *Mol. Neurobiol* **8:** 121.

Masison, D.C. and R.B. Wickner. 1995. Prion-inducing domain of yeast Ure2p and protease resistance of Ure2p in prion-containing cells. *Science* **270:** 93.

McKinley, M.P., D.C. Bolton, and S.B. Prusiner. 1983. A protease-resistant protein is a structural component of the scrapie prion. *Cell* **35:** 57.

McKinley, M.P., R.K. Meyer, L. Kenaga, F. Rahbar, R. Cotter, A. Serban, and S.B. Prusiner. 1991. Scrapie prion rod formation in vitro requires both detergent extraction and limited proteolysis. *J. Virol.* **65:** 1340.

Oesch, B., D. Westaway, M. Wälchli, M.P. McKinley, S.B. Kent, R. Aebersold, R.A. Barry, P. Tempst, D.B. Teplow, L.E. Hood, S.B. Prusiner, and C. Weissmann. 1985. A cellular gene encodes scrapie PrP 27-30 protein. *Cell* **40:** 735.

Pan, K.M., M. Baldwin, J. Nguyen, M. Gasset, A. Serban, D. Groth, I. Mehlhorn, Z. Huang, R.J. Fletterick, F.E. Cohen, and S.B. Prusiner. 1993. Conversion of alpha-helices into beta-sheets features in the formation of the scrapie prion proteins. *Proc. Natl. Acad. Sci.* **90:** 10962.

Prusiner, S.B. 1982. Novel proteinaceous infectious particles cause scrapie. *Science* **216:** 136.

———. 1989. Scrapie prions. *Annu. Rev. Microbiol.* **43:** 345.

———. 1991. Molecular biology of prion diseases. *Science* **252:** 1515.

———. 1993. Transgenetic investigations of prion diseases of humans and animals. *Philos. Trans. R. Soc. Lond. B Biol.* **339:** 239.

Prusiner, S.B., D.C. Bolton, D.F. Groth, K.A. Bowman, S.P. Cochran, and M.P. McKinley. 1982. Further purification and characterization of scrapie prions. *Biochemistry* **21:** 6942.

Prusiner, S.B., M. Scott, D. Foster, K.M. Pan, D. Groth, C. Mirenda, M. Torchia, S.L. Yang, D. Serban, G.A. Carlson, P.C. Hoppe, D. Westaway, and S.J. DeArmond. 1990. Transgenetic studies implicate interactions between homologous PrP isoforms in scrapie prion replication. *Cell* **63:** 673.

Riek, R., S. Hornemann, G. Wider, M. Billeter, R. Glockshuber, and K. Wüthrich. 1996. NMR structure of the mouse prion protein domain PrP(121-231). *Nature* **382:** 180.

Sailer, A., H. Büeler, M. Fischer, A. Aguzzi, and C. Weissmann. 1994. No propagation of prions in mice devoid of PrP. *Cell* **77:** 967.

Sakaguchi, S., S. Katamine, N. Nishida, R. Moriuchi, K. Shigematsu, T. Sugimoto, A. Nakatani, Y. Kataoka, T. Houtani, S. Shirabe, H. Okada, S. Hasegawa, T. Miyamoto, and T. Noda. 1996. Loss of cerebellar Purkinje cells in aged mice homozygous for a disrupted PrP gene. *Nature* **380:** 528.

Sakaguchi, S., S. Katamine, K. Shigematsu, A. Nakatani, R. Moriuchi, N. Nishida, K. Kurokawa, R. Nakaoke, H. Sato, K. Hishage, J. Kuno, T. Noda, and T. Miyamoto. 1995. Accumulation of proteinase K-resistant prion protein (PrP) is restricted by the expression level of normal PrP in mice inoculated with a mouse-adapted strain of the Creutzfeldt-Jakob disease agent. *J. Virol.* **69:** 7586.

Scott, M., D. Foster, C. Mirenda, D. Serban, F. Coufal, M. Wälchli, M. Torchia, D. Groth, G. Carlson, S.J. DeArmond, D. Westaway, and S.B. Prusiner. 1989. Transgenic mice expressing hamster prion protein produce species-specific scrapie infectivity and amyloid plaques. *Cell* **59:** 847.

Shyng, S.L., M.T. Huber, and D.A. Harris. 1993. A prion protein cycles between the cell surface and an endocytic compartment in cultured neuroblastoma cells. *J. Biol. Chem.* **268:** 15922.

Stahl, N., D.R. Borchelt, K. Hsiao, and S.B. Prusiner. 1987. Scrapie prion protein contains a phosphatidylinositol glycolipid. *Cell* **51:** 229.

Stahl, N., M.A. Baldwin, R. Hecker, K.M. Pan, A.L. Burlingame, and S. Prusiner. 1992. Glycosylinositol phospholipid anchors of the scrapie and cellular prion proteins contain sialic acid. *Biochemistry* **31:** 5043.

Stahl, N., M.A. Baldwin, D.B. Teplow, L. Hood, B.W. Gibson, A.L. Burlingame, and S.B. Prusiner. 1993. Structural studies of the scrapie prion protein using mass spectrometry and amino acid sequencing. *Biochemistry* **32:** 1991.

Tobler, I., S.E. Gaus, T. Deboer, P. Achermann, M. Fischer, T. Rulicke, M. Moser, B. Oesch, P.A. McBride, and J.C. Manson. 1996. Altered circadian activity rhythms and sleep in mice devoid of prion protein. *Nature* **380:** 639.

Weissmann, C. 1991. Spongiform encephalopathies. The prion's progress (news). *Nature* **349:** 569.

Weissmann, C., H. Büeler, M. Fischer, and M. Aguet. 1993. Role of the PrP gene in transmissible spongiform encephalopathies. *Intervirology* **35:** 164.

Whittington, M.A., K.C. Sidle, I. Gowland, J. Meads, A.F. Hill, M.S. Palmer, J.G. Jefferys, and J. Collinge. 1995. Rescue of neurophysiological phenotype seen in PrP null mice by transgene encoding human prion protein. *Nat. Genet.* **9:** 197.

Wilesmith, J.W., J.B. Ryan, W.D. Hueston, and L.J. Hoinville. 1992. Bovine spongiform encephalopathy: Epidemiological features 1985 to 1990. *Vet. Rec.* **130:** 90.

Will, R.G., J. W. Ironside, M. Zeidler, S.N. Cousens, K. Estibeiro, A. Alperovitch, S. Poser, M. Pocchiari, A. Hofman, and P.G. Smith. 1996. A new variant of Creutzfeld-Jakob disease in the UK. *Lancet* **347:** 921.

A New Variant of Creutzfeldt-Jakob Disease: Neuropathological and Clinical Features

J.W. Ironside, K. Sutherland, J.E. Bell, L. McCardle, C. Barrie, K. Estebeiro, M. Zeidler, and R.G. Will

CJD Surveillance Unit, Western General Hospital, Edinburgh, United Kingdom, EH4 2XU

Creutzfeldt-Jakob disease (CJD) is the commonest form of transmissible spongiform encephalopathy in man. Most cases are sporadic, but around 10–15% of CJD cases occur as familial disorders which are associated with pathogenic mutations or insertions in the prion protein gene (PRNP) on chromosome 20 (Prusiner 1993). CJD may also occur as an iatrogenic disorder, most cases of which have occurred in recipients of human cadaveric pituitary hormones (Brown et al. 1992). The PRNP contains a naturally polymorphic locus at codon 129 in Caucasians, where either methionine or valine may be encoded (Prusiner 1993). Homozygosity at this locus occurs in around 90% of both sporadic and iatrogenic cases of CJD, whereas only 49% of the normal Caucasian population are homozygous, indicating that homozygosity at codon 129 represents a risk factor for the development of this disease (Collinge et al. 1991; Palmer et al. 1991; Brown et al. 1992). Previous studies of CJD have not identified any other constant factors associated with an increased risk of developing this disease (Brown et al. 1987; Cousens et al. 1990).

Surveillance of CJD was reinstituted in the United Kingdom (UK) in 1990 to identify any changes in the nature and occurrence of this disease after the epidemic of bovine spongiform encephalopathy (BSE) in cattle, which was first identified pathologically in 1986 (Wells et al. 1987), although a novel spongiform encephalopathy had previously been reported in a captive nyala in the UK (Anon 1987). The population in the UK may have been exposed to the BSE agent through a number of potential routes, including occupational and dietary exposure. Studies on scrapie, the related spongiform encephalopathy in sheep, have indicated that there is no relationship between potential human exposure to the scrapie agent and the occurrence of CJD; CJD appears to occur at a similar incidence in countries where scrapie has never been detected or has been eradicated and in countries where the disorder is endemic in the sheep population (Brown et al. 1987). Surveillance of CJD in the UK has been carried out in previous decades; the results of these earlier studies provide important historical epidemiological and clinical data on CJD which antedate the discovery of BSE (Cousens et al. 1990). Parallel prospective studies on the incidence and clinicopathological features of CJD have been carried out in France, Italy, Germany, and the Netherlands (where BSE is either absent or present only at very low levels) between 1993 and 1995 with similar methodology to the UK study (Delasnerie-Laupretre et al. 1995).

The overall autopsy rate for suspected cases of CJD in the UK is greater than 70% (The National CJD Surveillance Unit 1995). The neuropathological material received for examination in the CJD Surveillance Unit laboratory includes brain biopsy specimens, fixed brains from autopsy cases, and paraffin-embedded tissue blocks and sections which are submitted with the collaboration of neuropathologists and general pathologists throughout the UK, without whom this study would not be possible.

Since 1995, we have identified 11 cases of CJD in the UK with clinical and neuropathological features that differ markedly from previous cases identified by the CJD Surveillance Unit (Will et al. 1996), from historical control material in UK, and from the comparable European studies. These cases appear to represent a new variant of CJD; a further case in France has recently been confirmed pathologically and reviewed in the CJD Surveillance Unit, Edinburgh (Chazot et al. 1996). Initial descriptive studies of the neuropathology of these 12 cases have now been supplemented by automated computerized morphometry (Sutherland et al. 1996), which confirms that the pathological changes in the brain are not only similar from case to case, but are also clearly distinguishable from other cases of sporadic CJD.

METHODS

Clinical features. Case ascertainment in the CJD surveillance project is largely by direct referral from physicians and pathologists throughout the UK; death certificates on which CJD is mentioned are also studied. Clinical details, including electroencephalogram (EEG) studies and neuroradiological investigations, are obtained on all referred cases and classified according to standardized criteria. Blood samples are obtained with informed consent for PRNP analysis by PCR techniques and direct sequencing, and detailed information on potential risk factors for CJD is obtained from patients' relatives by a standard questionnaire (The National CJD Surveillance Unit 1995).

Neuropathology. Since 1990, 207 cases of CJD have been examined neuropathologically in the CJD Surveillance Unit Laboratory. The Neuropathology Laboratory, University of Edinburgh at the Western General Hospital, has archival material from cases of CJD diagnosed before the outbreak of BSE. These have been used as control materials, along with additional historical control material from the earlier prospective CJD surveillance project in the UK during the period 1980–1984.

Six brain biopsy specimens and eleven brain autopsy specimens from the new variant CJD cases were examined in the CJD Surveillance Unit laboratory. In the autopsy cases, representative material was examined from the frontal, temporal, parietal, and occipital lobes; the hippocampus; basal ganglia; thalamus; hypothalamus; midbrain; pons; medulla; and optic nerve. Spinal cord tissue was available in four cases (some limited to the cervical cord). Biopsy specimens were fixed in 10% formalin for 24–48 hours. The autopsy tissues were fixed by immersion in 10% formalin for a minimum of 3 weeks and sampled for histology and immunocytochemistry. All tissue blocks were immersed in 96% formic acid for 1 hour before routine processing into paraffin wax. Serial sections were cut at 5 μm and stained by conventional histological techniques and immunocytochemistry for prion protein (PrP) using two monoclonal antibodies, KG9 and 3F4 (Goodbrand et al. 1995). Pretreatments for immunocytochemistry include hydrated autoclaving of sections at 121°C for 10 minutes, immersion in formic acid for 5 minutes followed by 4 mole/L guanidine thiocyanate for 2 hours (Goodbrand et al. 1995). Immunocytochemistry was also performed using a polyclonal antibody to glial fibrillary acidic protein (GFAP; Dako, UK). Further details of the immunocytochemical techniques are given in Table 1.

Image analysis. To assist in the investigation of the neuropathological features observed in cases of CJD, a dedicated, highly automated image analysis system has been developed at the CJD Surveillance Unit (Sutherland et al. 1996). This computer system is able to quantify objectively the pathological features of spongiform change, PrP deposition, and astrocytosis. The computing platform used is a UNIX-based Sun workstation that controls the modified Leitz microscope and the attached motorized slide scanning stage. To reduce any spurious lighting variations in the sampled images, a stablized tungsten light source has been used. The image analysis software which has been designed to recognize the fundamental features of CJD pathology makes use of a general purpose image processing function library provided by the Medical Research Council's Human Genetics Unit in Edinburgh.

When quantifying the pathology found in different brain areas, an interactive system of field placement is used to ensure that the anatomical areas analyzed from different tissue blocks are truly comparable. This is facilitated by showing the operator an image of the entire tissue section on the computer screen, which allows selection of precise anatomical landmarks for inclusion in the quantification process. To produce comparable results for the pathological features observed, a detailed sampling protocol for the brain has been established in previous work (Sutherland et al. 1996). For this study, analysis has been performed on tissue samples from the frontal, occipital, and temporal lobes and thalamus, basal ganglia, and cerebellum in 5 cases of the new variant of CJD.

The individual software modules incorporated in this system have been extensively validated prior to their use in the studies on the neuropathological phenotype in CJD (MacDonald et al. 1996). The recognition of spongiform change is based on tonal and morphological constraints encapsulated in the algorithm used to assess this feature. The computer system is able to produce either a count of the number of vacuoles or a value for the ratio of vacuolated tissue to the overall tissue area. In the quantification of prion protein deposits, the operator is required to set an image threshold to define the image intensity corresponding to immunopositivity within the image; the system is then able to produce a figure for the percentage tissue area occupied by this feature. For astrocytes, the computer produces a total count of the number of immunocytochemically defined cells observed in a predetermined unit of area.

RESULTS

The clinical features of these cases are summarized in Table 2. The most notable differences from typical cases of sporadic CJD in the period 1990–1994 in the surveillance study are a young age at clinical onset, a prolonged duration of illness, initial presenting features with prominent psychiatric symptoms and dysesthesia, and absence of typical EEG features of

Table 1. Details of Immunocytochemical Techniques

Antibody	Type	Source	Dilution	Incubation
PrP (KG9)	monoclonal	Dr. C. Birkett	1: 200	overnight
PrP (3F4)	monoclonal	Dr. R. Kascsak	1:1500	overnight
GFAP	polyclonal	Dako, UK	1:1500	30 min

Table 2. Summary of the Clinical Features in 12 Patients with the New Variant of CJD

Age at onset	Sex	Duration of illness (m)	Presenting symptom
16	F	24	dysesthesia
18	M	11	behavioral change
19	M	13	personality change
26	F	22.5	dysesthesia
26	M	23	dysesthesia
28	F	10	memory impairment
28	F	11	behavioral change
29	M	9	personality change
29	F	17	depression
29	M	7.5	foot pain
31	M	9.5	memory impairment
39	F	21	dysesthesia

sporadic CJD. These differences are summarized in Table 3. PRNP analysis showed no pathogenic mutations or insertions; all patients were homozygous for methionine at codon 129.

The 12 cases of CJD described above have neuropathological findings that clearly distinguish them from other cases examined in the CJD Surveillance Unit (Bell and Ironside 1993). One of the patients on whom a brain biopsy was performed is still alive (Will et al. 1996). In the 5 other patients on whom brain biopsy was performed, autopsy histology has been examined. All cases showed the typical neuropathological features of CJD—spongiform change, neuronal loss, and reactive astrocytosis (Budka et al. 1995). The most important distinguishing feature on routine microscopy was the presence of kuru-type PrP amyloid plaques surrounded by a corona or halo of spongiform change (Fig. 1). These plaques were distributed widely throughout the cerebral cortex, basal ganglia, and cerebellum (Fig. 2), but were most evident in the occipital lobe, particularly in the visual cortex. Spongiform change was most evident in the basal ganglia (Fig. 3); in typical cases of CJD it is most obvious in the cerebral cortex, although often in a variable distribution (Bell and Ironside 1993; Budka et al. 1995). Other neuropathological features characteristic of the new variant of CJD include marked thalamic gliosis (Fig. 4) and spongiform change in the cerebellar molecular layer.

Table 3. Comparison of Clinical Features of the New Variant of CJD with Cases of Sporadic CJD in the UK during 1990–1994

	New variant CJD	Typical sporadic CJD
Number of patients	12	186
Mean age at onset (y)	29.5	63.5
Mean duration of illness (m)	15	5
Sex ratio (M:F)	1:1	1: 1.7
Typical EEG changes (%)	0	65
Presentation with dementia (%)	0	86
MM at codon 129 in PRNP (%)	100	84

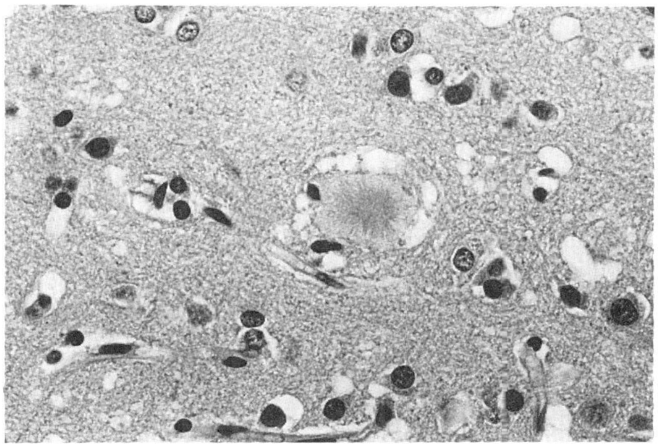

Figure 1. The cerebral cortex in a case of new variant CJD contains a large kuru-type amyloid plaque surrounded by a halo of spongiform change (*center*). Hematoxylin and eosin stain, 250x.

PrP immunocytochemistry in the new variant cases confirmed the presence of large kuru-type PrP plaques and also showed extensive deposition of PrP in all gray matter regions, particularly in the occipital cortex, basal ganglia, and cerebellum, where abundant PrP deposition occurred in the molecular layer (Fig. 5). In these regions, smaller plaque-like structures were clearly identifiable along with perivascular and pericellular PrP deposits. Occasional multifocal plaques were identified in the cerebellar molecular layer, and smaller plaques were present in the cerebellar white matter. The structure of the cerebellar PrP deposits differed substantially from those observed in the Gerstmann-Straussler-Scheinker syndrome (GSS) and in cases of iatrogenic CJD associated with growth hormone therapy (Bell and Ironside 1993; Billette de Villemeur et al. 1994; Budka et al. 1995).

Quantitative studies of PrP deposition confirmed these subjective impressions, and comparison with a

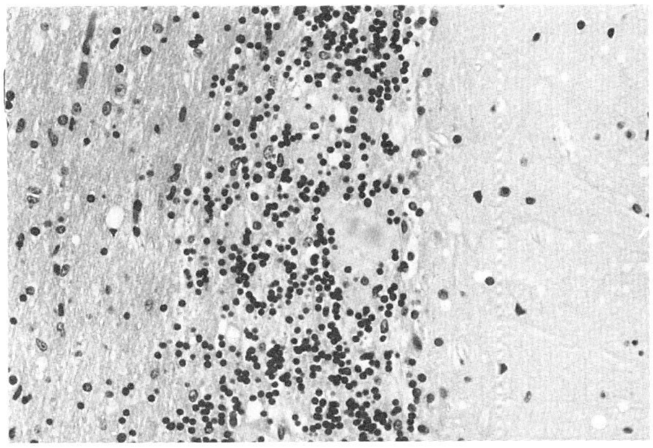

Figure 2. The cerebellar cortex in the same case as in Fig. 1 contains 2 kuru-type amyloid plaques in the granular layer (*center*). Spongiform change is present in the molecular layer (*right*). Hematoxylin and eosin stain, 120x.

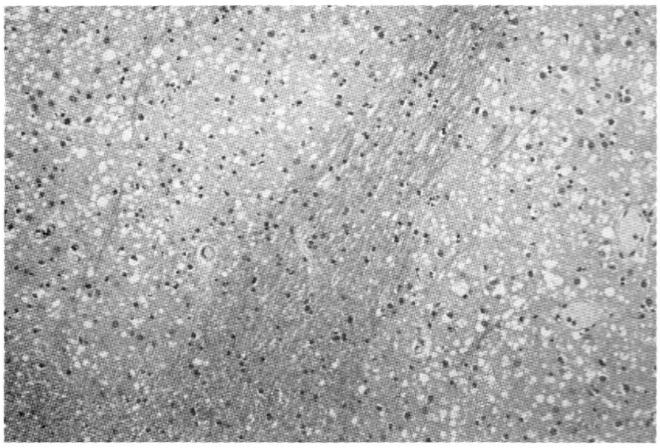

Figure 3. Spongiform change in the basal ganglia in new variant CJD is characterized by multiple small vacuoles within the gray matter. The white matter (*center*) is not involved. Hematoxylin and eosin stain, 90x.

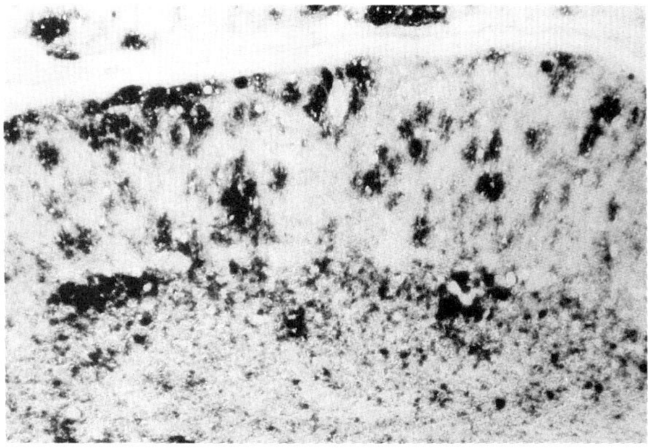

Figure 5. The cerebellum in new variant CJD after immunocytochemistry for PrP shows extensive PrP accumulation with numerous plaque-like structures and pericellular deposits, which are particularly evident in the molecular layer. KG9 monoclonal antibody, 90x.

series of cases of sporadic CJD in individuals of known PrP genotype at codon 129 (MacDonald et al. 1996) confirmed that the new variant has substantially larger areas of PrP deposition throughout the brain, particularly in the cerebellum and occipital lobe (Figs. 6,7). In addition, quantitative studies of astrocytosis using sections stained for GFAP showed extensive thalamic astrocytosis, with astrocytosis also marked in the basal ganglia (Fig. 8). Cerebral and cerebellar astrocytosis was less marked, in contrast to the overall pattern of PrP deposition. These changes were also distinguishable from patterns of astrocytosis observed in sporadic CJD in older individuals prior to 1995 in the UK (MacDonald et al. 1996).

DISCUSSION

The 12 cases included in this report exhibit clinical and pathological features markedly different from those encountered in typical cases of sporadic CJD in older individuals (Brown et al. 1987; Bell and Ironside 1993). The remarkably low age at onset, with a generally protracted and unusual clinical course including the absence of EEG changes typical of CJD, raises the possibility that these cases represent a new clinicopathological variant in the spectrum of human spongiform encephalopathies. This possibility is reinforced by the remarkably consistent neuropathological features, which appear never to have been identified previously in cases of CJD (Budka et al. 1995). Review of previously published reports on young patients with CJD worldwide has not revealed any descriptions of these unusual pathological features (Packer at al 1980; Monreal et al. 1981; Brown et al. 1985; Berman et al. 1988; Kulczycki et al. 1991). The previously described cases of CJD in young patients are usually isolated case reports, and in systematic surveys, the identification of CJD in patients aged less than 30 years old is extremely uncommon (Brown et al. 1987), making the diagnosis of these 12 cases over a period of around 1 year even more remarkable (Bateman et al. 1995; Britton et al. 1995; Chazot et al. 1996; Will et al. 1996).

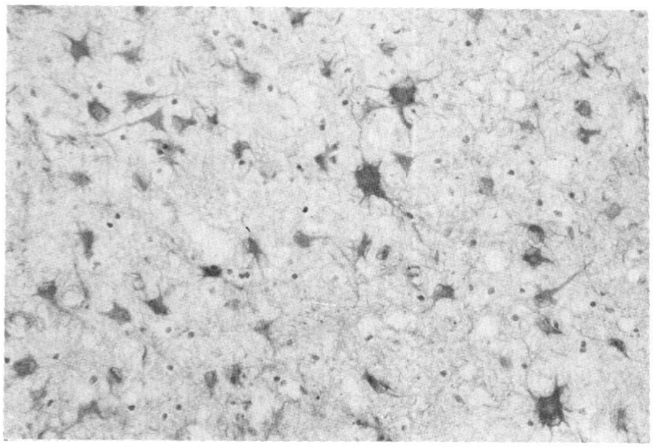

Figure 4. Astrocytic hypertrophy and hyperplasia are evident in the dorsomedial thalamic nucleus in a case of new variant CJD. Immunocytochemistry for GFAP, 200x.

Review of the earlier cases of CJD in the UK surveillance project, inspection of historical cases of CJD in the UK, review of the published literature (including a recent large series from the Corsellis Collection of brains in the Runwell Hospital, Essex [Bruton et al. 1995]), and identification of CJD patients under the age of 40 in the UK prior to 1990 and in France, Italy, Germany, and the Netherlands during 1993–1995 have not revealed any previous cases with a similar neuropathological phenotype.

No known genetic mutations have been identified in these cases. Direct sequencing of the PRNP gene has confirmed this finding, with all patients homozygous for methionine at codon 129. Amyloid plaques occur in around 10% of cases of sporadic CJD, but are usually confined to the cerebellum (Budka et al. 1995). In a previous study (de Silva et al. 1994), we investigated the relationship between PrP genotype and amyloid plaques in sporadic CJD in the UK, and found that

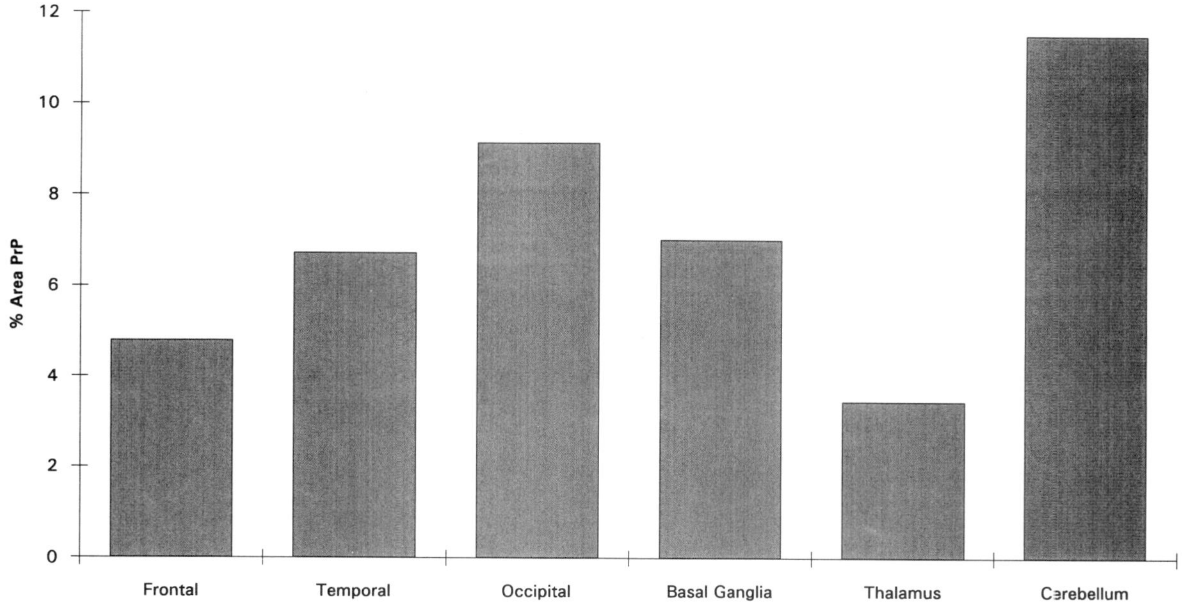

Figure 6. PrP deposition after immunocytochemistry in six brain areas in the new variant of CJD is measured as a percentage area of the total histological section. The findings confirm that PrP deposition is most marked in the cerebellum, followed by the occipital cortex.

most patients with PrP plaques prior to 1995 were either VV or MV at codon 129 in the PrP gene. The 12 cases under discussion are all MM at codon 129 and have widespread plaques throughout the brain.

The neuropathological features in this series of cases also differ from those in iatrogenic CJD, including cases associated with growth hormone therapy, where cerebellar pathology is most evident (Billette de Villemeur et al. 1994). The pathological features are also distinct from those of familial CJD and GSS,

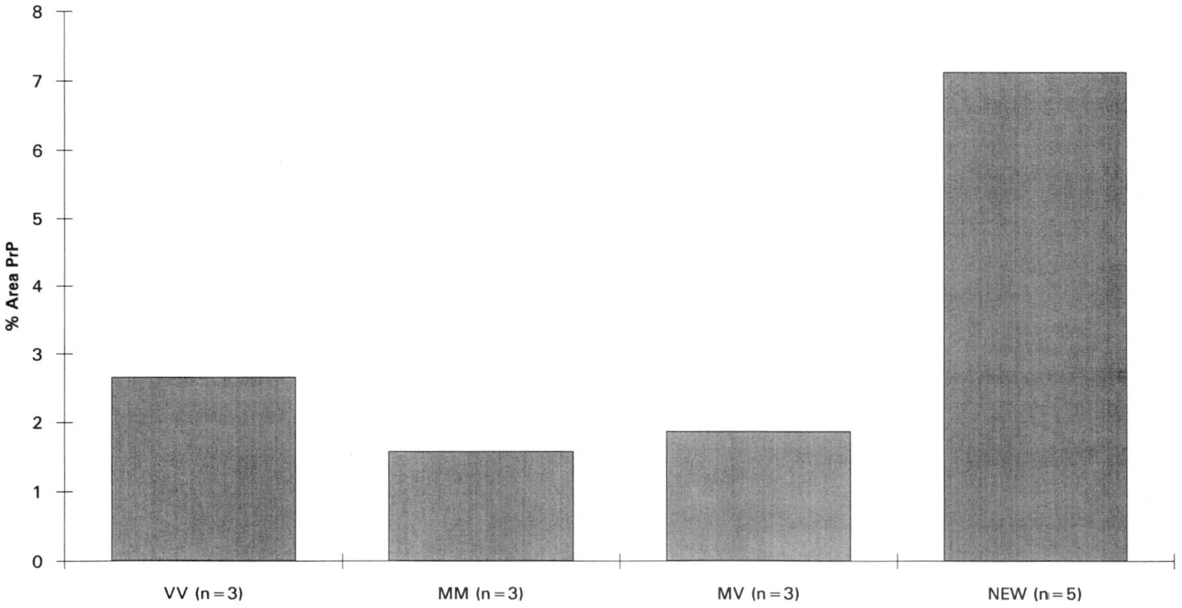

Figure 7. PrP staining in the new variant of CJD as a sum of the six brain areas in Fig. 5 is compared with a similar analysis in cases of sporadic CJD in older individuals of known PrP genotype at codon 129 (VV, MM, and MV). The level of PrP accumulation in the new variant cases is far greater than in any of the previous cases and, in particular, is approximately 4 times greater than the older MM patients identified prior to 1995.

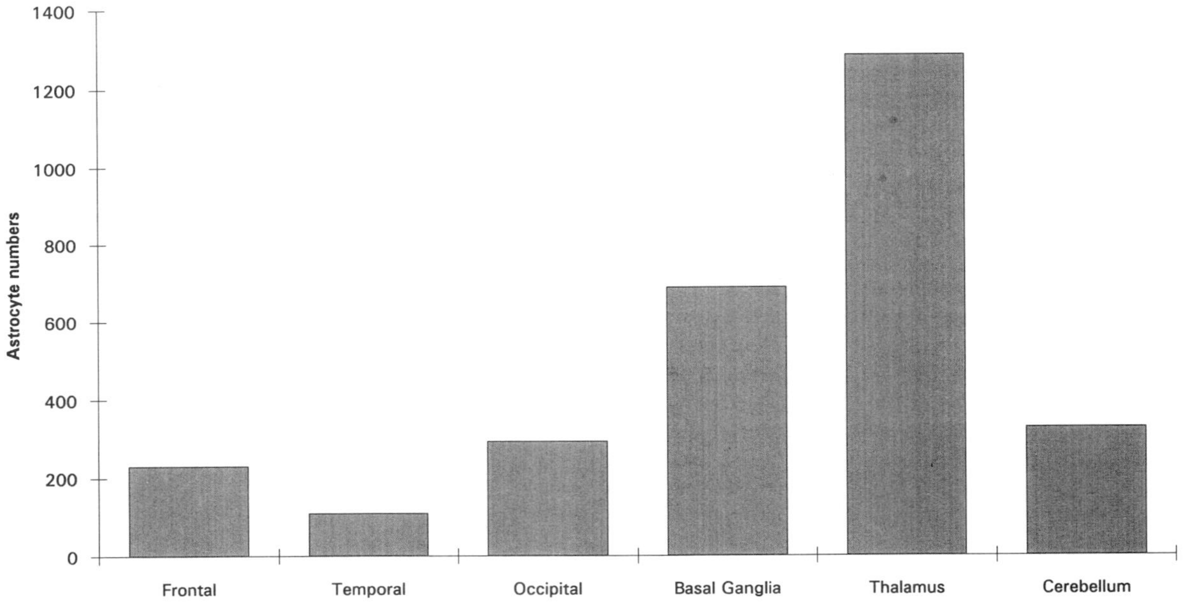

Figure 8. Astrocytosis in six brain areas has been quantified after immunocytochemistry for GFAP and expressed as numbers of astrocytes in a unit area. The findings confirm the presence of marked thalamic astrocytosis, with lesser degrees of astrocytosis present in the basal ganglia. The cerebral and cerebellar cortex, in contrast, show less astrocytosis, and in general, the level of astrocytosis appears inversely related to the level of PrP deposition in Fig. 6.

which are associated with characteristic PrP genetic mutations (Bell and Ironside 1993; Prusiner 1993; Budka et al. 1995). The thalamic gliosis in the new variant cases is reminiscent of that occurring in fatal familial insomnia, but the extensive PrP deposition and amyloid plaque formation in the new variant CJD cases are clearly distinct from the characteristic pathology in fatal familial insomnia (Medori et al. 1992).

The neuropathological features of the new variant CJD cases are similar to those described in kuru (Klatzo et al. 1959), although spongiform change and vacuolation around the amyloid plaques in kuru have not been described, and extensive studies of PrP immunocytochemistry have not yet been performed or published on kuru tissues. It will be important in the future to review the pathology of kuru material and to compare the findings with the new variant CJD cases, and to perform immunocytochemistry for PrP on any residual kuru tissues where possible.

Our earlier report on the first 10 patients with this new variant of CJD suggested that exposure to the BSE agent was the most plausible interpretation of this finding (Will et al. 1996). In the UK, exposure of the population to the BSE agent was likely to have been highest in the 1980s, particularly before the ban on the use of specified bovine offal in human foodstuffs. If this is the case, it is not certain why a previously unrecognized variant of CJD has been found only in persons under the age of 45 years; continued clinical and pathological surveillance will be required to identify any further cases occurring in older ages, especially in groups in which other causes of dementia are common.

The very recent identification in France, which has a low reported incidence of BSE, of a patient with this new variant of CJD has raised a question concerning the possible relationship of this disorder to BSE (Chazot et al. 1996). Although it is not known whether this patient could have been exposed to the BSE agent, a significant proportion of British foodstuffs are exported to France. The precise nature of the relationship of this new variant of CJD to BSE requires further clinical, pathological, and scientific investigations, with specific reference to transmission studies and strain typing in mice (Bruce et al. 1991). In a recent transmission study of BSE by intracerebral inoculation to three macaque monkeys, the neuropathological changes were found to closely resemble those in the new variant of CJD, with PrP plaques surrounded by spongiform change in the cerebral cortex (Lasmezas et al. 1996). Although this report does not provide proof of an association between BSE and the new variant of CJD, it reinforces both the hypothesis concerning such a link and the need for further investigative studies as indicated above. If a causal link with BSE is established, then the wide potential exposure of the UK and European population to the BSE agent and the long incubation period for this group of disorders suggest that further cases of this new variant of CJD are likely to be identified in a wider age group.

ACKNOWLEDGMENTS

This study would not have been possible without the support and cooperation of neurologists and neuropathologists throughout the UK; Professor I.V. Allen, Dr. S. Al Sarraj, Dr. D. Hilton, Professor N. Kopp, Professor P. Lantos, Professor S. Love, Dr. R. Perry, and Dr. H. Reid are thanked for access to tissues for study. We are grateful to Dr. C. Birkett, Institute for Animal Health, Compton, for the generous gift of the monoclonal PrP antibody KG9; to Professor P.G. Smith and Dr. S.N. Cousens, London School of Hygiene and Tropical Medicine, for assistance with epidemiological studies; and to Ms. A. Mackenzie for secretarial assistance. The authors acknowledge the help of Mr. S. MacDonald in providing some of the quantitative data. The CJD Surveillance Unit is supported by the Department of Health; Dr. K. Sutherland is supported by the Biotechnology and Biological Sciences Research Council (grant 15/BS204814).

REFERENCES

Anon. 1987. Scrapie-like disease in a captive nyala. In *Animal health.* Report of the Chief Veterinary Officer, p.69. HMSO, London.

Bateman, D., D. Hilton, S. Love, M. Zeidler, J. Beck, and J. Collinge. 1995. Sporadic Creutzfeldt-Jakob disease in a 18-year old in the UK. *Lancet* **346:** 1155.

Bell, J.E. and J.W. Ironside. 1993. Neuropathology of spongiform encephalopathies in humans. *Br. Med. Bull.* **49:** 738.

Berman, P., G.S. Davidson, and L.E. Becker. 1988. Progressive neurological deterioration in a 14-year-old girl. *Pediatr. Neurosci.* **14:** 42.

Billette de Villemeur, T., A. Gellott, J.P. Deslys, D. Dormont, C. Duyckaerts, L. Jardin, J. Denni, and O. Robain. 1994. Iatrogenic Creutzfeldt-Jakob disease in three growth hormone recipients: A neuropathological study. *Neuropathol. Appl. Neurobiol.* **20:** 111.

Britton, T.C., S. Al-Sarraj, C. Shaw, T. Campbell, and J. Collinge. 1995. Sporadic Creutzfeldt-Jakob disease in a 16-year old in the UK. *Lancet* **346:** 1155.

Brown, P., M.A.Preece, and R.G.Will. 1992. Friendly fire in medicine: Hormones, homografts, and Creutzfeldt-Jakob disease. *Lancet* **340:** 24.

Brown, P., F. Cathala, R.F. Roberts, D.C. Gajdusek, and P. Cataigne. 1987. The epidemiology of Creutzfeldt-Jakob disease: Conclusion of a 15-year investigation in France and review of the world literature. *Neurology* **37:** 895.

Brown, P., F. Cathala, R. Labauge, M. Pages, J.C. Alary, and H. Baron. 1985. Epidemiologic implications of Creutzfeldt-Jakob disease in a 19-year old girl. *Eur. J. Epidemiol.* **1:** 42.

Bruce, M.E., I. McConnell, H. Fraser, and A.G. Dickinson. 1991. The disease characteristics of different strains of scrapie in Sinc congenic mouse lines: Implications for the nature of the agent and host controls of pathogenesis. *J. Gen. Virol.* **72:** 595.

Bruton, C.J., R.K. Bruton, S.M. Gentleman, and G.W. Roberts. 1995. Diagnosis and incidence of prion (Creutzfeldt-Jakob) disease: A retrospective archival study with implications for future research. *Neurodegeneration* **4:** 357.

Budka, H., A. Aguzzi, P. Brown, J.-M. Brucher, O. Bugiani, F. Gullotta, M. Haltia, J.-J. Hauw, J.W. Ironside, K. Jellinger, H.A. Kretzschmar, P.L. Lantos, C. Masullo, W. Schlote, J. Tateishi, and R.O. Weller. 1995. Neuropathological diagnostic criteria for Creutzfeldt-Jakob disease (CJD) and other human spongiform encephalopathies (prion diseases). *Brain Pathol.* **5:** 459.

Chazot, G., E. Broussolle, C.L. Lapras, T. Blattler, A. Aguzzi, and N. Kopp. 1996. New variant of Creutzfeldt-Jakob disease in a 26-year-old French man. *Lancet* **347:** 1181.

Collinge, J., M.S. Palmer, and A.J. Dryden. 1991. Genetic predisposition to iatrogenic Creutzfeldt-Jakob disease. *Lancet* **337:** 1441.

Cousens, S.N., R. Harries-Jones, R. Knight, R. Will, P.G. Smith, and W.B. Matthews. 1990. Geographical distribution of cases of Creutzfeldt-Jakob disease in England and Wales 1970–84. *J. Neurol. Neurosurg. Psychiatry* **53:** 459.

de Silva, R., J.W. Ironside, L. McCardle, T.F.G. Esmonde, J.E. Bell, and R.G. Will. 1994. Neuropathological phenotype and "prion protein" genotype correlation in sporadic Creutzfeldt-Jakob disease. *Neurosci. Lett.* **179:** 50.

Delasnerie-Laupretre, N., S. Poser, M. Pocchiari, D.P.W.M. Wientjens, and R.G. Will. 1995. Incidence of Creutzfeldt-Jakob disease in Europe. *Lancet* **346:** 898.

Goodbrand, I.A., J.W. Ironside, D. Nicolson, and J. E. Bell. 1995. Prion protein accumulation in the spinal cords of patients with sporadic and growth hormone associated Creutzfeldt-Jakob disease. *Neurosci. Lett.* **183:** 127.

Klatzo, I., D.C. Gajdusek, and V. Zigas. 1959. Pathology of kuru. *Lab. Invest.* **8:** 799.

Kulczycki, J., H. Jedrzejowska, K. Gajkowski, E. Tarnowska-Dzidusko, and W. Lojkowska. 1991. Creutzfeldt-Jakob disease in young people. *Eur. J. Epidemiol.* **7:** 501.

Lasmezas, C.I., J.-P. Deslys, R. Demaimay, K.T. Adjou, F. Lamoury, D. Dormont, O. Roubain, J. Ironside, and J.-J. Hauw. 1996. BSE transmission to macaques. *Nature* **381:** 743.

MacDonald, S.T., K. Sutherland, and J.W. Ironside. 1996. Prion protein genotype and pathological phenotype studies in sporadic Creutzfeldt-Jakob disease. *Neuropathol. Appl. Neurobiol.* **22:** 285.

Medori, R., H.J. Trischler, A. LeBlanc, F. Villare, V. Manetto, H.Y. Chen, R. Xue, S. Leal, P. Montagna, P. Cortelli, P. Tinuper, P. Avoni, M. Mochi, A. Baruzzi, J.J. Hauw, J. Ott, E. Lugaresi, L. Autilio-Gambetti, and P. Gambetti. 1992. Fatal familial insomnia is a prion disease with a mutation at codon 178 of the prion gene. *N. Eng. J. Med.* **326:** 444.

Monreal, J., G.H. Collings, C.L. Masters, C. M. Fisher, C. Kim C.J. Gibbs Jr., and D.C. Gajdusek. 1981. Creutzfeldt-Jakob disease in an adolescent. *J. Neurol. Sci.* **52:** 341.

Packer, R.J., D.R. Cornblath, N.K. Gonatas, L.A. Bruno, and A.K. Asbury. 1980. Creutzfeldt-Jakob disease in a 20-year old woman. *Neurology* **30:** 492.

Palmer, M.S., A.J. Dryden, J.T. Hughes, and J. Collinge. 1991. Homozygous prion protein genotype predisposes to sporadic Creutzfeldt-Jakob disease. *Nature* **352:** 340.

Prusiner, S.B. 1993. Genetic and infectious prion diseases. *Arch. Neurol.* **50:** 1129.

Sutherland, K., S.T. Macdonald, and J.W. Ironside. 1996. Quantification and analysis of the neuropathological features of Creutzfeldt-Jakob disease. *J. Neurosci. Methods* **64:** 123.

The National CJD Surveillance Unit, and the Department of Epidemiology and Population Sciences, London School of Hygiene and Tropical Medicine. 1995. *Creutzfeldt-Jakob disease surveillance in the United Kingdom:* 4th Annual Report.

Wells, G.A.H., A.C. Scott, C.T. Johnson, R.F. Gunning, R.D. Hancock, M. Jeffrey, M. Dawson, and R. Bradley. 1987. A novel progressive spongiform encephalopathy in cattle. *Vet. Rec.* **121:** 419.

Will, R.G., J.W. Ironside, M. Zeidler, S.N. Cousens, K. Estebeiro, A. Alperovitch, S. Poser, M. Pocchiari, A. Hofman, and P.G. Smith. 1996. A new variant of Creutzfeldt-Jakob disease in the UK. *Lancet* **347:** 921.

Abnormal Plasma Membrane Properties and Functions in Prion-infected Cell Lines

S.J. DeArmond,[1] Y. Qiu,[2] K. Wong,[2] R. Nixon,[1] W. Hyun,[3]
S.B. Prusiner,[4,5] and W.C. Mobley[5]

[1]*Department of Pathology,* [3]*Department of Research and Specialized Laboratory Medicine,* [4]*Department of Biochemistry and Biophysics,* [5]*Department of Neurology, University of California at San Francisco, California 94143;* [2]*Department of Defense, Armed Forces Institute of Pathology, Washington, DC 20306*

Following the discoveries that highly purified preparations of the scrapie agent consist almost exclusively of a single protease-resistant isoform of the prion protein (PrP), designated PrP^{Sc} (Prusiner 1982), and that PrP^{Sc} is derived from a normal, constitutively expressed, protease-sensitive isoform, designated PrP^{C}, which is encoded by a single-copy host gene (Oesch et al. 1985), came the first generation of PrP-specific antibodies (Bendheim et al. 1984) and oligonucleotide probes (Oesch et al. 1985). With these advances, Stanley Prusiner invited our Neuropathology Research Laboratory to provide a neurohistological component to his studies. A fruitful collaboration resulted which has continued for more than 12 years In our first immunohistochemical study, we discovered that the amyloid plaques in experimental scrapie react strongly and specifically with PrP-specific antibodies (Bendheim et al. 1984). That finding convinced us that we had a unique opportunity to obtain a better understanding of the pathogenesis of scrapie in animals and the related human disorders, sporadic, iatrogenic, and familial Creutzfeldt-Jakob disease (CJD) and the rare familial disorder Gerstmann-Sträussler-Scheinker syndrome (GSS). Our overall objective has been to test whether PrP^{Sc} accumulation in the brain causes the clinically relevant neuronal dysfunction, vacuolation, and death characteristic of prion diseases. The combined results of studies from our laboratory and from Stanley Prusiner's laboratory have led to a unifying hypothesis that all aspects of spontaneous, infectious, and genetic prion diseases are due to abnormalities of the prion protein.

The purpose of this paper is to review the data which support the hypothesis that PrP^{Sc} accumulation in the brain causes neuronal dysfunction, vacuolation, and death. More recent data from studies of scrapie-infected cell lines suggest cellular mechanisms of dysfunction. Our overall goal has been to generate testable hypotheses to explain the pathogenesis of prion diseases by correlating what is known about the conversion of PrP^{C} to PrP^{Sc} with known scrapie-associated cellular abnormalities.

PrP^{Sc} ACCUMULATION CAUSES NEURONAL DYSFUNCTION AND DEGENERATION

The first indication that PrP^{Sc} is pathogenic was the finding that amyloid plaques in scrapie-infected animals and in human prion diseases are composed of protease-resistant PrP (Bendheim et al. 1984; DeArmond et al. 1985; Snow et al. 1989). Amyloid plaques were relatively easy to immunostain with PrP-specific antibodies by standard immunohistochemical techniques; however, the location of PrP^{Sc} and, for that matter, PrP^{C}, in the brain parenchyma, away from the plaques and their association with neuropathological changes, were significantly more problematic. Before immunohistochemical results could be accepted, it was necessary to verify them by an independent method such as quantitative Western analysis (DeArmond et al. 1987). In addition, before it was possible to test whether or not the neuronal vacuolation and the reactive astrocytic gliosis of prion diseases are causally related to PrP^{Sc}, it was necessary to develop methods that distinguish PrP^{C} from PrP^{Sc}, since no PrP-specific antibodies to date can do this. The criterion used to distinguish the two isoforms has been their differential susceptibility to proteinase K (PK) digestion: PrP^{C} is rapidly and completely digested whereas only the amino-terminal ~67 amino acids of PrP^{Sc} are digested, yielding PrP 27-30 without loss of infectivity (Oesch et al. 1985). PrP immunohistochemistry on aldehyde-fixed brain sections from normal hamsters and from those terminally ill with scrapie were difficult to interpret because of the uncertainty that PrP^{C} was completely eliminated by pretreatment of sections with PK and because of the great variation of the intensity of the PrP^{Sc} signal following aldehyde fixation (DeArmond et al. 1987). The reason for the capriciousness of PrP^{Sc} immunostaining in situ was revealed a few years later by a dot-blot study of brain homogenates, which showed that PrP^{Sc} must first be denatured in order to react with existing PrP-specific antibodies (Serban et al. 1990). In the meantime, we were able to confirm that the neuroanatomical distribution of PrP^{Sc} accumulation in aldehyde-fixed brain sections revealed by immunohistochemistry is accurate by electrophoresis and Western analysis of PK-digested homogenates of dissected brain regions. Those initial studies showed that the spongiform degeneration and reactive astrocytosis colocalize with sites of PrP^{Sc} accumulation and, therefore, supported a cause-effect relationship (DeArmond et al. 1987).

Subsequently, we examined the temporal pattern of PrP^{Sc} accumulation in PK-treated homogenates of dissected brain regions obtained throughout the course of scrapie in Syrian hamsters inoculated intrathalamically with the Sc237 scrapie prion strain (Fig. 1) (Jendroska et al. 1991). Four relevant observations were made: First, PrP^{Sc} accumulates exponentially in many, but not all, brain regions beginning with the site of inoculation in the thalamus. Second, the pattern of spread of PrP^{Sc} from brain region to brain region suggested that it occurred by anterograde and retrograde axonal transport in most instances; however, spread to some brain regions, such as the septum, also appeared to result from diffusion of nascent PrP^{Sc} released from sites of formation into the extracellular space of the central nervous system (CNS). The fact that a limited number of regions appeared to be affected as a result of release of nascent PrP^{Sc} was the first indication that the structure of PrP^{Sc} plays a central role in selective and differential targeting of neurons, which is one of the phenotypic characteristics that define strains of scrapie prions (DeArmond and Prusiner 1993; DeArmond et al. 1993). Third, spongiform degeneration and reactive astrocytic gliosis developed 1–2 weeks after the start of PrP^{Sc} accumulation in a region. Fourth, the total brain PrP^{Sc} at each time point during the course of scrapie,

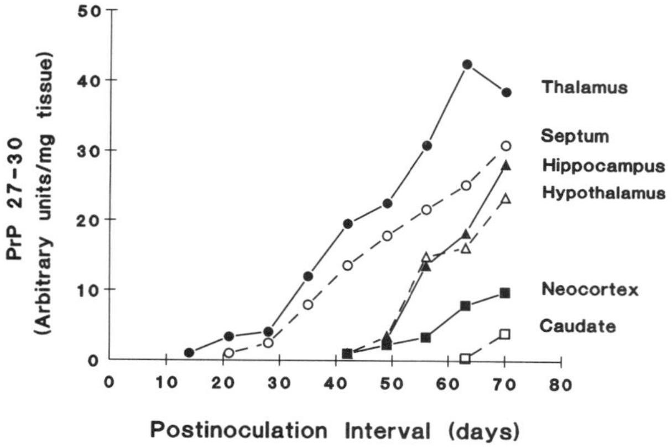

Figure 1. Protease-resistant prion protein (PrP 27-30) increases exponentially in brain regions in a pattern and sequence characteristic for each scrapie prion strain beginning at the site of inoculation in the thalamus. The concentration of PrP 27-30 (PrP^{Sc}) was determined by reflectance densitometry of Western transfers of regional brain homogenates exposed to PK. Syrian hamsters were inoculated intrathalamically with Sc237 prions. (Reprinted, with permission, from Jendroska et al. 1991.)

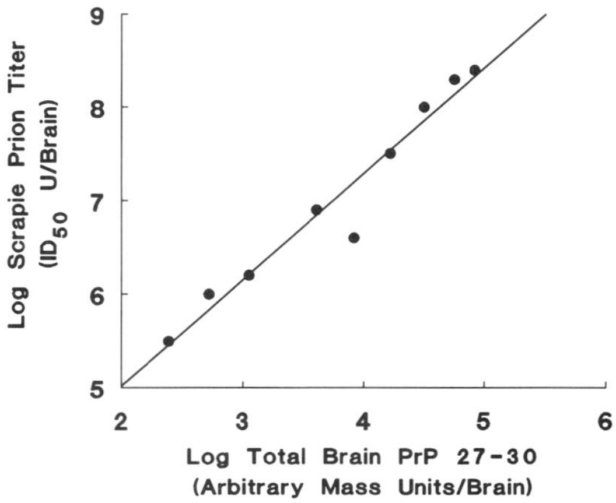

Figure 2. There is a strong correlation between the log of whole-brain PrP 27-30 concentration and log of whole-brain infectivity titer (R = 0.992). Whole-brain PrP 27-30 was calculated by summing the concentration in each brain region for each time point between 14 and 70 days postinoculation. Syrian hamsters were inoculated intrathalamically with Sc237 prions. (Reprinted, with permission, from Jendroska et al. 1991.)

based on the sum of PrP^{Sc} levels in each brain region, was directly proportional to the whole-brain scrapie infectivity titer (Fig. 2). Thus, our studies of PrP^{Sc} kinetics argued strongly for the unifying hypothesis that its accumulation in the brain is causally related to neuronal dysfunction and for the hypothesis that PrP^{Sc} is the main, if not sole, functional component of prions.

Subsequently, two immunological techniques that are able to differentiate PrP^{C} and PrP^{Sc} were developed. These have verified and extended our original findings. The histoblot technique, which was developed in our laboratory, combines the morphological advantages of histological sectioning with the neurochemical advantages of dot-blotting to distinguish PrP^{C} from PrP^{Sc} based on their differential susceptibility to PK digestion and their relative reactivity with PrP antibodies in their natural and denatured states (Taraboulos et al. 1992b). Histoblots are made by transferring (blotting) frozen sections of unfixed brain tissue to nitrocellulose paper, where PrP^{C} can be completely eliminated with certainty by treatment with PK digestion. The undigested portion of PrP^{Sc}, PrP 27-30, which is poorly antigenic in its native configuration, is then exposed to 4 M guanidinium (Gdn) which greatly enhances binding of PrP-specific antibodies. The result is an intense immunostaining signal with little or no background which is quantifiable and reveals the neuroanatomic location of PrP^{Sc}. Because PrP^{Sc} shows little or no reaction with the current PrP-specific antibodies, the location of PrP^{C} can be determined in histoblots that are not treated with PK or Gdn. Histoblotting has verified the earlier biochemical study of PrP^{Sc} kinetics, which showed that PrP^{Sc} deposition precedes the development of histopathology and that spongiform degeneration and reactive astrocytic gliosis localize precisely with PrP^{Sc}. An example of the precision of the relationship between sites of PrP^{Sc} deposition and pathological changes was seen in the cerebral cortex of Syrian hamsters inoculated with two different scrapie strains (Fig. 3) (Hecker et al. 1992). With the Sc237 prion strain, PrP^{Sc} accumulation tends to remain localized to the deeper layers of the cerebral cortex: Spongiform degeneration and reactive astrocytic gliosis are localized to the same region. In contrast, with the 139H strain, PrP^{Sc} is distributed to all layers of the cerebral cortex, as are the pathological changes. A similar correlation between sites of PrP^{Sc} accumulation and neuropathological changes was obtained by Bruce and her colleagues (Bruce et al. 1989).

The second advance in PrP^{Sc} immunostaining was made in Tateishi's laboratory, in Japan, and has been named hydrolytic autoclaving (Muramoto et al. 1992). Aldehyde-fixed, paraffin-embedded tissue sections are autoclaved in dilute hydrochloric acid before immunohistochemical staining. This technique takes advantage of the relative resistance of PrP^{Sc} to acid hydrolysis. There are advantages and disadvantages to both techniques. Histoblots allow quantitation and subregional localization of both PrP^{C} and PrP^{Sc} in serial sections of the CNS, but do not show cellular localization. Hydrolytic autoclaving is less sensitive, appears to be selective for PrP^{Sc} based on comparison with histoblots, and reveals the cellular localization of PrP^{Sc} (DeArmond and Prusiner 1995).

The results of immunohistochemistry, Western transfer analysis, and histoblotting have provided strong indirect evidence that PrP^{Sc} accumulation in the brain causes the neuropathological features characteristic of prion diseases. Negative evidence for this causal relationship is the failure of intracerebral prion inoculation to cause disease or neuropathological changes in PrP knockout mice, which do not express PrP^{C} and, therefore, do not form PrP^{Sc} (Büeler et al. 1992, 1993; Prusiner et al. 1993). Although this review focuses on prion diseases acquired by infection with prions, investigations of dominantly inherited prion diseases provide the strongest direct argument that abnormal PrP is pathogenic. Thus, more than 15 mutations of the human PrP gene have been genetically linked to the spontaneous development of a variety of clinically and neuropathologically defined prion diseases, including several forms of familial CJD, GSS, and fatal familial insomnia (FFI) (DeArmond and Prusiner 1995). The codon 102 mutation, which was linked to the original GSS family (Kretzschmar et al. 1991), results in a leucine-for-proline substitution (Hsiao et al. 1989). When this mutation is made at the homologous site in a mouse PrP transgene, the resulting transgenic (Tg)-GSS mice develop a neurodegenerative disease spontaneously with widespread vacuolation of gray matter, astrocytic gliosis, and GSS-type amyloid plaque formation (Hsiao et al. 1994). In summary, whether abnormal PrP is formed as a consequence of infection with prions or as a consequence of a dominantly inherited PrP gene mutation, the result is neuronal dysfunction and death.

NEURONAL VACUOLATION SUGGESTS DYSFUNCTIONAL WATER AND ION REGULATION

The principal neuropathological change common to all prion diseases is vacuolation of nerve cell processes (spongiform degeneration) (Masters and Richardson 1978; Beck and Daniel 1987). Vacuolation occurs primarily in the region of synapses and is characterized by focal neuritic swelling, loss of internal organelles, and accumulation of abnormal membranes (Lampert et al. 1972; Chou et al. 1980). Because spongiform degeneration resembles the neuropathological change associated with abnormal receptor-mediated ion channel function (Olney 1986), we examined receptor-mediated Ca^{++} regulation in two cell lines chronically infected with scrapie prions, designated ScN_2a and ScHaB, and in their uninfected counterparts, N_2a and HaB cells (Kristensson et al. 1993). Exposure of N_2a and HaB cells to bradykinin (Bk) produced a transient increase in intracellular Ca^{++} concentration ($[Ca^{++}]_i$) as the result of release of Ca^{++} from internal stores (Fig. 4). Prion infection of both cell lines markedly reduced or eliminated Bk-activated increases in $[Ca^{++}]_i$. The ScHaB clonal cell line subsequently lost scrapie infectivity and has resisted reinfection with scrapie prions. The loss of PrP^{Sc} and infectivity from these cells was a particularly important event in the original study, because a robust Bk-stimulated Ca^{++} response returned. This argues that the attenuated response in scrapie-infected cells was related specifically to scrapie infection and the presence of PrP^{Sc} and not an inherent characteristic of the ScHaB clonal line. The results also support the possibility that neuronal dysfunction and vacuolation may be due to abnormal ion channel regulation.

AN ATTENUATED INOSITOL TRIPHOSPHATE RESPONSE LOCALIZES ONE SCRAPIE ABNORMALITY TO THE PLASMA MEMBRANE

The goal of our next series of studies was to learn more about dysfunction of receptor-mediated Ca^{++} regulation in ScN_2a cells (Wong et al. 1996). The cascade of events during Bk-stimulated release of calcium from intracellular stores includes: (1) binding of Bk to cell membrane Bk receptors, (2) coupling of the Bk receptor with its ligand to a G_p complex and to phospholipase C (PLC) in the cell membrane, (3) formation of the inositol triphosphate (IP_3) second messenger, (4) diffusion and binding of IP_3 to IP_3 receptors on the endoplasmic reticulum (ER), (5) opening of calcium channels in ER membranes, and (6) release of Ca^{++} into the cytoplasm (Berridge 1987). To localize the defect to a cellular compartment, we focused first on the IP_3 second-messenger response to

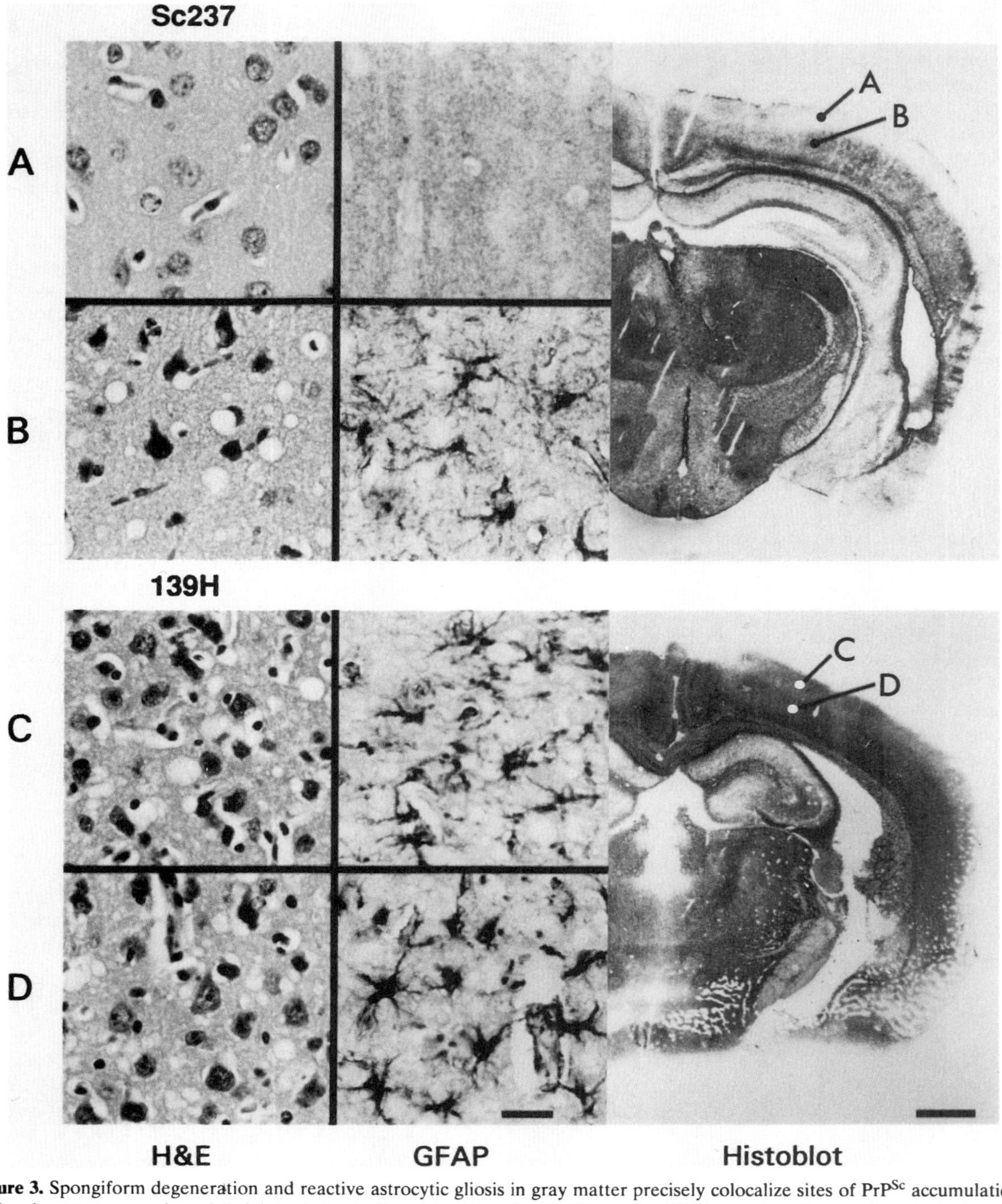

Figure 3. Spongiform degeneration and reactive astrocytic gliosis in gray matter precisely colocalize sites of PrP^{Sc} accumulation. Syrian hamsters were inoculated intrathalamically with either the Sc237 or the 139H scrapie prion strains. Animals were sacrificed when clinical signs of scrapie presented: 70 days postinoculation for Sc237 prions and 168 days for 139H prions. (*Left panels*) Hematoxylin and eosin (H&E) stains to assess the degree of vacuolization (spongiform degeneration). (*Middle panels*) Glial fibrillary acidic acid immunohistochemistry (GFAP) to evaluate the degree of reactive astrocytic gliosis. (*Right panels*) Histoblots treated with PK and Gdn and immunostained with PrP-specific antibodies show the sites of PrP^{Sc} accumulation. The lettered black dots on the histoblots show the approximate locations of the respective photomicrographs in the *left* and *middle* panels. Bar for histoblots, 1 mm. Bar for histological sections, 50 μm. (Reprinted, with permission, from Hecker et al. 1992.)

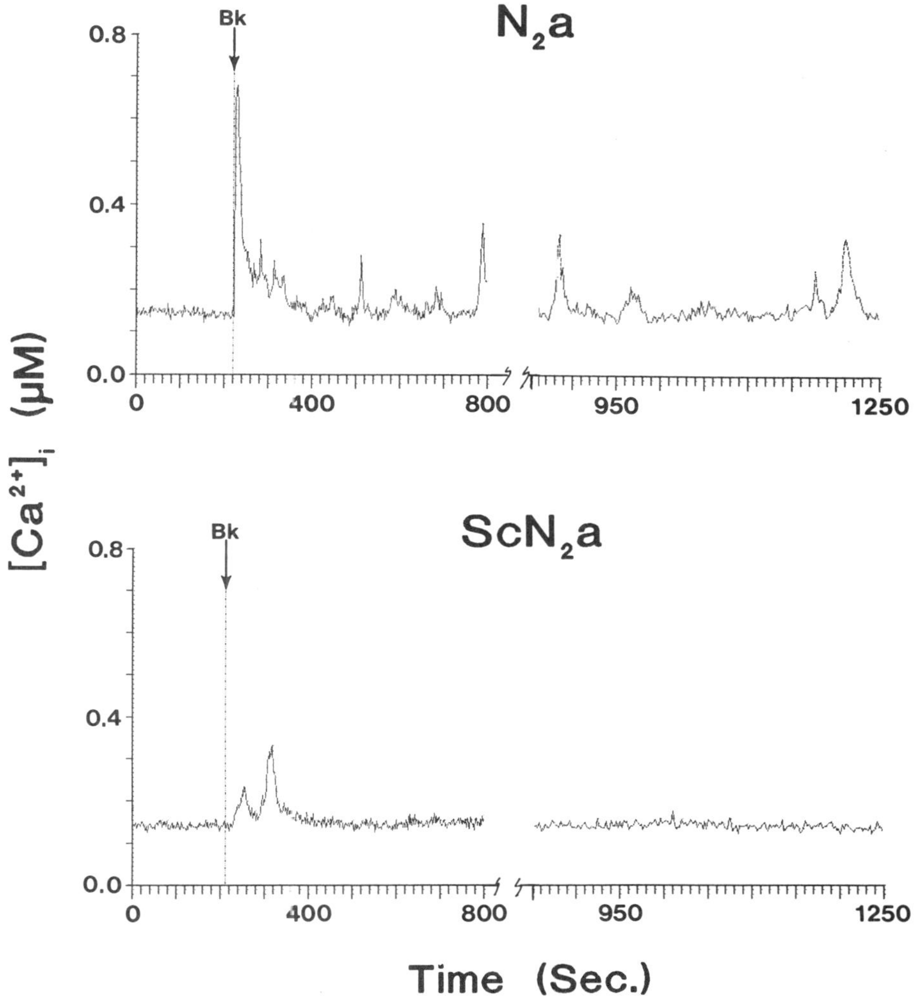

Figure 4. Intracellular calcium $[Ca^{++}]_i$ responses to 20 μM bradykinin (Bk) in N_2a and ScN_2a cells. The immediate calcium peak was greatly attenuated in ScN_2a cells and was not followed by afterdischarges seen in N_2a cells. (Reprinted, with permission, from Kristensson et al. 1993.)

Bk stimulation. A normal IP_3 response would argue that the dysfunction is localized to the Ca^{++} release mechanisms of the ER, whereas a decreased IP_3 response would argue that abnormalities originate within the plasma membrane where IP_3 is generated.

We found that the Bk-stimulated IP_3 second-messenger response was decreased by 90% in ScN_2a cells relative to N_2a cells (Fig. 5). A small increase in IP_3 concentration in ScN_2a cells 20 seconds after exposure to Bk was not statistically different from background resting levels. Furthermore, the decreased Ca^{++} responses were not due to delayed IP_3 release, since concentrations approaching background levels were found at 30 seconds and 40 seconds. The attenuated intracellular Ca^{++} response in ScN_2a cells correlated temporally with the weak IP_3 response, since increased $[Ca^{++}]_i$ reached a peak about 20–30 seconds after Bk exposure and was near background levels at 40 seconds. We concluded that the decreased IP_3 response accounted for the attenuated Bk-stimulated intracellular Ca^{++} response.

DECREASED Bk-STIMULATED IP_3 RESPONSE CORRELATES WITH DECREASED Bk RECEPTOR BINDING AFFINITY

Competitive binding assays suggested that the attenuated IP_3 and Ca^{++} responses were not due to loss of Bk receptors. Saturation binding assays indicated there were 3–4 times more Bk receptors on ScN_2a cells based on the B_{max} calculations (Fig. 6). These results argue that the decreased IP_3 and Ca^{++} responses were due to alteration of Bk receptors, rather than loss of Bk receptors. Saturation binding assays showed that the decreased IP_3 and Ca^{++} responses were related to an alteration of the Bk-receptor-binding affinity since

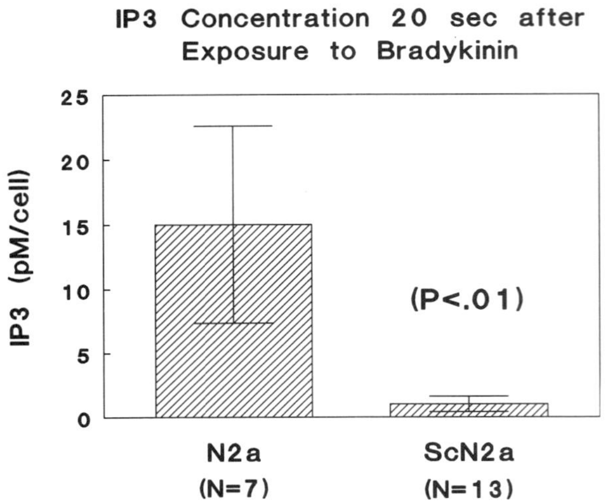

Figure 5. The IP_3 second-messenger response 20 sec after exposure of ScN_2a cells to 20 μM bradykinin was significantly reduced compared to N_2a cells. (Reprinted, with permission, from Wong et al. 1996.)

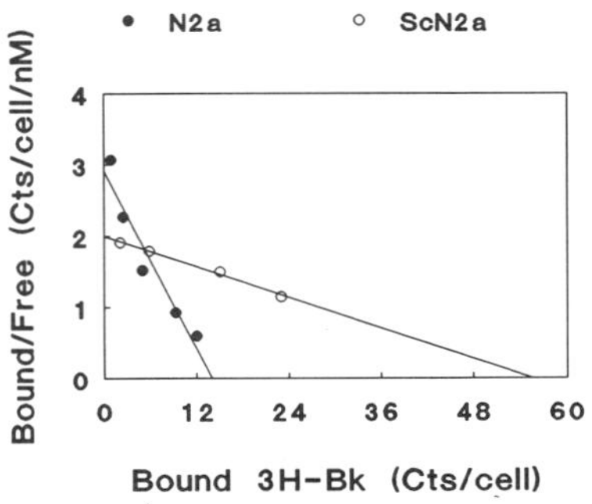

Figure 6. Scatchard analysis of a bradykinin (Bk) saturation binding assay shows that the slope of the line ($-1/K_d$) is less and the x-intercept (B_{max}) is greater for ScN_2a cells. Each data point is the mean of three culture wells. (Reprinted, with permission, from Wong et al. 1996.)

calculations of its dissociation constant, K_d, indicated that it was decreased 5- to 13-fold.

PLASMA MEMBRANE FLUIDITY IS MARKEDLY DECREASED IN SCRAPIE-INFECTED CELLS

The marked reduction in Bk-receptor-binding affinity in the setting of an increased number of Bk receptors raised the possibility that plasma membrane fluidity is also abnormal in scrapie-infected cells. To test this possibility, membrane fluidity was measured by the fluorescence recovery after photobleaching (FRAP) method using the fluorescent lipid probe, nitrobenzoxadiazole-labeled phosphocholine (NBD-C6-PC), which provides a measure of the degree of lateral fluidity (rate of lateral diffusion of the probe) in the outer leaflet of the plasma membrane. The underlying premise is that the major components of cell membranes, including proteins, lipids, and polysaccharides, are in a continual state of dynamic interaction with each other, with the result that changes in any membrane component influence membrane fluidity and, in turn, any change in membrane fluidity influences the interactions of its components and their functions (Szolosi 1994).

In five experiments, lateral membrane fluidity was consistently less in ScN_2a cells. Typical results from a single N_2a and ScN_2a cell are presented in Figure 7. The vertical axis represents the inverse of fluorescence intensity. At time zero, a 2.6-μm-diameter spot on the cell surface was bleached, and the lowest fluorescence intensity was recorded, represented by the highest value on the vertical axis. Subsequent measurements made for up to 40 seconds after bleaching show a decrease in the curve as unbleached lipid probe diffused into the bleached area. Visual inspection of the fluorescence intensity recovery curves shows that diffusion of the lipid probe was prolonged in the ScN_2a cell. The mobility measurements from 18 N_2a and 22 ScN_2a cells in three separate experiments showed a significant difference. The mean and standard deviation for N_2a cells was 8.04 ± 6 and for ScN_2a cells was 1.13 ± 1 ($cm^2/sec \times 10^{-9}$) ($p < .01$).

PHYSIOLOGICAL EFFECTS OF DECREASED MEMBRANE FLUIDITY

Factors that profoundly affect plasma membrane fluidity include temperature, membrane potential, fatty acid, and protein composition; in turn, fluidity changes profoundly alter the function of plasma membrane components (Szolosi 1994). The effects of experimentally induced membrane fluidity changes on the functions of numerous enzyme, receptor, and transport systems have been reported previouly (Solomonson et al. 1976; Szamel and Resch 1981; Brasitus et al. 1985, 1988; Tsakiris 1985; Minocha et al. 1988; Suzuki et al. 1988; Field et al. 1990; Kuo et al. 1990). A threefold change was considered significant in those studies. In our study, FRAP analysis revealed a sevenfold decrease in fluidity in scrapie-infected cells compared to noninfected N_2a cells. This degree of change, therefore, has a profound effect on the activity of a variety of plasma membrane enzymes, receptors, and ion channels and could explain the change in Bk-receptor-binding affinity.

The question raised by our findings is whether decreased membrane fluidity is the central physiological abnormality in prion-infected nerve cells. The reasonableness of this possibility is that all of the known clinical and neuropathological features of prion diseases could be explained by decreased neuronal membrane fluidity. It could alter release of transmitters from the presynaptic neuron and could markedly decrease the postsynaptic response to transmitters. Both abnormalities could result in failure of synaptic

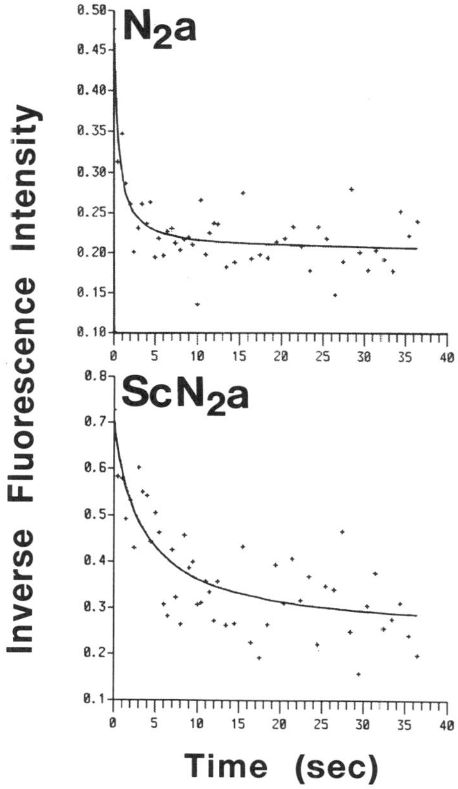

Figure 7. Examples of fluorescence recovery after FRAP analysis curves from a single N_2a and ScN_2a cell. The rate of diffusion of NBD-C6-PC into the bleached area on the plasma membrane was more rapid in N_2a cells. (Reprinted, with permission, from Wong et al. 1996.)

transmission and lead to functional disconnection of affected neuron populations. This could explain why some patients with CJD are profoundly demented but show only minimal vacuolation of neurons, no nerve cell loss, and no reactive astrocytic gliosis. Decreased membrane fluidity could also alter ion and water balance across the neuronal cell membrane and lead to focal vacuolation. Finally, it could alter the responsiveness of neurons to neurotrophic factors and result in nerve cell death.

ORIGIN AND DISPOSITION OF PrP^{Sc}

The membrane fluidity hypotheses, or any other hypothesis about the mechanisms of cell dysfunction in prion diseases, must be placed into context with what is known about the conversion of PrP^C to PrP^{Sc} and the subsequent accumulation of PrP^{Sc} in and around cells, since, ultimately, they are the driving forces that create the physiological abnormalities in prion diseases as described above. Most of our knowledge about the metabolism and trafficking of PrP^C and PrP^{Sc} comes from investigations in the normal and scrapie-infected mouse N_2a neuroblastoma cell line. Once infected with scrapie prions, the resulting ScN_2a cell line retains infectivity chronically and on all subsequent passages in culture (Butler et al. 1988). PrP^C is constitutively expressed in both N_2a and ScN_2a cells. Ninety percent of the cell's PrP^C becomes attached to the outer surface of the cells by its glycosyl-phosphatidylinositol (GPI) anchor following its synthesis and passage through the Golgi complex (Borchelt et al. 1990). Like other GPI-anchored proteins, PrP^C re-enters the cell through caveolae (Ying et al. 1992); however, it also appears to be capable of internalization via clathrin-coated pits (Shyng et al. 1994). About 10% of the endocytosed PrP^C is degraded while the remainder is recycled to the cell surface along with other proteins and lipids of the endosome. In pulse-chase experiments, PrP^C in uninfected cells is rapidly labeled by a radioactive amino acid tracer and appears to be completely degraded with loss of the tracer in about 6 hours (Caughey et al. 1989; Borchelt et al. 1990). In scrapie-infected ScN_2a cells, labeling of PrP^{Sc} is delayed by about 1 hour after the pulse and increases to a maximum during the time period when the PrP^C pool loses its tracer (Borchelt et al. 1990). Over the next 24 hours, there is little or no loss of tracer from the PrP^{Sc} pool. These results argue that PrP^{Sc} is derived from PrP^C, but, unlike PrP^C, PrP^{Sc} is not degraded and accumulates in the cell. The PrP^C precursor pool from which PrP^{Sc} is formed must first reach the cell surface, since blocking of PrP^C export from the ER-Golgi complex to the plasma membrane inhibits formation of PrP^{Sc} (Taraboulos et al. 1992a), and since exposure of scrapie-infected cells to phosphatidylinositol-specific phospholipase C (PIPLC), which releases PrP^C from the cell surface, also inhibits formation of PrP^{Sc} (Caughey and Raymond 1991). The distribution of PrP^{Sc} in cells is still being determined. Immunoelectron microscopy indicates that most PrP^{Sc} accumulates in structures containing "myelin" figures (e.g., layers of phospholipid-rich membranes) believed to be secondary lysosomes (McKinley et al. 1991). The only other location in the cell culture definitely known to contain PrP^{Sc} is the conditioned culture medium, which appears to accumulate PrP^{Sc} as a result of excretion from infected cells or, more likely, as a result of death of infected cells. The site where PrP^C is converted to PrP^{Sc} is not known, although it is suspected to occur in a cholesterol-rich endosomal compartment.

The same process of PrP^C conversion to PrP^{Sc} in scrapie-infected cells appears to occur in vivo. The highest rate of PrP^C conversion to PrP^{Sc} probably occurs in CNS neurons, since they express the highest levels of PrP mRNA (Kretzschmar et al. 1986; DeArmond et al. 1992). Following intracerebral inoculation of an animal with prions, PrP^{Sc} begins to accumulate exponentially in the brain (Jendroska et al. 1991). Even in the CNS, PrP^{Sc} appears to accumulate both within neurons and in the extracellular space surrounding neurons (DeArmond et al. 1987; DeArmond and Prusiner 1995).

MECHANISM OF CELL DYSFUNCTION: HYPOTHESES

Hypotheses about the mechanism of cell dysfunction in prion diseases must take into account all of the known cellular abnormalities. Three classes of relevant abnormalities have been identified. First, and most importantly, when a susceptible cell is exposed to PrP^{Sc} in the form of prions, a self-perpetuating process is set in motion. It begins with an interaction of PrP^{Sc} with the constitutively expressed normal prion protein isoform, PrP^{C}, after which the latter is converted into an identical conformer of the former. Ultimately, it is the conversion of PrP^{C} to PrP^{Sc}, and/or the accumulation of PrP^{Sc}, which generates the physiological abnormalities. Second, we have identified a number of plasma membrane abnormalities which, by themselves, can account for all of the functional and morphological abnormalities of neurons observed in prion diseases, as described above. Third, heat shock protein responses in ScN_2a cells are also abnormal including (1) the absence of inducible Hsp72 and Hsp28 responses, (2) granular deposits of Hsp73 in unstressed ScN_2a cells, and (3) failure of Hsp73 redistribution to the nucleus with heat shock (Tatzelt et al. 1995).

From the above, it is reasonable to ask how conversion of PrP^{C} to PrP^{Sc} might cause plasma membrane and stress protein abnormalities and whether the latter two are interrelated. Two pathogenic pathway hypotheses are currently being investigated. The first suggests that the conversion of PrP^{C} to PrP^{Sc} alters lipid and protein trafficking in and out of the plasma membrane which, in turn, affects the composition, fluidity, and function of plasma membrane components. The second suggests that the accumulation of abnormally folded and protease-resistant PrP^{Sc} in the cell sequesters stress proteins (chaperones) and/or alters their compartmentalization and regulation. In case of the latter, it is possible that proteins targeted to the plasma membrane, such as the Bk receptor, are misfolded during synthesis as a result of chaperone abnormalities. The arrival of abnormally folded Bk-receptor protein in the plasma membrane might explain why its binding constants are markedly decreased. It could also explain decreased membrane fluidity, particularly if many membrane proteins are abnormally folded during their synthesis. An intriguing variation on this possibility has been suggested by Liautard to explain the origin of the three forms of prion diseases: infectious, genetic, and sporadic (Liautard 1993). The foundation of the argument is that a misfolded chaperone can induce misfolding of proteins and, in the case of autofolding (auto-chaperone), may lead to new misfolded chaperones. From some structural similarities between the prion protein and chaperones and from the effects of pathogenic mutations of the prion protein on its structure, Liautard proposes that PrP may itself be a chaperone and perform an auto-chaperone function.

The known abnormal Hsp responses and the possibility that the prion protein is itself an auto-chaperone are particularly interesting because the conversion of PrP^{C} to PrP^{Sc} involves a change in molecular conformation from an α-helical configuration to β-sheet (Caughey et al. 1991; Gasset et al. 1993; Pan et al. 1993; Safar et al. 1993) and because one of the main functions of molecular chaperones is to control protein folding. Chaperones may directly or indirectly contribute to the conversion of PrP^{C} to PrP^{Sc} and, therefore, participate in the propagation of prions. The relationship between decreased plasma membrane fluidity and abnormal Hsp responses in ScN_2a cells is not known. However, modulation of membrane fluidity in dimorphic fungi by exposure to unsaturated or saturated fatty acids has a profound effect on the transcription of the Hsp70 and Hsp82 genes (Maresca and Kobayashi 1993); therefore, they may be secondary to a primary effect on plasma membrane fluidity in scrapie. An association of membrane fluidity with Hsp regulation could also be via abnormal Ca^{++} signaling, given that the calcium ionophore, A23187, induces the 80-kD and 100-kD heat shock proteins in tracheal epithelium (Smith et al. 1982).

SUMMARY

A long trail of evidence indicates that the formation of PrP^{Sc} or its accumulation causes the neuronal dysfunction and clinical features of prion diseases. The results of our current line of studies argue that the main neuropathological and clinical features of prion diseases are explained by altered ion channel function secondary to decreased plasma membrane fluidity. This kind of mechanism has the potential to functionally disconnect neuronal networks and cause neuronal vacuolation. Our laboratory is currently focusing its investigations on pathogenic mechanisms that have the potential to link the formation of PrP^{Sc} with plasma membrane abnormalities in prion diseases.

In summary, the first hypothesis suggests that the conversion of PrP^{C} to PrP^{Sc} affects plasma membrane fluidity directly, which secondarily alters the properties and functions of its components. In contrast, the second hypothesis argues that PrP^{Sc} accumulation alters the ability of chaperones to correctly fold plasma membrane proteins during their synthesis, which directly affects the properties of nascent proteins and secondarily affects membrane fluidity. Our current investigations are attempting to determine which of these mechanisms are plausible and, then, which is primary.

ACKNOWLEDGMENTS

The authors thank Ms. Marlyna Stewart for her help with preparing the manuscript. This study was supported by grants from the National Institutes of Health (NS-14069, AGO-8967, AG-02132, and NS-22786) and the American Health Assistance Foundation, as well as gifts from the Sherman Fairchild and Bernard Osher Foundations.

REFERENCES

Beck, E. and P.M. Daniel. 1987. Neuropathology of slow transmissible encephalopathies. In *Prions—Novel infectious pathogens causing scrapie and Creutzfeldt-Jakob disease* (ed. S.B. Prusiner and M.P. McKinley), p. 331. Academic Press, Orlando, Florida.

Bendheim, P.E., R.A. Barry, S.J. DeArmond, D.P. Stites, and S.B. Prusiner. 1984. Antibodies to a scrapie prion protein. *Nature* **310:** 418.

Berridge, M.J. 1987. Inositol trisphosphate and diacylglycerol: Two interacting second messengers. *Annu. Rev. Biochem.* **56:** 159.

Borchelt, D.R., M. Scott, A. Taraboulos, N. Stahl, and S.B. Prusiner. 1990. Scrapie and cellular prion proteins differ in their kinetics of synthesis and topology in cultured cells. *J. Cell Biol.* **110:** 743.

Brasitus, T.A., N.O. Davidson, and D. Schachter. 1985. Variations in dietary triacylglycerol saturation alter the lipid composition and fluidity of rat intestinal plasma membranes. *Biochim. Biophys. Acta* **812:** 460.

Brasitus, T.A., R. Dahiya, P.K. Dudeja, and B.M Bissonnette. 1988. Cholesterol modulates alkaline phosphatase activity of rat intestinal microvillus membranes. *J. Biol. Chem.* **263:** 8592.

Bruce, M.E., P.A. McBride, and C.F. Farquhar 1989. Precise targeting of the pathology of the sialoglycoprotein, PrP, and vacuolar degeneration in mouse scrapie. *Neurosci. Lett.* **102:** 1.

Büeler, H., A. Aguzzi, A. Sailer, R.-A. Greiner, P. Autenried, M. Aguet, and C. Weissmann. 1993. Mice devoid of PrP are resistant to scrapie. *Cell* **73:** 1339.

Büeler, H., M. Fischer, Y. Lang, H. Bluethmann, H.-P. Lipp, S.J. DeArmond, S.B. Prusiner, M. Aguet, and C. Weissmann. 1992. Normal development and behaviour of mice lacking the neuronal cell-surface PrP protein. *Nature* **356:** 577.

Butler, D.A., M.R.D. Scott, J.M. Bockman, D.R. Borchelt, A. Taraboulos, K.K. Hsiao, D.T. Kingsbury, and S.B. Prusiner. 1988. Scrapie-infected murine neuroblastoma cells produce protease-resistant prion proteins. *J. Virol.* **62:** 1558.

Caughey, B. and G.J. Raymond. 1991. The scrapie-associated form of PrP is made from a cell surface precursor that is both protease- and phospholipase-sensitive. *J. Biol. Chem.* **266:** 18217.

Caughey, B., R.E. Race, D. Ernst, M.J. Buchmeier, and B. Chesebro. 1989. Prion protein biosynthesis in scrapie-infected and uninfected neuroblastoma cells. *J. Virol.* **63:** 175.

Caughey, B.W., A. Dong, K.S. Bhat, D. Ernst, S.F. Hayes, and W.S. Caughey. 1991. Secondary structure analysis of the scrapie-associated protein PrP 27-30 in water by infrared spectroscopy. *Biochemistry* **30:** 7672.

Chou, S.M., W.N. Payne, C.J. Gibbs, Jr., and D.C. Gajdusek. 1980. Transmission and scanning electron microscopy of spongiform change in Creutzfeldt-Jakob disease. *Brain* **103:** 885.

DeArmond, S.J. and S.B. Prusiner. 1993. The neurochemistry of prion diseases. *J. Neurochem.* **61:** 1589.

———. 1995. Etiology and pathogenesis of prion diseases. *Am. J. Pathol.* **146:** 785.

DeArmond, S.J., M.P. McKinley, R.A. Barry, M.B. Braunfeld, J.R. McColloch, and S.B. Prusiner. 1985. Identification of prion amyloid filaments in scrapie-infected brain. *Cell* **41:** 221. DeArmond, S.J., W.C. Mobley, D.L. DeMott, R.A. Barry, J.H. Beckstead, and S.B. Prusiner. 1987. Changes in the localization of brain prion proteins during scrapie infection. *Neurology* **37:** 1271.

DeArmond, S.J., S.-L. Yang, A. Lee, R. Bowler, A. Taraboulos, D. Groth, and S.B. Prusiner. 1993. Three scrapie prion isolates exhibit different accumulation patterns of the prion protein scrapie isoform. *Proc. Natl. Acad. Sci.* **90:** 6449.

DeArmond, S.J., K. Jendroska, S.-L. Yang, A. Taraboulos, R. Hecker, K. Hsiao, L. Stowring, M. Scott, and S.B. Prusiner. 1992. Scrapie prion protein accumulation correlates with neuropathology and incubation times in hamsters and transgenic mice. In *Prion diseases of humans and animals* (ed. S.B. Prusiner et al.), p. 483. Ellis Horwood, London.

Field, C.J., E.A. Ryan, A.B. Thomson, and M.T. Clandinin. 1990. Diet fat composition alters membrane phospholipid composition, insulin binding, and glucose metabolism in adipocytes from control and diabetic animals. *J. Biol. Chem.* **265:** 11143.

Gasset, M., M.A. Baldwin, R.J. Fletterick, and S.B. Prusiner. 1993. Perturbation of the secondary structure of the scrapie prion protein under conditions associated with changes in infectivity. *Proc. Natl. Acad. Sci.* **90:** 1.

Hecker, R., A. Taraboulos, M. Scott, K.-M. Pan, M. Torchia, K. Jendroska, S.J. DeArmond, and S.B. Prusiner. 1992. Replication of distinct prion isolates is region specific in brains of transgenic mice and hamsters. *Genes Dev.* **6:** 1213.

Hsiao, K., H.F. Baker, T.J. Crow, M. Poulter, F. Owen, J.D. Terwilliger, D. Westaway, J. Ott, and S.B. Prusiner. 1989. Linkage of a prion protein missense variant to Gerstmann-Sträussler syndrome. *Nature* **338:** 342.

Hsiao, K.K., D. Groth, M. Scott, S.-L. Yang, H. Serban, D. Rapp, D. Foster, M. Torchia, S.J. DeArmond, and S.B. Prusiner. 1994. Serial transmission in rodents of neurodegeneration from transgenic mice expressing mutant prion protein. *Proc. Natl. Acad. Sci.* **91:** 9126.

Jendroska, K., F.P. Heinzel, M. Torchia, L. Stowring, H.A. Kretzschmar, A. Kon, A. Stern, S.B. Prusiner, and S.J. DeArmond. 1991. Proteinase-resistant prion protein accumulation in Syrian hamster brain correlates with regional pathology and scrapie infectivity. *Neurology* **41:** 1482.

Kretzschmar, H.A., S.B. Prusiner, L.E. Stowring, and S.J. DeArmond. 1986. Scrapie prion proteins are synthesized in neurons. *Am. J. Pathol.* **122:** 1.

Kretzschmar, H.A., G. Honold, F. Seitelberger, M. Feucht, P. Wessely, P. Mehraein, and H. Budka. 1991. Prion protein mutation in family first reported by Gerstmann, Sträussler, and Scheinker. *Lancet* **337:** 1160.

Kristensson, K., B. Feuerstein, A. Taraboulos, W.C. Hyun, S.B. Prusiner, and S.J. DeArmond. 1993. Scrapie prions alter receptor-mediated calcium responses in cultured cells. *Neurology* **43:** 2335.

Kuo, P., M. Weinfeld, and J. Loscalzo. 1990. Effect of membrane fatty acyl composition on LDL metabolism in Hep G2 hepatocytes. *Biochemistry* **29:** 6626.

Lampert, P.W., D.C. Gajdusek, and C.J. Gibbs, Jr. 1972. Subacute spongiform virus encephalopathies. Scrapie, kuru and Creutzfeldt-Jakob disease: A review. *Am. J. Pathol.* **68:** 626.

Liautard, J.-P. 1993. Prions and molecular chaperones. *Arch. Virol. (suppl.)* **7:** 227.

Maresca, B. and G. Kobayashi. 1993. Changes in membrane fluidity modulate heat shock gene expression and produced attenuated strain in the dimorphic fungus *Histoplasma capsulatum. Arch. Med. Res.* **24:** 247.

Masters, C.L. and E.P. Richardson, Jr. 1978. Subacute spongiform encephalopathy Creutzfeldt-Jakob disease—The nature and progression of spongiform change. *Brain* **101:** 333.

McKinley, M. P., A. Taraboulos, L. Kenaga, D. Serban, A. Stieber, S.J. DeArmond, S.B. Prusiner, and N. Gonatas. 1991. Ultrastructural localization of scrapie prion proteins in cytoplasmic vesicles of infected cultured cells. *Lab. Invest.* **65:** 622.

Minocha, R., S.N. Sanyal, A. Wali, K. Gumbhir, and S. Majumdar. 1988. Effect of cholesterol and temperature perturbations on membrane hydrolases and transport of calcium and glucose in guinea pig brush border membrane vesicles. *Biochem. Int.* **16:** 1019.

Muramoto, T., T. Kitamoto, J. Tateishi, and I. Goto. 1992. The sequential development of abnormal prion protein accumulation in mice with Creutzfeldt-Jakob disease. *Am. J. Pathol.* **140:** 1411.

Oesch, B., D. Westaway, M. Wälchli, M.P. McKinley, S.B.H. Kent, R. Aebersold, R.A. Barry, P. Tempst, D.B. Teplow, L.E. Hood, S.B. Prusiner, and C. Weissmann. 1985. A cellular gene encodes scrapie PrP 27-30 protein. *Cell* **40:** 735.

Olney, J.W. 1986. Inciting excitotoxic cytocide among central neurons. *Adv. Exp. Med. Biol.* **203:** 631.

Pan, K.-M., M. Baldwin, J. Nguyen, M. Gasset, A. Serban, D. Groth, I. Mehlhorn, Z. Huang, R.J. Fletterick, F.E. Cohen, and S.B. Prusiner. 1993. Conversion of α-helices into β-sheets features in the formation of the scrapie prion proteins. *Proc. Natl. Acad. Sci.* **90:** 10962.

Prusiner, S.B. 1982. Novel proteinaceous infectious particles cause scrapie. *Science* **216:** 136.

Prusiner, S.B., D. Groth, A. Serban, R. Koehler, D. Foster, M. Torchia, D. Burton, S.-L. Yang, and S.J. DeArmond. 1993. Ablation of the prion protein (PrP) gene in mice prevents scrapie and facilitates production of anti-PrP antibodies. *Proc. Natl. Acad. Sci.* **90:** 10608.

Safar, J., P.P. Roller, D.C. Gajdusek, and C.J. Gibbs, Jr. 1993. Conformational transitions, dissociation, and unfolding of scrapie amyloid (prion) protein. *J. Biol. Chem.* **268:** 20276.

Serban, D., A. Taraboulos, S.J. DeArmond, and S.B. Prusiner. 1990. Rapid detection of Creutzfeldt-Jakob disease and scrapie prion proteins. *Neurology* **40:** 110.

Shyng, S.-L., J.E. Heuser, and D.A. Harris. 1994. A glycolipid-anchored prion protein is endocytosed via clathrin-coated pits. *J. Cell Biol.* **125:** 1239.

Smith, P.L., M.J. Welsh, J.S. Stoff, and R.A. Frizzell. 1982. Chloride secretion by canine tracheal epithelium: I. Role of intracellular cAMP levels. *J. Membr. Biol.* **70:** 217.

Snow, A.D., R. Kisilevsky, J. Willmer, S.B. Prusiner, and S.J. DeArmond. 1989. Sulfated glycosaminoglycans in amyloid plaques of prion diseases. *Acta Neuropathol.* **77:** 337.

Solomonson, L.P., V.A. Liepkalns, and A.A. Spector. 1976. Changes in (Na^{++} K^{+})-ATPase activity of Ehrlich ascites tumor cells produced by alteration of membrane fatty acid composition. *Biochemistry* **15:** 892.

Suzuki, M., Y. Kawaguchi, M. Momose, T. Morita, K. Yokoyama, and T. Miyahara. 1988. 1,25-Dihydroxyvitamin D stimulates sodium-dependent phosphate transport by renal outer cortical brush-border membrane vesicles by directly affecting membrane fluidity. *Biochem. Biophys. Res. Commun.* **150:** 1193.

Szamel, M. and K. Resch. 1981. Modulation of enzyme activities in isolated lymphocyte plasma membranes by enzymatic modification of phospholipid fatty acids. *J. Biol. Chem.* **256:** 11618.

Szolosi, J. 1994. Fluidity/viscosity of biological membranes. In *Mobility and proximity in biological membranes.* (ed. S. Damjanovich), p. 137. CRC Press, Boca Raton, Flordia.

Taraboulos, A., A.J. Raeber, D.R. Borchelt, D. Serban, and S.B. Prusiner. 1992a. Synthesis and trafficking of prion proteins in cultured cells. *Mol. Biol. Cell* **3:** 851.

Taraboulos, A., K. Jendroska, D. Serban, S.-L. Yang, S.J. DeArmond, and S.B. Prusiner. 1992b. Regional mapping of prion proteins in brains. *Proc. Natl. Acad. Sci.* **89:** 7620.

Tatzelt, J., J. Zuo, R. Voellmy, M. Scott, U. Hartl, S.B. Prusiner, and W.J. Welch. 1995. Scrapie prions selectively modify the stress response in neuroblastoma cells. *Proc. Natl. Acad. Sci.* **92:** 2944.

Tsakiris, S. 1985. Control of the activity of brain synaptosome-associated acetylcholinesterase by acidic phospholipids. *Z. Naturforsch.* **40:** 97.

Wong, K., Y. Qiu, W. Hyun, R. Nixon, J. VanCleff, J. Sanchez-Salazar, S. Prusiner, and S. DeArmond. 1996. Decreased receptor-mediated calcium response in prion-infected cells correlates with decreased membrane fluidity and IP3 release. *Neurology* **47:** (in press.)

Ying, Y.-S., R.G.W. Anderson, and K.G. Rothberg. 1992. Each caveola contains multiple glycosyl-phosphatidylinositol-anchored membrane proteins. *Cold Spring Harbor Symp. Quant. Biol.* **57:** 593.

Prions of Yeast, [PSI] and [URE3], as Models for Neurodegenerative Diseases

R.B. WICKNER, D.C. MASISON, H.K. EDSKES, AND M.-L. MADDELEIN
Section on Genetics of Simple Eukaryotes, National Institute of Diabetes, Digestive, and Kidney Diseases, National Institutes of Health, Bethesda, Maryland 20892-0830

Among neurodegenerative diseases are several characterized by accumulation of abnormal forms of normal proteins, the amyloidoses. These include Alzheimer's disease, transthyretin amyloidotic polyneuropathy, and senile amyloidoses. The spongiform encephalopathies are in some ways the best-understood members of this group, and include scrapie of sheep, mad cow disease, kuru, Creutzfeldt-Jakob disease (GJD), Gerstmann-Sträussler syndrome (GSS), and fatal familial insomnia of man. These spongiform encephalopathies are all essentially the same disease and are thought to be due to a self-propagating change of a normal cellular protein (PrP^C) to an abnormal form (PrP^{Sc}) (Alper et al. 1967; Griffith 1967; Prusiner 1982 and this volume; Weissmann et al., this volume). Although Alper had provided evidence against nucleic acid involvement in the scrapie agent (Alper et al. 1967), and Griffith suggested an infectious protein (Griffith 1967), it was Prusiner who purified the scrapie agent and first identified PrP as its major constituent, then coining the term "prion" (Prusiner 1982) to designate such infectious proteins (Table 1). The evidence is steadily mounting that the scrapie group of PrP diseases are, in fact, prion diseases with no nucleic acid component of the infectious process, but there remain some paradoxical results and more than a few skeptics.

We have proposed that two non-Mendelian genetic elements of the yeast, *Saccharomyces cerevisiae*, are not nucleic acid replicons, but are actually infectious proteins, analogous (but not homologous) to the PrP diseases of mammals (Wickner 1994). We proposed that [URE3] is a prion form of Ure2p, and [PSI] is a prion form of Sup35p. The genetic evidence that these are yeast prions is perhaps better than that for the mammalian case (for review, see Wickner 1996b), but the biochemical evidence is not as complete.

We foresee the utility of the yeast prions in studies of the mechanisms of prion formation and propagation, and in the design of simple assays, analogous to the Ames mutagen tests, to test both for prion-inducing substances and conditions and for prion-curing agents. These systems may also be useful in pointing the way to surrogate studies, where the mammalian components themselves are studied directly in yeast, analogous to the two-hybrid system. Finally, it may be possible to find yet other prions using the tools of yeast molecular genetics, and thereby to assess the likely breadth of the prion phenomenon.

In the 1960s and 1970s, yeast non-Mendelian genetic elements were a focus of attention because it was expected that they would correspond to small nucleic acid replicons whose analysis was within reach. During this era, mitochondrial DNA markers, 2μ DNA, the killer character (a satellite dsRNA of the L-A dsRNA virus), and 20S RNA were described. However, several non-Mendelian elements did not fulfill this expectation and remained unassociated with nucleic acid replicons. Most prominent among these, because of the care with which they were documented, were [PSI] and [URE3].

[PSI] was discovered by Brian Cox (1965) as a non-Mendelian element enhancing the efficiency of the weak ochre suppressor, *SUQ5*. *SUQ5* is a serine-inserting classic tRNA suppressor mutation, but the tRNA itself is not modified by [PSI] (Leibman et al. 1975; Waldron et al. 1981). [PSI] also increases the action of strong tRNA suppressors, making them lethal, and some frameshift suppressors as well (Cox 1971; Cummins et al. 1980). Paromomycin suppression of UAG, UGA, and UAA mutations is also increased by the presence of [PSI] (Palmer et al. 1979).

[URE3] was found by Francois Lacroute in 1971 in a search for mutants allowing cells blocked in pyrimidine biosynthesis at aspartate transcarbamylase to take up ureidosuccinate, the product of the reaction (Fig. 1) (Lacroute 1971). Yeast growing on a good nitrogen source, like ammonia, represses synthesis of proteins needed to utilize poor nitrogen sources (for review, see Cooper 1982; Magasanik 1992). Dal5p, a transporter normally devoted to the poor nitrogen source, allantoate, also recognizes the similar compound, ureidosuccinate (Turoscy and Cooper 1987), but on media containing ammonia, Dal5p is repressed. The negative element in this control system is Ure2p, which acts by inhibiting the positive transcription regulator, Gln3p (Fig. 1).

METHODS

Genetic methods and plasmid constructions. These were carried out as described previously (Wickner 1994; Masison and Wickner 1995). The phenotype of [URE3] strains can be assessed in two ways. We usually use uptake of ureidosuccinate (100 μg/ml) in the

Table 1. Early History of the Prion Concept

1732	Scrapie described in Britain
1936	Transmission from sheep to sheep by Cuille and Chelle (France)
1957	Zigas and Gajdusek describe kuru
1959	Hadlow points out similarity of pathology of kuru and scrapie
1963–1975	Gajdusek transmits kuru, CJD, GSS (including familial cases) to monkeys
1966	Alper shows UV-resistance of scrapie agent; suggests it has no nucleic acid
1967	Griffith suggests the prion model for scrapie (without the word prion)
1982	Prusiner purifies scrapie agent, finds one predominant protein component, PrP
1982	Prusiner coins the term prion "to denote a small *pro*teinaceous *in*fectious particle which is resistant to inactivation by most procedures that modify nucleic acids"
1985	Clones of PrP show it is a host-encoded protein (Weissmann and Prusiner; Chesebro)

presence of ammonia as nitrogen source (SD medium) in a strain blocked in aspartate transcarbamylase (*ura2*) as shown by growth of the strain in the absence of uracil. An alternative assay is based on the ability of a [URE3] strain to take up ureidosuccinate and secrete uracil, thereby allowing growth in a halo around the [URE3] strain of a lawn of a *ura2* strain.

Preparation of extracts and proteinase K digestion. Cells were lysed by agitation with glass beads, and unbroken cells were removed by a 10-second centrifugation at 12,000*g* (Masison and Wickner 1995). The extracts were centrifuged 15 minutes at 15,000*g* and the supernatant fraction was retained. Each reaction included 150 μg of protein in 60 μl. Of this, 8 μl was removed at t = 0 and added to sample buffer, and a second aliquot was incubated at 37°C for 25 minutes before addition of sample buffer. To the remaining 44 μl was added 1 μl of proteinase K (2 mg/ml). Aliquots of 8 μl were removed at the indicated times (Fig. 3), added to sample buffer (63 mM, Tris-HCl, pH 6.8, 2% SDS, 10% glycerol, 0.7 M 2-mercaptoethanol, 0.025% bromphenol blue, and 3 mM phenylmethyl sulfonyl fluoride) and placed on dry ice. Samples were boiled for 2 minutes, analyzed by electrophoresis on 15% polyacrylamide/SDS gels or 4–20% gradient gels, and probed with affinity-purified antibody to a GST-Ure2p fusion protein (Wickner 1994).

RESULTS AND DISCUSSION

Expected Properties of a Yeast Prion

We have proposed genetic criteria for a yeast prion (Wickner 1994). Since a prion is an infectious protein, it should, like other infectious elements of *S. cerevisiae*, be a non-Mendelian genetic element. The yeast

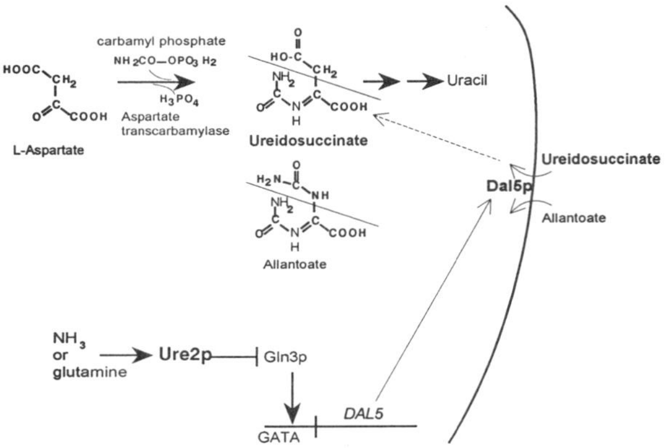

Figure 1. Role of Ure2p in the regulation of nitrogen metabolism. When supplied with a good nitrogen source, such as ammonia or glutamine, yeast shuts off synthesis of enzymes involved in utilization of poor nitrogen sources (for review, see Cooper 1982; Magasanik 1992). This shutoff is mediated in part by Ure2p blocking the action of Gln3p, a positive transcription factor for many of the regulated genes. Allantoate is a poor nitrogen source for yeast, and its permease (*DAL5*) is regulated by Ure2p. Allantoate is structurally similar to ureidosuccinate, the product of aspartate transcarbamylase in the uracil biosynthesis pathway, and so ureidosuccinate is taken up by the Dal5p permease (Turoscy and Cooper 1987). Thus, normal cells cannot take up ureidosuccinate if ammonia is present, but *ure2* mutants (and [URE3] strains) can do so.

dsRNA viruses and ssRNA replicons resemble the core particles of their mammalian homologs, lacking the outer shells needed for extracellular transit, but having a similar replicative apparatus. Yeast retroviruses (retrotransposons) lack the Env protein needed for extracellular particle formation, but have Gag and Gag-Pol and an intracellular replication cycle nearly identical to that of mammalian retroviruses. These infectious elements are nonetheless widespread among yeast strains. Whether because they cannot or need not leave and reenter cells (because the frequent mating of yeast cells in nature makes extracellular passage unnecessary), these yeast viruses use only the mating process to pass from cell to cell (for review, see Wickner 1996c). Similarly, a yeast prion should be a non-Mendelian genetic element. This is illustrated for [URE3] and [PSI] in Figure 2.

Reversible curability of yeast prions. Once cured, a nucleic acid replicon, such as mitochondrial DNA or the yeast dsRNA viruses, will not reappear unless introduced from another cell. In contrast, a prion can arise spontaneously, at some low frequency. The change of the normal form to the altered (prion) form is a stochastic process that can occur in the absence of any of the prion form, although its rate is dramatically stimulated by the prion form. Thus, even if the prion is cured by some treatment of the cells, and the cured strain is carefully purified and grown up, there should arise, among these cells, some that have spontaneously acquired the prion.

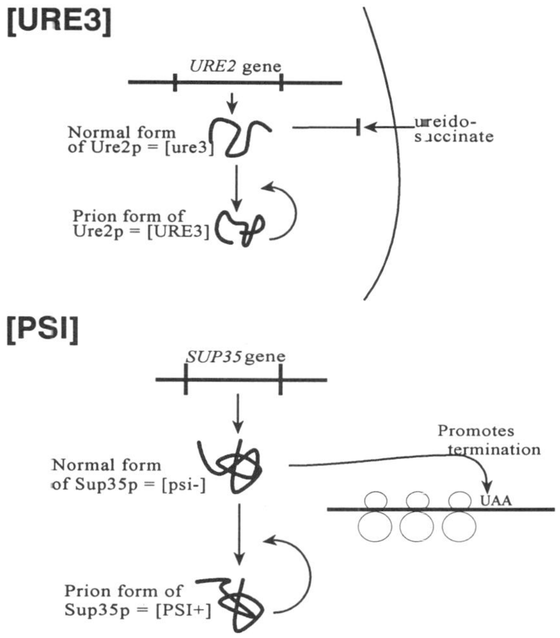

Figure 2. [URE3] and [PSI] as prions of Ure2p and Sup35p, respectively (Wickner 1994). The prion form of Ure2p (Sup35p) cannot carry out its normal function of blocking ureidosuccinate uptake (termination of translation), but it can catalyze the conversion of the normal form of the protein into this same altered form. Thus, the phenotype of *ure2* mutants is the same as that of [URE3] strains, because both lack the normal protein. The *ure2* mutants fail to propagate [URE3] because, without a new supply of Ure2p to convert to the prion form, the prion form is diluted out and lost. Similarly for [PSI] and Sup35p. Transmission of some of the prion form to a new cell results in conversion of the normal form in that cell to the prion form, thus transmitting the trait as a non-Mendelian genetic element.

Overproduction of the normal form induces appearance of the prion form. If there is more of the normal form present in the cell, then the stochastic process has more targets. Once one nidus of the prion change has arisen in a cell, the change should propagate throughout the cell, converting all of the normal form to the prion form.

Genetic relationship of the normal form gene to the prion. Prion propagation requires a steady supply of the normal form of the protein. Deletion of the normal form's gene should result in failure to propagate the prion, and such a mutation would show up in genetic analysis as a chromosomal gene needed for the propagation of the non-Mendelian element. Notably, either the presence of the prion form (a dominant trait) or mutation of the chromosomal gene results in the *same* phenotype, namely, the phenotype of the absence of an active gene product (Table 2). In contrast, the presence of a nucleic acid replicon such as mitDNA and chromosomal mutants in factors necessary for its propagation result in *opposite* phenotypes (ability and inability to grow on ethanol as a carbon source, in the case of mitochondrial DNA).

[URE3] Has the Genetic Properties of a Prion Form of Ure2p

[URE3] can be cured by growing cells on rich medium in the presence of 5 mM guanidine HCl (M. Aigle, cited in Cox et al. 1988; Wickner 1994). From such a cured strain, however, can be isolated [URE3] derivatives at a frequency of about 10^{-6} (Wickner 1994). We emphasize that it is not the curability of [URE3] by guanidine that points to its being a prion, because similar concentrations of guanidine block replication of poliovirus (Tamm and Eggers 1963). Rather, it is the *reversibility* of the curing, the reappearance of the genetic element after it has been cured, that is a predicted feature of prions.

Overexpression of the normal Ure2p, either from its own promoter on a high-copy plasmid, or from the strong *GAL1,10* promoter, leads to a 20- to 100-fold increase in the frequency with which [URE3] arises (Table 3) (Wickner 1994; Masison and Wickner 1995). As discussed below, certain deletion mutants of *URE2*, when overexpressed, produce even higher frequencies of [URE3] (Masison and Wickner 1995).

The product of the URE2 gene is necessary for the propagation of [URE3] (Table 4) (Aigle and Lacroute 1975; Wickner 1994), and yet *ure2* mutants and [URE3] strains have the *same* phenotype; namely, ability to take up ureidosuccinate in the presence of ammonia (and other phenotypes related to release of nitrogen catabolite repression) (Lacroute 1971; Drillien and Lacroute 1972; Drillien et al. 1973).

It is remarkable that simply introducing the Ure2p-overproducing plasmid into a cell results in the generation of the [URE3] genetic element (Wickner 1994;

Table 2. Relation of Prion to the Chromosomal Gene Encoding the Protein: How to Discover a Prion

Non-Mendelian element	Phenotype due to presence of the dominant element	Phenotype of maintenance gene mutant	Relation of A and B
mitDNA	growth on glycerol	no growth on glycerol	opposite
M dsRNA satellite	killer toxin made	no toxin made	opposite
Theoretical prion	defective	defective	same
[URE3]	nitrogen derepressed	nitrogen derepressed	same
[PSI]	ter readthrough	ter readthrough	same

Table 3. Overexpression of Ure2p Increases Frequency of [URE3]

Plasmid	C-source	[URE3]/ 10^6 cells	Fold
Experiment 1			
YEp351G	dextrose	7	1
YEp351G	galactose	30	4
YEp351G-URE2	dextrose	9	1
YEp351G-URE2	galactose	2101	233

Data from Wickner (1994).

Masison and Wickner 1995). Introduction of a plasmid overproducing one of several deletion mutants lacking part of the carboxy-terminal domain of Ure2p results in even more efficient induction of [URE3] (see below; Masison and Wickner 1995). The comparable experiments in scrapie are the overproduction of PrP from a transgene and overproduction of the P101L mutant of mouse PrP—homologous to a human mutation that produces GSS, one of the inherited forms of human prion disease (Hsiao et al. 1990; Westaway et al. 1994). In each case, a disease with some similarity to scrapie was produced, but only tiny amounts of infectivity were detected, on the order of 10^{-5} of the normal amount (Hsiao et al. 1994).

Protease Resistance of Ure2p in [URE3] Strains

The protease resistance of PrP^{Sc} compared to PrP^{C} was one of the early pieces of evidence pointing to PrP as the protein responsible for scrapie infectivity (Bolton et al. 1982; Oesch et al. 1985). We found tha Ure2p in extracts of [URE3] cells was resistant tc proteinase K compared to the same protein in extracts of isogenic wild-type cells (Fig. 3) (Masison and Wickner 1995). Cells cured of [URE3] had Ure2p which had recovered its protease sensitivity, and independent [URE3] isolates all had proteinase K-resistant Ure2p. These results indicate that there was some change in the Ure2p protein in [URE3] cells compared to the wild type. It is also clear from Figure 3 that the amount of Ure2p did not change as a result of the [URE3] change, a result that rules out some alternative models of [URE3].

Prion-inducing Domain of Ure2p: Interactions with Nitrogen-repression Domain

We expressed various parts of the *URE2* gene from a *GAL1,10* promoter and determined which parts of the gene were necessary to complement a deletion of the gene (*ure2*Δ) and which part was necessary, when overproduced in a wild-type strain, to stimulate the generation of [URE3] (Fig. 4) (Masison and Wickner 1995). We found that deletion of even a few residues from the carboxyl terminus results in loss of ability to complement the *ure2*Δ mutation, but induction of

Table 4. *URE2* Is Needed for Propagation of [URE3]

Manipulation	Chromosome	DNA plasmid	[ure] or [URE3]	Growth on ureidosuccinate
A. Starting strain→	*ure2*Δ	none	[ure3-o]	+
B. Transform with pURE2	*ure2*Δ	pURE2	[ure3-o]	–
C. Select [URE3]	*ure2*Δ	pURE2	[URE3]	+
D. Allow loss of pURE2	*ure2*Δ	none	????	+
E. Retransform with pURE2	*ure2*Δ	pURE2	[ure3-o]	–

Strain	Chromosomal *URE2* genotype	[URE3] isolate	Ure phenotype of D
3422	*ure2*Δ	[URE3]U1	–
	*ure2*Δ	[URE3]U2	–
	*ure2*Δ	[URE3]U2	–
	*ure2*Δ	[URE3]U4	–
3423	*ure2*Δ	[URE3]U2	–
	*ure2*Δ	[URE3]U3	–
3389	*URE2*	[URE3]U22	+
3389	*URE2*	[ure3]	–

The *ure2*Δ strains 3422 and 3423 were transformed with YEp351-URE2 to make them phenotypically Ure^- (unable to take up ureidosuccinate). [URE3] derivatives were then selected on SD+his+ureidosuccinate. Each purified [URE3] derivative was tested for stability by subcloning on the same medium, and each of 20 subclones were still Ure^+. After purification of the [URE3] clones, they were allowed to lose YEp351-URE2 by subcloning on YPAD. These Leu^- clones were purified on YPAD, YEp351-URE2 was then reintroduced, and four transformants from each original [URE3] isolate were purified and tested for the Ure phenotype. As controls, [URE3] and [ure3-o] derivatives of strain 3389 (*MAT***a** *kar1 ura2 leu2 his*$^-$ YEp351-URE2 [ure3-o]) carrying the same YEp351-URE2 were treated similarly starting at step B in the scheme above.

[URE3] is not only maintained, but increased about 100-fold (Fig. 4) (Masison and Wickner 1995). The same result is found for larger carboxy-terminal deletions, and deletion of all but the amino-terminal 65 amino acid residues leaves [URE3] induction at the same high level (Masison and Wickner 1995). In contrast, as previously reported (Coschigano and Magasanik 1991), the amino-terminal 65 residues are dispensable for complementation of a *ure2Δ* mutation. However, deletion of this amino-terminal region prevents the spontaneous [URE3] events from being observed (Fig. 4). We suggest that this amino-terminal domain is necessary *in cis* for a molecule to be recruited into the

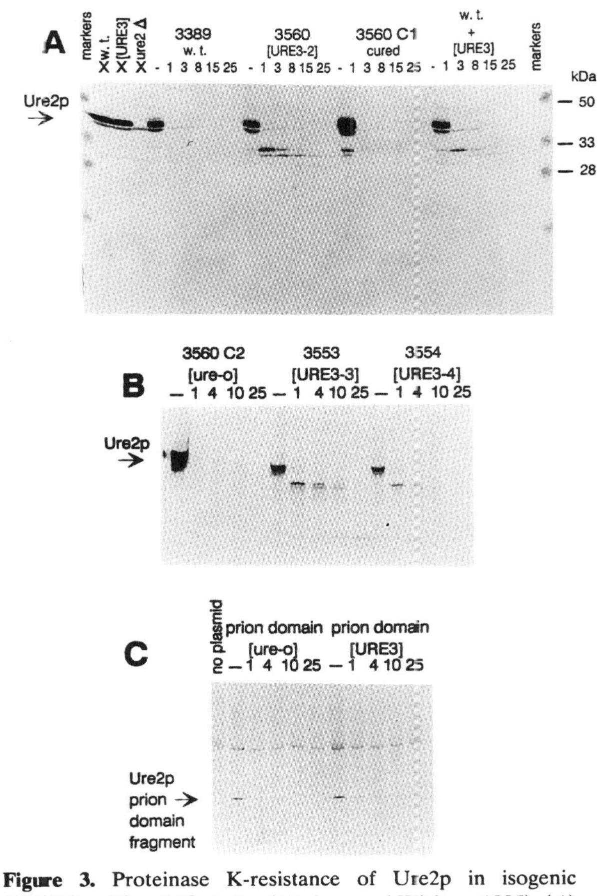

Figure 3. Proteinase K-resistance of Ure2p in isogenic [URE3] and [ure3-0] strains (Masison and Wickner 1995). (*A*) Comparison of wild-type strain 3389 ([ure-o]), [URE3] strain 3560, guanidine-cured [ure-o] strain 3560 C1 and a mixture of strains 3389 and 3560. Lanes marked X are samples removed at 0 time. Lanes marked "–" were incubated at 37°C for 25 min but without added proteinase K. Lanes labeled with a number were incubated with proteinase K for that many minutes at 37°C (see Methods). (*B*) Comparison of guanidine-cured strain 3560 C2 with two other independent [URE3] isolates from strain 3389, strains 3553 and 3554. (*C*) Comparison of protease sensitivity of the prion domain fragment (Ure2p residues 1–65) expressed from p680 in strain 44445-27D (MATα *leu2 ura2 trp1 pep4* [ure-o] and a [URE3] derivative.

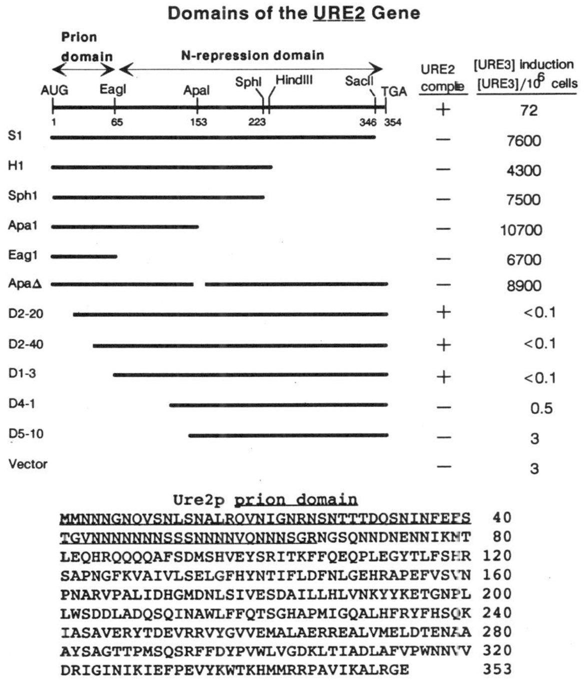

Figure 4. Prion-inducing domain of Ure2p. Deletion mutants of *URE2* were expressed from a *GAL1,10* promoter in a *ure2Δ* strain to assess complementation ability, or in a wild-type strain to measure ability to induce [URE3]. For the complementation test, ability to block growth of the *ura2 ure2Δ* host when ureidosuccinate is supplied in place of uracil (ammonia as nitrogen source) indicates ability to complement. For the [URE3] induction assay, overexpression is induced for 5 days on minimal medium with galactose and uracil and then plated on dextrose minimal medium with ureidosuccinate. The number of colonies able to grow on ureidosuccinate per 10^6 cells plated is shown. The solid bar indicates the part of the Ure2p expressed.

prion event. We refer to this amino-terminal 65-amino-acid residue domain of Ure2p as the prion-inducing domain. This part of the protein is 40% asparagine and is also rich in serine and threonine (Fig. 4).

Our results suggest that there is a specific interaction between the amino-terminal prion-inducing domain and the carboxy-terminal nitrogen regulation domain (Fig. 5). (1) The amino-terminal domain must be present for inactivation of the carboxy-terminal domain. (2) Deletion of the amino-terminal domain weakens the nitrogen regulation activity of the carboxy-terminal domain. (3) Deletion of the carboxy-terminal domain apparently destabilizes the amino-terminal domain, increasing the frequency of the prion change by about 100-fold. (4) Fusing the amino-terminal prion-inducing domain of Ure2p to lacZ did not make the β-galactosidase subject to inactivation in cells that had become [URE3], indicating that there is some specificity in what protein the prion domain will act on (Masison and Wickner 1995).

The involvement of the amino-terminal domain in

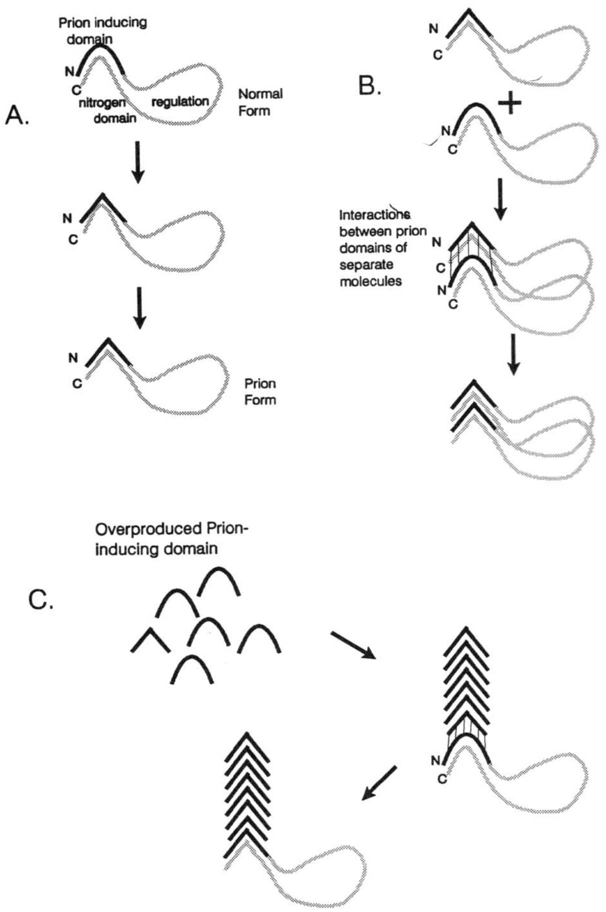

Figure 5. Model of [URE3] generation and propagation. Our data indicate that the amino-terminal 65 amino acid residues (the prion-inducing domain) is sufficient to induce [URE3] when overexpressed, and is necessary for the carboxy-terminal nitrogen regulatory domain to be inactivated by the [URE3] change (Fig. 3) (Masison and Wickner 1995). The prion-inducing domain has both a *trans* action in inducing [URE3] when overexpressed, and a *cis* action in being required for susceptibility of the carboxy-terminal part to the [URE3] change. We propose that the transmission of the prion effect is via this amino-terminal domain as shown here. A similar model can explain the transmission of [PSI] by the amino-terminal domain of Sup35p. In this case, aggregation of Sup35p specifically in [PSI]-containing strains has been demonstrated (Paushkin et al. 1996).

prion induction suggests that this part of the molecule should be altered when the cells acquire [URE3]. Indeed, we found that this domain was protease-resistant in cells that acquired [URE3] (Fig. 3C) (Masison and Wickner 1995).

[PSI] Has the Genetic Properties of a Prion Form of Sup35p

[PSI] can be efficiently cured by growth in high-osmotic-strength medium (Singh et al. 1979) or, like [URE3], by growth of cells on rich media containing 5 mM guanidine HCl (Tuite et al. 1981). Curing of [PSI] by either agent is, as for [URE3], reversible in the sense that [PSI]-containing derivatives can again be isolated from cured clones (Tuite et al. 1981; Chernoff et al. 1993).

Overexpression of Sup35p increases the frequency with which [PSI] arises about 100-fold over the background rate (Chernoff et al. 1993). The *SUP35* gene is required for the propagation of [PSI] (Ter-Avanesyan et al. 1994; Doel et al. 1994). The *sup35* mutants were first described as omnipotent suppressors, like [PSI] itself, able to promote the suppression of amber, opal, or ochre termination mutations (Mortimer and Hawthorne 1966; Hawthorne and Mortimer 1968). Sup35p is now known to be one of the two subunits of the translation termination release factor (Stansfield et al. 1995; Zhouravleva et al. 1995).

We reinterpreted these results to suggest that [PSI] is a prion, an altered form of Sup35p (Wickner 1994). The logical parallel between [URE3] and [PSI] is reflected in the symmetry between the two systems in Figure 2.

Prion-propagation Domain of Sup35p

The carboxy-terminal part of Sup35p is essential for cell growth, being the part that carries out the translation termination action with Sup45p (Fig. 6) (Kushnirov et al. 1988; Wilson and Culbertson 1988). Ter-Avanesyan and coworkers have tested various fragments of Sup35p for their ability to support the propagation of [PSI] in a strain with a carboxy-terminal domain expressed from the chromosomal copy of *SUP35*. They found that the amino-terminal 123 residues were sufficient for this activity (Fig. 6) (Ter-Avanesyan et al. 1994). Although the authors propose that "the Sup35p serves as a trans-acting factor required for the maintenance of [*psi*$^+$]" (Ter-Avanesyan et al. 1994), our prion model better explains the results.

Sup35p Is Aggregated and Partially Inactive in [PSI] Strains

Using the yeast in vitro translation system, Tuite et al. (1983) found that readthrough of termination codons by known suppressor tRNAs was efficient in extracts of [PSI$^+$] strains, but undetectable in extracts from [psi$^-$] strains. This was the expected result, because it corresponded with the in vivo phenotypes of [PSI$^+$] and [psi$^-$] strains. What was unexpected was that mixtures of extracts of [PSI$^+$] and [psi$^-$] cells showed the characteristics of the extract of the [psi$^-$] cells—[psi$^-$] was dominant in vitro even though [PSI$^+$] is dominant in vivo (Tuite et al. 1983). The factor in [psi$^-$] extracts blocking readthrough by [PSI$^+$] extracts was purified and found to be in the ribosome salt wash (Tuite et al. 1987), the same localization as defined by others for Sup35p (Eustice et al. 1986; Didichenko et al. 1991). This result was not explained satisfactorily

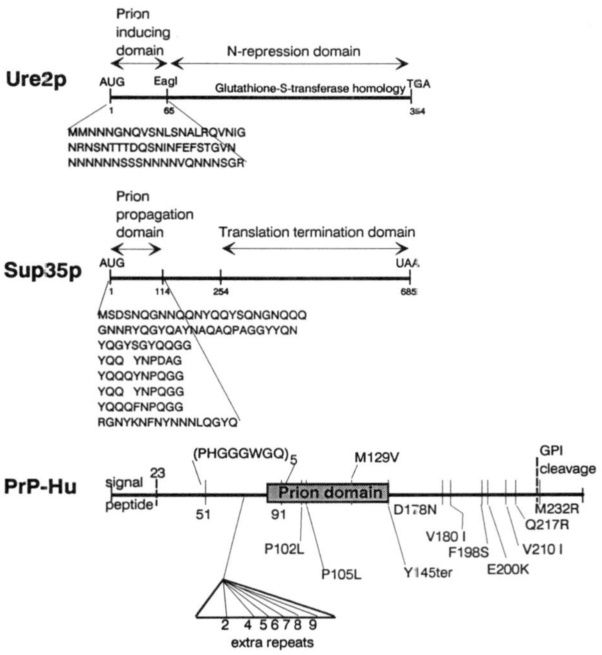

Figure 6. Comparison of Ure2p, Sup35p, and PrP. The prion-inducing domain of Ure2p is that part of the protein which when overproduced in a strain with a normal chromosomal *URE2* induces [URE3] formation. The prion propagation domain of Sup35p is necessary for prion propagation, but the carboxy-terminal part of the molecule is necessary for cell growth, and so cannot be separately tested for involvement in [PSI] propagation. The critical region of PrP has been delimited by an amber mutation at residue 145 (Kitamoto et al. 1993), which causes GSS, and amino-terminal truncations of residues 32–80 (Fischer et al. 1996), which restore susceptibility to *Prnp*$^{o/o}$ mice.

until our prion model for [PSI] (Wickner 1994) led us to reinterpret this result. We suggested that the [psi$^-$] extract contained excess Sup35p to act in translation termination, whereas the [PSI$^+$] extract contained only the inactive form (Fig. 7) (Wickner and Masison 1996). Thus, presence of the active form ([psi$^-$]) was dominant over the presence of the inactive prion form ([PSI$^+$]) in vitro, although in vivo, the prion form would convert the normal form into the prion form, so that [PSI$^+$] would be dominant.

Sup35p, in extracts of normal strains, sediments at the rate expected of a Sup35p-Sup45p heterodimer. In support of our prion hypothesis for [PSI], it has now been found that in extracts of a strain carrying [PSI], Sup35p is found as a rapidly sedimenting species (Paushkin et al. 1996). Paushkin et al. show that this aggregation is mediated via the amino-terminal domain that they previously showed was necessary for propagation of [PSI] (Paushkin et al. 1996). Thus, it appears that the aggregation of Sup35p is the [PSI] state. Sup35p is essential for cell growth, so it is likely that either the aggregated Sup35p is partially active or there remains a small amount of normal soluble Sup35p even in [PSI$^+$] cells.

Hsp104 Levels Are Critical to [PSI] Propagation

Either elevated expression of Hsp104 or deletion of the *HSP104* gene results in loss of [PSI] (Chernoff et al. 1995). The authors suggest that Hsp104 participates in the reaction of altered molecules of Sup35p with the normal molecules to alter the latter. Hsp104 is specifically needed for recovery of cells from heat shock but is otherwise dispensable. This heat-shock protein is capable of disaggregating and reactivating luciferase in vivo without affecting its turnover (Parsell et al. 1994). In light of their finding a correlation of aggregation of Sup35p with the presence of [PSI], Paushkin et al. suggest that high levels of Hsp104 eliminate [PSI] by completely disaggregating Sup35p, and normal levels of Hsp104 ensure inheritance (propagation) of [PSI] by preventing all of the aggregated Sup35p from being retained by one cell as a lump (Paushkin et al. 1996).

Comparison of Yeast "Prions" with Mammalian Spongiform Encephalopathies

One can compare the genetic criteria we proposed for yeast prions to what is known about PrP:

1. Reversible curing is not possible for mammalian prion diseases, but it is conceptually similar to the spontaneous occurrence of CJD. But is spontaneous CJD really spontaneous? Could it actually be due to somatic mutation or an unrecognized exposure? "Somatic mutation" cannot be the origin of [URE3] or [PSI] because the cured strain demonstrably has a normal *URE2* or *SUP35* gene, and cured strains regain the prion with the same frequency as the wild-type parent strain.
2. Remarkably, simply introduction of a plasmid overproducing the normal protein induces the prion states in yeast (Chernoff et al. 1993; Wickner 1994; Masison and Wickner 1995). However, the scrapie-like syndrome in mice resulting from overproduction of the normal or the GSS-like PrP are associated with almost no infectious material (Hsiao et al. 1990, 1994; Westaway et al. 1994). This is a puzzle.
3. Relation of phenotypes: The fact that the *ure2* mutants and [URE3] strains have the same phenotype, as do *sup35* mutants and [PSI] strains, serves both to help identify the chromosomal gene for the normal form (along with the requirement of the respective wild-type alleles for propagation of the prions), and also to support the idea that [URE3] and [PSI] are indeed prions. Although deletion of PrP produces little or no phenotype (Büeler et al. 1992), the P101L mice die of a scrapie-like syndrome (Hsiao et al. 1990), showing that it is dysfunction of PrP that produces the disease.

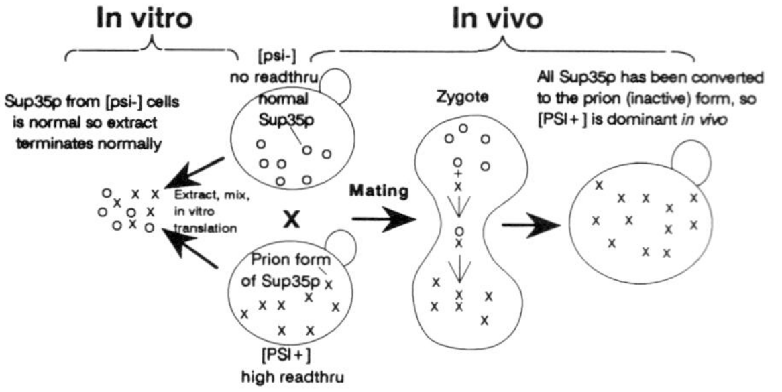

Figure 7. The prion hypothesis explains why [PSI+] is dominant in vivo, but [psi−] is dominant in in vitro protein synthesis (see text).

Overall, the genetic evidence for a prion is better for yeast, as all predictions are realized. However, the biochemical aspects have been far better studied for PrP. Most critical here is the need to purify Ure2p and Sup35p and to infect cells with the isolated material; this was the original basis for identification of PrP as the scrapie agent (Bolton et al. 1982; Diringer et al. 1983). Of course, demonstration of in vitro conversion of normal to prion form in a reaction dependent on prion form, such as has been shown by Caughey and Lansbury and coworkers for PrP (Kocisko et al. 1994, 1995; Bessen et al. 1995), would be strong support for the prion model.

Disease in [URE3] and [PSI] is produced by inactivation of the normal protein. In the case of PrP, recent work shows that the PrP^{Sc} positively gums up the works (Brandner et al. 1996). It is neither the absence of the normal form, PrP^{C}, nor the extracellular deposition of the altered form, PrP^{Sc}, that induces pathology (Brandner et al. 1996), but perhaps the PrP^{Sc} that has been recycled back into the cell (for review, see Caughey 1991) that has deleterious effects.

In yeast, other infectious elements can actually benefit the host. L-A is a dsRNA virus found in most yeast strains. A satellite of L-A, called M dsRNA, encodes a secreted protein toxin that can kill other strains not carrying M dsRNA (for review, see Wickner 1996a). Similarly, it is possible that wild-type yeast may find [PSI] or [URE3] useful under some conditions (other than the artificial conditions used to select them).

What Are the Genetic Properties Expected of a Non-PrP Human Prion Disease?

Our work broadens the prion concept and should encourage those who have been seeking evidence that other degenerative diseases follow the prion model. Among the expected characteristics of such diseases are:

1. Genetic (dominant) and spontaneous forms of the same disease
2. Onset generally late in life
3. Absence of an immune response
4. Increased gene dosage increases the probability of disease

CONCLUSIONS

Our work supports the prion concept with stronger genetic evidence than is yet available for the mammalian systems. As is often the case in yeast, the genetic work is well ahead of the biochemical aspects, and in this regard, yeast prions are not as well documented as are those of mammals.

We have shown that prions are not unique to one mammalian protein, but are a widespread phenomenon. We expect other prions to be found in many different systems, and the genetic criteria we have established for yeast may aid in this process.

Finally, we have shown that prions can be the basis for inheritance, as well as for infection. In yeast and other fungi, these are essentially the same thing, since yeast viruses are spread horizontally largely through mating and hyphal fusion. It is possible that some maternally inherited traits of higher organisms may be found to be based on prions.

REFERENCES

Aigle, M. and F. Lacroute. 1975. Genetical aspects of [URE3], a non-Mendelian, cytoplasmically inherited mutation in yeast. *Mol. Gen. Genet.* **136:** 327.

Alper, T., W.A. Cramp, D.A. Haig, and M.C. Clarke. 1967. Does the agent of scrapie replicate without nucleic acid? *Nature* **214:** 764.

Bessen, R. A., D.A. Kocisko, G.J. Raymond, S. Nandan, P.T. Landsbury, and B. Caughey. 1995. Non-genetic propagation of strain-specific properties of scrapie prion protein. *Nature* **375:** 698.

Bolton, D.C., M.P. McKinley, and S.B. Prusiner. 1982. Identification of a protein that purifies with the scrapie prion. *Science* **218:** 1309.

Brandner, S., S. Isenmann, A. Raeber, M. Fischer, A. Sailer, Y. Kobayashi, S. Marino, C. Weissmann, and A. Aguzzi. 1996. Normal host prion protein necessary for scrapie-induced neurotoxicity. *Nature* **379:** 339.

Büeler, H., M. Fischer, Y. Lang, H. Bluethmann, H.P. Lipp, S.J. DeArmond, S.B. Prusiner, M. Aguet, and C. Weissmann. 1992. Normal·development and behavior of mice lacking the neuronal cell-surface PrP protein. *Nature* **356:** 577.

Caughey, B. 1991. Cellular metabolism of normal and scrapie-associated forms of PrP. *Semin. Virol.* **2:** 189.

Chernoff, Y.O., I.L. Derkach, and S.G. Inge-Vechtomov. 1993. Multicopy SUP35 gene induces de-novo appearance of psi-like factors in the yeast *Saccharomyces cerevisiae. Curr. Genet.* **24:** 268.

Chernoff, Y.O., S.L. Lindquist, B.-I. Ono, S.G. Inge-Vechtomov, and S.W. Liebman. 1995. Role of the chaperone protein Hsp104 in propagation of the yeast prion-like factor [psi+]. *Science* **268:** 880.

Cooper, T.G. 1982. Nitrogen metabolism in *Saccharomyces cerevisiae.* In *The molecular biology of the yeast* Saccharomyces: *Metabolism and gene expression* (ed. J.N.

Strathern et al.), p. 39. Cold Spring Harbor Laboratory, Cold Spring Harbor, New york.

Coschigano, P.W. and B. Magasanik. 1991. The *URE2* gene product of *Saccharomyces cerevisiae* plays an important role in the cellular response to the nitrogen source and has homology to glutathione S-transferases. *Mol. Cell. Biol.* **11:** 822.

Cox, B.S. 1965. PSI, a cytoplasmic suppressor of super-suppressor in yeast. *Heredity* **20:** 505.

———. 1971. A recessive lethal super-suppressor mutation in yeast and other PSI phenomena. *Heredity* **26:** 211.

Cox, B.S., M.F. Tuite, and C.S. McLaughlin. 1988. The Psi factor of yeast: A problem in inheritance. *Yeast* **4:** 159.

Cummins, C.M., R.F. Gaber, M.R. Culbertson, R. Mann, and G.R. Fink. 1980. Frameshift suppression in *Saccharomyces cerevisiae*. III. Isolation and genetic properties of group III suppressors. *Genetics* **95:** 855.

Didichenko, S.A., M.D. TerAvanesyan, and V.N. Smirnov. 1991. Ribosome-bound EF-1 alpha-like protein of yeast *Saccharomyces cerevisiae*. *Eur. J. Biochem.* **198:** 705.

Diringer, H., H. Gelderblom, H. Hilmert, M. Ozel, C. Edelbluth, and R.H. Kimberlin. 1983. Scrapie infectivity, fibrils and low molecular weight protein. *Nature* **306:** 476.

Doel, S.M., S.J. McCready, C.R. Nierras, and B.S. Cox. 1994. The dominant *PNM2*⁻ mutation which eliminates the [PSI] factor of *Saccharomyces cerevisiae* is the result of a missense mutation in the *SUP35* gene. *Genetics* **137:** 659.

Drillien, R. and F. Lacroute. 1972. Ureidosuccinic acid uptake in yeast and some aspects of its regulation. *J. Bacteriol.* **109:** 203.

Drillien, R., M. Aigle, and F. Lacroute. 1973. Yeast mutants pleiotropically impaired in the regulation of the two glutamate dehydrogenases. *Biochem. Biophys. Res. Commun.* **53:** 367.

Eustice, D.C., L.P. Wakem, J.M. Wilhelm, and F. Sherman. 1986. Altered 40S ribosomal subunits in omnipotent suppressors of yeast. *J. Mol. Biol.* **188:** 207.

Fischer, M., T. Rulicke, A. Raeber, A. Sailer, M. Moser, B. Oesch, S. Brandner, A. Aguzzi, and C. Weissmann. 1996. Prion protein (PrP) with amino-terminal deletions restoring susceptibility of PrP knockout mice to scrapie. *EMBO J.* **15:** 1255.

Griffith, J.S. 1967. Self-replication and scrapie. *Nature* **215:** 1043.

Hawthorne, D.C. and R.K. Mortimer. 1968. Genetic mapping of nonsense suppressors in yeast. *Genetics* **60:** 735.

Hsiao, K.K., M. Scott, D. Foster, D.F. Groth, S.J. DeArmond, and S.B. Prusiner. 1990. Spontaneous neurodegeneration in transgenic mice with mutant prion protein of Gerstmann-Sträussler syndrome. *Science* **250:** 1587.

Hsiao, K.K., D. Groth, M. Scott, S.-L. Yang, H. Serban, D. Rapp, D. Foster, M. Torchia, S.J. DeArmond, and S.B. Prusiner. 1994. Serial transmission in rodents of neurodegeneration from transgenic mice expressing mutant prion protein. *Proc. Natl. Acad. Sci.* **91:** 9126.

Kitamoto, T., R. Iizuka, and J. Tateishi. 1993. An amber mutation of prion protein in Gerstmann-Sträussler syndrome with mutant PrP plaques. *Biochem. Biophys. Res. Commun.* **192:** 525.

Kocisko, D.A., S.A. Priola, G.J. Raymond, B. Chesebro, P.T. Landsbury, and B. Caughey. 1995. Species specificity in the cell-free conversion of prion protein to protease-resistant forms: A model for the scrapie species barrier. *Proc. Natl. Acad. Sci.* **92:** 3923.

Kocisko, D.A., J.H. Come, S.A. Priola, B. Chesebro, G.J. Raymond, P.T. Lansbury, and B. Caughey. 1994. Cell-free formation of protease-resistant prion protein. *Nature* **370:** 471.

Kushnirov, V.V., M.D. Ter-Avanesyan, M.V. Telckov, A.P. Surguchov, V.N. Smirnov, and S.G. Inge-Vechtomov. 1988. Nucleotide sequence of the *SUP2(SUP35)* gene of *Saccharomyces cerevisiae*. *Gene* **66:** 45.

Lacroute, F. 1971. Non-Mendelian mutation allowing ureidosuccinic acid uptake in yeast. *J. Bacteriol.* **106:** 519.

Leibman, S.W., J.W. Stewart, and F. Sherman. 1975. Serine substitutions caused by an ochre suppressor in yeast. *J. Mol. Biol.* **94:** 595.

Magasanik, B. 1992. Regulation of nitrogen utilization. In *The molecular and cellular biology of the yeast* Saccharomyces: *Gene expression* (ed. E.W. Jones et al.), p. 283. Cold Spring Harbor Laboratory Press, Cold Spring Harbor, New York.

Masison, D.C. and R.B. Wickner. 1995. Prion-inducing domain of yeast Ure2p and protease resistance of Ure2p in prion-containing cells. *Science* **270:** 93.

Mortimer, R.K. and D.C. Hawthorne. 1966. Genetic mapping in *Saccharomyces*. *Genetics* **53:** 165.

Oesch, B., D. Westaway, M. Wälchli, M.P. McKinley, S.B. Kent, R. Aebersold, R.A. Barry, P. Tempst, D.B. Teplow, L.E. Hood, S.B. Prusiner, and C. Weissmann. 1985. A cellular gene encodes scrapie PrP 27-30 protein. *Cell* **40:** 735.

Palmer E., J. Wilhelm, and F. Sherman. 1979. Phenotypic suppression of nonsense mutants in yeast by aminoglycoside antibiotics. *Nature* **277:** 148.

Parsell, D.A., A.S. Kowal, M.A. Singer, and S. Lindquist. 1994. Protein disaggregation mediated by heat-shock protein Hsp104. *Nature* **372:** 475.

Paushkin, S.V., V.V. Kushnirov, V.N. Smirnov, and M.D. Ter-Avanesyan. 1996. Propagation of the yeast prion-like [psi⁺] determinant is mediated by oligomerization of the *SUP35*-encoded polypeptide chain release factor. *EMBO J.* **15:** 3127.

Prusiner, S.B. 1982. Novel proteinaceous infectious particles cause scrapie. *Science* **216:** 136.

Singh, A.C., C. Helms, and F. Sherman. 1979. Mutation of the non-Mendelian suppressor [PSI] in yeast by hypertonic media. *Proc. Natl. Acad. Sci.* **76:** 1952.

Stansfield, I., K.M. Jones, V.V. Kushnirov, A.R. Dagkesamanskaya, A.I. Poznyakovski, S.V. Paushkin, C.R. Nierras, B.S. Cox, M.D. Ter-Avanesyan, and M.F. Tuite. 1995. The products of the *SUP45* (eRF1) and *SUP35* genes interact to mediate translation termination in *Saccharomyces cerevisiae*. *EMBO J.* **14:** 4365.

Tamm, I. and H.J. Eggers. 1963. Specific inhibition of replication of animal viruses. *Science* **142:** 24.

Ter-Avanesyan, A., A.R. Dagkesamanskaya, V.V. Kushnirov, and V.N. Smirnov. 1994. The *SUP35* omnipotent suppressor gene is involved in the maintenance of the non-Mendelian determinant [psi⁺] in the yeast *Saccharomyces cerevisiae*. *Genetics* **137:** 671.

Tuite, M.F., B.S. Cox, and C.S. McLaughlin. 1983. In vitro nonsense suppression in [psi⁺] and [psi⁻] cell-free lysates of *Saccharomyces cerevisiae*. *Proc. Natl. Acad. Sci.* **80:** 2824.

———. 1987. A ribosome-associated inhibitor of in vitro nonsense suppression in [psi⁻] strains of yeast. *FEBS Lett.* **225:** 205.

Tuite, M.F., C.R. Mundy, and B.S. Cox. 1981. Agents that cause a high frequency of genetic change from [psi⁺] to [psi⁻] in *Saccharomyces cerevisiae*. *Genetics* **98:** 691.

Turoscy, V. and T.G. Cooper. 1987. Ureidosuccinate is transported by the allantoate transport system in *Saccharomyces cerevisiae. J. Bacteriol.* **169:** 2598.

Waldron, C., B.S. Cox, N. Wills, R.F. Gesteland, P.W. Piper, D. Colby, and C. Guthrie. 1981. Yeast ochre suppressor SUQ5-o1 is an altered $tRNA^{ser}{}_{UCA}$. *Nucleic Acids Res.* **9:** 3077.

Westaway, D., S.J. DeArmond, J. Cayetano-Canlas, D. Groth, D. Foster, S.-L. Yang, M. Torchia, G.A. Carlson, and S.B. Prusiner. 1994. Degeneration of skeletal muscle, peripheral nerves, and the central nervous system in transgenic mice overexpressing wild-type prion proteins. *Cell* **76:** 117.

Wickner, R.B. 1994. Evidence for a prion analog in *S. cerevisiae*: The [URE3] non-Mendelian genetic element as an altered *URE2* protein. *Science* **264:** 566.

———. 1996a. Double-stranded RNA viruses of yeast. *Microbiol. Rev.* **60:** 250.

———. 1996b. Prions and RNA viruses of *Saccharomyces cerevisiae. Annu. Rev. Genet.* **30:** (in press).

———. 1996c. Viruses of yeasts, fungi and parasitic microorganisms. *Fields virology* (ed. B.N. Fields et al.), p. 557. Raven Press, New York.

Wickner, R.B. and D.C. Masison. 1996. Evidence for two prion diseases in yeast: [URE3] and [PSI]. *Curr. Top. Microbiol. Immunol.* **207:** 147.

Wilson, P.G. and M.R. Culbertson. 1988. *SUF12* suppressor protein of yeast: A fusion protein related to the EF-1 family of elongation factors. *J. Mol. Biol.* **199:** 559.

Zhouravleva, G., L. Frolova, X. LeGoff, R. LeGuellec, S. Inge-Vectomov, L. Kisselev, and M. Philippe. 1995. Termination of translation in eukaryotes is governed by two interacting polypeptide chain release factors, eRF1 and eRF3. *EMBO J.* **14:** 4065.

The Role of Presenilin 1 in the Genetics of Alzheimer's Disease

R.F. Clark,[1] M. Hutton,[2] C. Talbot,[1] M. Wragg,[1] C. Lendon,[1] F. Busfield,[1] S.W. Han,[1] J. Perez-Tur,[2] M. Adams,[3] R. Fuldner,[3] G. Roberts,[4] E. Karran,[4] J. Hardy,[2] and A. Goate[1]
[1]*Department of Psychiatry, Washington University School of Medicine, St. Louis, Missouri 63110;* [2]*Mayo Clinic, Jacksonville, Florida 32224;* [3]*The Institute for Genomic Research, Rockville, Maryland 20878;* [4]*Department of Molecular Neuropathology, SmithKline Beecham Pharmaceuticals, Essex, United Kingdom*

Many epidemiological surveys have been carried out to identify risk factors for AD. However, apart from advanced age and Down's syndrome, the only variable consistently found to have an effect is the presence of a positive family history of the disease (van Duijn et al. 1991). The most striking evidence suggesting the importance of genetic factors in the etiology of AD is the existence of pedigrees in which the disease segregates in a manner consistent with fully penetrant autosomal dominant transmission (Nee et al. 1983). The disease in these families is often referred to as familial Alzheimer's disease (FAD). However, most cases of AD do not appear to be familial and are classified as sporadic, although sporadic AD does not necessarily imply a nongenetic etiology. Two subsets of FAD have been recognized on the basis of age of onset: late onset (LOAD) with age of onset over 65 years and early onset (EOAD) with age of onset under 65 years.

The observation of AD neuropathology in all Down's syndrome individuals over the age of 30 years (Heston and Mastri 1977) led researchers to test for genetic linkage between AD and markers on the long arm of chromosome 21 (St. George-Hyslop et al. 1987). At about the same time, the gene encoding the β-amyloid precursor protein (βAPP) was cloned and localized to the same region of chromosome 21 (Goldgaber et al. 1987; Tanzi et al. 1987). Sequencing of the βAPP gene in FAD families showing evidence for linkage to chromosome 21 led to the identification of five point mutations that segregate with disease (Table 1) (Chartier-Harlin et al. 1991; Goate et al. 1991; Murrell et al. 1991; Hendriks et al. 1992; Mullan et al. 1992a). The first of these mutations to be described was the V717I mutation, which has subsequently been observed in eleven other families, strongly supporting the hypothesis that this mutation is pathogenic (Naruse et al. 1991; Yoshioka et al. 1991; Fidani et al. 1992; Karlinsky et al. 1992; Sorbi et al. 1993). The description of five other mutations, all in exons 16 and 17, supports the hypothesis that these mutations are pathogenic (Table 1). Two of the mutations are at the same codon as the first mutation, APP717, but change the valine to glycine or phenylalanine (Chartier-Harlin et al. 1991; Murrell et al. 1991). A double point mutation in exon 16 leads to the substitution of two consecutive amino acids, at codons 670 and 671 (Mullan et al. 1992a). All the families found with the APP717 and 670/671 mutations show the classic pathology of AD and have an early age of onset of disease, with age of onset for APP717 ranging from 39 to 55 years and for APP670/671 ranging from 45 to 61 years. Inheritance is dominant with complete penetrance by the early 60s.

The first mutation to be reported in the βAPP gene was a point mutation at APP693 that leads to a glutamine for glutamic acid substitution (Table 1). This mutation was reported in a family with a rare autosomal dominant disorder, hereditary cerebral hemorrhage with amyloidosis-Dutch type (HCHWA-D) (Levy et al. 1990). Patients with this disease die as a result of multiple cerebral hemorrhages in their 40s and 50s. Neuropathological examination has revealed the presence of large numbers of β-amyloid (Aβ) deposits in the cerebral blood vessels and diffuse plaques within the parenchyma. This disease could therefore be described as a vascular form of AD. A second family highlighting the link between these disorders was described by Hendriks et al. (1992). Four individuals have the symptoms of cerebral hemorrhage with onset around 40 years, whereas seven others present with presenile dementia at about 49 years of age. All affected individuals have an amino acid substitution at codon 692.

Two normal proteolytic pathways for βAPP have been identified. A constitutive secretory pathway (α-secretase) involves cleavage at Aβ amino acid 16 (Esch et al. 1990; Sisodia et al. 1990), an event that results in the release of a large soluble βAPP derivative and retention of an 8.7-kD membrane-bound peptide. This endoproteolytic cleavage destroys the Aβ peptide and thus cannot contribute to amyloid generation. A second proteolytic pathway leads to the generation of Aβ. The activities responsible for these processing events are termed β-secretase and γ-secretase.

The AD-causing mutations appear to flank the Aβ sequence, suggesting that they may interfere with the degradation of βAPP by modulating the β- and γ-secretase pathways, thus causing an increase in the concentration of amyloidogenic fragments. Fibroblast cultures from patients with the APP670/671 mutation secrete threefold more Aβ than control fibroblasts; this

Table 1. APP Mutations Associated with Disease

Exon	Codon	Mutation	Phenotype	# of families
16	670/671	KM/NL	AD	1
17	692	A→G	CH/AD	1
17	693	E→Q	CH	1
17	717	V→I	AD	11
17	717	V→G	AD	1
17	717	V→F	AD	1

increase in secretion was seen in cultures from both affected and presymptomatic carriers (Citron et al. 1994). In cells transfected with the APP717 mutation, the ratio of Aβ1-42 to Aβ1-40 is increased (Suzuki et al. 1994). Aβ1-42 forms amyloid fibrils more readily than Aβ1-40 and is thus postulated to be more pathogenic. It has therefore been hypothesized that βAPP mutations cause disease by modifying βAPP processing in a way that results in increased Aβ deposition. Further evidence in support of the hypothesis has recently come from the introduction of an APPV717F transgene into mice (Games et al. 1995). These mice develop an age-related neurodegeneration and deposit large amounts of Aβ peptide in their brains. The hypothesis also predicts that other mutations which lead to AD will be in genes involved in the regulation or processing of βAPP.

The second gene to be implicated in AD pathogenesis is apolipoprotein E (APOE). The protein is found bound to Aβ in cerebrospinal fluid and colocalizes to senile plaques and neurofibrillary tangles in AD brains (Namba et al. 1989; Strittmatter et al. 1993). The APOE gene is part of an apolipoprotein gene cluster at chromosome 19q13.2, a region previously implicated in LOAD through genetic linkage studies (Pericak-Vance et al. 1991). The relevance of APOE to LOAD was examined by genotyping patients from LOAD kindreds for APOE protein polymorphisms. In Caucasian controls, the allele frequencies for the ε2, ε3, and ε4 alleles are 0.08, 0.78, and 0.14, respectively. A strong allelic association between AD and the ε4 allele of APOE was reported in LOAD families with an increase in the ε4 allele to 0.52 (Strittmatter et al. 1993). The APOE ε4 association with AD has been confirmed in many studies of LOAD, including familial samples (Saunders et al. 1993), autopsy series (Rebeck et al. 1993), clinic-based cases (Poirier et al. 1993), and population-based studies (Mayeux et al. 1993). The association has also been reported in a number of different ethnic groups, including Japanese (Noguchi et al. 1993), African-Americans (Hendrie et al. 1995; Maestre et al. 1995), and Hispanics (Maestre et al. 1995). The ε4 allele also appears to act as a dose-dependent age-of-onset modifier (Corder et al. 1993). The highest risk is associated with the ε4/ε4 genotype, with intermediate risk associated with the ε3/ε4 genotype. In many studies, the ε2 allele frequency in AD patients is lower than controls, suggesting that ε2 may be protective against AD (Corder et al. 1994; Talbot et al. 1994).

In 1992, genetic linkage was reported between early-onset FAD and markers on the long arm of chromosome 14 (Schellenberg et al. 1992). This first report was quickly followed by three others confirming the observation (Mullan et al. 1992b; St. George-Hyslop et al. 1992; Van Broeckhoven et al. 1992). Linkage was first reported to D14S43 and localized to a region of about 23 cM between D14S52 and D14S53. The isolation of additional genetic markers led to the candidate region being narrowed to a distance of 6.4 cM between D14S289 and D14S61 (Cruts et al. 1995a). Complete yeast artificial chromosome (YAC) contigs were developed between these flanking markers (Clark et al. 1995a; Cruts et al. 1995a). A positional cloning strategy led, last year, to the identification of five missense mutations in a novel gene from this region in seven families multiply affected by EOAD (Sherrington et al. 1995). The gene, S182 or presenilin 1 (PS-1), appears to code for an integral membrane protein of 467 amino acids with 6–9 transmembrane (TM) domains.

RESULTS AND DISCUSSION

Mapping and Sequencing of the PS-1 Gene

Full-length cDNA clones for the PS-1 gene were isolated and sequenced. Analysis of the sequence revealed that it was identical in predicted amino acid sequence to that previously reported, with the exception of the absence of the amino acid sequence VRSQ at position 26-29. Identification of the intron-exon boundaries of the PS-1 gene showed that the coding region of PS-1 is encoded by 10 exons (Clark et al. 1995b) and that the presence or absence of these amino acids is due to the presence of two 5′ donor splice sites 12 bp apart at the 3′ end of exon 3. These alternative transcripts are expressed at approximately equal levels in all tissues analyzed. The functional significance of this alternative splicing is at present unknown. We developed sequence tagged sites (STSs) for the 5′ and 3′ UTRs and for exons within the PS-1 gene. These STSs were used to localize the PS-1 gene within our YAC contig of chromosome 14q24.3. The PS-1 gene maps just telomeric to D14S77 and is localized within a 75-kb region, oriented 5′–3′ centromere-telomere (Clark et al.1995b).

Mutations within the PS-1 Gene

Thirty-two different mutations have been found in more than 50 families, including families of Caucasian, Japanese, Ashkenazi-Jewish, and Hispanic origins (Table 2) (Campion et al. 1995; Clark et al. 1995b; Cruts et al. 1995b; Perez-Tur et al. 1995; Rogaev et al. 1995; Sherrington et al. 1995; Wasco et al. 1995; Boteva et al. 1996; Hutton et al. 1996; Rossor et al. 1996). The distribution of the mutations suggests clustering at TM2, encoded by exon 5, and the large hydrophilic loop, encoded by exons 8 and 9 (Hutton et al. 1996), that is likely to occur between TM6 and TM7. All of the mutations except one are missense mutations, suggesting that mutations in the PS-1 gene lead to a dysfunction, rather than loss of function, of the PS-1 protein. The one exception is a splice site mutation (Perez-Tur et al. 1995) that results in an amino acid substitution at codon 290 followed by the deletion of exon 9 and a protein that remains in frame until the normal stop codon.

Studies of the clinical and neuropathological features of PS-1 families show that AD in these families is severe. Onset can occur as early as 30 years of age, and disease duration is often shorter than observed in late-onset AD. The clinical features characteristic of AD in these families include prominent seizures, myoclonus, and paratonia, all features that usually occur later in the course of the disease in other forms of AD. For the most part, however, the clinical and neuropathological phenotypes of PS-1 families overlap those observed in other forms of AD. Inheritance is autosomal dominant and fully penetrant by the age of 50 in many families and by the late 50s in others. The mean age of onset of disease in PS-1 mutation families is generally earlier than in βAPP mutation families, but considerable overlap does exist (PS-1 range 33–60 years, βAPP range 43–62 years). When the same mutation is present in several families, the mean age of onset is very similar.

Linkage studies had suggested that this locus was the major cause of autosomal dominant early-onset FAD. Mutation analysis in families large enough for linkage studies supports this view; 50–70% carry PS-1 mutations. However, large-scale screening of EOAD cases with more limited family history, but still consistent with autosomal dominant inheritance, has yielded a much lower incidence of mutations (M. Wragg, unpubl.).

Table 2. Mutations in the Presenilin Genes Associated with AD

Exon	Codon	Mutation	No. of families	Mean onset (yrs)
PS-2				
5	141	N→1	1 (7)[a]	51
7	239	M→V	1	50
PS-1				
4	82	V→L	1	55
4	96	V→F	1	52.5
5	115	Y→H	1	36
5	120	E→K	1	36
5	139	M→V	2	41
		M→T	1	49
5	143	I→T	1	35
		I→F	1	55[b]
5	146	M→V	3	38
		M→L	2	43
			3[c]	40
6	163	H→R	4	47
		H→Y	1	47
7	213	I→T	1	45
7	231	A→T	1	51
7	246	A→E	1	53
	250	L→S	1	53
8	260	A→V	1	45
8	263	C→R	1	50
8	264	P→L	2	52
	267	P→S	1	35
8	269	R→G	1	47
8	269	R→H	1	51
8	280	E→A	1(7)[a]	47
8		E→G	2	42
8	285	A→V	1	55
8	286	L→V	1	48
8/9	290	S→Y [X9 spl out]		43
11	384	G→A	1	34
11	392	L→V	2	46
11	410	C→Y	2	49
11	436	P→S	1	52

[a]A founder effect was observed in the Volga German (NI41I) and Colombian families (E280A) carrying these mutations.
[b]One individual with this mutation is unaffected at age 68 years.
[c]Method of analysis did not distinguish between M→V/L.

Association between a Polymorphism in the PS-1 Gene and LOAD

As yet, PS-1 mutations have only been identified in families with EOAD. However, since some mutations result in a later age of onset, perhaps due to a milder effect on PS-1 function, it cannot be excluded that PS-1 mutations may also result in LOAD. Recently, using a biallelic polymorphism in intron 8 of the PS-1 gene, we observed an association between homozygosity for one allele of this PS-1 polymorphism and LOAD (Wragg et al. 1996). A statistically significant difference in both allele frequency ($p = 0.006$) and genotype distribution ($p = 0.007$) was observed between LOAD cases and controls in a Caucasian population (Table 3). The effect was due to a higher proportion of AD patients who were homozygous for the absence of the artificial *Bam*HI site (allele 1). Homozygosity of allele 1 in the PS-1 gene was associated with a doubling of risk for LOAD compared with 12 and 22 genotypes. The association between the PS-1 [11] genotype and AD was present and of similar magnitude for cases with onset above and below age 65 years. Furthermore, there was no evidence by linear regression analyses that PS-1 genotype predicted age of onset of dementia. Since our initial report of this study, three papers have replicated our observation and two others have been unable to

Table 3. PS-1 Genotype and Allele Frequencies

	Genotypes			Alleles		
	11	12	22	12/22	1	2
Controls	0.27	0.52	0.21	0.73	0.54	0.46
Cases	0.43	0.41	0.16[a]	0.57[b]	0.63	0.37[c]

Cases vs. controls, c2: [a]$p = 0.007$, [b]$p = 0.0017$ (odds ratio 1.97, 95% CI 1.29–3.00), and [c]$p = 0.006$.

replicate the observation (Bouras et al. 1996; Higuchi et al. 1996; Kehoe et al. 1996; Perez-Tur et al. 1996; Scott et al. 1996). The reasons for these discrepancies are not yet clear.

Presenilin 2, a Homolog of the PS-1 Gene

The presenilin 1 gene shows substantial homology with three expressed sequence tags (ESTs) in the public databases which were subsequently mapped to chromosome 1 (presenilin 2). At about the same time, genetic linkage was established in Volga German FAD kindreds between AD and markers on the distal long arm of chromosome 1 (Levy-Lahad et al. 1995a). Sequencing of the presenilin 2 (PS-2) cDNA from AD cases from these families led to the identification of a single point mutation that causes a substitution of N141I (Table 2) (Levy-Lahad et al. 1995b). A second missense mutation, M239V, has been found in an Italian FAD family (Rogaev et al. 1995).

Both presenilin proteins have roughly 450 amino acids and share an overall homology of 67%. The homology between PS-1 and PS-2 is particularly high over regions encoding the putative TM domains (Fig. 1). Indeed, all of the amino acids that cause AD when mutated in PS-1 or PS-2 are conserved (Fig. 1). The PS-2 gene may therefore encode a subunit isoform of PS-1, a different subunit of a protein complex, or a closely related protein.

Expression and Alternative Splicing of the Presenilin Genes

Both presenilin genes are ubiquitously expressed with alternative spliced forms identified in different tissues. Alternative splicing of exon 8 in PS-2 results in a shorter isoform that is more prominent in leukocytes than in brain (Rogaev et al. 1995). Since many of the PS-1 mutations are clustered in exon 8, and there is an association between an intronic polymorphism in intron 8 and LOAD, this domain may be of particular significance to the function or pathogenicity of the presenilins. A splice form of exon 3 of PS-1, which uses an alternate splice donor site, deletes the four amino acids VRSQ (Clark et al. 1995b). The functional significance of this is undetermined. Recently, another splice form of PS-1 was reported in liver, spleen, and kidney, where insertion of an additional 92-bp exon between exons 10 and 11 of the major brain transcripts results in a frameshift to produce a truncated PS-1 of 374 amino acids (Sahara et al. 1996).

Function of the Presenilins

It is, at this stage, premature to be definite about the role of the presenilins PS-1 and PS-2 and their relationship, if any, to the amyloidogenesis of AD. However, Younkin and colleagues (Scheuner et al. 1996) have reported an increase in the ratio of Aβ1-42:Aβ1-40 in the culture medium of fibroblasts and in plasma from chromosome 14 and chromosome 1 FAD cases. Such an observation is very similar to the effect of the APP717 mutations and may suggest an abnormality in the γ-secretase processing pathway.

The PS-1 protein (or a carboxyl fragment) has been immunologically localized to the amyloid plaques in patients with Aβ-related amyloidoses, including sporadic AD and PS-1-linked FAD patients (Wisniewski et al. 1995). Recently, the presenilin proteins have been localized in the endoplasmic reticulum and Golgi bodies in cells transfected in vitro with tagged presenilin constructs (Kovacs et al. 1996).

Recently, yet another function has been proposed for the presenilin protein using *Caenorhabditis elegans* as the model organism. In *C. elegans*, *lin-12* and *glp-1* genes are members of the Notch family of receptors. The Notch family of proteins mediates the specification of numerous cell fates during development and has been studied extensively in *Drosophila* and *C. elegans*. When Levitan and Greenwald screened for mutations in *C. elegans* that would suppress *lin-12* gain-of-function mutations, a new gene was identified (*sel-12*) that appears to function by facilitating, in receiving cells, the signaling mediated by *lin-12* and *glp-1* (Levitan and Greenwald 1995). This *sel-12* gene is remarkably homologous to PS-1 and PS-2 in humans, mice, and rats (Fig. 1) (50% amino acid identity between human PS-1 and SEL-12 over the length of the sequence). Furthermore, of the 30 known mutations in PS-1 or PS-2 that lead to EOAD, 24 alter amino acids that are identical in SEL-12 and human and mouse PS-1 and PS-2. This high degree of conservation suggests that the function of the SEL-12 and presenilin proteins may also be conserved.

In a recent study, using a "death-trap" assay to identify genes that protect against T-cell-receptor-induced apoptosis in a T-cell hybridoma, a mouse clone showing 98% homology with the carboxy-

```
1 Human PS-2 MLTFMASDSEEEVCD ERTSLMSAESPTPRS CQEGRQGPEDGENTA QWRSQENEEDGEEDP DRYVCSGVPGRPPGL EEELTLKYGAKHVIM    90
3 Mouse PS-1 -----MTEIPAPLSY FQNAQMSEDSHSSSA IRSQNDSQERQQQHD RQRLDNPEPISNGRP QS-NSRQVVEQDEEE DEELTLKYGAKHVIM    84
4 Rat PS-1   -----MTEIPAPLSY FQNAQMSEDSHSSS- VRSQNDNQERQQHHD RQRLDNPESISNGRP QSNFTRQVIEQDEEE DEELTLKYGAKHVIM    84
5 Human PS-1 -----MTELPAPLSY FQNAQMSEDNHLSNT VRSQNDNRERQEHND RRSLGHPEPLSNGRP QG-NSRQVVEQDEEE DEELTLKYGAKHVIM    84
6 SEL-12     --------------- -----------MPST RRQQEGGGADAETHT VYGTNLITNRNSQ-- ED----------ENV VEEAELKYGASHVIH    52

1 Human PS-2 LFVPVTLCMIVVVAT IKSVRFYTEKNG-QL IYTTFTEDTPSVGQR LLNSVLNTLIMISVI VVMTIFLVVLYKYRC YKFIHGWLIMSSLML   179
3 Mouse PS-1 LFVPVTLCMVVVVAT IKSVSFYTRKDG-QL IYTPFTEDTETVGQR ALHSILNAAIMISVI VIMTILLVVLYKYRC YKVIHAWLIISSLLL   173
4 Rat PS-1   LFVPVTLCMVVVVAT IKSVSFYTRKDG-QL IYTPFTEDTETVGQR ALHSILNAAIMISVI VVMTILLVVLYKYRC YKVIHAWLIVSSLLL   173
5 Human PS-1 LFVPVTLCMVVVVAT IKSVSFYTRKDG-QL IYTPFTEDTETVGQR ALHSILNAAIMISVI VVMTILLVVLYKYRC YKVIHAWLIISSLLL   173
6 SEL-12     LFVPVSLCMALVVFT MNTITFYSQNNGRHL LYTPFVRETDSIVEK GLMSLGNALVMLCVV VLMTVLLIVFYKYKF YKLIHGWLIVSSFLL   142

1 Human PS-2 LFLFTYIYLGEVLKT YNVAMDYPTLLLTVW NFGAVGMVCIHWKGP LVLQQAYLIMISALM ALVFIKYLPEWSAWV ILGAISVYDLVAVLC   269
3 Mouse PS-1 LFFFSFIYLGEVFKT YNVAVDYVTVALLIW NFGVVGMIAIHWKGP LRLQQAYLIMISALM ALVFIKYLPEWTAWL ILAVISVYDLVAVLC   263
4 Rat PS-1   LFFFSFIYLGEVFKT YNVAVDYITVALLIW NFGVVGMIAIHWKGP LRLQQAYLIMISALM ALVFIKYLPEWTAWL ILAVISVYDLVAVLC   263
5 Human PS-1 LFFFSFIYLGEVFKT YNVAVDYITVALLIW NFGVVGMISIHWKGP LRLQQAYLIMISALM ALVFIKYLPEWTAWL ILAVISVYDLVAVLC   263
6 SEL-12     LFLFTTIYVQEVLKS FDVSPSALLVLFGLG NYGVLGMMCIHWKGP LRLQQFYLITMSALM ALVFIKYLPEWTVWF VLFVISVWDLVAVLT   232

1 Human PS-2 PKGPLRMLVETAQER NEPIFPALIYSSAMV WTVGMAKLDPSSQGA LQLP------YDPEM EED--SYDSFGEP-- -SYPEVFEPPLTGYP   348
2 Mouse PS-2 --------------- --------------- --------------- --------------- --------------- ------------GYP     3
3 Mouse PS-1 PKGPLRMLVETAQER NETLFPALIYSSTMV WLVNMAEGDPEAQRR VPKNPK----YNTQR AER-ETQDSGSGNDD GGFSEEWEAQRDSHL   348
4 Rat PS-1   PKGPLRMLVETAQER NETLFPALIYSSTMV WLVNMAEGDPEAQRR VPKNPK----YSTQG TEREETQDTGTGSDD GGFSEEWEAQRDSHL   349
5 Human PS-1 PKGPLRMLVETAQER NETLFPALIYSSTMV WLVNMAEGDPEAQRR VSKNSK----YNAES TER-ESQDTVAENDD GGFSEEWEAQRDSHL   348
6 SEL-12     PKGPLRYLVETAQER NEPIFPALIYSSGVI YPYVLVTAVENTTDP REPTSSDSNTSTAFP GEASCSSETPKRPKV KRIPQKVQIESNTTA   322

1 Human PS-2 G-------------- ---EEL-------EE EEERGVKLGLGDFIF YSVLVGKAAATGSGD WNTTLACFVAILIGL CLTLLLLAVFKKALP   414
2 Mouse PS-2 G-------------- ---EEL-------EE EEERGVKLGLGDFIF YSVLVGKAAATGNGD WSTTLACFIAILIGL CLTLLLLAVFKKALP    69
3 Mouse PS-1 GPH-----RSTPESR AAVQELSGSILTSED PEERGVKLGLGDFIF YSVLVGKASATASGD WNTTIACFVAILIGL CLTLLLLAIFKKALP   433
4 Rat PS-1   GPH-----RSTPESR AAVQELSGSILTSED PEERGVKLGLGDFIF YSVLVGKASATASGD WNTTIACFVAILIGL CLTLLLLAIFKKALP   434
5 Human PS-1 GPH-----RSTPESR AAVQELSSSILAGED PEERGVKLGLGDFIF YSVLVGKASATASGD WNTTIACFVAILIGL CLTLLLLAIFKKALP   433
6 SEL-12     STTQNSGVRVERELA AERPTVQDANFHRHE EEERGVKLGLGDFIF YSVLLGKASSY--FD WNTTIACYVAILIGL CFTLVLLAVFKRALP   410

1 Human PS-2 ALPISITFGLIFYFS TDNLVRPFMDTLASH QLYI   448
2 Mouse PS-2 ALPISITFGLIFYFS TDNLVRPFMDTLASH QLYI   103
3 Mouse PS-1 ALPISITFGLVFYFA TDYLVQPFMDQLAFH QFYI   467
4 Rat PS-1   ALPISITFGLIFYFA TDYLVQPFMDQLAFH QFYI   468
5 Human PS-1 ALPISITFGLVFYFA TDYLVQPFMDQLAFH QFYI   467
6 SEL-12     ALPISIFSGLIFYFC TRWIITPFVIQVSQK CLLY   444
```

Figure 1. Alignment of the putative peptide sequences for the presenilin genes and SEL-12. Protein sequences (Levitan and Greenwald 1995; Levy-Lahad et al. 1995b; Sherrington et al. 1995) were aligned to maximize homology with BLAST. The SEL-12 sequence was amended using Genbank sequence U41540 (R. Wilson, pers. comm.). All known FAD mutations are to underlined amino acids (Campion et al. 1995; Cruts et al. 1995b; Clark et al. 1995b; Levy-Lahad et al. 1995b; Rogaev et al. 1995; Sherrington et al. 1995; Wasco et al. 1995; Boteva et al. 1996; Hutton et al. 1996; Rossor et al. 1996).

terminal 103 amino acids of human PS-2 was identified (Vito et al. 1996). Since it was not demonstrated that protein was actually expressed from this partial cDNA, it was not clear whether the protective effect was due to protein or RNA. Therefore, one can only speculate on what the function of the presenilins might be, with functions as a receptor, ligand channel, or membrane structural protein as good initial candidates.

SUMMARY

Approximately 75% of AD patients have an onset of the disease after the age of 60 years, and 60% of AD patients have no family history of the disease. Some cases of EOAD are clearly inherited in an autosomal-dominant manner. The βAPP gene on chromosome 21, the PS-1 gene on chromosome 14, and the PS-2 gene on chromosome 1 have all been characterized as genes in which mutations lead to familial EOAD. For LOAD, the work on ApoE indicates that the ε4 allele is a risk factor for developing AD. However, 35–50% of all AD patients do not have an ε4 allele. Other loci contributing to LOAD remain to be mapped and characterized. As in other complex disorders, these additional loci may involve genetic interactions with the known AD loci. Identification of all susceptibility loci for AD is a major goal in resolving the pathogenesis of AD.

ACKNOWLEDGMENTS

Work in A.G.'s laboratory is supported by a career development award from the National Institutes of Health (AG-00634), a Zenith Award from the Alzheimer's Association, and a grant from the Western-Southern Foundation. Work in J.H.'s laboratory was supported by National Institutes of Health project grants (AG-11871 and AG-12028) and the American

Health Assistance Foundation. The Metropolitan Life Foundation and SmithKline Beecham Advanced Technologies in Genetics provided support to A.G. and J.H. Human Genome Sciences and SmithKline Beecham Advanced Technologies in Genetics provided support to the Institute for Genomic Research.

REFERENCES

Boteva, K., M. Vitek, H. Mitsuda, H. de Silva, P.-T. Xu, G. Small, and J.R. Gilbert. 1996. Mutation analysis of presenilin 1 gene in Alzheimer's disease. *Lancet* **347**: 130.

Bouras, C., P. Giannakouplos, J. Shioi, N. Tezapsidis, and N. Robakis. 1996. Presenilin 1 polymorphism and Alzheimer's disease. *Lancet* **347:** 1185.

Campion, D., J.-M. Flaman, A. Brice, D. Hannequin, B. Dubois, C. Martin, V. Moreau, F. Charbonnier, O. Didierjean, S. Tardieu, C. Penet, M. Puel, F. Pasquier, F. Le Doze, G. Bellis, A. Calenda, R. Heilig, M. Martinez, J. Mallet, M. Bellis, F. Clerget-Darpoux, Y. Agid, and T. Frebourg. 1995. Mutations of the presenilin 1 gene in families with early-onset Alzheimer's disease. *Hum. Mol. Genet.* **4:** 2373.

Chartier-Harlin, M.-C., F. Crawford, H. Houlden, A. Warren, D. Hughes, L. Fidani, A. Goate, M. Rossor, P. Roques, J. Hardy, and M. Mullan. 1991. Early onset Alzheimer's disease caused by mutations at codon 717 of the β-amyloid precursor protein gene. *Nature* **353:** 844.

Citron, M., C. Vigo-Pelfrey, D.B. Teplow, C. Miller, D. Schenk, J. Johnston, B. Winblad, N. Venizelos, L. Lannfelt, D.J. Selkoe. 1994. Excessive production of amyloid beta-protein by peripheral cells of symptomatic and presymptomatic patients carrying the Swedish familial Alzheimer disease mutation. *Proc. Natl. Acad. Sci.* **91:** 11993.

Clark, R.F., M. Cruts, K. Korenblat, C. He, C. Talbot, C. Van Broeckhoven, and A. M. Goate. 1995a. A yeast artificial chromosome contig from human chromosome 14q24 spanning the Alzheimer's disease locus, AD3. *Hum. Mol. Genet.* **4:** 1347.

Clark, R.F., M. Hutton, R.A. Fuldner, S. Froelich, E. Karran, C. Talbot, R. Crook, C. Lendon, G. Prihar, C. He, K. Korenblat, A. Martinez, M. Wragg, F. Busfield, M. I. Behrens, A. Myers, J. Norton, J.C. Morris, N. Mehta, C. Pearson, S. Lincoln, M. Baker, K. Duff, C. Zehr, J. Perez-Tur, H. Houlden, A. Ruiz, J. Ossa, F. Lopera, M. Arcos, L. Madrigal, J. Collinge, C. Humphreys, T. Asworth, S. Sarner, N. Fox, R. Harvey, A. Kennedy, P. Roques, R.T. Cline, C.A.Philips, J.C. Venter, L. Forsell, K. Axelman, L. Lilius, J. Johnston, R. Cowburn, M. Viitanen, B. Winblad, K. Kosik, M. Haltia, M. Poyhonen, D. Dickson, D. Mann, D. Neary, J. Snowden, P. Lantos, L. Lannfelt, M. Rossor, G.W. Roberts, M.D. Adams, J. Hardy, and A.M. Goate. 1995b. The structure of the presenilin 1 (S182) gene and identification of six novel mutations in early onset AD families. *Nat. Genet.* **11:** 219.

Corder, E.H., A.M. Saunders, W.J. Strittmatter, D.E. Schmechel, P.C. Gaskell, G.W. Small, A.D. Roses, J.L. Haines, and M.A. Pericak-Vance. 1993. Gene dose of apolipoprotein E type 4 allele and the risk of Alzheimer's disease in late onset families. *Science* **261:** 921.

Corder, E.H., A.M. Saunders, N.J. Risch, W.J. Strittmatter, D.E. Schmechel, P.C. Gaskel, Jr., J.B. Rimmler, P.A. Locke, P.M. Conneally, K.E. Schmader, G.W. Small, A. D. Roses, J.L. Haines, and M.A. Pericak-Vance. 1994. Protective effect of apolipoprotein E type 2 allele for late onset Alzheimer disease. *Nat. Genet.* **7:** 180.

Cruts, M., H. Backhovens, J. Theuns, R.F. Clark, D. Le Paslier, J. Weissenbach, A.M. Goate, J.-J. Martin, and C. Van Broeckhoven. 1995a. Genetic and physical characterization of the early-onset Alzheimer's disease AD3 locus on chromosome 14q24.3. *Hum. Mol. Genet.* **4:** 1355.

Cruts, M., H. Backhovens, S.-Y. Wang, G. Van Gassen, J. Theuns, C. De Jonghe, A. Wehnert, J. De Voecht, G. De Winter, P. Cras, M. Bruyland, N. Datson, J. Weissenbach, J.T. den Dunnen, J-J. Martin, L. Hendriks, and C. Van Broeckhoven. 1995b. Molecular genetic analysis of familial early-onset Alzheimer's disease linked to chromosome 14q24.3. *Hum. Mol. Genet.* **4:** 2363.

Esch, F.S., P.S. Keim, E.C. Beattie, R.W. Blacher, A. Culwell, T. Oltersdorf, D. McClure, and P.J. Ward. 1990. Cleavage of amyloid beta peptide during constitutive processing of its precursor. *Science* **248:** 1122.

Fidani, L., K. Rooke, M.-C. Chartier-Harlin, D. Hughes, R. Tanzi, M. Mullan, P. Roques, M. Rossor, J. Hardy, and A.M. Goate. 1992. Screening for mutations in the open reading frame and promoter of the β-amyloid precursor protein gene in familial Alzheimer's disease: Identification of a further family with APP717 Val→ Ile. *Hum. Mol. Genet.* **1:** 165.

Games, D., D. Adams, R. Alessandrini, R. Barbour, P. Berthelette, C. Blackwell, T. Carr, J. Clemens, T. Donaldson, F. Gillespie, T. Guido, S. Hagopian, K. Johnson-Wood, K. Khan, M. Lee, P. Leibowitz, I. Lieberburg, S. Little, E. Masliah, M. Montoya-Zavala,. L. Mucke, L. Paganini, E. Penniman, M. Power, D. Schenk, P. Seubert, B. Snyder, F. Soriano, H. Tan, J. Vitale, S. Wadsworth, B. Wolozin, and J. Zhao. 1995. Alzheimer-type neuropathology in transgenic mice overexpressing V717F β-amyloid precursor protein. *Nature* **373:** 523.

Goate, A.M., M.-C. Chartier Harlin, M. Mullan, J. Brown, F. Crawford, L. Fidani, L. Giuffra, A. Haynes, N. Irving, L. James, R. Mant, P. Newton, K. Rooke, P. Roques, C. Talbot, M. Pericak-Vance, A. Roses, R. Williamson, M. Rossor, M. Owen, and J. Hardy. 1991. Segregation of a missense mutation in the amyloid precursor protein gene with familial Alzheimer's disease. *Nature* **349:** 704.

Goldgaber, D., M.I. Lerman, O.W. McBride, U. Saffiotti, and D.C. Gajdusek. 1987. Characterization and chromosomal localization of a cDNA encoding brain amyloid of Alzheimer's disease. *Science* **235:** 877.

Hendrie, H.C., K.S. Hall, S. Hui, F.W. Unverzagt, C.E. Yu, D.K. Lahiri, A. Sahota, M. Farlow, B. Musick, C.A. Class, A. Brashear, V. E. Burdine, B.O. Osuntokun, A.O. Ogunniyi, O. Gureje, O. Baiyewu, and G.D. Schellenberg. 1995. Apolipoprotein E genotypes and Alzheimer's disease in a community study of elderly African Americans. *Ann. Neurol.* **37:** 118.

Hendriks, L., C. van Duijn, P. Cras, M. Cruts, W. Van Hul, F. van Harskamp, A. Warren, M. McGinnis, S. Antonorakis, and C. Van Broeckhoven. 1992. Presenile dementia and cerebral haemorrhage linked to a mutation at codon 692 of the β-amyloid precursor protein gene. *Nat. Genet.* **1:** 218.

Heston, L. and A. Mastri. 1977. The genetics of Alzheimer's disease: Associations with hematologic malignancy and Down syndrome. *Arch. Gen. Psychiatry* **34:** 976.

Higuchi, S., T. Muramatsu, S. Matsushita, H. Arai, and H. Sasaki. 1996. Presenilin 1 polymorphism and Alzheimer's disease. *Lancet* **347:** 1185.

Hutton, M., F. Busfield, M. Wragg, R. Crook, J. Perez-Tur, R.F. Clark, G. Prihar, C. Talbot, H. Phillips, K. Wright, M. Baker, C. Lendon, K. Duff, A. Martinez, H. Houlden, J.C. Morris, N. Fox, R. Harvey, A. Kennedy, P. Roques, P. Lantos, A. Nichols, E. Karran, G. Roberts, J.C. Venter, M. Adams, R.T. Cline, C.A. Philips, R. Fuldner, M. Rossor, J. Hardy, and A.M. Goate. 1996. A complete analysis of the presenilin 1 gene in a series of families with Alzheimer's disease with a mean age of onset below 60 years: Identification of further mutations. *NeuroReport* **7:** 801.

Karlinsky, H., G.Vaula, J.L. Haines, J. Ridgley, C. Bergeron, M. Mortilla, R.G. Tupler, M.E. Percy, Y. Robitaille, N.E. Noldy, T. Yip, R.E. Tanzi, J.F. Gusella, R.Becker, J.M. Berg, D.R. Crapper-McLachlan, and P.H. St. George-Hyslop. 1992. Molecular and prospective phenotypic characterization of a pedigree with familial Alzheimer's disease and a missense mutation in codon 717 of the β-amyloid precursor protein gene. *Neurology* **42:** 1445.

Kehoe, P., J. Williams, S. Lovestone, G. Wilcock, and M. J. Owen. 1996. Presenilin 1 polymorphism and Alzheimer's disease. *Lancet* **347:** 1185.

Kovacs, D.M., H.J. Fausett, K.J. Page, T.-W. Kim, R.D. Moir, D.E. Merriam, R.D. Hollister, O.G. Hallmark, R. Mancini, K.M. Felsenstein, B.T. Hyman, R.E. Tanzi, and W. Wasco. 1996. Alzheimer-associated presenilins 1 and 2: Neuronal expression in brain and localization to intracellular membranes in mammalian cells. *Nat. Med.* **2:** 224.

Levitan, D. and I. Greenwald. 1995. Facilitation of *lin-12*-mediated signalling by *sel-12*, a *Caenorhabditis elegans* S182 Alzheimer's disease gene. *Nature* **377:** 351.

Levy, E., M.D. Carman, I.J. Fernandez Madrid, M.D. Power, I. Lieberburg, S.G. van Duinen, G.T. Bots, W. Luyendijk, and B. Frangione. 1990. Mutation of the Alzheimer's disease amyloid gene in hereditary cerebral hemorrhage, Dutch type. *Science* **248:** 1124.

Levy-Lahad, E., E.M. Wijsman, E. Nemens, L. Anderson, K.A.B. Goddard, J.L. Weber, T.D. Bird, and G.D. Schellenberg. 1995a. A familial Alzheimer's disease locus on chromosome 1. *Science* **269:** 970.

Levy-Lahad, E., W. Wasco, P. Poorkaj, D.M. Romano, J. Oshima, W.H. Pettingell, C. Yu, P.D. Jondro, S.D. Schmidt, K. Wang, A.C. Crowley, Y-H. Fu, S.Y. Guenette, D. Galas, E. Nemens, E.M. Wijsman, T.D. Bird, G.D. Schellenberg, and R.E.Tanzi. 1995b. Candidate gene for the chromosome 1 familial Alzheimer's disease locus. *Science* **269:** 973.

Maestre, G., R. Ottmann, Y. Stern, B. Gurland, M. Chun, M-X. Tang, M. Shelanski, B. Tycko, and R. Mayeux. 1995. Apolipoprotein E and Alzheimer's disease: Ethnic variation in genotypic risk. *Ann. Neurol.* **37:** 254.

Mayeux, R., Y. Stern, R. Ottman, T.K. Tatemichi, M. Tang, G. Maestre, C. Nagai, B. Tycko, and H. Ginsberg. 1993. The apolipoprotein epsilon 4 allele in patients with Alzheimer's disease. *Ann. Neurol.* **34:** 752.

Mullan, M., F. Crawford, K. Axelman, H. Houlden, L. Lilius, B. Winblad, and L. Lannfelt. 1992a. A pathogenic mutation for probable Alzheimer's disease in the APP gene at the N-terminus of β-amyloid. *Nat. Genet.* **1:** 345.

Mullan, M., H. Houlden, M. Windelspecht, L. Fidani, C. Lombardi, P. Diaz, M. Rossor, R. Crook, J. Hardy, K. Duff, and F. Crawford. 1992b. A locus for familial early-onset Alzheimer's disease on the long arm of chromosome 14, proximal to the a1-antichymotrypsin gene. *Nat. Genet.* **2:** 340.

Murrell, J., M. Farlow, B. Ghetti, and M. Benson. 1991. A mutation in the amyloid precursor protein associated with hereditary Alzheimer's disease. *Science* **254:** 97.

Namba, Y., M. Tomonaga, H. Kawasaki, E. Otomo, and K. Ikeda. 1989. Apolipoprotein E immunoreactivity in cerebral amyloid deposits and neurofibrillary tangles in Alzheimer's disease and kuru plaque amyloid in Creutzfeldt Jacob disease. *Brain Res.* **541:** 163.

Naruse, S., S. Igarashi, H. Kobayashi, K. Aoki, T. Inuzuka, K. Kaneko, T. Shimizu, K. Iihara, T. Kojima, T. Miyatake, and S. Tsuji. 1991. Mis-sense mutation Val→Ile in exon 17 of amyloid precursor protein gene in Japanese familial Alzheimer's disease. *Lancet* **337:** 978.

Nee, L.E., R.J. Polinsky, R. Eldridge, H. Weingartner, S. Smallberg, and M. Ebert. 1983. A family with histologically confirmed Alzheimer's disease. *Arch. Neurol.* **40:** 203.

Noguchi, S., K. Murakami, and N. Yamada. 1993. Apolipoprotein E genotype and Alzheimer's disease. *Lancet* **342:** 737.

Perez-Tur, J., F. Wavrantdevrieze, J. Lambert, and M.-C. Chartier-Harlin. 1996. Presenilin 1 polymorphism and Alzheimer's disease. *Lancet* **347:** 1560.

Perez-Tur, J., S. Froelich, G. Prihar, R. Crook, M. Baker, K. Duff, M. Wragg, F. Busfield, C. Lendon, R.F. Clark, P. Roques, R.A. Fuldner, J. Johnston, R. Cowburn, C. Forsell, K. Axelman, L. Lilius, H. Houlden, E. Karran, G.W. Roberts, M. Rossor, M.D. Adams, J. Hardy, A. Goate, L. Lannfelt, and M. Hutton. 1995. A mutation in Alzheimer's disease destroying a splice acceptor site in the presenilin-1 gene. *NeuroReport* **7:** 297.

Pericak-Vance, M.A., J. Bebout, P. Gaskell, L. Yamaoka, W. Hung, M. Alberts, A. Walker, R. Bartlett, C. Haynes, K. Welsh, and A. Roses. 1991. Genetic linkage studies in late onset familial Alzheimer's disease. *Am. J. Hum. Genet.* **48:** 1034.

Poirier, J., J. Davignon, D. Bouthillier, S. Kogan, P. Bertrand, and S. Gauthier. 1993. Apolipoprotein E polymorphism and Alzheimer's disease. *Lancet* **342:** 697.

Rebeck, G.W., J. Reiter, D. Strickland, and B. Hyman. 1993. Apolipoprotein E in sporadic Alzheimer's disease: Allelic variation and receptor interactions. *Neuron* **11:** 575.

Rogaev, E.I., R. Sherrington, E. Rogaeva, G. Levesque, M. Ikeda, Y. Liang, H. Chi, C. Lin, K. Holman, T. Tsuda, L. Mar, S. Sorbi, B. Nacmias, S. Placentini, L. Amaducci, I. Chumakov, D. Cohen, L. Lannfelt, P. Fraser, J. Rommens, and P.H. St. George-Hyslop. 1995. Familial Alzheimer's disease in kindreds with missense mutations in a gene on chromosome 1 related to the Alzheimer's disease type 3 gene. *Nature* **376:** 775.

Rossor, M., N. Fox, J. Beck, T. Campbell, and J. Collinge. 1996. Incomplete penetrance of FAD in a pedigree with a novel PS-1 gene mutation. *Lancet* **347:** 1560.

Sahara, N., Y. Yahagi, H. Takagi, T. Kondo, M. Okochi, M.Usami, T. Shirasawa, and H. Mori. 1996. Identification and characterization of presenilin I-467, I-463 and I-374. *FEBS Lett.* **381:** 7.

Saunders, A.M., W. Strittmatter, D. Schmechel, P. St. George-Hyslop, M. Pericak-Vance, S. Joo, B. Rosi, J. Gusella, D. Crapper-MacLachlan, M. Alberts, C. Hulette, B. Crain, D. Goldgaber, and A. Roses. 1993. Association of apolipoprotein E allele E4 with late-onset familial and sporadic Alzheimer's disease. *Neurology* **43:** 1467.

Schellenberg, G.D., T. Bird, E.Wijsman, H. Orr, L. Anderson, E. Nemens, J. White, L. Bonnycastle, J. Weber, M.

Alonso, H. Potter, L. Heston, and G. Martin. 1992. Genetic linkage evidence for a familial Alzheimer's disease locus on chromosome 14. *Science* **258:** 668.

Scheuner, D., C. Eckman, M. Jensen, X. Song, M. Citron, N. Suzuki, T. Bird, J. Hardy, M. Hutton, W. Kukull, L. Lannfelt, E. Larson, E. Levy-Lahad, E. Poskind, P. Poorkaj, G. Schellenberg, R. Tanzi, M. Viltanen, W. Wasco, D. Selkoe, and S. Younkin. 1996. The extracellular concentration of amyloid β-protein (Aβ) ending at Aβ42(43) is increased in vivo by the presenilin 1/2 and amyloid β-protein precursor mutations linked to familial Alzheimer's disease. *Nat. Med.* **2:** 1.

Scott, W., J. Growdon, A. Roses, J. Haines, and M. Pericak-Vance. 1996. Presenilin 1 polymorphism and Alzheimer's disease. *Lancet* **347:** 1186.

Sherrington, R., E. Rogaev, Y. Liang, E. Rogaeva, G. Levesque, M. Ikeda, H. Chi, C. Lin, K. Holman, T. Tsuda, L. Mar, J-F. Foncin, A. Bruni, M. Montesi, S. Sorbi, I. Rainero, L. Pinessi, L. Nee, I. Chumakov, D. Pollen, A. Brookes, P. Sanseau, R. Polinsky, W. Wasco, H. da Silva, J. Haines, M. Pericak-Vance, R. Tanzi, A. Roses, P. Fraser, J. Rommens, and P. St. George-Hyslop. 1995. Cloning of a gene bearing mis-sense mutations in early-onset familial Alzheimer's disease. *Nature* **375:** 754.

Sisodia, S., E. Koo, K. Beyreuther, A. Unterbeck, and D. Price. 1990. Evidence that beta-amyloid protein in Alzheimer's disease is not derived by normal processing. *Science* **248:** 492.

Sorbi, S., B. Nacmias, P. Forleo, S. Piacentini, and L. Amaducci. 1993. APP717 and Alzheimer's disease in Italy. *Nat. Genet.* **4:** 10.

St. George-Hyslop, P.H., R.E. Tanzi, R. Polinsky, J. Haines, L. Nee, P. Watkins, R. Myers, R. Feldman, D. Pollen, D. Drachman, J. Growdon, A. Bruni, J.-F. Foncin, D. Salmon, P. Frommelt, L. Amaducci, S. Sorbi, S. Piacantini, G. Stewart, W. Hobbes, P.M. Conneally, and J. Gusella. 1987. The genetic defect causing familial Alzheimer's disease maps on chromosome 21. *Science* **235:** 885.

St. George-Hyslop, P., J. Haines, E. Rogaev, M. Mortilla, G. Vaula, M. Pericak-Vance, J.-F. Foncin, M. Montesi, A. Bruni, S. Sorbi, I. Rainero, L. Pinessi, D. Pollen, R. Polinsky, L. Nee, J. Kennedy, F. Macciardi, E. Rogaeva, Y. Liang, N. Alexandrova, W. Lukiw, K. Schlumpf, R. Tanzi, T. Tsuda, L. Farrer, J.-M. Cantu, R. Duara, L. Amaducci, L. Bergamini, J. Gusella, A. Roses, and D. Crapper-McLachlan. 1992. Genetic evidence for a novel familial Alzheimer's disease locus on chromosome 14. *Nat. Genet.* **2:** 330.

Strittmatter, W.J., A. Saunders, D. Schmechel, M. Pericak-Vance, J. Enghild, G. Salvesen, and A. Roses. 1993. High-avidity binding to β-amyloid and increased frequency of type 4 allele in late-onset familial Alzheimer disease. *Proc. Natl. Acad. Sci.* **90:** 1977.

Suzuki, N., T. Cheung, X-D. Cai, A. Odaka, L. Otvos, C. Eckman, T. Golde, and S. Younkin. 1994. An increased percentage of long amyloid β protein secreted by familial amyloid β protein precursor (βAPP717) mutants. *Science* **264:** 1336.

Talbot, C., C. Lendon, N. Craddock, S. Shears, J.C. Morris, and A. Goate. 1994. Protection against Alzheimer's disease with apoE epsilon 2. *Lancet* **343:** 1432.

Tanzi, R.E., J. Gusella, P. Watkins, G. Bruns, P. St. George-Hyslop, M. Van Keuren, D. Patterson, S. Pagan, D. Kurnit, and R. Neve. 1987. Amyloid beta protein gene: cDNA, mRNA distribution, and genetic linkage near the Alzheimer locus. *Science* **235:** 880.

Van Broeckhoven, C., H. Backhovens, M. Cruts, G. De Winter, M. Bruyland, P. Cras, and J.-J. Martin. 1992. Mapping of a gene predisposing to early-onset Alzheimer's disease to chromosome 14q24.3. *Nat. Genet.* **2:** 335.

van Duijn, C.M., D. Clayton, V. Chandra, L. Fratiglioni, A. Graves, A. Heyman, A. Jorm, E. Kokmen, K. Kondo, J. Mortimer, W. Rocca, S. Shalat, H. Soininen, and A. Hofman. 1991. Familial aggregation of Alzheimer's disease and related disorders: A collaborative re-analysis of case-control studies. *Int. J. Epidemiol.* (suppl. 2) **20:** S13.

Vito, P., E. Lacana, and L. D'Adamio. 1996. Interfering with apoptosis: Ca^{2+}-binding protein ALG-2 and Alzheimer's disease gene ALG-3. *Science* **271:** 521.

Wasco, W., W. Pettingell, P. Jondro, S. Schmidt, S. Gurubhagavatula, L. Rodes, T. DiBlasi, D. Romano, S. Guenette, D. Kovacs, J. Growdon, and R. Tanzi. 1995. Familial Alzheimer's chromosome 14 mutations. *Nat. Med.* **1:** 848.

Wisniewski, T., J. Palha, J. Ghiso, and B. Frangione. 1995. S182 protein in Alzheimer's disease neuritic plaques. *Lancet* **346:** 1366.

Wragg, M., M. Hutton, C. Talbot, F. Busfield, S.W. Han, C. Lendon, R.F. Clark, J.C. Morris, D. Edwards, E. Pfeiffer, R. Crook, G. Prihar, H. Phillips, M. Baker, M. Rossor, H. Houlden, E. Karran, G. Roberts, N. Craddock, A. Goate, and J. Hardy. 1996. Genetic association between intronic polymorphism in presenilin-1 gene and late-onset Alzheimer's disease. *Lancet* **347:** 509.

Yoshioka, K, T. Miki, T. Katsuya, T. Ogihara, and Y. Sakaki. 1991. The 717Val→Ile substitution in amyloid precursor protein is associated with familial Alzheimer's disease regardless of ethnic groups. *Biochem. Biophys. Res. Commun.* **178:** 1141.

Two Homologous Genes Causing Early-onset Familial Alzheimer's Disease

P.H. St. George-Hyslop,[1] G. Levesque,[1] L. Levesque,[1] J. Rommens,[2] D. Westaway,[1] and P.E. Fraser[1]
[1]Department of Medicine (Division of Neurology), University of Toronto; Department of Medicine (Division of Neurology), The Toronto Hospital; The Centre for Research in Neurodegenerative Diseases, University of Toronto Toronto, Ontario, Canada, M5S 3H2; [2]Department of Molecular and Medical Genetics, University of Toronto, Department of Genetics, The Hospital for Sick Children, Toronto, Ontario, Canada

The etiology of Alzheimer's disease (AD) is unarguably complex. Genetic studies early on had indicated that even among the apparently familial cases of AD, more than one genetic etiology must exist (St. George-Hyslop et al. 1991). Nevertheless, recent application of molecular genetic strategies has led to the identification of four different genes associated with inherited susceptibility to AD.

The first of these genes, the β-amyloid precursor protein (βAPP) gene, was identified from several intersecting lines of evidence. The first of these lines of evidence was the cloning and mapping to chromosome 21 of the gene that encodes the precursor of a 40- to 42-amino acid β-peptide (Aβ), which forms a principal component of the amyloid plaque, one of the neuropathological hallmarks of AD (Goldgaber et al. 1987; Kang et al. 1987; Robakis et al. 1988). Second, patients with Down's syndrome (trisomy 21) almost invariably develop the neuropathological hallmarks of AD by the age of 40 years (Mann et al. 1984, 1989). Third, several pedigrees multiply affected with early-onset AD had shown suggestive evidence for linkage to genetic markers on chromosome 21 near the βAPP gene (St. George-Hyslop et al. 1987; Goate et al. 1989). Finally, mutations within the βAPP gene had been discovered in another disease (hereditary cerebral hemorrhage with amyloidosis-Dutch type) which is characterized by profound β-peptide deposition in cerebral blood vessels (Levy et al. 1990). These converging lines of evidence strongly suggested that the βAPP gene might be the site of mutations in some cases of familial AD. Sequencing studies subsequently confirmed that a small proportion of pedigrees were indeed associated with a cluster of mutations at the amino terminus, in the center, or at the carboxyl terminus of the β-peptide domain encoded in exons 16 and 17 of the βAPP gene (Chartier-Harlin et al. 1991; Goate et al. 1991; Murrell et al. 1991; Hendricks et al. 1992; Karlinsky et al. 1992; Mullan et al. 1992). These mutations are thought to alter the processing of the βAPP precursor, thereby augmenting the production of various different β-peptide derivatives, but especially the longer isoforms ending at residue 42 of the β-peptide (Cai et al. 1992; Citron et al. 1992; Haass et al. 1994; Suzuki et al. 1994; Tamaoka et al. 1994).

Shortly after the discovery of these mutations, it became clear that mutations in βAPP were a relatively infrequent cause of AD (only ~20 pedigrees have been identified to date). A genome search in the non-βAPP pedigrees was undertaken and led to the discovery of suggestive linkage at a cluster of genetic markers on chromosome 19q13 (Pericak-Vance et al. 1991). Subsequently, Strittmater et al., while searching for proteins in the cerebrospinal fluid (CSF) that were capable of binding the β-peptide, isolated apolipoprotein E (ApoE) and noted that ApoE was encoded on chromosome 19q13 (Strittmatter et al. 1993, 1994a,b). Although it was already known that ApoE was deposited in amyloid plaques of AD (Wisniewski and Frangione 1992), the importance of ApoE to the pathogenesis of AD became clear when the group of Roses et al. made the observation that the ε4 allele of ApoE (Cys112Arg) was associated with a dose-dependent increase in risk and a reduction in age of onset of AD. Significantly, the association between the ε4 allele of ApoE and AD held not only for familially aggregated cases as would be expected, but also for apparently sporadic forms of the disease (Saunders et al. 1993). In addition, less robust evidence suggests that the ε2 allele may have a protective effect against AD and may promote longevity (Corder et al. 1993, 1994). The mechanisms by which various alleles of the ApoE gene lead to increased or decreased risk of AD remains unclear. It has been suggested that the ε4 allele might bind the β-peptide more easily. Alternatively, the ε3 allele might bind microtubule-associated proteins such as τ, thereby protecting them from hyperphosphorylation (which is thought to be important in the conversion of τ into the paired helical filament structures in neurofibrillary tangles). It has also been suggested that the β-peptide and ApoE may compete for clearance through the LDL receptor protein (also known as the α2 macroglobulin receptor). Finally, the effect of various ApoE alleles might be conferred through a differential effect on response to repair and regeneration after selected types of neuronal injury. Although the ApoE association accounts for a significant proportion of the risk for sporadic and familially clustered late-onset AD, it is important to note that not all subjects who are homozygous for the ε4 allele necessarily develop AD, thus indicating that other factors are likely to be necessary for the development of

AD in ε4 carriers. Conversely, there is a significant proportion of cases where no ε4 is present, indicating that ε4 is not a necessary condition for AD.

One particular subset of cases that were not explained by the ε4 allele of ApoE or by missense mutations in the βAPP gene were a group of pedigrees segregating a very aggressive early-onset form of autosomal dominant AD (Goudsmit et al. 1981; Nee et al. 1983; Foncin et al. 1985; Frommelt et al. 1991; Pollen 1993). Genetic linkage studies mapped the locus associated with this AD3 subtype to chromosome 14q24.3 (Schellenberg et al. 1992; St. George-Hyslop et al. 1992; Van Broeckhoven et al. 1992). The obvious candidate genes on chromosome 14 were rapidly excluded either by virtue of their location outside the obligate recombinational boundaries defined by the genetic linkage studies, or because sequencing of their open reading frame failed to discover any mutations in subjects with the AD3 phenotype (Rogaev et al. 1993; Wong et al. 1993). Consequently, a positional cloning strategy was undertaken. These studies led to the identification of a novel gene, presenilin 1 (PS1) (Sherrington et al. 1995). The open reading frame for PS1 suggested that it would encode 467 amino acids and would be organized into several hydrophobic domains, implying that the PS1 protein is likely to be a multispanning transmembrane (TM) protein. The PS1 protein is also predicted to have highly acidic hydrophilic domains at the amino terminus and between the putative sixth and seventh TM domains. Mutational analysis of the open reading frame of this gene has led to the discovery of at least 25 different missense mutations, including one which arises from a splice site mutation causing the exclusion of exon 10 and the in-frame fusion of exon 9 to exon 11 (Campion et al. 1995; Cruts et al. 1995; The Alzheimer's Disease Collaborative Group 1995; Van Broeckhoven 1995; Sato et al. 1996; S. Froelich et al.; R. Sherrington et al.; both in prep.).

During the cloning of the PS1 gene on chromosome 14, a highly similar but not quite identical sequence was identified in an expressed sequenced tag site (EST) in the public nucleotide sequence database (Rogaev et al. 1995). The exact significance of this similar sequence was not immediately apparent, because it could have been a sequencing artifact, a pseudogene, or a homologous gene. Consequently, after we had completed the sequencing and analysis of the chromosome 14 PS1 gene, we returned to this EST and were able to establish that it was part of a spliced transcript, contained a long open reading frame, had a different pattern of transcription compared to PS1, and encoded a putative polypeptide that had overall a 67% amino acid sequence identity and an almost identical predicted structure (Rogaev et al. 1995). The principal differences between the two genes were in the predicted amino acid sequences of the hydrophilic amino terminus and the loop domain between TM6 and TM7. Once again, mutation screening identified the presence of two different missense mutations (Levy-Lahad et al. 1995; Rogaev et al. 1995). This gene, which was termed presenilin 2 (PS2), was mapped to chromosome 1.

METHODS

Ascertainment of the genomic structure. Genomic clones corresponding to the human PS1 gene were obtained by screening of the total human genomic DNA CEPH YAC library, the Los Alamos National Laboratory human chromosome-14-specific cosmid library, and the Roswell Park Cancer Institute human PAC total human genomic DNA libraries as described previously (Rogaev et al. 1996). A series of genomic subclones were obtained, and these in turn were reiteratively screened with fragments of the PS1 cDNA in order to identify progressively smaller subclones containing single exons. These small subclones containing single exons were then sequenced to determine flanking in intronic sequences as well as the intron-exon boundaries for each exon (Rogaev et al. 1996).

Isolation of the PS2 cDNA. During the isolation of cDNA fragments using a direct cDNA selection method with immobilized chromosome 14 genomic DNA clones as the trapping target, we isolated a cDNA subclone (cDNAY-788-170) that turned out to be a part of the PS1 cDNA. When the nucleotide sequence of this PS1 subclone was used to investigate the EST and the other nucleotide sequence databases, a similar but not identical sequence was retrieved (initially T03796 and subsequently R14600 and R05907). These sequences showed sufficient similarities to the PS1 gene to raise the question as to whether the sequence was partially in error or whether the second sequence reflected a homolog or a pseudogene. Consequently, as indicated earlier, after we had completed the analysis of the PS1 gene, we returned to investigate these issues by creating a series of oligonucleotide primers corresponding to the sequences from these ESTs and used these to generate probes to screen cDNA libraries. These initial smaller clones were then hybridized to Southern blots of restricted genomic DNA, Northern blots, and additional cDNA libraries in order to respectively provide evidence for intron-exon boundaries and transcription in brain, and to identify full-length transcripts (Rogaev et al. 1995).

Generation of anti-presenilin antibodies. To generate antibodies with which to investigate the subcellular distribution and trafficking of the presenilin proteins, we constructed GST-fusion proteins as well as short synthetic peptides to various regions of the PS1 and PS2 protein sequences that were predicted to be particularly antigenic. These proteins were then used to immunize rabbits and mice as described previously (L. Levesque et al., in prep.). A series of antibodies were therefore generated which identified peptide sequences at the amino terminus (TOR1142), in the hydrophilic loop between TM1 and TM2 (TOR519), or in the hydrophilic loop domain between TM6 and TM7 (TOR520, CDGN7, TOR1143). Additional amino-terminal antibodies were obtained from S.E. Gandy (14.2), and carboxy-terminal antibodies from D.J. Selkoe (BOS4624, BOS4627).

Immunohistochemistry. Fluorescent and nonfluorescent immunohistochemistry was performed on both transfected and native cells bearing either wild-type or mutant human presenilin cDNA sequences as described previously (L. Levesque et al., in prep.). These antibodies were also used to investigate the protein expression of the presenilins in mammalian brain (specifically the macaque cerebellum) at both the light microscopic and electron microscopic levels, as described previously (L. Levesque et al., in prep.).

RESULTS

Screening of the cDNA clones recovered from the 14q24.3 region of chromosome 14 led to the discovery of missense mutations in the open reading frame of one cDNA identified by clone S182 (Sherrington et al. 1995). The open reading frame of the cDNA, which was subsequently named presenilin 1 (PS1), encoded a polypeptide containing approximately 467 amino acids in its longest isoform. Subsequent studies of the genomic structure of the PS1 gene have revealed that it contains 13 different transcribed exons (Rogaev et al. 1996). Exons 1 and 2 represent alternate initial nontranslated exons. The upstream nontranscribed sequences 5′ to exon 1 contain a number of putative transcriptional elements including STAT and AP1 consensus sequences. This region upstream of exon 1 also contains putative TATA and CAAT boxes. In contrast, the region immediately upstream of exon 2 is particularly GC-rich and lacks a TATA box. Analysis of multiple transcripts from brain revealed that the majority of the transcripts begin in exon 1. In contrast, however, a small proportion of transcripts in nonneural tissues, such as colon, contain exon 2 as the initial transcribed sequence. Both types of transcripts are spliced to exon 3 as the second exon. The ATG start codon is contained in exon 4, which also shows alternate use of a splice site at the 3′ end of exon 4, which results in the variable presence of 12 base pairs encoding the amino acids valine, arginine, serine, and glutamine. The second site of alternate splicing involves exon 9, which encodes residues which, in a seven transmembrane model, would be predicted to be located at the carboxyl terminus of TM6 and the beginning of the exposed loop domain between TM6 and TM7. Removal of this sequence would allow exon 10 to reconstitute the hydrophobic domain of TM6 and would shorten the TM6-TM7 loop domain. The majority of tissues contain transcripts bearing exon 9 as the major isoform. However, in leukocytes, transcripts with and transcripts without exon 9 are found in approximately equal abundance.

Analysis of the genomic structure for the PS2 gene shows a very similar structure to that of the PS1 gene (R. Sherrington et al., in prep.). Alternative splicing of PS2 transcripts is associated with a variable presence of Glu-325 as a result of alternate use of splice sites between exons encoding residues in the TM6 and TM7 loop domain. In addition, a low level of alternative splicing of the exon equivalent to PS1 exon 9 is occasionally observed in several different tissues.

Characterization of the Presenilin Proteins

Antibodies specific to various domains of PS1, as well as antibodies generated against peptide sequences conserved in both PS1 and PS2, were used to investigate Western blots containing lysates of native cultured human cells such as normal fibroblasts, lysates of human brain, and lysates from brain of transgenic mice bearing PS1 cDNAs under the control of either the prion or platelet-derived growth factor receptor-β subunit gene promoter elements. In cultured cells such as fibroblasts, these studies revealed that amino-terminal-directed antibodies detected a low-intensity band of approximately 45 kD and a more intense 35-kD band. In contrast, antibodies directed to the apex of the TM6-TM7 loop domain (e.g., antibody TOR520) detect a weak approximately 45-kD band and a more intense 18-kD band. A similar picture was also observed with carboxy-terminal-directed antibodies such as BOS4627. In lysates from human brain, the intensity of the high-molecular-weight bands was generally decreased in comparison to cultured cells. Western blots containing lysates of brain from mice bearing PS1 transgenes revealed that in nontransgenic littermates, the predominant immunoreactive bands were also those of the 35-kD and 18-kD cleavage products. In contrast, lysates from brains of PS1 transgenic littermates contained the cleavage products from the endogenous murine gene, but they also contained additional bands representing cleavage of the human transgene product, which were of a slightly different molecular weight than the endogenous murine gene (suggesting cleavage at a slightly different site). Furthermore, in transgenes expressing the highest levels of human cDNA and PS1 protein, it was apparent that full-length PS1 protein of approximately 45 kD was observed. Similar observations have been reported by others (Thinkaran et al. 1996).

Immunolocalization

Antibodies specific for the amino terminus of PS1 detect immunoreactivity predominantly localized in the perinuclear membrane, endoplasmic reticulum, early Golgi apparatus, and in some as-yet-unidentified cytoplasmic vesicular structures in both transfected and native cultured cells. An essentially identical picture is identified with antibodies directed at the carboxyl terminus or the exposed domain between TM1 and

TM2, both of which are conserved between PS1 and PS2. It should be noted, however, that both amino-terminal- and carboxy-terminal-directed antibodies have a predilection for identification of the presenilin cleavage products. Studies with antibodies directed to the TM6-TM7 loop domain in the vicinity of the cleavage product, which would be expected to identify only full-length presenilin proteins, are currently under way.

To explore the localization of presenilin proteins in mammalian brain, we have examined presenilin immunolocalization using the amino-terminal-directed antibody BOS4627. In primate cerebellum, the predominant localization at the light microscopic level is in the granular cell layer and in the large Purkinje fibers. At the electron microscopic level, immunoreactivity can be clearly seen associated with perinuclear envelope and with the intracellular membranous structures such as the endoplasmic reticulum (L. Levesque et al., in prep.).

Transgenic Animals

To date, a limited series of mice bearing wild-type and mutant PS1 transgenes under the control of the hamster prion protein gene promoter or the human platelet-derived growth factor receptor β subunit gene promoter have been analyzed up to 3 months of age. Analysis of Western blots from these animals (see above) suggests that there is a pathway for cleavage of the PS1 holoprotein to two subunits (a 35-kD amino-terminal fragment and an 18-kD amino-terminal fragment) and that both the endogenous and transgenic presenilin proteins are processed. However, at the current time, no definite clinical, behavioral, or neuropathological changes have been observed in the brains of mice bearing mutant PS1 transgenes.

CONCLUSIONS

The cloning of two genes with strong structural and amino acid sequence similarities strongly argues that both the PS1 gene on chromosome 14, and the PS2 gene on chromosome 1, may subserve related or overlapping activities. This view is further supported by the fact that mutations in both genes lead to the AD phenotype.

The natural function of the presenilins remains unclear. Three different hypotheses have been proposed. First, on the basis of similarities in sequence and structure to the *Caenorhabditis elegans* SPE-4 gene which is thought to play a role in membrane and protein trafficking in the Golgi-derived fibrous body-membranous organelle in spermatocytes or *C. elegans* (L'Hernault and Arduengo 1992), it is conceivable that the presenilins may have a similar function in membrane and protein trafficking. Partial support for this observation has been provided by preliminary data suggesting that fibroblasts from patients with PS1 and PS2 mutations display an abnormal handling of the βAPP protein, which in turn results in an increased secretion of Aβ isoforms such as $A\beta_{1\text{-}42}$ (Martin et al. 1995; Scheuner et al. 1995).

An alternate proposal for presenilin function is that they may play a role in intracellular signal transduction. This hypothesis is based on the observation that mutants in the *sel*12 homolog of presenilins in *C. elegans* have a suppressor effect on activated Notch/lin12 mutants (Levitan and Greenwald 1995). These *sel*12 mutations lead to defects in vulva cell fate decisions mediated through the Notch/lin12 intracellular signaling pathway. The suppressor effect of *sel*12 on the Notch/lin12 pathway could arise either because *sel*12 has a downstream signal transduction role or because *sel*12 plays some role in the intracellular trafficking of transmembrane proteins such as Notch/lin12. A similar function, therefore, could be envisaged for the presenilins with respect to the processing function and intracellular trafficking events related to βAPP, which is also a cell-surface transmembrane protein.

A final and somewhat more speculative function for presenilins is a role in protection from apoptosis. This preliminary observation is derived from experiments attempting to isolate genes that protect T-cells from apoptotic cell death arising from receptor-mediated activation of apoptosis. In one of these experiments, a cDNA potentially encoding the carboxyl terminus of PS2 was found to rescue cells from apoptosis.

The current data bearing on processing and the intracellular localization of PS1 and PS2 do not allow any of the above hypotheses to be excluded, although localization within the endoplasmic reticulum Golgi and some as-yet-uncharacterized intracytoplasmic vesicles provides an argument in favor of the hypothesis that the presenilins play some role in intracellular protein and membrane trafficking.

In addition to the unresolved question of the function of the PS1 and PS2 genes, it is also unclear how mutations that are often very conservative missense substitutions lead to the activation of a pathway which culminates in the development of AD. The conservative nature of the majority of the *sel*12 missense substitutions, together with their distribution across the entire PS1 protein, suggests that the mutations may have either a novel function effect or a loss-of-function effect. Few clues can be garnered from the known mutations in the *C. elegans sel*12 gene beyond the fact that the majority of mutations caused a truncated and therefore presumably unstable protein with a loss-of-function effect.

REFERENCES

Cai, X.D., T.E. Golde, and S.G. Younkin. 1992. Release of excess amyloid β protein from a mutant β protein precursor. *Science* **259:** 514.

Campion, D., J.-aM. Flaman, A. Brice, D. Hannequin, B. Dubois, C. Martin, V. Moreau, F. Charbonnier, O. Didierjean, S. Tardieu, J. Mallet, M. Bellis, C. Clerget-Darpoux, Y. Agid, and T. Frebourg. 1995. Mutations of the Presenilin-1 gene in families with early onset Alzheimer's disease. *Hum. Mol. Genet.* **4:** 2373.

Chartier-Harlin, M.-C., F. Crawford, H. Holden, A. Warren, D. Hughes, L. Fidani, A. Goate, M. Rossor, J. Hardy, and M. Mullan. 1991. Early-onset Alzheimer's disease caused by mutations at codon 717 of the β-amyloid precursor gene. *Nature* **353:** 844.

Citron, M., T. Oltersdorf, C. Haass, C. McConlogue, A.Y. Hung, P. Seubert, C. Vigo-Pelfrey, I. Lieberburg, and D.J. Selkoe. 1992. Mutation of the β-amyloid precursor protein in familial Alzheimer's disease increases β-protein production. *Nature* **360:** 672.

Corder, E.H., A.M. Saunders, W.J. Strittmatter, D.E. Schmechel, P.C. Gaskell, G.W. Small, A D. Roses, J.L. Haines, and M.A. Pericak-Vance. 1993. Gene dosage of apolipoprotein E type 4 allele and the risk for Alzheimer's disease in late onset families. *Science* **261:** 921.

Corder, E.H., A.M. Saunders, N.J. Risch, and W.J. Strittmatter, D.E. Schmechel, P.C. Gaskell, Jr., J.B. Rimmler, P.A. Locke, P.M. Conneally, K.E. Schmader, G.W. Small, A.D. Roses, J.L. Haines, and M.A. Pericak-Vance. 1994. Protective effect of apolipoprotein E type 2 allele for late-onset Alzheimer disease. *Nat. Genet.* **7:** 180.

Cruts, M., J.-J. Martin, and C. Van Broeckhoven. 1995. Molecular genetic analysis of familial early-onset Alzheimer's disease linked to chromosome 14q24.3. *Hum. Mol. Genet.* **4:** 2363.

Foncin, J.-F., D. Salmon, V. Supino-Viterbo, R.G. Feldman, G. Macchi, P. Mariotti, C. Scopetta, G. Caruso, and A.C. Bruni. 1985. Alzheimer's presenile dementia transmitted in an extended kindred. *Rev. Neurol.* **141:** 194.

Frommelt, P., R. Schnabel, W. Kuhne, L.E. Nee, and R.J. Polinsky. 1991. Familial Alzheimer disease: A large multigenerational German kindred. *Alzheimer Dis. Assoc. Disord.* **5:** 36.

Goate, A.M., M.-C. Chartier-Harlin, M. Mullan, J. Brown, F. Crawford, L. Fidani, L. Guiffra, A. Haynes, and J.A. Hardy. 1991. Segregation of a missense mutation in the amyloid precursor protein gene with familial Alzheimer disease. *Nature* **349:** 704.

Goate, A., A.R. Haynes, M.J. Owen, M. Farrall, L.A. James, L.Y. Lai, M. Mullan, M. Rossor, and J. Hardy. 1989. Predisposing locus for Alzheimer disease on chr. 21. *Lancet* **I:** 352.

Goldgaber, D., M.I. Lerman, O.W. McBride, U. Safiotti, and D.C. Gajdusek. 1987. Characterization and chromosomal localization of a cDNA encoding brain amyloid of Alzheimer's disease. *Science* **235:** 877.

Goudsmit, J., B.J. White, L.R. Weitkamp, B.J. Keats, C.H. Morrow, and D.C. Gadjusek. 1981. Familial Alzheimer's disease in two kindreds of the same geographic origin: A clinical and genetic study. *J. Neurol. Sci.* **49:** 78.

Haass, C., A.Y. Hung, D.J. Selkoe, and D.B. Teplow. 1994. Mutations associated with a locus for familial Alzheimer's disease result in alternative processing of amyloid β-protein precursor. *J. Biol. Chem.* **269:** 17741.

Hendricks, M., C.M. van Duijn, P. Cras, J.-J. Martin, and C. Van Broeckhoven. 1992. Presenile dementia and cerebral hemorrhage linked to a mutation at codon 692 of the β-amyloid precursor protein gene. *Nat. Genet.* **1:** 218.

Kang, J., H.G. Lemaire, A. Unterbeck, J.M Salbaum, C.L. Masters, G. Multhap, K. Beyreuther, and B. Muller-Hill. 1987. The precursor of Alzheimer disease amyloid A4 protein resembles a cell surface receptor. *Nature* **325:** 733.

Karlinsky, H., G. Vaula, J.L. Haines, J. Ridgley, C. Bergeron, M. Mortilla, R. Tupler, M. Percy, Y. Robitaille, D.R. Crapper-MacLachlan, and P. St. George-Hyslop. 1992. Molecular and prospective phenotypic characterization of a pedigree with familial Alzheimer disease and a missense mutation in codon 717 of the β-amyloid precursor protein (APP) gene. *Neurology* **42:** 1445.

Levitan, D. and I. Greenwald. 1995. Facilitation of lin-12-mediated signalling by sel-12, a *Caenorhabditis elegans* S182 Alzheimer's disease gene. *Nature* **377:** 351.

Levy, E., M.D. Carman, I.J. Fernandez-Madrid, M.D. Power, I. Lieberburg, G. Sjoerd, S.G. van Duinen, G. Bots, W. Luyendijk, and B. Frangione. 1990. Mutation of the Alzheimer's disease amyloid gene in hereditary cerebral hemorrhage-Dutch type. *Science* **248:** 1124.

Levy-Lahad, E., E.M. Wijsman, E. Nemens, L. Anderson, T. Bird, G. Martin, and G. Schellenberg. 1995. A familial Alzheimer's disease locus on chromosome 1. *Science* **269:** 970.

L'Hernault, S.W.L. and P.M. Arduengo. 1992. Mutation of a putative sperm membrane protein in *Caenohabditis elegans* prevents sperm differentiation but not its associated meiotic divisions. *J. Cell Biol.* **119:** 55.

Mann, D.M.A., P.O. Yates, and B. Marcyniuk. 1984. Alzheimer's presenile dementia, senile dementia of the Alzheimer type, and Down's syndrome in middle age form a continuum of pathologic changes. *Neuropathol. Appl. Neurobiol.* **10:** 185.

Mann, D.M., A. Brown, D. Prinja, C.A. Davies, M. Landen, C.L. Masters, and K. Beyreuther. 1989. An analysis of the morphology of senile plaques in Down's syndrome patients of different ages using immunocytochemical and lectin histochemical techniques. *Neuropathol. Appl. Neurobiol.* **15:** 317.

Martin, R.N., B.A. Turner, R.T. Carroll, D. Sweeney, K.S. Kim, H.M. Wisniewski,, J.P. Blass, G.E. Gibson, and S.E. Gandy. 1995. High levels of amyloid β-protein from S182 (Glu246) familial Alzheimer's cells. *NeuroReport* **7:** 217–220.

Mullan, M.J., F. Crawford, K. Axelman, A. Goate, L. Lannfelt, and J. Hardy. 1992. A pathogenic mutation for probable Alzheimer's disease in the APP gene at the N-terminus of β-amyloid. *Nat. Genet.* **1:** 345.

Murrell. J., M. Farlow, B. Ghetti, and M.D. Benson. 1991. A mutation in the amyloid precursor protein associated with hereditary Alzheimer's disease. *Science* **254:** 97.

Nee, L., R.J. Polinsky, R. Eldridge, H. Weingartner, S. Smallberg, and M. Ebert. 1983. A family with histologically confirmed Alzheimer disease. *Arch. Neurol.* **40:** 203.

Pericak-Vance, M.A., J.L. Bedout, P.C. Gaskell, and A.D. Roses. 1991. Linkage studies in familial Alzheimer disease—Evidence for chromosome 19 linkage. *Am. J. Hum. Genet.* **48:** 1034.

Pollen, D. 1993. Hannah's heirs: The quest for the genetic origins of Alzheimer's disease. Oxford University Press, Oxford, United Kingdom.

Robakis, N.K., D.K. Lahiri, H.R. Brown, R. Rubenstein, B. Mehta, H. Wisniewski, and N. Goller. 1988. Expression studies of the gene encoding the Alzheimer's disease and Down syndrome amyloid peptide. In *Disorders of the developing nervous system: Changing views on their origins, diagnoses and treatments*, p. 183. A.R. Liss, New York.

Rogaev, E.I., W.J. Lukiw, G. Vaula, J.L. Haines, E.A. Rogaeva, T. Tsuda, N. Alexandrova, and P. St. George-Hyslop. 1993. Analysis of the cFOS gene on chr. 14 and the 5′promoter of the amyloid precursor protein gene in familial Alzheimer's disease. *Neurology* **43:** 2275.

Rogaev, E.I., R. Sherrington, C. Wu, G. Levesque, Y. Liang, E.A. Rogaeva, H. Chi, M. Ikeda, K. Holman, C. Lin, W.J. Lukiw, P.J. de Jong, P.E. Fraser, J.M. Rommens, and P.H. St. George-Hyslop. 1996. Analysis of the 5′ sequence, genomic structure and alternative splicing of the presenilin 1 gene associated with early onset Alzheimer's disease. *Genomics* (in press).

Rogaev, E.I., R. Sherrington, E.A. Rogaeva, G. Levesque, M. Ikeda, Y. Liang, H. Chi, C. Lin, K. Holman, T. Tsuda, L. Mar, S. Sorbi, B. Nacmias, S. Piacentini, L. Amaducci, I. Chumakov, D. Cohen, L. Lannfelt, P.E. Fraser, J.M. Rommens, and P. St. George-Hyslop. 1995. Familial Alzheimer's disease in kindreds with missense mutations in a novel gene on chromosome 1 related to the Alzheimer's disease type 3 gene. *Nature* **376:** 775.

Sato, S., K. Kamino, T. Miki, A. Doi, K. Li, P. St. George-Hyslop, T. Ogihara, and Y. Sakaki. 1996. Splicing mutation of presenilin 1 gene for early onset familial Alzheimer's disease. *Hum. Mutat.* (in press).

Saunders, A., W.J. Strittmatter, S. Schmechel, P. St. George-Hyslop, M. Pericak-Vance, S.H. Joo, B.L. Rosi, J.F. Gusella, D. Crapper-McLachlan, J. Growden, M.J. Alberts, C. Hulette, B. Crain, D. Goldgaber, and A.D. Roses. 1993. Association of apoliprotein E allele e4 with the late-onset familial and sporadic Alzheimer disease. *Neurology* **43:** 1467.

Schellenberg, G.D., T.D. Bird, E.M. Wijsman, H.T. Orr, L. Anderson, E. Nemens, J.A. White, and L. Bonnycastle. 1992. Genetic linkage evidence for a familial Alzheimer's disease locus on chr. 14. *Science* **258:** 668.

Scheuner, D., T. Bird, M. Citron, L. Lannfelt, G. Schellenberg, D. Selkoe, M. Viitanen, and S.G. Younkin. 1995. Fibroblasts from carriers of familial AD linked to chromosome 14 show increased Aβ production. *Soc. Neurosci. Abstr.* **21:** 1500.

Sherrington, R., E. Rogaev, Y. Liang, E. Rogaeva, G. Levesque, M. Ikeda, H. Chi, C. Lin, K. Holman, T. Tsuda, L. Mar, P. Fraser, J.M. Rommens, and P. St. George-Hyslop. 1995. Cloning of a gene bearing missense mutations in early onset familial Alzheimer's disease. *Nature* **375:** 754.

St. George-Hyslop, P.H., R.E. Tanzi, R.J. Polinsky, J.L. Haines, L. Nee, P.C. Watkins, R.H. Myers, P.M. Conneally, and J.F. Gusella. 1987. The genetic defect causing familial Alzheimer disease maps on chromosome 21. *Science* **235:** 885.

St. George-Hyslop, P., J. Haines, E. Rogaev, M. Mortilla, G. Vaula, M. Pericak-Vance, J.-F. Foncin, M. Montesi, A. Bruni, S. Sorbi, I. Rainero, I. Pinessi, D. Pollen, R. Polinsky, L. Nee, J. Kennedy, F. Macciardi, E. Rogeava, Y. Liang, N. Alexandrova, W. Lukiw, K. Schlumpf, T. Tsuda, L. Farrer, J.-M. Cantu, R. Duara, L. Amaducci, L. Bergamini, J. Gusella, A. Roses, and D. Crapper-MacLachlan. 1992. Genetic evidence for a novel familial Alzheimer disease gene on chromosome 14. *Nat. Genet.* **2:** 330.

St. George-Hyslop, P.H., J.L. Haines, L.A. Farrer, R. Polinsky, C. van Broeckhoven, A. Goate, D.R. Crapper-McLachlan, and more than 25 others. 1991. Genetic linkage studies suggest that Alzheimer's disease is not a single homogeneous disorder. *Nature* **347:** 194.

Strittmatter, W.J., A.M. Saunders, M. Pericak-Vance, G.S. Salvesen, J. Enghild, and A.D. Roses. 1993. Apolipoprotein E: High avidity binding to Aβ amyloid and increased frequency of type 4 isoform in familial Alzheimers disease. *Proc. Natl. Acad. Sci.* **90:** 1977.

Strittmatter, W.J., A.M. Saunders, M. Goedert, K.H. Weisgraber, L.M. Dong, R. Jakes, D. Huang, M. Pericak-Vance, D. Schmechel, and A. Roses. 1994. Isoform-specific interactions of ApoE with microtubule associated protein tau: Implications for Alzheimer disease. *Proc. Natl. Acad. Sci.* **91:** 11183.

Strittmatter, W.J., K.H. Weisgraber, M. Goedert, A.M. Saunders, D. Huang, E.H. Corder, L.-M. Dong, R. Jakes, M.J. Alberts, J.R. Gilbert, D.E. Schmechel, M.A. Pericak-Vance, and A.D. Roses. 1994. Hypothesis: Microtubule instability and paired helical filament formation in the Alzheimer disease brain as a function of apolipoprotein E genotype. *Exp. Neurol.* **125:** 163.

Suzuki, N., T.T. Cheung, X.-D. Cai, A. Odaka, L. Otvos, C. Eckman, T. Golde, and S.G. Younkin. 1994. An increased percentage of long amyloid β protein secreted by familial amyloid β protein precursor (βAPP717) mutants. *Science* **264:** 1336.

Tamaoka, A., A. Odaka, Y. Ishibashi, M. Usami, N. Sahara, N. Suzuki, N. Nukina, H. Mizusawa, S. Shoji, I. Kanazawa, and H. Mori. 1994. APP717 missense mutation affects the ratio of amyloid β protein species (Aβ1-42/43 and aβ1-40) in familial Alzheimer's disease brain. *J. Biol. Chem.* **269:** 32721.

The Alzheimer's Disease Collaborative Group. 1995. The structure of the presenilin I gene and the identification of six mutations in early onset AD pedigrees. *Nat. Genet.* **11:** 219.

Thinkaran, G., D.R. Borchelt, M.K. Lee, H.H. Slunt, L. Spitzer, G. Kim, T. Ratovisky, F. Davenport, C. Nordstedt, M. Seeger, A.I. Levey, S.E. Gandy, N.A. Jenkins, N. Copeland, D.L. Price, and S.S. Sisodia. 1996. Endoproteolysis of presenilin 1 and accumulation of processed derivatives in vivo. *Neuron* **17:** 181–190.

Van Broeckhoven, C. 1995. Presenilins and Alzheimer disease. *Nat. Genet.* **11:** 230.

Van Broeckhoven, C, H. Backhovens, M. Cruts, G. De Winter, M. Bruyland, P. Cras, and J.-J. Martin. 1992. Mapping of a gene predisposing to early-onset Alzheimer's disease to chromosome 14q24.3. *Nat. Genet.* **2:** 335.

Wisniewski, T, and B. Frangione. 1992. Apolipoprotein E: A pathological chaperone protein in patients with cerebral and systemic amyloid. *Neurosci. Lett.* **135:** 235.

Wong, L., Y. Liang, T. Tsuda, Q. Fong, G. Galway, N. Alexandrova, E. Rogeava, W. Lukiw, J. Smith, E. Rogaev, D. Crapper-MacLachlan, and P. St. George-Hyslop. 1993. Mutation of the gene for the human lysosomal serine protease cathepsin G is not the cause of aberrant APP processing in familial Alzheimer disease. *Neurosci. Lett.* **152:** 96.

Molecular Dissection of the Neurofibrillary Lesions of Alzheimer's Disease

M. GOEDERT, M.G. SPILLANTINI, M. HASEGAWA, R. JAKES, R.A. CROWTHER, AND A. KLUG
Medical Research Council Laboratory of Molecular Biology, Cambridge CB2 2QH, United Kingdom

Alzheimer's disease (AD) is characterized clinically by a progressive loss of memory and other cognitive functions, resulting in a severe dementia. The intellectual decline is accompanied by the progressive accumulation in the brain of insoluble fibrous material, extracellularly in the form of plaques made of amyloid protein Aβ, and intracellularly in the form of neurofibrillary lesions. Most cases of AD are sporadic, and familial cases are genetically heterogeneous, with different primary causes leading to the same phenotype and neuropathology. It is therefore likely that the activation of several distinct pathological pathways can lead to the disease, with neuritic plaques and neurofibrillary lesions representing the points of convergence of these events. A study of the mechanisms that lead to the formation of plaques and neurofibrillary lesions is essential for an understanding of the pathogenesis of all forms of AD.

In this paper, we deal exclusively with the neurofibrillary pathology. The extent and topographical distribution of neurofibrillary lesions provide a reliable pathological correlate of the degree of dementia (Braak and Braak 1991). The formation of neurofibrillary lesions is therefore believed to lead to the symptoms of AD, which result most probably from the degeneration of nerve cells in cerebral cortex and hippocampal formation, with ensuing neuronal cell loss and reduction in synapse numbers. The finding of large numbers of amyloid deposits in some cognitively normal individuals (also known as pathological aging) has shown that amyloid deposits are not sufficient for dementia (Dickson et al. 1991). In contrast, large numbers of neurofibrillary lesions in hippocampus and/or cerebral cortex are accompanied by dementia.

Neurofibrillary lesions are found in nerve cell bodies and apical dendrites as neurofibrillary tangles, in distal dendrites as neuropil threads, and in the abnormal neurites that are associated with some amyloid plaques (Fig. 1) (for review, see Goedert 1993; Lee 1995). Ultrastructurally, all three lesions contain paired helical filaments (PHFs) as major fibrous components and straight filaments (SFs) as minor components (Fig. 2). Neurofibrillary lesions develop in the vast majority of nerve cells that undergo degeneration in AD. Their relative insolubility enables them to survive after the death of affected nerve cells as extracellular tangles that accumulate in the neuropil.

During the past decade, significant progress has been made in unraveling the molecular composition of the PHF and in deducing possible mechanisms that may lead to its assembly. It is well established that the PHF is made of microtubule-associated protein tau in a hyperphosphorylated state and that, as a consequence, tau is unable and unavailable to bind to microtubules and to promote microtubule assembly. A large number of normal and abnormal phosphorylation sites in tau have been identified, and there is some evidence to suggest that proline-directed protein kinases and/or protein phosphatase 2A may be instrumental in leading to tau hyperphosphorylation. However, it is not known whether hyperphosphorylation of tau is either necessary or sufficient for PHF formation. An understanding of the mechanisms that lead to PHF assembly requires the ability to make synthetic paired helical-like filaments from full-length tau protein. Our recent work on in vitro filament assembly suggests that an interaction between tau protein and sulfated glycosaminoglycans may be sufficient for PHF assembly.

STRUCTURE OF THE PHF

The PHF, as its name suggests, consists of two strands of subunits that twist around one another in a helical fashion (Fig. 2). When viewed in the electron microscope, the helical twist and relative disposition of the two strands give rise to images in which the width alternates between 8 nm and 20 nm, with an apparent period of 80 nm (Crowther and Wischik 1985).

PHFs can be isolated either in the form of tangle fragments (Kondo et al. 1988; Wischik et al. 1988) or as dispersed filaments (Greenberg and Davies 1990; Lee et al. 1991). The two types of PHFs have tau sequences in common but differ in their properties. Whereas most dispersed PHFs are soluble in guanidine or sodium dodecylsulfate, most tangle fragment PHFs are insoluble in these reagents. Both types of PHFs differ also in their sensitivity to proteases. Pronase treatment of tangle preparations removes a fuzzy coat from the PHF and leaves behind a pronase-resistant core. When dispersed filaments are treated with pronase under the same conditions, they are completely degraded (Goedert et al. 1992c), illustrating the differing protease sensitivities of tangle fragment and dispersed PHFs. The morphology of the PHF core is similar to

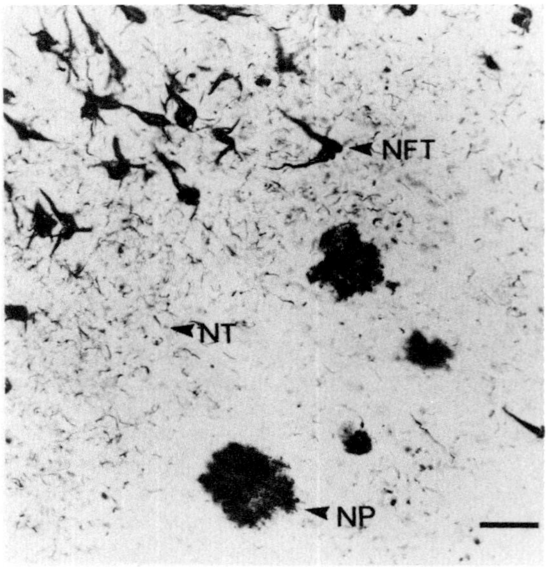

Figure 1. Neurofibrillary pathology in the entorhinal cortex from the brain of an AD patient. The section was stained with an anti-tau serum. (NFT) Neurofibrillary tangle; (NT) Neuropil thread; (NP) Neuritic plaque. Bar, 100 μm.

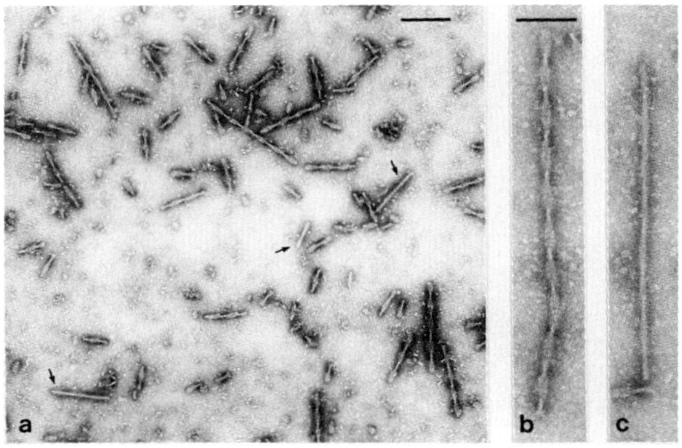

Figure 2. Electron micrographs of negatively stained abnormal filaments from the brain of an AD patient. (*a*) Low-power view showing predominantly paired helical filaments, but with a few straight filaments (*arrows*). (*b,c*) High-power view of a paired helical filament (*b*) and a straight filament (*c*). Bars: *a*, 200 nm; *b,c*, 100 nm.

that of untreated PHFs, but structural details are seen more clearly, because the disordered coat has been removed. From electron micrographs, it is possible to compute a map of the cross-sectional density in the core. The structural subunit seen in image reconstructions shows three domains arranged in a C-shape, and the filament consists of a double-helical stack of such subunits (Crowther and Wischik 1985).

SFs represent a minority species, both in tangle fragment and dispersed filament preparations. Images of SFs show approximately the same periodicity as PHFs, but a much less marked modulation in width (Fig. 2) (Crowther 1991). SFs and PHFs have common tau sequences and behave in a similar manner when treated with pronase. Rarely, hybrid filaments are observed that show a sharp transition from a segment of PHF into a segment of SF. This indicates that PHFs and SFs contain identical or closely related subunits that are arranged differently in the two types of filaments. This is supported by the computed cross-section of the SF, which shows two C-shaped subunits very similar to those seen in the PHF, but arranged back-to-back rather than base-to-base (Crowther 1991). The SF is thus a structural variant of the PHF, in that both contain two strands of closely related subunits, but the relative arrangement of the two strands differs in the two types of filaments.

TAU PROTEIN IN NORMAL BRAIN

Tau is an abundant protein in both the central and peripheral nervous systems. In brain it is found predominantly in nerve cells, where it is concentrated in nerve cell axons. This contrasts with the distribution of the neurofibrillary lesions in AD, which are found in nerve cell bodies, dendrites, and axons. Tau isoforms are produced from a single gene through alternative mRNA splicing (Goedert et al. 1988, 1989; Lee et al. 1988). In adult human brain six isoforms are found, which range from 352 to 441 amino acids and differ from each other by the presence or absence of three inserts (Fig. 3). The most striking feature of the tau sequences is the presence of three or four tandem repeats of 31 or 32 amino acids located in the carboxy-terminal half (Goedert et al. 1989), which constitute microtubule-binding domains (Butner and Kirschner 1991; Goode and Feinstein 1994). Microtubules assembled in the presence of tau show arms projecting from the microtubule surface (Hirokawa et al. 1988). Tau thus consists of a carboxy-terminal microtubule-binding domain and an amino-terminal projection domain. Besides being distinguished by the presence of three or four tandem repeats, some tau isoforms contain 29 or 58 amino acid inserts located near the amino terminus (Fig. 3). Isoforms with a large additional insert in the amino-terminal half have been described in the peripheral nervous system (Couchie et al. 1992; Goedert et al. 1992a). In immature human brain, only the shortest isoform with three repeats is expressed. The developmental shift of human tau bands from a simple fetal pattern to a more complex adult pattern thus involves the transition from the expression of the isoform with three repeats, containing no inserts, to the expression of all six isoforms.

Tau is a phosphoprotein, and phosphorylation is a also developmentally regulated. Thus, tau from immature brain is phosphorylated at more sites than tau from adult brain, implying selective dephosphorylation of the shortest tau isoform during brain maturation. Phosphorylation sites have been identified by mass spectrometry and peptide sequencing (Watanabe et al.

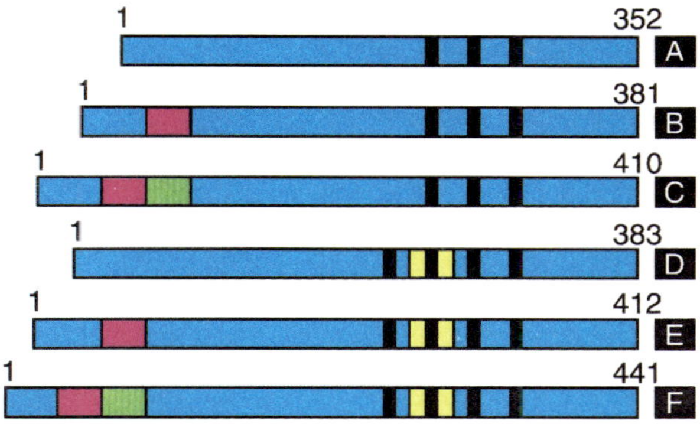

Figure 3. Schematic representation of the six human brain tau isoforms (A–F). The region common to all isoforms is shown in blue, and the inserts that distinguish them are shown in red, green and yellow. The three (in isoforms A–C) or four (in isoforms D–F) tandem repeats are shown by black bars. The number of amino acids is indicated. The 352-amino-acid isoform (A) is expressed in fetal brain, whereas all six isoforms (A–F) are expressed in adult brain.

1993) and through the use of phosphorylation-dependent anti-tau antibodies (for review, see Lee 1995). Tau from developing brain is phosphorylated at 15 known sites in the shortest isoform, whereas tau from adult brain is phosphorylated at at least 9 sites in the six isoforms (Fig. 4). With the exception of S262, which is located at the beginning of the first repeat, all the known phosphorylation sites in tau are located outside the microtubule-binding repeat region. Phosphorylation is heterogeneous, implying that a given tau molecule is partially phosphorylated at some, but not all, of these sites. Many of these sites are serine or threonine residues that are followed by a proline, suggesting that proline-directed protein kinases may phosphorylate tau in normal brain. Accordingly, mitogen-activated protein (MAP) kinase, glycogen synthase kinase-3 (GSK3), and neuronal cdc2-like kinase (NCLK) phosphorylate tau at many of the above S/T-P sites in vitro (Drewes et al. 1992; Hanger et al. 1992; Paudel et al. 1993). Moreover, the MAP kinase-related stress-activated protein (SAP) kinases SAP kinase-1 (or JNK) and SAP kinase-3 also phosphorylate tau at many of these S/T-P sites (our unpublished observations). In addition, GSK3 in the presence of heparin, as well as cAMP-dependent protein kinase and Ca^{++}/calmodulin-dependent protein kinase II, phosphorylate S262 in tau in vitro, as does a 110-kD protein kinase from brain (Yang et al. 1994; Drewes et al. 1995; Litersky et al. 1996). Tau phosphorylation by a number of protein kinases is markedly stimulated in a substrate-dependent manner by sulfated glycosaminoglycans, such as heparin and heparan sulfate (Fig. 5) (Mawal-Dewan et al. 1992; Brandt et al. 1994; Yang et al. 1994).

The phosphorylation state of a protein is the result of a balance between protein kinase and protein phos-

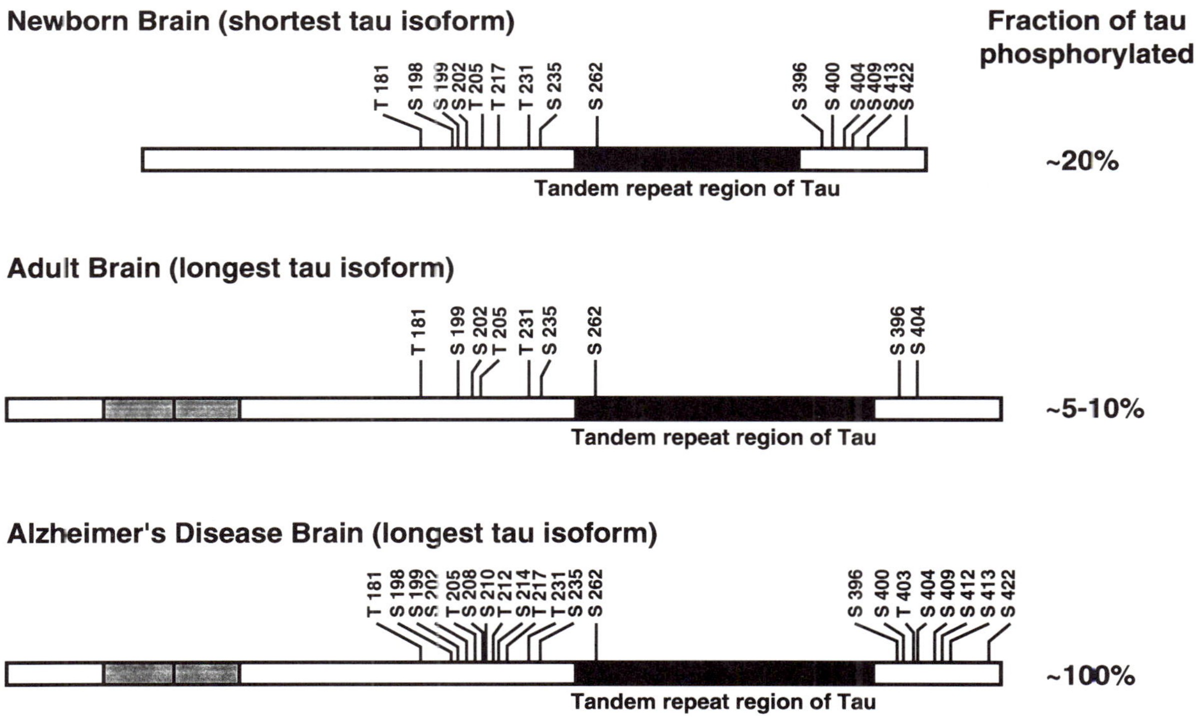

Figure 4. Identified phosphorylation sites in tau from newborn brain, adult brain, and AD brain. In newborn brain, only the shortest tau isoform is expressed, whereas six isoforms are expressed in adult human brain. In adult brain and AD brain, all six isoforms are phosphorylated on the residues shown here for the longest isoform. The approximate fraction of tau that is phosphorylated at the sites shared between newborn brain, adult brain, and AD brain is shown on the right.

phatase activities. Of the major phosphatase activities in a crude brain extract, tau phosphorylated by MAP kinase, GSK3, NCLK, or cAMP-dependent protein kinase is dephosphorylated predominantly by the trimeric form of protein phosphatase 2A (PP2A) (Goedert et al. 1992b; 1995). PP2A has also been shown to play an important role in the dephosphorylation of tau in cultured nerve cells (Fleming and Johnson 1995). Treatment of these cells with microtubule-depolymerizing agents leads to the PP2A-mediated dephosphorylation of tau (Merrick et al. 1996). The finding that a substantial pool of PP2A from a number of neuronal and nonneuronal cell lines is associated with microtubules (Sontag et al. 1995) indicates that it is well positioned to regulate tau phosphorylation in vivo. Upon treatment of cultured nerve cells with a Ca^{++} ionophore, PP2B has also been shown to participate in the dephosphorylation of tau (Fleming and Johnson 1995).

TAU PROTEIN IN THE PHF

Protein chemistry and molecular cloning established directly that tau forms an integral component of the PHF (Goedert et al. 1988; Kondo et al. 1988; Wischik et al. 1988), thereby putting more indirect immunohistochemical studies (Brion et al. 1985) on a solid basis. The tau sequences obtained from pronase-treated PHFs have shown that both three- and four-repeat isoforms contribute to the core of the PHF, but that a length of protein containing only three repeats is protected (Jakes et al. 1991). These results were obtained using PHFs extracted from tangle fragments. Because of the insolubility of these filaments, it was not possible to conclude that tau is the only component of the PHF or to show whether there are other components. This situation changed with the development

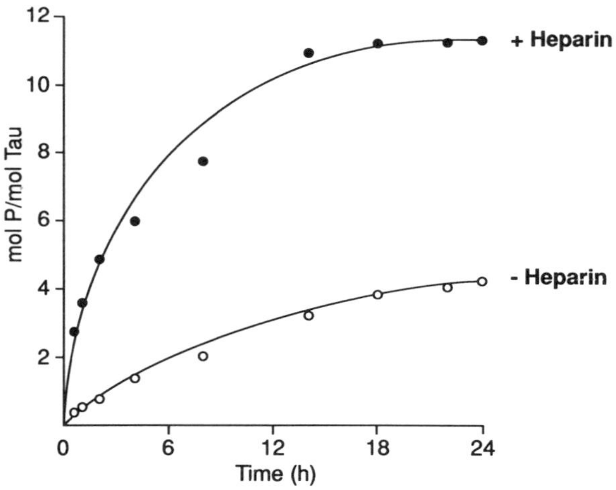

Figure 5. Heparin-induced stimulation of tau phosphorylation by NCLK. Recombinant htau40 (441-amino-acid isoform of human tau) was incubated with recombinant reconstituted NCLK in the presence or absence of 100 μg/ml heparin.

of extraction techniques for dispersed PHFs (Greenberg and Davies 1990). A study involving purification of these filaments to apparent homogeneity has provided strong evidence that tau forms the PHF (Lee et al. 1991). Unlike tangle fragment PHFs, a large proportion of dispersed PHFs contains intact tau (Lee et al. 1991; Goedert et al. 1992c). This is consistent with the view that dispersed filaments constitute an earlier stage of PHFs than the bulk of filaments isolated from tangle fragments.

Tau protein extracted from dispersed PHFs runs as three major bands of 60, 64, and 68 kD apparent molecular mass, with a variable amount of background smear (Flament et al. 1989; Greenberg and Davies 1990), which results from partially proteolyzed and cross-linked PHFs. These PHF-tau bands run more slowly on gels than normal or recombinant tau. They contain the whole of tau, as they stain with antibodies directed against the amino and carboxyl termini of tau. After treatment with alkaline phosphatase at high temperature, the three PHF-tau bands electrophorese as six bands that align with the recombinant tau isoforms (Goedert et al. 1992c; Greenberg et al. 1992). The relative proportions of the six bands are similar to those of soluble tau from normal adult brain (Goedert and Jakes 1990). Thus, PHFs contain all six adult brain tau isoforms in a hyperphosphorylated state. PHF-tau has a greatly reduced ability to bind to microtubules and to promote microtubule assembly; this functional impairment results entirely from hyperphosphorylation, since dephosphorylated PHF-tau binds as well to microtubules as does normal tau (Bramblett et al. 1993; Yoshida and Ihara 1993).

PHF-tau is both abnormally phosphorylated and hyperphosphorylated (Fig. 4). Abnormal phosphorylation means that more residues are phosphorylated in PHF-tau than in normal brain tau, whereas hyperphosphorylation means that, for a given site, a higher proportion of tau molecules is phosphorylated in PHF-tau than in normal brain tau. A large number of these sites have been identified by protein sequencing and mass spectrometry (Hasegawa et al. 1992; Morishima-Kawashima et al. 1995) and through the use of phosphorylation-dependent anti-tau antibodies (for review, see Lee 1995). Some of these sites are also phosphorylated in tau from developing rat brain, but to a lesser extent than in PHF-tau (Fig. 4). Although similar sites of phosphorylation were not detected in tau from adult human autopsy brain, studies of adult human brain tau obtained from fresh cortical biopsy samples suggest that a number of these sites are also phosphorylated in tau from adult human brain, but to a smaller extent than in tau from developing brain (Matsuo et al. 1994).

However, a number of additional sites have been identified as phosphorylation sites in PHF-tau by mass spectrometry that have so far not been found in rapidly isolated fetal rat tau or in biopsy-derived adult human brain tau. It remains to be seen whether these sites are truly abnormally phosphorylated in PHF-tau. This will depend on the production of novel phosphorylation-dependent anti-tau antibodies and on future mass spectrometric studies performed on rapidly isolated fetal and adult human brain tau. AP422, which is specific for phosphoserine 422 in tau, is such an antibody; it strongly recognizes PHF-tau but is virtually unreactive with biopsy-derived adult human brain tau, implying that S422 is abnormally phosphorylated in PHF-tau (Hasegawa et al. 1996). MAP kinase is the only known enzyme that phosphorylates S422 in tau, suggesting that MAP kinase or a MAP kinase-like enzyme may be involved in this abnormal phosphorylation (Hasegawa et al. 1996). About half of the known phosphorylation sites in PHF-tau are S/T-P sites. With the exception of S262, they are all located outside the microtubule-binding repeat region.

It is unclear whether the defect underlying hyperphosphorylation of tau results from an increased protein kinase activity, a decreased protein phosphatase activity, or from a combination of both. The finding that nonassembled soluble tau is more prone to postmortem dephosphorylation than assembled PHF-tau has led to the suggestion that the reduced activity of protein phosphatases may be responsible for the hyperphosphorylation of tau in AD (Matsuo et al. 1994). A recent study on adult rat using chronic intraventricular infusion of okadaic acid sufficient to inhibit PP2A has demonstrated that tau becomes localized to the somatodendritic compartment in nerve cells, where it is hyperphosphorylated (Arendt et al. 1995). A similar distribution of hyperphosphorylated tau was obtained in transgenic mice expressing the longest human brain tau isoform (Götz et al. 1995). However, no PHFs have as yet been observed using either experimental paradigm. Interestingly, the okadaic acid treatment also led to the formation of Aβ-containing extracellular deposits (Arendt et al. 1995).

SYNTHETIC PHFS

The PHF constitutes the ultrastructural hallmark of the neurofibrillary lesions of AD. Although analytical studies have shown that it is made of hyperphosphorylated tau protein, they have so far failed to provide any significant insights into the mechanisms that lead to PHF formation. An understanding of these mechanisms requires the ability to form paired helical-like filaments from defined components under in vitro conditions. Over the past 5 years, the availability of large quantities of recombinant tau isoforms and the ease with which tau fragments can be expressed have facilitated studies aimed at producing synthetic PHFs. It has been shown that paired helical-like filaments can be assembled in vitro from bacterially expressed nonphosphorylated three-repeat fragments of tau (Crowther et al. 1992; Wille et al. 1992). Filaments with dimensions similar to Alzheimer PHFs were produced by dialysis or by hanging-drop equilibration of the fragments against high concentrations of Tris at acidic pH. These filaments lend strong support to the view that the repeat region of tau is the only component necessary for the morphological appearance of the PHF. However, they fail to provide any insight into filament formation in vivo, since they are only obtained with truncated tau under nonphysiological conditions. This contrasts with dispersed PHFs from AD brain which consist of full-length tau protein. We have previously described the formation of a small number of twisted filaments from full-length tau in high salt in the presence of protease inhibitors (Crowther et al. 1994). However, the significance of these filaments remains unclear, as their formation may depend on an ill-defined interaction between tau and pepstatin, and the accompanying "mini-filaments" observed consist of pepstatin (Mothes et al. 1990). Thus, these findings, which indicate that only repeat region fragments of tau reproducibly form paired helical-like filaments in vitro, suggest that the amino- and carboxy-terminal regions of tau are inhibitory toward self-assembly.

During the course of recent experiments using sulfated glycosaminoglycans to stimulate phosphorylation of full-length recombinant tau, we noticed the presence of high-molecular-weight aggregates of tau that formed in a glycosaminoglycan-dependent, but phosphorylation-independent, manner. Electron microscopy revealed the presence of many filaments, with differing morphologies for tau isoforms with three or four microtubule-binding repeats (Goedert et al. 1996). Tau isoforms with three repeats give filaments with a typical paired-helical morphology, when incubated with heparin (Fig. 6A) or heparan sulfate (Fig. 6B), whereas tau isoforms with four repeats give filaments with a straight appearance (Fig. 6C). Tau protein phosphorylated with MAP kinase or NCLK prior to incubation with heparin or heparan sulfate forms filaments that are indistinguishable from those formed by nonphosphorylated tau, indicating that tau phosphorylation is neither stimulatory nor inhibitory for in vitro filament formation. Each of the six recombinant human brain tau isoforms forms either paired-helical or straight filaments in the presence of sulfated glycosaminoglycans under physiological conditions.

Similar results are obtained with truncated tau proteins consisting of three or four microtubule-binding repeats only and with proteins comprising the repeat region and the carboxyl terminus of tau. In contrast, a truncated form consisting of the amino-terminal domain of tau up to but excluding the repeat region fails to give filaments. By immunoelectron microscopy, the paired helical-like filaments are decorated by antibodies directed against the amino and carboxyl termini of tau, but not by an antibody against the microtubule-binding repeat region (Fig. 7) (Goedert et al. 1996). These results, which indicate that in the filaments the repeat region of tau is inaccessible to the antibody, are identical to those previously obtained with PHFs from AD brain (Goedert et al. 1992c). They establish that the microtubule-binding repeat region of tau is essen-

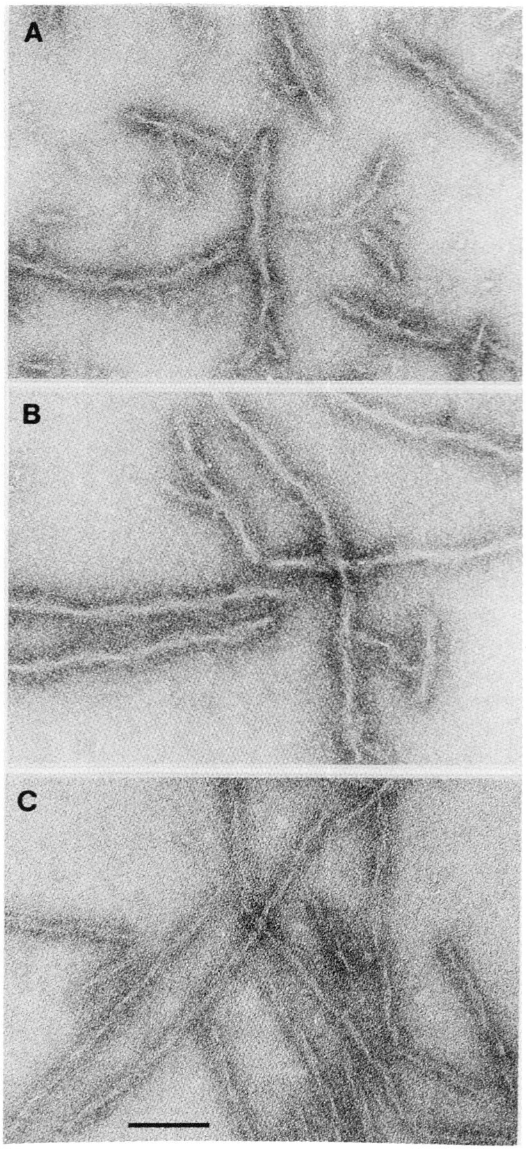

Figure 6. Sulfated glycosaminoglycan-induced filament assembly. (*A*) Recombinant three-repeat htau37 (381-amino-acid isoform of human tau) was incubated with heparin; (*B*) htau37 was incubated with heparan sulfate; (*C*) recombinant four-repeat htau40 (441-amino-acid isoform of human tau) was incubated with heparin. Note the presence of paired helical-like filaments in *A* and *B* and straight filaments in *C*. Bar, 100 nm.

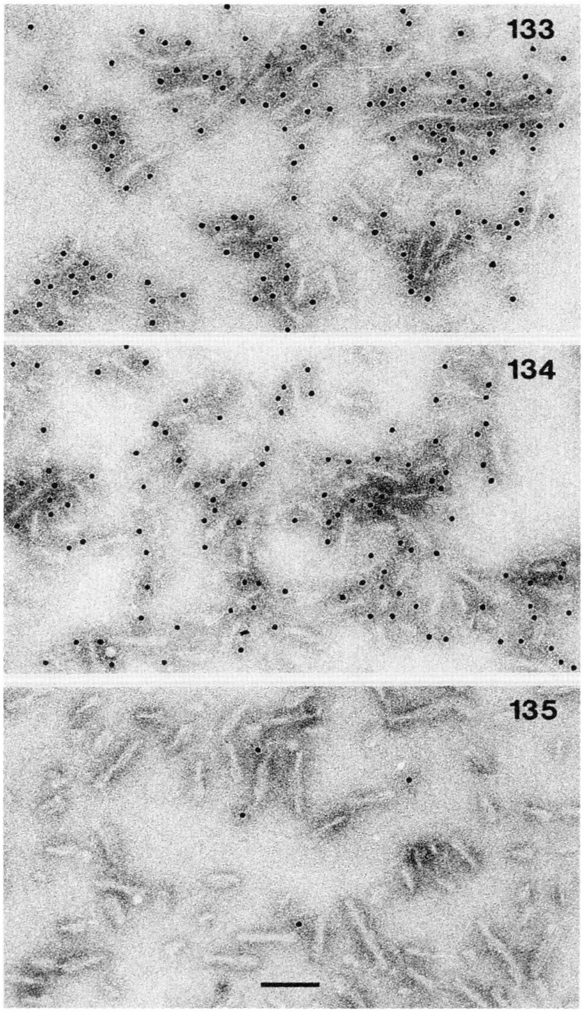

Figure 7. Immunoelectron microscopy of paired helical-like filaments with antibodies directed against the amino terminus (antiserum 133), the carboxyl terminus (antiserum 134), and the microtubule-binding repeats (antiserum 135) of human tau. Gold labeling is seen with 133 and 134 but not 135, as for Alzheimer filaments (Goedert et al. 1992c). Bar, 100 nm.

tial for sulfated glycosaminoglycan-induced filament formation. It is well known that three microtubule-binding repeats of tau form the core of the PHF from AD brain (Wischik et al. 1988; Jakes et al. 1991), thus supporting the evidence for a similar organization of the two types of filaments. The dimensions of tau filaments formed in the presence of sulfated glycosaminoglycans are similar to those of filaments extracted from AD brain, with a diameter of approximately 20 nm for twisted and 15 nm for straight filaments, with a crossing-over spacing of approximately 80 nm for paired helical-like filaments, although their twist is in general less regular than in Alzheimer filaments (Goedert et al. 1996).

The six recombinant tau isoforms and all truncated proteins examined bind to heparin-Sepharose in a salt-dependent manner, indicating the presence of multiple heparin-binding sites that are distributed throughout the tau sequence. This binding is probably mediated by electrostatic interactions between negative charges in heparin and positive charges in tau. Tau is positively charged in the repeat region and in the region upstream of the repeats, whereas its amino-terminal region of 125 amino acids is negatively charged overall.

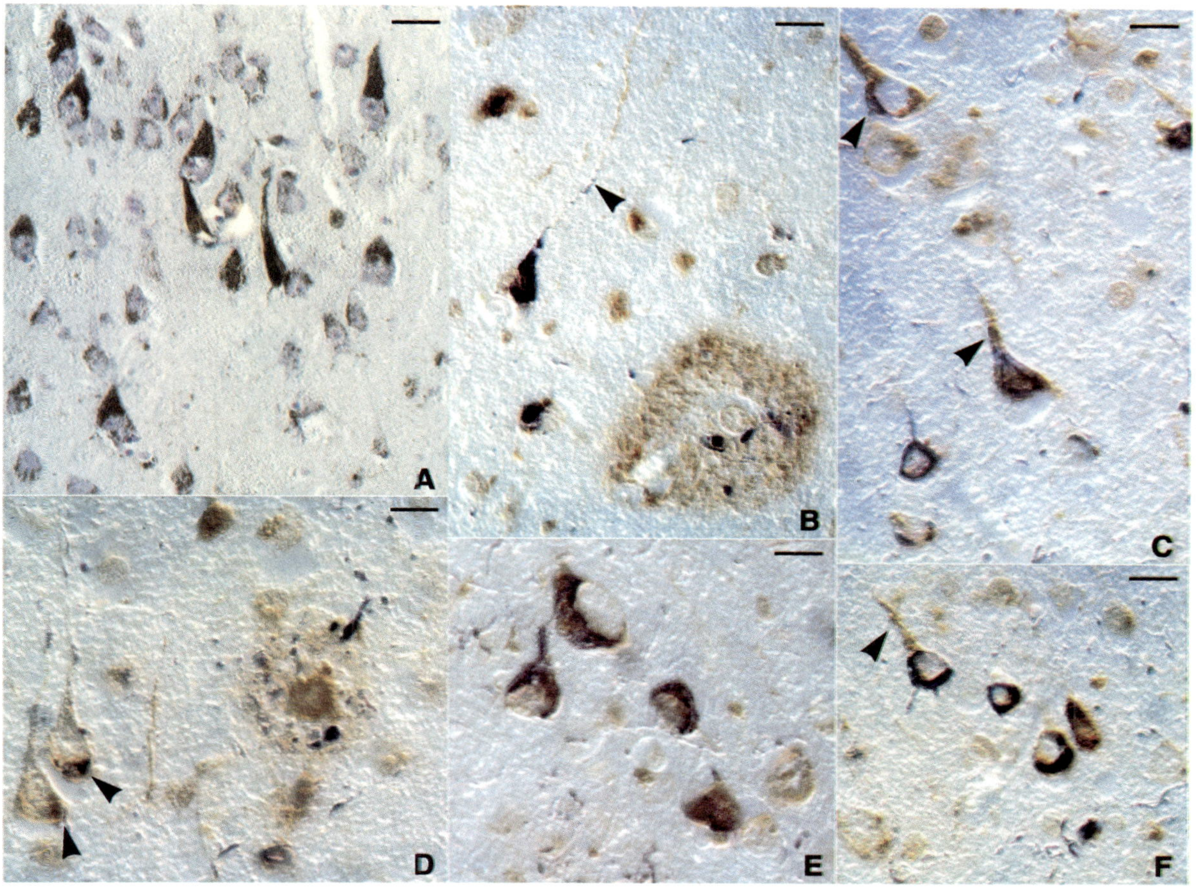

Figure 8. Staining of hippocampal formation from AD brain with the anti-heparan sulfate antibody 10E4 (*A*) and double-labeling with 10E4 and the phosphorylation-dependent anti-tau antibody AT8 (*B–F*). 10E4 staining is shown in brown and AT8 staining in blue (Nomarski optics). Note staining of some pyramidal cells with 10E4 in *A* and double-labeling of many nerve cells in *B–F*. Pyramidal cells with partially double-labeled cell bodies or neurites are arrowed in *B*, *C*, *D*, and *F*. The section in *A* was counterstained with thionin, with no counterstaining in *B–F*. Bars: *A*, 45 μm; *B*, 34 μm; *C*, 30 μm; *D,E*, 24 μm; and *F*, 43 μm.

The presence of heparin prevents tau from binding to taxol-stabilized microtubules, and microtubules assembled in the presence of tau rapidly depolymerize upon addition of heparin. This indicates that heparin prevents tau from promoting microtubule assembly and stability.

Previous experiments on AD brain have shown staining of heparan sulfate in neurofibrillary lesions (Snow et al. 1989, 1990: Kato et al. 1991; Perry et al. 1991). However, it had not been investigated whether heparan sulfate and hyperphosphorylated tau coexist in the earliest known stages of neurofibrillary pathology, where nerve cells stain diffusely with phosphorylation-dependent anti-tau antibodies ("pre-tangle" stage of AD) (Braak et al. 1994). We have therefore performed single- and double-labeling immunohistochemistry on hippocampal formation from AD brain using the anti-heparan sulfate antibody 10E4 (David et al. 1992) and the phosphorylation-dependent anti-tau antibody AT8. As shown in Figure 8A, a subset of pyramidal cells is strongly immunoreactive with 10E4; these include cells with overt neurofibrillary tangles, as well as non-tangle-bearing cells. Double-labeling immunohistochemistry shows that nerve cells that stain diffusely with AT8 also stain with 10E4 (Fig. 8B–F). In most cells, the brown 10E4 and the blue AT8 staining are intermixed. However, in some nerve cells, the heparan sulfate staining is more extensive than the tau staining (arrowed cells in Fig. 8C,F). In addition, small patches of tau staining are seen in cell bodies and neurites of some pyramidal cells with diffuse heparan sulfate staining (arrowed cells in Fig. 8C,D). Moreover, some tau-negative nerve cells are heparan-sulfate-positive, suggesting that the accumulation of heparan sulfate may precede hyperphosphorylation of tau.

Taken together, these findings indicate that an interaction between tau protein and sulfated glycosaminoglycans may lead to the formation of the neurofibrillary lesions of AD. These lesions consist of PHFs containing hyperphosphorylated tau protein that is unable to bind to microtubules. Sulfated glycosaminoglycans are known to stimulate tau phosphorylation by a number of protein kinases in a substrate-dependent manner (Mawal-Dewan et al. 1992; Brandt et al. 1994; Yang et al. 1994). The results presented here show that a phosphorylation-independent interaction between full-length tau and sulfated glycosaminoglycans leads to the formation of filaments closely resembling those found in AD brain. In the presence of sulfated glycosaminoglycans, three repeat-containing tau isoforms give rise to paired helical-like filaments, whereas four repeat isoforms give straight filaments, thus suggesting a mechanism for the two tau assemblies present in AD brain. The interaction between tau and sulfated glycosaminoglycans prevents tau from binding to microtubules and from promoting microtubule assembly. Moreover, heparan sulfate and hyperphosphorylated tau colocalize in nerve cells in AD brain prior to the formation of overt neurofibrillary lesions. These findings suggest that an increase in sulfated glycosaminoglycans within the cytoplasm of nerve cells may lead to the neurofibrillary pathology of AD by triggering the hyperphosphorylation of tau, by destabilizing microtubules, and by inducing assembly of PHFs. They also provide a simple assay for the identification of compounds that interfere with PHF formation.

REFERENCES

Arendt, T., M. Holzer, R. Fruth, M.K. Brückner, and U. Gärtner. 1995. Paired helical filament-like phosphorylation of tau, deposition of β/A4-amyloid and memory impairment in rat induced by chronic inhibition of phosphatase 1 and 2A. *Neuroscience* **69:** 691.

Braak, H. and E. Braak. 1991. Neuropathological staging of Alzheimer-related changes. *Acta Neuropathol.* **82:** 239.

Braak, E., H. Braak, and E.M. Mandelkow. 1994. A sequence of cytoskeleton changes related to the formation of neurofibrillary tangles and neuropil threads. *Acta Neuropathol.* **87:** 554.

Bramblett, G.T., M. Goedert, R. Jakes, S.E. Merrick, J.Q. Trojanowski, and V.M.-Y. Lee. 1993. Abnormal tau phosphorylation at Ser^{396} in Alzheimer's disease recapitulates development and contributes to reduced microtubule binding. *Neuron* **10:** 1089.

Brandt, R., G. Lee, D.B. Teplow, D. Shalloway, and M. Abdel-Ghany. 1994. Differential effect of phosphorylation and substrate modulation on tau's ability to promote microtubule growth and nucleation. *J. Biol. Chem.* **269:** 11776.

Brion, J.P., H. Passareiro, J. Nunez, and J. Flament-Durand. 1985. Mise en évidence immunologique de la protéine tau au niveau des lésions de dégénérescence neurofibrillaire de la maladie d'Alzheimer. *Arch. Biol.* **95:** 229.

Butner, K.A. and M.W. Kirschner. 1991. Tau protein binds to microtubules through a flexible array of distributed weak sites. *J. Cell Biol.* **115:** 717.

Couchie, D., C. Mavilia, I.S. Georgieff, R.K.H. Liem, M.L. Shelanski, and J. Nunez. 1992. Primary structure of high molecular weight tau present in the peripheral nervous system. *Proc. Natl. Acad. Sci.* **89:** 4378.

Crowther, R.A. 1991. Straight and paired helical filaments in Alzheimer disease have a common structural unit. *Proc. Natl. Acad. Sci.* **88:** 2288.

Crowther, R.A. and C.M. Wischik. 1985. Image reconstruction of the Alzheimer paired helical filament. *EMBO J.* **4:** 3661.

Crowther, R.A., O.F. Olesen, R. Jakes, and M. Goedert. 1992. The microtubule-binding repeats of tau protein assemble into filaments like those found in Alzheimer's disease. *FEBS Lett.* **309:** 199.

Crowther, R.A., O.F. Olesen, M.J. Smith, R. Jakes, and M. Goedert. 1994. Assembly of Alzheimer-like filaments from full-length tau protein. *FEBS Lett.* **337:** 135.

David, G., X.M. Bai, B. Van der Schueren, J.J. Cassiman, and H. Van den Berghe. 1992. Developmental changes in heparan sulfate expression: In situ detection with mAbs. *J. Cell Biol.* **119:** 961.

Dickson, D.W., H.A. Crystal, L.A. Mattiace, D.M. Masur, A.D. Blau, P. Davies, S.-H. Yen, and M.K. Anderson. 1991. Identification of normal and pathological aging in prospectively studied non-demented elderly humans. *Neurobiol. Aging* **13:** 179.

Drewes, G., B. Lichtenberg-Kraag, F. Döring, E.M. Mandelkow, J. Biernat, M. Dorée, and E. Mandelkow. 1992. Mitogen-activated protein (MAP) kinase transforms tau protein into an Alzheimer-like state. *EMBO J.* **11:** 2131.

Drewes, G., B. Trinczek, S. Illenberger, J. Biernat, G. Schmitt-Ulms, H.E. Meyer, E.M. Mandelkow, and E. Mandelkow. 1995. Microtubule-associated protein/microtubule affinity-regulating kinase. *J. Biol. Chem.* **270:** 7679.

Flament, S., A. Delacourte, B. Hémon, and A. Défossez. 1989. Characterization of two pathological tau protein variants in Alzheimer's disease. *J. Neurol. Sci.* **92:** 133.

Fleming, L.M. and G.V.W. Johnson. 1995. Modulation of the phosphorylation state of tau in situ: The roles of calcium and cyclic AMP. *Biochem. J.* **309:** 41.

Goedert, M. 1993. Tau protein and the neurofibrillary pathology of Alzheimer's disease. *Trends Neurosci.* **16:** 460.

Goedert, M. and R. Jakes. 1990. Expression of separate isoforms of human tau protein: Correlation with the tau pattern in brain and effects on tubulin polymerization. *EMBO J.* **9:** 4225.

Goedert, M., M.G. Spillantini, and R.A. Crowther. 1992a. Cloning of a big tau microtubule-associated protein characteristic of the peripheral nervous system. *Proc. Natl. Acad. Sci.* **89:** 4378.

Goedert, M., E.S. Cohen, R. Jakes, and P. Cohen. 1992b. p42 MAP kinase phosphorylation sites in microtubule-associated protein tau are dephosphorylated by protein phosphatase $2A_1$: Implications for Alzheimer's disease. *FEBS Lett.* **312:** 95.

Goedert, M., M.G. Spillantini, N.J. Cairns, and R.A. Crowther. 1992c. Tau proteins of Alzheimer paired helical filaments: Abnormal phosphorylation of all six brain isoforms. *Neuron* **8:** 159.

Goedert, M., R. Jakes, Z. Qi, J.H. Wang, and P. Cohen. 1995. Protein phosphatase 2A is the major enzyme in brain that dephosphorylates tau protein phosphorylated by proline-directed protein kinases or cAMP-dependent protein kinase. *J. Neurochem.* **65:** 2804.

Goedert, M., M.G. Spillantini, R. Jakes, D. Rutherford, and R.A. Crowther. 1989. Multiple isoforms of human microtubule-associated protein tau. Sequences and localization in neurofibrillary tangles of Alzheimer's disease. *Neuron* **3:** 519.

Goedert, M., C.M. Wischik, R.A. Crowther, J.E. Walker, and A. Klug. 1988. Cloning and sequencing of the cDNA encoding a core protein of the paired helical filament of

Alzheimer disease. Identification as the microtubule-associated protein tau. *Proc. Natl. Acad. Sci.* **85:** 4051.

Goedert, M., R. Jakes, M.G. Spillantini, M. Hasegawa, M.J. Smith, and R.A. Crowther. 1996. Assembly of microtubule-associated protein tau into Alzheimer-like filaments induced by sulphated glycosaminoglycans. *Nature* **383:** 550.

Götz, J., A. Probst, M.G. Spillantini, T. Schäfer, R. Jakes, K. Bürki, and M. Goedert. 1995. Somatodendritic localization and hyperphosphorylation of tau protein in transgenic mice expressing the longest human brain tau isoform. *EMBO J.* **14:** 1304.

Goode, B.L. and S.C. Feinstein. 1994. Identification of a novel microtubule binding and assembly domain in the developmentally regulated inter-repeat region of tau. *J. Cell Biol.* **124:** 769.

Greenberg, S.G. and P. Davies. 1990. A preparation of Alzheimer paired helical filaments that displays distinct tau proteins by polyacrylamide gel electrophoresis. *Proc. Natl. Acad. Sci.* **87:** 5827.

Greenberg, S.G., P. Davies, J.D. Schein, and L.I. Binder. 1992. Hydrofluoric acid-treated PHF proteins display the same biochemical properties as normal tau. *J. Biol. Chem.* **267:** 564.

Hanger, D.P., K. Hughes, J.R. Woodgett, J.P. Brion, and B.H. Anderton. 1992. Glycogen synthase kinase-3 induces Alzheimer's disease-like phosphorylation of tau: Generation of paired helical filament epitopes and neuronal localization of the kinase. *Neurosci. Lett.* **147:** 58.

Hasegawa, M., R. Jakes, R.A. Crowther, V.M.-Y. Lee, Y. Ihara, and M. Goedert. 1996. Characterization of mAb AP422, a novel phosphorylation-dependent monoclonal antibody against tau protein. *FEBS Lett.* **384:** 25.

Hasegawa, M., M. Morishima-Kawashima, K. Takio, M. Suzuki, K. Titani, and Y. Ihara. 1992. Protein sequence and mass spectrometric analyses of tau in the Alzheimer's disease brain. *J. Biol. Chem.* **267:** 17047.

Hirokawa, N., Y. Shiomura, and S. Ogabe. 1988. Tau proteins: The molecular structure and mode of binding on microtubules. *J. Cell Biol.* **107:** 1449.

Jakes, R., M. Novak, M. Davison, and C.M. Wischik. 1991. Identification of 3- and 4-repeat tau isoforms within the PHF in Alzheimer's disease. *EMBO J.* **10:** 2725.

Kato, T., H. Sasaki, T. Katagiri, H. Sasaki, K. Koiwai, H. Youki, S. Totsuka, and T. Ishii. 1991. The binding of basic fibroblast growth factor to Alzheimer's neurofibrillary tangles and senile plaques. *Neurosci. Lett.* **122:** 33.

Kondo, J., T. Honda, H. Mori, Y. Hamada, R. Miura, H. Ogawara, and Y. Ihara. 1988. The carboxyl third of tau is tightly bound to paired helical filaments. *Neuron* **1:** 827.

Lee, G., N. Cowan, and M. Kirschner. 1988. The primary structure and heterogeneity of tau protein from mouse brain. *Science* **239:** 285.

Lee, V.M.-Y. 1995. Disruption of the cytoskeleton in Alzheimer's disease. *Curr. Opin. Neurobiol.* **5:** 663.

Lee, V.M.-Y., B.J. Balin, L. Otvos, and J.Q. Trojanowski. 1991. A68—A major subunit of paired helical filaments and derivatized forms of normal tau. *Science* **251:** 675.

Litersky, J.M., G.V.W. Johnson, R. Jakes, M. Goedert, M. Lee, and P. Seubert. 1996. Tau protein is phosphorylated by cAMP-dependent protein kinase and Ca^{2+}/calmodulin-dependent protein kinase II within its microtubule-binding domains at Ser^{262} and Ser^{356}. *Biochem. J.* **316:** 655.

Matsuo, E.S., R.-W. Shin, M.L. Billingsley, A. Van de Voorde, M. O'Connor, J.Q. Trojanowski, and V.M.-Y. Lee. 1994. Biopsy-derived adult human brain tau is phosphorylated at many of the same sites as Alzheimer's disease paired helical filament tau. *Neuron* **13:** 989.

Mawal-Dewan, M., P.C. Sen, M. Abdel-Ghany, D. Shalloway, and E. Racker. 1992. Phosphorylation of tau protein by purified $p34^{cdc28}$ and a related protein kinase from neurofilaments. *J. Biol. Chem.* **267:** 19705.

Merrick, S.E., D.C. Demoise, and V.M.-Y. Lee. 1996. Site-specific dephosphorylation of tau protein at Ser/Thr 202/205 in response to microtubule depolymerization in cultured human neurons involves protein phosphatase 2A. *J. Biol. Chem.* **271:** 5589.

Morishima-Kawashima, M., M. Hasegawa, K. Takio, M. Suzuki, H. Yoshida, K. Titani, and Y. Ihara. 1995. Proline-directed and non-proline-directed phosphorylation of PHF-tau. *J. Biol. Chem.* **270:** 823.

Mothes, E., R.L. Shoeman, R.R. Schröder, and P. Traub. 1990. Polymerizing properties of pepstatin A. *J. Struct. Biol.* **105:** 80.

Paudel, H.K., J. Lew, A. Zenobia, and J.H. Wang. 1993. Brain proline-directed kinase phosphorylates tau on sites that are abnormally phosphorylated in tau associated with Alzheimer's paired helical filaments. *J. Biol. Chem.* **268:** 23512.

Perry, G., S.L. Siedlak, P. Richey, M. Kawai, P. Cras, R.N. Kalaria, P.G. Galloway, J.M. Scardina, B. Cordell, B.D. Greenberg, S.R. Ledbetter, and P. Gambetti. 1991. Association of heparan sulfate proteoglycan with the neurofibrillary tangles of Alzheimer's disease. *J. Neurosci.* **11:** 3679.

Snow, A.D., S. Lara, D. Nochlin, and T.N. Wight. 1989. Cationic dyes reveal proteoglycans structurally integrated within the characteristic lesions of Alzheimer's disease. *Acta Neuropathol.* **78:** 113.

Snow, A.D., H. Mar, D. Nochlin, R.T. Sekiguchi, K. Kimata, S. Koike, and T.N. Wight. 1990. Early accumulation of heparan sulfate in neurons and in the beta-amyloid protein-containing lesions of Alzheimer's disease and Down's syndrome. *Am. J. Pathol.* **137:** 1253.

Sontag, E., V. Nunbhadki-Craig, G.S. Bloom, and M.C. Mumby. 1995. A novel pool of protein phosphatase 2A is associated with microtubules and is regulated during the cell cycle. *J. Cell Biol.* **128:** 1131.

Watanabe, A., M. Hasegawa, M. Suzuki, K. Takio, M. Morishima-Kawashima, K. Titani, T. Arai, K.S. Kosik, and Y. Ihara. 1993. In vivo phosphorylation sites in fetal and adult rat tau. *J. Biol. Chem.* **268:** 25712.

Wille, H., G. Drewes, J. Biernat, E.M. Mandelkow, and E. Mandelkow. 1992. Alzheimer-like paired helical filaments and antiparallel dimers formed from microtubule-associated protein tau in vitro. *J. Cell Biol.* **118:** 573.

Wischik, C.M., M. Novak, H.C. Thøgersen, P.C. Edwards, M.J. Runswick, R. Jakes, J.E. Walker, C. Milstein, M. Roth, and A. Klug. 1988. Isolation of a fragment of tau derived from the core of the paired helical filament of Alzheimer disease. *Proc. Natl. Acad. Sci.* **85:** 4506.

Yang, S.-D., J.-S. Yu, S.-G. Shiah, and J.J. Huang. 1994. Protein kinase F_A/glycogen synthase kinase-3 alpha after heparin potentiation phosphorylates tau on sites abnormally phosphorylated in Alzheimer's disease brain. *J. Neurochem.* **63:** 1416.

Yoshida, H. and Y. Ihara. 1993. Tau in paired helical filament is functionally distinct from fetal tau: Assembly incompetence of paired helical filament tau. *J. Neurochem.* **61:** 1183.

Neuronal Sorting and Processing of Amyloid Precursor Protein: Implications for Alzheimer's Disease

P.J. TIENARI,[1,2,5] B. DE STROOPER,[3] E. IKONEN,[2] N. IDA,[1] M. SIMONS,[1,2]
C.L. MASTERS,[4] C.G. DOTTI,[2] AND K. BEYREUTHER[1]

[1]*Center for Molecular Biology (ZMBH), University of Heidelberg, INF 282, D-69120, Heidelberg, Germany;* [2]*Cell Biology Programme, European Molecular Biology Laboratories (EMBL), D-69012, Heidelberg, Germany;* [3]*Center for Human Genetics, B-3000 Leuven, Belgium;* [4]*Department of Pathology, University of Melbourne, Parkville, Victoria 3052, Australia*

Alzheimer's disease (AD) is the most common cause of dementia, with a prevalence of more than 5% among people over the age of 65. It is a disease of the brain affecting especially temporal and parietal cortex, hippocampus, and amygdala. The distinguishing histopathological features are the senile plaques and neurofibrillary tangles. The main proteinaceous component of the senile plaques is aggregated β-amyloid (βA4) (Glenner and Wong 1984; Masters et al. 1985). βA4 is produced by proteolytic cleavages of the amyloid precursor protein (APP). The prototype βA4 peptide is 42 amino acids long, but it shows some amino- and carboxy-terminal raggedness in biological fluids as well as in senile plaques. The length of βA4 is considered critical in its ability to aggregate, since the peptide ending at residue 42 is more aggregating in vitro than the peptide ending at residue 40 (Hilbich et al. 1991; Jarrett et al. 1993).

Three lines of evidence support a causal role of βA4 in AD pathogenesis. First, mutations in the APP gene cause familial early-onset AD with autosomal dominant inheritance (chromosome 21). These mutations have been shown to increase either the overall amount or the length of βA4 (Citron et al. 1992; Cai et al. 1993; Iwatsubo et al. 1994; Suzuki et al. 1994). Furthermore, transgenic mice expressing one of the APP mutations exhibit similar amyloid pathology in the brain as is found in AD (Games et al. 1995). The second line of evidence for the amyloid hypothesis comes from studies on Down's syndrome. Subjects with Down's syndrome have an extra copy of the APP gene because of chromosome 21 trisomy, and they almost invariably develop early-onset AD with massive βA4 deposition in the brain. Importantly, amyloid pathology precedes the onset of AD by decades, suggesting that it would be a cause of the disease rather than its consequence (Rumble et al. 1989; Teller et al. 1996). Third, mutations in the newly identified familial early-onset AD genes, presenilin 1 and 2 (Levy-Lahad et al. 1995; Rogaev et al. 1995; Sherrington et al. 1995), located on chromosomes 14 and 1, respectively, have been found to increase the amount of carboxy-terminally elongated βA4 species both in vivo and in vitro (Scheuner et al. 1996). This suggests a functional link between the mutated presenilins and βA4 formation. Since cerebral βA4 deposition is a common feature of all forms of AD (sporadic, familial, and Down's syndrome cases), a common pathway involving increased βA4 formation or deposition is well supported by the available data.

APP, the precursor of βA4, resembles a cell-surface receptor, but its function remains unclear. It consists of a large extracellular domain, a single transmembrane domain, and a short cytoplasmic tail (Kang et al. 1987). APP has several alternatively spliced isoforms; the 695-amino-acid isoform (APP_{695}) is predominantly expressed in neurons (Sandbrink et al. 1994). Studies in neuronal and nonneuronal cells have demonstrated that APP may be either secreted via the constitutive secretory pathway or inserted into cellular membranes as a transmembrane holoprotein (Weidemann et al. 1989). Further cleavages can occur during endocytosis (Selkoe 1994). The "α-cleavage" occurs at the middle part of βA4, thus precluding amyloid formation, whereas the amyloidogenic "β-cleavage" occurs at the amino-terminus of βA4 (see Fig. 1). A third cleavage, "γ-cleavage," occurs in the transmembrane domain of the α- or β-cleaved carboxy-terminal fragment and releases the 3- to 4-kD p3 and βA4 peptides from the cell. The enzymes generating these cleavages remain unidentified.

To understand the pathogenetic cascade of AD, knowledge about the metabolism of APP in the affected cells, i.e., central nervous system neurons, is required. Here we summarize our recent studies on intracellular trafficking of APP with special emphasis on its polarized sorting in hippocampal neurons. Additionally, we have analyzed proteolytic processing of APP in these cells, focusing on the neuronal mechanisms of βA4 generation.

MATERIALS AND METHODS

DNA constructs and preparation of recombinant Semliki Forest Virus (SFV). A c-myc epitope (EQKLISEEDL) was introduced to APP_{695} sequence at sites corresponding to the amino terminus or car-

[5]Present address: Department of Neurology, University of Helsinki, Haartmaninkatu 4, FIN-00290 Helsinki, Finland.

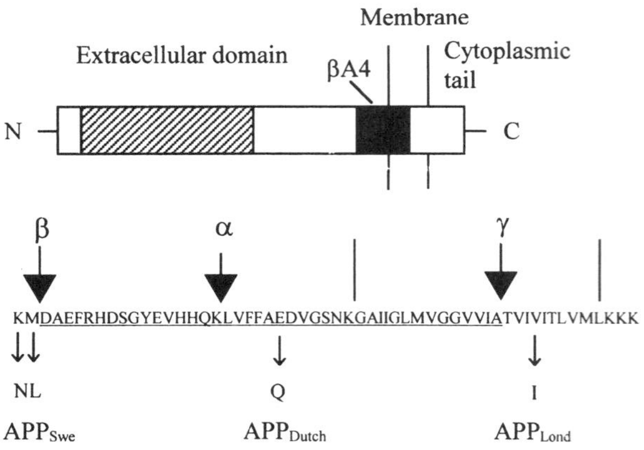

Figure 1. Schematic presentation of proteolytic cleavage sites and clinical mutations of APP. The amino acid sequence of βA4 (1–42) is underlined (one-letter code for amino acids). The major cleavage sites are indicated by arrows on the top of the sequence; the three mutations analyzed in this study are shown below the sequence.

boxyl terminus of APP. Mutagenesis and cloning into the expression vector pSFV1 (Liljeström and Garoff 1991) was carried out as described previously (Tienari et al. 1996). pSFV1/APP and pSFV-helper DNAs were in vitro transcribed as described previously (Liljeström and Garoff 1991). The pSFV1/APP transcription mix was cotransfected into baby hamster kidney cells with pSFV-helper transcription mix using electroporation, and the secreted SFV particles were subsequently concentrated and titrated (Olkkonen et al. 1993).

Neuronal culture, infections, and immunofluorescence. Dissociated hippocampal neuron cultures were prepared from rat embryos as described previously (Goslin and Banker 1991). The cells were maintained in culture in serum-free N_2-medium in the presence of astrocytes. Infections, immunofluorescence, and the assay for quantification of the axonal and dendritic distribution of protein have been described previously (De Hoop et al. 1995; Tienari et al. 1996).

Antibodies. The following primary antibodies were used in immunofluorescence: a monoclonal c-myc antibody 9E10 (Evan et al. 1985) for the detection of the amino- or carboxy-terminally inserted c-myc epitope; a human specific monoclonal antibody (W2-2) against the residues 1–16 of βA4; a polyclonal antibody, anti-FdAPP, against APP ectodomain (Weidemann et al. 1989); a polyclonal antibody against MAP2, generously provided by Dr. Diez-Guerra, Centro de Biologia Molecular, Madrid, Spain; and a monoclonal antibody against MAP2 (clone AP20) from Boehringer Mannheim Biochemica, Mannheim, Germany. The secondary antibodies in immunofluorescence were goat anti-mouse IgG and goat anti-rabbit IgG (Cappel, Durham, North Carolina). In immunoprecipitation of metabolically labeled cells, the anti-FdAPP was used to detect secreted APP and holoAPP; a polyclonal antibody 692 raised against βA4 synthetic peptide 1–40 was used to precipitate βA4 and p3. Monoclonal antibodies W0-2 (epitope between residues 5 and 8 of βA4) as well as βA4 carboxyl terminus-specific antibodies G2-10 and G2-11 were used to detect total βA4 and its carboxy-terminal variants in immunoblots (Ida et al. 1996).

Biochemical analyses. For metabolic labeling, the culture medium was exchanged to methionine-free MEM containing 300–500 μCi/ml of $[^{35}S]$methionine and 1/10 of N_2-supplement with 15 mg/l of methionine. Conditioned medium and cells were harvested and immunoprecipitated as described previously (Simons et al. 1996). Immunoprecipitated material was analyzed as described by Tienari et al. (1996). For immunoblotting, neurons cultured on 3-cm dishes were infected with SFV/APP, and the cells (in 0.7 ml lysis buffer) and the conditioned medium (1 ml) were harvested at 6–7 hours postinfection as described previously (Simons et al. 1996). For detection of total βA4 as well as APP_{sec} and holoAPP, the conditioned media and cell lysates were immunoprecipitated with W0-2 in the presence of protein G-agarose (Boehringer Mannheim, Germany). The carboxy-terminal variants of βA4, β40, and β42 were detected by precipitating the samples with G2-10 and G2-11 (Ida et al. 1996), respectively, in the presence of protein G-agarose.

RESULTS

Analysis of Axonal Sorting Signals of APP Reveals a Function for the βA4 Domain

In neurons, APP undergoes fast anterograde axonal transport (Koo et al. 1990) and has been detected in both pre- and postsynaptic sites, in vesicular elements in the cell body, axon, and dendrites, as well as on the surface of axons and dendrites (Schubert et al. 1991; Ferreira et al. 1993; Allinquant et al. 1994; Caporaso et al. 1994; Simons et al. 1995; Yamazaki et al. 1995). We have previously shown, using the SFV expression system in hippocampal neurons, that newly synthesized APP is intially targeted to the axon and is only later found in the dendrites (Simons et al. 1995). Two experimental procedures supported the concept that the dendritic APP is at least partially derived from the axon via transcytosis: (1) Protein synthesis inhibition at the time of axonal expression did not block the dendritic appearance of APP, and (2) anti-myc antibody bound to APP at the axonal surface was later found in the dendrites (Simons et al. 1995).

Since newly synthesized APP is initially transported to the axon, we analyzed the sorting signals responsible for this polarized delivery. We analyzed the intracellular distribution of human wild-type APP (APP_{wt}) and several APP mutants in mature synaptically active hippocampal neurons in culture using immunofluorescence microscopy. To specifically follow the fate of newly synthesized protein rather than the steady-state distribution of endogenous APP, we used a viral expression system for expression of c-myc-tagged APP. We chose the SFV system (Liljeström and Garoff 1991) because it permits rapid initiation of protein synthesis after a 1-hour infection and does not produce major cytopathic effects during the first 8 hours postinfection (Olkkonen et al. 1993). Based on the initial distribution of the protein, the cells were grouped into three categories: (1) axonal, (2) dendritic, and (3) mixed; i.e., axonal and dendritic. Axons and dendrites were distinguished by both morphological and immunocytochemical criteria. Morphologically, an axon appears as a long, thin process with uniform diameter, whereas dendrites are more numerous, thicker, and tapering in diameter. Immunocytochemically, microtubule associated protein-2 (MAP2) can be used to distinguish between these processes, since only dendrites (and the soma) are MAP2-positive in mature hippocampal neurons.

Clinical APP mutations. We first analyzed whether pathogenic mutations of human APP would affect its sorting. Two APP mutations implicated in early-onset familial AD were tested (Fig. 1) (Goate et al. 1991; Mullan et al. 1992). A third type of mutation ("Dutch"), which has been implicated in brain amyloidosis with hemorrhage, was also tested (Fig. 1) (Levy et al. 1990). Start of the SFV-driven protein synthesis could be visualized in tubular structures in the cell body at 2–2.5 hours postinfection in both APP_{wt} and the clinical mutants. At 3–4 hours postinfection, both APP_{wt} and the clinical mutants started to appear preferentially in the axon (Fig. 2). Similar distribution of protein was found with the anti-myc antibody recognizing amino- or carboxy-terminally inserted myc epitope. The observed predominantly axonal distribution demonstrates that the clinical mutations do not alter the polarized trafficking of APP.

Contribution of ectodomain and cytoplasmic tail. We next tested the contribution of the cytoplasmic tail and the ectodomain to the observed axonal delivery of APP. Similar to APP_{wt}, the cytoplasmic tail deletion mutant (ΔCT) was distributed preferentially to the axon at 3.5–4 hours postinfection (Fig. 3). The ectodomain deletion mutant (SPC99), on the other hand, showed a striking effect on the polarity of transport. The protein polarity was virtually reversed with a predominantly somatodendritic localization (Fig. 3). Expression of the ectodomain only as a soluble mutant ($APP_{s\alpha}$) also resulted in a somatodendritic distribution of the protein (Fig. 3). These results demonstrate that the ectodomain, but not the cytoplasmic tail, is required for axonal sorting of APP, and that APP ectodomain has to be membrane-inserted for correct sorting.

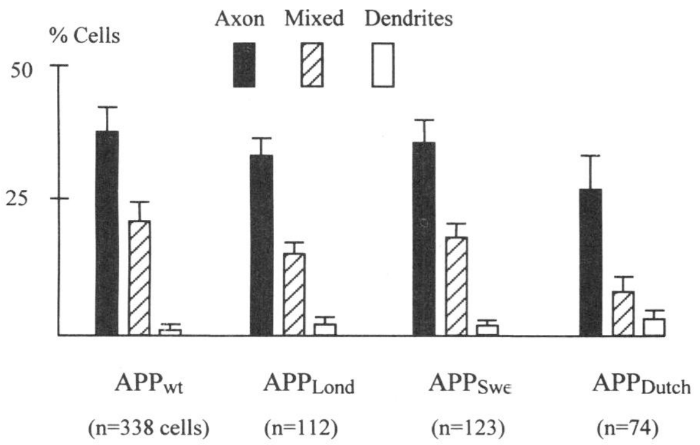

Figure 2. Axonal targeting of wild-type APP and the clinical mutants. Quantitative analysis of the distribution of APP_{wt} and clinical APP mutants at an early phase of transport (3.5–4 hr postinfection). The cells with exclusive cell body labeling (41–62% of the cells) are not indicated by a column. Quantitation was based on at least three independent experiments; error bars represent S.E.M. APP_{wt} as well as APP_{Lond} and APP_{Swe} were visualized with an antibody against either amino- or carboxy-terminally inserted *c-myc* epitope; APP_{Dutch} was visualized with the W2-2 antibody.

Ectodomain determinants. To map the ectodomain region(s) needed for axonal sorting, we designed a set of deletions that encompass 99% of the amino acid residues in the APP_{695} ectodomain (Fig. 4). Deletion of the amino acids 4–392 (ΔCys) had no effect on axonal sorting. A mild decrease in axonal sorting was observed with the carbohydrate domain deletion mutant (residues 392–598, ΔCHO) which exhibited a mixed, i.e., axonal and dendritic, distribution in the majority of cells. The most significant effect was detected with the deletion of the extracellular portion of βA4 (ΔA4), which showed a somatodendritic predominance in its distribution. Virtually no cells transported ΔA4 exclusively to the axon. Surface labeling with antibodies W2-2 (ΔCys and ΔCHO) and anti-FdAPP (ΔA4) demonstrated that all of these truncated proteins reached the plasma membrane (not shown), suggesting that the transmembrane topology of APP was maintained in these mutants. The profound effect on APP sorting found with the ΔA4 mutant suggests that the extracellular part of the βA4 domain would play an important role in axonal delivery. To further analyze the contribution of the βA4 domain, we tested a mutant SPC111 containing only βA4 plus 12 adjacent amino-terminal residues in the ectodomain. This mutant carries a slight amino-terminal elongation as compared to the SPC99 mutant, which was somatodendritically sorted (see Fig. 4). We tested whether this short elongation present in SPC111 but not in SPC99 could induce wild-type APP-like sorting. Expression of SPC111 mutant resulted in a mixed (axonal and dendritic) distribution of the protein in the majority of the cells (Fig. 4). Thus, although expression of this construct resulted in a significantly increased axonal

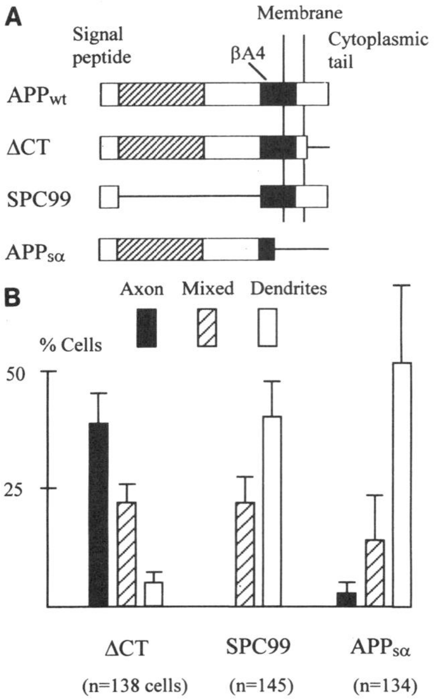

Figure 3. Membrane-bound ectodomain of APP but not the cytoplasmic tail is needed for its axonal sorting. (*A*) Scheme of the mutations. (*B*) Quantitative analysis of the distribution of the deletion mutants ΔCT (3.5–4 hr postinfection), SPC99 (6.5 hr postinfection), and APPsα (4 hr postinfection). ΔCT was visualized with an antibody against an amino-terminal c-myc epitope. SPC99 was visualized with antibodies against a carboxy-terminal myc epitope as well as with the W2-2 antibody. APPsα was visualized with an antibody against an amino-terminal c-myc epitope. Cells with exclusive cell body labeling are not indicated by a column. Quantitation was based on three independent experiments; error bars represent S.E.M.

delivery as compared to the SPC99 expressing cells, this ectodomain region (βA4 plus 12 adjacent amino-terminal residues) per se was not sufficient to restore full axonal sorting. This implies that the axonal delivery of APP is mediated by at least two determinants, neither of which is alone sufficient. One of the determinants would be dependent on an intact βA4 domain, the others would be located upstream (amino-terminally) from it. The upstream determinants should reside in the region encoded by exons 11–15, which was absent in both ΔCHO and SPC111 mutants. This region contains two N-glycosylation motifs. Since N-glycans have been shown to contain sorting information in epithelial cells (Sheiffele et al. 1995), we tested the effect of tunicamycin, an N-glycosylation inhibitor, on the sorting of APP_{wt}. In tunicamycin-treated cells, a mixed, axonal and dendritic, distribution of APP_{wt} was found (Fig. 4). Moreover, the pattern of transport in tunicamycin-treated cells was virtually identical to the pattern observed in the ΔCHO mutant (Fig. 4), suggesting that deletion of the N-glycosylation sites in ΔCHO led to its missorting.

Taken together, these results indicate that both an intact βA4 domain and N-glycosylation are required for axonal sorting of APP. The membrane-proximal βA4-dependent signal would be the major contributor to axonal sorting, whereas the N-glycosylation-dependent signal would have a weaker effect.

Mechanisms of βA4 Generation in Cultured Hippocampal Neurons

Although the metabolism of APP has been studied in detail in many cell types, information on the mechanisms of βA4 production in the cells that are affected in AD, i.e. hippocampal neurons, is lacking. One rea-

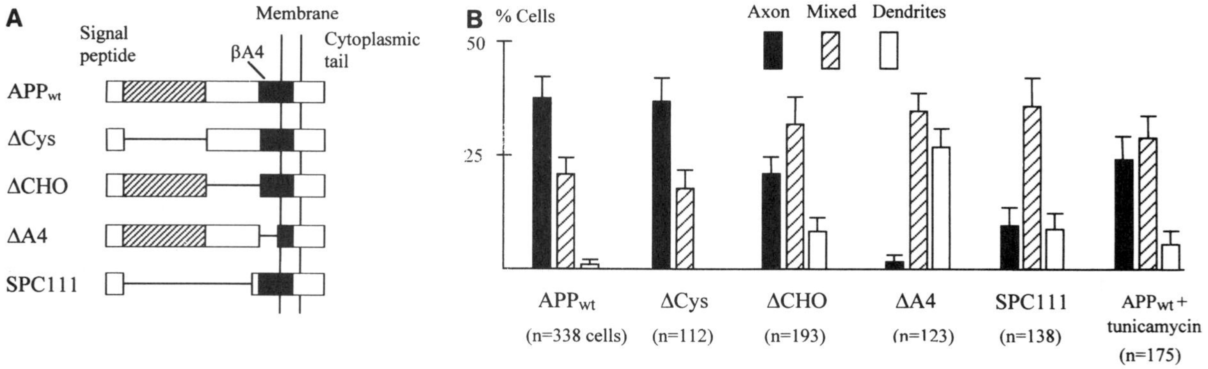

Figure 4. Effect of serial ectodomain deletions and tunicamycin treatment on the axonal sorting of APP. (*A*) Scheme of the mutations. (*B*) Quantitative analysis of the distribution of the ectodomain deletions at 3.5–4 hr postinfection. Each mutant was detected with an antibody recognizing a carboxy-terminally inserted c-myc epitope. ΔA4 was additionally detected with the anti-FdAPP against APP ectodomain. Cells with exclusive cell body labeling are not indicated by a column. Tunicamycin treatment was started at 0 hr or 0.5 hr postinfection and the cells were fixed at 4 hr postinfection. Difference in the proportion of cells with exclusive axonal labeling in wild-type versus ΔCHO: $p<0.01$; APP_{wt} and tunicamycin^{+} versus tunicamycin^{-} $p<0.025$ (Student's t-test, 2-tailed).

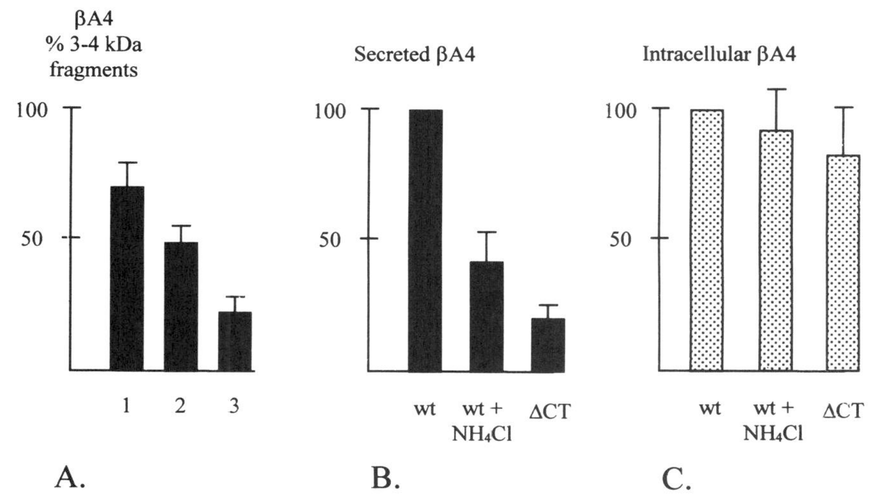

Figure 5. βA4 production in hippocampal neurons. (*A*) Relative amount of βA4 among the secreted 3- to 4-kD peptides. Lanes: (*1*) Hippocampal neurons labeled in MEM/[^{35}S]Met+N_2-supplement. (*2*) Hippocampal neurons labeled in MEM/[^{35}S]Met only. (*3*) Primary cultures of mouse fibroblasts labeled in MEM/[^{35}S]Met. (*B*) Effect of NH_4Cl treatment and expression of the ΔCT mutant on the secreted βA4 after normalizing to the levels of APP_{sec}. The amount of βA4 in APP_{wt} is fixed to 100. (*C*) Effect of NH_4Cl treatment and expression of the ΔCT mutant on the intracellular βA4 after normalizing to the levels of APP_{sec}.

son for this is the difficulty in recovering enough protein from cultured neurons for biochemical analyses. In order to obtain sufficient amounts of protein for these analyses, we expressed APP via the SFV system; this also allowed us to analyze the processing of APP mutants in hippocampal neurons. Here we focus on the generation of βA4 and p3, the amino termini of which are the products of β and α cleavages, respectively (see Fig. 1). Typically, immunoprecipitation of these peptides from the conditioned medium of a variety of nonneuronal cells recovers higher amounts of p3 than βA4 (Haass et al. 1992, 1993; Hartmann et al. 1996). This was also the case when we analyzed βA4 and p3 that were secreted from primary cultures of mouse fibroblasts expressing human APP via the SFV system. In these cells (labeled in MEM/[^{35}S]Met), βA4 constituted 20–25% of the immunoprecipitated 3- to 4-kD peptides (Fig. 5A). In contrast, when human APP was expressed in hippocampal neurons, βA4 constituted approximately 70% of the immunoprecipitated 3- to 4-kD peptides when the cells were labeled in MEM in the presence of N_2-supplement (insulin, progesterone, transferrin) and 45–50% when the experiment was carried out in MEM/[^{35}S]Met only (Fig. 5A).

Neurons are the only cells that have been shown to produce substantial amounts of cell-lysate-associated βA4 (Wertkin et al. 1993). In agreement with this study using a neuronal teratocarcinoma cell line, we were able to precipitate βA4 (but not p3) from the cell lysates of hippocampal neurons expressing human APP_{wt}. Two procedures support the conclusion that the cell-lysate-associated βA4 mostly (>80%) represents a de-novo-synthesized pool of molecules: (1) In pulse-chase experiments, βA4 was found in the cells before it appeared in the medium, and (2) when metabolically labeled βA4-containing medium was transferred onto nonlabeled cells, only trace amounts of radiolabeled βA4 recovered from the nonlabeled cells after 3–12 hours incubation (not shown).

Previous studies in other cell types have demonstrated that secreted βA4, but not p3, is produced by a pH-sensitive and endocytosis-dependent mechanism (Haass et al. 1993; Koo and Squazzo 1994). Whether this mechanism also operates in neurons is not known. Therefore, we tested the effect of NH_4Cl, an alkalizing agent widely used in previous studies, on the production of the 3- to 4-kD peptides in hippocampal neurons. In agreement with studies in nonneuronal cells, the secretion of βA4 was relatively decreased as compared to p3 upon NH_4Cl treatment (Fig. 5B). However, the production of intracellular βA4 was not significantly inhibited by NH_4Cl (Fig. 5C). Endocytosis dependence of βA4 production was tested by expressing a mutant (ΔCT) lacking the cytoplasmic tail of APP, and thereby the endocytosis signals. Expression of this mutant in hippocampal neurons resulted in marked down-regulation of βA4 secretion but, again, this effect was not observed in intracellular βA4 (Fig. 5B,C). These results indicate that in hippocampal neurons the intracellular and secreted βA4 species are generated by distinct mechanisms. The secreted species is clearly NH_4Cl-sensitive and endocytosis-dependent as reported in other cells, whereas the intracellular species is generated via an alternate mechanism.

Effect of APP Clinical Mutants on the Secreted and Intracellular Pools of βA4

We analyzed the production of secreted and intracellular βA4 species of two APP mutations, APP_{Swe}

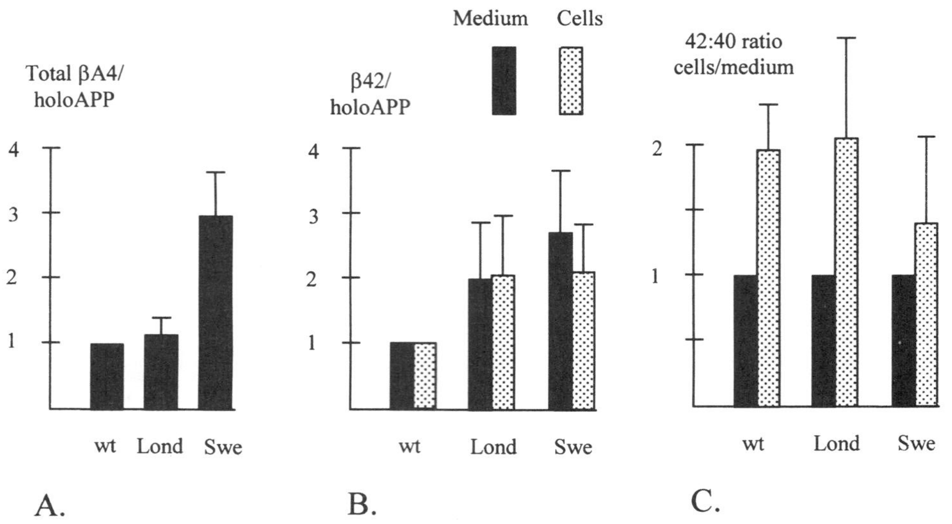

Figure 6. Effect of APP clinical mutants on the production of βA4 and its carboxy-terminal variants β40 and β42. (*A*) Total βA4 in the media after normalizing to holoAPP levels in neurons expressing APP_{wt}, APP_{Lond}, and APP_{Swe} (n=8 each). Medium and cells were harvested at 6–7 hr postinfection. Quantification was based on pairwise comparisons between APP_{wt} and the clinical mutants within each experiment. (*B*) β42 levels in APP_{wt} and the clinical mutants after normalizing to holoAPP. Medium and cell lysates were analyzed separately, and both are fixed to 1 in APP_{wt}. APP_{Lond} versus APP_{wt} $p<0.02$ (medium), $p<0.02$ (cells); APP_{Swe} versus APP_{wt} $p<0.001$ (medium), $p<0.01$ (cells); APP_{Lond} versus APP_{Swe} p=n.s. Student's t-test for pairwise comparisons (n=8 each). (*C*) 42:40 ratios in cells versus medium of neurons expressing APP_{wt}, APP_{Lond}, and APP_{Swe}. 42:40 ratio in the medium of each dish is fixed to 1. Cells versus medium difference was analyzed by Student's t-test for pairwise comparisons (n=9 each): APP_{wt} $p<0.001$; APP_{Lond} $p<0.02$; APP_{Swe} p=n.s. (2-tailed p-values).

and APP_{Lond} (Fig. 1), implicated in early-onset familial AD (Goate et al. 1991; Mullan et al. 1992). APP_{Swe} has been demonstrated to favor β-cleavage at the expense of α-cleavage, thus secreting more βA4 than APP_{wt} (Citron et al. 1992; Cai et al. 1993). On the other hand, APP_{Lond} has been shown to generate more carboxy-terminally elongated βA4 species (β42/43) in relation to APP_{wt} (Suzuki et al. 1994).

Here we expressed APP_{wt}, APP_{Swe}, and APP_{Lond} in hippocampal neurons and measured total βA4, β40, and β42 in the secreted and intracellular pools. Expression of APP_{Swe} resulted in an increased secretion of total βA4 compared to APP_{wt}, as has been previously shown in neuronal (De Strooper et al. 1995b) and non-neuronal cells (Citron et al. 1992; Cai et al. 1993), whereas APP_{Lond} had no effect on the secretion of total βA4 (Fig. 6A). The level of intracellular βA4 followed that of the secreted species (not shown). Next we analyzed the production of β42 by the clinical mutants as compared to APP_{wt}. In APP_{Lond} there was a 2-fold increase in β42 both in the media and cell lysates; a similar or slightly higher increase of β42 was found in APP_{Swe} (Fig. 6B). This illustrates that the overall increased production of βA4 in APP_{Swe} translates also into increased β42 levels. Finally, we tested whether the 42:40 ratios differ in the intracellular versus extracellular compartments. The 42:40 ratio of the cell lysate versus medium of each dish, expressing APP_{wt} or the clinical mutants, was compared. There was a 1.9- to 2.0-fold mean increase in the 42:40 ratio in the cell lysates compared to the media upon expression of APP_{wt} and APP_{Lond} (Fig. 6C), demonstrating a significantly increased recovery of β42 from the cell lysates. This effect was, however, not significant upon expression of APP_{Swe} (Fig. 6C).

These results demonstrate that a common feature of APP_{Lond} and APP_{Swe} is their increased generation of β42 both in the secreted and intracellular pools of βA4. Furthermore, the cell lysates of neurons expressing APP_{wt} and APP_{Lond} harbored a significantly higher fraction of β42 compared to the respective conditioned media, indicating that β42 would be overrepresented in the intracellular pool of βA4.

DISCUSSION

A Hierarchy of APP Sorting

The hierarchical appearance of newly synthesized APP first in the axon and later in the dendrites raises questions as to how this process is regulated. We and other workers have provided evidence for the involvement of transcytosis (Simons et al. 1995; Yamazaki et al. 1995). Ligand-induced transcytosis of polymeric immunoglobulin receptor from basolateral to apical domain has been described in epithelial cells (Aoreti and Mostov 1994 and references therein), and a similar process from somatodendritic to axonal domain has been documented in neurons as well (Ikonen et al. 1993; De Hoop et al. 1995). Ligand binding could thus be one factor regulating the polarized distribution of APP in neurons.

When considering APP transcytosis as a sorting problem, it appears that neurons should utilize more than one sorting station in regulating polarized distribution of APP. The first sorting station would be at the *trans*-Golgi network (TGN), responsible for initial axonal delivery, and further sorting would occur subsequently during endocytosis and transcytosis. Our analysis of the APP-deletion mutants revealed three principal patterns of polarity: axonal, mixed, and somatodendritic. Thus, the polarity could be reversed with some of the mutations, indicating that APP contains both axonal and somatodendritic sorting signals that can be sequentially decoded. The emergence of the somatodendritic pattern in the SPC99 mutant suggests that the (recessive) somatodendritic signals are most likely located in the cytoplasmic tail of APP. In epithelial cells, the same cytoplasmic sorting signals can be decoded in both the TGN and endosomes (Matter et al. 1993; Aoreti and Mostov 1994). Hence, it is possible the same signals that direct the SPC99 mutant to the dendrites would also mediate the axonal-dendritic transcytosis of APP_{wt}. This would provide a physiological explanation to the hierarchy of axonal and somatodendritic signals on APP as well as to the hierarchy of APP transport: initially axonal, later dendritic.

βA4 Domain Is Essential for Axonal Sorting of APP

Our data suggest that the membrane-proximal βA4-dependent signal would be the major contributor to axonal sorting, whereas the N-glycosylation-dependent signal would have a weaker effect. That βA4 domain is required for axonal sorting of APP reveals a somewhat surprising biological function for this juxtamembranous portion of the molecule. Furthermore, βA4 domain is not involved in polarized sorting of APP in epithelial MDCK cells (De Strooper et al. 1995a,c; Haass et al. 1995), indicating a neuron-specific function for it. An attractive hypothesis for the role of the βA4 domain in intraneuronal sorting would be that APP interacts directly via this domain with a sorting receptor in the TGN in order to get packaged into axonal transport vesicles. Although the three-dimensional structure of APP is not known, βA4 domain should be physically accessible for interactions with other molecules, since it represents the region where the major proteolytic cleavages of APP occur. Furthermore, interaction of βA4 with the sorting machinery could modulate the relative usage of the α- and β-cleavages at the βA4 domain. It is conceivable that the high secretion of βA4 in relation to p3 we observed in hippocampal neurons partially arises from interactions between βA4 domain and sorting machinery, resulting in down-regulation of α-cleavage. It is also of note that we did not detect any p3 among the intracellular 3- to 4-kD peptides, suggesting that virtually no α-cleavage occurs in the compartment that generates intracellular βA4. Thus, interactions of the βA4-domain with the sorting machinery form an interesting novel parameter that could regulate the relative utility of α- and β-cleavages and would provide a link between neuronal type of sorting and neuronal type of processing of APP.

APP Sorting in Neurons Versus Nonneuronal Cells

A comparison of APP sorting in hippocampal neurons versus that in MDCK cells illustrates that these cell types decode different signals from APP. The APP holoprotein transport is regulated by ectodomain determinants in neurons, as shown here, whereas in MDCK cells it is regulated by signals in the cytoplasmic tail (De Strooper et al. 1995a; Haass et al. 1995). This implies that either there are specific molecules present in neurons, which are able to recognize the axonal signals on APP ectodomain, or there are different posttranslational modifications of APP in these cells. Newly synthesized APP is sorted axonally in neurons and basolaterally in epithelial cells. Hence, APP represents an interesting exception to the proposed axonal/apical and somatodendritic/basolateral parallel between neurons and epithelial cells (Dotti and Simons 1990; Craig and Banker 1994). In our study, only the ectodomain deletion mutant SPC99 and the soluble mutant $APP_{s\alpha}$ were sorted in a parallel manner (somatodendritic/basolateral) as compared to MDCK cells expressing similar mutants (De Strooper et al. 1995a,c; Haass et al. 1995).

Distinct Pathways for the Generation of Intracellular and Secreted βA4

The cellular source of βA4 in AD plaques has been unclear. Our studies in hippocampal neurons revealed that these cells process APP in an amyloidogenic manner characterized by high βA4-to-p3 ratio in contrast to various nonneuronal cells studied to date (Haass et al. 1992, 1993; Hartmann et al. 1996). This suggests that neurons could be an important source of βA4 in AD brains. In addition to the high βA4-to-p3 ratio, an intriguing aspect of neurons is that these are the only cells that have been found to produce substantial amounts of intracellular βA4 and also the main victims in the AD disease process. We demonstrated that the intracellular and secreted βA4 species derive by distinct pathways as judged by their different NH_4Cl-sensitivity and endocytosis-dependence. This is a conceptually important finding, since it raises questions on the relative contribution of these dual pathways in AD. Moreover, these pathways might be differently modulated by pharmacological strategies.

Clinical APP Mutants and βA4 Production

Our analysis of the clinical APP mutants demonstrated that the common feature of APP_{Lond} and

APP_{Swe} is that they both increase β42 in the intra- and extracellular compartments. That two different APP mutations exhibit this same effect strengthens the hypothesis that β42 would play a central role in AD. The analysis of β42 contribution of APP_{Lond} and APP_{Swe} revealed that these mutants would generate 2.0- and 2.7-fold more of this peptide in the medium, and 2.0- and 2.1-fold more in the cell lysates, respectively, as compared to APP_{wt}. Hence, the β42 loads generated by these mutants are close to each other. Interestingly, the mean age of onset of carriers of these mutations is also very similar: APP_{Lond}, 57 years and APP_{Swe}, 53 years (Goate et al. 1991; Mullan et al. 1992).

A Role of Intracellular βA4 in AD?

It is clear that the intracellular and extracellular pools of βA4 are not completely separate, since the intracellular βA4 is known to eventually become secreted (Fuller et al. 1995; Turner et al. 1996). In our system, the amount of intracellular βA4 was roughly 15% of that found in the medium. Considering the minimal volume of the cells (<1/1000) compared to the medium, the concentration of βA4 is apparently several orders of magnitude (>150-fold) higher intracellularly than in the conditioned medium. This is of importance, since high local concentrations of βA4 are known to increase its aggregation and pathogenicity. Concentrations of 10–40 mM have been shown to be toxic to cell cultures (Selkoe 1994). This is, however, much higher than the nanomolar concentrations found in biological fluids in vivo and in vitro. In addition to the total concentration of βA4, the concentration of ions, such as Zn^{++}, and the presence of "pathological chaperones" influence its aggregation in vitro (Bush et al. 1994; Ma et al. 1994). A third factor, which is believed to be a critical player in neurodegeneration, is the amount of β42 (Iwatsubo et al. 1994; Selkoe 1994; Suzuki et al. 1994; Scheuner et al. 1996; Teller et al. 1996). This view is further supported by our finding that both APP_{Lond} and APP_{Swe} increase this particular fraction of βA4 and suggests a shared disease mechanism for these two mutations. We observed a slightly increased recovery of β42 in relation to β40 from the cell lysates compared to the media of APP_{wt}- and APP_{Lond}-expressing neurons, suggesting that β42 would constitute a larger fraction in the intracellular than in the secreted pool. This could obviously strengthen the pathogenic effects of intracellular βA4. An alternative explanation to the increased recovery of β42 from the cell lysates could be its increased cell surface association or internalization. However, if this were the case, we would have expected to find the same in APP_{Swe}-expressing cells, which had the highest absolute levels of β42, but this was not observed.

A role of intracellular βA4 in AD has been, for technical reasons, difficult to address. Some insights into the potential role of intracellular βA4 have been gained from studies in mice with a transgenic βA4 (1–42) minigene (LaFerla et al. 1995). These mice exhibit neurodegeneration with apoptotic features. This is of interest, since several groups have reported apoptotic features also in AD brains (Lassmann et al. 1995; Andersson et al. 1996) and in cultures of Down's syndrome neurons (Busciglio and Yankner 1995). A link between apoptosis and AD is also supported by the finding that a partial cDNA of the mouse homolog of the early-onset AD gene, presenilin-2, functions as an apoptosis inhibitor (Vito et al. 1996). Furthermore, an enhanced rate of apoptosis has been reported in cells transfected with APP_{695} Val-642 mutations (such as APP_{Lond}) compared to APP_{wt} transfected cells, which could not be induced by addition of extracellular β42 (Yamatsuji et al. 1996). This suggests that extracellular βA4 does not explain this finding and provides a challenge to the amyloid hypothesis. However, the Val-642 mutant clearly produces a higher fraction of β42 than APP_{wt}, both in the secreted and intracellular pools. Hence, it is possible that this peptide actually exerts its effects in a specific intracellular compartment. A role of intracellular amyloid has been raised in the context of another type of amyloidosis, the pancreatic amylin deposition of type 2 diabetes mellitus. Intracellular amylin deposition has been found to precede extracellular deposition in human insulinomas (O'Brien et al. 1994), and overexpression of amylin leads to intracellular amyloid formation and cytotoxicity in COS cells (O'Brien et al. 1995). Furthermore, the cytotoxic effect of amylin requires conformational changes, as has also been found with βA4, and the affected cells exhibit apoptotic features (Lorenzo et al. 1994), revealing an interesting parallel between these two amyloid peptides.

Neuron-specific Features in APP Metabolism

APP represents an interesting, ubiquitously expressed model molecule whose metabolism has been studied in detail in several types of cells. Intriguing differences have been found in its metabolism in neuronal versus nonneuronal cells. First, as shown here, the β-secretase pathway is more prominent in neurons than in nonneuronal cells. Second, the neuronal and nonneuronal splice variants exhibit different post-translational modifications and intracellular transport (Hartmann et al. 1996 and references therein). Third, the polarized transport of holoAPP is controlled by different sorting signals in neurons compared to epithelial cells, with the βA4 domain being involved only in neurons (De Strooper et al. 1995a,c; Haass et al. 1995; Tienari et al. 1996). Fourth, neurons represent the only cell type that has been found to produce abundant intracellular βA4, and as shown here, neurons are able to generate this intracellular βA4 via an alternate pathway. These differences in metabolism between neurons and other cells may have more general impact in explaining why mutations in many ubiquitously expressed proteins result in diseases manifested only in the nervous system, e.g. APP/AD, cystatin B/epilepsy (Pennachio et al. 1996), and prion protein/spongiform encephalopathies (Prusiner 1996). Selective vulnerability of neurons has been considered as one explanation; the insights gained from studies on APP suggest that neuron-specific metabolic pathways of a protein could be an additional factor resulting in nervous-system-specific diseases.

ACKNOWLEDGMENTS

We thank Liane Meyn for preparing the hippocampal cultures. P.J.T. and B.D.S. have been supported by European Molecular Biology Organization fellowships, E.I. by a European Community Human Capital and Mobility fellowship, K.B. by a Bundesminister für Bildung, Wissenschaft Forschung und Technologie grant, and K.B. and C.G.D. by Deutsche Forschungsgemeinschaft (SFB 317) grants.

REFERENCES

Allinquant, B., K. Moya, C. Bouillot, and A. Prochiantz. 1994. Amyloid precursor protein in cortical neurons: Coexistence of two pools differently distributed in axons and dendrites and association with cytoskeleton. *J. Neurosci.* **14:** 6842.

Andersson, A.J., J.H. Su, and C.W. Cotman. 1996. DNA damage and apoptosis in Alzheimer's disease: Colocalization with c-Jun immunoreactivity, relationship to brain area, and effect of postmortem delay. *J. Neurosci.* **15:** 1710.

Aoreti, B. and K. Mostov. 1994. Polarized sorting of polymeric immunoglobulin receptor in the exocytic and endocytic pathways is controlled by the same amino acids. *EMBO J.* **13:** 2297.

Busciglio, J. and B.A. Yankner. 1995. Apoptosis and increased generation of reactive oxygen species in Down's syndrome neurons in vitro. *Nature* **378:** 776.

Bush, A.I., W.H. Pettingell, G. Multhaup, M. de Paradis, J.-P. Vonsattel, J.F. Gusella, K. Beyreuther, C.L. Masters, and R.E. Tanzi. 1994. Rapid induction of Alzheimer Aβ amyloid formation by zinc. *Science* **265:** 1464.

Cai, X.D., T.E. Golde, and S.G. Younkin. 1993. Release of excess amyloid β protein from a mutant amyloid β protein precursor. *Science* **259:** 514.

Caporaso, G.L., K. Takei, S.E. Gandy, M. Matteoli, O. Mundigl, P. Greengard, and P. de Camilli. 1994. Morphological and biochemical analysis of the intracellular trafficking of the Alzheimer's β/A4 amyloid precursor protein. *J. Neurosci.* **14:** 3122.

Citron, M., T. Oltersdorf, C. Haass, L. McConlogue, A.Y. Hung, P. Seubert, C. Vigo-Pelfrey, I. Lieberburg, and D.J. Selkoe. 1992. Mutation of the β-amyloid precursor protein in familial Alzheimer's disease increases β-protein production. *Nature* **360:** 672.

Craig, A.M. and G. Banker. 1994. Neuronal polarity. *Annu. Rev. Neurosci.* **17:** 267.

De Hoop, M., C. von Poser, C. Lange, E. Ikonen, W. Hunziker, and C.G. Dotti. 1995. Intracellular routing of wild-type and mutated polymeric immunoglobulin receptor in hippocampal neurons in culture. *J. Cell Biol.* **130:** 1447.

De Strooper, B., K. Craessaerts, F. Van Leuven, and H. Van Den Berghe. 1995a. Exchanging the extracellular domain of amyloid precursor protein for horseradish peroxidase does not interfere with alpha-secretase cleavage of the beta-amyloid region, but randomizes secretion in Madin-Darby canine kidney cells. *J. Biol. Chem.* **270:** 30310.

De Strooper, B., M. Simons, G. Multhaup, F. Van Leuven, K. Beyreuther, and C.G. Dotti. 1995b. Production of intracellular amyloid-containing fragments in hippocampal neurons expressing human amyloid precursor protein and protection against amyloidogenesis by subtle amino acid substitutions in the rodent sequence. *EMBO J.* **14:** 4932.

De Strooper, B., K. Craessaerts, I. Dewachter, D. Moechars, B. Greenberg, F. Van Leuven, and H. Van Den Berghe. 1995c. Basolateral secretion of amyloid precursor protein in Madin-Darby canine kidney cells is disturbed by alterations of intracellular pH and by introducing a mutation associated with familial Alzheimer's disease. *J. Biol. Chem.* **270:** 4058.

Dotti, C.G. and K. Simons. 1990. Polarized sorting of viral glycoproteins to the axon and dendrites of hippocampal neurons in culture. *Cell* **62:** 63.

Evan, G., G.K. Lewis, G. Ramsay, and J.M. Bishop. 1985. Isolation of monoclonal antibodies specific for c-*myc* proto-oncogene product. *Mol. Cell. Biol.* **5:** 3610.

Ferreira, A., A. Caceres, and K. Kosik. 1993. Intraneuronal compartments of amyloid precursor protein. *J. Neurosci.* **13:** 3112.

Fuller, S.J., E. Storey, Q.X. Li, A.I. Smith, K. Beyreuther, and C.L. Masters. 1995. Intracellular production of beta A4 amyloid of Alzheimer's disease: Modulation by phosphoramidon and lack of coupling to the secretion of the amyloid precursor protein. *Biochemistry* **34:** 8091.

Games, D., D. Adams, R. Alessandrini, R. Barbour, P. Berthelette, C. Blackwell, T. Carr, J. Clemens, T. Donaldson, F. Gillespie, T. Guido, S. Hagopian, K. Johnsoamino-Wood, K. Khan, M. Lee, P. Leibowitz, I. Lieberburg, S. Little, E. Masliah, L. McConlogue, M. Montoya-Zavala, L. Mucke, L. Paganini, E. Penniman, M. Power, D. Schenk, P. Seubert, B. Snyder, F. Soriano, H. Tan, J. Vitale, S. Wadsworth, B. Wolozin, and J. Zhao. 1995. Alzheimer-type neuropathology in transgenic mice overexpressing V717F β-amyloid precursor protein. *Nature* **373:** 523.

Glenner, G.C. and C.W. Wong. 1984. Alzheimer's disease: Initial report of the purification and characterisation of a novel cerebrovascular amyloid protein. *Biochem. Biophys. Res. Commun.* **120:** 885.

Goate, A., M.C. Chartier-Harlin, M. Mullan, J. Brown, F. Crawford, L. Fidani, L. Giufra, A. Haynes, N. Irwing, L. James, R. Mant, P. Newton, K. Rooke, P. Roques, C. Talbot, M. Pericak-Vance, A. Roses, R. Williamson, M. Rossor, M. Owen, and J. Hardy. 1991. Segregation of a missense mutation in the amyloid precursor protein gene with familial Alzheimer's disease. *Nature* **349:** 704.

Goslin, K. and G.A. Banker. 1991. Rat hippocampal neurons in low density culture. In *Culturing nerve cells* (ed. G.A. Banker and K. Goslin.), p. 251. MIT Press, Cambridge, Massachusetts.

Haass, C., E.H. Koo, D. Teplow, and D.J. Selkoe. 1995. Polarized secretion of β-amyloid precursor protein and β-amyloid peptide in MDCK cells. *J. Cell Biol.* **128:** 537.

Haass, C., A.Y. Hung, M.G. Schlossmacher, D.B. Teplow, and D.J. Selkoe. 1993. β-amyloid peptide and a 3-kDa fragment are derived by distinct cellular mechanisms. *J.*

Biol. Chem. **268:** 3021.

Haass, C., M.G. Schlossmacher, A.Y. Hung, C. Vigo-Pelfrey, A. Mellon, B.L., Ostaszewski, I. Lieberburg, E.H. Koo, D. Schenk, D.B. Teplow, and D.J. Selkoe. 1992. Amyloid β-peptide is produced by cultured cells during normal metabolism. *Nature* **359:** 322.

Hartmann, T., C. Bergsdorf, R. Sandbrink, P.J. Tienari, G. Multhaup, N. Ida, S. Bieger, T. Dyrks, A. Weidemann, C.L. Masters, and K. Beyreuther. 1996. Alzheimer's disease βA4 protein release and amyloid precursor protein sorting are regulated by alternative splicing. *J. Biol. Chem.* **271:** 13208.

Hilbich, C., B. Kister-Woike, J. Reed, C.L. Masters, and K. Beyreuther. 1991. Aggregation and secondary structure of synthetic amyloid beta A4 peptides of Alzheimer's disease. *J. Mol. Biol.* **218:** 149.

Ida, N., T. Hartmann, J. Pantel, J. Schröder, R. Zirfass, H. Förstel, R. Sandbrink, C.L. Masters, and K. Beyreuther. 1996. Analysis of heterogeneous βA4 peptides in human cerebrospinal fluid and blood by a newly-developed sensitive Western blot assay. *J. Biol. Chem.* **271:** 22908.

Ikonen, E., R.G. Parton, W. Hunziker, K. Simons, and C.G. Dotti. 1993. Transcytosis of the polymeric immunoglobulin receptor in cultured hippocampal neurons. *Curr. Biol.* **3:** 635.

Iwatsubo, T., A. Odaka, N. Suzuki, H. Mizusawa, N. Nukina, and Y. Ihara. 1994. Visualization of Aβ42(43) and Aβ(40) in senile plaques with end-specific Aβ monoclonals: Evidence that an initially deposited species is Aβ42(43). *Neuron* **13:** 45.

Jarrett, J.T., E.P. Berger, and P.T. Landsbury. 1993. The carboxy terminus of the beta amyloid protein is critical for the seeding of amyloid formation: Implications for the pathogenesis of Alzheimer's disease. *Biochemistry* **32:** 4693.

Kang, J., H.G. Lemaire, A. Unterbeck, J.M. Salbaum, C.L. Masters, K.H. Grzeschik, G. Multhaup, K. Beyreuther, and B. Müller-Hill. 1987. The precursor of Alzheimer's disease amyloid A4 protein resembles a cell-surface receptor. *Nature* **325:** 733.

Koo, E.H. and S.L. Squazzo. 1994. Evidence that production and release of amyloid beta-protein involves the endocytic pathway. *J. Biol. Chem.* **269:** 17386.

Koo, E.H., S.S. Sisodia, D.A. Archer, L.J. Martin, A. Weidemann, K. Beyreuther, C.L. Masters, and D.L. Price. 1990. Precursor of amyloid precursor protein in Alzheimer's disease undergoes fast anterograde axonal transport. *Proc. Natl. Acad. Sci.* **87:** 1561.

LaFerla, F.M., B.T. Tinkle, C.J. Biedrich, C.C. Haudenschild, and G. Jay. 1995. The Alzheimer's Aβ peptide induces neurodegeneration and apoptotic cell death in transgenic mice. *Nat. Genet.* **9:** 21.

Lassmann, H., C. Bancher, H. Breitschopf, J. Wiegel, M. Bobinski, K. Jellinger, and H.M. Wisniewski. 1995. Cell death in Alzheimer's disease evaluated by DNA fragmentation in situ. *Acta Neuropathol.* **89:** 35.

Levy, E., M.D. Carman, I.J. Fernandez-Madrid, M.D. Power, I. Lieberburg, S.G. van Duinen, G.T.A.M. Bots, W. Luyendijk, and B. Frangione. 1990. Mutation of the Alzheimer's disease amyloid gene in hereditary cerebral amyloidosis, Dutch type. *Science* **248:** 1124.

Levy-Lahad, E., W. Wasco, P. Poorkaj, D.M. Romano, J. Oshima, W.H. Pettingell, C.E. Yu, P.D. Jondro, S.D. Schmidt, K. Wang, A.C. Crowley, Y.H. Fu, S.Y. Guenette, D. Galas, E. Nemens, E.M. Wijsman, T.D. Bird, G.D. Schellenberg, and R.E. Tanzi. 1995. Candidate gene for the chromosome 1 familial Alzheimer's disease locus. *Science* **269:** 973.

Liljeström, P. and H. Garoff. 1991. A new generation of animal cell expression vectors based on the Semliki forest virus replicon. *Bio/Technology* **9:** 1356.

Lorenzo, A., R. Razzaboni, G.C. Weir, and B.A. Yankner. 1994. Pancreatic islet cell toxicity of amylin associated with type-2 diabetes mellitus. *Nature* **368:** 756.

Ma, J., A. Yee, B. Brewer, Jr., S. Das, and H. Potter. 1994. Amyloid-associated proteins alpha 1-antichymotrypsin and apolipoprotein E promote assembly of Alzheimer beta protein into filaments. *Nature* **372:** 92.

Masters, C.L., G. Multhaup, G. Simms, J. Pottgiesser, R.N. Martins, and K. Beyreuther. 1985. Amyloid core protein in Alzheimer's disease and Down syndrome. *Proc. Natl. Acad. Sci.* **82:** 4245.

Matter, K., J.A. Whitney, E.M. Yamamoto, and I. Mellman. 1993. Common signals control LDL receptor sorting in endosomes and the Golgi complex of MDCK cells. *Cell* **74:** 1053.

Mullan, M., F. Crawford, K. Axelman, H. Houlden, L. Lilius, B. Winnblad, and L. Lannfelt. 1992. A pathogenic mutation for probable Alzheimer's disease in the APP-gene at the N-terminus of β-amyloid. *Nat. Genet.* **1:** 345.

O'Brien, P.C., A.E. Butler, K. Johson, and P.C. Butler. 1994. Islet amyloid polypeptide (IAPP) in human insulinomas: Evidence for intracellular amyloidogenesis. *Diabetes* **43:** 329.

O'Brien, T., P.C. Butler, D.K. Kreutter, L.A. Kane, and L. Eberhardt. 1995. Human islet amyloid polypeptide expression in cos-1 cells. A model of intracellular amyloidogenesis. *Am. J. Pathol.* **147:** 609.

Olkkonen, V.M., P. Liljeström, H. Garoff, K. Simons, and C.G. Dotti. 1993. Expression of heterologous proteins in cultured rat hippocampal neurons using Semliki forest virus vector. *J. Neurosci. Res.* **35:** 445.

Pennachio, L.A., A.-E. Lehesjoki, N.E. Stone, V.L. Willour, K. Virtaneva, J. Miao, E. D'Amato, L. Ramirez, M. Faham, M. Koskiniemi, J.A. Warrington, R. Norio, A. de la Chapelle, D.R. Cox, and R.M. Myers. 1996. Mutations in the gene encoding cystatin B in progressive myoclonus epilepsy (EPM1). *Science* **271:** 1731.

Prusiner, S.B. 1996. Human prion diseases and neurodegeneration. *Curr. Top. Microbiol. Immunol.* **207:** 1.

Rogaev, E.I., R. Sherrington, E.A. Rogaeva, G. Levesque, M. Ikeda, Y. Liang, H. Chi, C. Lin, K. Holman, T. Tsuda, L. Mar, S. Sorbi, B. Nacmias, S. Placentini, L. Amaducci, I. Chumakov, D. Cohen, L. Lannfelt, P.E. Fraser, J.M. Rommens, and P.H. St. George-Hyslop. 1995. Familial Alzheimer's disease in kindred with missense mutations in a gene on chromosome 1 related to the Alzheimer's disease type 3 gene. *Nature* **376:** 775.

Rumble, B., R. Retallack, C. Hilbich, G. Simms, G. Multhaup, R. Martins, A. Hockey, P. Montgomery, K. Beyreuther, and C.L. Masters. 1989. Amyloid A4 protein and its precursor in Down's syndrome and Alzheimer's disease. *N. Engl. J. Med.* **320:** 1446.

Sandbrink, R., C.L. Masters, and K. Beyreuther. 1994. βA4 amyloid protein precursor mRNA isoforms without exon 15 are ubiquitously expressed in rat tissues including brain, but not in neurons. *J. Biol. Chem.* **269:** 1510.

Scheiffele, P., J. Peränen, and K. Simons. 1995. N-glycans as apical sorting signals in epithelial cells. *Nature* **387:** 96.

Scheuner, D., X. Song, M. Citron, N. Suzuki, T.D. Bird, J.

Hardy, M. Hutton, L. Lannfelt, E. Levy-Lahad, E.R. Pekind, P. Poorkaj, G.D. Schellenberg, R.E. Tanzi, M. Viitanen, W. Wasco, D.J. Selkoe, and S.G. Younkin. 1996. The S182 and STM2 mutations linked to familial Alzheimer's disease increase the extracellular concentration of amyloid β protein (Aβ) ending at Aβ42(43). *Nat. Med.* **2:** 864.

Schubert, W., R. Prior, A. Weidemann, H.G. Lemaire, C.L. Masters, and K. Beyreuther. 1991. Localization of Alzheimer's βA4 amyloid presursor protein at central and peripheral synaptic sites. *Brain Res.* **563:** 184.

Selkoe, D.J. 1994. Amyloid β-protein presursor: New clues to the genesis of Alzheimer's disease. *Curr. Opin. Neurobiol.* **4:** 708.

Sherrington, R., E.I. Rogaev, Y. Liang, E.A. Rogaeva, G. Levesque, M. Ikeda, H. Chi, G. Li, K. Holman, T. Tsuda, L. Mar, J.F. Foncin, A.C. Bruni, M.P. Montesi, S. Sorbi, I. Rainero, L. Pinessi, L. Nee, I. Chumakov, D. Pollen, A. Brookes, P. Sanseau, R.J. Polinsky, W. Wasco, H.A. Da Silva, J.L. Haines, M.A. Pericak-Vance, R.E. Tanzi, A.D. Roses, P.E. Fraser, J.M. Rommens, and P.H. St. George-Hyslop. 1995. Cloning of a gene bearing missense mutations in early-onset familial Alzheimer's disease. *Nature* **375:** 754.

Simons, M., B. De Strooper, G. Multhaup, P.J. Tienari, C.G. Dotti, and K. Beyreuther. 1996. Amyloidogenic processing of the human amyloid precursor protein in primary cultures of rat hippocampal neurons. *J. Neurosci.* **16:** 899.

Simons, M., E. Ikonen, P.J. Tienari, A. Cid-Arregui, U. Mönning, K. Beyreuther, and C.G. Dotti. 1995. Intracellular routing of human amyloid protein precursor: Axonal delivery followed by transport to the dendrites. *J. Neurosci. Res.* **41:** 121.

Suzuki, N., T.T. Cheung, X.-D. Cai, A. Odaka, L. Otvos Jr., C. Eckman, T.E. Golde, and S.G. Younkin. 1994. An increased percentage of long amyloid β protein secreted by familial amyloid β protein precursor (βAPP717) mutants. *Science* **264:** 1336.

Teller, J.K., C. Russo, L.M. DeBusk, G. Angelini, D. Zaccheo, F. Dagna-Bricarelli, P. Scartezzini, S. Bertolini, D.M.A. Mann, M. Tabaton, and P. Gambetti. 1996. Presence of soluble amyloid β-peptide precedes amyloid plaque formation in Down's syndrome. *Nat. Med.* **2:** 93.

Tienari, P.J., B. De Strooper, E. Ikonen, M. Simons, A. Weidemann, C. Czech, T. Hartmann, N. Ida, G. Multhaup, C.L. Masters, F. Van Leuven, K. Beyreuther, and C.G. Dotti. 1996. The β-amyloid domain is essential for axonal sorting of amyloid precursor protein. *EMBO J.* **16:** 5218.

Turner, R.S., N. Suzuki, A.S.C. Chyung, S.G. Younkin, and V.M.-Y Lee. 1996. Amyloid β40 and β42 are generated intracellularly in cultured human neurons and their secretion increases with maturation. *J. Biol. Chem.* **271:** 8966.

Weidemann, A., G. König, D. Bunke, P. Fischer, C.L. Masters, and K. Beyreuther. 1989. Identification, biogenesis and localization of precursors of Alzheimer's disease A4 amyloid protein. *Cell* **57:** 115.

Wertkin, A.M., R.S. Turner, S.J. Pleasure, S.G. Golde, J.Q. Trojanowski, and V.M.Y. Lee. 1993. Human neurons derived from a teratocarcinoma cell line express solely the 695-amino acid amyloid precursor and produce intracellular β-amyloid or A4 peptides. *Proc. Natl. Acad. Sci.* **90:** 9513.

Vito, P., E. Lacana, and L. D'Adamio. 1996. Interfering with apoptosis: $Ca2^{+}$-binding protein ALG-2 and Alzheimer's disease gene ALG-3. *Science* **271:** 521.

Yamatsuji, T., T. Okamoto, S. Takeda, Y. Murayama, N. Tanaka, and I. Nishimoto. 1996. Expression of V642 APP mutant causes cellular apoptosis as Alzheimer trait-linked phenotype. *EMBO J.* **15:** 498.

Yamazaki, T., D.J. Selkoe, and E.H. Koo. 1995. Trafficking of cell surface β-amyloid precursor protein: Retrograde and transcytotic transport in cultured neurons. *J. Cell Biol.* **129:** 431.

Cell Biology of the β-Amyloid Precursor Protein and the Genetics of Alzheimer's Disease

D.J. SELKOE
Department of Neurology and Program in Neurosciences, Harvard Medical School, and Center for Neurologic Diseases, Brigham and Women's Hospital, Boston, Massachusetts 02115

Progressive cerebral deposition of the 40- to 42-residue amyloid β-protein (Aβ) is an invariant feature of Alzheimer's disease (AD). Myriad spherical deposits of Aβ occur in limbic and association cortices. Many of these are intimately associated with dystrophic axons and dendrites, activated microglia, and reactive astrocytes (the neuritic plaques). Aβ is derived by constitutive proteolytic processing from a large type I integral membrane glycoprotein, the β-amyloid precursor protein (βAPP), which is encoded in humans by a gene on chromosome 21q (Kang et al. 1987). Patients born with trisomy 21 (Down's syndrome) overexpress βAPP throughout life and begin to develop cortical Aβ deposits as early as the second decade of life, followed by the gradual development of the full histopathological features of AD over the next three to four decades (Mann et al. 1989; Lemere et al. 1996a).

AD represents the most common basis for late-life memory and cognitive failure in most developed countries. Although a small proportion of cases experience onset of symptoms prior to age 60, most cases appear with increasing frequency after the mid 60s, and patients can present with symptoms as late as the 90s and beyond. The strong association of clinical AD with aging is reflected in the fact that cognitively unimpaired or minimally impaired older humans frequently develop small or moderate numbers of amorphous Aβ deposits in the cortex that are associated with little or no neuritic and glial dystrophy (the diffuse plaques). This association of cerebral Aβ deposition with aging also occurs in virtually all nonhuman primates, as well as in cats, dogs, and certain other higher mammals. Therefore, cerebral β-amyloidosis is not restricted to AD but is a feature of aging in a number of mammals. Because mild amnesiac and cognitive symptoms in the elderly have been associated with Aβ deposition and early neuritic plaque formation that are less robust than those usually seen in clinically typical AD (Morris et al. 1996), the development of pharmacological inhibitors of the neuropathology of AD may ultimately have import for the treatment of mild cognitive impairment in the elderly.

In addition to immature Aβ deposits (diffuse plaques) and mature (neuritic) plaques, AD subjects almost always develop large numbers of intraneuronal neurofibrillary tangles in selected neurons of the hippocampus, amygdala, neocortex, and certain subcortical nuclei. These tangles consist of paired, helically wound approximately 10-nm filaments (PHF) which exist in large non-membrane-bound bundles in the perinuclear cytoplasm and are also found in dystrophic cortical neurites, both within and between the neuritic plaques. The combined presence of neuritic plaques and neurofibrillary tangles in numbers exceeding those found in normal aged individuals establishes a final neuropathological diagnosis of AD.

Extensive morphological, biochemical, and molecular genetic studies of AD during the last decade have resulted in the identification of at least four genes, mutations or polymorphisms of which are associated with the accelerated development of the disease (for review, see Selkoe 1996). The first familial AD (FAD) gene to be identified was the β*APP* gene itself. Six missense mutations in βAPP, all clustered within exons 16 and 17 that encode the Aβ region of the precursor, have been identified in a small number of families worldwide. Subjects bearing one of these mutations develop early-onset but otherwise relatively typical AD, often beginning in the 50s. The second identified FAD gene is that coding for apolipoprotein E on chromosome 19. In this case, the naturally occurring ε4 polymorphism confers a substantially greater risk of developing AD than do the ε2 and ε3 polymorphisms, and ε4 also lowers the age of onset of the late-onset, common form of AD into the 60s and early 70s (Corder et al. 1993). The third and fourth genes linked to AD are the recently cloned *presenilin 1* (Sherrington et al. 1995) and *presenilin 2* (Levy-Lahad et al. 1995; Rogaev et al. 1995) genes on chromosomes 14 and 1, respectively. Patients with missense mutations in one or the other of these presenilin genes (~30 mutations have been identified to date) develop very early onset, dominantly transmitted AD, with symptoms appearing in the 40s or 50s or sometimes earlier. In summary, there are three known causative genes showing virtually full penetrance (β*APP, PS1, PS2*) and one major genetic risk factor (the ApoE ε4 allele).

Knowledge of the specific proteins comprising the histological lesions found in all AD cases, and of the altered gene products causing familial forms of the disease, has enabled rapid progress in deciphering the biochemical and cell biological mechanisms that underlie the development of the AD phenotype. Progress in this area has in turn provided important new information of interest to cell biologists and biochemists in general. In this chapter, I focus particularly on genotype-to-phenotype relationships in FAD and how understanding the cellular trafficking and proteolytic processing of βAPP has provided evidence of a common pathogenic mechanism for all forms of AD.

RESULTS

βAPP Trafficking and Proteolytic Processing

We have investigated the trafficking and processing of βAPP in several nonneural cell types, including polarized Madin Darby canine kidney (MDCK) cells, and in primary neurons (for review, see Selkoe 1994). An understanding of βAPP metabolic pathways is needed to elucidate the genotype-to-phenotype relationships of the known FAD genes. βAPP is a heterogeneous group of polypeptides that undergo alternative splicing (the longest transcript being 770 amino acids) and complex posttranslational processing, including N- and O-linked glycosylation, phosphorylation, and sulfation (Weidemann et al. 1989; Oltersdorf et al. 1990). The most important aspect of the posttranslational modification of βAPP for both its function and dysfunction relates to its endoproteolysis at several sites to release a variety of secreted derivatives from the cell. βAPP is expressed in virtually all neural and nonneural cell types examined to date, with the highest transcription generally found in the brain and kidney. The βAPP sequence is highly conserved in mammals, and close homologs have been found in *Drosophila* and *Caenorhabditis elegans*.

βAPP polypeptides are cotranslationally translocated into the endoplasmic reticulum (ER) via their signal peptide and then matured through the central vacuolar pathway, where the N- and O-linked glycosylation and phosphorylation of the ectodomain occur. βAPP can also undergo secretory cleavages within the late Golgi, *trans*-Golgi network (TGN), secretory vesicles budding off the TGN, and at the cell surface. The principal secretory cleavage—first identified at the cell surface but now known to occur also in the intracellular secretory pathway—is a scission at residue 687 of βAPP_{770} to create a large soluble ectodomain derivative and a membrane-retained carboxy-terminal fragment (Fig. 1). The unknown protease(s) that effects this cleavage is designated α-secretase(s). βAPP molecules that reach the cell surface but escape cleavage by α-secretase can subsequently be reinternalized via clathrin-coated pits and vesicles and targeted to endosomes and lysosomes. Some early endosomes containing βAPP have been shown to recycle to the cell surface (Yamazaki et al. 1996). It is within the latter pathway that wild-type βAPP molecules are principally converted to Aβ peptides. The first step involves an endoproteolytic cleavage of membrane-anchored βAPP_{770} at residue 671, generating a truncated form of APP_s designated APP_s-β and a 12-kD membrane-retained carboxyl-terminal fragment (CTF) (Fig. 1). During the recycling of early endosomes, the 12-kD CTF may undergo one of two cleavages, at residues 711 or 713, by an activity referred to as γ-secretase(s) to generate, respectively, the 40- or the 42-residue form of Aβ. The resultant ~7- to 8-kD CTF is unstable and is assumed to be rapidly degraded. The 10-kD CTF, which arises from α-secretase cleavage of βAPP after residue 687 (= residue 16 of Aβ), can also undergo γ-secretase cleavages at the Aβ40 and Aβ42 sites, giving rise to a peptide designated p3, which can thus be Aβ residue 17–40 or 17–42 (Fig. 1). Exactly how the 10-kD and 12-kD CTFs can undergo cleavage at residues within their transmembrane domains remains enigmatic. It should be noted that β-secretase cleavage is a less common event than α-secretase cleavage of the precursor in most cell types. In addition, γ-secretase cleavage at βAPP residue 711 (Aβ residue 40) is a far more common event than γ-secretase cleavage at residue 713 (Aβ residue 42), so that the ratio of $A\beta_{40}$ to $A\beta_{42}$ peptides in the conditioned media of most βAPP-expressing cells is generally in the range of 10:1 to 20:1.

The various secretory fragments just described have been detected not only in the conditioned media of cultured cells, but also in vivo. Human cerebrospinal fluid (CSF) generally contains 2- to 6-nM levels of Aβ peptides ending at residue 40 ($A\beta_{40}$), and approximately 1/10 or 1/20 of this amount of Aβ peptides ending at residue 42 ($A\beta_{42}$). In human plasma, both peptides are present at considerably lower concentrations than in CSF, generally in the 100 pM range. Therefore, it is to be emphasized that all known secreted derivatives of βAPP, including $A\beta_{40}$ and $A\beta_{42}$ peptides, are *normal* products of cellular metabolism throughout life (Selkoe 1994).

Although the β- and γ-secretase cleavages that generate Aβ are currently believed to occur principally in early endosomes at mildly acidic pH (Table 1), Aβ can also be generated in the secretory pathway. Specifically, βAPP molecules bearing the so-called "Swedish" FAD-linked double missense mutation immediately amino-terminal to the β-secretase cleavage site have been shown to undergo the latter cleavage in secretory vesicles budding off the TGN (Haass et al. 1995). Several pharmacological agents that disrupt trafficking of membrane proteins through the central vacuolar pathway or alter vesicular pH gradients have been shown to inhibit Aβ secretion (for review, see Selkoe 1994).

Mechanisms of AD-linked Missense Mutations in βAPP

On the basis of this current understanding of βAPP trafficking/processing from work in our laboratory and numerous other laboratories, we have undertaken studies of the effects of the FAD-linked βAPP missense mutations on Aβ production. The Swedish βAPP

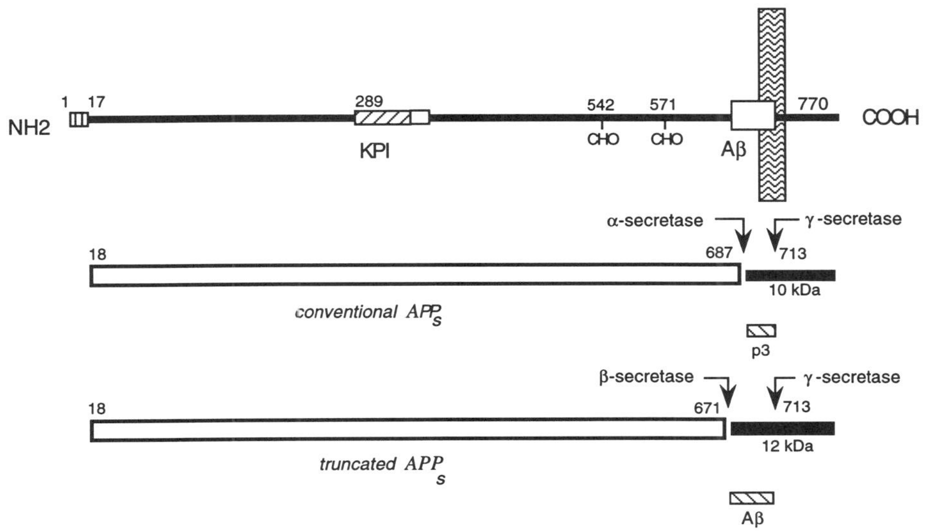

Figure 1. Schematic diagrams of the β-amyloid precursor protein and its principal metabolic derivatives. The upper diagram depicts the largest of the known βAPP alternate transcripts, comprising 770 amino acids. Regions of interest are indicated at their correct relative positions. A 17-residue signal peptide occurs at the amino terminus (*box with vertical lines*). Two alternatively spliced exons of 56 and 19 amino acids are inserted at residue 289; the first contains a serine protease inhibitor domain of the Kunitz type (KPI). Two sites of N-glycosylation (CHO) are found at residues 542 and 571. A single membrane-spanning domain at amino acids 700–723 is indicated by the vertical hatched bar. The amyloid β-protein (Aβ) fragment (*white box*) includes 28 residues just outside the membrane plus the first 12–14 residues of the transmembrane domain. In the middle diagram, the arrow indicates the site (after residue 687) of a constitutive proteolytic cleavage, made by an unknown protease(s) designated α-secretase, that enables secretion of the large, soluble ectodomain of APP (APP_s) into the medium and retention of the 83-residue carboxy-terminal fragment (~10 kD) in the membrane. The 10-kD fragment can undergo cleavage by an unknown protease(s) called γ-secretase at residues 711 or 713 to release the p3 peptide. The lower diagram depicts the alternative proteolytic cleavage after residue 671 by an unknown enzyme(s) called β-secretase that results in the secretion of a truncated APP_s molecule and the retention of a 99-residue (~12 kD) carboxy-terminal fragment. The 12-kD fragment can also undergo cleavage by γ-secretase at residues 711 or 713 to release $A\beta_{40}$ or $A\beta_{42}$, respectively.

double mutation, whether expressed in transfected cells or examined in primary skin fibroblasts of gene carriers, results in a substantial (3- to 6-fold) increase in the secretion of Aβ peptides, those ending both at residue 40 and at residue 42 (Citron et al. 1992; Cai et al. 1993). We performed site-directed mutagenesis at and around the β-secretase cleavage site (residue 671–672) of βAPP, which showed that substitution of the wild-type methionine at 671 by the Swedish mutant leucine results in increased generation of the 12-kD CTF (the immediate precursor of Aβ), whereas placing virtually any other amino acid in this position sharply decreases 12-kD (and hence Aβ) production (Citron et al. 1995).

Table 1. Data Supporting Early Endosomes as the Principal Site of Aβ Generation

Deleting βAPP cytoplasmic domain (GYENPTY) lowers Aβ production
Mild alkalinization lowers Aβ production
Altering vesicular H^+ transport lowers Aβ production
Late endosome/lysosome fractions do not contain Aβ
Endocytosis of surface-labeled βAPP molecules leads directly to release of labeled Aβ
Kinetics of labeled Aβ release are slightly slower than those of APP_s release and consistent with those of recycling endosomes
Depleting cellular K^+ inhibits clathrin-mediated endocytosis and lowers Aβ production

The next missense mutation we investigated was that at βAPP692 (Aβ residue 21) (Haass et al. 1994). This mutation occurs in an extended Flemish family in which members develop early-onset AD or severe cerebral amyloid angiopathy with hemorrhages, or both. We found that this mutant form of βAPP, expressed in transfected cells, leads to an increased ratio of Aβ to p3 peptide production and an increased amino-terminal heterogeneity of Aβ, effects that would tend to promote amyloidogenesis (Aβ filament formation). Studies of synthetic Aβ peptides containing the Flemish mutation have not clearly shown that this peptide is significantly more prone to aggregate into polymers (i.e., filaments) than wild-type Aβ. A missense mutation at the next codon, βAPP693, occurs in two Dutch families and results in a phenotype of severe cerebral amyloid angiopathy with hemorrhages (accompanied by numerous diffuse plaques in the cortex). Studies by Frangione and colleagues with Dutch synthetic Aβ peptides have demonstrated an increased propensity for aggregation and fibrillogenesis (Wisniewski et al. 1991). Recently, we have expressed the Dutch mutant βAPP isoform in transfected cells and shown that it increases the Aβ/p3 ratio in a fashion similar to the adjacent Flemish mutation (D. Watson et al., unpubl.).

Younkin and colleagues (Suzuki et al. 1994) have clearly demonstrated that the mutations at codon βAPP717 found in several different FAD families of European or Japanese descent result in increased γ-secretase-mediated cleavage of βAPP at position 713, leading to a selective increase in the secretion of the $A\beta_{42}$ peptide. Why mutations occurring four residues carboxy-terminal to the 713 cleavage site lead to increased cleavage there is not clear, because so little is known about the nature and the mechanism of γ-secretase.

The initial mechanistic findings on βAPP missense mutations described above were conducted in stably transfected cells, but it has been possible to confirm the effects in primary cultured fibroblasts and plasma obtained from the Swedish and βAPP717 mutation-bearing families. In the case of the Swedish mutation, even fibroblast media (Citron et al. 1994) and plasmas (Scheuner et al. 1996) from mutant gene carriers who were a number of years younger than the predicted age of onset showed the increases in Aβ peptide production. It now appears clear that all of the known βAPP missense mutations that produce FAD act by increasing the production of Aβ peptides, particularly the more hydrophobic and highly aggregation-prone $A\beta_{42}$ peptides.

Apolipoprotein ε4 in AD

Although a number of in vitro studies about the possible mechanisms of the ApoE4 isoform in promoting the development of late-onset AD have been published, a definitive understanding of the pathogenicity of this protein awaits further research. The most consistently confirmed phenotypic alteration in AD subjects harboring one or two ε4 alleles compared to those with only ε2 and ε3 alleles is an ε4-dosage-dependent increase in the number and density of Aβ plaques and vascular deposits (Rebeck et al. 1993; Schmechel et al. 1993; Hyman et al. 1995). It has also been shown that the principal neuronal receptor capable of binding and internalizing apolipoprotein E, the low-density lipoprotein receptor-related protein (LRP), can be immunocytochemically localized to neurites within amyloid plaques (Rebeck et al. 1993), and other known soluble ligands for LRP are also found within the plaques. Assays of Aβ production in cells doubly transfected with βAPP and each of the human ApoE isoforms, cells which secrete both Aβ and the ApoE proteins at levels comparable to those in human CSF, show no significant elevation of Aβ production (Biere et al. 1995). Several in vitro studies of Aβ-ApoE interactions, generally employing supraphysiological doses of one or both proteins and purified non-lipidated ApoE, have suggested that ApoE 4 promotes, or is at least more permissive for, Aβ aggregation into filaments (see, e.g., Ma et al. 1994; Evans et al. 1995). Besides this putative mechanism, there is interest in determining whether ApoE4, which cannot undergo dimerization because it lacks cysteines, binds extracellular Aβ less well and thus participates in its clearance less effectively, resulting in excessive extracellular Aβ buildup. Other roles for ApoE in the inflammatory process associated with amyloid deposits and as the ApoE isoform that supports neurite outgrowth and maintenance least well have been proposed. However, such mechanisms would not necessarily account for the simple increase in the number of Aβ deposits in the brains of ε4-bearing subjects (Hyman et al. 1995), making it appear more likely that Aβ aggregation and/or clearance is at issue here.

The Presenilin Proteins: Pathogenic Mechanism

The cloning of the *presenilin 1 (PS1)* and *presenilin 2 (PS2)* genes and the discovery of missense mutations that link strongly with AD have provided a genetic explanation for the most aggressive known form of the disease. However, even prior to the identification of these genes, Younkin and colleagues undertook analyses of Aβ production in fibroblasts from patients known to have gene defects on chromosomes 14 or 1. A multicenter collaborative study showed that these patients incurred a selective increase in the extracellular levels of $A\beta_{42}$ peptide, with little or no accompanying increase in the $A\beta_{40}$ peptides (Scheuner et al. 1996). Some of the plasma samples were obtained from presymptomatic individuals, clearly demonstrating that the selective rise in the $A\beta_{42}$ production cannot be considered an effect of the disease but rather preceded it. To confirm this finding and to begin to explore its mechanism, we have established stably presenilin-transfected human 293 cell lines and have collaborated with Jimin Zhang and Edward Koo to analyze stable CHO transfectants that they have produced. The cells were allowed to reach confluence, and media were conditioned for about 24 hours, after which two methods of Aβ quantitation were performed. First, the media were divided into two aliquots, and one of these was immunoprecipitated with an antibody (prepared by Peter Seubert, Dale Schenk, and colleagues) that is highly specific for the free carboxyl terminus of the $A\beta_{42}$ peptide and does not detect the $A\beta_{40}$ species. The other aliquot was precipitated with an antibody recognizing both forms, to measure total Aβ production. The second method of quantitation was the use of sandwich ELISAs developed by Seubert and Schenk to measure $A\beta_{42}$ and total Aβ. In studies performed to date, both methods have been applied to several CHO cell lines stably expressing either wild-type or mutant PS1 or PS2, whereas only the ELISA method has been used on the 293 lines expressing wild-type or mutant PS1. In all cases, we have observed statistically significant ~1.3- to 2.5-fold increases in the $A\beta_{42}/A\beta_{40}$ ratios in the FAD-linked mutant PS1 and PS2 cell lines compared to PS wild-type lines. The degree of increase is closely similar to that observed by Younkin and collaborators (Scheuner et al. 1996) in primary fibroblast media and plasma samples from PS patients. The effect clearly required the expression of the mutant PS molecules; in certain CHO clones that lost expression over time, the $A\beta_{42}/A\beta_{40}$ ratio declined to normal. However, the phenotypic effect did not appear to vary quantitatively as a function of the level of PS expression. We also found no significant change in the levels of βAPP holoprotein in cell lysates or the APP_s-α or APP_s-β secreted derivatives in culture media. Our results therefore support those of the plasma and fibroblast media assays and indicate that a direct effect of the expression of mutant PS1 and PS2 is to increase the cellular production of the highly amyloidogenic 42-residue form of Aβ. Therefore, the effect of presenilin mutants on βAPP processing appears to be closely similar to that observed with the βAPP717 codon mutations; indeed, a direct side-by-side comparison of the respective cell lines demonstrates an indistinguishable pattern of $A\beta_{42}$, but not $A\beta_{40}$, elevation. In accord with the higher levels of $A\beta_{42}$ found in extracellular fluids, immunocytochemical analysis of the brains of patients dying with a PS1 (Glu280Ala) mutation demonstrates a selective and highly significant increase in the amount of $A\beta_{42}$ immunoreactive deposits in hippocampus, cerebral cortex, cerebellum, and other brain regions (Lemere et al. 1996b).

The Presenilin Proteins: Initial Characterization

The primary structure of PS1 deduced from its DNA sequence predicts a 467-residue polypeptide with 7–9 putative transmembrane domains (Sherrington et al. 1995). Messenger RNA analyses indicate that the protein is expressed in many mammalian tissues, with particularly high levels in the brain (Kovacs et al. 1996). Establishing the normal and pathological roles of the presenilins in the nervous system requires the identification and detailed characterization of the PS polypeptides in human brain tissue. We have produced a panel of antibodies specific for different regions of the PS1 and/or PS2 proteins and have used these to detect the protein and its proteolytic derivatives in stably transfected human cell lines, primary neurons and glia, and the brains of mice and monkeys, as well as normal, sporadic AD, and PS1-linked FAD subjects. Our antibodies were raised to various synthetic peptides or a recombinant fusion protein from several regions of the PS1 protein: the amino terminus, the proximal and the distal portions of the putative TM6-7 hydrophilic loop (assuming that PS1 is a 7-transmembrane protein), and the carboxyl terminus. When tested by immunoprecipitation of transiently PS1-transfected COS cells, antibody 4624 to the TM6/7 loop and antibody 4627 to the carboxyl terminus detected full-length PS1 as two closely spaced proteins of 43–45 kD: a tightly focused upper band and a broader, fuzzy lower band. Both bands were abolished by preabsorbing these antisera with their respective immunogens and were not detected in nontransfected COS cells. In COS cells transiently transfected with PS2 cDNA, 4627 specifically detected two similar bands that migrated slightly ahead of the PS1 polypeptides on 10% SDS-PAGE gels, in keeping with the high degree of sequence conservation between the carboxyl termini of PS1 and the slightly smaller size of PS2. Antibody 4624 failed to detect the overexpressed PS2, in accord with the substantial sequence divergence in this proportion of the TM6/7 loop. Polyclonal antibody X81 to the first 81 residues comprising the PS1 amino terminus also precipitated the two 43- to 45-kD proteins in PS1 transfectants, but recognized the PS2 polypeptides very weakly, again as expected from their amino-terminal sequence divergence.

In addition to recognizing these PS monomers, all three antibodies specifically precipitated higher-molecular-weight bands at about 95 kD, about 140 kD, and more than 180 kD. Experiments reported by our collaborators and us (J. Walter et al., in prep.) have shown that PS1 does not undergo posttranslational modification by addition of sugar, sulfate, or phosphate groups. The immunoprecipitated high-molecular-weight proteins could be directly immunoblotted with the PS antibodies, and their ratio to the 43- to 45-kD monomers was constant at different levels of PS1 expression. We conclude that the higher-molecular-weight bands represent SDS-stable PS oligomers, as also observed by other laboratories in high-expressing PS1-transfected cells. We have directly radiosequenced the amino termini of the 43-kD and 45-kD immunoprecipitated monomers and confirmed that they each begin with the methionine at position 1 of the predicted PS1 sequence. Their slightly different sizes, despite the absence of demonstrable posttranslational modifications, suggest that the two bands represent SDS-stable conformers.

Our initial attempts to detect endogenous PS proteins in brain and nontransfected cultured cells by direct immunoblotting or immunoprecipitation suggested that the holoprotein was present at very low levels. A protocol with greater sensitivity was therefore developed by covalently coupling polyclonal IgG of antibodies X81 (amino terminus) or 4627 (carboxyl terminus) to protein A–Sepharose beads; immunoprecipitating PS proteins from unlabeled cell lysates or frozen mouse, monkey, or human brain tissues; and immunoblotting the precipitates with these and other PS1 antibodies. Using this method, stably PS1-transfected 293 cells show the characteristic 43- to 45-kD PS1 polypeptides. In untransfected 293 cells, we detected small amounts of endogenous 43- to 45-kD PS1 monomers that comigrated with those overexpressed in the transfectants. However, both the untransfected and the transfected cells contained a group of four or five strongly labeled smaller proteins of ~18–22 kD precipitable by both loop and carboxy-terminal PS1 antibodies. An additional band at ~14 kD was brought down solely by the 4627 (carboxy-terminal) antibody and detected by that and other carboxy-terminal antibodies but not by loop antibodies, suggesting that this species begins after the latter domain.

In view of this evidence for the existence of a set of carboxy-terminal proteolytic fragments of PS1, we used coupled antibody X81 for both precipitation and blotting and observed a strongly labeled ~27-kD protein (plus a slightly larger minor band) that was present in both untransfected and transfected 293 cells. Because the relative sizes of the major amino- and carboxy-terminal immunoreactive bands (27 kD and 18 kD) were consistent with the ~45-kD size of the sequenced holoprotein in these cells, we postulated that the fragments arose by an endoproteolytic cleavage. Surprisingly, these various fragments were only modestly increased in amount in the transfected cells, despite the very substantial increase in the PS1 holoprotein over endogenous levels.

We next carried out pulse-chase experiments on the transfected 293 cell lines. The 43- to 45-kD holoprotein declined rather rapidly in amount, with a half-life of about 60 minutes. The 27-kD and 18-kD amino- and carboxy-terminal proteolytic fragments, respectively, appeared at about 20 minutes of chase and increased modestly in the next 40 minutes, after which they remained essentially unchanged for up to 6 hours. We interpret this result to indicate that there is a precursor/product relationship between the holoprotein and the amino- and carboxy-terminal fragments. Nonetheless, the large majority of PS1 holoprotein is apparently degraded by another pathway, presumably to individual amino acids, and only a small portion of the precursor is converted into the specific amino- and carboxy-terminal fragments under the pulse-chase conditions of our experiments.

To confirm unequivocally that the smaller PS1-immunoreactive species arose from a specific endoproteolytic cleavage, we performed radiosequencing of the free amino terminus of the major 18-kD carboxy-terminal fragment precipitated from metabolically labeled PS1 transfectants. Sequence with [^{35}S]methionine and [^{3}H]valine produced a pattern of radioactive peaks that was consistent with the 18-kD protein having a principal start site at residue 299 of PS1, with minor species beginning at residues 292 and 298. Therefore, even the major carboxy-terminal-reactive fragment, when cut out of gels and sequenced, shows some amino-terminal heterogeneity.

We used the combined immunoprecipitation/Western blot method to substantially enrich presenilin proteins from freshly frozen monkey or mouse brains. Even amounts of starting tissue as high as 20 mg (wet weight) failed to reveal any specifically immunoreactive holoprotein in the ~45-kD range. However, we consistently detected a major 18-kD carboxy-terminal fragment and minor flanking proteins, as well as a major ~27-kD amino-terminal fragment and minor flanking proteins in brain tissue. The two major bands comigrated with the corresponding bands in untransfected and PS1-transfected 293 cells. We next performed similar experiments on homogenates of frozen human cerebral cortex. Again, no full-length PS polypeptides could be detected, despite a large amount of starting tissue. The amino- and carboxy-terminal fragments obtained were highly similar to those in mouse brain. To determine whether missense mutations in PS1 altered this polypeptide profile, we obtained postmortem brain tissue from four different patients of the FAD3 family (Sherrington et al. 1995) harboring the Cys410Tyr mutation in PS1 and compared the fragments obtained to those found in identically prepared samples from four sporadic AD brains and four aged nondemented brains. We observed no consistent differences in the multiple carboxy- and amino-terminal fragments of presenilin; again, no full-length presenilin polypeptides were detected under these conditions.

Finally, we examined primary neuronal and glial cultures established from E18 mouse brains. Using the immunoprecipitation/Western blot technique, the major amino- and carboxy-terminal PS1 fragments were observed in a pattern closely similar to that described above in brain tissue. PS polypeptides appeared to be more abundant in neurons than in glia. We next surveyed six different mouse organs (brain, muscle, liver, kidney, spleen, and lung) and found the expected amino- and carboxy-terminal fragment patterns in all these tissues; however, the carboxy-terminal proteins were somewhat smaller (~13–18 kD), and the major amino-terminal fragment was correspondingly larger, in kidney. In general, the PS1 fragment patterns were relatively similar in all neural-derived material, including primary neurons, primary glia, and mouse, monkey, and human brains.

DISCUSSION

The Presenilin Polypeptides

We interpret the above results to indicate that there are very low levels of endogenous presenilin holoproteins in both neural cells and brain tissue. This appears to be the case, as well, for several peripheral tissues, although we were able to detect low levels of full-length PS1 in human kidney 293 cells. However, there are readily detectable amino- and carboxy-terminal proteolytic fragments that we have shown to arise from single endoproteolytic cleavages around residue 299 in the proximal part of the TM6/7 hydrophilic loop. The prominence of the fragments versus the very low abundance of the holoprotein and the rapid turnover of transfected presenilin shown in our pulse-chase experiments is consistent with a model in which the amount of full-length presenilin is tightly regulated at a low level, and any excess precursor arising from overexpression is rapidly degraded by an alternate, nonspecific pathway. At steady-state levels in brain and other tissues, it appears that virtually all presenilin molecules exist as endoproteolytic fragments. The functional implications of this interesting processing will require much further study; almost nothing is known about the putative activities of the presenilins.

Regarding their dysfunction in FAD, we postulate on the basis of the data reported above that mutant PS1 and PS2 subtly but significantly alter the proteolysis of βAPP by γ-secretase to favor the cleavage at residue 42 of the Aβ region over the more common cleavage at residue 40. Recent studies of other laboratories have suggested that the presenilin proteins are overwhelmingly localized to the endoplasmic reticulum in both transfected and nontransfected cells. Some localization to the Golgi compartment has been described. βAPP resides in considerable part in the Golgi, but the β- and γ-secretase cleavages that generate Aβ are believed (as described above) to be carried out principally in the reinternalization/endosomal pathway and also in the TGN and secretory vesicles derived therefrom. On the other hand, some granulovesicular staining in neurons in addition to the principal ER pattern has been described which suggests that presenilin molecules may reach small vesicular compartments closer to the cell surface. We have been unable to coprecipitate PS1 and βAPP molecules in doubly transfected cells. At this juncture, we postulate that presenilin, when mutant, may affect the trafficking or processing of γ-secretase or another protein involved in its regulation rather than directly binding to the βAPP holoprotein.

To date, we have noticed no significant change in the level of the amino- and carboxy-terminal fragments of PS1 either in the brains of four subjects bearing the Cys410Tyr PS1 mutation or in several transfected mutant cell lines in which we quantitated Aβ42/40 ratios. However, recent data we have obtained suggest that a cell line with another PS1 mutation currently under study may show some decrease in fragments compared to wild-type PS1 transfectants. In one FAD-linked mutation shown to increase the 42/40 Aβ ratio, namely an intronic mutation that results in the deletion of exon 9 (residues 290–319), Thinakaran et al. (1996) have reported a marked decrease in the fragment amount in primary lymphoblasts from subjects with this mutation. Their result is consistent with our radiosequencing data showing that the principal site of proteolysis (residue 299) is within exon 9.

It will be of interest to recombinantly express in cells just the carboxy- or just the amino-terminal fragments of PS1, each bearing a naturally occurring missense mutation, in order to see whether just the mutant fragment will confer the Aβ42/40 phenotype in the absence of full-length mutant PS1. Analogous studies expressing wild-type fragments, particularly in cells and mice in which the endogenous PS1 gene has been knocked out, will provide insights into the function of PS1 and the role of proteolytic processing therein.

Toward a Common Pathogenetic Pathway in FAD

Evidence summarized above indicates that all four known genes that underlie familial forms of AD produce a phenotype of either increased cellular $A\beta_{42}$ production or (in the case of ApoE4) increased steady-state levels of parenchymal and vascular Aβ deposits in the brain. This strong genetic support for an early role of $A\beta_{42}$ in FAD is supported by numerous morphological and immunocytochemical studies which show that $A\beta_{42}$ peptides are the first to be deposited in Down's syndrome (Iwatsubo et al. 1995; Lemere et al. 1996a), in normal age-related amyloidosis, and, by implication, in AD. Moreover, a transgenic mouse strongly overexpressing the Val717Phe missense mutation in βAPP develops diffuse and neuritic Aβ deposits in an age-related fashion, and these lesions are associated with activated microglia, a brisk reactive astrocytosis, and dystrophic dendrites (Games et al. 1995). Indeed, neuritic plaques in these mice show a striking resemblance to those observed in humans, including the presence of fibrillar Aβ seen by electron microscopy.

On the basis of these and other data, we hypothesize that AD is a syndrome in which different gene defects can lead—either directly or indirectly—to increased expression or altered proteolytic processing of βAPP or to changes in Aβ aggregation and clearance in the extracellular space (Fig. 2). These changes gradually result in a chronic imbalance between Aβ production and clearance, leading first to the progressive accumulation of soluble and insoluble Aβ oligomers and polymers in forms that are not morphologically detectable, and later to the development of discrete, microscopically visible plaques. The development of such Aβ aggregates initiates a complex, multistep cascade that includes gliosis, inflammatory changes, neuritic/synaptic changes, neurofibrillary tangles, and transmitter loss.

Extensive in vitro and some in vivo studies of the pathobiological effects of Aβ peptides have demonstrated toxicity to neurons and activation of microglia and astrocytes when aggregated, fibrillar Aβ is used, but not when soluble, monomeric Aβ is used (see, e.g., Pike et al. 1993; Lorenzo and Yankner 1994). These findings, together with those in the Val717Phe transgenic mouse summarized above (Games et al. 1995), strongly suggest that the accumulation first of aggregated $A\beta_{42}$ and later of aggregated $A\beta_{40}$ in plaques can lead to associated microglial activation, local inflammatory changes such as cytokine release, triggering of the classic complement pathway, local astrocytosis, and acute-phase protein release. Whether this

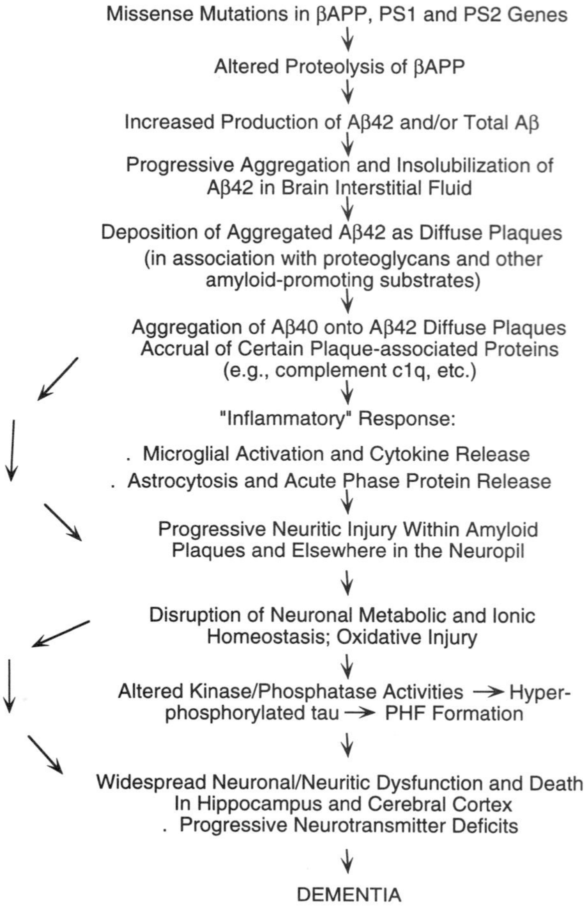

Figure 2. Hypothetical sequence of the molecular pathogenesis of familial forms of AD.

inflammatory response is required for subsequent neuritic/neuronal injury, or whether the latter can occur as a direct effect of the accumulation of first nonfibrillar and then fibrillar Aβ, remains to be determined. It is likely that certain features of this amyloid-induced inflammatory and neuritotoxic process can lead to altered metabolic and ionic homeostasis in neurons which, in turn, triggers changes in intraneuronal phosphorylation/dephosphorylation cascades that result in excessively phosphorylated forms of the microtubule-associated protein, tau. It is believed that such forms are the principal or sole constituent of the paired helical filaments that comprise the neurofibrillary tangles which develop in selected neurons. Such a scenario would be consistent with the well-documented neuropathological evidence that neurofibrillary tangles indistinguishable from those found in AD can arise in at least a dozen etiologically distinct neurological disorders, almost all of which (besides AD) have no β-amyloidosis. For example, a latent, late-measles encephalitis (subacute sclerosing panencephalitis) occurs rarely in teenagers previously affected with measles and can produce profound neurofibrillary-tangle formation in the absence of any β-amyloid. Thus, PHF formation can reasonably be viewed as a somewhat nonspecific, albeit cytopathologically important, response to a variety of neural insults.

The gradual progression of the hypothetical but supportable cascade described above would lead to the profound changes in neuronal form, metabolism, and function, including deficits in multiple neurotransmitter systems, that are now well known to characterize clinical AD. A mechanism of this type can most clearly be supported at this time in the relatively rare cases of autosomally dominant FAD caused by missense mutations in the βAPP, PS1, or PS2 genes. In those patients, current data strongly support a very early role for altered βAPP processing and excessive $A\beta_{42}$ production. The enhanced amyloid deposition associated with an inheritance of one or two ApoE ε4 alleles could be operating at the level of the aggregation of $A\beta_{42}$ and/or $A\beta_{40}$ during early plaque formation or via a failure to clear these peptides. As regards the more than 50% of AD which is not currently explained by any of these four genetic diatheses, one cannot yet say whether the model described here will apply. However, the neuropathological and clinical phenotypes of these many cases are, in general, substantially overlapping with those caused by the identified gene defects.

CONCLUSION

The hypothetical scheme for the mechanism of familial forms of AD offered here can serve as a model for how the seemingly disparate molecular, biochemical, and neuropathological features of AD could be integrated into a temporal sequence of events. A great deal more study is needed. Nonetheless, there appears to be a sufficient consensus that a cascade initiated by Aβ accumulation and deposition is operative in at least some cases of AD so that the search for therapeutic approaches to inhibit this cascade is now well under way. Such approaches include (1) inhibiting the amyloid-forming β-secretase and/or γ-secretase enzymes; (2) diverting βAPP from its amyloidogenic processing pathway to increased cleavage by α-secretase; (3) preventing the aggregation of extracellular Aβ into fibrils; (4) interfering with the toxic response of neurons to amyloid or its associated proteins; and (5) inhibiting the inflammatory process that occurs around amyloid plaques.

Among these specific options for therapy based on an Aβ-mediated cascade, it is likely that inhibitors of γ-secretase and/or β-secretase will be among the first agents to be advanced to clinical trials. A particularly attractive target on theoretical grounds is that of inhibiting Aβ aggregation. The reasons for this conclusion include the facts that only aggregated, not monomeric, Aβ appears to be associated with local neuritic toxicity and glial activation in vitro and in vivo; that inhibitors of this process could act in the extracellular space rather than requiring uptake into neurons and glia; and, most importantly, that such inhibitors would be affecting a purely pathological event, because there is no current evidence that Aβ aggregation into filaments is contributing to normal brain function. The anti-inflammatory approach and related attempts to reduce oxidative injury to neurons are also highly worthy of pursuit, given rapidly expanding information about these processes in AD brain tissue. In the final analysis, it appears that multiple distinct therapeutic modalities, including many not discussed here, will need to be offered to patients with this devastating disorder at various stages during its currently inexorable progression.

ACKNOWLEDGMENTS

I thank the members of my laboratory for their many contributions to the concepts and data summarized here. This work was supported in part by National Institutes of Health grants AG-12749 and AG-06173.

REFERENCES

Biere, A.L., B. Ostaszewski, H. Zhao, S. Gillespie, S.G. Younkin, and D.J. Selkoe. 1995. Co-expression of β-amyloid precursor protein (βAPP) and apolipoprotein E in cell culture: Analysis of βAPP processing. *Neurobiol. Dis.* **2:** 177.

Cai, X.-D., T.E. Golde, and G.S. Younkin. 1993. Release of excess amyloid β protein from a mutant amyloid β protein precursor. *Science* **259:** 514.

Citron, M., D.B. Teplow, and D.J. Selkoe. 1995. Generation of amyloid β-protein from its precursor is sequence specific. *Neuron* **14:** 661.

Citron, M., T. Oltersdorf, C. Haass, L. McConlogue, A.Y. Hung, P. Seubert, C. Vigo-Pelfrey, I. Lieberburg, and D.J. Selkoe. 1992. Mutation of the β-amyloid precursor protein in familial Alzheimer's disease increases β-protein production. *Nature* **360:** 672.

Citron, M., C. Vigo-Pelfrey, D.B. Teplow, C. Miller, D. Schenk, J. Johnston, B. Winblad, N. Venizelos, L. Lannfelt, and D.J. Selkoe. 1994. Excessive production of amyloid β-protein by peripheral cells of symptomatic and presymptomatic patients carrying the Swedish familial Alzheimer's disease mutation. *Proc. Natl. Acad. Sci.* **91:** 11993.

Corder, E.H., A.M. Saunders, W.J. Strittmatter, D.E. Schmechel, P.C. Gaskell, Jr., G.W. Small, A.D. Roses, J.L. Haines, and M.A. Pericak-Vance. 1993. Gene dose of apolipoprotein E type 4 allele and the risk of Alzheimer's disease in late onset families. *Science* **261:** 921.

Evans, K.C., E.P. Berger, C.-G. Cho, K.H. Weisgraber, and P.T. Lansbury, Jr. 1995. Apolipoprotein E is a kinetic but not a thermodynamic inhibitor of amyloid formation: Implications for the pathogenesis and treatment of Alzheimer disease. *Proc. Natl. Acad. Sci.* **92:** 763.

Games, D., D. Adams, R. Alessandrini, R. Barbour, P. Berthelette, C. Blackwell, T. Carr, J. Clemens, T. Donaldson, F. Gillespie, T. Guido, S. Hagopian, K. Johnson-Wood, K. Khan, M. Lee, P. Leibowitz, I. Lieberburg, S. Little, E. Masliah, L. McConlogue, M. Montoya-Zavala, L. Mucke, L. Paganini, E. Penniman, M. Power, D. Schenk, P. Seubert, B. Snyder, F. Soriano, H. Tan, J. Vitale, S. Wadsworth, B. Wolozin, and J. Zhao. 1995. Alzheimer-type neuropathology in transgenic mice overexpressing V717F β-amyloid precursor protein. *Nature* **373:** 523.

Haass, C., A.Y. Hung, D.J. Selkoe, and D.B. Teplow. 1994. Mutations associated with a locus for familial Alzheimer's disease result in alternative processing of amyloid β-protein precursor. *J. Biol. Chem.* **269:** 17741.

Haass, C., C.A. Lemere, A. Capell, M. Citron, P. Seubert, D. Schenk, L. Lannfelt, and D.J. Selkoe. 1995. Swedish mutation causes early-onset AD by β-secretase cleavage within the secretory pathway. *Nat. Med.* **1:** 1291.

Hyman, B.T., H.L. West, G.W. Rebeck, S.V. Buldyrev, R.N. Mantegna, M. Ukleja, S. Havlin, and H.E. Stanley. 1995. Quantitative analysis of senile plaques in Alzheimer's disease: Observation of log-normal size distribution and molecular epidemiology of differences associated with apolipoprotein E genotype and trisomy 21 (Down syndrome). *Proc. Natl. Acad. Sci.* **92:** 3586.

Iwatsubo, T., A. Odaka, N. Suzuki, H. Mizwa, N. Nukina, and Y. Ihara. 1995. Visualization of Aβ42(43) and Aβ40 in senile plaques with end-specific Aβ monoclonals: Evidence that an initially deposited species is Aβ42(43). *Neuron* **13:** 45.

Kang, J., H.-G. Lemaire, A. Unterbeck, J.M. Salbaum, C.L. Masters, K.-H. Grzeschik, G. Multhaup, K. Beyreuther, and B. Muller-Hill. 1987. The precursor of Alzheimer's disease amyloid A4 protein resembles a cell-surface receptor. *Nature* **325:** 733.

Kovacs, D. M., H.J. Fausett, K.J. Page, T.-W. Kim, R.D. Moir, D.E. Merriam, R.D. Hollister, O.G. Hallmark, R. Mancini, K.M. Felsenstein, B.T. Human, R.E. Tanzi, and W. Wasco. 1996. Alzheimer-associated presenilins 1 and 2: Neuronal expression in brain and localization to intracellular membranes in mammalian cells. *Nat. Med.* **2:** 224.

Lemere, C.A., J.K. Blustzjan, H. Yamaguchi, T. Wisniewski, T.C. Saido, and D.J. Selkoe. 1996a. Sequence of deposition of heterogeneous amyloid β-peptides and Apo E in Down syndrome: Implications for initial events in amyloid plaque formation. *Neurobiol. Dis.* **3:** 16.

Lemere, C.A., F. Lopera, K.S. Kosik, C.L. Lendon, J. Ossa, T.C. Saido, H. Yamaguchi, A. Ruiz, A. Martinez, L. Madrigal, L. Hincapie, J.C. Arango L., L.D.C. Anthony, E.H. Koo, A.M. Goate, D.J. Selkoe, and J.C. Arango V. 1996b. The E280A presenilin 1 mutation leads to a distinct Alzheimer's disease phenotype: Increased Aβ42 deposition and severe cerebellar pathology. *Nat. Med.* **2:** 1146.

Levy-Lahad, E., W. Wasco, P. Poorkaj, D.M. Romano, J. Oshima, H. Pettingell, C. Yu, P.D. Jondro, S.D. Schmidt, K. Wang, A.C. Crowley, Y.-H. Fu, S.Y. Guenette, D. Galas, E. Nemens, E.M. Wijsman, T.D. Bird, G.D. Schellenberg, and R.E. Tanzi. 1995. Candidate gene for the chromosome 1 familial Alzheimer's disease locus. *Science* **269:** 973.

Lorenzo, A. and B. Yankner. 1994. β-amyloid neurotoxicity requires fibril formation and is inhibited by Congo red. *Proc. Natl. Acad. Sci.* **91:** 12243.

Ma, J., A. Yee, H.B. Brewer, Jr., S. Das, and H. Potter. 1994. The amyloid-associated proteins α1-antichymotrypsin and apolipoprotein E promote the assembly of the Alzheimer β-protein into filaments. *Nature* **372:** 92.

Mann, D.M.A., A. Brown, D. Prinja, C.A. Davies, M. Landon, C.L. Masters, and K. Beyreuther. 1989. An analysis of the morphology of senile plaques in Down's syndrome patients of different ages using immunocytochemical and lectin histochemical techniques. *Neuropathol. Appl. Neurobiol.* **15:** 317.

Morris, J.C., M. Storandt, D.W. McKeel, Jr., E.H. Rubin, J.L. Price, E.A. Grant, and L. Berg. 1996. Cerebral amyloid deposition and diffuse plaques in "normal" aging: Evidence for presymptomatic and very mild Alzheimer's disease. *Neurology* **46:** 707.

Oltersdorf, T., P.J. Ward, T. Henriksson, E.C. Beattie, R. Neve, I. Lieberburg, and L.C. Fritz. 1990. The Alzheimer amyloid precursor protein. Identification of a stable intermediate in the biosynthetic/degradative pathway. *J. Biol. Chem.* **265:** 4492.

Pike, C.J., D. Burdick, A.J. Walencewicz, C.G. Glabe, and C.W. Cotman. 1993. Neurodegeneration induced by β-amyloid peptides in vitro: The role of peptide assembly state. *J. Neurosci.* **13:** 1676.

Rebeck, G.W., J.S. Reiter, D.K. Strickland, and B.T. Hyman. 1993. Apolipoprotein E in sporadic Alzheimer's disease: Allelic variation and receptor interactions. *Neuron* **11:** 575.

Rogaev, E.I., R. Sherrington, E.A. Rogaeva, G. Levesque, M. Ikeda, Y. Liang, H. Chi, C. Lin, K. Holamn, T. Tsuda, L. Mar, S. Sorbi, B. Nacmias, S. Piacentini, L. Amaducci, I. Chumakov, D. Cohen, L. Lannfelt, P.E. Fraser, J.M. Rommens, and P.H. St. George-Hyslop. 1995. Familial Alzheimer's disease in kindreds with missense mutations in a gene on chromosome 1 related to the Alzheimer's disease type 3 gene. *Nature* **376:** 775.

Scheuner, D., X. Song, M. Citron, N. Suzuki, T.D. Bird, J. Hardy, M. Hutton, E.L. Lannfelt, E. Levy-Lahad, E.R. Peskind, P. Poorkaj, G.D. Schellenberg, R.E. Tanzi, M. Viitanen, W. Wasco, D.J. Selkoe, and S.G. Younkin. 1996. The presenilin 1 and 2 mutations linked to familial Alzheimer's disease increase the extracellular concentration of amyloid β protein (Aβ) ending at Aβ42(43). *Nat. Med.* **2:** 864.

Schmechel, D.E., A.M. Saunders, W.J. Strittmatter, B.J. Crain, C.M. Hulette, S.H. Joo, M.A. Pericak-Vance, D. Goldgaber, and A.D. Roses. 1993. Increased amyloid β-peptide deposition in cerebral cortex as a consequence of apolipoprotein E gentoype in late-onset Alzheimer disease. *Proc. Natl. Acad. Sci.* **90:** 9649.

Selkoe, D.J. 1994. Cell biology of the amyloid β-protein precursor and the mechanism of Alzheimer's disease. *Annu. Rev. Cell Biol.* **10:** 373.

———. 1996. Amyloid β-protein and the genetics of Alzheimer's disease. *J. Biol. Chem.* **271:** 18295.

Sherrington, R., E.I. Rogaev, Y. Liang, E.A. Rogaeva, G. Levesque, M. Ikeda, H. Chi, C. Lin, G. Li, K. Holman, T. Tsuda, L. Mar, J.-F. Foncin, A.C.Bruni, M.P. Montesi, S. Sorbi, I. Rainero, L. Pinessi, L. Nee, I. Chumakov, D.A. Pollen, A.D. Roses, P.E. Fraser, J.M. Rommens, and P.H. St. George-Hyslop. 1995. Cloning of a novel gene bearing missense mutations in early onset familial Alzheimer disease. *Nature* **375:** 754.

Suzuki, N., T.T. Cheung, X.-D. Cai, A. Odaka, L. Otvos, Jr., C. Eckman, T.E. Golde, and S.G. Younkin. 1994. An increased percentage of long amyloid β protein secreted by familial amyloid β protein precursor (βAPP717) mutants. *Science* **264:** 1336.

Thinakaran, G., D.R. Borchelt, M.K. Lee, H.H. Slunt, L. Spitzer, G. Kim, T. Rotovitsky, F. Davenport, C. Nordstedt, M. Seeger, J. Hardy, A.I. Levey, S.E. Gandy, N.A. Jenkins, N.G. Copeland, D.L. Price, and S.S. Sisodia. 1996. Endoproteolysis of presenilin 1 and accumulation of processed derivatives in vivo. *Neuron* **17:** 181.

Weidemann, A., G. Konig, D. Bunke, P. Fischer, J.M. Salbaum, C.L. Masters, and K. Beyreuther. 1989. Identification, biogenesis and localization of precursors of Alzheimer's disease A4 amyloid protein. *Cell* **57:** 115.

Wisniewski, T., J. Ghiso, and B. Frangione. 1991. Peptides homologous to the amyloid protein of Alzheimer's disease containing a glutamine for glutamic acid substitution have accelerated amyloid fibril formation. *Biochem. Biophys. Res. Commun.* **179:** 1247.

Yamazaki, T., E.H. Koo, and D.J. Selkoe. 1996. Trafficking of cell-surface amyloid β-protein precursor. II. Endocytosis, recycling and lysosomal targeting detected by immunolocalization. *J. Cell Sci.* **109:** 999.

Protein:Protein Interactions in Alzheimer's Disease and the CAG Triplet Repeat Diseases

W.J. STRITTMATTER,[1,2] J.R. BURKE,[1] V.S. DESERRANO,[1] D.Y. HUANG,[1,2]
W. MATTHEW,[2] A.M. SAUNDERS,[1] B.L. SCOTT,[1] J.M. VANCE,[1]
K.H. WEISGRABER,[3] AND A.D. ROSES[1,2]

[1]*Deane Laboratory, Division of Neurology, and* [2]*Department of Neurobiology, Duke University Medical Center, Durham, North Carolina 27710;*
[3]*Gladstone Institute of Cardiovascular Disease, San Francisco, California 94141*

The genetic association of the apolipoprotein (apoE) E4 allele with late-onset familial and sporadic Alzheimer's disease (AD) implicates isoform-specific interactions of apoE in the pathogenesis of this disease. We have identified isoform-specific interactions of apoE with several molecules important in disease pathology and, potentially, disease pathogenesis. Binding of Aβ peptide, τ, MAP2c, laminin, and growth factors by apoE may modify their function or metabolism. apoE quantitatively alters Aβ deposition in vitro and in situ in an isoform-specific manner. Microtubule metabolism is also altered by apoE. apoE bound to laminin increases neurite extension. Identification of the isoform-specific interactions of apoE that influence the pathogenesis of AD is critical for developing therapeutic strategies.

At least five adult-onset neurodegenerative diseases, including Huntington's disease (HD) and dentatorubral-pallidoluysian atrophy (DRPLA), are produced by genes containing a variably increased CAG repeat within the coding region. The size range of the repeats is similar in all diseases; unaffected individuals have fewer than 30 CAG repeats, and affected patients usually have more than 40 repeats. The size of the inherited CAG repeat correlates with the severity and age at disease onset. As shown by other investigators, the CAG triplet repeat produces a polyglutamine domain in the expressed proteins. Each of these diseases is inherited as a dominant trait. A pathological gain of function in gene carriers has been proposed as a genetic explanation, but with many possible functional hypotheses. We sought to identify proteins in brain that selectively interact with polyglutamine-domain proteins, hypothesizing that the polyglutamine domain may determine protein-protein interactions. Glyceraldehyde-3-phosphate dehydrogenase (GAPDH) in brain homogenate selectively binds a synthetic 60-glutamine peptide and not a 20-glutamine peptide. The DRPLA and Huntington proteins in normal brain bind GAPDH. Interactions between mutant and normal glutamine-repeat proteins with GAPDH may alter the enzymatic or structural roles of GAPDH.

PROTEIN:PROTEIN INTERACTIONS IN AD

apoE Alleles and AD

Inheritance of specific apoE alleles determines, in large part, the risk and age-of-onset distribution of late-onset familial and sporadic AD (Corder et al 1993; Saunders et al. 1993, 1996; Roses et al. 1994). The mechanism by which the apoE isoforms differentially contribute to disease expression is unknown, however. Several isoform-specific interactions of apoE have been identified; for example, with the microtubule-associated protein τ, which forms the paired helical filament and neurofibrillary tangles, and with Aβ peptide, a major component of the neuritic plaque. Identification of isoform-specific interactions of apoE give rise to testable hypotheses for the mechanism of pathogenesis of AD. An unresolved issue of increasing importance is the relationship between the structural pathological lesions and the cellular pathogenesis responsible for the clinical disease phenotype of progressive dementia.

apoE in the Central Nervous System

apoE may perform multiple metabolic functions in the brain. apoE is in the extracellular space, as a free and as a bound protein. It is also found within some neurons, both in the cytoplasm and in the intravesicular space of endosomes, lysosomes, and peroxisomes. Multiple sites suggest several, perhaps distinct, metabolic functions. Not all of the functions of apoE may be relevant to its role in the ADs. Interactions that are qualitatively or quantitatively different involving the apoE isoforms are candidates for developing hypotheses of how the various apoE alleles differentially regulate disease expression.

Intraneuronal Localization of apoE

In situ hybridization studies on brain have indicated that apoE mRNA is expressed in astrocytes and microglia, and not in neurons. However, recent immunohistochemical studies on AD brain have shown apoE in both tangle-bearing and tangle-free nerve cells, indicating that apoE may play a role in neuronal metabolism and in neuronal degeneration or regeneration in the central nervous system (Strittmatter et al. 1993a; Han et al. 1994a,b). Immunoreactive apoE was demonstrated in hippocampal neurons, independent of apoE genotype (Han et al. 1994a). Immunoreactive apoE was also observed in hippocampal granule cells of Parkinson disease patients, several patients with other neurodegenerative diseases, and some aged controls without known brain disease (Han et al. 1994b). Only a small proportion of the apoE immunoreactive neurons in AD patients also contained neurofibrillary tangles, suggesting that apoE accumulation precedes development of neurofibrillary changes (Han et al. 1994a). apoE immunoreactivity is identified in specific subsets of neurons, with punctate staining around soma, diffuse cytoplasmic staining, and granular staining. Ultrastructural studies of human and prosimian brain confirmed the cytoplasmic localization of apoE immunoreactivity (Han et al. 1994a).

The mechanism of apoE entry into the cytoplasmic compartment of nerve cells is not yet understood. The major apoE receptor on neurons is the low-density-lipoprotein receptor-related protein (LRP), a receptor with multiple known interactions (Rebeck et al. 1993). Other proteins, including the bacterial toxins pertussis and botulinum, and lactoferrin, are also capable of crossing cellular membranes, gaining access to the cytoplasm from the extracellular space.

The apoE Isoforms

The most common isoform of apoE in the general population, apoE3, is secreted as a 299-amino-acid protein containing a single cysteine residue at position 112. The other two common isoforms, apoE2 and apoE4, differ at one of two positions (residues 112 and 158) from apoE3 by cysteine-arginine interchanges: apoE2 contains a cysteine at position 158 and apoE4 contains an arginine at 112 (for review, see Weisgraber 1994). The single amino acid differences among the common isoforms of apoE result in significant differences in the biochemistry and cellular metabolism of these proteins, and in marked differences in the risk of AD. The single cysteine in apoE3 permits disulfide bond formation with other molecules, including itself (Weisgraber and Shinto 1991). apoE3 forms heterodimers with apolipoprotein A-II and homodimers with another apoE3 molecule (Weisgraber and Mahley 1978). apoE4 lacks a cysteine and cannot form these disulfide-mediated complexes.

Isoform-specific Interactions of apoE in Cholesterol Transport and Receptor Binding

The apoE isoforms differ in their interactions with the low-density lipoprotein (LDL) receptor and in binding cholesterol containing lipid particles Gregg et al. 1983). apoE3 and apoE4 bind the LDL receptor with high affinity, whereas apoE2 binds with very low affinity (~ 1% of apoE3). Severe atherosclerosis is common in some individuals homozygous for apoE2 and is thought to be due to decreased receptor-mediated apoE endocytosis. apoE binds other cell-surface receptors, including LRP, the very-low-density lipoprotein receptor (VLDL-receptor), and a scavenger receptor, but the interactions of the various isoforms of apoE with these receptors have not yet been extensively investigated. The ability of apoE to bind phospholipid particles is isoform-specific, with apoE2 and apoE3 preferentially associating with high-density lipoprotein (HDL) particles and apoE4 preferentially associating with VLDL particles.

apoE contains two functionally important domains, one that binds the LDL receptor and the other that binds lipoprotein particles (VLDL or HDL). Thrombin cleaves apoE at residues 191 and 215, yielding a 22-kD amino-terminal fragment and a 10-kD carboxy-terminal fragment. The region of apoE that binds the LDL receptor is contained in the amino-terminal domain (residues 1–191) (Bradley et al. 1982); the major lipid-binding region of apoE resides in the carboxy-terminal domain, with residues carboxy-terminal to 244 playing a major role (Weisgraber 1990). The cysteine:arginine interchange at position 112, which distinguishes apoE3 from apoE4, is not contained in the major lipid-binding region of apoE yet influences the distribution of these isoforms among the various lipoprotein particle classes. apoE3 and apoE2 preferentially bind HDL, and apoE4 binds the triglyceride-rich lower-density lipoprotein particles, both VLDL and IDL. A domain:domain interaction has been suggested to account for the distribution effect. The determination of the three-dimensional structure of the receptor-binding domain of apoE has helped model isoform-specific functional properties, including the differences in LDL receptor binding and lipid particle binding.

Irreversible, Isoform-specific Binding of apoE3 with the Microtubule-binding Proteins τ and MAP-2

Neurofibrillary tangles (NFT) are dense bundles of long unbranched filaments in the cytoplasm of some neurons (Arriagada et al. 1992). These filamentous structures are aggregations of paired helical filaments. The filaments consist primarily of the microtubule-associated protein (MAP) τ that is highly phosphorylated. Each filament is 10 nm in width, and two filaments are helically twisted about each other with a periodic full twist every 160 nm. NFTs may be so dense they distort the neuronal cell body and displace the nucleus. Paired helical filaments may also be found in neurites undergoing degeneration (for review, see Kosik 1992; Crowther 1993).

τ normally binds and stabilizes microtubules and

promotes the assembly of microtubules by polymerizing tubulin. Microtubules are necessary for neurite extension and maintenance and for the transport of materials along the axon and dendrites in both orthograde and retrograde directions. In AD, τ becomes abnormally phosphorylated and self-assembles into the pathological paired helical filaments forming NFTs (Liu et al. 1991; Goedert et al. 1992; Nixon et al. 1993).

Because of the genetic relevance of apoE4 and the presence of immunoreactive apoE in neurons containing NFTs, isoform-specific interactions of apoE with τ are being studied. In vitro, human apoE3 binds τ, forming a molecular complex that resists dissociation by boiling in 2% sodium dodecyl sulfate (SDS) (Strittmatter et al. 1994a,b). apoE4 does not irreversibly bind τ under identical conditions. The SDS-stable apoE3/τ complex is dissociated by boiling in the reducing agent β-mercaptoethanol. However, the apoE3/τ was probably not complexed through disulfide bond formation, since τ binds both the monomer and the homodimer of apoE3. There is only insignificant SDS-stable binding of τ by apoE4 under a variety of conditions, including increased duration of incubation, increased concentration of apoE4, or pH values 4.6–7.6. τ binds the 22-kD amino-terminal fragment of apoE3, which contains the LDL-receptor-binding domain.

Paired helical filament τ is phosphorylated at a number of serine/threonine–proline sites. At least some of these sites are phosphorylated by incubating recombinant τ with a crude rat brain extract and ATP. Recombinant τ-40 phosphorylated in this manner does not bind either apoE3 or apoE4, even with a prolonged 12-hour incubation. In AD, hyperphosphorylated τ is believed to self-assemble into the paired helical filament by formation of antiparallel dimers of the microtubule-binding repeat region. In vitro, these microtubule-binding repeats of τ self-assemble into paired helical-like filaments (Crowther et al. 1994). It is unclear whether hyperphosphorylation steps occur early or late in paired helical filament formation. In vitro, apoE3 irreversibly binds these microtubule-binding repeat regions of τ, whereas apoE4 does not bind with this avidity (Strittmatter et al. 1994a).

We have used synthetic peptides corresponding to the 18-amino-acid microtubule-binding region from each of the four τ repeats (designated repeat peptides I–IV) to study the interactions between τ and apoE. Each synthetic peptide bound apoE3 and resisted boiling in 2% SDS. Each microtubule-binding repeat is capable of binding apoE3 independently, and the complete microtubule-binding domain is not required. Of the four peptides, only those from repeats II and III contain a cysteine residue, indicating that disulfide bond formation beween τ and apoE3 cannot be the sole reason for these in vitro interactions. In contrast to the binding observed with apoE3, τ repeat peptides I, II, and IV did not bind to apoE4, even at 10^{-5} M. Repeat peptide III showed binding to apoE4 down to 10^{-6} M. These results indicate that apoE3 has an affinity for the microtubule-binding peptide repeats of τ that is at least two orders of magnitude higher than that of apoE4 (Huang et al. 1995b).

Ser-262 is the only residue within the repeat region that is known to be phosphorylated in PHF-τ, and its phosphorylation reduces the ability of τ to bind to microtubules (Biernat et al. 1993). We therefore investigated the influence of phosphorylation of Ser-262 on the interactions between τ and apoE3. Phosphorylation of repeat peptide I, at a position equivalent to Ser-262, completely abolished its ability to bind apoE3 (Huang et al. 1995a).

Another microtubule-associated protein, MAP2c, which is localized to dendrites, interacts with the apoE isoforms in a similar manner. MAP2c and τ are both members of a group of MAPs that bind microtubules and promote their assembly, and stabilize their polymerized structure (Goedert et al. 1991). In vitro, apoE3 also irreversibly binds MAP2c, similar to its isoform-specific interaction with τ (Huang et al. 1994). apoE4 does not bind MAP2c under identical conditions. Binding of MAP2c by apoE3, forming a complex stable in SDS, is detectable within 1 hour. However, no such binding of MAP2c by apoE4 is observed. apoE also interacts with the cytoskeletal proteins neurofilament protein and actin with isoform specificity (Fleming et al. 1996).

Isoform-specific interactions of apoE with τ and MAP2c may regulate intraneuronal metabolism in AD and alter the rate of formation of paired helical filaments and NFTs. Such isoform-specific interactions of apoE with τ and MAP2c might alter their metabolism, affecting the dynamic instability of tubular plasticity or specific aspects of microtubule assembly and stabilization. These apoE isoform-specific interactions may be central to disease mechanism.

Irreversible, Isoform-specific Binding of apoE with Aβ Peptide

Neuritic plaques are extracellular structures with complex molecular and cellular constituents required, by definition, for the diagnosis of definite AD. Plaques contain Aβ, a peptide of 39–43 amino acids, which is produced by proteolytic cleavage of the amyloid precursor protein (APP) in its normal metabolism. Other proteins found in the neuritic plaque include apoE (Namba et al. 1991; Strittmatter et al. 1993a), α_1-antichymotrypsin, IgG, several complement proteins, amyloid P, glycosaminoglycans, Sp40,40, and laminin. apoE binds laminin, thereby increasing neuronal attachment and altering the morphology of cultured neurons (Huang et al. 1995a). The complete molecular composition of the fibrillar structures in the plaque, the mechanism of assembly, and their role in the disease are unknown.

apoE accumulates extracellularly in the senile plaque and congophilic angiopathy of AD (Namba et al. 1991; Strittmatter et al. 1993a). In vitro, apoE3 and apoE4 irreversibly bind Aβ peptide, resisting dissociation by SDS or guanidine hydrochloride (Strittmatter et al. 1993a,b). apoE4 binds Aβ peptide more rapidly, and with a different pH-dependence than does apoE3. The apoE3/Aβ peptide complex is first detectable after 2 hours' incubation, and increases over the next 24 hours. In contrast, the apoE4/Aβ complex is detected after 5 minutes' incubation. LaDu et al. (1995) have demonstrated that such isoform-dependent interactions depend on the state of the protein, including the presence of bound lipid particles.

Binding of Aβ by apoE seems to require the oxidation of apoE and can be prevented or reversed by reduction with dithiothreitol or β-mercaptoethanol. Oxygen-saturated buffer increases, and nitrogen-saturated buffer decreases, the rate of this SDS-stable binding (Strittmatter et al. 1993b). The domain of apoE that binds Aβ peptide was determined by examining various recombinantly expressed apoE fragments (Strittmatter et al. 1993b). Aβ binding to apoE seems to require the domain of apoE between amino acids 244 and 272, within the region of apoE previously shown to mediate binding to lipoprotein particles.

After days of in vitro incubation, apoE and Aβ peptide form unique fibrils, with apoE4 forming more abundant fibrils than apoE3 (Sanan et al. 1994). Aβ(1–28) or Aβ(1–40) incubated with apoE forms simple 10-nm fibrils that are distinctly different from the twisted ribbons formed by Aβ alone. The presence of apoE on or in these simple fibrils was demonstrated using several monoclonal antibodies, each specific for a different region of apoE. Immunogold labeling showed that apoE associates with these fibrils along their full length, suggesting that apoE may be adsorbed to the outside of the simple fibrils or intercalated between the Aβ peptide monomers, perhaps forming a hybrid fibril.

In vitro differences in the binding of these apoE isoforms with Aβ peptide are paralleled by differences in vivo. In a study of brain tissue from AD patients homozygous for APOE4 or APOE3, immunostaining of Aβ in senile plaques was greatly increased in APOE4 patients (Schmechel et al. 1993). In addition, Aβ immunoreactivity in plaques was also increased in APOE4 homozygotes. Although patients homozygous for APOE4 have denser and larger amyloid plaques, their duration of disease is not different from patients with the same age of onset who are homozygous for APOE3. Therefore, deposition of Aβ relates to the APOE4 allele as a phenotypic variable that appears to be independent of the course of the disease.

Cross-linking and Adducation of apoE Isoforms by Products of Lipid Peroxidation

One consequence of oxidative damage to cells is lipid peroxidation, an autocatalytic process that damages lipid-containing structures and yields reactive by-products, primarily malondialdehyde (MDA) and 4-hydroxy-2-nonenal (HNE). MDA and HNE are electrophilic species that can covalently modify cellular macromolecules; each reacts with nucleophilic groups in amino acid residues to form monoadducts as well as intra- and intermolecular cross-links. We tested the hypothesis that two products of lipid peroxidation, MDA and HNE, covalently modify apoE and alter its metabolism. We have shown that apoE is covalently modified by products of lipid peroxidation, MDA and HNE, both in vitro and in vivo. Compared to MDA, HNE more effectively cross-linked apoE3 than apoE4 in vitro.

In vitro, both HNE and MDA cross-linked purified apoE3 and apoE4. HNE was a more potent cross-linker than MDA, and purified apoE3 was more susceptible to cross-linking by HNE than was purified apoE4 (Montine et al. 1996b). In P19 neuroglial cultures, oxidative stress with lipid peroxidation led to increased intracellular accumulation of anti-HNE and anti-apoE immunoreactive proteins of approximately 50 kD (Montine et al. 1996a). Intracellular accumulation of the 50-kD apoE-immunoreactive protein (apoE-50) was not prevented by cycloheximide, suggesting formation by posttranslational mechanisms. In cerebrospinal fluid (CSF), a 50-kD apoE-immunoreactive protein comigrated with proteins most immunoreactive for HNE and MDA adducts, and containing NaB_3H_4-reducible bonds. These proteins were in CSF from adult subjects (with or without dementia), and in AD patients homozygous for APOE3 or APOE4 alleles. These data suggest that HNE covalently cross-links apoE in P19 neuroglial cultures to form a 50-kD protein and that similar modifications of apoE appear to occur in vivo.

Reactive oxygen species are generated primarily from mitochondria during normal aerobic metabolism, and aerobic organisms have evolved a variety of antioxidant strategies. Lipid peroxidation, an important consequence of oxidative damage, increases with age in brain and is further increased in patients with AD. Our results suggest that apoE may be especially vulnerable to covalent modification by electrophilic species generated from lipid peroxidation, likely because it is a major lipid transporting apolipoprotein. The resulting altered metabolism of apoE provides a potential link between processes of aging, viz., brain lipid peroxidation, and a protein critical to the pathogenesis of late-onset AD.

Future Directions

Since the alleles of apoE determine the risk of developing AD, as well as the average age of onset, identification of the specific isoform-specific metabolism of apoE in disease pathogenesis is of central importance. Several isoform-specific interactions of apoE with other molecules have been identified, which include interactions with two molecules responsible for disease pathology, τ, which forms the NFT, and Aβ peptide, the primary constituent of the neuritic plaque. Adduction and cross-linking of the apoE isoforms by peroxidized lipids may contribute to the relevant isoform-specific metabolism in AD. Identification of additional isoform-specific protein interactions, and other isoform-specific posttranslational modifications, will produce new hypotheses of the role of apoE in AD.

PROTEIN:PROTEIN INTERACTIONS IN THE CAG TRIPLET REPEAT DISEASES

Five neurodegenerative, late-onset diseases that are caused by expansion of CAG trinucleotide repeats producing large polyglutamine domains in the expressed proteins are HD, DRPLA, spinocerebellar ataxia I (SCA1), spinobulbar muscular atrophy (SBMA), and Machado-Joseph disease. The normal function of most of these proteins is unknown, as is their role in pathogenesis. These disorders share a number of similarities, suggesting that they may share a pathogenetic mechanism. The common features include overlapping clinical phenotype, restriction of pathology to the central nervous system, selectivity of neuronal destruction, and delay in symptom onset until long after birth. Other than the polyglutamine repeat, however, the disease proteins are not homologous. This has led to the proposal that the polyglutamine domain may be responsible for pathogenesis.

Although there are many possible interactions of expanded polyglutamine repeats that could mediate neuronal degeneration, we have studied the role of the repeat itself in determining repeat-specific protein-protein interactions. Polyglutamine domains interact with other proteins by forming pleated sheet structures termed polar zippers. We hypothesize that CAG trinucleotide repeat disease pathogenesis is mediated through abnormal protein interactions via the polyglutamine repeat and that these interactions are modified by the size of the repeat.

General Features of CAG Repeat Diseases Suggesting Common Molecular Pathogenesis

The CAG trinucleotide repeat diseases may share a common pathogenetic mechanism because (1) all cause inherited neurodegenerative diseases with pathology almost exclusively restricted to the CNS; (2) the neuronal target population is remarkably focal for each disease; (3) development is normal even in individuals expressing an expanded repeat (Onodera et al. 1995); (4) symptoms typically do not begin for decades after birth; (5) the repeat size has a similar normal (~5–35) and expanded (~ 40 to <100) range in each of the diseases (Willems 1994); (6) the age of onset of symptoms and disease severity correlate with size of the repeat (LaSpada et al. 1992; Andrew et al. 1993; Orr et al. 1993); and (7) pathogenesis is the result of a gain of function of the expressed protein rather than loss of activity.

The evidence that these diseases result from a gain of function comes primarily from three observations. SBMA, also known as Kennedy's disease, is caused by expansion of the CAG repeat in the androgen receptor gene on the X chromosome. Numerous mutations and even deletion of the androgen receptor gene cause androgen insensitivity, but none, other than expansion of the CAG repeat, is associated with the motor neuron cell death characteristic of this disease (Quigley and French 1994). SBMA does not result from impaired or absent androgen receptor function. Similarly, knockout mice with a deletion of the entire HD gene are clinically and pathologically normal (Duyao et al. 1995). Transgenic mice containing the SCA1 gene with the normal-sized repeat are clinically and pathologically normal, whereas those with an expanded repeat display clinical and pathological features of SCA1 (Burright et al. 1995).

Intraneuronal Localization of Polyglutamine Domain Proteins

HD and DRPLA protein are found only in the cytoplasm (DeFiglia et al. 1995; Yazawa et al. 1995). Ataxin 1, the protein responsible for SCA1, may be a transcriptional regulator, as it is found primarily in the nucleus in most tissues; but in the target cells, cerebellar Purkinje neurons, it is also found in the cytoplasm (Servadio et al. 1995). The intracellular location of the Machado-Joseph protein is unknown.

Polyglutamine Domains May Mediate Protein-protein Interactions

Perutz and colleagues demonstrated that polyglutamine peptides self-associate, forming sheets strongly held together by hydrogen bonds, and suggested that polyglutamine interacts with other proteins by forming polar zippers in β-pleated sheet domains (Perutz et al. 1994; Stott et al. 1995). This polar zipper interaction is analogous to the well-known leucine zipper interaction responsible for protein interactions between the transcription factors c-jun and c-fos. Stott et al. (1995) confirmed the ability of polyglutamine-domain-containing proteins to interact by synthesizing an artificial polyglutamine domain into a truncated chymotrypsin inhibitor 2 protein (CI-2). The polyglutamine-containing CI-2 formed oligomers mediated through β-sheet structures, as predicted. These oligomers demonstrated marked stability with no change in structure, as measured by circular dichroism on heating to 70°C despite the fact that the added domains were only 10 glutamines in length. Stability of longer complexes has not been studied. Increasing the length of the polyglutamine domain may result in excessively "tight" binding of normally interacting proteins or may cause new interactions that result in novel properties.

Interactions of Polyglutamine with GAPDH

To determine whether polyglutamine domains could bind other protein, we developed an in vitro assay. Cortical brain homogenate was incubated with synthetic polyglutamine peptides containing either 20 or 60 glutamines immobilized on polystyrene beads. The 20-glutamine peptide represents the size of the polyglutamine domain in the normal protein, and the 60-glutamine peptide represents the size in the mutant disease-associated form. A small subset of brain proteins bound preferentially to the 60-glutamine peptide. The major protein bound to the 60-glutamine peptide had a molecular size of approximately 37 kD and was identified by microsequencing to be GAPDH (Burke et al. 1996). The identity of this protein was confirmed on Western blot with anti-GAPDH antibody.

GAPDH was then immobilized to an agarose resin to determine if CAG repeat disease proteins in brain homogenate would bind to this protein. Silver stain of proteins eluted following binding to GAPDH showed that few brain proteins were retained. Among the proteins bound by GAPDH were DRPLA protein and HD and some lower-molecular-weight protein immunologically reactive with the DRPLA or HD antibodies. The observation that GAPDH binds preferentially to "expanded" glutamine peptide (60-mers), and GAPDH binds polyglutamine-containing peptides, suggests that this interaction may be biologically relevant.

GAPDH (EC 1.2.1.18)

GAPDH is a 37-kD protein with many enzymatic and binding activities. The two major enzymatic activities are in glycolysis/gluconeogenesis, and as a uracil DNA glycosylase (Meyer-Siegler et al. 1991). Other functions of GAPDH include binding tRNA (Singh and Green 1993), AU-rich regions of RNA (Nagy and Rigby 1995), ATP (Nakai et al. 1991), and calcyclin (Zeng et al. 1993); and complexing with the carboxy-terminal region of the amyloid precursor protein (Schulze et al. 1993). GAPDH also binds the erythrocyte glucose transporter (Lachaal et al. 1990), actin (Mejean et al. 1989), and tubulin (Somers et al. 1990). GAPDH is a highly duplicated gene in humans with more than 100 pseudogenes and one functional gene located on chromosome 12p13 (Piechaczyk et al. 1984; Tso et al. 1985). GAPDH is found throughout the cell, with the major fraction in the cytoplasm associated with cytoskeletal proteins and membranes and small amounts in the nucleus (Morgenegg et al. 1986; Ronai 1993). The crystalline structure of GAPDH shows that the NAD^+-binding domain consists of a core of pleated sheets surrounded by α helices, raising the possibility that complex formation between GAPDH and polyglutamine domains may involve the NAD^+-binding region.

GAPDH and Polyglutamine Repeat Diseases

Interactions of polyglutamine-repeat proteins with GAPDH could result in neurodegeneration by altering any of the enzymatic and structural roles of GAPDH.

Impairment of energy generation. Impairment of energy generation has long been considered a potential mechanism for pathogenesis in neurodegenerative diseases, especially HD (Beal 1992). Consistent with this hypothesis, numerous studies of HD patients and individuals at risk for disease have demonstrated decreased glucose utilization by positron emission tomography (PET scan) (Mazziotta et al. 1987; Grafton et al. 1992). Although impairment in glucose utilization may be a nonspecific effect of neuronal dysfunction, studies in at-risk individuals demonstrate that glucose metabolism is decreased long before signs of gross brain atrophy. Additionally, reduction in glucose metabolism extends beyond the basal ganglia structures most severely affected in HD, suggesting a generalized impairment (Martin et al. 1992). Impaired energy metabolism may also be responsible for the increase in basal ganglia and cerebral cortex lactate seen in vivo by nuclear magnetic resonance (NMR) spectroscopy in patients with HD (Jenkins et al. 1993).

DNA repair. DNA is damaged continually with estimated frequencies of spontaneous depurination occurring 10,000 times daily in each cell and 20,000–40,000 single-strand breaks occurring per cell per day (Rao 1993). DNA damage occurs in all cells, including postmitotic neurons. Any event that interferes with repair could have long-lasting consequences, such as turning genes on or off, or synthesis of aberrant mRNA, leading to dysfunctional proteins. Chronic defects in DNA repair have been postulated for a number of neurodegenerative diseases (Rao 1993).

GAPDH was recently identified as identical to an enzyme previously characterized as a uracil DNA glycosylase (UDG) (Meyer-Siegler et al. 1991). UDG removes uracil when it occurs in DNA due to misincorporation of deoxyuridine triphosphate or from deamination of cytosine. Spontaneous deamination occurs at a rate of 100–300 events per cell per day (Lindahl and Nyberg 1974), implying a continual need for UDG activity. UDG function in CAG trinucleotide repeat diseases is unknown. More difficult to explain is how cytoplasmic proteins such as HD and DRPLA can interfere with nuclear-based DNA repair proteins. Polyglutamine-repeat protein binding may prevent transport of GAPDH to the nucleus, or the GAPDH-repeat protein complex may be transported but dysfunctional.

Cytoskeletal integrity. The cytoskeleton is essential to maintain neuronal morphology and maintenance of processes. Susceptible striatal neurons in HD exhibit marked proliferation of dendrites prior to dendritic pruning and neuronal loss (Graveland et al. 1985; Ferrante et al. 1991). GAPDH promotes tubulin polymerization (Muronetz et al. 1994), the major constituent of microtubules. If stimulation of tubulin polymerization by GAPDH is modified by expanded polyglutamine repeat proteins, then aberrant control of the cytoskeleton could cause neuronal dysfunction and death.

Ubiquitous GAPDH and Expanded Polyglutamine Repeat Proteins, and Focal Neuronal Degeneration

How could interactions between two proteins present in all cells, GAPDH and polyglutamine proteins, cause focal pathology? Both the mutant and normal isoforms of the polyglutamine proteins are translated widely throughout the brain and body in HD (Li et al. 1993; Jou and Myers 1995), DRPLA (Onodera et al. 1995; Yazawa et al. 1995), SCA1 (Servadio et al. 1995), and SBMA. The brain may be the target in these five polyglutamine repeat diseases because neurons are postmitotic cells, increasing susceptibility to chronic accumulation of damage. Damage to dividing cells, in contrast, can be compensated by allowing the damaged cell to die and replacing it with a daughter cell from an adjacent healthy cell.

The hypothesis underlying these studies is that interactions between expanded polyglutamine domain proteins and GAPDH are responsible for pathogenesis of the CAG trinucleotide repeat diseases. Our evidence suggesting a role for GAPDH includes: (1) Few proteins from brain homogenate bind to immobilized polyglutamine peptide; (2) of the bound proteins, few show preferential binding to 60-mer glutamine ("pathological length") over 20-mer glutamine ("normal length"); (3) the major species preferentially bound to the 60-glutamine peptide is GAPDH; (4) few proteins in brain homogenate bind GAPDH immobilized on agarose beads; (5) interactions between GAPDH and polyglutamine repeat proteins may be relevant to pathogenesis by modifying an existing function, or by generating a novel function, for either the polyglutamine protein or GAPDH.

REFERENCES

Arriagada, P.V., J.H. Growdon, T. Hedley-White, and B.T. Hyman. 1992. Neurofibrillary tangles but not senile plaques parallel duration and severity of Alzheimer's disease. *Neurology* **42:** 631.

Andrew, S.E., Y.P. Goldberg, B. Kremer, H. Telenius, J. Theilmann, S. Adam, E. Starr, F. Squitieri, B. Lin, M.A. Kalchman, R.K. Graham, and M.R. Hayden. 1993. The relationship between trinucleotide (CAG) repeat length and clinical features of Huntington's disease. *Nat. Genet.* **4:** 398.

Beal, M.F. 1992. Does impairment of energy metabolism result in excitotoxic neuronal death in neurodegenerative illnesses? *Ann. Neurol.* **31:** 119.

Biernat, J., N. Gustke, G. Drewes, E.-M. Mandelkow, and E. Mandelkow. 1993. Phosphorylation of Ser-262 strongly reduces binding of tau to microtubules: Distinction between PHF-like immunoreactivity and microtubule binding. *Neuron* **11:** 153.

Bradley, W.A., E.B. Gilliam, A.M. Gotto, Jr., and S.H. Gianturco. 1982. Apolipoprotein E degradation in human very low density lipoporoteins by plasma protease(s): Chemical and biological consequences. *Biochem. Biophys. Res. Commun.* **109:** 1360.

Burke, J.R., J. Enghild, M.E. Martin, Y.-S. Jou, R.M. Myers, A.D. Roses, J.M. Vance, and W.J. Strittmatter. 1996. Huntingtin and DRPLA proteins selectively interact with the enzyme GAPDH. *Nat. Med.* **2:** 347.

Burright, E.N., H.B. Clark, A Servadio, T. Matilla, R.M. Fedderson, W.S. Yunis, L.A. Duvick, H.Y. Zoghbi, and H.T. Orr. 1995. SCA1 transgenic mice: A model for neurodegeneration caused by CAG trinucleotide expansion. *Am. J. Hum. Genet.* (suppl.) **57:** 8.

Corder, E.H., A.M. Saunders, W.J. Strittmatter, D. Schmechel, P. Gaskell, G.W. Small, A.D.Roses, J.L. Haines, and M.A. Pericak-Vance. 1993. Apolipoprotein E gene dose affects the risk of Alzheimer's diease. *Science* **261:** 921.

Crowther, R.A. 1993. Tau protein and paired helical filaments of Alzheimer's disease. *Curr. Opin. Struct. Biol.* **3:** 202.

Crowther, R.A., O.F. Olesen, M.J. Smith, R. Jakes, and M. Goedert. 1994. Assembly of Alzheimer-like filaments from full-length tau protein. *FEBS Lett.* **337:** 135.

DiFiglia, M., E. Sapp, K. Chase, C. Schwarz, A. Meloni, C. Young, E. Martin, J-P. Vonsattel, R. Carraway, S.A. Reeves, F.M. Boyce, and N. Aronin. 1995. Huntingtin is a cytoplasmic protein associated with vesicles in human and rat brain neurons. *Neuron* **14:** 1075.

Duyao, M.P., A.B. Auerbach, A. Ryan, F. Persichetti, G.T. Barnes, S.M. McNeil, P. Ge, J-P. Vonsattel, J.F. Gusella, A.L. Joyner, and M.E. MacDonald. 1995. Inactivation of the mouse Huntington's disease gene homolog Hdh. *Science* **269:** 407.

Ferrante, R.J., N.W. Kowall, and E.P. Richardson, Jr. 1991. Proliferative and degenerative changes in striatal spiny neurons in Huntington's disease: A combined study using the section-Golgi method and calbindin D28k immunocytochemistry. *J. Neurosci.* **11:** 3877.

Fleming, L., K.H. Weisgraber, W.J. Strittmatter, J.C. Troncoso, and G.V.W. Johnson. 1996. Differential binding of apoE isoforms to tau and other cytoskeletal proteins. *Exp. Neurol.* **138:** 252.

Goedert, M., R.A. Crowther, and C.C. Garner. 1991. Molecular characterization of microtubule-associated proteins tau and MAP 2. *Trends Neurosci.* **14:** 193.

Goedert, M., M.G. Spillantini, N.J. Cairns, and R.A. Crowther. 1992. Tau proteins of Alzheimer paired helical filaments: Abnormal phosphorylation of all six brain isoforms. *Neuron* **8:** 159.

Grafton, S.T., J.C. Mazziotta, J.J. Pahl, P. St. George-Hyslop, J.L. Haines, J.M. Hoffman, L.R. Baxter, and M.E. Phelps. 1992. Serial changes of cerebral glucose metabolism and caudate size in persons at risk for Huntington's disease. *Arch. Neurol.* **49:** 1161.

Graveland, G.A., R.S. Williams, and M. DiFiglia. 1985. Evidence for degenerative and regenerative changes in neostriatal spiny neurons in Huntington's disease. *Science* **227:** 770.

Gregg, R.E., G. Ghiselli, and H.B. Brewer, Jr. 1983. Apolipoprotein $E_{Bethesda}$: A new variant of apolipoprotein E associated with type III hyperlipidemia. *J. Clin. Endocrinol. Metab.* **57:** 969.

Han, S.-H., G. Einstein, K.H. Weisgraber, W.J. Strittmatter, A. Saunders, M. Pericak-Vance, A.D. Roses, and D.E. Schmechel. 1994a. Apolipoprotein E is localized to the cytoplasm of human cortical neurons: A light and electron microscopic study. *J. Neuropathol. Exp. Neurol.* **53:** 535.

Han, S.-H., C. Hulette, A.M. Saunders, G. Einstein, V.M. Pericak, W.J. Strittmatter, A.D. Roses, and D.E. Schmechel. 1994b. Apolipoprotein E is present in hippocampal neurons without neurofibrillary tangles in Alzheimer's diease and in age-matched controls. *Exp. Neurol.* **128:** 13.

Huang, D.Y., K.H. Weisgraber, W.J. Strittmatter, and W. Matthew. 1995a. apoE interacts with laminin, increases neuron attachment and alters morphology. *Exp. Neurol.* **136:** 251.

Huang, D.Y., K.H. Weisgraber, M. Goedert, A.M. Saunders, A.D. Roses, and W.J. Strittmatter. 1995b. apoE3 binding to tau tandem repeat I is abolished by tau serine 262 phosphorylation. *Neurosci. Lett.* **192:** 209.

Huang, D.Y., M. Goedert, R. Jakes, K.H. Weisgraber, C. Garner, A.M. Saunders, M. Pericak-Vance, D. Schmechel, A.D. Roses, and W.J. Strittmatter. 1994. Isoform-specific interactions of apolipoprotein E with the microtubule-associated protein MAP 2c: Implications for Alzheimer's disease. *Neurosci. Lett.* **182:** 55.

Jenkins, B.G., W.J. Koroshetz, M.F. Beal, and B.R. Rosen. 1993. Evidence for impairment of energy metabolism in vivo in Huntington's disease using localized 1H NMR spectroscopy. *Neurology* **43:** 2689.

Jou, Y.S. and R.M. Myers. 1995. Evidence from antibody studies that the CAG repeat in the Huntington disease gene is expressed in the protein. *Hum. Mol. Genet.* **4:** 465.

Kosik, K.S. 1992. Tau protein and neurodegeneration. *Mol. Neurobiol.* **4:** 171.

Lachaal, M., C.J. Berenski, J. Kim, and C.Y. Jung. 1990. An ATP-modulated specific association of glyceraldehyde-3-phosphate dehydrogenase with human erythrocyte glucose transporter. *J. Biol. Chem.* **265:** 15449.

LaDu, M.J., T.M. Pederson, D.E. Frail, C.A. Reardon, G.S. Getz, and M.T. Falduto. 1995. Purification of apolipoprotein E attenuates isoform-specific binding to β-amyloid. *J. Biol. Chem.* **270:** 9039.

LaSpada, A.R., D.B. Roling, A.E. Harding, C.L. Warner, R. Spiegel, W.C. Yee, and K.H. Fischbeck. 1992. Meiotic stability and genotype-phenotype correlation of the trinucleotide repeat in X-linked spinal and bulbar muscular atrophy. *Nat. Genet.* **2:** 301.

Li, S-H, G. Schilling, W.S. Young, X-J. Li, R.L. Margolis, O.C. Stine, M.V. Wagster, M.H. Abbott, M.L. Franz, N.G. Ranen, S.E. Folstein, J.C. Hedreen, and C.A. Ross. 1993. Huntington's disease gene (IT15) is widely expressed in human and rat tissues. *Neuron* **11:** 985.

Lindahl, T. and B. Nyberg. 1974. Heat-induced deamination of cytosine residues in deoxyribonucleic acid. *Biochemistry* **13:** 3405.

Liu, W-K., H. Ksiezak-Reding, and S-H. Yen. 1991. Abnormal tau proteins from Alzheimer's disease brains. Purification and amino acid analysis. *J. Biol. Chem.* **266:** 21723.

Martin, W.R., C. Clark, W. Ammann, A.J. Stoessl, W. Shtybel, and M.R. Hayden. 1992. Cortical glucose metabolism in Huntington's disease. *Neurology* **42:** 223.

Mazziotta, J.C., M.E. Phelps, J.J. Pahl, S.C. Huang, L.R. Baxter, W.H. Riege, J.M. Hoffman, D.E. Kuhl, A.B. Lanto, J.A. Wapenski, and C.H. Markham. 1987. Reduced cerebral glucose metabolism in asymptomatic subjects at risk for Huntington's disease. *N. Engl. J. Med.* **316:** 357.

Mejean, C., F. Pons, Y. Benyamin, and C. Roustan. 1989. Antigenic probes locate binding sites for the glycolytic enzymes glyceraldehyde-3-phosphate dehydrogenase, aldolase and phosphofructokinase on the actin monomer in microfilaments. *Biochem. J.* **264:** 671.

Meyer-Siegler, K., D.J. Mauro, G. Seal, J. Wurzer, J.K. deRiel, and M.A. Sirover. 1991. A human nuclear uracil DNA glycosylase is the 37-kDa subunit of glyceraldehyde-3-phosphate dehydrogenase. *Proc. Natl. Acad. Sci.* **88:** 8460.

Montine, T.J., V. Amarnath, M.E. Martin, W.J. Strittmatter, and D.G. Graham. 1996a. E-4-hydroxy-2-nonenal, is cytotoxic and covalently crosslinks cytoskeletal proteins in P19 neuroglial cells. *Am. J. Pathol.* **148:** 89.

Montine, T.J., D.Y. Huang, W.M. Valentine, V. Amarnath, A.M. Saunders, K.H. Weisgraber, D.G. Graham, and W.J. Strittmatter. 1996b. Crosslinking of apolipoprotein E by products of lipid peroxidation. *J. Neuropathol. Exp. Neurol.* **55:** 202.

Morgenegg, G., G.C. Winkler, U. Hübscher, C.W. Heizmann, J. Mous, and C.C. Kuenzle. 1986. Glyceraldehyde-3-phosphate dehydrogenase is a nonhistone protein and a possible activator of transcription in neurons. *J. Neurochem.* **47:** 54.

Muronetz, V.I., Z.X. Wang, T.J. Keith, H.R. Knull, and D.K. Srivastava. 1994. Binding constants and stoichiometries of glyceraldehyde 3-phosphate dehydrogenase-tubulin complexes. *Arch. Biochem. Biophys.* **313:** 253.

Nagy, E. and W.F. Rigby. 1995. Glyceraldehyde-3-phosphate dehydrogenase selectively binds AU-rich RNA in the NAD(+)-binding region (Rossmann fold). *J. Biol. Chem.* **270:** 2755.

Nakai, A., M. Satoh, K. Hirayoshi, and K. Nagata. 1991. Identification of the ATP-binding heat-inducible protein of M_R = 37,000 as glyceraldehyde-3-phosphate dehydrogenase. *Biochem. Biophys. Res. Commun.* **176:** 59.

Namba, Y., M. Tomonaga, H. Kawasaki, E. Otomo, and K. Ikeda. 1991. Apolipoprotein E immunoreactivity in cerebral amyloid deposits and neurofibrillary tangles in Alzheimer's disease and kuru plaque amyloid in Creutzfeldt-Jakob disease. *Brain Res.* **541:** 163.

Nixon, R.A. 1993. The regulation of neurofilament protein dynamics by phosphorylation: Clues to neurofibrillary pathobiology. *Brain Pathol.* **3:** 29.

Onodera, O., M. Oyake, H. Takano, T. Ikeuchi, S. Igarashi, and S. Tsuji. 1995. Molecular cloning of a full-length cDNA for dentatorubral-pallido luysian atrophy and regional expression of the expanded alleles in the CNS. *Am. J. Hum. Genet.* **57:** 1050.

Orr, H.T., M.Y. Chung, S. Banfi, T.J. Kwiatkowski, Jr., A. Servadio, A.L. Beaudet, L.A. Duvick, L.P. Ranum, and H.Y. Zoghbi. 1993. Expansion of an unstable trinucleotide CAG repeat in spinocerebellar ataxia type 1. *Nat. Genet.* **4:** 221.

Perutz, M.F., T. Johnson, M. Suzuki, and J.T. Finch. 1994. Glutamine repeats as polar zippers: Their possible role in inherited neurodegenerative diseases. *Proc. Natl. Acad. Sci.* **91:** 5355.

Piechaczyk, M., J.M. Blanchard, S. Riaad-El Sabouty, C. Dani, L. Marty, and P. Jeanteur. 1984. Unusual abundance of vertebrate 3-phosphate dehydrogenase pseudogenes. *Nature* **312:** 469.

Quigley, C.A. and F.S. French. 1994. Androgen insensitivity

syndromes. *Curr. Ther. Endocrinol. Metab.* **5:** 342.

Rao, K.S. 1993. Genomic damage and its repair in young and aging brain. (Review). *Mol. Neurobiol.* **7:** 23.

Rebeck, G.W., J.S. Reiter, D.K. Strickland, and B.T. Hyman. 1993. Apolipoprotein E in sporadic Alzheimer's disease: Allelic variation and receptor interactions. *Neuron* **11:** 575.

Ronai, Z. 1993. Glycolytic enzymes as DNA binding proteins. (Review). *Int. J. Biochem.* **25:** 1073.

Roses, A.D., W.J. Strittmatter, M.A. Pericak-Vance, E.H. Corder, A.M. Saunders, and D.E. Schmechel. 1994. Clinical application of apolipoprotein E genotyping to Alzheimer's disease. *Lancet* **343:** 1564.

Sanan, D., K.H. Weisgraber, R.W. Mahley, D.Y. Huang, S.J. Russell, A. Saunders, D. Schmechel, T. Wisniewski, B. Frangione, A.D. Roses, and W.J. Strittmatter. 1994. Apolipoprotein E associates with Aβ amyloid peptide to form novel monofibrils in vitro: Isoform apoE4 associates more efficiently than apoE3. *J. Clin. Invest.* **94:** 860.

Saunders, A.M., C. Hulette, K.A. Welsh, D.E. Schmechel, B. Crain, J.R. Burke, M.J. Alberts, W.J. Strittmatter, J.C. Breitner, C. Rosenberg, S.V. Scott, P.C. Gaskell, Jr., M.A. Pericak-Vance, and A.D. Roses. 1996. Specificity, sensitivity, and predictive value of apolipoprotein E genotyping in a consecutive autopsy series of sporadic Alzheimer's disease patients. *Lancet* **348:** 90.

Saunders, A.M., W.J. Strittmatter, D. Schmechel, P.H. St. George-Hyslop, M.A. Pericak-Vance, S.H. Joo, B.L. Rosi, J.F. Gusella, D.R. Crapper-MacLachlan, J. Growden, M.J. Alberts, C. Hulette, B. Crain, D.Goldgaber, and A.D. Roses. 1993. Association of apolipoprotein E allele c4 with late-onset familial and sporadic Alzheimer's disease. *Neurology* **43:** 1467.

Schmechel, D.E., A.M. Saunders, W. J. Strittmatter, S.H. Joo, C. Hulette, B. Crain, D. Goldgaber, and A.D. Roses. 1993. Increased vascular and plaque Aß4 amyloid deposits in sporadic Alzheimer's disease patients with apolipoprotein E-e4 allele. *Proc. Natl. Acad. Sci.* **90:** 9649.

Schulze, H., A. Schuler, D. Stuber, H. Dobeli, H. Langen, and G. Huber. 1993. Rat brain glyceraldehyde-3-phosphate dehydrogenase interacts with the recombinant cytoplasmic domain of Alzheimer's beta-amyloid precursor protein. *J. Neurochem.* **60:** 1915.

Servadio, A., B. Koshy, D. Armstrong, B. Antalffy, H.T. Orr, and H.Y. Zoghbi. 1995. Expression analysis of the ataxin-1 protein in tissues from normal and spinocerebellar ataxia type 1 individuals. *Nat. Genet.* **10:** 94.

Singh, R. and M.R. Green. 1993. Sequence-specific binding of transfer RNA by glyceraldehyde-3-phosphate dehydrogenase. *Science* **259:** 365.

Somers, M., Y. Engelborghs, and J. Baert. 1990. Analysis of the binding of glyceraldehyde-3-phosphate dehydrogenase to microtubules, the mechanism of bundle formation and the linkage effect. *Eur. J. Biochem.* **193:** 437.

Stott, D., J.M. Blackburn, P.J.G. Butler, and M. Perutz. 1995. Incorporation of glutamine repeats makes protein oligomerize: Implications for neurodegenerative diseases. *Proc. Natl. Acad. Sci.* **92:** 6509.

Strittmatter, W.J., A.M. Saunders, M. Pericak-Vance, G.S. Salvesen, J. Enghild, and A.D. Roses. 1993a. Apolipoprotein E: High avidity binding to Aβ amyloid and increased frequency of type 4 isoform in familial Alzheimer's disease. *Proc. Natl. Acad. Sci.* **90:** 1977.

Strittmatter, W.J., A.M. Saunders, M. Goedert, K. Weisgraber, L.-M. Dong, R. Jakes, D.Y. Huang, M. Pericak-Vance, D. Schmechel, and A.D. Roses. 1994a. Isoform-specific interactions of apolipoprotein E with microtubule-associated protein tau: Implications for Alzheimer's disease. *Proc. Natl. Acad. Sci.* **91:** 11183.

Strittmatter, W.J., K.H.Weisgraber, D. Huang, L.-M. Dong, G.S. Salvesen, M. Pericak-Vance, D. Schmechel, A.M. Saunders, D.M. Goldgaber, and A.D. Roses. 1993b. Binding of human apolipoprotein E to Aβ4 peptide: Isoform-specific effects and implications for late-onset Alzheimer's disease. *Proc. Natl. Acad. Sci.* **90:** 8098.

Strittmatter, W.J., K.H. Weisgraber, M. Goedert, A.M. Saunders, D. Huang, E.H. Corder, L.-M. Dong, R. Jakes, M.J. Alberts, J.R. Gilbert, D.E. Schmechel, M.A. Pericak-Vance, and A.D. Roses. 1994b. Hypothesis: Microtubule instability and paired helical filament formation in the Alzheimer's disease brain as a function of apolipoprotein E genotype. *Exp. Neurol.* **125:** 163.

Tso, J.Y., X.H. Sun, T.H.Kao, K.S. Reece, and R. Wu. 1985. Isolation and characterization of rat and human glyceraldehyde-3-phosphate dehydrogenase cDNAs: Genomic complexity and molecular evolution of the gene. *Nucleic Acids Res.* **13:** 2485.

Weisgraber, K.H. 1990. Apolipoprotein E distribution among human plasma lipoproteins: Role of the cysteine-arginine interchange at residue 112. *J. Lipid Res.* **31:** 1503.

———. 1994. Apolipoprotein E: Structure-function relationships. *Adv. Protein Chem.* **45:** 249.

Weisgraber, K.H. and R.W. Mahley. 1978. Apoprotein (E--A-II) complex of human plasma lipoproteins. I. Characterization of this mixed disulfide and its identification in a high density lipoprotein subfraction. *J. Biol. Chem.* **253:** 6281.

Weisgraber, K.H. and L.H. Shinto. 1991. Identification of the disulfide-linked homodimer of apolipoprotein E3 in plasma. *J. Biol. Chem.* **266:** 12029.

Willems, P.J. 1994. Dynamic mutations hit double figures. *Nat. Genet.* **8:** 213.

Yazawa, I., N. Nukina, H. Hashida, J. Goto, M. Yamada, and I. Kanazawa. 1995. Abnormal gene product identified in hereditary dentatorubral-pallidoluysian atrophy (DRPLA) brain. *Nat. Genet.* **10:** 99.

Zeng, F.Y., V. Gerke, and H.J. Gabius. 1993. Identification of annexin II, annexin VI and glyceraldehyde-3-phosphate dehydrogenase as calcyclin-binding proteins in bovine heart. *Int. J. Biochem.* **25:** 1019.

Myotonic Dystrophy: Discussion of Molecular Mechanism

C.T. CASKEY,[1] M.S. SWANSON,[2] AND L.T. TIMCHENKO[3]

[1]*Merck Research Laboratories, West Point, Pennsylvania 19486;* [2]*Department of Molecular Genetics and Microbiology and Center for Mammalian Genetics, University of Florida College of Medicine, Gainesville, Florida 32610;* [3]*Department of Medicine, Section of Cardiology, Baylor College of Medicine, Houston, Texas 77030*

Myotonic dystrophy (DM) is a neuromuscular disorder with autosomal dominant inheritance, associated with muscle weakness and myotonia, dilated cardiomyopathy, cataracts, and mental and endocrine abnormalities (Wieringa 1994; Harper 1995; Monckton and Caskey 1995; Timchenko et al. 1995a). Features of DM include the unusual phenomenon of anticipation, characterized by earlier onset and increased severity of the disease in successive generations (Howeler et al. 1989). Intensive searches for the gene and mutation responsible for DM resulted in discovery of the myotonin-protein kinase (*Mt-PK*) gene, which contains a track of CTG trinucleotide repeats in the 3′-untranslated region (Aslanidis et al. 1992; Brook et al. 1992; Buxton et al. 1992; Fu et al. 1992; Harley et al. 1992; Mahadevan et al. 1992). The size of the CTG trinucleotide repeat region varies in the normal population, from 5 to 30 repeats, but in affected individuals it increases dramatically, sometimes up to several hundreds or even several thousands of repeats. There is a clear correlation between the size of the CTG expansion and the severity of the clinical symptoms (Hunter et al. 1992; Tsilfidis et al. 1992; Redman et al. 1993).

Certain properties of the CTG trinucleotide repeat region in the *Mt-PK* gene, such as mitotic and meiotic instability, explained unusual inheritance patterns and variations in the clinical manifestation of DM. Identification of the mutation causing DM allowed fast and relatively inexpensive molecular diagnostic methods. However, important problems remain unsolved, especially the question of how expansion of CTG trinucleotide repeats leads to the clinical pathology. The protein product of the *Mt-PK* gene was predicted to be a serine-threonine kinase because of high homology with the serine-threonine kinase family (Fig. 1). Therefore, after discovery of the *Mt-PK* gene, a major focus of the research into the molecular basis of DM concerned the gene product and its kinase activity.

THE Mt-PK PROTEIN IS A SERINE-THREONINE KINASE

To study the Mt-PK protein, a number of different antibodies were generated (Fu et al. 1993; van der Ven et al. 1993; Brewster et al. 1994; Koga et al. 1994), which interact on immunoblots with a 52- to 55-kD protein from skeletal muscle and heart tissue. This protein was recognized as a product of the *Mt-PK* gene; however, additional antibodies were produced that interacted with 72- to 82-kD proteins (Maeda et al. 1995; Timchenko et al. 1995b; Whiting et al. 1995). It was therefore suggested that the 52- to 55-kD protein is a truncated form of the full-length kinase, or another protein that cross-reacts with Mt-PK antibodies. Comparison of the kinase specificities of the full-length and truncated isoforms indicated that they phosphorylate different amino acid residues. The 52- to 55-kD protein phosphorylates at tyrosine residues (Etongue-Mayer et al. 1994), whereas the 72-kD protein phosphorylates at serine and threonine residues (Fig. 2) (Dunne et al. 1994; Timchenko et al. 1995b). Moreover, when tissue protein extracts were prepared from engineered mice lacking the *Mt-PK* gene, only the full-length isoform was absent (Jansen et al. 1996). These data indicate that the full-length isoforms are products of the *Mt-PK* gene, and that the 52- to 55-kD protein is a different protein that is immunocrossreactive with Mt-PK.

Little is known about substrates for Mt-PK. Since DM patients are characterized by defects in muscle excitation after voluntary contraction, it was suggested that ion channels might be excellent candidates for Mt-PK substrates. Two reports so far have demonstrated a probable involvement of Mt-PK in the phosphorylation

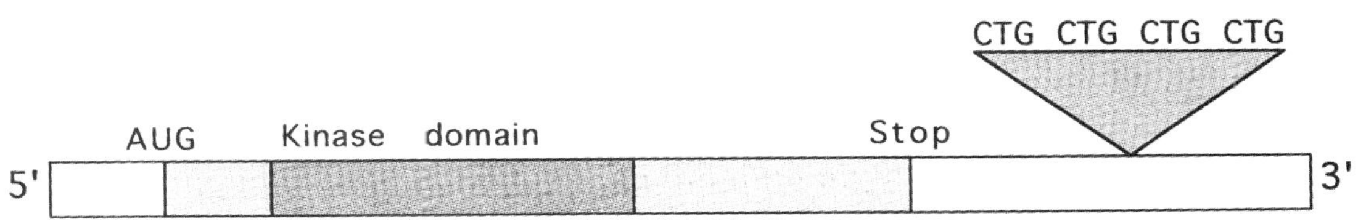

Figure 1. Diagram of the structure of the *Mt-PK* mRNA. One of the domains of *Mt-PK* is homologous to the kinase family. The position of CTG repeats in the 3′-untranslated region is indicated.

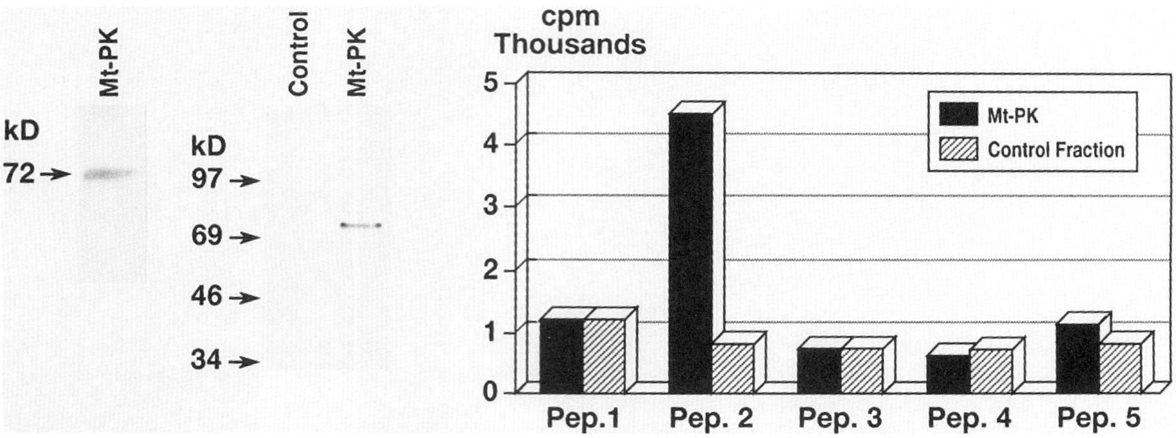

Figure 2. Phosphorylation of Mt-PK protein in vivo and in vitro. Electrophoretic analysis on the left shows phosphorylated Mt-PK protein precipitated from human fibroblasts grown with [^{32}P]orthophosphate. Electrophoretic analysis in the middle panel shows autophosphorylation of the recombinant Mt-PK protein. The diagram on the right indicates the levels of phosphorylation of the synthetic peptides by purified fusion Mt-PK. Mt-PK significantly phosphorylates peptide 2 (Gly-Arg-Gly-Leu-Ser-Leu-Ser-Arg), which contains a serine residue at the phosphorylation site but not peptides for Tyr kinase (peptide 1), Ca^{++}/calmodulin-dependent kinase (peptide 3), protein kinase C (peptide 4), or a peptide containing homoserine (peptide 5).

of voltage-dependent Ca^{++} release and Na^{+} channels (Mounsey et al. 1995; Timchenko et al. 1995b). Further investigation should indicate the significance of these findings.

TRINUCLEOTIDE REPEAT EXPANSION RESULTS IN DECREASED Mt-PK EXPRESSION

A second direction of research into cellular mechanisms that cause DM was the determination of how expanded CTG repeats affect expression of the *Mt-PK* gene. Location of the CTG repeat in the 3′-untranslated region of the *Mt-PK* gene suggests that CTG trinucleotide repeats may affect the efficiency of transcription of the *Mt-PK* gene, or the stability, polyadenylation, or transport of Mt-PK mRNA. Both negative (Carango et al. 1993; Fu et al. 1993; Hofmann-Radvanyi and Junien 1993; Hofmann-Radvanyi et al. 1993; Novelli et al. 1993; Koga et al. 1994; Krahe et al. 1995) and positive (Sabourin et al. 1993) effects of the CTG expansion on expression of the *Mt-PK* gene have been reported. Experimental data indicated that CTG expansion results in reduction of Mt-PK steady-state mRNA and protein levels, except for one report that describes the identification of a congenital DM patient with increased expression of the *Mt-PK* gene (Sabourin et al. 1993).

To verify the effect of the CTG expansion on the expression of *Mt-PK* gene, the steady-state levels of Mt-PK mRNA and full-length protein were studied in a severely affected patient who was homozygous for the DM mutation. An advantage of using cells from homozygous patients is the complete absence of the normal *Mt-PK* allele, which might otherwise mask, or compensate for, expression from the mutant allele. Northern and immunoblot analyses demonstrated that both Mt-PK mRNA and 72-kD protein levels were significantly reduced in cultured cells derived from a homozygous DM patient (Fig. 3) (L. Timchenko et al., unpubl.). On the basis of these observations, we and other workers conclude that the CTG expansion has a negative effect on *Mt-PK* expression.

Recent progress in the generation of *Mt-PK* "gene knockout" mice confirmed that loss of Mt-PK protein is involved in the development of muscle weakness and myopathy and is a part of the DM phenotype (Jansen et al. 1996; Reddy et al. 1996). However, loss of Mt-PK function is probably only one of the important com-

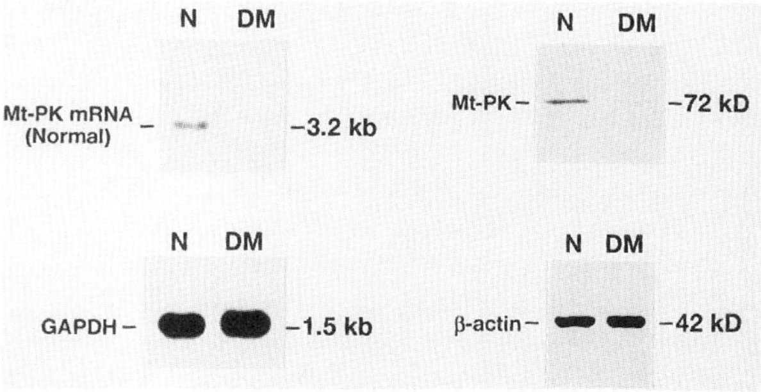

Figure 3. Reduction of *Mt-PK* expression in a homozygous DM patient with a severe clinical phenotype. Northern analysis on the left shows Mt-PK mRNA (3.2 kb) in cultured muscle cells derived from a normal control (N). Mutant Mt-PK mRNA is undetectable because of significantly decreased *Mt-PK* expression in DM cells. GAPDH (glyceraldehyde-3-phosphate dehydrogenase) was expressed equally in normal and DM cells. Immunoblot analysis (*right* panel) of the same cultured cells shows reduction of the 72-kD Mt-PK protein in the DM patient.

ponents in DM pathology, since heterozygous *Mt-PK* knockout mice are phenotypically normal (Reddy et al. 1996). This observation suggests that other genes or factors may be crucial for development of this disorder. One suggestion has been that CTG expansion has a negative effect on the expression of genes adjacent to *Mt-PK* (Jansen et al. 1995; Harris et al. 1996). Alternatively, it has been proposed that CTG/CUG trinucleotide repeats may be binding sites for specific DNA- or RNA-binding proteins, and that expansion of the repeats in DM patients may result in these proteins being sequestered or their function being disturbed (Wang et al. 1995; Timchenko et al. 1996).

The precise mechanism of Mt-PK reduction is unknown, although a few hypotheses have been suggested: (1) CTG repeats may affect the efficiency of *Mt-PK* transcription, since CTG expansion is a site of preferential nucleosome assembly (Wang et al. 1994; Wang and Griffith 1995); (2) CTG expansion may lead to abnormal polyadenylation of Mt-PK mRNA and other RNAs (Wang et al. 1995), suggesting that mutant Mt-PK mRNA has a "dominant-negative" pleiotropic effect; and (3) CTG trinucleotide expansion may also result in the abnormal transfer of mutant messages from the nucleus to the cytoplasm, since abnormally high concentrations of expanded Mt-PK mRNAs have been detected in the nuclei of DM cells (Taneja et al. 1995).

To study the effect of excess expression of the *Mt-PK* gene, mice overexpressing *Mt-PK* were generated (Jansen et al. 1996). These animals developed hypertrophic cardiomyopathy and greater neonatal mortality, showing a good correlation between the number of copies of the *Mt-PK* gene and the severity of the cardiac defects. These data indicate that Mt-PK is involved in the development of cardiomyopathy in individuals affected by DM, although the mechanism of this involvement remains to be investigated. Even when the *Mt-PK* genes in these mice contain a normal number of CTG repeats, an increase in the number of gene copies leads to overproduction of CTG repeats. We hypothesize that CTG/CUG repeats may be binding sites for DNA- or RNA-binding proteins, whose function could be disrupted by both CTG expansion and overproduction of CTG repeats.

IDENTIFICATION OF THE CUG TRIPLET REPEAT RNA-BINDING PROTEIN

As a first step toward testing the hypothesis presented above, we searched for DNA- and RNA-binding proteins that exhibited CTG or CUG triplet repeat-binding activities (Timchenko et al. 1996). Using double- or single-stranded DNA fragments containing CTG repeats, and a CUG oligoribonucleotide, we have identified a family of proteins that bind specifically to CTG/CUG repeats. Study of the binding specificities of the identified proteins with specific and nonspecific competitors indicated that HeLa cells contain at least three proteins recognizing double-stranded CTG trinucleotide repeats. These proteins were localized exclusively in the nucleus, suggesting a possible function in the regulation of transcription of the *Mt-PK* gene or of other genes adjacent to *Mt-PK*. Another protein, the single-stranded CTG-repeat-recognizing protein (ssCRRP), was identified predominantly in the cytoplasm of HeLa cells (Fig. 4). This protein does not bind single-stranded CAG or CGG oligonucleotides, nor a double-stranded DNA fragment containing CTG repeats, but it does recognize with equal affinity single-stranded CTG and CUG oligonucleotides. In addition to ssCRRP, a CUG-binding protein (CUG-BP) was identified, which exclusively recognizes the CUG repeat oligoribonucleotide (Fig. 4). This protein was found in both the cytoplasm and the nucleus (see below) and displayed RNA-binding activity specific for CUG repeats, but not RNA CGG repeats, single-stranded DNA CTG, CAG, or CGG repeats, or double-stranded CTG repeats. Both RNA-binding proteins, ssCRRP and CUG-BP, were suggested as candidates involved in the regulation of Mt-PK mRNA processing and transfer.

The identification of a group of proteins that bind to DNA or RNA trinucleotide repeats suggests that they may play an important role in DM pathology. Therefore, the next step in investigating these triplet repeat-binding proteins was to analyze their binding activities in cells derived from normal control and DM patients. Binding activities associated with double-stranded CTG-binding proteins and ssCRRP protein did not change in DM patients, although RNA-binding activity of CUG-BP was altered in DM cells, suggesting that this protein might be involved in DM pathology (Fig. 5) (L. Timchenko et al., unpubl.).

CUG-BINDING PROTEIN IS A NOVEL HUMAN RIBONUCLEOPROTEIN, hNab50

To understand the nature of CUG-BP, this protein was purified to homogeneity for microsequencing to determine if CUG-BP was a known protein (L. Timchenko et al., unpubl.). Purification of CUG-BP yielded two protein isoforms, with molecular masses of 49 kD and 51 kD, that exhibited specific RNA CUG-binding activities. Immunoblot analysis of these proteins with antibodies against different RNA-binding proteins indicated that CUG-BP interacts with monoclonal antibody (MAb) 3B1, which is specific for a novel RNA-binding protein, hNab50, recently identified by interaction with a yeast protein Nab2p in vivo (J. Miller et al., unpubl.).

The yeast protein Nab2p might be an essential factor for the regulation of poly(A) tail length and/or nucleoplasmic export of RNAs (Anderson et al. 1993 and unpubl.), since depletion of, or mutations in, this protein result in hyperpolyadenylation of mRNAs and accumulation of poly$(A)^+$ RNAs within the nucleus. Several human proteins, including hNab50, were isolat-

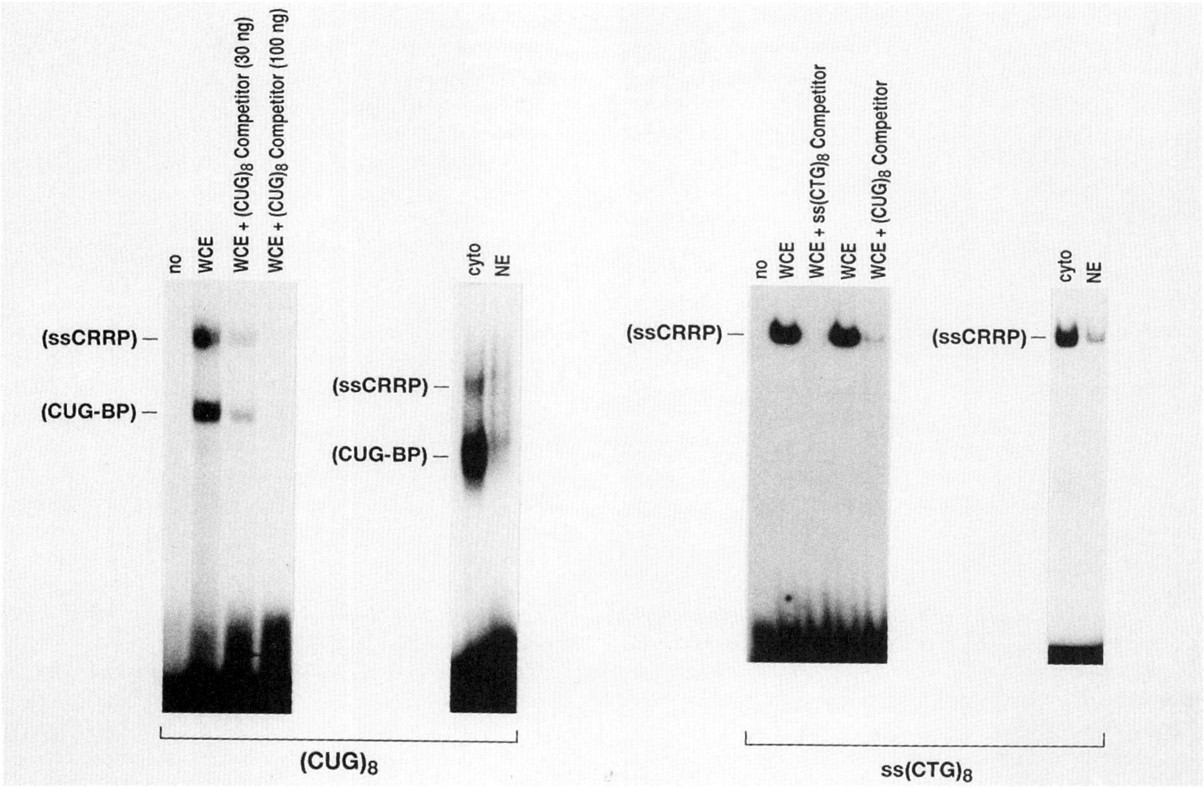

Figure 4. Identification of the RNA CUG triplet repeat-binding proteins. Bandshift analyses indicate two eukaryotic proteins (CUG-BP and ssCRRP) specifically bound to the RNA probe containing eight CUG repeats. CUG-BP protein is bound to RNA $(CUG)_8$ oligonucleotide but not to single-stranded DNA $(CTG)_8$. Both CUG-BP and ssCRRP proteins are present in the cytoplasm and nucleus.

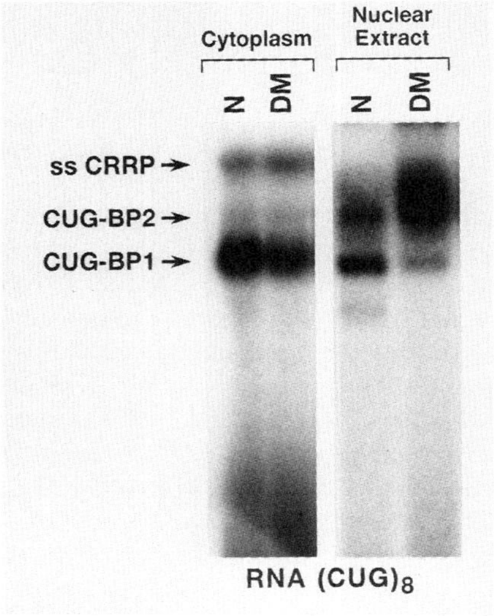

Figure 5. RNA-binding activity of CUG-BP is altered in DM patients. Bandshift analysis of nuclear and cytoplasmic protein extracts indicates an increase of RNA $(CUG)_n$ binding activity associated with CUG-BP2 in DM patients. In contrast, the RNA-binding activity of ssCRRP is unchanged.

ed from a HeLa cell cDNA-activation domain library and designated "*p*roteins that *i*nteract with *N*ab2p" (Pin). Three cDNAs encoding the hPin21 protein were identified out of eight cDNA clones isolated. In agreement with our previous results that Nab2p functions in RNA export from the nucleus, a database search revealed that hPin21 was identical to the human Rab protein. The Rab protein was characterized recently as a factor that binds the HIV-1 Rev protein activation domain, and it has been suggested that Rab is a cofactor for Rev-mediated RNA export (Bogerd et al. 1995). Quantitative β-galactosidase enzyme assays indicated that the interaction of yeast Nab2p with human Rab was very strong (Fig. 6). Four additional cDNA clones encoding hPin22 (hNab50), hPin23, hPin24, and hPin25 proteins were also identified in this screen. In vivo interaction of hNab50 and Nab2p suggests that hNab50 is involved in RNA processing and/or transport.

Analysis of the sequence data indicated that hNab50 is a member of a family of nuclear RNA-binding proteins that contains three RNA-binding motifs termed ribonucleoprotein consensus sequence RNA-binding domains (RBDs) (Fig. 7). A search of databases demonstrated that hNab50 was nearly identical

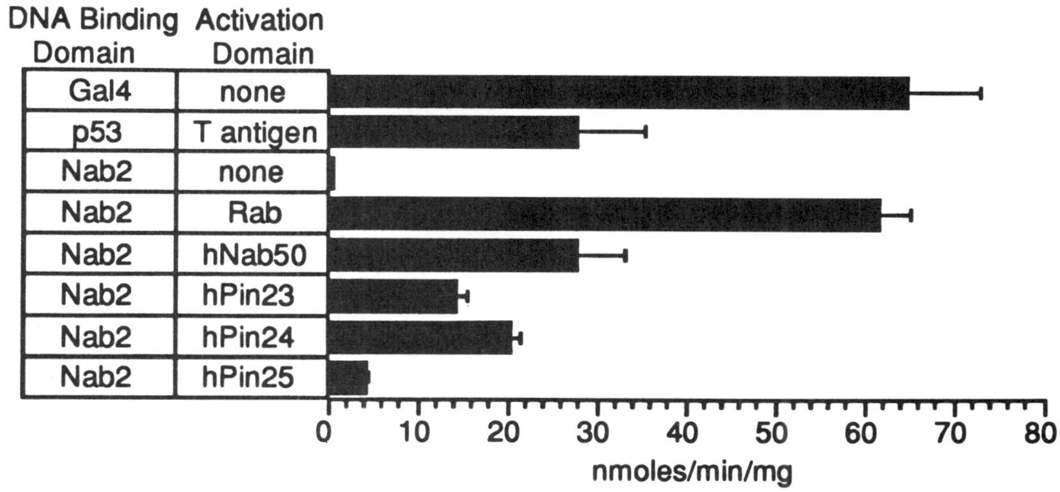

Figure 6. Isolation of hNab50. The β-galactosidase activities of the His^+/β-gal^+ yeast strains isolated using a two-hybrid interaction system (Clontech) are shown. Positive controls include intact Gal4p and the interaction between human p53 and SV40 large-T antigen.

(98% identity from amino acid residues 127 to 362) to a partially sequenced mouse protein that is expressed in the brain, and very similar (44% identity from amino acid residues 11 to 482) to a protein from *Xenopus laevis* that is expressed specifically in the nervous system and activated during gastrulation (Richter et al. 1988; Kato 1992). Although the anti-hNab50 MAb 3B1 detected 50-kD proteins in several different types of

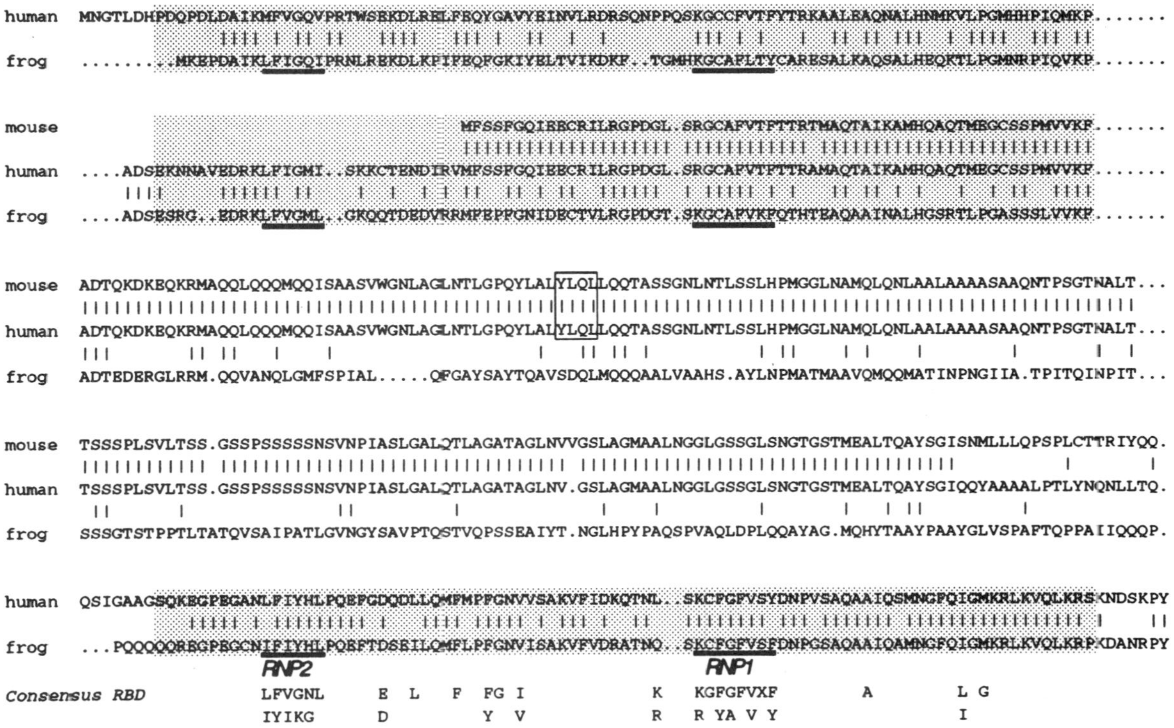

Figure 7. Sequence of hNab50 and similarity to related proteins differentially expressed in the vertebrate nervous system. Amino acid sequence of hNab50 is compared to a partially sequenced mouse homolog and a similar protein isolated from *X. laevis*. The boxed tetrapeptide (YLQL) is present in a subset of HeLa cell cDNA clones. The ribonucleoprotein consensus sequence RNA-binding domains (RBDs) are stippled and the most conserved motifs within RBD, RNP1 and RNP2, are underlined. The consensus RBD is from Bandziulis et al. (1989).

vertebrate tissue-culture cells (L. Timchenko et al., unpubl.), a larger protein exists in mouse tissues. Three proteins of 49, 51, and 52 kD were detectable in mouse 3T3 cells with MAb 3B1 (L. Timchenko et al., unpubl.), but only the two smaller proteins were present in the mouse tissues examined, whereas the 70-kD polypeptide was detectable in all tissues. Furthermore, the relative amounts of the 3B1-reactive polypeptides varied between different tissues, with the 49/51-kD polypeptides most abundant in brain, and the 70-kD protein the predominant form in heart. This latter result suggested a precursor/product relationship between the 49/51-kD and 70-kD proteins, and the possibility that the various polypeptides recognized by MAb 3B1 are isoforms generated by alternative pre-mRNA splicing and/or posttranslational modification.

Several hnRNPs have been shown to possess both sequence-specific and transcript-specific binding preferences (for review, see Dreyfuss et al. 1993; Swanson 1995). If CUG-BP/hNab50 plays a role in DM pathogenesis, then this hnRNP might bind to the 3′-untranslated region of Mt-PK mRNA. Using an in vitro photocrosslinking assay, we have demonstrated that the CUG-BP/hNab50 present in HeLa cell nuclear extract binds to RNAs that include the 3′-untranslated region of Mt-PK mRNA, but not actin mRNA (L. Timchenko et al., unpubl.).

Study of the biological role of the CUG-BP/hNab50 protein is only at the initial stage, and future work must determine if this protein is associated with DM pathology. However, some preliminary conclusions may guide future research directions related to the physiological role of this protein. So far, two of the most important properties of CUG-BP/hNab50 have been identified and associated with its RNA-binding activity: (1) the ability of CUG-BP/hNab50 to bind to CUG trinucleotide repeats and the 3′-untranslated region of Mt-PK mRNA in vitro and to poly(A)$^+$ mRNA in vivo; and (2) alterations of the RNA-binding activity of CUG-BP/hNab50 in DM patients. In studying the significance of the interaction of this protein with CUG trinucleotide repeats, the next step must be investigation of the binding of the CUG-BP/hNab50 protein and Mt-PK mRNA in vivo. Altered RNA-binding activity of CUG-BP/hNab50 in DM cells suggests that CUG-BP/hNab50 is abnormal in DM patients. To understand the nature of these alterations, the function of this protein in normal cells should first be determined. Since the hNab50 protein was identified in a yeast two-hybrid screen using a protein that plays a role in the polyadenylation and nuclear exit of mRNAs in yeast, it is possible that CUG-BP/hNab50 is one of the components of the RNA/protein complex responsible for mRNA processing and/or transport. Abnormalities of Mt-PK mRNA polyadenylation (Wang et al. 1995) and nuclear exit (Taneja et al. 1995) may be associated with the altered function of CUG-BP/hNab50.

It is important to understand the mechanism of the

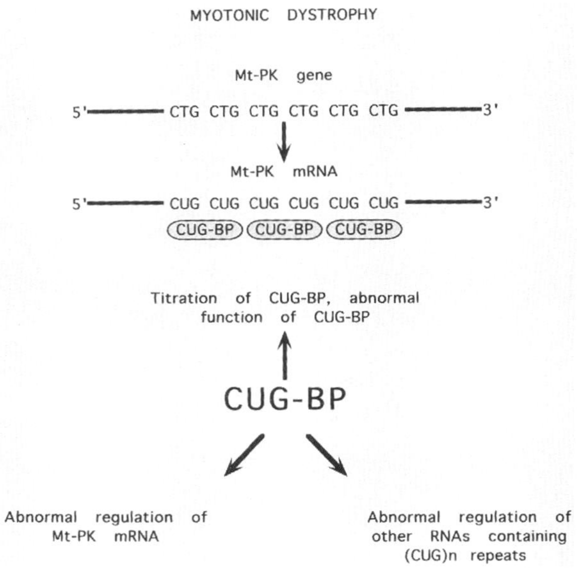

Figure 8. Hypothetical model for DM. In normal cells, CUG-BP protein may regulate the processing and/or transport of Mt-PK mRNA, as well as other mRNAs with CUG trinucleotide repeats. In DM patients, RNA trinucleotide repeats are expanded and Mt-PK mRNA therefore contains an increased number of RNA-binding sites for CUG-BP. We hypothesize that binding of free CUG-BP by expanded CUG repeats leads to reduced levels of the CUG-BP or alteration of its activity. Thus, regulation of Mt-PK mRNA expression, and other $(CUG)_n$-containing mRNAs, is abnormal in DM patients.

regulation of the RNA-binding activity of CUG-BP/hNab50. Analysis of the amino acid sequence of CUG-BP/hNab50 revealed a few phosphorylation sites for serine/threonine kinases. Preliminary data (L. Timchenko et al., unpubl.) indicate that CUG-BP1 and CUG-BP2 are two protein isoforms with different levels of phosphorylation. Therefore, RNA binding activity of CUG-BP/hNab50 may be regulated by phosphorylation/dephosphorylation. Since the CTG expansion in DM is located in a gene that encodes a kinase, it is possible that perturbations in Mt-PK levels are critical for the CUG-BP/hNab50 RNA-binding activity.

A PUTATIVE ROLE FOR CUG-BP/hNab50 IN DM PATHOGENESIS

We propose a hypothetical model for DM (Fig. 8). According to this model, the Mt-PK $(CUG)_n$ trinucleotide repeat expansion acts as a binding site for CUG-BP/hNab50, and expansion of the repeat results in three important events. First, the number of CUG-BP/hNab50 proteins sequestered on the mutant Mt-PK mRNA is dependent on the number of $(CUG)_n$ repeats, and large expansions lead to a loss of CUG-BP/hNab50 from other RNA-binding sites. Second, a reduction in the amount of CUG-BP/hNab50 might affect the processing and/or export of other mRNAs if

CUG-BP/hNAB50 is important for the biogenesis of other mRNAs. Third, abnormal function of CUG-BP/hNab50 leads to a reduction of Mt-PK mRNA and protein, resulting in reduced phosphorylation of substrate proteins. If CUG-BP/hNab50 is phosphorylated by Mt-PK mRNA in vivo, then the $(CUG)_n$ RNA-binding activity of CUG-BP/hNab50 may be altered. In DM, a large number of CUG-BP proteins bind to the expanded CUG repeat of Mt-PK mRNA. As a result, the transport of Mt-PK mRNA to the cytoplasm is blocked and the levels of mature mRNA and Mt-PK protein are significantly reduced. It is interesting to note that Taneja et al. (1995) have found an increased concentration of Mt-PK mRNA in the nuclei of DM patients, an observation that agrees with our hypothesis. This model predicts that patients with DM without abnormal expansion of the Mt-PK $(CTG)_n$ trinucleotide repeat (Thornton et al. 1994) may have mutations in the CUG-BP/hNab50 gene that alter the mRNA-binding properties of this human hnRNP. The genetic and biochemical linking of Mt-PK functions to an RNA-binding protein that is phosphorylated and binds CUG repeats suggests the model proposed above. More importantly, this linkage provides a new experimental pathway to resolve the pathogenesis of the DM trinucleotide repeat expansion.

REFERENCES

Anderson, J.T., S.M. Wilson, K.V. Datar, and M.S. Swanson. 1993. NAB2: a yeast nuclear polyadenylated RNA-binding protein essential for cell viability. *Mol. Cell. Biol.* **13:** 2730.

Aslanidis, C., G. Jansen, C. Amemiya, G. Shutler, M. Mahadevan, C. Tsilfidis, C. Chen, J. Alleman, N.G. Wormskamp, M. Vooijs, J. Buxton, K. Johnson, H.J.M. Sweets, G.G. Lennon, A.V. Carrano, R.G. Korneluk, B. Wieringa, and P.J. de Jong. 1992. Cloning of the essential myotonic dystrophy region and mapping of the putative defect. *Nature* **355:** 548.

Bandziulis, R.G., M.S. Swanson, and G. Dreyfuss. 1989. RNA-binding proteins as developmental regulators. *Genes Dev.* **3:** 431.

Bogerd, H.P., R.A. Fridell, S. Madore, and B R. Cullen. 1995. Identification of a novel cellular cofactor for the Rev/Rex class of retroviral regulatory proteins. *Cell* **82:** 485.

Brewster, B.S., S. Jeal, and P.N. Strong. 1994. Identification of a protein product of the myotonic dystrophy gene using peptide specific antibodies. *Biochem. Biophys. Res. Commun.* **194:** 1256.

Brook, J.D., M.E. McCurrach, H.G. Harley, A.J. Buckler, D. Church, H. Aburatani, K. Hunter, V.P. Stanton, J.-P. Thirion, T. Hudson, R. Sohn, B. Zemelman, R.G. Snell, S.A. Rundle, S. Crow, J. Davies, P. Shelbourne, J. Buxton, C. Jones, V. Juvonen, K. Johnson, P.S. Harper, D.J. Shaw, and D.E. Housman. 1992. Molecular basis of myotonic dystrophy: Expansion of a trinucleotide (CTG) repeat at the 3′ end of a transcript encoding a protein kinase family member. *Cell* **68:** 799.

Buxton, J., P. Shelbourne, J. Davies, C. Jones, T. Van Tongeren, C. Aslanidis, P. de Jong, G. Jansen, M. Anvret, B. Riley, B. Williamson, and K. Johnson. 1992. Detection of an unstable fragment of DNA specific to individuals with myotonic dystrophy. *Nature* **355:** 547.

Carango, P., J.E. Noble, H.G. Marks, and V.L. Funange. 1993. Absence of myotonic dystrophy protein kinase (DMPK) mRNA as a result of a triplet expansion in myotonic dystrophy. *Genomics* **18:** 340.

Dreyfuss, G., M.J. Matunis, S. Pinol-Roma, and C.G. Burd. 1993. hnRNP proteins and the biogenesis of mRNA. *Annu. Rev. Biochem.* **62:** 289.

Dunne, P.W., E.T. Walch, and H.F. Epstein. 1994. Phosphorylation reactions of recombinant human myotonic dystrophy protein kinase and their inhibition. *Biochemistry* **33:** 10809.

Etongue-Mayer, P., R. Faure, J.-P. Bouchard, M.-C. Thibault, and J. Puymurat. 1994. The myotonin-protein kinase phosphorylates tyrosine residues in normal human skeletal muscle. *Biochem. Biophys. Res. Commun.* **199:** 89.

Fu, Y.-H., D.L. Friedman, S. Richards, J.A. Pearlman, R.A. Gibbs, A. Pizzuti, T. Ashizawa, M.B. Perryman, G. Scarlato, R.G. Fenwick, Jr., and C.T. Caskey. 1993. Decreased expression of myotonin-protein kinase messenger RNA and protein in adult form of myotonic dystrophy. *Science* **260:** 235.

Fu, Y.-H., A. Pizzuti, R.G. Fenwick, Jr., J. King, S. Rajnarayan, P.W. Dunne, J. Dubel, G.A. Nasser, T. Ashizawa, P. de Jong, B. Wieringa, R. Korneluk, M.B. Perryman, H.F. Epstein, and C.T. Caskey. 1992. An unstable triplet repeat in a gene related to myotonic dystrophy. *Science* **255:** 1256.

Harley, H.G., J.D. Brook, S.A. Rundle, S. Crow, W. Reardon, A.J. Buckler, P.S. Harper, D.E. Housman, and D.J. Shaw. 1992. Expansion of an unstable DNA region and phenotypic variation in myotonic dystrophy. *Nature* **355:** 545.

Harper, P.S. 1995. Myotonic dystrophy and other autosomal muscular disorders. In *The metabolic and molecular bases of inherited disease* (ed. C.R. Scriver et al.), vol. 3, p. 4227. McGraw-Hill, New York.

Harris, S., C. Moncrieff, and K. Johnson. 1996. Myotonic dystrophy: Will the real gene please step forward! *Hum. Mol. Genet.* **5:** 1417.

Hofmann-Radvanyi, H. and C. Junien. 1993. Myotonic dystrophy: Over-expression or/and under-expression? A critical review on a controversial point. *Neuromusc. Disorders* **3:** 497.

Hofmann-Radvanyi, H., C. Lavedan, J.-P. Rabes, D. Savoy, C. Duros, K. Johnson, and C. Junien. 1993. Myotonic dystrophy: Absence of CTG enlarged transcript in congenital forms, and low expression of the normal allele. *Hum. Mol. Genet.* **2:** 1263.

Howeler, C.J., H.F.M. Busch, J.P.M. Geraedts, M.F. Niermeijer, and A. Stall. 1989. Anticipation in myotonic dystrophy: Fact or fiction? *Brain* **122:** 779.

Hunter, A., C. Tsilfidis, G. Mettler, P. Jacob, M. Mahadevan, L. Surh, and R. Korneluk. 1992. The correlation of age of onset with CTG trinucleotide repeat amplification in myotonic dystrophy. *J. Med. Genet.* **29:** 774.

Jansen, G., D. Bachner, M. Coerwinkel, N. Wormsamp, H. Hameister, and B. Wieringa. 1995. Structural organization and developmental expression pattern of the mouse WD-repeat gene DMR-N9 immediately upstream of the myotonic dystrophy locus. *Hum. Mol. Genet.* **4:** 843.

Jansen, G., P.J.T.A. Croenen, D. Bachner, P.H.K. Jap, M. Coerwinkel, F. Oerlemans, W. van den Broek, B. Gohlsch, D. Pette, J.J. Plomp, P.C. Molenaar, M.G.J. Nederhoff,

C.J.A. van Echteld, M. Dekker, A. Berns, H. Hameister, and B. Wieringa. 1996. Abnormal myotonic dystrophy protein kinase levels produce only mild myopathy in mice. *Nat. Genet.* **13:** 316.

Kato, K. 1992. Finding new genes in the nervous system by cDNA analysis. *Trends Neurosci.* **15:** 319.

Koga, R., Y. Nakao, Y. Kurano, T. Tsukahara, A. Nakamura, S. Ishiura, I. Nonaka, and K. Arahata. 1994. Decreased myotonin-protein kinase in the skeletal and cardiac muscle in myotonic dystrophy. *Biochem. Biophys. Res. Commun.* **202:** 577.

Krahe, R., T. Ashizawa, C. Abbruzzese, E. Roeder, P. Carango, M. Giacenelli, V.L. Funanage, and M.J. Siciliano. 1995. Effect of myotonic dystrophy trinucleotide repeat expansion on DMPK transcription and processing. *Genomics* **28:** 1.

Maeda, M., C.S. Taft, E.W. Bush, E. Holder, W.M. Bailey, H. Neville, M.B. Perryman, and R.D. Bies. 1995. Identification, tissue-specific expression, and subcellular localization of the 80- and 71-kD forms of myotonic dystrophy kinase protein. *J. Biol. Chem.* **270:** 20246.

Mahadevan, M., C. Tsilfidis, L. Sabourin, G. Shutler, C. Amemiya, G. Jansen, C. Neville, M. Narang, J. Barcelo, and K. O'Hoy. 1992. Myotonic dystrophy mutation: An unstable CTG repeat in the 3′ untranslated region of the gene. *Science* **255:** 1253.

Monckton, D.G. and C.T. Caskey. 1995. Unstable triplet repeat diseases. *Circulation* **91:** 1.

Mounsey, J.P., P. Xu, J.E. John III, L.T. Horne, J. Gilbert, A.D. Roses, and J.R. Moorman. 1995. Modulation of skeletal muscle sodium channels by human myotonin protein kinase. *J. Clin. Invest.* **95:** 2379.

Novelli, G., N.M. Gennarelli, G. Zelano, A. Pizzuti, C. Fattorini, C.T. Caskey, and B. Dallapiccola. 1993. Failure in detecting mRNA transcripts from the mutated allele in myotonic dystrophy muscle. *Biochem. Mol. Biol. Int.* **29:** 291.

Reddy, S., D.B.J. Smith, M.M. Rich, J.M. Leferovich, P. Reily, B.M. Davis, K. Tran, H. Rayburn, R. Bronson, D. Cros, R.J. Balice-Gordon, and D. Housman. 1996. Mice lacking the myotonic dystrophy protein kinase develop a late onset progressive myopathy. *Nat. Genet.* **13:** 325.

Redman, J.B., R.G. Fenwick, Y.-H. Fu, A. Pizzuti, and C.T. Caskey. 1993. Relationship between parental trinucleotide CTG repeat length and severity of myotonic dystrophy in offspring. *J. Am. Med. Assoc.* **269:** 1960.

Richter, K., H. Grunz, and I.B. Dawid. 1988. Gene expression in the embryonic nervous system of *Xenopus laevis*. *Proc. Natl. Acad. Sci.* **85:** 8086.

Sabourin, L.A., M.S. Mahadevan, M. Narang, D.S.C. Lee, L.C. Surh, and R.G. Korneluk. 1993. Effect of the myotonic dystrophy (DM) mutation on mRNA levels of the DM gene. *Nat. Genet.* **4:** 233.

Swanson, M.S. 1995. Functions of nuclear pre-mRNA/mRNA-binding proteins. In *Pre-mRNA processing* (ed. A.I. Lamond), p. 17. Springer-Verlag, New York.

Taneja, K.L., M. McCurrach, M. Schalling, D. Housman, and R.H. Singer. 1995. Foci of trinucleotide repeat transcripts in nuclei of myotonic dystrophy cells and tissues. *J. Cell Biol.* **128:** 995.

Thorton, C.A., R.C. Griggs, and R.T. Moxley. 1994. Myotonic dystrophy with no trinucleotide repeat expansion. *Ann. Neurol.* **35:** 269.

Timchenko, L., D.G. Monckton, and C.T. Caskey. 1995a. Myotonic dystrophy: An unstable CTG repeat in a protein kinase gene. *Semin. Cell Biol.* **6:** 13.

Timchenko, L.T., N.A. Timchenko, C.T. Caskey, and R. Roberts. 1996. Novel proteins with binding specificity for DNA CTG repeats and RNA CUG repeats. *Hum. Mol. Genet.* **5:** 115.

Timchenko, L., W. Nastainczyk, T. Schneider, B. Patel, F. Hofmann, and C.T. Caskey. 1995b. Full-length myotonin protein kinase (72kDa) displays serine kinase activity. *Proc. Natl. Acad. Sci.* **92:** 5366.

Tsilfidis, C., A.E. MacKenzie, G. Mettler, J. Barcelo, and R.G. Korneluk. 1992. Correlation between CTG trinucleotide repeat length and frequency of severe congenital myotonic dystrophy. *Nat. Genet.* **1:** 192.

van der Ven, P.F.M., G. Jansen, T.H.M.S.M. van Kuppevelt, M.B. Perryman, M. Lupa, P.W. Dunne, H.J. ter Laak, J.H. Veerkamp, H.F. Epstein, and B. Wieringa. 1993. Myotonic dystrophy kinase is a component of neuromuscular junctions. *Hum. Mol. Genet.* **2:** 1889.

Wang, J., E. Pegoraro, E. Menegazzo, M. Gennarelli, R.C. Hoop, C. Angelini, and E.P. Hoffman. 1995. Myotonic dystrophy: Evidence for a possible dominant-negative RNA mutation. *Hum. Mol. Genet.* **4:** 599.

Wang, Y. and J. Griffith. 1995. Expanded CTG triplet blocks from the myotonic dystrophy gene create the strongest known natural nucleosome positioning elements. *Genomics* **25:** 570.

Wang, Y., S. Amirhaeri, S. Kang, R.D. Wells, and J.D. Griffith. 1994. Preferential nucleosome assembly at DNA triplet repeats from myotonic dystrophy gene. *Science* **265:** 669.

Whiting, E.J., J.D. Waring, K. Tamai, M.J. Somerville, M. Hincke, W.A. Staines, J.-E. Ikeda, and R.G. Korneluk. 1995. Characterization of myotonic protein kinase (DMK) protein in human and rodent muscle and central nervous tissue. *Hum. Mol. Genet.* **4:** 1063.

Wieringa, B. 1994. Myotonic dystrophy reviewed: Back to the future. *Hum. Mol. Genet.* **3:** 1.

Huntington's Disease

J.F. Gusella,[1,2] S. McNeil,[1] F. Persichetti,[1] J. Srinidhi,[1] A. Novelletto,[3] E. Bird,[4]
P. Faber,[1] J.-P. Vonsattel,[5] R.H. Myers,[6] and M.E. MacDonald[1]
[1]*Molecular Neurogenetics Unit, Massachusetts General Hospital, Charlestown, Massachusetts 02129;*
[2]*Department of Genetics, Harvard Medical School, Boston, Massachusetts 02114;*
[3]*Department of Biology, University of Rome "Tor Vergata," Rome, Italy;*
[4]*Brain Tissue Resource Center, McLean Hospital, Belmont, Massachusetts 02178;*
[5]*Laboratory for Molecular Neuropathology, Massachusetts General Hospital, Charlestown, Massachusetts 02129;*
[6]*Department of Neurology, Boston University Medical School, Boston, Massachusetts 02118*

Huntington's disease (HD) is an inherited disorder involving selective degeneration of neurons in the brain (Martin and Gusella 1986). It is named for George Huntington, a family physician on Long Island, New York, who recognized the familial nature of the disorder and provided the first graphic description of it in 1872. HD is inherited in an autosomal dominant fashion and has a prevalence of about 1 in 10,000 in Caucasian populations, but HD also affects other races, albeit at lower frequency (Harper 1992). Persons carrying the HD defect are usually neurologically and behaviorally normal for many years prior to any disease manifestations. Onset of HD may occur at any time in life, from early in childhood until the ninth decade, but in most cases, symptoms begin in middle age, after the gene defect may already have been transmitted to children. Initially, the disorder is manifested as minor adventitious movements, abnormal eye saccades, awkward gait, and clumsiness. These motor abnormalities become progressively more exaggerated, eventually encompassing the entire body in a characteristic chorea: writhing, uncontrolled, "dance-like" movements. As the disease progresses, the patient gradually loses the capacity to function in daily life and, ultimately, to communicate. A course of 10–20 years of inexorable decline, often marked by extreme weight loss, ends in death, usually as a result of aspiration pneumonia, heart disease, or some other complication of the disorder. In patients who have early onset of HD in the juvenile years, the disorder is more severe and the movement disorder progresses rapidly beyond chorea to extreme rigidity. In a seeming deviation from the expectations of Mendelian inheritance, the preponderance of juvenile-onset HD cases inherit their defective allele from their father rather than from their mother.

HD was originally known as Huntington's chorea because of the prominence and peculiarity of the abnormal movements, until it was recognized that the disorder also exhibits psychiatric and cognitive disturbances. Indeed, chronic depression, impulsiveness, and erratic behavior, although not diagnostic of HD, may in some cases precede the onset of the movement disorder by several years. Later, the increase in motor dysfunction is paralleled by intellectual decline and sometimes by severe psychiatric changes.

The HD genetic defect causes this peculiar constellation of motor, psychiatric, and intellectual features by selectively killing a subset of neurons in the brain. Most severely affected is the striatum, where medium spiny GABAergic projection neurons disappear in a gradient progressing along postero-anterior, dorso-ventral, and medio-lateral axes (Vonsattel et al. 1985). These cells may dysfunction for some time prior to their death, as they can appear in postmortem brain to have wilted, recurved dendritic endings and changes in the density, shape, and size of spines (Graveland et al. 1985). Cell loss eventually decimates the caudate and putamen, leaving an expanded ventricle that appears as an empty hole in brain scans. However, although cell loss is most easily recognized in the basal ganglia where tissue architecture is totally destroyed, it is not limited to these regions. There is extensive cell loss in the cortex, as evidenced by an overall reduction in brain weight of 20% or more, but the precise cell populations that are affected have yet to be delineated.

The cause of the selective neuronal death in HD and the consequent clinical manifestations of the disorder remained a mystery until 1993, when a location cloning effort based on the mapping of the HD locus to chromosome 4p16.3 came to fruition (Gusella and MacDonald 1993). The HD defect was identified as an expanded and unstable trinucleotide repeat in a gene encoding a novel protein (Huntington's Disease Collaborative Research Group 1993). The discovery of the HD gene and the mutation that causes the disorder have explained some of the peculiarities of inheritance of this disorder and have suggested that it shares a similar mechanism of pathogenesis with several other neurodegenerative disorders.

MATERIALS AND METHODS

Human tissues and DNAs. Lymphoblast cell lines from HD families have been established in the Molecular Neurogenetics Unit during the past 16 years for use in genetic and biochemical studies (Anderson and Gusella 1984). Human brain tissue collected at autopsy and stored frozen by the Brain Tissue

Resource Center, McLean Hospital, Belmont, Massachusetts was used for preparation of DNA (Persichetti et al. 1995b). For each brain, one hemisphere was fixed and used for confirmation of HD neuropathology using the grading system of Vonsattel et al. (1985).

DNA was prepared from cultured cells and from postmortem cerebellar brain tissue as described previously (Gusella et al. 1983). The length of HD CAG alleles was assessed using polymerase chain reaction (PCR) to amplify only the CAG stretch (Warner et al. 1993), excluding the slightly polymorphic CCG repeat adjacent to the CAG stretch (Rubinsztein et al. 1993b). Additional data concerning CAG repeat lengths in HD and other disorders were collected from published literature reports as noted.

Data analysis. Nonlinear curve fitting and calculation of coefficient of determination were performed using SigmaPlot (Jandel Scientific).

RESULTS AND DISCUSSION

The HD Gene and Its Defect

The HD defect was first mapped to chromosome 4 by genetic linkage with the anonymous DNA markers *D4S10* in 1983 (Gusella et al. 1983). A decade of genetic and physical mapping studies confined the locus to a 2-Mb region of band 4p16.3, extending to within 2 Mb of the short-arm telomere (Gusella and MacDonald 1993). Although this region could not be narrowed further by recombination events in HD kindreds, haplotype analysis of HD chromosomes with multiallele markers suggested that about one-third of all HD chromosomes descend from a common founder (MacDonald et al. 1992). Investigation of this subset eventually indicated a segment of about 150 kb as the most likely location of the disease gene (Gusella and MacDonald 1995). Indeed, the defect was discovered when a CAG trinucleotide repeat in this region was found to be expanded and unstable on HD chromosomes (Huntington's Disease Collaborative Research Group 1993).

The CAG repeat, whose length can be readily monitored by PCR, is located in exon 1 of a 67-exon gene encoding a novel protein of unknown function (Fig. 1). On normal chromosomes, the CAG stretch is polymorphic, displaying 6–34 repeat units that are inherited in a strictly Mendelian fashion. On HD chromosomes, the CAG segment is expanded to 36 to more than 100 units (Fig. 2). The expanded alleles are

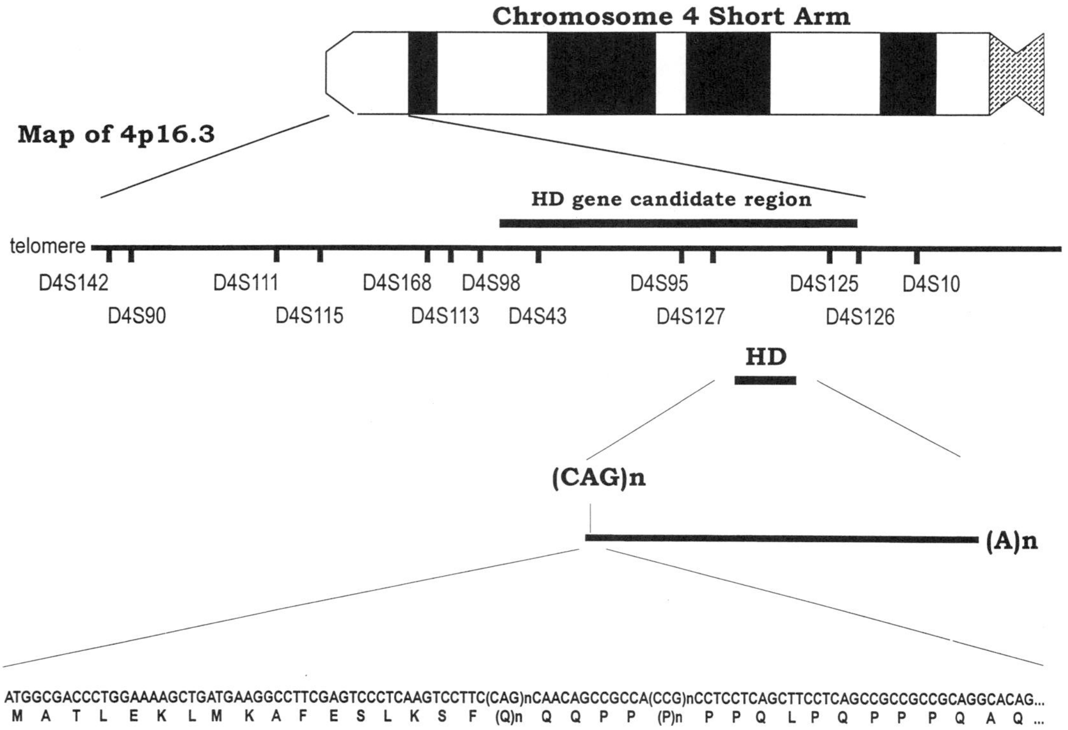

Figure 1. Site of the HD mutation. A schematic diagram of the short arm of chromosome 4 is shown above an expanded physical map of the 4p16.3 band, extending from the short-arm telomere to *D4S10*. The formal HD candidate region defined by recombination events in HD kindreds is shown above the map, with the location of the HD gene noted below the map. The HD gene, comprising 67 exons, produces an mRNA with a polymorphic CAG stretch near its 5′ end. The disease mutation involves expansion and meiotic instability of this CAG segment. At the bottom of the diagram, the DNA sequence encoding the amino terminus of huntingtin is shown above the corresponding protein sequence. Normal chromosomes show polymorphic variability both in the CAG segment encoding polyglutamine and in a downstream CCG segment encoding polyproline.

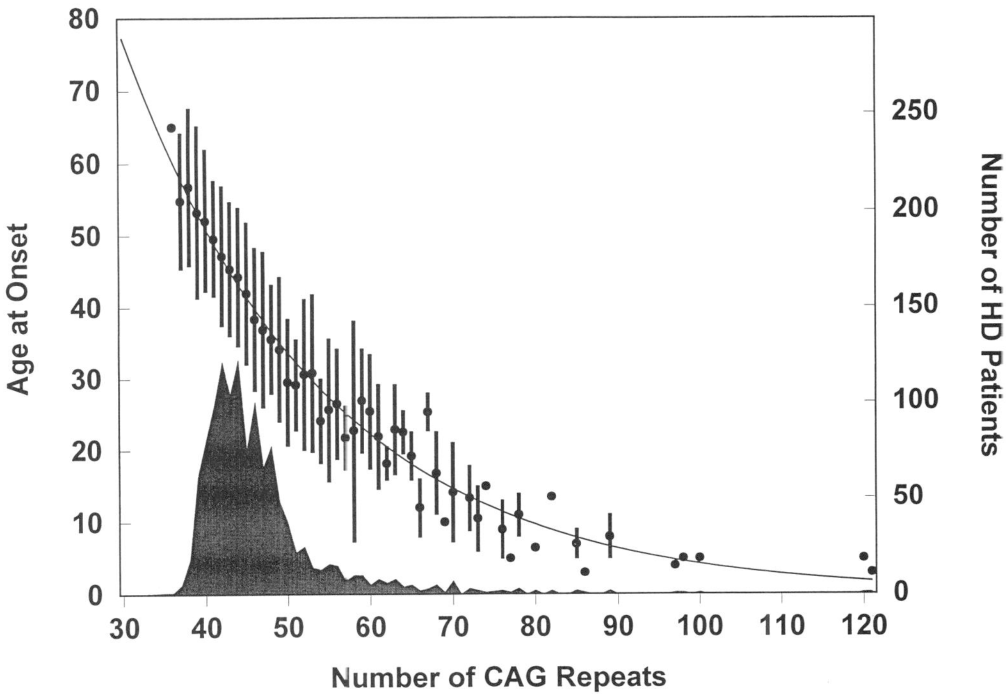

Figure 2. Relationship between age at neurological onset and number of consecutive CAG triplets. Data compiled from published reports involving 1226 HD patients (Andrew et al. 1993; Barron et al. 1993; Craufurd and Dodge 1993; De Rooij et al. 1993; Duyao et al. 1993; Huntington's Disease Collaborative Research Group 1993; Kremer et al. 1993; Norremolle et al. 1993, 1994; Rubinsztein et al. 1993a; Snell et al. 1993; Stine et al. 1993; Zuhlke et al. 1993; Illarioshkin et al. 1994; Kieburtz et al. 1994; Lucotte et al. 1994; Claes et al. 1995; Persichetti et al. 1995b) permitted the determination of mean age at neurological onset (*filled circles* ± S.D., left Y axis) associated with different numbers of CAG repeats in the disease allele. A line shows the fit of the data (r^2=.95)to an exponential decay model. The shaded area below shows the number of HD patients (right Y axis) possessing each number of CAG repeats.

extremely unstable in intergenerational transmission and change in length in the vast majority of meioses, indicating a mutation rate approaching 1. In contrast, the repeats are quite stable through mitosis, with little somatic mosaicism exhibited except by the largest alleles.

The intergenerational size changes in most alleles are small, 1–5 CAG units, with a bias toward expansion, although contractions are also frequent. In some cases, larger increases in CAG repeat number occur, resulting in a doubling or more of the length of the parental allele. These larger increases occur preferentially in male transmissions, indicating that whereas the mutation rate is similar in oogenesis and spermatogenesis, the magnitude of the mutation can be far greater in the latter (MacDonald et al. 1993). This instability in spermatogenesis can be visualized directly by examining allele lengths in DNA from sperm. Whereas somatic DNA from an HD male exhibits discrete lengths for the normal and mutant alleles, sperm DNA often shows a homogeneous PCR product only for the normal allele. In contrast, the disease allele yields a heterogeneous array of products spanning a size range both smaller and larger than the somatic disease allele. The average magnitude of the size changes appears to increase with increasing initial CAG allele length.

Clinical Correlations with CAG Repeat Length

There are no proven cases of HD caused by any mutation other than an expanded CAG segment, and all sporadic HD patients who represent new mutations to the disease possess an expanded allele (Goldberg et al. 1993; Myers et al. 1993; Davis et al. 1994; Bozza et al. 1995; Durr et al. 1995). Indeed, our extensive study of pathologically confirmed HD brains suggests that all individuals with clinical manifestations and neuropathological changes characteristic of HD possess an expanded CAG repeat (Persichetti et al. 1995b).

The variability of age at onset of HD is largely explained by the nature of the mutation and the behavior of the CAG repeat. Many studies have reported a strong inverse correlation between age at onset of neurological symptoms and the number of CAG units in the mutant allele (Gusella and MacDonald 1995). There is a similar inverse correlation of CAG repeat length and age at psychiatric onset (Persichetti et al. 1995b). As most HD chromosomes have allele lengths in the range of 40–50 CAG units, most patients have neurological onset between 35 and 55 years of age. Those persons who suffer onset of HD in childhood typically possess repeat lengths greater than 65 CAG units. The fact that these larger alleles can be generated more readily through spermatogenesis than through oogenesis explains the previously noted preponderance of paternal inheritance in cases of juvenile onset.

Although increasing CAG repeat length is associated on average with earlier onset, the allele length is not predictive in any individual case, as there is wide variation that probably results from the actions of modifying factors, either genetic, environmental, or stochastic (Fig. 2). This is most noteworthy for alleles with 36–39 CAGs, generally associated with onset of HD later in life. Some persons with alleles in this size range live to old age without displaying any manifestations of HD, suggesting that in such cases modifying factors can determine whether the disease allele is penetrant. The same factors, which remain to be identified, may operate in individuals with longer CAG repeat lengths to delay onset of symptoms.

Some investigators have attributed the inverse correlation between CAG repeat length and age at onset largely to juvenile-onset cases, but by combining the data from several published reports, it can be demonstrated that the correlation holds throughout the spectrum of onset ages (Fig. 2). Indeed, calculating the mean age of onset associated with the various CAG repeat lengths from the combined data sets should eliminate most of the variation in age at onset attributable to non-CAG length-related factors. In this circumstance, the data provide an excellent fit (r^2=.95) to an exponential decay model, indicating that in absolute terms, the contribution of each additional CAG unit to reducing age at onset becomes progressively smaller as the CAG length increases. This is consistent with a model in which the length of the CAG segment determines the rate of neuronal dysfunction or loss, with onset of symptoms occurring when remaining neuronal capacity of some crucial neuronal population falls below a critical threshold.

Despite variability in the immediate cause of death in HD patients, age at death is also inversely correlated with the length of the CAG repeat, indicating that the presence of the disease allele is the initial critical determinant of the patient's ultimate demise (Fig. 3). On average, there is a 15-year span between age at neurological onset and age at death. Assuming that neurological onset is a direct result of the loss of neurons in the brain, one might expect that an increasing rate of loss of neurons with increasing CAG length might produce more rapid death. This does not appear to be the case, as shown in Figure 4, where a collection

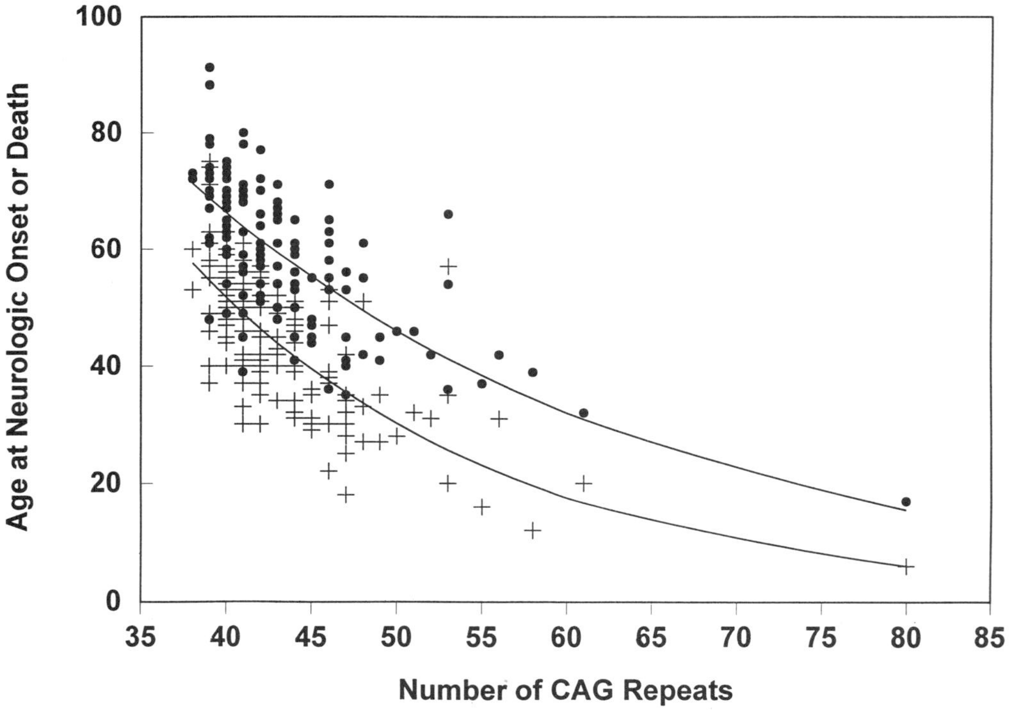

Figure 3. Age at neurological onset and age at death versus number of CAG repeats. Age at neurological onset (*crosses*) and age at death (*filled circles*) are plotted against the number of CAG repeats for 146 patients whose brains were subjected to postmortem analysis to confirm HD neuropathology (Persichetti et al. 1995b). On the basis of the relationship shown in Fig. 2, each set of data was fitted to an exponential decay curve (r^2 = .53 and .49, respectively).

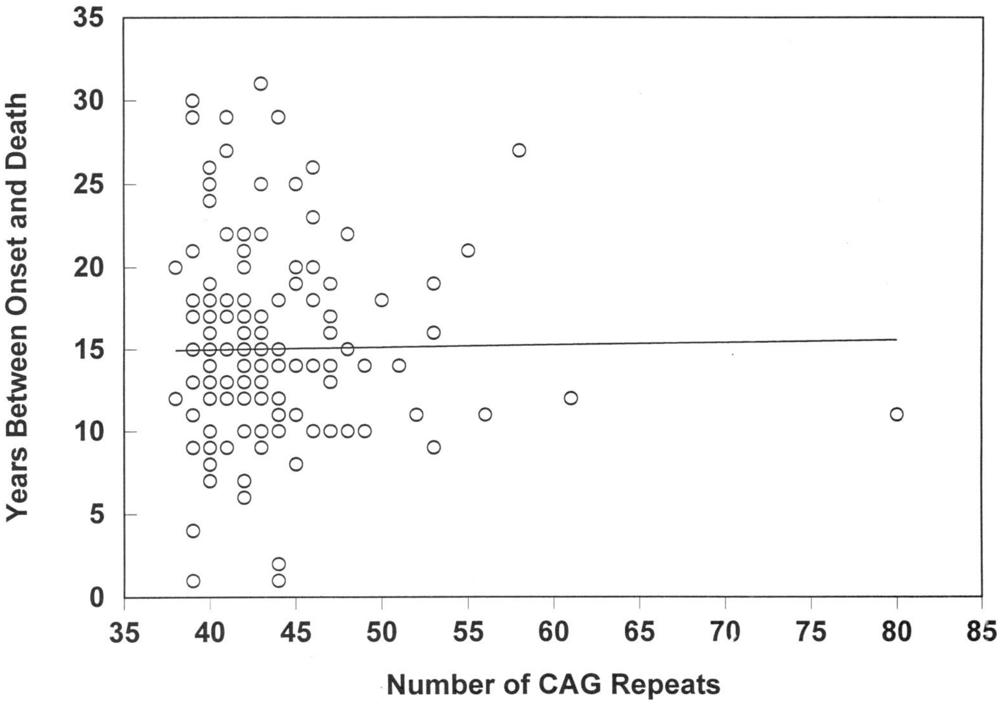

Figure 4. Lack of an effect of CAG repeat length on rate of progression to death. The difference between age at death and age at neurological onset is plotted against number of CAG repeats in the disease allele for the patients from Fig. 3. Linear regression analysis (*line*) failed to identify any relationship between the two parameters.

of 146 autopsy-proven HD cases displayed no correlation between life span after onset and CAG repeat length. It is conceivable that with additional data, such a correlation will be found, but it is already clear that the strength of any such correlation will not approach that of the correlation with age at onset. This suggests that the factors that lead from onset to death are not as tightly dependent on CAG repeat length as is onset itself.

Comparison with Other Trinucleotide Repeat Disorders

Several other neurodegenerative disorders have recently been attributed to the actions of expanded CAG repeats in the coding sequence of genes, suggesting that these disorders might all share a common pathogenic mechanism (Gusella and MacDonald 1996).

In Kennedy's disease, spinal bulbar muscular atrophy (SBMA) (Brooks and Fischbeck 1995; Fischbeck 1995), the expanded CAG segment alters the androgen receptor encoded at Xq11.2-q12 and, in males, causes a progressive loss of anterior horn cells in the spinal cord with consequent progressive muscular weakness. Mental retardation, androgen insensitivity, and variable endocrine abnormalities can be associated features. It should be noted that inactivating mutations in the androgen receptor gene do not mimic SBMA, but rather produce testicular feminization, indicating that the neurodegenerative actions of the expanded CAG repeat are not due to simple inactivation of the androgen receptor. Spinocerebellar ataxia 1 (SCA1) (Zoghbi 1995) is a progressive cerebellar ataxia with neuronal loss most prominent in the cerebellum, including both Purkinje cells and dentate nucleus neurons, in the inferior olive, and in cranial nerve nuclei III, IV, IX, X, and XII. SCA1 is caused by an expanded CAG repeat on 6p, located in the first third of the coding sequence of ataxin-1, a protein of unknown function. Dentatorubral-pallidoluysian atrophy (DRPLA) (Koide et al. 1994; Nagafuchi et al. 1994; Ikeuchi et al. 1995a,b) is characterized by neuronal death in the dentatofugal and pallidofugal systems, producing ataxia and choreoathetosis, along with myoclonus, epilepsy, and dementia. The expanded CAG repeat in DRPLA is located on chromosome 12p in the coding sequence of atrophin, another protein of unknown function. Expansion of the same CAG stretch is the cause of Haw River syndrome, a DRPLA-like disorder described in a single African-American family in North Carolina (Burke et al. 1994). Finally, Machado-Joseph disease (MJD) is another genetic ataxia that has proved to be allelic with spinocerebellar ataxia 3 (SCA3) (Kawaguchi et al.

1994; Cancel et al. 1995; Haberhausen et al. 1995; Matilla et al. 1995; Schols et al. 1995a,b; Durr et al. 1996; Higgins et al. 1996). Both are caused by an expanded CAG segment in the coding sequence of a novel gene on chromosome 14q32.1. MJD/SCA3 involves progressive degeneration of the spinocerebellar tracts, with relative sparing of the inferior olive and cerebellar cortex relative to SCA1.

In each of these trinucleotide repeat disorders, the normal alleles are polymorphic and the expanded alleles are unstable, each within a size range comparable to the normal and disease alleles in HD. Similarly, in these other disorders, CAG instability is most important in gametogenesis, although somatic changes in the expanded alleles have sometimes been observed. In several of these disorders, a similar relationship has been reported between CAG repeat length and age at onset of neurological symptoms to that demonstrated in HD. Moreover, in the more severe young-onset cases, the neuronal pathology extends beyond the regions most characteristic of each disorder to parts of the brain that degenerate in one or more of the other CAG repeat disorders. Although this might indicate that loss of neurons is occurring through a common pathogenic mechanism, detailed examination of the data reveals that there are differences between the disorders. In Figure 5, published data are compiled and summarized for direct comparison. The age-at-onset data for SCA1 superimpose on the HD curve when plotted against CAG repeat length. The data for DRPLA and MJD display similar slopes but are displaced to the right, requiring a greater degree of CAG expansion to cause a detectable neurological deficit at any given age. This may reflect differences in the extent of neuronal loss required in different neuronal populations before symptoms are elicited, or it could be due to fundamental differences in the pathogenic mechanism.

Another difference between HD and these other disorders is in the phenotype of homozygotes for the mutant allele. We have previously reported that HD appears to be a completely dominant disorder, with HD homozygotes not being significantly different from typical heterozygotes (Wexler et al. 1987; Myers et al. 1989). This is illustrated in Figure 6, where the age at onset of an HD homozygote is plotted against the CAG repeat length of the larger of the person's two disease alleles, falling quite close to the curve for typical HD heterozygotes. In contrast, reported homozygotes for DRPLA and MJD/SCA3 (Lang et al. 1994; Sato et al. 1995; Takiyama et al. 1995) show more severe symptoms than heterozygotes for these diseases, indicating a clear, although not completely additive, effect of the second disease allele (Fig. 6). The lack of a significant effect of a second disease allele in HD suggests that the presence of a single mutant gene is sufficient to saturate the pathogenic process. On the other hand, in DRPLA and MJD/SCA3, the pathogenic mechanism is not saturated in typical heterozygotes, as the capacity to accelerate the process with a second disease allele remains.

The HD Gene Product, Huntingtin

The HD gene encodes an approximately 350-kD protein dubbed huntingtin. This large protein does not show similarity to any previously reported sequences except in the low-complexity region encoded by the CAG repeat (consecutive glutamine residues) and adjacent degenerate CCG repeat (interrupted runs of proline residues), both of which are found in a variety of functionally unrelated proteins. The polyglutamine segment, which is lengthened in the disorder by the CAG expansion mutation, is located near huntingtin's amino terminus, 17 amino acids downstream from the initiator methionine. Although these first 17 amino acids are highly conserved in evolution, the subsequent polyglutamine-polyproline segment is not and may be largely dispensable with respect to huntingtin's normal biochemical function.

We and other workers have produced antisera for the specific detection of huntingtin from both normal and mutant alleles (DiFiglia et al. 1995; Gutekunst et al. 1995; Ide et al. 1995; Jou and Myers 1995; Persichetti et al. 1995a; Sharp et al. 1995; Trottier et al. 1995). Use of these reagents has revealed that huntingtin is a cytoplasmic protein found predominantly in the cytosol and only loosely associated with pelletable material. Detection of the protein with antisera directed against the initial 17 amino acids and against regions downstream from the predicted polyglutamine stretch have indicated that the CAG segment is indeed translated and that protein is produced from the disease allele. Interestingly, the abnormal protein product is distinguishable from normal huntingtin based on its reduced mobility on SDS-polyacrylamide gels, indicating an effect of the extra glutamines disproportionate to the molecular weight that they add. Longer CAG repeats may cause reduced expression of the disease allele relative to its normal counterpart, but this reduction is not due to destabilization of the protein which in lymphoblasts has a half-life of more than 24 hours (Persichetti et al. 1996). Huntingtin protein is widely expressed in both neuronal and nonneuronal cells, and no correlation has been detected within the brain between either the level or pattern of expression and subsequent cell death.

Mechanism of Pathogenesis

The mechanism whereby the HD mutation triggers the premature death of neurons in the brain is not yet understood. It has not been formally excluded that presence of the expanded CAG repeat acts by altering chromatin structure and transcription of genes in the HD region. Similarly, the possibility that the HD disease allele transcript interferes with normal mechanisms of nuclear RNA processing, export to the cyto-

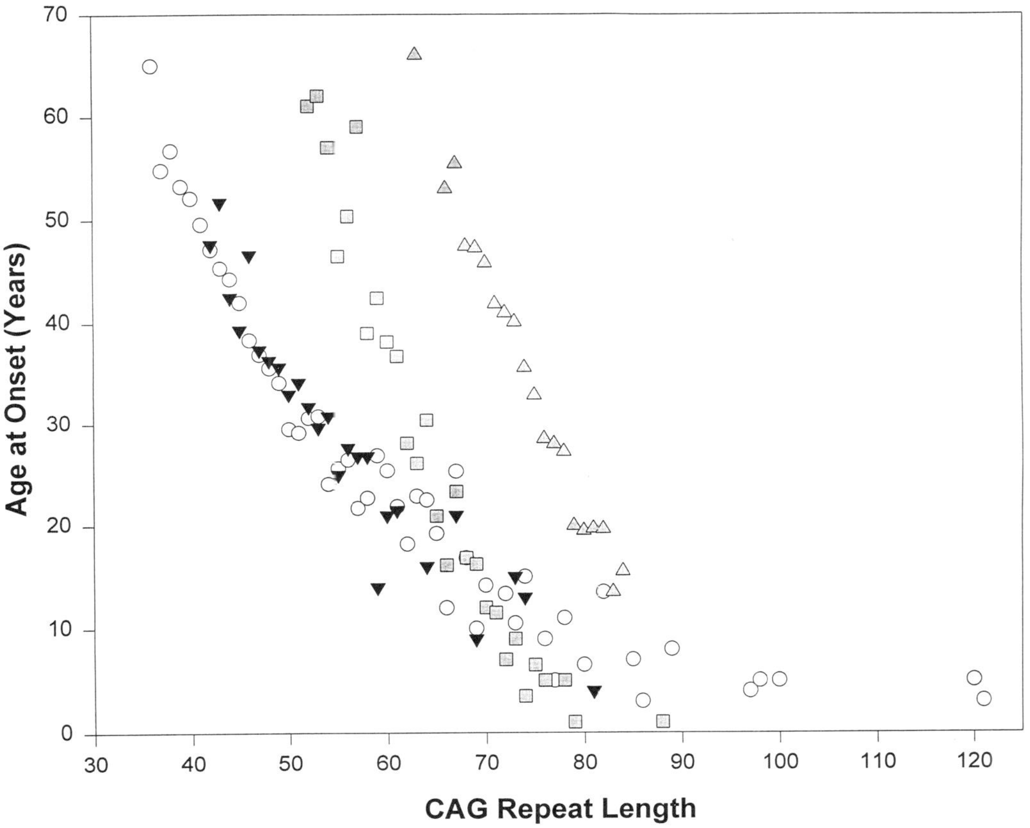

Figure 5. Onset and repeat length in CAG repeat disorders. Data compiled from published reports were used to calculate mean age at neurological onset (as in Fig. 2) associated with different CAG repeat lengths in the disease alleles of 1226 HD cases (*open circles*) (Andrew et al. 1993; Barron et al. 1993; Craufurd and Dodge 1993; De Rooij et al. 1993; Duyao et al. 1993; Huntington's Disease Collaborative Research Group 1993; Kremer et al. 1993; Norremolle et al. 1993; Rubinsztein et al. 1993a; Snell et al. 1993; Stine et al. 1993; Zuhlke et al. 1993; Illarioshkin et al. 1994; Kieburtz et al. 1994; Lucotte et al. 1994; Novelletto et al. 1994; Claes et al. 1995; Persichetti et al. 1995b), 42 SCA1 cases (*filled inverted triangles*) (Matilla et al. 1993; Ranum et al. 1994; Dubourg et al. 1995), 149 DRPLA cases (*shaded squares*) (Nagafuchi et al. 1994; Komure et al. 1995; Norremolle et al. 1995; Warner et al. 1995), and 332 MJD/SCA3 cases (*shaded triangles*) (Cancel et al. 1995; Maciel et al. 1995; Maruyama et al. 1995; Matilla et al. 1995; Ranum et al. 1995; Schols et al. 1995a).

plasm, or mRNA translation has not been conclusively eliminated. However, it seems most likely that the HD defect acts at the level of huntingtin protein, via a deleterious consequence of the expanded polyglutamine segment. The similarities with the other CAG repeat disorders suggest that a common mechanism of toxicity of expanded glutamine segments exists in neurons, but that the precise pattern and timing of neuronal death are determined by the protein context in which the polyglutamine segment is presented. Because each of the proteins in these disorders is unrelated to the others, loss of normal protein function is probably not the primary cause of pathogenesis, although it could certainly contribute to aspects of the disease phenotype. For example, reduced androgen receptor function has been implicated in some SBMA cases. Because the function of the HD protein is unknown, the potential participation of huntingtin's normal activity in the disease process cannot be ascertained at present. It is certainly conceivable that the expanded glutamine segment has no effect on the capacity of mutant huntingtin to fulfill its normal physiological role, but rather confers a novel additional property on the protein that results in neuronal death.

If the genetic defect acts at the protein level, then the amount of huntingtin produced from a single disease allele appears sufficient to fully trigger pathogenesis, with the maximal rate of neuronal loss determined largely by the CAG repeat length of the disease allele. Differences in the capacity of the proteins in the other disorders to trigger the same or a related disease process may depend on factors such as protein concentration, localization, normal function, and constraints imposed by the protein's structure and the relative location of the polyglutamine segment within it.

It has been suggested that mutant huntingtin could act as a substrate for transglutamination, thereby form-

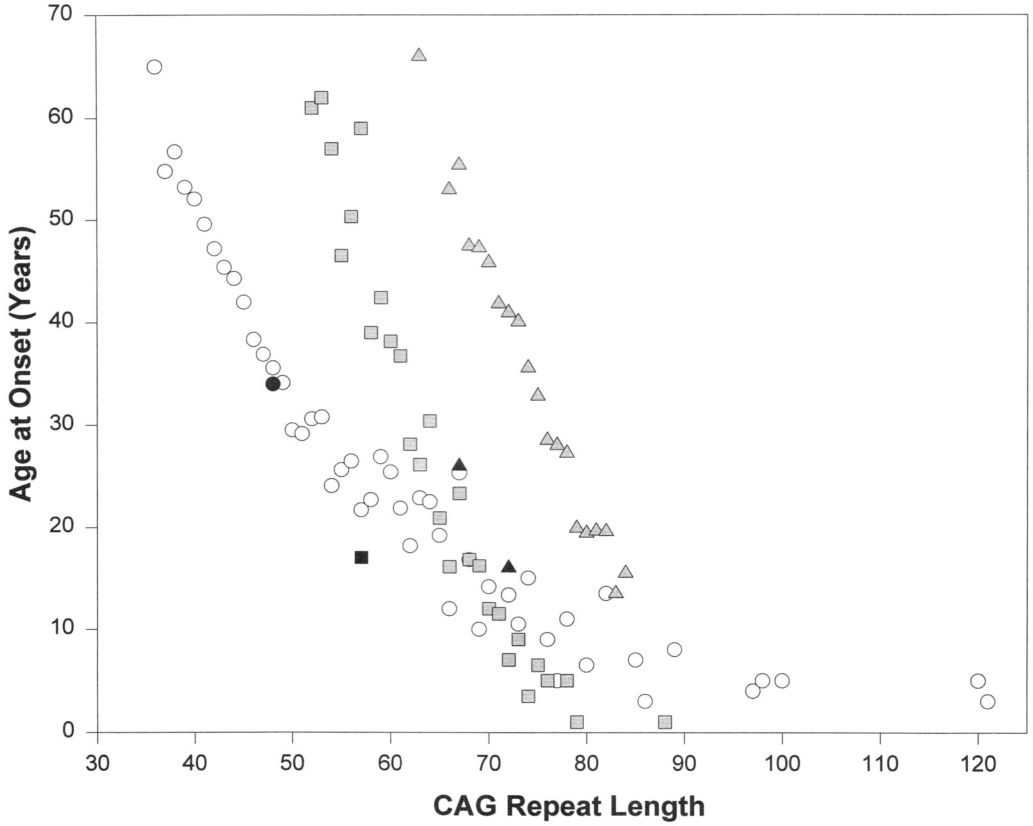

Figure 6. Onset in disease allele homozygotes. The data from Fig. 5 for HD (*open circles*), DRPLA (*shaded squares*), and MJD/SCA3 (*shaded triangles*) are replotted for comparison with the ages of onset of homozygotes for the corresponding disease alleles (*filled symbols*) (Wexler et al. 1987; Myers et al. 1989; Lang et al. 1994; Sato et al. 1995; Takiyama et al. 1995). In each case, the age at onset for the disease homozygote was plotted against the number of CAG repeats in the larger of the two disease alleles. A second dose of the disease allele did not displace the age at onset in HD from the distribution observed for HD heterozygotes, whereas the age at onset in each of DRPLA and MJD/SCA3 was significantly reduced relative to the corresponding heterozygotes.

ing a toxic by-product (Green 1993). Similarly, animal studies with chemicals that cause excitotoxicity by acting as agonists for types of neuronal glutamate receptors, and with agents that poison energy metabolism, have suggested that these biochemical processes could be involved in the progressive, selective neuronal loss of HD and these other neurodegenerative disorders (Beal 1994a,b). In any event, it seems likely that the mechanism of action of expanded polyglutamine segments requires physical interaction of the mutant proteins with other cellular components and that the selectivity of such interactions could also account for differences in the pattern and timing of neuronal loss. Consequently, we and other workers have isolated a number of proteins that interact with huntingtin in either its normal or mutant forms, or both (Li et al. 1995; Bao et al. 1996; Burke et al. 1996). None of these investigations has provided unequivocal evidence for the mechanism of disease pathogenesis. However, this approach remains one of the most attractive potential strategies to delineate huntingtin's normal function and to identify the abnormality that leads to the characteristic neuropathology of the disorder.

CONCLUSION

Molecular genetic investigations of HD have identified the primary defect in the disorder and have placed HD among a group of neurodegenerative disorders that appear to share a related mode of pathogenesis. However, molecular biological investigations have not yet elucidated the biochemical processes underlying the neuropathological effects of these mutations. The primary target of our current studies is the huntingtin protein, whose abnormal form has an expanded polyglutamine segment that may define its neurotoxicity. It is hoped that delineation of huntingtin's normal function and of the cell-biological and biochemical consequences of expanding huntingtin's polyglutamine segment will provide the knowledge necessary to develop a rational treatment for this devastating disorder. Given the similarities involved, it is likely that such progress in any of the neurodegenerative disorders involving translated CAG repeats would have a beneficial impact that would extend to each of these other afflictions.

ACKNOWLEDGMENTS

The authors' work has been supported by National Institutes of Health grants NS-16367 and NS-32765, and by grants from Bristol-Myers Squibb Inc., the Hereditary Disease Foundation, the Huntington's Disease Society of America, and the Foundation for the Care and Cure of Huntington's Disease (FCCHD). This paper is dedicated to the memory of Mr. Dennis Shea, the founder of the FCCHD, in recognition of his many critical contributions to the research effort directed at finding a cure for HD.

REFERENCES

Anderson, M.A. and J.F. Gusella. 1984. Use of cyclosporin A in establishing Epstein-Barr virus-transformed human lymphoblastoid cell lines. *In Vitro* **20:** 856.

Andrew, S.E., Y.P. Goldberg, B. Kremer, H. Telenius, J. Theilmann, S. Adam, E. Starr, F. Squitieri, B. Lin, M.A. Kalchman, R.K. Graham, and M.R. Hayden. 1993. The relationship between trinucleotide (CAG) repeat length and clinical features of Huntington's disease. *Nat. Genet.* **4:** 398.

Bao, J., A.H. Sharp, M.V. Wagster, M. Becher, G. Schilling, C.A. Ross, V.L. Dawson, and T.M. Dawson. 1996. Protein-protein interaction of huntingtin involves calmodulin. *Proc. Natl. Acad. Sci.* **93:** 5037.

Barron, L.H., J.P. Warner, M. Porteous, S. Holloway, S. Simpson, R. Davidson, and D.J. Brock. 1993 A study of the Huntington's disease associated trinucleotide repeat in the Scottish population. *J. Med. Genet.* **30:** 1003.

Beal, M.F. 1994a. Huntington's disease, energy, and excitotoxicity. *Neurobiol. Aging* **15:** 275.

———. 1994b. Neurochemistry and toxin models in Huntington's disease. *Curr. Opin. Neurol.* **7:** 542.

Bozza, A., S. Malagu, E. Calzolari, A. Novelletto, M. Pavoni, and L. del Senno. 1995. Expansion of a (CAG)n repeat region in a sporadic case of HD. *Acta Neurol. Scand.* **92:** 132.

Brooks, B.P. and K.H. Fischbeck. 1995. Spinal and bulbar muscular atrophy: A trinucleotide-repeat expansion neurodegenerative disease. *Trends Neurosci.* **18:** 459.

Burke, J.R., J.J. Enghild, M.E. Martin, Y.S. Jou, R.M. Myers, A.D. Roses, J.M. Vance, and W.J. Strittmatter. 1996. Huntingtin and DRPLA proteins selectively interact with the enzyme GAPDH. *Nat. Med.* **2:** 347.

Burke, J.R., M.S. Wingfield, K.E. Lewis, A.D. Roses, J.E. Lee, C. Hulette, M.A. Pericak-Vance, and J.M. Vance. 1994. The Haw River syndrome: Dentatorubropallidoluysian atrophy (DRPLA) in an African-American family. *Nat. Genet.* **7:** 521.

Cancel, G., N. Abbas, G. Stevanin, A. Durr, H. Chneiweiss, C. Neri, C. Duyckaerts, C. Penet, H.M. Cann, Y. Agid, and A. Brice. 1995. Marked phenotypic heterogeneity associated with expansion of a CAG repeat sequence at the spinocerebellar ataxia 3/Machado-Joseph disease locus. *Am. J. Hum. Genet.* **57:** 809.

Claes, S., K. Van Zand, E. Legius, R. Dom, M. Malfroid, F. Baro, J. Godderis, and J.J. Cassiman. 1995. Correlations between triplet repeat expansion and clinical features in Huntington's disease. *Arch. Neurol.* **52:** 749.

Craufurd, D. and A. Dodge. 1993. Mutation size and age at onset in Huntington's disease. *J. Med. Genet.* **30:** 1008.

Davis, M.B., D. Bateman, N.P. Quinn, C.D. Marsden, and A.E. Harding. 1994. Mutation analysis in patients with possible but apparently sporadic Huntington's disease. *Lancet* **344:** 714.

De Rooij, K.E., P.A. De Koning Gans, M.I. Skraastad, R.D. Belfroid, M. Vegter-Van Der Vlis, R.A. Roos, E. Bakker, G.J. Van Ommen, J.T. Den Dunnen, and M. Losekoot. 1993. Dynamic mutation in Dutch Huntington's disease patients: Increased paternal repeat instability extending to within the normal size range. *J. Med. Genet.* **30:** 996.

DiFiglia, M., E. Sapp, K. Chase, C. Schwarz, A. Meloni, C. Young, E. Martin, J.-P. Vonsattel, R. Carraway, S.A. Reeves, F.M. Boyce, and N. Aronin. 1995. Huntingtin is a cytoplasmic protein associated with vesicles in human and rat brain neurons. *Neuron* **14:** 1075.

Dubourg, O., A. Durr, G. Cancel, G. Stevanin, H. Chneiweiss, C. Penet, Y. Agid, and A. Brice. 1995. Analysis of the SCA1 CAG repeat in a large number of families with dominant ataxia: Clinical and molecular correlations. *Ann. Neurol.* **37:** 176.

Durr, A., C. Dode, V. Hahn, C. Pecheux, B. Pillon, J. Feingold, J.C. Kaplan, Y. Agid, and A. Brice. 1995. Diagnosis of "sporadic" Huntington's disease. *J. Neurol. Sci.* **129:** 51.

Durr, A., G. Stevanin, G. Cancel, C. Duyckaerts, N. Abbas, O. Didierjean, H. Chneiweiss, A. Benomar, O. Lyon-Caen, J. Julien, M. Serdaru, C. Penet, Y. Agid, and A. Brice. 1996. Spinocerebellar ataxia 3 and Machado-Joseph disease: Clinical, molecular, and neuropathological features. *Ann. Neurol.* **39:** 490.

Duyao, M., C. Ambrose, R. Myers, A. Novelletto, F. Persichetti, M. Frontali, S. Folstein, C. Ross, M. Franz, M. Abbott, J. Gray, P. Conneally, A. Young, J. Penney, Z. Hollingsworth, I. Shoulson, A. Lazzarini, A. Falek, W. Koroshetz, D. Sax, E. Bird, J. Vonsattel, E. Bonilla, J. Alvir, J. Bickham Conde, and 17 others. 1993. Trinucleotide repeat length instability and age of onset in Huntington's disease. *Nat. Genet.* **4:** 387.

Fischbeck, K.H. 1995. The expanded trinucleotide repeat in Kennedy's disease. *Proc. Assoc. Am. Physicians* **107:** 228.

Goldberg, Y.P., B. Kremer, S.E. Andrew, J. Theilmann, R.K. Graham, F. Squitieri, H. Telenius, S. Adam, A. Sajoo, E. Starr, A. Heiberg, G. Wolff, and M.R. Hayden. 1993. Molecular analysis of new mutations for Huntington's disease: Intermediate alleles and sex of origin effects. *Nat. Genet.* **5:** 174.

Graveland, G.A., R.S. Williams, and M. DiFiglia. 1985. Evidence for degenerative and regenerative changes in neostriatal spiny neurons in Huntington's disease. *Science* **227:** 770.

Green, H. 1993. Human genetic diseases due to codon reiteration: Relationship to an evolutionary mechanism. *Cell* **74:** 955.

Gusella, J.F. and M.E. MacDonald. 1993. Hunting for Huntington's disease. *Mol. Genet. Med.* **3:** 139.

———. 1995. Huntington's disease. *Semin. Cell Biol.* **6:** 21.

———. 1996. Trinucleotide instability: A repeating theme in human inherited disorders. *Annu. Rev. Med.* **47:** 201.

Gusella, J.F., N.S. Wexler, P.M. Conneally, S.L. Naylor, M.A.

Anderson, R.E. Tanzi, P.C. Watkins, K. Ottina, M.R. Wallace, A.Y. Sakaguchi, A.B. Young, I. Shoulson, E. Bonilla, and J.B. Martin. 1983. A polymorphic DNA marker genetically linked to Huntington's disease. *Nature* **306:** 234.

Gutekunst, C.A., A.I. Levey, C.J. Heilman, W.L. Whaley, H. Yi, N.R. Nash, H.D. Rees, J.J. Madden, and S.M. Hersch. 1995. Identification and localization of huntingtin in brain and human lymphoblastoid cell lines with anti-fusion protein antibodies. *Proc. Natl. Acad. Sci.* **92:** 8710.

Haberhausen, G., M.S. Damian, F. Leweke, and U. Muller. 1995. Spinocerebellar ataxia, type 3 (SCA3) is genetically identical to Machado-Joseph disease (MJD). *J. Neurol. Sci.* **132:** 71.

Harper, P.S. 1992. The epidemiology of Huntington's disease. *Hum. Genet.* **89:** 365.

Higgins, J.J., L.E. Nee, O. Vasconcelos, S.E. Ide, C. Lavedan, L.G. Goldfarb, and M.H. Polymeropoulos. 1996. Mutations in American families with spinocerebellar ataxia (SCA) type 3: SCA3 is allelic to Machado-Joseph disease. *Neurology* **46:** 208.

Huntington's Disease Collaborative Research Group. 1993. A novel gene containing a trinucleotide repeat that is expanded and unstable on Huntington's disease chromosomes. *Cell* **72:** 971.

Ide, K., N. Nukina, N. Masuda, J. Goto, and I. Kanazawa. 1995. Abnormal gene product identified in Huntington's disease lymphocytes and brain. *Biochem. Biophys. Res. Commun.* **209:** 1119.

Ikeuchi, T., O. Onodera, M. Oyake, R. Koide, H. Tanaka, and S. Tsuji. 1995a. Dentatorubral-pallidoluysian atrophy (DRPLA): Close correlation of CAG repeat expansions with the wide spectrum of clinical presentations and prominent anticipation. *Semin. Cell Biol.* **6:** 37.

Ikeuchi, T., R. Koide, O. Onodera, H. Tanaka, M. Oyake, H. Takano, and S. Tsuji. 1995b. Dentatorubral-pallidoluysian atrophy (DRPLA). Molecular basis for wide clinical features of DRPLA. *Clin. Neurosci.* **3:** 23.

Illarioshkin, S.N., S. Igarashi, O. Onodera, E.D. Markova, N.N. Nikolskaya, H. Tanaka, T.Z. Chabrashwili, N.G. Insarova, K. Endo, I.A. Ivanova-Smolenskaya, and S. Tsuji. 1994. Trinucleotide repeat length and rate of progression of Huntington's disease. *Ann. Neurol.* **36:** 630.

Jou, Y.S. and R.M. Myers. 1995. Evidence from antibody studies that the CAG repeat in the Huntington disease gene is expressed in the protein. *Hum. Mol. Genet.* **4:** 465.

Kawaguchi, Y., T. Okamoto, M. Taniwaki, M. Aizawa, M. Inoue, S. Katayama, H. Kawakami, S. Nakamura, M. Nishimura, I. Akiguchi, J. Kimura, S. Narumiya, and A. Kakizuka. 1994. CAG expansions in a novel gene for Machado-Joseph disease at chromosome 14q32.1. *Nat. Genet.* **8:** 221.

Kieburtz, K., M. MacDonald, C. Shih, A. Feigin, K. Steinberg, K. Bordwell, C. Zimmerman, J. Srinidhi, J. Sotack, J. Gusella, and I. Shoulson. 1994. Trinucleotide repeat length and progression of illness in Huntington's disease. *J. Med. Genet.* **31:** 872.

Koide, R., T. Ikeuchi, O. Onodera, H. Tanaka, S. Igarashi, K. Endo, H. Takahashi, R. Kondo, A. Ishikawa, T. Hayashi, M. Saito, A. Tomoda, T. Miike, H. Naito, F. Ikuta, and S. Tsuji. 1994. Unstable expansion of CAG repeat in hereditary dentatorubral-pallidoluysian atrophy (DRPLA). *Nat. Genet.* **6:** 9.

Komure, O., A. Sano, N. Nishino, N. Yamauchi, S. Ueno, K. Kondoh, N. Sano, M. Takahashi, N. Murayama, I. Kondo, S. Nagafuchi, M. Yamada, and I. Kanazawa. 1995. DNA analysis in hereditary dentatorubral-pallidoluysian atrophy: Correlation between CAG repeat length and phenotypic variation and the molecular basis of anticipation. *Neurology* **45:** 143.

Kremer, B., F. Squitieri, H. Telenius, S.E. Andrew, J. Theilmann, N. Spence, Y.P. Goldberg, and M.R. Hayden. 1993. Molecular analysis of late onset Huntington's disease. *J. Med. Genet.* **30:** 991.

Lang, A.E., E.A. Rogaeva, T. Tsuda, J. Hutterer, and P. St. George-Hyslop. 1994. Homozygous inheritance of the Machado-Joseph disease gene. *Ann. Neurol.* **36:** 443.

Li, X.J., S.H. Li, A.H. Sharp, F.C. Nucifora, Jr., G. Schilling, A. Lanahan, P. Worley, S.H. Snyder, and C.A. Ross. 1995. A huntingtin-associated protein enriched in brain with implications for pathology. *Nature* **378:** 398.

Lucotte, G., A. Aouizerate, O. Loreille, N. Gerard, and J.C. Turpin. 1994. Trinucleotide repeat elongation in the huntingtin gene in Huntington's disease patients from 85 French families. The French HD Research Group. *Genet. Couns.* **5:** 321.

MacDonald, M.E., G. Barnes, J. Srinidhi, M.P. Duyao, C.M. Ambrose, R.H. Myers, J. Gray, P.M. Conneally, A. Young, J. Penney, I. Shoulson, Z. Hollingsworth, W. Koroshetz, E. Bird, J.P. Vonsattel, E. Bonilla, C. Moscowitz, G. Penchaszadeh, L. Brzustowicz, J. Alvir, J. Bickham Conde, J.-H. Cha, L. Dure, F. Gomez, M. Ramos-Arroyo, and 8 others. 1993. Gametic but not somatic instability of CAG repeat length in Huntington's disease. *J. Med. Genet.* **30:** 982.

MacDonald, M.E., A. Novelletto, C. Lin, D. Tagle, G. Barnes, G. Bates, S. Taylor, B. Allitto, M. Altherr, R. Myers, H. Lehrach, F.S. Collins, J.J. Wasmuth, M. Frontali, and J.F. Gusella. 1992. The Huntington's disease candidate region exhibits many different haplotypes. *Nat. Genet.* **1:** 99.

Maciel, P., C. Gaspar, A.L. DeStefano, I. Silveira, P. Coutinho, J. Radvany, D.M. Dawson, L. Sudarsky, J. Guimaraes, J.E. Loureiro, M.M. Nezarati, L.I. Corwin, I. Lopes-Cendes, K. Rooke, R. Rosenberg, P. MacLeod, L.A. Farrer, J. Sequeiros, and G.A. Rouleau. 1995. Correlation between CAG repeat length and clinical features in Machado-Joseph disease. *Am. J. Hum. Genet.* **57:** 54.

Martin, J.B. and J.F. Gusella. 1986. Huntington's disease. Pathogenesis and management. *N. Engl. J. Med.* **315:** 1267.

Maruyama, H., S. Nakamura, Z. Matsuyama, T. Sakai, M. Doyu, G. Sobue, M. Seto, M. Tsujihata, T. Oh-i, T. Nishio, N. Sunohara, R. Takahashi, M. Hayashi, I. Nishino, T. Ohtake, T. Oda, M. Nishimura, T. Saida, H. Matsumoto, M. Baba, Y. Kawaguchi, A. Kakizuka, and H. Kawakami. 1995. Molecular features of the CAG repeats and clinical manifestation of Machado-Joseph disease. *Hum. Mol. Genet.* **4:** 807.

Matilla, T., A. McCall, S.H. Subramony, and H.Y. Zoghbi. 1995. Molecular and clinical correlations in spinocerebellar ataxia type 3 and Machado-Joseph disease. *Ann. Neurol.* **38:** 68.

Matilla, T., V. Volpini, D. Genis, J. Rosell, J. Corral, A. Davalos, A. Molins, and X. Estivill. 1993. Presymptomatic analysis of spinocerebellar ataxia type 1 (SCA1) via the expansion of the SCA1 CAG-repeat in a large pedigree displaying anticipation and parental male bias. *Hum. Mol. Genet.* **2:** 2123.

Myers, R.H., J. Leavitt, L.A. Farrer, J. Jagadeesh, H. McFarlane, C.A. Mastromauro, R.J. Mark, and J.F. Gusella. 1989. Homozygote for Huntington disease. *Am. J. Hum.*

Genet. **45:** 615.

Myers, R.H., M.E. MacDonald, W.J. Koroshetz, M.P. Duyao, C.M. Ambrose, S.A. Taylor, G. Barnes, J. Srinidhi, C.S. Lin, W.L. Whaley, A.M. Lazzarini, M. Schwarz, G. Wolff, E.D. Bird, J.-P.G. Vonsattel, and J.F. Gusella. 1993. De novo expansion of a (CAG)n repeat in sporadic Huntington's disease. *Nat. Genet.* **5:** 168.

Nagafuchi, S., H. Yanagisawa, K. Sato, T. Shirayama, E. Ohsaki, M. Bundo, T. Takeda, K. Tadokoro, I. Kondo, N. Murayama, Y. Tanaka, H. Kikishuma, K. Umino, H. Kurosawa, T. Furukawa, K. Nihei, T. Inoue, A. Sano, O. Komure, M. Takahashi, T. Tozikawa, I. Kanazawa, and M. Yamada. 1994. Dentatorubral and pallidoluysian atrophy expansion of an unstable CAG trinucleotide on chromosome 12p. *Nat. Genet.* **6:** 14.

Norremolle, A., J.E. Nielsen, S.A. Sorensen, and L. Hasholt. 1995. Elongated CAG repeats of the B37 gene in a Danish family with dentato-rubro-pallido-luysian atrophy. *Hum. Genet.* **95:** 313.

Norremolle, A., O. Riess, J.T. Epplen, K. Fenger, L. Hasholt, and S.A. Sorensen. 1993. Trinucleotide repeat elongation in the Huntingtin gene in Huntington disease patients from 71 Danish families. *Hum. Mol. Genet.* **2:** 1475.

Novelletto, A., F. Persichetti, G. Sabbadini, P. Mandich, E. Bellone, F. Ajmar, M. Pergola, L. Del Senno, M.E. MacDonald, J.F. Gusella, and M. Frontali. 1994. Analysis of the trinucleotide repeat expansion in Italian families affected with Huntington disease. *Hum. Mol. Genet.* **3:** 93.

Persichetti, F., L. Carlee, P.W. Faber, S.M. McNeil, C.M. Ambrose, J. Srinidhi, M.A. Anderson, G.T. Barnes, J.F. Gusella, and M.E. MacDonald. 1996. Differential expression of normal and mutant Huntington's disease gene alleles. *Neurobiol. Dis.* **3:** 183.

Persichetti, F., J. Srinidhi, L. Kanaley, P. Ge, R.H. Myers, K. D'Arrigo, G.T. Barnes, M.E. MacDonald, J.P. Vonsattel, J.F. Gusella, and E.D. Bird. 1995a. Huntington's disease CAG trinucleotide repeats in pathologically confirmed post-mortem brains. *Neurobiol. Dis.* **1:** 159.

Persichetti, F., C.M. Ambrose, P. Ge, S.M. McNeil, J. Srinidhi, M.A. Anderson, B. Jenkins, G.T. Barnes, M.P. Duyao, L. Kanaley, N.S. Wexler, R.H. Myers, E.D. Bird, J.-P. Vonsattel, M.E. MacDonald, and J.F. Gusella. 1995b. Normal and expanded Huntington's disease gene alleles produce distinguishable proteins due to translation across the CAG repeat. *Mol. Med.* **1:** 374.

Ranum, L.P., M.Y. Chung, S. Banfi, A. Bryer, L.J. Schut, R. Ramesar, L.A. Duvick, A. McCall, S.H. Subramony, L. Goldfarb, C. Gomez, L.A. Sandkuijl, H.T. Orr, and H.Y. Zoghbi. 1994. Molecular and clinical correlations in spinocerebellar ataxia type I: Evidence for familial effects on the age at onset. *Am. J. Hum. Genet.* **55:** 244.

Ranum, L.P., J.K. Lundgren, L.J. Schut, M.J. Ahrens, S. Perlman, J. Aita, T.D. Bird, C. Gomez, and H.T. Orr. 1995. Spinocerebellar ataxia type 1 and Machado-Joseph disease: Incidence of CAG expansions among adult-onset ataxia patients from 311 families with dominant, recessive, or sporadic ataxia. *Am. J. Hum. Genet.* **57:** 603.

Rubinsztein, D.C., D.E. Barton, B.C. Davison, and M.A. Ferguson-Smith. 1993a. Analysis of the huntingtin gene reveals a trinucleotide-length polymorphism in the region of the gene that contains two CCG-rich stretches and a correlation between decreased age of onset of Huntington's disease and CAG repeat number. *Hum. Mol. Genet.* **2:** 1713.

Rubinsztein, D.C., J. Leggo, D.E. Barton, and M.A. Ferguson-Smith. 1993b. Site of (CCG) polymorphism in the HD gene. *Nat. Genet.* **5:** 214.

Sato, K., K. Kashihara, S. Okada, T. Ikeuchi, S. Tsuji, T. Shomori, K. Morimoto, and T. Hayabara. 1995. Does homozygosity advance the onset of dentatorubral-pallidoluysian atrophy? *Neurology* **45:** 1934.

Schols, L., A.M. Vieira-Saecker, S. Schols, H. Przuntek, J.T. Epplen, and O. Riess. 1995a. Trinucleotide expansion within the MJD1 gene presents clinically as spinocerebellar ataxia and occurs most frequently in German SCA patients. *Hum. Mol. Genet.* **4:** 1001.

Schols, L., G. Amoiridis, M. Langkafel, T. Buttner, H. Przuntek, O. Riess, A.M. Vieira-Saecker, and J.T. Epplen. 1995b. Machado-Joseph disease mutations as the genetic basis of most spinocerebellar ataxias in Germany. *J. Neurol. Neurosurg. Psychiatry* **59:** 449.

Sharp, A.H., S.J. Loev, G. Schilling, S.H. Li, X.J. Li, J. Bao, M.V. Wagster, J.A. Kotzuk, J.P. Steiner, A. Lo, J. Hedreen, S. Sisodia, S.H. Snyder, T.M. Dawson, D.K. Ryugo, and C.A. Ross. 1995. Widespread expression of Huntington's disease gene (IT15) protein product. *Neuron* **14:** 1065.

Snell, R.G., J.C. MacMillan, J.P. Cheadle, I. Fenton, L.P. Lazarou, P. Davies, M.E. MacDonald, J.F. Gusella, P.S. Harper, and D.J. Shaw. 1993. Relationship between trinucleotide repeat expansion and phenotypic variation in Huntington's disease. *Nat. Genet.* **4:** 393.

Stine, O.C., N. Pleasant, M.L. Franz, M.H. Abbott, S.E. Folstein, and C.A. Ross. 1993. Correlation between the onset age of Huntington's disease and length of the trinucleotide repeat in IT-15. *Hum. Mol. Genet.* **2:** 1547.

Takiyama, Y., S. Igarashi, E.A. Rogaeva, K. Endo, E.I. Rogaev, H. Tanaka, R. Sherrington, K. Sanpei, Y. Liang, M. Saito, T. Tsuda, H. Takano, M. Ikeda, C. Lin, H. Chi, J.L. Kennedy, A.E. Lang, J.R. Wherrett, M. Segawa, Y. Nomura, T. Yuasa, J. Weissenbach, M. Yoshida, N. Nishizawa, K.K. Kidd, S. Tsuji, and P.H. St. George-Hyslop. 1995. Evidence for inter-generational instability in the CAG repeat in the MJD1 gene and for conserved haplotypes at flanking markers amongst Japanese and Caucasian subjects with Machado-Joseph disease. *Hum. Mol. Genet.* **4:** 1137.

Trottier, Y., D. Devys, G. Imbert, F. Saudou, I. An, Y. Lutz, C. Weber, Y. Agid, E.C. Hirsch, and J.L. Mandel. 1995. Cellular localization of the Huntington's disease protein and discrimination of the normal and mutated form. *Nat. Genet.* **10:** 104.

Vonsattel, J.P., R.H. Myers, T.J. Stevens, R.J. Ferrante, E.D. Bird, and E.P. Richardson, Jr. 1985. Neuropathological classification of Huntington's disease. *J. Neuropathol. Exp. Neurol.* **44:** 559.

Warner, J.P., L.H. Barron, and D.J. Brock. 1993. A new polymerase chain reaction (PCR) assay for the trinucleotide repeat that is unstable and expanded on Huntington's disease chromosomes. *Mol. Cell. Probes* **7:** 235.

Warner, T.T., L.D. Williams, R.W. Walker, F. Flinter, S.A. Robb, S.E. Bundey, M. Honavar, and A.E. Harding. 1995. A clinical and molecular genetic study of dentatorubropallidoluysian atrophy in four European families. *Ann. Neurol.* **37:** 452.

Wexler, N.S., A.B. Young, R.E. Tanzi, H. Travers, S. Starosta-Rubinstein, J.B. Penney, S.R. Snodgrass, I. Shoulson, F. Gomez, M.A. Ramos Arroyo, G.K. Penchaszadeh, H. Moreno, K. Gibbons, A. Faryniarz, W. Hobbs, M.A. Anderson, E. Bonilla, P.M. Conneally, and J.F.

Gusella. 1987. Homozygotes for Huntington's disease. *Nature* **326:** 194.
Zoghbi, H.Y. 1995. Spinocerebellar ataxia type 1. *Clin. Neurosci.* **3:** 5.
Zuhlke, C., O. Riess, K. Schroder, I. Siedlaczck, J.T. Epplen, W. Engel, and U. Thies. 1993. Expansion of the (CAG)n repeat causing Huntington's disease in 352 patients of German origin. *Hum. Mol. Genet.* **2:** 1467.

Targeted Inactivation of the Mouse Huntington's Disease Gene Homolog *Hdh*

M.E. MacDonald,[1] M. Duyao,[1,2] T. Calzonetti,[1] A. Auerbach,[3] A. Ryan,[1] G. Barnes,[1] J.K. White,[1] W. Auerbach,[3] J.-P. Vonsattel,[4] J.F. Gusella,[1,5] and A.L. Joyner[3]

[1]*Molecular Neurogenetics Unit, Massachusetts General Hospital, Charlestown, Massachusetts 02129;* [3]*Developmental Genetics Program, Skirball Institute for Biomolecular Medicine, N.Y.U. Medical Center, New York, New York 10016;* [4]*Laboratory for Molecular Neuropathology, Massachusetts General Hospital, Charlestown, Massachusetts 02129;* [5]*Department of Genetics, Harvard Medical School, Boston, Massachusetts 02114*

Huntington's disease (HD), with its characteristic constellation of motor, psychiatric, and cognitive abnormalities, is a dominantly inherited neurodegenerative disorder that occurs worldwide, although it is most prevalent (1 in 10,000 individuals) in populations of Western European ancestry (Martin and Gusella 1986; Harper 1992). HD can strike at any age, but typically symptoms begin in mid-life after the defect has been transmitted to the next generation. As the disease progresses, symptoms worsen to profound depression, dementia, and a complete loss of voluntary and involuntary motor control that is apparent from the dance-like choreiform movements that are the hallmark of HD. The juvenile form of the disease is characterized by a more severe clinical course that includes dystonic movements and rigidity, whereas late-onset HD is often associated with predominantly psychiatric and cognitive impairments rather than motor abnormalities.

The defect appears not to affect peripheral tissues, and clinical symptoms result from the gradual loss of neuronal cell populations in the brain, particularly large neurons in layer VI of the cerebral cortex and γ-aminobutyric acid (GABA), enkephalin, and substance P containing medium-sized spiny projection neurons in the basal ganglia (Graveland et al. 1985; Martin and Gusella 1986). Indeed, the pattern of neuronal cell death in the striatum, a gradient that begins in the tail of the caudate nucleus, gradually encompassing and destroying the entire structure, forms the basis for the neuropathological classification of HD (Vonsattel et al. 1985). The dramatic impact of the defect on the brain is evident from its shrunken appearance and about 20–30% reduction in weight in end-stage disease.

The underlying biochemical lesion in HD remains to be elucidated. Efforts to find selective biochemical and physiological deficits have failed to yield an effective therapeutic strategy, although neurotransmission, energy metabolism, and neuronal cell survival have been selected as potential targets (Martin 1995). Indeed, it is likely that those alterations observed in transmitters, receptors, and metabolites are secondary to the neurodegeneration that accompanies the disease process (Martin and Gusella 1986).

Several general hypotheses of neuronal cell death which provide working models to explore the mechanism of pathology in HD have emerged from lesioning in experimental animals, including excitatory amino acid toxicity, metabolic stress, free-radical-induced damage, and programmed cell death (for review, see Beal 1995; Sharp and Ross 1996). Populations of medium spiny projection neurons in the rodent and monkey striatum are sensitive to the effects of glutamate, kainate, and quinolinic acid after injection into the basal ganglia and to the action of inhibitors of mitochondrial function such as malonate or 3-nitropropionic acid following systemic administration. The apparently selective neuronal cell death in these lesion models is thought to be a consequence of the activation of NMDA receptors, either directly or indirectly as a result of abnormalities in energy metabolism. The inappropriate influx of Ca^{++} may ultimately kill the affected neurons via oxidative free radicals or trigger apoptotic cell death pathways.

In 1993, a new phase of HD research began with the discovery of the *HD* gene and its mutation, an expanded CAG repeat in a novel 4p16.3 gene (Huntington's Disease Collaborative Research Group 1993). Knowledge of the defect does not immediately reveal a particular biochemical lesion, but it places HD with other inherited neurodegenerative disorders caused by triplet repeat arrays which may ultimately share a common pathogenic mechanism (Gusella and MacDonald 1996). Moreover, the discovery accounts for many of the puzzling features of HD (Gusella and MacDonald 1995a), and it has laid the foundation for the generation of valid genetic models of the disorder in experimental animals.

The *HD* CAG repeat is polymorphic (6–34 units) on normal chromosomes, and these arrays are inherited in a Mendelian fashion. In contrast, on disease chromosomes the expanded repeat (37 to >100 units) is unstable, changing in size in most intergenerational transmissions. The length of the expanded CAG repeat is critical to the disease mechanism as it is the primary

[2]Present address: Sequana Therapeutics, La Jolla, California 92037.

determinant of the age of onset of symptoms and severity of the disorder. Thus, adult-onset HD is caused by CAG repeat lengths in the 40–50 unit range, whereas the relatively rare cases of juvenile-onset disease are due to repeat lengths greater than 60 units, and very late onset occurs typically with repeats in the 37–40 unit range. Another observation that must be explained is that HD homozygotes who have inherited two expanded *HD* CAG alleles of 40–50 repeats develop HD that is indistinguishable from the typical adult-onset disorder (Wexler et al. 1987; Myers et al. 1989), suggesting that a single expanded CAG array is sufficient to saturate the pathogenic mechanism. A further constraint on any genetic model is the observation that the inactivation of one allele by a chromosomal rearrangement involving the *HD* gene does not cause any abnormal phenotype (Ambrose et al. 1994; Persichetti et al. 1996).

It is not obvious how the CAG expansion causes the neuropathology of the disease, because the gene's function is not readily inferred from its sequence and its pattern of expression does not account for the selective impact of the mutation on neuronal populations in the basal ganglia (Gusella and MacDonald 1995b; Sharp and Ross 1996). The *HD* gene produces two mRNA species of 10.5 kb and 13.5 kb that both encode a single novel approximately 350-kD polypeptide dubbed huntingtin. The HD protein resides in the cytosol of a variety of cell types in the periphery and brain, where it may be loosely associated with a number of cell constituents including cytoskeletal or membranous components such as microtubules or synaptic vesicles.

The *HD* defect does not eliminate production of huntingtin mRNA and does not change the gross pattern of mRNA or protein in HD brain, although in the most severe cases it may affect expression of the abnormal allele (Persichetti et al. 1996). However, because the polymorphic CAG repeat is translated, the expanded CAG repeat produces an elongated polyglutamine segment that affects the structure of the abnormal protein, altering its migration on SDS-PAGE (Gutekunst et al. 1995; Ide et al. 1995; Persichetti et al. 1995; Sharp et al. 1995; Trottier et al. 1995a) and promoting its interaction with an anti-TBP monoclonal antibody reagent (Trottier et al. 1995b), suggesting that the defect acts at the level of protein activity.

The CAG expansion could simply eliminate huntingtin activity, or it could confer a new property on the protein which might affect its inherent physiological function by increasing it, by decreasing it in a dominant negative fashion, or by subtly altering its expression pattern. Alternatively, the new property might be unrelated to its inherent activity. Transgenic technology, particularly targeted mutagenesis of *Hdh*, the murine *HD* homolog, offers a route to investigate huntingtin's physiological function and explore the mechanism of neuropathology of the disorder in man.

METHODS

Predicted amino-terminal huntingtin sequences encoded by* HD *gene homologs. Amino-terminal huntingtin amino acid sequences shown in Figure 1 are taken from the literature, with the exception of amino acids 1–7 of the rat homolog. These have been added at the amino terminus of the cDNA sequence predicted by Schmitt et al. (1995) (GenBank # U18650) as rat reverse transcriptase-polymerase chain reaction (RT-PCR) products have been found by Ms. Pamela Foye and Dr. Gregor Sutcliffe (The Scripps Research Institute) to lack the 2-bp insertion contained in the published cDNAs. These investigators generated 178-bp RT-PCR products from adult rat striatal mRNA using oligonucleotide primers 5′-GGCTGAGCGCCTTG GTTCCGCT-3′ and 5′-CGCACTTGAGGGACTCG AAAGCCTTC-3′ that were then cloned and sequenced. These data were kindly provided before publication. The human *HD* sequence is described in Huntington's Disease Collaborative Research Group (1993) (GenBank #L12392) and Ambrose et al. (1994); the murine *Hdh* sequence is from Barnes et al. (1994) (GenBank #L28827), not those reported in Lin et al. (1994) (GenBank #L23312 and #L23313), which contain a number of unresolved sequence discrepancies including two that predict nonconserved amino acids at positions 2 and 28; and the sequence of the pufferfish *HD* homolog is reported in Baxendale et al. (1995) (GenBank #X82939).

Targeting* Hdh *in embryonic stem cells and generation of mutant mice. The details of the molecular and phenotypic characterization of the inactivating *Hdh* mutations shown in Tables 1 and 2 are taken from the literature. Construction of the $Hdh^{ex4/5}$ targeting vector, screening for successfully targeted R1 embryonic stem (ES) cell clones, characterization of the mutant allele, and generation of lines of mutant mice are described in Duyao et al. (1995). The generation and characterization of Hdh^{prex1} mutant CCE-3 ES cell lines and mice are detailed in Zeitlin et al. (1995), and the creation and phenotypic analysis of mice with the *HdhEx5* mutation are reported in Nasir et al. (1995). The genetic background of these lines of *Hdh* mutant mice is a mixture of 129Sv and either C57BL6 or CD1. F_1 offspring representing a single original ES cell line were typically used to produce homozygous progeny in the F_2 generation by intercrossing mutant heterozygote animals.

Histology. Histology of E7.5 embryos was performed by sectioning uteri that were fixed in Bouin's solution, paraffin-embedded, dewaxed, and rehydrated. Hematoxylin and eosin-stained sections were examined to determine whether each deciduum (usually 12–14 per uterus) contained a conceptus, and the developmental stage displayed by each embryo was documented with photomicrographs taken with EPY 64 or 160 tungsten film.

```
Human  MATLEKLMKAFESLKSFQQQQQQQQQQQQQQQQQQQQPPPPPPPPPPP...   48
Mouse  MATLEKLMKAFESLKSF.............QQQQQQQPPQPPPPPPPPPPP   38
Rat    MATLEKLMKAFESLKSF............QQQQQQQQPPQPPPPPPPPPP.   38
Fugu   MATMEKLMKAFESLKSF................QQQQGPP...........   24

Human  QLPQPPPQAQPLLPQPQPPPPPPPPPPPGPAVAEEPLHRP—KKELSATKKDRVN 10
Mouse  QPPQPPPQGQ........PPPPPPPLPGPA..EEPLHRP—KKELSATKKDRVN 80
Rat    QPPQPPPQGQ.........PPPPPPLPGPA..EEPLHRP—KKELSATKKDRVN 79
Fugu   ..............................TAEEIVQRQ—KKEQATTKKDRVS 4
```

Figure 1. Comparison of the amino-terminal 100 amino acids of human huntingtin with the homologous region of the mouse, rat, and pufferfish (Fugu) proteins. Amino acid residues identical in three or more of the species are shown in filled boxes, and those amino acids common to two are boxed. The location of intron 1 in the human gene is indicated by the horizontal bar.

Whole mount and RNA in situ analysis. Embryos were removed from uteri of euthanized females by dissection of decidual tissue and subsequent removal of Reichert's membrane and the ectoplacental cone when appropriate. Pregnancies for the collection of "staged" embryos were timed using the day that the vaginal plug was observed as E0.5. The embryos undergoing gastrulation were staged or classified by the presence of morphological landmarks as suggested previously (Downs and Davies 1993), and those in the process of organogenesis using morphological criteria (Theiler 1989). RNA in situ hybridization of dissected embryos was performed as described previously (Conlon and Herrmann 1993), using a digoxigenin-labeled antisense or sense *Hdh* RNA probe synthesized from a 1852-bp *Pst*I restriction fragment (7819–9670 of mouse Hdh cDNA, GenBank #L28827) subcloned into the pBluescript vector.

RESULTS

HD Gene Homologs

Huntingtin's approximately 3144-amino-acid sequence does not contain significant regions of homology with previously reported proteins, but the existence of highly related *HD* homologs in other organisms argues that it performs an essential cellular function. The mouse and rat sequences are highly related to each other and share about 90% amino acid

Table 1. Summary of the Characterization of Mutant *Hdh* Alleles

	Hdh allele[a]		
Parameter	$Hdh^{ex4/5}$	Hdh^{prex1}	Hdh^{ex5}
Targeting strategy			
deletes	3.8 kb	3.8 kb	0.6 kb
replaced with orientation	*neo* opposite	*neo* opposite	*neo* ?
alters	exons 4–5	5′ region	exon 5
	introns 3–6	exon 1 intron 1	intron 4
ES cell line targeted	R1	CCE-33	R1?
neo integrations	one	one	?
Hdh DNA tested	5′ and 3′ flank internal	3′ flank internal	3′ flank internal
predicted products[b]	splice 3–6	none	splice 4–6
	165 aa, 18 kD		185 AA, 20 kD
observed products	none	none	splice 4–6
	immunoblot	in situ	20 kD
ES cell phenotype	none	none	?
mice			
genetic background 129Sv	CD1,C57BL6	MFI,C57BL6	?
phenotype heterozygote	none	none	subtle[c]
phenotype homozygote	~E7.5 lethal	~E7.5 lethal	~E7.5 lethal

(?) Not reported; (aa) amino acids.
[a]Duyao et al. (1995); Zeitlin et al. (1995); Nasir et al. (1995).
[b]Products from mutant allele if *neo* removed by splicing.
[c]Reactive to handling, cognitive impairment, reduced volume of subthalamic nucleus.

Table 2. Summary of Genotypes and Phenotypes in Progeny of *Hdh* $^{+/-}$ Intercrosses

		Genotypes and Phenotypes							
		+/+		+/–		–/–		All genotypes	
Age	Mutant line	N[a]	A[b]	N	A	N	A	N	A
Liveborn	$Hdh^{ex4/5}$	76	0	160	0	0	0	236	0
Liveborn	Hdh^{prex1}	21	0	39	0	0	0	60	0
Liveborn	Hdh^{ex5}	81	0	0	144[c]	0	0	81	144[c]
	total	178	0	199	144[c]	0	0	377	144[c]
E9.5	$Hdh^{ex4/5}$	6	0	9	0	0	5	15	5
E9.5	Hdh^{ex5}	9	0	16	1	0	9	25	10
	total	15	0	25	1	0	14	40	15[d]
E8.5	$Hdh^{ex4/5}$	12	0	21	0	0	9	33	9
E8.5	HdV^{rex1}	3	0	4	0	0	8	32[c]	12[e]
E8.5	Hdh^{ex5}	16	1	46	1	2	12	64	14
	total	31	1	71	1	2	29	129	35[d]
E7.5	$Hdh^{ex4/5}$	14	0	28	0	0	12	42	12
E7.5	Hdh^{prex1}	4	0	10	0	0	5	26[c]	6[e]
E7.5	Hdh^{ex5}	23	2	24	1	2	2	49	5
	total	41	2	62	1	2	19	117	23[d]
E7.0	$Hdh^{ex4/5}$	9	0	7	0	0	6	14	6
E6.5	Hdt^{prex1}	0	0	6	0	0	3	6	3
E7.0/E6.5	total	9	0	13	0	0	9	20	9[d]
E9.5-E6.5	total	96	3	171	3	4	71	306	82[d]

[a]Phenotype within normal variation.
[b]Characteristic abnormal phenotype.
[c]Reactive to handling.
[d]Resorption sites, resorbing embryos, abnormal morphology.
[e]Not all typed.

sequence identity with the human version, whereas most segments of the pufferfish homolog are predicted to be about 65–80% identical. One striking exception, as shown in Figure 1, is the amino-terminal polyglutamine/polyproline-rich stretch encoded by the CAG repeat and adjacent CCG-rich segments. Normal human huntingtin has 13–36 consecutive glutamines encoded by the polymorphic $(CAG)_n(CAA)_2$ segment, and the murine homolog encodes seven glutamines in an imperfect repeat, $(CAG)_2CAA(CAG)_4$, the rat sequence $(CAG)_2CAA(CAG)_5$ predicts eight residues, and the pufferfish protein has four glutamines encoded by $(CAG)_2(CAA)_2$. Similarly, the degenerate polyproline-rich stretch is not conserved in length or composition, varying from 37 to 43 amino acids in man (Rubinsztein et al. 1993), to 30–31 in the mouse (Barnes et al. 1994; Lin et al. 1994) and 29 residues in the rat (Schmitt et al. 1995), to as few as 2 prolines in the pufferfish homolog (Baxendale et al. 1995). In contrast, the flanking sequences are strikingly conserved, particularly the 17 amino acids at the extreme amino terminus, which are identical in the rodent and human homologs (P. Foye and G. Sutcliffe, pers. comm.), including the rat protein that was initially predicted from sequence analysis to lack the first 7 amino acids (Schmitt et al. 1995). Thus, the CAG repeat stretch, which is critical for the mechanism of pathogenesis in HD, may not actually be required for huntingtin's inherent activity.

The identification and cloning of the various *HD* homologs provides the opportunity to explore huntingtin's physiological function in experimental animals. Of these, the mouse is the most attractive for creating a valid genetic model of the human disease. The ability to introduce targeted alterations in the mouse genome by homologous recombination in ES cells makes it possible to create new lines of mice with specific *Hdh* mutations to assess the likelihood of hypothetical scenarios for the mechanism of pathogenesis in HD.

Hdh, the Murine *HD* homolog

The mouse *HD* homolog, *Hdh*, is located in a segment of mouse chromosome 5 that displays synteny conservation with 4p16.3 but does not contain reported mutations causing any phenotype comparable to the human disorder (Grosson et al. 1994; Nasir et al. 1994). *Hdh*, by analogy with its human counterpart, is expected to comprise 67 exons with the amino-terminal polyglutamine/polyproline segment located in exon 1 (Barnes et al. 1994). The precise length of this exon is not known, as the *Hdh/HD* promoter has not been characterized except for speculation that upstream conserved sequence elements may act as SP1- and AP2-binding sites (Lin et al. 1995) and that a 120-bp segment of the region may affect the success of expression constructs (Goldberg et al. 1996a). Clearly, functional characterization of the promoter will provide key information about the precise location of the transcriptional start site(s) and the identification of sequences that determine the gene's broad temporal and spatial pattern of expression.

Like the human gene, *Hdh* is widely expressed in most cells and tissues as two mRNAs of about 10.5 kb and 13.5 kb that reflect the use of alternative polyadenylation signals in the 3′-untranslated region of exon 67. The ratio of the two mRNAs varies in different tissues with the 13.5-kb product predominating in fetal brain. The significance of this observation is not known, as both mRNA species encode the same approximately 350-kD polypeptide. There is no reliable evidence for the generation of alternative forms of huntingtin in rodent or normal human cells and tissues by alternative mRNA splicing (Barnes et al. 1994; Duyao et al. 1995; Persichetti et al. 1996). A careful investigation of the mouse gene reveals that the putative "alternative" *Hdh* mRNA splice variant reported in Lin et al. (1994) (GenBank # L23313) is probably the consequence of a cDNA cloning artifact.

Targeted *Hdh* Inactivation in ES Cells

Huntingtin's broad pattern of expression does not provide clues to its function or explain the apparently specific impact of the CAG expansion mutation on populations of neuronal cells in the cerebral cortex and basal ganglia. One relatively straightforward strategy for investigating both issues is the experimental elimination of huntingtin expression by specific disruption of *Hdh* so that the consequences of the reduced levels of expression can be assessed at the level of the whole organism. Three targeted *Hdh* inactivating mutations generated by homologous recombination in ES cells have been reported (Duyao et al. 1995; Nasir et al. 1995; Zeitlin et al. 1995), and the molecular and phenotypic characterization of these mutant ES cell *Hdh* alleles is summarized in Table 1.

We used cloned segments of 129Sv mouse genomic *Hdh* DNA and the pPNT plasmid to create pPNT-$Hdh^{ex4/5}$, a positive-negative selection targeting vector designed to remove 3.8 kb of the gene, eliminating sequences extending from intron 3 to intron 5, removing exons 4 and 5 and the fourth intron in their entirety, and inserting in their place (in reverse transcriptional orientation) the bacterial *neo* gene driven by the phosphoglycerate kinase 1 promoter (Duyao et al. 1995). The construct was introduced into the R1 line of ES cells, and successfully targeted clones were determined to have a single integration of the pPNT-$Hdh^{ex4/5}$ vector by hybridization with a *neo* probe; the integrity of the mutated allele was assessed using DNA probes located 5′ and 3′ to the sequences represented in the targeting vector (flanking probes). Moreover, the integrity of the targeted event was confirmed in clones of homozygous mutant ES cells, selected by growth in high concentrations of G418, with two mutant $Hdh^{ex4/5}$ alleles.

Hdh mRNA expression is disrupted by transcription of *neo* from the opposite strand, and removal of the *neo* insertion from the targeted allele by novel mRNA splicing events would juxtapose exons 3 and 6 of *Hdh*, entailing a frameshift that truncates the protein 30 non-huntingtin amino acids after the 135 huntingtin residues encoded by exons 1–3. As expected, the $Hdh^{ex4/5}$ mutation eliminated expression of the altered allele, and no full-length huntingtin or stable truncated products were detected in the homozygous mutant $Hdh^{ex4/5}$ ES cells using a panel of characterized amino-terminal and carboxy-terminal anti-huntingtin antisera (Persichetti et al. 1995, 1996), although the approximately 350-kD huntingtin protein is observed in wild-type R1 and heterozygous $Hdh^{ex4/5}$ mutant ES cells. Despite the altered levels of huntingtin, these ES cell clones were indistinguishable from each other and from wild-type ES cells, demonstrating that huntingtin activity is not required for the normal growth of ES cells in culture.

A second inactivating mutation, Hdh^{prex1}, was created by homologous recombination in the CCE-33 line of ES cells, targeting *Hdh* to replace about 3.8 kb of sequence, including a large portion of sequence upstream of the ATG codon, all of exon 1, and 600 bp of the first intron, with the *neo* gene inserted in the opposite transcriptional orientation (Zeitlin et al. 1995). Hybridization of Southern blots of genomic DNA from the targeted clones was used to demonstrate a single integration of the targeting vector, and 3′-flanking sequences confirmed the integrity of the successfully targeted mutant allele. This mutation eliminates *Hdh* mRNA expression, as demonstrated by RNA in situ hybridization of homozygous mutant embryos, presumably because DNA sequence elements required for transcription are removed, and/or by interference from *neo* transcription on the opposite DNA strand.

Homozygous mutant Hdh^{prex1} ES cell clones, derived by growth in high concentrations of G418, were also isolated and analyzed extensively for the effects of the elimination of huntingtin expression on ES cell growth. The wild-type, heterozygous Hdh^{prex1} and homozygous Hdh^{prex1} ES cell clones were indistinguishable, confirming that huntingtin is not required for normal growth in vitro. Furthermore, a quantitative analysis of the in vitro outgrowth of blastocysts from the heterozygous and homozygous lines of Hdh^{prex1} mutant ES cells was used to determine that the absence of huntingtin protein does not affect the capacity of these totipotent cells to spontaneously differentiate into cell types of the three germ-layer lineages in culture.

The molecular analysis of the third targeted *Hdh* mutation, *Hdh*^{Ex5}, is not described in detail (Nasir et al. 1995), but the targeting vector was designed to replace a 600-bp segment of DNA, including intron 4 sequences and a portion of exon 5 with *neo* (Table 1). The impact of the mutation on *Hdh* expression was evaluated by RT-PCR amplification of RNA from a heterozygous mutant mouse tissue. This analysis demonstrated that the *Hdh*^{Ex5} mutation does not eliminate transcription. Rather, it produces a novel mRNA splice product, presumably by exon skipping of the *neo* gene. The juxtaposition of exons 4 and 6 is expected to encode a novel huntingtin polypeptide consisting of 155 amino acids (~20 kD) encoded by exons 1–4 followed by 30 novel amino acids before creating an in-frame stop codon in exon 6. Immunoblot analysis revealed a new 20-kD polypeptide in heterozygous mutant *Hdh*^{Ex5} mouse brain tissue extracts (Nasir et al. 1995). A more complete molecular characterization of the disrupted *Hdh*^{Ex5} allele in ES cell clones and mouse tissue, including an evaluation of products that may include intervening *neo* sequences, will be necessary to understand the phenotypic consequences of this mutation. However, despite its more complex nature, the *Hdh*^{Ex5} mutation dramatically reduces or eliminates expression of the full-length huntingtin protein.

Heterozygous *Hdh* Inactivation Does Not Cause HD-like Pathology

In man, inactivation of one copy of the *HD* gene does not cause HD-like symptoms or any other abnormality (Ambrose et al. 1994; Persichetti et al. 1996), and the analysis of mutant *Hdh* mice created from the targeted ES cell lines described above provides experimental support for the notion that the human disease does not occur by the simple elimination of huntingtin expression. A summary of the characterization of the phenotypic consequences of the mutant *Hdh* alleles is shown in Tables 1 and 2. In each case, mutant ES cell clones were used to generate chimeric founder mice that were tested for germ-line transmission of the disrupted *Hdh* allele in a mixed genetic background including the targeted 129/Sv genome and another mouse strain (CD1, MF1, or C57BL6). All of the targeted *Hdh* alleles are inherited in a Mendelian fashion, and there is no evidence for segregation bias based on sex or age of the transmitting parent. Table 2 provides a summary of the genotypes and phenotypes exhibited by *Hdh*$^{ex4/5}$, *Hdh*^{prex1}, and *Hdh*^{ex5} animals generated by intercrossing, which also reveals the Mendelian inheritance of the mutant alleles when all progeny from this type of cross are analyzed.

Heterozygous *Hdh*$^{ex4/5}$ mutant mice express 50% of the huntingtin protein produced by their wild-type littermates (and only the full-length ~350-kD polypeptide). These heterozygous mutant animals do not, at any age, display a discernible abnormal phenotype on two mixed genetic backgrounds (129Sv/CD1 and 129Sv/C57BL6/J) and cannot be distinguished from wild-type littermates by appearance, including stature and weight, movement, or behaviors related to normal handling procedures and breeding. Heterozygous loss of huntingtin activity also does not affect breeding capacity or the life span of the animal.

Similarly, *Hdh* inactivation as a result of the *Hdh*^{prex1} mutation also does not provoke a heterozygous phenotype (Zeitlin et al. 1995). Although it is not evident from the data summarized in Table 2, these investigators state that the routine handling of hundreds of *Hdh*^{prex1} heterozygote mice generated from *Hdh*^{prex1} mutant ES cell clones on a mixed 129 Sv/MF 1 or 129Sv/C57BL6/J genetic background failed to distinguish the heterozygous mutant mice from their wild-type littermates. Thus, like the *Hdh*$^{ex4/5}$ heterozygotes, these mice do not develop abnormal behaviors (Tables 1 and 2).

The most telling finding for the human disease, however, is the observation that the simple elimination of 50% of huntingtin does not result in anatomical or pathological defects in the brain or periphery of *Hdh*$^{ex4/5}$ and *Hdh*^{prex1} mutant animals. Blinded neuropathological examination of serial sections of the brains of several mutant mice and sex-matched wild-type littermates revealed no evidence of anatomical abnormalities, neuronal degeneration, or other signs of pathology in the regions most affected in HD, the cerebral cortex, caudate putamen, globus pallidus, amygdala, substantia nigra reticulata and compacta, and subthalamic nucleus, or in any other area of the brain (Duyao et al. 1995; Zeitlin et al. 1995). This careful analysis was extended in the *Hdh*^{prex1} mutant animals to a morphometric analysis, which also failed to find evidence of neuroanatomical alterations, neuronal cell loss, or other cellular defects in the cortex or regions of the basal ganglia (Zeitlin et al. 1995). Thus, the evaluation of these heterozygous mutant *Hdh* mice provides experimental data in support of the observation that inactivation of one *HD* allele does not cause any abnormal phenotype in man.

In contrast, the more complex *Hdh*^{Ex5} mutation is reported to be associated with a subtle heterozygous phenotype (Tables 1 and 2) (Nasir et al. 1995). *Hdh*^{Ex5} mutant mice can be distinguished from their littermates because they are more reactive to handling. Quantitative analysis revealed a significant deficit in the reversal phase of the Morris water maze test, suggesting that the animals exhibit a cognitive impairment. Examination of the brains of two of the most compromised mice did not reveal frank anatomical or pathological aberrations, but subtle changes in the volume and number of neurons in the subthalamic nucleus were reported to be of significance. The molecular basis of these alterations is not understood, because the *Hdh*^{Ex5} mutation is complex, both reducing *Hdh* expression and generating novel protein products, making it difficult to determine the basis of the phenotype. Therefore, it is not yet apparent whether these findings have any bearing on the mechanism of the human disorder where no novel mRNA or polypeptides have been observed.

Homozygous *Hdh* Inactivation Causes Embryonic Lethality

An alternative scenario for the mode of action of the defect that involves huntingtin's inherent activity is a simple "dominant negative" model which postulates that the *HD* defect eliminates the activity of the mutated protein and also confers upon it the ability to interfere with the normal physiological function of the protein produced by the wild-type allele. This possibility has been tested by interbreeding heterozygous *Hdh* mutant mice to produce animals that do not express any huntingtin protein. The results reveal that, rather than displaying an HD-like phenotype, homozygous mutant animals die during embryogenesis.

As shown in Table 2, no homozygous mutant $Hdh^{ex4/5}$, Hdh^{prex1}, or Hdh^{Ex5} animals are represented in more than 500 liveborn offspring of parents that are both heterozygous *Hdh* mutants. However, the expected proportion of wild-type, heterozygote, and homozygote genotypes, predicted by Mendelian inheritance of the *Hdh* alleles to be a 1:2:1 ratio, is observed when embryos about E7.5–E9.5 are typed. The exception is the odd inheritance of the Hdh^{Ex5} allele in E7.5 embryos (25 wild type; 25 heterozygotes; 4 homozygotes), which is not explained but may reflect difficulties with the PCR genotyping assay and the preferential loss of homozygous mutant embryos from the analysis. Combining the transmission data of all three targeted alleles about E7.5–E 9.5, however, yields approximately the expected 1:2:1 ratio of genotypes (99 wild-type; 174 heterozygotes; 75 homozygotes), demonstrating that the failure to recover homozygous animals after birth is explained by the selective death of these embryos in utero. Indeed, morphological and microscopic examination of the homozygote mutants reveals a unique abnormal phenotype that is common to all three targeted *Hdh* alleles.

Homozygote $Hdh^{ex4/5}$ and *Hdhex1* mutant embryos are abnormally small at E6.5, but fail obviously at about E7.5–E8.5. As shown in Figure 2A, the wild-type embryo taken at about E7.5 has reached the late headfold stage of development, with the node and foregut pocket visible. In contrast, the typical homozygous mutant $Hdh^{ex4/5}$ embryo in Figure 2B is clearly abnormal. The egg cylinder is reduced in size and disorganized, the embryonic ectoderm is smooth and featureless, and the extraembryonic endoderm is folded and sags down around the small embryo which has not expanded properly. Histological examination of wild-type and mutant embryos is shown in Figure 2C and D, respectively. This examination reveals that, like its wild-type littermate, the mutant embryo has elaborated both extraembryonic and embryonic mesoderm (although it is abnormally thickened and disorganized), blood islands have formed, the amnion is present and closure is complete, the allantois is developing, extending into an expanded exocoelomic cavity, and the ectoplacental cavity is visible. Additionally, the elegant analysis of the Hdh^{prex1} embryos points out abnormalities in Reichert's membrane (Zeitlin et al. 1995) that have not been evaluated in the $Hdh^{ex4/5}$. Thus, homozygous mutant embryos achieve many developmental milestones but fail to undergo the initial morphological changes that signal the remodeling of the embryonic ectoderm and mesoderm during establishment of the anterior-posterior axis including a fully extended primitive streak and the formation of a node or anterior neurectoderm, headprocess, neural plate, headfold, or neural tube. Furthermore, the embryonic ectoderm, but not other germ layers, of the $Hdh^{ex4/5}$ and *Hdhex1* homozygous mutant embryos is replete with pyknotic and fragmented nuclei, especially in the anterior region. TUNEL analysis of the mutant *Hdhex1* embryos at about E7.5 demonstrates high levels of staining in the embryonic ectoderm, coincident with the pyknotic nuclei, suggesting that these cells are undergoing apoptotic cell death (Zeitlin et al. 1995). Nevertheless, mitotic activity in these mutant embryos appears grossly normal or is perhaps elevated so that many dividing cells are intermingled with those that are dying.

Another striking feature is the abnormal appearance of the extraembryonic endoderm. Rather than being composed of smooth columnar epithelial cells, the outermost cell layer of the mutant embryos is composed of rounded cells that are disorganized and "heaped up" around the embryo. These gross morphological abnormalities, however, do not appear to impair endocytosis, a function of this germ cell layer, which is normal in the mutant E7.5 embryos (Zeitlin et al. 1995).

In order to assess the $Hdh^{ex4/5}$ mutant phenotype in more detail, we examined the expression of *Brachyury T*, *gsc*, *HNF-3*β, and *fgf8*, genes with spatially and temporally restricted patterns of expression that act as markers of developing embryonic ectoderm and mesoderm. This preliminary analysis confirms the impression gained by whole-mount and section histological examination. A primitive streak is apparent and contains *Brachyury T* and *HNF-3*β expressing cells, although it is not fully extended to the distal pole. The embryonic ectoderm and mesoderm contain *gsc*, *HNF-3*β, and *fgf8* positive cells, but these cells are not located in discrete regions of the embryo in recognizable morphological structures. It is not clear whether this disorganization represents a failure of appropriate cell migration or reflects inappropriate cellular differentiation in response to the lack of huntingtin activity.

Hdh^{Ex5} homozygote embryos fail at about E7.5–E8.0 with a gross morphological phenotype that closely resembles that described above for the $Hdh^{ex4/5}$ and Hdh^{ex1} mutations. However, the reported characterization suggests that it produces a less severe

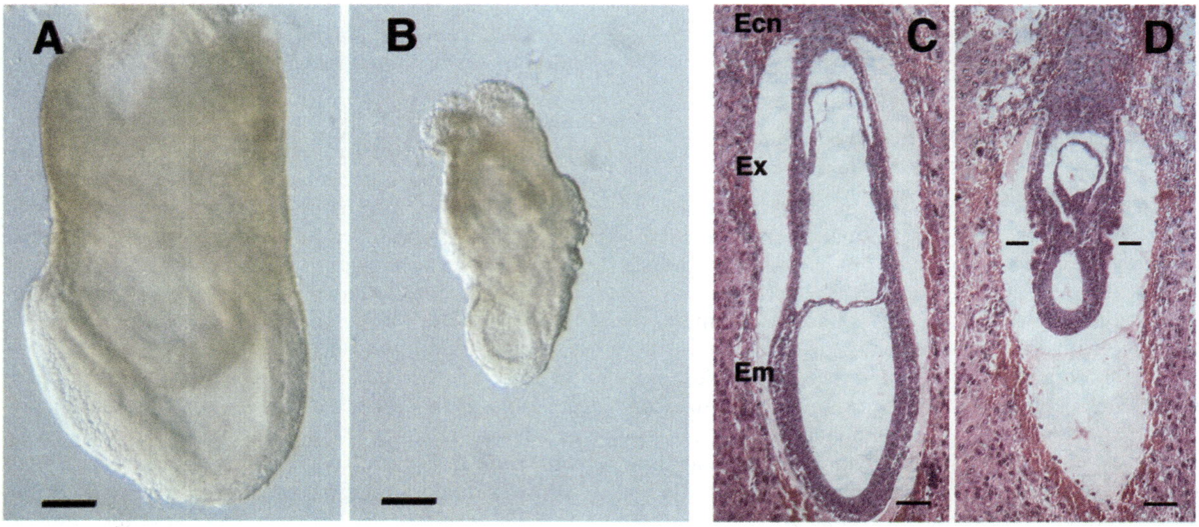

Figure 2. Morphology and histology of E7.5 wild-type and homozygous *Hdhex4/5* mutant embryos. Examples of wild-type (*A*,*C*) and homozygous mutant (*B*,*D*) E7.5 embryos are shown as whole embryos (*A*,*B*) with the ectoplacental cone and parietal endoderm removed and as sagittal (*C*,*D*) hematoxylin and eosin-stained sections. The bar beside the mutant embryo in *D* indicates junction of the extraembryonic and embryonic portions of the embryo. (Ecn) Ectoplacental cone; (Ex) extraembryonic portion of the embryo; (Em) embryonic portion of the embryo. Bars: *A*, *B*, 100 μM; *C*,*D*, 50 μM.

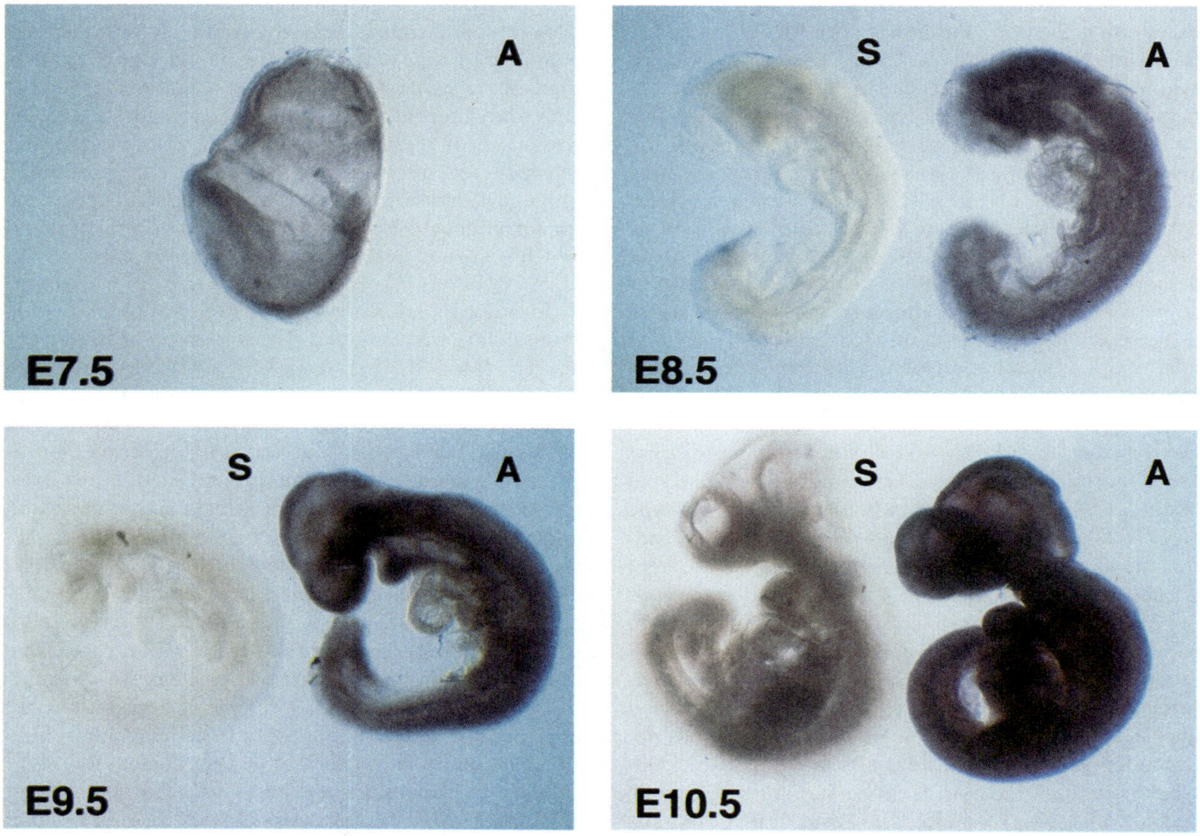

Figure 3. Whole-mount analysis of *Hdh* RNA expression. Whole-mount RNA of normal CD1 embryos was analyzed for *Hdh* expression by RNA in situ hybridization at E7.5, E8.5, E9.5, and E10.5 with an antisense (A) or control sense (S) *Hdh* cRNA probe. Blue staining indicates the presence of *Hdh* mRNA.

homozygous phenotype. As shown in Table 2, the homozyous mutant genotype was observed in morphologically normal embryos at E7.5 and E8.5 when neurulation is well advanced, whereas others appear to fail later, leaving resorption sites at E12.5. In contrast, $Hdh^{ex4/5}$ and Hdh^{ex1} mutant embryos could not be recovered at about E9.5–E10.5, and resorption sites consisting of extraembryonic membranes were used for genotyping. The distinct consequences of Hdh^{Ex5} mutant alleles have not been explained but may be related to the expression of a novel protein product that includes a portion of the amino terminus of huntingtin.

Hdh Expression in the Developing Embryo

The pattern of *Hdh* expression does not provide a satisfactory explanation for the dramatic impact of the absence of huntingtin on the extraembryonic endoderm and embryonic ectoderm in the homozygous mutant embryos. Huntingtin is expressed in ES cells (Duyao et al. 1995) and throughout embryonic development, although a detailed analysis at the cellular level, particularly during the time when the homozygous mutant embryos are failing at about E7.0–E7.5, has not been reported. In situ hybridization analysis at about E7.5 suggests either a broad pattern of expression (Duyao et al. 1995) or a more restricted location primarily in cells of the ectoderm/mesoderm (Zeitlin et al. 1995).

Figure 3 shows the results of whole-mount in situ hybridization with an anti-sense *Hdh* cRNA probe on dissected representative morphologically normal embryos from litters taken at E7.5, E8.5, E9.5, and E10.5, all exhibiting morphological features that are not achieved by homozygous mutant $Hdh^{ex4/5}$ or Hdh^{prex1} animals (early headfold stage E7.5 through organogenesis, which is well advanced at E10.5). The blue deposit indicates the presence of *Hdh* mRNA, and the results obtained on age-matched littermates with a sense cRNA control probe are shown for comparison (except for the E7.5 embryo). It is clear that at all stages represented in this analysis, *Hdh* mRNA is detected throughout the embryo and in the extraembryonic tissues observed in the early headfold stage E7.5 embryo.

Unlike developmentally regulated genes such as *Brachyury T*, *HNF-3*β, and *fgf8*, which are also expressed at discrete times in certain tissues in the adult, *Hdh* expression is not absolutely restricted either spatially or temporally during embryonic development; rather, it is present in a wide variety of cell types throughout the life span of the organism. Elimination of huntingtin activity, therefore, may lead to the abnormal homozygous *Hdh* mutant phenotype due to deficits in a variety of cell types, including those in germ layers that are grossly normal in the mutant embryo.

DISCUSSION

The pathogenic mechanism by which an expanded CAG repeat in the *HD* gene causes the characteristic neuropathology of HD remains to be discovered. Among human trinucleotide repeat disorders, the mode of action of the defect is known only in Fragile X mental retardation where *FMR1* activity is eliminated (Gusella and MacDonald 1996), permitting a useful model to be generated by inactivation of the mouse homolog (Dutch-Belgian Fragile X Consortium 1994). In contrast, the *HD* CAG expansion does not eliminate gene expression; rather, it is translated into a polymorphic stretch of polyglutamine residues at the amino terminus of huntingtin. The impact of the mutation on huntingtin's physiological function is not known, and its broad pattern of expression does not explain the specific pathology of the disease. The mode of action of the CAG repeat has been tested by eliminating huntingtin expression in the mouse. *Hdh* inactivation does not cause an HD-like pathology, but it has shed light on huntingtin's inherent activity and places empirical limitations on the theoretical scenarios that are invoked to explain the mechanism of pathogenesis in HD.

Three different disrupted *Hdh* alleles, $Hdh^{ex4/5}$, Hdh^{prex1}, and Hdh^{Ex5}, generated by homologous recombination in ES cells, have been reported. A comparison of the published data reveals that all three mutations eliminate the expression of huntingtin with similar phenotypic consequences. Characterization of the targeted ES cells demonstrates that huntingtin is expressed from the earliest stages of development, as well as in the developing embryo, extending previous studies that demonstrated mRNA expression in fetal mouse (Barnes et al. 1994; Lin et al. 1994), rat (Schmitt et al. 1995; P. Foye and G. Sutcliffe, pers. comm.), and human (Ambrose et al. 1994; Dure et al. 1994; Landwehrmeyer et al. 1995; Li et al. 1995) tissue. Moreover, the elimination of huntingtin expression in the $Hdh^{ex4/5}$ and Hdh^{prex1} mutant ES cell clones does elicit an overt phenotype, demonstrating that huntingtin's physiological activity is not required for cell growth or differentiation under standard culture conditions.

The characterization of mice heterozygous for two independent *Hdh* mutations that completely eliminate expression from the targeted allele, $Hdh^{ex4/5}$ and Hdh^{ex1}, demonstrates that levels of huntingtin protein can be reduced to 50% without overt behavioral or pathological consequences to the organism. Heterozygous mutant $Hdh^{ex4/5}$ and Hdh^{ex1} mice do not exhibit HD-like neuropathology or any other abnormal phenotype. However, the more complex Hdh^{Ex5} mutation produces a behavioral and subtle pathological phenotype in the subthalamic nucleus in the presence of huntingtin expressed from the wild-type allele. These phenotypes, which are not HD-like, are perhaps explained by the expression of novel gene products, including a novel 20-kD polypeptide that is predicted to contain the amino-terminal 155 amino acids of huntingtin and 30 non-huntingtin amino acids generated by aberrant mRNA splicing. It is not clear whether either the novel phenotype or its underlying molecular defect is of importance to the mechanism of pathogenesis in HD.

The dramatic impact of the complete elimination of huntingtin achieved by intercrossing heterozygous *Hdh* mutant mice, lethality at about E7.5–E9.5, clearly demonstrates that huntingtin has a critical role early in embryonic development. Thus, *Hdh* inactivation has provided a functional role for huntingtin's inherent physiological activity, and investigators have hypothesized that it is involved in neurulation (Nasir et al. 1995) or normal and abnormal developmental programmed cell death (Zeitlin et al. 1995). The phenotype of the homozygous *Hdh* mutants is unique. Other targeted mutations that inactivate genes with restricted expression patterns, such as the transcription factors *HNF-4* and *HNF-3*β, result in greater developmental heterogeneity of embryonic lethality (E6.5–E10.5). *fugl*, a broadly expressed gene inactivated by transgene insertion, also produces rapid cell death between E6.5 and E8.5, but these embryos do not elaborate mesoderm. Thus, huntingtin may provide an opportunity to study cellular and molecular events in embryonic development, before the emergence at E8.0–E8.5 of the neural tube, the precursor of the HD defect's target tissue in man.

The results of the targeted inactivation of *Hdh* fail to provide evidence in favor of a mode of action of the expanded CAG repeat mutation which involves a simple loss of huntingtin activity from the mutant allele. They also place crucial empirical limitations on other scenarios that postulate a loss of huntingtin function in the mechanism of HD pathogenesis. First, the absence of an HD-like phenotype in heterozygous *Hdh* mutant mice provides experimental support for the observation in man of a 50% reduction in huntingtin in a phenotypically normal individual (Ambrose et al. 1994; Persichetti et al. 1996). Therefore, if loss of huntingtin function is key to the pathogenic mechanism of HD, then the CAG expansion must decrease total huntingtin activity to below 50% of normal.

Second, the pathogenic mechanism in HD is dominant, and the defect may therefore operate in a dominant negative manner by inhibiting the activity of normal huntingtin. However, targeted inactivation of *Hdh* causes early embryonic lethality in homozygous mutant animals; heterozygotes either exhibit no abnormal phenotype (Duyao et al. 1995; Zeitlin et al. 1995) or may have subtle behavioral and neuroanatomical abnormalities (Nasir et al. 1995). In man, homozygotes for the *HD* gene defect are viable and have the same phenotype as HD heterozygotes (Wexler et al. 1987; Myers et al. 1989). If the CAG expansion acts in a dominant negative manner, then the defect must reduce huntingtin's activity below a critical threshold without eliminating it entirely. Based on the heterozygous *Hdh* mutant mice and on the phenotypically normal t(4;12) individuals, this activity threshold must be below 50%. Thus, in the loss-of-function scenario, the net huntingtin activity associated with causing HD pathogenesis must fall somewhere between 0 and 50% of normal. An additional limitation on this model is the correlation between disease severity and CAG repeat length, which predicts that levels of huntingtin activity must be reduced in a graded fashion with increasing CAG repeat length.

The empirical limits set on the loss of function model by the results of *Hdh* inactivation, and the constraints imposed by the dominant phenotype and the correlation between CAG repeat length and disease severity, are strict, but they do not exclude this mechanism. However, the alternative and more attractive gain-of-function model proposes that the expanded polyglutamine segment confers a new property on huntingtin that need not involve its normal physiological activity. The new property must be peculiarly detrimental to specific adult neurons and must act in a dominant fashion so that the pathogenic mechanism is insensitive to increases in the concentration of mutant protein beyond that produced by a single HD allele.

Several general gain-of-function models that involve altered protein/protein interactions have been advanced to explain HD and other CAG repeat diseases caused by polyglutamine. These include the accumulation of a toxic product as a result of inappropriate clearance of abnormal products resulting from transglutamination (Green 1993), β-pleated sheet conformers (Perutz et al. 1994; Perutz 1995), or amino-terminal fragments generated by cysteine protease cleavage (Goldberg et al. 1996b). Other traditional models, based on animal lesioning studies, favor an involvement of excitotoxic pathways of cell death that involve NMDA receptor-mediated glutamate toxicity, oxidative stress, free radical damage, and Ca^{++}-induced apoptosis. There is no compelling experimental data to support any of these models in HD pathogenesis in man. Indeed, in lymphoblastoid cell lines, normal huntingtin is not rapidly turned over or processed to a smaller product and, similarly, mutant huntingtin is not destabilized in HD heterozygotes and homozygotes. As predicted from the stability of both normal and mutant huntingtin, no disease-allele-specific processing or degradation products have been observed with multiple anti-huntingtin antisera. Clearly, it will be important to establish whether abnormal huntingtin products are found in the neuronal cells that are the targets of the mutation.

Because the HD defect is dominant, expression of mutant huntingtin protein ectopically in transgenic mice would be expected to provoke HD pathology if expressed in the appropriate tissues. Indeed, Purkinje cells in the cerebellum die when ataxin-1 (Burright et al. 1995) or a truncated version of the MJD1 protein (Ikeda et al. 1996) with elongated polyglutamine segments is expressed from a Purkinje-cell-specific promoter, producing profound ataxia in transgenic lines of mice. Expression of mutant huntingtin protein in the neurons of the cerebral cortex and basal ganglia would be expected, therefore, to provoke neuronal cell death that resembles HD neuropathology. However, it will be important to assess the impact of the mutant huntingtin when it is expressed in a wide variety of cells and tissues in order to establish whether the neuronal cell death is achieved by the same selective pathogenic mechanism that is operating in the human disorder. Targeting *Hdh* by homologous recombination in ES cells to introduce an expanded CAG segment at the appropriate location in the mouse gene will create an accurate genetic mouse model of HD. These mutant animals can be used to evaluate whether the elongated amino-terminal polyglutamine segment affects huntingtin's newly discovered physiological function in embryonic development and, importantly, will permit an exploration of the mechanism of pathogenesis in the human disease in the hopes of devising an effective therapeutic strategy.

ACKNOWLEDGMENTS

We thank S. Chui for his help with histology and acknowledge the support of the National Institutes of Health (grants NS-32765 and NS-16367), Bristol Myers Squibb (J.F.G. and A.L.J.), the Huntington's Disease Foundation, and the Hereditary Disease Foundation. J.K.W. is supported by the Huntington's Disease Foundation, and M.D. was supported by a fellowship from the Hereditary Disease Foundation. During the course of the work, A.L.J. was a Medical Research Council of Canada Scientist and International Scholar of the Howard Hughes Medical Institute. The additional support of the Foundation for the Care and Cure of Huntington's Disease (FCCHD) to help defray the costs associated with maintaining the $Hdh^{ex4/5}$ mutant mice is gratefully acknowledged. This paper is dedicated to the memory of Mr. Dennis Shea, founder of the FCCHD, in recognition of his many critical contributions to the research effort directed at finding a cure for HD.

REFERENCES

Ambrose, C.M., M.P. Duyao, G. Barnes, G.P. Bates, C.S. Lin, J. Srinidhi, S. Baxendale, H. Hummerich, H. Lehrach, M. Altherr, J.J. Wasmuth, A. Buckler, D. Church, D. Housman, M. Berks, G. Micklem, R. Durbin, A. Dodge, A. Read, J.F. Gusella, and M.E. MacDonald. 1994. Structure and expression of the Huntington's disease gene: Evidence against simple inactivation due to an expanded CAG repeat. *Somatic Cell Mol. Genet.* **20:** 27.

Barnes, G.T., M.P. Duyao, C.M. Ambrose, S. McNeil, F. Persichetti, J. Srinidhi, J.F. Gusella, and M.E. MacDonald. 1994. Mouse Huntington's disease gene homolog (Hdh). *Somatic Cell Mol. Genet.* **20:** 87.

Baxendale, S., S. Abdulla, G. Elgar, D. Buck, M. Berks, G. Micklem, R. Durbin, G. Bates, S. Brenner, S. Beck, et al. 1995. Comparative sequence analysis of the human and pufferfish Huntington's disease genes. *Nat. Genet.* **10:** 67.

Beal, M.F. 1995. Aging, energy, and oxidative stress in neurodegenerative diseases. *Ann. Neurol.* **38:** 357.

Burright, E.N., H.B. Clark, A. Servadio, T. Matilla, R.M. Feddersen, W.S. Yunis, L.A. Duvick, H.Y. Zoghbi, and H.T. Orr. 1995. SCA1 transgenic mice: A model for neurodegeneration caused by an expanded CAG trinucleotide repeat. *Cell* **82:** 937.

Conlon, R.A. and B.G. Herrmann. 1993. Detection of messenger RNA by in situ hybridization to postimplantation embryo whole mounts. *Methods Enzymol.* **225:** 373.

Downs, K.M. and T. Davies. 1993. Staging of gastrulating mouse embryos by morphological landmarks in the dissecting microscope. *Development* **118:** 1255.

Dure, L.S.T., G.B. Landwehrmeyer, J. Golden, S.M. McNeil, P. Ge, H. Aizawa, Q. Huang, C.M. Ambrose, M.P. Duyao, E.D. Bird, M. DiFiglia, J.F. Gusella, M.E. MacDonald, J.B. Penney, A.B. Young, and J.-P. Vonsattel. 1994. IT15 gene expression in fetal human brain. *Brain Res.* **659:** 33.

Dutch-Belgian Fragile X Consortium. 1994. Fmr1 knockout mice: A model to study fragile X mental retardation. *Cell* **78:** 23.

Duyao, M.P., A.B. Auerbach, A. Ryan, F. Persichetti, G.T. Barnes, S.M. McNeil, P. Ge, J.P. Vonsattel, J.F. Gusella, A.L. Joyner, and M.E. MacDonald. 1995. Inactivation of the mouse Huntington's disease gene homolog Hdh. *Science* **269:** 407.

Goldberg, Y.P., M.A. Kalchman, M. Metzler, J. Nasir, J. Zeisler, R. Graham, H.B. Koide, J. O'Kusky, A.H. Sharp, C.A. Ross, F. Jirik, and M.R. Hayden. 1996a. Absence of disease phenotype and intergenerational stability of the CAG repeat in transgenic mice expressing the human Huntington disease transcript. *Hum. Mol. Genet.* **5:** 177.

Goldberg, Y.P., D.W. Nicholson, D.M. Rasper, M.A. Kalchman, H.B. Koide, R.K. Graham, M. Bromm, P. Kazemi-Esfarjani, N.A. Thornberry, J.P. Vaillancourt, and M.R. Hayden. 1996b. Cleavage of huntingtin by apopain, a proapoptotic cysteine protease, is modulated by the polyglutamine tract. *Nat. Genet.* **13:** 442.

Graveland, G.A., R.S. Williams, and M. DiFiglia. 1985. Evidence for degenerative and regenerative changes in neostriatal spiny neurons in Huntington's disease. *Science* **227:** 770.

Green, H. 1993. Human genetic diseases due to codon reiteration: Relationship to an evolutionary mechanism (letter). *Cell* **74:** 955.

Grosson, C.L., M.E. MacDonald, M.P. Duyao, C.M. Ambrose, S. Roffler-Tarlov, and J.F. Gusella. 1994. Synteny conservation of the Huntington's disease gene and surrounding loci on mouse chromosome 5. *Mamm. Genome* **5:** 424.

Gusella, J.F. and M.E. MacDonald. 1995a. Huntington's disease. *Semin. Cell Biol.* **6:** 21.

———. 1995b. Huntington's disease: CAG genetics expands neurobiology. *Curr. Opin. Neurol.* **5:** 656.

———. 1996. Trinucleotide instability: A repeating theme in human inherited disorders. *Ann. Rev. Med.* (in press.)

Gutekunst, C.A., A.I. Levey, C.J. Heilman, W.L. Whaley, H. Yi, N.R. Nash, H.D. Rees, J.J. Madden, and S.M. Hersch. 1995. Identification and localization of huntingtin in brain and human lymphoblastoid cell lines with anti-fusion protein antibodies. *Proc. Natl. Acad. Sci.* **92:** 8710.

Harper, P.S. 1992. The epidemiology of Huntington's disease. *Hum. Genet.* **89:** 365.

Huntington's Disease Collaborative Research Group. 1993. A novel gene containing a trinucleotide repeat that is expanded and unstable on Huntington's disease chromosomes. *Cell* **72:** 971.

Ide, K., N. Nukina, N. Masuda, J. Goto, and I. Kanazawa. 1995. Abnormal gene product identified in Huntington's disease lymphocytes and brain. *Biochem. Biophys. Res. Commun.* **209:** 1119.

Ikeda, H., M. Yamaguchi, S. Sugai, Y. Aze, S. Narumiya, and A. Kakizuka. 1996. Expanded polyglutamine in the Machado-Joseph disease protein indices cell death in vitro and in vivo. *Nat. Genet.* **13:** 196.

Landwehrmeyer, G.B., S.M. McNeil, L.S.T. Dure, P. Ge, H. Aizawa, Q. Huang, C.M. Ambrose, M.P. Duyao, E.D. Bird, E. Bonilla, M. deYoung, A.J. Avila-Gonzales, N.S. Wexler, M. DiFiglia, J.F. Gusella, M.E. MacDonald, P.B. Penny, A.B. Young, and J.-P. Vonsattel. 1995. Huntington's disease gene: Regional and cellular expression in brain of normal and affected individuals. *Ann. Neurol.* **37:** 218.

Li, X.J., S.H. Li, A.H. Sharp, F.C. Nucifora, Jr., G. Schilling, A. Lanahan, P. Worley, S.H. Snyder, and C.A. Ross. 1995. A huntingtin-associated protein enriched in brain with implications for pathology. *Nature* **378:** 398.

Lin, B., J. Nasir, M.A. Kalchman, H. McDonald, J. Zeisler, Y.P. Goldberg, and M.R. Hayden. 1995. Structural analysis of the 5′ region of mouse and human Huntington disease genes reveals conservation of putative promoter region and di- and trinucleotide polymorphisms. *Genomics* **25:** 707.

Lin, B., J. Nasir, H. MacDonald, G. Hutchinson, R.K. Graham, J.M. Rommens, and M.R. Hayden. 1994. Sequence of the murine Huntington disease gene: Evidence for conservation, alternate splicing and polymorphism in a triplet (CCG) repeat (corrected) (published erratum appears in *Hum. Mol. Genet.* [1994] **3:** 530). *Hum. Mol. Genet.* **3:** 85.

Martin, J.B. 1995. Gene therapy and pharmacological treatment of inherited neurological disorders. *Trends Biotechnol.* **13:** 28.

Martin, J.B. and J.F. Gusella. 1986. Huntington's disease. Pathogenesis and management. *N. Engl. J. Med.* **315:** 1267.

Myers, R.H., J. Leavitt, L.A. Farrer, J. Jagadeesh, H. McFarlane, C.A. Mastromauro, R.J. Mark, and J.F. Gusella. 1989. Homozygote for Huntington disease. *Am. J. Hum. Genet.* **45:** 615.

Nasir, J., B. Lin, M. Bucan, T. Koizumi, J.H. Nadeau, and M.R. Hayden. 1994. The murine homologues of the Huntington disease gene (Hdh) and the alpha-adducin gene (Add1) map to mouse chromosome 5 within a region of conserved synteny with human chromosome 4p16.3. *Genomics* **22:** 198.

Nasir, J., S.B. Floresco, B., J.R. O'Kusky, V.M. Diewert, J.M. Richman, J. Zeisler, A. Borowski, J.D. Marth, A.G. Phillips, and M.R. Hayden. 1995. Targeted disruption of the Huntington's disease gene results in embryonic lethality and behavioral and morphological changes in heterozygotes. *Cell* **81:** 811.

Persichetti, F., C.M. Ambrose, P. Ge, S.M. McNeil, J. Srinidhi, M.A. Anderson, B. Jenkins, G.T. Barnes, M.P. Duyao, L. Kanaley, N.S. Wexler, R.H. Myers, E.D. Bird, J.-P. Vonsattel, M.E. MacDonald, and J.F. Gusella. 1995. Normal and expanded Huntington's disease gene alleles produce distinguishable proteins due to translation across the CAG repeat. *Mol. Med.* **1:** 374.

Persichetti, F., L. Carlee, P.W. Faber, S.M. McNeil, C.M. Ambrose, J. Srinidhi, M.A. Anderson, G.T. Barnes, J.F. Gusella, and M.E. MacDonald. 1996. Differential expression of normal and mutant Huntington's disease gene alleles. *Neurobiol. Dis.* (in press).

Perutz, M.F. 1995. Polar zippers: Their role in human disease. *Pharm. Acta Helv.* **69:** 213.

Perutz, M.F., T. Johnson, M. Suzuki, and J.T. Finch. 1994. Glutamine repeats as polar zippers: Their possible role in inherited neurodegenerative diseases. *Proc. Natl. Acad. Sci.* **91:** 5355.

Rubinsztein, D.C., D.E. Barton, B.C. Davison, and M.A. Ferguson-Smith. 1993. Analysis of the huntingtin gene reveals a trinucleotide-length polymorphism in the region of the gene that contains two CCG-rich stretches and a correlation between decreased age of onset of Huntington's disease and CAG repeat number. *Hum. Mol. Genet.* **2:** 1713.

Schmitt, I., D. Bachner, D. Megow, P. Henklein, H. Hameister, J.T. Epplen, and O. Riess. 1995. Expression of the Huntington disease gene in rodents: Cloning the rat homologue and evidence for downregulation in non-neuronal tissues during development. *Hum. Mol. Genet.* **4:** 1173.

Sharp, A.H. and C.A. Ross. 1996. Neurobiology of Huntington's Disease. *Neurobiol. Dis.* **3:** 3.

Sharp, A.H., S.J. Loev, G. Schilling, S.H. Li, X.J. Li, J. Bao, M.V. Wagster, J.A. Kotzuk, J.P. Steiner, A. Lo, J. Hedreen, S. Sisodia, S.H. Snyder, T.M. Dawson, D.K. Ryugo, and C.A. Ross. 1995. Widespread expression of Huntington's disease gene (IT15) protein product. *Neuron* **14:** 1065.

Theiler, K. 1989. *The house mouse: Atlas of embryonic development*. Springer-Verlag, New York.

Trottier, Y., D. Devys, G. Imbert, F. Saudou, I. An, Y. Lutz, C. Weber, Y. Agid, E.C. Hirsch, and J.L. Mandel. 1995. Cellular localization of the Huntington's disease protein and discrimination of the normal and mutated form. *Nat. Genet.* **10:** 104.

Trottier, Y., Y. Lutz, G. Stevanin, G. Imbert, D. Devys, G. Cancel, F. Saudou, C. Weber, G. David, L. Tora, Y. Agid, A. Brice, and J.L. Mandel. 1995. Polyglutamine expansion as a pathological epitope in Huntington's disease and four dominant cerebellar ataxias. *Nature* **378:** 403.

Vonsattel, J.P., R.H. Myers, T.J. Stevens, R.J. Ferrante, E.D. Bird, and E.P. Richardson, Jr. 1985. Neuropathological classification of Huntington's disease. *J. Neuropathol. Exp. Neurol.* **44:** 559.

Wexler, N.S., A.B. Young, R.E. Tanzi, H. Travers, S. Starosta-Rubinstein, J.B. Penney, S.R. Snodgrass, I. Shoulson, F. Gomez, M.A. Ramos-Arroyo, G. Penchaszadeh, R. Moreno, K. Gibbons, A. Faryniarz, W. Hobbs, M.A. Anderson, E. Bonilla, P.M. Conneally, and J.F. Gusella. 1987. Homozygotes for Huntington's disease. *Nature* **326:** 194.

Zeitlin, S., J.P. Liu, D.L. Chapman, V.E. Papaioannou, and A. Efstratiadis. 1995. Increased apoptosis and early embryonic lethality in mice nullizygous for the Huntington's disease gene homologue. *Nat. Genet.* **11:** 155.

Polyglutamine Expansions and Neurodegenerative Diseases

F. SAUDOU,[1,4] D. DEVYS,[1] Y. TROTTIER,[1] G. IMBERT,[1] M.-E. STOECKEL,[2] A. BRICE,[3] AND J.-L. MANDEL[1]
[1]*Institut de Génétique et de Biologie Moléculaire et Cellulaire (IGBMC), CNRS/INSERM/ULP, Illkirch-Strasbourg, France;* [2]*URA CNRS 1446, Strasbourg, France;* [3]*INSERM U.289, Hôpital de la Salpêtrière, Paris, France*

Positional cloning has allowed in recent years the identification of genes and mutations responsible for many neurodegenerative diseases. This has generated many surprises and raised many novel questions. Some of the most unexpected findings concern the implication of unstable expansions of trinucleotide repeats in a dozen diseases. The CGG expansions in the fragile X mental retardation (FMR1) gene, the CTG expansions at the myotonic dystrophy locus, and the recently discovered GAA expansions in Friedreich's ataxia, all untranslated, cause pleiotropic pathological or clinical manifestations affecting very different organs, even though the corresponding diseases are considered primarily neurological (Campuzano et al. 1996; Paulson and Fischbeck 1996; Eberhart and Warren; Caskey et al., both this volume). On the contrary, the expansions of CAG repeats coding for polyglutamines appear as purely neurodegenerative diseases, as all clinical manifestations can be ascribed to selective late-onset neuronal death (with the exception of the usually mild symptoms of androgen resistance in Kennedy disease). These mutations have previously been found in five diseases (Table 1), including Huntington's disease (HD), the most frequent and best known of all (Paulson and Fischbeck 1996; Gusella et al., this volume), and we recently reported evidence that two additional forms of spinocerebellar ataxia are caused by the same mechanism (Trottier et al. 1995b and see below). Spino-bulbar muscular atrophy (SBMA, or Kennedy disease) is caused by expansions of polyglutamines in the amino-terminal region of the androgen receptor (La Spada et al. 1991). The function of the proteins implicated in the other diseases is unknown, as they show no similarity among themselves, or to proteins of identified function.

Polyglutamine expansion diseases share very similar characteristics. In all of them, there is selective "programmed" death of neurons in different brain regions, and it is the nature of the affected neurons that accounts for the different clinical symptoms (Ross 1995; Paulson and Fischbeck 1996). Other cells or tissues do not appear affected. The number of glutamines in the normal form is variable, always in the same range of about 10–35 (Table 1). Past the pathological threshold (36–40 glutamines for HD, SBMA, and SCA1), there is a correlation between polyglutamine length and severity (longer repeats causing earlier age of onset). All these diseases show to various degrees the anticipation phenomenon: i.e., children tend to be affected at an earlier age than their affected parent. This is due to a further increase in the number of repeats that occurs often when a father (at least for HD, SCA1, or dentatorubropallidolysian atrophy [DRPLA]) transmits the mutation to some of his children (Paulson and Fischbeck 1996). The parental bias of instability is less obvious in SCA3 (Dürr et al. 1996; Igaraschi et al. 1996).

The characteristics of these diseases led to the conclusion that the expansion mutation does not cause a loss of function of the gene (as in the vast majority of genetic diseases), but confers a novel property (a gain of function) to the affected protein, which is responsible for neuronal death. A major problem is to understand why these proteins can tolerate, in their normal forms, a very wide variation in the number of glutamines, whereas a few more will cause the disease, and even more glutamines will accelerate its course. What is the nature of the "gain of function?" The other puzzling question is what causes the selectivity of the brain lesions, as the proteins implicated are found very widely in the brain and in many other organs of the body.

RESULTS

Localization of Huntingtin

The protein implicated in Huntington's disease is a very large (350 kD) protein of unknown function. We have previously characterized four monoclonal antibodies raised against fusion proteins corresponding to four regions of the protein. This allowed us to establish, concurrently with other groups, that the mutant protein can be distinguished from the normal one on the basis of size, indicating that the polyglutamine expansion is indeed present in the mature protein (Trottier et al. 1995a). Initial immunohistochemical analysis of postmortem brain tissue showed a localization in the cytoplasm of some neurons and a punctate pattern suggestive of an association with nerve endings; similar results were reported by Sharp et al. (1995). A more

[4]Present address: Division of Neuroscience, Children's Hospital, Department of Neurobiology, Harvard Medical School, Boston, Massachusetts 02115.

Table 1. Characteristics of the Polyglutamine Expansion Diseases

Disease	Protein	Function localization	Neuropathology[a]	Polyglutamine size	
				normal	disease
SBMA	androgen receptor	transcription factor (N)	anterior horn cells, brain stem motor neuron, dorsal root ganglia	11–33	40–62
HD	huntingtin	? (C)	striatum (medium spiny neurons) cerebral cortex	11–35	36–121
DRPLA	atrophin	? (C)	dentate, red and subthalamic nuclei, globus pallidus	7–35	49–79
SCA1	ataxin-1	? (N,C)	Purkinje cells, spino-cerebellar system	9–39*	40–81
SCA2	ataxin-2	? (C)	substantia nigra, pontine nuclei, inferior olives, cerebellar peduncles	17–29*	37–50
SCA3/MJD	ataxin-3	? (C)	dentate, red, subthalamic and pontine nuclei, globus pallidus	12–40	61–84
SCA7/ADCA II	(130 kD)	? (N)		not cloned	

(C) Cytoplasmic; (N) nuclear; (*) interrupted CAG repeats. For references see Ross (1995), Paulson and Fischbeck (1996), and Imbert et al. (1996) for SCA2.

[a]Primary sites.

prominent cytoplasmic labeling of cell bodies and dendrites was found by DiFiglia et al. (1995), who also reported partial association with membranes of vesicles. Gutekunst et al. (1995) also reported a cytosolic localization in somatodendritic regions of large neurons, but noted an association with microtubules in dendrites and rarer labeling of axon terminals.

We have recently performed an analysis of a fresh cortex sample (adjacent to a tumor). This showed enhanced staining of neurons in cerebral cortex (compared to postmortem brain), especially for large pyramidal neurons. The staining is cytoplasmic, excluding the nucleus, and concerns perikaryon, dendrites, and some axons (Fig. 1). Nerve terminals were only exceptionally and weakly stained (Fig. 1D). Staining in dendrites suggested an association with microtubules (Fig. 1B), whereas diffuse staining of the cytoplasm indicated a cytosolic localization. Analysis of the subcellular localization of huntingtin by fractionation of differentiated mouse NG108-15 neuroblastoma cells showed that huntingtin is enriched in the 140,000*g* fraction which contains synaptophysin (Fig. 2), as reported for rat brain by DiFiglia et al. (1995) and Sharp et al. (1995). However, the majority of huntingtin was present in the cytosolic fraction, in agreement with the immunohistochemistry and electron microscopy results.

All these results indicate that, unlike the androgen receptor (implicated in SBMA) and many other polyglutamine-containing proteins (Gerber et al. 1994), huntingtin is not a transcription factor. The localization of huntingtin may be consistent with a putative role in intracellular trafficking (DiFiglia et al. 1995; Gutekunst et al. 1995).

Selective Recognition of Proteins with Pathological Polyglutamine Tracts by a Monoclonal Antibody

Polyglutamine stretches are present in many other eukaryotic proteins, including a number of transcription factors (Gerber et al. 1994), and in proteins of unknown function identified by screens for CAG repeats in cDNA libraries (Li et al. 1993; Jiang et al. 1995; Neri et al. 1996). In humans, the most common allelic form of the TATA-binding protein (TBP), a basic transcription factor, has a stretch of 38 uninterrupted glutamines (Gostout et al. 1993; Imbert et al. 1994), and rare variants have 42 glutamines. This represents the longest polyglutamine stretch in a human protein not known to be associated with a neurodegenerative disease. A monoclonal antibody (1C2) raised against TBP was previously shown to recognize the polyglutamine-containing region (Lescure et al. 1995). We found that this antibody possesses the unexpected property of recognizing selectively the mutated proteins involved in HD and in other polyglutamine expansion diseases (Trottier et al. 1995b). The ability of this antibody to detect mutated huntingtin depends strikingly on the length of the polyglutamine stretch. HD proteins having a large pathological number of glutamines (associated with an early-onset disease) are detected much more efficiently than those having

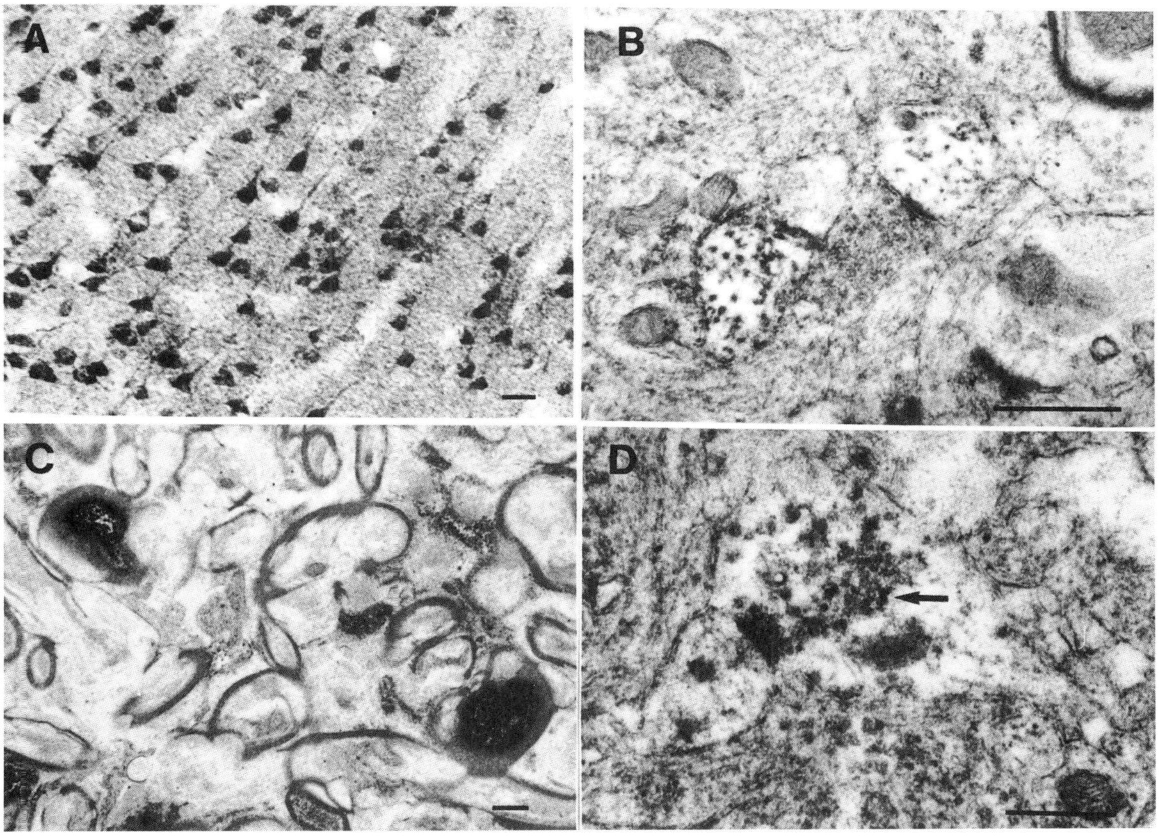

Figure 1. Immunohistochemical localization of huntingtin in normal human cortex. Frozen sections from a cortex biopsy were fixed in paraformaldehyde and analyzed with the 4E6 MAb, using immunoperoxidase. (*A*) Light microscopy showing dense staining of the pyramidal cells and their dendrites. (*B–D*) Electron microscopy. (*B*) In a cross-section of a dendrite, DAB reaction product is associated with microtubules. (*C*) Strong labeling of two myelinized axons. (*D*) Rare axon terminals contain DAB reaction product associated with the synaptic vesicles (*arrow*). Bars: (*A*) 20 μm, (*B–D*) 0.5 μm. (Methods as in Stoeckel et al. 1994.)

fewer repeats (Fig. 3). A semi-quantitative comparison showed that the intensity of signal for huntingtin with 85 glutamines is 2–4 times higher than that with 60 glutamines, and the latter is 10–20 times higher than for huntingtin having 39 glutamines (not shown). Under the pathological threshold of 38 glutamines, the protein is barely detectable (and not at all under 30 glutamines) (Fig. 3). The efficiency of the detection thus parallels the severity of the disease.

This antibody is also able to detect specifically in Western blot analysis the pathological proteins (but not the normal ones) present in lymphoblastoid cells of patients with spinocerebellar ataxias type 1 and type 3 (Trottier et al. 1995b). Even for TBP against which this monoclonal antibody was raised, the allelic forms with 38–42 glutamines are recognized more strongly in a whole protein extract than those with 32–33 glutamines, and those with 29–30 glutamines were barely detectable. This confirms that the 1C2 monoclonal antibody detects with high sensitivity a specific conformation epitope that appears in repeats of more than about 35 repeats, and that might be stabilized or more predominant in longer repeats.

We then tested this antibody in other inherited neurodegenerative diseases for which the genes (and corresponding proteins) have not been yet identified, and that show a strong anticipation phenomenon. Indeed, this antibody detected specifically two different proteins in two other diseases: spinocerebellar ataxia type 2 (a disease indistinguishable clinically from SCA1 and SCA3, but affecting a different gene, linked to chromosome 12; Gispert et al. 1993), and spinocerebellar ataxia with retinal degeneration (SCA7), a clinical entity showing linkage to chromosome 3 in all families tested (Benomar et al. 1995; Holmberg et al. 1995). This demonstrated that polyglutamine expansions are also responsible for these two other neurodegenerative diseases. Furthermore, we showed that the SCA2 protein is in the cytoplasm of cells, whereas the SCA7 protein is in the nucleus (Trottier et al. 1995b). This confirms that the various proteins implicated in the seven known polyglutamine diseases have

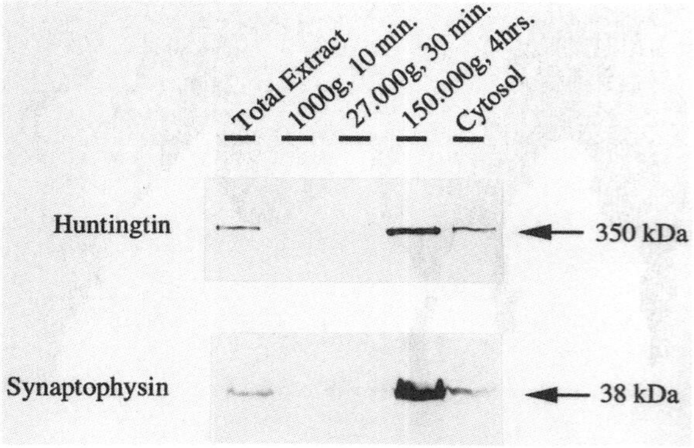

Figure 2. Subcellular localization of huntingtin. Rodent neuroblastoma cell line NG108-15 was differentiated by cAMP treatment (DMEM plus 1% inactivated FCS, isobutylmethylxanthine 100 μM, forskolin 10 μM, 6 days) and subjected to subcellular fractionation by successive centrifugation steps. 50 μg of each fraction was analyzed by Western blotting and immunoprobed with the 4C8 MAb raised against huntingtin (Trottier et al. 1995a) or an anti-synaptophysin MAb (SVP-38, Sigma Immuno Chemicals). The cytosolic fraction contained about 40% of the cell proteins, and the synaptic vesicle fraction (150,000*g*) about 7%. (Adapted from Linstedt and Kelly 1991.)

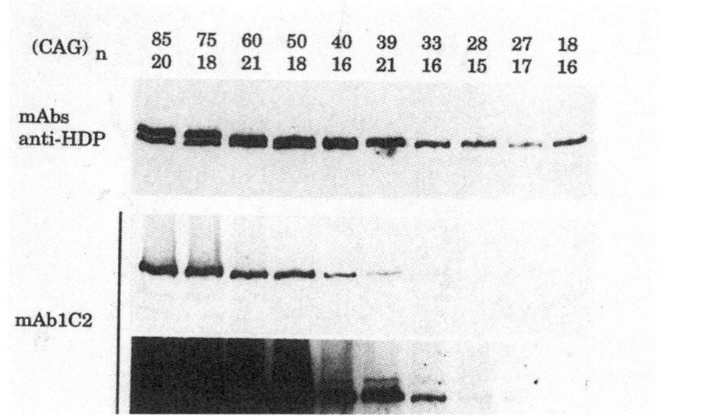

Figure 3. Selective detection of huntingtin with expanded polyglutamine. Lymphoblastoid cell extracts from HD and normal individuals are ordered by decreasing length of polyglutamine with respect to the larger allele. Using specific anti-huntingtin MAb, allelic huntingtins show equivalent signal intensities. With the MAb 1C2, the intensity of signal of the mutated huntingtins increases with the length of the polyglutamine stretch, from 39 to 85 glutamines. A gross overexposure of the blot shows a detectable signal of huntingtins with 28–33 glutamines (*bottom*). (Reprinted, with permission, from Trottier et al. 1995b [copyright Macmillan].)

very little in common with respect to their normal function in the cell.

We have more recently used the 1C2 monoclonal antibody to screen two cDNA expression libraries derived from lymphoblasts from a SCA2 and a SCA7 patient, respectively. Under the bacteriophage plaque screening conditions used (no SDS treatment as in Western blots), we observed that 1C2 is able to recognize shorter glutamine repeats (above 11 glutamines), and we thus identified five new polyglutamine coding cDNAs, including one that corresponds to a normal allele of the SCA2 gene (Imbert et al. 1996).

This antibody may be a useful tool for identifying new proteins/genes involved in other glutamine repeat neurodegenerative diseases and, in particular, for testing whether the same mechanism may be involved in other diseases with suggested anticipation. These include certain families with schizophrenia, manic depressive illness, rare familial forms of Parkinson's disease, etc. (Ross et al. 1993). It should be emphasized that the presence of anticipation in psychiatric diseases is rather controversial, as anticipation is a clinical observation that can also be caused by ascertainment bias (McInnis et al. 1993). In any case, given the high genetic heterogeneity of these diseases, expansion mutations are very unlikely to constitute a major factor. The antibody may also be used to selectively follow the localization and fate of the abnormal proteins in brain samples from patients deceased from a polyglutamine expansion disease, or in suitable animal models (such as the SCA1 mouse model recently constructed by Burright et al. 1995; see also Orr and Zoghbi, this volume). This may help us to understand the pathological mechanisms leading to neuronal death.

Toward Cellular and Animal Models for HD

To gain insight into the mechanism of toxicity of the mutated huntingtin, we generated clonal cell lines expressing either the normal or the mutated huntingtin. We used the NG108-15 neuroblastoma cell line (a hybrid between mouse neuroblastoma and rat glioma cells), which can be morphologically differentiated upon cAMP exposure. These cells then stop dividing, extend long neurite-like processes, and express neuronal markers. Using the whole HD cDNA under the control of the cytomegalovirus (CMV) promoter, we established NG108-15 stable cell lines expressing, in addition to the endogenous rodent huntingtin, either a normal huntingtin with 15 glutamines (HD-15) or a mutated huntingtin with 73 glutamines (HD-73) (Fig. 4A). The latter corresponds to a juvenile-onset form of the disease. In normal culture condition, there was no apparent effect of the expression of the mutated huntingtin. Upon 4–6 days of cAMP treatment, we noticed an increased cellular mortality in three independent clones expressing HD-73 compared to wild-type cells or HD-15 transformed cells. However, upon prolonged passage of the HD-73 cells, this effect was lost (Fig. 4B). An analysis of the cell line showed that this correlated with a loss of expression of the mutated protein at higher passages (Fig. 4A). This confirms that the toxicity is due to the presence of the mutated huntingtin and suggests that these cells will be useful as a cellular model for HD. The presence of specific DNA laddering in HD-73 cAMP-treated cells suggests that the toxicity occurs through an apoptotic mecha-

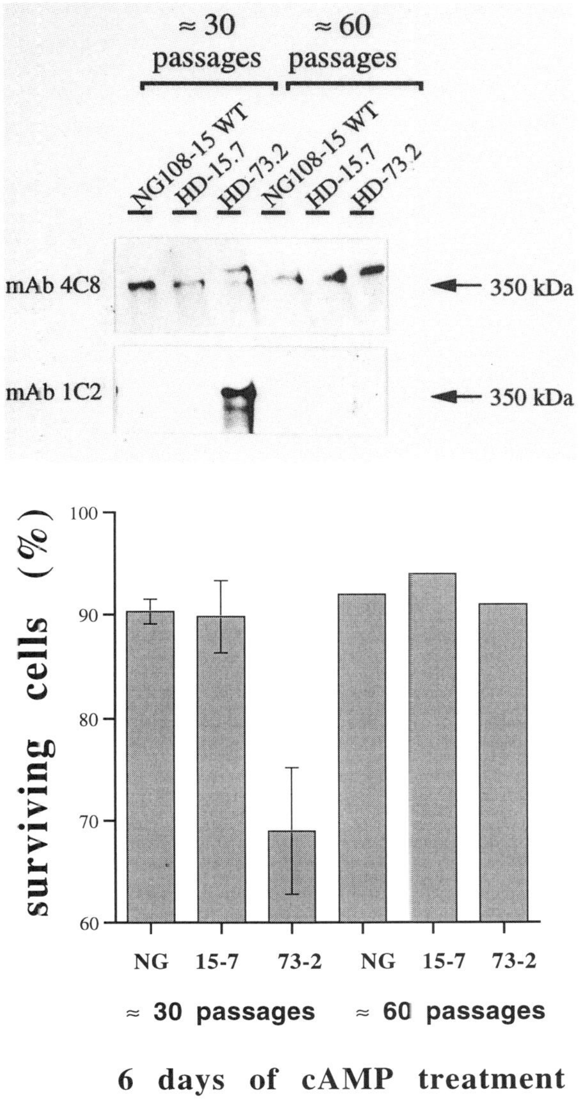

Figure 4. Increased cell death in NG108-15 expressing the mutated huntingtin. (*A*) Generation of rodent neuroblastoma cell lines expressing the normal huntingtin with 15 glutamines (HD-15) or the mutated huntingtin with 73 glutamines (HD-73). NG108-15 cells were transformed with the HD cDNA having 15 CAGs or 73 CAGs under the control of the CMV promoter by the calcium phosphate method and selected by G418 (0.5 mg/ml). Clones HD-15.7 and HD-73.2 were analyzed for the expression of huntingtin by Western blotting (cells at 30 passages). Note the presence of a doublet for the HD-73.2 cells, the upper band corresponding to the mutated huntingtin. The mutated huntingtin is also detected with the MAb 1C2 that recognize expanded polyglutamine, whereas there is no signal for the wild-type NG108-15 or the HD-15.7 cells. After 60 passages in normal culture conditions, expression of the mutated huntingtin was lost. (*B*) Cells were treated during 6 days by cAMP in a 1% FCS-containing medium, and MTT (0.5 mg/ml, Sigma) was added to the plates (3 hr). Toxicity was assayed by visual counting of viable and dead cells and is expressed as a percentage of surviving cells. The data are means ± S.E.M. for at least three independent experiments.

nism (not shown). Interestingly, cell death is correlated to the presence of a 90-kD (apparent m.w.) breakdown product containing the polyglutamine stretch (F. Saudou, in prep.).

These constructs were also used to generate transgenic mice. Four founders carrying the HD-73 transgene were obtained. Low levels of expression were detected in the offspring. Indeed, in brain extracts, mutated huntingtin was only detected by the 1C2 monoclonal antibody but not by anti-huntingtin monoclonal antibody, and the levels of expression of the transgene were about 30- to 100-fold lower than for the endogenous huntingtin. The founder mice and some of the positive offspring expressed from 4 to 6 months of age a puzzling behavioral phenotype characterized by the tendency for the mice, when taken from their cage, to go back rapidly and climb into the cage. In the founders (C57BL/6–DBA/2 heterozygous mice), the intensity of this phenotype appeared to correlate with the level of expression of the transgene; however, this phenotype was lost in almost all the offspring (backcrossed to C57BL/6). We are currently investigating the possibility that this phenotype is dependent on the DBA background. Immunohistochemistry analyses are being performed in these mice to determine if any neuropathology can be detected, particularly concerning striatal neurons, but the low expression of the transgene indicates that these mice will probably not provide an optimum model for the analysis of HD mechanisms. More efficient promoters are required to drive the expression of the mutated huntingtin. Using a strong Purkinje-cell-specific promoter, it has been shown by other workers that a mutated ataxin-1 protein (with 82 glutamines) and a truncated mutated ataxin-3 (but not the corresponding full-length protein) can indeed elicit impressive Purkinje cell degeneration (Burright et al. 1995; Ikeda et al. 1996; Orr and Zoghbi, this volume).

DISCUSSION

The mechanisms by which expanded polyglutamines cause specific neuronal death constitute a fascinating but unsolved problem. It seems clear that this occurs through a gain of toxic properties or function. This was demonstrated for HD and SBMA. Patients homozygous for the expansion in the HD gene show no increased severity compared to heterozygous individuals with the same expansion size (Gusella et al., this volume). However, it should be noted that although based on the analysis of very rare individuals, an increased severity was observed in patients homozygous for DRPLA and SCA3 expanded alleles (Sato et al. 1995; Takiyama et al. 1995; Lerer et al. 1996). More strikingly, patients with testicular feminization syndrome or partial androgen resistance show total or partial loss of function of the androgen receptor (AR), respectively, but have no neurological phenotype. Very mild symptomatology of androgen resistance in SBMA patients indicates that a long polyglutamine tract may slightly decrease AR function, but this cannot account for the symptoms of neuronal degeneration (Brooks and Fischbeck 1995).

Many hypotheses have been proposed to explain the toxicity of expanded polyglutamines. All models need to account for (1) the narrow and similar pathological threshold observed in at least four diseases: 36–40 glutamines for HD, SBMA, SCA1, and SCA2, where 30–35 glutamines are normal; (2) the correlation between increased polyglutamine length and increased severity or decreased age at onset; (3) the absence of apparent correlation between the region-specific neuronal death and the wide expression pattern (with the exception of SBMA, where toxicity to motoneurons seems to correlate with higher expression of the AR in these cells). We briefly review and discuss the various current hypotheses.

Because the only target protein with a known function is the AR, and because many transcription factors contain polyglutamine stretches, it was suggested that increased polyglutamine length could lead to abnormal *trans*-activation properties and abnormal expression of some target genes. Whereas cotransfection and in vitro studies showed that polyglutamine length may indeed modulate activity of the AR or of chimeric transcription factors (Chamberlain et al. 1994; Gerber et al. 1994; Kazemi-Esfarjani et al. 1995), the fact that the proteins implicated in HD, SCA3, and DRPLA are not nuclear indicates that they are not transcription factors.

Preferential DNA expansion in affected brain regions was suggested as a possible mechanism, based on the observation that in early-onset HD patients with a very large expansion, the size of the polyglutamine tract was smaller in the unaffected cerebellum than in other brain regions (Telenius et al. 1994). However, a smaller size was also observed in cerebellum in a SCA1 patient, suggesting that this phenomenon is unrelated to the region-specific pathology (Chong et al. 1995). Additionally, in the vast majority of patients, the observed somatic mosaicism for repeat length appears extremely limited and thus of doubtful functional significance. However, as suggested by J. Gusella (pers. comm.), one cannot exclude that further elongation of the repeat may occur in some neurons in a stochastic manner; for instance, as a result of a DNA repair mechanism, and would not be detected if it leads to preferential death of the affected neuron.

Green (1993) suggested that long polyglutamine could constitute an abnormal target for neuronal transglutaminases, generating cross-links and toxic degradation products. It seems difficult, however, to see how a change in a few glutamine residues could alter sensitivity to transglutaminases, especially given the large number of other polyglutamine-containing proteins present in the cells, unless there is a conformational change above the pathological threshold that alters sensitivity to transglutaminases (see below). In addition, the regional specificity of neurodegeneration would not to be accounted for with such an hypothesis.

A change in conformation past the pathological threshold would be consistent also with two current hypotheses: (1) the existence of abnormal interactions between the mutant proteins and proteins preferentially present in the neurons susceptible to degenerate; (2) an abnormality of processing generating toxic products, dependent on the presence/activity of relevant proteases in specific neurons. Our results with the 1C2 antibody indeed indicate that such a conformational change occurs, and the striking correlation between increased polyglutamine length and increased affinity for the monoclonal antibody, past the pathological threshold, suggests that the epitope recognized by 1C2 is directly involved in the disease mechanisms. Perutz and colleagues showed that even rather short glutamine repeats may favor protein/protein interactions and oligomerization by forming β-pleated sheets ("polar zippers") (Perutz et al. 1994; Stott et al. 1995). It is not clear, however, how such a structure could account for the narrow threshold and for the dramatic effect of increased polyglutamine length. A direct structural analysis of the conformation of long polyglutamine is thus warranted. We have initiated a project to analyze by crystallography the amino-terminal region of TBP (38 Gln) complexed to the FAb fragment of the 1C2 antibody.

Proteins interacting with the polyglutamine tract, or whose interaction with huntingtin, ataxin, or atrophin is modulated by polyglutamine length, are now being identified. These include the brain-specific HAP-1 protein, calmodulin, or the very abundant protein GAPDH (Li et al. 1995; Bao et al. 1996; Burke et al. 1996; Koshy et al. 1996). HAP-1 interaction with huntingtin is enhanced by expanded polyglutamine (Li et al. 1995), and this protein shows a rather specific pattern of expression in neurons, but that does not seem to correlate well with HD pathology (Li et al. 1996). Although GAPDH interacts in experimental systems with the proteins implicated in HD, DRPLA, SBMA, and SCA1, an effect of polyglutamine length has not been demonstrated (Burke et al. 1996; Koshy et al. 1996), and it is difficult to think that such an abundant protein may be affected by the quantitatively very minor proteins subject to polyglutamine expansion. Thus, other interacting proteins must be sought. The example of the 1C2 antibody suggests that other proteins with similar recognition properties may exist.

Abnormal processing of proteins with expanded polyglutamine may be another way to explain toxicity (Cha and Dure 1994). Goldberg et al. (1996) have recently shown an increased sensitivity of mutated huntingtin to a cysteine protease (apopain) implicated in apoptotic processes, with appearance of specific cleavage products of 80–90 kD apparent molecular weight containing the polyglutamine. In our stably transformed lines expressing a huntingtin with 73 repeats, we found both increased apoptosis and increased presence of a similar 90-kD polyglutamine-containing product. Whether presence of the 90-kD product in these cells is a cause or a consequence of apoptosis remains to be elucidated. A cascade mechanism can be imagined, whereby a mutated protein could facilitate the initiation of an apoptotic process that would then accelerate the generation of toxic processing products. Indeed, experiments with truncated mutated SCA3 constructs have shown, in both transfected cells and transgenic mice, that shorter polyglutamine-containing proteins may be much more toxic than the complete protein (Ikeda et al. 1996). A modulating effect of the remaining protein might also account for the higher pathological threshold observed for SCA3, and to a lesser extent for DRPLA.

In conclusion, although initially it might seem doubtful whether one might obtain cellular or mouse models for such diseases, characterized by a rather late onset in humans, recent work shows that useful models can indeed be obtained that should help to decipher the mechanisms of polyglutamine expansion diseases. Pathways of neuronal death may be better studied in cellular models, but the problem of why different neurons are affected in different diseases will require construction of transgenic mice that express different mutated proteins under the same promoter, or the same protein under different promoters, in order to distinguish whether it is the nature of the target proteins, their mode of expression, or a conjunction of both that determines the specific neuropathology.

ACKNOWLEDGMENTS

We thank C. Weber for her most efficient help, Dr L. Tora and Y. Lutz for the monoclonal antibodies, and Dr. M. LeMeur and the mouse facility for establishing transgenic mice. This work was supported by grants from Association Française Contre les Myopathies, CNRS, INSERM, Groupement de Recherches et d'Etudes sur les Génomes, and Centre Hospitalier Régional Universitaire de Strasbourg. G.I. and Y.T. were supported by Association Huntington France, Ecole Polytechnique, Medical Research Council of Canada, and the Hereditary Disease Foundation.

REFERENCES

Bao, J., A.H. Sharp, M.V. Wagster, M. Becher, G. Schilling, C.A. Ross, V.L. Dawson, and T.M. Dawson. 1996. Expansion of polyglutamine repeat in huntingtin leads to abnormal interactions involving calmodulin. *Proc. Natl. Acad. Sci.* **93:** 5037.

Benomar, A., L. Krols, G. Stevanin, G. Cancel, E. Leguern, G. David, H. Ouhabi, J.J. Martin, A. Durr, A. Zaim, N. Ravise, C. Busque, C. Penet, N. Vanregemorter, J. Weissenbach, M. Yahyaoui, T. Chkili, Y. Agid, C. Vanbroeckhoven, and A. Brice. 1995. The gene for autosomal dominant cerebellar ataxia with pigmentary macular dystrophy maps to chromosome 3p12-p21.1. *Nat. Genet.* **10:** 84.

Brooks, B.P. and K.H. Fischbeck. 1995. Spinal and bulbar muscular atrophy: A trinucleotide-repeat expansion neurodegenerative disease. *Trends Neurosci.* **18:** 459.

Burke, J.R., J.J. Enghild, M.E. Martin, Y.S. Jou, R.M. Myers, A.D. Roses, J.M. Vance, and W.J. Strittmatter. 1996. Huntingtin and DRPLA proteins selectively interact with the enzyme GAPDH. *Nature Med.* **2:** 347.

Burright, E.N., H.B. Clark, A. Servadio, T. Matilla, R.M. Feddersen, W.S. Yunis, L.A. Duvick, H.Y. Zoghbi, and H.T. Orr. 1995. SCA1 transgenic mice: A model for neurodegeneration caused by an expanded CAG trinucleotide repeat. *Cell* **82:** 937.

Campuzano, V., L. Montermini, M.D. Molto, L. Pianese, M. Cossee, F. Cavalcanti, E. Monros, F. Rodius, F. Duclos, A. Monticelli, F. Zara, J. Canizares, H. Koutnikova, S.I. Bidichandani, C. Gellera, A. Brice, P. Trouillas, G. De Michele, A. Filla, R. De Frutos, P. Francisco, P.I. Patel, S. Di Donato, J.-L. Mandel, S. Cocozza, M. Koenig, and M. Pandolfo. 1996. Friedreich's ataxia: Autosomal recessive disease caused by an intronic GAA triplet repeat expansion. *Science* **271:** 1423.

Cha, J.H. and L.S. Dure. 1994. Trinucleotide repeats in neurologic diseases: An hypothesis concerning the pathogenesis of Huntington's disease, Kennedy's disease, and spinocerebellar ataxia type I. *Life Sci.* **54:** 1459.

Chamberlain, N.L., E.D. Driver, and R.L. Miesfeld. 1994. The length and location of CAG trinucleotide repeats in the androgen receptor N-terminal domain affect transactivation function. *Nucleic Acids Res.* **22:** 3181.

Chong, S.S., A.E. McCall, J. Cota, S.H. Subramony, H.T. Orr, M.R. Hughes, and H.Y. Zoghbi. 1995. Gametic and somatic tissue-specific heterogeneity of the expanded SCA1 CAG repeat in spinocerebellar ataxia type 1. *Nat. Genet.* **10:** 344.

DiFiglia, M., E. Sapp, K. Chase, C. Schwarz, A. Meloni, C. Young, E. Martin, J.-P. Vonsattel, R. Carraway, S.A. Reeves, F.M. Boyce, and N. Aronin. 1995. Huntingtin is a cytoplasmic protein associated with vesicules in human and rat brain neurons. *Neuron* **14:** 1075.

Dürr, A., G. Stevanin, G. Cancel, C. Duyckaerts, N. Abbas, O. Didierjean, H. Chneiweiss, Ali. Benomar, and O. LyonCaen. 1996. Spinocerebellar ataxia 3 and Machado-Joseph disease: Clinical, molecular, and neuropathological features. *Ann. Neurol.* **39:** 490.

Gerber, H.P., K. Seipel, O. Georgiev, M. Hofferer, M. Hug, S. Rusconi, and W. Schaffner. 1994. Transcriptional activation modulated by homopolymeric glutamine and proline stretches. *Science* **263:** 808.

Gispert, S., R. Twells, G. Orozco, A. Brice, J. Weber, L. Heredero, K. Scheufler, B. Riley, R. Allotey, C. Nothers, R. Hillermann, A. Lunkes, C. Khati, G. Stevanin, A. Hernandez, C. Magarino, T. Klockgether, A. Durr, H. Chneiweiss, J. Enczmann, M. Farrall, J. Beckmann, M. Mullan, P. Wernet, Y. Agid, H.-J. Freund, R. Williamson, G. Auburger, and S. Chamberlain. 1993. Chromosomal assignment of the second locus for autosomal dominant cerebellar ataxia (SCA2) to chromosome 12q23-24.1. *Nat. Genet.* **4:** 295.

Goldberg, Y.P., D.W. Nicholson, D.M. Rasper, M.A. Kalchman, H.B. Koide, R.K. Graham, M. Bromm, P. Kazemi-Esfarjani, N.A. Thornberry, J.P. Vaillancourt, and M.R. Hayden. 1996. Cleavage of huntingtin by apopain, a proapoptotic cysteine protease, is modulated by the polyglutamine tract. *Nat. Genet.* **13:** 442.

Gostout, B., Q. Liu, and S.S. Sommer. 1993. "Cryptic" repeating triplets of purines and pyrimidines (cRRY(i)) are frequent and polymorphic: Analysis of coding cRRY(i) in the proopiomelanocortin (POMC) and TATA-binding protein (TBP) genes. *Am. J. Hum. Genet.* **52:** 1182.

Green, H. 1993. Human genetic diseases due to codon reiteration: Relationship to an evolutionary mechanism [letter]. *Cell* **74:** 955.

Gutekunst, C.A., A.I. Levey, C.J. Heilman, W.L. Whaley, H. Yi, N.R. Nash, H.D. Rees, J.J. Madden, and S.M. Hersch. 1995. Identification and localization of huntingtin in brain and human lymphoblastoid cell lines with anti-fusion protein antibodies. *Proc. Natl. Acad. Sci.* **92:** 8710.

Holmberg, M., J. Johansson, L. Forsgren, J. Heijbel, O. Sandgren, and G. Holmgren. 1995. Localization of autosomal dominant cerebellar ataxia associated with retinal degeneration and anticipation to chromosome 3p12-p21.1. *Hum. Mol. Genet.* **4:** 1441.

Igaraschi, S., Y. Takiyama, G. Cancel, EA. Rogaeva, H. Sasaki, A. Wakisaka, and Y.X. Zhou. 1996. Intergenerational instability of the CAG repeat of the gene for Machado-Joseph (MJD1) is affected by the genotype of normal chromosome: Implications for the molecular mechanisms of the instability of the CAG repeat. *Hum. Mol. Genet.* **5:** 923.

Ikeda, H., M. Yamaguchi, S. Sugai, Y. Aze, S. Narumiya, and A. Kakizuka. 1996. Expanded polyglutamine in the Machado-Joseph disease protein induces cell death in vitro and in vivo. *Nat. Genet.* **13:** 196.

Imbert, G., Y. Trottier, J. Beckman, and J.-L. Mandel. 1994. The gene for the TATA-binding protein (TBP) that contains a highly polymorphic protein coding CAG repeat maps to 6q27. *Genomics* **21:** 667.

Imbert, G., F. Saudou, G. Yvert, D. Devys, Y. Trottier, J.M. Garnier, C. Weber, J.L. Mandel, G. Cancel, N. Abbas, A. Dürr, O. Didierjean, G. Stevanin, Y. Agid, and A. Brice. 1996. Cloning of the gene for spinocerebellar ataxia 2 reveals a locus with high sensitivity to expanded CAG/glutamine repeats and high instability. *Nat. Genet.* **14:** 285.

Jiang, J.-X., R. Lekanne Deprez, E. Zwarthoff, and P. Riegman. 1995. Characterization of four novel CAG repeat-containing cDNAs. *Genomics* **30:** 91.

Kazemi-Esfarjani, P., M.A. Trifiro, and L. Pinsky. 1995. Evidence for a repressive function of the long polyglutamine tract in the human androgen receptor: Possible pathogenetic relevance for the (CAG)(n)-expanded neuronopathies. *Hum. Mol. Genet.* **4:** 523.

Koshy, B., T. Matilla, E.N. Burright, D.E. Merry, K.H. Fischbeck, H.T. Orr, and H.Y. Zoghbi. 1996. Spinocerebellar ataxia type-1 and spinobulbar muscular atrophy gene products interact with glyceraldehyde-3-phosphate dehydrogenase. *Hum. Mol. Genet.* **5:** 1311.

La Spada, A.R., E.M. Wilson, D.B. Lubahn, A.E. Harding, and K.H. Fischbeck. 1991. Androgen receptor gene mutations in X-linked spinal and bulbar muscular atrophy. *Nature* **352:** 77.

Lerer, I., D. Merims, D. Abeliovich, J. Zlotogora, and N. Gadoth. 1996. Machado-Joseph disease: Correlation between the clinical features, the CAG repeat length and homozygosity for the mutation. *Eur. J. Hum. Genet.* **4:** 3.

Lescure, A., Y. Lutz, D. Eberhard, X. Jacq, A. Krol, I. Grummt, I. Davidson, P. Chambon, and L. Tora. 1995. The N-terminal domain of the human TATA-binding protein plays a role in transcription from TATA-containing RNA polymerase II and III promoters. *EMBO J.* **13:** 1166.

Li, S.H., M.G. McInnis, R.L. Margolis, S.E. Antonarakis, and C.A. Ross. 1993. Novel triplet repeat containing genes in human brain: Cloning, expression, and length polymorphisms. *Genomics* **16:** 572.

Li, X.J., A.H. Sharp, S.H. Li, T.M. Dawson, S.H. Snyder, and C.A. Ross. 1996. Huntingtin associated protein (HAP1): Discrete neuronal localizations in the brain resemble those of neuronal nitric oxide synthase. *Proc. Natl. Acad. Sci.* **93:** 4839.

Li, X.J., S.H. Li, A.H. Sharp, F.C. Nucifora, Jr., G. Schilling, A. Lanahan, P. Worley, S.H. Snyder, and C.A. Ross. 1995. A huntingtin-associated protein enriched in brain with implications for pathology. *Nature* **378:** 398.

Linstedt, A.D. and R.B. Kelly. 1991. Synaptophysin is sorted from endocytotic markers in neuroendocrine PC12 cells but not transfected fibroblasts. *Neuron* **7:** 309.

McInnis, M.G., F.J. McMahon, G.A. Chase, S.G. Simpson, C.A. Ross, and J.R. De Paulo, Jr. 1993. Anticipation in bipolar affective disorder [see comments]. *Am. J. Hum. Genet.* **53:** 385.

Neri, C., V. Albanese, A.S. Lebre, S. Holbert, C. Saada, L. Bougueleret, S. Meier-Ewert, I. LeGall, P. Millasseau, H. Bui, C. Giudicelli, C. Massart, and S. Guillou. 1996. Survey of CAG/CTG repeats in human cDNAs representing new genes: Candidates for inherited neurological disorders. *Hum. Mol. Genet.* **5:** 1001.

Paulson, H.L. and K.H. Fischbeck. 1996. Trinucleotide repeats in neurogenetic disorders. *Annu. Rev. Neurosci.* **19:** 79.

Perutz, M.F., T. Johnson, M. Suzuki, and J.T. Finch. 1994. Glutamine repeats as polar zippers: Their possible role in inherited neurodegenerative diseases. *Proc. Natl. Acad. Sci.* **91:** 5355.

Ross, C. 1995. When more is less: Pathogenesis of glutamine repeat neurodegenerative diseases. *Neuron* **15:** 493.

Ross, C.A., M.G. McInnis, R.L. Margolis, and S.-H. Li. 1993. Genes with triplets: Candidate mediators of neuropsychiatric disorders. *Trends Neurosci.* **16:** 254.

Sato, K., K. Kashihara, S. Okada, T. Ikeuchi, S. Tsuji, T. Shomori, K. Morimoto, and T. Hayabara. 1995. Does homozygosity advance the onset of dentatorubral-pallidoluysian atrophy? *Neurology* **45:** 1934.

Sharp, A.H., S.J. Loev, G. Schilling, S.H. Li, X.J. Li, J. Bao, M.V. Wagster, J.A. Kotzuk, J.P. Steiner, A. Lo, J. Hedreen, S. Sisodia, S.H. Snyder, T.M. Dawson, D.K. Ryugo, and C.A. Ross. 1995. Widespread expression of Huntington's disease gene (IT15) protein product. *Neuron* **14:** 1065.

Stoeckel, M.E., C. Hindelang, M.J. Klein, M. Poissonnier, and J.M. Felix. 1994. Expression of the alpha-subunit of glycoprotein hormones in the pars tuberalis-specific glandular cells in rat, mouse and guinea-pig. *Cell Tissue Res.* **278:** 617.

Stott, K., J.M. Blackburn, P.J.G. Butler, and M. Perutz. 1995. Incorporation of glutamine repeats makes protein oligomerize: Implication for neurodegenerative diseases. *Proc. Natl. Acad. Sci.* **92:** 6509.

Takiyama, Y., S. Igarashi, E.A. Rogaeva, K. Endo, E.I. Rogaev, H. Tanaka, R. Sherrington, K. Sanpei, Y. Liang, M. Saito, T. Tsuda, H. Takano, M. Ikeda, C. Lin, H. Chi, J.L. Kennedy, A.E. Lang, J.R. Wherrett, M. Segawa, Y. Nomura, T. Yuasa, J. Weissenbach, M. Yoshida, M. Nishizawa, K.K. Kidd, S. Tsuji, and P.H. St. George-Hyslop. 1995. Evidence for inter-generational instability in the CAG repeat in the MJD1 gene and for conserved haplotypes at flanking markers amongst Japanese and

Caucasian subjects with Machado-Joseph disease. *Hum. Mol. Genet.* **4:** 1137.

Telenius, H., B. Kremer, Y.P. Goldberg, J. Theilmann, S.E. Andrew, J. Zeisler, S. Adam, C. Greeberg, E.J. Ives, L.A. Clarke, and M.R. Hayden. 1994. Somatic and gonodal mosaicism of the Huntington disease gene CAG repeat in brain and sperm. *Nat. Genet.* **6:** 409.

Trottier, Y., D. Devys, G. Imbert, F. Saudou, I. An, Y. Lutz, C. Weber, Y. Agid, E.C. Hirsch, and J.L. Mandel. 1995a. Cellular localization of the Huntington's disease protein and discrimination of the normal and mutated form. *Nat. Genet.* **10:** 104.

Trottier, Y., Y. Lutz, G. Stevanin, G. Imbert, D. Devys, G. Cancel, F. Saudou, C. Weber, G. David, L. Tora, Y. Agid, A. Brice, and J.-L. Mandel. 1995b. Polyglutamine expansion as a pathological epitope in Huntington's disease and four dominant cerebellar ataxias. *Nature* **378:** 403.

Toward Understanding Polyglutamine-induced Neurological Disease in Spinocerebellar Ataxia Type 1

H.T. ORR[1] AND H.Y. ZOGHBI[2]

[1]*Departments of Laboratory Medicine and Pathology, Biochemistry, and Institute of Human Genetics, University of Minnesota, Minneapolis, Minnesota 55455;* [2]*Department of Human and Molecular Genetics, Pediatrics, Neurology, and Howard Hughes Medical Institute, Baylor College of Medicine, Houston, Texas 77030*

Autosomal dominantly inherited spinocerebellar ataxias (SCAs) are a complex group of disorders, each with a variable degree of neurodegeneration, causing dysfunction of the cerebellum, spinal tracts, and brain stem (Greenfield 1954). Since there is considerable overlap in clinical presentation among the various SCAs, the development of a clinical classification scheme has been very difficult and controversial. The recent advent of molecular genetic approaches to disease classification has resulted in gradual formation of a genetic classification scheme for the SCAs.

Spinocerebellar ataxia type 1 (SCA1) is one form of SCA that has been classified based on its genetic mapping to the short arm of human chromosome 6 (Yakura et al. 1974: Jackson et al. 1977). Clinical features of early stage SCA1 include gait ataxia, dysarthria, and nystagmus. As the disease worsens, ataxia progresses and other cerebellar signs develop, including dysmetria and hypotonia. In later stages of SCA1, muscle atrophy, decreased deep tendon reflexes, and loss of proprioception and vibration sense become common. The final stage of SCA1 is characterized by facial weakness and loss of bulbar functions including severe dysarthria and dysphagia which result in frequent choking and coughing spells, a poor cough reflex, food aspiration, and recurrent pneumonia, which usually results in death.

Typically, SCA1 is an adult-onset disease usually with symptoms developing in the third or fourth decade. In a few instances, juvenile onset of SCA1 has been reported (Schut 1950; Zoghbi et al. 1988). Interestingly, each of these juvenile SCA1 patients inherited the disease from an affected father. In most cases, the disease progresses over a period of 10–15 years. However, in juvenile cases, disease progression is much more rapid (Currier et al. 1982; Zoghbi et al. 1988). Neuropathological studies at autopsy reveal considerable atrophy of the cerebellar cortex with severe degeneration of Purkinje cells and dentate nuclei neurons. In addition, neuronal degeneration is found within the inferior olive and cranial nerve nuclei III, IV, IX, X, and XII. Demyelination of the spinocerebellar tracts and dorsal columns is also noted.

The location of the *SCA1* gene was first determined to be the short arm of chromosome 6 through linkage to the human leukocyte antigen (HLA) complex (Yakura et al. 1974). The *SCA1* locus was next determined to lie distal to the HLA complex on chromosome 6p (Rich et al. 1987). Subsequently, the genetic position of the *SCA1* gene was refined with the demonstration of very close linkage to a polymorphic DNA marker, D6S89 (Ranum et al. 1991; Zoghbi et al. 1991; Kwiatkowski et al. 1993). This marker maps distal to the HLA complex in chromosomal band 6p22-p23. The combined analysis of about 120 affected individuals using D6S89 revealed a single individual in which a chromosomal recombination event had occurred between SCA1 and the marker D6S89. This indicated that, in fact, marker D6S89 is located very close to the *SCA1* gene at a genetic distance of less than 1 cM distal or telomeric to the *SCA1* gene. The next step in the genetic definition of the *SCA1* locus was accomplished with the identification of marker D6S274 as lying proximal or on the centromeric side of the *SCA1* gene. Again, in a large population of SCA1-affected individuals, a single individual with a recombination between *SCA1* and D6S274 was found. Importantly, the genetic distance between the markers flanking the *SCA1* gene, D6S89 and D6S274, was determined to be less than 2.0 cM. This genetic distance roughly corresponds to a physical distance of less than 2.0 Mb of DNA, an amount of DNA that can be fairly readily cloned in overlapping yeast artificial chromosomes (YACs). Thus, the *SCA1* region, from D6S274 to D6S89, was isolated in a series of overlapping YAC clones which formed a contig of 1.2 Mb (Banfi et al. 1993). For the isolation of the *SCA1* gene itself, these YAC clones were subsequently converted into cosmid clones.

Remembering the observation of anticipation in families with SCA (Schut 1950; Zoghbi et al. 1988), we hypothesized that the mutational mechanism causing SCA1 could be an unstable trinucleotide repeat. Therefore, to test this hypothesis, cosmid clones from the *SCA1* candidate region were probed with oligonucleotides representing various permutations of trinucleotide repeats, starting with a CAG-containing oligonucleotide probe (Orr et al. 1993). Twenty-three cosmids from the *SCA1* candidate region hybridized to this CAG-containing probe and shared a common 3.2-kb *Eco*RI fragment. Sequence analysis of this fragment revealed it contained a CAG repeat with a configuration of $(CAG)_{12}CATCAGCAT(CAG)_{15}$. This 3.2-kb *Eco*RI fragment was subsequently used to examine Southern blots of DNAs from members of families with a juvenile case of SCA1. This analysis revealed an enlarged fragment in DNA from the juvenile patients. Moreover, further Southern analyses indicated that an enlarged restriction fragment was present in the DNA of all SCA1 patients but in none of the DNA from unaffected individuals. Oligonucleotide primers flanking the CAG repeat were synthesized for the development of a polymerase chain reaction (PCR)-based test of repeat expansion. This analysis revealed that the *SCA1* CAG repeat is highly polymorphic and that unaffected individuals carry two *SCA1* alleles, each with a repeat size ranging from 6 to 39 CAGs. In contrast, individuals affected with SCA1 have one allele with a repeat number within the unaffected range and a second allele of the *SCA1* gene with 40–82 CAG triplet repeats. So far, the analysis of every ataxia family known to have SCA1 by linkage analysis revealed an expanded allele in each of the affected individuals examined. These data indicate that CAG triplet expansion to a size of 40 or greater is the mutational cause of SCA1 and that other types of mutations within the *SCA1* gene are less likely to have occurred. An important observation regarding the relationship between the CAG repeat and development of disease is that the number of triplet units correlates inversely with the age of onset and disease severity (Orr et al. 1993; Ranum et al. 1994).

The intergenerational stability of the CAG repeat size at *SCA1* has been examined for both unaffected and expanded affected alleles. In over 1000 examples of parent-to-offspring transmission, there have been no reported instances of instability for the CAG repeat on unaffected alleles. On the other hand, the CAG repeat number on expanded *SCA1* alleles is unstable upon transmission from affected parent to offspring. Both decreases and increases in the number of CAG repeats have been noted in transmissions from an affected parent. Interestingly, a significant difference in the type and size of repeat number change has been found in maternal versus paternal transmission of an affected allele (Chung et al. 1993). Of the 16 paternal transmissions examined, 63% resulted in an increase in the number of *SCA1* CAG triplets, with an average increase of 3.3 repeats. In contrast, in 28 cases of maternal transmission of an affected allele, 69% of the transmissions resulted in no change or a decrease in the number of CAG triplets, with an average change of -0.4 triplets. This difference in the intergenerational stability of the CAG repeat between maternal and paternal transmissions is statistically significant ($p<0.005$) and explains the fact that all juvenile cases of SCA1 reported to date have been the result of the transmission of an affected allele from a father to offspring. Moreover, the most dramatic intergenerational increase in *SCA1* CAG repeat number found, an increase of 28 CAG triplets, was in a paternal transmission (Orr et al. 1993).

The presence of CAT trinucleotides interposed between two tracts of CAG triplet repeats on an unaffected *SCA1* allele suggested that this interruption may have a role in the stability of the CAG repeat. To test this hypothesis, the sequence configuration of the CAG repeat was examined on both unaffected and affected *SCA1* alleles using a combination of direct sequence analysis and digestion of PCR products with the restriction enzyme *Sfa*NI which cleaves $GCATC(N)_5$, allowing a determination of the presence of at least one CAT interruption within the CAG repeat. Analysis of 126 chromosomes with an unaffected allele of *SCA1* revealed an interrupted repeat configuration with one, two, or three CAT triplets in 123 out of 126 chromosomes studied (Chung et al. 1993). The only 3 chromosomes with an unaffected allele that lacked the CAT interruption were the 2 smallest unaffected alleles found, one with 19 CAG triplets and 2 chromosomes with 21 CAG repeats. Thus, 98% of the unaffected and stable alleles of *SCA1* had a CAG repeat configuration containing at least one CAT trinucleotide interruption within the CAG repeat tract. In contrast, of the 30 affected *SCA1* chromosomes examined, every single one had a perfect, uninterrupted tract of CAG triplet repeats. Perfect CAG repeat tracts were found on all affected chromosomes from seven unrelated kindreds, with at least four different haplotypes at D6S288 and D6S274. In addition, perfect repeats have also been reported for all of the affected *SCA1* alleles in 19 other SCA1 families (Jodice et al. 1994). These data indicate that the loss of the CAT interruption in alleles of 21 or more repeats renders the CAG repeat unstable and susceptible to subsequent intergenerational expansion (Chung et al. 1993). More recently, comparative analysis of a large normal allele with 39 interrupted midstream CAT interspersions in stabilizing $(CAG)_n$ tracts within the *SCA1* gene (Chong et al. 1995) CAG repeats, and a small affected allele with 40 uninterrupted CAG repeats, revealed that the interrupted allele was somatically stable, whereas the allele with a perfect stretch of CAGs was unstable. These data provide further support for a role of midstream CAT interspersions in stabilizing $(CAG)_n$ tracts within the *SCA1* gene (Chong et al. 1995).

The transcript expressed from the *SCA1* gene is 10,660 bp and is found in a wide variety of different cell and tissue types (Orr et al. 1993; Banfi et al. 1994). The coding region is 2448 bp long and encodes a protein, ataxin-1, of 792–829 amino acids, depending on the number of CAG repeats that encode a polyglutamine tract within the protein. The *SCA1*-encoded protein, designated ataxin-1, is a novel protein without any detectable homologies to previously identified genes or proteins in the databases. Both the 5′-untranslated and 3′-untranslated region of the *SCA1* transcript are extremely long, 935 bp and 7277 bp, respectively.

At the genomic level, the *SCA1* gene spans about 450 kb of DNA and consists of nine exons (Banfi et al.

1994). An unusual feature of the structure of the *SCA1* gene is that the 5′-untranslated region is found in the first seven exons, the region encoding the ataxin-1 protein is located within two large exons, 8 and 9, of 2079 and 7805 bp, respectively. The murine *Sca1* gene has a very similar organization to that of the human gene, and the coding regions of the two genes are highly similar (88% identity at the amino acid level). The only major difference is the virtual absence of the CAG repeat in the mouse sequence, suggesting that the polyglutamine stretch is not critical for the normal function of ataxin-1 in the mouse. RNA in situ expression analysis in the mouse revealed that *Sca1* is widely expressed in the central nervous system postnatally, with the highest expression in hippocampal granular cells and cerebellar Purkinje cells. It is interesting to note that there is a transient burst in *Sca1* expression in Purkinje cells at postnatal day 14, when the cerebellar cortex becomes physiologically functional (Banfi et al. 1996).

Toward a further understanding of the mechanisms underlying SCA1 pathogenesis, our laboratories have pursued studies directed at an examination of the ataxin-1 protein and the development and characterization of a transgenic mouse model of neurodegeneration induced by an expanded allele of *SCA1*.

EXPANDED *SCA1* ALLELES ARE TRANSLATED INTO PROTEIN

Recently, polyclonal antibodies have been generated against the ataxin-1 protein (Servadio et al. 1995). These antisera were used to determine that ataxin-1 is also found in a wide variety of cell and tissue types. When these antibodies were used to probe Western blots of cellular extracts prepared from lymphoblastoid cells established from SCA1 patients with differing numbers of *SCA1* CAG repeats, two bands were detected. One band, about 100 kD in size, is identical in size to the band found in extracts prepared from unaffected individuals. The second ataxin-1 band found in extracts from SCA1-affected individuals is increased in size by an amount proportional to the number of CAG repeats found on their affected *SCA1* allele. These results confirmed that the CAG repeat is located within the coding region of the ataxin-1 protein, and that an expansion of CAG repeat number leads to the production of an ataxin-1 protein with an increased number of amino acids. Since the size of the mutant ataxin-1 protein inversely correlates with the age of onset of SCA1, the change in size of the mutant protein must determine the extent of its abnormal function.

Numerous observations support the concept that the pathogenesis of the CAG-mediated neurodegenerative diseases is due to a gain-of-function mechanism rather than a loss-of-function mechanism. Most notable among these is the fact that males with a deletion of the androgen receptor (AR) do not develop motor neuron disease as do individuals with an expanded number of glutamine repeats in the AR, who develop spinobulbar muscular atrophy (Quigley et al. 1992). Moreover, individuals with a heterozygous deletion of the Huntington disease (HD) gene lack HD-like symptoms (Gusella et al. 1985), and disruption of the *HD* gene in mice is embryonically lethal in null mutant mice and results in no evidence of HD-like symptoms or neuropathology in heterozygote mice with a targeted *HD* gene (Duyao et al. 1995; Nasir et al. 1995; Zeitlin et al. 1995). The fact that in each of the CAG-based diseases the trinucleotide repeat is located within the coding region of the gene and encodes a polyglutamine tract suggests that the pathogenesis is mediated by the expression of the mutant protein.

SUBCELLULAR LOCALIZATION OF ATAXIN-1

Using antisera directed to the carboxy-terminal region of ataxin-1, immunolocalization studies were performed on brain tissue (Servadio et al. 1995). Ataxin-1 protein is detectable in a wide variety of cell types both from individuals affected with SCA1 and from unaffected individuals. Within nonneuronal cells, immunohistochemical studies reveal that ataxin-1 expression is most notable in the cytoplasm. In contrast, in brain cells from SCA1 patients and unaffected individuals, ataxin-1 has a nuclear localization. Purkinje cells in the cerebellar cortex, a cell type exhibiting prominent pathology in SCA1, like other neurons of the CNS exhibit strong nuclear expression of ataxin-1. However, in contrast to the other neuronal cell types, Purkinje cells also have detectable levels of ataxin-1 within their cytoplasm. Thus, by both Western blot analysis and immunohistochemical studies, it is clear that the cerebellum expresses the ataxin-1 protein encoded by an expanded, mutant allele of *SCA1*. Furthermore, subcellular localization studies indicate no gross difference in the cellular compartmentalization of ataxin-1 produced from a normal allele versus a mutant allele of *SCA1*.

SCA1 TRANSGENIC MICE

Given that all available evidence supports a gain-of-function mechanism for SCA1 pathogenesis, transgenic mice carrying either a normal unexpanded or mutant expanded protein were established to test the gain-of-function hypothesis directly (Burright et al. 1995). In these studies, expression of the *SCA1* transgenes was directed specifically to Purkinje cells of the cerebellar cortex using regulatory elements from the *Pcp-2/L7* gene. We and other workers have demonstrated that promoter elements from the *Pcp-2/L7* gene can effectively direct gene expression to Purkinje cells in transgenic mice (Oberdick et al. 1990; Vandaele et al. 1991). *Pcp-2/SCA1* transgenes were constructed carrying either an interrupted 30-CAG repeat (PS-30) or 82 uninterrupted CAG repeats (PS-82). The translational integrity of each construct was verified using transfections in COS cells.

Seven transgenic lines were established for the PS-30 *SCA1* transgene construct, and six transgenic lines were generated carrying the PS-82 *SCA1* transgene. As assessed by reverse transcriptase (RT) PCR and Northern blots, three of the PS-30 lines expressed the transgene at levels between 50 and 100 times that of endogenous murine *Sca1*. Three of the remaining PS-30 lines expressed transgene RNA at a level substantially less than *Sca1*, and one PS-30 line failed to express detectable levels of the transgene. Five of the PS-82 transgenic lines expressed the *SCA1* transgene at a level between 10 and 100 times that of *Sca1*. One PS-82 line failed to express detectable levels of transgene product. None of the PS-30 transgenic animals developed an abnormal neurological phenotype or cerebellar pathology. In contrast, all five of the PS-82 transgenic lines expressing detectable levels of transgene product developed an abnormal neurological phenotype, ataxia, characterized by an initial reduction in cage activity, a gentle swaying of the head while walking, and incoordination. These symptoms progressed in severity until animals were clearly ataxic and often fell while attempting to stand on their hind legs. Transgenic lines with the most severe neurological phenotype exhibited the most severe neuropathological alterations. Evidence of substantial loss of Purkinje cells was found in cerebella from two lines of transgenic mice, B04 and B05. In addition, numerous ectopic Purkinje cells were found within the molecular layer. The dendritic arboration of Purkinje cells from these animals was also very abnormal. Examination of cerebella from several of the PS-30 transgenic lines failed to reveal any gross or microscopic evidence of pathology. Likewise, the single PS-82 line that failed to express the transgene also lacked cerebellar pathology. Thus, all pathological changes found were specific to those transgenic animals expressing a PS-82 transgene.

At the protein level, ataxin-1 encoded by the transgene was readily detectable by Western blot analysis in cerebellar extracts prepared from the three PS-30 transgenic lines expressing high levels of transgene RNA. In contrast, Western blot analysis of cerebellar extracts prepared from each of the high-expressing PS-82 transgenic lines failed to reveal detectable protein product from the expanded allele (Burright et al. 1995). These Western blots were performed on cerebellar extracts from mice at different ages (5–40 weeks), which by Northern analysis, expressed high levels of *SCA1* transgene mRNA. To examine transgene ataxin-1 expression further, we have performed immunohistochemical studies on PS-30 and PS-82 transgenic cerebella using the same anti-ataxin-1 antibodies used for the Western analyses. As predicted from the Western blot studies, immunohistochemical studies using the ataxin-1 antibodies used for the Western analyses, diluted to a concentration that resulted in little or no staining of nontransgenic cerebella (Fig. 1A), revealed substantial nuclear staining for ataxin-1 and some cytoplasmic staining of Purkinje cells in cerebellum from a PS-30 transgenic animal (Fig. 1B). Interestingly, a similar immunohistochemical analysis of ataxin-1 expression in sections of cerebellum from a PS-82 transgenic animal revealed intense nuclear staining and little or no cytoplasmic staining for ataxin-1 (Fig. 1C). Thus, the protein product of an expanded *SCA1* allele is detectable immunohistochemically but not by Western blot. In contrast, ataxin-1 protein encoded by a normal, unexpanded allele is detectable by both immunohistochemical and Western blot analyses. This observation raises the intriguing possibility that the product of an expanded, mutant allele of *SCA1* is in some fashion specifically altered within Purkinje cells, a prominent cellular site of SCA1 pathology.

In an attempt to correlate the pathological alterations with neurological changes, we have initiated a more detailed examination of the time course of events in the PS-82 transgenic line B05. Cerebellar development in B05 animals is normal at least up through postnatal day 16. As evident by Northern analysis, transgene expression is first detectable around postnatal day 10. The first histological abnormality detected in B05 animals is the appearance of intracellular vacuoles within Purkinje cells at postnatal day 25. The first signs of abnormal neurological function, impaired performance on a RotaRod, is seen at 5 weeks of age (Fig. 2). At 8 weeks of age there is a noticeable dwindling of the proximal arborations of Purkinje cell dendritic trees (Fig. 3). Onset of ataxia, as evident by cage behavior, begins in B05 animals at about 12 weeks of age. By 16 weeks of age, there is mild loss of Purkinje cells and the appearance of an occasional ectopic Purkinje cell within the molecular layer. From 20 weeks of age to 14 months, the loss of Purkinje cells, dwindling of their dendritic trees, and presence of ectopic Purkinje cells becomes progressively more extensive. It is important to note that there is a substantial degree of neurological dysfunction in B05 transgenic animals prior to significant loss of Purkinje cells from the cerebellar cortex.

ATAXIN-1/GAPDH INTERACTIONS

To examine the hypothesis that a gain-of-function mechanism mediated by protein-protein interactions involving the expanded glutamine repeat of ataxin-1 is the basis of SCA1 pathogenesis, we have used the yeast two-hybrid system to identify proteins that interact with ataxin-1. Among the clones identified in a screen of a mouse embryonic library was the glycolytic enzyme glyceraldehyde-3-phosphate dehydrogenase (GAPDH) (Koshy et al. 1996). Interaction between ataxin-1 and GAPDH was demonstrated at the protein level in vitro as well. In addition, it was demonstrated that another polyglutamine-containing protein, the AR, also is capable of interacting with GAPDH. The

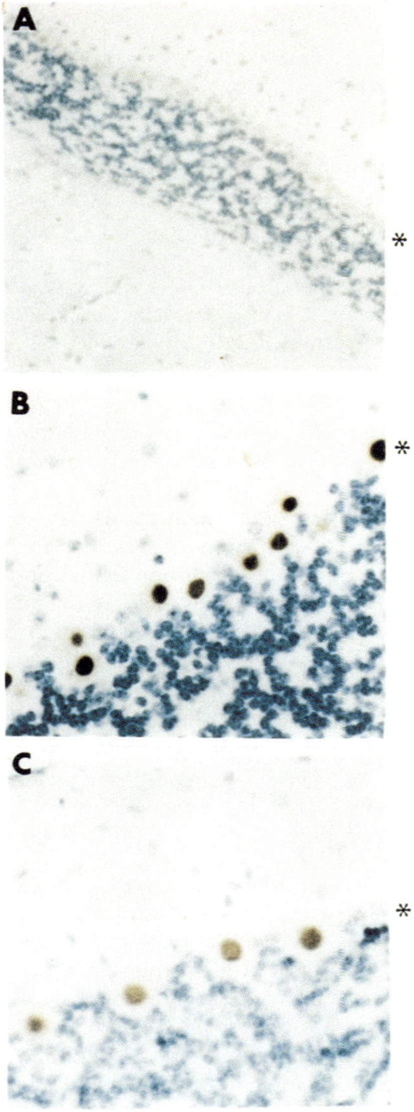

Figure 1. Immunohistochemical detection of ataxin-1 in Purkinje cells of *SCA1* transgenic mice. The Purkinje cell layer is indicated by (*). (*A*) Absence of ataxin-1 immunoreactivity in Purkinje cells of nontransgenic mouse (160x). The antibodies have been diluted to a point where murine ataxin-1 reactivity is not seen. (*B*) Ataxin-1 immunoreactivity in Purkinje cells from a PS-30 transgenic mouse (400x). (*C*) Immunoreactivity to ataxin-1 in Purkinje cells of the PS-82 transgenic B05 animal (400x).

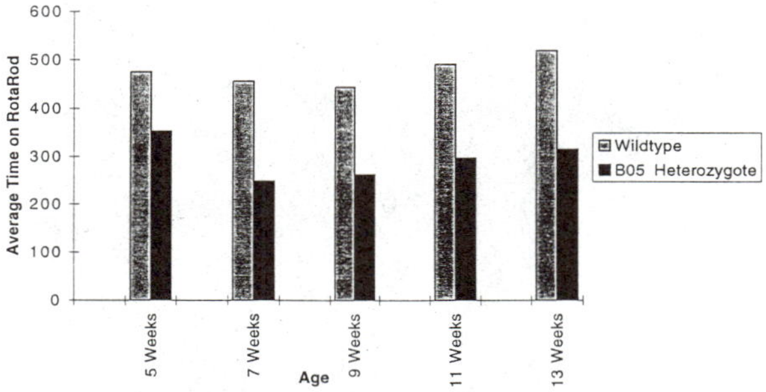

Figure 2. Impaired neurological ability of B05 *SCA1* transgenic mice as assessed by their ability to remain on the RotaRod. The average time B05 and nontransgenic littermates were able to stay on a rotating rod is depicted for several ages. Ataxia, as determined by an abnormal cage behavior, develops at 12 weeks for B05 transgenic mice.

polyglutamine tract within the AR becomes unstable and expands to cause the neuromuscular disorder spinobulbar muscular atrophy. However, for both ataxin-1 and the androgen receptor, the interaction with GAPDH was found not to be affected by the length of the polyglutamine tract. In both instances, products of expanded alleles interacted with GAPDH to the same degree as products of unexpanded alleles.

DISCUSSION

Five neurodegenerative diseases have been characterized to date and shown to be due to the expansion of an unstable CAG repeat that encodes a polyglutamine tract within the coding region of each respective gene. In addition to SCA1, these disorders include spinobulbar muscular atrophy (SBMA) caused by the expansion of a polyglutamine tract within the androgen receptor, HD, dentatorubropallidolysian atrophy (DRPLA) and its allelic disorder Haw-River syndrome, and Machado-Joseph disease and its allelic disorder SCA3. The vast preponderance of evidence obtained for these diseases supports a gain-of-function mechanism rather than a loss-of-function mechanism of pathogenesis. Each disease appears to develop as a result of the expression of the gene product encoded by an expanded, mutant allele. Furthermore, the numerous genetic similarities among the CAG-based disorders has led to the suggestion of a common mechanism of pathogenesis.

In this light, it was very provocative when investigators found that the gene products of four of these CAG disorders interact with the glycolytic enzyme GAPDH (Burke et al. 1996; Koshy et al. 1996). Intriguingly, the interaction with GAPDH seemed to be through the polyglutamine tracts of the HD, DRPLA, SCA1, and AR gene products. Although GAPDH has been implicated with several cellular functions, it has two well-characterized enzymatic activities. GAPDH is a critical regulatory step in glycolysis, where it catalyzes the oxidation and phosphorylation of D-glyceraldehyde-3-phosphate to 1,3-diphosphoglycerate and is involved in the conversion of glucose to pyruvic acid. In addition, GAPDH has uracil DNA glycosylase activity. It has been suggested that the impairment of neuronal energy metabolism is an attractive mechanism for the induction of neurodegenerative disease (Beal 1992). Thus, the finding that the gene products of four different CAG-based neurodegenerative diseases interact with GAPDH suggested that the impairment

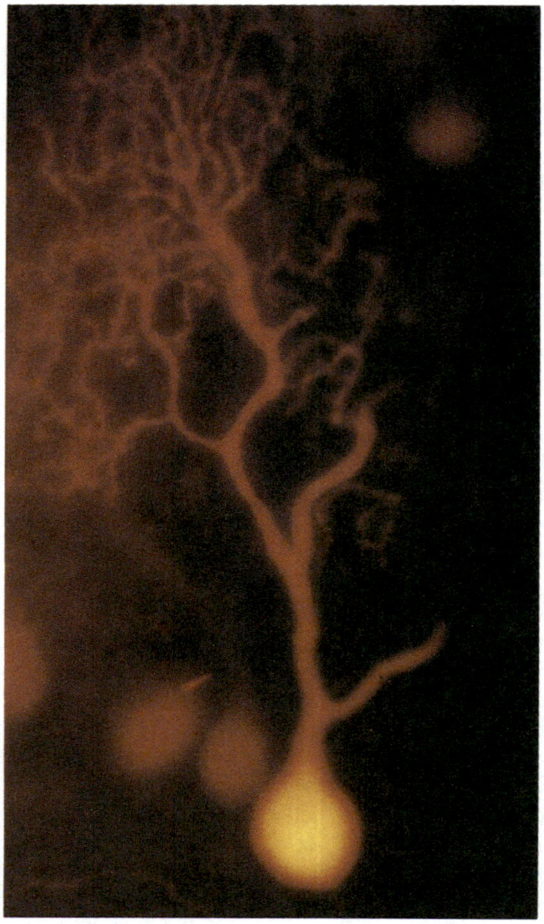

Figure 3. Atrophic Purkinje cell dendritic tree seen in a cerebellum from a 1-week-old B05 transgenic mouse. The Purkinje cells were immunostained with an antibody directed against calbindin.

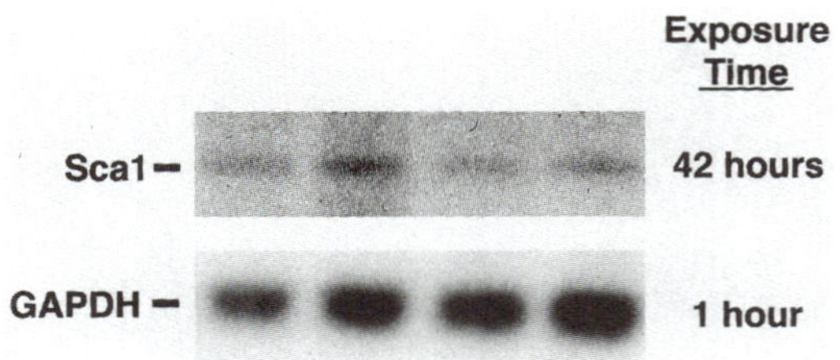

Figure 4. *Sca1* and GAPDH mRNA levels in murine cerebellar RNA. A Northern blot of 10 μg of total mouse cerebellar RNA was probed simultaneously with *Sca1* and GAPDH cDNA clones and exposed for 42 hr and 1 hr for *Sca1* and GAPDH, respectively.

of this enzyme may be a common means of pathogenesis.

There are several points regarding GAPDH impairment as a common modality of polyglutamine disorders that remain to be addressed, however. Whereas Burke et al. (1996) reported that GAPDH preferentially bound to a 60-glutamine peptide and not to a 20-glutamine peptide, these investigators found that GAPDH bound only to a fragment of the HD protein and could not demonstrate binding to full-length HD protein. More recently, Koshy et al. (1996) found that in the yeast two-hybrid system, ataxin-1 and AR binding to GAPDH was not altered by the length of the polyglutamine tracts. In addition, the relative cellular abundance of the polyglutamine proteins and GAPDH is not stoichiometrically favorable for a one-to-one interaction having much of an effect on GAPDH function. This imbalance is most dramatically demonstrated by a Northern blot of cerebellar RNA probed for both ataxin-1 and GAPDH RNA (Fig. 4). Thus, there remain important questions regarding the physiological and pathological relevance of polyglutamine/GAPDH interactions for the induction of neurodegenerative disease.

Are there any other features of the polyglutamine proteins, and ataxin-1 in particular, that might provide insights into how the expansion of the polyglutamine tract leads to disease symptoms? Immunohistochemical analysis of the subcellular localization of ataxin-1 clearly demonstrates a predominant nuclear localization. This is potentially noteworthy since the AR, the SBMA gene product, is well known to be a transcription factor. Furthermore, polyglutamine tracts are a common feature of other regulators of transcription (Courey et al. 1989). Thus, expansion of the polyglutamine tracts may uniformly cause disruption of nuclear function.

The demonstration that HD protein and the DRPLA protein are predominantly cytoplasmic (Gutekunst et al. 1995; Persichetti et al. 1995; Sharp et al. 1995; Yazawa et al. 1995) questions the disruption of nuclear function as a common mechanism of pathogenesis. However, before a nuclear disruption model is completely removed from further consideration, there are some points worth mentioning. There is a report that the HD gene product is present in both the cytoplasm and nucleus of neurons (Hoogeveen et al. 1993). Moreover, Bessert et al. (1995) identified a functional nuclear localization signal peptide within the HD protein, and within the DRPLA gene product two peptide motifs associated with nuclear function have been identified (Nagafuchi et al. 1994). These motifs in the DRPLA protein are arginine-serine dipeptides that are found in several proteins colocalized with the spliceosomes (Fu 1995) and arginine-aspartic acid dipeptides that are found in a family of nuclear RNA-binding proteins (Surowy et al. 1990). It is intriguing to speculate that a nuclear localization may be an important aspect of polyglutamine protein-induced neurodegeneration, and that nuclear localization is cell-specific and occurs only under given physiological conditions.

That transgenic mice expressing an expanded allele of *SCA1* undergo neurological and neuropathological changes clearly demonstrates that murine neurons are susceptible to the adverse effects of an expanded polyglutamine tract. Why should there be any doubt regarding this point? First of all, murine homologs of the AR, HD, and SCA1 genes (He et al. 1990; Lin et al. 1994; Banfi et al. 1996), while highly homologous to their human counterparts, have only two to four glutamines at the site of the polyglutamine tract in the human proteins. In addition, transgenic mice carrying an expanded allele of the AR (Bingham et al. 1995), or an expanded allele of the HD gene (Goldberg et al. 1996), failed to develop motor neuron disease and signs of HD, respectively. An important aspect of the AR and HD transgenic studies is that, in both cases, only a low level of transgene expression was achieved. Moreover, the expanded alleles consisted of 45 and 44 repeats, respectively. Obtaining neurological alterations in the *SCA1* mice where a high-level transgene expression was achieved of an expanded allele of 82 repeats indicates that murine neurons are more resistant to polyglutamine-induced pathogenesis.

Regardless, the *SCA1* transgenic mice do provide a useful model for determining factors that might be important for the induction of neurological disease by the expansion of polyglutamine tracts. Possibly the most relevant point determined to date from our analysis of the *SCA1* transgenic mice relates to a prevailing concept that these neurological disorders develop as a result of the death of a specific population of neurons. In fact, the time point of neurological alteration in the *SCA1* mice is substantially well before there is apparent neuronal cell loss. Two well-characterized models of ataxia in the mouse where an abnormal neurological phenotype is clearly due to the loss of Purkinje cells from the cerebellar cortex are the *pcd* mutant mouse strain (Mullen et al. 1976) and Purkinje cell death due to the expression of SV40 T antigen in transgenic mice (Feddersen et al. 1992). In both of these cases, ataxia develops only after there has been a greater than 50% loss of Purkinje cells. This is in dramatic contrast to the development of ataxia in the *SCA1* transgenic mice (Fig. 5). Ataxia in the *SCA1* mice develops in the absence of a significant loss of Purkinje cells. Thus, the data argue that emphasis should not be placed on neuronal cell death as the mechanism for neurological disease in SCA1, and in possibly the other CAG disorders. Rather, the data indicate that other pathophysiological processes in neurons expressing mutant proteins may be sufficient to produce the disease state. Furthermore, preventing neuronal cell death alone may not be sufficient to alter the development of the abnormal neurological phenotype found in these "neurodegenerative" diseases.

Are there any clues from the *SCA1* transgenic animals that might be suggestive of pathophysiological processes important for disease development? To date, two morphological changes are routinely seen in Purkinje cells from transgenic mice expressing an expanded allele of *SCA1*. The first pathological change found in Purkinje cells is the appearance of intracellular vacuoles. The vacuoles appear in Purkinje cells of mice from the B05 transgenic line by 25 days of age, before any other morphological or physiological alteration is noted. Interestingly, vacuoles similar to these have been noted in models of neuronal cell death due to an ion imbalance (Treinin and Chalfie 1995).

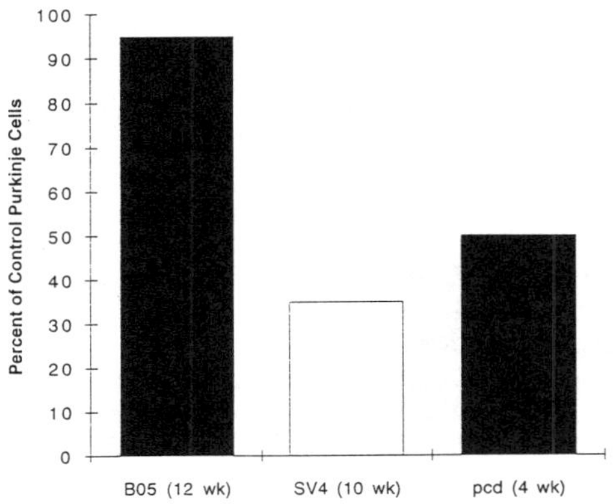

Figure 5. Purkinje cell numbers in cerebella from three types of ataxic mice. The number of Purkinje cells represents the percentage of the number found in a midsagittal section from the cerebellar cortex of a normal adult mouse. The ataxic animals, *SCA1* B05 transgenic animals, SV40 T antigen SV4 transgenic mice, and *Pcd* mutant mice were analyzed at the time of onset of ataxia as determined by cage behavior.

A second morphological alteration that has been seen in Purkinje cells of *SCA1* transgenic animals is the dwindling of Purkinje cell dendrites. Detectable in B05 mice by about 8 weeks of age, this dwindling appears to initiate in the proximal portion of the Purkinje cell dendritic tree. It will be important to determine the specific physiological abnormalities that may be occurring within Purkinje cells of B05 at a time when these morphological abnormalities are apparent.

ACKNOWLEDGMENTS

Work in the authors' laboratories was supported by grants from the National Institute of Neurological Disease and Stroke, the National Institutes of Health (NS-22920 and NS-33718 to H.T.O. and NS-27699 to H.Y.Z.). H.Y.Z. is an Investigator of the Howard Hughes Medical Institute. Portions of this work were supported by core facilities of the Mental Retardation Research Center and the Child Health Research Center at Baylor College of Medicine.

REFERENCES

Banfi, S., M.-Y. Chung, T.J. Kwiatkowski, L.P.W. Ranum, A.E. McCall, A.C. Chinault, H.T. Orr, and H.Y. Zoghbi. 1993. Mapping and cloning the critical region for the spinocerebellar ataxia type 1 gene in a yeast artifical chromosome contig spanning 1.2 Mb. *Genomics* **18:** 627.

Banfi, S., A. Servadio, M.-Y. Chung, F. Capozzoli, L.A. Duvick, R. Elde, H.Y. Zoghbi, and H.T. Orr. 1996. Cloning and developmental expression analysis of the murine homolog of the spinocerebellar ataxia type 1 gene (*Sca1*). *Hum. Mol. Genet.* **5:** 33.

Banfi, S., A. Servadio, M.-Y. Chung, T.J. Kwiatkowski, A.E. McCall, L.A. Duvick, Y. Shen, E.J. Roth, H.T. Orr, and H.Y. Zoghbi. 1994. Identification and characterization of the gene causing type 1 spinocerebellar ataxia. *Nat. Genet.* **7:** 513.

Beal, M.F. 1992. Does impairment of energy metabolism result in excitotoxic neuronal death in neurodegenerative illnesses? *Ann. Neurol.* **31:** 119.

Bessert, D.A., K.L. Gutridge, J.C. Dunbar, and L.R. Carlock. 1995. The identification of a functional nuclear localization signal in the Huntington disease protein. *Mol. Brain Res.* **33:** 165.

Bingham, P.M., M.O. Scott, S. Wang, M.J. McPaul, E.M. Wilson, J.Y. Garbern, D.E. Merry, and K.H. Fishbeck. 1995. Stability of an expanded trinucleotide repeat in the androgen receptor gene in transgenic mice. *Nat. Genet.* **7:** 513.

Burke, J.R., J.J. Enghild, M.E. Martin, Y.-S. Jou, R.M. Myers, A.D. Roses, J.M. Vance, and W.J. Strittmatter. 1996. Huntington and DRPLA proteins selectively interact with the enzyme GAPDH. *Nat. Med.* **2:** 347.

Burright, E.N., H.B. Clark, A. Servadio, T. Matilla, R.M. Feddersen, W.S. Yunis, L.A. Duvick, H.Y. Zoghbi, and H.T. Orr. 1995. SCA1 transgenic mice: a model for neurodegeneration caused by an expanded CAG trinucleotide repeat. *Cell* **82:** 937.

Chong, S.S., A.E. McCall, J. Cota, S.H. Subramony, H.T. Orr, M.R. Hughes, and H.Y. Zoghbi. 1995. Gametic and somatic tissue-specific heterogeneity of the expanded SCA1 CAG repeat in spinocerebellar ataxia type 1. *Nat. Genet.* **10:** 344.

Chung, M.-Y., L.P.W. Ranum, L.A. Duvick, A. Servadio, H.Y. Zoghbi, and H.T. Orr. 1993. Analysis of the CAG repeat expansion in spinocerebellar ataxia type 1 (SCA1): Evidence for a possible mechanism predisposing to intergeneration instability. *Nat. Genet.* **5:** 254.

Courey, A.J., D.A. Holtzman, S.P. Jackson, and R. Tjian. 1989. Synergistic activation by the glutamine-rich domains of human transcription factor Sp1. *Cell* **59:** 827.

Currier, R.D., J.F. Jackson, and E.F. Meydrech. 1982. Progression rate and age at onset are related in autosomal dominant neurologic diseases. *Neurology* **32:** 260.

Duyao, M.P., A.B. Auerbach, A. Ryan, F. Perischetti, G.T. Barnes, S.M. McCeil, P. Ge, J.-P Vonsattel, J.F. Gusella, A.L. Joyner, and M.E. MacDonald. 1995. Inactivation of the mouse Huntington's disease gene homolog *Hdh*. *Nature* **269:** 407.

Feddersen, R.M., R. Ehlenfeldt, W.S. Yunis, H.B. Clark, and H.T. Orr. 1992. Disrupted cerebellar cortical development and progressive degeneration of Purkinje cells in SV40 T antigen transgenic mice. *Neuron* **9:** 955.

Fu, X.-D. 1995. The superfamily of arginine/serine-rich splicing factors. *RNA* **1:** 663.

Goldberg, Y.P., M.A. Kalchman, M. Metzler, J. Nasir, J. Zeisler, R. Graham, H.B. Koide, J. O'Kusky, A.H. Sharp, C.A. Ross, F. Jirik, and M.R. Hayden. 1996. Absence of disease phenotype and intergenerational stability of the CAG repeat in transgenic mice expressing the human Huntington disease transcript. *Hum. Mol. Genet.* **5:** 177.

Greenfield, J.G. 1954. *The spino-cerebellar degenerations*. Charles C. Thomas, Springfield, Illinois.

Gusella, J.F., R.E. Tanzi, P.I. Bader, M.C. Phelan, R. Stevenson, M.R. Hayden, K.J. Hofman, A.G. Faryniarz, and K. Gibbons. 1985. Deletion of Huntington's disease-linked G8 (D4S10) locus in Wolf-Hirschorn syndrome. *Nature* **318:** 75.

Gutekunst, C.-A., A.I. Levey, C.J. Heilman, W.L. Whaley, H. Yi, N.R. Nash, H.D. Rees, J.J. Madden, and S.M. Hersch. 1995. Identification and localization of huntingtin in brain and human lymphoblastoid cell lines with anti-fusion protein antibodies. *Proc. Natl. Acad. Sci* **92:** 8710.

He, W.W., L.M. Fischer, S. Sun, D.L. Bilhartz, X.P. Zhu, C.Y. Young, D.B. Kelly, and D.J. Tindall. 1990. Molecular cloning of androgen receptors from divergent species with polymerase chain reaction technique: Complete cDNA sequence of the mouse androgen receptor and isolation of androgen receptor cDNA probes from dog, guinea pig, and clawed frog. *Biochem. Biophys. Res. Commun.* **171:** 697.

Hoogeveen, A.T., R. Willemsen, N. Meyer, K.E. de Rooji, R.A.C. Roos, G.-J.B. van Ommen, and H. Galjaard. 1993. Characterization and localization of the Huntington disease gene product. *Hum. Mol. Genet.* **2:** 2069.

Jackson, J.F., R.D. Currier, P.I. Terasaki, and N.E. Morton. 1977. Spinocerebellar ataxia and HLA linkage: Risk prediction by HLA typing. *N. Engl. J. Med.* **296:** 1138.

Jodice, C., P. Malaspina, F. Persichetti, A. Novelletto, M. Spardaro, P. Giunti, C. Morocutti, L. Terrenato, A.E. Harding, and M. Frontali. 1994. Effect of trinucleotide repeat length and parental sex on phenotypic variation in spinocerebellar ataxia 1. *Am. J. Hum. Genet.* **54:** 959.

Koshy, B., T. Matilla, E.N. Burright, D.E. Merry, K.H. Fishbeck, H.T. Orr, and H.Y. Zoghbi. 1996. Spinocerebellar ataxia type-1 and spinobulbar muscular atrophy gene products interact with glyceraldehyde-3-phosphate dehydrogenase. *Hum. Mol. Genet.* (in press).

Kwiatkowski, T.J., Jr., H.T. Orr, S. Banfi, A.E. McCall, C. Jodice, F. Persichetti, A. Novelletto, F. LeBorgne-DeMarquoy, M. Frontali, S.H. Subramony, A.L. Beaudet, L. Terrenato, H.Y. Zoghbi, and L.P.W. Ranum. 1993. The gene for autosomal dominant spinocerebellar ataxia (SCA1) maps centromeric to D6S89 and shows no recombination, in nine large kindreds, with a dinucleotide repeat at the AM10 locus. *Am. J. Hum. Genet.* **53:** 391.

Lin, B., J. Nasir, H. MacDonsald, G. Hutchinson, R.K. Graham, J.M. Rommens, and M.R. Hayden. 1994. Sequence of the murine Huntington disease gene; evidence for conservation, and polymorphism in a triplet (CCG) repeat alternate splicing. *Hum. Mol. Genet.* **3:** 85.

Mullen, R.J., E.M. Eicher, and R.L. Sidman. 1976. Purkinje cell degeneration, a new neurological mutation in the mouse. *Proc. Natl. Acad. Sci.* **73:** 208.

Nagafuchi, S., H. Yanagisawa, E. Ohsaki, T. Shirayama, K. Tadokoro, T. Inoue, and M. Yamada. 1994. Structure and expression of the gene responsible for the triplet repeat disorder, dentatorubral and pallidoluysian atrophy (DRPLA). *Nat. Genet.* **8:** 177.

Nasir, J., S.B. Floresco, J.R. O'Kusky, V.M. Diewert, J.M. Richman, J. Zeisler, A. Borowski, J.D. Marth, A.G. Phillips, and M.R. Hayden. 1995. Targeted disruption of the Huntington's disease gene results in embryonic lethality and behavioral and morphological changes in heterozygotes. *Cell* **81:** 811.

Oberdick, J., R.J. Smeyne, J.R. Mann, S. Zackson, and J.I. Morgan. 1990. A promoter that drives transgene expression in cerebellar Purkinje and retinal bipolar cells. *Science* **248:** 223.

Orr, H.T., M.-Y. Chung, S. Banfi, T.J. Kwiatkowski, A. Servadio, A.L. Beaudet, A.E. McCall, L.A. Duvick, L.P.W. Ranum, and H.Y. Zoghbi. 1993. Expansion of an unstable trinucleotide CAG repeat in spinocerebellar ataxia type 1. *Nat. Genet.* **4:** 221.

Persichetti, F., C.M. Ambrose, P. Gei, S.M. McNeirl, J. Srinidhi, M.A. Anderson, B. Jenkins, G.T. Barnes, M.P. Duyao, L. Kanaley, N.S. Wexler, R.H. Meyers, E.D. Bird, J.-P. Vonsattel, M.E. MacDonald, and J. F. Gusella. 1995. Normal and expanded Huntington's disease gene alleles produce distinguishable proteins due to translation across the CAG repeat. *Mol. Med.* **1:** 374.

Quigley, C.A., K.J. Friedman, A. Johnson, R.G. Lafrenierre, L.M. Silverman, D.B. Lubahn, T.R. Brown, E.M. Wilson, H.F. Willard, and F.S. French. 1992. Complete deletion of the androgen receptor gene: Definition of the null phenotype of the androgen insensitivity syndrome and determination of carrier status. *J. Clin. Endocrinol. Metab.* **74:** 927.

Ranum, L.P.W., L.A. Duvick, S.S. Rich, L.J. Schut, M. Litt, and H.T. Orr. 1991. Localization of the autosomal dominant, HLA-linked spinocerebellar ataxia (SCA1) locus in two kindreds within an 8.0 cM subregion of chromosome 6p. *Am. J. Hum. Genet.* **49:** 31.

Ranum, L.P.W., M.-Y. Chung, S. Banfi, A. Bryer, L.J. Schut, R. Ramesar, L.A. Duvick, A. McCall, S.H. Subramony, L. Goldfarb, C. Gomez, L.A. Sandkuijl, H.T. Orr, and H.Y. Zoghbi. 1994. Molecular and clinical correlations in spinocerebellar ataxia type 1 (SCA1): Evidence for familial effects on the age of onset. *Am. J. Hum. Genet.* **55:** 244.

Rich, S.S., P. Wilkie, L. Schut, G. Vance, and H.T. Orr. 1987. Spinocerebellar ataxia: Localization of an autosomal dominant locus between two markers on human chromosome 6. *Am. J. Hum. Genet.* **41:** 524.

Schut, J.W. 1950. Hereditary ataxia: Clinical study through six generations. *Arch. Neurol. Psych.* **63:** 535.

Servadio, A., S. Banfi, H.T. Orr, and H.Y. Zoghbi. 1995. SCA1 alleles with CAG expansions produce proportionately lengthened proteins of normal abundance. *Nat. Genet.* **10:** 94.

Sharp, A.H., S.J. Loev, G. Schilling, S.-H. Li, X.-J. Li, J. Bao, M.V. Wagster, J.A. Kotzuk, J.P. Steiner, A. Lo, J. Hedreen, S. Sisodia, S.H. Synder, T.M. Dawson, D.K. Ryugo, and C.A. Ross. 1995. Widespread expression of Huntington's disease gene (IT15) protein product. *Neuron* **14:** 1065.

Surowy, C., G. Hoganson, J. Gosink, K. Strunk, and R.A. Spritz. 1990. The human "RD" protein is closely related to a number of nuclear RNA-binding proteins and has been highly conserved. *Gene* **90:** 299.

Treinin, M. and M. Chalifie. 1995. A mutated acetylcholine receptor subunit casuses neuronal degeneration in *C. elegans. Neuron* **14:** 871.

Vandaele, S., D.T. Nordquist, R.M. Feddersen, I. Tretjakoff, A.C. Perteson, and H.T. Orr. 1991. Purkinje cell protein-2 regulatory regions and transgene expression in cerebellar compartments. *Genes Dev.* **5:** 1136.

Yakura, H., A. Wakisaka, S. Fujimoto, and K. Itakura. 1974. Hereditary ataxia and HLA genotypes. *N. Engl. J. Med.* **291:** 154.

Yazawa, I., N. Nukina, H. Hashida, J. Goto, M. Yamada, and I. Kanazawa. 1995. Abnormal gene product identified in hereditary dentatorubral-pallidoluysian atrophy (DRPLA) brain. *Nat. Genet.* **10:** 99.

Zeitlin, S., J.-P. Liu, D.L. Chapman, V.E. Papaioannou, and A. Efstratiadis. 1995. Increased apoptosis and early embryonic lethality in mice nullizygous for the Huntington's disease gene homologue. *Nat. Genet.* **11:** 155.

Zoghbi, H.Y., M.S. Pollack, L.A. Lyons, R.E. Ferell, S.P. Daiger, A.L. Beaudet. 1988. Spinocerebellar ataxia: Variable age of onset and linkage to human leukocyte antigen in a large kindred. *Ann. Neurol.* **23:** 580.

Zoghbi, H.Y., C. Jodice, L.A. Sandkuijl, T.J. Kwiatkowski, Jr., A.E. McCall, S.A. Huntoon, P. Lulli, M. Spadaro, M. Litt, H.M. Cann, M. Frontali, and L. Terrenato. 1991. The gene for autosomal dominant spinocerebellar ataxia (SCA1) maps telomeric to HLA complex and is closely linked to the D6S89 locus in three large kindreds. *Am. J. Hum. Genet.* **49:** 23.

Molecular Mechanisms for Charcot-Marie-Tooth Disease and Related Demyelinating Peripheral Neuropathies

L.E. WARNER,[1] L.T. REITER,[1] T. MURAKAMI,[1] AND J.R. LUPSKI[1-3]
[1]*Department of Molecular and Human Genetics,* [2]*Department of Pediatrics, and* [3]*Human Genome Center, Baylor College of Medicine, Houston, Texas 77030*

Myelin permits the rapid conduction of neuronal impulses and is an essential component of both the peripheral nervous system (PNS) and central nervous system (CNS). A condensed myelin sheath in the PNS consists of an extension of the plasma membrane from Schwann cells that repeatedly wraps and compacts around an axon in a 1:1 arrangement. This spiraling of the Schwann cell creates two different repeating layers as visualized by electron microscopy, the major dense line and the intraperiod line, formed by the apposition of the intracellular and extracellular regions, respectively (Lemke 1988; Snipes and Suter 1995). Although much is known about the overall structure and makeup of mature peripheral myelin, the process of myelin assembly remains largely a mystery. Unraveling this phenomenon will require a better understanding of the various myelin proteins involved and how they interact to form and maintain myelin. An excellent way to do this is through the study of myelin dysfunction. Many human inherited peripheral neuropathies are a manifestation of peripheral myelin dysfunction and have long been suspected to result from abnormalities in Schwann cells and their myelin sheath. Hereditary motor and sensory neuropathies (HMSN), the largest class of hereditary neuropathies, includes hereditary neuropathy with liability to pressure palsies (HNPP), Charcot-Marie-Tooth disease (CMT), Dejerine-Sottas syndrome (DSS), and congenital hypomyelination (CH). In this review, we highlight some of the remarkable recent advances that have been made in the elucidation of the molecular etiology of these neuropathies with emphasis on what this knowledge reveals about the process of myelination and the function of the genes involved.

CLINICAL SYMPTOMS AND PATHOGENESIS

Initially, insight into the role the peripheral myelin proteins play in myelination was drawn from analyzing the clinical and pathological findings of these disorders. These findings suggest that HMSN can sometimes be difficult to separate into distinct clinical categories, but instead may represent a spectrum of related clinical findings resulting from an underlying defect in myelination or a "myelinopathy."

Symptoms of HNPP include periodic episodes of numbness, muscular weakness, atrophy, and sometimes palsies following minor compression or trauma to the peripheral nerve (Lupski et al. 1993a). Electrophysiological studies sometimes show mild slowing of nerve conduction velocities (NCV) and may reveal conduction blocks in affected individuals and clinically asymptomatic individuals who carry a mutation. Both segmental demyelination and remyelination with tomacula or sausage-like focal thickenings of the myelin sheath, and inner uncompacted myelin lamellae due to a separation of major dense lines, are characteristic findings on nerve biopsy (Yoshikawa and Dyck 1991). These pathological findings suggest the involvement of a protein important to the maintenance of myelin compaction.

CMT, the most common inherited peripheral neuropathy, is characterized by progressive atrophy of the distal muscles which usually manifests within the first two decades of life. Electrophysiological studies separate CMT into two major forms. CMT type 1 (CMT1), the hypertrophic form, has been divided into subtypes based on genetic linkage: CMT1A at 17p11.2-p12 (Vance et al. 1989), CMT1B at 1q21.2-q23 (Hayasaka et al. 1993b); and CMTX at Xq13.1 (Bergoffen et al. 1993a). CMT1 is a demyelinating neuropathy with mildly to severely reduced NCV (Kaku et al. 1993a; Lupski et al. 1993a). There is marked uniformity of the conduction slowing, which argues for an intrinsic Schwann cell abnormality (Kaku et al. 1993b). Peripheral nerve biopsies of CMT1 patients show segmental demyelination/remyelination and hypertrophic changes due to onion bulb formation. Onion bulbs are formed by circumferentially flattened Schwann cells and their processes (Lupski and Garcia 1992). These pathological findings for CMT1 support a predominant defect in the synthesis or maintenance of myelin. In contrast, CMT type 2 (CMT2), the neuronal form, exhibits normal or only mildly reduced motor NCV of decreased amplitudes, suggestive of an underlying axonal lesion (Lupski et al. 1991a; Dyck et al. 1993).

DSS is a related demyelinating neuropathy with pathological features and clinical symptoms which overlap CMT1, but which tends to be more severe and have an earlier age of onset (Dyck et al. 1993). However, since the finding of allelic mutations in the genes associated with CMT1A and CMT1B (Hayasaka et al. 1993a; Roa et al. 1993a), DSS can no longer be regarded as a separate entity. Instead, CMT1 and DSS represent a spectrum of clinical findings in which the variations in severity are likely related to the effects different mutations in the same protein have on its function.

CH is characterized clinically by early onset in infancy of hypotonia, areflexia, distal muscle weakness, and very slow NCV (Harati and Butler 1985). It is considered to result from a congenital impairment in myelin formation based on the lack of active myelin breakdown and hypomyelination of most or all fibers as indicated by nerve biopsy (Harati and Butler 1985). There is variation in the prognosis which correlates with the presence or absence of onion bulbs (Harati and Butler 1985). This variation is probably due to genetic heterogeneity with mutations in an essential early myelin gene(s) resulting in a severe prognosis, whereas mutations in a later acting gene(s) lead to a milder outcome.

DNA REARRANGEMENTS ASSOCIATED WITH CMT1A AND HNPP

Molecular genetic analysis demonstrated a novel disease-causing mechanism involving large inherited DNA rearrangements as the basis for both CMT1A and HNPP. CMT1A is associated with a 1.5-Mb tandem DNA duplication in 17p11.2-p12 that is transmitted in a stable manner in both mitosis and meiosis (Lupski et al. 1991b, 1993b; Raeymaekers et al. 1991; Pentao et al. 1992), whereas HNPP is associated with the reciprocal 1.5-Mb deletion at the same position (Fig. 1) (Chance et al. 1993, 1994). The frequency of the CMT1A duplication among unrelated CMT1 patients is approximately 70%, increases to 85% when pedigrees demonstrate male-to-male transmission, and ranges from 76% to 90% when only de novo cases are considered (Hoogendijk et al. 1992; Wise et al. 1993; Nelis et al. 1996a). The HNPP deletion frequency among unrelated HNPP patients is estimated at 84%, and the de novo HNPP deletion accounts for 86% of the sporadic HNPP cases (Nelis et al. 1996a). The finding that a consistently sized DNA duplication or deletion occurs repeatedly at the 17p11.2-p12 region, as evidenced by the detection of duplication- or deletion-specific junction fragments by pulsed field gel electrophoresis, strongly indicates that a precise recombination event generates the duplication and deletion (Roa et al. 1995).

The high frequency of new mutation (Hoogendijk et al. 1992; Blair et al. 1996) and uniformity of junction fragment size in de novo duplication/deletion cases of CMT1A and HNPP, respectively, suggest the presence of an intrinsic structural property of the genome that predisposes the region to discrete DNA rearrangements. Physical mapping studies identified the presence of two, approximately 30-kb, low-copy direct repeats (CMT1A-REPs) that flank the 1.5-Mb region duplicated in CMT1A (Pentao et al. 1992) and deleted in HNPP (Chance et al. 1994). Furthermore, the duplication/deletion boundaries were found to lie at the CMT1A-REPs, resulting in three copies on the duplicated chromosome (Pentao et al. 1992) and only one copy on the deleted chromosome (Fig. 1) (Chance et al. 1994). Segregation of marker genotypes from within the duplicated region suggested a mechanism of unequal crossing-over for the generation of the CMT1A duplication (Raeymaekers et al. 1991). On the basis of these findings, a model of homologous recombination between misaligned CMT1A-REP elements was proposed as a mechanism for the generation of both the CMT1A duplication (Pentao et al. 1992) and the HNPP deletion (Fig. 1) (Chance et al. 1994). This model predicts that individuals mosaic for the duplication should not be identified unless they represent somatic reversion events (Liehr et al. 1996).

Interestingly, both the de novo CMT1A duplication (Raeymaekers et al. 1991; Palau et al. 1993; Wise et al. 1993; Hertz et al. 1994; Mancardi et al. 1994; Blair et al. 1996; Timmerman et al. 1996c) and the HNPP deletion (Chance et al. 1993; Mariman et al. 1994; Verhalle et al. 1994; Timmerman et al. 1996b,c) occur preferentially on the paternally inherited chromosome, indicating that male-specific factor(s) may operate during gametogenesis to generate the duplication or deletion (Table 1). However, the identification of de novo duplications (Mancardi et al. 1994; Blair et al. 1996) and deletions (Reisecker et al. 1994; LeGuern et al. 1996) of maternal origin indicates that this event is not solely associated with male meiosis (Table 1). The finding that one of the maternally derived HNPP deletions results from an intrachromosomal rearrangement suggests that the intrachromosomal rearrangement may be specific to maternal transmission (LeGuern et al. 1996) and could account for the observed decreased paternal origin for HNPP deletion versus CMT1A duplication (Table 1). Further studies will be required to determine if sex predilection for unequal crossing-over is a general phenomenon for the human genome.

MOLECULAR MECHANISM FOR RECIPROCAL RECOMBINATION

To map the recombination breakpoint within the CMT1A-REPs, restriction sites that were unique to either the proximal or distal CMT1A-REP were determined (Lopes et al. 1996; Reiter et al. 1996). An *Eco*RI site unique to the distal CMT1A-REP, which divides the 7.8 *Eco*RI fragment from the proximal CMT1A-REP into 1.8-kb and 6.0-kb *Eco*RI fragments, had previously been identified (Fig. 1) (Pentao et al. 1992). Dosage patterns of the 7.8/6.0 fragments observed in multiple unrelated CMT1A duplication patients (a gain of one copy of the 6.0 fragment) and HNPP deletion patients (the loss of one copy of the 6.0 fragment) indicated that in the majority of patients the crossover occurred distal to the unique *Eco*RI site (Chance et al. 1994; Kiyosawa et al. 1995; LeGuern et al. 1995; Loren-

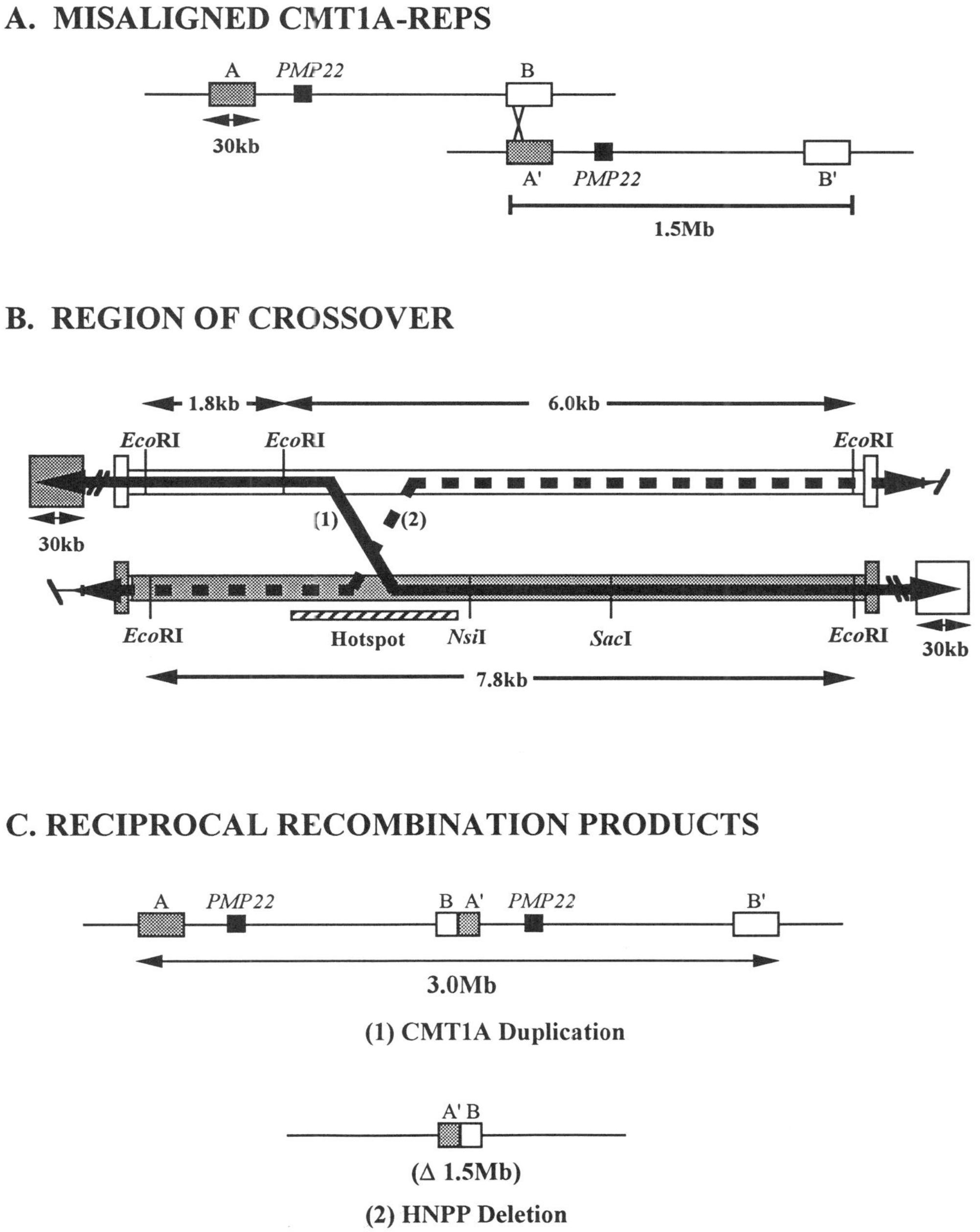

Figure 1. Proposed model of unequal crossing-over between misaligned repeats leading to the CMT1A duplication and the HNPP deletion. The shaded boxes represent the proximal CMT1A-REP, the open boxes represent the distal CMT1A-REP, and the black boxes represent the *PMP22* gene. (*A*) Misaligned CMT1A-REP elements. (*B*) The misaligned distal and proximal CMT1A-REPs are expanded to show the unique restriction sites and the hotspot for recombination. The 7.8-kb proximal *Eco*RI fragment and 1.8-kb and 6.0-kb distal *Eco*RI fragments are indicated by arrows. The thick black line (1) indicates the region of crossover in the majority of CMT1A duplication patients and the dashed black line (2) the region of crossover in the majority of HNPP deletion patients. The striped box indicates the hotspot region for homologous recombination which yields a 1.7-kb junction fragment in CMT1A duplication patients and a 7.8-kb junction fragment in HNPP deletion patients upon triple digestion with *Eco*RI, *Sac*I, and *Nsi*I. (*C*) Reciprocal recombination products resulting from the homologous recombination of misaligned CMT1A-REPs.

zetti et al. 1995; Lopes et al. 1996; Timmerman et al. 1996b). Restriction enzyme analysis and DNA sequencing of the proximal and distal CMT1A-REPs allowed the identification of two other unique restriction sites, *Nsi*I and *Sac*I, both of which map to the proximal CMT1A-REP (Reiter et al. 1996). Upon double digest-

Table 1. Parental Origin of CMT1A Duplication and HNPP Deletion

Rearrangement	Paternal (%)	Maternal (%)	Total
CMT1A duplication	26 (89.6)	3 (10.4)	29
HNPP deletion	5 (71.4)	2 (28.6)	7
Total	31 (86.1)	5 (13.9)	36

ion of CMT1A duplication and HNPP deletion patient genomic DNA with *Eco*RI and *Sac*I, putative junction fragments were identified—a 3.2-kb fragment in the CMT1A duplication patients and a 7.8-kb fragment in the deletion patients (Kiyosawa and Chance 1996; Lopes et al. 1996; Reiter et al. 1996; Timmerman et al. 1996c). This localized the crossover site to a 3.2-kb region between the unique *Eco*RI site in the distal CMT1A-REP and the unique *Sac*I site in the proximal CMT1A-REP (Fig. 1). After triple digestion with *Eco*RI, *Sac*I, and *Nsi*I, the predicted 1.7-kb *Eco*RI/*Nsi*I and 7.8-kb *Eco*RI/*Eco*RI junction fragments were observed in the majority of unrelated CMT1A duplication and HNPP deletion patients, respectively, indicating that there is a hotspot for recombination in the 1.7-kb region between *Eco*RI and *Nsi*I (Reiter et al. 1996; Timmerman et al. 1996c). A relative risk calculation in two independent studies indicated that the strand exchange event occurs in the 1.7-kb region with a preference of 53:1 (Reiter et al. 1996) or 52:1 (Timmerman et al. 1996c) over the surrounding approximately 28 kb of homology between the CMT1A-REP repeats. Figure 2 shows the placement of individual crossover events in CMT1A duplication and HNPP deletion patients from these two studies (Reiter et al. 1996; Timmerman et al. 1996c). The fact that a high percentage of both CMT1A duplication and HNPP deletion patients cross over in the same 1.7-kb region indicates a recombination hotspot and suggests that a specific feature of this region must be mediating the crossover event.

Only a few restriction sites within the 7.8-kb *Eco*RI/*Eco*RI region could be detected that were unique to either the proximal or distal CMT1A-REP, thus indicating a high degree of homology. Initially it was hypothesized that a region of identity within this region of homology could promote the initiation of strand exchange events at the hotspot (Kiyosawa et al. 1995; Reiter et al. 1996). Shotgun sequencing of the 7.8-kb region which contains the 1.7-kb hotspot junction fragment revealed that the CMT1A-REPs are

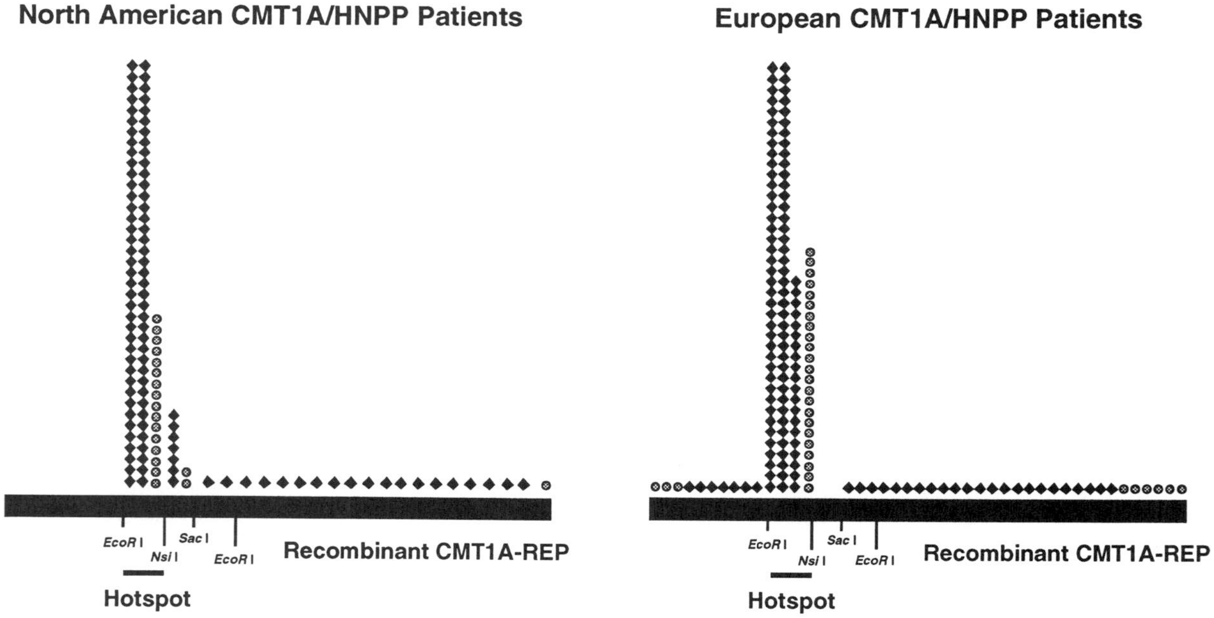

Figure 2. Placement of the crossover events in individual CMT1A/HNPP patients. The recombinant CMT1A-REP is shown. Each symbol indicates the crossover event of one patient. The black diamond represents the crossover event in CMT1A and the shaded circle represents the crossover event in HNPP. *Eco*RI, *Nsi*I, and *Sac*I are restriction sites present in the different recombinant CMT1A-REPs, and the black horizontal line indicates the hotspot for recombination between *Eco*RI and *Nsi*I. The placement of crossovers between the unique *Sac*I from the proximal CMT1A-REP and the unique *Eco*RI site from the distal CMT1A-REP was determined by the identification of junction fragments from the recombinant CMT1A-REP detected by Southern analysis after digestion of patient genomic DNA. The exact placement of crossovers outside these unique restriction site boundaries is unknown. Such crossovers are placed on either side of the hotspot region by examining dosage of alleles in patients who do not have junction fragments. The North American cohort contains 104 CMT1A duplication patients and 19 HNPP deletion patients (Reiter et al. 1996). The European cohort contains 130 CMT1A duplication patients and 32 HNPP deletion patients (Timmerman et al. 1996c).

>98% identical. The hotspot region is not, however, significantly more identical than the surrounding areas of homology and does not contain the longest stretch of identity in the 7.8-kb region (Reiter et al. 1996). These data implied that another DNA sequence characteristic or signal, present at or near the hotspot region, was initiating the strand exchange event.

Further sequence analysis of the 7.8-kb region, containing the novel junction fragment boundaries, identified a *mariner* transposon-like element near the hotspot for homologous recombination. This element has been designated MITE, for *Mariner insect transposon-like element* (Reiter et al. 1996). The MITE element is probably not active due to a number of premature stops found within the putative open reading frame. It has only been recently that *mariner* transposons have been reported in the human genome (Morgan 1995; Oosumi et al. 1995; Robertson et al. 1996; Smit and Riggs 1996), and even though an active version of the *mariner*-like elements has not been identified, the association of MITE with a hotspot of recombination argues that there may be an active *mariner* transposase somewhere in the human genome (Reiter et al. 1996). In support of this prediction, an apparently testis-specific signal was detected on a Northern blot using the 1.8-kb *Eco*RI/*Eco*RI fragment from the distal CMT1A-REP which spans the MITE element (Kiyosawa and Chance 1996; Reiter et al. 1996). The identification of an apparent testis-specific signal is intriguing, since it could explain the preferential occurrence of the de novo duplication/deletion event during male gametogenesis. A preliminary consensus sequence for the irritans subfamily of *mariners*, of which MITE is a member, has recently been described and could potentially be used to identify active human *mariners* (Robertson et al. 1996). Our proposed model (Reiter et al. 1996) of how the transposon-like MITE element could be mediating an increase in homologous recombination between the CMT1A-REPs suggests that a functional *mariner* transposase from somewhere in the genome could completely or partially excise the MITE element, generating the double-strand break which is the signal for initiating strand exchange events (Fig. 3).

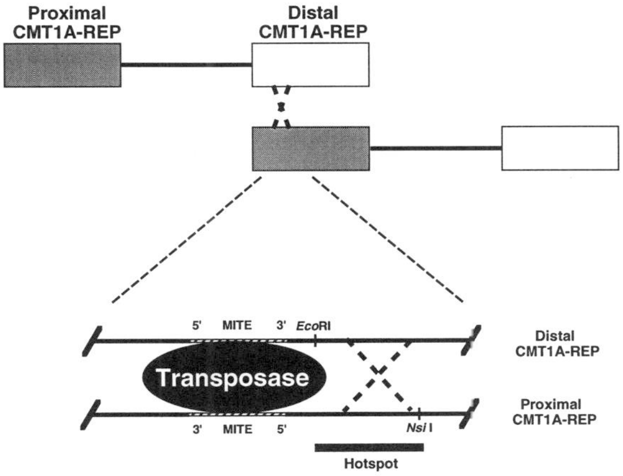

Figure 3. Model of how MITE element could mediate homologous recombination. Shaded boxes indicate proximal CMT1A-REP and white boxes indicate distal CMT1A-REP. The black oval depicts an active transposase from elsewhere in the genome which performs a partial or complete excision of the MITE element (*striped boxes*) resulting in a double strand break. During repair of the break, a holliday junction is formed (one for partial and two for complete excision). This junction can then migrate and consistently resolve within the 1.7-kb hotspot region flanked by an *Eco*RI site in the distal CMT1A-REP and a *Nsi*I site in the proximal CMT1A-REP.

TWO ALTERNATIVE MECHANISMS FOR CMT1A: GENE DOSAGE AND POINT MUTATION

Two alternative mechanisms result in the same clinical and electrophysiological phenotype of CMT1A: gene dosage resulting from the duplication of a particular region and point mutations within the dosage-sensitive gene in nonduplication patients. An intriguing question is how these two distinct mechanisms result in the same phenotype. One hypothesis that could explain both mechanisms is that each could cause the disruption of the formation and/or functioning of a multimeric protein complex (Roa et al. 1993b).

A number of mechanisms (gene interruption, position effect, and gene dosage) were initially proposed to explain the causative mechanism of the CMT1A duplication (Lupski et al. 1991b). However, the present evidence overwhelmingly supports the gene dosage model in which increased expression of a critical gene or genes within the duplication causes the disease phenotype. This evidence includes rare homozygous CMT1A duplication patients who exhibit a more severe clinical phenotype (Lupski et al. 1991b; Kaku et al. 1993a) and the identification of partial trisomy patients who exhibit NCVs similar to CMT1A duplication patients (Lupski et al. 1992; Roa et al. 1996b). The finding of patients with either partial trisomy of chromosome 17p or duplications smaller than the common 1.5-Mb duplication (Ionasescu et al. 1993; Palau et al. 1993; Valentijn et al. 1993), who exhibit the electrophysiological abnormalities observed in CMT1, essentially rules out the position effect and gene interruption models, since the DNA rearrangement endpoints are distinct from each other as well as from the typical 1.5-Mb CMT1A duplication.

The *PMP22* (*peripheral myelin protein-22kD*) gene was initially proposed as the dosage-sensitive gene within the CMT1A duplication region, based on its identification as the mutated gene in the *Trembler* (Tr) and *Trembler-J* mice (Suter et al. 1992a,b). The *Pmp-22* gene maps to mouse chromosome 11 which is syntenic to human chromosome 17p, and *Trembler* is the animal model for CMT based on similarities in electrophysiological and neuropathological findings. Since its initial proposal as the dosage-sensitive gene, a considerable amount of evidence has been generated that further supports the dosage sensitivity of *PMP22* in demyelinating peripheral neuropathy: (1) PMP22 is highly expressed predominantly in the PNS (Patel et al. 1992; Snipes et al. 1992); (2) the entire *PMP22* gene maps within both the common 1.5-Mb duplication (Matsunami et al. 1992; Patel et al. 1992; Pentao et al. 1992; Timmerman et al. 1992; Valentijn et al. 1992b) and three smaller duplications (Ionasescu et al. 1993; Palau et al. 1993; Valentijn et al. 1993); (3) *PMP22* point mutations are found in some non-duplication patients (Valentijn et al. 1992a; Roa et al. 1993b), but not within CMT1A duplication patients (Warner et al. 1996a); (4) elevated *PMP22* mRNA is detected in nerve biopsies from CMT1A duplication patients (Yoshikawa et al. 1994); and (5) *PMP22* transgenic rats/mice that overexpress PMP22 develop a peripheral neuropathy that closely resembles CMT1 (Huxley et al. 1996; Sereda et al. 1996). A direct role for *PMP22* in HNPP pathogenesis is clearly documented by a rare patient, without the HNPP deletion, who instead has a *PMP22* frameshift mutation that causes a nonsense codon. Therefore, a loss-of-function allele is an alternative mechanism for the haploinsufficiency resulting from the HNPP deletion (Nicholson et al. 1994).

At present, the function of PMP22 is unknown. However, its apparent dosage sensitivity suggests its involvement in a multimeric complex within myelin in which the exact macromolecular stoichiometry is critical to proper functioning. A number of functions have been proposed for PMP22. PMP22 may function in adhesion between myelin membranes based on evidence that it carries an L2/HNK-1 epitope, which has been implicated in the adhesive process (Snipes et al. 1993), and the observation of uncompacted myelin in HNPP patients who are deleted for one copy of *PMP22* (Yoshikawa and Dyck 1991). A dual function in myelin compaction and early myelin development has also been speculated for PMP22 based on its proposed adhesive properties, its original identification as a growth-arrest-specific gene (Manfioletti et al. 1990), and its structural resemblance to PLP, the major CNS myelin protein. PLP is also dosage sensitive, as indicated by duplications or deletions of *PLP* that are associated with Pelizaeus-Merzbacher disease (PMD) (Cremers et al. 1987; Raskind et al. 1991; Ellis and Malcolm 1994; Carango et al. 1995; Inoue et al. 1996). In addition, overexpression of *plp* in transgenic mice leads to severe hypomyelination in the CNS (Kagawa et al. 1994; Readhead et al. 1994). PLP is speculated to play a dual role in CNS myelin compaction and early myelin development based on the different phenotypes of the mouse mutants *jimpy* and *rumpshaker* (Dautigny et al. 1986; Schneider et al. 1992). Others propose PLP and PMP22 may be components of an adhesive ion pore (Suter and Snipes 1995). Each of these potential functions involves precise protein-protein interactions and is thus consistent with the evidence that altered dosage of PMP22 results in a phenotype.

These potential structural functions that require the interaction of a number of proteins not only could account for *PMP22* gene dosage sensitivity, but also could explain the effect of point mutations. Point mutations in *PMP22* that are associated with CMT1A or DSS (Roa and Lupski 1994; Ionasescu et al. 1995a; Valentijn et al. 1995; Navon et al. 1996) are all found within the transmembrane domain and are thought to lead to a gain-of-function effect (Fig. 4 and Table 2). This is again similar to *PLP*, since point mutations in *PLP* are associated with PMD (Hudson et al. 1989) and spastic paraplegia (Kobayashi et al. 1994; Saugier-Veber et al. 1994). Interestingly, studies have shown that the mutations in *PLP* affecting amino acids in the transmembrane domains cause the mutant protein to remain in the endoplasmic reticulum (ER) and subsequently cause oligodendrocyte cell death by the accumulation of misfolded protein in the ER (Gow et al. 1994).

Retinitis pigmentosa, associated with mutations in the *rhodopsin* gene (Nathans 1994), is another disorder that exemplifies the relationship between gene dosage and point mutation. The findings of retinal degeneration in transgenic mice with a *rhodopsin* mutation, Pro23His, suggests that these mutations are gain-of-function or dominant-negative mutations (Olsson et al. 1992). Like *PLP*, mutations in *rhodopsin* accumulate in the ER (Sung et al. 1991). Moreover, transgenic mice overexpressing normal rhodopsin also have photoreceptor degeneration indicating a gene-dosage effect (Olsson et al. 1992). Interestingly, these three dosage-sensitive genes, *PMP22*, *PLP*, and *rhodopsin,* are all abundantly expressed and encode apparently integral membrane proteins.

GENES ASSOCIATED WITH OTHER SUBTYPES OF CMT1 AND RELATED NEUROPATHIES

The fact that CMT shows dominant, recessive, and X-linked inheritance suggests the involvement of a family of genes whose products have similar functions or are involved in a final common pathway. This seems to be true for CMT1, since all the identified mutations involve genes encoding myelin proteins. This observation and the hypothesis that PMP22 is part of a multimeric complex can easily explain the genetic heterogeneity seen in CMT and its related neuropathies, since mutations in different proteins can produce similar phenotypes if they perform similar functions or are part of the same protein complex (Roa and Lupski 1994; Nicholson 1995).

P_0, encoded by the *MPZ* gene, is the major structural component of the peripheral nerve myelin (Lemke 1988). It is important to the formation and compaction of the intraperiod and major dense lines of the peripheral nerve myelin (D'Urso et al. 1990; Filbin

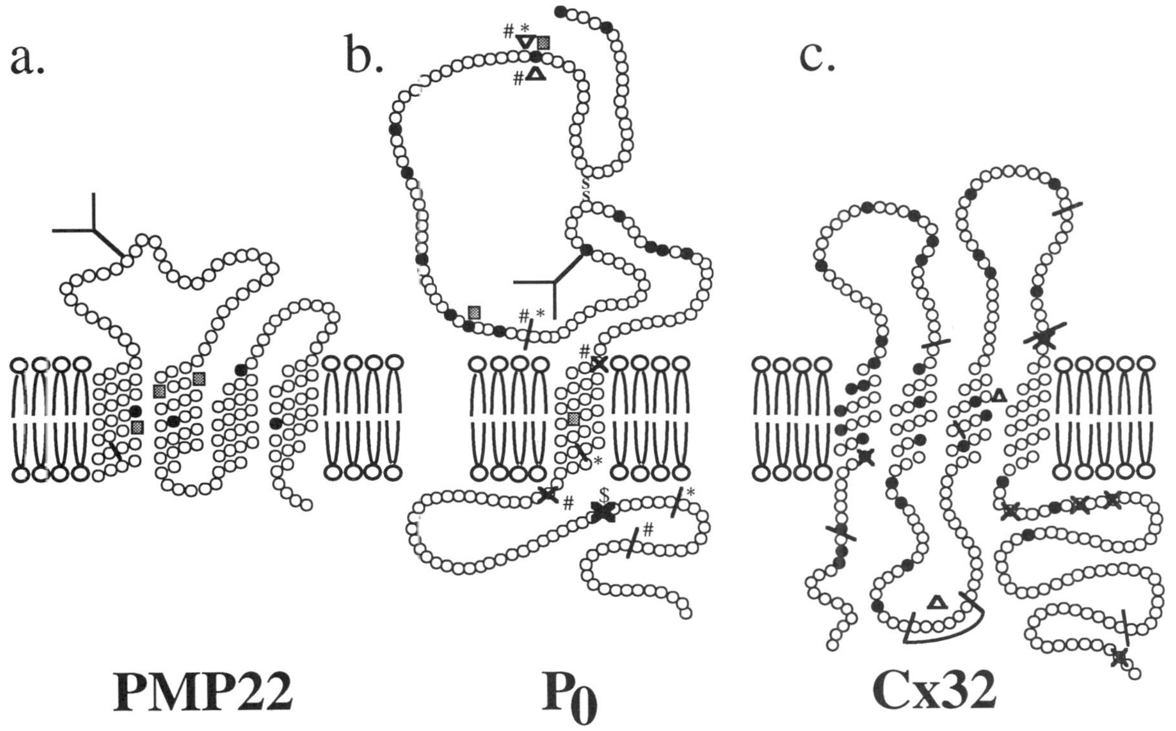

Figure 4. Structural models of the PMP22, P_0, and Cx32 membrane-associated myelin proteins and mutations associated with inherited peripheral neuropathies. Individual amino acid residues in each protein are indicated by circles and the glycosylation sites are shown for PMP22 and P_0. (*a*) Mutations affecting PMP22 are associated with CMT1A (*filled circles*), DSS (*shaded squares*), and HNPP (slash indicating a frameshift mutation). (*b*) Mutations affecting P_0 are associated with CMT1B (*filled circles* or #), DSS (*shaded squares* or *), and congenital hypomyelination (thick X with $). (*c*) Mutations affecting *Cx32* lead to CMTX. For all three proteins, filled circles or squares represent amino acid substitutions, nonsense mutations are indicated by an X, deletions are indicated by the Δ beside the specific amino acid(s) deleted, and frameshift mutations are indicated by a slash preceding the first amino acid affected in the reading frame. The individual mutations associated with human disease phenotypes are listed in Table 2.

et al. 1990; Ding and Brunden 1994). Allelic point mutations in *MPZ* are associated with CMT1B, DSS, and recently CH (Fig. 4 and Table 2) (Warner et al. 1996b). Analysis of these mutations has led to a hypothesis regarding genotype/phenotype correlations. It is hypothesized that loss-of-function alleles, as evidenced by the nonsense mutations at positions 125 and 152, result in the less severe CMT1B phenotype, whereas alleles that potentially act as dominant-negative mutations result in the more severe DSS or CH phenotypes (Warner et al. 1996b). For example, cysteine substitutions at positions 34 and 69 that are postulated to form disulfide aggregates in the extracellular space and disturb the normal confirmation and function of the P_0 protein complex may be dominant-negative mutations (Shapiro et al. 1996; Warner et al. 1996b). Different missense amino acid substitutions at the identical positions (Ser34Phe, Arg69His, and Arg69Ser) result in a less severe CMT phenotype and are thought to represent loss-of-function alleles. This hypothesis is further substantiated by the fact that loss-of-function nonsense codons result in CMT1. The analysis of *MPZ* mutations in demyelinating neuropathies also suggests that the intracellular domain is crucial to proper function, as patients with mutations involving the P_0 intracellular domain display severe phenotypes (Warner et al. 1996b).

X-linked CMT (CMTX) results from mutations in the connexin-32 (*Cx32*) gene (Fig. 4 and Table 2) (Bergoffen et al. 1993b). *Cx32* mutations appear to be the most common cause of non-duplication CMT1 (Nelis et al. 1996a), with mutations occurring throughout the protein and leading to single amino acid substitutions, codon deletions, frameshift, or nonsense mutations (Fig. 4 and Table 2). Connexins are a group of related membrane-spanning proteins that assemble to form intercellular channels for the transport of ions and small molecules. Connexin 32 is located at the nodes of Ranvier and Schimdt-Lanterman incisures in areas of noncompacted myelin and may modulate Schwann cell and axon interactions (Bergoffen et al. 1993b). This could explain the mixed axonal and demyelinating features seen in CMTX. It is perhaps because of the axonal component and the fact that affected females are asymptomatic or less severely af-

Table 2. Myelin Gene Mutations Associated with Inherited Peripheral Neuropathies

Gene/ disease	Mutation	Ref.*	Mutation	Ref.*	Mutation	Ref.*	Gene/ disease	Mutation	Ref.*	Mutation	Ref.*	Mutation	Ref.*	Mutation	Ref.*
PMP22							*MPZ*								
CMT1A	L16P	1	S79C	1	T118M	1	CMT1B	I1M	5	Y53C	5	306delA	10	I106L	6
	L147R	2						T5I	6	D61E	5	N93S	11	G108S	5
								ΔS34	5,6	K67E	5	K101R	6,12	Y125X	5
DSS	H12Q	3	M69K	1	S72L	1,4		S34F	7	R69H	5,6	D105E	5	Y152X	5
								ΔF35	8	R69S	10	D105N	5	697del4	11
HNPP	19delAG	1						S49L	5,9	W72C	9	I106T	5		
							DSS	S34C	5	R69C	6,10	G138R	5	521del4	13
								660insGC	5						
							CH	Q186X	10						
Cx32															
CMT1X	G12S	14	L25F	11	S49Y	18		Q80R	16	W133R	14	R164W	16,19	E208K	14
	V13L	14	S26L	11	L56F	11		P87A	11	410delT	14	P172S	14	Y211X	17
	R15W/45del11	15	I30N	14	C60F	14		M93V	11	V139M	11,14	524insA	14	R215W	13,14
	R15Q	11,14	M34T	17	V63I	14		V95M	14,15	R142W	11,14	S182T	14	C217X	14
	R15W	11,15	V35M	14	Y65C	14		E102G	13,14	ΔL143	14	556insG	16	R220X	14
	R22X	14	V38M	14	217delC	14		R107W	17	L156R	14	E186X	14	R238H	11
	R22Q	11,16	A40V	11	R75Q	17		331del18	14,16	P158A	14	E186K	14	791del29	16
														S281X	11

CMT = Charcot-Marie-Tooth; DSS = Dejerine-Sottas syndrome; HNPP = hereditary neuropathy with liability to pressure palsies; CH = congenital hypomyelination; del/Δ = deletion; ins = insertion; X = nonsense. Standard abbreviations for amino acid residues are used; nucleotide numbering starts at the translation initation site; amino acid numbering in *MPZ* refers to the processed or mature protein. References: (1) for review, see Roa and Lupski 1994; (2) Navon et al. 1996; (3) Valentijn et al. 1995; (4) Ionasescu et al. 1995a; (5) for review, see Roa et al. 1996a; (6) Gabreëls-Festen et al. 1996; (7) Blanquet-Grossard et al. 1995; (8) Ikegami et al. 1996; (9) Latour et al. 1995; (10) Warner et al. 1996b; (11) Nelis et al. 1996a; (12) Tachi et al. 1996; (13) L.E. Warner and J.R. Lupski, unpubl.; (14) for review, see Bone et al. 1995; (15) Nelis et al. 1996b; (16) Ionasescu et al. 1995b; (17) Tan et al. 1996; (18) Timmerman et al. 1996a; (19) Oterino et al. 1996.

fected than males that some females with *Cx32* mutations have been misdiagnosed with CMT2 (Timmerman et al. 1996a; L.E. Warner and J.R. Lupski, unpubl.).

As illustrated in Figure 4, there is allelic heterogeneity for point mutations associated with demyelinating neuropathy phenotypes, suggesting there are no specific point mutation hotspot regions in any of the three genes, *PMP22*, *MPZ*, or *Cx32*. One well-known point mutation hotspot in humans is at CpG dinucleotides and results from the deamination of 5-methylcytosine to thymine. Of the 87 identified point mutations in Table 2, 34.5% occur at CpG dinucleotides. The percentage of mutations at CpG dinucleotides occurring at each individual gene is: *PMP22* (25%), *MPZ* (27.6%), and *Cx32* (40%). This is similar to the percentages both Cooper and Youssoufian (35%) (1988) and Cooper and Krawczak (38%) (1993) state are responsible for single base-pair substitutions within coding regions that cause human genetic disease. The percentage of point mutations occurring at CpG dinucleotides is not higher than that seen throughout the human genome, and only 9% in *PMP22*, 27% in *MPZ*, and 55% in *Cx32* of the potential CpG dinucleotides available were actually identified to be mutated. Therefore, the methylation-mediated deamination model is an important mutational mechanism in demyelinating peripheral neuropathy, but does not constitute a mutation hotspot region in these three myelin genes that is significantly different from other disease-associated genes.

CONCLUSIONS

Molecular analysis of CMT and its related peripheral neuropathies has led to new insights into their molecular etiology and the function of various genes encoding peripheral myelin constituents. CMT1A is usually associated with a tandem 1.5-Mb duplication on 17p11.2-p12. Gene dosage of *PMP22* is the causative mechanism of the neuropathy in patients with the CMT1A duplication. It is intriguing that CMT1 is one of the most common autosomal dominant conditions affecting humans, and yet for the overwhelming majority of patients there is no mutant gene. *PMP22* appears to be dosage-sensitive, since both overexpression (CMT1A) and underexpression (HNPP) result in a neurological phenotype. Therefore, the exact macromolecular stoichiometry must be critical to its proper functioning. Alternatively, in the absence of the duplication, CMT1A can be caused by point mutations in *PMP22*. The pathological findings of uncompacted myelin and demyelination, along with the association of both these alternative mechanisms with the CMT1 phenotype, suggest PMP22 functions as part of a multimeric protein complex required for the maintenance of myelin compaction. The discovery that mutations involving three different myelin genes, *PMP22*, *MPZ*, and *Cx32*, are all associated with a similar phenotype also argues for complex protein interaction or similar functions within the myelin sheath.

The finding that different mutations involving the same locus (i.e., mutations in *MPZ* result in CMT1B, DSS, or CH, whereas mutations involving *PMP22* may result in CMT1A, HNPP, or DSS) can lead to different disease phenotypes indicates that these inherited peripheral neuropathies constitute a spectrum of phenotypes with a common underlying defect in myelination. The identification of multiple independent point mutations has permitted genotype-phenotype correlations which are crucial to understanding the functions of the protein(s). The severity of the disease seems to reflect the extent of the mutation's effect on the protein's function in myelination, with missense amino acid substitutions being more detrimental than null alleles by having a dominant-negative or a gain-of-function effect on a multimeric complex. The molecular findings in CMT and its related neuropathies have important ramifications for diagnosis (Lupski 1996), prognosis (Graf et al. 1996; Killian et al. 1996), genetic counseling, and rational approaches to therapy (Lupski et al. 1993a) for affected individuals. Furthermore, several authors have advocated that these conditions should be reclassified on the basis of molecular studies (Harding 1995; Ouvrier 1996).

Many of the findings in CMT also have far-reaching implication for other genetic disorders. The observation that a consistently sized DNA duplication or deletion was mediated by homologous recombination of misaligned repeats makes it conceivable that other genetic disorders may also prove to arise from recombination events mediated by specific structural features of the genome. The identification of *PMP22* as the dosage-sensitive gene within the duplication/deletion region has blurred the artificial boundaries that separate "single gene" disorders from chromosomal syndromes. Consequently, the clinical phenotype in chromosomal aneuploidy syndromes, like trisomy 21, may result from the effect of a small subset of dosage-sensitive genes mapping within the region of aneuploidy. Furthermore, the extreme variability of clinical expression observed in disorders resulting from gene dosage effects may reflect the fact that there is no abnormal gene product and that dosage of a protein may be more subject to the effects of modifier genes and/or other environmental influences (Garcia et al. 1995). Finally, the observation that the majority of all CMT1 cases are caused by the CMT1A duplication, despite the fact that mutations involving at least six loci can also result in a CMT1 phenotype, suggests DNA rearrangements may be a more frequent mutational mechanism than structural gene alteration at some loci (Lupski et al. 1996).

ACKNOWLEDGMENTS

We appreciate the cooperation of the CMT patients and their families. This work was supported in part by grants from the National Institute of Neurological Disorders and Stroke of the National Institutes of Health (R01 NS27042), the Muscular Dystrophy Association, and the Baylor Human Genome Center.

REFERENCES

Bergoffen, J., J. Trofatter, M.A. Pericak-Vance, J.L. Haines, P.F. Chance, and K.H. Fischbeck. 1993a. Linkage localization of X-linked Charcot-Marie-Tooth disease. *Am. J. Hum. Genet.* **52:** 312.

Bergoffen, J., S.S. Scherer, S. Wang, M.O. Scott, L.J. Bone, D.L. Paul, K. Chen, M.W. Lensch, P.F. Chance, and K.H. Fischbeck. 1993b. Connexin mutations in X-linked Charcot-Marie-Tooth disease. *Science* **262:** 2039.

Blair, I.P., J. Nash, M.J. Gordon, and G.A. Nicholson. 1996. Prevalence and origin of de novo duplications in Charcot-Marie-Tooth disease type 1A: First report of a de novo duplication with a maternal origin. *Am. J. Hum. Genet.* **58:** 472.

Blanquet-Grossard, F., D. Pham-Dinh, A. Dautigny, P. Latour, C. Bonnebouche, E. Corbillon, G. Chazot, and A. Vandenberghe. 1995. Charcot-Marie-Tooth type 1B neuropathy: Third mutation of serine 63 codon in the major peripheral myelin glycoprotein P0 gene. *Clin. Genet.* **48:** 281.

Bone, L.J., N. Dahl, M.W. Lensch, P.F. Chance, T. Kelly, E. Le Guern, S. Magi, G. Parry, H. Shapiro, S. Wang, and K.H. Fischbeck. 1995. New connexin32 mutations associated with X-linked Charcot-Marie-Tooth disease. *Neurology* **45:** 1863.

Carango, P., V.L. Funanage, R.E. Quirós, C.S. Debruyn, and H.G. Marks. 1995. Overexpression of DM20 messenger RNA in two brothers with Pelizaeus-Merzbacher disease. *Ann. Neurol.* **38:** 610.

Chance, P.F., N. Abbas, M.W. Lensch, L. Pentao, B.B. Roa, P.I. Patel, and J.R. Lupski. 1994. Two autosomal dominant neuropathies result from reciprocal DNA duplication/deletion of a region on chromosome 17. *Hum. Mol. Genet.* **3:** 223.

Chance, P.F., M.K. Alderson, K.A. Leppig, M.W. Lensch, N. Matsunami, B. Smith, P.D. Swanson, S.J. Odelberg, C.M. Disteche, and T.D. Bird. 1993. DNA deletion associated with hereditary neuropathy with liability to pressure palsies. *Cell.* **72:** 143.

Cooper, D.N. and M. Krawczak. 1993. *Human gene mutation.* BIOS Scientific, Oxford.

Cooper, D.N. and H. Youssoufian. 1988. The CpG dinucleotide and human genetic disease. *Hum. Genet.* **78:** 151.

Cremers, F.P.M., R.A. Pfeiffer, T.J.R. van de Pol, M.H. Hofker, T.A. Kruse, B. Wieringa, and H.H. Ropers. 1987. An interstitial duplication of the X chromosome in a male allows physical fine mapping of probes from the Xq13-q22 region. *Hum. Genet.* **77:** 23.

Dautigny, A., M.-G. Mattei, D. Morello, P.M. Alliel, D. Pham-Dinh, L. Amar, D. Arnaud, D. Simon, J.-F. Mattei, J.-L. Guenet, P. Jollès, and P. Avner. 1986. The structural gene coding for myelin-associated proteolipid protein is mutated in *jimpy* mice. *Nature* **321:** 867.

Ding, Y. and K.R. Brunden. 1994. The cytoplasmic domain of myelin glycoprotein P_0 interacts with negatively charged phospholipid bilayers. *J. Biol. Chem.* **269:** 10764.

D'Urso, D., P.J. Brophy, S.M. Staugaitis, C.S. Gillespie, A.B. Frey, J.G. Stempak, and D.R. Colman. 1990. Protein zero of peripheral nerve myelin: Biosynthesis, membrane insertion, and evidence for homotypic interaction. *Neuron* **2:** 449.

Dyck, P.J., P. Chance, R. Lebo, and J.A. Carney. 1993. Hereditary motor and sensory neuropathies. In *Peripheral neuropathy* (ed. P.J. Dyck et al.), p. 1094. W.B. Saunders, Philadelphia.

Ellis, D. and S. Malcolm. 1994. Proteolipid protein gene dosage effect in Pelizaeus-Merzbacher disease. *Nat. Genet.* **6:** 333.

Filbin, M.T., F.S. Walsh, B.D. Trapp, J.A. Pizzey, and G.I. Tennekoon. 1990. Role of myelin P_0 protein as a homophilic adhesion molecule. *Nature* **344:** 871.

Gabreëls-Festen, A.A.W.M., J.E. Hoogendijk, P.H.S. Meijerink, F.J.M. Gabreëls, P.A. Bolhuis, S. van Beersum, T. Kulkens, E. Nelis, F.G.I. Jennekens, M. de Visser, B.G.M. van Engelen, C. Van Broeckhoven, and E.C.M. Mariman. 1996. Two divergent types of nerve pathology in patients with different P_0 mutations. *Neurology* (in press).

Garcia, C.A., R.E. Malamut, J.D. England, G.S. Parry, P. Liu, and J.R. Lupski. 1995. Clinical variability in two pairs of identical twins with the Charcot-Marie-Tooth disease type 1A duplication. *Neurology* **45:** 2090.

Gow, A., V.L. Friedrich, Jr., and R.A. Lazzarini. 1994. Many naturally occurring mutations of myelin proteolipid protein impair its intracellular transport. *J. Neurosci. Res.* **37:** 574.

Graf, W.D., P.F. Chance, M.W. Lensch, L.J. Eng, H.P. Lipe, and T.D. Bird. 1996. Severe vincristine neuropathy in Charcot-Marie-Tooth disease type 1A. *Cancer* **77:** 1356.

Harati, Y. and I.J. Butler. 1985. Congenital hypomyelinating neuropathy. *J. Neurol. Neurosurg. Psychiatry* **48:** 1269.

Harding, A.E. 1995. From the syndrome of Charcot, Marie and Tooth to disorders of peripheral myelin proteins. *Brain* **118:** 809.

Hayasaka, K., M. Himoro, Y. Sawaishi, K. Nanao, T. Takahashi, G. Takada, G.A. Nicholson, R.A. Ouvrier, and N. Tachi. 1993a. *De novo* mutation of the myelin P_0 gene in Dejerine-Sottas disease (hereditary motor and sensory neuropathy type III). *Nat. Genet.* **5:** 266.

Hayasaka, K., M. Himoro, Y. Wang, M. Takata, S. Minoshima, N. Shimizu, M. Miura, K. Uyemura, and G. Takada. 1993b. Structure and chromosomal localization of the gene encoding the human myelin protein zero (MPZ). *Genomics* **17:** 755.

Hertz, J.M., A.D. Børglum, C.A. Brandt, T. Flint, and C. Bisgaard. 1994. Charcot-Marie-Tooth disease type 1A: The parental origin of a *de novo* 17p11.2-p12 duplication. *Clin. Genet.* **46:** 291.

Hoogendijk, J.E., G.W. Hensels, A.A.W.M. Gabreëls-Festen, F.J.M. Gabreëls, E.A.M. Janssen, P. De Jonghe, J.-J. Martin, C. Van Broeckhoven, L.J. Valentijn, F. Baas, M. De Visser, and P.A. Bolhuis. 1992. De novo mutation in hereditary motor and sensory neuropathy type 1. *Lancet* **339:** 1081.

Hudson, L.D., C. Puckett, J. Berndt, J. Chan, and S. Gencic. 1989. Mutation of the proteolipid protein gene *PLP* in a human X chromosome-linked myelin disorder. *Proc. Natl. Acad. Sci.* **86:** 8128.

Huxley, C., E. Passage, A. Manson, G. Putzu, D. Figarella-Branger, J.F. Pellissier, and M. Fontés. 1996. Construction of a mouse model of Charcot-Marie-Tooth disease type 1A by pronuclear injection of human YAC DNA. *Hum. Mol. Genet.* **5:** 563.

Ikegami, T., G. Nicholson, H. Ikeda, A. Ishida, H. Johnston,

G. Wise, R. Ouvrier, and K. Hayasaka. 1996. A novel homozygous mutation of the myelin Po gene producing Dejerine-Sottas disease (hereditary motor and sensory neuropathy type III). *Biochem. Biophys. Res. Commun.* **222:** 107.

Inoue, K., H. Osaka, N. Sugiyama, C. Kawanishi, H. Onishi, A. Nezu, K. Kimura, S. Kimura, Y. Yamada, and K. Kosaka. 1996. A duplicated *PLP* gene causing Pelizaeus-Merzbacher disease detected by comparative multiplex PCR. *Am. J. Hum. Genet.* **59:** 32.

Ionasescu, V.V., R. Ionasescu, C. Searby, and D.F. Barker. 1993. Charcot-Marie-Tooth neuropathy type 1A with both duplication and non-duplication. *Hum. Mol. Genet.* **2:** 405.

Ionasescu, V.V., R. Ionasescu, C. Searby, and R. Neahring. 1995a. Dejerine-Sottas disease with de novo dominant point mutation of the PMP22 gene. *Neurology* **45:** 1766.

Ionasescu, V., C. Searby, R. Ionasescu, and W. Meschino. 1995b. New point mutations and deletions of the connexin 32 gene in X-linked Charcot-Marie-Tooth neuropathy. *Neuromusc. Disord.* **5:** 297.

Kagawa, T., K. Ikenaka, Y. Inoue, S. Kuriyama, T. Tsujii, J. Nakao, K. Nakajima, J. Aruga, H. Okano, and K. Mikoshiba. 1994. Glial cell degeneration and hypomyelination caused by overexpression of myelin proteolipid protein gene. *Neuron* **13:** 427.

Kaku, D.A., G.J. Parry, R. Malamut, J.R. Lupski, and C.A. Garcia. 1993a. Nerve conduction studies in Charcot-Marie-Tooth polyneuropathy associated with a segmental duplication of chromosome 17. *Neurology* **43:** 1806.

———. 1993b. Uniform slowing of conduction velocities in Charcot-Marie-Tooth polyneuropathy type 1. *Neurology* **43:** 2664.

Killian, J.M., P.S. Tiwari, S. Jacobson, R.D. Jackson, and J.R. Lupski. 1996. Longitudinal studies of the duplication form of Charcot-Marie-Tooth polyneuropathy. *Muscle Nerve* **19:** 74.

Kiyosawa, H. and P. Chance. 1996. Primate origin of the CMT1A-REP repeat and analysis of a putative transposon-associated recombinational hotspot. *Hum. Mol. Genet.* **5:** 745.

Kiyosawa, H., M.W. Lensch, and P.F. Chance. 1995. Analysis of the CMT1A-REP repeat: Mapping crossover breakpoints in CMT1A and HNPP. *Hum. Mol. Genet.* **4:** 2327.

Kobayashi, H., E.P. Hoffman, and H.G. Marks. 1994. The *rumpshaker* mutation in spastic paraplegia. *Nat. Genet.* **7:** 351.

Latour, P., F. Blanquet, E. Nelis, C. Bonnebouche, F. Chapon, P. Diraison, E. Ollagnon, A. Dautigny, D. Pham-Dinh, G. Chazot, M. Boucherat, C. Van Broeckhoven, and A. Vandenberghe. 1995. Mutations in the myelin protein zero gene associated with Charcot-Marie-Tooth disease type 1B. *Hum. Mutat.* **6:** 50.

LeGuern, E., R. Gouider, N. Ravisé, J. Lopes, S. Tardieu, M. Gugenheim, N. Abbas, P. Bouche, Y. Agid, and A. Brice. 1996. A *de novo* case of hereditary neuropathy with liability to pressure palsies (HNPP) of maternal origin: A new mechanisn for deletion in 17p11.2? *Hum. Mol. Genet.* **5:** 103.

LeGuern, E., R. Gouider, J. Lopes, N. Abbas, M. Gugenheim, S. Tardieu, N. Ravisé, J.-M. Léger, J.-M. Vallat, P. Bouche, Y. Agid, A. Brice, and the French CMT Collaborative Research Group. 1995. Constant rearrangement of the CMT1A-REP sequences in HNPP patients with a deletion in chromosome 17p11.2: A study of 30 unrelated cases. *Hum. Mol. Genet.* **4:** 1673.

Lemke, G. 1988. Unwrapping the genes of myelin. *Neuron* **1:** 535.

Liehr, T., B. Rautenstrauss, H. Grehl, K.D. Bathke, A. Ekici, A. Rauch, and H.-D. Rott. 1996. Mosaicism for the Charcot-Marie-Tooth disease type 1A duplication suggests somatic reversion. *Hum. Genet.* **98:** 22.

Lopes, J., E. LeGuern, R. Gouider, S. Tardieu, N. Abbas, N. Birouk, M. Gugenheim, P. Bouche, Y. Agid, A. Brice, and the French CMT Collaborative Research Group. 1996. Recombination hot spot in a 3.2-kb region of the Charcot-Marie-Tooth type 1A repeat sequences: New tools for molecular diagnosis of hereditary neuropathy with liability to pressure palsies and of Charcot-Marie-Tooth type 1A. *Am. J. Hum. Genet.* **58:** 1223.

Lorenzetti, D., D. Pareyson, A. Sghirlanzoni, B.B. Roa, N.E. Abbas, M. Pandolfo, S. Di Donato, and J.R. Lupski. 1995. A 1.5-Mb deletion in 17p11.2-p12 is frequently observed in Italian families with hereditary neuropathy with liability to pressure palsies. *Am. J. Hum. Genet.* **56:** 91.

Lupski, J.R. 1996. DNA diagnostics for Charcot-Marie-Tooth disease and related inherited neuropathies. *Clin. Chem.* **42:** 1.

Lupski, J.R. and C.A. Garcia. 1992. Molecular genetics and neuropathology of Charcot-Marie-Tooth disease type 1A. *Brain Pathol.* **2:** 337.

Lupski, J.R., P.F. Chance, and C.A. Garcia. 1993a. Inherited primary peripheral neuropathies: Molecular genetics and clinical implications of CMT1A and HNPP. *J. Am. Med. Assoc.* **270:** 2326.

Lupski, J.R., J.R. Roth, and G.M. Weinstock. 1996. Chromosomal duplications in bacteria, fruit flies, and humans. *Am. J. Hum. Genet.* **58:** 21.

Lupski, J.R., C.A. Garcia, G.J. Parry, and P.I. Patel. 1991a. Charcot-Marie-Tooth polyneuropathy syndrome: Clinical, electrophysiologic, and genetic aspects. In *Current neurology* (ed. S. Appel), p. 1. Mosby-Yearbook, Chicago.

Lupski, J.R., L. Pentao, L.L. Williams, and P.I. Patel. 1993b. Stable inheritance of the CMT1A DNA duplication in two patients with CMT1 and NF1. *Am. J. Med. Genet.* **45:** 92.

Lupski, J.R., C.A. Wise, A. Kuwano, L. Pentao, J.T. Parke, D.G. Glaze, D.H. Ledbetter, F. Greenberg, and P.I. Patel. 1992. Gene dosage is a mechanism for Charcot-Marie-Tooth disease type 1A. *Nat. Genet.* **1:** 29.

Lupski, J.R., R. Montes de Oca-Luna, S. Slaugenhaupt, L. Pentao, V. Guzzetta, B.J. Trask, O. Saucedo-Cardenas, D.F. Barker, J.M. Killian, C.A. Garcia, A. Chakravarti, and P.I. Patel. 1991b. DNA duplication associated with Charcot-Marie-Tooth disease type 1A. *Cell* **66:** 219.

Mancardi, G.L., A. Uccelli, E. Bellone, A. Sghirlanzoni, P. Mandich, D. Pareyson, A. Schenone, M. Abbruzzese, and F. Ajmar. 1994. 17p11.2 duplication is a common finding in sporadic cases of Charcot-Marie-Tooth type 1. *Eur. Neurol.* **34:** 135.

Manfioletti, G., M.E. Ruaro, G. Del Sal, L. Philipson, and C. Schneider. 1990. A growth arrest-specific (*gas*) gene codes for a membrane protein. *Mol. Cell. Biol.* **10:** 2924.

Mariman, E.C.M., A.A.W.M. Gabreëls-Festen, S.E.C. van Beersum, L.J. Valentijn, F. Baas, P.A. Bolhuis, P.J.H. Jongen, H.H. Ropers, and F.J.M. Gabreëls. 1994. Prevalence of the 1.5-Mb 17p deletion in families with hereditary neuropathy with liability to pressure palsies. *Ann. Neurol.* **36:** 650.

Matsunami, N., B. Smith, L. Ballard, M.W. Lensch, M. Robertson, H. Albertsen, C.O. Hanemann, H.W. Müller, T.D. Bird, R. White, and P.F. Chance. 1992. Peripheral myelin protein–22 gene maps in the duplication in chromosome 17p11.2 associated with Charcot-Marie-Tooth 1A. *Nat. Genet.* **1:** 176.

Morgan, G.T. 1995. Identification in the human genome of mobile elements spread by DNA-mediated transposition. *J. Mol. Biol.* **254:** 1.

Nathans, J. 1994. In the eye of the beholder: Visual pigments and inherited variation in human vision. *Cell* **78:** 357.

Navon, R., B. Seifried, N.S. Gal-On, and M. Sadeh. 1996. A new point mutation affecting the fourth transmembrane domain of PMP22 results in a severe, de novo Charcot-Marie-Tooth disease. *Hum. Genet.* **97:** 685.

Nelis, E., C. Van Broeckhoven, and the European CMT Consortium. 1996a. Estimation of the mutation frequencies in Charcot-Marie-Tooth disease type 1 and hereditary neuropathy with liability to pressure palsies: A European collaborative study. *Eur. J. Hum. Genet.* **4:** 25.

Nelis, E., L.E. Warner, E. De Vriendt, P.F. Chance, J.R. Lupski, and C. Van Broeckhoven. 1996b. Comparison of single-strand conformation polymorphism (SSCP) and heteroduplex analysis (HA) for detection of mutations in CMT1 and related peripheral neuropathies. *Eur. J. Hum. Genet.* (in press).

Nicholson, G. 1995. Myelin gene dosage and mutation in the hereditary motor and sensory neuropathies: A review. *J. Neurol. Neurosurg. Psychiatry* **58:** 523.

Nicholson, G.A., L.J. Valentijn, A.K. Cherryson, M.L. Kennerson, T.L. Bragg, R.M. DeKroon, D.A. Ross, J.D. Pollard, J.G. Mcleod, P.A. Bolhuis, and F. Baas. 1994. A frame shift mutation in the *PMP22* gene in hereditary neuropathy with liability to pressure palsies. (Erratum *Nat. Genet.* **7:** 113) *Nat. Genet.* **6:** 263.

Olsson, J.E., J.W. Gordon, B.S. Pawlyk, D. Roof, A. Hayes, R.S. Molday, S. Mukai, G.S. Cowley, E.L. Berson, and T.P. Dryja. 1992. Transgenic mice with a rhodopsin mutation (Pro23His): A mouse model of autosomal dominant retinitis pigmentosa. *Neuron* **9:** 815.

Oosumi, T., W.R. Belknap, and B. Garlick. 1995. *Mariner* transposons in humans. *Nature* **378:** 672.

Oterino, A., F.I. Montón, V.M. Cabrera, F. Pinto, A. Gonzalez, and N.R. Lavilla. 1996. Arginine-164-tryptophan substitution in connexin32 associated with X linked dominant Charcot-Marie-Tooth disease. *J. Med. Genet.* **33:** 413.

Ouvrier, R. 1996. Correlation between the histopathologic, genotypic, and phenotypic features of hereditary peripheral neuropathies in childhood. *J. Child Neurol.* **11:** 133.

Palau, F., A. Löfgren, P. De Jonghe, S. Bort, E. Nelis, T. Sevilla, J.-J. Martin, J. Vilchez, F. Prieto, and C. Van Broeckhoven. 1993. Origin of the *de novo* duplication in Charcot-Marie-Tooth disease type 1A: Unequal nonsister chromatid exchange during spermatogenesis. *Hum. Mol. Genet.* **2:** 2031.

Patel, P.I., B.B. Roa, A.A. Welcher, R. Schoener-Scott, B.J. Trask, L. Pentao, G.J. Snipes, C.A. Garcia, U. Francke, E.M. Shooter, J.R. Lupski, and U. Suter. 1992. The gene for the peripheral myelin protein PMP-22 is a candidate for Charcot-Marie-Tooth disease type 1A. *Nat. Genet.* **1:** 159.

Pentao, L., C.A. Wise, A.C. Chinault, P.I. Patel, and J.R. Lupski. 1992. Charcot-Marie-Tooth type 1A duplication appears to arise from recombination at repeat sequences flanking the 1.5 Mb monomer unit. *Nat. Genet.* **2:** 292.

Raeymaekers, P., V. Timmerman, E. Nelis, P. De Jonghe, J.E. Hoogendijk, F. Baas, D.F. Barker, J.J. Martin, M. De Visser, P.A. Bolhuis, C. Van Broeckhoven, and the HMSN Collaborative Research Group. 1991. Duplication in chromosome 17p11.2 in Charcot-Marie-Tooth neuropathy type 1a (CMT1a). *Neuromusc. Disord.* **1:** 93.

Raskind, W.H., C.A. Williams, L.D. Hudson, and T.D. Bird. 1991. Complete deletion of the proteolipid protein gene (*PLP*) in a family with X-linked Pelizaeus-Merzbacher disease. *Am. J. Hum. Genet.* **49:** 1355.

Readhead, C., A. Schneider, I. Griffiths, and K.-A. Nave. 1994. Premature arrest of myelin formation in transgenic mice with increased proteolipid protein gene dosage. *Neuron* **12:** 583.

Reisecker, F., F. Leblhuber, R. Lexner, G. Radner, W. Rosenkranz, and K. Wagner. 1994. A sporadic form of hereditary neuropathy with liability to pressure palsies: Clinical, electrodiagnostic, and molecular genetic findings. *Neurology* **44:** 753.

Reiter, L.T., T. Murakami, T. Koeuth, L. Pentao, D.M. Muzny, R.A. Gibbs, and J.R. Lupski. 1996. A recombination hotspot responsible for two inherited peripheral neuropathies is located near a *mariner* transponson-like element. *Nat. Genet.* **12:** 288.

Roa, B.B. and J.R. Lupski. 1994. Molecular genetics of Charcot-Marie-Tooth neuropathy. *Adv. Hum. Genet.* **22:** 117.

Roa, B.B., U. Ananth, C.A. Garcia, and J.R. Lupski. 1995. Molecular diagnosis of CMT1A and HNPP. *LabMedica Int.* **12:** 22.

Roa, B.B., P.J. Dyck, H.G. Marks, P.F. Chance, and J.R. Lupski. 1993a. Dejerine-Sottas syndrome associated with point mutation in the peripheral myelin protein 22 (*PMP22*) gene. *Nat. Genet.* **5:** 269.

Roa, B.B., L.E. Warner, C.A. Garcia, D. Russo, R. Lovelace, P.F. Chance, and J.R. Lupski. 1996a. Myelin protein zero (*MPZ*) gene mutations in nonduplication type 1 Charcot-Marie-Tooth disease. *Hum. Mutat.* **7:** 36.

Roa, B.B., F. Greenberg, P. Gunaratne, C.M. Sauer, M.S. Lubinsky, C. Kozma, J.M. Meck, R.E. Magenis, L.G. Shaffer, and J.R. Lupski. 1996b. Duplication of the *PMP22* gene in 17p partial trisomy patients with Charcot-Marie-Tooth type 1A neuropathy. *Hum. Genet.* **97:** 642.

Roa, B.B., C.A. Garcia, U. Suter, D.A. Kulpa, C.A. Wise, J. Mueller, A.A. Welcher, G.J. Snipes, E.M. Shooter, P.I. Patel, and J.R. Lupski. 1993b. Charcot-Marie-Tooth disease type 1A: association with a spontaneous point mutation in the *PMP22* gene. *N. Engl. J. Med.* **329:** 96.

Robertson, H.M., K.L. Zumpano, A.R. Lohe, and D.L. Hartl. 1996. Reconstructing the ancient *mariners* of humans. *Nat. Genet.* **12:** 360.

Saugier-Veber, P., A. Munnich, D. Bonneau, J.-M. Rozet, M. Le Merrer, R. Gil, and O. Boespflug-Tanguy. 1994. X-linked spastic paraplegia and Pelizaeus-Merzbacher disease are allelic disorders at the proteolipid protein locus. *Nat. Genet.* **6:** 257.

Schneider, A., P. Montague, I. Griffiths, M. Fanarraga, P. Kennedy, P. Brophy, and K.-A. Nave. 1992. Uncoupling of hypomyelination and glial cell death by a mutation in the proteolipid protein gene. *Nature* **358:** 758.

Sereda, M., I. Griffiths, A. Pühlhofer, H. Stewart, M.J. Rossner, F. Zimmermann, J.P. Magyar, A. Schneider, E. Hund, H.-M. Meinck, U. Suter, and K.-A. Nave. 1996. A transgenic rat model of Charcot-Maire-Tooth disease. *Neuron* **16:** 1049.

Shapiro, L., J.P. Doyle, P. Hensley, D.R. Colman, and W. Hendrickson. 1996. Crystal structure of the extrcellular domain from P_0, the major structural protein of peripheral nerve myelin. *Neuron* (in press).

Smit, A.F.A. and A.D. Riggs. 1996. *Tiggers* and other DNA transposon fossils in the human genome. *Proc. Natl. Acad. Sci.* **93:** 1443.

Snipes, G.J. and U. Suter. 1995. Molecular anatomy and genetics of myelin proteins in the peripheral nervous system. *J. Anat.* **186:** 483.

Snipes, G.J., U. Suter, and E.M. Shooter. 1993. Human peripheral myelin protein-22 carries the L2/HNK-1 carbohydrate adhesion epitope. *J. Neurochem.* **61:** 1961.

Snipes, G.J., U. Suter, A.A. Welcher, and E.M. Shooter. 1992. Characterization of a novel peripheral nervous system myelin protein (PMP-22/SR13). *J. Cell Biol.* **117:** 225.

Sung, C.-H., B.G. Schneider, N. Agarwal, D.S. Papermaster, and J. Nathans. 1991. Functional heterogeneity of mutant rhodopsins responsible for autosomal dominant retinitis pigmentosa. *Proc. Natl. Acad. Sci.* **88:** 8840.

Suter, U. and G.J. Snipes. 1995. Peripheral myelin protein 22: Facts and hypotheses. *J. Neurosci. Res.* **40:** 145.

Suter, U., J.J. Moskow, A.A. Welcher, G.J. Snipes, B. Kosaras, R.L. Sidman, A.M. Buchberg, and E.M. Shooter. 1992a. A leucine-to-proline mutation in the putative first transmembrane domain of the 22-kDa peripheral myelin protein in the *trembler-J* mouse. *Proc. Natl. Acad. Sci.* **89:** 4382.

Suter, U., A.A. Welcher, T. Özcelik, G.J. Snipes, B. Kosaras, U. Francke, S. Billings-Gagliardi, R.L. Sidman, and E.M. Shooter. 1992b. *Trembler* mouse carries a point mutation in a myelin gene. *Nature* **356:** 241.

Tachi, N., N. Kozuka, K. Ohya, S. Chiba, K. Sasaki, K. Uyemura, and K. Hayasaka. 1996. A new mutation of the Po gene in patients with Charcot-Marie-Tooth disease type 1B: Screening of the Po gene by heteroduplex analysis. *Neurosci. Lett.* **204:** 173.

Tan, C.C., P.J. Ainsworth, A.F. Hahn, and P.M. MacLeod. 1996. Novel mutations in the connexin 32 gene associated with X-linked Charcot-Marie-Tooth disease. *Hum. Mutat.* **7:** 167.

Timmerman, V., P. De Jonghe, P. Spoelders, S. Simokovic, A. Löfgren, E. Nelis, J. Vance, J.-J. Martin, and C. Van Broeckhoven. 1996a. Linkage and mutation analysis of Charcot-Marie-Tooth neuropathy type 2 families with chromosomes 1p35-p36 and Xq13. *Neurology* **46:** 1311.

Timmerman, V., A. Löfgren, E. Le Guern, P. Liang, P. De Jonghe, J.-J. Martin, D. Verhalle, W. Robberecht, R. Gouider, A. Brice, and C. Van Broeckhoven. 1996b. Molecular genetic analysis of the 17p11.2 region in patients with hereditary neuropathy with liability to pressure palsies (HNPP). *Hum. Genet.* **97:** 26.

Timmerman, V., B. Rautenstrauss, L. Reiter, T. Koeuth, A. Löfgren, T. Liehr, E. Nelis, K.D. Bathke, P. DeJonghe, H. Grehl, J.-J. Martin, J.R. Lupski, and C. Van Broeckhoven. 1996c. Detection of the CMT1A/HNPP recombination hotspot in unrelated patients of European decent. *J. Med. Genet.* (in press).

Timmerman, V., E. Nelis, W. Van Hul, B.W. Nieuwenhuijsen, K.L. Chen, S. Wang, K. Ben Othman, B. Cullen, R.J. Leach, C.O. Hanemann, P. De Jonghe, P. Raeymaekers, G.-J.B. van Ommen, J.-J. Martin, H.W. Müller, J.M. Vance, K.H. Fischbeck, and C. Van Broeckhoven. 1992. The peripheral myelin protein gene *PMP22* is contained within the Charcot-Marie-Tooth disease type 1A duplication. *Nat. Genet.* **1:** 171.

Valentijn, L.J., F. Baas, I. Zorn, G.W. Hensels, M. de Visser, and P.A. Bolhuis. 1993. Alternatively sized duplication in Charcot-Marie-Tooth disease type 1A. *Hum. Mol. Genet.* **2:** 2143.

Valentijn, L.J., R.A. Ouvrier, N.H.A. van den Bosch, P.A. Bolhuis, F. Baas, and G.A. Nicholson. 1995. Déjérine-Sottas neuropathy is associated with a de novo PMP22 mutation. *Hum. Mutat.* **5:** 76.

Valentijn, L.J., F. Baas, R.A. Wolterman, J.E. Hoogendijk, N.H.A. van den Bosch, I. Zorn, A.A.W.M. Gabreëls-Festen, M. de Visser, and P.A. Bolhuis. 1992a. Identical point mutations of *PMP22* in *Trembler-J* mouse and Charcot-Marie-Tooth disease type 1A. *Nat. Genet.* **2:** 288.

Valentijn, L.J., P.A. Bolhuis, I. Zorn, J.E. Hoogendijk, N. van den Bosch, G.W. Hensels, V.P. Stanton, Jr., D.E. Housman, K.H. Fischbeck, D.A. Ross, G.A. Nicholson, E.J. Meershoek, H.G. Dauwerse, G.-J.B. van Ommen, and F. Baas. 1992b. The peripheral myelin gene *PMP22/GAS-3* is duplicated in Charcot-Marie-Tooth disease type 1A. *Nat. Genet.* **1:** 166.

Vance, J.M., G.A. Nicholson, L.H. Yamaoka, J. Stajich, C.S. Stewart, M.C. Speer, W.-Y. Hung, A.D. Roses, D. Barker, and M.A. Pericak-Vance. 1989. Linkage of Charcot-Marie-Tooth neuropathy type 1a to chromosome 17. *Exp. Neurol.* **104:** 186.

Verhalle, D., A. Löfgren, E. Nelis, I. Dehaene, P. Theys, M. Lammens, R. Dom, C. Van Broeckhoven, and W. Robberecht. 1994. Deletion in the CMT1A locus on chromosome 17p11.2 in hereditary neuropathy with liability to pressure palsies. *Ann. Neurol.* **35:** 704.

Warner, L.E., B.B. Roa, and J.R. Lupski. 1996a. Absence of *PMP22* coding region mutations in CMT1A duplication patients: Further evidence supporting gene dosage as a mechanism for Charcot-Marie-Tooth disease type 1A. *Hum. Mutat.* **8:** (in press).

Warner, L.E., M.J. Hilz, S.H. Appel, J.M. Killian, E.H. Kolodny, G. Karpati, S. Carpenter, G.V. Watters, C. Wheeler, D. Witt, A. Bodell, E. Nelis, C. Van Broeckhoven, and J.R. Lupski. 1996b. Clinical phenotypes of different *MPZ* (P_0) mutations may include Charcot-Marie-Tooth type 1B, Dejerine-Sottas, and congenital hypomyelination. *Neuron* (in press).

Wise, C.A., C.A. Garcia, S.N. Davis, Z. Heju, L. Pentao, P.I. Patel, and J.R. Lupski. 1993. Molecular analyses of unrelated Charcot-Marie-Tooth (CMT) disease patients suggest a high frequency of the CMT1A duplication. *Am. J. Hum. Genet.* **53:** 853.

Yoshikawa, H. and P.J. Dyck. 1991. Uncompacted inner myelin lamellae in inherited tendency to pressure palsy. *J. Neuropath. Exp. Neurol.* **50:** 649.

Yoshikawa, H., T. Nishimura, Y. Nakatsuji, H. Fujimura, M. Himoro, K. Hayasaka, S. Sakoda, and T. Yanagihara. 1994. Elevated expression of messenger RNA for peripheral myelin protein 22 in biopsied peripheral nerves of patients with Charcot-Marie-Tooth disease type 1A. *Ann. Neurol.* **35:** 445.

Connexin32 and X-linked Charcot-Marie-Tooth Disease

K.H. Fischbeck, S.M. Deschênes, L.J. Bone, and S.S. Scherer
Neurology Department, University of Pennsylvania School of Medicine, Philadelphia, Pennsylvania 19104

A common theme in the Symposium is that the identification of defective genes in hereditary neurological disease can give new insight into basic mechanisms of cellular structure and function. This paper deals with the genetic defect responsible for the X-linked form of Charcot-Marie-Tooth disease.

X-LINKED CHARCOT-MARIE-TOOTH DISEASE AND CONNEXIN32

Charcot-Marie-Tooth disease (CMT) causes progressive weakness, atrophy, and sensory loss in the feet, lower legs, and hands. Overall, CMT is a relatively common hereditary disorder, affecting about 1 in 2500 individuals, more than 100,000 Americans. The cause of the manifestations of CMT is degeneration of the peripheral nerves. In different families, the degenerative process can affect the axons, the myelin, or both.

CMT is genetically heterogeneous. It is classified first according to whether the pathology is primarily demyelinative or axonal, and second according to the specific genetic defect (Chance and Fischbeck 1994). The most common form, CMT1A, and a less common form, CMT1B, are caused by defects in the genes for myelin proteins PMP22 and P_0, respectively. The X-linked form of the disease (CMTX) is caused by mutations in the gap junction protein, connexin32 (Bergoffen et al. 1993b).

CMTX accounts for about 10% of patients with CMT and is probably the second most common cause of hereditary neuropathy after CMT1A. It is most often considered an X-linked dominant disease (Fischbeck et al. 1990; Deschênes et al. 1996). The disease is commonly passed from generation to generation, affecting both males and females as with autosomal dominant transmission, except that there is no father-to-son transmission. Heterozygous females are variably involved and in some families may be asymptomatic. Nerve conduction velocities tend to be slow, in an intermediate range, and nerve biopsies may show signs of both demyelination and axonal degeneration.

Several years ago, we and other workers set out to identify the CMTX disease gene by positional cloning, and the disease locus was eventually narrowed to a small segment of the proximal long arm of the X chromosome, at Xq13.1 (Bergoffen et al. 1993a). The interval to which CMTX was mapped contained three previously identified genes, including the gene for connexin32. We evaluated connexin32 as a candidate gene, first by determining whether or not it is expressed in peripheral nerve. Northern blots show that connexin32 is expressed in peripheral nerve, and that it follows the same pattern of expression as other myelin-related genes, decreasing in nerve that is degenerating after transection and increasing in nerve that is regenerating after a crush (Scherer et al. 1995). This pattern differs from that of nerve growth factor receptor and the housekeeping gene glyceraldehyde phosphate dehydrogenase. In cultured Schwann cells, connexin32 is expressed with other myelin genes when the cells are treated with forskolin, an agent that increases cAMP levels.

Connexin32 is encoded by a relatively simple gene with two promoters, and the translated sequence is contained in a single exon (Fig. 1). The first promoter, P1, drives expression in the liver, where connexin32 was first identified, and elsewhere in the body. The second promoter, P2, is nervous-system-specific and drives expression in peripheral nerve in a pattern similar to other myelin genes. Once we knew that the connexin32 gene is expressed in peripheral nerve and mapped to the same location as CMTX on the X chromosome, we set out to look for mutations in CMTX patients. We found that the large majority of CMTX patients have mutations in the translated portion of the gene (Bone et al. 1995). Since 1993, over 70 different mutations have been identified.

Many of the known CMTX mutations are shown in Figure 2, where connexin32 is shown in its likely topographic orientation, as an integral membrane protein with four transmembrane domains and amino and carboxyl termini within the cell. There are two extracellular loops with highly conserved cysteine residues that are thought to be involved in intramolecular disulfide bonds that ultimately stabilize

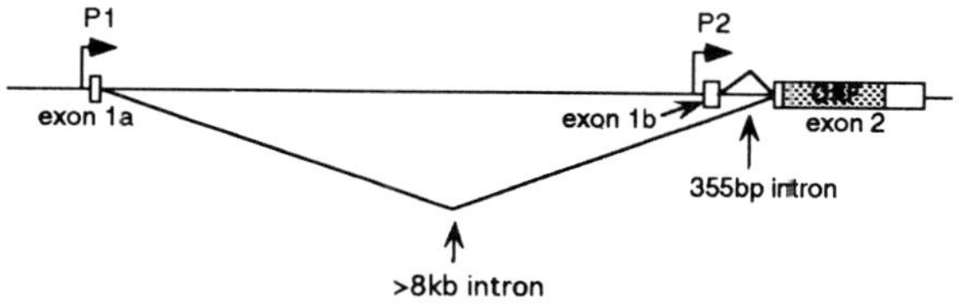

Figure 1. Structure of the human connexin32 gene. (ORF) Open reading frame.

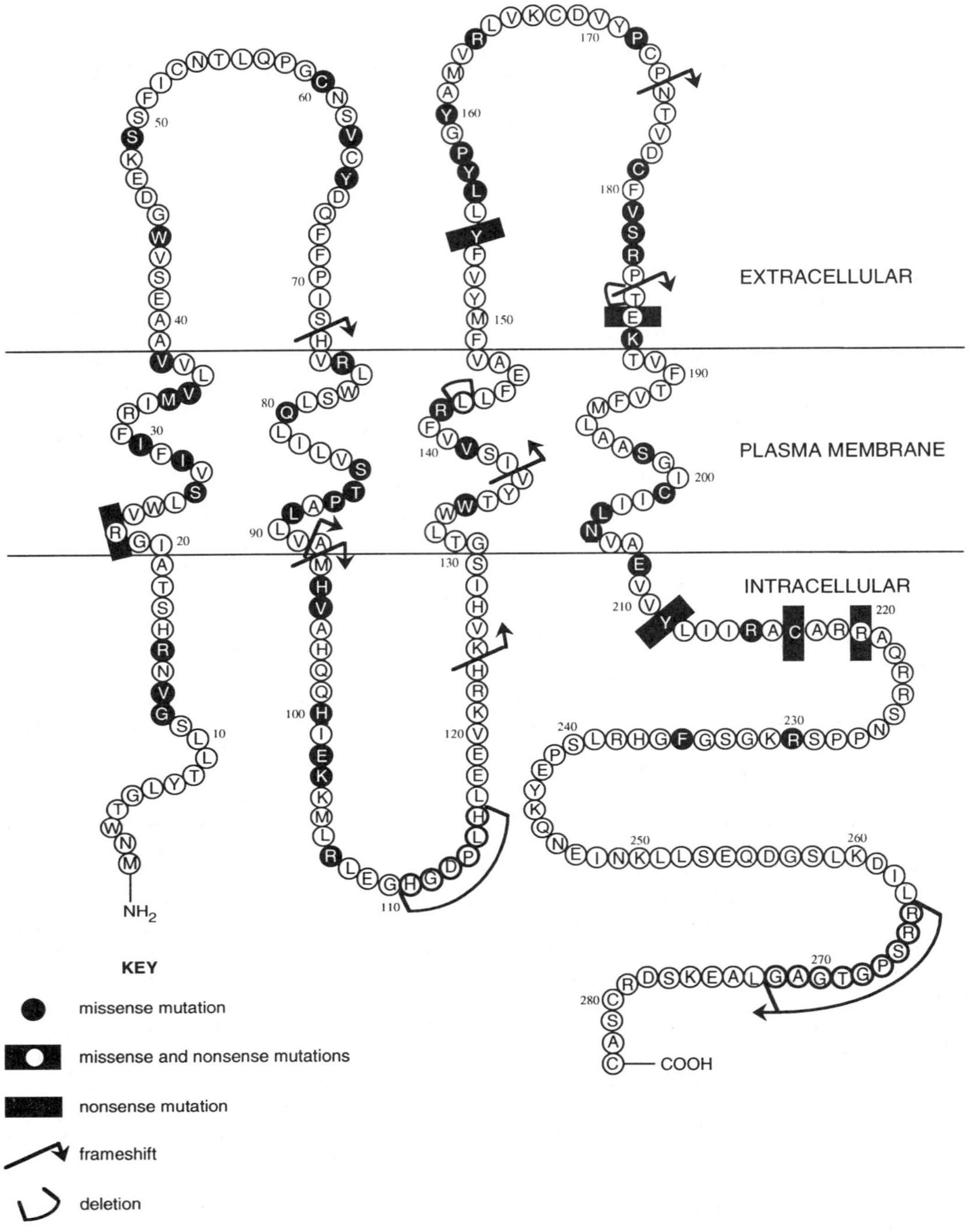

Figure 2. Diagram showing the topographic orientation of connexin32 with the locations of known CMTX mutations. 74 different mutations have been identified in 91 families.

the gap junction structure. The transmembrane domains are also highly conserved across species and among different members of the connexin gene family. The CMTX mutations are mostly missense (amino acid substitutions), although deletions, frameshifts, and premature stop mutations are also seen. Mutations have been found in every portion of the protein.

CONNEXIN32 STRUCTURE AND FUNCTION

Connexin32, like other members of the connexin family, is a channel protein. Six identical subunits cluster in the plasma membrane to form a hemichannel or connexon. This structure docks with a similar structure in another membrane to form a complete channel.

The channel has a central pore that allows passage of ions and other small molecules up to 1000 daltons in size from one cell to another. An array of individual channels makes up a gap junction.

Connexin32 is found in a variety of cells and tissues, including liver, secretory epithelium, and brain. Until it was implicated in CMTX, connexin32 was not known to be expressed in peripheral nerve, nor were gap junctions known to play a role in peripheral nerve structure and function.

What effect do the CMTX mutations have on the function of connexin32? Roberto Bruzzone in David Paul's laboratory at Harvard addressed this question by introducing wild-type and mutant connexin32 into *Xenopus* oocytes and assaying the formation of gap junctions electrophysiologically (Bruzzone et al. 1994). Normal connexin32, but not mutant connexin32, forms functional gap junctions in this system. Furthermore, mutant connexin32 interferes with the formation of gap junctions by co-injected wild-type cDNA, suggesting a dominant-negative effect.

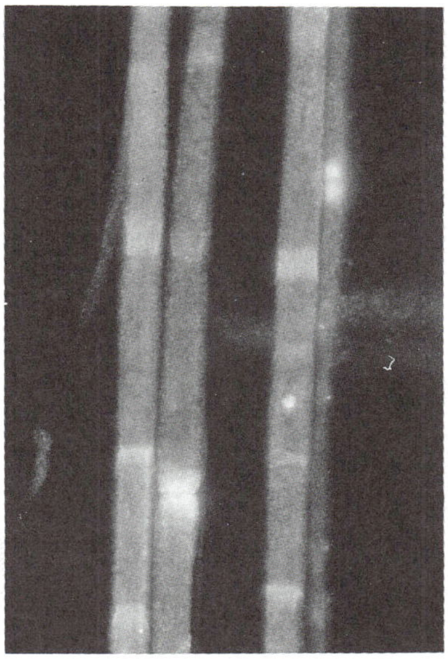

Figure 4. Teased fiber preparation of rat sciatic nerve, showing immunofluorescent staining of connexin32 at nodes of Ranvier and Schmidt-Lanterman incisures.

INTRACELLULAR TRAFFICKING OF MUTANT CONNEXIN32

We have gone on to investigate the fate of mutant connexin32 in stably transfected mammalian (PC12J) cells. Here the wild-type connexin32 protein forms aggregates at points of cell-cell contact (Fig. 3A). These are not seen in nontransfected cells. Immunohistochemistry of cells transfected with connexin32 cDNA derived from a CMTX patient shows that the mutant protein "hangs up" in the cytoplasm, most prominently in the endoplasmic reticulum and Golgi apparatus, and is not properly routed to the plasma membrane (Fig. 3B).

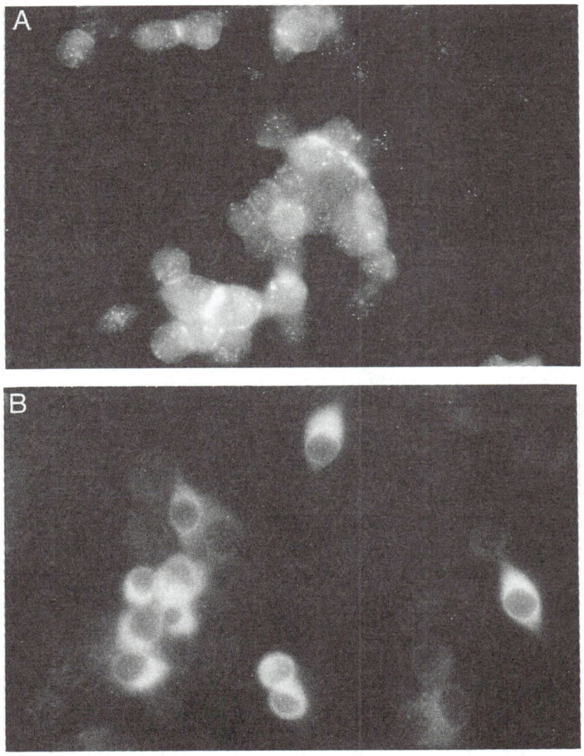

Figure 3. Immunofluorescence of connexin32 in stably transfected PC12J cells. (*A*) Wild-type connexin32, which localizes to the plasma membrane at points of cell-cell contact. (*B*) Mutant connexin32, which remains in the cytoplasm.

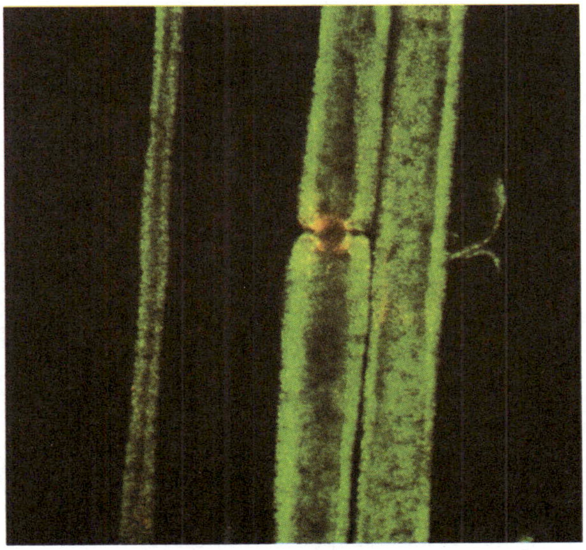

Figure 5. Confocal image of myelinated nerve fibers showing immunofluorescent staining of P_0 (*green*) and connexin32 (*orange*).

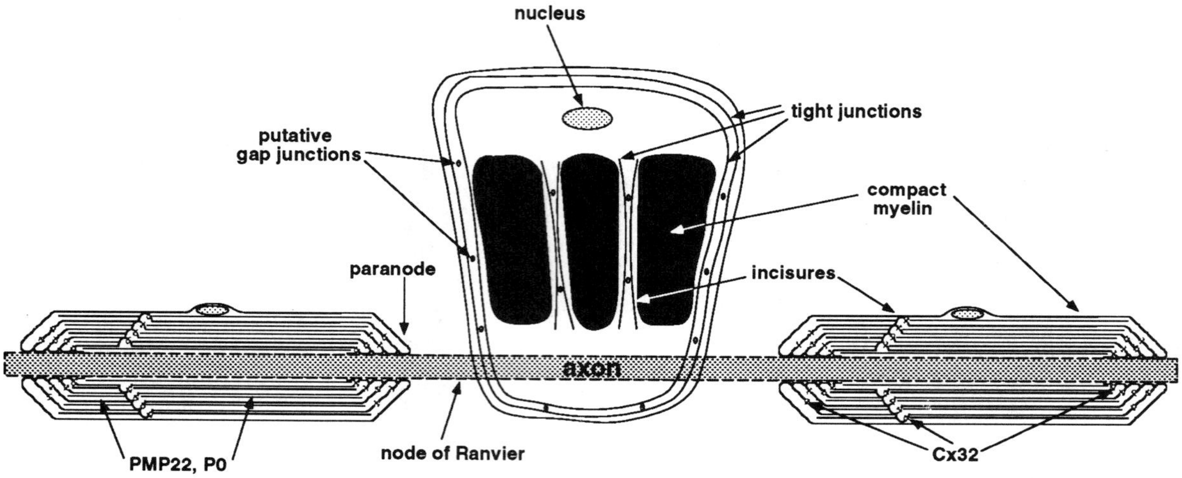

Figure 6. Schematic diagram of myelinated nerve, with the Schwann cell "unwound." Shown are the relative distributions of connexin32 and other myelin proteins and the location of putative gap junctions.

We have looked at seven different mutations and have found different effects on intracellular trafficking. In one case, the mutant cDNA is expressed at the mRNA but not the protein level; perhaps this protein is degraded too rapidly to give signal by immunofluorescence and Western blot. In several cases, some plasma membrane signal is seen. However, with most mutations, particularly those affecting residues within and adjacent to the transmembrane domains, the protein accumulates in the cytoplasm. It may be that misrouted connexin32 protein has a toxic effect on Schwann cells and axons, beyond the direct effects of loss of the protein's function. We plan to sort out toxic or dominant-negative effects in vivo by studying transgenic mice.

We are using transgenic constructs with the P_0 promoter to introduce two different mutant forms of connexin32 into mice. These mice are being bred with connexin32 knockout mice to observe the effects of the mutations on a null background. The knockout mice were produced by Dr. Klaus Willecke in Bonn, and have a relatively mild phenotype, consistent with a dominant-negative or toxic effect of the mutant protein on peripheral nerve.

CONNEXIN32 FUNCTION IN NORMAL NERVE

What is connexin32 doing in peripheral nerve? We can begin to answer that question by looking to see where connexin32 is normally located. We have done immunohistochemistry and have found connexin32 to be present in noncompacted myelin around the nodes of Ranvier and at Schmidt-Lanterman incisures (Bergoffen et al. 1993b; Scherer et al. 1995). This is a different distribution from other proteins implicated in hereditary neuropathy, PMP22 and P_0, which are located in compact myelin. The incisures and paranodes where connexin32 is located are residual folds of noncompacted Schwann cell cytoplasm that remain after the Schwann cell wraps itself around the axon to form the myelin sheath.

Figure 4 shows a teased fiber preparation demonstrating connexin32 staining in noncompacted myelin at the nodes and incisures. Figure 5 is a confocal image of myelinated nerve fibers with P_0 stained green in the compact myelin, and connexin32 stained orange at the node of Ranvier. There is no overlap between the distributions of P_0 and connexin32. Figure 6 shows the locations of connexin32 and other myelin proteins in peripheral nerve. David Paul proposed that connexin32 forms "reflexive" gap junctions at these sites, connecting different parts of the same Schwann cell rather than two different cells, and forming a path for diffusion of ions and other small molecules across the myelin sheath. This path perhaps provides nutritional support to the innermost layers of Schwann cell cytoplasm and indirectly to the axon, as well.

Preliminary results with injection of different dyes into myelinating Schwann cells of peripheral nerve indicate that such a path does indeed exist (R. Balice-Gordon et al., unpubl.). Low-molecular-weight dyes pass rapidly through incisures to the inner layers of Schwann cell cytoplasm, whereas high-molecular-weight dyes do not. We suspect that a loss of this pathway and perhaps additional toxic effects of misrouted protein account for the myelin loss and axonal degeneration of X-linked Charcot-Marie-Tooth disease.

The connexin32-CMTX story demonstrates how, when the interests of basic research and clinical medicine are coincident, we are brought to a better understanding not only of disease mechanisms, but also of the essentials of normal nervous system structure and function.

ACKNOWLEDGMENTS

This work was supported by grants from the Muscular Dystrophy Association and the National Institutes of Health (grant number NS-08075).

REFERENCES

Bergoffen, J., J. Trofatter, M.A. Pericak-Vance, J. Haines, P.F. Chance, and K.H. Fischbeck. 1993a. Linkage localization of X-linked Charcot-Marie-Tooth disease. *Am. J. Hum. Genet.* **52:** 312.

Bergoffen, J., S.S. Scherer, S. Wang, M.O. Scott, L.J. Bone, D.L. Paul, K. Chen, M.W. Lensch, P. Chance, and K.H. Fischbeck. 1993b. Connexin mutations in X-linked Charcot-Marie-Tooth disease. *Science* **262:** 2039.

Bone, L.J., N. Dahl, M.W. Lensch, P.F. Chance, T. Kelly, E. Le Guern, S. Magi, G. Parry, H. Shapiro, S. Wang, and K.H. Fischbeck. 1995. New connexin32 mutations associated with X-linked Charcot-Marie-Tooth disease. *Neurology* **45:** 1863.

Bruzzone, R., T.W. White, S.S. Scherer, K.H. Fischbeck, and D.L. Paul. 1994. Null mutations of connexin32 in patients with X-linked Charcot-Marie-Tooth disease. *Neuron* **13:** 1253.

Chance, P.F., and K.H. Fischbeck. 1994. Molecular genetics of Charcot-Marie-Tooth disease and related neuropathies. *Hum. Molec. Genet.* **3:** 1503.

Deschênes, S.M., L.J. Bone, K.H. Fischbeck, and S.S. Scherer. 1996. Connexin32 and X-linked Charcot-Marie-Tooth disease. In *The biology of gap junctions* (ed. D. Spray and R. Dermetziel), p. 213. R.G. Landes, Austin, Texas.

Fischbeck, K.H., A. Ritter, Y. Shi, M.P. Rozear, M.A. Pericak-Vance, A.D. Roses, P. Chance, and B. Burton. 1990. X-linked recessive and X-linked dominant Charcot-Marie-Tooth disease. In *Charcot-Marie-Tooth disorders: Pathophysiology, molecular genetics, and therapy* (ed. R.E. Lovelace and H.K. Shapiro), p. 335. Wiley-Liss, New York.

Scherer, S.S., S. M. Deschênes, Y. Xu, J.B. Grinspan, K.H. Fischbeck, and D.L. Paul. 1995. Connexin32 is a myelin-related protein in the PNS and CNS. *J. Neurosci.* **15:** 8281.

The Molecular Basis of Fragile X Syndrome

D.E. EBERHART AND S.T. WARREN
Howard Hughes Medical Institute and Departments of Biochemistry and Pediatrics, Emory University School of Medicine, Atlanta, Georgia 30322

Fragile X syndrome is one of the most common forms of inherited mental retardation. The disease is caused by the massive expansion and concomitant methylation of a CGG repeat located in the 5′-untranslated region of the *FMR1* gene, which results in transcriptional silencing of the gene. Since the absence of the fragile X mental retardation protein (FMRP) leads to mental retardation and FMRP is abundantly expressed in the neurons of the hippocampus and cerebellum, determining the normal function of the protein would not only provide information about the pathogenesis of fragile X syndrome, but should also provide insight into the mechanisms involved in cognition, memory, and behavior. Until recently there had been limited progress in elucidating the function of FMRP other than showing that FMRP can selectively bind RNA. Recent reports suggest that FMRP may be involved in the nuclear export and ribosome presentation of specific transcripts.

CLINICAL FEATURES AND INHERITANCE PATTERN

Fragile X syndrome, originally known as Martin-Bell syndrome, was found to cosegregate with a marker X chromosome characterized by a folate-sensitive fragile site at Xq27.3. The prevalence of fragile X syndrome has been estimated at 1 in 2000 males, making it the most common form of X-linked mental retardation. Fragile X patients show mild to severe mental retardation, with IQs generally between 20 and 60; mild facial dysmorphia, generally more prominent in males, including long, narrow facies and large ears; and macroorchidism (increased testicular volume) in postpubescent males. Many fragile X patients display additional clinical features which can include connective tissue abnormalities, hyperactivity and attention deficit disorder, and autistic-like behaviors (for reviews, see Warren and Nelson 1994; Warren and Ashley 1995).

Fragile X syndrome is an X-linked dominant disorder with reduced penetrance that shows an unusual inheritance pattern, referred to as the Sherman paradox (Sherman et al. 1984, 1985). It was observed that daughters of obligate carrier males were not at risk for inheriting fragile X syndrome, but grandsons of transmitting males were at risk when the allele was passed from the daughter. Thus, fragile X syndrome has only been observed when the mutant allele is maternally inherited. In addition, the risk of an individual having fragile X syndrome is influenced by his position in the pedigree, with risk increasing through the generations. The molecular basis of this unusual inheritance pattern was revealed upon cloning of the *FMR1* gene.

THE *FMR1* GENE

A positional cloning approach was taken to clone the gene responsible for fragile X syndrome (for review, see Warren and Ashley 1995). The molecular basis of fragile X syndrome was shown to be the expansion of the CGG repeat located in the 5′-untranslated region of the *f*ragile X *m*ental *r*etardation *1* (*FMR1*) gene (Fig. 1) (Kremer et al. 1991; Verkerk et al. 1991; Yu et al. 1991; Ashley et al. 1993b). The CGG repeat is highly polymorphic in normal individuals with sizes of 6 to 54 repeats and a mode of 30 repeats (Jacobs et al. 1993; Snow et al. 1993). The repeat is cryptic with interspersed AGG repeats most often found at repeat positions 10 and 20 (Eichler et al. 1994; Kunst and Warren 1994). In fragile X families, the CGG repeat is unstable and exists in premutation and full mutation forms. Carrier males and females have premutation alleles with CGG repeats ranging from 54 to about 200, whereas fragile X patients have full mutation alleles with repeats of more than 230 and often greater than 1000 (Fu et al. 1991). When the CGG repeat is expanded into the full mutation range, virtually the entire *FMR1* gene, including the CGG repeat and CpG island, is abnormally methylated (Oberlé et al. 1991; Hornstra et al. 1993), resulting in transcriptional silencing of the *FMR1* gene (Pieretti et al. 1991; Sutcliffe et al. 1992).

The correlation of CGG repeat size with penetrance for fragile X syndrome made it possible to resolve the Sherman paradox. Nonpenetrant males have CGG repeats in the premutation range, and the risk of expansion into the full mutation range is directly related to repeat length (Fu et al. 1991). However, it is not clear why expansion from premutation to full mutation is only seen when the fragile X allele is maternally inherited. The unusual inheritance pattern of fragile X syndrome can be described in terms of genetic anticipation, which refers to increasing severity or decreasing age of onset in subsequent generations, although penetrance, not expressivity, is increased in subsequent generations in fragile X syndrome.

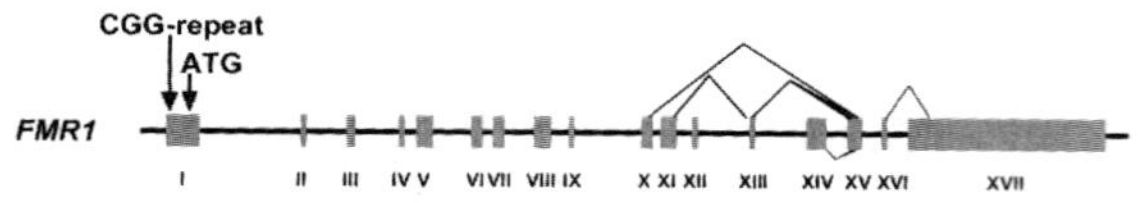

Figure 1. The *FMR1* gene. Exons 1–17 are shown as boxes connected by lines representing introns with alternative splicing depicted in the 3′end. The CGG repeat in the 5′-untranslated region that undergoes expansion in fragile X individuals is indicated, along with the ATG start codon. (Adapted from Eichler et al. 1993.)

Other Trinucleotide Repeat Expansion Diseases

Since the cloning of *FMR1*, it has been demonstrated that trinucleotide repeat expansions result in nine other neurological diseases (Table 1) (see Ashley and Warren 1995; Warren 1996). Until the recent discovery that Friedreich's ataxia is caused by a trinucleotide repeat expansion, all known repeat expansion diseases showed a dominant inheritance pattern and had repeats located in exons (Warren 1996). In contrast to the other repeat expansion diseases, Friedreich's ataxia is a recessive disease that does not show genetic anticipation and is caused by the expansion of a GAA repeat in an intron (Campuzano et al. 1996). It seems likely that numerous other diseases result from trinucleotide repeat expansion, given that there are other diseases that exhibit genetic anticipation, that uncharacterized human repeat loci have been detected (Riggins et al. 1992; Schalling et al. 1993), and that recessive diseases can be caused by trinucleotide repeat expansions.

Methylation of the *FMR1* Gene

Expansion of the CGG repeat into the full mutation range is accompanied by abnormal methylation of the *FMR1* gene. Molecular diagnosis of fragile X syndrome is most often made using Southern blot analysis of genomic DNA digested with *Eco*RI and a methylation-sensitive enzyme (*Eag*I or *Bss*HII) to allow detection of methylation status and repeat size (Fig. 2). In addition, amplification of the CGG repeat region using the polymerase chain reaction can be utilized to determine more precisely the size of the CGG repeat tract (Fig. 3) (for review of molecular diagnostics, see Warren and Nelson 1994).

For individuals with repeats in the 200–300 size range, methylation seems to be the best indicator of penetrance. Several individuals have been identified who are mosaic for the full fragile X mutation with repeats of 200–400 but show little or no methylation of the *FMR1* locus and are phenotypically normal (Loesch et al. 1993). Conversely, some individuals with repeats in the 200–300 range along with partial methylation have mild clinical symptoms of fragile X syndrome (McConkie-Rosell et al. 1993). Approximately half of females with a full mutation repeat display mental impairment (Rousseau et al. 1991). Nonpenetrant females with a full mutation may escape clinical involvement due to X-inactivation patterns that would affect the number of cells expressing *FMR1* in key regions of the brain (Kirchgessner et al. 1995).

One might conclude that removal of the aberrant methylation associated with full mutation size repeats would be a possible treatment for fragile X syndrome. However, an expanded and unmethylated CGG repeat tract (266 repeats) appears to inhibit translation of the corresponding *FMR1* message, resulting in very low levels of protein (Feng et al. 1995). Therefore, even if methylation is removed to alleviate transcriptional silencing, *FMR1* mRNAs containing multiple CGG repeats may be poorly translated due to stalling of the ribosomal initiation complex (Feng et al. 1995).

Table 1. Trinucleotide Repeat Expansions in Humans

Locus	Disorder	Repeat	Repeat location	Consequence of repeat expansion
FMR1 (FRAXA)	fragile X syndrome	CGG	5′UTR	loss of function/fragile site
FRAXE	fragile XE mental retardation	GCC	5′UTR	loss of function/fragile site
FRA11B	predisposition to Jacobsen (11q-) syndrome in offspring	CGG	5′UTR	fragile site
FRAXF	none	GCC	n.d.[a]	fragile site
FRA16A	none	CGG	n.d.	fragile site
AR	spinal and bulbar muscular atrophy	CAG	coding	gain and partial loss-of-function
SCA1	spinocerebellar ataxia type 1	CAG	coding	gain of function
Hdh (IT15)	Huntington's disease	CAG	coding	gain of function
B37 (DRPLA)	Dentatorubral-pallidoluysian atrophy Haw River syndrome (phenotypic variant)	CAG	coding	gain of function
MJD1 (SCA3)	Machado-Joseph disease	CAG	coding	gain of function
DMPK	myotonic dystrophy	CTG	3′UTR	abnormal processing of *DMPK* message?
FRDA	Friedreich's ataxia	GAA	intron	disruption of RNA splicing

[a]n.d. = not determined.

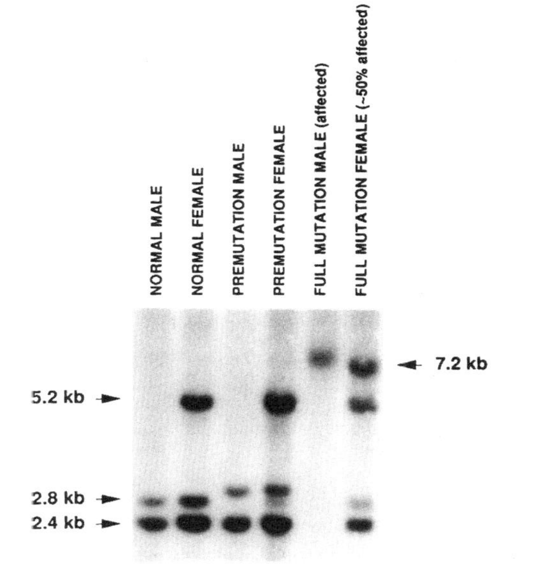

Figure 2. Molecular detection of the *FMR1* gene. Southern blot of genomic DNA digested with *Eco*RI and the methylation-sensitive enzyme, *Bss*HII, run on an agarose gel, blotted onto nylon membrane, and probed with radiolabeled *FMR1* fragment pE5.1. An examination of band size allows estimation of repeat size and determination of methylation status. (Reprinted, with permission, from Warren and Nelson 1994 [copyright American Medical Association].)

Altered Chromatin Conformation at the Fragile X Locus

The mechanism by which CGG repeat expansion and subsequent methylation results in the transcriptional silencing of *FMR1* and the fragile site formation seen in fragile X syndrome is unclear. It has been reported that CGG repeats can form unusual DNA structures in vitro (Gacy et al. 1995), but these data have not been confirmed in vivo. Since expanded premutation and full mutation repeats have proven refractory to cloning, an in vivo approach was taken to assess chromatin structure at the fragile X locus (D.E. Eberhart and S.T. Warren, in prep.). Lymphoblastoid cells from normal, premutation, or fragile X individuals were permeabilized and incubated with endonucleases to allow cleavage of the DNA in vivo as a means of assessing chromatin accessibility. Whereas DNA from normal and premutation cells was completely digested in vivo, DNA from full mutation fragile X individuals was not cleaved at the fragile locus but was completely digested at another locus on the X chromosome. Therefore, it appears that CGG repeat expansion and methylation may lead to the formation of an altered chromatin structure that results in the transcriptional silencing of *FMR1*.

It has been suggested that methylation of CpG islands can result in altered chromatin structure, which either directly inhibits transcription due to structural changes (Antequera et al. 1990) or indirectly inhibits transcription via proteins that bind to methylated CpGs (Boyes and Bird 1991). An increase in the number of CTG repeats, as seen in myotonic dystrophy, increases the efficiency of nucleosome formation which could affect transcription (Wang et al. 1994; Wang and Griffith 1995), and it is possible that expanded CGG repeat tracts undergo a similar phenomenon. One documented change following repeat expansion and methylation is delayed timing of replication of the *FMR1* locus (Hansen et al. 1993), which may be the molecular basis for cytogenetic fragile site expression. Although repeat expansion seems to precede methylation (Sutcliffe et al. 1992), further work is necessary to characterize the changes that occur following repeat expansion and methylation and to determine the mechanism by which these changes lead to the transcriptional silencing that results in fragile X syndrome.

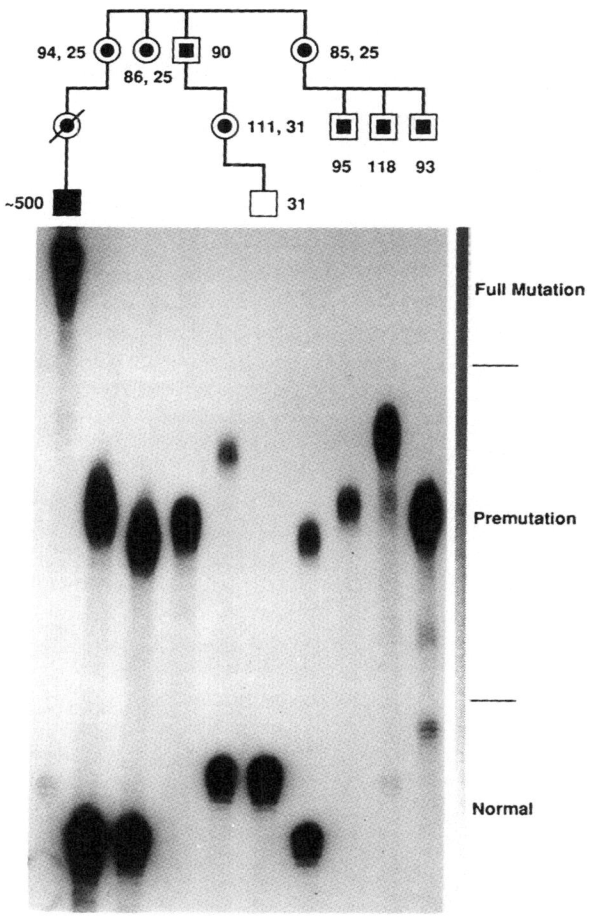

Figure 3. PCR amplification of the *FMR1* CGG repeat by using primers flanking the repeat allows precise estimation of repeat size. (Reprinted, with permission, from Warren and Nelson 1994 [copyright American Medical Association].)

CGG Repeat Expansion in the *FMR1* Gene

The mechanism and timing of CGG repeat expansion in fragile X syndrome have not been defined.

Analysis of fragile X pedigrees has failed to detect any new mutations that result in fragile X syndrome (Rousseau et al. 1991; Smits et al. 1993). Consistent with this observation, linkage disequlibrium has been observed between normal and fragile X chromosomes via haplotype analysis with flanking polymorphisms (Richards et al. 1992), suggesting that a subset of normal chromosomes are predisposed to CGG repeat expansion at the fragile X locus. Certain haplotypes that contain more nearly pure CGG repeat tracts (with fewer AGG repeats) are overrepresented on fragile X chromosomes, leading to the suggestion that alleles with long, perfect repeat tracts are predisposed to expansion (Hirst et al. 1994; Kunst and Warren 1994; Snow et al. 1994). Accordingly, it was reported that intergenerational instability correlates with uninterrupted repeat tracts of 34–38 repeats (Eichler et al. 1994). *FMR1* CGG repeat tracts tend to be smaller or more cryptic in nonhumans (Ashley et al. 1993b; Eichler et al. 1995) and presumably more stable, which may partially explain why trinucleotide repeat instability has only been observed in humans. Sequence analysis of *FMR1* repeats has identified a distinct polarity in the repeat tracts with all length variation occurring in the 3′end (Kunst and Warren 1994). On the basis of these observations, several groups have proposed models of repeat expansion based on slippage during lagging-strand DNA synthesis (Eichler et al. 1994; Kunst and Warren 1994; Richards 1994).

The timing of the CGG repeat expansion in fragile X syndrome is unclear. Several observations have led to the hypothesis that repeat instability is limited to a brief window during embryonic development. Somatic mosaicism is often observed in fragile X males who contain both premutation and multiple full mutation alleles (Fu et al. 1991), and expanded CGG repeats are mitotically stable (Wohrle et al. 1993). In addition, only premutation size repeats are found in sperm from males with full mutation alleles in their somatic tissue, suggesting that expansion occurs after segregation of the germ cells in embryonic development, or that *FMR1* expression might be vital to sperm viability (Reyniers et al. 1993). However, *FMR1* knockout mice are fertile (Dutch-Belgian Fragile X Consortium 1994), suggesting that there is no selection against full mutation sperm.

FMR1 Gene Structure and Expression

The *FMR1* gene has 17 exons and shows extensive alternative splicing at the 3′end (Fig. 1) (Ashley et al. 1993b; Eichler et al. 1993). Zoo blot analysis using a *FMR1* probe shows that the gene is conserved in numerous species, suggesting that it has an important function (Verkerk et al. 1991). When compared to human *FMR1*, the murine, chicken, and *Xenopus* genes show amino acid identities of 97%, 91%, and 86%, respectively (Ashley et al. 1993b; Siomi et al. 1995; Price et al. 1996). The CGG repeat is located in the 5′-untranslated region of exon 1 and is 250 bp downstream from the CpG island located in the putative *FMR1* promoter region (Ashley et al. 1993b; Eichler et al. 1993). Hergersberg et al. (1995) report that a 2.8-kb *FMR1* fragment, including the CpG island and the CGG repeat, can direct tissue-specific expression of a reporter gene. It has been reported that nuclear proteins can specifically bind to the CGG repeat (Richards et al. 1993). Further work is needed to define the *cis*-regulatory elements directing *FMR1* expression, but evolutionary conservation of the CGG repeat in mammals is consistent with the repeat's being important for gene expression (Ashley et al. 1993b; Eichler et al. 1995). In contrast to mammals, the chicken *fmr1* gene contains a CCT repeat (Price et al. 1996), and no repeat was noted in 125 bp of 5′-untranslated region in the *Xenopus fmr1* gene (Siomi et al. 1995).

FMR1 is widely expressed, both in the tissues affected by fragile X syndrome and in tissues showing no phenotypic involvement. Northern analysis of human tissue detected abundant expression of a 4.4-kb *FMR1* message in brain, testes, placenta, lung, and kidney (Hinds et al. 1993). RNA in situ hybridization in the adult mouse revealed abundant *fmr1* expression in brain, testes, ovary, esophageal epithelium, thymus, eye, and spleen, with moderate expression in colon, uterus, thyroid, and liver, and no expression in the heart, aorta, or muscle (Hinds et al. 1993). An examination of cross sections of mouse brain or sections of a 25-week-old human fetal brain revealed strong *fmr1* expression in the neurons of the hippocampus and granular layer of the cerebellum with sparse glial staining (Abitbol et al. 1993; Hinds et al. 1993). Using antibodies directed against the *FMR1* gene product, FMRP, analysis of protein levels in the brain revealed high levels of FMRP in neurons with little staining in white matter (Devys et al. 1993). In addition, a *FMR1/lacZ* transgene shows high levels of β-galactosidase expression in the neurons of the hippocampus and the granular layer of the cerebellum (Hergersberg et al. 1995). In summary, *FMR1* shows widespread expression during development with neuronal expression becoming localized to the areas of the hippocampus and cerebellum that are involved in cognition, memory, and behavior, a finding that is consistent with the fragile X phenotype.

THE FRAGILE X MENTAL RETARDATION PROTEIN

Initially, it was not clear whether the absence of FMRP, the protein encoded by *FMR1*, was solely responsible for fragile X syndrome. Since nearly all cases of fragile X syndrome are caused by repeat expansion, it seemed possible that other genes in the region might be inactivated by the methylation that accompanies repeat expansion. However, no additional genes have been located near *FMR1,* and several *FMR1* deletions and a point mutation result in the mental retardation and characteristic phenotype of fragile X syndrome (Hirst et al. 1995; Lugenbeel et al. 1995 and references therein). In addition, targeted inactivation of the murine *fmr1* gene results in mice with cognitive deficits, hyperactivity, and increased testicular volume, a phenotype similar to fragile X syndrome (Dutch-Belgian Fragile X Consortium 1994). Therefore, the absence of functional FMRP is responsible for the fragile X syndrome phenotype.

FMR1 shows extensive alternative splicing at the 3′ end, resulting in multiple FMRP isoforms with distinct carboxyl termini (Ashley et al. 1993b). FMRP isoforms of distinct molecular weights are apparent on protein immunoblot analysis from a variety of tissues, although isoforms are sometimes present at different quantitative levels (Khandjian et al. 1995; Verheij et al. 1995). Both the chicken and *Xenopus fmr1* genes do not contain exon 11 or 12 (Siomi et al. 1995; Price et al. 1996). Since no FMRP isoform-specific antibodies have been reported, there is no information regarding functional diversity or distinct tissue distributions among isoforms.

FMRP Is an RNA-binding Protein

Initial homology searches with *FMR1* and FMRP sequences revealed no homology with known genes or proteins. However, searches with smaller portions of FMRP amino acid sequence revealed the presence of motifs, two KH domains and a RGG box, which are found in proteins that interact with RNA (Fig. 4) (Ashley et al. 1993a; Siomi et al. 1993). Ashley et al. (1993a) demonstrated that FMRP can bind to its own message in vitro with high affinity and can bind to a subset of human brain mRNAs. FMRP also binds homopolymer RNA in vitro (Siomi et al. 1993). In addition, FMRP can be UV-crosslinked to mRNA in vivo (Eberhart et al. 1996). Given the selective RNA binding ability of FMRP, it has been suggested that FMRP might play a role in RNA metabolism (see below).

The region of FMRP responsible for RNA binding has not been precisely delineated. An isoleucine-to-asparagine mutation in a highly conserved residue in the second KH domain of FMRP was observed in a severely affected fragile X syndrome patient (De Boulle et al. 1993), and this mutation was shown to eliminate binding to poly(U) RNA under high-salt conditions (Siomi et al. 1994). Three-dimensional solution structure analysis suggests that the Ile-Asn mutation disrupts the structure of the KH domain fold (Musco et al. 1996). Attempts to define the region of FMRP responsible for RNA binding have demonstrated the importance of the carboxyl terminus, which includes the RGG box. FMRP constructs with truncated carboxyl termini cannot bind mRNA (Siomi et al. 1993; Price et al. 1996). Thus, at least a portion of the carboxyl terminus of FMRP, encoded by exons 14–17, is necessary for FMRP-RNA binding, whereas the KH domains may play a role in modulating binding.

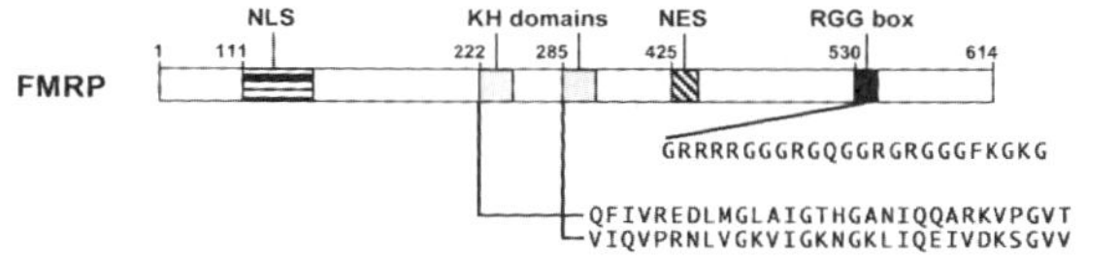

Figure 4. Schematic representation of FMRP with the nuclear localization signal (NLS), KH domains, nuclear export signal (NES), and RGG box indicated. Amino acid numbers are labeled according to Ashley et al. (1993b).

FMRP Is Associated with Ribosomes

Immunolocalization studies with antibodies directed against FMRP have revealed that FMRP is predominantly localized in the cytoplasm with a diffuse granular staining pattern (Devys et al. 1993; Verheij et al. 1993). Recent reports have indicated that FMRP is associated with translating ribosomes (Eberhart et al. 1996; Khandjian et al. 1996; Tamanini et al. 1996). FMRP is associated with ribosomes in an RNA-dependent manner (Eberhart et al. 1996; Tamanini et al. 1996). EDTA treatment, which dissociates ribosomal subunits, releases FMRP from ribosomes into messenger ribonucleoprotein (mRNP) particles (Eberhart et al. 1996). Taken as a whole, these data suggest that FMRP associates with ribosomes as a component of a mRNP particle.

The localization of FMRP in neurons has been analyzed using immunogold electron microscopy with an antibody directed against FMRP (S. Hersch et al., in prep.). The highest concentration of immunogold particles was seen in the cell body in regions rich in ribosomes, but immunogold particles were also seen in dendritic spines at sites where ribosomes are customarily found. Neuronal FMRP was also found in synaptosomes associated with ribosomes. It has been established that synaptic plasticity, as reflected by hippocampal long-term potentiation (LTP), requires protein synthesis (Frey et al. 1991), and it has been suggested that regulated translation occurs in hippocampal processes (Miyashiro et al. 1994; Steward 1994). Therefore, since FMRP is associated with ribosomes and the hippocampus is rich in FMRP (Abitbol et al. 1993; Hinds et al. 1993), FMRP could conceivably be involved in modulating translation, which appears to play a crucial role in learning and memory.

FMRP Could Be Involved in RNA Export

Although FMRP is predominantly localized in the cytoplasm, nuclear staining has been reported (Devys et al. 1993; Verheij et al. 1993). Since FMRP seems to associate with ribosomes as a component of mRNP particles, and most RNP particles are formed in the nucleus, and given the fact that other RNA-binding proteins can shuttle between the nucleus and cytoplasm, it is intriguing to consider that FMRP might enter the nucleus as a part of its normal function. Eberhart et al. (1996) utilized FMRP deletion and fusion

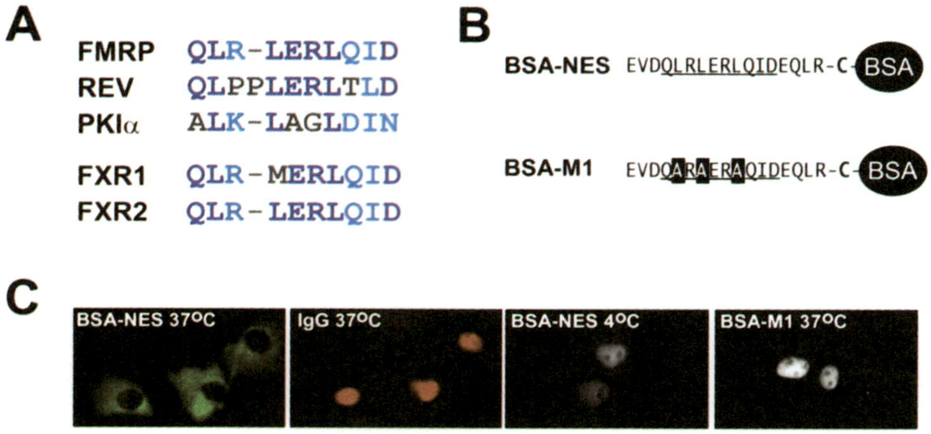

Figure 5. FMRP contains a functional NES. (*A*) NES sequences of FMRP, Rev, and PKI are shown with identical residues in dark blue and similar residues in light blue. The putative NES sequences of FXR1 and FXR2 are also shown. (*B*) Schematic representation of NES and M1 peptides conjugated to bovine serum albumin (BSA) via the carboxy-terminal cysteine. The putative NES sequence is underlined. In M1, leucine residues that were mutated from leucine to alanine are indicated by black boxes. (*C*) Fluorescent micrographs of COS7 cells 1 hour after nuclear microinjection of BSA-peptide conjugates. Fluorescein isothiocyanate-labeled BSA-NES (*green*) and lissamine rhodamine-labeled IgG (*red*) were coinjected. The IgG served as a control for injection site and leakage. BSA-NES is efficiently exported, whereas the IgG is retained in the nucleus. BSA-NES injected and incubated at 4°C was not exported. BSA-M1 was not exported. (Adapted from Eberhart et al. 1996.)

constructs to delineate a nuclear localization signal (NLS) in the amino terminus of FMRP and a nuclear export signal (NES) encoded by exon 14 (Fig. 4). The FMRP NES resembles the NES motifs recently described for the HIV-1 Rev protein (Fischer et al. 1995) and protein kinase inhibitor α (PKI) (Fig. 5A) (Wen et al. 1995). A 17-amino-acid peptide containing the FMRP NES can direct temperature-dependent nuclear export of a microinjected protein conjugate, whereas a mutant peptide cannot direct export (Fig. 5B,C). Im-

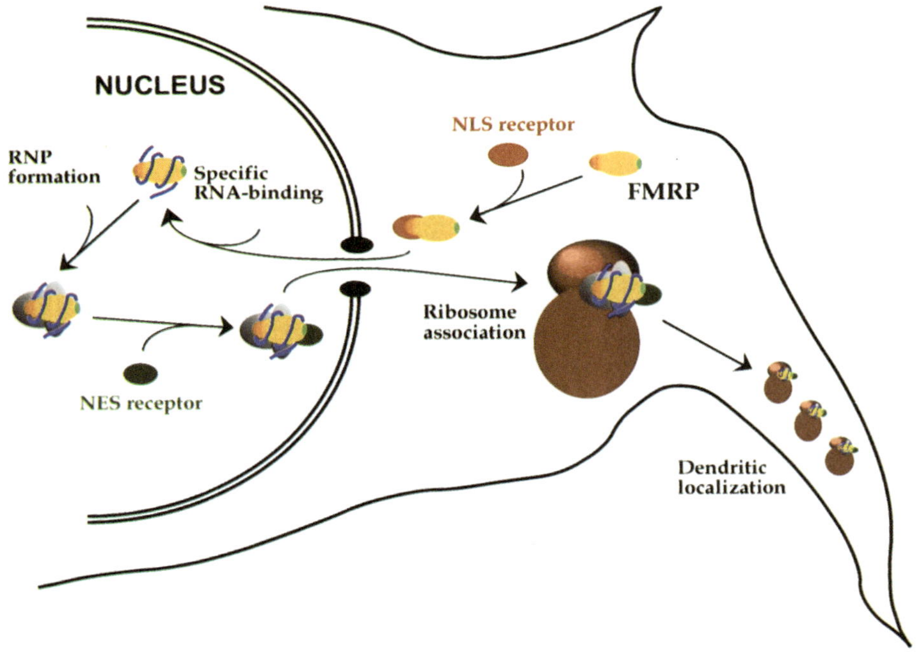

Figure 6. Model for FMRP cellular behavior. The NLS (*blue*) and NES (*red*) regions of FMRP are shown along with their appropriate receptors, which mediate transport across the nuclear pore. It is speculated that nascent FMRP enters the nucleus, selectively binds mRNA(s) within a mRNP particle, and then mediates export of the mRNP particle from the nucleus via its NES. In the cytoplasm, the FMRP-mRNP particle associates with ribosomes and may modulate translation of the mRNA(s) to which it binds. Given the presence of FMRP in dendritic spines of neurons, FMRP may play some role in localized translation at the postsynaptic junction.

munogold electron microscopy provides further evidence that FMRP is capable of shuttling between the nucleus and the cytoplasm. Whereas FMRP occurs predominantly in the cytoplasm of neurons, FMRP is detected in the nucleus and in transit through the nuclear pore (S. Hersch et al., in prep.).

The process of nuclear export is poorly understood, but the discovery of NESs has provided a great deal of insight into RNA export (Gerace 1995; Gorlich and Mattaj 1996). It has been suggested that protein-based NESs may be a common feature of nuclear RNA export (Gerace 1995). Rev binds and directs export of viral mRNAs containing the Rev response element binding site (Fischer et al. 1995). TFIIIA, which has been implicated in the export of 5S rRNA, contains a putative leucine-rich NES which can substitute for the Rev NES (Fischer et al. 1995; Gorlich and Mattaj 1996). hnRNP A1, which is associated with poly(A) RNA in both the nucleus and cytoplasm, contains the M9 domain, which allows shuttling between the two compartments (Michael et al. 1995). Other proteins that resemble hnRNP A1, such as the predominantly cytoplasmic hrp36 protein of *Chironomous tentans* (Visa et al. 1996), have also been implicated in RNA export. Although further analysis is necessary to determine the export characteristics of FMRP, the identification of domains that mediate nucleocytoplasmic shuttling suggests that FMRP may be involved in RNA export.

FMRP Homologs

Two autosomal homologs of *FMR1* have recently been described. Both FXR1 (Coy et al. 1995; Siomi et al. 1995) and FXR2 (Zhang et al. 1995) proteins show significant homology with FMRP, especially in the NLS region, the KH domains, and the NES (Fig. 5A). Like FMRP, FXR1 and FXR2 can bind RNA in vitro and are predominantly localized to the cytoplasm (Siomi et al. 1995; Zhang et al. 1995). The nucleocytoplasmic shuttling ability and ribosome association of FXR1 and FXR2 have not been tested. The tissue distribution of *FXR1* appears distinct from that of *FMR1* (Coy et al. 1995). An extensive analysis of the *FXR2* expression pattern has not been published, but expression is found in the brain and was detected in HeLa cells (Zhang et al. 1995) suggesting that *FXR2* may be expressed in some of the same tissues as *FMR1*. The tissue distribution of the three proteins is important, since it has been reported that FMRP, FXR1, and FXR2 can all form heteromers as well as homomers (Zhang et al. 1995). Heteromer formation does not require the carboxyl terminus but does require the presence of the central portion of FMRP, which contains the KH domains. The ability to form heteromers with FXR1 and FXR2, as well as the ability to form homomers, could have significant implications for the regulation of FMRP function.

Implications for Fragile X Syndrome

Taken as a whole, recent data suggest that nascent FMRP may enter the nucleus and bind specific mRNAs as part of a ribonucleoprotein (RNP) particle prior to being exported back into the cytoplasm via the NES (Fig. 6). In the cytoplasm, the FMRP-mRNP particle can associate with ribosomes, where FMRP may somehow modulate translation of the mRNA(s) to which it is bound. It is possible that FMRP plays some role in localized translation in neuronal dendrites, which may influence cognition. Thus, the emerging view is that fragile X syndrome results from the anomalous nuclear export and translational control of specific transcripts, leading to their inappropriate translation.

ACKNOWLEDGMENTS

S.T.W. is an investigator with the Howard Hughes Medical Institute and a National Alliance for Research on Schizophrenia and Depression Established Investigator.

REFERENCES

Abitbol, M., C. Menini, A.-L. Delezoide, T. Rhyner, M. Vekemans, and J. Mallet. 1993. Nucleus basalis magnocellularis and hippocampus are the major sites of *FMR-1* expression in the human fetal brain. *Nat. Genet.* **4:** 147.

Antequera, F., J. Boyes, and A. Bird. 1990. High levels of de novo methylation and altered chromatin structure at CpG islands in cell lines. *Cell* **62:** 503.

Ashley, C.T. and S.T. Warren. 1995. Trinucleotide repeat expansion and human disease. *Annu. Rev. Genet.* **29:** 703.

Ashley, C.T., K.D. Wilkinson, D. Reines, and S.T. Warren. 1993a. *FMR1* protein: Conserved RNP family domains and selective RNA binding. *Science* **262:** 563.

Ashley, C.T., J.S. Sutcliffe, C.B. Kunst, H.A. Leiner, E.E. Eichler, D.L. Nelson, and S.T. Warren. 1993b. Human and murine *FMR-1:* Alternative splicing and translational initiation downstream of the CGG repeat. *Nat. Genet.* **4:** 244.

Boyes, J. and A. Bird. 1991. DNA methylation inhibits transcription indirectly via a methyl-CpG binding protein. *Cell* **64:** 1123.

Campuzano, V., L. Montermini, M.D. Molto, L. Pianese, M. Cossee, F. Cavalcanti, E. Monros, F. Rodius, F. Duclos, A. Monticelli, F. Zara, J. Canizares, H. Koutnikova, S.I. Bidichandani, C. Gellera, A. Brice, P. Trouillas, G.D. Michele, A. Filla, R.D. Frutos, F. Palau, P.I. Patel, S.D. Donato, J.-L. Mandel, S. Cocozza, M. Koenig, and M. Pandolfo. 1996. Friedreich's ataxia: Autosomal recessive disease caused by an intronic GAA triplet repeat expansion. *Science* **271:** 1423.

Coy, J.F., Z. Sedlacek, D. Bachner, H. Hameister, S. Joos, P. Lichter, H. Delius, and A. Poustka. 1995. Highly conserved 3′UTR and expression pattern of FXR1 points to a divergent gene regulation of FXR1 and FMR1. *Hum. Mol. Genet.* **4:** 2209.

De Boulle, K., A.J.M.H. Verkerk, E. Reyniers, L. Vits, J. Hendrickx, B. Van Roy, F. Van den Bos, E. de Graaff, B.A. Oostra, and P.J. Willems. 1993. A point mutation in the *FMR-1* gene associated with fragile X mental retarda-

tion. *Nat. Genet.* **3:** 31.
Devys, D., Y. Lutz, N. Rouyer, J.-P. Bellocq, and J.-L. Mandel. 1993. The *FMR-1* protein is cytoplasmic, most abundant in neurons, and appears normal in carriers of the fragile X premutation. *Nat. Genet.* **4:** 335.
Dutch-Belgian Fragile X Consortium. 1994. FMR1 knockout mice: A model to study fragile X mental retardation. *Cell* **78:** 23.
Eberhart, D.E., H.E. Malter, Y. Feng, and S.T. Warren. 1996. The fragile X mental retardation protein is a ribonucleoprotein containing both nuclear localization and nuclear export signals. *Hum. Mol. Genet.* **5:** 1083.
Eichler, E.E., S. Richards, R.A. Gibbs, and D.L. Nelson. 1993. Fine structure of the human *FMR1* gene. *Hum. Mol. Genet.* **2:** 1147.
Eichler, E.E., C.B. Kunst, K.A. Lugenbeel, O.A. Ryder, D. Davison, S.T. Warren, and D.L. Nelson. 1995. Evolution of the cryptic *FMR1* CGG repeat. *Nat. Genet.* **11:** 301.
Eichler, E.E., J.J.A. Holden, B.W. Popovich, A.L. Reiss, K. Snow, S.N. Thibodeau, C.S. Richards, P.A. Ward, and D.L. Nelson. 1994. Length of uninterrupted CGG repeats determines instability in the *FMR1* gene. *Nat. Genet.* **8:** 88.
Feng, Y., F. Zhang, L.K. Lokey, J.L. Chastain, L. Lakkis, D. Eberhart, and S.T. Warren. 1995. Translational suppression by trinucleotide repeat expansion at *FMR1*. *Science* **268:** 731.
Fischer, U., J. Huber, W.C. Boelens, I.W. Mattaj, and R. Luhrmann. 1995. The HIV-1 Rev activation domain is a nuclear export signal that accesses an export pathway used by specific cellular RNAs. *Cell* **82:** 475.
Frey, S., C. Schweigert, M. Krug, and B. Lossner. 1991. Long-term potentiation induced changes in protein synthesis of hippocampal subfields of freely moving rats: Time-course. *Biomed. Biochim. Acta* **50:** 1231.
Fu, Y.-H., D.P. Kuhl, A. Pizzuti, M. Pieretti, J.S. Sutcliffe, S. Richards, A.J.M.H. Verkerk, J.J.A. Holden, R.G. Fenwick Jr., S.T. Warren, B.A. Oostra, D.L. Nelson, and C.T. Caskey. 1991. Variation of the CGG repeat at the fragile X site results in genetic instability: Resolution of the Sherman paradox. *Cell* **67:** 1047.
Gacy, A.M., G. Goellner, N. Juranic, S. Macura, and C.T. McMurray. 1995. Trinucleotide repeats that expand in human disease form hairpin structures in vitro. *Cell* **81:** 533.
Gerace, L. 1995. Nuclear export signals and the fast track to the cytoplasm. *Cell* **82:** 341.
Gorlich, D. and I. Mattaj. 1996. Nucleocytoplasmic transport. *Science* **271:** 1513.
Hansen, R.S., T.K. Canfield, M.M. Lamb, S.M. Gartler, and C.D. Laird. 1993. Association of fragile X syndrome with delayed replication of the *FMR1* gene. *Cell* **73:** 1403.
Hergersberg, M., K. Matsuo, M. Gassman, W. Schaffner, B. Luscher, T. Rulicke, and A. Aguzzi. 1995. Tissue-specific expression of a *FMR1*/β-galactosidase fusion gene in transgenic mice. *Hum. Mol. Genet.* **4:** 359.
Hinds, H.L., C.T. Ashley, D.L. Nelson, S.T. Warren, D.E. Housman, and M. Schalling. 1993. Tissue specific expression of *FMR1* provides evidence for a functional role in fragile X syndrome. *Nat. Genet.* **3:** 36.
Hirst, M.C., P.K. Grewal, and K.E. Davies. 1994. Precursor arrays for triplet repeat expansion at the fragile X locus. *Hum. Mol. Genet.* **3:** 1553.
Hirst, M., P. Grewal, A. Flannery, R. Slatter, E. Maher, D. Barton, J.-P. Fryns, and K. Davies. 1995. Two new cases of *FMR1* deletions associated with mental impairment. *Am. J. Hum. Genet.* **56:** 67.
Hornstra, I.K., D.L. Nelson, S.T. Warren, and T.P. Yang. 1993. High resolution methylation analysis of the *FMR1* gene trinucleotide repeat region in fragile X syndrome. *Hum. Mol. Genet.* **2:** 1659.
Jacobs, P.A., H. Bullman, J. Macpherson, S. Youings, V. Rooney, A. Watson, and N.R. Dennis. 1993. Population studies of the fragile X: A molecular approach. *J. Med. Genet.* **30:** 454.
Khandjian, E.W., F. Corbin, S. Woerly, and F. Rousseau. 1996. The fragile X mental retardation protein is associated with ribosomes. *Nat. Genet.* **12:** 91.
Khandjian, E.W., A. Fortin, A. Thibodeau, S. Tremblay, F. Cote, D. Devys, J.-L. Mandel, and F. Rousseau. 1995. A heterogeneous set of *FMR1* proteins is widely distributed in mouse tissues and modulated in cell culture. *Hum. Mol. Genet.* **4:** 783.
Kirchgessner, C.U., S.T. Warren, and H.L. Willard. 1995. X inactivation of the *FMR1* fragile X mental retardation gene. *J. Med. Genet.* **32:** 925.
Kremer, E.J., M. Pritchard, M. Lynch, S. Yu, K. Holman, E. Baker, S.T. Warren, D. Schlessinger, G.R. Sutherland, and R.I. Richards. 1991. Mapping of DNA instability at the fragile X to a trinucleotide repeat sequence p(CGG)*n*. *Science* **252:** 1711.
Kunst, C.B. and S.T. Warren. 1994. Cryptic and polar variation of the fragile X repeat could result in predisposing normal alleles. *Cell* **77:** 853.
Loesch, D.Z., R. Huggins, D.A. Hay, A.K. Gedeon, J.C. Mulley, and G.R. Sutherland. 1993. Genotype-phenotype relationships in fragile X syndrome: A family study. *Am. J. Hum. Genet.* **53:** 1064.
Lugenbeel, K.A., A.M. Peier, N.L. Carson, A.E. Chudley, and D.L. Nelson. 1995. Intragenic loss of function mutations demonstrate the primary role of *FMR1* in fragile X syndrome. *Nat. Genet.* **10:** 483.
McConkie-Rosell, A., A.M. Lachiewicz, G.A. Spiridigliozzi, J. Tarleton, S. Schoenwald, M.C. Phelan, P. Goonewardena, X. Ding, and W.T. Brown. 1993. Evidence that methylation of the FMR-1 locus is responsible for variable phenotypic expression of the fragile X syndrome. *Am. J. Hum. Genet.* **53:** 800.
Michael, W.M., M. Choi, and G. Dreyfuss. 1995. A nuclear export signal in hnRNP A1: A signal-mediated, temperature-dependent nuclear protein export pathway. *Cell* **83:** 291.
Miyashiro, K., M. Dichter, and J. Eberwine. 1994. On the nature and differential distribution of mRNAs in hippocampal neurites: Implications for neuronal functioning. *Proc. Natl. Acad. Sci.* **91:** 10800.
Musco, G., G. Stier, C. Joseph, M. Antonietta, C. Morelli, M. Nilges, T.J. Gibson, and A. Pastore. 1996. Three-dimensional structure and stability of the KH domain: Molecular insights into the fragile X syndrome. *Cell* **85:** 237.
Oberlé, I., F. Rousseau, D. Heitz, C. Kretz, D. Devys, A. Hanauer, J. Boué, M.F. Bertheas, and J.-L. Mandel. 1991. Instability of a 550-base pair DNA segment and abnormal methylation in fragile X syndrome. *Science* **252:** 1097.
Pieretti, M., F. Zhang, Y.H. Fu, S.T. Warren, B.A. Oostra, C.T. Caskey, and D.L. Nelson. 1991. Absence of expression of the *FMR-1* gene in fragile X syndrome. *Cell* **66:** 817.
Price, D.K., F. Zhang, C.T. Ashley, and S.T. Warren. 1996. The chicken *FMR1* gene is highly conserved with a CCT 5′ untranslated repeat and encodes an RNA-binding

protein. *Genomics* **31:** 3.

Reyniers, E., L. Vits, K. De Boulle, B. Van Roy, D. Van Velzen, E. de Graaff, A.J.M.H. Verkerk, H.Z.J. Jorens, J.K. Darby, B. Oostra, and P.J. Willems. 1993. The full mutation in the *FMR-1* gene of male fragile X patients is absent in their sperm. *Nat. Genet.* **4:** 143.

Richards, R. I. 1994. Simple repeat DNA is not replicated simply. *Nat. Genet.* **6:** 114.

Richards, R.I., K. Holman, and G.R. Sutherland. 1993. Fragile X syndrome unstable element, p(CCG)n, and other simple tandem repeats sequences are binding sites for specific nuclear proteins. *Hum. Mol. Genet.* **2:** 1429.

Richards, R.I., K. Holman, K. Friend, E. Kremer, D. Hillen, A. Staples, W.T. Brown, P. Goonewardena, J. Tarleton, C. Schwartz, and G.R. Sutherland. 1992. Evidence of founder chromosomes in fragile X syndrome. *Nat. Genet.* **1:** 257.

Riggins, G.J., L.K. Lokey, J.L. Chastain, H.A. Leiner, S.L. Sherman, K.D. Wilkinson, and S.T. Warren. 1992. Human genes containing polymorphic trinucleotide repeats. *Nat. Genet.* **2:** 186.

Rousseau, F., D. Heitz, V. Biancalana, S. Blumenfield, C. Kretz, J. Boué, N. Tommerup, C. van der Hagen, C. DeLozier-Blanchet, M.F. Croquette, S. Gilgenkrantz, P. Jalbert, M.A. Voelckel, I. Oberlé, and J.-L. Mandel. 1991. Direct diagnosis by DNA analysis of the fragile X syndrome of mental retardation. *N. Engl. J. Med.* **325:** 1673.

Schalling, M., T.J. Hudson, K.H. Buetow, and D.E. Housman. 1993. Direct detection of novel expanded trinucleotide repeats in the human genome. *Nat. Genet.* **4:** 135.

Sherman, S.L., N.E. Morton, P.A. Jacobs, and G. Turner. 1984. The marker (X) syndrome: A cytogenetic and genetic analysis. *Ann. Hum. Genet.* **48:** 21.

Sherman, S.L., P.A. Jacobs, N.E. Morton, U. Froster-Iskenius, P.N. Howard-Peebles, K.B. Nielson, M.W. Partington, G.R. Sutherland, G. Turner, and M. Watson. 1985. Further segregation analysis of the fragile X syndrome with special reference to transmitting males. *Hum. Genet.* **69:** 289.

Siomi, H., M.C. Siomi, R.L. Nussbaum, and G. Dreyfuss. 1993. The protein product of the fragile X gene, *FMR1*, has characteristics of an RNA binding protein. *Cell* **74:** 291.

Siomi, H., M. Choi, M.C. Siomi, R.L. Nussbaum, and G. Dreyfuss. 1994. Essential role for KH domains in RNA binding: Impaired RNA binding by a mutation in the KH domain of *FMR1* that causes fragile X syndrome. *Cell* **77:** 33.

Siomi, M., H. Siomi, W.H. Sauer, S. Srinivasan, R.L. Nussbaum, and G. Dreyfuss. 1995. *FXR1*, an autosomal homolog of the fragile X mental retardation gene. *EMBO J.* **14:** 2401.

Smits, A.P.T., J.C.F.M. Dreesen, J.G. Post, D.F.C.M. Smeets, C. de Die-Smulders, T. Spaans-van der Bijl, L.C.P. Govaerts, S.T. Warren, B.A. Oostra, and B.A. van Oost. 1993. The fragile X syndrome: No evidence for any recent mutations. *J. Med. Genet.* **30:** 94.

Snow, K., D.J. Tester, K.E. Kruckeberg, D.J. Schaid, and S.N. Thibodeau. 1994. Sequence analysis of the fragile X trinucleotide repeat: Implications for the origin of the fragile X mutation. *Hum. Mol. Genet.* **3:** 1543.

Snow, K., L.K. Doud, R. Hagerman, R.G. Pergolizzi, S.H. Erster, and S.N. Thibodeau. 1993. Analysis of a CGG sequence at the FMR-1 locus in fragile X families and in the general population. *Am. J. Hum. Genet.* **53:** 1217.

Steward, O. 1994. Dendrites as compartments for macromolecular synthesis. *Proc. Natl. Acad. Sci. USA* **91:** 10766.

Sutcliffe, J.S., D.L. Nelson, F. Zhang, M. Pieretti, C.T. Caskey, D. Saxe, and S.T. Warren. 1992. DNA methylation represses *FMR-1* transcription in fragile X syndrome. *Hum. Mol. Genet.* **1:** 397.

Tamanini, F., N. Meijer, C. Verheij, P.J. Willems, H. Galjaard, B.A. Oostra, and A.T. Hoogeveen. 1996. FMRP is associated to the ribosomes via RNA. *Hum. Mol. Genet.* **5:** 801.

Verheij, C., C.E. Bakker, E. de Graaff, J. Keulemans, R. Willemsen, A.J.M.H. Verkerk, H. Galjaard, A.J.J. Reuser, A.T. Hoogeveen, and B.A. Oostra. 1993. Characterization and localization of the *FMR-1* gene product associated with fragile X syndrome. *Nature* **363:** 722.

Verheij, C., E. de Graaff, C.E. Bakker, R. Willemsen, P.J. Willems, N. Meijer, H. Galjaard, A.J.J. Reuser, B.A. Oostra, and A.T. Hoogeveen. 1995. Characterization of *FMR1* proteins isolated from different tissues. *Hum. Mol. Genet.* **4:** 895.

Verkerk, A.J.M.H., M. Pieretti, J.S. Sutcliffe, Y.-H. Fu, D.P.A. Kuhl, A. Pizutti, O. Reiner, S. Richards, M.F. Victoria, F. Zhang, B.E. Eussen, G.J.B. van Ommen, L.A.J. Blonden, G.J. Riggins, J.L. Chastain, C.B. Kunst, H. Galjaard, C.T. Caskey, D.L. Nelson, B.A. Oostra, and S.T. Warren. 1991. Identification of a gene (*FMR-1*) containing a CGG repeat coincident with a breakpoint cluster region exhibiting length variation in fragile X syndrome. *Cell* **65:** 905.

Visa, N., A.T. Alzhanova-Ericsson, X. Sun, E. Kiseleva, B. Bjorkroth, T. Wurtz, and B. Daneholt. 1996. A pre-mRNA-binding protein accompanies the RNA from the gene through the nuclear pores and into polysomes. *Cell* **84:** 253.

Wang, Y.-H. and J. Griffith. 1995. Expanded CTG triplet blocks from the myotonic dystrophy gene create the strongest known natural nucleosome positioning elements. *Genomics* **25:** 570.

Wang, Y.-H., S. Amirhaeri, S. Kang, R.D. Wells, and J.D. Griffith. 1994. Preferential nucleosome assembly at the DNA triplet repeat from the myotonic dystrophy gene. *Science* **265:** 669.

Warren, S.T. 1996. The expanding world of trinucleotide repeats. *Science* **271:** 1374.

Warren, S.T. and C.T. Ashley. 1995. Triplet repeat expansion mutations: The example of fragile X syndrome. *Annu. Rev. Neurosci.* **18:** 77.

Warren, S.T. and D.L. Nelson. 1994. Advances in molecular analysis of fragile X syndrome. *J. Am Med. Assoc.* **271:** 536.

Wen, W., J.L. Meinkoth, R.Y. Tsien, and S.S. Taylor. 1995. Identification of a signal for rapid export of proteins from the nucleus. *Cell* **82:** 463.

Wohrle, D., I. Hennig, W. Vogel, and P. Steinbach. 1993. Mitotic stability of fragile X mutations in differentiated cells indicates early post-conceptional trinucleotide repeat expansion. *Nat. Genet.* **4:** 140.

Yu, S., M. Pritchard, E. Kremer, M. Lynch, J. Nancarrow, E. Baker, K. Holman, J.C. Mulley, S.T. Warren, D. Schlessinger, G.R. Sutherland, and R.I. Richards. 1991. Fragile X genotype characterized by an unstable region of DNA. *Science* **252:** 1179.

Zhang, Y., J.P. O'Connor, M.C. Siomi, S. Srinivasan, A. Dutra, R.L. Nussbaum, and G. Dreyfuss. 1995. The fragile X mental retardation syndrome protein interacts with novel homologs FXR1 and FXR2. *EMBO J.* **14:** 5358.

Molecular Characterization of the Protein Products of the Fragile X Syndrome Gene and the Survival of Motor Neurons Gene

Q. Liu, H. Siomi, M.C. Siomi, U. Fischer, Y. Zhang, L. Wan, and G. Dreyfuss
Howard Hughes Medical Institute and Department of Biochemistry, University of Pennsylvania School Of Medicine, Philadelphia, Pennsylvania 19104-6148

RNA-binding proteins play critical roles in many cellular processes, and their involvement in posttranscriptional regulation of the pathway of gene expression in eukaryotic cells is particularly well documented (Burd and Dreyfuss 1994). There is increasing interest in the role of RNA-binding proteins during the development of the nervous system, since the aberrant expression of several RNA-binding proteins has been shown to result in defects in neuronal development and function (Table 1). Through our studies of hnRNP proteins, the major proteins that interact with pre-mRNAs (hnRNAs) and mRNAs (Dreyfuss et al. 1993), we have identified motifs and interacting proteins which, in turn, spawned new and interesting observations on important human neurogenetic diseases. These include studies, described below, on fragile X syndrome and on the protein product of the survival of motor neurons gene, the likely disease gene of spinal muscular atrophy.

FRAGILE X SYNDROME

Fragile X syndrome is the most common form of inherited mental retardation and second only to Down's syndrome as a known chromosomal cause of mental retardation (Nussbaum and Ledbetter 1995; Oostra and Willems 1995). Affected individuals suffer from moderate to severe mental retardation (average IQ of 20–60) and display a myriad of usually mild physical symptoms including elongated facial features, large, everted ears, and in male adults, an enlargement of the testes (macroorchidism). As the name implies, this syndrome is an X-linked genetic disorder and is frequently associated with a fragile site, or a gap, observed in metaphase stains of the X chromosomes of affected individuals.

The fragile site has been mapped to region Xq27.3 on the long arm of the human X chromosome. Using a positional cloning strategy, the FMR1 gene was isolated (Verkerk et al. 1991) and the mutational basis of the syndrome was determined to be the expansion of a trinucleotide repeat $(CGG)_n$ present in the 5′-untranslated region of the identified gene (for review, see Oostra and Willems 1995; Warren and Ashley 1995). Whereas in normal individuals the CGG repeat length is polymorphic, ranging from 5 to 50 copies, in fragile X patients hundreds and occasionally thousands of repeats are observed. This finding has led to the discovery of a new dynamic mutation mechanism, trinucleotide repeat expansion, which is responsible for a growing number of human neurogenetic diseases (Warren and Ashley 1995). A consequence of this

Table 1. Examples of Genes That Encode RNA-binding Proteins Implicated in Neuronal Development

Gene	Comments	RNA-binding motif	References
elav (*Drosophila*)	required for correct differentiation and maintenance of neurons	RNP	Robinow et al. (1988)
musashi (*Drosophila*)	involved in external sensory-organ specification	RNP	Nakamura et al. (1994)
couch potato (*Drosophila*)	mutations result in hypoactive behavior in adults	RNP	Bellen et al. (1992)
nonA (*Drosophila*)	required for vision and courtship song	RNP	Jones and Rubin (1990); von Besser et al. (1990)
quaking (mouse)	mutations result in a deficiency of myelin in the central nervous system that is accompanied by a characteristic tremor	KH	Ebersole et al. (1996)
HuD (human)	implicated in paraneoplastic sensory neuropathy	RNP	Szabo et al. (1991)
Nova (human)	implicated in paraneoplastic opsoclonus-ataxia	KH	Buckanovich et al. (1993)

amplification is that the CGG repeats as well as the CpG island near the FMR1 gene become methylated (Pieretti et al. 1991). As a result, the FMR1 locus reportedly becomes silent or attenuated at both the transcriptional and translational levels (Pieretti et al. 1991; Siomi et al. 1993b; Verheij et al. 1993). Numerous lines of evidence suggest that the lack of expression of FMR1 is responsible for the pathogenesis of fragile X syndrome (for review, see Oostra and Willems 1995; Warren and Ashley 1995). Finally, mice containing an inactivated *fmr1* gene displayed typical, albeit mild, symptoms of fragile X syndrome including learning and memory deficits, aberrant behavior, and macro-orchidism (The Dutch-Belgian Fragile X Consortium 1994). This animal model supports the central role of FMR1 in fragile X syndrome, and it should serve as a valuable tool for the elucidation of the physiological role of FMR1.

An understanding of the function of FMR1 would provide great insight into the molecular basis of fragile X syndrome and possibly into the processes that underlie memory, learning, and intelligence. Analysis of the amino acid sequence of FMR1 revealed the presence of two types of RNA-binding motifs, one RGG box and two KH domains (Figs. 1 and 2B). Both of these motifs were initially characterized in hnRNP proteins, a class of abundant nuclear proteins that bind pre-mRNA and play important roles in pre-mRNA processing and in the biogenesis of mRNA (Kiledjian and Dreyfuss 1992; Siomi et al. 1993a; for review, see Burd and Dreyfuss 1994). The RNA-binding domains in FMR1 appear to be functional, as FMR1 was demonstrated to directly bind RNA in vitro (Ashley et al. 1993; Siomi et al. 1993b). RNA binding was impaired by substitution of a conserved residue in the KH domain (Siomi et al. 1994). Significantly, the RNA-binding activity of a mutant protein (Ile-304→Asn change in the second KH domain) originally identified in a severely affected fragile X patient (De Boulle et al. 1993) was also severely impaired (Siomi et al. 1994). These findings suggest a strong connection between fragile X syndrome and the RNA-binding activity of FMR1. However, the cognate RNA target of FMR1 has not yet been identified.

Recently, two FMR1-related genes, FXR1 and FXR2, have been cloned and characterized (Coy et al. 1995; Siomi et al. 1995; Zhang et al. 1995). The amino acid sequence of FMR1 is highly related to those of FXR1 and FXR2 (86% and 70% identity, respectively) throughout the amino-terminal region (Fig. 2B). This region encompasses the RNA-binding domains and, consistent with this, both FXR1 and FXR2 bind RNA in vitro similarly to FMR1 (Siomi et al. 1995; Zhang et al. 1995). The carboxy-terminal region of all three proteins, however, is highly divergent, sharing only around 6% similarity. Like FMR1, FXR1 and FXR2 are found almost exclusively in the cytoplasm. In contrast to FMR1, both FXR1 and FXR2 are encoded by autosomal genes (located at 3q28 and 17p13.1, respectively) and they do not seem to have trinucleotide repeats in their 5′ UTR. It is not yet known if there are mental retardation genes in these regions of the genome. Expression of FXR1 and FXR2 is unchanged in fragile X patients (Siomi et al. 1995; Zhang et al. 1995). Interestingly, FMR1 is found to interact with FXR1 and with FXR2 both in vitro and in vivo (Zhang et al. 1995). In addition, FXR1 is capable of interacting with FXR2. All three proteins are also capable of

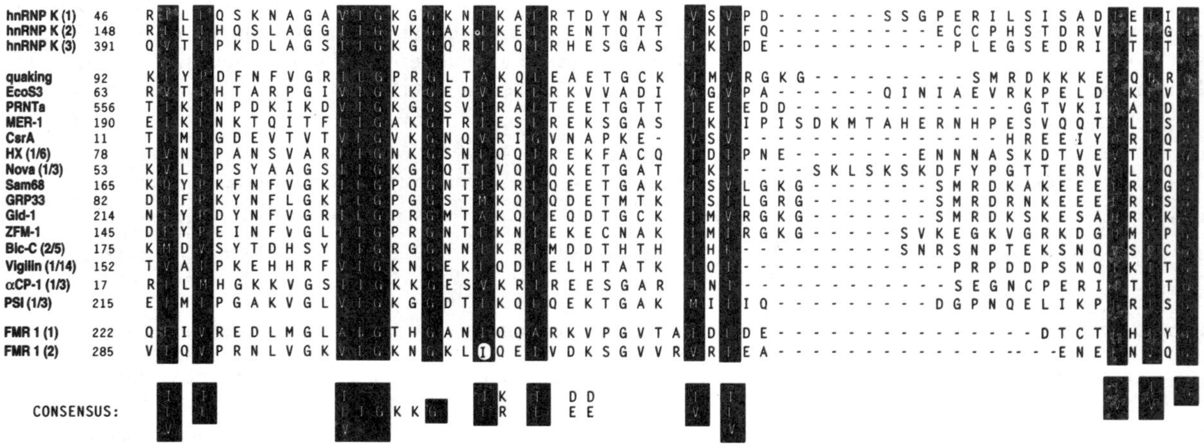

Figure 1. Sequence alignment of the KH domain-containing proteins. Highly conserved positions are highlighted in black. The sequences are from various species and the alignment and the numbering shown were taken from Siomi et al. (1993a,b) and Musco et al. (1996). Secondary structure indicated for the KH-6 domain of human vigilin (Musco et al. 1996) is also shown at the bottom. The position of a single point mutation in FMR1 resulting in an Ile-367→Asp found in a very severe fragile X syndrome patient (De Boulle et al. 1993) is circled.

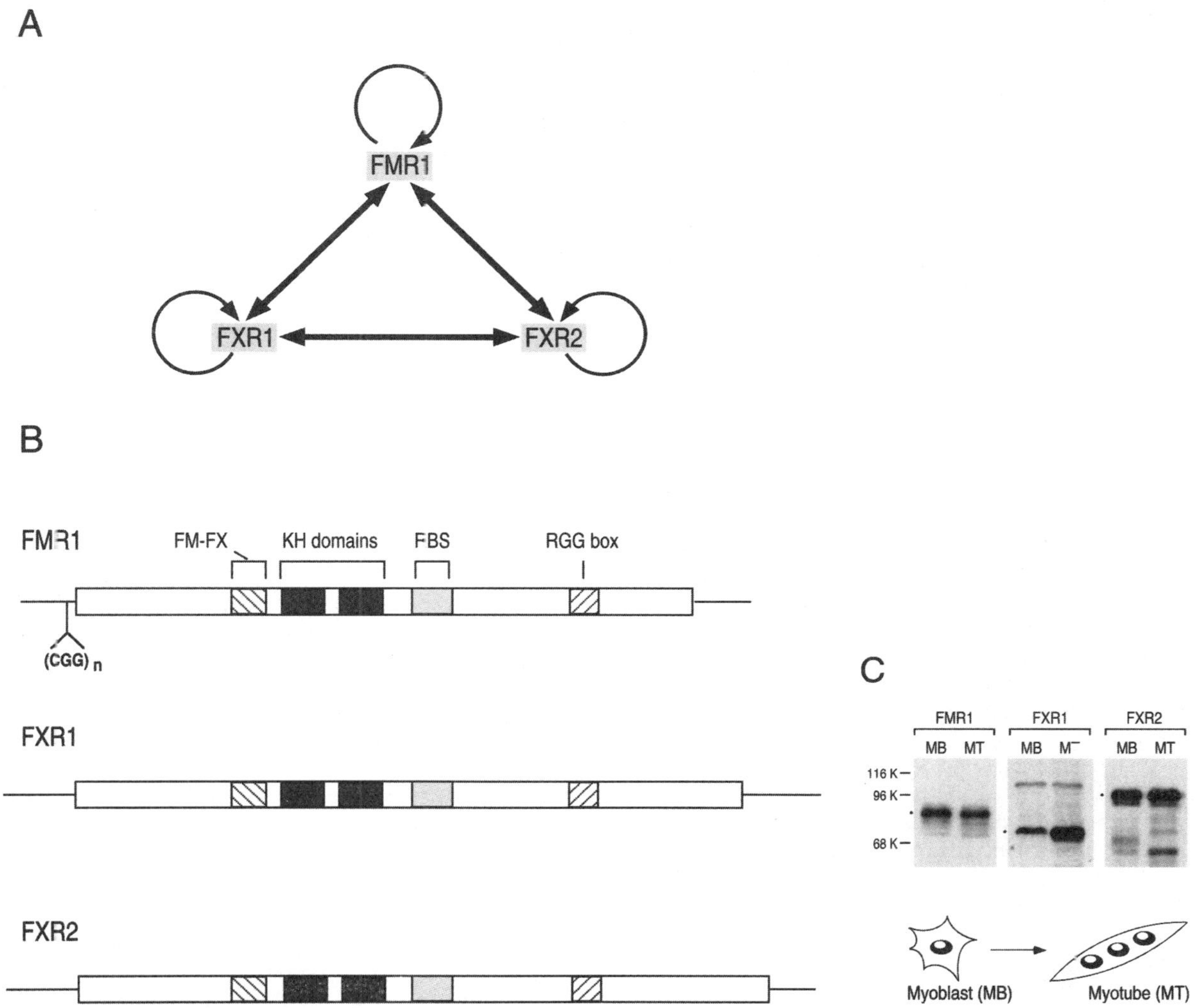

Figure 2. FMR1/FXRs are members of a gene family. (*A*) Model summarizing the observed interactions among the FMR1, FXR1, and FXR2 proteins. The data are based on the findings described in Zhang et al. (1995). (*B*) Schematic diagrams of FMR1, FXR1, and FXR2 proteins. The structural organization of the FMR1 and the FXR proteins is schematically represented with functional domains that have been mapped previously. Functional domains are indicated by KH (hnRNP K homology), RGG (a stretch rich in glycine and arginine residues), RBS (ribosome binding site), and FM-FX (FMR1-FXR interaction domain). The polymorphic triplet repeats associated with the fragile X syndrome are also shown in the 5′ UTR of FMR1. (*C*) Differential induction of FMR1, FXR1, and FXR2 proteins during muscle differentiation. Total protein was isolated from mouse Sol 8 cells (Montarras et al. 1989) reaching confluence in medium containing 20% FCS and from 3 days after switching cells to medium supplemented with 10% horse serum (differentiation medium). Protein blots of extracts prepared as described above were detected with anti-FMR1 antibody, anti-FXR1 antibody, or anti-FXR2 antibody. After induction of differentiation, FXR1 protein levels increase approximately fivefold while FMR1 and FXR2 seem to stay constant during this period. (MB) Myoblast. (MT) Myotube.

homotypic interactions (Zhang et al. 1995). These three proteins thus form a small gene family of proteins related by structure and most likely by function (Fig. 2A). It is likely that FXR1 and FXR2 play important roles in the function of FMR1 and in the development of the fragile X syndrome. Transgenic mice studies that either inactivate or enhance FXR1 and/or FXR2 function should greatly assist in establishing their specific roles in fragile X syndrome. Whatever the outcome of this relationship, FMR1 can no longer be considered to function alone but likely has, in FXR1 and FXR2, partners for the development of intelligence. It is possible that FXR1 and FXR2 could modulate RNA binding specificity through a direct interaction with FMR1.

FMR1 and FXR1 gene expression has been studied in a variety of human and murine tissues. During embryonic development, expression of these genes is widespread and at a high level. However, the high level of expression becomes more localized in adult: High expression levels persist into adulthood in the brain and in the testes (Abitbol et al. 1993; Bächner et al. 1993; Hinds et al. 1993; Coy et al. 1995). The precise site of high expression levels of the two genes, however, differs within brain and testis. For example, whereas FMR1 is highly expressed in proliferating spermatogonia, the expression of FXR1 is enhanced in postmeiotic spermatids (Bächner et al. 1993; Coy et al. 1995). This pattern of expression of the two genes in pre- and postmeiotic cells may result from FMR1 being X-linked and FXR1 being autosomal. FMR1 and FXR1 are also differentially regulated during terminal differentiation of muscle cells (Fig. 2C). After induction of differentiation by serum deprivation, FXR1 protein levels increase approximately fivefold. In contrast, the levels of FMR1 protein appear to remain constant during this period. These expression patterns indicate that although the functions of these proteins are likely to be similar, they do not complement each other in more specific functions. The degree of possible functional complementation of these gene products could be resolved by generating double knockout mice for these distinct loci.

Recent experiments indicate that FMR1 and the FXR proteins are associated with ribosomes, predominantly with 60S ribosomal subunits (Khandjian et al. 1996; Siomi et al. 1996). These findings suggest a biochemical function for FMR1, FXR1, and FXR2 proteins that is related to the function of ribosomes, including translational regulation or mRNA stability. We have delineated the region of FMR1 that mediates its binding to 60S ribosomal subunits (Siomi et al. 1996). This region, which corresponds to exons 13 and 14 of the FMR1 gene, is highly conserved among the FMR1-FXR family (Fig. 3A). Part of this region is predicted to have a high propensity to form a coiled-coil motif, which is known to be involved in protein-protein interactions between two amphipathic α-helices. Thus, exons 13 and 14 are likely to participate in mediating the direct interaction of FMR1 with 60S ribosomal subunits through the predicted coiled-coil domain. Interestingly, the predicted amphipathic α-helix contains an amino acid sequence that is reminiscent of the recently discovered Rev/PKI-type nuclear export signal sequences (Fig. 3B) (Fischer et al. 1995; Wen et al. 1995). In vitro translated FMR1 (Fig. 3C, lanes 3, 4) and FXR1 proteins (not shown) are indeed exported to the cytoplasm upon injection into the nucleus of *Xenopus laevis* oocytes whereas a deletion mutant of FMR1 comprising the first 12 exons only, and therefore lacking the NES region, remains restricted to the nucleus (Fig. 3C, lanes 1, 2). The export is saturable by an excess of Rev-NES peptides coupled to BSA, indicating that the FMR1 sequence mediates this transport by the same nuclear export pathway that is used by Rev and PKI (Fig. 3, lanes 5, 6). Thus, these and other data show that FMR1 contains a sequence that can serve as a nuclear export signal and indicate that this protein may also have, at some stage, a function in the nucleus and that it may serve to transport RNAs between the nucleus and the cytoplasm. In agreement with this notion, it has been reported that the amino terminus of FMR1 contains a nuclear localization signal (NLS) (Devys et al. 1993). However, we note that when we inject a mutant of FMR1 that lacks the NES into the cytoplasm of *Xenopus* oocytes, we do not observe any import even when we block the potential export of injected FMR1 protein by prior nuclear injections of saturating amounts of Rev-NES peptides coupled to BSA (Fig. 3C, lanes 7–10 and data not shown). It is, therefore, not certain whether native FMR1 actually shuttles between the nucleus and the cytoplasm, or whether its apparent nuclear export results simply as a coincidence from the fact that the leucine-rich ribosome-binding sequence can mediate interaction with the Rev/PKI export machinery when artificially placed in the nucleus. Alternatively, FMR1 may shuttle in somatic cells but have a NLS that is not functional in the amphibian oocyte.

What then may the function of FMR1 and the FXR proteins be? Since they are ubiquitously expressed in tissues and their amino acid sequences are highly conserved among divergent organisms, they may have a housekeeping role. A likely function of FMR1 and the FXRs that is suggested by their association with ribosomes is a function in the regulation of translation of specific brain and testis mRNAs. The next important and crucial step toward understanding the function of these proteins as well as the molecular basis of fragile X syndrome will be to identify the cellular RNA molecules with which these proteins interact.

THE SURVIVAL OF MOTOR NEURONS PROTEIN AND THE IDENTIFICATION OF GEMS, A NOVEL NUCLEAR STRUCTURE

Spinal muscular atrophy (SMA) is a common, often fatal autosomal recessive disease affecting approximately 1 in 6000 newborns. It is characterized by degeneration of anterior horn cells of the spinal cord leading to progressive muscle wasting and paralysis. The disease is classified into three types based on the age of onset and the clinical course (Pearn 1980; Munsat and Davies 1992). All three forms of childhood SMA have been mapped to chromosome 5q13 (Brzustowicz et al. 1990; Melki et al. 1990). This chromosomal locus is highly unstable and contains a 500-kb inverted repeat. Recently, two genes, one of them survival of motor neurons (SMN) (Lefebvre et al. 1995) and the other neuronal apoptosis inhibitory protein (NAIP) (Roy et al. 1995), have been identified within this repeat, and both have been suggested as the gene responsible for SMA (Lewin 1995). The telomeric copy of SMN is absent in more than 98% of the patients regardless of the severity of the SMA phenotype. The SMN gene encodes a novel protein with 294 amino acids and no significant homology with any other protein in the database.

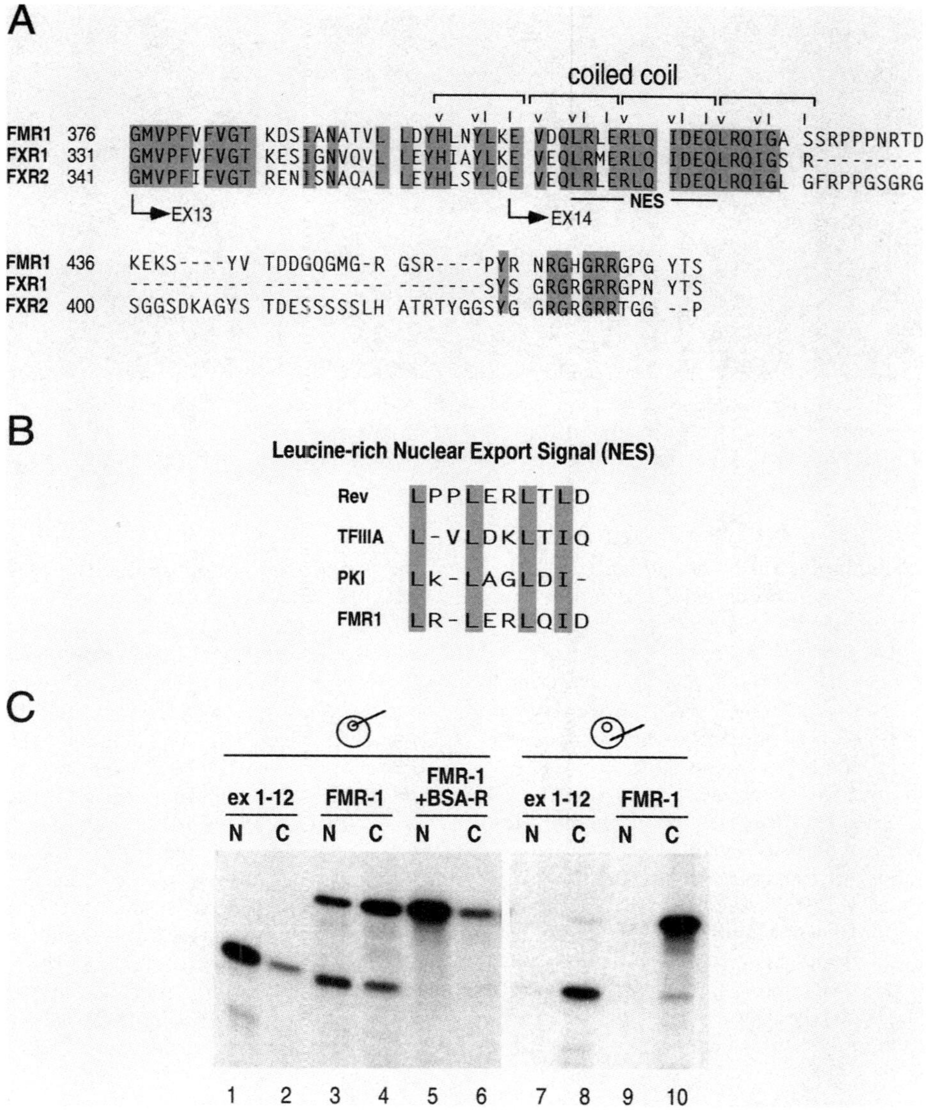

Figure 3. Sequences of the FMR1 protein that mediates interaction with 60S ribosomal subunits and nuclear export. (*A*) Sequences in exons 13 and 14 of FMR1 mediate the association with 60S ribosomal subunits. The data are based on the findings described in Siomi et al. (1996). The putative coiled-coil motif corresponding to a region within exons 13 and 14 is highly conserved among FMR1/FXR proteins. (*B*) Comparison of nuclear export signal sequences from HIV-1 Rev, transcription factor IIIA (TFIIIA) of *X. laevis*, cAMP-dependent protein kinase inhibitor with the coiled-coil regions of FMR1/FXR proteins. (*C*) Nucleocytoplasmic transport of in vitro translated FMR1 protein and a deletion mutant thereof. In vitro translated ^{35}S-labeled full-length human FMR1 and a deletion mutant that comprises the first 12 exons only (exons *1–12*) were injected into the nucleus of oocytes either alone (lanes *1–4*) or along with a 20 µg/µl solution of BSA-NES conjugate. Export was analyzed 3 hr later by manual dissection of nuclei and cytoplasm followed by SDS-PAGE and fluorography. In lanes *7–10*, the same in vitro translated proteins were injected into the cytoplasm of oocytes and the nuclear import was analyzed 12 hr later as described above.

During the process of studying proteins that interact with hnRNP U (Kiledjian and Dreyfuss 1992), we found that the carboxyl terminus of the hnRNP U protein interacts with the SMN protein. Further experiments showed that SMN interacts with itself and with several other RNA-binding proteins such as the small nucleolar RNAs-associated protein fibrillarin (Lischwe et al. 1985; Tollervey et al. 1991). Immunofluorescence microscopy localization experiments using monoclonal antibodies against SMN show that SMN is found in both the nucleus and the cytoplasm. It is diffusely distributed in the cytoplasm and is highly concentrated in several intense dot-like structures in the nucleus termed gems (Liu and Dreyfuss 1996). Gems are novel nuclear structures which are related to, yet clearly distinct from, another subnuclear structure, coiled bodies (for reviews on coiled bodies, see Lamond and Carmo-Fonseca 1993; Wu et al. 1993; Roth 1995). The coiled

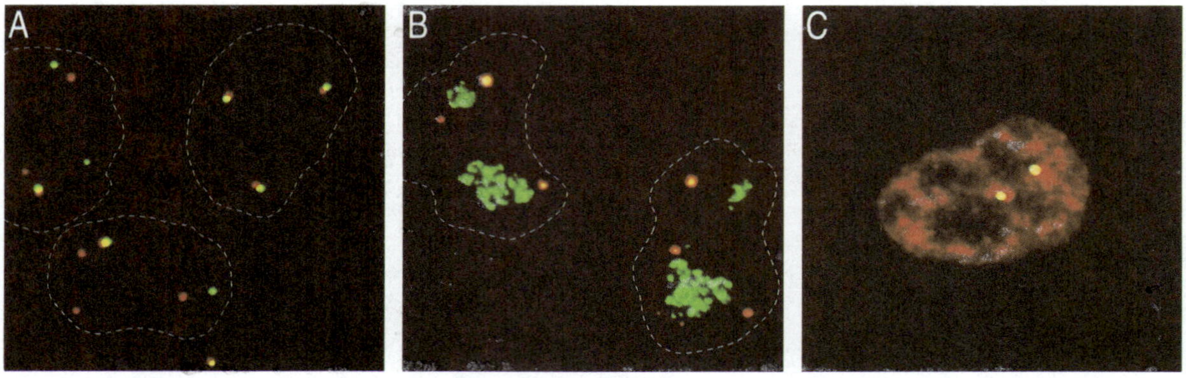

Figure 4. Gems are novel nuclear structures related to coiled bodies. The computer superimposed confocal images of indirect double immunofluorescence experiments using HeLa cells with anti-SMN antibody 2B1 (*green*) and anti-p80-coilin antibody Pδ (*red*) in *A*, anti-SMN antibody 2B1 (*red*) and anti-fibrillarin antibody 1881 (*green*) in *B*, anti-SMN antibody 2B1 (*green*) and anti-sm antibody Y12 (*red*) in *C*.

body is an evolutionarily conserved subnuclear structure found in both plants and animals. It contains p80-coilin, a protein detectable only in the coiled body; fibrillarin, Nopp140, and several snoRNAs such as U3, found also in nucleoli; snRNA U7; and spliceosomal snRNPs. Mutational analysis of p80-coilin indicated that there is a functional interaction between coiled bodies and the nucleolus (Bohmann et al. 1995). However, the exact function of coiled bodies is still not clear, although it has been suggested that they are involved in the biogenesis, recycling, or storage of snRNPs (Lamond and Carmo-Fonseca 1993; Wu and Gall 1993; Gall et al. 1995). Figure 4 shows double-label immunofluoresence staining using antibodies against SMN (green) and against p80-coilin (Fig. 4A, red), fibrillarin (Fig. 4B, green; SMN—red), and Y12 (Fig. 4C, red), respectively. These experiments demonstrate that gems are related to coiled bodies; frequently these two bodies are positioned very close to each other, other times they are completely separate. Sometimes gems and coiled bodies appear to colocalize. The close association of gems with coiled bodies indicates that gems are probably functionally associated with coiled bodies and may therefore also be involved in RNA metabolism. This idea is further strengthened by the observation that SMN also interacts with fibrillarin, which is one of the components of coiled bodies (Liu and Dreyfuss 1996).

Coiled bodies are dynamic structures that disassemble during mitosis and re-form in daughter cell nuclei (Carmo-Fonseca et al. 1993). Gems behave similarly during mitosis (Liu and Dreyfuss 1996). However, there is a striking difference in the timing of their re-formation in daughter nuclei. Using anti p80-coilin as a marker for coiled bodies, p80-coilin becomes concentrated in the daughter nucleus and then becomes

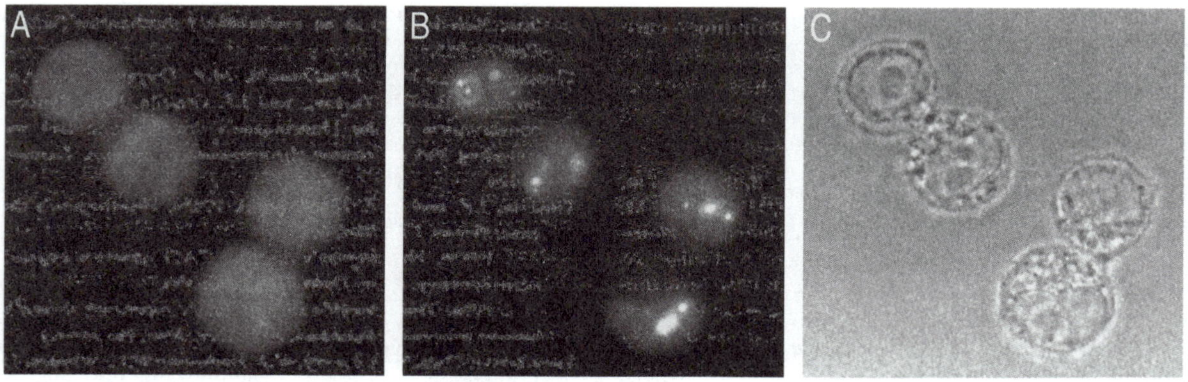

Figure 5. Coiled bodies re-form earlier than gems after mitosis. (*A*) Localization pattern of SMN proteins at early interphase immediately after mitosis. The SMN proteins were visualized by immunofluorescence analysis in a Zeiss light microscope with 63x objective using monoclonal antibody 2B1. SMN protein mostly exists in the cytoplasm. (*B*) Localization pattern of p80-coilin visualized by anti-p80 coilin antibody pδ in the same cell. (*C*) Phase contrast image of the same cell. The nucleolus is already visible in the daughter nucleus.

concentrated within coiled bodies (Fig. 5B). At these early times post-mitosis, the SMN protein, on the other hand, is absent from the nucleus and is only detectable in the cytoplasm (Fig. 5A). Gems are detectable only later after coiled bodies have re-formed. Carmo-Fonseca et al. (1993) have shown that there is a lag period after mitosis during which coiled bodies are not detected. Here we show that this lag period is much longer for gems. The relocalization of SMN and coilin to the nucleus after mitosis is reminiscent of the behavior of hnRNP proteins, as some of them (e.g., hnRNP C and U) return into the nucleus immediately after mitosis whereas others (mainly shuttling proteins such as the hnRNP A and B groups) are imported much later, only after the reinitiation of transcription (Piñol-Roma and Dreyfuss 1991). It will be interesting to find out whether the entry of SMN into the nucleus is transcription-dependent.

The sequence of the SMN protein does not provide any functional information. However, since gems are related to coiled bodies and possibly involved in RNA metabolism, we were interested in determining if SMN has nucleic acid binding activity. To test this, we performed ribohomopolymer binding experiments at different salt concentrations using in vitro translated SMN (Siomi et al. 1994). As shown in Figure 6, in vitro translated myc-tagged full-length SMN binds to poly r(G) and poly r(U) efficiently (lanes 1–7). For poly r(U) the binding is resistant even to 0.5 M NaCl concentration (lane 7), suggesting that the SMN protein has considerable avidity for RNA. This binding has at least some hallmarks of specificity since, under the same conditions, it does not bind to poly r(A) and poly r(C) at all (data not shown).

The telomeric and the centromeric copies of SMN are identical except for five silent base changes (Lefebvre et al. 1995). However, the centromeric copy undergoes alternative splicing of exon 7, resulting in a protein with a different carboxy-terminal end (Gennarelli et al. 1995; Lefebvre et al. 1995). Interestingly, patient studies suggest that exon 7 is important for SMN function. For those patients in whom the telomeric copy of SMN is retained, most lacked exon 7 but retained exon 8. Some of them have a gene conversion event that causes the replacement of telomeric exon 7 with centromeric exon 7. Some patients have mutations in intron 6, causing the deletion of exon 7 (Lefebvre et al. 1995). These findings suggest that the telomeric exon 7 is important for SMN function. To see if this region affects the nucleic acid binding capacity of the SMN protein, we carried out the same binding experiments using myc-tagged SMN lacking exon 7 (myc-Cd16) and myc-tagged SMN with a deletion of the first 27 amino acids (exon 1), myc-Nd27. The capacity of SMN to bind to poly r(G) and r(U) is severely impaired for truncated SMN lacking exon 7 (Fig. 6, lanes 8–14). Whereas full-length SMN binds to poly r(G) at 0.25 M and to poly r(U) at 0.5 M salt concentration (lanes 3 and 7), the truncated version binds very weakly at 100 mM (lanes 9 and 12). This effect is specific for exon 7, since the deletion of exon 1 from the amino-terminal end of the protein has no such effect (Fig. 6, lanes 15–21). We conclude that the SMN protein has the capacity to bind RNA and that exon 7 of the protein is important for this activity. However, it is unclear whether this capacity reflects a significant function of SMN and whether the SMN protein binds a specific, or indeed any, RNA in vivo.

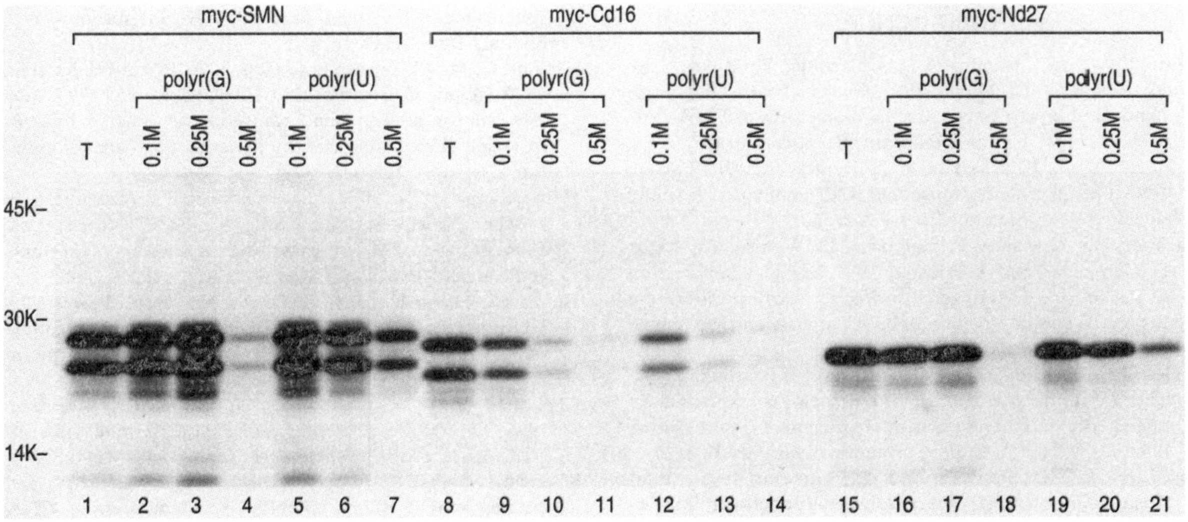

Figure 6. SMN protein has nucleic acid binding characteristics. In vitro translated myc-tagged full-length SMN, myc-tagged SMN with exon 7 deleted (myc-Cd16), and myc-tagged SMN with exon 1 deleted (myc-Nd27) were incubated with poly r(G) and r(U) at different NaCl concentrations indicated above each lane. The bound fraction was analyzed on a 12.5% SDS-polyacrylamide gel.

In conclusion, the study of SMN protein has led us to the discovery of a novel nuclear structure that is related to coiled bodies and possibly involved in RNA metabolism. Recent experiments raise the possibility that SMN binds to RNA in vivo. The specific function of SMN and of gems remains the subject of intense study in this laboratory. These studies are directed at determining what are other components of gems, what proteins interact with SMN and how these proteins are involved in RNA metabolism, and, last, why deletions or mutations of this protein lead to motor neuron degeneration. The association of RNA-binding proteins with several distinct neurological disorders demonstrated that interference with the function of RNA-binding proteins can result in severe neurological disease. One of the challenges for this area of research in the future will be to understand the normal functions of these proteins and to explain how mutations or defective expression of these proteins leads to disease.

ACKNOWLEDGMENTS

We thank Dr. Eng M. Tan for the anti-coilin and anti-fibrillarin antibodies, Dr. Maria Carmo-Fonseca for the anti-coilin monoclonal antibody, Dr. Joan. A. Steitz for the anti-Sm Y12 monoclonal antibody, and Dr. Joseph Craft for anti-fibrillarin antibodies. We thank Dr. Peter Bannerman and Tracy Oliver for help with the confocal microscopy. We are grateful to members of our laboratory for stimulating discussions and, in particular, to Dr. W. Matthew Michael for critical comments on this manuscript. This work was supported by the Howard Hughes Medical Institute and by a grant from the National Institutes of Health.

REFERENCES

Abitbol, M., I.C. Menin, A.L. Delezoide, T. Rhyner, M. Vekemans, and J. Mallet. 1993. Nucleus basalis magnocellularis and hippocampus are the major sites of FMR-1 expression in the human fetal brain. *Nat. Genet.* **4:** 147.

Ashley, C.T., Jr., K.D. Wikinson, D. Reines, and S.T. Warren. 1993. FMR1 protein: Conserved RNP family domains and selective RNA binding. *Science* **262:** 563.

Bächner, D., A. Manca, P. Steinbach, D. Wohrle, W. Vogel, H. Hameister, and A. Poustka. 1993. Enhanced expression of the murine FMR1 gene during germ cell proliferation suggests a special function in both the male and the female gonad. *Hum. Mol. Genet.* **2:** 2043.

Bellen, H.J., S. Kooyer, D. D'Evelyn, and J. Pearlman. 1992. The *Drosophila* couch potato protein is expressed in nuclei of peripheral neuronal precursors and shows homology to RNA-binding proteins. *Genes Dev.* **6:** 2125.

Bohmann, K., J.A. Ferreira, and A.I. Lamond. 1995. Mutational analysis of p80 coilin indicates a functional interaction between coiled bodies and the nucleolus. *J. Cell Biol.* **131:** 817.

Brzustowicz, L.M., T. Lehner, L.H. Castilla, G.K. Penchaszadeh, K. Wilhelmsen, R. Daniels, K.E. Davies, M. Leppert, F. Ziter, D. Wood, V. Dubowitz, J. Ott, T.L. Munsat, and T.C. Gilliam. 1990. Genetic mapping of chronic childhood-onset spinal muscular atrophy to chromosome 5q11.2-13. *Nature* **344:** 540.

Buckanovich, R.J., J.B. Posner, and R.B. Darnell. 1993. Nova, the paraneoplastic Ri antigen, is homologous to an RNA-binding protein and is specifically expressed in the developing motor system. *Neuron* **11:** 657.

Burd, C.G. and G. Dreyfuss. 1994. Conserved structures and diversity of functions of RNA-binding proteins. *Science* **265:** 615.

Carmo-Fonseca, M., J. Ferreira, and A.I. Lamond. 1993. Assembly of snRNP-containing coiled bodies is regulated in interphase and mitosis—Evidence that the coiled body is a kinetic nuclear structure. *J. Cell Biol.* **120:** 841.

Coy, J.F., Z.-S. Sedlacek, D. Bachner, H. Hameister, S. Joos, P. Lichter, H. Delius, and A. Poustka. 1995. Highly conserved 3′ UTR and expression pattern of FXR1 points to a divergent gene regulation FXR1 and FMR1. *Hum. Mol. Genet.* **4:** 2209.

De Boulle, K., A.J.M.H. Verkerk, E. Reyniers, L. Vits, J. Hendrickx, B. Van Roy, F. van den Bos, E. de Graff, B.A. Oostra, and P.J. Willems. 1993. A point mutation in the FMR-1 gene associated with fragile X mental retardation. *Nat. Genet.* **3:** 31.

Devys, D., Y. Lutz, N. Rouyer, J.P. Bellocq, and J.L. Mandel. 1993. The FMR-1 protein is cytoplasmic, most abundant in neurons and appears normal in carriers of a fragile X premutation. *Nat. Genet.* **4:** 335.

Dreyfuss, G., M.J. Matunis, S. Piñol-Roma, and C.G. Burd. 1993. HnRNP proteins and the biogenesis of mRNA. *Annu. Rev. Biochem.* **62:** 289.

Ebersole, T.A., Q. Chen, M.J. Justice, and K. Artzt. 1996. The quaking gene product necessary in embryogenesis and myelination combines features of RNA binding and signal transduction proteins. *Nat. Genet.* **12:** 260.

Fischer, U., J. Huber, W.C. Boelens, I.W. Mattaj, and R. Luhrmann. 1995. The HIV-I Rev activation domain is a nuclear export signal that accesses an export pathway used by specific cellular RNAs. *Cell* **82:** 475.

Gall, J.G., A. Tsvetkov, Z.A. Wu, and C. Murphy. 1995. Is the sphere organelle coiled body a universal nuclear component? *Dev. Genet.* **16:** 25.

Gennarelli, M., M. Lucarelli, F. Capon, A. Pizzuti, L. Merlini, C. Angelini, G. Novelli, and B. Dallapiccola. 1995. Survival motor neuron gene transcript analysis in muscles from spinal muscular atrophy patients. *Biochem. Biophys. Res. Commun.* **213:** 342.

Hergersberg, M., K. Matsuo, M. Gassmann, W. Schaffner, B. Luscher, T. Rülicke, and A. Aguzzi. 1995. Tissue-specific expression of a *FMR1* β-galactosidase fusion gene in transgenic mice. *Hum. Mol. Genet.* **4:** 359.

Hinds, H., C. Ashley, J. Sutcliffe, D. Nelson, S. Warren, D. Housman, and M. Schalling. 1993. Tissue specific expression of FMR-1 provides evidence for a functional role in fragile X syndrome. *Nat. Genet.* **3:** 36.

Khandjian, E.W., F. Corbin, S. Woerly, and F. Rousseau. 1996. The fragile X mental retardation protein is associated with ribosomes. *Nat. Genet.* **12:** 91.

Kiledjian, M. and G. Dreyfuss. 1992. Primary structure and binding activity of the hnRNP U protein: Binding RNA through RGG box. *EMBO J.* **11:** 2655.

Jones, K.R. and G.M. Rubin. 1990. Molecular analysis of no-on-transit A, a gene required for normal vision in *Drosophila. Neuron* **4:** 711.

Lamond, A.I. and M. Carmo-Fonseca. 1993. The coiled body.

Trends Cell Biol. **3:** 198.

Lefebvre, S., L. Burglen, S. Reboullet, O. Clermont, P. Burlet, L. Viollet, B. Benichou, C. Cruaud, P. Millasseau, M. Zeviani, D.L. Paslier, J. Frezal, D. Cohen, J. Weissenbach, A. Munnich, and J. Melki. 1995. Identification and characterization of a spinal muscular atrophy-determining gene. *Cell* **80:** 155.

Lewin, B. 1995. Genes for SMA: In parvo. *Cell* **80:** 1.

Lischwe, M.A., R.L. Ochs, R. Reddy, R.G. Cook, L.C. Yeoman, E.M. Tan, M. Reichlin, and H. Busch. 1985. Purification and partial characterization of a nucleolar scleroderma antigen. *J. Biol. Chem.* **260:** 14304.

Liu, Q. and G. Dreyfuss. 1996. A novel nuclear structure containing the survival of motor neurons protein. *EMBO J.* **15:** 3555.

Melki, J., S. Abdelhak, P. Sheth, M.F. Bachelot, P. Burlet, A. Marcadet, J. Aicardi, A. Barois, J.P. Carriere, M. Fardeau, D. Fontan, G. Ponsot, T. Billette, C. Angelini, C. Barbosa, G. Ferriere, G. Lanzi, A. Ottolini, M.C. Babron, D. Cohen, A. Hanauer, F. Clerget-Darpoux, M. Lathrop, A. Munnich, and J. Frezal. 1990. Gene for chromic proximal spinal muscular atrophies maps to chromosome 5q. *Nature* **344:** 767.

Montarras, D., C. Pinset, J. Chelly, A. Kahn, and F. Gros. 1989. Expression of MyoD1 coincides with terminal differentiation in determined but inducible muscle cells. *EMBO J.* **8:** 2203.

Munsat, T.L. and K.E. Davies. 1992. Meeting report: International Consortium meeting. *Neuromusc. Disorders* **2:** 423.

Musco, G., G. Stier, C. Joseph, M.A.C. Morelli, M. Nilges, T.J. Gibson, and A. Pastore. 1996. Three-dimensional structure and stability of the KH domain: Molecular insights into the fragile X syndrome. *Cell* **85:** 237.

Nakamura, M., H. Okano, J.A. Blendy, and C. Montell. 1994. Musashi, a neuronal RNA-binding protein required for *Drosophila* adult external sensory organ development. *Neuron* **13:** 67.

Nussbaum, R.L. and D.H. Ledbetter. 1995. In *Fragile-X syndrome.* In *Metabolic basis of inherited disease*, 7th edition (ed. C.R. Scriver et al.), p. 795. McGraw-Hill, New York.

Oostra, B.A. and P.J. Willems. 1995. A fragile gene. *BioEssays* **17:** 941.

Pearn, J. 1980. Classification of spinal muscular atrophies. *Lancet* **1:** 919.

Pieretti, M., F. Zhang, Y. Fu, S. Warren, B. Oostra, C. Caskey, and D.L. Nelson. 1991. Absence of expression of the FMR-1 gene in fragile X syndrome. *Cell* **66:** 817.

Piñol-Roma, S. and G. Dreyfuss. 1991. Transcription-dependent and transcription-independent nuclear transport of hnRNP proteins. *Science* **253:** 312

Robinow, S., A.R. Campos, K.-M. Yao, and K. White. 1988. The *elav* gene product of *Drosophila*, required in neuron, has three RNP consensus motifs. *Science* **242:** 1570.

Roth, M.B. 1995. Spheres, coiled bodies and nuclear bodies. *Curr. Opin. Cell Biol.* **7:** 325.

Roy, N., M.S. Mahadevan, M. McLean, G. Shutler, Z. Yaraghi, R. Farahani, S. Barid, A. Besner-Johnston, C. Lefebvre, X. Kang, M. Salih, H. Aubry, K. Tamai, X. Guan, P. Ioannou, T.O. Crawford, P.J. de Jong, L. Surh, J.-E. Ikeda, R.G. Korneluk, and A. Mackenzie. 1995. The gene for neuronal apoptosis inhibitory protein is partially deleted in individuals with spinal muscular atrophy. *Cell* **80:** 167.

Siomi, H., M. Choi, M. Siomi, and G. Dreyfuss. 1994. Essential role for KH domains in RNA binding: Impaired RNA binding by a mutation in the KH domains of FMR1 that cause fragile X syndrome. *Cell* **77:** 33.

Siomi, H., M.J. Matunis, W.M. Michael, and G. Dreyfuss. 1993a. The pre-mRNA binding K protein contains a novel evolutionarily conserved motif. *Nucleic Acids Res.* **21:** 1193.

Siomi, H., M.C. Siomi, R.L. Nussbaum, and G. Dreyfuss. 1993b. The protein product of the fragile X gene, FMR1, has characteristics of an RNA-binding protein. *Cell* **74:** 291.

Siomi, C.M., Y. Zhang, H. Siomi, and G. Dreyfuss. 1996. Specific sequences in the fragile X syndrome protein FMR1 and the FXR proteins mediate their binding to 60s ribosomal subunits and the interactions among them. *Mol. Cell. Biol.* **16:** 3825.

Siomi, C.M., H. Siomi, W. Sauer, S. Srinivasan, R. Nussbaum, and G. Dreyfuss. 1995. FXR1, an autosomal homolog of the fragile X mental retardation gene. *EMBO J.* **14:** 2401.

Szabo, A., J. Dalmau, G. Manley, M. Rosenfeld, E. Wong, J. Henson, J.B. Posner, and H.M. Furneaux. 1991. HuD, a paraneoplastic encephalomyelitis antigene, contains RNA-binding domains and is homologous to Elav and Sex-lethal. *Cell* **67:** 325.

The Dutch-Belgian Fragile X Consortium. 1994. FMR1 Knockout mice: A model to study fragile X mental retardation. *Cell* **78:** 23.

Tollervey, D., H. Lehtonen, M. Carmo-Fonseca, and E.C. Hurt. 1991. The small nucleolar RNP protein NOP1 (fibrillarin) is required for pre-rRNA processing in yeast. *EMBO J.* **10:** 573.

Verheij, C., C. Bakker, E. de Graaf, J. Keulemans, R. Willemsen, A.J.M.H. Verkerk, H. Galjaard, A.J.J. Reuser, A.T. Hoogeveen, and B.A. Oostra. 1993. Characterization and localization of the FMR-1 gene product associated with fragile X syndrome. *Nature* **363:** 722.

Verkerk, A.J.M.H., M. Pieretti, J. Sutcliffe, Y. Fu, D. Kuhl, A. Pizzuti, O. Reiner, S. Richards, M.F. Victoria, F. Zhang, B.E. Eussen, G.-J.B. van Ommen, L.A.J. Blonden, G.J. Riggins, J.L. Chastain, C.B. Kunst, H. Galjaard, C.T. Caskey, D.L. Nelson, B.A. Oostra, and S.T. Warren. 1991. Identification of a gene (FMR-1) containing a CGG repeat coincident with a breakpoint cluster region exhibiting length variation in fragile X syndrome. *Cell* **65:** 905.

von Besser, H., P. Schnabel, C. Wieland, E. Fritz, R. Stanewsky, and H. Saumweber. 1990. The puff-specific *Drosophila* protein Bj6, encoded by the gene no-on transit A, shows homology to RNA-binding proteins. *Chromosoma* **100:** 37.

Warren, S and C.T. Ashley, Jr. 1995. Triple repeat expansion mutations: The example of fragile X syndrome. *Annu. Rev. Neurosci.* **18:** 77.

Wen, W., J.L. Meinkoth, R.Y. Tsien, and S. Taylor. 1995. Identification of a signal for rapid export of proteins from the nucleus. *Cell* **82:** 463.

Wu, C.H.H. and J.G. Gall. 1993. U7 small nuclear RNA in C snurposomes of the *Xenopus* germinal vesicle. *Proc. Natl. Acad. Sci.* **90:** 6257.

Wu, Z., C. Murphy, C.H.H. Wu, A. Tsvetkov, and J.G. Gall. 1993. Snurposomes and coiled bodies. *Cold Spring Harbor Symp. Quant. Biol.* **58:** 747.

Zhang, Y., P. O'Connor, M. Siomi, S. Srinivasan, A. Dutra, R.L. Nussbaum, and G. Dreyfuss. 1995. The fragile X mental retardation syndrome protein interacts with novel homologs FXR1 and FXR2. *EMBO J.* **14:** 5358.

ALS: Molecular Clues to the Jigsaw Puzzle of Neuronal Degeneration

T. SIDDIQUE
Department of Neurology, Department of Cell and Molecular Biology, and Northwestern Institute of Neuroscience, Northwestern University Medical School, Chicago, Illinois 60611

Amyotrophic lateral sclerosis (ALS), also called motor neuron disease (MND), is an age-dependent and fatal paralytic disorder, caused by degeneration of motor neurons in the motor cortex, brain stem, and spinal cord. ALS usually begins asymmetrically with involvement of the muscles of one or more limbs, speech, or deglutition in middle adult life. The involvement appears to spread in an anatomically contiguous manner and eventually becomes bilateral and symmetrical, progressing to paralysis and death. Mean survival is 3 years after the onset of symptoms (Mulder et al. 1986).

ALS occurs as an apparently sporadic disease (SALS) in 90% of cases; however, in 10% of ALS patients, a family history of the disease can be documented, and this subset of patients is classified as familial ALS (FALS). Multigenerational familial cases are usually genetic, but complex environmental and genetic interaction cannot be ruled out in duplex clusters. Genetically inherited FALS is transmitted either as an autosomal dominant (DFALS) or an autosomal recessive (RFALS) trait (Emery and Holloway 1982; Siddique et al. 1989).

DFALS is the most common form of FALS and is clinically indistinguishable from SALS. The mean age at onset of symptoms is 46 years, which is about 10 years earlier than SALS (Tandan and Bradley 1985; Siddique 1991). Studies of ALS families suggest that the penetrance of DFALS is age-dependent: 50% of the gene carriers develop disease by the age of 46 years and 90% by the age of 70 years (Siddique 1991). Although the age at onset of symptoms within DFALS families is commonly variable, no apparent genetic anticipation has been observed (Applebaum et al. 1992).

Current ALS research is focused on chromosome 21-linked FALS because of the identification of mutations in the gene for Cu,Zn superoxide dismutase (*SOD1*) (Deng et al. 1993; Rosen et al. 1993). In this review, we summarize the most recent developments in FALS research, which may give insight into the possible mechanisms of pathogenesis underlying this disease.

FALS AND SUPEROXIDE DISMUTASE

Chromosomal mapping of a locus for FALS on chromosome 21q22.1 was an important development, because it directly led to the identification of mutations in *SOD1* as a hitherto undiscovered cause of ALS (Siddique et al. 1991). The power of linkage analysis is demonstrated by the fact that even though SOD1 was a well studied and characterized ubiquitous enzyme, the connection between ALS and SOD1 had not been made until genetic linkage was established (Siddique et al. 1991). The other two isoforms of SOD are MnSOD (SOD2), coded on chromosome 6q25 and located in mitochondria, and extracellullar SOD (SOD3), coded on chromosome 4p15.2 (H.X. Deng and T. Siddique, unpubl.) and secreted into extracellular fluid. The genes for these two forms of SOD are not linked to FALS.

SUPEROXIDE AND CU/ZN SUPEROXIDE DISMUTASE

Superoxide ($O_2{\bullet}^-$) is an unstable and highly active molecule that causes oxidation of cell constituents either directly or through toxic and stable derivatives. $O_2{\bullet}^-$ is produced during normal aerobic metabolism. The major superoxide dismutase activity in cytoplasm is from SOD1, which consists of 153 highly conserved amino acids with a molecular mass of about 16 kD. SOD1 is a homodimer, and within each monomer there is a cave-like active site containing one ion each of copper and zinc. The major known function of this enzyme is to detoxify $O_2{\bullet}^-$ to form O_2 and H_2O_2. H_2O_2 in turn is detoxified by either glutathione peroxidase or catalase. The interface between the monomers of SOD1 is strongly hydrophobic, resulting in a stable dimer formation; dimerization doubles the dismutase activity of SOD1. $O_2{\bullet}^-$ is guided to the Cu(II)-containing active site through a positively charged electrostatic guidance channel, the positive charges being provided by the amino acids Lys-122, Lys-136, and Arg-143. The latter allows the docking of the negatively charged $O_2{\bullet}^-$ in close proximity to the copper atom. Twenty-one highly conserved amino acid residues coded by exons 3 and 5 contribute to the active channel. The channel narrows down in a stepwise fashion from a large shallow depression about 24 Å across to a deeper well about 10 Å wide and 5 Å deep, which further narrows to less than 4 Å above the copper atom (Tainer et al. 1982; Getzoff et al. 1989). The sphere radius accessible to the copper atom in wild-type SOD1 is about 1.7 Å (Tainer et al. 1983; Getzoff et al. 1992). The dismutase reaction proceeds at a very rapid rate of $2 \times 10^9\ \text{M}^{-1}\text{sec}^{-1}$ and is most likely only limited by substrate (Klug et al. 1972). The electrostatic guidance channel thus provides a funneling of $O_2\cdot^-$ molecule from a wide area to a small and size-matched active site. Access to the active site is limited by size and charge, which favors the negatively charged $O_2\cdot^-$ and excludes molecules of larger size. The two-step dismutase reaction proceeds as follows:

$$O_2\cdot^- + \text{Enz-Cu(II)} + H^+ \rightarrow O_2 + \text{Enz-Cu(I)} \quad (1)$$
$$O_2\cdot^- + \text{Enz-Cu(I)} + H^+ \rightarrow H_2O_2 + \text{Enz-Cu(II)} \quad (2)$$
$$2O_2\cdot^- + 2H^+ \xrightarrow{\text{SOD1}} H_2O_2 + O_2 \quad (3)$$

Besides the dismutase activity, SOD1 has a marginal peroxidase activity (Fridovich 1975; Yim et al. 1990; Yim et al. 1993), and a role in Cu and Zn homeostasis has also been attributed to SOD1. H_2O_2, one of the products of the dismutase reaction, is thought to inactivate SOD1 (Symonyan and Nalbandyan 1972). The inactivation of SOD1 by its own H_2O_2 production and peroxidase activity is as follows:

$$H_2O_2 + \text{Enz-Cu(II)} \longleftrightarrow O_2\cdot^- + \text{Enz-Cu(I)} + 2H^+ \quad (4)$$
$$\text{Enz-Cu(I)} + H_2O_2 \longleftrightarrow \text{Enz-Cu(II)-OH}\cdot + OH^- \quad (5)$$
$$\text{Enz-Cu(II)-OH}\cdot + \text{ImHis63} \rightarrow \text{Enz-Cu(II)} + \text{ImHis}\cdot + H_2O \quad (6)$$

Enz is the SOD1 enzyme and ImH63 is the imidazole moiety of the histidine residue at position 63 of the SOD1 polypeptide. In vivo, the peroxidase activity could be significant in the presence of an excess production of H_2O_2, which may result from a burst of $O_2\cdot^-$ molecules (Yim et al. 1993).

SOD1 AND CHROMOSOME 21-LINKED FALS

In the SOD1 gene, 53 mutations have been identified in FALS families linked to chromosome 21q, of which 51 are given in Table 1. These mutations segregate with ALS (Deng et al. 1993). Among these 51 mutations, there are 45 missense mutations, a stop codon mutation (Zu et al. 1997), a deletion mutation, two intronic mutations in intron 4 that alter the splicing site, and two insertion mutations that also result in a truncated protein. One of the intronic mutation changes an A to G, 11 bp upstream of the splicing site (Zu et al. 1997), and the other intronic mutation changes a T to G, 10 bp upstream of the splicing site (Sapp et al. 1995). All of the reported mutations are in exons 1, 2, 4, and 5, except for one unidentified mutation in exon 3, which contributes to the lower rim of the electrostatic guidance channel and the Cu- and Zn-binding sites.

When the initial mutations identified in FALS were mapped to the crystallographic structure of SOD1, they were found to be clustered in the loops joining the β barrel (Deng et al. 1993). The mutated side chains cluster near the two Greek key connections closing off the ends of the β barrel, in the dimeric interface, and at the base of the active side loop. These side chains, which are structurally conserved in the wild type of SOD1 structures from different species, appear to be critical for the structural integrity of this dimeric enzyme. Some of the side-chain mutations, such as A4V, L38V, L106V, and V148A, would also be expected to destabilize the subunit folding or the dimer contact. Three mutations, H46R, L84V, and D90A, occur outside of the β strand and the loop forming the β barrel. The mutations H46R and H48Q directly affect the ligation of the Cu atom in the protein, since H46 and H48 are two of the four histidines that bind to Cu in SOD1. The mutation L84V occurs at the end of the Zn-binding loop where it joins the β barrel, whereas D90A is expected to have only local effects and to cause few changes in the protein structure (Deng et al. 1993, 1995; Själander et al. 1995). Most mutations in *SOD1* can be predicted to destabilize the protein, resulting in a less active, rather than an inactive, SOD1 protein. D90A is expected to be relatively stable without apparent decrease in enzyme activity (Deng et al. 1993, 1995; Själander et al. 1995). Our studies of purified SOD1 mutant proteins show that most mutations have decreased activity. This is different from some results of other investigators, where normal activity was found. One reason for this difference may be the different methods used for measuring SOD1 activity. We used the direct KO_2 method of Marklund, whereas others used indirect assays requiring xanthine/xanthine oxidase. In the latter assay, if xanthine interacted directly with mutant SOD1, formazon formation may have been reduced, resulting in the false interpretation of increased dismutase activity.

The analysis of the SOD1 enzyme activity supports the structural prediction of loss of activity in most instances due to structural instability. The cytosolic superoxide dismutase activity assayed in red blood cells, transformed lymphoblastoid cells, and brain tissues from FALS patients with mutations in the SOD1 gene was found to be between 30% and 70% of normal activity (Bowling et al. 1993; Deng et al. 1993; Robberecht et al. 1994). FALS patients homozygous for D90A mutation have near normal SOD1 activity (Andersen et al. 1995; Själander et al. 1995). The intrinsic activity of mutated SOD polypeptide expressed in COS-1 cells and in yeast is between 0 and 70% of the normal polypeptide (Borchelt et al. 1994, 1995; Rabizadeh et al. 1995). These observations support the hypothesis that a decrease in SOD activity in FALS patients may result from instability of the mutant and wild-type heterodimers and mutant homodimers. The random dimerization of mutant and wild-type monodimers would predict that 25% of the SOD are wild-type homodimers, 25% are mutant homodimers, and 50% are mutant/wild heterodimers. However, in some mutations, mutant SOD1 monomers were not found to have a dominant negative effect on the dis-

Table 1. *SOD1* Mutations in FALS

Amino acid substitution	Mutation symbol	Nucleotide substitution	Reference
Exon 1			
Ala-4→Val	A4V	GCC→GTC	Deng et al. (1993)
Ala-4→Thr	A4T	GCC→ACC	Nakano et al. (1994)
Val-7→Glu	V7E	GTG→GAG	Hirano et al. (1994)
Leu-8→Gln	L8Q	CTG→CAG	Bereznai et al. (1995)
Val-14→Met	V14M	GTG→ATG	Deng et al. (1995)
Gly-16→Ser	G16S	GGC→AGC	Kawamata et al. (1996)
Glu-21→Lys	E21K	GAG→AAG	Jones et al. (1994b)
Glu-21→Gly	E21G	GAG→GGG	Moulard et al. (1995)
Exon 2			
Gly-37→Arg	G37R	GGA→AGA	Rosen et al. (1993)
Leu-38→Val	L38V	CTG→GTG	Rosen et al. (1993)
Gly-41→Ser	G41S	GGC→AGC	Rosen et al. (1993)
Gly-41→Asp	G41D	GGC→GAC	Rosen et al. (1993)
His-43→Arg	H43R	CAT→CGT	Rosen et al. (1993)
His-46→Arg	H46R	CAT→CGT	Aoki et al. (1993)
His-48→Gln	H48Q	CAT→CAG	Orrell et al. (1997)
Exon 3: Point mutation reported but not identified			Hansen et al. (1996)
Exon 4			
Leu-84→Val	L84V	TTG→GTG	Aoki et al. (1995); Deng et al. (1995)
Gly-85→Arg	G85R	GGC→CGC	Rosen et al. (1993)
Asp-90→Ala	D90A	GAC→GCC	Andersen et al. (1995); Själander et al. (1995)
Gly-93→Ala	G93A	GGT→GCT	Rosen et al. (1993)
Gly-93→Cys	G93C	GGT→TGT	Rosen et al. (1993)
Gly-93→Arg	G93R	GGT→CGT	Elshafey et al. (1994)
Gly-93→Asp	G93D	GGT→GAT	Esteban et al. (1994)
Gly-93→Ser	G93S	GGT→AGT	Kawamata et al. (1994)
Gly-93→Val	G93V	GGT→GTT	Orrell et al. (1997)
Glu-100→Gly	E100G	GAA→GGA	Rosen et al. (1993)
Glu-100→Lys	E100K	GAA→AAA	H.X. Deng et al. (unpubl.)
Asp-101→Asn	D101N	GAT→AAT	Jones et al. (1994a)
Asp-101→Gly	D101G	GAT→GGT	Orrell et al. (1997)
Ile-104→Phe	I104F	ATC→TTC	Ikeda et al. (1996)
Leu-106→Val	L106V	CTC→GTC	Rosen et al. (1993)
Gly-108→Val	G108V	GGA→GTA	Orrell et al. (1997)
Ile-112→Thr	I112T	ATC→ACC	Esteban et al. (1994)
Ile-113→Thr	I113T	ATT→ACT	Rosen et al. (1993)
Arg-115→Gly	R115G	CGC→GGC	Kostrzewa et al. (1994)
Exon 5			
Asp-124→Val	D124V	GAT→GTT	N. Laing (unpubl.)
Asp-125→His	D125H	GAC→CAC	Orrell et al. (1997)
Leu-126→stop	L126stop	TTG→TAG	Zu et al. (1997)
Ser-134→Asn	S134N	AGT→AAT	Watanabe et al. (1996)
Asn-139→Lys	N139K	AAC→AAA	Pramatarova et al. (1995)
Leu-144→Phe	L144F	TTG→TTC	Deng et al. (1993)
Leu-144→Ser	L144S	TTG→TCG	Sapp et al. (1995)
Ala-145→Thr	A145T	GCT→ACT	Sapp et al. (1995)
Cys-146→Arg	C146R	TGT→CGT	Kawamata et al. (1996)
Val-148→Gly	V148G	GTA→GGA	Deng et al. (1993)
Val-148→Ile	V148I	GTA→ATA	Ikeda et al. (1995)
Ile-149→Thr	I149T	ATT→ACT	Pramatarova et al. (1995)
Deletion			
Leu	GAC T*T*GGC126-GAC GGC		
(with stop codon at Lys-130,23 aa deleted)			Nakashima et al. (1995)
Insertion			
	AAT GAT*-^{132} TAG		
(with stop codon at 133)			Orrell et al. (1997)
	TTG-^{126} G*G*G* G*GG		
(with stop codon at 133)			Hansen et al. (1996)
Splice junction			
+Phe-Leu-Glu	T→G 10 bp before exon 5		Sapp et al. (1995)
+Phe-Phe-Thr-Gly-Pro-stop	A→G 11 bp before exon 5 (all exon 5 deleted)		Zu et al. (1997)

mutase activity of normal monodimers. A contrary result was shown in mutant SOD1 from *Drosophila* (Phillips et al. 1995). Thus, the effect of mutations may differ in producing a dominant negative effect.

Another reason for reduction in SOD1 activity in the red blood cells of FALS patients is due to the destabilized SOD1 protein, resulting in a shorter half-life of mutant SOD1 protein. For example, in a COS-1 cell-culture system, the half-life for A4V is about 7 hours, whereas for the normal SOD1 protein, it is about 30 hours (Borchelt et al. 1994). Quantitative analysis of SOD1 protein in FALS patients showed a reduction in SOD amount by 35–75% of the normal value (T. Siddique et al., unpubl.); no decrease in SOD1 protein was observed in non-chromosome-21 FALS patients.

Different mutations in *SOD1* do not seem to have significant influence on the age at onset of symptoms. Half of FALS patients develop symptoms by 46 years of age. However, some mutations affect the progression of disease. The mean duration for FALS patients with A4V mutation is 1.2 years, which is significantly shorter than the mean duration observed in patients with E100G mutation, which is 4.7 years (Juneja et al. 1997). Duration for most of the FALS patients with SOD1 mutations ranges from 3 to 5 years; H46R and G37R have the longest duration of about 18–20 years (Aoki et al. 1995; Deng et al. 1995).

Two mutations are worth mentioning because of their specificity. The D90A mutation was previously described as a polymorphism with a relatively high frequency of 2.5% in the Northern Swedish/Finnish population; Prevalence of ALS is not significantly increased in this population (Beckman et al. 1973). It has been recently observed that homozygotes for the D90A mutation develop ALS (Andersen et al. 1995; Själander et al. 1995). The penetrance is estimated to be 38%, suggesting that D90A is a recessive mutation for ALS (Andersen et al. 1995). It is intriguing, however, that heterozygotes of this mutation do develop ALS in the non-Swedish population (W. Robberecht, pers. comm.). Another interesting mutation, I113T, has been reported in several apparently sporadic cases (Jones et al. 1994a,b). We identified an apparently sporadic ALS case with the I113T mutation, but detailed family history and analysis of family DNA indicated that this mutation was actually inherited. The D90A and I113T mutations suggest that some cases of SALS are genetic but have penetrance of the inherited gene, strongly arguing for modifying factors.

OTHER FORMS OF FALS

FALS is a disorder with genetic heterogeneity (Siddique 1991; Hentati et al. 1994). Both DFALS and RFALS have more than one locus in the genome. RFALS is rare and observed with relatively high prevalence in Tunisia (Ben Hamida et al. 1990). RFALS families of Pakistani origin and other ethnicities have also been identified (T. Siddique, unpubl.). The penetrance of RFALS is 100% by the age of 20. The mean age at onset of symptoms in RFALS is 12.03 (range 3–23 years), and the duration of the disease ranges from 15 to 20 years. RFALS is a juvenile form of ALS, but not the only juvenile form, because symptoms can occur early in some patients with SALS or with DFALS (T. Siddique et al., unpubl.). In most cases, the symptoms of SALS and DFALS do not occur before the age of 10 years and rarely before the age of 20. Bulbar involvement almost always occurs in juvenile ALS.

Three clinical variants of RFALS are known (Ben Hamida et al. 1990). The more common variant, RFALS type 1, is characterized by the relative predominance of lower motor neuron involvement early in the disease, accompanied by atrophy and weakness in hand and foot muscles. The tongue is affected in later stages and bulbar involvement occurs, but is usually slowly progressive. Upper motor neuron involvement is moderate in early stages and becomes more apparent as the disease progresses. In RFALS type 3, the symptoms of upper motor neuron degeneration predominate. Patients with RFALS type 3 show spasticity of limb and facial muscles, spastic and slurred speech usually leading to anarthria, and uncontrolled weeping and laughter. Lower motor neuron involvement occurs later in the disease and affects both hands and feet. In RFALS type 2, symptoms are confined to the lower limbs, which is most likely a form of autosomal recessive familial spastic paraplegia.

A large inbred Tunisian family with RFALS type 3 (genetic nomenclature symbol ALS2) has been linked to chromosome 2q33-35 (Hentati et al. 1994). The ALS2 locus was subsequently refined to 2q33 (A. Hentati et al., unpubl.). The genetic analysis of families with RFALS type 1 did not show linkage to markers on either chromosome 2q33 or chromosome 21q, demonstrating genetic locus heterogeneity in RFALS (Hentati et al. 1994). The locus for RFALS type 1 (ALS4) has now been identified, but not published (A. Hentati et al., unpubl.).

Some cases of ALS with dementia can also be familial; several pedigrees with dominant inheritance have been described previously (Emery and Holloway 1982). We studied three multigenerational families in which either frontal lobe dementia or ALS was prominent or in which both coexisted in the same individual. In three individuals in one family, we observed pathological changes that were identical to those seen in ALS. In addition, a spongiform change with neuronal loss and gliosis in the superficial layer of the cortex was also noted. Positive LOD scores (logarithm of the odds of linkage) in the range of 1 were obtained with chromosome 17q markers, but linkage could not be established (T. Siddique et al., unpubl.).

Disinhibition-dementia-Parkinsonism-amyotrophy-complex (DDPAC) is a condition characterized by association of frontal lobe dementia, with Parkinsonism, and amyotrophy (Wilhelmsen et al. 1994). The variability of clinical symptoms between patients is a striking feature of DDPAC. The most common features are disinhibition and frontal lobe dementia. Amyotrophy is absent in some patients but is the most prominent clinical feature in other patients. The pathological hallmark of DDPAC is spongiform change and neuronal loss with gliosis affecting mostly the superficial layer of the brain. There is also a marked loss of motor neurons in the spinal cord. The gene locus for DDPAC is on chromosome 17q21-22 (Wilhelmsen et al. 1994).

TRANSGENIC MOUSE MODEL FOR FALS

Three transgenic mouse lines were initially made immediately after *SOD1* mutations in FALS were identified: two lines expressing mutant SOD1 (A4V and G93A) and the other line expressing wild-type SOD1 (Gurney et al. 1994). The mice overexpressing the G93A mutation developed symptoms similar to human ALS at 3–4 months of age, whereas mice overexpressing wild-type human SOD1 at a comparable age were not affected (Gurney et al. 1994). Similar results have been reported in transgenic mice overexpressing the human *SOD1* gene with the G37R mutation and mouse *SOD1* gene with the G86R mutation that corresponds to G85R mutation in humans (Ripps et al. 1995; Wong et al. 1995). A clear dosage effect of the mutant gene has been observed in the mice, where the higher the copy number of the mutant gene, the earlier the onset of the disease (Gurney et al. 1994; Wong et al. 1995). The two lines of mice with low copy number of the A4V mutation, the most frequent SOD1 mutation identified in human FALS, developed disease phenotype after 700 days of age (T. Siddique et al., unpubl.). This is at least 200–500 days later than the mice with higher expression of mutant SOD1.

The observations from the various lines of mice expressing different mutations suggest that it is unlikely that disease phenotype is caused by a position effect of the integration of the mutant SOD1 gene (McCord 1994). Rather, it is likely to be a toxic effect of mutant SOD1 on motor neurons leading to their death. Such a toxic mechanism may also underlie FALS in humans. One major question regarding these transgenic mice with extraordinary overexpression of mutant SOD1 is whether these mice are ideal models for FALS in humans. This question arises due to the following differences between transgenic mice and humans: (1) *Genetic background.* FALS patients have one copy each of the normal and mutant SOD1 genes, whereas mice have two copies of endogenous murine SOD1 and several copies of human mutant SOD1. The copy number and expression level significantly affect the phenotype of the mice (Gurney et al. 1994; Wong et al. 1995). (2) *Pathology.* The pathology in transgenic mice is different in mice with different mutations and also differs in mice with varying levels of expression of SOD1 (Dal Canto and Gurney 1994, 1995; Wong et al. 1995). (3) *Age at onset.* The disease phenotype in high copy number transgenic mice is around 3–4 months of age, which in mouse chronobiology is earlier than that of FALS patients (Gurney et al. 1994; Ripps et al. 1995; Wong et al. 1995). Additionally, pathological changes have been identified in the nervous system of the transgenic mice overexpressing wild-type SOD1 (Epstein et al. 1987; Dal Canto and Gurney 1994, 1995). However, the pathology in the mice with lower overexpression of mutant SOD1 has greater similarity to that seen in ALS patients (Dal Canto and Gurney 1994, 1995). Thus, to date, this mouse model is the most proximate to human ALS.

POSSIBLE MOLECULAR MECHANISMS FOR ALS

Explanations of mechanisms by which mutant SOD causes motor neuron degeneration have focused on the exaggerated or disturbed known functions of SOD1. The known functions of SOD1 are (1) dismutase, (2) peroxidase, and possibly (3) metal binding.

Loss of Dismutase Function

SOD1 is an antioxidant defense which catalyzes the conversion of superoxide free radical anion ($O_2 \cdot^-$) to hydrogen peroxide (H_2O_2) and oxygen (O_2). However, the biological effects of the conversion of $O_2 \cdot^-$ to H_2O_2 by SOD1 on the viability of the cells may be double-edged. H_2O_2 and its derivatives are directly toxic to the cell and may signal apoptosis. Mapping of the mutation sites to the crystallographic structure of wild-type SOD1 predicted that these mutations destabilize the protein structure, leading to a less active enzyme rather than a completely inactive or a more active SOD1 in FALS (Deng et al. 1993). This prediction has been confirmed by enzymatic assay of SOD1 activity in red blood cells, lymphoblastoid cells, and brain tissues from FALS patients (Bowling et al. 1993; Deng et al. 1993; Robberecht et al. 1994). These observations exclude the possibility that a more active SOD1 is involved in FALS and support the hypothesis that a decrease of SOD1 activity, and therefore an increase of $O_2 \cdot^-$, may be responsible for the disease. This hypothesis is supported by in vitro studies; reduction of SOD1 activity by chronic application of SOD1 antisense oligonucleotides triggers neuronal death. This death process can be averted by agents that enhance intracellular antioxidant defense (Rabizadeh et al. 1995). However, this hypothesis is not fully defensible for the following two reasons: (1) Although most mutations in the SOD1 gene cause a decrease in the steady state of cytosolic SOD1 activity, there are at least two exceptions, G37R and D90A, which appear to have no significant decrease in SOD1 activity. (2) Transgenic mice overexpressing FALS-linked mutations in the SOD1 gene on a normal mouse background develop disease similar to ALS in humans, whereas those overexpressing normal SOD1 remain phenotypically unaffected (Gurney et al. 1994; Ripps et al. 1995; Wong et al. 1995). These observations from overexpression transgenic mouse models and from SOD1 knockout mice (Reaume et al. 1996) strongly disagree with "loss of function" but support a "gain of toxic function" hypothesis (Gurney et al. 1994; Ripps et al. 1995; Wong et al. 1995; Reaume et al. 1996). Firm conclusions for these two hypotheses are not possible yet, although gain of a toxic function appears more likely.

SOD1 as a Free Radical Generator

It is known that SOD1 has some peroxidase activity in addition to the major superoxide dismutase activity (Fridovich 1975; Yim et al. 1990). Our studies of 16 different SOD1 mutant lymphoblastoid cell lines from FALS patients have shown an increased detection of H_2O_2 in FALS cell lines but not in normal controls (M.S. Ahmed et al., unpubl.). It has also been reported that FALS-associated mutant SOD1 enzyme catalyzes the reduction of H_2O_2, therefore acting as a peroxidase; this process occurs more rapidly with mutant than wild-type SOD1 (Wiedau-Pazos et al. 1996; Yim et al. 1996). These results, although derived from in vitro studies, support the gain of a toxic function mechanism and indicate that increased peroxidase activity of mutant SOD1 may play a critical role in the pathogenesis of SOD1-linked FALS. Recently, screening of potential therapeutics in our transgenic mouse model expressing a G93A mutation indicated that dietary supplementation with vitamin E delayed onset of clinical disease and slowed progression, although it did not prolong survival (Gurney et al. 1996). This supports the hypothesis that the pathogenesis of SOD1-related FALS may in part be due to oxidative damage to cellular components.

SOD1 Complexes

With one exception (D90A; Själander et al. 1995), FALS-associated mutated SOD1 molecules are unstable. These unstable mutants would have altered conformations that may precipitate to form aggregates in motor neurons which, in turn, could disturb normal cell function and lead to cell death. A high concentration of unstable mutant SOD1 in the nervous system may facilitate the formation of inclusions such as Lewy body-like inclusions recently reported in FALS patients with an A4V mutation. These inclusions are positive with antibody against SOD1 (Deng et al. 1995; Shibata et al. 1996).

Rim Distortion Hypothesis

Crystallographic structural mapping studies predict that FALS mutations will lead to a structural change of mutant SOD1 (Deng et al. 1993). If these changes distort the electrostatic guidance channel and allow the catalytic site to become exposed and more shallow, molecules normally excluded may gain access to the catalytic reactive site. Beckman and colleagues (1993) proposed that mutant SOD1 may react with peroxynitrite formed from superoxide and nitric oxide and facilitate nitration of tyrosine residues of critical cytosolic proteins, thus injuring cells. The access of peroxynitrite would be in keeping with the model of a promiscuous accessibility of the Cu site. Our preliminary studies on protein structure using antibodies against SOD1 suggest that a common conformational change occurs in the mutants A4V, G37R, and H46R that may affect the lower rim of the electrostatic guidance channel coded by exon 3. The rim distortion hypothesis is also favored by our newly identified truncation mutations. These mutations result in a truncated SOD1 by deleting exon-5-encoded polypeptide, which constitutes a part of the upper rim of the electrostatic channel (Zu et al. 1997). These truncation mutations remove the entire upper rim of the electrostatic guidance channel and have no dismutase activity. They are thus instructive in separating the FALS-associated toxic property of mutant SOD1 from the dismutase activity. The distortion of the molecule is expected, as the sphere size accessible to the copper atom in these mutants is enhanced. This opening up of the electrostatic guidance channel would allow spheres up to a radius of 5.7 Å to access the active site, as opposed to only 1.7 Å radius in the wild type (Zu et al. 1997).

Mutant SOD1 possibly exhibits metal-mediated cytotoxicities by disrupting the intracellular homeostasis of Cu and Zn. It is well known that Cu and Zn are potential neurotoxins (Koh and Choi 1988; Scheinberg 1988). Sudden and en masse release of Zn from SOD1 aggregates in motor neurons may lead to cell death.

The current hypotheses for the pathogenesis of FALS are focused on free radical damage to motor neurons, but many questions remain unanswered. Elucidation of the pathogenesis of FALS may benefit patients with other forms of ALS or other neurodegenerative disorders that share similar mechanisms of disease.

SPORADIC ALS

SALS is clinically identical to familial ALS and pathologically very similar, but the mechanism of disease in ALS is not related to mutations in SOD1. This suggests that the phenotype of ALS can result from multiple pathways underlining the genetic and etiological heterogeneity of both familial and sporadic ALS. λ_S is a measure of risk to relatives of the proband as compared to the general population. In general, larger estimates of λ_S correspond to larger genetic control of trait variation. The risk to siblings of ALS patients or (λ_S) is not low and was calculated to be between 40 and 133, based on the epidemiological studies of Murros and Fugelhom (1983) and McGuire et al.

(1996) suggesting a significant genetic contribution (M. Pericak-Vance and J. Haines, pers. comm.). FALS associated with SOD1 represents a large genetic effect in a small ALS population (2.5% of ALS cases). On the contrary, SALS may result from a genetic predisposition due to multiple small effects in larger ALS populations. Thus, the newer techniques of identifying these effects, such as transmission disequilibrium testing (TDT) (Ewens and Spielman 1997), could be applied to SALS. The optimum study population would be SALS patients and their parents, where the controls are the nontransmitted alleles of the parents. The obvious limitation of this method is that disequilibrium in outbred populations can only be detected in a very small segment of DNA flanking the gene producing the putative effect. Because hyperdense maps of the human genome with markers less than 0.25 cM apart are not yet available, TDT is currently restricted to those loci that are postulated to be involved in the pathogenesis of ALS. Examples of such genes would include genes for glutamate transporters, calcium homeostasis, apoptosis, and intracellular protein cargo transport.

SOD1 AND SALS

Because of the similarity between FALS and SALS, we investigated the connection between FALS and SOD1. We reasoned that if in human SOD1-linked ALS, the pathogenesis is indeed due to gain of a toxic function (as in the transgenic mouse model), then there should be a final common pathway present in all the 50 or so known SOD1 mutations. The only known commonality in these mutations is an alteration of the conformation of the SOD1 molecule. We further reasoned that although SOD1 is normally tolerated by the immune system, anti-SOD1 antibodies may be produced if the immune system is presented with novel epitopes of SOD1 due to altered conformation. To investigate this further, we tested SALS sera for SOD1-specific antibodies, and detected them in 15% of SALS cases as opposed to their presence in less than 2% of controls (J. Zu and T. Siddique, unpubl.). Measurement of SOD1 activity and SOD1 protein in red blood cells (RBCs) of 100 SALS patients and 100 age-matched controls showed a statistically significant increase in both activity and protein in the SALS group (J. Zu et al., unpubl.). To test if the observed increase in the SOD1 protein and activity was genetically influenced, we measured those parameters in 48 parents of 24 SALS patients. The SOD1 protein and activity were also significantly increased in the RBCs of this group of parents. This study suggests that SOD1 concentration in RBCs, and by inference in the nervous system, is associated with SALS and may be genetically determined. This appears to be an example of the effect of a genetic predisposition associated with ALS discussed above. Thus, with the continuing development of statistical genetic methods, it is not unreasonable to predict that TDT-type methods will be successfully applied to genetically complex disorders of neurodegeneration such as ALS.

REFERENCES

Andersen, P.M., P. Nilsson, V. Ala-Hurula, M.L. Keranen, I. Tarvainen, T. Haltia, L. Nilsson, M. Binzer, L. Forsgren, and S.L. Marklund. 1995. Amyotrophic lateral sclerosis associated with homozygosity for an Asp90Ala mutation in Cu/Zn-superoxide dismutase. *Nat. Genet.* **10:** 61.

Aoki, M., M. Ogasawara, Y. Matsubara, K. Narisawa, S. Nakamura, Y. Itoyama, and K. Abe. 1993. Mild ALS in Japan associated with novel SOD mutation. *Nat. Genet.* **5:** 323.

Aoki, M., K. Abe, K. Houi, M. Ogasawara, Y. Matsubara, T. Kobayashi, S. Mochio, K. Narisawa, and Y Itoyama. 1995. Variance of age at onset in a Japanese family with amyotrophic lateral sclerosis associated with a novel Cu/Zn superoxide dismutase mutation. *Ann. Neurol.* **37:** 676.

Applebaum, J.S., R.P. Roos, E.F. Salazar-Grueso, A. Buchman, S. Iannaccone, R. Glantz, T. Siddique, and R. Maselli. 1992. Intrafamilial heterogeneity in hereditary motor neuron disease. *Neurology* **42:** 1488.

Beckman, G., L. Beckman, and L.-O. Nilsson. 1973. A rare homozygous phenotype of superoxide dismutase, SOD2. *Hereditas* **75:** 138.

Beckman, J.S., M. Carson, C.D. Smith, and W.H. Koppenol. 1993. ALS, SOD and peroxynitrite. *Nature* **364:** 584.

Ben Hamida, M., F. Hentati, and C. Ben Hamida. 1990. Hereditary motor system diseases (chronic juvenile amyotrophic lateral sclerosis) conditions combing a bilateral pyramidal syndrome with limb and bulbar amyotrophy. *Brain* **113:** 347.

Bereznai, B., G.D. Borasio, A. Winkler, and T. Gasser. 1995. SOD1 punkmutation in einer familie mit ALS. In *Abstracts from the Annual Meeting of the German Society of Neuro-genetics*, Munich, Germany.

Borchelt, D.R., M. Guarnieri, P.C. Wong, M.K. Lee, H.S. Slunt, Z.S. Xu, S.S. Sisodia, D.L. Price, and D.W. Cleveland. 1995. Superoxide dismutase 1 subunits with mutations linked to familial amyotrophic lateral sclerosis do not affect wild-type subunit function. *J. Biol. Chem.* **270:** 3234.

Borchelt, D.R., M.K. Lee, H.S. Slunt, M. Guarnieri, Z.S. Xu, P.C. Wong, R.H. Brown, Jr., D.L. Price, S.S. Sisodia, and D.W. Cleveland. 1994. Superoxide dismutase 1 with mutations linked to familial amyotrophic lateral sclerosis possesses significant activity. *Proc. Natl. Acad. Sci.* **91:** 8292.

Bowling, A.C., J.B. Schulz, R.H. Brown, Jr., and M.F. Beal. 1993. Superoxide dismutase activity, oxidative damage and mitochondrial energy metabolism in familial and sporadic amyotrophic lateral sclerosis. *J. Neurochem.* **61:** 2322.

Dal Canto, M.C. and M.E. Gurney. 1994. The development of central nervous system pathology in a murine transgenic model of human amyotrophic lateral sclerosis. *Am. J. Pathol.* **145:** 1271.

———. 1995. Neuropathological changes in two lines of mice carrying a transgene for mutant human Cu,Zn SOD, and in mice overexpressing wild type human SOD: A model of familial lateral sclerosis (FALS). *Brain Res* **676:** 25.

Deng, H.X., J.A. Tainer, H. Mitsumoto, A. Ohnishi, X. He, W.Y. Hung, Y. Zhao, T. Juneja, A. Hentati, and T. Siddique. 1995. Two novel SOD1 mutations in patients with familial amyotrophic lateral sclerosis. *Hum. Mol. Genet.* **4:** 1113.

Deng, H.X., A. Hentati, J.A. Tainer, Z. Iqbal, A. Cayabyab, W.Y. Hung, E.D. Getzoff, H. Ping, B. Herzfeldt, R.P. Roos, C. Warner, G. Deng, E. Soriano, C. Smyth, H.E. Parge, A. Ahmed, A.D. Roses, R.A. Hallewell, M.A. Pericak-Vance, and T. Siddique. 1993. Amyotrophic lateral sclerosis and structural defects in Cu,Zn superoxide dismutase. *Science* **261:** 1047.

Elshafey, A., W.G. Lanyon, and J.M. Connor. 1994. Identification of a new missense point mutation in exon 4 of the Cu/Zn superoxide dismutase (SOD-1) gene in a family with amyotrophic lateral sclerosis. *Hum. Mol. Genet.* **3:** 363.

Emery, A.E.H. and S. Holloway. 1982. Familial motor neuron disease. In *Human motor neuron diseases* (ed. L.P. Rowland), p. 139. Raven Press, New York.

Epstein, C.J., K.B. Avraham, M. Lovett, S. Smith, O. Elroy-Stein, G. Rotman, C. Bry, and Y. Groner. 1987. Transgenic mice with increased Cu/Zn-superoxide dismutase activity: Animal model of dosage effects in Down syndrome. *Proc. Natl. Acad. Sci.* **84:** 8044.

Esteban, J., D.R. Rosen, A.C. Bowling, P. Sapp, D. McKenna-Yasek, J.P. O'Regan, M.F. Beal, H.R. Horvitz, and R.H. Brown, Jr. 1994. Identification of two novel mutations and a new polymorphism in the gene for Cu/Zn superoxide dismutase in patients with amyotrophic lateral sclerosis. *Hum. Mol. Genet.* **3:** 997.

Ewens, W.J. and R.S. Spielman. 1997. Transmission/disequilibrium test with many marker alleles: Testing for linkage and testing for association. *Am. J. Hum. Genet.* (in press).

Fridovich, I. 1975. Superoxide dismutases. *Annu. Rev. Biochem.* **44:** 147.

Getzoff, E.D., J.A. Tainer, M.M. Stempien, G.I. Bell, and R.A. Hallewell. 1989. Evolution of Cu/Zn superoxide dismutase and the Greek key beta-barrel structural motif. *Proteins* **5:** 322.

Getzoff, E.D., D.E. Cabelli, C.L. Fisher, H.E. Parge, M.S. Viezzoli, L. Banci, and R.A. Hallewell. 1992. Faster superoxide dismutase mutants designed by enhancing electrostatic guidance. *Nature* **358:** 347

Gurney, M.E., F.B. Cutting, P. Zhai, A. Doble, C.P. Taylor, P.K. Andrus, and E.D. Hall. 1996. Benefit of vitamin E riluzole, and gabapentin in a transgenic model of familial amyotrophic lateral sclerosis. *Ann. Neurol.* **39:** 147.

Gurney, M.E., H. Pu, A.Y. Chiu, M.C. Dal Canto, C.Y. Polchow, D.D. Alexander, J. Caliendo, A. Hentati, Y.W. Kwon, H.X. Deng, W. Chen, P. Zhai, R.L. Sufit, and T. Siddique. 1994. Motor neuron degeneration in mice that express a human Cu,Zn superoxide dismutase mutation. *Science* **264:** 1772.

Hansen, C., O. Gredal, M. Karlsborg, L. Werdelin, P.M. Andersen, P. Nilson, S.L. Marklund, and K.B. Nielsen. 1996. Two new SOD1 mutations in ALS: A four base pair insertion in exon 5 and a missense mutation in exon 3. In *Abstracts from the 7th International Symposium on ALS/MND*, Chicago, Illinois.

Hentati, A., K. Bejaoui, M.A. Pericak-Vance, F. Hentati, M.C. Speer, W.Y. Hung, D.A. Figlewicz, J. Haines, J. Rimmler, C. Ben Hamida, M. Ben Hamida, R.H. Brown, and T. Siddique. 1994. Linkage of recessive familial amyotrophic lateral sclerosis to chromosome 2q33-q35. *Nat. Genet.* **7:** 425.

Hirano, M., J. Fujii, Y. Nagai, M. Sonobe, K. Okamoto, H. Araki, N. Taniguchi, and S. Ueno. 1994. A new variant Cu/Zn superoxide dismutase (Val7→Glu) deduced from lymphocyte mRNA sequences from Japanese patients with familial amyotrophic lateral sclerosis. *Biochem. Biophys. Res. Commun.* **204:** 572.

Ikeda, M., K. Abe, M. Aoki, M. Ogasawara, T. Kameya, M. Watanabe, M. Shoji, S. Hirai, and Y. Itoyama. 1995. A novel point mutation in the Cu/Zn superoxide dismutase gene in a patient with familial amyotrophic lateral sclerosis. *Hum. Mol. Genet.* **4:** 491.

Ikeda, M., K. Abe, M. Aoki, M. Sahara, M. Watanabe, M. Shoji, P.H. St. George-Hyslop, S. Hirai, and Y. Itoyama. 1996. Variable clinical symptoms in the pedigrees of familial amyotrophic lateral sclerosis with novel missense point mutations in the Cu/Zn superoxide dismutase gene. In *Amyotrophic lateral sclerosis: Progress and perspectives in basic research and clinical application* (ed. I. Nakano and A. Hirano), p. 285. Elsevier, The Netherlands.

Jones, C.T., R.J. Swingler, and D.J. Brock. 1994a. Identification of a novel SOD1 mutation in an apparently sporadic amyotrophic lateral sclerosis patient and the detection of Ile113Thr in three others. *Hum. Mol. Genet.* **3:** 649.

Jones, C.T., P.J. Shaw, G. Chari, and D.J. Brock. 1994b. Identification of a novel exon 4 SOD1 mutation in a sporadic amyotrophic lateral sclerosis patient. *Mol. Cell. Probes* **8:** 329.

Juneja, T., M. Pericak-Vance, N.G. Laing, S. Dave, and T. Siddique. 1997. Prognosis in familial ALS: Progression and survival in patients with E100G and A4V mutations in Cu,Zn superoxide dismutase. *Neurology* **48:** 55.

Kawamata, J., H. Hasegawa, S. Shimohama, J. Kimura, S. Tanaka, and K. Ueda. 1994. KLeu106→Val (CTC→GTC) mutation of superoxide dismutase-1 gene in patient with familial amyotrophic lateral sclerosis in Japan. *Lancet* **343:** 1501.

Kawamata, J., S. Shimohama, H. Hasegawa, T. Imura, J. Kimura, and K. Ueda. 1996. Deletion and point mutations in superoxide dismutase-1 gene in amyotrophic lateral sclerosis. In *Amyotrophic lateral sclerosis: Progress and perspectives in basic research and clinical application* (ed. I. Nakano and A. Hirano), p. 276. Elsevier, The Netherlands.

Klug, D., J. Rabani, and I. Fridovich. 1972. A direct demonstration of the catalytic action of superoxide dismutase through the use of pulse radiolysis. *J. Biol. Chem.* **247:** 4839.

Koh, J.Y. and D.W. Choi. 1988. Zinc alters excitatory amino acid neurotoxicity on cortical neurons. *J. Neurosci.* **8:** 2164.

Kostrzewa, M., U. Burck-Lehmann, and U. Muller. 1994. Autosomal dominant amyotrophic lateral sclerosis: A novel mutation in the Cu/Zn superoxide dismutase-1 gene. *Hum. Mol. Genet.* **3:** 2261.

McCord, J.M. 1994. Mutant mice, Cu,Zn superoxide dismutase, and motor neuron degeneration. *Science* **266:** 1586.

McGuire, V., W.T. Longstreth, Jr., T.D. Koepsell, and G. van Belle. 1996. Incidence of amyotrophic lateral sclerosis in three counties in western Washington State. *Neurology* **47:** 571.

Moulard, B., W. Camu, A. Brice, F. Salachos, V. Mcininger, and A. Mallafossc. 1995. A previously undescribed mutation in the *SOD1* gene in a French family with atypical ALS. In *Abstracts from the 6th International Symposium on ALS/MND*, Dublin, Ireland.

Mulder, D.W., L.T. Kurland, K.P. Offord, and C.M. Beard.

1986. Familial adult motor neuron disease: Amyotrophic lateral sclerosis. *Neurology* **36:** 511.

Murros, K. and R. Fogelholm. 1983. Amyotrophic lateral sclerosis in middle-Finland: An epidemiological study. *Acta Neurol. Scand.* **67:** 41.

Nakano, R., S. Sato, T. Inuzuka, K. Sakimura, M. Mishina, H. Takahashi, F. Ikuta, Y. Honma, J. Fujii, N. Taniguchi, and S. Tsuji. 1994. A novel mutation in Cu/Zn superoxide dismutase gene in Japanese familial amyotrophic lateral sclerosis. *Biochem. Biophys. Res. Commun.* **200:** 695.

Nakashima, K., Y. Watanabe, N. Kuno, E. Nanba, and K. Takahashi. 1995. Abnormality of Cu/Zn superoxide dismutase (SOD1) activity in Japanese familial amyotrophic lateral sclerosis with two base pair deletion in the SOD1 gene. *Neurology* **45:** 1019.

Orrell, R.W., J.J. Habgood, I. Gardiner, A.W. King, F.A. Bowe, R.A. Hallewell, S.L. Marklund, J. Greenwood, and J. de Belleroche. 1997. Clinical and functional investigation of 10 missense mutations and a novel frameship insertion mutation of the gene for copper-zinc superoxide dismutase in UK families with amyotrophic lateral sclerosis. *Neurology* **48:** 746.

Phillips, J.P., J.A. Tainer, E.D. Getzoff, G.L. Boulianne, K. Kirby, and A.J. Hilliker. 1995. Subunit-destabilizing mutations in *Drosophila* copper/zinc superoxide dismutase: Neuropathology and a model of dimer dysequilibrium. *Proc. Natl. Acad. Sci.* **92:** 8574.

Pramatarova, A., D.A. Figlewicz, A. Krizus, F.Y. Han, I. Ceballos-Picot, A. Nicole, M. Dib, V Meininger, R.H. Brown, and G.A. Rouleau. 1995. Identification of new mutations in the Cu/Zn superoxide dismutase gene of patients with familial amyotrophic lateral sclerosis. *Am. J. Hum. Genet.* **56:** 5926.

Rabizadeh, S, E.B. Gralla, and D.R. Borchelt, R. Gwinn, J.S. Valentine, S. Sisoda, P. Wong, M. Lee, H. Hahn, and D.E. Bredesen. 1995. Mutations associated with amyotrophic lateral sclerosis convert superoxide dismutase from an antiapoptotic gene to a proapoptotic gene: Studies in yeast and neural cells. *Proc. Natl. Acad. Sci.* **92:** 3024.

Reaume, A.G., J.L. Elliott, E.K. Hoffman, N.W. Kowall, R.J. Ferrante, D.F. Siwek, H.M. Wilcox, D.G. Flood, M.F. Beal, R.H. Brown, Jr., R.W. Scott, and W.D. Snider. 1996. Motor neurons in Cu/Zn superoxide dismutase-deficient mice develop normally but exhibit enhanced cell death after axonal injury. *Nat. Genet.* **13:** 43.

Ripps, M.E., G.W. Huntley, P.R. Hof, J.H. Morrison, and J.W. Gordon. 1995. Transgenic mice expressing an altered murine superoxide dismutase gene provide an animal model of amyotrophic lateral sclerosis. *Proc. Natl. Acad. Sci.* **92:** 689.

Robberecht, W., P. Sapp, M.K. Viaene, D. Rosen, D. McKenna-Yasek, J. Haines, R. Horvitz, P. Theys, and R.H. Brown, Jr. 1994. Cu/Zn superoxide dismutase, activity in sporadic and familial amyotrophic lateral sclerosis. *J. Neurochem.* **62:** 384.

Rosen, D.R., T. Siddique, D. Patterson, D.A. Figlewicz, P. Sapp, A. Hentati, D. Donaldson, J. Goto, J.P. O'Regan, H.X. Deng, Z. Rahmani, A. Krizus, D. McKenna-Yasek, A. Cayabyab, S. Gaston, M. Berger, R.E. Tanzi, J.J. Halperin, B. Herzfeldt, R. Van den Bergh, W.Y. Hung, T. Bird, G. Deng, D.W. Mulder, C. Smyth, N.G. Laing, E. Soriano, M.A. Pericak-Vance, J. Haines, G.A. Rouleau, J.S. Gusella, H.R. Horvitz, and R.H. Brown, Jr. 1993. Mutations in Cu/Zn superoxide dismutase gene are associated with familial amyotrophic lateral sclerosis. *Nature* **362:** 59.

Sapp, P.C., D.R. Rose, B.A. Hosler, J. Esteban, D. McKenna-Yasek, J.P. O'Regan, H.R. Horvitz, and R.H. Brown, Jr. 1995. Identification of three novel mutations in the gene for Cu/Zn superoxide dismutase in patients with familial amyotrophic lateral sclerosis. *Neuromusc. Disord.* **5:** 353.

Scheinberg, H. 1988. The neurotoxicity of copper. In *Metal neurotoxicity* (S.C. Bondy and K.N. Prasad), p. 55. CRC Press, Boca Raton, Florida.

Shibata, N., A. Hirano, M. Kobayashi, T. Siddique, T. Kato, and K. Asayama. 1996. Intense SOD1 immunoreactivity in intracytoplasmic hyaline inclusion of familial ALS with posterior column involvement. *J. Neuropathol. Exp. Neurol.* **55:** 481.

Siddique, T. 1991. Molecular genetics of familial amyotrophic lateral sclerosis. *Adv. Neurol.* **56:** 227.

Siddique, T., M.A. Pericak-Vance, B.R. Brooks, R.P. Roos, W.Y. Hung, J.P. Antel, T.L. Munsat, K. Phillips, K. Warner, M. Speer, W.B. Bias, N.A. Siddique, and A.D. Roses. 1989. Linkage analysis in familial amyotrophic lateral sclerosis. *Neurology* **39:** 919.

Siddique, T., D.A. Figlewicz, M.A. Pericak-Vance, J.L. Haines, G. Rouleau, A.J. Jeffers, P. Sapp, W.Y. Hung, J. Bebout, D. McKenna-Yasek, G. Deng, H.R. Horvitz, J.F. Gusella, R.H. Brown, Jr., A.D. Roses, et al. 1991. Linkage of a gene causing familial amyotrophic lateral sclerosis to chromosome 21 and evidence of genetic locus heterogeneity. *N. Engl. J. Med.* **324:** 1381.

Själander, A., G. Beckman, H.X. Deng, Z. Iqbal, J.A. Tainer, and T. Siddique. 1995. The D90A mutation results in a polymorphism of Cu,Zn superoxide dismutase that is prevalent in northern Sweden and Finland. *Hum. Mol. Genet.* **4:** 1105.

Symonyan, M.A. and R.N. Nalbandyan. 1972. Interaction of hydrogen peroxide with superoxide dismutase from erythrocyte. *FEBS Lett.* **28:** 22.

Tainer, J.A., E.D. Getzoff, K.M. Beem, J.S. Richardson, and D.C. Richardson. 1982. Determination and analysis of the 2Å structure of copper, zinc superoxide dismutase. *J. Mol. Biol.* **160:** 181.

Tainer, J.A., E.D. Getzoff, J.S. Richardson, and J.R. Richardson. 1983. Structure and mechanism of copper, zinc superoxide dismutase. *Nature* **306:** 284.

Takahashi, H., T. Makifuchi, R. Nakano, S. Sato, T. Inuzuka, K. Sakimura, M. Mishina, Y. Honma, S. Tsuji, and F. Ikuta. 1994. Familial amyotrophic lateral sclerosis with a mutation in the Cu/Zn superoxide dismutase gene. *Acta Neuropathol.* **88:** 185.

Tandan, R. and W.G. Bradley. 1985. Amyotrophic lateral sclerosis: Part 1. Clinical features, pathology, and ethical issues in management. *Ann. Neurol.* **18:** 271.

Watanabe, Y., Y. Kono, E. Nanba, K. Nakashima, S. Kato, E. Ohama, and K. Takahashi. 1996. The absence of abnormal Cu/Zn superoxide dismutase (SOD1) in familial amyotrophic lateral sclerosis with two basepair deletion in the SOD1 gene. In *Amyotrophic lateral sclerosis: Progress and perspectives in basic research and clinical application* (ed. I. Nakano and A. Hirano), p. 281. Elsevier, The Netherlands.

Wiedau-Pazos, M., J.J. Goto, S. Rabizadeh, E.B. Gralla, J.A. Roe, and M.K. Lee. 1996. Altered reactivity of superoxide dismutase in familial amyotrophic lateral sclerosis. *Science* **271:** 515.

Wilhelmsen, K.C., T. Lynch, E. Pavlou, M. Higgins, and T.G. Nygaard. 1994. Localization of disinhibition-dementia-parkinsonism-amyotrophy complex to 17q21-22. *Am. J. Hum. Genet.* **55:** 1159.

Wong, P.C., C.A. Pardo, D.R. Borchelt, M.K. Lee, N.G. Copeland, N.A. Jenkins, S.S. Sisodia, D.W. Cleveland, and D.L. Price. 1995. An adverse property of a familial ALS-linked SOD1 mutation causes motor neuron disease characterized by vacuolar degeneration of mitochondria. *Neuron* **14:** 1105.

Yim, M.B., P.B. Chock, and E.R. Stadtman. 1990. Copper, zinc superoxide dismutase catalyzes hydroxyl radical production from hydrogen peroxide. *Proc. Natl. Acad. Sci.* **87:** 5006.

———. 1993. Enzymatic function of Cu,Zn superoxide dismutase as a free radical generator. *J. Biol. Chem.* **268:** 4099.

Yim, M.B., J.H. Kang, H.S. Yim, H.S. Kwak, P.B. Chock, and E.R. Stadtman. 1996. Again of function of an amyotrophic lateral sclerosis-associated Cu,Zn-superoxide dismutase mutant: An enhancement of free radical formation due to a decrease in K_m for hydrogen peroxide. *Proc. Natl. Acad. Sci.* **93:** 5709.

Yulug, I.G., N. Katsanis, J. de Belleroche, J. Collinge and E.M. Fisher. 1995. An improved protocol for the analysis of SOD1 gene mutations, and a new mutation in exon 4. *Hum. Mol. Genet.* **4:** 1101.

Zu, J., H.X. Deng, H. Mitsumoto, M.S. Ahmed, W.Y. Hung, Z.J. Cai, T.P. Lo, J.A. Tainer, and T. Siddique. 1997. Exon 5 encoded domain is not required for the toxic function of mutant SOD1 but essential for the dismutase activity: Identification and characterization of two new FALS associated SOD1 mutations. *Neurogenetics* **1:** (in press).

Neurofilaments, Radial Growth of Axons, and Mechanisms of Motor Neuron Disease

T.L. WILLIAMSON,[1] J.R. MARSZALEK,[2] J.D. VECHIO,[1] L.I. BRUIJN,[1] M.K. LEE,[4] Z. XU,[5] R.H. BROWN, JR.,[6] AND D.W. CLEVELAND[1-3]

[1]*Ludwig Institute for Cancer Research,* [2]*Division of Cellular and Molecular Medicine, and* [3]*Departments of Medicine and Neuroscience, University of California at San Diego, La Jolla, California 92093;* [4]*Neuropathology Laboratory, Johns Hopkins University School of Medicine, Baltimore, Maryland 21205;* [5]*Worcester Foundation for Biomedical Research, Shrewsbury, Massachusetts 01545;* [6]*Day Laboratory for Neuromuscular Research, Massachusetts General Hospital, Boston, Massachusetts 02114*

Neurons are highly asymmetric cells, and this asymmetry is generated in two phases: neurite elongation and radial growth. In the first phase, neurons extend processes that navigate long distances through the embryo, ultimately stably attaching to their targets. After synapse formation, the second phase initiates concomitant with myelination. During this radial growth phase, neurofilaments accumulate to become the most abundant cytoskeletal elements. Radial growth represents the major growth phase in terms of increase in neuronal cell volume, resulting in up to an order of magnitude increase in axonal diameters (Fig. 1A) (Berthold 1978). This increase in diameter is important for correct neuronal function, since the conduction velocity of nerve fibers is directly proportional to their diameter (Hursh 1939). In the case of the meter-long human motor and sensory neurons of the peripheral nervous system, radial growth results in a cell with >10^3 times the volume of most animal cells, and 99.9% of this volume is in the axon (see Fig. 1A).

Since the initial visualization of neurofilaments by the great neuroanatomists of the 19th century (see, e.g., Cajal 1903), mounting evidence has pointed to their importance as the primary determinants of radial growth. The first direct evidence that neurofilaments are the primary determinant of axonal caliber came from the identification of a mutant Japanese quail (quiver or Quv) that accumulates no neurofilaments in its axons (Yamasaki et al. 1991) due to a premature translation termination in NF-L (Ohara et al. 1993). This results in no detectable NF-L protein, total absence of neurofilaments, and axons that fail to grow radially and that have reduced conduction velocity (Sakaguchi et al. 1993). Additional evidence comes from a transgenic mouse line expressing the NF-H subunit with almost the entire 120-kD β-galactosidase polypeptide attached to its carboxy-terminal tail. Expression of this mutant NF-H blocks transport of all neurofilaments into axons and severely inhibits radial growth (Eyer and Peterson 1994).

From these efforts, it can be concluded that assembly and accumulation of axonal neurofilaments are essential components for the up to 100-fold volume increase that occurs during radial growth. This highlights a key general question in neurobiology: What are the principles specifying axonal volume and how does a structural scaffolding, such as an array of neurofilaments, mediate axonal architecture so as to determine and maintain axonal volume?

What we attempt here is review of the evidence for what neurofilaments are, how neurofilaments mediate radial growth of axons, and how disruption of normal axonal architecture, caused by misaccumulation and/or disorganization of either normal or mutant neurofilament subunits, can be direct causes of selective motor neuron death that mimics the most frequent human motor neuron disease, amyotrophic lateral sclerosis (ALS).

METHODS

Production and screening of transgenic mice. DNAs containing the MSV-NF-L, MSV-NF-M, or NF-H transgenes were purified by electroelution following agarose gel electrophoresis (for details of transgenes, see Lee et al. 1994; Marszalek et al. 1996; Xu et al. 1996). The DNA was microinjected into pronuclei of one-cell mouse embryos obtained by mating C57B6 x C3 F_1 females with C57B6 males. Mouse pups were analyzed for the presence of the transgene by DNA blotting of mouse tail DNA as described previously (Monteiro et al. 1990; Xu et al. 1993). Tail DNAs were digested with *Eco*RI (for MSV-NF-L or MSV-NF-M Δ50) or *Eco*RV (for NF-H), separated on 0.8% agarose gels, and transferred to GeneScreen Plus membranes (New England Biolabs). The membrane was incubated with 1 x 10^6 cpm/ml of probe prepared by random primer extension using [α-^{32}P]dATP and a fragment from the 3′-flanking region of the transgene.

SDS-PAGE and detection of neurofilament proteins by immunoblotting. Sciatic nerves and spinal cords were homogenized (with a polytron homogenizer) in a buffer containing 25 mM sodium phosphate, pH 7.2, 5 mM EDTA, pH 8, and 1% SDS. The homogenates were boiled for 5 minutes, clarified by centrifugation at 16,000*g* for 5 minutes, and super-

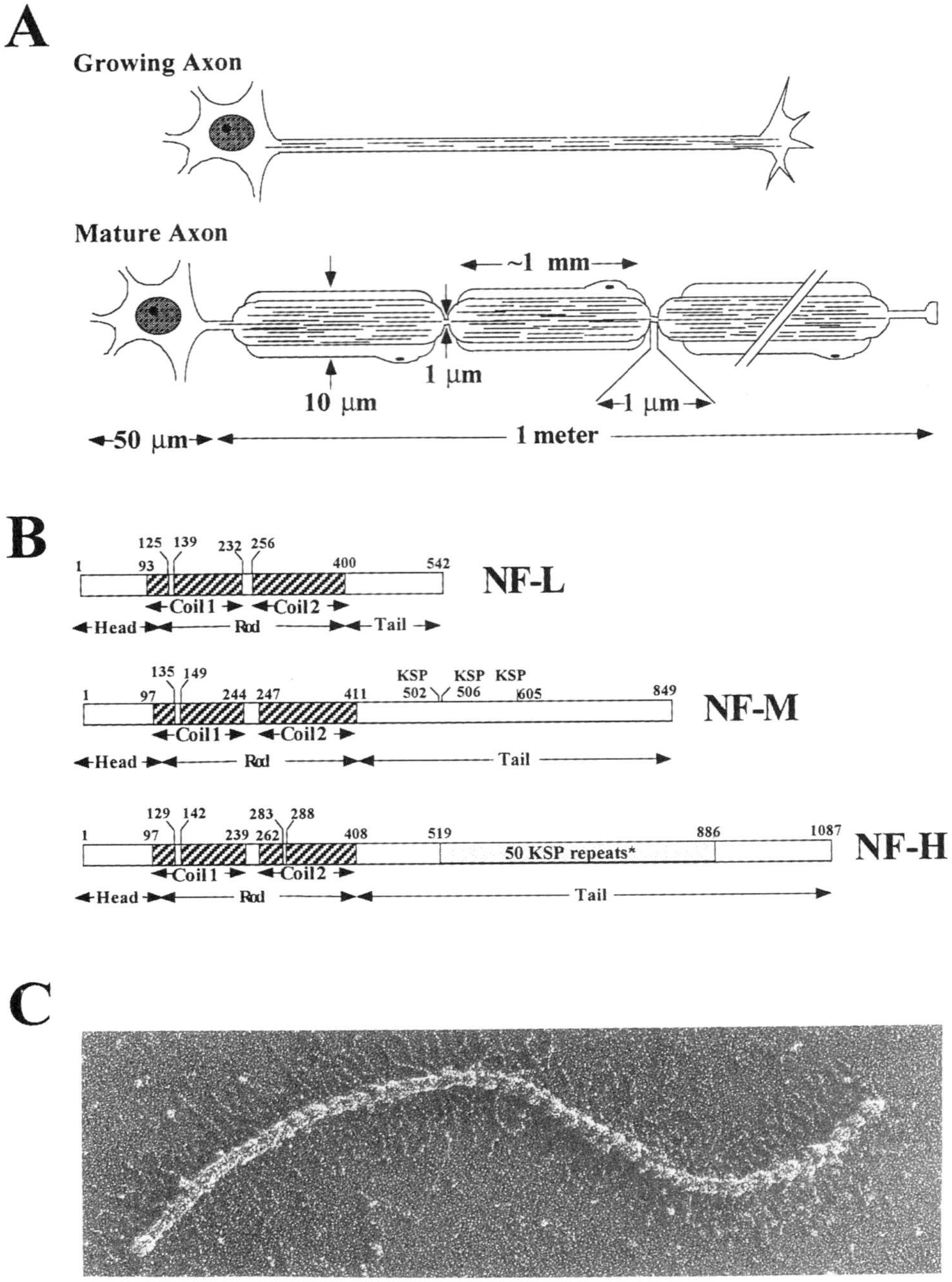

Figure 1. Neurofilaments and radial growth. (*A*) Schematic representation of the structural features and asymmetry of a human motor neuron. The enlarged portion shows neurofilament arrays in the ~10-μm-diameter segments (internodes) myelinated by single Schwann cells and in the ~1-μm-diameter unmyelinated nodes of Ranvier. (*B*) Schematic represention of the structure of the neurofilament proteins NF-L, NF-M, and NF-H. (*C*) Rotary-shadowed view of a native neurofilament showing the tail domains of NF-M and NF-H extending from the core of the filament. (Micrograph kindly provided by U. Aebi.)

natants were transferred to new tubes. Protein concentration was determined using the bicinchoninic acid (BCA) assay kit (Pierce Chemical Company). Protein extracts, as well as known amounts of neurofilament standards, were separated by SDS-PAGE using gels containing 6% or 7.5% polyacrylamide. Proteins separated by SDS-PAGE were transferred to nitrocellulose where neurofilament proteins and tubulin were immunologically detected (Lopata and Cleveland 1987). Immunoreactive bands were visualized by autoradiography using Kodak XAR film. Quantification was performed by phosphorimaging (Molecular Dynamics) using known amounts of purified mouse spinal cord neurofilaments as standards.

Tissue preparation and morphological analysis. Transgenic and littermate control animals were anesthetized by intraperitonial injection of (0.02 cc/g) Avertin. Both sciatic nerves, as well a 0.5-cm segment of tail, were removed for biochemical analyses. Mouse tissues were then fixed by intracardial perfusion with 4% paraformaldehyde and 2.5% glutaldehyde in 0.1 M sodium phosphate, pH 7.6. The paraformaldehyde/glutaldehyde-fixed tissues were postfixed in the same fixative for 24 hours at 4°C followed by 2% osmium tetroxide in 0.1 M phosphate buffer, dehydrated in alcohols, and embedded in Epon-Araldite resin. For light microscopy, 1-μm sections were stained with toludine blue. Thin sections for electron microscopy were stained with uranyl acetate and lead citrate and examined with a Hitachi H-600 transmission electron microscope.

Morphometric analysis. To determine the diameters of myelinated axons, L5 ventral roots were embedded in Epon, 1-μm sections were cut and stained with toluidine blue, and sections were viewed under 100x magnification. The images were digitized and converted to a 512 x 512 pixel video display using a video camera and frame-grabber video board. All myelinated axons were identified, and areas were determined by morphometric software program (Bioquant MegX, R & M Biometrics, Nashville, Tennessee). The entire nerve was measured using contiguous nonoverlapping fields with center-of-gravity exclusion to avoid double counting or size bias in the counts. Light level and optimal threshold on a 256 gray-scale were determined for each field independently. The cross-sectional area of each axon was measured and converted to a diameter of a circle of equivalent area.

Axonal transport analysis. The velocity of axonally transported neurofilaments was determined in 8-week-old transgenic and nontransgenic littermates. To metabolically label newly synthesized neurofilaments, 300 μCi of [^{35}S]methionine was injected into the ventral horn of the lumbar spinal cord. Fourteen days following the injection, the L5 roots, dorsal root ganglia, and approximately 3 cm of sciatic nerve were removed and cut into 3-mm segments. Each segment was homogenized in a buffer containing 50 mM sodium phosphate, pH 7.15, 150 mM NaCl, 1 mM EDTA, 1% Triton X100, and 0.9 M sucrose, and centrifuged at 12,000*g* for 30 minutes. Essentially all of the neurofilament proteins (NF-L, NF-M, and NF-H), along with cold insoluble tubulin and actin, were recovered in the pellet fraction. The entire pellet was resolubilized in 2% SDS-containing gel sample buffer and the proteins were separated by SDS-PAGE. The distribution of [^{35}S]methionine-labeled proteins was visualized by fluorography. The radioactivity associated with each of the neurofilament subunits was determined by phosphorimaging.

Single-strand conformation polymorphism analysis. A series of overlapping primer pairs spanning the entire coding regions for each of the three neurofilament subunits, NF-L, NF-M, and NF-H, was synthesized. Primers ranged in length from 15 to 21 bases, with predicted melting temperatures ranging from 56°C to 64°C. In most cases, primers were 50% G-C, 50% A-T, and began and ended with a G or a C. Primer sequences were checked using MacVector OLIGO™ to ensure that sequences were not recognized multiple times in the gene and that they did not form hairpins or anneal to one another. Primers were specifically selected at the intron/exon borders such that little or no intron sequence was amplified, beyond that contained in the primers. In some cases it was necessary, due to the G-C-rich content of some areas, to include a small segment of intron. This intron sequence was usually restricted to only the length of a primer.

Genomic DNAs were prepared from nuclei of lymphocytes or lymphoblastoic cell lines by lysis in 10 mM Tris, 100 mM NaCl, 1 mM EDTA followed by protein removal by digestion with proteinase K, SDS, and sequential phenol and chloroform extraction and ethanol precipitation. Approximately 20 ng of total genomic DNA from immortalized lymphocyte cell lines was amplified for a given region of either NF-L, NF-M, or NF-H. Resultant polymerase chain reaction (PCR) products averaged 269 bp in length, with the largest product 456 bp. Samples were denatured at 95°C for 2 minutes and cooled to room temperature in the heating block, then 3–4 μl was loaded onto a 35 x 43 cm, 0.4-mm-thick gel composed of 15 ml of Hydrolink MDE™ Gel (JT Baker, No. 4739.00), 3 ml glycerol, 1.8 ml 20x TBE (108 g Tris base, 55 g boric acid, 40 ml 0.5 mM EDTA, pH 8.0, in 1000 ml) in a final volume of 60 ml. Running buffer used was 0.6x TBE. Electrophoresis was at 4 watts for 17 hours at room temperature. Gels were then dried and exposed on Kodak XAR-5 film at –80°C for 2–16 hours.

For the 1041- or 1069-base (depending on 43 or 44 repeats) KSP repeat domain of NF-H, the entire domain was amplified and then doubly digested with *Pvu*II and *Pst*I to produce four smaller fragments (162, 172, 260, and 446 bp; see Fig. 4), which are within the range of sensitivity for detection of mutations by single-strand conformation polymorphism (SSCP). Products were denatured by mixing with 190 μl of denaturing solution at incubation at 95°C for 2 minutes and cooled to room temperature in the heating block, then 6–8 μl was loaded onto an SSCP gel. To verify which of the radiolabeled fragments represented products corresponding to each of the four DNA fragments, samples were also run on an 8% native polyacrylamide gel along with DNA markers. The gel was ethidium-bromide-stained, visualized under UV, and each of the four expected restriction fragments was recovered by electroelution overnight, ethanol-precipitated, and individually analyzed by SSCP.

Perkin Elmer AmpliCycle™ Sequencing (N808-0175) was used to sequence all of the polymorphisms detected by SSCP analysis. Sequencing was performed both on the initial (heterozygous) PCR fragments and following subcloning into pCR™ II using the TA Cloning® Kit (Invitrogen K2000-01).

RESULTS

Neurofilaments Are Obligate Heteropolymers of NF-L, NF-M, and NF-H

Easily purified by their rapid sedimentation under physiological salt, neurofilaments are composed of three closely related protein subunits (Fig. 1B): NF-L (68 kD), NF-M (95 kD), and NF-H (115 kD), each of which consists of globular head and tail domains separated by a 310-amino-acid coiled-coil domain characteristic of the family of intermediate filament proteins (Fuchs and Weber 1994). One or more members of this family, including proteins such as keratins, GFAP, vimentin, peripherin, and desmin, are present in the cytoplasm of most animal cells. Expression of neurofilament subunits by DNA transfection (Ching and Liem 1993; Lee et al. 1993) reveals that the filaments are obligate heteropolymers requiring NF-L and NF-M or NF-H, although there is no fixed stoichiometry of the individual subunits. Where neurofilaments differ most strikingly from other intermediate filament subunits is in the presence of long tail domains on both NF-M and NF-H (Fig. 1B). These extend up to 25 nm from the surface of the 10-nm-diameter assembled filament (Fig. 1C) (Hisanaga and Hirokawa 1988; Troncoso et al. 1990; for review, see Heins and Aebi 1994), and in the case of NF-H (see Fig. 1B), a large portion of this tail domain comprises a lysine-serine-proline (KSP)-containing motif repeated 40–50 times (depending on species), the serine of which is phosphorylated nearly stoichiometrically in myelinated axonal segments.

Neurofilaments as Determinants of Radial Growth

Since neurofilaments are required for axonal growth and there is a linear correlation between neurofilament number and axonal cross-sectional area in a wide variety of nerve settings (Friede and Samorajski 1970; Hoffman et al. 1984, 1985), an initial simple view of how neurofilaments specify radial growth is that interactions between adjacent filaments or between filaments and other axonal components form a three-dimensional array of cross-linked filaments in which axonal cross-sectional area expands or contracts so as to keep a constant density of neurofilaments (i.e., filaments per cross-sectional area). To examine whether the number of neurofilaments can specify growth in caliber, transgenic mice were constructed that synthesize elevated levels of completely wild-type murine NF-L (Monteiro et al. 1990). Compared with nontransgenic animals, immunoblotting revealed a twofold increase in wild-type NF-L, with constant levels of NF-M and NF-H (Fig. 2A, compare lanes 1 and 2; quantified in Fig. 2B, lanes W [wild type] and L [NF-L transgenic]). Electron microscopy confirmed a doubling in neurofilament number in the NF-L transgenic mice. However, despite this increase, quantitative morphometry on axons of the sciatic nerve revealed that radial growth of the large caliber axons was inhibited (Fig. 2C, dashed curve) compared with nontransgenic, littermate control mice (Fig. 2C, stippled curve). These results disprove the view that filament number alone is sufficient to mediate radial growth.

To test whether increasing the content of the long tail domains of the NF-M or NF-H subunits could stimulate radial growth (perhaps by promoting an increase in filament-filament spacing), transgenic mice were constructed that synthesized increased levels of NF-M or NF-H. For NF-M, the transgene chosen encoded a wild-type murine NF-M subunit in which the final 50 amino acids were substituted with an 11-amino-acid myc epitope tag (Wong et al. 1995a). For NF-H, the transgene used was a 23-kb segment that encoded completely wild-type mouse NF-H.

In the highest expressing NF-M line, NF-M content was doubled. This did not affect the total neurofilament subunit content in motor and sensory axons, but increases in NF-M were offset by proportionate decreases in NF-H (not shown), and this severely inhibited growth in axonal cross-sectional area (Fig. 2C, top, solid curve) compared with normal axons (Fig. 2C, top, stippled line). Increase in NF-M did not affect the level of phosphorylation of NF-H, as judged by its mobility on SDS-polyacrylamide gels or by immunoreactivity to phosphorylation-sensitive antibodies. Similarly, synthesizing NF-H at twice the normal rate (Xu et al. 1996) led to a twofold increase in axonal NF-H and a selective reduction in axonal NF-M (Fig. 2A, lane 3; Fig. 2B, lane H), as well as a small reduction in the number of neurofilaments (see reduction in total subunit content; Fig. 2B, lane H). This, in turn, severely inhibited radial growth in axons greater than 2 μm in diameter (Fig. 2C, bottom, solid line). In other transgenic lines, further increases in NF-H synthesis (up to 4.5-fold the normal level) reduced axonal subunit content even further with a corresponding loss in neurofilament number and even more complete inhibition of radial growth (Marszalek et al. 1996). Thus, increasing the level of any single neurofilament subunit inhibits radial growth.

Moreover, measurement of nearest-neighbor filament-filament spacing in NF-M (Wong et al. 1995a) or NF-H (Marszalek et al. 1996) -overexpressing mice revealed very little difference from that present in normal animals, despite the marked inhibition of radial growth, whereas in mice accumulating excessive NF-L there was a modest (15%) reduction in filament spacing (Xu et al. 1996). Since radial growth can be markedly inhibited in NF-M and NF-H transgenic

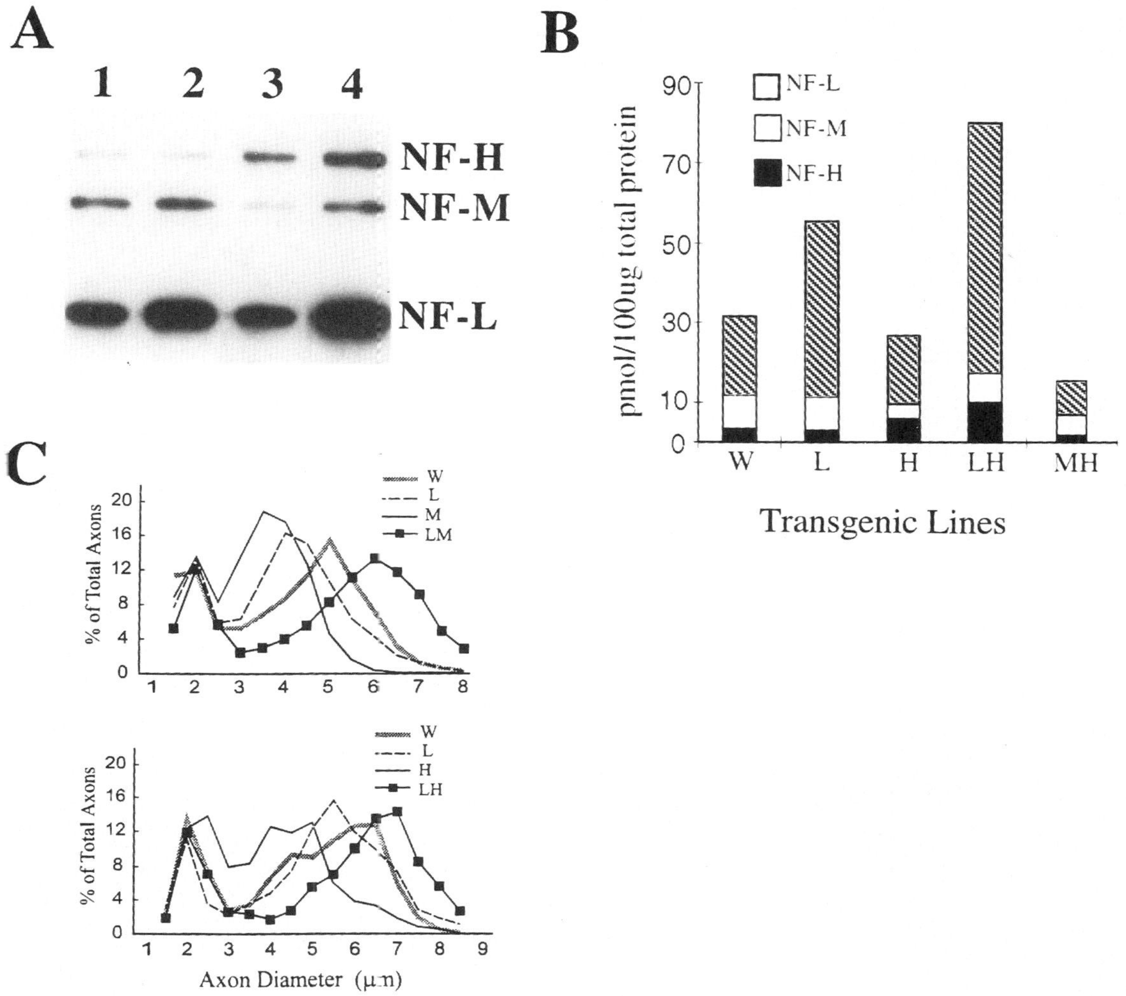

Figure 2. Changes in neurofilament subunit content in 8-week-old mice generated by crossing mice overexpressing NF-L with mice overexpressing NF-M or NF-H. (*A*) Immunoblot of 2.5 μg of total proteins extracted from sciatic nerve of 8-week-old mice using antibodies specific to each of the neurofilament subunits. (Lane *1*) Wild-type mice; (lane *2*) L mice; (lane *3*) NF-H transgenic mice; (lane *4*) NF-L/NF-H doubly transgenic mice. (*B*) The average NF content was quantified by phosphorimaging. (W) normal mice; (L) NF-L, (H) NF-H, (LH) NF-L/NF-H doubly transgenic mice, and (MH) NF-M/NF-H doubly transgenic mice. (*C*) A combined increase in NF-L and NF-H, or NF-L and NF-M, stimulates radial axonal growth. The average size distribution of axons in L5 ventral roots is shown from wild type, NF-L, NF-M, NF-H, NF-L/NF-M doubly transgenic mice, and NF-L/NF-H doubly transgenic mice. (Reprinted, with permission, from Xu et al. 1996.)

mice, despite no change in interfilament distance, we conclude that interactions between nearest-neighbor filaments cannot be sufficient to specify radial growth.

To test whether simultaneous elevation of any pair of neurofilament subunits would affect axonal architecture and/or enhance radial growth, the initial NF-L, NF-M, and NF-H transgenic mice were mated to each other. Increase in NF-L and NF-M or NF-L and NF-H combined to yield an increase in total axonal neurofilament subunit content (e.g., Fig. 2B, lane LH) and an increase in axonal neurofilament number. In both cases, this stimulated radial growth (Fig. 2C, curves LM and LH). On the other hand, although it was plausible that an increased synthesis of the tail domains of NF-M and NF-H would enhance the ability of neurofilaments to organize axoplasm so as to mediate growth in caliber, increasing both NF-M and NF-H simultaneously severely inhibited neurofilament accumulation in axons (Fig. 2B, lane MH), presumably by blocking neurofilament transport out of the cell bodies. This was accompanied by a correspondingly severe inhibition of radial growth, with few axons growing larger than 3 μm in diameter (Xu et al. 1996). Curiously, despite axons with sparsely packed neurofilaments in these MH mice, the remaining neurofilaments were found in pairs or clusters with nearly normal nearest-neighbor spacing, demonstrating that there must be attractive forces between axonal neurofilaments.

These results demonstrate that NF-M and NF-H play complementary roles along with NF-L in determining normal axonal calibers. The most abundant subunit, NF-L, provides most of the building blocks necessary for filament assembly, whereas the NF-M and NF-H tails link neurofilaments to surrounding axonal elements. In addition, in the LH and MH doubly transgenic animals, the ratio of the sum of NF-M plus NF-H to NF-L remains the same (Fig. 2B) (Xu et al. 1996). This demonstrates that NF-M and NF-H compete with each other for assembly and/or transport with a limiting amount of NF-L. Mechanistically, spacing between adjacent neurofilaments cannot represent a key property for radial growth, since the nearest-neighbor distances between filaments are nearly unchanged in axons that differ markedly in radial growth and neurofilament subunit content. Rather, it seems most likely that NF-M- and NF-H-dependent radial growth arises by interactions between neurofilaments that are not nearest neighbors, or between neurofilaments and other axonal components.

Neurofilaments and Axonal Transport

A central component of radial growth is the delivery of neurofilaments and other proteins into the axon by axonal transport. Axonal transport comprises two components: transport of vesicles and mitochondria by kinesin and related proteins (fast transport) and movement of the major structural components of the neuron, enzymes, and other cytosolic proteins (slow transport). Slow transport can be divided into two components, based on their rates of movement: SCa (~0.5 mm/day), containing the neurofilament proteins, tubulin, and actin, and SCb (~1 mm/day), containing tubulin, actin, and other cytosolic proteins. The mechanism of slow transport is not known, although it has been studied over the past 20 years.

The rate of neurofilament transport decreases over development, and it has been proposed that this decrease is responsible for radial growth (Hoffman et al. 1983, 1985; Willard and Simon 1983). Developmentally, the slowing of transport occurs concomitantly with increasing NF-H expression, and it has been suggested that it is the increased NF-H expression that slows neurofilament transport (Willard and Simon 1983). To test this directly, transgenic mice synthesizing 4.5 times the normal level of wild-type mouse NF-H have been constructed, and the effect on neurofilament composition, radial growth, and axonal transport has been determined. The transport of newly synthesized polypeptides along the motor axons was examined by analyzing the distribution of radiolabeled polypeptides in the ventral root and sciatic nerve at 14 days following the injection of [^{35}S]methionine into the ventral horn of the spinal cord (Fig. 3). In the transgenic mice expressing increased levels of NF-H, transported NF-H and NF-L were primarily in the insoluble fraction, as was also the case for nontransgenic animals, but the rate of transport was markedly retarded. In the normal mouse (Fig. 3A), a peak of radioactivity for NF-L, NF-M, and NF-H was found at segment 2, a distance about 8 mm from the cell bodies, corresponding to a transport rate of 0.6 mm/day. In the NF-H transgenic mice (Fig. 3B), neurofilament transport was decreased both in amount and in speed (by 2 weeks postinjection, the peak had not yet entered the segments available for analysis, indicating a slowing by at least 2- or 3-fold). This was a selective retardation of neurofilament subunits, as transport of other components in the insoluble phase was unaltered. Moreover, increased synthesis of NF-H resulted in a selective reduction (~2-fold compared to NF-L) in the amount of NF-M transported (e.g., see cytoskeletal phases of Fig. 3A,B), consistent with the lower axonal content of NF-M. Further inspection of the transported proteins in the soluble phase revealed that the amount of other cargoes moved in slow axonal transport, such as tubulin and actin (and an unidentified protein marked with an asterisk in Fig. 3A,B), was undiminished while its velocity was modestly elevated (especially apparent for tubulin; Fig. 3B, right). Thus, in motor axons, increased synthesis of NF-H leads to selective reduction in the amount and rate of transport of neurofilament subunits, while transport of other components of slow transport is accelerated in transit rate.

Neurofilaments and Motor Neuron Disease

In addition to the role of neurofilaments in radial growth, abnormal accumulations of neurofilaments are a common early pathological hallmark in patients with the motor neuron disease ALS (Carpenter 1968; Chou and Fakadej 1971; Hirano et al. 1984a,b; Hirano 1991). These observations led to the hypothesis that abnormalities in neurofilament organization may be involved in the pathogenesis of ALS. Initial direct evidence for the role of neurofilaments in motor neuron disease comes from transgenic mice expressing 3–4 times the normal levels of wild-type mouse NF-L (Xu et al. 1993) or wild-type human NF-H (Cote et al. 1993). In both cases, this resulted in abnormal masses of neurofilaments accumulated in perikarya and axons, and motor neuron dysfunction and neurogenic atrophy of skeletal muscle. However, the relevance of these mice to human disease was questionable, since neither set of mice exhibits the extensive motor neuron death (Xu et al. 1993; Collard et al. 1995) associated with human motor neuron disease.

To examine directly if aberrant neurofilament subunits could be a direct cause of motor neuron disease that mimicked the selective killing of motor neurons found in human disease, especially ALS, the most abundant adult human motor neuron disorder, several lines of transgenic mice were constructed expressing a point mutant at the end of the rod domain of NF-L (Fig. 4A) (Lee et al. 1994). Since mutations in keratins, the intermediate filament proteins of skin, were known

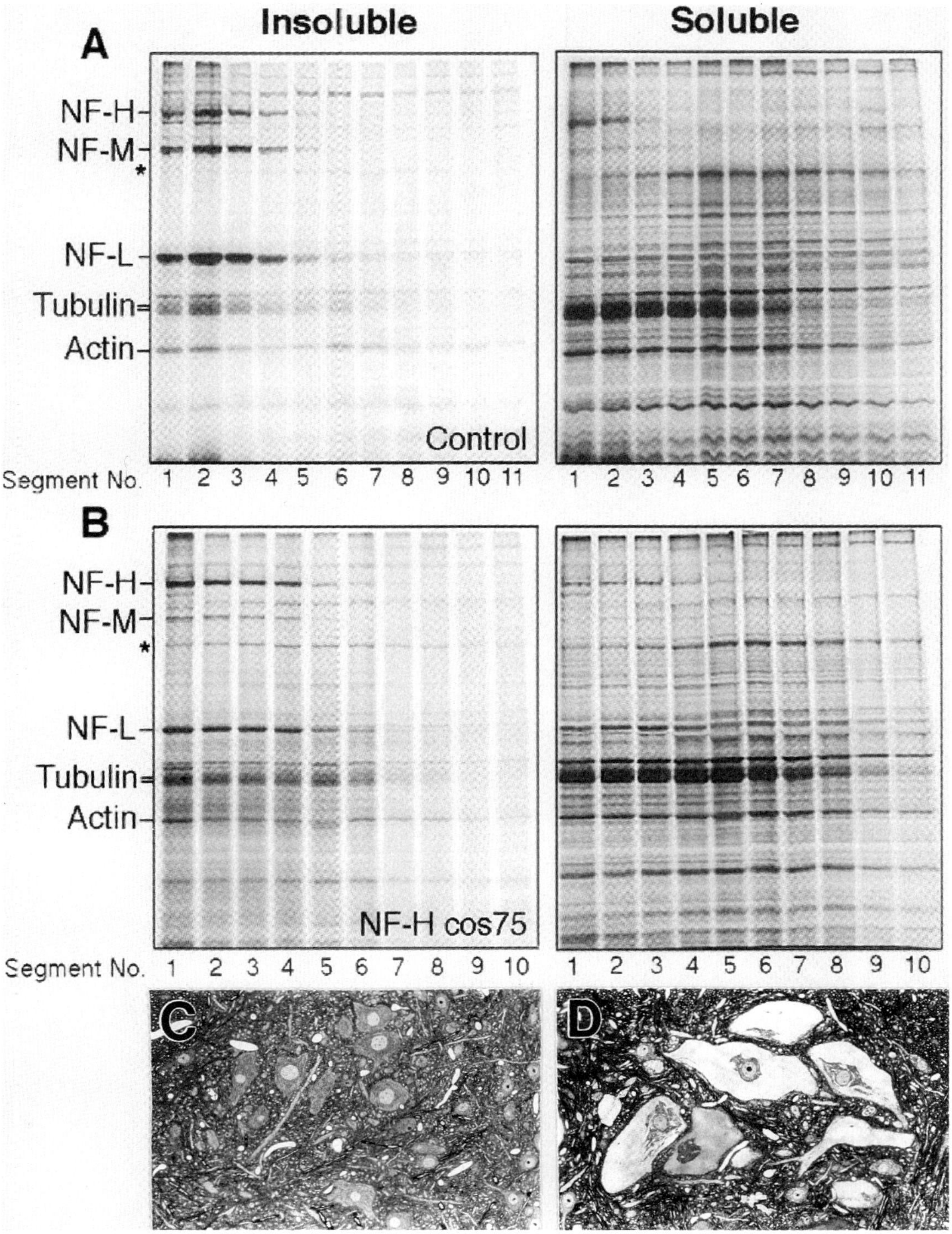

Figure 3. Overexpression of NF-H causes selective slowing of neurofilament transport. Transport of radiolabeled proteins in sciatic nerve motor neurons of (*A*) control and (*B*) NF-H cos75 mice. (*C*) Ventral horn of wild-type mouse showing motor neuron cell bodies. (*D*) Ventral horn of NF-H cos75 mouse, which expresses 4.5 times the normal level of wild-type NF-H. Motor neuron cell bodies are very swollen and contain huge accumulations of neurofilaments. (Reprinted, with permission, from Marszalek et al. 1996.)

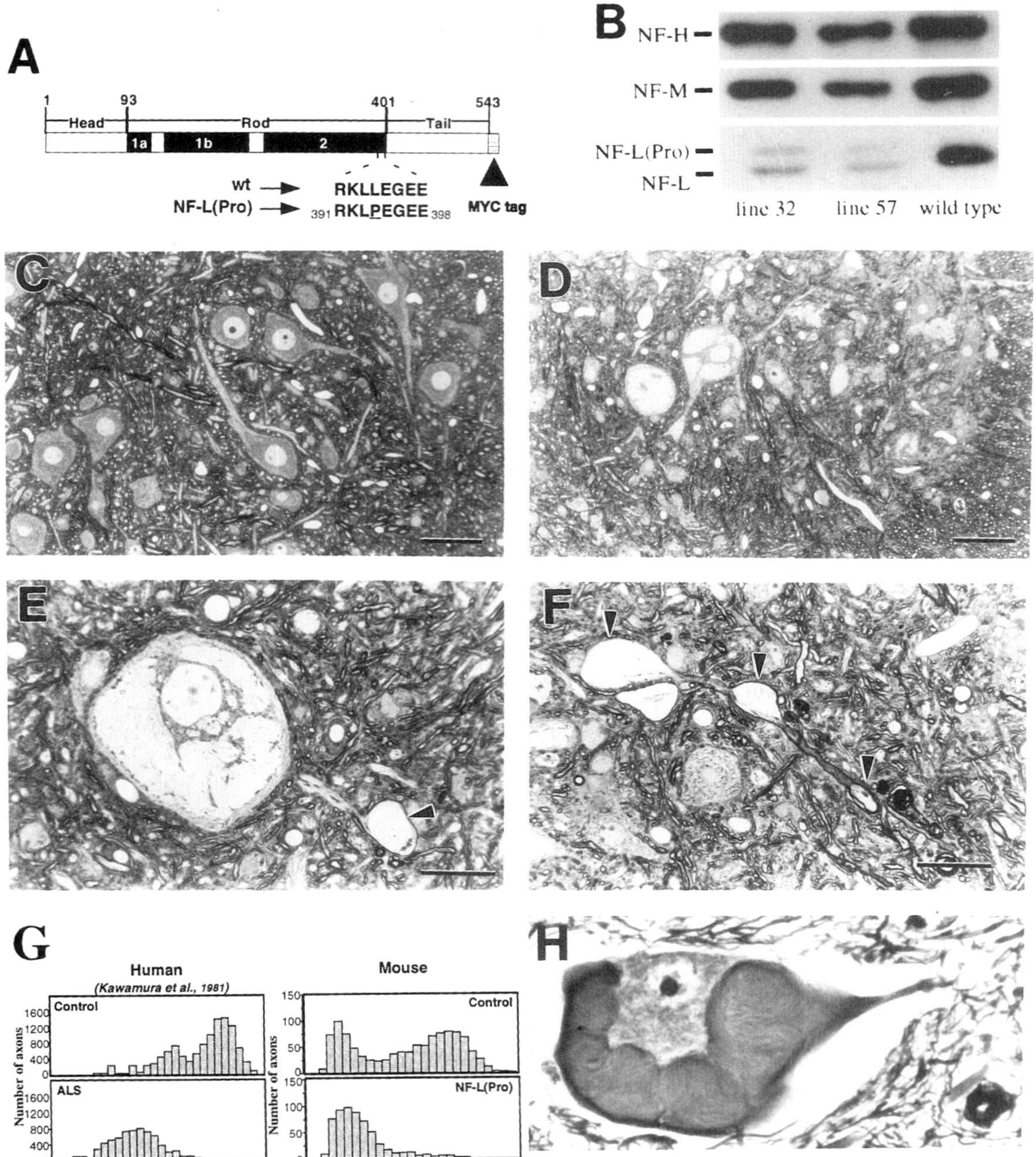

Figure 4. Expression of NF-L containing a point mutation causes motor neuron cell death. (*A*) Schematic representation of the structure of the transgenic NF-L protein, showing a leucine to proline mutation at the end of the rod domain. (*B*) Immunoblot showing that modest levels of mutant NF-L (NF-L(Pro)) accumulate in the sciatic nerves of transgenic mice. (*C*) Ventral horn of wild-type mouse, showing normal motor neurons. (*D*) Ventral horn of transgenic mouse, showing degenerating motor neurons and axonal swellings. High-power micrographs show (*E*) a swollen cell body with a proximal axonal swelling (*arrowhead*), and (*F*) a single axon containing multiple axonal swellings (*arrowheads*). (*G*) Graph showing the selective loss of large caliber motor neurons in human ALS and in mice expressing the NF-L(Pro) transgene. The human data are replotted from Kawamura et al. (1981). The mouse data are replotted from Lee et al. (1994). (*H*) High-power micrograph showing neurofilament accumulations in a motor neuron from an ALS patient (from Hirano 1988). Parts *A–F* are reproduced with permission from Lee et al. (1994); part *H* is reproduced with permission from Hirano (1991). Bars: *C,D*, 50 µm; *E,F*, 20 µm.

to cause two dominantly inherited skin-blistering diseases (Coulombe et al. 1991; Chipev et al. 1992; Lane et al. 1992; Rothnagel et al. 1992), a mutation analogous to one of the frequently occurring keratin mutations was engineered into the end of the conserved helical region of the mouse NF-L subunit. Codon 394 was mutated to introduce a leucine to proline substitution, and a carboxy-terminal 11-amino-acid epitope was also added so that the mutant protein could be followed independent of the endogenous wild-type NF-L subunits. Microinjection of the resultant gene yielded 12 transgenic lines that as early as 18 days after birth displayed abnormal gait, reduced activity, and weakness in both the upper and lower limbs. These abnormalities progressively increased in severity and, in most lines, progressed to death. Quantitative immunoblot analysis revealed that even the most strikingly affected animals, with earliest onsets, accumulated the transgene product only to a level equivalent to wild-type NF-L (Fig. 4B). The levels of the endogenous wild-type NF-L, NF-M, and NF-H subunits were reduced by about 50% compared with normal mice (Fig. 4B, compare lines 32 and 57 with wild type; note the mutant subunit migrates a little slower as a consequence of the epitope tag), a feature arising from death of a corresponding number of motor neurons (Fig. 4G, right).

Examination of spinal cords from animals expressing this mutant NF-L subunit revealed loss of motor neurons of the lumbar (Fig. 4D) and cervical spinal cord, when compared with nontransgenic littermates (Fig. 4C). As in many ALS cases (e.g., see silver-stained example of a rapidly progressing case of ALS in Fig. 4H), the surviving ventral horn motor neurons were chromatolytic and were grossly distended with material that stained lightly with toluidine blue (Fig. 4D,E) but very strongly with silver (Lee et al. 1994). Moreover, cords at all levels displayed severe perikaryal, dendritic, and axonal abnormalities. Cell bodies containing distorted nuclei and microglial nodules indicative of invasion and phagocytosis of degenerating neuronal cell bodies by glial cells were frequently seen. Moreover, as reported frequently for ALS (see, e.g., Carpenter 1968; Hirano et al. 1984a,b), neurofilament-rich swellings of proximal axons (axonal spheroids) were frequently found in the initial unmyelinated segment and in the root exit zones (e.g., arrowheads in Fig. 4E,F).

Examination of spinal white matter did not reveal striking abnormalities in the cortical region, although occasional degenerating axons were seen in the dorsal lateral region as well as in the ventral funiculus containing descending motor axons of the rubrospinal and reticulospinal tracts (Brown 1971). The degeneration of descending fibers demonstrates that at least some upper motor neurons are affected in the transgenic animals, although the cortical spinal tract, most prominently affected in human disease, did not contain any degenerating axons.

To determine whether the NF-L mutant protein resulted in permanent loss of axons, the number of surviving axons was measured in the ventral roots of one transgenic line (line 61) that accumulated among the lowest levels of the mutant NF-L. Motor neuron degeneration in this line is obvious at 6 weeks, but not 6 months, of age as a consequence of an unexplained silencing of transgene expression as the animals age. Comparison of the number of ventral root axons from 12-month-old mice revealed that there is a permanent loss of motor axons (50% from the largest [L5] root) from all levels of the lumbar cord (Fig. 4G, right). As is also the case in ALS (Fig. 4G, left) (Kawamura et al. 1981), the large neurofilament-rich axons are lost, while smaller axons with naturally lower neurofilament content are spared.

A Search for Mutations in NF-L, NF-M, and NF-H as Primary Causes of ALS

The production of transgenic mice that develop motor neuron disease as the consequence of expression of a mutant NF-L subunit suggested that similar mutations could represent the primary cause of a proportion of human ALS, particularly familial ALS, which is inherited as an autosomal dominant. Although mutations in the soluble, ubiquitously expressed enzyme superoxide dismutase 1 (SOD1) are known to cause about 20% of cases of familial ALS (Bowling et al. 1993; Brown 1995), the cause(s) of most (~80%) instances of familial disease (and all causes of sporadic disease) is unknown.

To determine whether mutation in neurofilament subunits causes or predisposes to ALS, SSCP (see Methods), coupled with DNA sequencing, was used (Fig. 5) (Vechio et al. 1996) to search for mutations in the entirety of the human NF-L, NF-M, and NF-H genes from 100 familial ALS patients, as well as from 75 sporadic ALS patients. This revealed six polypeptide sequence variants in the rod and tail domains of NF-L, NF-M, and NF-H (one in the NF-L tail [D469N], one each in the NF-M rod [I129M] and tail [A474T], and three in the NF-H tail [E460K, P615L, and A805E]). However, all were found at comparable frequency in DNA from normal individuals, and no variant cosegregated with disease. No additional polymorphisms were identified in the sporadic ALS samples. Deletions of 1 or 34 codons in the KSP repeat domain of NF-H reported previously in 5 of 356 sporadic ALS patients (Figlewicz et al. 1994) were not found in any of the familial or sporadic ALS samples examined here or in a separate analysis of the KSP domain of NF-H in 100 familial ALS DNAs (Rooke et al. 1996). These results indicate that if neurofilament mutations do cause any cases of ALS, it is highly unlikely that they can account for more than a very small proportion.

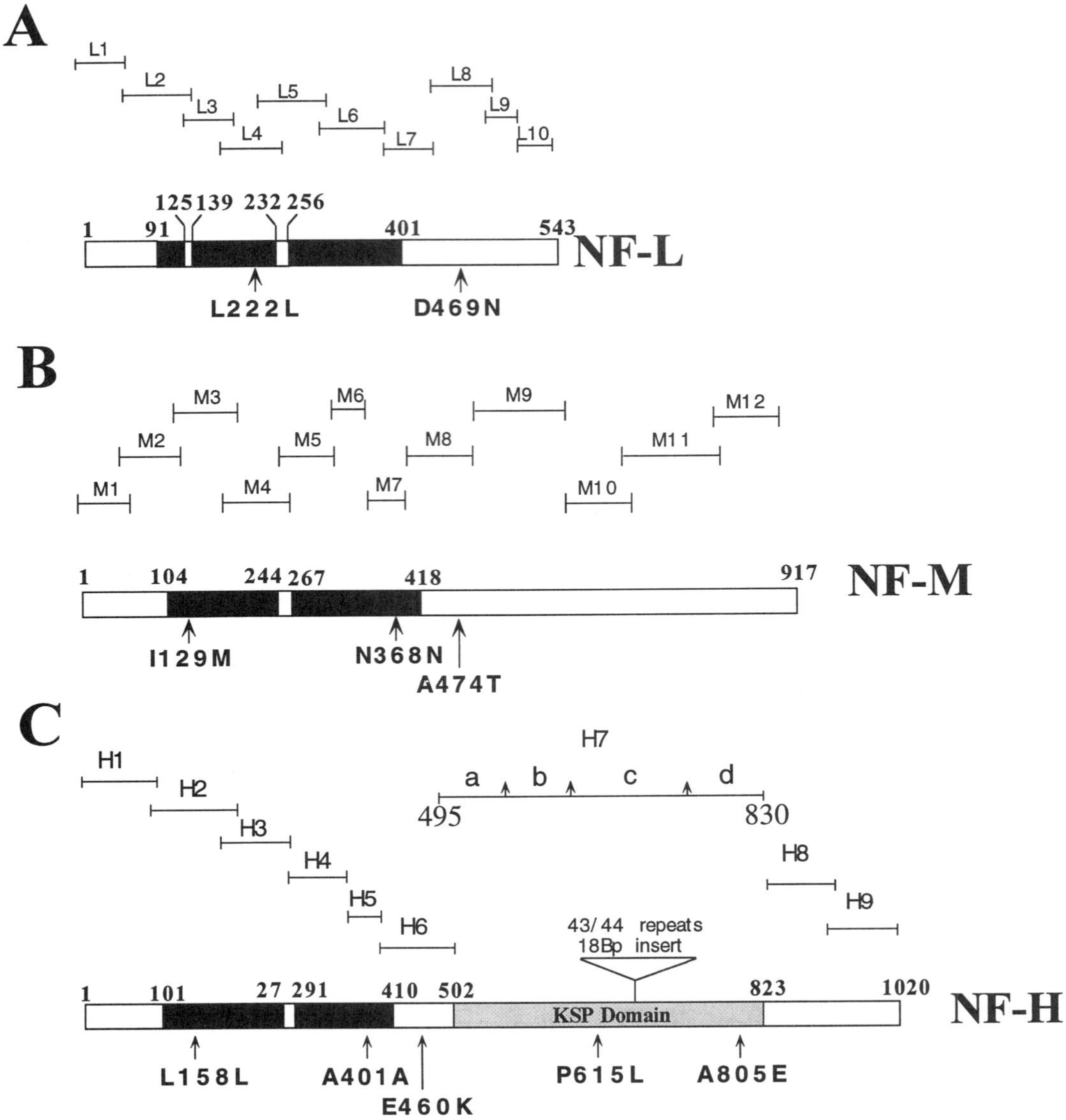

Figure 5. Use of SSCP and DNA sequencing to search for mutations in NF-L, NF-M, and NF-H in DNAs from familial and sporadic ALS patients. Schematic diagram of the (*A*) NF-L, (*B*) NF-M, and (*C*) NF-H polypeptides. Coding regions amplified using PCR primers are displayed at the top. Positions of SSCP shifts are shown by the arrows, along with changes in the encoded polypeptide. Data are redrawn from Vechio et al. (1996).

Increase in Wild-type Mouse NF-H Synthesis Does Not Result in Disease or Motor Neuron Degeneration or Death

In transgenic mice expressing wild-type human NF-H mRNA at 2-fold over the endogenous murine NF-H mRNA levels, perikaryal and axonal accumulations of neurofilaments in neurons, slowing of axonal neurofilament transport, and reduction in caliber of large myelinated motor axons have been reported. These changes are accompanied by development of overt clinical abnormalities beginning as early as 3–4 months of age and characterized by fine tremors, forelimb weakness, and neurogenic muscle atrophy (Cote et al. 1993; Collard et al. 1995). Transgenic mice expressing murine NF-H show similar increase in NF-H expression, cytoskeletal abnormalities, and decrease in axonal neurofilament transport. However, none of five murine NF-H transgenic lines develops any obvious phenotype, even at more than 2 years of age. To determine whether there are presymptomatic changes that are consistent with the early stages of disease development, the three lines expressing the highest levels of mouse NF-H (lines 35, 61, and 75) were examined at up to 2 years of age for any significant loss of motor neurons and for development of muscle atrophy. In contrast to the human NF-H transgenic mice, detailed microscopic examination of sections from multiple skeletal muscles failed to show any signs of neurogenic atrophy of the muscle fibers in any of the lines of murine NF-H transgenic mice. Even very aged (2-year-old) animals of the highest expressing line revealed no statistically significant loss in motor neurons (as determined by counting the number of surviving axons in the L4 and L5 ventral roots), nor did they display any muscle atrophy, despite chronically decreased axonal caliber and continuous perikaryal accumulations in motor neurons that resulted in much more grossly distended cell bodies (Fig. 3D) than seen in mice developing disease from increased expression of murine NF-L (Xu et al. 1993) or human NF-H (Cote et al. 1993). Proximal axonal swellings containing masses of neurofilaments were found in the transgenic mice expressing increased levels of mouse NF-H, but these were less frequent than in the NF-L (Xu et al. 1993) transgenic animals. In the NF-H mice, not only was there absence of neuronal loss, but other markers (e.g., reactive astrocytosis) frequently found in neurodegenerative disease were also absent. Unlike the situation reported following expression of human NF-H (Collard et al. 1995), there was not a loss of mitochondria in axons from mice expressing high levels of mouse NF-H; rather, morphologically normal mitochondria were found in the transgenic axons at the same frequency per axonal cross-sectional area as present in wild-type axons.

DISCUSSION

Mechanism of Neurofilament-dependent Radial Growth: Transport and Phosphorylation

In combination with earlier transgenic mice expressing elevated levels of murine NF-L (Monteiro et al. 1990; Xu et al. 1993) and epitope-tagged NF-M (Wong et al. 1995a), it is now clear that significant increases in any single neurofilament subunit inhibit growth in caliber. On the other hand, modest increases in both NF-L and either NF-M or NF-H significantly promote radial growth (Xu et al. 1996). As proposed earlier (Xu et al. 1996), the simplest view is that radial growth requires all three subunits: NF-L to support filament assembly, and a scaffolding of NF-M and NF-H tails cross-bridged between neurofilaments and/or other axonal components. What is clear, however, is that changing the content of NF-H (with a corresponding reduction in NF-M) does not affect nearest-neighbor spacing of neurofilaments, a finding that goes hand in hand with the identical situation following doubled axonal NF-M and a corresponding loss in NF-H (Wong et al. 1995a). Since radial growth can be markedly inhibited despite no change in interfilament distance, this gives further weight to the argument that interactions between nearest-neighbor filaments do not specify radial growth. The key property(ies) needed to stimulate caliber growth must include longer-range interactions between neurofilaments that are not nearest neighbors or between neurofilaments and other axonal components.

Interactions between filaments are almost certainly regulated by phosphorylation of the highly repetitive KSP domain in the tail of NF-H. The ~ 50 repeats are highly phosphorylated (Geisler et al. 1987; Lee et al. 1988) only after the filaments have entered the axon (Sternberger and Sternberger 1983; Lee et al. 1986; Glicksman et al. 1987; Nixon et al. 1987; Oblinger 1987). NF-H phosphorylation correlates with an increased interfilament distance, as shown, e.g., in mouse optic nerve (Nixon et al. 1994) and the relatively long unmyelinated initial segment of the primary sensory neurons in the dorsal root ganglia (Hsieh et al. 1994). Similarly, in mice with defects in myelination (e.g., the trembler mouse [deWaegh et al. 1992] or mice with transgene-induced peripheral hypomyelination [Cole et al. 1994]), the failure of myelination results in decreased phosphorylation of NF-H and NF-M, increased neurofilament density, and inhibition of radial growth.

One probable mechanism through which elevated synthesis of NF-H (and possibly NF-M) levels affects caliber is by retarding neurofilament transport, possibly by shifting an equilibrium toward assembly of stationary neurofilaments. Two pools of neurofilaments (and/or neurofilament subunits) are known in axons, one moving at the traditionally measured slow axonal transport rate and the other essentially stationary (Nixon and Logvinenko 1986; Lasek et al. 1992), although there is disagreement over the magnitude of the stationary phase. An obvious possibility would be that NF-H (or NF-M) tail-dependent cross-bridging between filaments and/or to other axonal components yields a shift to the immobile (or less mobile) phase in the axons, whereas in the cell bodies, similar cross-linking may block access of oligomers and/or polymers as initial substrates for entering the transport machinery, hence resulting in perikarya swollen with assembled neurofilaments.

Evidence for Structuring Axoplasm by Cross-linking Neurofilaments to Actin

The finding that NF-H and NF-M are essential for regulating radial growth, but not by changing interfilament distance, leads to the proposal that interactions between neurofilaments and other structures (such as microtubules or actin filaments) may represent the key interactions sufficient for stimulating radial growth. One candidate protein for linking neurofilaments to actin filaments is BPAG1 (bullous pemphigoid antigen 1). BPAG1 was first identified as an epidermal protein (now referred to as BPAG1e) with antisera from patients with the autoimmune disorder bullous pemphigoid (Stanley 1993). In skin-cell precursors, BPAG1e localizes to the intracellular portion of the hemidesmosome, a region where the keratin filament network interacts with the underlying basement membrane. The surprising initial finding was that although mice develop a skin-blistering disease following disruption of the BPAG1 gene, the loss of BPAG1 results in a severe dystonia and sensory nerve degeneration that culminates in death at about 1 month of age (Guo et al. 1995). Mating of the BPAG1-deleted mice to the classic sensory mouse mutant, dystonia musculorum (dt), as well as cloning of the dt locus (Brown et al. 1995), proved that BAPG1 and dt are the same locus. This led to the discovery of a pair of neuronal forms, named BAPG1n (Yang et al. 1996) or dystonin (Brown et al. 1995), each of which contains the same intermediate filament-binding domain present in the carboxy-terminal tail of epidermal BPAG1, but which also contain a novel amino terminus possessing a spectrin-like actin-binding domain that does indeed bind in vitro to actin with an affinity typical for other actin-binding proteins (Yang et al. 1996). BPAG1n is expressed by sensory neurons, but not motor neurons, and is localized along the length of the axons. Moreover, when BPAG1n was cotransfected into cells with neurofilaments, the BPAG1n reorganized and co-aligned the neurofilament network with the endogenous actin network (Guo et al. 1995). NF-H can also be coimmunoprecipitated from these cells with a BPAG1 antibody.

It seems all but certain, therefore, that BPAG1n does cross-link neurofilaments to actin in sensory neurons. Obviously, this could play a role either in mediating radial growth or in transporting neurofilaments. The major mystery is why BPAG1 should be specific to sensory neurons. These results beg the question: Is there an equivalent molecule in motor neurons and if so (as seems highly likely), could its disruption or altered function play a role in radial growth and in motor neuron disease?

Evidence That Aberrant Axonal Neurofilaments Do Contribute to Motor Neuron Disease

Despite the absence of examples of mutations in neurofilament genes as the primary cause of ALS, several lines of evidence offer strong support for aberrant accumulation of axonal neurofilaments as an important contributor to disease progression. Neurofilament accumulation is prominent in familial ALS caused by mutations in SOD1 (for mutation A4V, see Hirano et al. 1984b; and for mutation I113T, see Rouleau et al. 1996). Moreover, transgenic mice that express SOD1 mutations develop motor neuron disease characterized by axonal swellings composed of neurofilament aggregates and/or vacuoles (Gurney et al. 1994; Wong et al. 1995b; Tu et al. 1996).

Furthermore, whereas the absence of disease, motor neuron death, or denervation atrophy of skeletal muscle even in aged animals expressing wild-type mouse NF-H at up to 4.5 times its normal rate demonstrates that motor neurons are remarkably tolerant of misaccumulated neurofilaments assembled from wild-type subunits, this contrasts sharply with the situation arising from expressing two times lower levels of human NF-H (Cote et al. 1993). The human NF-H subunit, which differs from mouse NF-H in more than 160 amino acid positions scattered throughout the polypeptide backbone (counting the many sequence differences in the long KSP repeat domain as only a single difference [Julien et al. 1988; Lee et al. 1988]), results in progressive neuronopathy (Cote et al. 1993), inhibition of radial growth, and increased frequency of axonal degeneration (Collard et al. 1995), albeit without significant decrease in axon number even in aged animals (see, e.g., total wild-type and transgenic axon number in Fig. 1b of Collard et al. [1995]).

Disease developed by animals accumulating human NF-H led to the initial proposal that modest up-regulation of NF-H cross-linkers impairs neurofilament transport, causing neuronal swellings with ensuing axonopathy and muscle atrophy (Cote et al. 1993; Collard et al. 1995). However, the absence of disease in any mice expressing varying amounts of mouse NF-H shows that the wild-type NF-H cannot provoke similar disease, despite slowing of neurofilament transport to a comparable extent (Fig. 3). The combined data instead strongly support the view that human NF-H causes disease in mice by acting as an aberrant, mutant subunit. A similar situation has already emerged from analysis of mice expressing wild-type or mutant NF-L subunits. A doubling of murine NF-L content (and a corresponding increase in axonal neurofilaments) does not result in disease (Monteiro et al. 1990; Xu et al. 1993), whereas accumulation of one fourth as much of a point mutant in NF-L reproduces most features of ALS, including selective death of motor neurons (Lee et al. 1994). Wild-type NF-L produces disease only when expressed at a level that yields four times the normal number of axonal neurofilaments (Xu et al. 1993), ten times more than required to produce disease from accumulation of the mutant NF-L subunit, and even at this level, the wild-type protein does not cause motor neuron death.

The combined findings offer strong support for the view that neurofilament-dependent dysfunction, degeneration, and/or death of motor neurons in mice is mediated through disorganized arrays of filaments impeding axonal transport, not only of neurofilaments (as seen in the mice expressing wild-type mouse NF-H presented here), but also of other components in both anterograde and/or retrograde movement (as seen in mice expressing human NF-H [Collard et al. 1995]).

Regarding familial ALS caused by mutation in the enzyme SOD1 (Rosen et al. 1993), disease (at least in mice) has been shown to arise from a toxic property of the mutant subunit (Gurney et al. 1994; Wong et al. 1995b). Although the toxic property(ies) is not yet identified, two plausible proposals are mutant enzyme-mediated nitration of protein-bound tyrosines (Beckman et al. 1993) or action of the mutants as peroxidases (Wiedau-Pazos et al. 1996). Neurofilaments, as abundant and long-lived proteins, are attractive candidates for progressively accumulating such chemical damage, which in turn may cause aberrant assembly and/or organization of neurofilaments that can choke overall axonal transport. Consistent with this proposal, neurofilament accumulations are hallmarks of sporadic (Hirano et al. 1984a) and familial (Hirano et al. 1984b) disease, and are especially conspicuous in disease mediated by SOD mutations (e.g., for mutations A4V, see Hirano et al. 1984a; Shibata et al. 1996; and for I113T, see Rouleau et al. 1996). In conjunction with the earlier evidence from Julien and colleagues (Cote et al. 1993; Collard et al. 1995), the sum of the evidence thus strongly supports the view that aberrant accumulations of altered axonal neurofilaments, whether primary or secondary insults, mediate neuronal failure through strangulation of the axonal transport so crucial to these large asymmetric cells.

CONCLUSION

Results from transgenic mouse studies suggest that NF-H regulates radial growth, but that this does not correlate with neurofilament nearest-neighbor distance. NF-M may dictate interfilament distance, but the data suggest that NF-H interacts with linker proteins (e.g., BPAG1n) to facilitate radial growth. NF-M and NF-H appear to compete for assembly and/or transport, since increasing one subunit results in a decrease in axonal levels of the other subunit. Although mutations in the proteins do cause motor neuron degeneration in mice, mutations in neurofilament proteins do not appear as a major cause of ALS. Overexpression of normal human NF-H in mice causes motor neuron dysfunction, apparently due to a slowing of neurofilaments, tubulin, actin, and other components of slow axonal transport. In contrast, mice that overexpress 4.5 times the normal level of *mouse* NF-H show no motor deficits (even at 2 years of age) and have a selective slowing of neurofilament transport. These results suggest that motor neuron dysfunction in mice overexpressing NF-H is a consequence of the reduced transport of components other than neurofilaments. Whether a similar mechanism underlies the pathogenesis of ALS remains to be determined.

ACKNOWLEDGMENTS

We thank Drs. Asao Hirano and Ueli Aebi for allowing us to reproduce images from their work. This work has been supported by grants to D.W.C. from the National Institutes of Health (grant NS-27036) and the ALS Association. T.L.W. and L.I.B. are recipients of postdoctoral fellowships from the Muscular Dystrophy Association.

REFERENCES

Beckman, J.S., M. Carson, C.D. Smith, and W.H. Koppenol. 1993. ALS, SOD and peroxynitrite. *Nature* **364:** 584.

Berthold, C.H. 1978. Morphology of normal peripheral axons. In *Physiology and pathobiology of axons* (ed. S.G. Waxman), p. 3. Raven Press, New York.

Bowling, A.C., J.B. Schulz, R.H. Brown, Jr., and M.F. Beal. 1993. Superoxide dismutase activity, oxidative damage, and mitochondrial energy metabolism in familial and sporadic amyotrophic lateral sclerosis. *J. Neurochem.* **61:** 2322.

Brown, A., G. Bernier, M. Mathieu, J. Rossant, and R. Kothary. 1995. The mouse dystonia musculorum gene is a neural isoform of bullous pemphigoid antigen 1. *Nat. Genet.* **10:** 301.

Brown, L.T. 1971. Projection and termination of the cortospinal tract in rodents. *Exp. Brain Res.* **13:** 432.

Brown, R.H. 1995. Amyotrophic lateral sclerosis: Recent insights from genetics and transgenic mice. *Cell* **80:** 687.

Cajal, S.R. 1903. Embryogenesis of neurofibrils. *Trab. Lab. Invest. Biol. Univ. Madrid* **2:** 219.

Carpenter, S. 1968. Proximal axonal enlargement in motor neuron disease. *Neurology* **18:** 841.

Ching, G.Y. and R.K. Liem. 1993. Assembly of type IV neuronal intermediate filaments in nonneuronal cells in the absence of preexisting cytoplasmic intermediate filaments. *J. Cell Biol.* **122:** 1323.

Chipev, C.C., B.P. Korge, N. Markova, S.J. Bale, J.J. DiGiovanna, J.G. Compton, and P.M. Steinert. 1992. A leucine–proline mutation in the Hi subdomain of keratin 1 causes epidermolytic hyperkeratosis. *Cell* **70:** 821.

Chou, S.M. and A.V. Fakadej. 1971. Ultrastructure of chromatolytic motor neurons and anterior spinal roots in a case of Werdnig-Hoffman disease. *J. Neuropathol. Exp. Neurol.* **30:** 42.

Cole, J.S., A. Messing, J.Q. Trojanowski, and V.M.Y. Lee. 1994. Modulation of axon diameter and neurofilaments by hypomyelinating Schwann cells in transgenic mice. *J. Neurosci.* **14:** 6956.

Collard, J.F., F. Cote, and J.P. Julien. 1995. Defective axonal transport in a transgenic mouse model of amyotrophic lateral sclerosis. *Nature* **375:** 61.

Cote, F., J.F. Collard, and J.P. Julien. 1993. Progressive neuronopathy in transgenic mice expressing the human neurofilament heavy gene: A mouse model of amyotrophic lateral sclerosis. *Cell* **73:** 35.

Coulombe, P.A., M.E. Hutton, A. Letai, A. Hebert, A.S. Paller, and E. Fuchs. 1991. Point mutations in human keratin 14 genes of epidermolysis bullosa simplex patients: Genetic and functional analyses. *Cell* **66:** 1301.

de Waegh, S.M., V.M. Lee, and S.T. Brady. 1992. Local modulation of neurofilament phosphorylation, axonal caliber, and slow axonal transport by myelinating Schwann cells. *Cell* **68:** 451.

Eyer, J. and A. Peterson. 1994. Neurofilament-deficient axons and perikaryal aggregates in viable transgenic mice expressing a neurofilament-β-galactosidase fusion protein. *Neuron* **12:** 389.

Figlewicz, D.A., A. Krizus, M.G. Martinoli, V. Meininger, M. Dib, G.A. Rouleau, and J.-P. Julien. 1994. Variants of the heavy neurofilament subunit are associated with the development of amyotrophic lateral sclerosis. *Hum. Mol. Genet.* **3:** 1757.

Friede, R.L. and T. Samorajski. 1970. Axon caliber related to

neurofilaments and microtubules in sciatic nerve fibers of rats and mice. *Anat. Rec.* **167:** 379.
Fuchs, E. and K. Weber. 1994. Intermediate filaments: Structure, dynamics, function and disease. *Annu. Rev. Biochem.* **63:** 345.
Geisler, N., J. Vandekerckhove, and K. Weber. 1987. Location and sequence characterization of the major phosphorylation sites of the high molecular mass neurofilament proteins M and H. *FEBS Lett.* **221:** 403.
Glicksman, M.A., D. Soppet, and M.B. Willard. 1987. Posttranslational modification of neurofilament polypeptides in rabbit retina. *J. Neurobiol.* **18:** 167.
Guo, L., L. Degenstein, J. Dowling, Q.C. Yu, R. Wollmann, B. Perman, and E. Fuchs. 1995. Gene targeting of BPAG1: Abnormalities in mechanical strength and cell migration in stratified epithelia and neurologic degeneration. *Cell* **81:** 233.
Gurney, M.E., H. Pu, A.Y. Chiu, M.C. Dal Canto, C.Y. Polchow, D.D. Alexander, J. Caliendo, A. Hentati, Y.W. Kwon, and H.X. Deng. 1994. Motor neuron degeneration in mice that express a human Cu,Zn superoxide dismutase mutation. *Science* **264:** 1772.
Heins, S. and U. Aebi. 1994. Making heads and tails of intermediate filament assembly, dynamics and networks. *Curr. Opin. Cell Biol.* **6:** 25.
Hirano, A., Ed. 1988. Argentophilic intracytoplasmic inclusions. In *Color atlas of pathology of the nervous system*, p. 99. Igako-Shoin, Tokyo.
———. 1991. Cytopathology of amyotrophic lateral sclerosis. *Adv. Neurol.* **56:** 91.
Hirano, A., H. Donnenfeld, S. Sasaki, and I. Nakano. 1984a. Fine structural observations of neurofilamentous changes in amyotrophic lateral sclerosis. *J. Neuropathol. Exp. Neurol.* **43:** 461.
Hirano, A., I. Nakano, L.T. Kurland, D.W. Mulder, P.W. Holley, and G. Saccomanno. 1984b. Fine structural study of neurofibrillary changes in a family with amyotrophic lateral sclerosis. *J. Neuropathol. Exp. Neurol.* **43:** 471.
Hisanaga, S. and N. Hirokawa. 1988. Structure of the peripheral domains of neurofilaments revealed by low angle rotary shadowing. *J. Mol. Biol.* **202:** 297.
Hoffman, P.N., J.W. Griffin, and D.L. Price. 1984. Control of axonal caliber by neurofilament transport. *J. Cell Biol.* **99:** 705.
Hoffman, P.N., J.W. Griffin, B.G. Gold, and D.L. Price. 1985. Slowing of neurofilament transport and the radial growth of developing nerve fibers. *J. Neurosci.* **5:** 2920.
Hoffman, P.N., R.J. Lasek, J.W. Griffin, and D.L. Price. 1983. Slowing of the axonal transport of neurofilament proteins during development. *J. Neurosci.* **3:** 1694.
Hsieh, S.-T., G.J. Kidd, T.O. Crawford, Z.-S. Xu, B.D. Trapp, D.W. Cleveland, and J.W. Griffin. 1994. Regional modulation of neurofilament organization by myelination in normal axons. *J. Neurosci* **14:** 6392.
Hursh, J.B. 1939. Conduction velocity and diameter of nerve fibers. *Am. J. Physiol.* **127:** 131.
Julien, J.P., F. Cote, L. Beaudet, M. Sidky, D. Flavell, F. Grosveld, and W. Mushynski. 1988. Sequence and structure of the mouse gene coding for the largest neurofilament subunit. *Gene.* **68:** 307.
Kawamura, Y., P. Dyck, M. Shimono, H. Okazaki, J. Tateishi, and H. Doi. 1981. Morphometric comparison of the vulnerability of peripheral motor and sensory neurons in amyotrophic lateral sclerosis. *J. Neuropathol. Exp. Neurol.* **40:** 667.
Lane, E.B., E.L. Rugg, H. Navsaria, I.M. Leigh, A.H. Heagerty, A. Ishida-Yamamoto, and R.A. Eady. 1992. A mutation in the conserved helix termination peptide of keratin 5 in hereditary skin blistering. *Nature* **356:** 244.
Lasek, R.J., P. Paggi, and M.J. Katz. 1992. Slow axonal transport mechanisms move neurofilaments relentlessly in mouse optic axons. *J. Cell Biol.* **117:** 607.
Lee, M.K., J.R. Marszalek, and D.W. Cleveland. 1994. A mutant neurofilament subunit causes massive, selective motor neuron death: Implications for the pathogenesis of human motor neuron disease. *Neuron* **13:** 975.
Lee, M.K., Z. Xu, P.C. Wong, and D.W. Cleveland. 1993. Neurofilaments are obligate heteropolymers in vivo. *J. Cell Biol.* **122:** 1337.
Lee, V.M., M.J. Carden, and J.Q. Trojanowski. 1986. Novel monoclonal antibodies provide evidence for the in situ existence of a nonphosphorylated form of the largest neurofilament subunit. *J. Neurosci.* **6:** 850.
Lee, V.M., L. Otvos, Jr., M.J. Carden, M. Hollosi, B. Dietzschold, and R.A. Lazzarini. 1988. Identification of the major multiphosphorylation site in mammalian neurofilaments. *Proc. Natl. Acad. Sci.* **85:** 1998.
Lopata, M.A. and D.W. Cleveland. 1987. In vivo microtubules are copolymers of available beta-tubulin isotypes: Localization of each of six vertebrate beta-tubulin isotypes using polyclonal antibodies elicited by synthetic peptide antigens. *J. Cell Biol.* **105:** 1707.
Marszalek, J.R., T.L. Williamson, M.K. Lee, Z. Xu, T.O. Crawford, P.N. Hoffman, and D.W. Cleveland. 1996. Neurofilament subunit NF-H modulates axonal diameter by affecting the rate of neurofilament transport. *J. Cell Biol.* (in press).
Monteiro, M.J., P.N. Hoffman, J.D. Gearhart, and D.W. Cleveland. 1990. Expression of NF-L in both neuronal and nonneuronal cells of transgenic mice: Increased neurofilament density in axons without affecting caliber. *J. Cell Biol.* **111:** 1543.
Nixon, R.A. and K.B. Logvinenko. 1986. Multiple fates of newly synthesized neurofilament proteins: Evidence for a stationary neurofilament network distributed nonuniformly along axons of retinal ganglion cell neurons. *J. Cell Biol.* **102:** 647.
Nixon, R.A., S.E. Lewis, and C.A. Marotta. 1987. Posttranslational modification of neurofilament proteins by phosphate during axoplasmic transport in retinal ganglion cell neurons. *J. Neurosci.* **7:** 1145.
Nixon, R.A., P.A. Paskevich, R.K. Sihag, and C.Y. Thayer. 1994. Phosphorylation on carboxyl terminus domains of neurofilament proteins in retinal ganglion cell neurons in vivo: Influences on regional neurofilament accumulation, interneurofilament spacing, and axon caliber. *J. Cell Biol.* **126:** 1031.
Oblinger, M.M. 1987. Characterization of posttranslational processing of the mammalian high-molecular-weight neurofilament protein in vivo. *J. Neurosci.* **7:** 2510.
Ohara, O., Y. Gahara, T. Miyake, H. Teraoka, and T. Kitamura. 1993. Neurofilament deficiency in quail caused by nonsense mutation in neurofilament-L gene. *J. Cell Biol.* **121:** 387.
Rooke, K., D.A. Figlewicz, F. Han, and G.A. Rouleau. 1996. Analysis of the KSP repeat of the neurofilament heavy-subunit in familial amyotrophic lateral sclerosis. *Ann. Neurol.* **46:** 789.
Rosen, D.R., T. Siddique, D. Patterson, D.A. Figlewicz, P. Sapp, A. Hentati, D. Donaldson, J. Goto, J.P. O'Regan,

H.X. Deng, and R. Brown. 1993. Mutations in Cu/Zn superoxide dismutase gene are associated with familial amyotropic lateral sclerosis. *Nature* **362:** 59.

Rothnagel, J.A., A.M. Dominey, L.D. Dempsey, M.A. Longley, D.A. Greenhalgh, T.A. Gagne, M. Huber, E. Frenk, D. Hohl, and D.R. Roop. 1992. Mutations in the rod domains of keratins 1 and 10 in epidermolytic hyperkeratosis. *Science* **257:** 1128.

Rouleau, G.A., A.W. Clark, K. Rooke, A. Pramatarova, A. Krizus, O. Suchowersky, J.-P. Julien, and D. Figlewicz. 1996. SOD1 mutation is associated with accumulation of neurofilaments in amyotrophic lateral sclerosis. *Ann. Neurol.* **39:** 128.

Sakaguchi, T., M. Okada, T. Kitamura, and K. Kawasaki. 1993. Reduced diameter and conduction velocity of myelinated fibers in the sciatic nerve of a neurofilament-deficient mutant quail. *Neurosci. Lett.* **153:** 65.

Shibata, N., A. Hirano, M. Kobayashi, T. Siddique, H.-X. Deng, W.-Y Hung, T. Kato, and K. Asayama. 1996. Intense superoxide dismutase-1 immunoreactivity in intracytoplasmic hyaline inclusions of familial amyotrophic lateral sclerosis with posterior column involvement. *J. Neuropathol. Exp. Neurol.* **55:** 481.

Stanley, J.R. 1993. Cell adhesion molecules as targets of autoantibodies in pemphigus and pemphigoid, bullous diseases due to defective epidermal adhesion. *Adv. Immunol.* **53:** 291.

Sternberger, L.A. and N.H. Sternberger. 1983. Monoclonal antibodies distinguish phosphorylated and nonphosphorylated forms of neurofilaments in situ. *Proc. Natl. Acad. Sci.* **80:** 6126.

Troncoso, J.C., J.L. March, M. Haner, and U. Aebi. 1990. Effect of aluminum and other multivalent cations on neurofilaments in vitro: An electron microscopic study. *J. Struct. Biol.* **103:** 2.

Tu, P.H., P. Raju, K.A. Robinson, M.E. Gurney, J.Q. Trojanowski, and V.M.-Y. Lee. 1996. Transgenic mice carrying a human mutant superoxide dismutase transgene develop neuronal cytoskeletal pathology resembling human amyotrophic lateral sclerosis lesions. *Proc. Natl. Acad. Sci.* **93:** 3155.

Vechio, J.V., L.I. Bruijn, Z.-S. Xu, R.H. Brown, Jr., and D.W. Cleveland. 1996. Identification of variants in human neurofilament genes: Absence of linkage to familial ALS. *Ann. Neurol.* (in press).

Wiedau-Pazos, M., J.J. Goto, S. Rabizadeh, E.D. Gralla, J.A. Roe, J.S. Valentine, and D.E. Bredesen. 1996. Altered reactivity of superoxide dismutase in familial amyotrophic lateral sclerosis. *Science* **271:** 515.

Willard, M. and C. Simon. 1983. Modulations of neurofilament axonal transport during the development of rabbit retinal ganglion cells. *Cell* **35:** 551.

Wong, P.C. and D.W. Cleveland. 1990. Characterization of dominant and recessive assembly-defective mutations in mouse neurofilament NF-M. *J. Cell Biol.* **111:** 1987.

Wong, P.C., J. Marszalek, T.O. Crawford, Z. Xu, S.T. Hsieh, J.W. Griffin, and D.W. Cleveland. 1995a. Increasing neurofilament subunit NF-M expression reduces axonal NF-H, inhibits radial growth, and results in neurofilamentous accumulation in motor neurons. *J. Cell Biol.* **130:** 1413.

Wong, P.C., C.A. Pardo, D.R. Borchelt, M.K. Lee, N.G. Copeland, N.A. Jenkins, S.S. Sisodia, D.W. Cleveland, and D.L. Price. 1995b. An adverse property of a familial ALS-linked SOD1 mutation causes motor neuron disease characterized by vacuolar degeneration of mitochondria. *Neuron* **14:** 1105.

Xu, Z., L.C. Cork, J.W. Griffin, and D.W. Cleveland. 1993. Increased expression of neurofilament subunit NF-L produces morphological alterations that resemble the pathology of human motor neuron disease. *Cell* **73:** 23.

Xu, Z., J.R. Marszalek, M.K. Lee, P.C. Wong, T.O. Crawford, S.-T. Hsieh, J.W. Griffin, and D.W. Cleveland. 1996. Subunit composition of neurofilaments specifies axonal diameter. *J. Cell Biol.* **133:** 1061.

Yamasaki, H., C. Itakura, and M. Mizutani. 1991. Hereditary hypotrophic axonopathy with neurofilament deficiency in a mutant strain of the Japanese quail. *Acta Neuropathol.* **82:** 427.

Yang, Y., J. Dowling, Q.-C. Yu, P. Kouklis, D. Cleveland, and E. Fuchs. 1996. A new type of cytoskeletal protein: Connecting actin microfilaments to intermediate filaments. *Cell* **86:** 655.

Neurodegenerative Diseases and Model Systems

D.L. Price,[1–4] D.R. Borchelt,[1,4] P.C. Wong,[1,4] C.A. Pardo,[1,4] G. Thinakaran,[1,4] M.K. Lee,[1,4] D.W. Cleveland,[5] and S.S. Sisodia[1,3,4]

Departments of [1]Pathology, [2]Neurology, [3]Neuroscience, and [4]The Neuropathology Laboratory, The Johns Hopkins University School of Medicine, Baltimore, Maryland 21205; [5]Ludwig Institute, Departments of Medicine and Neuroscience, University of California at San Diego, La Jolla, California 92093-0660

The neurodegenerative disorders, including amyotrophic lateral sclerosis (ALS) and Alzheimer's disease (AD), are among the most puzzling and devastating illnesses in medicine. These two diseases, which are associated with a variety of etiological/risk factors, including age and the presence of mutations in specific genes, have many features in common (Table 1). Familial ALS (FALS) and familial AD (FAD) are autosomal dominant, age-related disorders linked to mutations in superoxide dismutase 1 (SOD1) and amyloid precursor protein (APP) presenilin genes (PS1/PS2), respectively, which affect vulnerable populations of nerve cells. In ALS, progressive weakness and muscle atrophy reflect the vulnerability of motor neurons; in AD, dementia results from the involvement of populations of neurons in the neocortex, hippocampus, and basal forebrain cholinergic system. The mechanisms leading to the dysfunction/death of these subsets of nerve cells are not well understood, and, unfortunately, no specific therapies are available. However, because of new advances in genetics, cellular/molecular biology, and transgenic (Tg) technologies, investigators are now in a position to model these disorders with a high degree of fidelity (Fig. 1). The availability of these models will promote rapid progress in understanding the mechanisms of many neurodegenerative disorders and will eventually allow the testing of new therapies that target these mechanisms.

AMYOTROPHIC LATERAL SCLEROSIS

Clinical Manifestations

Patients with ALS and FALS develop weakness, muscular atrophy, spasticity, and a variety of other motor signs (Williams and Windebank 1993; Rowland 1994) that are attributed to damage to large α-motor neurons of the brain stem and spinal cord and to upper motor neurons in the neocortex (Oppenheimer and Esiri 1992).

Genetics of SOD1-linked FALS

Approximately 10% of adult-onset cases of ALS are familial and inherited as autosomal dominant disorders (Siddique et al. 1989; 1991). SOD1 mutations account for about 20% of families with the autosomal dominant form of FALS (Deng et al. 1993; Rosen et al. 1993), and to date, more than 40 different missense SOD1 mutations have been documented in these early-onset cases (Rosen et al. 1993; Carri et al. 1994). Because SOD1 acts as a free radical scavenger by catalyzing the formation of H_2O_2 through the dismutation of $\cdot O_2$ (Fridovich 1986; Halliwell 1992), it protects molecules and organelles that would otherwise be damaged by free radicals (Halliwell and Gutteridge 1985; Beckman et al. 1990). Although it was initially thought that SOD1 mutations reduced enzyme activity (Deng et al. 1993), it is now clear that significant reductions in levels of free radical scavenging do not necessarily occur in many cases of SOD1-linked FALS, and available evidence now favors the hypothesis that mutant SOD1 gains toxic properties (see below).

Neuropathology

In sporadic ALS, motor neurons show a variety of inclusions, including ubiquitinated and phosphorylated neurofilament (NF) immunoreactivities in cell bodies; fragmentation of the Golgi apparatus; axonal spheroids (i.e., maloriented skeins of NF in greatly enlarged proximal axons); distal axonal atrophy; dying back (fewer axons distally than proximally); reduced numbers of large myelinated fibers; and Wallerian degeneration of motor axons (Smith 1955; Clark et al. 1984; Schmidt et al. 1987; Hirano 1991; Chou 1992; Gonatas et al. 1992; Hirano and Kato 1992; Oppenheimer and Esiri 1992; Shibata et al. 1993; Lowe 1994). In some cases of FALS, SOD1, ubiquitin, and NF-immunoreactive intracytoplasmic inclusions are seen in motor neurons (Shibata et al. 1993, 1996; Rouleau et al. 1996), and NF may accumulate in cell bodies and neuronal processes (Takahashi et al. 1972; Mizusawa et al. 1989; Rouleau et al. 1996). At the end stage of both ALS and FALS, the numbers of motor neurons are reduced in spinal cord and brain stem nuclei (Kato et al. 1993), and astrogliosis is evident at these sites. Motor axons undergo Wallerian degeneration, and there is grouped atrophy and fiber type grouping of skeletal muscles (Tandan and Bradley 1985; Oppenheimer and Esiri 1992).

Animal Models of Motor Neuron Disease

Because observations made in tissues from cases of ALS are biased toward end-stage disease, early patho-

Table 1. Features Shared by FALS and FAD

Onset in mid-to-late life
Progressive course
Genetic heterogeneity
Linked to several loci/mutations in specific genes
Mutant proteins gain toxic properties
Selective vulnerability (death) of subsets of neurons
Cytoskeletal and axonal abnormalities
Oxidative damage
No effective therapies
Tg mice reproduce disease

genic events are not well understood. Critical questions (i.e., organelles and macromolecules targeted by the disease, the character and evolution of pathogenic processes, and, most importantly, primary and secondary molecular/biochemical mechanisms that lead to dysfunction/death of motor neurons) can be investigated in model systems. Over the past decade, studies of a variety of animal models of ALS have provided important information about the processes implicated in the dysfunction and death of motor neurons

β,β′-Iminodipropionitrile (IDPN)-induced NF axonopathy. This experimentally induced animal model has proved extraordinarily valuable for the analyses of mechanisms that lead to the formation of NF axonal spheroids. The systemic administration of IDPN to rodents causes limb weakness and the development of enormous swellings of proximal axons that are filled with maloriented arrays of NF (Fig. 2); distal axons become atrophic (Chou and Hartmann 1964; Griffin et al. 1978, 1982b, 1983c; Clark et al. 1980; Griffin and Price 1981a,b; Gold et al. 1986). Radiolabeling studies have demonstrated that IDPN selectively impairs the slow transport of NF proteins, perhaps by dissociating NF from microtubules and causing transported NF to accumulate in proximal segments of axons (Griffin et al. 1978; Griffin et al. 1983a,b).

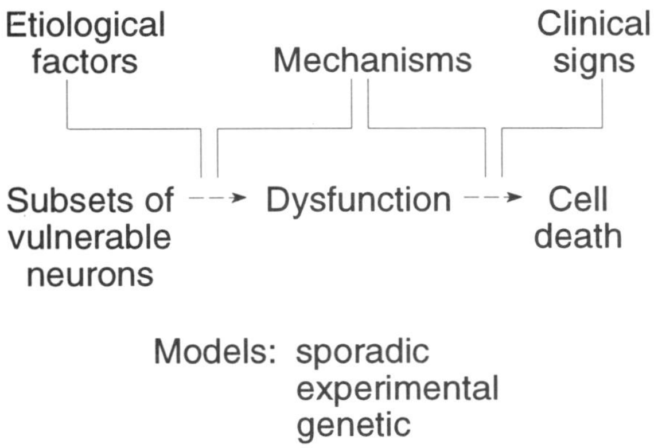

Figure 1. Neurodegenerative diseases. Schematic showing the relationships of etiologies, selective vulnerabilities, mechanisms of disease/cell death with clinical phenotypes, and models of disease.

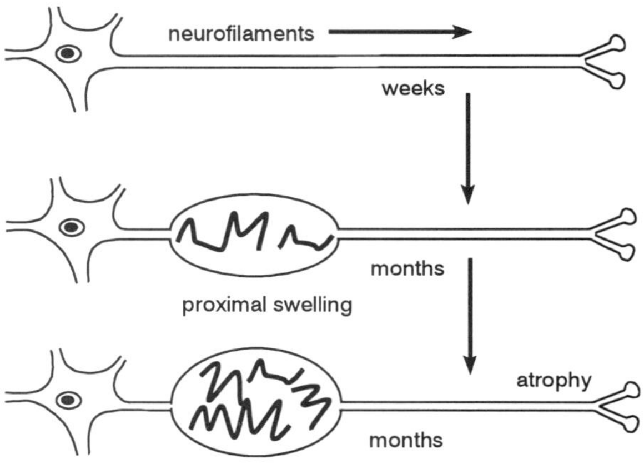

Figure 2. IDPN intoxication. This schematic depicts the nature and evolution of NF axonal pathology (axonal swellings) and axonal atrophy.

Hereditary canine spinal muscular atrophy (HCSMA). This disease, occurring in Brittany spaniels, exhibits three phenotypes—accelerated, intermediate, and chronic (Table 2) (Cork et al. 1979; Lorenz et al. 1979; Sack et al. 1984). Electromyography and muscle biopsies disclose patterns consistent with denervation atrophy. Many motor neurons develop NF-filled swellings of the proximal axon (Cork et al. 1979, 1982). In these cells, the transport of the NF proteins (and possibly tubulin) is impaired (Griffin et al. 1982a). NF-L mRNA is selectively decreased (Muma and Cork 1993); altered stoichiometry of NF subunits could impair NF assembly and transport, leading to swollen axons. The weakness in HCSMA may be related to four processes: conduction failure through swollen NF-filled axons denuded of myelin sheaths (Cork et al. 1989a,b; Pinter et al. 1995); functional deficits involving the distal parts of motor axons (Pinter et al. 1995); disconnection of neurons from muscle leading to difficulties in maintaining force output of motor units (Pinter et al. 1995); and eventual degeneration of motor neurons.

Tg mice with the G37R HuSOD1 mutation. Tg mice with different SOD1 mutations (Table 3) develop motor neuron disease (Gurney et al. 1994; Ripps et al. 1995; Wong et al. 1995), whereas wild-type (wt) human (Hu)SOD1 Tg mice with similar levels of enzyme in

Table 2. Three Phenotypes of HCSMA

Phenotype	Age of onset	Clinical course
Accelerated	6 weeks	rapid; quadriparesis by 16 weeks of age
Intermediate	6 months to 1 year	gradual; quadriparesis by 2–3 years of age
Chronic	6 months to 1 year	slow; relatively benign course extending >6 years of age

Table 3. HuSOD1 Tg Mice

Mutant	Line #	Strain	SODI activity cord	SODI activity brain	SOD1 protein in cord	Onset of motor neuron disease (months)
HuG37R	42	B6/C3	14	n.d.	12	3.5–4
	9	B6/C3	9	n.d.	6	5–6
	106	B6/C3	7	n.d.	5	5.5–7.5
	29	B6/C3	7	n.d.	5	6–8
	50	B6/C3	n.d.	n.d.	3	11
	1	B6/C3	n.d.	n.d.	1	none at 20
Hu wt	76		10		10	none
	30		8		7	none
HuG93A	G1	B6/SJL	n.d.	4	5	4–6
MoG85R	M1	FVB	n.d.	1	n.d.	3–4

n d. indicates not determined.

identical tissue distributions do not develop clinical signs (Wong et al. 1995). When transfection experiments demonstrated that some mutations did not reduce SOD1 activities (Borchelt et al. 1994, 1995), we questioned whether all cases of SOD1-linked FALS could be explained by reductions in SOD1 activity and hypothesized that autosomal dominant FALS was caused by a toxic effect of mutant SOD1. Based on studies of the activities and stabilities of mutant SOD1 in vitro (Borchelt et al. 1994), we chose to introduce the G37R, A4V, and G85R HuSOD1 transgenes into mice because in vitro gel assays disclosed that these mutations are associated with high (G37R), intermediate (A4V), and low (G85R) levels of SOD1 activities. In this review, we focus on the G37R HuSOD1 Tg mice.

From many founders expressing G37R HuSOD1, we produced multiple lines of mice that expressed G37R HuSOD1 at 3–12 times the levels of endogenous SOD1 in the spinal cord; gels show a comparable increase in SOD1 activity, confirming that the G37R mutation synthesized in vivo retains full specific activity (Wong et al. 1995). Significantly, Tg mice with the highest levels of mutant SOD1 developed the most aggressive forms of the disease.

At 4 months of age, G37R SOD1 Tg mice showed reduced spontaneous movements, difficulty moving their hind limbs, muscle wasting, and electromyographic patterns consistent with motor neuron disease. Subsequently, the forelimbs became weak, and hindlimbs were completely paralyzed.

At 5–7 weeks (i.e., long before clinical signs), these Tg mice began to accumulate SOD1 in swollen motor axons that contain very small vacuoles (D.R. Borchelt et al., in prep.). Metabolic radioalabeling methods have demonstrated that both endogenous mouse SOD1 and G37R HuSOD1 are transported anterograde, as part of slow component *b*, into motor axons of the sciatic nerve (D.R. Borchelt et al., in prep.). Small vacuoles are also present in dendrites (as disclosed by staining with antibodies recognizing microtubule-associated protein-2 [MAP-2]). By 2 months of age, the vacuoles, usually associated with swollen mitochondria in various stages of degeneration, are conspicuous in axons and dendrites more than in cell bodies (Wong et al. 1995). Mitochondria in adjacent nonneuronal cells are unaffected. The patterns of NF and MAP-2 immunoreactivities in axons and dendrites, respectively, are altered; cell bodies and dendrites exhibit ubiquitin and phosphorylated NF immunoreactivities. Astrogliosis is present in proximity to these abnormal neurons. Motor axons in intraspinal segments and roots exhibit a series of abnormalities including vacuoles and cytoskeletal alterations; eventually, Wallerian degeneration occurs, and the number of end plates is reduced. Changes in muscle fibers are consistent with denervation.

These observations are consistent with the idea that HuSOD1 gains adverse properties (Wong et al. 1995), triggering a cascade of pathological events that leads to degeneration of motor neurons. Several additional findings are consistent with this hypothesis: The onset and progression of FALS do not necessarily correlate with levels of SOD1 activity (Cleveland et al. 1995); some mutant SOD1s are associated with near-normal levels of enzyme activity/stability in vitro (Borchelt et al. 1994); SOD1 mutations do not act in a dominant negative fashion on wt SOD1 (Borchelt et al. 1995); and some mutant SOD1s restore SOD1 null yeast to the wt phenotype (Rabizadeh et al. 1995) yet cause the death of nerve cells in vitro (Rabizadeh et al. 1995; Wiedau-Pazos et al. 1996). These results, in conjunction with the finding that several lines of Tg mice with different SOD1 mutations develop disease, despite the presence of normal SOD1 activity (Gurney et al. 1994; Ripps et al. 1995; Wong et al. 1995), indicate that SOD1-linked motor neuron disease is not the result of reduced enzyme activity, but rather mutant SOD1 gains a toxic property that damages motor neurons.

Among the mysteries of the neurodegenerative diseases is the problem of "selective vulnerability," a term used to describe the disease-characteristic involvements of specific populations of neurons. The vulnerability of specific cells determines the clinical phenotypes of each disease. Selectivity also exists in the biochemical mechanisms of disease, because different diseases alter target discrete processes in neurons. A number of features of motor neurons could enhance the vulnerability of these cells to SOD1 mutations (Fig. 3). SOD1 is abundant in neural tissues (representing 0.7% of soluble protein in spinal cord) and is enriched in motor neurons (Powell et al. 1978). The relative abundance of SOD1 in motor neurons is one of the factors that contribute to the selective vulnerability of these cells in SOD1-linked FALS. However, other properties of motor neurons must also play significant roles in determining susceptibility to SOD1 mutations. These large cells have long, large-caliber, NF-rich axons; cytoskeletal and other constituents must be actively transported to maintain their axons, imposing a metabolic burden on these cells. If trans-

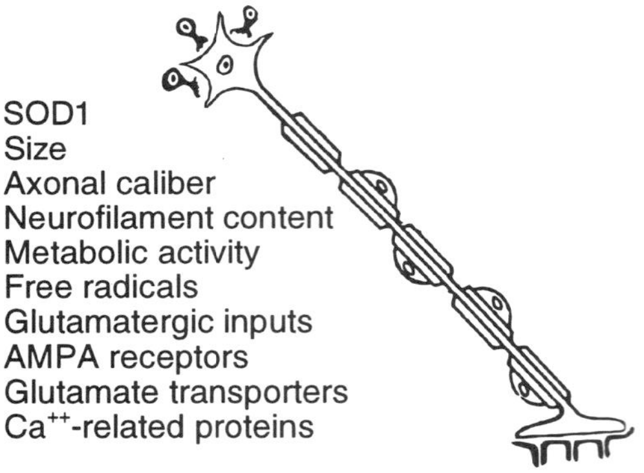

Figure 3. Motor unit with excitatory and inhibitory inputs. The factors listed are postulated to influence the vulnerability of motor neurons in FALS.

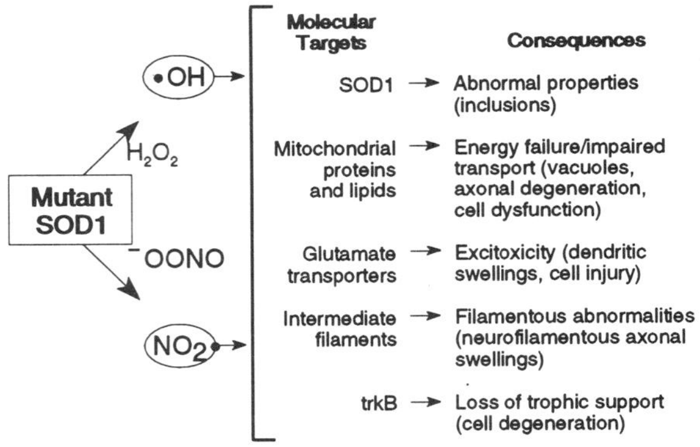

Figure 4. Possible mechanisms of SOD1 toxicity, molecular targets, and consequences for motor neurons.

port is compromised, the axons develop a series of abnormalities, the character of which depends on the nature and time course of the impairment in transport. The metabolic activity of mitochondria in motor neurons generates free radicals that, if not adequately scavenged, could damage cellular processes (see below) (Beal 1996). Moreover, motor neurons receive a variety of glutamatergic inputs that utilize different types of receptors, including AMPA receptors (Martin et al. 1993), in synaptic transmission (Rothstein et al. 1994). Levels of glutamate are dramatically influenced by glutamate transporters (Rothstein et al. 1994), and increases in levels of glutamate would promote excitotoxicity (Rothstein 1996b), which increases the energy demands on the cells. In parallel, levels of intracellular calcium may increase, exacerbating toxicity (Beal 1996). It has been argued that levels of protective calcium-binding protein influence cell vulnerability, and it may be significant that motor neurons have reduced levels of calbindin (Morrison et al. 1996). Finally, motor neurons are, in part, dependent on trophic factors derived from the periphery (Oppenheim et al. 1992; Sendtner et al. 1992; Yan et al. 1992; Koliatsos et al. 1993; Clatterbuck et al. 1994; Koliatsos et al. 1994; Ehlers et al. 1995), and changes in the retrograde transport of trophic receptors (Ehlers et al. 1995) could compromise the viability of motor neurons.

Mutant SOD1 could damage cellular/molecular targets by a variety of mechanisms (Fig. 4). Dale Bredesen and colleagues have proposed, on the basis of in vitro studies (Wiedau-Pazos et al. 1996), that mutant SOD1 acts as a peroxidase that oxidizes a variety of targets; chelating agents abolish this oxidation, implicating Cu^{++} in this process. Beckman and colleagues (Beckman et al. 1993) have hypothesized that mutant SOD1 can utilize peroxynitrate to form nitronium ions that can nitrate tyrosine residues. The nitration of proteins important in the biology of motor neurons could have a significant impact on the structure/functions/viability of these cells. Oxidation or nitration reactions involving some of these targets (i.e., proteins and lipids of mitochondria, glutamate transporters, trkB, NF) (Fig. 4) could initiate a cascade of events that lead to a series of structural/functional abnormalities and, eventually, the death of motor neurons. Consistent with this idea are preliminary studies from Tg mice with HuSOD1 mutations that show early accumulation of mutant SOD1 in mildly abnormal axons; swollen mitochondria; increased levels of free nitrotyrosine in the spinal cords (F. Beal et al., pers. comm.); morphological features of excitotoxicity (dendritic swellings); and reductions in levels of glutamate transporters (L. Bruijn et al., pers. comm.). The oxidation of SOD1 or the oxidation/nitration of other proteins (mitochondrial constituents, cytoskeletal elements, glutamate transporters, trophic receptors) could lead to altered protein-protein interactions and/or protein aggregates (inclusions); compromised energy levels; impaired axonal transport; enhanced excitotoxicity; and reduced levels of trophic support. Antioxidants, in combination with other agents (anti-excitotoxic compounds, growth factors) may attenuate these processes (Elliott and Snider 1996; Rothstein 1996a; Yuen and Mobley 1996). Support for this idea is provided by a recent study showing the modest effects of antioxidant and anti-excitotoxic treatments in a line of H93A HuSOD1 Tg mice (Gurney et al. 1996).

ALZHEIMER'S DISEASE

Clinical Manifestations

AD, the most common cause of dementia occurring in mid-to-late life, affects 7–10% of individuals over 65 years of age and perhaps 40% of persons over 80 years of age (Evans et al. 1989). Clinical signs include loss of memory, impairments of higher cortical functions, behavioral/psychiatric abnormalities, and, eventually, profound dementia (Price et al. 1996). Increases in life expectancy will inevitably lead to a significantly increased prevalence and cost of AD. Clearly, AD will be one of the most important public health problems of the next century.

Genetics

Approximately 10% of cases of AD are familial and show autosomal dominant inheritance (Bird 1994; Schellenberg 1995); subsets of these cases are linked to mutations of specific genes (Bondi et al. 1994; Schellenberg 1995), including APP and PS1/PS2. Late-onset disease is associated with the presence of copies of the apolipoprotein E (apoE) allele (Roses 1995). Below is given a brief summary of the biology of APP and PS1 and 2, which are relevant to work on Tg mice.

APP. A gene on chromosome 21 encodes this type-I integral membrane glycoprotein (Glenner and Wong 1984a,b; Masters et al. 1985a,b; Kang et al. 1987). The Aβ amyloid region is composed of 28 amino acids of the ectodomain and 11–14 amino acids of the transmembrane domain (Kang et al. 1987). APP is expressed in many cells, including neurons that transport proteins in axons by the rapid transport system (Koo et al. 1990a,b; Martin et al. 1991; Sisodia et al. 1993). In a small fraction of FAD cases, mutations have been documented in the APP gene (Chartier-Harlin et al. 1991; Goate et al. 1991; Naruse et al. 1991; Hendricks et al. 1992; Mullan et al. 1992). Clustered around the Aβ domain, the mutation is associated with more Aβ, a greater proportion of large Aβ peptides (i.e., Aβ42), an increase in the microheterogeneity/hydrophobicity of secreted Aβ species, or an increase in the propensity to aggregate into fibrils (Wisniewski et al. 1991; Citron et al. 1992; Cai et al. 1993; Haass et al. 1994; Suzuki et al. 1994; Thinakaran et al. 1996a).

PS1/2. The PS (1 and 2), encoded by genes on chromosomes 14 and 1, respectively, show mutations in cases of FAD. These highly homologous proteins (Sherrington et al. 1995) are predicted to contain 7–9 transmembrane helices (Sherrington et al. 1995; Slunt et al. 1995). Recent studies of the topology of PS1 suggest a protein with eight transmembrane domains, a cytoplasmic loop interacting with cytosolic constituents, and carboxy- and amino-terminal domains that are also cytoplasmic (Fig. 5) (Doan et al. 1996b). PS1 mRNA protein is expressed in the brain, particularly in neurons (Kovacs et al. 1996; Lee et al. 1996). In cultured cells and brains (human, monkey, and mouse), PS1 is endoproteolytically processed to tau as a ~28-kD amino-terminal fragment and a ~18-kD carboxy-terminal fragment (Thinakaran et al. 1996a). Because of the paucity of accumulated full-length PS and the generality of PS processing across tissues, we have suggested that the two PS fragments may act as functional units (Thinakaran et al. 1996a). Although the biological functions of PS are not yet well understood, the finding of significant homology between PS and sel-12, a gene product that plays a role in the determination of cell fates during development in *Caenorhabditis elegans* (Levitan and Greenwald 1995), suggests that PS may be important in developmental processes in mammalian tissues. This issue can be examined by gene-targeting strategies.

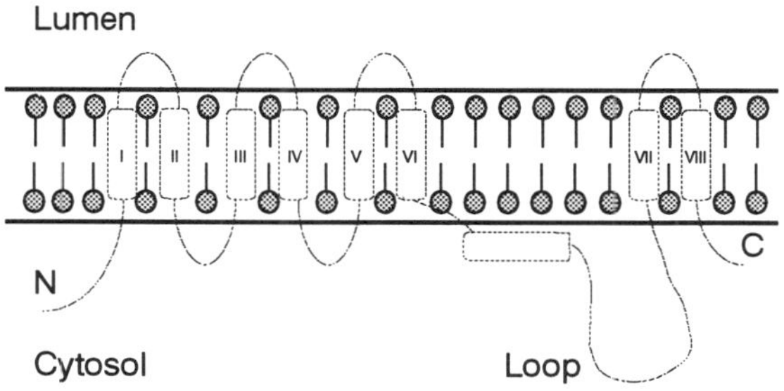

Figure 5. Topology of PS1. This protein has eight hydrophobic transmembrane domains (rectangles I-VIII in plasma membrane) and one hydrophobic domain that does not span the plasma membrane. Note the cytoplasmic location of the carboxyl and amino termini and the loop. PS1 undergoes endoproteolytic cleavage (*dotted line*) generating carboxy- and amino-terminal fragments. More than 50% of mutations involve transmembrane domains II, VI, and the region between VI and the carboxy-terminal portion of the loop. The diagram is based on the topology studies of Doan et al. (1996a,b).

The majority (~70%) of cases of early-onset FAD are linked to mutations in the PS1 gene located on chromosome 14 (St. George-Hyslop et al. 1992; Alzheimer's Disease Collaborative Group 1995; Sherrington et al. 1995). Approximately 50% of mutations occur within or immediately adjacent to the predicted loop domain (Fig. 5) (Alzheimer's Disease Collaborative Group 1995; Sherrington et al. 1995; Doan et al. 1996a). The PS2 gene, localized on chromosome 1, shows substantial homology with PS1, and mutations in PS2 cause an autosomal dominant AD in Volga German kindreds and in an Italian pedigree (Levy-Lahad et al. 1995a,b; Li et al. 1995; Rogaev et al. 1995).

The mechanisms by which mutations in PS1/2 predispose individuals to FAD are not clear. However, the absence of deletions or truncation mutations in PS1/2 leads to the suggestion that early-onset FAD in these affected pedigrees is the result of mutant PS protein influenced by toxic effects perhaps mediated by Aβ42. Lines of evidence favoring this hypothesis include: Plasma and conditioned media from fibroblasts obtained from carriers of PS mutations have elevated levels of Aβ42 species (Scheuner et al. 1996); in vitro studies of transfected cell lines expressing PS1 mutations have increased ratios of Aβ42/Aβ40 (Borchelt et al. 1996); and, as outlined below, the brains of young Tg mice coexpressing a chimeric APP and an FAD-linked PS1 variant show elevated Aβ42/AB40 ratios as compared to ratios in the brains of Tg mice expressing APP alone or Tg mice coexpressing wt HuPS1 and APP (Borchelt et al. 1996).

Neuropathology

AD selectively affects neurons in certain brain regions and populations of neurons, including those in the hippocampus, neocortex, and basal forebrain cholinergic system (Arnold et al. 1991; Braak and Braak 1994; Price et al. 1996). Many vulnerable nerve cells show accumulations of straight and paired helical filaments as neurofibrillary tangles (cell bodies and proximal dendrites), dystrophic neurites (axons/terminals), and neuropil threads (distal dendrites) (Lee 1995). These filaments are composed principally of phosphorylated tau, a low-molecular-weight, microtubule-associated protein. In neurofibrillary tangles, tau is hyperphosphorylated, a state in which it is unable to bind microtubules. Eventually, tangle-bearing cells die, possibly by mechanisms that involve apoptotic pathways (Su et al. 1994; Troncoso et al. 1996).

The brains of cases of AD are characterized by the deposition of an ~4-kD Aβ peptide derived from APP, a type-I integral membrane glycoprotein encoded by a gene on chromosome 21 (Glenner and Wong 1984a,b; Masters et al. 1985a,b; Kang et al. 1987). The Aβ region is composed of 28 amino acids of the ectodomain and 11–14 amino acids of the adjacent transmembrane domain of APP.

α-Secretase, a presumed membrane-bound endoprotease (whose specificity is independent of primary structure of the substrate but depends on α-helical conformation and distance of the hydrolyzable bond from the membrane [Sisodia 1992]), cleaves APP between positions 16 and 17 of Aβ (Esch et al. 1990; Sisodia et al. 1990; Anderson et al. 1991; Wang et al. 1991), a cleavage that precludes the formation of Aβ (Fig. 6). β- and α-secretase cleave at the amino- and carboxy-terminal portions of Aβ, respectively (Citron et al. 1992, 1993; Shoji et al. 1992, 1993). Aβ42 is the most common Aβ peptide species in diffuse and compact amyloid plaques (Iwatsubo et al. 1994, 1995; Shinkai et al. 1995; Lemere et al. 1996). Aβ42 is deposited early (Burdick et al. 1992) and provides a substrate for additional amyloid deposits (Jarrett and Lansbury 1993; Jarrett et al. 1993). Moreover, aggregated forms of Aβ peptide are neurotoxic (Pike et al. 1993; Cotman and Pike 1994; Simmons et al. 1994; Busciglio et al. 1995). Thus, multiple lines of evidence indicate that Aβ plays a critical role in the pathogenesis of AD (Table 4).

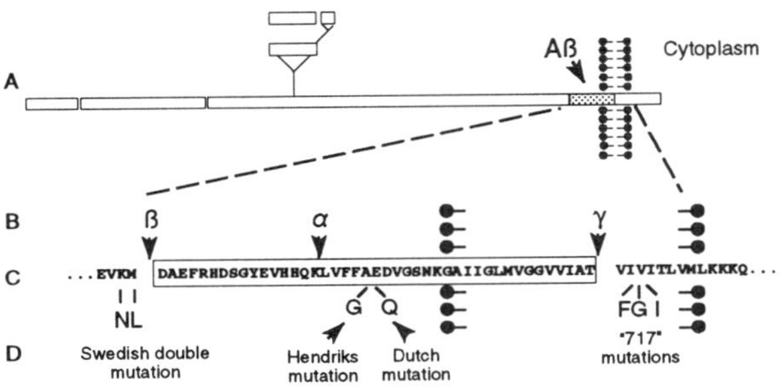

Figure 6. APP isoforms (*A*); α-, β-, and γ-secretase cleavage sites (*B*); Aβ42 (*C*); and positions of mutations linked to FAD (*D*). (Modified from Price et al. 1997.)

Models of Aging and AD: Aged Nonhuman Primate Models

Many nonhuman primate species live for several decades and, with age, some individuals develop behavioral impairments and brain abnormalities, including amyloid deposits (Fig. 7). Aged monkeys provide excellent models exhibiting some of the behavioral and brain abnormalities (Fig. 8) that occur in aged humans and, to a lesser extent, individuals with AD (Wisniewski and Terry 1973b; Bartus et al. 1978, 1979, 1980; Brizzee et al. 1980; Goldman-Rakic and Brown 1981; Struble et al. 1982, 1985; Kitt et al. 1984; Davis 1985; Ridley et al. 1986; Selkoe et al. 1987; Walker et al. 1987, 1988b, 1990; Abraham et al. 1989; Rapp and Amaral 1989; Rosen et al. 1989; Wenk et al. 1989; Cork et al. 1990; Heilbroner and Kemper 1990; Wagster et al. 1990; Bachevalier et al. 1991; Beal et al. 1991; Martin et al. 1991; Walker 1991; Bowling et al. 1993).

With a life span of 37–40 years (Tigges et al. 1988), *Macaca mulatta* develop age-associated impairments in performance on cognitive and memory tasks. In our colony of macaques, behavioral tasks were used to assess the integrity of specific brain regions/circuits in animals ranging from 4 to 35 years of age (Presty et al. 1987; Bachevalier et al. 1991). Deficits first appear late in the second decade, become more evident after the mid-20s, and progress with increasing age (Presty et al. 1987; Bachevalier et al. 1991). Initial impairments occur in the performance of certain spatial abilities at 16–19 years of age; however, in other test categories, behavior (i.e., recognition memory) was not altered until late in the third decade of life. Monkeys that performed poorly on one task were frequently quite successful on another. Chronological peers showed significant differences in performance on behavioral tasks. These variations in performance among aged animals and among tasks were similar to those observed in aged humans.

Aged rhesus monkeys also develop many of the brain abnormalities observed in older humans (Sussman et al. 1966; Wisniewski and Terry 1973a,b; Brizzee et al. 1980; Goldman-Rakic and Brown 1981; Struble et al. 1982; Kitt et al. 1984; Selkoe et al. 1987;

Table 4. Aβ and Alzheimer's Disease

Aβ42 deposited early (AD and Down's syndrome)
Aβ42 forms fibrillar aggregates in vitro (nidus for other peptides)
APP mutations increase amount, length, or aggregation of Aβ
PS mutations increase ratios of Aβ42/Aβ40 in:
media of cultures from cases of PS1 and PS2 mutations
sera from affected family members
media of transfected cells expressing APP and mutant PS1
brains of Tg mice coexpressing APPswe and mutant PS1
APP mutant mice have behavioral deficits and amyloid
Aβ42 hypothesized to have toxic properties

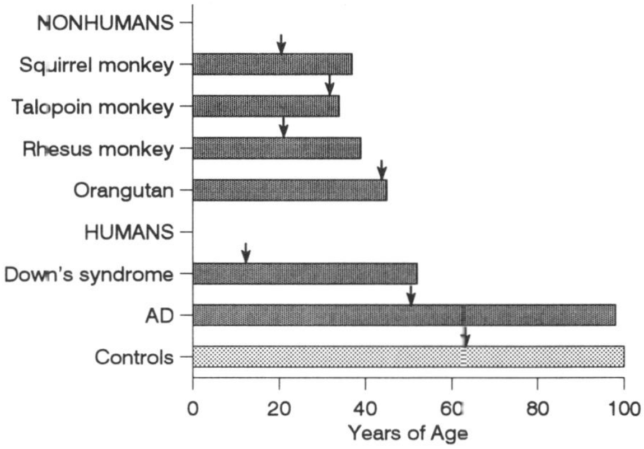

Figure 7. Life spans of primates and average time of appearance of senile plaques (*arrows*).

Walker et al. 1987, 1988a, 1990; Abraham et al. 1989; Wenk et al. 1989; Cork et al. 1990; Heilbroner and Kemper 1990; Wagster et al. 1990; Beal et al. 1991; Martin et al. 1991; Poduri et al. 1994; Rapp et al. 1994; Walker 1994). At about 20–25 years of age, these animals show dystrophic neurites (i.e., distal axons, nerve terminals, dendrites) derived from cholinergic, monoaminergic, serotoninergic, GABAergic, and peptidergic populations of neurons (Kitt et al. 1984, 1985, 1989; Struble et al. 1984; Walker et al. 1985, 1987, 1988a; Martin et al. 1991, 1994). Dystrophic neurites

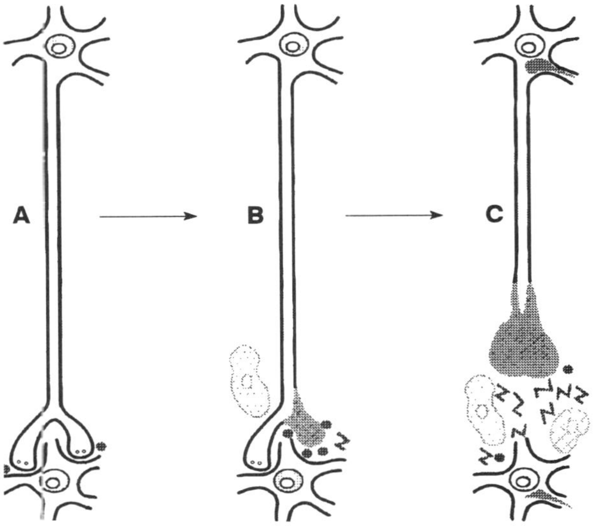

Figure 8. Evolution of cellular abnormalities in aged nonhuman primates. (*A*) Normal neuron synapsing on target cell. A small amount of Aβ (*dots*) is present in the extracellular space. (*B*) Aβ42 (*"Z" shapes*) begins to accumulate in the extracellular space near synapses. Dystrophic neurites retract from the target. Astrocytes are evident at these sites. (*C*) A mature senile plaque consists of Aβ42, dystrophic neurites, astrocytes, and microglial cells. Inputs to the target cell are reduced. Note intracellular tangle-like structure in cell bodies of both neurons.

are in immediate proximity to Aβ42>Aβ40 deposits present in diffuse plaques, in compact plaques, and in vessel walls (congophilic angiopathy) (Walker et al. 1987, 1990; Walker 1991; Levy et al. 1995; Morelli et al. 1996). APP-immunoreactive neurites may be one source for some of the Aβ deposited in the brains of these aged animals, but astrocytes and microglia, which are always present in mature plaques, may also participate in the formation of Aβ (Masters et al. 1985a; Martin et al. 1991; Miyakawa et al. 1992; Wisniewski et al. 1992). In addition, smooth muscle cells of the vessel wall may serve as a source for Aβ deposits in congophilic angiopathy (Wisniewski and Terry 1973b; Struble et al. 1982, 1985; Selkoe et al. 1987; Walker et al. 1987, 1988a; Cork et al. 1990). In a number of older animals, the cell bodies of a small number of large cortical neurons exhibit phosphorylated epitopes of NF proteins and tau immunoreactivities. The formation of "forme fruste" neurofibrillary tangles occurs at a later stage than Aβ42 deposition.

Aged macaques also show reductions in neurotransmitter markers (Goldman-Rakic and Brown 1981; Walker et al. 1988b; Wenk et al. 1989; Wagster et al. 1990; Beal et al. 1991), which may be related to the cognitive/memory impairments in some aged animals. Variations in the performances of individual animals on specific behavioral tasks presumably reflect the patterns of these lesions in different animals.

TG Mice Relevant to FAD

Many groups have attempted to create Tg mouse models of AD (Lamb et al. 1993; Higgins et al. 1994; Price and Sisodia 1994; Games et al. 1995; Howland et al. 1995; Hsiao et al. 1995, 1996; LaFerla et al. 1995; Moran et al. 1995; Oster-Granite et al. 1996). Two lines of Tg mice with two different APP mutations have been demonstrated to show elevated levels of the APP transgene product, behavioral deficits, increased levels of Aβ42, and Aβ deposits associated with dystrophic neurites in hippocampus and cerebral cortex (Games et al. 1995; Hsiao et al. 1996). Features that distinguish these APP Tg animals from other APP Tg mice are not fully understood, but it appears, as is the case with SOD1 Tg mice, that achieving high levels of expression of the mutant APP transgene in nervous tissue is very important.

Tg mice with high levels of expression of wt or mutant HuPS1 transgenes show two PS1 fragments, as has been observed in several species, including humans (Thinakaran et al. 1996b). As of this writing, Tg mice expressing PS1 mutations have not developed a FAD phenotype. To determine whether PS1 mutations influence APP/Aβ processing, particularly levels of the toxic Aβ42, mutant PS1 Tg mice were mated with Tg animals expressing mutant APP. The brains of young Tg animals that coexpress mutant PS1 and APP with the Swedish double mutation (APPswe) showed elevated ratios of Aβ42:Aβ40 as compared to Tg mice that coexpress wt PS1 and APPswe or that express APPswe alone (Borchelt et al. 1996). Similarly, Tg mice expressing mutant PS1 alone (but not mice expressing wt PS1) also have increased levels of Aβ42 (Duff et al. 1996). In concert, these findings indicate that one mechanism by which mutant PS1 can cause amyloidogenesis in AD is the acquisition (or enhancement) of properties that influence APP processing in a manner that leads to increased extracellular concentrations of toxic Aβ42. To examine the effects of apoE3 or E4 alleles on these processes, similar Tg approaches can be used to introduce the apoE transgene into wt or mutant APP or PS Tg mice.

CONCLUSIONS

ALS and AD are prototypic neurodegenerative diseases that involve certain brain regions/specific populations of neurons and are associated with characteristic cellular abnormalities. In ALS, motor neurons dysfunction/die, whereas in AD, neuronal degeneration occurs in cortex, hippocampus, and several subcortical nuclear groups. Some cases of FALS are linked to mutations in SOD1, whereas some cases of FAD are linked to mutations in PS1 and PS2 genes or the APP gene. Investigators have used spontaneously occurring, experimentally produced, or genetically engineered models of disease to examine the mechanisms of these diseases in vivo. Models of ALS have been used to show that NF-filled swellings of axons are the result of impaired transport. Tg mice with SOD1 mutations develop the clinical features of FALS and exhibit selective degeneration of motor neurons, which is the consequence of the acquisition of toxic properties by mutant SOD1. Aged monkeys that develop cognitive/memory deficits and cellular abnormalities (i.e., amyloid deposits and cytoskeletal abnormalities) represent the best spontaneously occurring model of aging/AD. Tg mice expressing mutant APP and PS1 genes show some of the features of FAD, including increased levels of Aβ42, a peptide toxic to the nervous system. These animal models are proving to be of extraordinary importance for investigations of the mechanisms of dysfunction/death of neurons in vivo and will be of great value for testing new therapies.

ACKNOWLEDGMENTS

The authors thank Drs. Mark Becher, Edward Koo, Andrew Doan, Lucie Bruijn, Linda Cork, Lee Martin, John Griffin, Cheryl Kitt, Lary Walker, Paul Hoffman, Vassilis Koliatsos, Mortimer Mishkin, Jacqueline Bachevalier, Robert Struble, Neal Copeland, and Nancy Jenkins for their contributions to some of the work discussed in this review. This work was supported by grants from the U.S. Public Health Service (National Institutes of Health NS-20471, AG-05146) as well as the Metropolitan Life Foundation, the Adler Foundation, the Alzheimer's Association, Merck, Sharp & Dohme, Ltd., the American Health Assistance Foundation, the DeVelbiss Fund, and the Amyotrophic Lateral Sclerosis Association. Dr. Price is the recipient of a Javits Neuroscience Investigator Award (NIH NS-10580), and a Leadership & Excellence in Alzheimer's Disease (LEAD) Award (NIH AG-07914). Dr. Sisodia is the recipient of a Zenith Award from the Alzheimer's Association.

REFERENCES

Abraham, C.R., D.J. Selkoe, H. Potter, D.L. Price, and L.C. Cork. 1989. α_1-antichymotrypsin is present together with the β-protein in monkey brain amyloid deposits. *Neuroscience* **32:** 715.

Alzheimer's Disease Collaborative Group. 1995. The structure of the presenilin 1 (*S182*) gene and identification of six novel mutations in early onset AD families. *Nat. Genet.* **11:** 219.

Anderson, J.P., F.S. Esch, P.S. Keim, K. Sambamurti, I. Lieberburg, and N.K. Robakis. 1991. Exact cleavage site of Alzheimer amyloid precursor in neuronal PC-12 cells. *Neurosci. Lett.* **128:** 126.

Arnold, S.E., B.T. Hyman, J. Flory, A.R. Damasio, and G.W. Van Hoesen. 1991. The topographical and neuroanatomical distribution of neurofibrillary tangles and neuritic plaques in the cerebral cortex of patients with Alzheimer's disease. *Cereb. Cortex* **1:** 103.

Bachevalier, J., L.S. Landis, L.C. Walker, M. Brickson, M. Mishkin, D.L. Price, and L.C. Cork. 1991. Aged monkeys exhibit behavioral deficits indicative of widespread cerebral dysfunction. *Neurobiol. Aging* **12:** 99.

Bartus, R.T., R.L. Dean, and B. Beer. 1980. Memory deficits in aged Cebus monkeys and facilitation with central cholinomimetics. *Neurobiol. Aging* **1:** 145.

Bartus, R.T., R.L. Dean, III, and D.L. Fleming. 1979. Aging in the rhesus monkey: Effects on visual discrimination learning and reversal learning. *J. Gerontol.* **34:** 209.

Bartus, R.T., D. Fleming, and H.R. Johnson. 1978. Aging in the rhesus monkey: Debilitating effects on short-term memory. *J. Gerontol.* **33:** 858.

Beal, M.F. 1996. Mitochondria, free radicals, and neurodegeneration. *Curr. Opin. Neurobiol.* **6:** 661.

Beal, M.F., L.C. Walker, E. Storey, L. Segar, D.L. Price, and L.C. Cork. 1991. Neurotransmitters in neocortex of aged rhesus monkeys. *Neurobiol. Aging* **12:** 407.

Beckman, J.S., M. Carson, C.D. Smith, and W.H. Koppenol. 1993. ALS, SOD and peroxynitrite. *Nature* **364:** 584.

Beckman, J.S., T.W. Beckman, J. Chen, P.A. Marshall, and B.A. Freeman. 1990. Apparent hydroxyl radical production by peroxynitrite: Implications for endothelial injury from nitric oxide and superoxide. *Proc. Natl. Acad. Sci.* **87:** 1620.

Bird, T.D. 1994. Clinical genetics of familial Alzheimer disease. In *Alzheimer disease.* (ed. R.D. Terry et al.), p. 65. Raven Press, New York.

Bondi, M.W., D.P. Salmon, and N.M. Butters. 1994. Neuropsychological features of memory disorders in Alzheimer disease. In *Alzheimer disease.* (ed. R.D. Terry et al.), p. 41. Raven Press, New York.

Borchelt, D.R., M. Guarnieri, P.C. Wong, M.K. Lee, H.S. Slunt, Z. Xu, S.S. Sisodia, D.L. Price, and D.W. Cleveland. 1995. Superoxide dismutase 1 subunits with mutations linked to familial amyotrophic lateral sclerosis do not affect wild-type subunit function. *J. Biol. Chem.* **270:** 3234.

Borchelt, D.R., M.K. Lee, H.H. Slunt, M. Guarnieri, Z.-S. Xu, P.C. Wong, R.H. Brown, Jr., D.L. Price, S.S. Sisodia, and D.W. Cleveland. 1994. Superoxide dismutase 1 with mutations linked to familial amyotrophic lateral sclerosis possesses significant activity. *Proc. Natl. Acad. Sci.* **91:** 8292.

Borchelt, D.R., G. Thinakaran, C.B. Eckman, M.K. Lee, F. Davenport, T. Ratovitsky, C.-M. Praca, G. Kim, S. Seekins, D. Yager, H.H. Slunt, R. Wang, M. Seeger, A.I. Levey, S.E. Gandy, N.G. Copeland, N.A. Jenkins, D.L. Price, S.G. Younkin, and S.S. Sisodia. 1996. Familial Alzheimer's disease-linked presenilin 1 variants elevate Aβ1-42/1-40 ratio in vitro and in vivo. *Neuron* **17:** 1005.

Bowling, A.C., E.M. Mutisya, L.C. Walker, D.L. Price, L.C. Cork, and M.F. Beal. 1993. Age-dependent impairment of mitochondrial function in primate brain. *J Neurochem.* **60:** 1964.

Braak, H. and E. Braak. 1994. Pathology of Alzheimer's disease. In *Neurodegenerative diseases* (ed. D.B. Calne), p. 585. W.B. Saunders, Philadelphia.

Brizzee, K.R., J.M. Ordy, and R.T. Bartus. 1980. Localization of cellular changes within multimodal sensory regions in aged monkey brain: Possible implications for age-related cognitive loss. *Neurobiol. Aging* **1:** 45.

Burdick, D., B. Soreghan, M. Kwon, J. Kosmoski, M. Knauer, A. Henschen, J. Yates, C. Cotman, and C. Glabe. 1992. Assembly and aggregation properties of synthetic Alzheimer's A4/β amyloid peptide analogs. *J. Biol. Chem.* **267:** 546.

Busciglio, J., A. Lorenzo, J. Yeh, and B.A. Yankner. 1995. β-amyloid fibrils induce tau phosphorylation and loss of microtubule binding. *Neuron* **14:** 879.

Cai, X.-D., T.E. Golde, and S.G. Younkin. 1993. Release of excess amyloid β protein from a mutant amyloid β protein precursor. *Science* **259:** 514.

Carri, M.T., A. Battistoni, F. Polizio, A. Desideri, and G. Rotilio. 1994. Impaired copper binding by the H46R mutant of human Cu,Zn superoxide dismutase, involved in amyotrophic lateral sclerosis. *FEBS Lett.* **356:** 314.

Chartier-Harlin, M.-C., F. Crawford, H. Houlden, A. Warren, D. Hughes, L. Fidani, A. Goate, M. Rossor, P. Roques, J. Hardy, and M. Mullan. 1991. Early-onset Alzheimer's disease caused by mutations at codon 717 of the β-amyloid precursor protein gene. *Nature* **353:** 844.

Chou, S.M. 1992. Pathology-light microscopy of amyotrophic lateral sclerosis. In *Handbook of amyotrophic lateral sclerosis* (ed. R.A. Smith), p. 133. Marcel Dekker, New York.

Chou, S.-M. and H.A. Hartmann. 1964. Axonal lesions and waltzing syndrome after IDPN administration in rats. With a concept—"Axostasis". *Acta Neuropathol.* **3:** 428.

Citron, M., T. Oltersdorf, C. Haass, L. McConlogue, A.Y. Hung, P. Seubert, C. Vigo-Pelfrey, I. Lieberburg, and D.J. Selkoe. 1992. Mutation of the β-amyloid precursor protein in familial Alzheimer's disease increases β-protein production. *Nature* **360:** 672.

Clark, A.W., J.W. Griffin, and D.L. Price. 1980. The axonal pathology in chronic IDPN intoxication. *J. Neuropathol. Exp. Neurol.* **39:** 42.

Clark, A.W., I.M. Parhad, J.W. Griffin, and D.L. Price. 1984. Neurofilamentous axonal swellings as a normal finding in the spinal anterior horn of man and other primates. *J. Neuropathol. Exp. Neurol.* **43:** 253.

Clatterbuck, R.E., D.L. Price, and V.E. Koliatsos. 1994. Further characterization of the effects of brain-derived neurotrophic factor and ciliary neurotrophic factor on axotomized neonatal and adult mammalian motor neurons. *J. Comp. Neurol.* **342:** 45.

Cleveland, D.W., N. Laing, P.V. Hurse, and R.H. Brown, Jr. 1995. Toxic mutants in Charcot's sclerosis. *Nature* **378:** 342.

Cork, L.C., C. Masters, K. Beyreuther, and D.L. Price. 1990. Development of senile plaques. Relationships of neuronal abnormalities and amyloid deposits. *Am. J. Pathol.* **137:** 1383.

Cork, L.C., J.W. Griffin, C. Choy, C.A. Padula, and D.L. Price. 1982. Pathology of motor neurons in accelerated hereditary canine spinal muscular atrophy. *Lab. Invest.* **46:** 89.

Cork, L.C., J.W. Griffin, J.F. Munnell, M.D. Lorenz, R.J. Adams, and D.L. Price. 1979. Hereditary canine spinal muscular atrophy. *J. Neuropathol. Exp. Neurol.* **38:** 209.

Cork, L.C., R.G. Struble, B.G. Gold, C. DiCarlo, K.E. Fahnestock, J.W. Griffin, and D.L. Price. 1989a. Changes in size of motor axons in hereditary canine spinal muscular atrophy. *Lab. Invest.* **61:** 333.

Cork, L.C., R.J. Altschuler, P.J. Bruha, J.M. Morris, D.G. Lloyd, H.L. Loats, J.W. Griffin, and D.L. Price. 1989b. Changes in neuronal size and neurotransmitter marker in hereditary canine spinal muscular atrophy. *Lab. Invest.* **61:** 69.

Cotman, C.W. and C.J. Pike. 1994. β-amyloid and its contributions to neurodegeneration in Alzheimer disease. In *Alzheimer disease* (ed. R.D. Terry et al.), p 305. Raven Press, New York.

Davis, R.T. 1985. The effects of aging on the behavior of rhesus monkeys. In *Behavior and pathology of aging in rhesus monkeys* (ed. R.T. Davis and C.W. Leathers), p. 57. A.R. Liss, New York.

Deng, H.-X., A. Hentati, J.A. Tainer, Z. Iqbal, A. Cayabyab, W.-Y. Hung, E.D. Getzoff, P. Hu, B. Herzfeldt, R.P. Roos, C. Warner, G. Deng, E. Soriano, C. Smyth, H.E. Parge, A. Ahmed, A.D. Roses, R.A. Hallewell, M.A. Pericak-Vance, and T. Siddique. 1993. Amyotrophic lateral sclerosis and structural defects in Cu,Zn superoxide dismutase. *Science* **261:** 1047.

Doan, A., G. Thinakaran, A. Lanahan, D.L. Price, S.S. Sisodia, and P.E. Worley. 1996a. Identification and characterization of a presenilin 1 interacting protein. *Soc. Neurosci. Abstr.* **22:** 728.

Doan, A., G. Thinakaran, D.R. Borchelt, H.H. Slunt, T. Ratovitsky, M. Podlisny, D.J. Selkoe, M. Seeger, S.E. Gandy, D.L. Price, and S.S. Sisodia. 1996b. Protein topology of presenilin 1. *Neuron* **17:** 1023.

Duff, K., C. Eckman, C. Zehr, X. Yu, C.-M. Prada, J. Perez-Tur, M. Hutton, L. Buee, Y. Harigaya, D. Yager, D. Morgan, M.N. Gordon, L. Holcomb, L. Refolo, B. Zenk, J. Hardy, and S. Younkin. 1996. Increased amyloid-β42(43) in brains of mice expressing mutant presenilin 1. *Nature* **383:** 710.

Ehlers, M.D., D.R. Kaplan, D.L. Price, and V.E. Koliatsos. 1995. NGF-stimulated retrograde transport of trkA in the mammalian nervous system. *J. Cell Biol.* **130:** 149.

Elliott, J.L. and W.D. Snider. 1996. Motor neuron growth factors. *Neurology* **47:** S47.

Esch, F.S., P.S. Keim, E.C. Beattie, R.W. Blacher, A.R. Culwell, T. Oltersdorf, D. McClure, and P.J. Ward. 1990. Cleavage of amyloid β peptide during constitutive processing of its precursor. *Science* **248:** 1122.

Evans, D.A., H.H. Funkenstein, M.S. Albert, P.A. Scherr,

N.R. Cook, M.J. Chown, L.E. Hebert, C.H. Hennekens, and J.O. Taylor. 1989. Prevalence of Alzheimer's disease in a community population of older persons. Higher than previously reported. *J. Am. Med. Assoc.* **262:** 2551.

Fridovich, I. 1986. Superoxide dismutases. *Adv. Enzymol. Relat. Areas Mol. Biol.* **58:** 61.

Games, D., D. Adams, R. Alessandrini, R. Barbour, P. Berthelette, C. Blackwell, T. Carr, J. Clemens, T. Donaldson, F. Gillespie, T. Guido, S. Hagopian, K. Johnson-Wood, K. Khan, M. Lee, P. Leibowitz, I. Lieberburg, S. Little, E. Masliah, L. McConlogue, M. Montoya-Zavala, L. Mucke, L. Paganini, E. Penniman, M. Power, D. Schenk, P. Seubert, B. Snyder, F. Soriano, H. Tan, J. Vitale, S. Wadsworth, B. Wolozin, and J. Zhao. 1995. Alzheimer-type neuropathology in transgenic mice overexpressing V717F β-amyloid precursor protein. *Nature* **373:** 523.

Glenner, G.G. and C.W. Wong. 1984a. Alzheimer's disease: Initial report of the purification and characterization of a novel cerebrovascular amyloid protein. *Biochem. Biophys. Res. Commun.* **120:** 885.

———. 1984b. Alzheimer's disease and Down's syndrome: Sharing of a unique cerebrovascular amyloid fibril protein. *Biochem. Biophys. Res. Commun.* **122:** 1131.

Goate, A., M.-C. Chartier-Harlin, M. Mullan, J. Brown, F. Crawford, L. Fidani, L. Giuffra, A. Haynes, N. Irving, L. James, R. Mant, P. Newton, K. Rooke, P. Roques, C. Talbot, M. Pericak-Vance, A. Roses, R. Williamson, M. Rossor, M. Owen, and J. Hardy. 1991. Segregation of a missense mutation in the amyloid precursor protein gene with familial Alzheimer's disease. *Nature* **349:** 704.

Gold, B.G., J.W. Griffin, D.L. Price, L.C. Cork, and H.E. Lowndes. 1986. Structural correlates of physiological abnormalities in β,β′-iminodipropionitrile. *Brain Res.* **362:** 205.

Goldman-Rakic, P.S. and R.M. Brown. 1981. Regional changes of monoamines in cerebral cortex and subcortical structures of aging rhesus monkeys. *Neuroscience* **6:** 177.

Gonatas, N.K., A. Stieber, Z. Mourelatos, Y. Chen, J.O. Gonatas, S.H. Appel, A.P. Hays, W.F. Hickey, and J.-J. Hauw. 1992. Fragmentation of the Golgi apparatus of motor neurons in amyotrophic lateral sclerosis. *Am. J. Pathol.* **140:** 731.

Griffin, J.W. and D.L. Price. 1981a. Demyelination in experimental IDPN and hexacarbon neuropathies: Evidence for an axonal influence. *Lab. Invest.* **45:** 130.

———. 1981b. Schwann cell and glial responses in β,β′-iminodipropionitrile intoxication. I. Schwann cell and oligodendrocyte ingrowths. *J. Neurocytol.* **10:** 995.

Griffin, J.W., D.L. Price, and P.N. Hoffman. 1983a. Neurotoxic probes of the axonal cytoskeleton. *Trends Neurosci.* **6:** 490.

Griffin, J.W., L.C.. Cork, R.J. Adams, and D.L. Price. 1982a. Axonal transport in hereditary canine spinal muscular atrophy (HCSMA). *J. Neuropathol. Exp. Neurol.* **41:** 370.

Griffin, J.W., K.E. Fahnestock, D.L. Price, and L.C. Cork. 1983b. Cytoskeletal disorganization induced by local application of β,β′-iminodipropionitrile and 2,5-hexanedione. *Ann. Neurol.* **14:** 55.

Griffin, J.W., K.E. Fahnestock, D.L. Price, and P.N. Hoffman. 1983c. Microtubule-neurofilament segregation produced by β,β′-iminodipropionitrile: Evidence for the association of fast axonal transport with microtubules. *J. Neurosci.* **3:** 557.

Griffin, J.W., B.G. Gold, L.C. Cork, D.L. Price, and H.E. Lowndes. 1982b. IDPN neuropathy in the cat: Coexistence of proximal and distal axonal swellings. *Neuropathol. Appl. Neurobiol.* **8:** 351.

Griffin, J.W., P.N. Hoffman, A.W. Clark, P.T. Carroll, and D.L. Price. 1978. Slow axonal transport of neurofilament proteins: Impairment by β,β′-iminodipropionitrile administration. *Science* **202:** 633.

Gurney, M.E., F.B. Cuttings, P. Zhai, A. Doble, C.P. Taylor, P.K. Andrus, and E.D. Hall. 1996. Benefit of vitamin E, riluzole, and gabapentin in a transgenic model of familial amyotrophic lateral sclerosis. *Ann. Neurol.* **39:** 147.

Gurney, M.E., H. Pu, A.Y. Chiu, M.C. Dal Canto, C.Y. Polchow, D.D. Alexander, J. Caliendo, A. Hentati, Y.W. Kwon, H.-X. Deng, W. Chen, P. Zhai, R.L. Sufit, and T. Siddique. 1994. Motor neuron degeneration in mice that express a human Cu,Zn superoxide dismutase mutation. *Science* **264:** 1772.

Haass, C., A.Y. Hung, D.J. Selkoe, and D.B. Teplow. 1994. Mutations associated with a locus for familial Alzheimer's disease result in alternative processing of amyloid β-protein precursor. *J. Biol. Chem.* **269:** 17741.

Haass, C., A.Y. Hung, M.G. Schlossmacher, D.B. Teplow, and D.J. Selkoe. 1993. β-amyloid peptide and a 3-kDa fragment are derived by distinct cellular mechanisms. *J. Biol. Chem.* **268:** 3021.

Haass, C., M.G. Schlossmacher, A.Y. Hung, C. Vigo-Pelfrey, A. Mellon, B.L. Ostaszewski, I. Lieberburg, E.H. Koo, D. Schenk, D.B. Teplow, and D.J. Selkoe. 1992, Amyloid β-peptide is produced by cultured cells during normal metabolism. *Nature* **359:** 322.

Halliwell, B. 1992. Oxygen radicals as key mediators in neurological disease: Fact or fiction? *Ann. Neurol.* **32:** S10.

Halliwell, B. and J.M.C. Gutteridge. 1985. Oxygen radicals and the nervous system. *Trends Neurosci.* **8:** 22.

Heilbroner, P.L. and T.L. Kemper. 1990. The cytoarchitectonic distribution of senile plaques in three aged monkeys. *Acta Neuropathol.* **81:** 60.

Hendricks, L., C.M. van Duijn, P. Cras, M. Cruts, W. Van Hul, F. van Harskamp, A. Warren, M.G. McInnis, S.E. Antonarakis, J.-J. Martin, A. Hofman, and C. Van Broeckhoven. 1992. Presenile dementia and cerebal haemorrhage linked to a mutation at codon 692 of the β-amyloid precursor protein gene. *Nat. Genet.* **1:** 218.

Higgins, L.S., D.M. Holtzman, J. Rabin, W.C. Mobley, and B. Cordell. 1994. Transgenic mouse brain histopathology resembles early Alzheimer's disease. *Ann. Neurol.* **35:** 598.

Hirano, A. 1991. Cytopathology of amyotrophic lateral sclerosis. In *Amyotrophic lateral sclerosis and other motor neuron diseases* (ed. L.P. Rowland), p. 91. Raven Press, New York.

Hirano, A. and S. Kato. 1992. Fine structural study of sporadic and familial amyotrophic lateral sclerosis. In *Handbook of amyotrophic lateral sclerosis* (R.A. Smith), p. 183. Marcel Dekker, New York.

Howland, D.S., M.J. Savage, F.A. Huntress, R.E. Wallace, D.A. Schwartz, T. Loh, R.H. Melloni, Jr., L.J. DeGennaro, B.D. Greenberg, R. Siman, M.E. Swanson, and R.W. Scott. 1995. Mutant and native human β-amyloid precursor proteins in transgenic mouse brain. *Neurobiol. Aging* **16:** 685.

Hsiao, K., P. Chapman, S. Nilsen, C. Eckman, Y. Harigaya, S. Younkin, F.S. Yang, and G. Cole. 1996. Correlative memory deficits, Aβ elevation, and amyloid plaques in transgenic mice. *Science* **274:** 99.

Hsiao, K.K., D.R. Borchelt, K. Olson, R. Johannsdottir, C.

Kitt, W. Yunis, S. Xu, C. Eckman, S. Younkin, D. Price, C. Iadecola, H.B. Clark, and G. Carlson. 1995. Age-related CNS disorder and early death in transgenic FVB/N mice overexpressing Alzheimer amyloid precursor proteins. *Neuron* **15:** 1203.

Iwatsubo, T., D.M.A. Mann, A. Odaka, N. Suzuki, and Y. Ihara. 1995. Amyloid β protein (Aβ) deposition: Aβ42(43) precedes Aβ40 in Down syndrome. *Ann. Neurol.* **37:** 294.

Iwatsubo, T., A. Odaka, N. Suzuki, H. Mizusawa, N. Nukina, and Y. Ihara. 1994. Visualization of Aβ42(43)-positive and Aβ40-positive senile plaques with end-specific Aβ-monoclonal antibodies: Evidence that an initially deposited Aβ species is Aβ1-42(43). *Neuron* **13:** 45.

Jarrett, J.T. and P.T. Lansbury, Jr. 1993. Seeding "one-dimensional crystallization" of amyloid: A pathogenic mechanism in Alzheimer's disease and scrapie? *Cell* **73:** 1055.

Jarrett, J.T., E.P. Berger, and P.T. Lansbury, Jr. 1993. The carboxy terminus of the β amyloid protein is critical for the seeding of amyloid formation: Implications for the pathogenesis of Alzheimer's disease. *Biochemistry* **32:** 4693.

Kang, J., H.-G. Lemaire, A. Unterbeck, J.M. Salbaum, C.L. Masters, K.-H. Grzeschik, G. Multhaup, K. Beyreuther, and B. Müller-Hill. 1987. The precursor of Alzheimer's disease amyloid A4 protein resembles a cell-surface receptor. *Nature* **325:** 733.

Kato, S., M. Oda, and H. Hayashi. 1993. Neuropathology in amyotrophic lateral sclerosis patients on respirators: Uniformity and diversity in 13 cases. *Neuropathology* **13:** 229.

Kitt, C.A., L.C. Walker, M.E. Molliver, and D.L. Price. 1989. Serotoninergic neurites in senile plaques in cingulate cortex of aged nonhuman primate. *Synapse* **3:** 12.

Kitt, C.A., D.L. Price, R.G. Struble, L.C. Cork, B.H. Wainer, M.W. Becher, and W.C. Mobley. 1984. Evidence for cholinergic neurites in senile plaques. *Science* **226:** 1443.

Kitt, C.A., R.G. Struble, L.C. Cork, W.C. Mobley, L.C. Walker, T.H. Joh, and D.L. Price. 1985. Catecholaminergic neurites in senile plaques in prefrontal cortex of aged nonhuman primates. *Neuroscience* **16:** 691.

Koliatsos, V.E., R.E. Clatterbuck, J.W. Winslow, M.H. Cayouette, and D.L. Price. 1993. Evidence that brain-derived neurotrophic factor is a trophic factor for motor neurons in vivo. *Neuron* **10:** 359.

Koliatsos, V.E., M.H. Cayouette, L.R. Berkemeier, R.E. Clatterbuck, D.L. Price, and A. Rosenthal. 1994. Neurotrophin 4/5 is a trophic factor for mammalian facial motor neurons. *Proc. Natl. Acad. Sci.* **91:** 3304.

Koo, E.H., S.S. Sisodia, L.C. Cork, A. Unterbeck, R.M. Bayney, and D.L. Price. 1990a. Differential expression of amyloid precursor protein mRNAs in case of Alzheimer's disease and in aged nonhuman primates. *Neuron* **2:** 97.

Koo, E.H., S.S. Sisodia, D.R. Archer, L.J. Martin, A. Weidemann, K. Beyreuther, P. Fischer, C.L. Masters, and D.L. Price. 1990b. Precursor of amyloid protein in Alzheimer disease undergoes fast anterograde axonal transport. *Proc. Natl. Acad. Sci.* **87:** 1561.

Kovacs, D.M., H.J. Fausett, K.J. Page, T.-W. Kim, R.D. Moir, D.E. Merriam, R.D. Hollister, O.G. Hallmark, R. Mancini, K.M. Felsenstein, B.T. Hyman, R.E. Tanzi, and W. Wasco. 1996. Alzheimer-associated presenilins 1 and 2: Neuronal expression in brain and localization to intracellular membranes in mammalian cells *Nat. Med.* **2:** 224.

LaFerla, F.M., B.T. Tinkle, C.J. Bieberich, C.C. Haudenschild, and G. Jay. 1995. The Alzheimer's Aβ peptide induces neurodegeneration and apoptotic cell death in transgenic mice. *Nat. Genet.* **9:** 21.

Lamb, B.T., S.S. Sisodia, A.M. Lawler, H.H. Slunt, C.A. Kitt, W.G. Kearns, P.L. Pearson, D.L. Price, and J.D. Gearhart. 1993. Introduction and expression of the 400 kilobase *precursor amyloid protein* gene in transgenic mice. *Nat. Genet.* **5:** 22.

Lee, M.K., H.H. Slunt, L.J. Martin, G. Thinakaran, G. Kim, S.E. Gandy, M. Seeger, E. Koo, D.L. Price, and S.S. Sisodia. 1996. Expression of presenilin 1 and 2 (PS1 and PS2) in human and murine tissues. *J. Neurosci.* **16:** 7513.

Lee, V.M.-Y. 1995. Disruption of the cytoskeleton in Alzheimer's disease. *Curr. Opin. Neurobiol.* **5:** 663.

Lemere, C.A., J.K. Blusztajn, H. Yamaguchi, T. Wisniewski, T.C. Saido, and D.J. Selkoe. 1996. Sequence of deposition of heterogeneous amyloid β-peptides and APO E in Down syndrome: Implications for initial events in amyloid plaque formation. *Neurobiol. Dis.* **3:** 16.

Levitan, D. and I. Greenwald. 1995. Facilitation of *lin-12*-mediated signalling by *sel-12*, a *Caenorhabditis elegans* S182 Alzheimer's disease gene. *Nature* **377:** 351.

Levy, E., A. Amorim, B. Frangione, and L.C. Walker. 1995. β-amyloid precursor protein gene in squirrel monkeys with cerebral amyloid angiopathy. *Neurobiol. Aging* **16:** 805.

Levy-Lahad, E., E.M. Wijsman, E. Nemens, L. Anderson, K.A.B. Goddard, J.L. Weber, T.D. Bird, and G.D. Schellenberg. 1995a. A familial Alzheimer's disease locus on chromosome 1. *Science* **269:** 970.

Levy-Lahad, E., W. Wasco, P. Poorkaj, D.M. Romano, J. Oshima, W.H. Pettingell, C.-E. Yu, P.D. Jondro, S.D. Schmidt, K. Wang, A.C. Crowley, Y.-H. Fu, S.Y. Guenette, D. Galas, E. Nemens, E.M. Wijsman, T.D. Bird, G.D. Schellenberg, and R.E. Tanzi. 1995b. Candidate gene for the chromosome 1 familial Alzheimer's disease locus. *Science* **269:** 973.

Li, J., J. Ma, and H. Potter. 1995. Identification and expression analysis of a potential familial Alzheimer disease gene on chromosome 1 related to *AD3*. *Proc. Natl. Acad. Sci.* **92:** 12180.

Lorenz, M.D., L.C. Cork, J.W. Griffin, R.J. Adams, and D.L. Price. 1979. Hereditary spinal muscular atrophy in Brittany spaniels: Clinical manifestations. *J. Am. Vet. Med. Assoc.* **175:** 833.

Lowe, J. 1994. New pathological findings in amyotrophic lateral sclerosis. *J. Neurol. Sci.* **124:** 38.

Martin, L.J., C.A. Pardo, L.C. Cork, and D.L. Price. 1994. Synaptic pathology and glial responses to neuronal injury precede the formation of senile plaques and amyloid deposits in the aging cerebral cortex. *Am. J. Pathol.* **145:** 1358.

Martin, L.J., C.D. Blackstone, A.I. Levey, R.L. Huganir, and D.L. Price. 1993. AMPA glutamate receptor subunits are differentially distributed in rat brain. *Neuroscience* **53:** 327.

Martin, L.J., S.S. Sisodia, E.H. Koo, L.C. Cork, T.L. Dellovade, A. Weidemann, K. Beyreuther, C. Masters, and D.L. Price. 1991. Amyloid precursor protein in aged nonhuman primates. *Proc. Natl. Acad. Sci.* **88:** 1461.

Masters, C.L., G. Multhaup, G. Simms, J. Pottgiesser, R.N. Martins, and K. Beyreuther. 1985a. Neuronal origin of a cerebral amyloid: Neurofibrillary tangles of Alzheimer's disease contain the same protein as the amyloid of plaque cores and blood vessels. *EMBO J.* **4:** 2757.

Masters, C.L., G. Simms, N.A. Weinman, G. Multhaup, B.L.

McDonald, and K. Beyreuther. 1985b. Amyloid plaque core protein in Alzheimer disease and Down syndrome. *Proc. Natl. Acad. Sci.* **82:** 4245.

Miyakawa, T., S. Katsuragi, K. Yamashita, and K. Ohuchi. 1992. Morphological study of amyloid fibrils and preamyloid deposits in the brain with Alzheimer's disease. *Acta Neuropathol.* **83:** 340.

Mizusawa, H., S. Matsumoto, S.-H. Yen, A. Hirano, R.R. Rojas-Corona, and H. Donnefeld. 1989. Focal accumulation of phosphorylated neurofilaments within anterior horn cell in familial amyotrophic lateral sclerosis. *Acta Neuropathol.* **79:** 37.

Moran, P.M., L.S. Higgins, B. Cordell, and P.C. Moser. 1995. Age-related learning deficits in transgenic mice expressing the 751-amino acid isoform of human β-amyloid precursor protein. *Proc. Natl. Acad. Sci.* **92:** 5341.

Morelli, L., L. Wei, A. Amorim, J. McDermid, C.R. Abee, B. Frangione, L.C. Walker, and E. Levy. 1996. Cerebrovascular amyloidosis in squirrel monkeys and rhesus monkeys: Apolipoprotein E genotype. *FEBS Lett.* **379:** 132.

Morrison, B.M., J.W. Gordon, M.E. Ripps, and J.H. Morrison. 1996. Quantitative immunocytochemical analysis of the spinal cord in G86R superoxide dismutase transgenic mice: Neurochemical correlates of selective vulnerability. *J. Comp. Neurol.* **373:** 619.

Mullan, M., F. Crawford, K. Axelman, H. Houlden, L. Lillius, B. Winblad, and L. Lannfelt. 1992. A pathogenic mutation for probable Alzheimer's disease in the APP gene at the N-terminus of β-amyloid. *Nat. Genet.* **1:** 345.

Muma, N.A. and L.C. Cork. 1993. Alterations in neurofilament mRNA in hereditary canine spinal muscular atrophy. *Lab. Invest.* **69:** 436.

Naruse, S., S. Igarashi, H. Kobayashi, K. Aoki, T. Inuzuka, K. Kaneko, T. Shimizu, K. Iihara, T. Kojima, T. Miyatake, and S. Tsuji. 1991. Mis-sense mutation Val→Ile in exon 17 of amyloid precursor protein gene in Japanese familial Alzheimer's disease. *Lancet* **337:** 978.

Oppenheim, R.W., Y. Qin-Wei, D. Prevette, and Q. Yan. 1992. Brain-derived neurotrophic factor rescues developing avian motoneurons from cell death. *Nature* **360:** 755.

Oppenheimer, D.R. and M.M. Esiri. 1992. Diseases of the basal ganglia, cerebellum and motor neurons. In *Greenfield's neuropathology* (ed .J.H. Adams and L.W. Duchen), p. 988. Oxford University Press, New York.

Oster-Granite, M.L., D.L. McPhie, J. Greenan, and R.L. Neve. 1996. Age-dependent neuronal and synaptic degeneration in mice transgenic for the C terminus of the amyloid precursor protein. *J. Neurosci.* **16:** 6732.

Pike, C.J., D. Burdick, A.J. Walencewicz, C.G. Glabe, and C.W. Cotman. 1993. Neurodegeneration induced by β-amyloid peptides *in vitro*: The role of peptide assembly state. *J. Neurosci.* **13:** 1676.

Pinter, M.J., R.F. Waldeck, N. Wallace, and L.C. Cork. 1995. Motor unit behavior in canine motor neuron disease. *J. Neurosci.* **15:** 3447.

Poduri, A., M. Gearing, G.W. Rebeck, S.S. Mirra, J. Tigges, and B.T. Hyman. 1994. Apolipoprotein E4 and beta amyloid in senile plaques and cerebral blood vessels of aged rhesus monkeys. *Am. J. Pathol.* **144:** 1183.

Powell, H.C., T. Koch, R. Garrett, and P.W. Lampert. 1978. Schwann cell abnormalities in 2,5-hexanedione neuropathy. *J. Neurocytol.* **7:** 517.

Presty, S.K., J. Bachevalier, L.C. Walker, R.G. Struble, D.L. Price, M. Mishkin, and L.C. Cork. 1987. Age differences in recognition memory of the rhesus monkey (*Macaca mulatta*). *Neurobiol. Aging* **8:** 435.

Price, D.L. and S.S. Sisodia. 1994. Cellular and molecular biology of Alzheimer's disease and animal models. *Annu. Rev. Med.* **45:** 435.

Price, D.L., C.H. Kawas, and S.S. Sisodia. 1997. Aging of the brain and dementia of the Alzheimer's type. In *Principles of neural science* (ed. E.R. Kandel et al.). Elsevier, New York.

Rabizadeh, S., E. Butler Gralla, D.R. Borchelt, R. Gwinn, J. Selverstone Valentine, S. Sisodia, P. Wong, M. Lee, H. Hahn, and D.E. Bredesen. 1995. Mutations associated with amyotrophic lateral sclerosis convert superoxide dismutase from an antiapoptotic gene to a proapoptotic gene: Studies in yeast and neural cells. *Proc. Natl. Acad. Sci.* **92:** 3024.

Rapp, P.R. and D.G. Amaral. 1989. Evidence for task-dependent memory dysfunction in the aged monkey. *J. Neurosci.* **9:** 3568.

Rapp, P.R., M.T. Kansky, J.A. Roberts, and H. Eichenbaum. 1994. New directions for studying cognitive decline in old monkeys. *Semin. Neurosci.* **6:** 369.

Ridley, R.M., T.K. Murray, J.A. Johnson, and H.F. Baker. 1986. Learning impairment following lesion of the basal nucleus of Meynert in the marmoset: Modification by cholinergic drugs. *Brain Res.* **376:** 108.

Ripps, M.E., G.W. Huntley, P.R. Hof, J.H. Morrison, and J.W. Gordon. 1995. Transgenic mice expressing an altered murine superoxide dismutase gene provide an animal model of amyotrophic lateral sclerosis. *Proc. Natl. Acad. Sci.* **92:** 689.

Rogaev, E.I., R. Sherrington, E.A. Rogaeva, G. Levesque, M. Ikeda, Y. Liang, H. Chi, C. Lin, K. Holman, T. Tsuda, L. Mar, S. Sorbi, B. Nacmias, S. Piacentini, L. Amaducci, I. Chumakov, D. Cohen, L. Lannfelt, P.E. Fraser, J.M. Rommens, and P.H. St. George-Hyslop. 1995. Familial Alzheimer's disease in kindreds with missense mutations in a gene on chromosome 1 related to the Alzheimer's disease type 3 gene. *Nature* **376:** 775.

Rosen, C.L., R.P. Bunge, M.D. Ard, and P.M. Wood. 1989. Type 1 astrocytes inhibit myelination by adult rat oligodendrocytes *in vitro*. *J. Neurosci.* **9:** 3371.

Rosen, D.R., T. Siddique, D. Patterson, D.A. Figlewicz, P. Sapp, A. Hentati, D. Donaldson, J. Goto, J.P. O'Regan, H.-X. Deng, Z. Rahmani, A. Krizus, D. McKenna-Yasek, A. Cayabyab, S.M. Gaston, R. Berger, R.E. Tanzi, J.J. Halperin, B. Herzfeldt, R. Van den Bergh, W.-Y. Hung, T. Bird, G. Deng, D.W. Mulder, C. Smyth, N.G. Laing, E. Soriano, M.A. Pericak-Vance, J. Haines, G.A. Rouleau, J.S. Gusella, H.R. Horvitz, and R.H. Brown, Jr. 1993. Mutations in Cu/Zn superoxide dismutase gene are associated with familial amyotrophic lateral sclerosis. *Nature* **362:** 59.

Roses, A.D. 1995. Apolipoprotein E genotyping in the differential diagnosis, not prediction, of Alzheimer's disease. *Ann. Neurol.* **38:** 6.

Rothstein, J.D. 1996a. Therapeutic horizons for amyotrophic lateral sclerosis. *Curr. Opin. Neurobiol.* **6:** 679.

———. 1996b. Excitotoxicity hypothesis. *Neurology* **47:** S19.

Rothstein, J.D., L. Martin, A.I. Levey, M. Dykes-Hoberg, L. Jin, D. Wu, N. Nash, and R.W. Kuncl. 1994. Localization of neuronal and glial glutamate transporters. *Neuron* **13:** 713.

Rouleau, G.A., A.W. Clark, K. Rooke, A. Pramatarova, A. Krizus, O. Suchowersky, J.-P. Julien, and D. Figlewicz.

1996. SOD1 mutation is associated with accumulation of neurofilaments in amyotrophic lateral sclerosis. *Ann. Neurol.* **39:** 128.

Rowland, L.P. 1994. Natural history and clinical features of amyotrophic lateral sclerosis and related motor neuron diseases. In *Neurodegenerative diseases* (ed. D.B. Calne), p. 507. W.B. Saunders, Philadelphia.

Sack, G.H., Jr., L.C. Cork, J.M. Morris, J.W. Griffin, and D.L. Price. 1984. Autosomal dominant inheritance of hereditary canine spinal muscular atrophy. *Ann. Neurol.* **15:** 369.

Schellenberg, G.D. 1995. Progress in Alzheimer's disease genetics. *Curr. Opin. Neurol.* **8:** 262.

Scheuner, D., C. Eckman, M. Jensen, X. Song, M. Citron, N. Suzuki, T.D. Bird, J. Hardy, M. Hutton, W. Kukull, E. Larson, E. Levy-Lahad, M. Viitanen, E. Peskind, P. Poorkaj, G. Schellenberg, R. Tanzi, W. Wasco, L. Lannfelt, D. Selkoe, and S. Younkin. 1996. Secreted amyloid β-protein similar to that in the senile plaques of Alzheimer's disease is increased *in vivo* by the presenilin 1 and 2 and *APP* mutations linked to familial Alzheimer's disease. *Nat. Med.* **2:** 864.

Schmidt, M.L., M.J. Carden, V.M.-Y. Lee, and J.Q. Trojanowski. 1987. Phosphate dependent and independent neurofilament epitopes in the axonal swellings of patients with motor neuron disease and controls. *Lab. Invest.* **56:** 282.

Selkoe, D.J., D.S. Bell, M.B. Podlisny, D.L. Price, and L.C. Cork. 1987. Conservation of brain amyloid proteins in aged mammals and humans with Alzheimer's disease. *Science* **235:** 873.

Sendtner, M., B. Holtmann, R. Kolbeck, H Thoenen, and Y.-A. Barde. 1992. Brain-derived neurotrophic factor prevents the death of motoneurons in newborn rats after nerve section. *Nature* **360:** 757.

Sherrington, R., E.I. Rogaev, Y. Liang, E.A. Rogaeva, G. Levesque, M. Ikeda, H. Chi, C. Lin, G. Li, K. Holman, T. Tsuda, L. Mar, J.-F. Foncin, A.C. Bruni, M.P. Montesi, S. Sorbi, I. Rainero, L. Pinessi, L. Nee, I. Chumakov, D. Pollen, A. Brookes, P. Sanseau, R.J. Polinsky, W. Wasco, H.A.R. Da Silva, J.L. Haines, M.A. Pericak-Vance, R.E. Tanzi, A.D. Roses, P.E. Fraser, J.M. Rommens, and P.H. St George-Hyslop. 1995. Cloning of a gene bearing missense mutations in early-onset familial Alzheimer's disease. *Nature* **375:** 754.

Shibata, N., M. Hirano, and K. Kobayashi. 1993. Immunohistochemical demonstration of Cu/Zn superoxide dismutase in the spinal cord of patients with familial amyotrophic lateral sclerosis. *Acta Histochem. Cytochem.* **26:** 619.

Shibata, N., A. Hirano, M. Kobayashi, T. Siddique, H.-X. Deng, W.-Y. Hung, T. Kato, and K. Asayama. 1996. Intense superoxide dismutase-1 immunoreactivity in intracytoplasmic hyaline inclusions of familial amyotrophic lateral sclerosis with posterior column involvement. *J. Neuropathol. Exp. Neurol.* **55:** 481.

Shinkai, Y., M. Yoshimura, Y. Ito, A. Odaka, N. Suzuki, K. Yanagisawa, and Y. Ihara. 1995. Amyloid β-proteins 1-40 and 1-42(43) in the soluble fraction of extra- and intracranial blood vessels. *Ann. Neurol.* **38:** 421.

Shoji, M., T.E. Golde, J. Ghiso, T.T. Cheung, S. Estus, L.M. Shaffer, X.-D. Cai, D.M. McKay, R. Tintner, B. Frangione, and S.G. Younkin. 1992. Production of the Alzheimer amyloid β protein by normal proteolytic processing. *Science* **258:** 126.

Siddique, T., M.A. Pericak-Vance, B.R. Brooks, R.P. Roos, W.-Y. Hung, J.P. Antel, T.L. Munsat, K. Phillips, K. Warner, M. Speer, W.B. Bias, N.A. Siddique, and A.D. Roses. 1989. Linkage analysis in familial amyotrophic lateral sclerosis. *Neurology* **39:** 919.

Siddique, T., D.A. Figlewicz, M.A. Pericak-Vance, J.L. Haines, G. Rouleau, A.J. Jeffers, P. Sapp, W.-Y. Hung, J. Bebout, D. McKenna-Yasek, G. Deng, H.B. Horvitz, J.F. Gusella, R.H. Brown, Jr., A.D. Roses, R.P. Roos, D.B. Williams, D.W. Mulder, P.C. Watkins, R. Noore, G. Nicholson, R. Reed, B.R. Brooks, B. Festoff, J.P. Antel, R. Tandan, T.L. Munsat, N.G. Laing, J.J. Halperin, F.H. Norris, R. Van den Bergh, L. Swerts, R.E. Tanzi, B. Jubelt, K.D. Mathews, and E.P. Bosch. 1991. Linkage of a gene causing familial amyotrophic lateral sclerosis to chromosome 21 and evidence of genetic-locus heterogeneity. *N. Engl. J. Med.* **324:** 1381.

Simmons, L.K., P.C. May, K.J. Tomaselli, R.E. Rydel, K.S. Fuson, E.F. Brigham, S. Wright, I. Lieberburg, G.W. Becker, D.N. Brems, et al. 1994. Secondary structure of amyloid beta peptide correlates with neurotoxic activity in vitro. *Mol. Pharmacol.* **45:** 373.

Sisodia, S.S. 1992. β-amyloid precursor protein cleavage by a membrane-bound protease. *Proc. Natl. Acad. Sci.* **89:** 6075.

Sisodia, S.S., E.H. Koo, K. Beyreuther, A. Unterbeck, and D.L. Price. 1990. Evidence that β-amyloid protein in Alzheimer's disease is not derived by normal processing. *Science* **248:** 492.

Sisodia, S.S., E.H. Koo, P.N. Hoffman, G. Perry, and D.L. Price. 1993. Identification and transport of full-length amyloid precursor proteins in rat peripheral nervous system. *J. Neurosci.* **13:** 3136.

Slunt, H.H., G. Thinakaran, M.K. Lee, and S.S. Sisodia. 1995. Nucleotide sequence of the chromosome 14-encoded *S182* cDNA and revised secondary structure prediction. *Int. J. Exp. Clin. Invest. (Amyloid)* **2:** 188.

Smith, M.C. 1955. Argyrophile bodies in the human spinal cord. *J. Neurol. Neurosurg. Psychiatry* **18:** 13.

St. George-Hyslop, P.H., P. Haines, E. Rogaev, M. Mortilla, G. Vaula, M. Pericak-Vance, J.-F. Foncin, M. Montesi, A. Bruni, S. Sorbi, I. Rainero, L. Pinessi, D. Pollen, R. Polinsky, L. Nee, J. Kennedy, F. Macciardi, E. Rogaeva, Y. Liang, N. Alexandrova, W. Lukiw, K. Schlumpf, R. Tanzi, T. Tsuda, L. Farrer, J.-M. Cantu, R. Duara, L. Amaducci, L. Bergamini, J. Gusella, A. Roses, and D. Crapper McLachlan. 1992. Genetic evidence for a novel familial Alzheimer's disease locus on chromosome 14. *Nat. Genet.* **2:** 330.

Struble, R.G., L.C. Cork, P.J. Whitehouse, and D.L. Price. 1982. Cholinergic innervation in neuritic plaques. *Science* **216:** 413.

Struble, R.G., J.C. Hedreen, L.C. Cork, and D.L Price. 1984. Acetylcholinesterase activity in senile plaques of aged macaques. *Neurobiol. Aging* **5:** 191.

Struble, R.G., D.L. Price, Jr., L.C. Cork, and D.L. Price. 1985. Senile plaques in cortex of aged normal monkeys. *Brain Res.* **361:** 267.

Su, J.H., A.J. Anderson, B.J. Cummings, and C.W. Cotman. 1994. Immunohistochemical evidence for apoptosis in Alzheimer's disease. *Neuroreport* **5:** 2529.

Sussman, S.J., R.L. Magoffin, E.H. Lennette, and J. Schieble. 1966. Cold agglutinins, Eaton agent, and respiratory infections of children. *Pediatrics* **38:** 571.

Suzuki, N., T.T. Cheung, X.-D. Cai, A. Odaka, L. Otvos, Jr., C. Eckman, T.E. Golde, and S.G. Younkin. 1994. An increased percentage of long amyloid β protein secreted by familial amyloid β protein precursor (βAPP_{717}) mutants. *Science* **264:** 1336.

Takahashi, K., H. Nakamura, and E. Okada. 1972. Hereditary amyotrophic lateral sclerosis. Histochemical and electron microscopic study of hyaline inclusions in motor neurons. *Arch. Neurol.* **27:** 292.

Tandan, R. and W.G. Bradley. 1985. Amyotrophic lateral sclerosis: Part 1. Clinical features, pathology, and ethical issues in management. *Ann. Neurol.* **18:** 271.

Thinakaran, G., D.B. Teplow, R. Siman, B. Greenberg, and S.S. Sisodia. 1996a. Metabolism of the "Swedish" APP variant in Neuro2A (N2a) cells: Evidence that cleavage at the "β-secretase" site occurs in the Golgi apparatus. *J. Biol. Chem.* **271:** 9390.

Thinakaran, G., D.R. Borchelt, M.K. Lee, H.H. Slunt, L. Spitzer, G. Kim, T. Ratovitski, F. Davenport, C. Nordstedt, M. Seeger, J. Hardy, A.I. Levey, S.E. Gandy, N. Jenkins, N. Copeland, D.L. Price, and S.S. Sisodia. 1996b. Endoproteolysis of presenilin 1 and accumulation of processed derivatives *in vivo*. *Neuron* **17:** 181.

Tigges, J., T.P. Gordon, H.M. McClure, E.C. Hall, and A. Peters. 1988. Survival rate and life span of rhesus monkeys at the Yerkes Regional Primate Research Center. *Am. J. Primatol.* **15:** 263.

Troncoso, J.C., R.R. Sukhov, C.H. Kawas, and V.E. Koliatsos. 1996. *In situ* labeling of dying cortical neurons in normal aging and in Alzheimer's disease: Correlations with senile plaques and disease progression. *J. Neuropathol. Exp. Neurol.* **55:** 1134.

Wagster, M.V., P.J. Whitehouse, L.C. Walker, K.J. Kellar, and D.L. Price. 1990, Laminar organization and age-related loss of cholinergic receptors in temporal neocortex of rhesus monkey. *J. Neurosci.* **10:** 2879.

Walker, L.C. 1991. Animal models of cerebral amyloidosis. *Bull. Clin. Neurosci.* **56:** 86.

———. 1994. The senescent primate brain. *Semin. Neurosci.* **6:** 379.

Walker, L.C., C. Masters, K. Beyreuther, and D.L. Price. 1990, Amyloid in the brains of aged squirrel monkeys. *Acta Neuropathol.* **80:** 381.

Walker, L.C., C.A. Kitt, L.C. Cork, R.G. Struble, T.L. Dellovade, and D.L. Price. 1988a. Multiple transmitter systems contribute neurites to individual senile plaques. *J. Neuropathol. Exp. Neurol.* **47:** 138.

Walker, L.C., C.A. Kitt, R.G. Struble, M.V. Wagster, D.L. Price, and L.C. Cork. 1988b. The neural basis of memory decline in aged monkeys. *Neurobiol. Aging* **9:** 657.

Walker, L.C., C.A. Kitt, E. Schwam, B. Buckwald, F. Garcia, J. Sepinwall, and D.L. Price. 1987. Senile plaques in aged squirrel monkeys. *Neurobiol. Aging* **8:** 291.

Walker, L.C., C.A. Kitt, R.G. Struble, D.E. Schmechel, W.H. Oertel, L.C. Cork, and D.L. Price. 1985. Glutamic acid decarboxylase-like immunoreactive neurites in senile plaques. *Neurosci. Lett.* **59:** 165.

Wang, R., J.F. Meschia, R.J. Cotter, and S.S. Sisodia. 1991. Secretion of the β/A4 amyloid precursor protein. Identification of a cleavage site in cultured mammalian cells. *J. Biol. Chem.* **266:** 16960.

Wenk, G.L., D.J. Pierce, R.G. Struble, D.L. Price, and L.C. Cork. 1989. Age-related changes in multiple neurotransmitter systems in the monkey brain. *Neurobiol. Aging* **10:** 11.

Wiedau-Pazos, M., J.J. Goto, S. Rabizadeh, E.B. Gralla, J.A. Roe, M.K. Lee, J.S. Valentine, and D.E. Bredesen. 1996. Altered reactivity of superoxide dismutase in familial amyotrophic lateral sclerosis. *Science* **271:** 515.

Williams, D.B. and A.J. Windebank. 1993. Motor neuron disease. In *Peripheral neuropathy* (ed. P.J. Dyck et al.), p. 1028. W.B. Saunders, Philadelphia.

Wisniewski, H.M. and R.D. Terry. 1973a. Morphology of the aging brain, human and animal. *Prog. Brain Res.* **40:** 167.

———. 1973b. Reexamination of the pathogeneisis of the senile plaque. In *Progress in neuropathology* (ed. H.M. Zimmerman), p. 1. Grune and Stratton, New York.

Wisniewski, H.M., J. Wegiel, K.C. Wang, and B. Lach. 1992. Ultrastructural studies of the cells forming amyloid in the cortical vessel wall in Alzheimer's disease. *Acta Neuropathol.* **84:** 117.

Wisniewski, T., J. Ghiso, and B. Frangione. 1991. Peptides homologous to the amyloid protein of Alzheimer's disease containing a glutamine for glutamic acid substitution have accelerated amyloid fibril formation. *Biochem. Biophys. Res. Commun.* **179:** 1247.

Wong, P.C., C.A. Pardo, D.R. Borchelt, M.K. Lee, N.G. Copeland, N.A. Jenkins, S.S. Sisodia, D.W. Cleveland, and D.L. Price. 1995. An adverse property of a familial ALS-linked SOD1 mutation causes motor neuron disease characterized by vacuolar degeneration of mitochondria. *Neuron* **14:** 1105.

Yan, Q., J. Elliott, and W.D. Snider. 1992. Brain-derived neurotrophic factor rescues spinal motor neurons from axotomy-induced cell death. *Nature* **360:** 753.

Yuen, E.C. and W.C. Mobley. 1996. Therapeutic potential of neurotrophic factors for neurological disorders. *Ann. Neurol.* **40:** 346.

Extracellular Proteases in Neuronal Function and Degeneration

S. STRICKLAND, A. GUALANDRIS, A.D. ROGOVE,
AND S.E. TSIRKA
Department of Pharmacology, University Medical Center at Stony Brook, New York 11794-8651

A central question in neuronal function concerns the activity-dependent modification of synapses, which can include both intracellular and extracellular changes. For the extracellular events, attention has been directed at the modulation of release and binding of neurotransmitters. However, in addition to neurotransmitters, a complex array of molecules is present in the extracellular space, as a result of constitutive or regulated secretion from pre- and postsynaptic cells. Regulation of any of these molecules could participate in synaptic modulation.

The identification of synaptic regulators is a daunting task, due to the cellular and architectural complexity of the nervous system and the subtlety of the changes that occur normally. One approach that has proven valuable is to induce pathological alterations in the nervous system, which may represent exaggerated forms of normal, subtle changes, and to analyze the consequences of these alterations. The study of experimentally induced, neurodegenerative situations has the additional benefit that a better understanding of the pathology might allow development of new therapeutic approaches.

Accumulating data indicate that the extracellular protease tissue plasminogen activator (tPA) plays an important role in the mammalian CNS. Here, we review the evidence that an extracellular proteolytic cascade contributes both to neuronal degeneration and to normal processes involved in learning and memory.

RESULTS

The Hippocampus and Neuronal Degeneration

The hippocampus, a bilateral structure in the temporal lobe of the brain, is where learning and memory are consolidated (Amaral 1994). Four main cell types are present in the hippocampus: neurons, oligodendrocytes, astrocytes, and microglia. In simple terms, the neurons provide the electrical activity of the region, the oligodendrocytes produce myelin, the astrocytes support the neurons in various ways (e.g., by producing growth factors), and the microglia are cells of nonneuronal origin, which have properties of tissue-specific macrophages (Altman 1994).

The function of the hippocampus was first discovered in patients who underwent bilateral removal of this region. These patients are unable to learn and/or retrieve new information, but their ability to recall old information remains intact (anterograde amnesia; Amaral 1994). Neurons in this crucial region of the brain are sensitive to degeneration in various neuropathologies such as stroke, epilepsy, and Alzheimer's disease, and a consequence of this degeneration is profound memory and cognitive impairment.

Tissue Plasminogen Activator

tPA is a serine protease that converts the inactive zymogen plasminogen to the active serine protease plasmin (Vassalli et al. 1991). This protease cascade is capable of generating potent proteolytic activity, which can be attenuated by inhibitors. tPA exists as a single gene in mammals, and the protein has been well-characterized biochemically. Although tPA was originally thought to be primarily a fibrinolytic protease, the enzyme is produced in a wide variety of tissues and situations that suggest it has additional functions, e.g., in the brain, maturing oocyte, oviduct, endocrine pancreas, pituitary, and adrenal medulla (Rickles and Strickland 1988).

Given the widespread expression of tPA, it was surprising that mice deficient for tPA develop normally and produce fertile adults (Carmeliet et al. 1994). This result prompted an intensified search for in vivo functions for the enzyme. In this respect, our finding that tPA mediates neuronal death in the mouse hippocampus (described below) provides a new experimental system to analyze the function of this enzyme in an in vivo context.

tPA in the Central Nervous System

Proteolytic activity has been correlated with various aspects of neurogenesis (for review, see Pittman 1990). Evidence suggests that tPA has a role in the function of mammalian CNS:

1. tPA mRNA is highly expressed in both neurons and microglial cells of the mouse hippocampus (Sappino et al. 1993; Qian et al. 1993; Tsirka et al. 1995, 1997).
2. tPA enzyme activity is high in the mouse hippocampus and hypothalamus. However, some regions that contain high mRNA levels showed little en-

zymatic activity. Analysis of this discrepancy suggests that protease inhibitors are attenuating the expressed activity (Sappino et al. 1993).

3. tPA mRNA is up-regulated in the rat and mouse hippocampus after experimentally induced seizures (Qian et al. 1993; Carroll et al. 1994).
4. Learning and memory involve increased sensitivity of synapses between active neurons. It is possible to model this change, known as long-term potentiation (LTP), by stimulating neuronal pathways and measuring subsequent synaptic enhancement (Bliss and Collingridge 1993). In $tPA^{-/-}$ mice, the late phase of LTP is abnormal (Frey et al. 1996; Huang et al. 1996), linking the enzyme to normal hippocampal functions.
5. $tPA^{-/-}$ mice are resistant to experimentally induced neuronal degeneration and seizure (Tsirka et al. 1995; described below).
6. In PC12 cells (a rat adrenal-derived pheochromocytoma cell line) and primary hippocampal neurons, tPA is stored inside the cells, and its secretion is induced by depolarization (Gualandris et al. 1996; Parmer et al. 1997). This regulated secretion, which is reminiscent of the release of neurotransmitters, implicates tPA in normal synaptic activity.
7. tPA mRNA levels were enhanced in Purkinje cells of the cerebellum in rats presented with a motor learning task (Seeds et al. 1995).

In summary, tPA expression appears to be involved in critical functions of the CNS, but there are many unanswered questions concerning the mechanism by which this enzyme affects neurons.

An Experimental Paradigm for Studying Neuronal Degeneration

In molecular terms, it is not known why hippocampal neurons die in neurodegenerative disorders, but many of these pathologies—including ischemic stroke, epilepsy, glaucoma, Huntington's disease, and perhaps Alzheimer's disease—are thought to involve the increased release of the excitatory amino acid glutamate (excitotoxicity, Lipton and Rosenberg 1994). We have therefore used injection of glutamate analogs into the mouse hippocampus as a model system to achieve excessive excitotoxin concentration and to effect neuronal degeneration.

In this model, mice are anesthetized and placed in a stereotaxic apparatus. Using published coordinates for brain anatomy, substances can be injected into defined regions of the brain. When glutamate or other potent glutamate analogs, such as kainate (which acts on the kainate type of glutamate receptors), are injected into the hippocampus, neurons are reproducibly destroyed in the injected region (Coyle et al. 1978; Andersson et al. 1991). The neuronal cell loss can be easily visualized by preparing sections of the brain one or more days after injection and staining the sections with cresyl violet. This dye stains ribosomal RNA, and the neurons, by virtue of their large size and abundant ribosomes, are more intensely stained than any other cell type in the brain. Thus, in an untreated mouse, the neuronal layers of the hippocampus are stained blue. In contrast, after kainate injection, the blue staining largely disappears in the hippocampal regions CA1, CA2, and CA3, confirming neuron loss. Serial sections can be examined by camera lucida drawings to quantitate the degree of degeneration (Tsirka et al. 1995).

We have used this system to investigate the function of tPA in the CNS. The model has several advantages: (1) By concentrating on the hippocampus, we can perform experiments in the whole animal. Since the cellular interactions in the CNS are extraordinarily complex and largely unknown, an in vivo approach is an important component of the analysis. (2) Since the experiments are performed primarily in mice, we can exploit the power of mouse genetics (e.g., transgenic animals, targeted mutants). (3) We can dramatically alter degeneration by delivery of exogenous proteases and protease inhibitors to the hippocampus, thus opening up a biochemical approach to the problem. Below, we summarize the results of applying this logic to the study of extracellular proteases in the mouse hippocampus.

tPA Mediates Neuronal Degeneration in the Mouse Hippocampus

We have two lines of evidence indicating that tPA plays a critical role in neuronal degeneration:

1. $tPA^{-/-}$ mice are resistant to excitotoxin-mediated neuronal degeneration. To determine if tPA has a function in neuronal degeneration, we analyzed neuronal destruction elicited by glutamate analogs in mice lacking tPA (Carmeliet et al. 1994). Mice deficient for tPA are highly resistant to neuronal degeneration after kainate injection (Fig. 1; quantitation shown in Table 1). The $tPA^{-/-}$ mice are also resistant to degeneration invoked by agonists whose action is mediated through the AMPA or NMDA subtype of glutamate receptors (Tsirka et al. 1995). Thus, the decrease in neuronal cell death in $tPA^{-/-}$ mice is observed with a wide range of glutamate analogs, which act through different receptor classes.
2. $tPA^{-/-}$ mice are resistant to chemically induced seizure. Since tPA is induced in the hippocampus after seizure (Qian et al. 1993), we analyzed the response of $tPA^{-/-}$ mice to seizure induction. The convulsants metrazol or kainate were injected i.p. Wild-type mice exhibited seizures soon after the drug administration. In contrast, the $tPA^{-/-}$ mice were resistant to seizure (Tsirka et al. 1995). The $tPA^{-/-}$ genotype affected both the dose of agent required to produce seizure and the time delay between drug delivery and seizure onset.

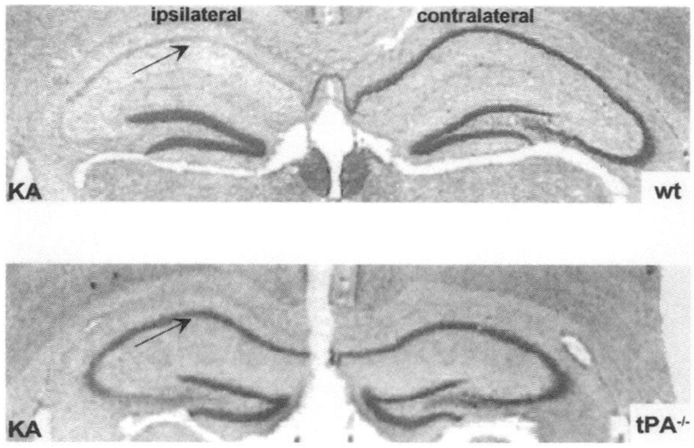

Figure 1. tPA$^{-/-}$ mice are resistant to excitotoxin-induced degeneration in the hippocampus. Low-magnification cresyl violet staining of coronal brain sections through the hippocampus. Kainate was injected into wild-type and tPA$^{-/-}$ mice. The top panel shows unilateral degeneration (loss of staining) on the injected side (ipsilateral) in wild-type mice, the bottom panel shows lack of degeneration in tPA$^{-/-}$ mice. (Reprinted, with permission, from Tsirka et al. 1995 [copyright Macmillan].)

An interesting possible connection to these results has emerged from studies on human epilepsy. Mutations in cystatin B, a cysteine protease inhibitor, lead to a familial progressive myoclonus epilepsy (Pennacchio et al. 1996). A conceptual link exists between these results in humans and our results in mice: too little protease, resistance to seizure; too little protease inhibitor, increased susceptibility to seizure. The connection is not direct, since cystatin B would not be expected to inhibit with high-affinity serine proteases like tPA. In addition, cystatin B is presumed to be intracellular, and tPA's role is thought to be extracellular. Nevertheless, it seems possible that these results, involving a balance between protease activity and inhibition, may be linked in ways that are not yet appreciated.

Plasminogen-deficient Mice Are Resistant to Neuronal Degeneration

The above results demonstrated using two distinct experimental systems that tPA functions in neuronal degeneration. The only known physiological substrate for tPA is the zymogen plasminogen, which tPA can activate to the active protease plasmin. To determine if tPA mediates neuronal destruction via activation of plasminogen, we analyzed neuronal degeneration in plasminogen-deficient (plg$^{-/-}$) mice (Bugge et al. 1995). These mice were equally resistant to degeneration as tPA$^{-/-}$ mice (Table 1). Our results suggest that activation of plasminogen is a critical step in tPA-mediated destruction of neurons.

There is another form of plasminogen activator in mammals designated urokinase-type plasminogen activator (uPA). Although uPA is produced in many tissues, it is not found in the hippocampus (Rickles and Strickland 1988; Sappino et al. 1993). To test if a reduction in systemic plasminogen activation might be contributing to the phenotype, we tested uPA$^{-/-}$ mice (Carmeliet et al. 1994) for kainate-mediated degeneration. These mice did not exhibit resistance. Given the role of tPA in fibrinolysis, we also analyzed whether fibrinogen or fibrin might be playing a role in degeneration. Fibrinogen-deficient mice (Suh et al. 1995) did not exhibit resistance to excitotoxins. These results are summarized in Table 2.

Table 1. Resistance to Neuronal Degeneration in Mice Deficient in Components of the Fibrinolytic System

Genotype	Resistance to kainate-induced neuronal degeneration
tPA$^{-/-a}$	yes[d]
Plasminogen$^{-/-b}$	yes[e]
uPA$^{-/-a}$	no[e]
Fibrinogen$^{-/-c}$	no[e]

[a]Carmeliet et al. 1994; [b]Bugge et al. 1995; [c]Suh et al. 1995; [d]Tsirka et al. 1995 [e]Tsirka et al. 1997.

tPA Is Expressed in the Hippocampus by Both Neurons and Microglial Cells, Whereas Plasminogen Is Expressed Exclusively by Neurons

Given the effects of tPA and plasminogen on neuronal degeneration, we examined whether these proteins were synthesized in the hippocampus. Although tPA is widely expressed in mammals (Rickles and Strickland 1988), plasminogen is an abundant serum protein synthesized primarily in the liver (Raum et al. 1980) and is too large to traverse the blood-brain barrier without a specialized transport system. Therefore, plasminogen in the hippocampus could be derived either from the blood-borne protein via leakage or transport, or from local synthesis (suggested by Sappino et al. 1993).

Table 2. Genotype and Administration of tPA and PAI-1 Modulate Sensitivity to Neuronal Degeneration in the Hippocampus

Material infused	% of CA1–CA3 region that remains intact after kainate injection into: wild-type mice	tPA$^{-/-}$ mice	plg$^{-/-}$ mice
Buffer[a]	12.2 ± 5.6 (n=15)	95.6 ± 1.1 (n=15)	93.3 ± 3.1 (n=4)
tPA	n.d.	9.7 ± 4.8 (n=3)	n.d.
PAI-1[b]	74.6 ± 5.8 (n=2)	n.d.	n.d.

This table gives a summary of the neuroprotection obtained. For more detailed quantitation, see Tsirka et al. (1996). (n.d.) Not determined.

[a]The infusion of buffer was performed as an experimental control for tPA and PAI-1 infusions and had no effect on neuronal degeneration when compared to non-infused animals.

[b]Similar results were obtained with α_2-antiplasmin and tPA-Stop.

To determine the sites of synthesis of tPA and plasminogen mRNA, in situ hybridization was used on control or kainate-injected brain sections. tPA mRNA was detected along the neuronal cell layers in the hippocampus as described previously (Qian et al. 1993; Sappino et al. 1993; Carroll et al. 1994). At higher magnification, the pattern of tPA mRNA along the neuronal cell layer was complex, suggesting that synthesis was occurring both in neurons and in perineuronal microglial cells. In addition, after destruction of neurons by kainate injection, the staining disappeared in the larger cells (neurons) but remained in the darker and smaller microglial cells. These results, coupled with extensive double-labeling experiments, demonstrate that tPA mRNA is produced both in neurons (the staining that disappears after injection of kainate) and in the microglia that overlie the neuronal cell layer (the staining that persists after kainate injection).

Plasminogen mRNA was also detected in the hippocampus along the neuronal cell layers. However, plasminogen mRNA was detected only in large neuronal cells. The mRNA staining was completely abolished by kainate destruction of neurons, demonstrating that the sole source of plasminogen expression is neurons.

It was also of interest to determine whether tPA and plasminogen proteins were present in the hippocampus. The presence of tPA protein was examined by immunohistochemistry (Tsirka et al. 1997) and by determining tPA activity on tissue sections (Sappino et al. 1993; Tsirka et al. 1995; Gualandris et al. 1996). tPA enzyme activity is primarily detected in CA2-3 and the dentate gyrus, and is not detected in the CA1 region.

We investigated the presence of plasminogen protein by immunohistochemistry (Tsirka et al. 1997). Although plasminogen mRNA is present in most hippocampal neurons, only a small subset of neurons stained for plasminogen protein. These results demonstrate that tPA and plasminogen are synthesized in the hippocampus and suggest that posttranscriptional regulation may control the expression of plasminogen protein.

Infusion of tPA Protein into tPA-deficient Mice Restores Sensitivity to Excitotoxin-mediated Neuronal Degeneration

$tPA^{-/-}$ and $plasminogen^{-/-}$ mice, which are both resistant to neuronal degeneration, develop normally (Carmeliet et al. 1994; Bugge et al. 1995) and do not exhibit any obvious hippocampal abnormalities (Tsirka et al 1995; Frey et al. 1996). However, the prenatal and postnatal development of these mice could have led to subtle alterations in brain architecture or circuitry, which could serve as an explanation for the resistance to excitotoxins.

One method of addressing this concern would be to reestablish the wild-type phenotype in an adult deficient mouse by restoration of the targeted gene product (see, e.g., Zhou et al. 1995). Therefore, we delivered buffer or recombinant tPA to $tPA^{-/-}$ mice via a subcutaneously placed minipump for 2 days, then injected kainate intracerebrally. After an additional 5 days, sections were examined for neuronal degeneration. If sensitivity to kainate was restored by tPA, it would demonstrate that the resistance in the $tPA^{-/-}$ mice is a consequence of lack of the enzyme at the time of excitotoxin administration.

$tPA^{-/-}$ mice infused with buffer did not exhibit significant neuronal degeneration after unilateral kainate injection, showing that the infusion protocol does not influence the resistant phenotype reported previously (Tsirka et al. 1995). In contrast, $tPA^{-/-}$ mice infused with tPA (either the human or mouse enzyme) exhibited dramatic neuronal degeneration in the CA1-CA3 regions of the hippocampus after injection of kainate (Table 1) (Tsirka et al. 1996). To verify that the infusion of tPA was generating proteolytic activity, cryostat brain sections of these mice were subjected to an in situ tPA activity assay (Sappino et al. 1993; Tsirka et al. 1995). Proteolytic activity was detected bilaterally over the hippocampus of the infused $tPA^{-/-}$ mice, whereas no tPA activity was observed in $tPA^{-/-}$ mice infused with buffer. The activity determinations further showed that tPA had been delivered equally to both cerebral hemispheres. Since degeneration was only observed in the kainate-injected side and not in the uninjected side, the conclusion can be drawn that tPA activity alone at this concentration is not sufficient to kill neurons.

These results indicate that tPA is acutely required for neuronal death at the time of excitotoxic insult. They also validate intra-hippocampal infusion as an experimental paradigm for intervention in the degeneration process (Tsirka et al. 1996).

Inhibition of tPA or Plasmin Confers Resistance to Excitotoxin-mediated Neuronal Degeneration in Wild-type Mice

Since tPA is required at the time of excitotoxin injection to mediate neuronal degeneration, it was possible that inhibition of enzymatic activity might retard neuronal cell death. For these experiments, protease inhibitors were delivered via minipump for 2 days into wild-type mice, and kainate was then injected intracerebrally. After a further 5 days, sections were examined for neuronal degeneration. To date, we have tested three inhibitors:

1. *Mouse plasminogen activator inhibitor-1(PAI-1).* PAI-1 is a serine protease inhibitor (serpin) that inhibits tPA and uPA (Hekman and Loskutoff 1988). Since uPA is not found in the mouse hippocampus (Rickles and Strickland 1988; Sappino et al. 1993), the only known target for PAI-1 in this tissue would be tPA. Mice were infused with PAI-1 (obtained

from American Diagnostica) and injected 2 days later with kainate. Then the status of neuronal cells in the hippocampus was evaluated. As expected, control, wild-type mice infused with buffer were sensitive to neuronal degeneration (Fig. 2, top). In contrast, mice infused with PAI-1 were resistant to kainate-induced neuronal death (Fig. 2, bottom). The resistance of these PAI-1-infused wild-type mice was comparable to that observed with untreated $tPA^{-/-}$ mice (Table 1). These data demonstrate that inhibition of tPA activity in the adult animal can retard hippocampal neuronal death (Tsirka et al. 1996).

2. α_2-*Antiplasmin.* To evaluate directly if plasmin, the product generated by the action of tPA on plasminogen, is mediating neuronal death, α_2-antiplasmin (from Sigma) was infused into wild-type mice. This specific plasmin inhibitor also retarded neuronal degeneration induced by kainate. Therefore, inhibition of either tPA or plasmin activity in the adult animal can protect against hippocampal neuronal death (Tsirka et al. 1997).
3. tPA-Stop (2,7-bis-[4-amidinobenzylidene]-cycloheptan-1-one]) (from American Diagnostica). This small-molecule inhibitor of tPA that is nontoxic also effectively protected neurons against kainate-induced injury.

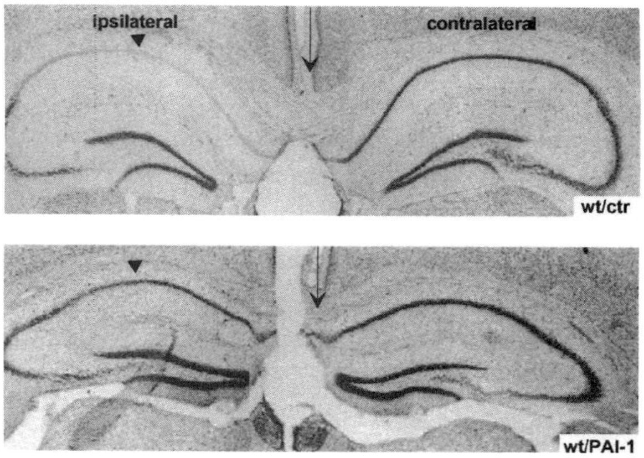

Figure 2. Plasminogen activator inhibitor-type 1 (PAI-1) can prevent kainate-induced neuronal degeneration. Cresyl violet-stained coronal sections through the hippocampus of wild-type mice. The mice were infused with buffer or mouse PAI-1 for 2 days, kainate was injected, the infusion was continued for 5 days further, and the mice were analyzed. (*Top*) Section from a wild-type mouse infused with buffer showing extensive kainate-induced degeneration. (*Bottom*) Section from a wild-type mouse infused with PAI-1, showing resistance to kainate-induced degeneration. Arrowheads point to the site of injection; arrows indicate the site of infusion. Similar results were obtained with α_2-antiplasmin or tPA-Stop. (Reprinted, with permission, from Tsirka et al. 1996 [copyright Macmillan].)

Possible Physiological Roles for Extracellular Proteolytic Cascades in Neurons: Regulated Secretion of tPA from PC12 Cells

To analyze the production of tPA by neurons, we have used PC12 cells as a model system (Gualandris et al. 1996). When these cultures were analyzed for tPA, the activity was exclusively associated with the cell extracts, and no activity was detectable in the conditioned medium. Various lines of evidence indicated that the cell-associated tPA activity was intracellular. This result was surprising, since in other cell lines tPA is constitutively secreted, and the conditioned medium contains the majority of the activity (e.g., in differentiated F9 cells) (Strickland and Mahdavi 1978).

PC12 cells exhibit regulated secretion from presynaptic vesicles. Neurotransmitter release can be induced by depolarization of the cells with external potassium. tPA secretion could also be induced in this manner, since increasing amounts of tPA activity were found in the conditioned medium as a function of increasing external K^+ (Fig. 3). This secretion was not affected by inhibiting RNA or protein synthesis but was inhibited by calcium channel blockers. These results demonstrate a neuronal activity-dependent mechanism that can rapidly increase the amount of tPA in the extracellular fluid by inducing secretion of previously synthesized enzyme.

The tPA/plasminogen extracellular proteolytic cascade, with components stemming from neighboring cell types, may have a normal function in mediating neuronal plasticity. The synthesis of tPA is induced in the rat hippocampus after protocols that promote neuronal remodeling (Qian et al. 1993), and in the rat cerebellum after complex motor learning (Seeds et al.

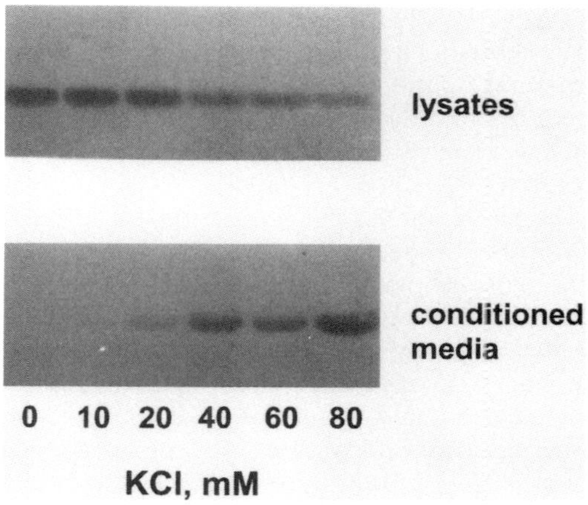

Figure 3. Secretion of tPA from PC12 cells is regulated by depolarization. Zymographic analysis of tPA activity in PC12 cells in response to increasing concentrations of the depolarizing agent KCl. tPA activity in cell lysates (100 μg, *upper* panel) and in conditioned media (about 50 μl normalized for protein, *lower* panel) of PC12 cells incubated for 1 hr with KCl. Lane *0* indicates the released or the cell-associated tPA activity detected in medium supplemented with 1% serum without KCl. (Reprinted, with permission, from Gualandris et al. 1996.)

1995). Furthermore, the release of tPA can be induced by depolarization from neuronal cells (Gualandris et al. 1996), where it may be stored in presynaptic vesicles (Parmer et al. 1997). Thus, the elaboration of proteolytic activity might be activity-dependent and thus constrain proteolytic neuronal restructuring to those situations in which it is advantageous.

DISCUSSION

A central hypothesis emerges from the above results and from work in other laboratories: An extracellular proteolytic cascade of tPA and plasmin participates in neuronal cell death in the mammalian CNS. This hypothesis can be formulated in the following working model:

Kainate → neurons/microglia → tPA
→ plasminogen/plasmin → substrate cleavage
→ degeneration

The synthesis of plasminogen by neuronal cells and of tPA by both neurons and microglia cells suggests that both cell types are necessary to effect neuronal degeneration in the hippocampus. One possible reason for this neuronal-microglial cross-talk would be to limit degeneration to those areas in which both cells had received the appropriate stimulus. For example, upon neuronal injury, macrophages infiltrate and accumulate in the brain; if these cells were solely responsible for neurotoxicity, they might cause extensive neuronal degeneration along their migration path. Instead, the participation of the injured neuronal cells in their own demise (by presenting the plasminogen component of the cascade) could provide a means to limit the destructive capacity of the microglia to those areas in which neurons have been injured. In this regard, intracerebral infusion of tPA does not cause neuronal degeneration in the side contralateral to kainate injection, presumably because increased plasminogen is also a necessary element in the pathway.

Another reason for the participation of adjacent cell types is that production of both tPA and plasminogen in the same cell could lead to intracellular proteolysis and cell death (Sandgren et al. 1991). It is tempting to speculate that this mechanism could contribute to neuronal death after excitotoxic injury. However, we do not think that intracellular generation of plasmin plays a significant role in this system, since administration of PAI-1 retards kainate-induced degeneration, and this serpin would presumably only inhibit proteases in the extracellular space. Although tPA and plasminogen mRNAs are expressed by neurons, it is possible that the two proteins are produced by different neuronal cell populations. Alternatively, if both tPA and plasminogen are synthesized in the same neurons, these cells may avoid intracellular damage either by translational control of the mRNAs (Huarte et al. 1987) or by sequestration of the protein products in vesicles (Parmer et al. 1997).

In most situations in which tPA and uPA have been studied, the enzymes require the presence of plasminogen to be effective, due to the catalytic amplification generated by zymogen activation. The absence of tPA attenuates microglial activation, but the absence of plasminogen does not (data not shown), indicating that this effect of tPA does not require plasminogen. Microglial activation thus represents the first example of a plasminogen-independent role for tPA.

Major causes of neuronal cell degeneration in humans include brain ischemia (e.g., caused by reduced blood flow to the brain following thrombotic stroke), epilepsy, and Alzheimer's disease. The correlation between tPA and neuronal destruction suggests that overexpression of tPA activity could contribute to neuronal destruction in neurodegenerative diseases. In this respect, Alzheimer amyloid β-peptide analogs have been found to stimulate tPA activity in vitro (Kingston et al. 1995), further suggesting that elevated protease activity may be related to this pathology.

One final point deserves mention with regard to tPA in the CNS. tPA has been evaluated for treating thrombotic stroke (Hacke et al. 1995; Marler et al. 1995) and is now approved for this use. The protease accelerates vascular reperfusion of the brain, but since the blood-brain barrier is often compromised in stroke, tPA may also leak into the brain parenchyma. Our work suggests that this excess tPA might contribute to neuronal degeneration and long-term damage. The fact that many stroke patients will soon be treated with tPA gives added impetus to understanding the role of the enzyme in the CNS.

REFERENCES

Altman, J. 1994. Microglia emerge from the fog. *Trends Neurosci.* **17:** 47.

Amaral, D.G. 1994. Hippocampal formation. *Encycl. Hum. Behav.* **2:** 509.

Andersson, P.-B., V.H. Perry, and S. Gordon. 1991. The kinetics and morphological characteristics of the macrophage-microglial response to kainic acid-induced neuronal degeneration. *Neuroscience* **42:** 201.

Bliss, T.V. and G.L. Collingridge. 1993. A synaptic model of memory: Long-term potentiation in the hippocampus. *Nature* **361**:31.

Bugge, T.H., M.J. Flick, C.C. Daugherty, and J.L. Degen. 1995. Plasminogen deficiency causes severe thrombosis but is compatible with development and reproduction. *Genes Dev.* **9:** 794.

Carmeliet, P., L. Schoonjans, L. Kieckens, B. Ream, J. Degen, R. Bronson, R. De Vos, J.J. van den Oord, D. Collen, and R.C. Mulligan. 1994. Physiological consequences of loss of plasminogen activator gene function in mice. *Nature* **368:** 419.

Carroll, P.M., S.E. Tsirka, W.G. Richards, M.A. Frohman, and S. Strickland. 1994. Regulatory sequences of the mouse tissue plasminogen activator gene direct appropriate expression in development and seizure-enhanced response in the CNS. *Development* **120:** 3173.

Coyle, J.T., Molliver, M.E., and Kuhar, M.J. 1978. *In situ* injection of kainic acid: A new method for selectively lesioning neural cell bodies while sparing axons of passage. *J. Comp. Neurol.* **180:** 301.

Frey, U., M. Müller, and D. Kuhl. 1996. A different form of long-lasting potentiation revealed in tissue plasminogen activator mutant mice. *J. Neurosci.* **16:** 2057.

Gualandris, A., T.E. Jones, S. Strickland, and S.E. Tsirka. 1996. Membrane depolarization induces calcium-dependent secretion of tissue plasminogen activator. *J. Neurosci.* **16:** 2220.

Hacke, W., M. Kaste, C. Fieschi, D. Toni, E. Lesaffre, R. von Kummer, G. Boysen, E. Bluhmki, G. Höxter, M.-H. Mahagne, and M. Hennerici (for the ECASS Study Group). 1995. Intravenous thrombolysis with recombinant tissue plasminogen activator for acute hemispheric stroke. *J. Am. Med. Assoc.* **274:** 1017.

Hekman, C.M. and D.J. Loskutoff. 1988. Kinetic analysis of the interactions between plasminogen activator inhibitor-1 and both urokinase and tissue plasminogen activator. *Arch. Biochem. Biophys.* **262:** 199.

Huang, Y.-Y., M.E. Bach, H.-P. Lipp, M. Zhuo, D.P. Wolfer, R.D. Hawkins, L. Schoonjans, E.R. Kandel, J.-M. Godfraind, R. Mulligan, D. Collen, and P. Carmeliet. 1996. Mice lacking the gene encoding tissue-type plasminogen activator show a selective interference with late-phase long-term potentiation in both Schaffer collateral and mossy fiber pathways. *Proc. Natl. Acad. Sci.* **93:** 8699.

Huarte, J., D. Belin, A. Vassalli, S. Strickland, and J.-D. Vassalli. 1987. Meiotic maturation of mouse oocytes triggers the translation and polyadenylation of dormant tissue-type plasminogen activator mRNA. *Genes Dev.* **1:** 1201.

Kingston, I.B., M.J.M. Castro, and S. Anderson. 1995. *In vitro* stimulation of tissue-type plasminogen activator by Alzheimer amyloid β-peptide analogues. *Nat. Med.* **1:** 138.

Lipton, S.A. and P.A. Rosenberg. 1994. Excitatory amino acids as a final common pathway for neurologic disorders. *New Engl. J. Med.* **330:** 613.

Marler, J.R. et al. (for the National Institute of Neurological Disorders and Stroke rt-PA Stroke Study Group). 1995. Tissue plasminogen activator for acute ischemic stroke. *New Engl. J. Med.* **333:** 1581.

Parmer, R.T., M. Mahata, S. Mahata, M.T. Sebald, D.T. O' Connor, and L.A. Miles. 1997. Tissue plasminogen activator (t-PA) is targeted to the regulated secretory pathway: Catecholamine storage vesicles as a reservoir for the rapid release of t-PA. *J. Biol. Chem.* **272:** (in press).

Pennacchio, L.A., A.E. Lehesjoki, N.E. Stone, V.L. Willour, K. Virtaneva, J. Miao, E. D'Amato, L. Ramirez, M. Faham, M. Kostiniemi, J.A. Warrington, R. Norio, A. de la Chapelle, D.R. Cox, and R.M. Myers. 1996. Mutations in the gene encoding cystatin B in progressive myoclonus epilepsy (EPM1). *Science* **271:** 1731.

Pittman, R.N. 1990. Developmental roles of proteases and inhibitors. *Semin. Dev. Biol.* **1:** 65.

Qian, Z., M.E. Gilbert, M.A. Colicos, E.R. Kandel, and D. Kuhl. 1993. Tissue-plasminogen activator is induced as an immediate-early gene during seizure, kindling and long-term potentiation. *Nature* **361:** 453.

Raum, D., D. Marcus, C.A. Alper, R. Levey, P.D. Taylor, and T.E. Starzl. 1980. Synthesis of human plasminogen by the liver. *Science* **208:** 1036.

Rickles, R. and S. Strickland. 1988. Tissue plasminogen activator mRNA in murine tissues. *FEBS Lett.* **229:** 100.

Sandgren, E.P., R.D. Palmiter, J.L. Heckel, C.C. Daugherty, R.L. Brinster, and J.L. Degen. 1991. Complete hepatic regeneration after somatic deletion of an albumin-plasminogen activator transgene. *Cell* **66:** 245.

Sappino, A.P., R. Madani, J. Huarte, D. Belin, J.Z. Kiss, A. Wohlwend, and J.-D. Vassalli. 1993. Extracellular proteolysis in the adult murine brain. *J. Clin. Invest.* **92:** 679.

Seeds, N.W., B.L. Williams, and P.C. Bickford. 1995. Tissue plasminogen activator induction in Purkinje neurons after cerebellar motor learning. *Science* **270:** 1992.

Strickland, S. and V. Mahdavi. 1978. The induction of differentiation in teratocarcinoma stem cells by retinoic acid. *Cell* **15:** 393.

Suh, T.T., K. Holmback, N.J.Jensen, C.C. Daugherty, K. Small, D.I. Simon, S. Potter, and J.L. Degen. 1995. Resolution of spontaneous bleeding events but failure of pregnancy in fibrinogen-deficient mice. *Genes Dev.* **9:** 2020.

Tsirka, S.E., A.D. Rogove, and S. Strickland. 1996. Neuronal death and tissue plasminogen activator. *Nature* **384:** 123.

Tsirka, S.E., A. Gualandris, D.G. Amaral, and S. Strickland. 1995. Excitotoxin-induced neuronal degeneration and seizure are mediated by tissue plasminogen activator. *Nature* **377:** 340.

Tsirka, S.E., A.D. Rogove, T.H. Bugge, J.L. Degen, and S. Strickland. 1997. An extracellular proteolytic cascade promotes neuronal degeneration in the mouse hippocampus. *J. Neurosci.* **17:** 543.

Vassalli, J.-D., A.P. Sappino, and D. Belin. 1991. The plasminogen activator/plasmin system. *J. Clin. Invest.* **88:** 1067.

Zhou, Q.-Y., C.J. Quaife, and R.D. Palmiter. 1995. Targeted disruption of the tyrosine hydroxylase gene reveals that catecholamines are required for mouse fetal development. *Nature* **374:** 640.

Molecular Analysis of Neurotransmitter Transport into Secretory Vesicles

Y. Liu, C. Waites, D. Krantz, P. Tan, and R.H. Edwards
Departments of Neurology and Physiology, University of California at San Francisco, School of Medicine, San Francisco, California 94143-0435

Synaptic transmission depends on the storage of neurotransmitter within secretory vesicles that undergo regulated exocytosis in response to stimulation. Since classic transmitters are either synthesized in the cytoplasm or appear there after re-uptake from the synapse, vesicular storage depends on transport from the cytoplasm, and distinct transport activities have been described for the different transmitters (Edwards 1992; Schuldiner et al. 1995). In contrast to plasma membrane transporters that terminate synaptic transmission by removing classic transmitters from the synapse and use the Na^+ gradient across the plasma membrane to drive active transport (Amara and Kuhar 1993), vesicular transport activities use the proton electrochemical gradient across the vesicular membrane that is generated by a vacuolar H^+-ATPase. In particular, the vesicular transport activities for monoamines and acetylcholine (ACh) depend on the chemical component of the gradient (ΔpH) and so act as proton exchangers (Anderson et al. 1982; Johnson 1988). In addition, different drugs inhibit the plasma membrane and vesicular transporters. In the case of monoamines, cocaine and antidepressant drugs inhibit the plasma membrane transporters, whereas reserpine and tetrabenazine inhibit the vesicular transporters. Since reserpine produces a syndrome that resembles depression and amphetamines may also interfere with the storage of monoamines (Sulzer and Rayport 1990; Rudnick and Wall 1992a), the regulation of vesicular transport in general and monoamine transport in particular has the potential to influence behavior. We have explored this possibility by characterizing the proteins responsible for vesicular transmitter transport.

VESICULAR AMINE TRANSPORT, MPTP TOXICITY, AND PARKINSON'S DISEASE

To identify the proteins that package neurotransmitters into secretory vesicles, we have used a genetic selection procedure. Systemic administration of 1-methyl-4-phenyl-1,2,3,6-tetrahydropyridine (MPTP) produces a clinical syndrome that strongly resembles severe idiopathic Parkinson's disease (PD) (Langston et al. 1983). Pathologically, MPTP toxicity involves the same dopamine neurons of the substantia nigra as PD. The striking similarity between MPTP toxicity and PD has further suggested that MPTP may help to understand the mechanisms involved in this type of neural degeneration. After penetrating the blood-brain barrier, glial monoamine oxidase B (MAO-B) converts MPTP to the active metabolite *N*-methyl-4-phenylpyridinium (MPP^+) (Heikkila et al. 1984; Langston et al. 1984). The plasma membrane transport activities selectively expressed by monoamine cells then accumulate the toxin (Javitch et al. 1985). Inside the cell, MPP^+ enters mitochondria (Ramsay and Singer 1986) and inhibits oxidative phosphorylation, apparently by binding to complex I of the respiratory chain (Nicklas et al. 1985; Krueger et al. 1990; Ramsay et al. 1991). Several features of idiopathic PD support the relevance of the MPTP model. The primary site of MPTP action is respiration, and mitochondrial abnormalities have been reported in idiopathic PD (Schapira et al. 1990; Shoffner et al. 1991). In addition, the MAO-B inhibitor deprenyl blocks the toxicity of MPTP and has been suggested to slow the progression of PD (Parkinson's Study Group 1989, 1993). However, an exogenous toxin has not yet been identified in PD (Tanner and Langston 1990), and we still do not understand aspects of the MPTP model, such as the selective vulnerability of dopamine neurons in the midbrain. Other monoamine cell populations in the brain stem, sympathetic ganglia, and adrenal medulla accumulate MPP^+ but show little toxicity (Johannessen et al. 1985). Some of these regions, such as the ventral tegmentum and locus coeruleus, show susceptibility to MPTP in primates but to a relatively minor degree (Mitchell et al. 1985; Deutch et al. 1986; German et al. 1992). Since PD similarly affects these populations to a lesser extent than the substantia nigra, the discrepancy has relevance for the idiopathic disorder as well.

To understand the differences in vulnerability to MPTP among cells that all accumulate the toxin, we have taken advantage of the observation that rat pheochromocytoma PC12 cells, which have been used as a model system to study the effects of MPP^+ because they express a plasma membrane norepinephrine transporter, show susceptibility only to relatively high concentrations of the toxin (Denton and Howard 1987). Interestingly, Chinese hamster ovary (CHO) fibroblasts, which lack a plasma membrane monoamine transporter, show greater sensitivity to MPP^+ than do PC12 cells. Thus, a neurotoxin causes more injury to a fibroblast than to a neuroendocrine cell.

Nonetheless, the relative resistance of PC12 cells to MPP^+ in vitro is actually consistent with the relative resistance of the adrenal medullary cells to MPTP in vivo. Using this paradigm to dissect the mechanism of PC12 cell resistance, we transfected the MPP^+-sensitive CHO cells with a cDNA library from PC12 cells. In contrast to wild-type CHO cells, which yielded no resistant colonies after growth in 500 μM MPP^+, the transfected cells selected in 1 mM MPP^+ yielded one extremely toxin-resistant clone. We then excluded compensation for a defect in respiration and a change in the properties of the mitochondria as the mechanisms of resistance (Liu et al. 1992a). Since chromaffin granules from adrenal medullary cells accumulate MPP^+ (Daniels and Reinhard 1988; Scherman et al. 1988), we next examined the possibility that a vesicular monoamine transporter might confer resistance to the toxin by sequestering it in a vesicular compartment, away from the primary site of action in mitochondria. Indeed, reserpine increased the sensitivity of the resistant cells to that of wild-type CHO cells (Liu et al. 1992a). Treatment of wild-type CHO cells with reserpine did not change their sensitivity even to lower concentrations of MPP^+, showing that this mechanism is unique to the transfected cells. Thus, apparent expression of vesicular amine transport in a nonneuronal cell line may be able to sequester MPP^+ even in the absence of regulated secretory vesicles and so protect the cell.

To assess transport activity directly, we loaded CHO cells with high concentrations of dopamine and used glyoxylic acid-induced histofluorescence to identify its intracellular distribution. Wild-type cells showed diffuse cytoplasmic fluorescence. In contrast, the drug-resistant cells showed strong staining of a perinuclear compartment and scattered particulate sites throughout the cytoplasm (Liu et al. 1992a). Furthermore, reserpine converted the particulate pattern observed in resistant cells to the wild-type pattern. Thus, vesicular monoamine transport appeared responsible for the resistance to MPP^+.

Retransfection of plasmids rescued from the genomic DNA of MPP^+-resistant cells identified a single clone responsible for resistance to the toxin. Stable transformants expressing this cDNA that were selected in the neomycin analog G418 also showed the particulate pattern of dopamine-loaded fluorescence (Liu et al. 1992b), indicating that selection in MPP^+ is not necessary for the expression of transport activity. The sequence predicted a protein of 521 amino acids, twelve transmembrane domains (TMDs), but no signal peptide, suggesting that both amino and carboxyl termini reside in the cytoplasm (Liu et al. 1992b). However, the sequence shows no significant similarity to the plasma membrane transmitter transporters. Indeed, a large hydrophilic loop predicted to reside in the lumen of the vesicle occurs between TMD1 and 2 rather than between TMD3 and 4 (as in the plasma membrane transporters). On the other hand, the amino-terminal half of the protein shows remote but definite similarity to a series of bacterial proteins. These include several tetracycline resistance genes and a multidrug resistance transporter unrelated to mammalian multidrug resistance transporters (Nguyen et al. 1983; Neal and Chater 1987; Neyfakh et al. 1991). Supporting the functional relevance of the sequence similarity, the vertebrate amine transporter and the bacterial proteins both mediate the efflux of toxins from the cell. In addition, both classes of proteins use ΔpH as the driving force and so act by proton exchange (Kaneko et al. 1985). Finally, reserpine inhibits the bacterial multidrug resistance transporter as well as the neurotransmitter transporter (Neyfakh et al. 1991). Molecular cloning has thus identified a novel mammalian gene family that seems to have evolved from ancient detoxification systems. Together with the ability to protect against MPP^+, the relationship to bacterial proteins suggests that vesicular transport may have two functions, one in packaging transmitter for release by regulated exocytosis and the other in protection. However, no exogenous toxin has been identified in idiopathic PD (Tanner and Langston 1990), and the epidemiology does not suggest toxic exposure (Eldridge and Rocca 1992).

Substantial evidence indicates that PD involves an increase in oxidative stress, but the cause remains unknown (Cohen 1990; Fahn and Cohen 1992). A variety of neurotoxins such as 6-OH-dopamine oxidize very easily and injure dopaminergic cells, but these compounds are not known to occur in vivo. Interestingly, MPTP toxicity can increase oxidative stress since overexpression of superoxide dismutase, converting highly reactive superoxide radical to hydrogen peroxide, protects against MPTP toxicity in transgenic mice (Przedborski et al. 1992). Thus, oxidative stress may result from toxic exposure, but the most compelling toxin in idiopathic PD appears to be the normal neurotransmitter dopamine itself. Like 6-OH-dopamine, dopamine oxidizes quite readily and produces substantial toxicity at low doses. Indeed, dopamine is much more toxic to cultured neural cells than similar concentrations of MPP^+ (Rosenberg 1988; Michel and Hefti 1990). Unlike excitotoxicity (Choi 1988), dopamine toxicity does not involve an interaction with specific receptors. Rather, metabolism of hydrogen peroxide by catalase protects against dopamine toxicity, indicating that a substantial part of the cellular injury derives from oxidation of dopamine to hydrogen peroxide (Rosenberg 1988). Thus, dopamine may act as an endogenous toxin to increase oxidative stress directly.

The action of dopamine as an endogenous toxin may contribute to the selective cell loss that occurs in PD. In addition to neurons in the substantia nigra, dopamine cells in the ventral tegmental area show considerable involvement. In contrast, norepinephrine and serotonin cell groups show much less involvement, presumably because these transmitters oxidize much less readily than dopamine. Furthermore, variation in the extent of degeneration may reflect additional factors, such as the amount of dopamine produced and its turnover.

The action of dopamine as an endogenous toxin in idiopathic PD predicts several differences from MPTP toxicity. First, in contrast to MPP^+, dopamine toxicity does not require transport into the cell that produces it. High-affinity plasma membrane uptake may influence cytoplasmic concentrations of the transmitter, but inhibitors would almost certainly have less effect on cytoplasmic dopamine than on MPP^+ toxicity. Second, free-radical damage due to the oxidation of dopamine presumably involves more than simply the mitochondria, possibly accounting for the failure to demonstrate a defect in respiration early in PD (Jenner et al. 1992). Third, dopamine neurons express MAO-A rather than MAO-B (Westlund et al. 1988). For this reason, inhibition of MAO-B with deprenyl would have little effect on endogenous dopamine toxicity and might help to explain the equivocal results of drug trials (Parkinson's Study Group 1989, 1993). Indeed, oxidation by MAO may actually have a protective role within dopamine neurons, since nonenzymatic oxidation has the potential to produce even more toxic compounds than enzymatic oxidation.

If dopamine acts as an endogenous toxin in idiopathic PD, the factors that determine its metabolism and distribution will have important roles. Since dopamine metabolism reflects the amount of transmitter produced and its turnover, neural activity should govern dopamine metabolism and so influence the susceptibility to PD. Importantly, glutamate receptor antagonists reduce MPTP toxicity (Turski et al. 1991). In addition, the loss of dopamine cells would require those remaining to increase their dopamine production, putting them at greater risk in a self-perpetuating cycle of accelerated degeneration. Supporting this possible mechanism, several individuals at first asymptomatic after exposure to MPTP have subsequently developed typical, slowly progressive PD (Vingerhoets et al. 1994).

The presumptive ability of vesicular amine transport to protect against dopamine as well as MPP^+ toxicity implies that cytoplasmic accumulation of the transmitter is toxic. Indeed, the apparent affinity of the vesicular amine transporter ($K_m \sim 0.2$ μM) greatly exceeds that of the vesicular transporters for other classic transmitters ($K_m \sim 1$ mM) (Schuldiner et al. 1995; Liu and Edwards 1996), suggesting that the transporter helps to maintain low cytoplasmic concentrations of monoamine. In addition to uptake into the vesicle, however, vesicular efflux may also contribute to cytoplasmic dopamine levels and toxicity. In the presence of the driving force for uptake $\Delta\mu_{H+}$, chromaffin granules show extremely little efflux of preloaded [^{3}H]serotonin even after dilution into buffer without transmitter that should promote redistribution (Johnson 1988). Originally attributed to the formation of an insoluble complex in the vesicle lumen, chromaffin ghosts prepared by repeated osmotic lysis show similarly low rates of efflux for up to 1 hour after dilution of the preloaded vesicles (Maron et al. 1983). However, dissipation of $\Delta\mu_{H+}$ through a variety of means causes rapid efflux, presumably by eliminating a kinetic barrier to flux reversal. Curiously, none of the uptake inhibitors has been shown to block efflux, suggesting that it may not involve the vesicular amine transport protein. Studies using synaptic vesicles also indicate transporter-independent efflux (Floor et al. 1995). However, reserpine and tetrabenazine do inhibit an exchange reaction promoted by the addition of unlabeled substrate to vesicles preloaded with [^{3}H] dopamine (Maron et al. 1983; Floor et al. 1995). The drugs thus inhibit exchange but not net efflux, suggesting either that the transporter participates only in exchange or that the conditions of efflux preclude drug inhibition. Since the cytoplasmic concentration of substrate may determine its toxicity, understanding the mechanism of efflux and, in particular, the role of the transport protein has special significance for the role of dopamine in PD. Interestingly, psychostimulants also promote the redistribution of stored monoamine to the cytoplasm and produce substantial toxicity.

Considerable evidence has shown that amphetamines increase synaptic concentrations of monoamine by reversing the direction of flux through plasma membrane amine transporters (Fisher and Cho 1979; Di Chiara and Imperato 1988; Hernandez et al. 1988; Carboni et al. 1989; Rudnick and Wall 1992a,b,c; Schuldiner et al. 1993b; Sulzer et al. 1993; Wall et al. 1995). However, the normal, low cytoplasmic concentrations of monoamine (0.1–1 μM) cannot sustain significant synaptic concentrations in the absence of substantial vesicular efflux. Net efflux may occur through exchange of the cytoplasmic amphetamine for luminal monoamine, followed by diffusion of the lipophilic drug back out of the vesicle for another round of exchange. Alternatively, amphetamine may act as a weak base, dissipate $\Delta\mu_{H+}$, and promote efflux in this way (Sulzer and Rayport 1990). Regardless of the exact mechanism, amphetamines produce considerable damage to monoamine terminals (Steele et al. 1994), consistent with the action of monoamines as endogenous toxins. Supporting this, a dye that images free radicals shows localized damage, presumably near sites of vesicular storage, within dopamine neurons exposed to amphetamines (Cubells et al. 1994). If the transport protein mediates this flux reversal, it may thus have a role in the pathogenesis of idiopathic PD as well as in psychostimulant toxicity. We have used the cDNA identified by selection in MPP^+ to assess the role in both neural degeneration and synaptic transmission.

To assess whether the vesicular monoamine transporters (VMATs) may contribute to human genetic disease, we have determined the chromosome location of the human genes. The human VMAT1 gene resides at 8p21 (Peter et al. 1993) and VMAT2 at 10q25

(Erickson and Eiden 1993; Peter et al. 1993; Surratt et al. 1993), regions not known to be linked to neurological or psychiatric disease. Furthermore, sequence analysis of the VMAT2 protein-coding region from 17 patients with affective disorders shows no changes, suggesting that an inherited defect in VMAT2 is not responsible for most forms of this illness (Lesch et al. 1994). However, the extent of VMAT2 involvement in hereditary neuropsychiatric disease remains unknown because linkage has failed to identify the chromosomal regions responsible for many human syndromes. In addition, acquired changes in transport activity may have a larger role than inherited differences.

MOLECULAR ANALYSIS OF VESICULAR AMINE TRANSPORT

Analysis of RNA from different tissues shows expression of the cloned VMAT sequences in the adrenal gland but not the adult brain (Liu et al. 1992b). Although lower levels of this putative protective activity in the brain might contribute to the increased vulnerability of dopamine cells in the midbrain relative to adrenal chromaffin cells, the absence of detectable mRNA suggested a distinct gene. Indeed, cDNAs from rat brain stem and basophilic leukemia cell libraries have predicted a closely related but distinct sequence now known as VMAT2 to distinguish it from VMAT1 expressed in the adrenal (Erickson et al. 1992; Liu et al. 1992b). In situ hybridization showed expression of VMAT2 in multiple central monoamine populations including the substantia nigra, ventral tegmental area, locus coeruleus, and raphe. Surprisingly, the transport protein purified from the bovine adrenal gland based on binding to reserpine shows stronger sequence similarity to rat VMAT2 than VMAT1 (Stern-Bach et al. 1992; Krejci et al. 1993; Howell et al. 1994), suggesting that both isoforms may occur in chromaffin cells and that VMAT2 may predominate in the bovine adrenal medulla.

A series of biochemical assays have been used to determine the functional properties of the two cloned VMATs. In fibroblast cell lines such as CHO, COS, and CV1 cells where the proteins are expressed either transiently or stably, the VMATs localize to endosomes where a proton electrochemical gradient provides the driving force for active transport (Liu et al. 1992b, 1994). To bypass the plasma membrane as a barrier to uptake by intracellular vesicles, the cells are either disrupted by homogenization (Liu et al. 1992b) or partially permeabilized with digitonin (Erickson et al. 1992), then incubated with the radiolabeled substrate for varying intervals before rapid dilution and filtration to remove the untransported material. MPP^+-resistant stable CHO transformants and other cells transiently expressing the VMATs exhibit time-dependent uptake of [^{3}H]serotonin that requires ATP and an intact proton electrochemical gradient, as anticipated for a known proton exchanger. Membrane vesicles generally indicate a higher apparent affinity than the semi-permeabilized cells, and both VMATs have the highest appparent affinity for serotonin (K_m ~ 0.2 mM for VMAT2), followed by dopamine, norepinephrine, and epinephrine (Peter et al. 1994). In addition, VMAT2 has an approximately threefold higher apparent affinity for most monoamine substrates (including MPP^+) than VMAT1 (Peter et al. 1994), suggesting a greater potential for detoxification. Histamine also inhibits serotonin transport by VMAT2 but not VMAT1, suggesting that mast cells and other histamine-containing cells express VMAT2 rather than VMAT1, consistent with the expression of VMAT2 by rat basophilic leukemia cells (Erickson et al. 1992). Although it remains unknown whether they interact directly or indirectly with the transporter to promote flux reversal, amphetamines also inhibit VMAT2 more potently than VMAT1, strongly suggesting that this effect does not result entirely from the dissipation of ΔpH as previously suggested. Human VMAT2 shows functional characteristics similar to rat VMAT2 (Erickson and Eiden 1993), consistent with the strong sequence similarity (Peter et al. 1993; Surratt et al. 1993).

In terms of pharmacology, reserpine inhibits serotonin transport by both VMAT1 and VMAT2 and binds to the transporters in the same way as previously described for chromaffin granules (Weaver and Deupree 1982; Scherman and Henry 1984; Rudnick et al. 1990). In particular, [^{3}H]reserpine binds with two affinities, $\Delta\mu_{H+}$ accelerates binding, and monoamines inhibit reserpine binding with potencies similar to their apparent affinity as substrate (Schuldiner et al. 1993a). Tetrabenazine, in contrast, inhibits VMAT2 much more potently than VMAT1 (Peter et al. 1994). Indeed, this result may account for the selective depletion of central rather than peripheral monoamine stores by tetrabenazine and the reduced side effect of hypotension with this drug compared to reserpine (Carlsson 1965). To characterize further the reduced potency of tetrabenazine for VMAT1, we examined the binding of [^{3}H]dihydrotetrabenazine and found that it does not interact with VMAT1 at high affinity.

Drug binding has also enabled us to determine the number of transporters. Using this number, we have calculated a turnover number for both VMAT1 and VMAT2 of about 400/min. Although higher than previously observed using chromaffin granules, this number still falls well below that required to fill synaptic vesicles (2–10,000) that recycle in 1–2 minutes (Betz and Bewick 1992; Ryan et al. 1993) if only 2–3 transport proteins occur per vesicle. Although the standard transport assay involves incubation at 29°C, and the turnover number at 37°C may be somewhat higher, this general transport rate might allow dense-core vesicles to fill completely, since they mature over minutes to hours, but synaptic vesicles loaded through this mechanism may contain different amounts of transmitter that reflect the speed of recycling and neural activity. The observations also suggest that

VMAT2 should protect against MPP^+ toxicity and related forms of degeneration at least as well as VMAT1, possibly because central monoamine populations use more toxic transmitters such as dopamine rather than the less toxic norepinephrine and epinephrine expressed by the adrenal gland.

The close similarity between the two VMATs suggested that chimeric transporters would retain function and so enable the identification of residues that modulate substrate recognition and drug sensitivity, properties that differ between VMAT1 and 2 (Peter et al. 1995). Using a large series of functional chimeras, biochemical analysis shows that the same domains interact in the same manner to determine recognition of the substrates serotonin and histamine and inhibition by tetrabenazine (Fig. 1). In particular, TMD5–8 and TMD9–12 of VMAT2 are both necessary for the high-affinity interactions of VMAT2. Surprisingly, the extreme amino terminus of VMAT2 alone confers a partial VMAT2 phenotype in terms of both substrate recognition and drug inhibition, raising the possibility that modification of the amino- and carboxyl termini, e.g., by phosphorylation, may regulate transport activity. In addition to these domains that influence both substrate recognition and tetrabenazine sensitivity, the analysis of chimeras has also revealed domains that interact selectively with the high-affinity substrate serotonin. TMD3–4 of VMAT2 increases the apparent affinity for serotonin, and TMD5–7 of VMAT2 paradoxically decreases serotonin affinity in the context of amino-terminal VMAT2 sequences but increases it in the context of carboxy-terminal VMAT2 sequences.

It is surprising that many of the same domains interact in the same way to influence both substrate recognition and sensitivity to tetrabenazine, a drug not considered to act at the site of substrate recognition. Indeed, high concentrations of monoamine are required to prevent tetrabenazine binding and, in contrast to reserpine, the imposition of ΔpH does not influence tetrabenazine binding (Darchen et al. 1989). However, tetrabenazine can prevent reserpine binding, suggesting that the two drug-binding sites may represent different conformations of the transport protein. Alternatively, the drugs may bind to overlapping sites, in which case tetrabenazine would bind near the site of substrate recognition. Interestingly, histamine is a relatively low-affinity substrate for VMAT2 and, in contrast to other monoamines, does not inhibit reserpine binding (Merickel and Edwards 1995), suggesting that it, like tetrabenazine, may interact with the transport protein at a site distinct from other, high-affinity substrates. Reserpine is a very weak inhibitor of histamine transport, further supporting the possibility of a distinct substrate recognition site. The identical pattern of histamine recognition and tetrabenazine sensitivity observed in the chimeras (Peter et al. 1996) now raises the possibility that tetrabenazine binds to the site of histamine recognition, adjacent to but distinct from the recognition site for high-affinity substrates. Further

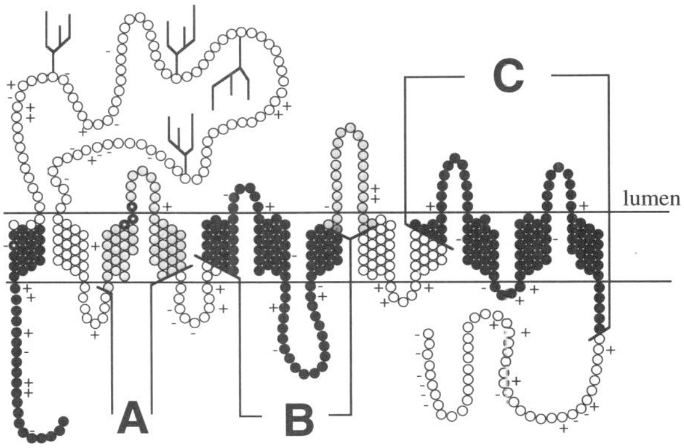

Figure 1. Site-directed mutagenesis and chimeric analysis of the VMATs identifies residues and domains that influence substrate recognition and sensitivity to tetrabenazine. Site-directed mutagenesis has implicated an aspartate in TMD1 and three serines in TMD3 in substrate recognition (*spheres*). In addition to these residues required for substrate recognition, three domains modulate substrate affinity and tetrabenazine sensitivity. TMD3–4 from VMAT2 (domain A) confers a higher affinity for serotonin but not histamine or tetrabenazine. TMD5–8 from VMAT2 (domain B) confers a higher affinity for both serotonin and histamine as well as a higher sensitivity to tetrabenazine but requires the presence of more carboxy-terminal VMAT2 sequences. Surprisingly, TMD5–7 from VMAT2 reduces the affinity for serotonin but not for the other compounds in the presence of more amino-terminal VMAT2 sequences. TMD8–12 (domain C) also increases affinity for both substrates and sensitivity to tetrabenazine, but only in the presence of more amino-terminal VMAT2 sequences. Thus, domains B and C require other regions (presumably each other) for high substrate affinity and drug sensitivity. Interestingly, the amino terminus of VMAT2 alone confers a partial VMAT2 phenotype. The circles denote amino acid residues from VMAT2, with black circles indicating those residues identical to VMAT1. The gray circles indicate conservative substitutions and white circles nonconservative differences between VMAT1 and 2. Acidic residues are indicated with a – and basic residues with a +.

analysis of point mutants within the domains identified by the chimeras will test this possibility.

In addition to the analysis of chimeras, site-directed mutagenesis has identified a role for specific residues in substrate recognition by the VMATs. Neutralization of an aspartate in TMD1 to asparagine and replacement of serines in TMD3 with alanine result in stable proteins still able to bind reserpine (Merickel et al. 1995). Indeed, $\Delta\mu_{H+}$ still accelerates reserpine binding to the mutants, indicating that they remain coupled to the driving force. However, serotonin no longer inhibits reserpine binding to the mutants, demonstrating a selective defect in substrate recognition. By analogy with monoamine receptors (Strader et al. 1989), the aspartate may bind to the amino group and the serines to the hydroxyl groups of the substrate. To understand how substrate translocation is driven by ΔpH, we and other investigators have also focused on the pathway for protons.

Residues at the carboxyl terminus of VMAT2 have been implicated in proton movement. Mutation of a histidine between TMD10 and 11, the only histidine conserved between VMAT1 and VMAT2, disrupts coupling to $\Delta\mu_{H+}$ as measured by reserpine binding (Shirvan et al. 1994). This histidine also shows conservation in VMATs from different species and in the vesicular ACh transporters from several species, but one member of the gene family contains a tyrosine at this site, raising the possibility of additional roles for this residue. Replacement of an aspartate in TMD10 by glutamate has a striking effect on sensitivity to bulk-phase pH (S. Schuldiner, pers. comm.). Surprisingly, substitution of an aspartate in TMD11 by glutamate eliminates transport activity despite normal coupling to $\Delta\mu_{H+}$ (S. Schuldiner, pers. comm.). One of these or other acidic residues predicted to reside within TMDs may also form a salt bridge with the sole basic residue predicted to reside within TMD2. However, the mechanism by which substrate translocation couples to proton movement requires information about the structural changes produced by interaction among the sites.

VESICULAR ACh TRANSPORT

The apparent relationship of two vesicular monoamine transport proteins to a class of bacterial antibiotic resistance proteins suggested that these transporters might be the first members of a novel eukaryotic gene family. Indeed, work in the nematode *Caenorhabditis elegans* subsequently identified a gene (*unc-17*) that shows considerable sequence similarity to the amine transporters (Alfonso et al. 1993). Since *unc-17* mutants are resistant to organophosphorus toxins that kill wild-type organisms by inhibiting acetylcholinesterase and producing lethal synaptic concentrations of ACh, *unc-17* mutants presumably survive as a result of defective ACh release. Immunocytochemistry showed localization of the *unc-17* protein in cholinergic cells and in synaptic vesicles, further supporting a role in vesicular ACh transport. Importantly, the bioenergetics of vesicular ACh transport had previously been shown to involve proton exchange and so to resemble vesicular amine transport.

To identify a vertebrate homolog of *unc-17*, the sequence was initially used to isolate a closely related cDNA from the heavily cholinergic *Torpedo* electric lobe. The *Torpedo* sequence in turn showed strong similarity to *unc-17* and the VMATs. Expression of the RNA in electric lobe but not electroplax or liver further supported a role in vesicular ACh transport (Roghani et al. 1994; Varoqui et al. 1994). Using the similarity between *unc-17* and the *Torpedo* homolog, a related cDNA was then isolated from rat (Erickson et al. 1994; Roghani et al. 1994). The rat protein contains acidic residues in putative TMDs 1, 6, 10, and 11 and a basic residue in TMD2, residues conserved in the VMATs (Bejanin et al. 1994; Erickson et al. 1994; Roghani et al. 1994). The putative VAChT cDNA also predicts a leucine-rich domain at the carboxyl terminus. In situ hybridization showed expression by cholinergic cell populations in the basal forebrain, septum, basal ganglia, and motor nuclei of the brain stem and spinal cord, a distribution corresponding exactly to that observed for the biosynthetic enzyme choline acetyltransferase (ChAT). Interestingly, the VAChT gene resides at the same genomic locus as ChAT in both *C. elegans* (Alfonso et al. 1994) and mammals (Erickson et al. 1994; Roghani et al. 1994). In addition, the VAChT gene undergoes coordinate regulation with the biosynthetic enzyme, presumably as a result of shared promoter elements (Berse and Blusztajn 1995). In further contrast to the VMATs, whose protein-coding domain derives from many exons, the protein-coding region of VAChT occurs in a single exon (Bejanin et al. 1994). Despite the evidence for coordinate gene regulation, ChAT declines in Alzheimer's disease, whereas VAChT (as measured by vesamicol binding) increases (Kish et al. 1990; Ruberg et al. 1990). The mechanism for this divergent regulation is presumably posttranscriptional but remains unknown.

Although classic studies using *Torpedo* synaptic vesicles had suggested that vesamicol binds to a distinct, associated protein rather than to the transporter itself (Bahr and Parsons 1992), rat VAChT binds to the potent inhibitor vesamicol with relatively high affinity in several heterologous expression systems (Varoqui et al. 1994). In further contrast to previous work showing weak inhibition of vesamicol binding by substrate, ACh competitively inhibits vesamicol binding to the transporter transiently expressed in COS cells, and with a potency very similar to the K_m reported for transport (~0.5 mM) (A. Roghani and R.H. Edwards, unpubl.). We have also generated anti-peptide antibodies that demonstrate high levels of protein expression by COS cells and, furthermore, indicate localization to endosomes, the membrane compartment in which VMAT2 appears in COS and which appears able to support transport activity. However, standard transport assays using either membrane vesicles or permeabilized cells have thus far failed to show functional transport. One group has reported uptake by nonpermeabilized cells expressing the protein and potent inhibition by vesamicol, but the low levels of transport and the apparent requirement for intact cells raise questions about the nature of the activity observed (Erickson et al. 1994). The ACh transporter in *Torpedo* synaptic vesicles has been suggested to associate with other vesicle proteins such as SV2 that may be required for function (Bahr and Parsons 1992), but coexpression experiments have thus far failed to demonstrate significant transport activity.

REGULATION AND LOCALIZATION

Vesicular amine transport may influence the amount of transmitter per vesicle and hence quantal size. In addition, vesicular transport sets the cytoplasmic concentration of transmitter and so determines the potential for toxicity. Previous work has shown that prolonged depolarization increases VMAT expression in bovine chromaffin cells (Desnos et al. 1992) and rat sympathetic neurons (Desnos et al. 1990). The increase appears to be transcriptional (Krejci et al. 1993), but more recent results suggest the possibility of short-term, posttranscriptional regulation. Activation of cAMP-dependent signaling pathways reduces VMAT activity (Nakanishi et al. 1995), presumably as a result of phosphorylation. However, the mechanism by which cAMP-dependent protein kinase affects neurotransmitter storage remains unclear: It may involve the vacuolar H^+-ATPase, a chloride conductance that affects the expression of the proton electrochemical as ΔpH or $\Delta\psi$, or VMAT. In addition, we have recently found that VMAT2 but not VMAT1 undergoes constitutive phosphorylation at the carboxyl terminus by a casein kinase (D. Krantz, R.H. Edwards, in prep.). Inducible phosphorylation of VMAT2 also occurs, although the functional significance of this modification remains to be demonstrated.

In addition to the regulation of intrinsic transport activity, the localization of vesicle transport proteins may have a dramatic influence on transmitter release. Most classic transmitters are stored in small, clear, synaptic vesicles (SVs) that cluster at the nerve terminal and mediate the extremely rapid, precise release of transmitter (Bennett and Scheller 1994; Jahn and Südhof 1994). In contrast, neural peptides (or hormones) are stored in larger dense-core vesicles (LDCVs) (or secretory granules in endocrine cells) that respond to different stimuli than synaptic vesicles, occur at the cell body and dendrites as well as the nerve terminal, and mediate the slower release characteristic of neuromodulators (Kelly 1993; Martin 1994). However, monoamines differ from most other classic transmitters and have been reported to occur in LDCVs as well as SVs (Smith 1972; Thureson-Klein 1983). In the adrenal medulla, monoamines are stored in chromaffin granules (LDCVs), whereas in the brain, they are stored in small vesicles that may contain a dense core depending on the mode of fixation but otherwise resemble SVs. Since localization of the VMATs determines the site of monoamine storage, and release from different secretory vesicles alters the function of monoamines as signaling molecules, we have raised antibodies to both VMATs and used these reagents to localize the proteins both in PC12 cells in vitro and in monoamine cells in vivo.

The existence of two VMATs, one expressed in the adrenal gland and the other in the brain, suggests that these proteins may localize differently: VMAT1 to LDCVs and VMAT2 to SVs. Indeed, both adrenal chromaffin cells and PC12 cells show preferential localization of the endogenous VMAT1 to LDCVs rather than the small, synaptic-like microvesicles present in these cells (Liu et al. 1994). Small amounts of VMAT1 occur in light vesicle populations, and at least some of these do appear to be SVs. However, heterologous expression of the central VMAT2 in PC12 cells also shows virtually exclusive localization of the introduced protein in LDCVs (Y. Liu et al., in prep.). Since PC12 cells may lack the cellular machinery present in neurons that is required for appropriate sorting to SVs, we have also used immunoelectron microscopy to localize VMAT2 in vivo. Surprisingly, higher levels of VMAT2 expression also occur in LDCVs than SVs in the nucleus tractus solitarius (Nirenberg et al. 1995). In the midbrain, VMAT2 labels a prominent population of tubulovesicular structures in the cell bodies and dendrites of dopamine neurons in the substantia nigra and ventral tegmental area (Nirenberg et al. 1996). Although the nature of this compartment remains unclear, it presumably accounts for the prominent reserpine-sensitive release of dopamine previously documented from the cell body or dendrites of midbrain neurons (Heeringa and Abercrombie 1995; Kalivas and Duffy 1993). Nonetheless, VMAT2 clearly occurs at significant levels on SVs in vivo, and the cause of the difference in membrane trafficking of VMAT2 between PC12 cells and monoamine neurons remains uncertain. However, PC12 cells clearly contain SVs and, in contrast to the VMATs, sort putative VAChT exclusively to SVs in both PC12 cells (Y. Liu and R.H. Edwards, in prep.) and in vivo (Gilmor et al. 1996).

The differences in membrane trafficking to LDCVs and SVs presumably reflect the different mechanisms by which these vesicles form. LDCVs bud from the *trans*-Golgi network (TGN) (Farquhar et al. 1978; Tooze and Tooze 1986), suggesting that the soluble contents of this regulated secretory pathway sort away from the constitutive secretory pathway at this site. Alternatively, constitutively released proteins may be removed from immature LDCVs by selective retrieval after the TGN (Kuliawat and Arvan 1992, 1994). In either case, the formation of the dense core appears critical for sorting to the regulated pathway. Rather than a specific signal, the general biophysical properties of proteins destined for LDCVs indeed appear to promote aggregation under the relevant conditions (Tooze et al. 1993). Nonetheless, the mechanism by which these aggregates sort into LDCVs remains unknown. Presumably, they bind to membrane receptors that in turn interact with a cytosolic sorting machinery. However, few if any integral membrane proteins restricted to LDCVs have been identified. As an integral membrane protein almost exclusively on LDCVs at least in PC12 cells, VMAT2 now provides an opportunity to characterize the sorting event that is crucial to the biogenesis of the regulated secretory pathway (Fig. 2). In contrast, membrane proteins destined for SVs enter the constitutive secretory pathway at the TGN and enter SVs only after retrieval from the cell surface (Kelly 1991; Regnier-Vigouroux et al. 1991). Thus, VMAT2 may not have the opportunity to enter SVs if it sorts

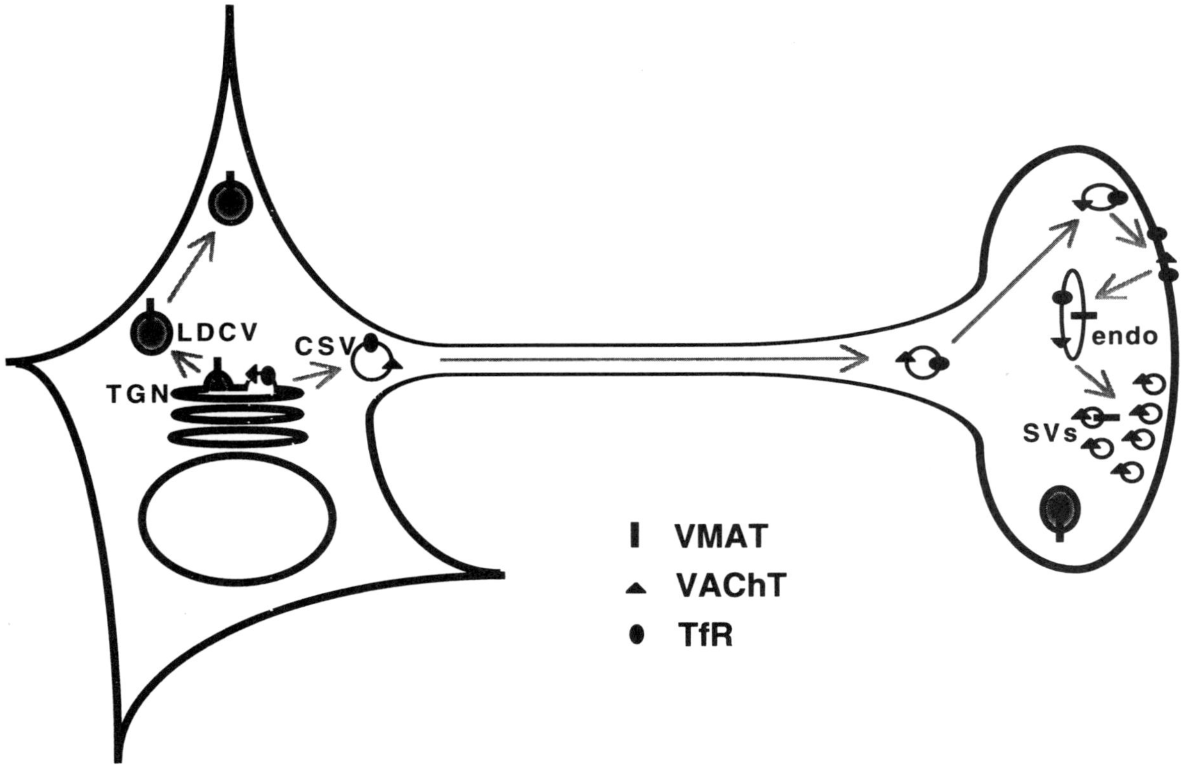

Figure 2. Differential sorting of the VMATs and VAChT. The VMATs (*rectangles*) localize preferentially to LDCVs, whereas the closely related VAChT (*triangle*) localizes almost exclusively to SVs. Localization at these sites makes several predictions about the sorting of these proteins that reflects the biogenesis of these secretory vesicles. LDCVs bud from the TGN and translocate to sites in the cell body and dendrites as well as the nerve terminal. Thus, proteins such as the VMATs that localize in LDCVs presumably sort to this regulated secretory pathway and away from the constitutive secretory pathway in the TGN. In contrast, proteins destined for SVs enter the constitutive secretory pathway (CSV) and after appearance at the cell surface, undergo internalization to an endosomal compartment and only then enter SVs. VMATs and VAChT thus diverge at the level of the TGN, suggesting a specific sorting event that presumably involves cytosolic machinery. The appearance of VMATs in SVs may occur through two distinct mechanisms. The proteins may sort incompletely at the TGN, with some entering the constitutive secretory pathway and, after internalization from the cell surface, SVs. Alternatively, VMATs may sort stringently to LDCVs and, after their fusion with the plasma membrane, undergo endocytosis and incorporation into SVs. Endo indicates endosomes and the sphere denotes transferrin receptors (TfR), which undergo endocytosis but do not enter SVs.

stringently to LDCVs and these LDCVs do not undergo constitutive exocytosis, preventing the recruitment of VMAT2 into endosomes and SVs.

SUMMARY

Molecular cloning of the transport proteins involved in packaging monoamines and ACh into secretory vesicles has implicated their activity in neural degeneration as well as signaling. Future studies will explore further the mechanism of active transport, its regulation, and the membrane trafficking of the proteins with the long-term goal of understanding how the regulation of transmitter release and, in particular, quantal size influences information processing and behavior. In addition, the bioenergetics of vesicular GABA and glutamate transport suggests that the proteins responsible for these activities may belong to a distinct gene family.

ACKNOWLEDGMENTS

This work was supported by grants from the National Institutes of Health, the National Institute of Mental Health, the National Institute for Drug Abuse, the Alzheimer's Program of the State of California, the American Parkinson's Disease Association, and the National Alliance for Research on Schizophrenia and Affective Disorders.

REFERENCES

Alfonso, A., K. Grundahl, J.S. Duerr, H.-P. Han, and J.B. Rand. 1993. The *Caenorhabditis elegans unc-17* gene: A putative vesicular acetylcholine transporter. *Science* **261:** 617.

Alfonso, A., K. Grundahl, J.R. McManus, J.M. Asbury, and J.B. Rand. 1994. Alternative splicing leads to two cholinergic proteins in *Caenorhabditis elegans*. *J. Mol. Biol.* **241:** 627.

Amara, S.G. and M.J. Kuhar. 1993. Neurotransmitter transporters: recent progress. *Annu. Rev. Neurosci.* **16:** 73.

Anderson, D.C., S.C. King, and S.M. Parsons. 1982. Proton gradient linkage to active uptake of 3H-acetylcholine by *Torpedo* electric organ synaptic vesicles. *Biochemistry* **21:** 3037.

Bahr, B.A. and S.M. Parsons. 1992. Purification of the vesamicol receptor. *Biochemistry* **31:** 5763.

Bejanin, S., R. Cervini, J. Mallet, and S. Berrard. 1994. A unique gene organization for two cholinergic markers, choline acetyltransferase and a putative vesicular transporter of acetylcholine. *J. Biol. Chem.* **269:** 21944.

Bennett, M.K. and R.H. Scheller. 1994. A molecular description of synaptic vesicle membrane trafficking. *Annu. Rev. Biochem.* **63:** 63.

Berse, B. and J.K. Blusztajn. 1995. Coordinated up-regulation of choline acetyltransferase and vesicular acetylcholine transporter gene expression by the retinoic acid receptor alpha, cAMP, and leukemia inhibitory factor/ciliary neurotrophic factor signaling pathways in a murine septal cell line. *J. Biol. Chem.* **270:** 22101.

Betz, W.J. and G.S. Bewick. 1992. Optical analysis of synaptic vesicle cycling at the frog neuromuscular junction. *Science* **255:** 200.

Carboni, E., A. Imperato, L. Perezzani, and G.D. Chiara. 1989. Amphetamine, cocaine, phencyclidine and nomifensine increase extracellular dopamine concentrations preferentially in the rat nucleus accumbens of freely moving rats. *Neuroscience* **28:** 653.

Carlsson, A. 1965. Drugs which block the storage of 5-hydroxytryptamine and related amines. *Handb. Exp. Pharmacol.* **19:** 529.

Choi, D.W. 1988. Glutamate neurotoxicity and diseases of the nervous system. *Neuron* **1:** 623.

Cohen, G. 1990. Monamine oxidase and oxidative stress at dopaminergic synapses. *J. Neural Transm. Suppl.* **32:** 229.

Cubells, J.F., S. Rayport, G. Rajendran, and D. Sulzer. 1994. Methamphetamine neurotoxicity involves vacuolation of endocytic organelles and dopamine-dependent intracellular oxidative stress. *J. Neurosci.* **14:** 2260.

Daniels, A.J. and J.F. Reinhard. 1988. Energy-driven uptake of the neurotoxin 1-methyl-4-phenylpyridinium into chromaffin granules via the catecholamine transporter. *J. Biol. Chem.* **263:** 5034.

Darchen, F., E. Scherman, and J.P. Henry. 1989. Reserpine binding to chromaffin granules suggests the existence of two conformations of the monoamine transporter. *Biochemistry* **28:** 1692.

Denton, T. and B.D. Howard. 1987. A dopaminergic cell line variant resistant to the neurotoxin 1-methyl-4-phenyl-1,2,3,6-tetrahydropyridine. *J. Neurochem.* **49:** 622.

Desnos, C., M. Laran, and D. Scherman. 1992. Regulation of the chromaffin granule catecholamine transporter in cultured bovine adrenal medullary cells-stimulus biosynthesis coupling. *J. Neurochem.* **59:** 2105.

Desnos, C., B. Raynaud, S. Vidal, M.J. Weber, and D. Scherman. 1990. Induction of the vesicular monoamine transporter by elevated potassium concentration in cultures of rat sympathetic neurons. *Dev. Brain Res.* **52:** 161.

Deutch, A.Y., J.D. Elsworth, M. Goldstein, K. Fuxe, D.E. Redmond, J.R. Sladek, and R.H. Roth. 1986. Preferential vulnerability of A8 dopamine neurons in the primate to the neurotoxin 1-methyl-4-phenyl-1,2,3,6-tetrahydropyridine. *Neurosci. Lett.* **68:** 51.

Di Chiara, G. and A. Imperato. 1988. Drugs abused by humans preferentially increase synaptic dopamine concentrations in the mesolimbic system of freely moving rats. *Proc. Natl. Acad. Sci.* **85:** 5274.

Edwards, R.H. 1992. The transport of neurotransmitters into synaptic vesicles. *Curr. Opin. Neurobiol.* **2:** 586.

Eldridge, R. and W.A. Rocca. 1992. Parkinson's disease. In *The genetic basis of common diseases* vol. 20, p. 775. Oxford University Press, New York.

Erickson, J.D. and L.E. Eiden. 1993. Functional identification and molecular cloning of a human brain vesicle monoamine transporter. *J. Neurochem.* **61:** 2314.

Erickson, J.D., L.E. Eiden, and B.J. Hoffman. 1992. Expression cloning of a reserpine-sensitive vesicular monoamine transporter. *Proc. Natl. Acad. Sci.* **89:** 10993.

Erickson, J.D., H. Varoqui, M.D. Schafer, W. Modi, M.F. Diebler, E. Weihe, J. Rand, L.E. Eiden, T.I. Bonner, and T.B. Usdin. 1994. Functional identification of a vesicular acetylcholine transporter and its expression from a "cholinergic" gene locus. *J. Biol. Chem.* **269:** 21929.

Fahn, S. and G. Cohen. 1992. The oxidant stress hypothesis in Parkinson's disease: Evidence supporting it. *Ann. Neurol.* **32:** 804.

Farquhar, M.G., J.J. Reid, and L.W. Daniell. 1978. Intracellular transport and packaging of prolactin: A quantitative electron microscope autoradiographic study of mamotrophs dissociated from rat pituitaries. *Endocrinology* **102:** 296.

Fisher, J.F. and A.K. Cho. 1979. Chemical release of DA from striatal homogenates: Evidence for an exchange diffusion model. *J. Pharmacol Exp. Ther.* **208:** 203.

Floor, E., P.S. Leventhal, Y. Wang, L. Meng, and W. Chen. 1995. Dynamic storage of dopamine in rat brain synaptic vesicles in vitro. *J. Neurochem.* **64:** 689.

German, D.C., K.F. Manaye, P.K. Sonsalla, and B.A. Brooks. 1992. Midbrain dopaminergic cell loss in Parkinson's disease and MPTP-induced parkinsonism: Sparing of calbindin-D28k-containing cells. *Ann. N.Y. Acad. Sci.* **648:** 42.

Gilmor, M.L., N.R. Nash, A. Roghani, R.H. Edwards, H. Yi, S.M. Hersch, and A.I. Levey. 1996. Expression of the putative vesicular acetylcholine transporter in rat brain and localization in cholinergic synaptic vesicles. *J. Neurosci.* **16:** 2179.

Heeringa, M.J. and E.D. Abercrombie. 1995. Biochemistry of somatodendritic dopamine release in substantia nigra: An in vivo comparison with striatal dopamine release. *J. Neurochem.* **65:** 192.

Heikkila, R.E., L. Manzino, F.S. Cabbat, and R.C. Duvoisin. 1984. Protection against the dopaminergic neurotoxicity of 1-methyl-4-phenyl-1,2,5,6-tetrahydropyridine by monoamine oxidase inhibitors. *Nature* **311:** 467.

Hernandez, L., F. Lee, and B.G. Hoebel. 1988. Microdialysis in the nucleus accumbens during feeding on drugs of abuse: Amphetamine, cocaine and phencyclidine. *Ann. N.Y. Acad. Sci.* **537:** 508.

Howell, M., A. Shirvan, Y. Stern-Bach, S. Steiner-Mordoch, J.E. Strasser, G.E. Dean, and S. Schuldiner. 1994. Cloning and functional expression of a tetrabenazine sensitive vesicular monoamine transporter from bovine chromaffin granules. *FEBS Lett.* **338:** 16.

Jahn, R. and T.C. Südhof. 1994. Synaptic vesicles and exocytosis. *Annu. Rev. Neurosci.* **17:** 219.

Javitch, J., R. D'Amato, J. Nye, and J. Javitch. 1985. Parkinsonism-inducing neurotoxin, N-methyl-4-phenyl-1,2,3,6-tetrahydropyridine: Uptake of the metabolite N-methyl-4-phenylpyridine by dopamine neurons explains selective toxicity. *Proc. Natl. Acad. Sci.* **82:** 2173.

Jenner, P., D.T. Dexter, J. Sian, A.H. Schapira, and C.D. Marsden. 1992. Oxidative stress as a cause of nigral cell death in Parkinson's disease and incidental Lewy body disease. *Ann. Neurol.* **32:** (suppl) 82.

Johannessen, J.N., C.C. Chiueh, R.S. Burns, and S.P. Markey. 1985. Differences in the metabolism of MPTP in the rodent and primate parallel differences in sensitivity to its neurotoxic effects. *Life Sci.* **36:** 219.

Johnson, R.G. 1988. Accumulation of biological amines into chromaffin granules: A model for hormone and neurotransmitter transport. *Physiol. Rev.* **68:** 232.

Kalivas, P.W. and P. Duffy. 1993. Time course of extracellular dopamine and behavioral sensitization to cocaine. II. Dopamine perikarya. *J. Neurosci.* **13:** 276.

Kaneko, M., A. Yamaguchi, and T. Sawai. 1985. Energetics of tetracycline efflux system encoded by *Tn*10 in *Escherichia coli. FEBS Lett.* **193:** 194.

Kelly, R.B. 1991. Secretory granule and synaptic vesicle formation. *Curr. Opin. Cell Biol.* **3:** 654.

———. 1993. Storage and release of neurotransmitters. *Cell* **72:** 43.

Kish, S.J., L.M. Distefano, S. Dozic, Y. Robitaille, A. Rajput, J.H.N. Deck, and O. Hornykiewicz. 1990. 3H-Vesamicol binding in human brain cholinergic deficiency disorders. *Neuroscience Lett.* **117:** 347.

Krejci, E., B. Gasnier, D. Botton, M.F. Isambert, C. Sagne, J. Gagnon, J. Massoulie, and J.P. Henry. 1993. Expression and regulation of the bovine vesicular monoamine transporter gene. *FEBS Lett.* **335:** 27.

Krueger, M.J., T.P. Singer, J.E. Casida, and R.R. Ramsay. 1990. Evidence that the blockade of mitochondrial respiration by the neurotoxin 1-methyl-4-phenylpyridinium (MPP^+) involves binding at the same site as the respiratory inhibitor, rotenone. *Biochem. Biophys. Res. Commun.* **169:** 123.

Kuliawat, R. and P. Arvan. 1992. Protein targeting via the "constitutive-like" secretory pathway in isolated pancreatic islets: Passive sorting in the immature granule component. *J. Cell Biol.* **118:** 521.

———. 1994. Distinct molecular mechanisms for protein sorting within immature secretory granules of pancreatic beta-cells. *J. Cell Biol.* **126:** 77.

Langston, J.W., P. Ballard, J.W. Tetrud, and I. Irwin. 1983. Chronic Parkinsonism in humans due to a product of meperidine analog synthesis. *Science* **219:** 979.

Langston, J.W., I. Irwin, E.G. Langston, and L.S. Forno. 1984. Pargyline prevents MPTP-induced Parkinsonism in primates. *Science* **225:** 1480.

Lesch, K.P., J. Gross, B.L. Wolozin, E. Franzek, D. Bengel, P. Riederer, and D.L. Murphy. 1994. Direct sequencing of the reserpine-sensitive vesicular monoamine transporter complementary DNA in unipolar depression and manic depressive illness. *Psychiatr. Genet.* **4:** 153.

Liu, Y. and R.H. Edwards. 1996. The role of vesicular transport proteins in synaptic transmission and neural degeneration. *Annu. Rev. Neurosci.* (in press).

Liu, Y., A. Roghani, and R.H. Edwards. 1992a. Gene transfer of a reserpine-sensitive mechanism of resistance to MPP^+. *Proc. Natl. Acad. Sci.* **89:** 9074.

Liu, Y., E.S. Schweitzer, M.J. Nirenberg, V.M. Pickel, C.J. Evans, and R.H. Edwards. 1994. Preferential localization of a vesicular monoamine transporter to dense core vesicles in PC12 cells. *J. Cell Biol.* **127:** 1419.

Liu, Y., D. Peter, A. Roghani, S. Schuldiner, G.G. Prive, D. Eisenberg, N. Brecha, and R.H. Edwards. 1992b. A cDNA that suppresses MPP^+ toxicity encodes a vesicular amine transporter. *Cell* **70:** 539.

Maron, R., Y. Stern, B.I. Kanner, and S. Schuldiner. 1983. Functional asymmetry of the amine transporter from chromaffin granules. *J. Biol. Chem.* **258:** 11476.

Martin, T.F.J. 1994. The molecular machinery for fast and slow neurosecretion. *Curr. Opin. Neurobiol.* **4:** 626.

Merickel, A. and R.H. Edwards. 1995. Transport of histamine by vesicular monoamine transporter-2. *Neuropharmacology* **34:** 1543.

Merickel, A., P. Rosandich, D. Peter, and R.H. Edwards. 1995. Identification of residues involved in substrate recognition by a vesicular monoamine transporter. *J. Biol. Chem.* **270:** 25798.

Michel, P.P. and F. Hefti. 1990. Toxicity of 6-hydroxydopamine and dopamine for dopaminergic neurons in culture. *J. Neurosci. Res.* **26:** 428.

Mitchell, I.J., A.J. Cross, M. A. Sambrook, and A.R. Crossman. 1985. Sites of the neurotoxic action of 1-methyl-4-phenyl-1,2,3,6-tetrahydropyridine in the macaque monkey include the ventral tegmental area and the locus coeruleus. *Neurosci. Lett.* **61:** 195.

Nakanishi, N., S. Onozawa, R. Matsumoto, H. Hasegawa, and S. Yamada. 1995. Effects of protein kinase inhibitors and protein phosphatase inhibitors on cyclic AMP-dependent down-regulation of vesicular monoamine transport in pheochromocytoma PC12 cells. *FEBS Lett.* **368:** 411.

Neal, R.J. and K.F. Chater. 1987. Nucleotide sequence analysis reveals similarities between proteins determining methylenomycin A resistance in streptomyces and tetracycline resistance in eubacteria. *Gene* **58:** 229.

Neyfakh, A.A., V.E. Bidnenko, and L.B. Chen. 1991. Efflux-mediated multidrug resistance in *Bacillus subtilis:* Similarities and dissimilarities with the mammalian system. *Proc. Natl. Acad. Sci.* **88:** 4781.

Nguyen, T.T., K. Postle, and K.P. Bertrand. 1983. Sequence homology between the tetracycline-resistance determinants of *Tn*10 and pBR322. *Gene* **25:** 83.

Nicklas, W.J., I. Vyas, and R.E. Heikkila. 1985. Inhibition of NADH-linked oxidation in brain mitochondria by 1-methyl-4-phenylpyridine, a metabolite of the neurotoxin 1-methyl-4-phenyl-1,2,3,6-tetrahydropyridine. *Life Sci.* **36:** 2503.

Nirenberg, M.J. J. Chan, Y. Liu, R.H. Edwards, and V.M. Pichel. 1996. Ultrastructural localization of the vesicular monoamine transporter-2 in midbrain dopaminergic neurons: Potential sites for somatodendritic storage and release of dopamine. *J. Neurosci.* **16:** 14135.

Nirenberg, M.J., Y. Liu, D. Peter, R.H. Edwards, and V.M. Pickel. 1995. The vesicular monoamine transporter-2 is present in small synaptic vesicles and preferentially localizes to large dense core vesicles in rat solitary tract nuclei. *Proc. Natl. Acad. Sci.* **92:** 8773.

Parkinson's Study Group. 1989. Effect of deprenyl on the progression of disability in early Parkinson's disease. *N. Engl. J. Med.* **321:** 1364.

———. 1993. Effects of tocopherol and deprenyl on the progression of disability in early Parkinson's disease. *N. Engl. J. Med.* **328:** 176.

Peter, D., T. Vu, and R.H. Edwards. 1996. Chimeric vesicular monoamine transporters identify structural domains that influence substrate affinity and sensitivity to tetrabenazine. *J. Biol. Chem.* **271:** 2979.

Peter, D., J. Jimenez, Y. Liu, J. Kim, and R.H. Edwards. 1994. The chromaffin granule and synaptic vesicle amine transporters differ in substrate recognition and sensitivity to inhibitors. *J. Biol. Chem.* **269:** 7231.

Peter, D., Y. Liu, C. Sternini, R. de Giorgio, N. Brecha, and R.H. Edwards. 1995. Differential expression of two vesicular monoamine transporters. *J. Neurosci.* **15:** 6179.

Peter, D., J.P. Finn, I. Klisak, Y. Liu, T. Kojis. C. Heinzmann, A. Roghani, R.S. Sparkes, and R.H. Edwards. 1993. Chromosomal localization of the human vesicular amine transporter genes. *Genomics* **18:** 720.

Przedborski, S., V. Kostic, V. Jackson-Lewis, A.B. Naini, S. Simonetti, S. Fahn, E. Carlson, C.J. Epstein, and J.L. Cadet. 1992. Transgenic mice with increased Cu/Zn-superoxide dismutase activity are resistant to N-methyl-4-phenyl-1,2,3,6-tetrahydropyridine-induced neurotoxicity. *J. Neurosci.* **12:** 1658.

Ramsay, R.R. and T. P. Singer. 1986. Energy-dependent uptake of N-methyl-4-phenylpyridinium, the neurotoxic metabolite of 1-methyl-4-phenyl-1,2,3,6-tetrahydropyridine, by mitochondria. *J. Biol. Chem.* **261:** 7585.

Ramsay, R.R., M.J. Krueger, S.K. Youngster, M.R. Gluck, J.E. Casida, and T.P. Singer. 1991. Interaction of 1-methyl-4-phenylpyridinium (MPP^+) and its analogs with the rotenone/piericidin binding site of NADH dehydrogenase. *J. Neurochem.* **56:** 1184.

Regnier-Vigouroux, A., S.A. Tooze, and W.B. Huttner. 1991. Newly synthesized synaptophysin is transported to synaptic-like microvesicles via constitutive secretory vesicles and the plasma membrane. *EMBO J.* **10:** 3589.

Roghani, A., J. Feldman, S.A. Kohan, A. Shirzadi, C.B. Gundersen, N. Brecha, and R.H. Edwards. 1994. Molecular cloning of a putative vesicular transporter for acetylcholine. *Proc. Natl. Acad. Sci.* **91:** 10620.

Rosenberg, P.A. 1988. Catecholamine toxicity in cerebral cortex in dissociated cell culture. *J. Neurosci.* **8:** 2887.

Ruberg, M., W. Mayo, A. Brice, C. Duyckaerts, J.J. Hauw, H. Simon, M. LeMoal, and Y. Agid. 1990. Choline acetyltransferase activity and 3H-vesamicol binding in the temporal cortex of patients with Alzheimer's disease, Parkinson's disease, and rats with basal forebrain lesions. *Neuroscience* **35:** 327.

Rudnick, G. and S.C. Wall. 1992a. The molecular mechanism of "ecstasy" [3,4-methylenedioxymethamphetamin (MDMA)]: Serotonin transporters are targets for MDMA-induced serotonin release. *Proc. Natl. Acad. Sci.* **89:** 1817.

———. 1992b. p-Chloroamphetamine induces serotonin release through serotonin transporters. *Biochemistry* **31:** 6710.

———. 1992c. Non-neurotoxic amphetamine derivatives release serotonin through serotonin transporters. *Mol. Pharmacol.* **43:** 271.

Rudnick, G., S.S. Steiner-Mordoch, H. Fishkes, Y. Stern-Bach, and S. Schuldiner. 1990. Energetics of reserpine binding and occlusion by the chromaffin granule biogenic amine transporter. *Biochemistry* **29:** 603.

Ryan, T.A., H. Reuter, B. Wendland, F.E. Schweizer, R.W. Tsien, and S.J. Smith. 1993. The kinetics of synaptic vesicle recycling measured at single presynaptic boutons. *Neuron* **11:** 713.

Schapira, A., J. Cooper, D. Dexter, J. Clark, P. Jenner, and C.D. Marsden. 1990. Mitochondrial complex I deficiency in Parkinson's disease. *J. Neurochem.* **54:** 823.

Scherman, D. and J.P. Henry. 1984. Reserpine binding to bovine chromaffin granule membranes. Characterization and comparison with dihydrotetrabenazine binding. *Mol. Pharmacol.* **25:** 113.

Scherman, D., F. Darchen, C. Desnos, and J.P. Henry. 1988. 1-Methyl-4-phenylpyridinium is a substrate of the vesicular monoamine transport system of chromaffin granules. *Eur. J. Pharmacol.* **146:** 359.

Schuldiner, S., Y. Liu, and R.H. Edwards. 1993a. Reserpine binding to a vesicular amine transporter expressed in Chinese hamster ovary fibroblasts. *J. Biol. Chem.* **268:** 29.

Schuldiner, S., A. Shirvan, and M. Linial. 1995. Vesicular neurotransmitter transporters: From bacteria to humans. *Physiol. Rev.* **75:** 369.

Schuldiner, S., S. Steiner-Mordoch, R. Yelin, S.C. Wall, and G. Rudnick. 1993b. Amphetamine derivatives interact with both plasma membrane and secretory vesicle biogenic amine transporters. *Mol. Pharmacol.* **44:** 1227.

Shirvan, A., O. Laskar, S. Steiner-Mordoch, and S. Schuldiner. 1994. Histidine-419 plays a role in energy coupling in the vesicular monoamine transporter from rat. *FEBS Lett.* **356:** 145.

Shoffner, J.M., R.L. Watts, J.L. Juncos, A. Torroni, and D.C. Wallace. 1991. Mitochondrial oxidative phosphorylation in Parkinson's disease. *Ann. Neurol.* **30:** 332.

Smith, A.D. 1972. Mechanisms involved in the release of noradrenaline from sympathetic nerve. *Br. Med. Bull.* **29:** 123.

Steele, T.D., U.D. McCann, and G.A. Ricaurte. 1994. 3,4-Methylenedioxymethamphetamine (MDMA, ecstasy): Pharmacology and toxicology in animals and humans. *Addiction* **89:** 539.

Stern-Bach, Y., J.N. Keen, M. Bejerano, S. Steiner-Mordoch, M. Wallach, J.B. Findlay, and S. Schuldiner. 1992. Homology of a vesicular amine transporter to a gene conferring resistance to 1-methyl-4-phenylpyridinium. *Proc. Natl. Acad. Sci.* **89:** 9730.

Strader, C.D., M.R. Candelore, W.S. Hill, I.S. Sigal, and R.A.F. Dixon. 1989. Identification of two serine residues involved in agonist activation of the beta-adrenergic receptor. *J. Biol. Chem.* **264:** 13572.

Sulzer, D. and S. Rayport. 1990. Amphetamine and other psychostimulants reduce pH gradients in midbrain dopaminergic neurons and chromaffin granules: A mechanism of action. *Neuron* **5:** 797.

Sulzer, D., N.T. Maidment, and S. Rayport. 1993. Amphetamine and other weak bases act to promote reverse transport of dopamine in ventral midbrain neurons. *J. Neurochem.* **60:** 527.

Surratt, C.K., A.M. Persico, X.-D. Yang, S.R. Edgar, G.S. Bird, A.L. Hawkins, C.A. Griffin, X. Li, E.W. Jabs, and G.R. Uhl. 1993. A human synaptic vesicle monoamine transporter cDNA predicts posttranslational modifications, reveals chromosome 10 gene localization and identifies TaqI RFLPs. *FEBS Lett.* **318:** 325.

Tanner, C.M. and J.W. Langston. 1990. Do environmental toxins cause Parkinson's disease? A critical review. *Neurology* **40:** 17.

Thureson-Klein, A. 1983. Exocytosis from large and small dense cored vesicles in noradrenergic nerve terminals. *Neuroscience* **10:** 245.

Tooze, J. and S.A. Tooze. 1986. Clathrin-coated vesicular transport of secretory proteins during the formation of ACTH-containing secretory granules in AtT20 cells. *J. Cell Biol.* **103:** 839.

Tooze, S.A., E. Chanat, J. Tooze, and W.B. Huttner. 1993. Secretory granule formation. In *Mechanisms of in-*

tracellular trafficking and processing of proproteins, p. 157. CRC Press, Boca Raton, Florida.

Turski, L., K. Bressler, K.-J. Rettig, P.-A. Loschmann, and H. Wachtel. 1991. Protection of substantia nigra from MPP^+ neurotoxicity by N-methyl-D-aspartate antagonists. *Nature* **349:** 414.

Varoqui, H., M.-F. Diebler, F.-M. Meunier, J.B. Rand, T.B. Usdin, T.I. Bonner, L.E. Eiden, and J.D. Erickson. 1994. Cloning and expression of the vesamicol binding protein from the marine ray *Torpedo*. Homology with the putative vesicular acetylcholine transporter UNC-17 from *Caenorhabditis elegans*. *FEBS Lett.* **342:** 97.

Vingerhoets, F.J., B.J. Snow, J.W. Tetrud, J.W. Langston, M. Schulzer, and D.B. Calne. 1994. Positron emission tomographic evidence for progression of human MPTP-induced dopaminergic lesions. *Ann. Neurol.* **36:** 765.

Wall, S.C., H. Gu, and G. Rudnick. 1995. Biogenic amine flux mediated by cloned transporters stably expressed in cultured cell lines: Amphetamine specificity for inhibition and efflux. *Mol. Pharmacol.* **47:** 544.

Weaver, J.H. and J.D. Deupree. 1982. Conditions required for reserpine binding to the catecholamine transporter on chromaffin granule ghosts. *Eur. J. Pharmacol.* **80:** 437.

Westlund, K.N., R.M. Denney, R.M. Rose, and C.W. Abell. 1988. Localization of distinct monoamine oxidase A and monoamine oxidase B cell populations in human brainstem. *Neuroscience* **25:** 439.

AIDS Dementia Complex: A Complex, Slow Virus "Model" of Acquired Genetic Neurodegenerative Disease

R.W. Price
Neurology Service, San Francisco General Hospital, and Department of Neurology, University of California, San Francisco, California 94110

The AIDS dementia complex (ADC) has a number of features in common with the neurodegenerative diseases: Its phenotype is that of a "system disease" with an hierarchical order of presenting symptoms and signs and subsequent progression (Nowak et al. 1991; Price 1995c); its pathology, although heterogeneous, also includes selective involvement of particular structures and regions of the nervous system (Kure et al. 1990; Kuchelmeister et al. 1993; Brew et al. 1995); its latency is long and its course protracted; and it may be clinically devastating, often lethally so (Neaton et al. 1994). It is also a genetic disease, albeit the result of the "acquired" exogenous genes of human immunodeficiency virus type one (HIV-1) (Feinberg 1996). On the other hand, it occurs in the setting of a general infection with primary involvement of another organ system rather than occurring as an isolated or predominating affliction of the central nervous system (CNS). It is a "slow" virus infection and a counterpart of one of the veterinary diseases, visna-maedi, studied by Sigurdsson, who first articulated the concept of slow infections more than 40 years ago (Sigurdsson et al. 1957). In this review, I focus on some of the salient issues of ADC pathogenesis and therapy. In the process, I also compare ADC to both acute viral infections and other neurodegenerative conditions with the hope that such a juxtaposition provides a useful perspective on both viral and neurodegenerative diseases.

Table 1 introduces some of these issues by comparing ADC with two other prototypic diseases: (1) poliomyelitis, an acute viral infection of the nervous system that preoccupied an earlier generation much as AIDS does our own era, and (2) spinocerebellar ataxia type 1 (SCA1), one of the trinucleotide repeat diseases that is used here as an example of a genetic neurodegenerative disorder and is the subject of other papers in this volume. The table outlines both differences and similarities, several of which are touched upon below. Clinically, the three diseases differ greatly in their temporal profiles, from acute evolution in the case of polio to the long latency and chronic evolution of SCA1, with ADC being somewhere in between. Both polio and ADC are caused by a transmitted "package" of exogenous genes, whereas SCA1 is passed vertically in sperm or ova. All have some features of selective vulnerability of certain CNS "systems," although ADC is perhaps the least fastidious in this regard, affecting certain gray matter nuclei more frequently, but the cortex and white matter more broadly as well. A major difference among the three conditions is degree of participation of the immune system. In SCA1 the immune system appears to have little or no role, whereas in poliomyelitis the immune system is critical both in curtailing infection so that its course is circumscribed and in preventing disease following immunization. In the case of ADC the relationship between the immune system and the causative virus is far more complex and, indeed, is central to both the long course and the eventual damage to the CNS. The immune system is both protector and pathological agonist. In fact, one of the principal differences between ADC and the other two diseases in the table is the complexity of the former's pathogenesis and the circuitous connection between the suspected etiology, HIV-1, and the clinical disease, ADC; the immune system is a central intermediary in disease production.

To consider this complexity, I first outline some of the fundamental features of the ADC and HIV-1 infection of the CNS, emphasizing clinical observations that bear on considerations of pathogenesis. As important background, I next consider selected facets of the biology of HIV-1 that are important in understanding neuropathogenesis before reviewing some of the critical changes in the immune system that set the stage for ADC development. I then discuss interactions of HIV-1 and the immune system within the CNS, drawing on both clinical and experimental observations, and from this consider a general model that is useful in formulating more detailed questions of pathogenesis and developing strategies for therapy.

ADC: A SUBCORTICAL DEMENTIA COMPLICATING LATE HIV-1 INFECTION

Late HIV-1 infection is complicated by an array of neurological disorders that contribute importantly to the morbidity and mortality of AIDS (Simpson et al. 1994; Price 1996). These include the more common CNS opportunistic infections of cerebral toxoplasmosis and progressive multifocal leukoencephalopathy (PML) caused by the otherwise benign papovavirus, JC; the opportunistic neoplasm, primary CNS lymphoma which relates to Epstein-Barr virus infection; and a number of other less common, but often

Table 1. Comparative Features of Poliomyelitis (an Acute Viral Infection), ADC (Result of a Slow Infection), and SCA1 (an Inherited Disease Related to a Trinucleotide Repeat Mutation of a Cell Gene, Ataxin)

	Poliomyelitis	ADC	SCA1
Time course	acute	slow	chronic
incubation	days	years	decades
evolution (after onset)	days	weeks–months	decades
"Abnormal" genes	yes	yes	yes
source	exogenous (infection)	exogenous (infection)	endogenous (host)
temporal profile of expression	phasic	augmentative (crescendo)	continuous
resultant complexity	moderate	high	low
System disease	yes	yes	yes
Principal (proximate) cause of neuronal (from without) damage	virus-induced cell modification (from within)	virus-driven immuno-pathology (from within)	mutant host gene product effect
Involvement of immune system in disease	yes	yes	no
in curtailing process	effective	ineffective	no
as pathological major agonist	no	yes	no

equally devastating, infections. However, perhaps the most common of the CNS diseases is ADC, which is caused not by another opportunistic pathogen, but by HIV-1 itself. This condition, which was recognized early in the AIDS epidemic, was described using a variety of terms, including, most recently, *HIV-associated cognitive/motor complex* (A.A.N.A.T.F. 1991). It also has a pediatric counterpart that is commonly called *HIV encephalopathy* (Belman 1994). There are a number of reasons to seek better understanding of ADC. First, it is a clinically important problem. Although controversy continues regarding its incidence, at least 10% of AIDS patients develop moderate to end-stage ADC (Stages 2–4), and the incidence is likely higher than this when one includes both milder cases and patients who reach the final phase of infection (Stage 1) (McArthur et al. 1993; Neaton et al. 1994). Given the prevalence of HIV-1 infection, this makes ADC the most common "neurodegenerative" disease afflicting young-middle age adults in which dementia is a principal feature. Its pediatric analog is, if anything, a more frequent complication of infection in childhood. In addition to being the source of considerable morbidity, it carries a high mortality. Stage 2–4 ADC is associated with one of the shortest survival times of AIDS-defining clinical diagnoses; in the experience of the Community Program for Clinical Research in AIDS (CPCRA), two-thirds of ADC patients were dead 6 months after diagnosis (Neaton et al. 1994). A second reason to elucidate ADC centers on its relation to HIV-1 infection of the CNS, and the fact that the latter is an integral part of the biology of this infection. The nervous system is exposed early to the virus and can be the site of florid productive infection during its final phase (Price 1995b); with the recent advent of potent antiretroviral therapy that can markedly suppress systemic infection, the possibility that the CNS may provide a critical "sanctuary" for infection and development of resistant mutants has become an important issue (Ho 1995; Feinberg 1996). Finally, the third reason to understand the pathogenesis of ADC, and one that provides some of the rationale for the approach taken in this review, is that this disorder may provide insight into the pathogenesis and therapy of other neurological diseases, including some classified as either neurodegenerative or immunopathological. It serves as a model, albeit in certain ways a caricature, of virus-induced neuropathogenesis in which endogenous host reactions, both immunological and neurotoxic, play a key role. Comparison with other neurodegenerative diseases also might, conversely, provide pathogenetic and therapeutic insight into ADC.

On the basis of its clinical phenotype, ADC is classified among the "subcortical" dementias (Benson 1987). At its core is psychomotor slowing: slowing of thought processes, difficulty with attention and concentration, and parallel slowing of rapid motor movements (Navia et al. 1986a; Price 1995c). These abnormalities are responsible for the early symptoms (trouble attending to tasks, or shifting mental "sets" quickly) and signs (slowed fine finger and eye movements), whereas with further progression, cognitive difficulty extends more broadly eventuating in vegetative mutism, and, likewise, motor dysfunction may evolve to spastic ataxia and finally to paraparesis or even quadraparesis-in-flexion. Abnormal reflexes appear early, with hyperactive deep tendon responses, and subsequently include "release" reflexes such as snout and grasp responses. Behavior usually parallels this psychomotor slowing with progressive dulling of the personality and apathy. These salient features are also reflected in the profile of abnormalities recorded by formal, quantitative neuropsychological testing in which timed motor tasks, quick reaction, and attention/concentration are characteristically altered (Tross et al. 1988; Sidtis 1994). Although usually not needed for diagnosis, this test profile is useful in further characterizing the phenotype of the condition and, in more practical application, for evaluating natural history and assessing response to therapy.

As alluded to above, in its stereotypy, bilateral symmetry, predominantly involving some components of the CNS while sparing others, ADC has some features of a system disease and in this way differs importantly from major opportunistic CNS infections that present with more randomly dispersed focal lesions (although also reflecting a different type of regional or cell selectivity: e.g., for gray matter in the case of toxoplasmosis; or oligodendrocytes and, hence, white matter in the case of PML). Neuroimaging of the brain in ADC often shows this symmetry. The most consistent finding is brain atrophy with reduced volume of both white and gray matter (Gelman and Guinto 1992; Aylward et al. 1993). Magnetic resonance imaging (MRI) may additionally show altered signal in the deeper white matter caused by increased water content, either in a diffuse or patchy pattern, and less commonly the diencephalic nuclei can show similar changes (Power et al. 1993). Functional imaging has shown metabolic abnormalities in ADC. These include abnormalities by magnetic resonance spectroscopy (MRS) with late depression of NAA levels and earlier increases in Cho and a peak that appears to correspond to a group of amino acids speculated to relate to early immune reaction to virus exposure (Jarvik et al. 1993; Paley et al. 1996; Tracey et al. 1996). Also of interest in defining the physiological basis of the clinical phenotype are observations of relative hypermetabolism of the basal ganglia and hypometabolism of cortex detected by positron emission tomography (PET) using ^{18}F-labeled deoxyglucose (Rottenberg et al. 1987).

Neuropathological analysis reveals several types of abnormalities, and there is some controversy regarding which of these correlate best with clinical findings and therefore point to the most important elements of pathogenesis (Navia et al. 1986b; Glass et al. 1993, 1995; Wiley and Achim 1994; Brew et al. 1995). The most common abnormality is pallor of the deep white matter associated with astrocytosis. This pallor is not true demyelination and likely reflects increased water content associated with altered blood-brain barrier (BBB) permeability (Power et al. 1993). The astrocytic reaction, accompanied also by microgliosis, clearly indicates that this is a pathogenic process, although its origin is not defined. Only some of these brains have detectable productive HIV-1 infection and often this is inconspicuous (Brew et al. 1995; Glass et al. 1995). In contrast, other cases exhibit more florid HIV-1 infection, warranting the term *HIV-1 encephalitis*. Many of these exhibit characteristic multinucleated cells and are also referred to as multinucleated-cell encephalitis; these multinucleated cells are derived from microglia-macrophages and are infected by HIV-1, which causes the cell fusion.

The distribution of infection in the brain is not homogeneous. Although there is considerable individual case variability, there is an hierarchical predilection for certain structures (Brew et al. 1995). Kure et al. (1990) have pointed out that this distribution resembles that of multisystem atrophy. The globus pallidus is the most commonly infected structure, followed by the striatum, substantia nigra, and deep white matter, whereas the cortex is relatively spared. This predilection reinforces the subcortical theme of the illness. The reason for this regional topography, however, remains enigmatic. Whether it relates to the preferred route of viral entry (e.g., entry via the choroid plexus in the lateral ventricles with spread into the adjacent brain, or because of selected entry of infected cells through the capillaries of certain regions) or to other local factors is unknown. One speculation is that infection is self-reinforcing: When infection damages local cells including neurons, this damage signals changes in local vessels that favor entry of both infected and susceptible cells (monocyte-macrophages) that are also activated, rendering them more permissive for HIV-1 replication, thereby establishing a vicious cycle. If this is important, the regional distribution would be determined by susceptibility of neurons to injury. A more heretical extension of this idea is that local HIV-1 infection is entirely secondary and that it merely follows pathology caused by something else (e.g., a blood-borne toxin) and serves as a marker for such injury rather than its cause. Although this seems unlikely or at least not fully sufficient, it cannot be lightly dismissed.

Neuropathological changes in AIDS patients also include morphological alterations of cortical neurons, with loss of neurons in some cortical regions (Masliah et al. 1996). Striking alterations of dendrites and reduction of synaptic density have been noted, and apoptosis of neurons and glia have also been reported. These observations indicate that although deeper structures are more notably infected, the cortex is also clearly involved in the disease process. Basal ganglion neurons are also reduced in number but have not been as extensively studied, particularly using quantitative, cytochemical, or ultrastructural methods. One other important pathology warrants inclusion, although it will not be considered further here. This is the vacuolar myelopathy found in some adult AIDS patients and included within the clinical ADC designation (Petito et al. 1985, 1994). This pathology, which can be severe, is indistinguishable from that of subacute combined degeneration resulting from cobalamine (vitamin B12) deficiency. The vacuolation does not correlate either with productive HIV-1 infection or with depressed serum B12 levels, but the similarity to subacute combined degeneration has raised speculation that it has a metabolic basis with a shared final pathway of myelin injury.

HIV-1: SELECTED CONSIDERATIONS BEARING ON ADC

HIV-1 not only is the cause of AIDS, but appears also to be the etiological agent "driving" ADC, although as discussed below, how it does this is uncertain. Table 2 outlines some of the biological properties of the virus that bear on its capacity to cause ADC. Since a detailed review of the biology of this complex virus is far beyond the scope of this paper, these properties are only discussed briefly. HIV-1 is a complex RNA virus that codes for a number of gene products which include the structural proteins and glycoproteins of the infectious virion; enzymes involved in reverse transcription, integration of the viral genome, and posttranscriptional processing, including the viral protease; and regulatory proteins controlling and modulating replication and gene expression (Greene 1991). It contains activation sequences that respond not only to viral signals (e.g., the *tat*-coded gene product), but also to physiological cell-coded signals. The latter are adaptively important in suppressing or augmenting replication in different settings of cell quiescence and activation which, in turn, permit both long-term latency and active viral replication depending on cell type and physiological signals.

HIV-1's principal targets are CD4$^+$ cells, including particularly helper T-lymphocytes expressing this receptor on their surface, but also macrophages and related microglia in the brain (Weiss 1996). Recently, a co-receptor has also been identified (Feng et al. 1996). These receptors are the principal determinants of cell tropism, particularly for productive infection. Infection has also been demonstrated in non-CD4$^+$ cells, both in cell culture and in vivo, including astrocytes and derivative cell lines and also perhaps neurons (Brack-Werner et al. 1991; Nuovo et al. 1994; Saito et al. 1994; Takahashi et al. 1996). A major characteristic of such infections is that they generally are "restricted," producing very limited or no progeny virus; infection is usually arrested at an early phase of replication with synthesis of regulatory gene products but failure of transition to production of the later structural genes needed to manufacture infectious progeny. The extent to which this type of infection contributes to in vivo brain dysfunction is uncertain. This paper focuses on the role of more indirect mechanisms of brain injury, but cytotoxicity related to this type of restricted viral gene expression in astrocytes or neurons remains an alternative explanation that requires further exploration.

Because of the poor fidelity of the virus-coded reverse transcriptase (RT), HIV-1 replication is accompanied by a high mutation rate. This results in continued evolution, diversification, and selection of the virus infecting the individual host; indeed, the host is infected by a "swarm" or quasispecies of viruses derived from common progenitors (Feinberg 1996). Resultant changes in viral antigens may be important in allowing evasion of antiviral surveillance until the host repertoire is exhausted. In the same way, alterations in the viral RT gene provide the substrate for

Table 2. Aspects of HIV-1 Bearing on CNS Infection, Brain Injury, and Treatment

HIV-1 characteristic	Potential implications for CNS infection and injury
Complex genome coding structural, enzyme, and regulatory products	produces infectious package (virion) to transmit and amplify its genome
	integrates into the cell genome, underlying long-term persistence
	adapted to exploit the variable physiological state of the host cell with responses to cell signals through activation sites
Infects CD4$^+$ cells	infects T-lymphocytes resulting in suppression of cell-mediated defenses
	productively infects macrophages and related cells, including microglia
Can infect non-CD4$^+$ cells	restricted infection of neuroectodermal cells, including astrocytes and perhaps neurons; also vascular endothelial cells
High mutation rate	allows it to evade immune surveillance
	phenotype alterations of the predominant quasispecies can include altered cell tropism and possibly neuropathogenicity
	underlies development of resistance to antiviral drugs
Some of its gene products are (potential) extracellular and intracellular signals and toxins	includes gp120, regulatory gene products of *tat*, *nef*, and *rev*

resistance to zidovudine (AZT) and other nucleoside as well as non-nucleoside RT inhibitors under the selective pressure of drug treatment (Richman 1996). Similarly, alterations in the viral protease confer resistant changes to the newer potent class of protease inhibitors.

Although more speculative, mutation and selective changes in the virus may also be important in determining the disease spectrum. Relevant to ADC, variants of the virus that have been identified in brains of patients with HIV-1 encephalitis exhibit the phenotypic property of macrophage tropism: They replicate well in monocyte-derived macrophages (and in microglia) but poorly in lymphocytic cell lines (O'Brien 1994). This is consonant with the limitation of productive brain infection to these bone marrow-derived cells, as discussed below. This tropism is associated principally with alterations in the gene coding for the external glycoprotein of HIV-1, gp120. However, macrophage tropism alone is insufficient to cause brain HIV-1 infection, since variants with this property are detected early in the infection and probably are present throughout infection in most patients, at least in certain organs. This has led to a search for particular mutations that might enhance the *neurovirulence* of the virus and explain why some patients develop ADC and others do not (Power et al. 1994). Such virulence might be conferred by changes in the virus that either favor brain replication or increase the stimulation of neurotoxic signals.

A final aspect of the virus that is seemingly important to ADC is the observation that some HIV-1 gene products serve as signal molecules, not only within infected cells, but also after extracellular release. For example, gp120 has been shown to have biological activity in a number of experimental systems beyond its role as a receptor ligand in viral infection. The putative role of this and other viral gene products is discussed further below.

THE IMMUNE SYSTEM IN ADC

One principal difference between ADC and SCA1 is the primary importance of the interaction of the disease-causing genes (the genes of HIV-1) with the immune system in ADC. Rather than being a primary affliction of the nervous system, ADC develops secondarily as a consequence of the underlying interaction of HIV-1 and the immune system. This interaction is what determines the development and the temporal course of clinical disease, and the balance between these two central agonists changes over time. During the initial phase of acute primary infection, a robust systemic viremia develops (virus predominance) but then subsides rapidly as specific immune defenses suppress infection. A period of immunodominant clinical latency follows, usually lasting for years and devoid of overt symptoms. However, as more recent studies have shown, infection is not silent during this time, but remains active and can be readily demonstrated in lymphatic tissue (Embretson et al. 1993; Pantaleo et al. 1993). The production of progeny virus and the turnover of $CD4^+$ cells is now known to be a very dynamic process: The plasma half-life of HIV-1 (as determined by viral RNA concentration) is approximately 6 hours and that of infected $CD4^+$ T cells is about 1.6 days (Ho et al. 1995; Wei et al. 1995; Ho 1996). With time, reserves of $CD4^+$ T-lymphocytes are reduced and their number in peripheral blood declines, until opportunistic complications develop and are eventually fatal. Two characteristics of this late phase appear important for ADC pathogenesis: the immunosuppression that allows brain infection to take place and immune activation which likely participates in the process of brain injury. These are two sides of the same coin resulting from the effects of the virus on immune reactions.

Clinical observations from both cross-sectional and longitudinal studies suggest that immunosuppression exerts a permissive effect on ADC. Both HIV-1 encephalitis and Stage 2–4 ADC are almost wholly disorders of patients with low blood $CD4^+$ T-lymphocyte counts (Bacellar et al. 1994). In early HIV-1 infection, minor inflammatory changes can be identified around blood vessels and in the leptomeninges (Gray et al. 1992; Bell et al. 1993). However, productive infection is not detected and, if the virus remains present in latent form, this likely is very limited since polymerase chain reaction (PCR) detects little proviral or no viral DNA. Likely, when virus enters, immune reactions in the brain control its replication and the infected cells either later exit or are eliminated. This CNS surveillance against local HIV-1 infection within brain is presumably why the epidemiologies of brain HIV-1 infection and ADC are very similar to those of other major neurological opportunistic disorders, including cerebral toxoplasmosis and primary CNS lymphoma (Neaton et al. 1994). In this sense, HIV-1 is an opportunistic brain infection that "creates its own opportunity" by first crippling immune defenses that suppress its own replication. However, immunosuppression alone is insufficient for the development of ADC, since many severely immunosuppressed patients with active viremia do not exhibit clinical ADC. Some other factor(s) must be involved, including perhaps changes in the behavior of the virus discussed earlier.

Whereas the case for the permissive effect of immunosuppression in ADC appears reasonably well founded, the importance of immune activation is more speculative. Before elaborating on this in the context of brain injury, it is worthwhile to emphasize that the late phase of HIV-1 infection is accompanied by a pattern of systemic immune activation which can be considered an intrinsic part of the dysregulation of immune responses induced by the virus (Pantaleo and Fauci 1995). Blood markers of immune activation, principally macrophage activation, have been shown to reflect stage of illness and prognosis independent of

CD4^{+} counts (Fahey et al. 1990). These include β_2-microglobulin (β_2M) and neopterin. Pathogenetically, these markers can be viewed as indicators of a switch to chronic production of a particular group of "proinflammatory" cytokines. Production of these cytokines is driven by HIV-1 infection and may originate in either infected macrophages or uninfected macrophages responding to signals from infected cells. As discussed below, this same activation occurs in the brain of ADC patients.

HIV-1 AND IMMUNE REACTIONS IN THE NERVOUS SYSTEM

A number of observations converge to implicate HIV-1 as the etiologic agent causing ADC. Others suggest that this involves indirect mechanisms rather than simply direct, virus-related alterations of the functional elements, particularly neurons (Table 3) (Price 1994). Perhaps foremost among the supporting clinical information is the fact that ADC and its associated pathologies are unique to HIV-1 infection and not seen as part of the spectrum of opportunistic complications of other immunosuppressed states. Additionally, no alternative etiology, and in particular no other organism, has been identified. Other circumstantial support is provided by animal models of lentivirus infection, most notably visna in sheep and simian human immunodeficiency virus (SIV), in which CNS infection and disease develop. More directly, a large number of studies have shown that the nervous system is exposed to HIV-1 early in the course of systemic infection (Resnick et al. 1988; Davis et al. 1992) and that productive and nonproductive brain infection occurs in its late phase (Nuovo et al. 1994; Saito et al. 1994; Brew et al. 1995; Takahashi et al. 1996). Although the association between brain infection and clinical disease is controversial, there is evidence suggesting that in overt HIV-1 encephalitis, cortical neuronal changes correlate with local productive infection (Wiley and Achim 1994). Viruses isolated from HIV-1 encephalitis also possess common features, particularly macrophage tropism (Koyangi et al. 1987; Li et al. 1992). Additionally, certain viral gene products have been shown to be neurotoxic in experimental models, either in cell culture or in animal models. Among these, most attention has been directed at the external glycoprotein, gp120, but the products of the *tat* gene and other regulatory genes have also been speculated to initiate neurotoxicity (for reviews, see Lipton and Gendelman 1995; Price 1995c). Perhaps the most elegant studies along these lines are those involving transgenic mice in which gp120 expression is controlled by the glial fibrillary acidic protein (GFAP) promoter, and astrocytosis similar to the human disease is accompanied by dendritic alterations virtually identical to those in man (Toggas et al. 1994; Mucke et al. 1995). Finally, antiviral therapy with AZT ameliorates ADC (Pizzo et al. 1988; Sidtis et al. 1993; Gray et al. 1994).

On the other hand, a number of observations also raise questions about HIV-1 as the cause of ADC, at least as the cause in the same way that poliovirus causes poliomyelitis. Among these is the fact that major *productive* infection is confined to cells of bone marrow origin, monocyte-derived macrophages and related microglia, rather than the principal "functional" cells of the CNS, neurons or macroglia (Michaels et al. 1988; Dickson and Lee 1995). Whereas recent studies suggest that HIV-1 brain infection is, in fact, more promiscuous and can include these cells, such infection is generally restricted with respect to viral gene expression as well as generally limited to severe cases (although more experience with combined PCR–in situ hybridization accompanied by clinical correlation is needed to more firmly address this issue) (Nuovo et al. 1994; Saito et al. 1994; Bagasra et al. 1996; Nuovo and Alfieri 1996; Takahashi et al. 1996). Additionally, the extent of productive infection does not always correlate fully with antemortem clinical severity, particularly, but not exclusively, in milder (Stage 1 and 2) cases; using traditional immunocytochemical methods to map infection, many of these are virus negative or show only very limited infection (Brew et al. 1995). A number of other studies have suggested that cell gene products, particularly those involved in cytokine pathways, may be important in mediating ADC. The first suggestions of this came from studies of CSF which showed that ADC severity correlates with concentrations of some of the activation markers, including β_2M and neopterin (Brew et al. 1990, 1992; Griffin et al. 1994). The endogenous excitatory neurotoxin, quinolinic acid, shows parallel activation with CSF levels in the neurotoxic range (Heyes et al. 1989). Similar observations have been made in the brains of ADC patients in which increased expression of tumor necrosis factor (TNF-α) mRNA has been noted to correlate with ADC (Tyor et al. 1992; Wesselingh et al. 1993). These human studies have been supplemented by cell culture studies showing that the neurotoxicity of gp120, at least in some test systems, may be indirectly mediated through its effects on other cells, including astrocytes and macrophages (Gelbard et al. 1994; Lipton and Gendelman 1995; Talley et al. 1995). Other viral gene products, either as specific signals or as components of a less specific reaction to cell injury, may similarly activate cellular genes in uninfected cells that eventuate in neuronal injury.

MODEL OF INFECTION AND STRATEGIES OF THERAPY

Models of Infection

Taking into account the observations reviewed above, I have configured a simple model isolating "functional" cell components as a step to dissecting the pathogenesis of this complex disease and developing therapeutic strategies (Fig. 1). This is a generic model

Table 3. Observations Supporting an Etiological Role for HIV-1 in ADC and Observations Suggesting That Pathogenesis Involves Indirect Mechanisms

	Supporting HIV-1 etiology	Suggesting indirect pathogenesis
Human studies		
clinical	ADC is unique to HIV-1 infection: not seen in other immunosuppressed patients no alternative etiology found responds to antiretroviral treatment	
CSF	HIV-1 reaches the CNS (at least CSF space) early in infection and probably throughout the course of infection, where it elicits local specific and nonspecific responses but without causing symptoms	general correlation of ADC severity with markers of immune activation (β_2M, neopterin, quinolinate) rather than with presence of virus
brain	virus can also reach the brain after acute exposure, but in the early phase of systemic infection the viral load in the brain is likely very low and local reactions are inconspicuous at a time when patients are neurologically asymptomatic	
	late in infection and in most patients with more severe ADC, HIV-1 encephalitis is demonstrable using a variety of techniques	ADC presence and severity does not always correlate with viral burden pathologically correlation may be better with cytokine expression (including TNF-α)
	infection has "system disease" distribution with predilection for subcortical structures, in line with clinical phenotype	productive infection occurs in macrophages and microglia rather than functional cells (although restricted infection involves the latter)
	alteration of cortical dendrites and reduction in synaptic density correlates with the local virus burden	
Animal models		
other lentiviruses	visna and SIV provide precedent for brain infection and brain disease associated with lentivirus infection	
transgenic mouse	gp120 transgenic driven by GFAP promotor develops astrocytosis and dendritic changes similar to man	gp120 neuronal changes blocked by memantine, suggesting NMDA agonist as toxin to neurons
cell culture	gp120 toxic to neurons	gp120 neuronal toxicity may require intermediary cells which are stimulated to produce host-coded toxin rather than acting directly
	other viral gene products are active signals and potentially toxic to neurons, including *tat*, *nef*, *rev*	infection provokes cytokine secretion and several are toxic to neurons, including TNF-α, PAF, quinolinate, and other identified and unidentified factors

that depicts some of the likely important cell interactions in functional terms but specifies neither the specific cells involved nor the chemical and molecular mediators effecting their interactions. In part, this is because these have not been specifically defined and also because there may, in fact, be redundancy in these interactions. More than one cell type may fulfill a certain role, and several mediators may act in parallel to contribute to the overall effect (Price 1995a,b).

The model is divided into two major compartments, the first encompassing infection and the second the subsequent steps leading to the characteristic neurological dysfunction of ADC, also referred to here as the neurotoxic pathway. The segregation of the first, or primary, compartment emphasizes that infection in the brain can be considered as a *metastatic* process, with both the productively infected cells (and yet to be infected targets) and the specifically reactive immune cells derived from the blood. The important aspects of this compartment relate to viral entry (likely principally with infected monocytes acting as "Trojan horses" that are signaled to enter as defenders but bring in the virus [Haase 1986]), specific and nonspecific host defenses that can modulate infection and probably the profile of immune activation as well, and the productively infected cells that initiate brain pathology. Notably, the kinetics of this infection may be different from those that contribute to the viral burden in plasma measured by RNA assays. It may be a component of the slower phase of viral replication (Ho et al. 1995), and, hence, although metastatic, it is "filtered" and differs in its principal components from

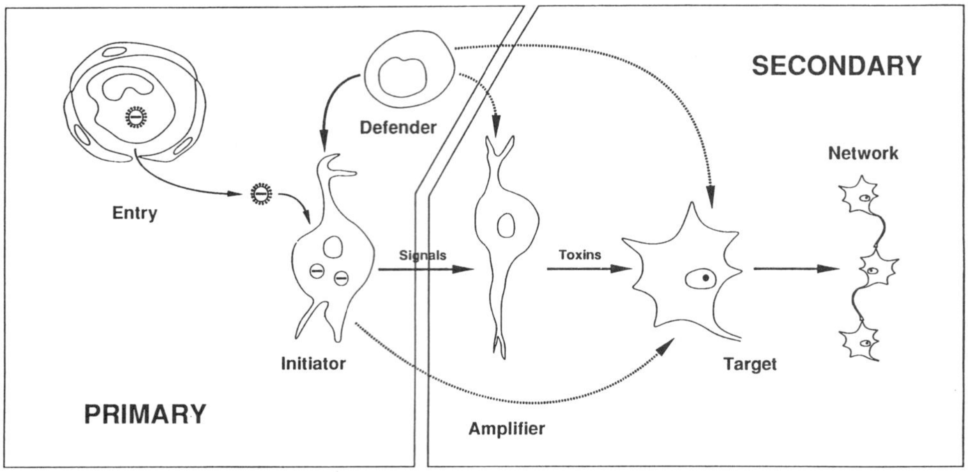

Figure 1. Two-compartment cell model of HIV-1 neuropathogenesis. The cells are intended to represent functional roles of various cells, and the arrows depict principal interactions of these cells.

the systemic, predominantly CD4+ T-lymphocyte infection. Among the differences are the cells supporting infection (macrophages and microglia) and the virus variants (macrophage-tropic) in the brain. This sequestered infection in the CNS is a potential focus of continued replication in the face of potent antivirals that suppress systemic replication and may enhance development of mutants which are more readily selected in the face of subtherapeutic drug concentrations (Richman 1994).

Additionally, these virus-infected macrophage-microglia not only support replication, but also release viral gene products (and perhaps cell-coded products as well) that drive events in the second compartment. Without infection, the neurotoxic pathway is not activated, unless a similar process can be provoked by systemic infection and blood-borne signals. The latter may indeed be the case and may provide an explanation for virus-negative brains in some ADC patients, but this parallel pathway will not be developed further here since the processes are similar, with the exception that the primary compartment is outside of the brain and the signals must breech the BBB. The second compartment hypothesizes a transducer-amplifier cell, or network of cells, that both converts the signal from the infected cell to a neurotoxic cascade and also expands this signal. This step is invoked to explain the extensive clinical dysfunction in the face of limited brain infection in some cases and is also in keeping with cell culture studies which suggest that intermediary cells are needed to induce neuronal toxicity from HIV-1 or gp120 (Gelbard et al. 1994; Lipton and Gendelman 1995). These intermediary cells likely include macrophages—microglia and astrocytes—both of which can produce cytokines and other neurotoxic products (Benveniste 1994). The profile of their production might be "set" by the background state of the immune system (and its dysregulation) resulting in chronic secretion without usual feedback inhibition. Vascular endothelial cells may also be seen as amplifiers if their response to local infection perturbs the integrity of the BBB, allowing entry of forbidden molecules from the blood (enhancing the toxicity of systemic infection hypothesized earlier) (Moses et al. 1995). Even neurons may be amplifiers; this was suggested to underlie one pathway involving NO production in HIV-1 infection (Dawson et al. 1993). These various mechanisms then converge on the target neuron where cell surface receptors, including NMDA receptors, and intracellular events lead up to dysfunction and death. The perturbation of these primary targets leads, in turn, to disturbed networks and the overall pattern of altered physiology that manifests as the ADC clinical phenotype.

A number of mediators have been hypothesized to be involved in this HIV-1-induced indirect pathogenesis. Indeed, as work in the field expands, a simple unifying pathway to brain injury becomes more difficult. However, instead of simply asking what mediators are involved, it may be more appropriate to ask what the critical mediator(s) is in HIV-1-related brain injury. Figure 2 diagrams theoretical events in the second compartment and includes some of the hypothetical signals and toxins. This figure emphasizes an important aspect of this issue: Both sides have a pyramidal shape, with the bases meeting at the amplifier step. Initiation of the process begins at the infected cell and *diverges and expands* through simultaneous elaboration of multiple mediators. These pathways, some of which represent reverberating and amplifying circuits, then eventually *converge* upon the target cell, likely using a final common mechanism at the cell surface and within the cell. This initial divergence and subsequent convergence have potentially important implications for prioritizing approaches to therapy discussed below. Additionally, in

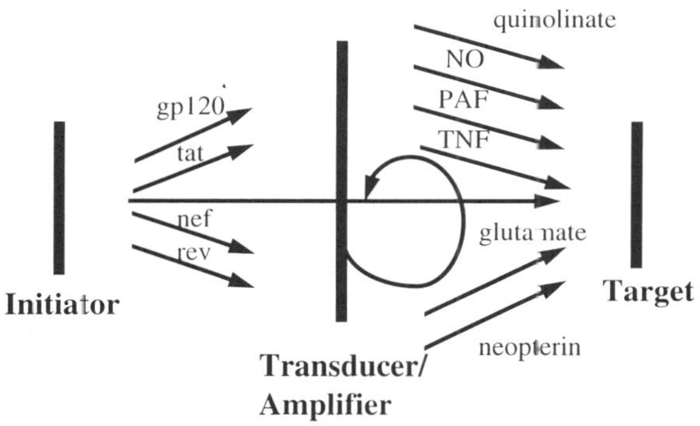

Figure 2. A simplified derivative of the cell model including some of the putative mechanisms linking infection with neuronal damage. Cells are represented by vertical bars, and some of the putative mediators and signals are identified as arrows. Pathways diverge from the initiator cell to the transducer/amplifier, and then converge on the target.

exploiting the final steps in this neurotoxic pathway, HIV-1 likely shares common mechanisms with other neurodegenerative diseases and might thereby point to common therapeutic interventions.

Therapeutic Targets

Each of the steps articulated in Figure 1 should be considered as a potential target for intervention (Price 1995a). Currently, *augmentation of host immune defenses* is being pursued in relation to systemic infection and, if successful, might apply in parallel to the brain, although modifications will be needed to assure brain access of immune cells or factors. Strategies to *restrict entry* of infected cells into the brain can also be considered, although they are presently largely theoretical and certainly not yet being pursued at the clinical level. In contrast, *antiviral therapy* of ADC is being actively pursued and, in the case of AZT, at least, has been shown to be effective in ameliorating ADC in both adults and children (Pizzo et al. 1988; Sidtis et al. 1993). This drug may also exert a preventative effect (Schmitt et al. 1988; Portegies et al. 1989). Whereas most of the newer nucleoside RT inhibitors, non-nucleoside RT inhibitors, and protease inhibitors have not been specifically tested with respect to efficacy in ADC, there has been a recent revival in interest in clinical assessment of some of the newer drugs including both nucleosides and protease inhibitors with favorable penetration into the CNS. As depicted in Figure 2, the emphasis on antiviral strategy seems appropriate, since infection is the initiating point of the divergent pathological mechanisms that eventuate in brain injury.

Therapeutic attention also is being directed at the second compartment. This might include several types of adjuvant strategies. Following the components of the cell model in Figure 1, therapies might include efforts aimed at the *amplifying*, chiefly cytokine-related, steps; inhibition of *neurotoxins* or their effects on the target cell; and modification of the "downstream" sequelae on modified *neural networks*. Addressing these mechanisms is somewhat more difficult or speculative, since there is less certainty regarding the relative importance of individual mechanisms and mediators. Nonetheless, several of the signals and toxins included in Figure 2 are being considered as therapeutic targets. For example, interruption of one of the principal cytokines, TNF-α, has been considered for inhibition using pentoxifylline or thalidomide, although a definitive study has not yet been carried out. Likewise, consideration of inhibitors of PAF, eicosinoids, and NO will all likely be entertained as drugs become available or as the relative importance of different pathways is more firmly established. However, consideration of the convergence on the effector side of Figure 2 might lead to early exploration of neuroprotective strategies that are already being tested or considered in other neurodegenerative disorders. In fact, this is also happening. On the basis of these general concepts and laboratory studies suggesting that gp120-induced neuronal toxicity, although indirectly mediated, involves NMDA receptor activation, an antagonist of this receptor, memantine, that is active in cell culture and in transgenic mice is being developed for clinical trial in ADC (Muller et al. 1992; Lipton 1994; Toggas et al. 1996). This drug has been shown to inhibit neuronal death in cell culture and to prevent the altered neuronal morphology found in the gp120 transgenic mouse model. The same rationale of inhibiting a "late" step in the neurotoxic pathway provided the rationale for a preliminary trial of therapy with the CNS-penetrating calcium channel blocker, nimodipine. Although this was only a Phase I trial, this drug did not show obvious dramatic efficacy (B. Navia et al., unpubl.).

Although not systematically explored, a compensatory strategy underlies the use of methylphenidate (Ritalin) and similar stimulants in ADC patients to overcome their psychomotor slowing (Fernandez and Levy 1994). Additionally, behavioral support is an important therapeutic adjunct for these patients to minimize their functional disability and provide optimal comfort (Boccellari and Zeifert 1994).

CONCLUSION

Finally, in returning to the initial comparison of ADC with poliomyelitis and SCA1, one can come back to the question of why it is a pathogenetically complex disorder and also why it pursues a slow course. The model in Figure 1 provides a simplified scheme outlining the complexity of ADC. Disease production is not only a matter of access and expression of the foreign pathogenic genes in the target cell; rather, it requires a series of complex cellular and molecular interactions. In addition, this action within the CNS must be preceded by a series of events outside of the nervous system involving interaction of HIV-1 with its principal target, the immune system. Through its adaptation to cause chronic infection of immune cells, HIV-1 eventually, usually after many years, wears down the immune system and begins a crescendo of increasing viral burden with eventual active replication in the brain. This, in concert with resetting of immune responses to favor production of a set of pro-inflammatory cytokines, leads to the release of signals and toxins that eventuate in progressive neurological dysfunction. Since these are physiological reactions, they may be only mildly neurotoxic, but in the face of uninterrupted exposure over a protracted period of time, cell products that are not meant to be present in the delicate extracellular environment of the brain lead first to functional, and later permanent, injury characteristic of ADC. Slowness then derives principally from the need for a preamble of chronic progressive systemic infection and complexity from the interaction of virus and immune system with only indirect effects on functional CNS cells.

ACKNOWLEDGMENTS

Our own studies of the AIDS dementia complex are supported by U.S. Public Health Service grant NS-25701. I thank Dr. John J. Sidtis for his valuable comments and for his help in conceptualizing and constructing Figure 1.

REFERENCES

American Academy of Neurology AIDS Task Force (A.A.N.A.T.F.). 1991. Nomenclature and research case definitions for neurologic manifestations of human immunodeficiency virus-type 1 (HIV-1) infection. Report of a Working Group of the American Academy of Neurology AIDS Task Force (review). *Neurology* **41:** 778.

Aylward, E.H., J.D. Henderer, J.C. McArthur, P.D. Brettschneider, G.J. Harris, P.E. Barta, and G.D. Pearlson. 1993. Reduced basal ganglia volume in HIV-1-associated dementia: Results from quantitative neuroimaging. *Neurology* **43:** 2099.

Bacellar, H., A. Munoz, E.N. Miller, B.A. Cohen, D. Besley, O.A. Selnes, J.T. Becker, and J.C. McArthur. 1994. Temporal trends in the incidence of HIV-1-related neurologic diseases: Multicenter AIDS Cohort Study, 1985–1992. *Neurology* **44:** 1892.

Bagasra, O., E. Lavi, L. Bobroski, K. Khalili, J. Pestaner, R. Tawadros, and R. Pomerantz. 1996. Cellular reservoirs of HIV-1 in the central nervous system of infected individuals: Identification by the combination of *in situ* polymerase chain reaction and immunohistochemistry. *AIDS* **10:** 573.

Bell, J.E., A. Busuttil, J.W. Ironside, S. Rebus, Y.K. Donaldson, P. Simmonds, and J.F. Peutherer. 1993. Human immunodeficiency virus and the brain: Investigation of viral load in pre-AIDS individuals. *J. Infect. Dis.* **168:** 818.

Belman, A.L. 1994. HIV-1-associated CNS disease in infants and children (review). *Res. Publ. Assoc. Res. Nerv. Ment. Dis.* **72:** 289.

Benson, D. 1987. The spectrum of dementia: A comparison of the clinical features of AIDS dementia and dementia of the Alzheimer's type. *Alzheimer Dis. Assoc. Disord.* **1:** 217.

Benveniste, E.N. 1994. Cytokine circuits in brain. Implications for AIDS dementia complex (review). *Res. Publ. Assoc. Res. Nerv. Ment. Dis.* **72:** 71.

Boccellari, A. and P. Zeifert. 1994. Management of neurobehavioral impairment in HIV-1 infection (review). *Psychiatr. Clin. N. Am.* **17:** 183.

Brack-Werner, R., A. Kleinschmidt, A. Ludvigsen, W. Mellert, M. Neuman, R. Herrman, M. Khim, A. Burny, N. Muller-Lantzsh, D. Stavrou, and V. Erfle. 1991. Infection of human brain cells by HIV-1: Restricted virus production in chronically infected human glial cell lines. *AIDS* **6:** 273.

Brew, B., M. Rosenblum, K. Cronin, and R. Price. 1995. The AIDS dementia complex and HIV-1 brain infection: Clinical-virological correlations. *Ann. Neurol.* **38:** 563.

Brew, B., R. Bhalla, M. Paul, H. Gallardo, J. McArthur, M. Schwartz, and R. Price. 1990. Cerebrospinal fluid neopterin in human immunodeficiency virus type 1 infection. *Ann. Neurol.* **28:** 556.

Brew, B.J., R.B. Bhalla, M. Paul, J.J. Sidtis, J.J. Keilp, A.E. Sadler, H. Gallardo, J.C. McArthur, M.K. Schwartz, and R.W. Price. 1992. Cerebrospinal fluid β_2-microglobulin in patients with AIDS dementia complex: An expanded series including response to zidovudine treatment. *AIDS* **6:** 461.

Davis, L.E., B.L. Hjelle, V.E. Miller, D.L. Palmer, A.L. Llewellyn, T.L. Merlin, S.A. Young, R.G. Mills, W. Wachsman, and C.A. Wiley. 1992. Early viral brain invasion in iatrogenic human immunodeficiency virus infection. *Neurology* **42:** 1736.

Dawson, V., T. Dawson, G. Uhl, and S. Snyder. 1993. Human immunodeficiency virus type 1 coat protein neurotoxicity mediated by nitric oxide in primary cortical cultures. *Proc. Natl. Acad. Sci.* **90:** 3256.

Dickson, D. and S. Lee. 1995. Microglia and HIV-related CNS neuropathology: An update. *J. Neuro-AIDS* **1:** 57.

Embretson, J., M. Zupanic, J.L. Ribas, A. Burk, P. Racz, K. Tenner-Racz, and A.T. Haase. 1993. Massive covert infection of helper T lymphocytes during the incubation period of AIDS. *Nature* **362:** 359.

Fahey, J., J. Taylor, R. Detels, B. Hofmann, R. Melmed, P. Nishanian, and J. Giorgi. 1990. The prognostic value of cellular and serologic markers in infection with human immunodeficiency virus type 1. *N. Engl. J. Med.* **322:** 166.

Feinberg, M. 1996. Changing the natural history of HIV disease. *Lancet* **348:** 239.

Feng, Y., C. Broder, P. Kennedy, and E. Berger. 1996. HIV-1 entry cofactor: Functional cDNA cloning of a seven-transmembrane G protein-coupled receptor. *Science* **272:** 872.

Fernandez, F. and J.K. Levy. 1994. Psychopharmacology in HIV spectrum disorders (review). *Psychiatr. Clin. N. Am.* **17:** 135.

Gelbard, H.A., H.S. Nottet, S. Swindells, M. Jett, K.A. Dzenko, P. Genis, R. White, L. Wang, Y.B. Choi, D. Zhang, S.A. Lipton, W.W. Tourtellotte, L.G. Epstein, and H.E. Gendelman. 1994. Platelet-activating factor: A candidate human immunodeficiency virus type 1-induced neurotoxin. *J. Virol.* **68:** 4628.

Gelman, B. and F.J. Guinto. 1992. Morphometry, histopathology, and tomography of cerebral atrophy in the acquired immunodeficiency syndrome. *Ann. Neurol.* **31:** 32.

Glass, J.D., H. Fedor, S.L. Wesselingh, and J.C. McArthur. 1995. Immunocytochemical quantitation of human immunodeficiency virus in the brain: Correlations with dementia. *Ann. Neurol.* **38:** 755.

Glass, J.D., S.L. Wesselingh, O.A. Selnes, and J.C. McArthur. 1993. Clinical-neuropathologic correlation in HIV-associated dementia. *Neurology* **43:** 2230.

Gray, F., M. Lescs, C. Keohane, F. Paraire, B. Marc, M. Durigon, and R. Gherardi. 1992. Early brain changes in HIV infection: Neuropathological study of 11 seropositive, non-AIDS cases. *J. Neuropathol. Exp. Neurol.* **51:** 177.

Gray, F., L. Belec, C. Keohane, P. De Truchis, B. Clair, M. Durigon, A. Sobel, and R. Gherardi. 1994. Zidovudine therapy and HIV encephalitis: A 10-year neuropathological survey. *AIDS* **8:** 489.

Greene, W. 1991. The molecular biology of human immunodeficiency virus type 1 infection. *N. Engl J. Med.* **324:** 308.

Griffin, D.E., S.L. Wesselingh, and J.C. McArthur. 1994. Elevated central nervous system prostaglandins in human immunodeficiency virus-associated dementia. *Ann. Neurol.* **35:** 592.

Haase, A. 1986. The pathogenesis of slow virus infections: Molecular analyses. *J. Infect. Dis.* **153:** 441.

Heyes, M.P., D. Rubinow, C. Lane, and S.P. Markey. 1989. Cerebrospinal fluid quinolinic acid concentrations are increased in acquired immune deficiency syndrome. *Ann. Neurol.* **26:** 275.

Ho, D.D. 1995. Time to hit HIV early and hard. *N. Engl. J. Med.* **333:** 450.

———. 1996. Viral counts count in HIV infection (perspectives). *Science* **272:** 1124.

Ho, D.D., A.U. Neumann, A.S. Perelson, W. Chen, J.M. Leonard, and M. Markowitz. 1995. Rapid turnover of plasma virions and CD4 lymphocytes in HIV-1 infection. *Nature* **373:** 123.

Jarvik, J.G., R.E. Lenkinski, R.I. Grossman, J.M. Gomori, M.D. Schnall, and I. Frank. 1993. Proton MR spectroscopy of HIV-infected patients: Characterization of abnormalities with imaging and clinical correlation. *Radiology* **186:** 739.

Koyangi, Y., S. Miles, R. Mitsuyasu, J. Merrill, H. Vinters, and I. Chen. 1987. Dual infection of the central nervous system by AIDS viruses with distinct cellular tropisms. *Science* **236:** 819.

Kuchelmeister, K., F. Gullotta, M. Bergmann, G. Angeli, and T. Masini. 1993. Progressive multifocal leukoencephalopathy (PML) in the acquired immunodeficiency syndrome (AIDS). A neuropathological autopsy study of 21 cases. *Pathol. Res. Pract.* **189:** 163.

Kure, K., K. Weidenhiem, W. Lyman, and D. Dickson. 1990. Morphology and distribution of HIV-1 gp41-positive microglia in subacute AIDS encephalitis. *Acta Neuropathol.* **80:** 393.

Li, Y., H. Hui, C.J. Burgess, R.W. Price, P.M. Sharp, B.H. Hahn, and G.M. Shaw. 1992. Complete nucleotide sequence, genome organization, and biological properties of human immunodeficiency virus type 1 in vivo: Evidence for limited defectiveness and complementation. *J. Virol.* **66:** 6587.

Lipton, S.A. 1994. Laboratory basis of novel therapeutic strategies to prevent HIV-related neuronal injury (review). *Res. Publ. Assoc. Res. Nerv. Ment. Dis.* **72:** 183.

Lipton, S.A. and H.E. Gendelman. 1995. Seminars in medicine of the Beth Israel Hospital, Boston. Dementia associated with the acquired immunodeficiency syndrome. (review). *N. Engl. J. Med.* **332:** 934.

Masliah, E., N. Ge, C. Achim, R. DeTeresa, and C. Wiley. 1996. Patterns of neurodegeneration in HIV encephalitis. *J. Neuro-AIDS* **1:** 161.

McArthur, J.C., D.R. Hoover, H. Bacellar, E.N. Miller, B.A. Cohen, J.T. Becker, N.M. Graham, J.H. McArthur, O.A. Selnes, L.P. Jacobson, B.R. Visscher, M. Concha, and A. Saah (for the Multicenter AIDS Cohort Study). 1993. Dementia in AIDS patients: Incidence and risk factors. Multicenter AIDS Cohort Study. *Neurology* **43:** 2245.

Michaels, J., R. Price, and M. Rosenblum. 1988. Microglia in the human immunodeficiency virus encephalitis of acquired immune deficiency syndrome: Proliferation, infection and fusion. *Acta Neuropathol.* **76:** 373.

Moses, A., S. Stenglein, and J. Nelson. 1995. HIV infection of the brain microvasculature and its contribution to the AIDS dementia complex. *J. Neuro-AIDS* **1:** 85.

Mucke, L., C.R. Abraham, M.D. Ruppe, E.M. Rockenstein, S.M. Toggas, M. Mallory, M. Alford, and E. Masliah. 1995. Protection against HIV-1 gp120-induced brain damage by neuronal expression of human amyloid precursor protein. *J. Exp. Med.* **181:** 1551.

Muller, W.E., H.C. Schroder, H. Ushijima, J. Dapper, and J. Bormann. 1992. gp120 of HIV-1 induces apoptosis in rat cortical cell cultures: Prevention by memantine. *Eur. J. Pharmacol.* **226:** 209.

Navia, B., B. Jordan, and R. Price. 1986a. The AIDS dementia complex. I. Clinical features. *Ann. Neurol.* **19:** 517.

Navia, B., E.-W. Cho, C. Petito, and R. Price. 1986b. The AIDS dementia complex. II. Neuropathology. *Ann. Neurol.* **19:** 525.

Neaton, J., D.N. Wentworth, F. Rhame, C. Hogan, D.I. Abrams, and L. Deyton. 1994. Considerations in choice of a clinical endpoint for AIDS clinical trials. *Stat. Med.* **13:** 2107.

Nowak, M., R. Anderson, and A. McLean. 1991. Antigenic diversity thresholds and the development of AIDS. *Science* **254:** 963.

Nuovo, G. and M. Alfieri. 1996. AIDS dementia is associated with massive, activated HIV-1 infection and concomitant expression of several cytokines. *Mol. Med.* **2:** 358.

Nuovo, G., F. Gallery, P. MacConnell, and A. Braun. 1994. In situ detection of polymerase chain reaction-amplified HIV-1 nucleic acids and tumor necrosis factor-alpha RNA in the central nervous system. *Am. J. Pathol.* **144:** 659.

O'Brien, W. 1994. Genetic and biologic basis of HIV-1 neurotropism. In *HIV, AIDS and the brain* (ed. R. Price and S. Perry), p. 47. Raven Press, New York.

Paley, M., P. Cozzone, J. Alonso, J. Vion-Dury, S. Confort-Gouny, I. Wilkinson, W. Chong, M. Hall-Craggs, M. Harrison, J. Gila, A. Rovira, J. Capellades, J. Rio, I. Ocana, F. Nicoli, C. Dhiver, J. Gastaut, K. Wicklow, and R. Sauter. 1996. Multicenter proton magnetic resonance spectroscopy study of neurological complications of AIDS. *AIDS Res. Hum. Retroviruses* **12:** 213.

Pantaleo, G. and A. Fauci. 1995. New concepts in the immunopathogenesis of HIV infection. *Ann. Rev. Immunol.* **13:** 487.

Pantaleo, G., C. Graziosi, J. Demarest, L. Butini, M. Montroni, C. Fox, J. Orenstein, D. Kotler, and A. Fauci. 1993. HIV infection is active and progressive in lymphoid tissue during clinically latent stages of the disease. *Nature* **362:** 355.

Petito, C.K., D. Vecchio, and Y.T. Chen. 1994. HIV antigen

and DNA in AIDS spinal cords correlate with macrophage infiltration but not with vacuolar myelopathy. *J. Neuropathol. Exp. Neurol.* **53:** 86.

Petito, C.K., B.A. Navia, E.-S. Cho, B.D. Jordan, D.C. George, and R.W. Price. 1985. Vacuolar myelopathy pathologically resembling subacute combined degeneration in patients with acquired immunodeficiency syndrome (AIDS). *N. Engl. J. Med.* **312:** 874.

Pizzo, P.A., J. Eddy, J. Falloon, F.M. Balis, R.F. Murphy, H. Moss, P. Wolters, P. Brouwers, P. Jarosinski, M. Rubin, S. Broder, R. Yarchoan, A. Bruntetti, M. Maha, S. Nusinoff-Lehrman, and D. Poplack. 1988. Effect of continuous intravenous infusion of zidovudine (AZT) in children with symptomatic HIV infection. *N. Engl. J. Med.* **319:** 889.

Portegies, P., J. de Gans, J.M. Lange, M.M. Derix, H. Speelman, M. Bakker, S. Danner, and J. Goudsmit. 1989. Declining incidence of AIDS dementia complex after introduction of zidovudine treatment (erratum in *Br. Med. J.* [1989] **299:** 1141). *Br. Med. J.* **299:** 819.

Power, C., P.A. Kong, T.O. Crawford, S. Wesselingh, J.D. Glass, J.C. McArthur, and B.D. Trapp. 1993. Cerebral white matter changes in acquired immunodeficiency syndrome dementia: Alterations of the blood-brain barrier. *Ann. Neurol.* **34:** 339.

Power, C., J.C. McArthur, R.T. Johnson, D.E. Griffin, J.D. Glass, S. Perryman, and B. Chesebro. 1994. Demented and nondemented patients with AIDS differ in brain-derived human immunodeficiency virus type 1 envelope sequences. *J. Virol.* **68:** 4643.

Price, R.W. 1994. Understanding the AIDS dementia complex (ADC). The challenge of HIV and its effects on the central nervous system (review). *Res. Publ. Assoc. Res. Nerv. Ment. Dis.* **72:** 1.

———. 1995a. AIDS dementia complex and HIV-1 brain infection: A pathogenetic framework for treatment and evaluation. *Curr. Top. Microbiol. Immunol.* **202:** 33.

———. 1995b. The cellular basis of central nervous system HIV-1 infection and the AIDS dementia complex: Introduction. *J. Neuro-AIDS* **1:** 1.

———. 1995c. Management of AIDS dementia complex and HIV-1 infection of the nervous system. *AIDS* **9:** S221.

———. 1996. Neurological complications of HIV infection. *Lancet* **348:** 445.

Resnick, L., J. Berger, P. Shapshak, and W. Tourtellotte. 1988. Early penetration of the blood-brain-barrier by HIV. *Neurology* **38:** 9.

Richman, D. 1994. Viral resistance to antiretroviral therapy. In *Textbook of AIDS medicine* (ed. S. Broder et al.), p. 795. Williams and Wilkins, Baltimore.

———.1996. HIV therapeutics (viewpoints). *Science* **272:** 1886.

Rottenberg, D.A., J.R. Moeller, S.C. Strother, J.J. Sidtis, B.A. Navia, V. Dhawan, J.Z. Ginos, and R.W. Price. 1987. The metabolic pathology of the AIDS dementia complex. *Ann. Neurol.* **22:** 700.

Saito, Y., L. Sharer, L. Epstein, J. Michaels, M. Mintz, M. Louder, K. Golding, T. Cvetkovich, and B. Blumberg. 1994. Overexpression of nef as a marker for restricted HIV-1 infection of astrocytes in postmortem pediatric central nervous system tissues. *Neurology* **44:** 474.

Schmitt, F.A., J.W. Bigleg, R. McKinnis, P.E. Logue, R.W. Evans, and J.L. Drucker. 1988. Neuropsychological outcome of azidothymidine (AZT) in the treatment of AIDS and AIDS-related complex: A double blind, placebo-controlled trial. *N. Engl. J. Med.* **319:** 1573.

Sidtis, J.J. 1994. Evaluation of the AIDS dementia complex in adults (review). *Res. Publ. Assoc. Res. Nerv. Ment. Dis.* **72:** 273.

Sidtis, J.J., C. Gatsonis, R.W. Price, E.J. Singer, A.C. Collier, D.D. Richman, M.S. Hirsch, F.W. Schaerf, M.A. Fischl, K. Kieburtz, D. Simpson, M.A. Koch, J. Feinberg, and the AIDS Clinical Trials Group. 1993. Zidovudine treatment of the AIDS dementia complex: Results of a placebo-controlled trial. AIDS Clinical Trials Group. *Ann. Neurol.* **33:** 343.

Sigurdsson, B., P. Palsson, and H. Grimson. 1957. Visna, a demyelinating transmissible disease of sheep. *J. Neuropathol. Exp. Neurol.* **16:** 389.

Simpson, D. and M. Tagliati. 1994 Neurologic manifestations of HIV infection. *Ann. Intern. Med.* **121:** 7769.

Takahashi, K., S. Wesselingh, D. Griffin, J. McArthur, R. Johnson, and J. Glass. 1996. Localization of HIV-1 in human brain using polymerase chain reaction/in situ hybridization and immunocytochemistry. *Ann. Neurol.* **39:** 705.

Talley, A.K., S. Dewhurst, S.W. Perry, S.C. Dollard, S. Gummuluru, S.M. Fine, D. New, L.G. Epstein, H.E. Gendelman, and H.A. Gelbard. 1995. Tumor necrosis factor α-induced apoptosis in human neuronal cells: Protection by the antioxidant *N*-acetylcysteine and the genes *bcl-2* and *crmA*. *Mol. Cell. Biol.* **15:** 2359.

Toggas, S., E. Masliah, and L. Mucke. 1996. Prevention of HIV-1 gp120-induced neuronal damage in the central nervous system of transgenic mice by the NMDA receptor antagonist memantine. *Brain Res.* **706:** 303.

Toggas, S.M., E. Masliah, E.M. Rockenstein, G.F. Rall, C.R. Abraham, and L. Mucke. 1994. Central nervous system damage produced by expression of the HIV-1 coat protein gp120 in transgenic mice (see comments). *Nature* **367:** 188.

Tracey, I., C. Carr, A. Guimaraes, J. Worth, B. Navia, and R. Gonzalez. 1996. Brain choline-containing compounds are elevated in HIV-positive patients before the onset of AIDS dementia complex: A proton magnetic resonance spectroscopic study. *Neurology* **46:** 783.

Tross, S., R. Price, B. Navia, H. Thaler, J. Gold, D. Hirsch, and J. Sidtis. 1988. Neuropsychological characterization of the AIDS dementia complex: A preliminary report. *AIDS* **2:** 81.

Tyor, W.R., J.D. Glass, J.W. Griffin, P.S. Becker, J.C. McArthur, L. Bezman, and D.E. Griffin. 1992. Cytokine expression in the brain during the acquired immunodeficiency syndrome. *Ann. Neurol.* **31:** 349.

Wei, X., S.K. Ghosh, M.E. Taylor, V.A. Johnson, E.A. Emini, P. Deutsch, J.D. Lifson, S. Bonhoefer, M.A. Nowak, B.H. Hahn, M.S. Saag, and G.M. Shaw. 1995. Viral dynamics in human immunodeficiency virus type 1 infection. *Nature* **373:** 117.

Weiss, R. 1996. HIV receptors and the pathogenesis of AIDS. *Science* **272:** 1885.

Wesselingh, S., C. Power, J. Glass, W. Tyor, J. McArthur, J. Farber, J. Griffen, and D. Griffen. 1993. Intracerebral cytokine mRNA expression in AIDS. *Ann. Neurol.* **33:** 576.

Wiley, C.A. and C. Achim. 1994. Human immunodeficiency virus encephalitis is the pathological correlate of dementia in acquired immunodeficiency syndrome (erratum appears in *Ann. Neurol.* [1995] **37:** 140). *Ann. Neurol.* **36:** 673.

Quantitative Trait Loci Mapping in Mouse Models of Complex Behavior

T.N. FERRARO AND W.H. BERRETTINI

Departments of Psychiatry and Human Behavior and Biochemistry and Molecular Pharmacology, Thomas Jefferson University, Philadelphia, Pennsylvania 19107

Quantitative trait loci (QTL) represent regions of the genome which contain genes that influence specific quantitative traits or phenotypes. Quantitative traits are defined as having an essentially continuous distribution of values across a population and result from complex interactions between multiple genes and the environment. Recently, the concept of localizing genes that determine quantitative traits has been revitalized as a result of the development of high-resolution genetic maps and mathematical constructs which can be used to correlate quantitative phenotype data in a population with DNA marker genotypes.

QTL mapping is a form of linkage analysis and, as such, it involves determining the probability that specific DNA marker loci are situated near genes that control expression of the phenotype in question. Like other forms of linkage analysis, QTL mapping involves the study of both parents and offspring. In the laboratory, QTL mapping is facilitated by studying strains of an organism that differ substantially in the trait to be analyzed, although a large strain difference is not an absolute requirement. The power to detect linkage in QTL analysis is determined by numerous factors, a crucial one being the overall effect size of a given QTL. It is possible that any given quantitative trait may be determined by a large number of QTLs, such that each one has only a very small effect in and of itself. In some cases, this obstacle can be overcome by studying many more individuals in an attempt to increase the level of sensitivity of the analysis. In extreme cases where there are a very large number of genes participating in expression of a quantitative trait, QTL mapping approaches may not be feasible.

The utility of modern QTL analysis was first demonstrated in studies of fruits and vegetables (Paterson et al. 1990). More recently, inbred strains of rodents have been shown to be amenable to this strategy, and a number of models have been developed to study phenotypes relevant to human disease, including cancer (Dietrich et al. 1993), obesity (Taylor and Phillips 1996), hypertension (Hilbert et al. 1991; Jacob et al. 1991), alcoholism (Melo et al. 1996), and diabetes (Todd et al. 1991). In this paper, we present results of recent work in our laboratory involving the use of QTL analysis to examine genetic contributions to epilepsy and opioid addiction in inbred mice.

DISSECTING GENETIC INFLUENCES ON MORPHINE PREFERENCE

Genetic predisposition to substance abuse has been suggested by family, twin, and adoption studies (Grove et al. 1990; Pickens et al. 1991; Rounsaville et al. 1991; Luther et al. 1992; Cadoret et al. 1995); however, the precise nature of this influence has been difficult to elucidate. Several experimental paradigms involving animals have been developed in an attempt to gain insight into the neurobiology underlying drug reinforcement and addiction. Such models include conditioned place preference, drug discrimination, and self-administration (Crabbe et al. 1994). We have adopted a morphine self-administration protocol to study the genetic influences on morphine preference in mice.

Morphine interacts with endogenous opioid receptors that help regulate a variety of complex physiological phenomena (in addition to reward and reinforcement) including analgesia, immune function, motor activity, thermoregulation, and stress responses (Mansour et al. 1988). One indication of genetic influences on opioid-related traits in animals is revealed by strain differences. C57BL/6J (B6) and DBA/2J (D2) mice have been shown to differ significantly in a number of opioid-related traits including analgesia, locomotor activity, hypothermia, and voluntary self-administration (Horowitz 1981; Belknap et al. 1989; Belknap and O'Toole 1991; Berrettini et al. 1994a). The large difference in morphine preference between these two strains of mice thus facilitates the use of QTL mapping as a strategy to probe the nature of the genetic influences involved in this trait.

Prior to mapping QTLs for morphine preference in these strains, we considered some potential pitfalls associated with oral self-administration of morphine. Pharmacokinetic experiments were conducted to determine plasma levels of morphine and its conjugated metabolites in both strains following oral consumption, and opioid antagonist experiments were conducted to establish that B6 preference is related to activation of opioid receptors in the central nervous system (Berrettini et al. 1994a). Genetic mapping was subsequently carried out using an F_2 intercross breeding scheme and the QTL strategy of intervals and extremes (Lander and Botstein 1989). Results revealed the presence of three QTLs. The strongest of these, on the proximal portion of chromosome 10, accounted for over 40% of the genetic variance in morphine consumption (Berrettini et al. 1994b). A compelling candidate gene for this QTL emerged when the μ opioid receptor gene was mapped to the region of the chromosome 10 QTL (Kozak et al. 1994). More recently, a QTL for morphine-induced analgesia was also localized to the proximal region of mouse chromosome 10, and this QTL was also associated with naloxone B_{max} in mouse brain (Belknap et al. 1995). We report here the fine mapping of a major morphine preference QTL on mouse chromosome 10.

Methods

Testing mice for voluntary morphine self-administration. B6 and D2 mice of both genders were purchased from The Jackson Laboratory, and all mice were housed individually prior to testing or breeding. Parental mice were cross-bred to produce F_1 offspring, which were intercrossed to produce a large F_2 population. Testing for voluntary morphine self-administration was carried out when mice were between the ages of 8 and 10 weeks. A two-bottle free-choice protocol was utilized for testing. Mice were offered a solution of morphine and a control solution of quinine for 8 consecutive days: days 1–4: 0.3 mg/ml morphine in 0.2% saccharin versus 0.2 mg/ml quinine in 0.2% saccharin; days 5–8: 0.7 mg/ml morphine in 0.2% saccharin versus 0.4 mg/ml quinine. Bottles were weighed daily, and their positions in the cages were alternated. Consumption during days 5–8 was averaged to obtain a morphine consumption index in mg/kg/day.

Genetic analysis of F_2 generation mice. F_2 mice exhibiting the lowest (n = 46) and highest (n = 49) levels of morphine consumption were selected for genotyping. DNA was extracted (Lahiri and Nurnberger 1991) from liver and used for typing microsatellite markers in standard PCR reactions coupled with polyacrylamide gel electrophoresis (Weber and May 1989). Initially, markers spaced at about 10-cM intervals across the genome were analyzed. Subsequently, additional markers were typed in the region of the chromosome 10 QTL. All autoradiograms were scored by two independent readers, and genotypes were entered into a database.

Allele distributions in the two groups of "low-consuming" and "high-consuming" F_2 mice were analyzed by chi-square analysis. Chromosomal regions in which markers yielded a significance level of $p < 0.01$ were analyzed using Mapmaker/QTL, a maximum likelihood software program for QTL studies (Lander et al. 1987; Lander and Botstein 1989). This program generates LOD scores over defined marker intervals on a genetic linkage map and provides estimates of the percentage of phenotypic variance explained by a QTL that exceeds a given LOD threshold. The program also compares different modes of inheritance (recessive, dominant, and additive) for each QTL, permitting some insight into the associated genetic mechanism.

Results

Voluntary morphine self-administration. Levels of morphine consumption for B6, D2, F_1, and F_2 mice are shown in Table 1. There were no gender differences in morphine consumption. The difference in the response variance between the F_2 and F_1 groups of mice indicates that about 70% of the total variance is genetic in origin. The distribution of morphine consumption values for the entire F_2 population is shown in Figure 1 along with an indication of extreme low- and high-consuming mice selected for genotyping.

Mapping loci for voluntary morphine consumption. Mapmaker/QTL analysis detected three loci influencing voluntary morphine consumption with LOD scores greater than 3.0 (Berrettini et al. 1994b). The strongest of these, *Mop2*, is found on chromosome 10 and yielded a maximum LOD score of 20.5. Figure 2 shows the linkage map for this QTL. Mapmaker analysis revealed that *Mop2* accounts for a large portion of the genetic variance (over 40%) but could not distinguish between dominant and additive modes of action. Indeed, having a B6 allele at marker D10Mit28 or D10Mit13 increases mean F_2 morphine consumption by 60%, and there was no significant difference between heterozygotes and homozygotes at these loci. Two other QTLs, *Mop1* on chromosome 1 and *Mop3* on chromosome 6, accounted for 10% and 36% of the genetic variance, respectively (Berrettini et al. 1994b). Taken together, and depending on the assumed mode of inheritance, these three QTLs accounted for 85–90% of the total genetic variance in morphine consumption.

Discussion

We have identified a major QTL for morphine preference on mouse chromosome 10 (Berrettini et al. 1994b). Fine mapping was carried out by studying several additional microsatellite markers on the proximal portion of this chromosome. Genotype

Table 1. Summary of Morphine Consumption by B6, D2, F_1, and F_2 Mice in a Two-bottle Choice Paradigm

Strain	N	Mean[a]	S.D.	Variance
B6	13	342	95	9025
D2	15	13	3	9
F1	20	97	35	1225
F2	606	112	63	3969

[a]Values given are mg morphine/kg body weight/day. Means for each animal were determined over a 4-day trial period during which time they had free access to both morphine (0.7 mg/ml in 0.2% saccharin) and quinine (0.4 mg/ml in 0.2% saccharin).

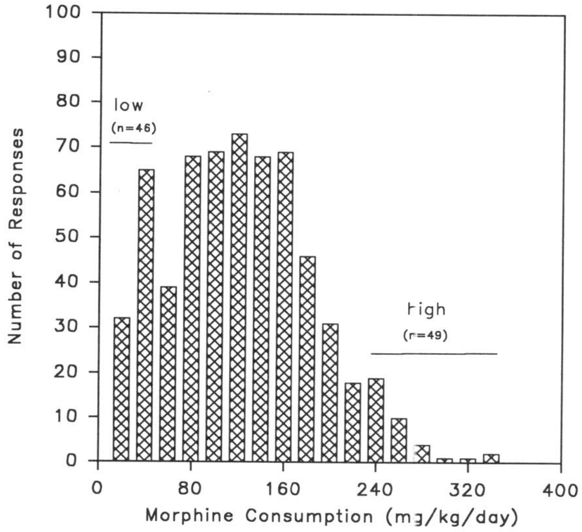

Figure 1. Distribution of morphine consumption values in B6 x D2 F_2 intercross mice. Mice were tested in a two-bottle choice paradigm as described in Methods. This distribution approximates a normal curve.

results showed that there were no low-morphine-preferring mice (out of 46) that were homozygous for the B6 allele at D10Mit75, D10Mit28, or D10Mit83, markers which span a distance of about 5 cM on the proximal arm of chromosome 10. Conversely, there were only 3 out of 49 high-morphine-preferring mice that were homozygous for the D2 allele at these markers. The maximal LOD score for this QTL occurred near D10Mit28. A strong candidate gene in this region is the μ opioid receptor gene, which maps just distal to the D10Mit28 (Kozak et al. 1994; Giros et al. 1995). Interestingly, a recent report of a QTL for another morphine-related phenotype, hot-plate analgesia, maps to this precise region in F_2 intercross progeny from the same two strains of mice, and this QTL also was associated with the number of binding sites for the opioid antagonist naloxone in the BXD RI strains (Belknap et al. 1995). Moreover, an earlier study using recombinant inbred strains derived from B6 and D2 mice described evidence for a QTL on the proximal region of chromosome 10 which significantly influenced morphine-induced hypothermia (Belknap and Crabbe 1992). Taken together, these studies indicate that this area of mouse chromosome 10 harbors a gene(s) that has a significant influence on differences in opioid-related behaviors between B6 and D2 mice. Studies are under way in our laboratory to determine if variation in the structure of the μ opioid receptor is involved in these differences.

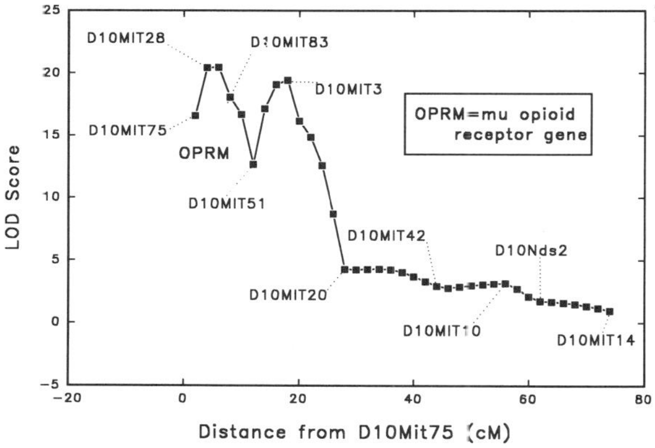

Figure 2. Genetic map of mouse chromosome 10 indicating interval LOD scores for linkage to loci controlling morphine preference in F_2 mice. LOD scores were determined using Mapmaker/QTL with morphine consumption as the trait measure. Extreme responders are indicated by horizontal lines. Mapping scores represent results of model-independent analyses.

The resolution of a second, slightly more distal peak in the Mapmaker analysis (between markers D10Mit51 and D10Mit3) suggests that there may be a second QTL in this region of chromosome 10 which also participates in regulation of voluntary morphine consumption in B6 and D2 mice. This peak was not observed in the original mapping study (Berrettini et al. 1994b) but was detected following the addition of data from the three newly typed markers in this region to the Mapmaker/QTL analysis. Other QTL studies have also shown linkage maps with more than one peak in a region (Flint et al. 1995; Ferraro et al. 1996; Melo et al. 1996), and it is very possible that these additional peaks are artifacts of the mapping procedures. Additional analyses are required to determine whether these represent multiple true QTLs (Zeng 1993, 1994).

In addition to a large QTL on chromosome 10, our original study on voluntary morphine consumption identified a second QTL of large effect (maximum LOD score = 15, 36% of genetic variance explained) on chromosome 6 in the vicinity of the *qui* locus (Berrettini et al. 1994b). It was concluded that part or all of this effect was related to the inclusion of the quinine/saccharin solution in the two-bottle choice paradigm, since significant differences had been documented between B6 and D2 mice in their preference for solutions containing quinine alone and saccharin alone (Lush 1984; Alexander et al. 1993; Belknap et al. 1993). The *qui* locus for quinine aversion has been mapped to chromosome 6 (Lush 1984) near the peak of the chromosome 6 QTL identified by Berrettini et al. (1994b), suggesting that this QTL may be due to quinine aversion rather than morphine preference. To test this hypothesis, a follow-up study was conducted to reevaluate the morphine preference QTLs on chromosomes 6 and 10. In the follow-up study, a smaller population of F_2 intercross progeny from B6 and D2 mice was tested in an experiment involving a free choice between a solution of morphine in saccharin and a solution of saccharin alone (Alexander et al. 1996). QTL mapping confirmed a locus of significant effect on the proximal part of chromosome 10 but provided no sup-

Table 2. Behavioral Seizures in D2 and B6 mice: Dose/Response Effects of KA and PTZ

	Percentage of mice with behavioral seizures[a]							
	KA				PTZ			
Dose	10	20	25	30	60	70	80	90
D2	0	20	80	100	0	14	90	86
B6	0	0	0[b]	25[b]	0	0	0[c]	14[d]

[a]Percentages for kainic acid (KA) represent animals experiencing at least a partial clonic seizure; percentages for pentylene tetrazole (PTZ) represent mice exhibiting a maximal seizure (tonic hindlimb extension).

[b]$p < 0.001$.

[c]$p < 0.002$.

[d]$p < 0.005$ vs. D2 strain at the respective dose (Fisher's exact test, $n = 6$–10 per strain).

port for a morphine-preference QTL on chromosome 6 (Alexander et al. 1996), indicating that the chromosome 10 QTL may be explained by the *qui* locus (Lush 1984).

The region of mouse chromosome 10 identified as containing a morphine-preference QTL exhibits substantial linkage homology with segments on the long arm of human chromosome 6 (DeBry and Seldin 1996). In fact, the gene for the human μ opioid receptor maps to this area (Giros et ai. 1995). Thus, the model of morphine preference in mice has the potential to address directly important questions in the genetics of human substance abuse. If μ opioid receptor variants explain differences in morphine-induced behavior in strains of mice, then this system would be especially important to examine in human opioid-dependent populations. Even if the μ opioid receptor gene is not the major gene underlying the effect of this chromosome 10 QTL in mice, the extensive sequence homology between species will enable studies in humans based on simple allele-sharing principles using anonymous DNA markers.

DISSECTING GENETIC INFLUENCES ON SEIZURE SENSITIVITY

Evidence continues to accumulate to support the hypothesis that certain types of human epilepsy have genetic components which are complex and heterogeneous (Greenberg et al. 1988; Leppert et al. 1989; Lewis et al. 1993; Whitehouse et al. 1993; Liu et al. 1995). Studies of animal models of seizure syndromes further support the heterogeneous nature of genetic influences on seizure susceptibility (Neumann and Seyfried 1990; Neumann and Collins 1991; Frankel et al. 1995; Ferraro et al. 1996) and promise to provide new clues for studying and treating human epilepsy.

Recent advances in mapping the murine genome (Dietrich et al. 1996) coupled with refinement of QTL methods for dissecting polygenic influences (Kruglyak and Lander 1995; Schork et al. 1995) have combined to permit detailed examination of the genetic determinants of various phenotypic characteristics such as those related to the initiation and propagation of seizure activity. Previous work has documented that mature DBA/2J (D2) mice are relatively seizure-sensitive, whereas C57BL/6J (B6) mice are relatively seizure-resistant (Engstrom and Woodbury 1988; Kosobud and Crabbe 1990; Ferraro et al. 1995). We have studied D2 and B6 mice utilizing an F_2 intercross QTL strategy in

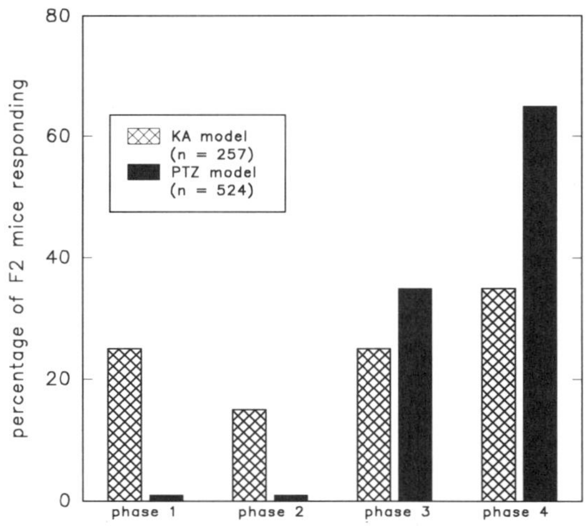

Figure 3. Maximal seizure responses observed in F_2 mice. F_2 mice were injected with KA (25 mg/kg, s.c.) and observed for 3 hr or with PTZ (80 mg/kg, s.c.) and observed for 1 hr. Maximum responses were defined as described in Methods. The top of each bar represents the fraction of the respective population for which the indicated response was observed to be the maximum response.

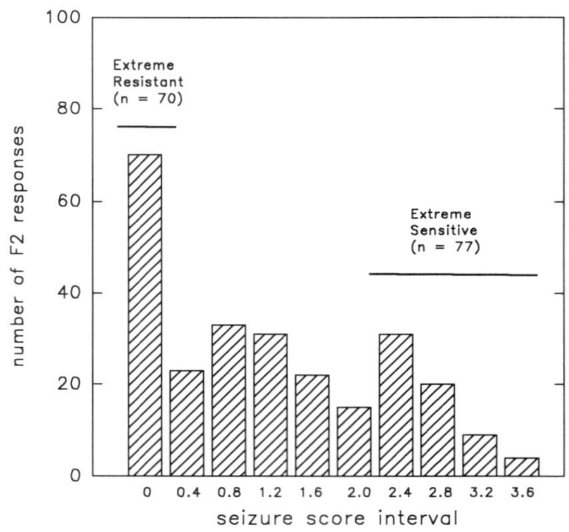

Figure 4. Distribution of seizure scores among F_2 mice treated with KA. F_2 mice were injected with KA (25 mg/kg, s.c.) and observed for 3 hr. Scores were calculated as described in Methods. The distribution is positively skewed (0.58) with negative kurtosis (–0.91) and deviates significantly from a normal distribution ($p < 0.01$, Kolmogorov-Smirnov Test).

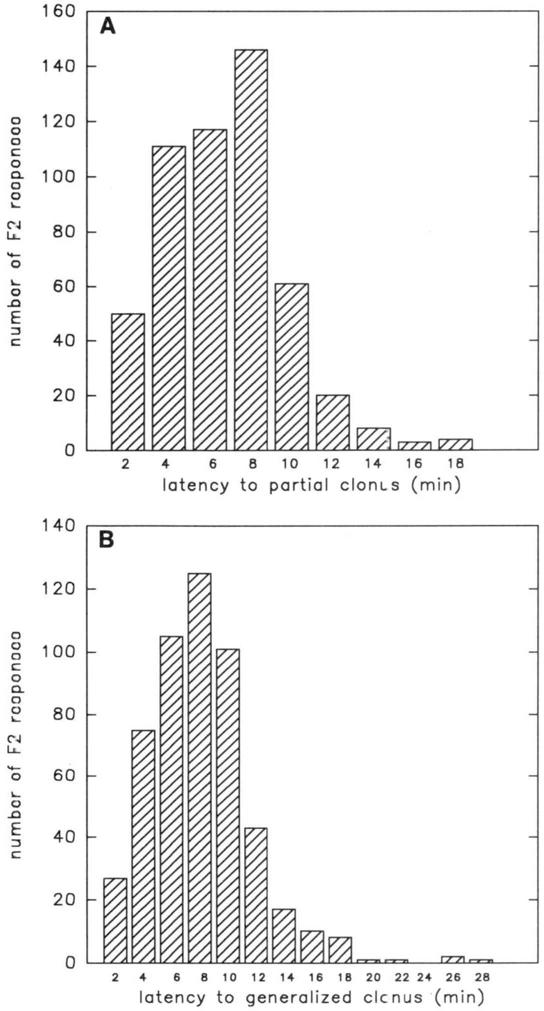

Figure 5. Distribution of seizure latencies among F_2 mice treated with PTZ. F_2 mice (n = 524) were injected with PTZ (80 mg/kg, s.c.) and observed for 1 hr. (*A*) Latency to partial clonus; (*B*) latency to generalized clonus.

an attempt to elucidate QTLs underlying sensitivity to seizures induced by systemic injection of kainic acid (KA) (Ferraro et al. 1997). In a follow-up study, we have tested D2 and B6 mice as well as their F_2 progeny for sensitivity to seizures induced by pentylenetetrazole (PTZ). Whereas KA induces seizures by activating specific subtypes of receptors for glutamic acid, the primary excitatory neurotransmitter in the CNS, PTZ induces seizures by blocking a specific subtype of receptors for GABA, the primary inhibitory neurotransmitter in the CNS. It is hypothesized that these complementary studies will point to common QTLs which are involved in the general seizure susceptibility of D2 mice relative to B6 mice.

We describe here evidence for several QTLs in the KA seizure model. The strongest of these, which we have termed *Kasz1*, resides on chromosome 1 and accounts for up to 20% of the strain difference in seizure response to KA (Ferraro et al. 1997). We also report preliminary confirmation of *Kasz1* in the PTZ model.

Methods

Screening mice with KA and PTZ. DBA/2J, C57BL/6J, B6D2F_1/J, and F_2 intercross progeny were tested between the ages of 8 and 10 weeks through injection of a single dose of KA (25 mg/kg, s.c.) or PTZ (80 mg/kg, s.c.). These doses were based on results of dose/response studies carried out in mice from each parental strain (Ferraro et al. 1995, 1997) and were chosen to optimize differences in strain response. Mice were observed for 1 hour (following PTZ injection) or 3 hours (following KA injection) and then killed by cervical dislocation.

There were several distinct phases to each seizure phenotype:

Phase 1. Hypoactivity: a progressive decrease in spontaneous motor activity resulting in the animal coming to rest in a crouched or prone position. In KA-treated mice, this led to rigidity, immobility, a fixed gaze, and postural abnormalities involving hyperflexion of body, neck, limbs, and tail.

Phase 2. Partial clonus: clonic seizure activity affecting face, head, and/or forelimbs.

Phase 3. Generalized clonus: sudden loss of upright posture; whole body clonus involving all four limbs

Table 3. Univariate Contingency Table Analysis of Allele Frequencies and Seizure Response in F_2 Mice Treated with KA

Marker	*p* Value[a]	Susceptibility allele	Mode[b]
D1Mit30	0.00003	D2	D
D1Mit16	0.00004	D2	D
D1Mit145	0.00008	D2	D
D4Mit9	0.013	B6	D
D11Mit14	0.004	B6	R
D11Mit224	0.001	B6	R
D15Mit6	0.001	D2	A
D15Mit46	0.018	D2	A
D16Mit5	0.012	B6	A
D18Mit9	0.0016	D2	A
D18Mit33	0.00004	D2	A
D18Mit8	0.00006	D2	A
D18Mit49	0.00006	D2	A

[a]Represents the association between genotypes and seizure status of F_2 generation low responders (phase 1 mice, n = 70) and high responders (phase 4 mice, n = 77).
[b]Mode of inheritance was determined by best fit regression analysis following marker recoding with seizure sensitive/resistant as the dependent variable (D=dominant, R=recessive, A=additive).

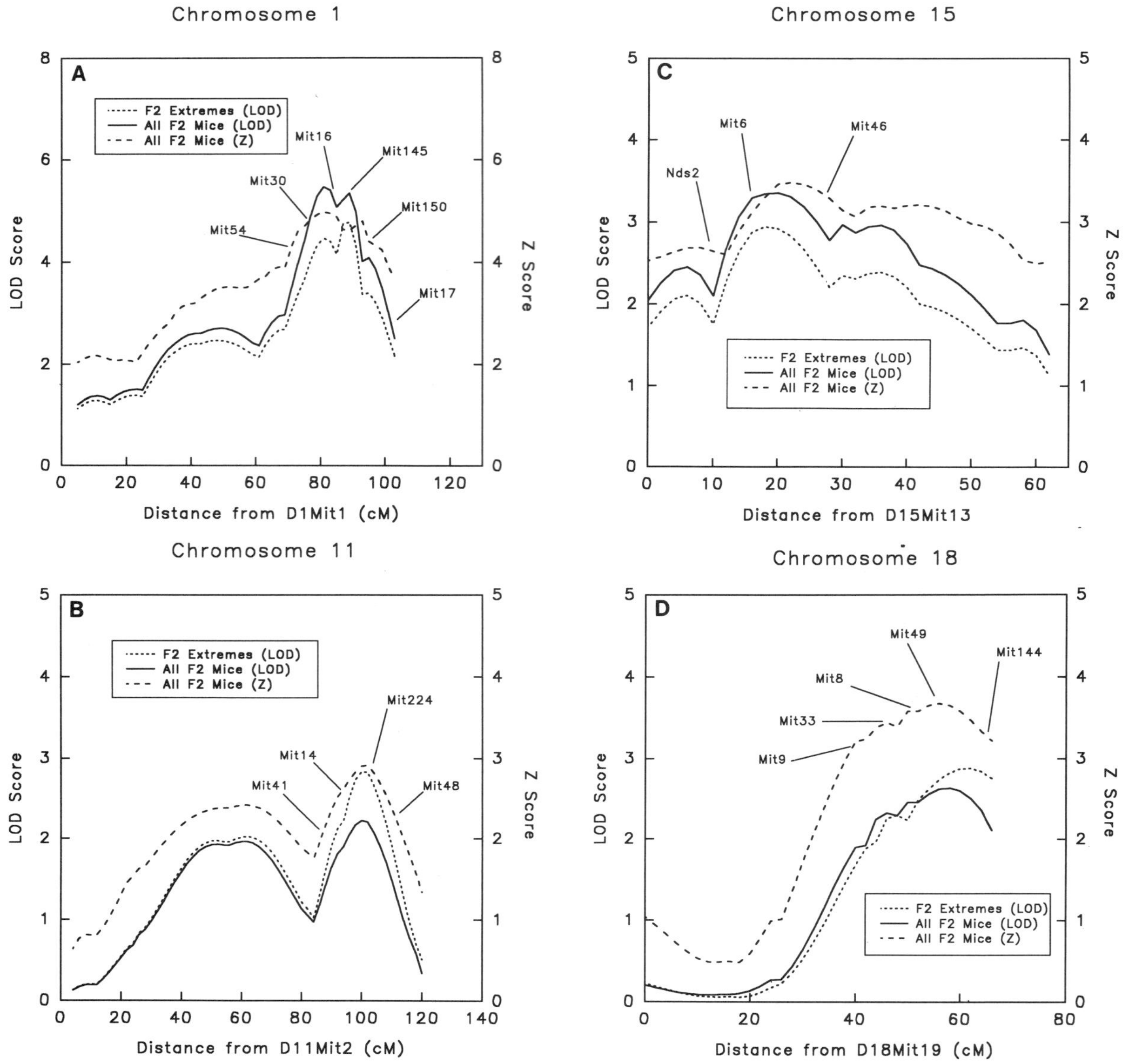

Figure 6. Genetic maps indicating interval LOD and Z scores for linkage to loci controlling sensitivity to KA-induced seizures in F_2 mice. LOD and Z values were determined using the standard and non-parametric versions of Mapmaker/QTL, respectively, with seizure score as the trait measure. Separate tests were carried out using genotypes from all F_2 mice or F_2 extreme responders only. Extreme responders are indicated by horizontal lines. Mapping scores represent results of model-independent analyses.

and tail; rearing and autonomic signs. Both KA- and PTZ-treated mice also frequently exhibited wild running and jumping.

Phase 4 (KA). Status epilepticus: continuous clonic or "limbic motor" seizure activity lasting at least 1 hour, or a series of intermittent clonic or limbic seizures without restoration of normal behavioral patterns during interictal periods.

Phase 4 (PTZ). Tonic/clonic (maximal) seizure: generalized clonic seizure accompanied by tonic hindlimb extension (THE). This response was specific for PTZ and not observed in any mice treated with KA. It was associated with death in most instances, although some mice recovered and even exhibited multiple tonic/clonic seizures within the 1-hour observation period.

A seizure score was generated for all KA-treated mice exhibiting behavioral seizures, and this score was used as a quantitative trait measure for mapping. The score was calculated using a weighted formula based on the latencies to the various components of the overall seizure syndrome. Latencies were taken as an inverse function and weighted according to a severity scale based on the specific seizure component represented. The scale was developed to account for the progressive nature of the KA seizure syndrome, treating status epilepticus as the most severe component of the phenotype (weight = 0.5), generalized clonus as the next most severe component (weight = 0.3), and partial clonus as the least severe component (weight = 0.2). Thus, the total seizure score for each mouse was calculated from the sum of each component (reciprocal of latency x 100) times its weight. Mice that did not exhibit a behavioral seizure during the observation period were given a score of 0. In separate statistical analyses, each of the individual latency components on which the seizure score was based was used directly as a quantitative trait measure for mapping.

***Genetic analysis of F_2* generation mice.** DNA was isolated from liver (Lahiri and Nurnberger 1991) taken at the time of death of all F_2 mice. Microsatellite (dinucleotide repeat) markers spanning the autosomal genome (~10-cM intervals) were amplified using standard PCR techniques and analyzed using polyacrylamide gel electrophoresis and ^{32}P autoradiography (Weber and May 1989) or agarose gel electrophoresis and ethidium bromide staining (Routman and Cheverud 1994), depending on the characteristics of the marker locus. Autoradiograms were scored by two independent readers, and genotypes were entered into a database.

Multiple analytic strategies were used for mapping seizure QTLs in F_2 mice screened with KA. First, associations were evaluated between genotypes determined at 150 marker loci and seizure responses in 257 F_2 progeny through use of ANOVA and contingency procedures. Simple genetic models were constructed using linear logistic regression analysis (McAleer et al. 1995; Schork et al. 1995). Seizure responses were analyzed separately as quantitative measures (seizure score) and qualitative measures (maximum response achieved; i.e., no seizure, partial clonus, generalized clonus, or status epilepticus). The second strategy used multivariate stepwise regression analysis to evaluate simultaneously the influence of multiple QTL (marker) effects which achieved a statistical significance level of $p < 0.02$ in the first strategy (Schork et al. 1995). The third strategy involved refining the position and effect of QTLs through interval mapping using the standard and non-parametric Mapmaker programs (Lander and Botstein 1989; Kruglyak and Lander 1995).

Analysis of data from F_2 mice screened with PTZ will be carried out using a similar panel of statistical tools; however, genotyping for this study has just begun and data for only a few loci are currently available for review. As in the KA experiment, the PTZ phenotype can be analyzed as both a quantitative and a qualitative response. Contingency analysis of PTZ F_2 data derived from chromosome-1 markers that were most significant in the KA study was carried out by defining the phenotype based on the presence or absence of a maximal seizure. Thus, in preliminary statistical mapping, expression of PTZ-induced tonic hindlimb extension was used to define seizure-sensitive F_2 mice for chi square analysis of chromosome-1 allele distributions.

Results

Behavioral seizure response to KA and PTZ. Dose/response studies were carried out in D2 and B6 mice to guide in the selection of an F_2 screening dose. These data are summarized in Table 2 for both KA and PTZ. Based on dose/response data, populations of F_2 intercross mice were generated and tested with either KA at a dose of 25 mg/kg ($n = 257$) or PTZ at a dose of 80 mg/kg ($n = 524$). Maximum qualitative responses for each convulsant are shown in Figure 3. Additionally, quantitative responses based on latency to each phase or behavioral component of the seizure phenotype were converted into a seizure score for KA-treated F_2 mice. The distribution of these scores is shown in Figure 4. Quantitative data on PTZ-induced seizures in F_2 mice are presented as raw latency distributions in Figure 5.

Mapping loci for seizure response to KA and PTZ. Genotype data were collected and analyzed in two stages in the KA study, first for the extreme responders ($n = 70$ seizure-resistant and $n = 77$ seizure-sensitive) and then for the remainder of the population. Univariate contingency analysis of allele frequencies revealed a number of marker loci (or groups of linked loci) that were associated with KA seizure-sensitive and -resistant phenotypes. These are listed in Table 3.

Markers passing liberal statistical thresholds in the univariate analysis were entered into multivariate logistic regression analysis. These regions of the genome were also scanned using the Mapmaker/QTL software, a maximum likelihood program that generates LOD scores over defined marker intervals on a genetic linkage map. LOD score results from Mapmaker/QTL are depicted in Figure 6. Markers retained in the final multivariate logistic regression model are shown in Table 4.

Quantitative analysis with the Mapmaker/QTL program was carried out using several different expressions of the KA phenotype data. Thus, the trait measure for mapping was defined as the total KA seizure score or as the inverse of the individual latencies (with non-seizing mice given a value of zero). Table 5 shows that LOD scores for KA-induced seizure QTLs are dependent on the definition of the quantitative trait, suggesting that different components of the KA-induced seizure syndrome are influenced by different genetic factors. This method of approaching the overall phenotype as a series of intermediate phenotypes has both advantages and disadvantages. On the positive side, it enables dissection of a complex phenotype into several more simple phenotypes, and in the KA model, it provides an opportunity to learn something about

Table 4. Multivariate Analysis of Marker Data for KA-induced Seizures in F_2 Mice

Marker[a]	Allele mode[b]		Chi-Sq	p Value[c]	Odds ratio[d]
D1Mit16	D2	D	19.16	0.0001	23.78
D4Mit9	B6	D	7.33	0.0068	5.77
D11Mit224	B6	R	7.13	0.0076	5.89
D18Mit49	D2	A	14.14	0.0002	35.71

Multivariate stepwise logistic regression was conducted by defining the dependent variable as seizure resistance (phase 1 mice; $n = 70$) or seizure susceptibility (phase 4; $n = 77$).

[a]Analyses utilized marker data recoded to reflect the best fitting mode of inheritance; results are given in terms of susceptibility allele.

[b]Mode of inheritance was determined by best-fit regression analysis (D=dominant, R=recessive, A=additive).

[c]Probability that the regression coefficient equals 0.00.

[d]Odds of expressing a KA-induced behavioral seizure when possessing the susceptible genotype at the indicated marker locus.

distinct genetic influences on initiation, propagation, and maintenance of abnormal neuronal excitability. Thus, QTL effects on chromosome 1 may be related to partial and generalized clonus; chromosome-15 QTL effects may be related to status epilepticus; and chromosome-18 QTL effects may be related to partial clonus. The downside of this approach relates to uncertainties about how to correct mathematically for the effects of running multiple statistical tests.

Genome scanning in the PTZ model is not complete; however, some genetic data have been collected for markers on chromosome 1. Univariate chi-square analysis of allele distributions for markers D1Mit30 and D1Mit16 confirms the existence of a QTL that influences the difference in seizure susceptibilities between D2 and B6 mice. D1Mit30 data (Fig. 7) were generated by grouping F_2 mice on the basis of whether they exhibited PTZ-induced THE. When focal and generalized clonic seizure latencies were compared in the two groups of F_2 mice distinguished by THE, latencies were documented to be significantly shorter in the THE group (data not shown), indicating an association between the two behavioral seizure components, THE and clonus.

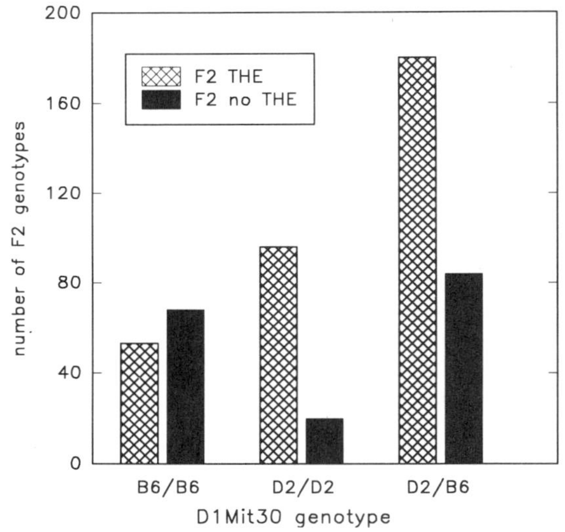

Figure 7. F_2 mice ($n = 524$) were injected with PTZ (80 mg/kg, s.c.) and observed for 1 hr. Mice were grouped according to the presence ($n = 339$) or absence ($n = 185$) of tonic hindlimb extension (THE), and genotypes were recorded at marker D1Mit30. Chi-square contingency analysis $p < 1 \times 10^{-8}$.

Table 5. Mapmaker/QTL LOD Scores as a Function of KA-induced Seizure Phenotype Specification

Phenotype (trait measure)	Marker interval	LOD[a]	Variance[b]
Total seizure score	D1Mit30-D1Mit16	5.47	17.2
	D15Mit6-D15Mit46	3.38	10.1
	D18Mit49-D18Mit144	2.50	7.7
Latency to partial clonus	D1Mit30-D1Mit16	6.01	20.1
	D15Mit6-D15Mit46	2.80	8.8
	D18Mit49-D18Mit144	3.46	11.2
Latency to generalized clonus	D1Mit30-D1Mit16	6.17	20.3
	D15Mit6-D15Mit46	2.28	7.2
	D18Mit49-D18Mit144	1.71	5.5
Latency to status epilepticus	D1Mit30-D1Mit145	2.49	6.8
	D15Mit6-D15Mit46	3.34	10.3
	D18Mit49-D18Mit144	1.58	4.9

[a]LOD scores were calculated using the full range of F_2 genotypes. Results of model-independent analyses are reported.

[b]Percentage of genetic variance explained.

Discussion

The large difference in seizure sensitivity between the D2 and B6 inbred mouse strains has been exploited in a QTL study. Using two chemoconvulsants that are known to induce seizures through different neurochemical mechanisms (and presumably different neuroanatomical pathways), we have begun to map QTLs that are fundamental in determining neuronal excitability. Using a panel of complementary analytic tools, several QTLs of significant effect have been characterized in an F_2 intercross population screened with KA. The QTL of greatest effect, *Kasz1*, resides on chromosome 1, most likely in the interval between markers D1Mit30 and D1Mit16, and meets the Lander and Kruglyak (1995) criteria for declaring significant linkage. Preliminary mapping in a separate group of F_2 mice screened with PTZ confirmed a QTL of significant effect near marker D1Mit30. Since collection of genotypes across the remainder of the genome for this group of mice is ongoing, the full range of genetic influences in the PTZ model remains to be determined. Nonetheless, the effect of the *Kasz1* appears strong in the PTZ model and will likely account for a substantial portion of the response variance.

The results of these experiments indicate that the region near D1Mit30 and D1Mit16 on mouse chromosome 1 includes a gene(s) which plays a fundamental role in the general seizure susceptibility of D2 mice relative to B6 mice. This genomic region has not been identified to contain genes involved in other mouse seizure models, with the possible exception of a study of ethanol-withdrawal seizures in the BXD RI strains (Crabbe and Belknap 1993). Candidate genes for *Kasz1* include both α (*Atp1a2*) and β (*Atp1b1*) subunits of the enzyme Na,K-ATPase (Kent et al. 1987). This region of mouse chromosome 1 is homologous to a portion of human chromosome 1q (DeBry and Seldin 1996). Proposing the involvement of Na,K-ATPase is particularly attractive, given the integral role of this membrane-bound ion pump in restoring membrane potential following neuronal depolarization and the ability of oubain, an inhibitor of Na,K-ATPase, to induce seizure activity (Bagetta et al. 1995; Brines et al. 1995). Additionally, evidence is accumulating that dysfunction of Na,K-ATPase can be a contributing factor in certain neurotoxicity paradigms and that it plays a role in neurodegeneration (Anderson et al. 1994; Brines et al. 1995), thus providing greater impetus to investigate the role of this enzyme and its genes in epilepsy.

Other provisional seizure-related QTLs were identified in the KA model; each was associated with a more modest influence on seizure susceptibility as compared to *Kasz1*. According to the recent Lander and Krugylak guidelines, the QTLs detected on chromosomes 11, 15, and 18 provide evidence for suggestive linkage (Lander and Kruglyak 1995). Thus, although these loci may be "statistically significant," they are potentially "false positive" results and best considered provisional until additional evidence can be generated to confirm their effects. In this regard, the QTL near D11Mit224 may be considered a confirmation of another recently described seizure-related QTL, *El6*, which localizes to the same region of chromosome 11 and also functions in a recessive fashion (Frankel et al. 1995). The QTLs identified on chromosomes 15 and 18, if real, appear to be novel seizure-related QTLs not previously reported in other complex mouse genetic seizure models (Neumann and Collins 1991; Frankel et al. 1994, 1995; Martin et al. 1995).

The strategy of testing D2 and B6 mice for seizure effects using different convulsant paradigms presents the opportunity to identify QTLs which are in common and therefore potentially most important for determining differences in neuronal excitability and susceptibility to behavioral seizures. The development of congenic strains derived from D2 and B6 mice, as well as use of these two strains in crosses with other inbred mouse strains, will help to further define the importance of seizure-related QTLs identified in these studies.

ACKNOWLEDGMENTS

This work was supported by National Institutes of Health grants DA-08041-01A3 and NS-33243-01.

REFERENCES

Alexander, R.C., J. Duda, D. Garth, W. Vogel, and W.H. Berrettini. 1993. Morphine and cocaine consumption in inbred mice. *Psychiatr. Genet.* **3:** 33.

Alexander, R.C., D. Heydt, T.N. Ferraro, W. Vogel, and W.H. Berrettini. 1996. Further evidence for a quantitative trait locus on murine chromosome 10 controlling morphine preference in inbred mice. *Psychiatr. Genet.* **6:** 29.

Anderson, W.R., J.E. Franck, W.L. Stahl, and A.A. Maki. 1994. Na,K-ATPase is decreased in hippocampus of kainate-lesioned rats. *Epilepsy Res.* **17:** 221.

Bagettap, G., M. Iannone, E. Palma, P. Rodino, T. Granato, and G. Nistico. 1995. Lack of involvement of nitric oxide in the mechanisms of seizures and hippocampal damage produced by kainate and oubain in rats. *Neurodegeneration* **4:** 43.

Belknap, J. and J. Crabbe. 1992. Chromosome mapping of gene loci affecting morphine and amphetamine responses in BXD recombinant inbred mice. *Ann. N.Y. Acad. Sci.* **654:** 311.

Belknap, J.K and L.A. O'Toole. 1991. Studies of genetic differences in response to opioid drugs. In *The genetic basis of alcohol and drug actions* (ed. J.C. Crabbe and R.A. Harris), p. 225. Plenum Press, New York.

Belknap, J.K, B. Noordewier, and M. Lame. 1989. Genetic dissociation of multiple morphine effects among C57BL/6J, DBA/2J and C3H/HeJ inbred mouse strains. *Physiol. Behav.* **46:** 69.

Belknap, J., J. Mogil, M. Helms, S. Richards, L. O'Toole, S. Bergeson, and K. Buck. 1995. Localization to chromosome 10 of a locus influencing morphine analgesia in crosses derived from C57BL/6 and DBA/2 strains. *Life Sci.* **57:** 117.

Berrettini, W.H., R.C. Alexander, T.N. Ferraro, and W.H. Vogel. 1994a. A study of oral morphine preference in inbred mouse strains. *Psychiatr. Genet.* **4:** 81.

Berrettini, W.H., T.N. Ferraro, R.C. Alexander, A.M. Buchberg, and W.H. Vogel. 1994b. Quantitative trait loci mapping of three loci controlling morphine preference using inbred mouse strains. *Nat. Genet.* **7:** 3.

Brines, M.L., A.O. Dare, and N.C. deLanerolle. 1995. The cardiac glycoside oubain potentiates excitotoxic injury of adult neurons in rat hippocampus. *Neurosci. Lett.* **191:** 145.

Cadoret, T.J., W.R. Yates, E. Troughton, G. Woodworth, and M.A. Stewart. 1995. Adoption study demonstrating two genetic pathways to drug abuse. *Arch. Gen. Psychiatr.* **52:** 42.

Crabbe, J.C., J.K. Belknap, and K.J. Buck. 1994. Genetic animal models of alcohol and drug abuse. *Science* **264:** 1715.

Crabbe, J.C. and J.K. Belknap. 1993. Behavior genetic analyses of drug withdrawal. *Alcohol Alcohol.* **2:** 477.

DeBry, R.W. and M.F. Seldin. 1996. Human/mouse homology relationships. *Genomics* **33:** 337.

Dietrich, W., J. Miller, R. Steen, M. Merchant, D. Damron-Boles, Z. Husain, R. Dredge, M. Daly, K., Ingalls, T. O'Connor, C. Evans, M. DeAngelis, D Levinson, L. Kruglyak, N. Goodman, N. Copeland, N. Jenkins, T. Hawkins, S. Lincoln, D. Page, and E. Lander. 1996. A comprehensive genetic map of the mouse genome. *Nature* **380:** 149.

Dietrich, W.F., E.S. Lander, J.S. Smith, A.R. Moser, K.A. Gould, C. Luongo, N. Borenstein, and W. Dove. 1993. Genetic identification of Mom-1, a major modifier locus affecting Min-induced intestinal neoplasia in the mouse. *Cell* **75:** 631.

Engstrom, F.L. and D.M. Woodbury. 1988. Seizure susceptibility in DBA and C57 mice: The effects of various convulsants. *Epilepsia* **29:** 389.

Ferraro, T.N., G.T. Golden, G.G. Smith, and W.H. Berrettini. 1995. Differential susceptibility to seizures induced by kainic acid. *Epilepsia* **36:** 301.

Ferraro, T.N., G.T. Golden, G.G. Smith, C. Ballas, H. Choi, N.J. Schork, P. St. Jean, and W.H. Berrettini. 1997. Mapping murine loci for seizure response to kainic acid. *Mamm. Genome* (in press).

Frankel, W.N., B.A. Taylor, J.L. Noebels, and C.M. Lutz. 1994. Genetic epilepsy model derived from common inbred mouse strains. *Genetics* **138:** 1.

Frankel, W.N., A. Valenzuela, C.M. Lutz, E.W. Johnson, W.F. Dietrich, and J.M. Coffin. 1995. New seizure frequency QTL and the complex genetics of epilepsy in EL mice. *Mamm. Genome* **6:** 830.

Giros, B., M. Pohl, J. Rochelle, and M. Seldin. 1995. Chromosomal localization of opioid peptide and receptor genes in the mouse. *Life Sci.* **56:** 369.

Greenberg, D.A., A.V. Delgado-Escueta, H. Widelitz, R.S. Sparkes, L. Treiman, H.M. Maldonado, M.S. Park, and P.I. Terasaki. 1988. Juvenile myoclonic epilepsy may be linked to the Bf and HLA loci on human chromosome 6. *Am. J. Med. Genet.* **31:** 185.

Grove, W.M., E.D. Eckert, L. Heston, T.J. Bouchard, Jr., N. Segal, and D.T. Lykken. 1990. Heritability of substance abuse and anti-social behavior: A study of monozygotic twins reared apart. *Biol. Psychiatry* **27:** 1293.

Hilbert, P., K. Lindpainter, J. Beckman, T. Serikawa, F. Soubrier, C. Dubay, P. Cartwright, B. DeGouyon, C. Julier, S. Takahasi, M. Vincent, D. Ganten, M. Georges, and G. Lathrop. 1991. Chromosomal mapping of two genetic loci associated with blood-pressure regulation in hereditary hypertensive rats. *Nature* **353:** 521.

Horowitz, G.P. 1981. Pharmacogenetic models and behavioral responses to opiates. In *Development of animal models as pharmacogenetic tools* (ed. J. McClearn), p. 209. NIAAA Research Monograph No. 6, USGPO, Washington, D.C.

Jacob, H., K. Lindpainter, S. Lincoln, K. Kusumi, R. Bunker, Y.-P. Mao, D. Ganten, and V. Dzau. 1991. Genetic mapping of a gene causing hypertension in the stroke-prone spontaneously hypertensive rat. *Cell* **67:** 213.

Kent, R.B., D.A. Fallows, E. Geissler, T. Glaser, J. Rettig Emanuel, P.A. Lalley, R. Levenson, and D.E. Houseman. 1987. Genes encoding α and β subunits of Na,K-ATPase are located on three different chromosomes in the mouse. *Proc. Natl. Acad. Sci.* **84:** 5369.

Kosobud, A.E. and J.C. Crabbe. 1990. Genetic correlations among inbred strain sensitivities to convulsions induced by 9 convulsant drugs. *Brain Res.* **526:** 8.

Kozak, C., J. Filie, M. Adamson, Y. Chen, and I. Yu. 1994. Murine chromosomal location of the mu and kappa opioid receptor genes. *Genomics* **21:** 659.

Krugylak, L. and E.S. Lander. 1995. A nonparametric approach for mapping quantitative trait loci. *Genetics* **139:** 1421.

Lahiri, D.K. and J.I. Nurnberger. 1991. A rapid nonenzymatic method for the preparation of high molecular weight DNA from blood for RFLP studies. *Nucleic Acids Res.* **19:** 5444.

Lander, E.S. and D. Botstein. 1989. Mapping Mendelian factors underlying quantitative traits using RFLP linkage maps. *Genetics* **121:** 185.

Lander, E.S. and L. Kruglyak. 1995. Genetic dissection of complex traits: Guidelines for interpreting and reporting linkage results. *Nat. Genet.* **11:** 241.

Lander, E.S., P. Green, J. Abrahamson, A. Barlow, M.J. Daly, S.E. Lincoln, and L. Newburg. 1987. MAPMAKER: An interactive computer package for constructing primary genetic linkage maps of experimental and natural populations. *Genomics* **1:** 174.

Leppert, M., V.E. Anderson, T. Quattlebaum, D. Stauffer, P. O'Connell, Y. Nakamura, J.-M. Lalouel, and R. White. 1989. Benign neonatal familial convulsions linked to genetic markers on chromosome 20. *Nature* **337:** 647.

Lewis, T.B., R.J. Leach, K. Ward, P. O'Connell, and S.G. Ryan. 1993. Genetic heterogeneity in benign familial neonatal convulsions: Identification of a new locus on chromosome 8q. *Am. J. Hum. Genet.* **53:** 670.

Liu, A.W., A.V. Delgado-Escueta, J.M. Serratosa, M.E. Alonso, M.T. Medina, M.N. Gee, S. Cordova, H.Z Zhao, J.M. Spellman, J.R. Ramos Peek, F. Rubio Donnadieu, and R.S. Sparkes. 1995. Juvenile myoclonic epilepsy locus in chromosome 6p21.2-p11: Linkage to convulsions and electroencephalography trait. *Am. J. Hum. Genet.* **57:** 368.

Lush, I. 1984. The genetics of tasting in mice: III: Quinine. *Genet. Res.* **44:** 151.

Luthar, S.S., S.F. Anton, K.R. Merikangas, and B.J. Rounsaville. 1992. Vulnerability to substance abuse and psychopathology among siblings of opioid abusers. *J. Nerv. Ment. Dis.* **180:** 153.

Mansour, A., H. Khachaturian, M.E. Lewis, H. Akil, and S.J. Watson. 1988. Anatomy of CNS opioid receptors. *Trends Pharmacol. Sci.* **11:** 308.

Martin, B., Y. Clement, P. Venault, G. Chapouthier. 1995. Mouse chromosomes 4 and 13 are involved in β-carboline-induced seizures. *J. Hered.* **86:** 274.

McAleer, M.A., P. Reifsnyder, S.M. Palmer, M. Prochazka, J.M. Love, J.B. Copeman, E.E. Powell, N.R. Rodrigues, J.-B. Prins, D.V. Serreze, N.H. DeLarato, L.S. Wicker, L.B. Peterson, N.J. Schork, J.A. Todd, and E.H. Leiter. 1995. Crosses of NOD mice with the related NON strain. *Diabetes* **44:** 1186.

Melo, J., J. Shendure, K. Pociask, and L. Silver. 1996. Identification of sex-specific quantitative trait loci controlling alcohol preference in C57BL/6 mice. *Nat. Genet.* **13:** 147.

Neumann, P.E. and R.L. Collins. 1991. Genetic dissection of susceptibility to audiogenic seizures in inbred mice. *Proc. Natl. Acad. Sci.* **88:** 5408.

Neumann, P.E. and T.N. Seyfried. 1990. Mapping of two genes that influence susceptibility to audiogenic seizures in crosses of C57BL/6J and DBA/2J mice. *Behav. Genet.* **20:** 307.

Paterson, A.H., J.W. Deverna, B. Lanini, and S.D. Tanksley. 1990. Fine mapping of quantitative trait loci using selected overlapping recombinant chromosomes in an interspecies cross of tomato. *Genetics* **124:** 735.

Pickens, R.W., D.S. Svikis, M. McGue, D.T. Lykken, L.L. Heston, and P.L. Clayton. 1991. Heterogeneity in the inheritance of alcoholism. *Arch. Gen. Psychiatr.* **48:** 19.

Rounsaville, B.J., T.R. Kosten, M.M. Weissman, B. Prusoff, D. Pauls, and S.F. Anton. 1991. Psychiatric disorders in relatives of probands with opiate addiction. *Arch. Gen. Psychiatr.* **46:** 33.

Routman, E. and J. Cheverud. 1994. A rapid method of scoring simple sequence repeat polymorphisms with agarose gel electrophoresis. *Mamm. Gen.* **5:** 187.

Schork, N.J., J.E. Krieger, M.R. Trolliet, K.G. Franchini, G. Koike, E.M. Krieger, E.S. Lander, V.J. Dzau, and H.J. Jacob. 1995. A biometrical genomic search in rats reveals the multigenic basis of blood pressure variation. *Genome Res.* **5:** 164.

Taylor, B.A. and S.J. Phillips. 1996. Detection of obesity QTLs on mouse chromosomes 1 and 7 by selective DNA pooling. *Genomics* **34:** 389.

Todd, J., T. Altman, R. Cornall, S. Ghosh, J. Hall, C. Hearne, A. Knight, J. Love, M. McAleer, J.-B. Prins, N. Rodrigues, M. Lathrop, A. Pressey, N. DeLarato, L. Peterson, and L. Wicker. 1991. Genetic analysis of autoimmune type 1 diabetes mellitus in mice. *Nature* **351:** 542.

Weber, J.L and P.E. May. 1989. Abundant class of human DNA polymorphisms which can be typed using the polymerase chain reaction. *Am. J. Hum. Genet.* **44:** 388.

Whitehouse, W.P., M. Rees, D. Curtis, A. Sundqvist, K. Parker, E. Chung, D. Baralle, and R.M. Gardiner. 1993. Linkage analysis of idiopathic generalized epilepsy (IGE) and marker loci on chromosome 6p in families of patients with juvenile myoclonic epilepsy: No evidence for an epilepsy locus in the HLA region. *Am. J. Hum. Genet.* **53:** 652.

Zeng, Z.-B. 1993. Theoretical basis of separation of multiple linked gene effects on mapping quantitative trait loci. *Proc. Natl. Acad. Sci.* **90:** 10972.

———. 1994. Precision mapping of quantitative trait loci. *Genetics* **136:** 1457.

Recent Developments in the Genetics of Bipolar Disorder

J.R. DEPAULO, JR. AND F.J. MCMAHON
Department of Psychiatry, Johns Hopkins University, Baltimore, Maryland 21287-7381

Ample evidence from twin and adoption studies supports an important genetic contribution to bipolar and to unipolar mood disorders (Mendlewicz and Rainer 1977). Segregation analyses conducted numerous times have revealed no consistent mode of inheritance (O'Rourke et al. 1983; Rice et al. 1987; Spence et al. 1993). At the same time, estimates of heritability are consistent in suggesting that genetic variation is the major etiologic factor for bipolar disorders.

Following the development of DNA-based marker technology as a tool for finding genes, psychiatric disorders, especially bipolar disorder, appeared to be particularly apt targets for these linkage studies. Several dramatic findings of linkage of the bipolar (Egeland et al. 1987; Baron et al. 1987) and the schizophrenia (Sherrington et al. 1988) phenotypes to chromosomal regions were reported, only to be "re-evaluated," "reduced" in significance, or otherwise withdrawn (Kelsoe et al. 1989; Baron 1993; Gurling and Sharma 1994). At a time when there is skepticism about the wisdom of doing linkage studies of complex psychiatric disorders, more powerful linkage methods are developing: More numerous and more informative genetic markers and more efficient "multi-point" statistical algorithms permit us to extract all, or nearly all, of the genetic information from a given family resource. Thus, the family resources become the crucial variables in the research. In the last 3 years, modest linkage findings have been published and, at least in a few cases, independently replicated. However, these findings are viewed with skepticism by some because the statistical tests of significance are marginal, the probability of false-positive findings is non-trivial, and the chromosomal regions are so broad as to make isolation of putative disease mutations a daunting task (Risch and Botstein 1996). Here, we review what we see as the areas of consistency from our studies and others' studies and the opportunities and challenges inherent in this research arena. As psychiatrists, we emphasize issues of the phenotype. We argue that phenotypic variations within and between families may provide crucial clues for locating genes and may speed the assessment of how they work.

The areas of consistency to be described in detail are as follows: (1) There appear to be one or possibly two regions of chromosome 18 that show linkage to some families with bipolar disorder (Berrettini et al. 1994; Stine et al. 1995; Freimer et al. 1996; Nothen et al. 1996); (2) there is an apparent linked region on chromosome 21q (Straub et al. 1994; Gurling et al. 1995; Detera-Wadleigh et al. 1996); and (3) there appears to be a parent-of-origin effect in the bipolar families based both on clinical grounds (McMahon et al. 1995; Gershon et al. 1996) and on several of the positive linkage results at these loci (Stine et al. 1995; Gershon et al. 1996; Detera-Wadleigh et al. 1996; T.C. Gilliam, pers. comm.).

The fundamental goal is to find the genes and the pathogenic mechanisms underlying bipolar disorders, which are prevalent and disabling, but may also convey some advantage in their milder forms. The challenges we face include the apparent facts that the disorders are etiologically and genetically heterogeneous, that multiple pathogenic alleles appear to be required to produce the phenotype in individuals, that the best phenotypic definition of the disorder is unclear, and that there is no known characteristic pathological lesion or pathophysiological marker for these disorders. At the same time, it should be remembered that these disorders, when diagnosed, can be considerably helped by a variety of medications. Thus, even partial understanding of the heretofore mysterious pathogenic mechanisms may have a dramatic clinical benefit for patients.

THE PHENOTYPES

Evidence for the Phenotypes: Which Are To Be Called Affected?

The notion of a spectrum of affective syndromes owes much to the family and case control family studies carried out in the 1970s and 1980s (Gershon et al. 1982; Winokur et al. 1982). These studies showed increased rates of bipolar and unipolar disorders in the relatives of bipolar, as compared to relatives of control, probands. However, there is some uncertainty about the inclusion of any phenotype other than bipolar I (classic manic depressive illness) as affected for purposes of genetic analyses. The phenotypes other than bipolar I most often considered as affected include bipolar II disorder, recurrent major depressive (or unipolar) disorder, and schizoaffective disorder, manic type. Milder affective states are sometimes included as affected in studies that analyze sequential sets of family members included in "narrow" to "broad" affection status categories. The conditions usually reserved for the broader definition of the phenotype include single-episode major depression, dysthymic disorder, minor depressions, depressive personality, hyperthymic personality, and cyclothymic personality.

Since the power of linkage studies of bipolar disorder (and schizophrenia) depends heavily on having families with many closely related and accurately diagnosed affected individuals, investigators would want to include all of the genetically related spectrum conditions as affected but would not want to call any individuals affected who do not share the affected genotype. In the absence of a priori knowledge, and with the scarcity of families we know to have many affected relatives all due to the same genotype, we face the dilemma of doing the studies with insufficient statistical power, or risk including as affected various spectrum conditions that may not share the affected genotype (phenocopies).

The Major Affective Disorders

The question of whether and how to include the family members with unipolar disorder is central in this regard. The rate of unipolar disorder, although higher in families with bipolar probands than in families with psychiatrically well probands, is so high in the control proband families that it is unlikely that all unipolar family members will have the same genetic diathesis as the bipolar proband. Thus, categorizing as affected all unipolars in families ascertained through severe bipolar probands (Blacker and Tsuang 1993; Baron et al. 1994) could increase to unacceptable levels the number of individuals who are called affected when they are not (phenocopies). Leaving them out reduces the number of persons called affected and the apparent statistical power of the sample. The field needs a way to distinguish which unipolars are genetically related to the bipolar probands and to include only these as affected (Blacker and Tsuang 1993; Baron 1994).

In bipolar II disorder, depressions predominate and the mild and brief elevations of mood and vitality, which define the condition as bipolar II, are not regularly reported or recognized (Endicott et al. 1985; Rice et al. 1986; Dunner and Tay 1993). Simpson and associates (1993) suggest that these cases represent many, if not most, of the "depression" cases which are related genetically to the bipolar I probands. In Simpson's analysis of the families of bipolar I probands, more relatives were diagnosed with bipolar II than with unipolar or bipolar I. Other studies in the field, however, consistently report that relatives with unipolar disorder outnumber those with bipolar disorder, leading to the conclusion that either the families studied by these groups were different or the threshold for diagnosis of bipolar II differed between studies. The latter interpretation is likely. Early family studies (Andreasen et al. 1981) that included the bipolar II diagnosis found unacceptably low levels of diagnostic reliability. However, they were based on interviews done mostly by non-clinician interviewers, and they were based on very few cases. Later studies (Dunner and Tay 1993; Simpson et al. 1996) have shown good diagnostic reliability when experienced clinicians did the interviews and made the diagnoses. The potential importance of the bipolar II diagnosis is supported further by reports that, at least at the loci on chromosome 18q where linkage was detected, the linkage finding was due substantially to the inclusion of bipolar II as an affected condition for all analyses (McMahon et al. 1996). The contributions of the bipolar II phenotype linkage to the linkage finding require prospective testing in an independent sample. If confirmed, it suggests a method for selecting relatives for study who share genetic determinants with the bipolar I probands.

Minor Affective Disorders and Possibly Related Nonaffective States

The so-called minor affective disorders, including minor depressions, dysthymic disorder (a chronic minor depression), and the temperamental variants, cyclothymia, hyperthymia, and depressive personality, have all been proposed (Kraepelin 1921) to represent a milder manifestation of the bipolar genotype. The close relationship of dysthymic disorder and major depression is very well established on clinical grounds (i.e., most dysthymic subjects have had or will have major depressive episodes). The association of bipolar II disorder with dysthymia has been strongly suggested (Wicki and Angst 1991; Akiskal 1994). Whether these clinical disorders all point to several different genotypes or are differing manifestations of the same genotype remains unknown.

Fewer consistent increases in the prevalence of various anxiety disorders and alcohol- and substance-abuse-related conditions have been reported in bipolar families (Winokur et al. 1971; Winokur 1979; Gershon et al. 1982), which leaves in doubt their relationships to the affected genotypes. Many, but not all, linkage studies consider family members with only the lesser variants of affective coloring and the anxiety disorders as unknown phenotypes for the purpose of linkage analysis. Once the genetic variants of bipolar disorder are defined, it will be of considerable interest to study the relationship of these conditions to the bipolar genotypes.

Age at Onset Variation

The utility of age at onset of bipolar disorder for discriminating between genetic subgroups or between genetic and nongenetic etiologies is unknown. However, several studies (Taylor and Abrams 1981; Ayuso-Gutierrez and Ramos-Brieva 1982), most done before a bipolar II classification was devised, and recent studies (McMahon et al. 1994) using bipolar I and II classes, demonstrate a narrow range of onset ages for all bipolar familial cases. In the McMahon et al. (1994) study, 80% of all bipolar subjects in 34 families fell ill by age 30. Thus, onset age is an unlikely basis for genetic subtyping of bipolar disorder. The McMahon et al. (1994) findings have shown that in a family sample ascertained through bipolar I probands, bipolar I and bipolar II relatives have indistinguishable distributions of onset age, whereas recurrent unipolar relatives have a broader range of onset ages. This suggests that bipolar II should be included with bipolar I relatives as affected in such families but that unipolar cases may be a more heterogeneous group etiologically. The age-at-onset research and the potential utility of onset age as a clue in the search for the pathogenic mechanisms involved in bipolar disorder have been reviewed recently (McMahon and DePaulo 1996).

Evidence for Familial Phenotypic Variation

Another important way to divide phenotypes is based on the variation between families rather than between individuals within families. In this arena, several important clinical observations may help unravel an apparently complicated situation. These include (1) parent-of-origin effects, which may reflect a role for imprinted genes and mitochondrial genes, and may produce atypical sex-related segregation of the disorder in some families; (2) familial comorbidity; and (3) the variation between generations within families (i.e., anticipation and cohort effects).

Parent of Origin Effects

During the last 30 years, a relative excess of apparent maternal, as opposed to paternal, transmission of the bipolar phenotype has been noted in several family studies (Winokur et al. 1969; Perris 1971; Mendlewicz et al. 1973). The initial interpretation was that bipolar disorder was, at least in part, a Mendelian X-linked disorder (Winokur et al. 1969; Mendlewicz et al. 1972; Risch and Baron 1982). There were linkage studies supporting this interpretation from several groups who reported that the bipolar disorder in such families was linked to the color-blindness loci and G6PD locus at the q telomere of the X chromosome (Reich et al. 1969; Mendlewicz et al. 1980; Baron et al. 1987). Recently, both the linkage studies and the interpretation of the apparent excess of maternal transmission have been revised. The linkage of bipolar disorder to DNA markers in the Xq28 region has not supported the earlier linkages using color blindness and G6PD, even in the same families where this was reported originally (Baron et al. 1993).

The pattern of transmission of the bipolar phenotype has been reassessed by McMahon et al. (1995). They found an excess of families with a maternal transmission pattern but also more affected relatives in the maternal line, including male and female relatives, and the absence of transmission from affected fathers to daughters as well as to sons in many families. The implications of this are that families should be divided into maternal and paternal subgroups for future linkage analyses of these families and that the hypotheses of mitochondrial inheritance or imprinting-influenced transmission should be tested. This observation of an excess of maternal transmission in bipolar families has been independently replicated (Gershon et al. 1996). It also has been employed to illuminate recent linkage reports that divide families on the basis of the apparent parental transmission pattern (Stine et al. 1995; Gershon et al. 1996; T.C. Gilliam, pers. comm.). Interestingly, in these studies it was linkage of the phenotype in so-called paternal families that revealed stronger evidence of linkage of the bipolar phenotype to markers on chromosome 18.

Familial Comorbidity Patterns

It seems intuitively obvious that comorbid conditions might reflect different causes of illness between those bipolar individuals and families who have or do not have the comorbid condition in question. However, the comorbid condition most often studied in bipolar disorder, alcoholism/substance abuse, predicted a poorer outcome but does not appear to predict differences in a familial loading or transmission pattern in families with bipolar and substance-related conditions. Recently, MacKinnon et al. (1997) have shown that panic attacks or panic disorder in bipolar probands predicts that their bipolar, but not unipolar or other relatives, will have an elevated rate of panic attacks or panic disorder. This suggests that bipolar families with comorbid panic attacks may be different in some aspect of pathogenesis from other bipolar families. About 15% of the families studied for our linkage analyses had probands with bipolar and comorbid panic attacks, which suggests that a sample of such families could be compared to families without panic in linkage studies. Other comorbid features that may help divide the families as well as panic disorder remain to be defined and tested.

Generational Differences as Possible Indicators of Genetic Subtypes

In 1992 when the genetic basis for myotonic dystrophy was discovered, a new mutation mechanism, the expansion in meiosis of a trinucleotide repeat sequence, was discovered. It had long been known that when families were ascertained for study or care, children affected with the illness tended to become ill at an earlier age than their parents. This clinical observation, called anticipation, was considered by Penrose (1948) to be an artifact of ascertainment. The most clear-cut bias is that families in which the parent has an early onset age, and the affected children have a late onset, are unlikely to be ascertained. The discovery of the trinucleotide repeat expansions and their correlation with age at onset and disease severity for several neuromuscular and neuropsychiatric phenotypes has encouraged both the analysis of family samples for anticipation and the search for expanded triplet repeats in the DNA of these and other patient samples. McInnis et al. (1993) authored the first modern report of anticipation in bipolar disorder. They found earlier onset age and more episodes of illness per year in the younger generation of their two-generation pedigrees. They employed multiple sampling schemes, including a careful clinical assessment procedure to reduce the likelihood of transmission through both parents (bilineality), and excluded the bipolar I probands to reduce the observation biases, the existence of which was never doubted. Several reports since then have confirmed, and a few have failed to find, a similar pattern of anticipation. However, the observation, no matter how carefully made, generates, but does not test, the hypothesis that triplet repeat expansions cause some familial forms of bipolar disorder.

In the last decade, a cohort effect was reported for unipolar and then for bipolar disorder (Gershon et al. 1987; Klerman and Weissman 1989). It was observed that there was a greater incidence and earlier onset of these disorders in persons born since 1945 and since 1960 compared to individuals born before those dates. No mechanism, genetic or otherwise, has been directly associated with the phenomenon, but it was surmised that increased prevalence of substance abuse may have caused the additional onset, or at least hastened it. After the reports of triplet repeat expansion and anticipation were published, a frequent question posed was whether the cohort effect might confound the analysis of anticipation or, alternately, be explained by anticipation. McInnis et al. (1993) did an analysis of covariance which detected an effect in the expected direction for the year of birth on onset age, but suggested that the generational or anticipation effect remained significant. Since a year of birth and generation are confounded variables, it is very difficult to disentangle their respective effects on onset age.

In summary, the clinical differences between individuals and between families affected by these disorders provide potential clues to help resolve the complex genetic origins of bipolar disorders. The painstaking clinical assessment of families is the rate-limiting step in the actual (as opposed to the nominal or calculated) power of genetic linkage analyses to detect linked loci for bipolar disorder and may suggest the types of genes or their mechanisms once the loci are found.

PROGRESS IN THE LABORATORY AND LINKAGE ANALYSES OF BIPOLAR DISORDER

Genome-wide Linkage Analyses

A few published linkage studies of bipolar disorder have used markers spanning all chromosomal arms (Coon et al. 1993; Ginns et al. 1996; Berrettini et al. 1997). These published studies have been limited by (1) very small samples, (2) the use of DNA markers that are less informative than the marker sets which are currently used, and (3) the use of parametric and nonparametric analytical methods that were not designed to maximize the information content of genome-wide studies. Only modestly positive results have been reported in these or other linkage studies, and few of these have been independently replicated. This suggests that major locus effects are uncommon in bipolar families or that they do not exist. In short, the worst-case scenarios of investigators engaged in this research have not been dispelled and loom larger now than before these studies were done. These include the possibility that no single locus (acting alone or in concert with a small number of other loci) accounts for more than 20% of the familial cases and the possibility that a substantial fraction of the phenotypes result from the inheritance of a combination of alleles which are so common in the population as to be normal variants.

In contrast, appropriately optimistic scenarios can be formulated based on three or four recent developments: First, two or three loci have been detected and independently confirmed at least at suggestive levels of statistical significance; second, the maps and analytic methods available for these studies are much more powerful than those of just a few years ago; third, the discovery of even one disease-related mutation may catalyze the more rapid discovery of the others (as has been occurring in Alzheimer's disease after the rare chromosome 21 locus was found); and fourth, very large samples needed to detect rare loci or loci of modest effect can be collected in collaborative style (as happened for breast cancer).

Review of Positive Linkage Claims

Following the reevaluation of the claims of linkage that could not be confirmed, the field has searched for ways to reduce the likelihood of further false-positive claims of linkage. The most visible result of this effort, besides the inevitable improvement in molecular and analytical tools, has been the tightening of the statistical standards for declaring linkage. This work is still being refined and promises more precise interpretation of genetic research data. However, given the less-than-overwhelming evidence supporting the presence of linkage to any locus, the field could find itself in a state of statistical limbo if it takes this effort as promising more than improved guidelines for communication of results. It is more than slightly ironic that all three of the most widely reported and apparently false-positive results (Baron et al. 1987; Egeland et al. 1987; Sherrington et al. 1988) would have met the new and very stringent statistical criteria recommended (Lander and Kruglyak 1996) for claiming linkage.

Chromosome-18 findings. Berrettini et al. (1994) reported modest evidence for linkage suggesting that a gene of small effect was located in the pericentromeric region of chromosome 18. Their study used 21 families ascertained by the psychiatric genetics group at the National Institute of Mental Health in Bethesda and a modest subset of the Amish pedigree (Egeland et al. 1987; Kelsoe et al. 1989).

Equivocal results of other groups at various chromosome-18 loci were interpreted alternately as supportive, as nonconfirming, and more cogently, as uninformative about linkage to the region reported by Berrettini. In 1995, investigators from John Hopkins (Stine et al. 1995) reported almost identical allele-sharing by affected sibs at some of the same markers previously reported and at other loci in the region cited above. However, in addition, a parent-of-origin effect was present in the Hopkins data so that evidence for linkage was concentrated in families with transmitting fathers, and a set of three markers at a distance of 40 cM on the q arm of the chromosome showed evidence for linkage also in paternal families.

Since then, the linkage to 18p pericentromeric region and the paternal parent of origin effect has been reported by two additional groups (Gershon et al. 1996; T.C. Gilliam, pers. comm.). Three other reports (Calzolari et al. 1996; DeBruyn et al. 1996; Freimer et al. 1996) have also suggested linkage to 18q loci within the 18q21-23 bands but find less evidence of linkage to the pericentromeric loci. Although opinions vary about whether these findings represent (1) a single poorly defined region of linkage somewhere on chromosome 18 or (2) two distinct linked regions (18p11 and 18q21-23), there is mounting evidence for at least one gene for bipolar disorder on chromosome 18.

Assuming linkage is established at one or two loci on 18, the route to delineation of the critical region or regions might be as difficult as establishing linkage. Analysis of haplotype may add little to the resolution of the locus, given uncertainties about which individuals in the families may be phenocopies and which families may have shared markers in the linked region by chance alone. Greater numbers of DNA markers will add very little, but more families will improve incrementally the likelihood of finding the critical crossovers. It would also be important to ensure that the families being used for this purpose are linked to the locus, although this may be an unrealistic expectation unless the families are large enough to demonstrate linkage individually. The other readily available but uncertain strategy for narrowing a linked region to a few megabases of DNA is to divide the phenotype into genetically meaningful subgroups at the level of individuals or families after the linkage is established.

Traditionally, it has been assumed that the more severe phenotype will be more likely to demonstrate linkage to a disease locus. However, empirical evidence for this is weak for bipolar disorder. In fact, we have argued that the milder phenotype (i.e., bipolar II) is genetically less complex and, for this reason, may prove to be the form of the phenotype most strongly correlated with one or more disease loci. This hypothesis is not without precedent; e.g., cafe au lait spots in neurofibromatosis (Riccardi and Lewis 1988).

Another powerful strategy would be to ascertain families from a genetically isolated population such as the Sardinians or the Lapps. These families are particularly useful for studies of linkage disequilibrium. Linkage disequilibrium exists between a marker and a disease locus when the two are in such close physical proximity that recombination events between them are very rare. This strategy was important in the localization of a susceptibility gene for insulin-dependent diabetes mellitus (Copeman et al. 1995).

Positive findings on chromosome 21. A more subtle but consistent (across three studies) finding has emerged on chromosome 21q. This finding was initially reported by Straub et al. (1994) as an LOD score (3.4) in only one of the 47 bipolar families being analyzed and supported by affected pedigree member analyses from the family set. The finding was not expected to be replicated in any modest-sized sample because, if true, it was a rare source of illness or it might have failed replication because it was a chance finding. Nonetheless, two recent papers supporting linkage at this locus have been published (Gurling et al. 1995; Detera-Wadleigh et al. 1996). The most persuasive is the finding of positive sib-pair analyses in the sample used in the original report on 18 (Detera-Wadleigh et al. 1996).

Recently Implicated Loci and Older Ones in Doubt

Several other loci recently implicated have not yet been replicated. The decision to tie this part of the saga into the older literature with reevaluated and recanted findings was made not because the newer work is problematic, but because independent replication is so central to the scientific task at hand and because at least two of the new findings are at loci very near the loci reported in the 1980s on chromosome 11p and Xq28.

Association studies of populations and linkage analyses of single large pedigrees are largely responsible for the current list of candidate loci that need to be tested for replication by the field at large. Single large-family studies have produced impressive LOD score results on chromosomes Xq26 and 4p (Pekkarinen et al. 1995; Blackwood et al. 1996). These are clear target loci for other studies. Associations and linkage results at the TH locus on 11p and the MAO locus on Xp have been inconsistent but also merit further study.

Several other chromosomal regions have been pointed to by other investigators as having suggestive evidence for linkage, but they and the loci noted above must be regarded as hypotheses in need of further testing. The genetic technology for finding genes of interest when applied to psychiatric disorders has very good prospects of locating important sources for these disorders. Determining which of the modest signals are truly relevant will be difficult—at least until we find and have a disease gene or mutation in hand and can employ it to reframe our search for the other genes involved in bipolar disorder.

REFERENCES

Akiskal, H.S. 1994. The temperamental borders of affective disorders. *Acta Psychiatr. Scand. Suppl.* **379:** 32.

Andreasen, N.C., W.M. Grove, R.W. Shapiro, M.B. Keller, R.M.A. Hirschfeld, and P. McDonald-Scott. 1981. Reliability of lifetime diagnosis: A multicenter collaborative perspective. *Arch. Gen. Psychiatry* **38:** 400.

Ayuso-Gutierrez, J.L. and J.A. Ramos-Brieva. 1982. The course of manic-depressive illness: A comparative study of bipolar I and bipolar II patients. *J. Affective Disord.* **4:** 9.

Baron, M. 1993. Manic-depression linkage to factor IX reconsidered (Letter; Comment). *Ann. Genet.* **36:** 187.

———. 1994. Novel strategies in molecular genetics of mental illness (Editorial). *Biol. Psychiatry* **35:** 757.

Baron, M., N. Risch, R. Hamburger, B. Mandel, S. Kushner, M. Newman, D. Drumer, and R.H. Belmaker. 1987. Genetic linkage between X-chromosome markers and bipolar affective illness. *Nature* **326:** 289.

Baron, M., N.F. Freimer, N. Risch, B. Lerer, J.R. Alexander, R.E. Straub, S. Asokan, K. Das, A. Peterson, J. Amos, J. Endicott, J. Ott, and T.C. Gilliam. 1993. Diminished support for linkage between manic depressive illness and X-chromosome markers in three Israeli pedigrees. *Nat. Genet.* **3:** 49.

Baron, M., J. Endicott, B. Lerer, J.E. Loth, J.R. Alexander, R. Simon, L. Sharpe, M. Gibbon, D. Hasin, B. Lilliston, S. Schacht, R. Blumenthal, J. Alexander, A. Verter, N. Tubi, R.R. Fieve, T.C. Gillian, T. Lehner, and J. Ott. 1994. A pedigree series for mapping disease genes in bipolar affective disorder: sampling, assessment, and analytic considerations. *Psychiatr. Genet.* **4:** 43.

Berrettini, W.H., T.N. Ferraro, L.R. Goldin, D.E. Weeks, S. Detera-Wadleigh, J.I. Nurnberger, Jr., and E.S. Gershon. 1994. Chromosome 18 DNA markers and manic-depressive illness: Evidence for a susceptibility gene. *Proc. Natl. Acad. Sci.* **91:** 5918.

Berrettini, W.H., T.N. Ferraro, L.R. Goldin, S.D. Detera-Wadleigh, H. Choi, D. Muniec, J.G. Guroff, D.M. Kazuba, J.I. Nurnberger, Jr., W.-T. Hsieh, M.R. Hoehe, and E.S. Gershon. 1997. A linkage study of bipolar illness. *Arch. Gen. Psychiatry* **54:** 27.

Blacker, D. and M.T. Tsuang. 1993. Unipolar relatives in bipolar pedigrees: Are they bipolar? *Psychiatr. Genet.* **3:** 5.

Blackwood, D.H.R., L. He, S.W. Morris, A. McLean, C. Whitton, M. Thompson, M.T. Walker, K. Woodburn, C.M. Sharp, A.F. Wright, Y. Shibasaki, D.M. St. Clair, D.J. Porteous, and W.J. Muir. 1996. A locus for bipolar affective disorder on chromosome 4p. *Nat. Genet.* **12:** 427.

Calzolari, E., V. Aiello, P. Palazzi, A. Sensi, S. Calzolari, D. Orrico, H. Holler, C. Marzi, S. Belli, F. Bernardi, and P. Patracchini. 1996. Psychiatric disorder in a familial 15-18 translocation and sublocalization of myelin basic protein to 18Q22.3. *Am. J. Med. Genet.* **67:** 154.

Coon, H., J. Jensen, M. Hoff, J. Holik, R. Plaetke, F. Reimherr, P. Wender, M. Leppert, and W. Byerley. 1993. A genome-wide search for genes predisposing to manic depression, assuming autosomal dominant inheritance. *Am. J. Hum. Genet.* **52:** 1234.

Copeman, J.B., F. Cucca, C.M. Hearne, R.J. Cornall, P.W. Reed, K.S. Rönningen, D.E. Undlien, L. Nistico, R. Buzzetti, R. Tosi, F. Pociot, J. Nerup, F. Cornélis, A.H. Barnett, S.C. Bain, and J.A. Todd. 1995. Linkage disequilibrium mapping of a type 1 diabetes susceptibility gene (*IDDM7*) to chromosome 2q31-q33. *Nat. Genet.* **9:** 80.

DeBruyn, A., D. Souery, K. Mendelbaum, J. Mendlewicz, and C. Vanbroeckhoven. 1996. Linkage analysis of families with bipolar illness and chromosome 18 markers. *Biol. Psychiatry* **39:** 679.

Detera-Wadleigh, S.D., J.A. Badner, L.R. Goldin, W.H. Berrettini, A.R. Sanders, D.Y. Rollins, G. Turner, T. Moses, H. Haerian, D. Muniec, J.I. Nurnberger, Jr., and E.S. Gershon. 1996. Affected-sib-pair analyses reveal support of prior evidence for a susceptibility locus for bipolar disorder, on 21q. *Am. J. Hum. Genet.* **58:** 1279.

Dunner, D.L. and L.K. Tay. 1993. Diagnostic reliability of the history of hypomania in bipolar II patients and patients with major depression. *Compr. Psychiatry* **34:** 303.

Egeland, J.A., D.S. Gerhard, D.L. Pauls, J.N. Sussex, K.K. Kidd, C.R. Allen, A.M. Hostetter, and D.E. Housman. 1987. Bipolar affective disorders linked to DNA markers on chromosome 11. *Nature* **325:** 783.

Endicott, J., J. Nee, N. Andreason, P. Clayton, M. Keller, and W. Coryell. 1985. Bipolar II: Combine or keep separate? *J. Affective Disord.* **8:** 17.

Freimer, N.B., V.I. Reus, M.A. Escamilla, L.A. McInnes, M. Spesny, P. Leon, S.K. Service, L.B. Smith, S. Silva, E. Rojas, A. Gallegos, L. Meza, E. Fournier, S. Baharloo, K. Blankenship, D.J. Tyler, S. Batki, S. Vinogradov, J. Weissenbach, S.H. Barondes, and L.A. Sandkuijl. 1996. Genetic mapping using haplotype, association and linkage methods suggests a locus for severe bipolar disorder (BPI) at 18q22-q23. *Nat. Genet.* **12:** 436.

Gershon, E.S., J.H. Hamovit, J.J. Guroff, and J.I. Nurnberger. 1987. Birth-cohort changes in manic and depressive disorders in relatives of bipolar and schizoaffective patients. *Arch. Gen. Psychiatry* **44:** 314.

Gershon, E.S., J.A. Badner, S.D. Detera-Wadleigh, T.N. Ferraro, and W.H. Berrettini. 1996. Maternal inheritance and chromosome 18 allele sharing in unilineal bipolar illness pedigrees. *Am. J. Med. Genet. (Neuropsychiatr. Genet.)* **67:** 202.

Gershon, E.S., J. Hamovit, J.J. Guroff, J.I. Nurnberger, L.R. Goldin, and W.E. Bunney. 1982. A family study of schizoaffective, bipolar I, bipolar II, unipolar and normal control probands. *Arch. Gen. Psychiatry* **39:** 1157.

Ginns, E.I., J. Ott, J.A. Egeland, C.R. Allen, C.S.J. Fann, D.L. Pauls, J. Weissenbach, J.P. Carulli, K.M. Falls, T.P. Keith, and S.M. Paul. 1996. A genome-wide search for chromosomal loci linked the bipolar affective disorder in the Old Order Amish. *Nat. Genet.* **12:** 431.

Gurling, H.M.D. and T. Sharma. 1994. Genetic linkage analysis and clinical approaches to the resolution of heterogeneity in the schizophrenias. In *Genetic approaches to mental disorders* (ed. E.S. Gershon and C.R. Cloninger), p. 231. American Psychiatric Press, Washington, D.C.

Gurling, H., C. Smyth, G. Kalsi, E. Moloney, L. Rifkin, J. O'Neill, P. Murphy, D. Curtis, H. Petursson, and J. Brynjolfsson. 1995. Linkage findings in bipolar disorder (Letter). *Nat. Genet.* **10:** 8.

Kelsoe, J.R., E.I. Ginns, J.A. Egeland, D.S. Gerhard, A.M. Goldstein, S.J. Bale, D.L. Pauls, R.T. Long, K.K. Kidd, and G. Conte. 1989. Re-evaluation of the linkage relationship between chromosome 11p loci and the gene for bipolar affective disorder in the Old Order Amish. *Nature*

342: 238.

Klerman, G.L. and M.M. Weissman. 1989. Increasing rates of depression (Comments; Review). *J. Am. Med. Assoc.* **261:** 2229.

Kraepelin, E. 1921. *Manic-depressive insanity and paranoia.* E. & S. Livingstone, Edinburgh, Scotland.

Lander, E. and L. Kruglyak. 1996. Genetic dissection of complex traits (reply). *Nat. Genet.* **12:** 357.

MacKinnon, D.F., F.J. McMahon, S.G. Simpson, M.G. McInnis, and J.R. DePaulo. 1997. Panic disorder with familial bipolar disorder. *Biol. Psychiatry* (in press).

McInnis, M.G., F.J. McMahon, G. Chase, S.G. Simpson, C.A. Ross, and J.R. DePaulo, Jr. 1993. Anticipation in bipolar affective disorder. *Am. J. Hum. Genet.* **53:** 385.

McMahon, F.J. and J.R. DePaulo. 1996. Genetics and age at onset. In *Mood disorders across the life span* (ed. K.I. Schulman et al.), p. 35. Wiley-Liss, New York.

McMahon, F.J., O.C. Stine, D.A. Meyers, S.G. Simpson, and J.R. DePaulo. 1995. Patterns of maternal transmission in bipolar affective disorder. *Am. J. Hum. Genet.* **56:** 1277.

McMahon, F.J., J. Xu, C. Stine, S.G. Simpson, and J.R. DePaulo, Jr. 1996. Clinical features of bipolar disorder linked to chromosome 18. In *Abstracts from the American Psychiatric Association Meeting* (NR651). American Psychiatric Association, Washington, D.C.

McMahon, F.J., G.A. Chase, S.G. Simpson, D.A. Meyers, O.C. Stine, S.E. Folstein, and J.R. DePaulo, Jr. 1994. Influence of clinical subtype, sex, and lineality on age at onset of major affective disorder in a family sample. *Am. J. Psychiatry* **151:** 210.

Mendlewicz, J. and J.D. Rainer. 1977. Adoption study supporting genetic transmission in manic-depressive illness. *Nature* **268:** 327.

Mendlewicz, J., J.L. Fleiss, and R.R. Fieve. 1972. Evidence for X-linkage in the transmission of manic-depressive illness. *J. Am. Med. Assoc.* **222:** 1624.

Mendlewicz, J., P. Linkoeski, and J. Wilmotte. 1980. Linkage between glucose-phosphate dehydrogenase deficiency and manic-depressive psychosis. *Br. J. Psychiatry.* **137:** 337.

Mendlewicz, J., R.R. Fieve, J.D. Rainer, and M. Cataldo. 1973. Affective disorder on paternal and maternal sides: Observations in bipolar (manic-depressive) patients with and without a family history. *Br. J. Psychiatry* **122:** 31.

Nothen, M.M., S. Cochon, N. Craddock, M. Albus, W. Maier, D. Lichtermann, B. Weigelt, E. Franzek, R. Rietschel, J. Korner, R. Fimmers, and P. Propping. 1996. Linkage studies of bipolar disorder to chromosome 18 markers. *Biol. Psychiatry* **39:** 501.

O'Rourke, D.H., P. McGuffin, and T. Reich. 1983. Genetic analysis of manic-depressive illness. *Am. J. Phys. Anthropol.* **62:** 51.

Pekkarinen, P., J. Terwilliger, P.E. Bredbacka, J. Lonnqvist, and L. Peltonen. 1995. Evidence of a predisposing locus to bipolar disorder on Xq24-q27 in an extended Finnish pedigree. *Genome Res.* **5:** 105.

Penrose, L.S. 1948. The problem of anticipation in pedigrees of dystrophia myotonica. *Ann. Eugen.* **14:** 125.

Perris, C. 1971. Abnormality on paternal and maternal sides: Observations in bipolar (manic-depressive) and unipolar depressive psychoses. *Br. J. Psychiatry* **118:** 207.

Reich, T., P.J. Clayton, and G. Winokur. 1969. Family history studies: V. The genetics of mania. *Am. J. Psychiatry* **125:** 1358.

Riccardi, V.M. and R.A. Lewis. 1988. Penetrance of von Recklinghausen neurofibromatosis: A distinction between predecessors and descendants. *Am. J. Hum. Genet.* **42:** 284.

Rice, J.P., J. Endicott, M.A. Knesevich, and N. Rochberg. 1987. The estimation of diagnostic sensitivity using stability data: An application to major depressive disorder. *J. Psychiatr. Res.* **21:** 337.

Rice, J.P., P. McDonald-Scott, J. Endicott, W. Coryell, W.M. Grove, M.B. Keller, and D. Altis. 1986. The stability of diagnosis with an application to bipolar II disorder. *Psychiatry Res.* **19:** 285.

Risch, N. and M. Baron. 1982. X-linkage and genetic heterogeneity in bipolar-related major affective illness: Reanalysis of linkage data. *Ann. Hum. Genet.* **46:** 153.

Risch, N. and D. Botstein. 1996. A manic depressive history. *Nat. Genet.* **12:** 351.

Sherrington, R., J. Brynjolfsson, H. Petursson, M. Potter, K. Dudleston, B. Barraclough, J. Wasmuth, M. Dobbs, and H. Gurling. 1988. Localization of a susceptibility locus for schizophrenia on chromosome 5. *Nature* **336:** 164.

Simpson, S.G., F.J. McMahon, M.G. McInnis, D.F. MacKinnon, and J.R. DePaulo, Jr. 1996. Reliability of the bipolar II diagnosis. *Psychiatr. Genet.* **5:** S92.

Simpson, S.G., S.E. Folstein, D.A. Meyers, F.J. McMahon, D.M. Busco, and J.R. DePaulo, Jr. 1993. Bipolar II: The most common phenotype? *Am. J. Psychiatry* **150:** 901.

Spence, A., H. Amali, A.D. Sadovnic, R.A. Remick, J.A. Bailey-Wilson, P. Flodman, and I.M.L. Yee. 1993. A single major locus is the best explanation for bipolar family data: Results of complex segregation analyses. *Psychiatr. Genet.* **3:** 143.

Stine, O.C., J. Xu, R. Koskela, F.J. McMahon, M. Gschwend, C. Friddle, C.D. Clark, M.G. McInnis, S.G. Simpson, T.S. Breschel, E. Vishio, K. Riskin, H. Feilotter, E. Chen, S. Chen, S.E. Folstein, D.A. Meyers, D. Botstein, T.G. Marr, and J.R. DePaulo. 1995. Evidence for linkage of bipolar disorder to chromosome 18 with a parent-of-origin effect. *Am. J. Hum. Genet.* **57:** 1384.

Straub, R.E., T. Lehner, Y. Luo, J.E. Loth, W. Shao, L. Sharpe, J.R. Alexander, K. Das, R. Simon, R.R. Fieve, B. Lerer, J. Endicott, J. Ott, T.C. Gilliam, and M. Baron. 1994. A possible vulnerability locus for bipolar affective disorder on chromosome 21q22.3. *Nat. Genet.* **8:** 291.

Taylor, M.A. and R. Abrams. 1981. Early- and late-onset bipolar illness. *Arch. Gen. Psychiatry* **38:** 58.

Wicki, W. and J. Angst. 1991. The Zurich study. X. Hypomania in a 28- to 30-year-old cohort. *Eur. Arch. Psychiatry Clin. Neurosci.* **240:** 339.

Winokur, G. 1979. Unipolar depression. Is it divisible into autonomous subtypes? *Arch. Gen. Psychiatry* **36:** 47.

Winokur, G., P.J. Clayton, and R. Reich. 1969. *Manic-depressive illness.* C.V. Mosby, St. Louis, Missouri.

Winokur, G., M. Tsuang, and R.R. Crowe. 1982. The Iowa 500: Affective disorder in relatives of manic and depressed patients. *Am. J. Psychiatry* **139:** 209.

Winokur, G., R. Cadoret, J. Dorzab, and M. Baker. 1971. Depressive disease. A genetic study. *Arch. Gen. Psychiatry* **24:** 135.

The Serotonin Transporter Gene and Affective Disorder

A.J. HARMAR,[1] A.D. OGILVIE,[1] S. BATTERSBY,[1] C.A.D. SMITH,[3] D.H.R. BLACKWOOD,[2]
W.J. MUIR,[2] G. FINK,[1] AND G.M. GOODWIN[2]
[1]*MRC Brain Metabolism Unit, Royal Edinburgh Hospital, Edinburgh EH10 5HF; Departments of* [2]*Psychiatry and* [3]*Pathology, University of Edinburgh, Edinburgh EH8 9JZ, Scotland*

Bipolar and unipolar affective disorder are commonly occurring, multifactorial diseases that are probably polygenic. Attempts to identify genetic factors contributing to susceptibility to affective disorder have utilized both linkage-based and candidate gene strategies, each of which has inherent advantages and disadvantages. We have adopted a candidate gene approach, drawing on evidence from a number of sources implicating dysfunction in serotonergic neurotransmission in the pathophysiology of depression. The duration of action of serotonin in the brain is limited by Na^+-dependent uptake via the serotonin transporter into the presynaptic terminal, where it is either repackaged or degraded by monoamine oxidase to its major metabolite, 5-hydroxyindoleacetic acid (5-HIAA). Initial evidence for a role for abnormal serotonin function in depression came from studies showing decreased levels of 5-HIAA in depressed patients, especially those likely to commit suicide (for review, see Meltzer and Lowy 1987). There is also evidence that plasma levels of tryptophan, the amino acid precursor of serotonin, are reduced in depression (Coppen and Wood 1978; DeMeyer et al. 1981) and that tryptophan depletion causes a lowering of mood in normal subjects and in recovered depressed patients (Salomon et al. 1993). In addition, the withdrawal of L-tryptophan treatment appears to precipitate relapse in chronically depressed patients (Ferrier et al. 1990). Reports of abnormalities in imipramine-binding sites in blood platelets and brain (Maj 1988; Boyer and Feighner 1991) suggest altered function and/or regulation of the serotonin transporter itself in affective disorder.

These findings suggesting a role for dysfunction of the serotonergic system in mood disorder are supported by evidence from drug treatment studies. One of the first drugs used convincingly to treat depressive illness was imipramine (Kuhn 1958), a tricyclic antidepressant that nonselectively inhibits the uptake of norepinephrine and serotonin. Evidence of its efficacy is now overwhelming (Davis and Glassman 1989). Serotonin-selective reuptake inhibitors (SSRIs) such as fluvoxamine, fluoxetine, and paroxetine target the serotonin transporter specifically. These drugs were developed in a successful strategy to retain the efficacy of the tricyclic compounds while reducing side effects and toxicity (Anderson and Tomenson 1994).

It is now possible to study the structure and function of the gene encoding the human serotonin transporter, the target of the SSRIs, at a molecular level. The transporter protein is encoded by a single gene located on chromosome 17q11.1-17q12 composed of 14 exons spanning approximately 31 kb (Ramamoorthy et al. 1993; Lesch et al. 1994). Studies of the serotonin transporter gene in affective disorder have been few and limited in scope. In one published study, variations in the coding region of the gene were analyzed in 17 patients with affective disorder. Only one base substitution, representing a silent polymorphism, was found in a single patient (Lesch et al. 1995).

Recently, a polymorphism in the second intron of the human serotonin transporter gene has been described (Fig. 1) (Lesch et al. 1994). This polymorphic region contains a 16- to 17-bp variable number tandem repeat (VNTR) element, close to a putative transcription factor (AP-1) binding site. We have analyzed allelic variations in the number of repetitive elements in this VNTR in 593 individuals and have identified three alleles, containing, respectively, 9, 10, and 12 repeats of the VNTR element, in our control and patient populations. Patients with a clear history of unipolar affective disorder are about four times more likely to carry the allele with 9 copies of the repeat element (Battersby et al. 1996; Ogilvie et al. 1996).

METHODS

Subjects. The design of the study was approved by the relevant committee for Medical Ethics. We compared 119 individuals with single or recurrent major depressive episodes and 128 individuals with bipolar disorder with a group of 346 controls. Patients with major affective disorder were recruited from the in-patient and out-patient population of the Royal Edinburgh Hospital. All patients met DSM III-R criteria for major depressive disorder or bipolar disorder and the probable Research Diagnostic Criteria (Spitzer et al. 1978) according to the Schedule for Affective Disorders and Schizophrenia (Lifetime version: SADS-LA) (Endicott and Spitzer 1978). We obtained control samples from two sources: 103 volunteers who were screened by a brief interview to exclude past psychiatric illness and 243 anonymous donors from the Scottish Blood Transfusion Service who met usual criteria for blood donation and were therefore not currently on any psychotropic medication.

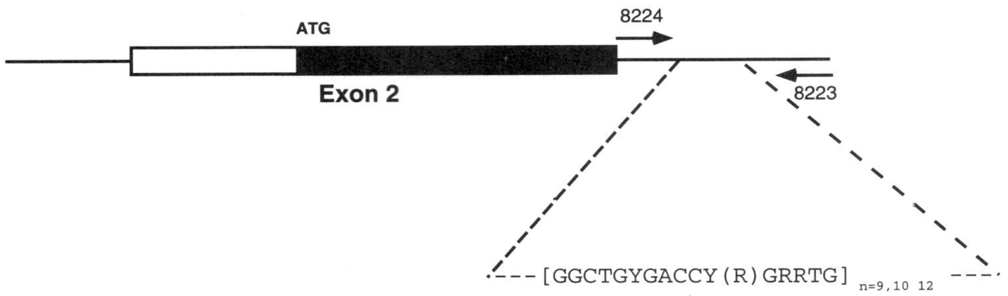

Figure 1. Schematic representation of the region of the serotonin transporter gene containing the VNTR. The consensus sequence of the VNTR and the locations of the forward (8224) and reverse (8223) primers used in PCR are indicated. The coding region of exon 2 is shaded. (Reprinted, with permission, from Ogilvie et al. 1996.)

DNA isolation. Genomic DNA was isolated from whole venous blood as described previously (Smith et al. 1992). 100 μl of whole blood was washed three times in TE buffer (10 mM Tris-HCl, pH 8, 1 mM EDTA). Peripheral blood leukocytes were harvested by centrifugation and resuspended in 100 μl of lysis buffer (50 mM KCl, 20 mM Tris-HCl, pH 8.3, 2.5 mM $MgCl_2$, 0.45% Nonidet P-40, 0.45% Tween 20) containing 200 μg ml^{-1} proteinase K. Lysis was completed by incubation for 20 minutes at 55°C. Crude lysates were diluted with an equal volume of sterile distilled water and heated to 96°C for 10 minutes to inactivate the proteinase. Samples were used immediately or stored at -20°C until required.

Polymerase chain reaction. PCR was carried out using two oligonucleotide primers (8224: 5′-GTCAGTATCACAGGCTGCGAG and 8223: 5′-TG TTCCTAGTCTTACGCCAGTG) flanking the VNTR in intron 2. Samples contained 50–100 ng of DNA; 1.5 units of *Taq* polymerase (Promega); 100 ng of each primer; 200 μM each dATP, dCTP, dGTP, and dTTP; 1% (v/v) DMSO; and 1.5 mM $MgCl_2$ in 50 μl of PCR buffer (Promega). PCR was carried out in a Hybaid Omnigene thermal cycler, using 35–43 cycles of primer annealing at 60°C (20 sec), polymerization at 72°C (20 sec), and denaturation at 94°C (30 sec). A final polymerization step of 120 sec was carried out to complete elongation of all amplified strands.

Identification of PCR products. PCR products were resolved on 5% nondenaturing polyacrylamide gels and visualized by ethidium bromide staining and UV transillumination (Fig. 2). The identity of the products was confirmed by digestion with restriction enzymes *Hae*III, *Bst*NI, and *Sma*I.

A minimum of 15 examples of each allele were sequenced. Amplified products were separated on 2% agarose gels, excised, and purified by the Wizard PCR DNA purification system (Promega), and concentrated with Microcon 100 columns (Amicon). Sequencing was accomplished using the Prism DyeDeoxy Terminator Cycle sequencing kit (Perkin Elmer) in a Perkin Elmer Cetus thermal cycler (30 cycles consisting of 30 sec at 96°C, 15 sec at 50°C, and 4 min at 50°C) with primers 8223 and 8224. Unincorporated nucleotides were removed by extraction with phenol:chloroform. Electrophoresis was carried out on an Applied Biosystems model 373 STRETCH DNA Sequencer at a constant power of 30 W for 12 hours using a 4.75% denaturing polyacrylamide gel.

For heteroduplex analysis, PCR products were denatured for 3 minutes at 95°C and allowed to cool to 37°C over 30 minutes. Samples (5 μl) were electrophoresed through MDE Hydrolink gels (AT Biochem) at 800 V overnight, and bands were visualized by silver staining.

Statistical methods. Analysis of genotype distribution was carried out on the raw frequencies by the chi-square test. Comparison of allele frequency distributions between the control and patient groups was by multiple analysis of variance (MANOVA) using the Statistical Package for the Social Sciences (SPSS Apple Macintosh version 4.0). Bonferroni correction was applied to allow for multiple comparisons when the chi-square test was employed to compare the affective subgroups with controls. Odds ratios and confidence limits were calculated by standard methods.

RESULTS

Characterization of VNTR Alleles

Three alleles of the VNTR region of intron 2 of the human serotonin transporter gene were identified when amplified fragments were resolved on 5% nondenaturing gels (Fig. 2) and by heteroduplex analysis (data not shown). Fifteen examples of each allele were sequenced and proved to be identical. The three alleles contained, respectively, 9 (STin2.9), 10 (STin2.10), and 12 (STin2.12) copies of a repetitive element that was present as seven variant motifs (indicated as A–G in Fig. 2). The repeating element conformed to the consensus sequence GGCTGYGACCY(R)GRRTG, where Y = T/C, R = G/A, with loss of the 12th base pair in motif D.

a

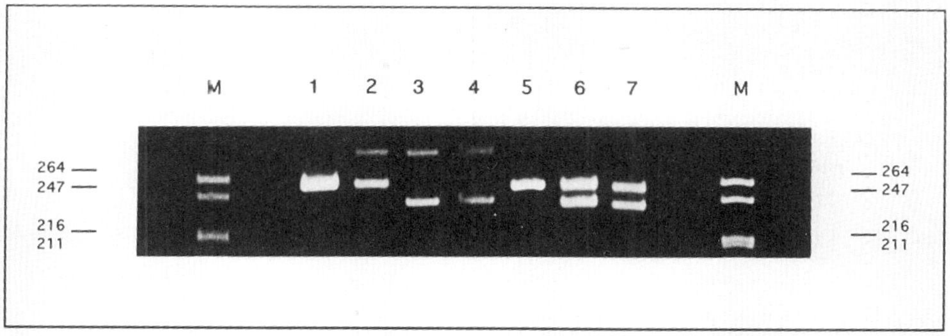

b

	1(A)	2(B)	3(C)	4(D)	5(E)
STin2.9	GGCTGTGACCCAGGGTG	GGCTGTGACCCGGAGTG	GGCTGTGACCCGGGGTG	GGCTGTGACCCGGGTG	GGCTGCGACCTGGGGTG
STin2.10	GGCTGTGACCCAGGGTG	GGCTGTGACCCGGAGTG	GGCTGTGACCCGGGGTG	GGCTGTGACCCGGGTG	GGCTGCGACCTGGGGTG
STin2.12	GGCTGTGACCCAGGGTG	GGCTGTGACCCGGAGTG	GGCTGTGACCCGGGGTG	GGCTGTGACCCGGGTG	GGCTGCGACCTGGGGTG

	6(F)	7(D)	8(G)	9(D)	10(G)
STin2.9	....	....	....	GGCTGTGACCCGGGTG	GGCTGTGACCTGGGGTG
STin2.10	GGCTGTGACCTGGGATG	....	....	GGCTGTGACCCGGGTG	GGCTGTGACCTGGGGTG
STin2.12	GGCTGTGACCTGGGATG	GGCTGTGACCCGGGTG	GGCTGTGACCTGGGGTG	GGCTGTGACCCGGGTG	GGCTGTGACCTGGGGTG

	11(D)	12(F)
STin2.9	GGCTGTGACCCGGGTG	GGCTGTGACCTGGGATG
STin2.10	GGCTGTGACCCGGGTG	GGCTGTGACCTGGGATG
STin2.12	GGCTGTGACCCGGGTG	GGCTGTGACCTGGGATG

Figure 2. (*a*) PCR analysis of VNTR in intron 2 of the serotonin transporter gene in seven individuals. Four different genotypes are shown: STin2.10/STin2.10 (267 bp: lanes *1,5*), STin2.10/STin 2.12 (267+300 bp: lane *2*), STin2.9/STin2.12 (250+300 bp: lanes *3,4*), and STin2.9/STin2.10 (250+267 bp: lanes *6,7*). 5% polyacrylamide gel stained with ethidium bromide. M indicates lanes containing DNA markers of the sizes indicated. (*b*) Sequences of STin2.9, 2.10, and 2.12 alleles of VNTR in intron 2 of human serotonin transporter gene. Seven variants of the 16/17-bp repetitive element (A–G) are seen. (Reprinted, with permission, from Battersby et al. 1996.)

Association Study

Allele frequencies for the VNTR were calculated for the control and patient groups (Table 1). Analysis by MANOVA showed a significant difference in overall allele distribution between the affective disorder group versus control group and the unipolar versus control group. There was a similar trend in the bipolar sample that did not reach statistical significance (p = 0.065, 2 d.f., two-tailed).

The difference between the patients with affective disorder and controls was largely explained by an increase in the proportion of individuals with genotypes containing the STin2.9 allele (Table 1). This was true for both unipolar and bipolar subgroups, although there appeared to be a larger effect in the unipolar group. For the risk of unipolar disorder given a single STin2.9 allele, the odds ratio was 4.44 (95% CI, 1.65–11.95) and for bipolar disorder 3.22 (95% CI, 1.15–9.09).

The mean age of the volunteer controls was 45 (S.D. 15) and of the patients 41 (S.D. 15). There was no significant sex difference in the distribution of STin2.9 allele between patient and control groups (chi-square = 0.99).

DISCUSSION

We have detected three novel alleles (STin2.9, STin2.10, and STin2.12) of the VNTR region of the serotonin transporter gene containing, respectively, 9, 10, and 12 copies of the VNTR element. There is a significant overall difference between affective disorder and control groups in the frequency distribution of alleles: The main finding is a significant increase in the frequency of the STin2.9 allele in patients with major affective disorder. Comparison of the sequences of the three alleles suggests that the shorter forms may have been generated by loss of central repeating elements. Evidence from VNTRs such as those in the collagen type II (COL2A1) and apolipoprotein B genes suggests that the secondary DNA structure may be important in the generation of new alleles (Berg and Olaisen 1993; Desmarais et al. 1993). The sequences of VNTRs may favor the formation of hairpins and loops, which could result in the generation of new alleles by replication slippage.

There are two alternative mechanisms that may explain the association between the STin2.9 allele and the risk of affective disorder. First, the VNTR may be in linkage disequilibrium with another more directly

Table 1. Distribution of Genotype and Allele Frequencies of VNTR in Control and Patient Groups

	N	Genotype distribution (%) 9+ 10 or 12	9 10	9 12	10 10	10 12	12 12	Allele frequency (%) STin2.9	STin2.10	STin2.12	F
Controls											
all controls	346	2.02	0.29	1.73	14.74	50.87	32.37	1.01	40.32	58.67	
B.T.S.	243	2.47	0.41	2.06	15.64	49.79	32.10	1.23	40.74	58.02	
screened	103	0.97	0.00	0.97	12.62	53.40	33.01	0.49	39.32	60.19	
Patients											
all affective disorder	247	7.29[a]	3.24	4.05	13.77	45.34	33.60	3.64	38.06	58.30	5.08[d]
bipolar	128	6.25[b]	2.34	3.91	14.06	48.44	31.25	3.13	39.45	57.42	2.74
unipolar	119	8.40[c]	4.20	4.20	13.45	42.02	36.13	4.20	36.55	59.24	5.42[e]

For description of B.T.S. (Blood Transfusion Service) and screened controls, see Methods. Significant differences from the combined control group in the total sample: [a]$\chi^2 = 9.89$, $p = 0.0017$, 1df; [b]$\chi^2 = 5.45$, $p = 0.0196$, 1df; [c]$\chi^2 = 10.23$, $p = 0.0014$, 1df; [d]MANOVA, 2df, $p = 0.006$; [e]MANOVA, 2df, $p = 0.005$.

relevant gene locus. Alternatively, it is possible that the level of serotonin transporter gene transcription may be influenced by the sequences of the repetitive elements in the VNTR themselves.

Linkage disequilibrium mapping (Jorde 1995) has been used to map a locus conferring susceptibility to Type I diabetes mellitus (the *IDDM2* locus) to a 14- to 15-bp VNTR located on chromosome 11p15.5 between the tyrosine hydroxylase and insulin genes and to demonstrate that other polymorphisms in the region, although in linkage disequilibrium with *IDDM2*, are unlikely to predispose to disease (Bennett et al. 1995). We are now conducting linkage disequilibrium mapping using markers upstream and downstream from the serotonin transporter VNTR. A recently described polymorphism in the 5′-flanking regulatory region of the serotonin transporter gene, with surprisingly large functional effects (Heils et al. 1996), will be included in this analysis.

VNTRs close to the insulin (*IDDM2* locus) (Catignani-Kennedy et al. 1995; Lucassen et al. 1995) and Harvey Ras-1 (Green and Krontiris 1993) genes bind transcription factors and show allelic variation associated with disease. These VNTRs regulate transcription in a cell- and promoter-specific way, small differences in nucleotide sequence influencing the level of transcriptional activity. At the *IDDM2* locus, it has been suggested that the absence of a single 14-bp repeat element designated "e" results in the loss of a protective effect against the development of insulin-dependent diabetes (Bennett et al. 1995). By analogy, the absence of the 16-bp element "F" near the center of the VNTR in the serotonin transporter gene may have functional consequences. Alternatively, it may simply be the overall length of the VNTR, which is adjacent to a putative transcription factor (AP-1) binding site, that is important. We are now investigating whether the VNTR influences the expression of the serotonin transporter in platelets, using reverse-transcriptase PCR, or in the living human brain, using single-photon emission tomography with 2β-carbomethoxy-3β-(4-[^{123}I]iodophenyl)tropane ([^{123}I]β-CIT), a ligand for the serotonin and dopamine transporters (Kuikka et al. 1995).

Our findings support the hypothesis that allelic variation in the serotonin transporter gene may contribute to susceptibility for both major depression and bipolar disorder. It remains to be established how far it accounts for the occurrence of affective disorder within families and whether there is a predictable association between particular alleles or combinations of alleles and individual patterns of illness.

ACKNOWLEDGMENTS

We thank Lilly Industries plc for financial support, Margaret van Beck for her help in data management, Norma Brearley for her assistance in preparation of the manuscript, Anne Ryman for help in the recruitment of patients, and Klaus Ebmeier and Alan Finlayson for statistical advice.

REFERENCES

Anderson I.M. and B.M. Tomenson. 1994. The efficacy of selective serotonin re-uptake inhibitors in depression: A meta-analysis of studies against tricyclic antidepressants. *J. Psychopharmacol.* **8:** 238.

Battersby, S., A.D. Ogilvie, C.A.D. Smith, D.H.R. Blackwood, W.J. Muir, J.P. Quinn, G. Fink, G.M. Goodwin, and A.J. Harmar. 1996. Structure of a VNTR of the serotonin transporter gene and association with affective disorder. *Psychiatr. Genet.* **6:** 1.

Bennett, S.T., A.M. Lucassen, S.C.L. Gough, E.E. Powell, D.E. Undlien, L.E. Pritchard, M.E. Merriman, Y. Kawaguchi, M.J. Dronsfield, F. Pociot, J. Nerup, N. Bouzekri, A. Cambon-Thomsen, K.S. Rønningen, A.H. Barnett, S.C. Bain, and J.A. Todd. 1995. Susceptibility to human type 1 diabetes at IDDM2 is determined by tandem repeat variation at the insulin gene minisatellite locus. *Nat. Genet.* **9:** 284.

Berg, E.S. and B. Olaisen. 1993. Characterization of the COL2A1 VNTR polymorphism. *Genomics* **16:** 350.

Boyer, W.F. and J.P. Feighner. 1991. The serotonin hypothesis: Necessary but not sufficient. In *Selective serotonin re-uptake inhibitors* (ed. J.P. Feighner and W.F. Boyer), p. 71. Wiley, Chichester, United Kingdom.

Catignani-Kennedy, G., M.S. German, and W.J. Rutter. 1995. The minisatellite in the diabetes susceptibility locus IDDM2 regulates insulin transcription. *Nat. Genet.* **9:** 293.

Coppen, A. and K. Wood. 1978. Tryptophan and depressive illness. *Psychol. Med.* **8:** 49.

Davis, J.M. and A.H. Glassman. 1989. Antidepressant drugs. In *Comprehensive textbook of psychiatry* (ed. H.I. Kaplan and B.J. Sadock), p. 1627. Williams and Wilkins, Baltimore, Maryland.

DeMeyer, M.K., P.A. Shea, H.C. Hendrie, and N.N. Yoshimura. 1981. Plasma tryptophan and five other amino acids in depressed and normal subjects. *Arch. Gen. Psychiatry* **38:** 642.

Desmarais, E., S. Vigneron, C. Buresi, F. Cambien, J.P. Cambou, and G. Roizes. 1993. Variant mapping of the Apo(B) AT rich minisatellite. Dependence on nucleotide sequence of the copy number variations. Instability of the non-canonical allelles. *Nucleic Acids Res.* **21:** 2179.

Endicott, J. and R.L. Spitzer. 1978. A diagnostic interview—The schedule for affective disorders and schizophrenia. *Arch. Gen. Psychiatry* **35:** 837.

Ferrier, I.N., D. Eccleston, P.B. Moore, and K.A. Wood. 1990. Relapse in chronic depressives on withdrawal of L-tryptophan. *Lancet* **336:** 380.

Green, M. and T.G. Krontiris. 1993. Allelic variation of reporter gene activation by the HRASI minisatellite. *Genomics* **17:** 429.

Heils, A., A. Teufel, S. Petri, G. Stober, P. Riederer, D. Bengel, and K.P. Lesch. 1996. Allelic variation of human serotonin transporter gene expression. *J. Neurochem.* **66:** 2621.

Jorde, L.B. 1995. Linkage disequilibrium as a gene-mapping tool. *Am. J. Hum. Genet.* **56:** 11.

Kuhn, R. 1958. The treatment of depressive states with G22355 (imipramine hydrochloride). *Am. J. Psychiatry* **115:** 459.

Kuikka, J.T., J. Tiihonen, K.A. Bergstrom, J. Karhu, P. Hartikainen, H. Vilnamaio, E. Lansimies, J. Lehtonen, and P. Hakola. 1995. Imaging of serotonin and dopamine transporters in the living human brain. *Eur. J. Nucl. Med.* **22:** 346.

Lesch, K.P., J. Gross, E. Franzek, B.L. Wolozin, P. Riederer, and D.L. Murphy. 1995. Primary structure of the serotonin transporter in unipolar depression and bipolar disorder. *Biol. Psychiatry* **37:** 215.

Lesch, K.P., U. Balling, J. Gross, K. Strauss, B.L. Wolozin, D.L. Murphy, and P. Riederer. 1994. Organization of the human serotonin transporter gene. *J. Neural Trans. Gen. Sect.* **95:** 157.

Lucassen, A.M., G.R. Screaton, C. Julier, T.J. Elliott, M. Lathrop, and J.I. Bell. 1995. Regulation of insulin gene expression by the IDDM associated, insulin locus haplotype. *Hum. Mol. Genet.* **4:** 501.

Maj, M. 1988. Changes in platelet ^{3}H-imipramine binding in depressed patients receiving electroconvulsive therapy. *Biol. Psychiatry* **24:** 469.

Meltzer, H.Y. and M.T. Lowy. 1987. The serotonin hypothesis of depression. In *Psychopharmacology, the third generation of progress* (ed. H. Meltzer), p. 513. Raven Press, New York.

Ogilvie, A.D., S. Battersby, V.J. Bubb, G. Fink, G.M. Goodwin, A.J. Harmar, and C.A.D. Smith. 1996. A polymorphism of the serotonin transporter gene is associated with susceptibility to major affective disorder. *Lancet* **347:** 731.

Ramamoorthy, S., A.L. Bauman, K.R. Moore, H. Han, T. Yang-Feng, A.S. Chang, V. Ganapathy, and R.D. Blakely. 1993. Antidepressant- and cocaine-sensitive human serotonin transporter: Molecular cloning, expression, and chromosomal localization. *Proc. Natl. Acad. Sci.* **90:** 2542.

Salomon, R.M., H.L. Miller, P.L. Delgado, and D. Charney. 1993. The use of tryptophan depletion to evaluate central serotonin function in depression and other neuropsychiatric disorders. *Int. Clin. Psychopharmacol.* **8:** 41.

Smith, C.A.D., A.C. Gough, P.N. Leigh, B.A. Summers, A.E. Harding, D.M. Maranganore, S.G. Sturman, A.H.V. Schapira, A.C. Williams, N.K. Spurr, and C.R. Wolf. 1992. Debrisoquine hydroxylase gene polymorphism and susceptibility to Parkinson's disease. *Lancet* **339:** 1375.

Spitzer, R.L., J. Endicott, and E. Robins. 1978. Research diagnostic criteria: Rationale and reliability. *Arch. Gen. Psychiatry* **35:** 773.

The Johns Hopkins University Collaborative Schizophrenia Study: An Epidemiologic-Genetic Approach to Test the Heterogeneity Hypothesis and Identify Schizophrenia Susceptibility Genes

A.E. Pulver,[1] P.S. Wolyniec,[1] D. Housman,[2] H.H. Kazazian,[3] S.E. Antonarakis,[4] G. Nestadt,[1] V.K. Lasseter,[1] J.A. McGrath,[1] B. Dombroski,[3] M. Karayiorgou,[5] C. Ton,[2] J.-L. Blouin,[4] and L. Kempf[1]

[1]*The Johns Hopkins University School of Medicine, Baltimore, Maryland 21205;* [2]*MIT Center for Cancer Research, Cambridge, Massachusetts 02139;* [3]*University of Pennsylvania Medical Center, Philadelphia, Pennsylvania 19104;* [4]*University of Geneva, Geneva, Switzerland;* [5]*The Rockefeller University, New York, New York 10021*

This paper is divided into two parts. Part I provides an overview of the epidemiology and genetics of schizophrenia and a description of the genetic strategies being pursued to identify schizophrenia susceptibility genes. Part II provides a description of the Johns Hopkins University Collaborative Schizophrenia Study that includes a summary of progress toward the identification and understanding of factors which contribute to schizophrenia susceptibility and to its heterogeneity.

PART I: OVERVIEW OF THE EPIDEMIOLOGY AND GENETICS OF SCHIZOPHRENIA

Epidemiology

Schizophrenia is a frequent and disabling disease of variable expression and unknown cause Symptoms include hallucinations, delusions, lack of motivation, and anhedonia. Prevalence of the disease is estimated to be about 1% worldwide (Eaton 1985). Ordinarily the illness develops in adolescence or early adulthood but has been observed to have onset in children as well as in later life (Gottesman and Shields 1982). Gender differences can be observed in prevalence, age at onset, premorbid characteristics, clinical expression, course of illness, response to treatment, and family morbidity risk (for review, see Goldstein et al. 1989). In all likelihood, schizophrenia is etiologically heterogeneous (for review, see Tsuang and Faraone 1995).

Risk Factors Associated with Etiology

What risk factors do we know may be associated with cause? Clearly, a family history of schizophrenia increases risk to relatives, and this is the basis for the search for genes involved in susceptibility (Gottesman and Shields 1982). For example, first-degree relatives (parents, siblings, and children) of schizophrenics who share on average 50% of their genes have approximately a 10% risk. Among first-degree relatives, the risk varies from 6% for parents, to 10% for siblings, and 13% for children. If one of the parents is also schizophrenic, the risk to the siblings increases to 17%. Children of two schizophrenics have a risk of 46% of developing the illness. Risk to second-degree relatives is approximately 3%. In addition, it has been repeatedly shown that concordance rates for schizophrenia are higher among monozygotic twins than among dizygotic twins (Gottesman and Shields 1982).

Initially, deficits in attention were shown to predict the later manifestation of schizophrenia among the offspring of schizophrenic parents (Erlenmeyer-Kimling et al. 1993). However, recently, data from a prospective study of a large birth cohort revealed that those individuals who later developed schizophrenia showed deficits in a range of behaviors as early as age four (Done et al. 1994; Jones et al. 1994). This finding implies that childhood and early adolescent behavioral and attentional deficits may be meaningful risk factors for schizophrenia in the general population (i.e., not just for the offspring of schizophrenic parents).

Other factors which may or may not have a genetic basis have been implicated as risk factors. These include season of birth, perinatal or obstetrical complications, and viral infection and/or extreme dietary restriction during the first trimester of pregnancy (for review, see Eaton 1991). With respect to season of birth, there is convincing evidence that a winter–spring birth date increases the risk for schizophrenia (for review, see Boyd et al. 1986). The basis for this association is unknown, but several hypotheses have been offered.

Without knowing the basis for the association between season of birth and the risk for schizophrenia, one can use season of birth to examine the hypothesis that schizophrenia is etiologically heterogeneous by looking for differences between winter-born and non-winter-born schizophrenics which may imply differences in causal mechanisms. Studies using an epidemiological sample of patients hospitalized in the greater Baltimore area have shown that schizophrenic patients who were born during the winter–spring months (February through May) differ from those born in other parts of the year by being more likely to have affected relatives (Pulver et al. 1992b). In addition, mothers of the winter–spring-born schizophrenic

  0-87969-071-2/96 $5+.00

patients were more likely to have a longer interval between their pregnancies than were the mothers of winter–spring-born controls (Pulver et al. 1992a). Other workers have reported that season of birth may be associated with specific clinical features of schizophrenia. For example, Katsanis et al. (1992) provide evidence that winter–spring-born schizophrenics are more prone to dysregulation of electrodermal activity than are winter-born controls. Non-winter-born schizophrenics did not differ from non-winter-born controls with respect to electrodermal activity. In addition, using a large sample of schizophrenic patients, Sacchetti et al. (1992) report that patients born during the winter–spring months show a higher frequency of enlargement of cerebral ventricles when compared to schizophrenic patients born during the rest of the year. The association between season of birth and ventricular enlargement was not present for patients diagnosed with affective disorders.

The role of obstetrical and perinatal events is unclear, but there is overwhelming consistency in the data obtained in retrospective studies that implicate them as risk factors for schizophrenia (for review, see McNeil 1995). More recently, data available from a prospective study of a large birth cohort did not find such an association (Sacker et al. 1995). It remains unclear what specific role these factors play and how they interact with other risk factors such as genetic susceptibility. Susser and colleagues (1996), in a study of a cohort born during the Dutch famine of 1944–45, found that exposure to extreme deficits in nutrition during the first trimester of pregnancy led to an increased risk for schizophrenia in the offspring.

One final association should be mentioned. As reviewed by Eaton et al. (1992), results from several studies suggest a lower than expected rate of rheumatoid arthritis among schizophrenics. The basis for the negative association between the two disorders is unknown. Several theories have been suggested, including nutritional, hormonal, and immunologic.

A Neurodevelopmental Hypothesis

It has been hypothesized that unspecified events, of genetic and/or environmental origin, acting early in fetal life may lead to aberrant development of cerebral structure and function, predisposing to schizophrenic illness later in life (Murray and Lewis 1987; Weinberger 1987; Lewis 1989; Lyon et al. 1989; Murray and O'Callaghan 1991). Although the literature on structural brain abnormalities is not altogether consistent, schizophrenic patients as a group have been reported to have significantly larger ventricles and/or atrophy of the frontal regions when compared to controls (see, e.g., Cannon and Marco 1994). Specific regional changes affecting frontal, temporal limbic, and basal ganglia have been reported (Gur and Pearlson 1993). Neuropathological studies indicate decreased cell numbers and/or cytoarchitectural abnormalities in certain brain regions that suggest disturbed brain-cell migration. The changes do not appear to be associated with degenerative or inflammatory processes and are most likely due to some neurodevelopmental lesion (Benes et al. 1986; Jakob and Beckmann 1986; Weinberger 1987; Jones and Murray 1991; Roberts 1991; Benes 1993; Keshavan et al. 1994; Marsh et al. 1994; Murray 1994; Ross and Pearlson 1996).

Additional evidence to support the neurodevelopmental hypothesis is that, in some cases, enlarged cerebral ventricles are present at or before the onset of the illness, whereas in others there is reduced volume of both temporal lobe and hippocampus (Weinberger 1987). Recent studies reported by Petty et al. (1995) have implicated the heteromodal cortex. Reversed asymmetry of the planum temporale was noted in a higher proportion of the schizophrenic subjects when compared to matched controls. In addition, both dermatoglyphic abnormalities and minor physical anomalies have been found at a higher rate among schizophrenic subjects than normal controls (Green et al. 1994). These findings provide additional support that differences between schizophrenics and the general population are present in utero.

A consensus is thus emerging that this illness occurs because of disturbances in intrauterine life that lead to structural and functional brain abnormalities. These could take the form of abnormalities of cell migration, failure to make connections, or reduced density of synapses, and clinical heterogeneity might vary according to the localization of the abnormality. There is reason to believe that the genetics of schizophrenia (or some forms of schizophrenia) is tied to the genetics of neurodevelopment, an observation that should help to focus efforts to pursue the elusive genetic basis of this devastating disease.

In summary, our understanding of the epidemiology of schizophrenia is far from complete. Additional studies with large numbers of subjects are needed to determine the interrelationships among risk factors and clinically descriptive variables. Most of the studies have emphasized one or two variables, perhaps because of limited numbers in study samples. Samples of sufficient size are necessary to resolve the remaining questions. The samples are only likely to be assembled through collaboration of several investigators. We have not been accustomed to such large-scale collaborative work; if we are to explore the heterogeneity of the disease by associations of constellations of genes with clusters of clinical variables and other risk factors, the assembly of large samples of patients and families is necessary.

Genetics

Twin, adoption, and family studies implicate genetic factors in the etiology of schizophrenia (for reviews, see Gottesman and Shields 1982; Murray et al. 1986; Tsuang et al. 1991). The mode of inheritance is not known (Risch and Baron 1984; Kendler and Diehl 1993). In all likelihood, inheritance of susceptibility is complex, involving both genes and experiences (see, e.g., McGue and Gottesman 1991). Schizophrenia shows familial co-aggregation with schizoaffective disorder, as well as with atypical psychotic disorders, schizotypal, avoidant, and paranoid personality disorders (Kendler et al. 1984, 1993). In some families, there is co-aggregation of both schizophrenia and bipolar disorder, which raises the possibility of some shared vulnerability (Taylor 1992).

Genetic Strategies to Identify Schizophrenia Susceptibility Genes

Linkage studies. Linkage studies test the association of a specific marker with disease status in a family. Linkage studies of schizophrenia date to as early as 1973 when Elston tested for linkage between schizophrenia and alleles of the Gc and Gm loci (Elston et al. 1973). Only within the past 6 years has a genome-wide search become possible due to the advances in recombinant DNA and other techniques that have led to the availability of an increasing number of highly polymorphic markers located throughout the genome. Although these markers have made it technically possible to complete the molecular analysis, other problems remain in studying complex diseases such as schizophrenia. The lack of sufficiently large numbers of well-characterized patients and their relatives, the need for more complex statistical analysis of the data, the requirement for new computer technology to allow efficient application of analyses to multiple variables, and the continuing need for even more markers in certain regions still limit the success of this work.

Two linkage paradigms have been used: the genome-wide scan and a candidate gene or region approach. (1) *Genome scan:* The genome-wide scan, which provided an early success in identifying the gene responsible for Huntington's disease (Gusella et al. 1983) is labor-intensive and costly. Results from several genome-wide scans have been reported (Barr et al. 1994; Coon et al. 1994b; Pulver et al. 1994c; Moises et al. 1995b). Despite the effort involved, none of these studies had enough families to establish conclusive evidence either for linkage and subsequent pursuit of more extensive cloning strategies or for rejecting linkage under heterogeneity. However, several regions of interest were identified. Cumulative evidence from different populations is now available to suggest that schizophrenia susceptibility genes may be found in regions on chromosome 22q (Coon et al. 1994a; Lasseter et al. 1995), chromosome 8p (Pulver et al. 1995), and chromosome 6p (Straub et al. 1995). Additional results from our group's genome-wide scan are reported in Part II of this paper. (2) *Candidate genes*: In schizophrenia, it is difficult to determine what genes should be considered candidates, given that the pathophysiology of schizophrenia is not known. Many hypothesized "candidate" genes have been tested in linkage studies. A list of hypothesized candidate genes that have been used in linkage and/or association studies is provided in Table 1. No consistent evidence has developed from this linkage approach. However, no candidate gene can be excluded and determined not to have a role in susceptibility to schizophrenia.

A *candidate region* approach may be more productive for schizophrenia. For example, structural chromosomal changes in affected individuals, including translocations and deletions, may lead to the identification of a specific region where a susceptibility gene may lie. This approach proved rewarding in neurofibromatosis, where reports of translocation in two affected individuals helped to localize the responsible gene (Fountain et al. 1989). There are several reports of structural chromosomal changes in schizophrenic subjects. A review of the literature was prepared by Ann Bassett (1992). Balanced and unbalanced translocations, inverted segments, deleted segments, and fragile sites were reported to occur in a single patient or several patients. They were found throughout the genome (i.e., 1q32.3 1q43, 2p11-2q13, 2q21, 2p21, 5p13-[5pter], 5q11.2-5q13.3, 6q14.2, 6q15, 7p12-[7pter], 8p23, 9p11-13, 9p22 10p12-10q21,11q25 [11qter] 13q21.2 13q31-13q32 17p12 18p 18q23 [18qter] 19p13,21) (Bassett 1992). Since her review, additional translocations in schizophrenic patients have been reported: 1p22 (Gordon et al. 1994), 2p11.29 (Maziade et al. 1993), 5p14.1 (Malaspina

Table 1. Hypothesized Candidate Genes for Schizophrenia Examined in Linkage or Association Studies

Candidate	Location
β-Amyloid precursor protein (APP)	21q21.3-q22.05
Catechol *O*-methyltransferase (COMT)	22q11
Debrisoquine hydroxylase (CYP2D6)	22q13.1
Dopamine receptor 1 (DRD1)	5q35.1
Dopamine receptor 2 (DRD2)	11q22-23
Dopamine receptor 3 (DRD3)	3q13.3
Dopamine receptor 4 (DRD4)	11p15.5
Dopamine receptor 5 (DRD5)	4p 15.1-16.1
Dopamine transporter (DAT)	5p15.3
$GABA_A$ receptor B	14p12-13
Glutamate receptor (GLUR5)	21q22.1
Neuropeptide Y (NPY)	7p15.1
Neurotrophin-3 (NT-3)	12p13
Porphobilogen deaminase (PBGD)	11q23.2-qter
Proopiomelanocortin (POMC)	2p25
Serotonin receptor 1A (HTR1A)	5q11.2-q13
Serotonin receptor 2A (HTR2A)	13q14-q21
Serotonin receptor 2C (HTR2C)	Xq24
Serotonin receptor 1D (HTR1DB)	1p36.3-p34.3
Tyrosine hydrogenase (TH)	11p15.5
Vesicular monoamine transporter (VMAT2)	10q25
Dopamine-β-hydroxylase (DBH)	9q34
Interleukin 2 (IL-2)	4q26-q27
Monoamine oxidase (MAO)	Xp11.23
Marfan	15q21.1
Human leukocyte antigens (HLA)(DQB1)	6p21.3

et al. 1992), 11q25 (Holland and Gosden 1990), an inversion on 4p15.2-q21.3 (Palmour et al. 1994), a trisomy of chromosome 5 (Rios et al. 1995), fragile sites at 8q24 10q24 (Garofalo et al. 1993), pericentric inversion of 9p11-9q13 (Nanko et al. 1993), and a deleted segment of 22q11.21-q11.23 (Bland 1982; Cannon-Spoor et al. 1982; Pulver et al. 1994b; Lindsay et al. 1996).

In addition to the candidate regions described above, there is also an hypothesis that the susceptibility to schizophrenia may be related to mutations specific to the sex chromosomes (for review, see Delisi et al. 1994a). Linkage/sib pair studies examining markers in the pseudo-autosomal region of the X chromosome have been reported (see, e.g., Collinge et al. 1991; Asherson et al. 1992; D'Amato et al. 1992, 1994; Wang et al. 1993; Barr et al. 1994; Crow et al. 1994; Delisi et al. 1994b; Kalsi et al. 1995; Maier et al. 1995; Okoro et al. 1995). The evidence from these studies is not conclusive; one cannot rule out the possibility of linkage of some region of the X chromosome with susceptibility to schizophrenia in some families.

Using a linkage strategy to identify schizophrenia susceptibility genes, one cannot expect to be able to identify a specific locus; rather, these studies may identify a region of interest within 1 cM of the gene (see, e.g., Devlin and Risch 1995). Using a combined linkage/association strategy (the association study strategy is described below) is likely to have more success (Ghosh 1995). The application of tests for linkage is not straightforward, given some of the properties of this disease. Difficulties include:

1. *Late age at onset:* Individuals may have the susceptibility gene but not exhibit the disease because they have not lived through the risk period.
2. *Variability in expression:* Uncertainty remains about the definition of a case of schizophrenia. Several diagnostic systems can be employed (see, e.g., Feighner et al. 1972; Endicott et al. 1975; American Psychiatric Association 1994), each with somewhat different criteria for schizophrenia. Pooling samples may cause confusion because of these diagnostic differences. Inter-rater reliability, even when using the same diagnostic system, cannot be assumed.
3. *Incomplete penetrance* has been assumed because concordance rates among monozygotic twins has been reported to vary between 40% and 60%. In addition, a study of the offspring of discordant monozygotic twins suggests that the rate of schizophrenia did not differ when the offspring of affected and nonaffected co-twins were compared, providing support for the hypothesis of incomplete penetrance (Kringlen and Cramer 1989). Using an "affecteds only" design where unaffected individuals have little impact on the analysis can circumvent this problem.
4. *Assortative mating* (i.e., the tendency for mated pairs to be more similar for some phenotypic trait than would be expected if the choice of a partner occurred at random) has been demonstrated to be present among schizophrenic patients (Rao et al. 1981; Parnas 1985, 1988). Nonrandom mating may result in a distortion of the distribution of genotypes in the offspring, and within family heterogeneity.
5. *Reduced fertility and shorter life span* in those who are affected with schizophrenia limits the availability of potentially informative pedigrees (see Rimmer and Jacobsen 1976; Black and Fisher 1992).
6. *Characteristics of affected individuals*, such as suspiciousness and social withdrawal, may decrease the probability that they and their relatives will participate in research.
7. *The mode of inheritance is not known:* Given the lack of knowledge about how schizophrenia is transmitted (see, e.g., Risch and Baron 1984) nonparametric approaches, which do not make assumptions as to mode of inheritance, in addition to parametric linkage analyses, are being conducted routinely by many groups (Fang et al. 1995).
8. Given the probable *etiological and genetic heterogeneity* in the populations studied so far (Garver et al. 1989), very large numbers of families are necessary if there is to be any statistical power in the tests for linkage and genetic heterogeneity (Kendler and Diehl 1993).

These complications, while increasing the difficulties of the studies, are not altogether insurmountable.

Association studies. In the study of complex diseases of unknown pathophysiology, linkage studies are useful for identifying regions of interest in multiplex families. Association studies can be helpful for testing known candidate genes and for narrowing regions of interest, once they are identified. No assumptions are made about the mode of inheritance. In this strategy, association of a specific allele of a polymorphic locus is tested with the occurrence of the disease in affected individuals compared to ethnically matched controls. This strategy has a practical advantage over that of linkage because relatively scarce multiplex families are not required, and it has considerable statistical power to detect genes of "small effect" (A. Chakravarti, pers. comm.). The Transmission Disequilibrium Test (TDT) is a further refinement of the association test (Spielman et al. 1993), which tests the transmission of a particular allele from a parent to the case, using the other untransmitted allele from the parent as the "control," and this test mitigates the need for ethnically well-matched controls. Differences in the distribution of alleles between cases and controls suggest that the marker may be involved with the cause or may be in linkage disequilibrium with the cause. Several groups have reported results from such tests using polymorphisms of genes presumed to have some role in determining susceptibility to other inherited traits such as blood groups, HLA serotypes, and group-specific components (see, e.g., Fananas et al. 1990, 1992; Saha

Table 2. Association Studies Which Provide Support for Further Investigations to Determine the Possible Role These Genes May Play in Schizophrenia Susceptibility

Candidate	Covariation detected	Reference
HLA DQB1 0303		Nimgaonkar et al. (1995)
HLA DQB1 0602		
HLA class II		Zamani et al. (1994)
HLA DQB1	ethnic	Nimgaonkar et al. (1993b)
Dopamine D-2 receptor gene	age and family history	Arinami et al. (1994); Itokawa et al. (1993)[a]
Dopamine D-3 receptor gene	sex and age difference family history	Griffon et al. (1996); Kennedy et al. (1995) Nimgaonkar et al. (1993a); Crocq et al. (1992)
Serontonin 2A receptor gene		Inayama et al (1996)
Neurotrophin-3 gene	sex severity	Dawson et al. (1995) Hattori and Nanko (1995); Nanko et al. (1994)
Prophobilinogen deaminase gene		Sanders et al. (1992)
Tyrosine hydroxylase gene		Wei et al. (1995)

[a]Structural change in DRD2-missense nucleotide mutation from C to G.

et al. 1990). At this time, no genes have been confirmed as either contributory or noncontributory to the risk for schizophrenia. In Table 2 we summarize investigations that have provided some preliminary evidence of an association between a candidate and the susceptibility to schizophrenia (or some forms of schizophrenia). These candidates should be studied further in other populations.

Summary: Part I

How are we most likely to make progress in understanding the etiology of schizophrenia? It is by a combined epidemiological and genetic approach in which we go from one discipline to the other as each new level of information is exposed. For example, risk factors may aggregate in such a way as to suggest a subtype of schizophrenia. Then, when genes are found, their presence in families may be tested in the context of previously described subtypes, as different risk factors may be associated with different mutations. Subtypes may be further refined by additional clinical description. Finally, as a result of this alternating approach, we expect to end up with well-characterized genes whose protein products have been identified and which have been shown to be associated with predictable constellations of clinical characteristics. It should be noted that in this analysis neither epidemiology nor molecular genetics is sufficient; both are necessary and both require equal care in the collection and management of the data. For example, failure in precision in the collection of the clinical data can confound the molecular work, however carefully that work may be done, and vice versa. In the remainder of this paper we describe such an approach.

PART 2: THE JOHNS HOPKINS UNIVERSITY COLLABORATIVE SCHIZOPHRENIA STUDY

The Maryland Epidemiology Sample

The Maryland Epidemiology Sample (MES) was developed to test the hypothesis that subtypes of schizophrenia represent the outcome of different causes rather than a variable response to the same provocation. The research goal was to describe the etiologic mechanism for the different subgroups, assuming that different mechanisms would call for different treatments. A combined epidemiologic–genetic approach was developed in 1983 (see Fig. 1). Such an approach had not previously been mounted, although a similar strategy has been followed by Kendler and his colleagues studying an epidemiological sample in Ireland (Kendler et al. 1993). The need for large-scale studies was evident, given that reports of evidence of schizophrenia susceptibility were often inconsistent and seldom replicated.

By screening all psychiatric admissions to 15 facilities in the greater Baltimore area between June 1983 and April 1989, 1670 patients were chosen to participate in the studies. Patients with a broad range of psychotic diagnoses were selected for a variety of reasons, including inevitable differences in diagnostic practices across facilities and the relevance of diagnosis to genetic susceptibility. Indeed, there is evidence that susceptibility genes may be shared across different diagnostic categories (Wildenauer et al., this volume).

Detailed clinical and family history information was acquired for the patients in the MES. Prior to discharge from the hospital, an in-person diagnostic interview was administered to the patients by a clinical psychologist or social worker. The interview examined both lifetime history and current episode. Patients were also asked to allow us to (1) contact them periodically after discharge from the hospital for additional information and enrollment in further studies, (2) obtain copies of their psychiatric records, (3) talk with at least two family members to ascertain the psychiatric status of their relatives, and (4) receive copies of their birth certificate and their birth records. A concern about the accuracy of a psychiatric diagnosis based solely on information reported by the patient during the diagnostic interview led us to develop a best-estimate diagnostic procedure. This diagnosis was made by a psychiatrist who (1) reviewed all of the information reported by the patient during the diagnostic interview, (2) reviewed all of the patient's psychiatric records, and (3) spoke with the patient or an informant 6 months after the patient's discharge from the hospital to obtain course and outcome information. The diagnosis was made according to DSM-III criteria.

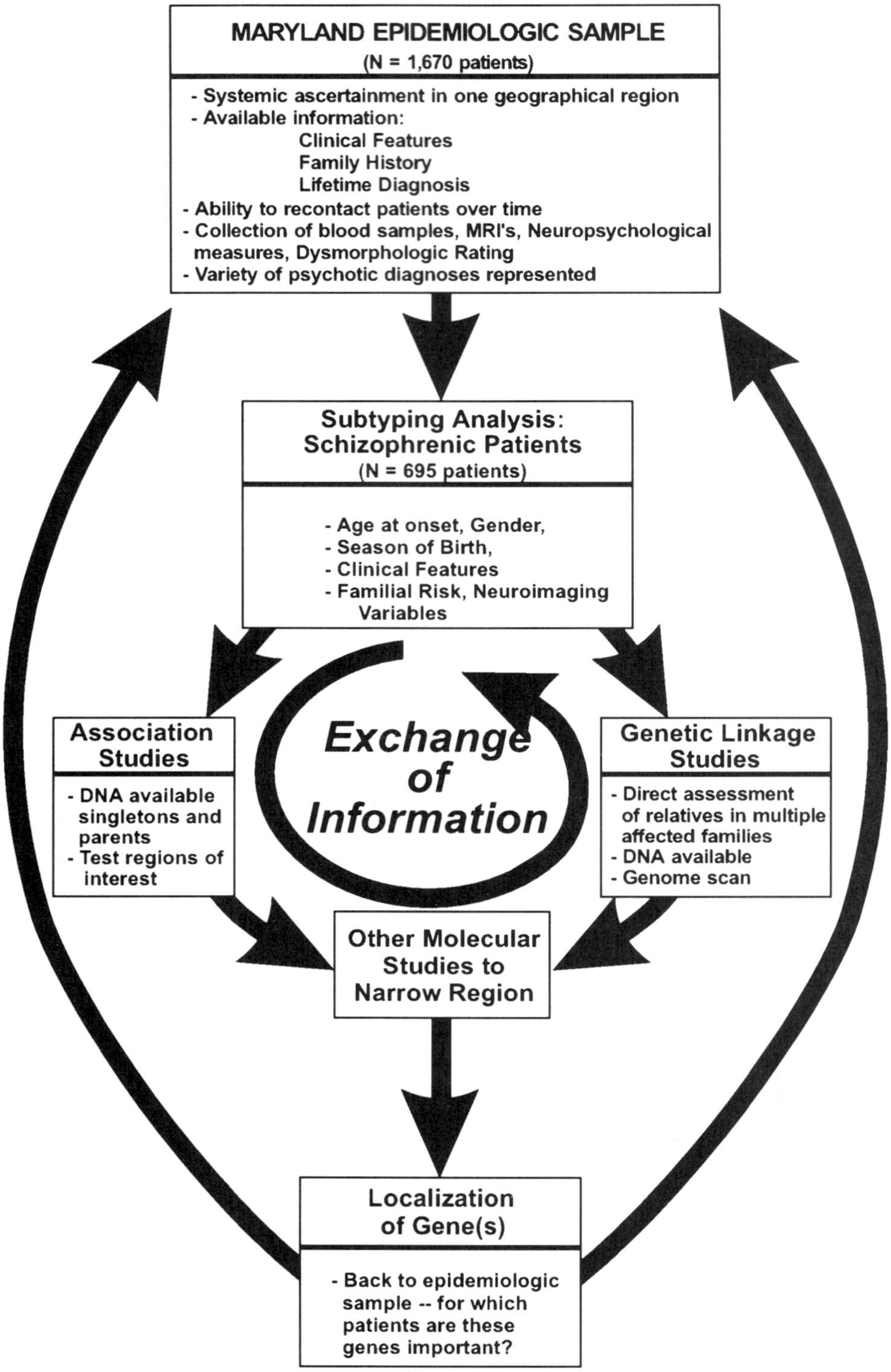

Figure 1. Schematic of epidemiologic/genetic approach.

For consenting patients in the MES (77% of the patients), a family history was obtained from two informants judged by the patient to be knowledgeable about his or her family. During a telephone interview, the informants were systematically questioned about the medical and psychiatric histories of the patient's first- and second-degree relatives. We used modified Family History Research Diagnostic Criteria to classify the relatives (Endicott et al. 1975). Since the family history method has been shown to be less accurate than directly assessing individuals for the identification of schizophrenia (Andreasen et al. 1977), we considered these data as preliminary to the collection of the data necessary to classify the relatives of probands for molecular studies. However, the family history data were used to determine whether patient characteristics delineate subtypes of schizophrenia that may differ in their etiologies. The results of these subtyping analyses are presented below.

Results of Initial Subtyping Analyses

The initial subtyping factors of interest were gender, age at onset, season of birth, and family history of schizophrenia. Utilizing family history information about the patients in the MES with a best-estimate diagnosis of schizophrenia, we have demonstrated the following: (1) first-degree relatives of female schizophrenics have a greater risk of developing schizophrenia than do first-degree relatives of male schizophrenics (Wolyniec et al. 1992); (2) first-degree relatives of schizophrenics with an early onset of illness (less than age 17) are at greater risk of developing schizophrenia than are first-degree relatives of schizophrenics with a later onset of illness (Pulver et al. 1990; Boyle et al. 1991); (3) first-degree relatives of schizophrenics born during the winter–spring months (specifically, February through May) are at higher risk of developing schizophrenia than are relatives of schizophrenics born during the other months of the year (Pulver et al. 1992b); (4) mothers of winter–spring-born schizophrenics have a greater spacing between their live births than do mothers of winter–spring-born controls (Pulver et al. 1992a); (5) the first-degree relatives of schizophrenic patients who also have a history of manic symptoms are at an increased risk for developing schizophrenia (Liang and Pulver 1996) than are the relatives of schizophrenic patients who do not have manic symptoms, and (6) the first-degree relatives of schizophrenic patients who also have a history of obsessive and compulsive symptoms are at a greater risk for depression and suicide than are the relatives of schizophrenics who do not have obsessive and compulsive symptoms (Samuels et al., in prep.).

On the basis of these results, we suggest that some individuals at an increased risk for schizophrenia due to genetic background may also be more vulnerable to some seasonally varying factor which further increases their risk (e.g., viral exposure in utero, pregnancy and birth complications). The greater spacing between the births of the mothers of winter–spring-born schizophrenic patients suggests that there might be other complicated pregnancies resulting in a nonviable outcome. It is important to determine whether the clinical features of schizophrenia which are associated with familial risk (i.e., age at onset, manic symptoms, obsessive-compulsive symptoms) characterize families, or some subset of families, or sibships. If this is the case, it will provide additional support for the idea that schizophrenia is etiologically heterogeneous, and these particular covariates may be helpful in discriminating between subgroups of patients in molecular studies.

Genetic Linkage Study

In 1989, a second phase of the work began. Here, the goal was to ascertain a set of families in which more than one individual was affected with schizophrenia (multiplex families) to be used to conduct a genome-wide search for genes and DNA markers associated with the risk for schizophrenia. The first source of such families was the MES. The families of schizophrenic patients who, on the basis of family history information, had at least one other living first- or second-degree relative with a diagnosis of either schizophrenia, schizoaffective disorder, or unspecified functional psychosis were considered eligible for this study. Less than one third of the schizophrenic patients in the MES had one or more affected relatives (for a description of the occurrence of schizophrenia in the relatives, see Pulver and Bale 1989). If direct assessment of the second affected family member confirmed a diagnosis of schizophrenia or schizoaffective disorder, complete ascertainment of the family was pursued. Complete ascertainment included direct psychiatric examinations and blood drawings for all of the proband's first- and second-degree relatives, as well as all of the first-degree relatives of other affected individuals in the family. Spouses of affected individuals were also included. Because of the need for greater statistical power in linkage studies, additional multiplex schizophrenic families were also recruited through physician referrals. The nonsystematically ascertained families were more likely to have at least three affected individuals.

Design features of the linkage study. It is our belief that quality control measures must be built into all aspects of data collection and analysis in a study of this kind. Some of the key design features of the linkage study include:

1. The majority of the families in the set used for the genome-wide scan were ascertained through a systematically selected group of patients (the MES). The set of families can be characterized by ascertainment class—either systematic or opportunistic.
2. The ascertainment strategy was specified in advance of data collection. We attempted to acquire information about all first- and second-degree relatives of affected individuals in each family. This information was gathered through any or all of the following: reports from family informants, review of psychiatric treatment records, direct psychiatric ex-

aminations, and reports from treating therapists and psychiatrists.

3. Rules for extending the pedigrees were specified; pedigrees were extended through affected individuals.
4. Direct psychiatric examinations of relatives were made by clinical psychologists or psychiatrists using standard psychiatric assessment instruments. The psychiatric assessments were designed to ascertain symptoms relevant to major mental disorders, as well as severe personality disorders. Information reported by the subject was supplemented by interviewing an informant identified by the subject. Examinations were audiotaped with the permission of the subject for quality control purposes.
5. To increase the accuracy of the assignment of affected status, final diagnoses were formulated through a consensus procedure. For each subject, two psychiatrists or psychologists independently reviewed all available information including the diagnostic interview, information reported by informants, psychiatric treatment records, and information reported by the subject's treating physician, and, after review, completed a DSM-III-R diagnostic assignment. If the two assignments agreed, the diagnosis was considered final. If there was disagreement, the case was discussed by the two raters until a consensus was reached. If a consensus could not be reached, additional information was sought and/or a third diagnostician was asked to review the case and to try to resolve the discrepancies. In some instances, this was not possible and the case was then classified as affected status unknown. Consensus was necessary not only for the diagnoses assigned, but also for age-at-onset ratings for each diagnosis.
6. The definition of affected and unknown phenotypes was specified prior to the analysis. This was done so that specific hypotheses could be tested rather than fishing for a positive result. For the analyses in the genome-wide search, individuals with a consensus diagnosis of either schizophrenia or schizoaffective disorder were considered affected; individuals with other psychotic disorders or schizotypal, schizoid, or paranoid personality disorder were classified as unknown.
7. To control for possible bias in coding genotyping data, molecular genetics laboratory personnel were blind to the affected status of all DNA samples in the laboratory, and all genotyping data were coded after consensus of two readers. Similarly, the diagnosticians were blind to the genotyping data. In addition, the genetic analysts were not involved in clinical or molecular assessments.
8. Given the variable age at onset of many psychiatric diseases, and the fact that many relatives have not lived through all the known risk periods for disease, a longitudinal study design was implemented to allow us to maintain current affected status of all individuals in the pedigree through regularly updated interviews.

Table 3. Description of 54 Pedigrees

Total number of individuals	456	
individuals genotyped	363	(80%)
Affected individuals	147	
age at onset		
<35	125	(85%)
≥35	17	(15%)
average	24.6	
sex		
male	90	(61%)
female	57	(39%)
DSM-III-R diagnosis		
schizophrenia	143	(97%)
schizoaffective	4	(3%)
average number of affecteds in each family	2.7	
Unaffected individuals	246	
age at assessment		
<35	30	(12%)
≥35	226	(88%)
Individuals with diagnosis "unknown"	63	
Linearity in pedigrees (re: proband)		
maternal	19	(35%)
paternal	8	(15%)
sibs only	27	(50%)

Description of the families being genotyped for the genome-wide scan. At this time, we have completed the diagnostic evaluations of more than 80 families. For the past 18 months, we have been genotyping 363 individuals in 54 pedigrees. Additional pedigrees are being added as we continue the research. However, at this time, all analyses are based on 54 families. Characteristics of the families are summarized in Table 3.

Strategy for the genome-wide search. Given the likelihood that no one gene will have a sufficient effect in all of the families, simulation studies revealed that the number of families we had available was insufficient to detect linkage for a gene contributing to liability in only a small proportion of families (under heterogeneity). We embarked on our studies knowing that collaborative efforts with other research groups were going to be necessary to detect genes that may be important to subsets of the schizophrenic families. Therefore, a three-stage strategy was developed; the first two stages involved typing markers in the families we ascertained, the third stage was to help facilitate the study of the regions that met criteria in other family samples (by other investigators) (see Table 4).

In analyses of our 54 families, low positive LOD scores were used as thresholds to detect regions of interest from a sparse linkage map. Additional markers were typed to create a dense map only at promising genomic regions. The staged approach was used to minimize the number of markers required for typing. An initial critical LOD score for stage I was selected that was highly likely to include any true linkage (LOD≥ 0.30). The strategy was to space markers every

Table 4. Three-stage Searching Strategy

Stage 1.	2-Point linkage analyses 54 JHU families Find markers where LRH ≥ 2.0 (LOD ≥ 0.30)
Stage 2.	2-Point linkage analyses 54 JHU families Find markers where LRH ≥ 10.0 (LOD ≥ 2.0)
Stage 3.	"Hot spot" Facilitate follow-up of region by other investigators in independent families

20 cM, adding additional markers (every 3 cM) to any selected regions of 40 cM. The critical LOD score for stage II was selected to be greater than or equal to 2.0. Any regions meeting the stage II criterion were then released to other investigators for independent replication (stage III).

Statistical analysis. Affected subjects for all statistical analyses were restricted to those satisfying DSM-III-R (American Psychiatric Association 1987) criteria for schizophrenia or schizoaffective disorder. Subjects with other psychotic disorders or "schizophrenia spectrum personality disorders" were classified as "unknown" phenotype with unknown liability. Both autosomal dominant and recessive models were used. Given that the concordance rate for schizophrenia among monozygotic twins has been reported to be between 50% and 65%, the classification of those who are unaffected is problematic. Therefore, the two parametric models are defined with "affecteds only" liability classes, where unaffected subjects were treated the same as unknown subjects; their genotypings are available, but their phenotype has no effect on the LOD score. In addition to linkage analyses using two models, nonparametric sib-pair analyses to test for sharing of alleles identical-by-descent were conducted. However, the results from linkage analyses using the autosomal dominant and recessive models were used to guide the laboratory through the two-stage strategy.

The programs MLINK, LODSCORE, ILINK (Lathrop and Lalouel 1984; Lathrop et al. 1984, 1986), and HOMOG (Ott 1991) were used, via the FAST-LINK versions (Cottingham et al. 1993; Schaffer et al. 1994) as implemented in the ANALYZE software (Terwilliger 1994) to compute 2-point maximum LOD scores under heterogeneity, for each locus tested. The ANALYZE software also estimates the proportion of alleles shared identical-by-descent in all available sib pairs (Kuokkanen et al. 1996; Satsangi et al. 1996). In addition, within the past several months, a novel and efficient way to run nonparametric multipoint analyses for many markers in a dense map has become available. Some of the data have been analyzed with these programs, known as MAPMAKER/SIBS (Kruglyak and Lander 1995) and GENEHUNTER (Kruglyak et al. 1996).

Results from the Genome Scan

We have typed and analyzed more than 650 markers, on all 22 autosomes, in the genome scan. We approximate that these markers cover 70% of the genome. Using the staged strategy, we have identified four regions which we felt were worthy of follow-up. These regions are 22q11-q13; 8p22- p21; 3p26-p24; and 13q14-q32. The results of analyses for each of these regions, as well as the data reported from other groups for these regions, are summarized below. In addition, we report the results of analyses of data generated to follow up a report from Straub et al. (1995), suggesting linkage on chromosome 6p24-p22.

Chromosome 22q. The region of interest on chromosome 22 is shown in Figure 2 (Pulver et al. 1994b). This is the first region identified in our genome scan, satisfying criteria for stage II. The maximum LOD score was obtained for the dominant model (LOD = 2.05) for the marker *D22S445* in 22q13. The highest LOD score obtained using the recessive model was 1.39 for *D22S685* mapped to 22q12. The most significant sib-pair sharing was found for the markers *D22S1268, D22S686* (p=.007) in 22q12-q13. The region

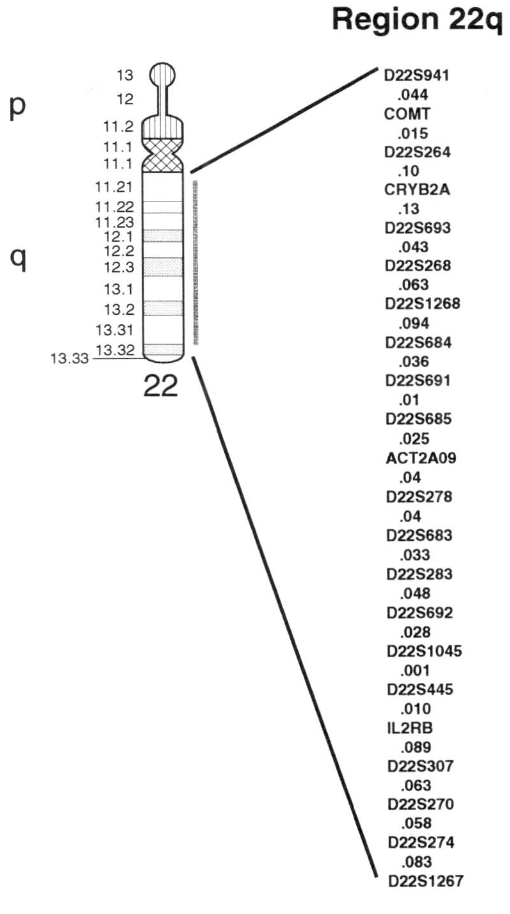

Figure 2. Ideogram of chromosome 22.

of allele sharing is relatively large. These data alone provide only suggestive evidence for a susceptibility gene somewhere in this region on chromosome 22. Recently completed multipoint analyses confirm that the region of interest is large and may, in fact, contain two separate regions of interest.

Prior to publishing the initial suggestive findings for this region, we organized a multicenter collaborative effort to investigate the region further. This was the first such effort to be taken in this field. Previous experience with a report "Localization of a Susceptibility Locus for Schizophrenia on Chromosome 5" (Sherrington et al. 1988), followed by a series of papers reporting no evidence for linkage (Kennedy et al. 1988; St. Clair et al. 1989; Aschauer et al. 1990; McGuffin et al. 1990; Crowe et al. 1991; Campion et al. 1992; Macciardi et al. 1992), was problematic for the field of psychiatric genetics (see, e.g., Owen 1992). The early pronouncement of a finding of a schizophrenia susceptibility gene followed by many failures to replicate caused disillusionment with the scientific goal and adversely affected the reputation of psychiatric genetics among the general scientific community. Prior to publication of our results on 22q (Pulver et al. 1994b), three research groups known to be genotyping families with schizophrenia were contacted in 1992 and advised of the findings; i.e., Kenneth Kendler and his colleagues, Michael Owen and Michael Gill and their colleagues, and Jacque Mallet and his colleagues. A collaboration was begun; interlaboratory reliability exercises were conducted for both the genotyping data and the diagnostic assignments.

As a result of the collaborative study, 217 additional families were genotyped for three markers on 22q (*D22S268*, *IL2RB*, and *D22S307*). The LOD score analyses for this independent sample of families did not support linkage (Pulver et al. 1994c). However, since power calculations showed that there was low power to detect linkage if 25% or less of the families were linked to markers in this region, we concluded that additional efforts needed to be mounted to test the hypothesis that there was a schizophrenia susceptibility gene in this region in some families. After we made our findings public, Coon and colleagues notified us that as part of their genome search using 9 families, they detected a LOD score of 2.09 for a recessive model toward the distal end of the chromosome at *D22S276*. Subsequently, their data were published (Coon et al. 1994a). Since then, several additional groups genotyped markers in the region. Although all of the reports have not supported linkage, none of them has been able to rule out the possibility of linkage for markers in this region for some subset of the schizophrenic families. Additional support has accrued: (1) Gill et al. (1996) reported their best evidence at *D22S278* in 22q12 (p<.01); (2) Schwab et al. (1995b) reported a mildly positive LOD (0.61) for *D22S304* which is approximately 3.5 cm centromeric to *D22S278*; (3) Polymeropoulos et al. (1994) reported greater than expected allele sharing for several markers in the region around *D22S278* (p<.02); (4) Moises et al. (1995a) reported some evidence for linkage disequilibrium between schizophrenia and allele #243 of *D22S278* (p=0.02) in 113 unrelated schizophrenic subjects and their 226 parents; and finally (5) a collaborative effort organized by Michael Gill and Homero Vallada et al. (Gill et al. 1996) employing an affected sib-pair analysis analyzed genotypings of one marker (*D22S278* in 22q12) typed by 11 research groups. From a pooled sample of more than 600 families, the analysis of the sub sample of 296 affected sib-pairs for whom parental data were available revealed a significant excess of alleles shared by affected individuals for the marker *D22S278* (p=.001).

In addition to the evidence for the region around *D22S278*, there is some evidence for a schizophrenia-related susceptibility locus centromeric to this region. The evidence is as follows: (1) Although for some time it had been observed that children with velo-cardio facial syndrome (VCFS), a congenital disorder associated with an interstitial deletion of 22q11, have a range of psychiatric and learning problems, a study using appropriate research methods found that by examining the psychiatric status of VCFS subjects who were between the ages of 16 and 25, a higher than expected rate of schizophrenia was found (Pulver et al. 1994a). (2) On the basis of the evaluation of 100 schizophrenic patients ascertained from the MES, we have reported a higher rate of the 22q11 deletion among the schizophrenics than would be expected based on estimated population prevalence (Karayiorgou et al. 1995; Lindsay et al. 1995). Details of this work as well as the results of additional work in this region are reported by Karayiorgou et al. (this volume).

Chromosome 8p22-p12. The region of interest on chromosome 8 (Pulver et al. 1995) is shown in Figure 3. The dominant model provided a maximum LOD score in this region for the marker *SFTP2* (2.40) in 8p21. The maximum LOD score for the recessive model was 2.10 for the marker *D8S136*, tightly linked to *SFTP2*. The most significant evidence for a susceptibility locus in this region from the analyses of allele sharing among sib pairs is for the marker *D8S258* (p<.001). Results of multipoint sib-pair analyses recently completed provide additional support for this region. A report of these analyses is currently being prepared for publication.

Given the strength and the consistency of these data, we requested that colleagues again join in a collaborative effort to study this region (stage III of our strategy). Douglas Levinson agreed to coordinate a study of 8p (and two other regions) using family data from 14 groups with a total of 567 informative pedigrees. The results of the analyses of five markers on 8p (*D8S261, D8S258, D8133, D8136,* and *D8S283)* have been completed and provide additional support for the presence of a schizophrenia susceptibility gene

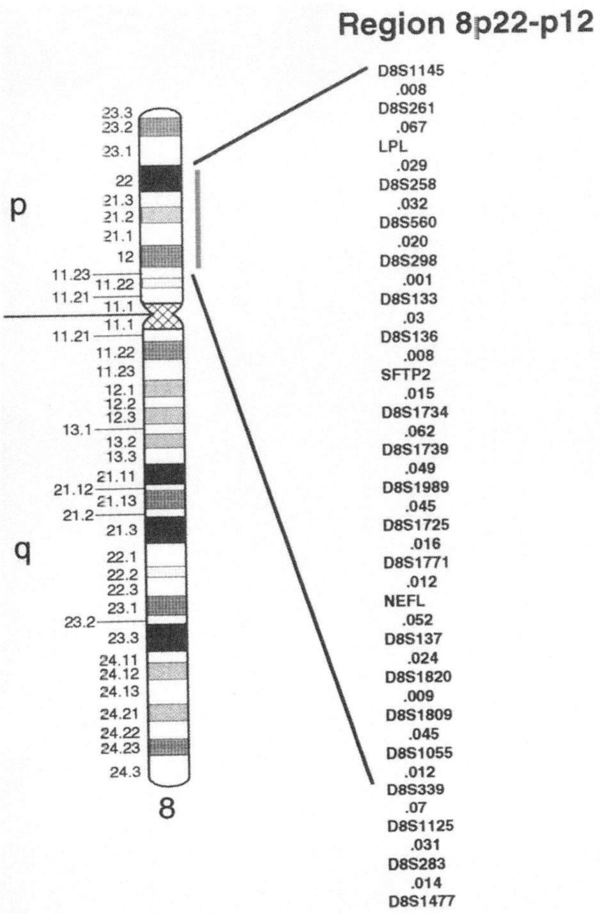

Figure 3. Ideogram of chromosome 8.

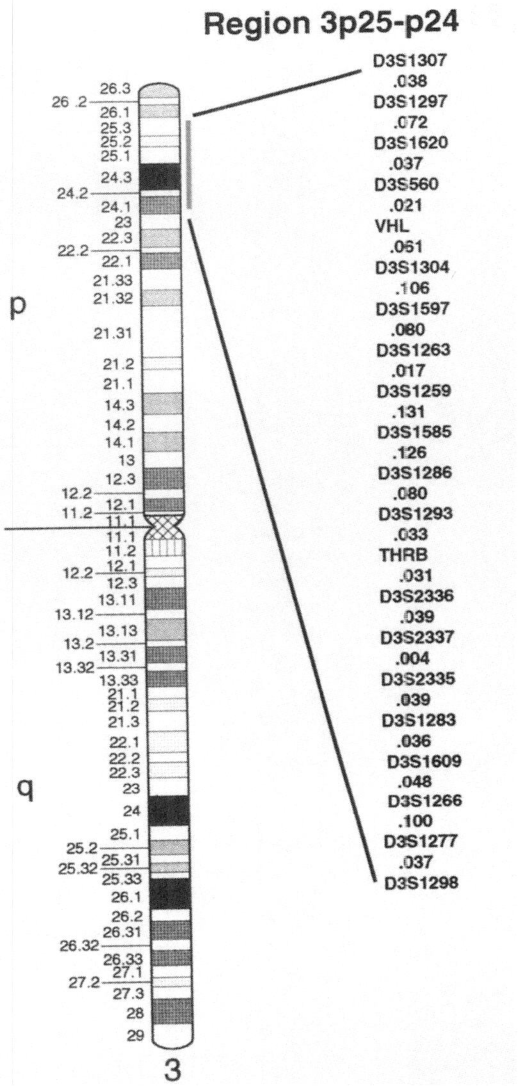

Figure 4. Ideogram of chromosome 3.

in this region (D. Levinson et al.; Schizophrenia Collaborative Linkage Group; both in prep.). The maximum LOD score 2.22 (p=.0014) for 13 groups (without our data) was obtained with a recessive model for locus *D8S261*, the most telomeric of the five markers tested. The nonparametric analyses report p<.005 for *D8S133* for allele sharing in the independent replication sample. Slightly positive LODs (>0.3) were observed in 10 of 13 groups.

Chromosome 3p26-p24. Figure 4 shows the region 3p26-p24, a region of approximately 60 cM mapped by 22-dinucleotide-repeat polymorphisms. The maximum LOD score in this region was obtained with an "affecteds only" dominant model for the marker *D3S1283* (LOD score 1.56). The maximum LOD score in this region using the affecteds-only recessive model was also at *D3S1283* (LOD score 1.75). Reanalyses with our current sample, and additional markers, now show that only one marker, *D3S1283*, shows evidence (p=.02) of excess sib-pair sharing. Markers in this region of chromosome 3 were also genotyped in the replication effort coordinated by Levinson. All heterogeneity LODs for four markers used in the follow-up effort *(D3S1293, D3S1283, D3S1266, D3S1298)* were less than 0.08 and the region was therefore considered negative. However, these data do not provide evidence to exclude the possibility of a schizophrenia susceptibility gene in the region in some individuals.

Chromosome 13q14-q32. The region of interest on the chromosome is 13q14-q32 and is shown in Figure 5. The greatest evidence for this region comes from the sib-pair analyses for the marker *D13S770* (p=.0002). The maximum LOD score in this region was obtained with a dominant model for the marker *D13S128* (LOD = 3.24). The maximum LOD score for the recessive model was 2.53 for the marker *D13S779.* Recently completed multipoint sib-pair sharing analyses for this region add support for a schizophrenia susceptibility locus in this region. A more dense map of this region is currently being genotyped.

Other evidence to support the existence of a susceptibility gene for schizophrenia in region 13q had pre-

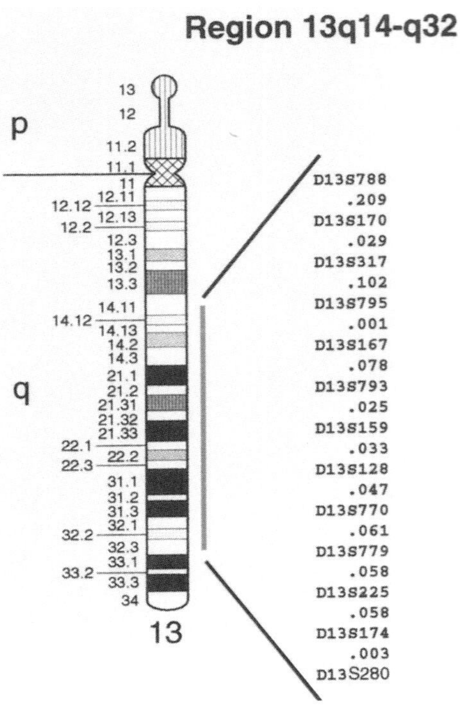

Figure 5. Ideogram of chromosome 13.

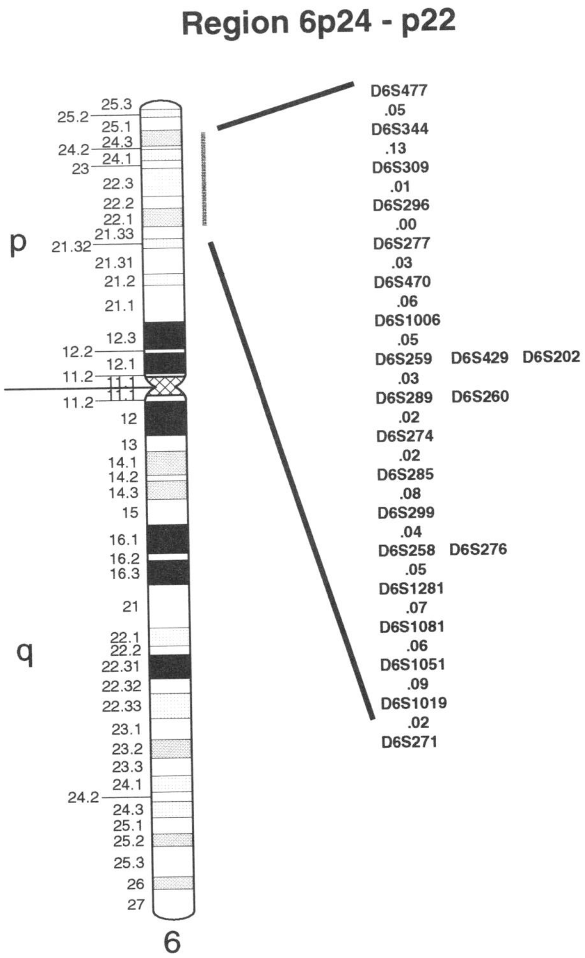

Figure 6. Ideogram of chromosome 6.

viously been reported by Lin et al. (1995) in their study of 13 schizophrenia pedigrees in the region 13q14.1-q32. LOD score analysis of markers in this region was moderately positive (*D13S144;* LOD=1.61). Multipoint results from a dominant model allowing for heterogeneity using a narrow definition of affected gave a maximum multipoint LOD score of 2.00 for *D13S128* in 13q32.

Chromosome 6p. As part of the 3-stage strategy, we also follow up reports of regions of interest from other groups. Kendler et al. informed us of their finding of a maximum LOD score of 3.51 for *D6S296* in their large Irish sample of nearly 300 pedigrees (Straub et al. 1995). There was also suggestive but weaker evidence for sib-pair sharing of alleles at *D6S296*. We have followed up this suggestion of linkage by typing markers in both 6p24-22 and in the more centromeric HLA region (6p21) (Antonarakis et al. 1995) (see Fig. 6). The strongest sib-pair sharing in the sample was seen for marker *D6S296* (p=.0003). The marker *D6S1006* gave the highest LOD for the dominant model (0.96) and also gave the highest recessive LOD (1.32).

Additional evidence supporting the existence of a schizophrenia susceptibility has also been obtained in several samples (Gurling et al. 1995; Schwab et al. 1995a; Wang et al. 1995) and the large collaborative effort organized by Levinson et al. (1996). These results of the analysis of the collaborative effort as well as additional work in this region by the Kendler group are reported by Straub et al. (this volume).

Summary: Part II

The results of our epidemiologic studies support the hypothesis that schizophrenia is etiologically heterogeneous. The true test of heterogeneity will only be possible when the specific etiologic mechanism(s) is delineated. The identification of schizophrenia susceptibility genes is an important step toward attaining this goal.

Over the last several years, significant progress has been made toward elucidating the genes associated with schizophrenia susceptibility. Our group has now reported four regions of interest from the genome scan (i.e., chromosomes 22q 11-13, 8p22-p12, 3p26-24, and 13q14-q32). Multicenter follow-up studies have now been completed for three of the regions (22q, 8p, and 3p), and evidence to support linkage has been obtained for two of the regions (22q and 8p). The region on 3p, although studied in a large collaborative follow-up study, did not provide evidence supporting linkage. This paper represents our first report of the region on chromosome 13q. We are hopeful that a collaborative follow-up will be organized to test this region. In addition to these regions, the cumulative evidence now available for the region of interest identified by Kendler and colleagues (Straub et al. 1995) on chromosome 6p24-p22 provides support for the existence of a susceptibility gene in this region as well.

In all likelihood, over the next several years we will learn of the existence of other regions of interest and other potential candidate genes. However, the identification of regions of interest is an initial step toward the next goal: the identification of the gene(s). The problem that we and others are now struggling with is how to move from a region of interest or a candidate region to the identification of a gene. Our group has articulated a plan, described below, to narrow the regions of interest. This plan requires an additional huge effort from scientists representing all of the disciplines in our multidisciplinary team.

Association/linkage disequilibrium tests. As a first step to follow up linkage results in family samples, association studies are conducted using a new sample of schizophrenic patients and their parents from simplex families in the epidemiologic sample; these families have not previously been analyzed in linkage studies. We are also planning a new data collection effort; i.e., to ascertain a sample of Ashkenazi Jewish schizophrenic patients and their families for both sib-pair studies and association studies. This new sample will be tested to determine if the previously identified regions of interest are important in this more homogeneous group, as well as to identify new regions of interest. In regions where the TDT and/or association studies confirm disequilibrium, family material can be used for molecular cloning strategies.

Refinement of disease definition/heterogeneity analyses. All of the analyses that we have reported thus far have been based on a strict definition of affected: i.e., a consensus diagnosis of schizophrenia or schizoaffective disorder. Additional analyses are planned that will expand the definition of affected to include what has previously been described as schizophrenia spectrum disease (schizotypal, schizoid, and paranoid personality disorders and unspecified psychotic disorders).

It has long been recognized that there is considerable clinical heterogeneity in schizophrenia. Recently, several independent studies employing multivariate techniques such as factor analysis and latent class analysis have consistently suggested that the symptoms of schizophrenia can be grouped into three dimensions: negative symptoms (affective flattening and negative thought disorder), disorganization (inappropriate affect and positive thought disorder), and positive psychotic symptoms (e.g., hallucinations) (for review, see Andreasen et al. 1995). The consistency of the findings across studies, and the presumed etiologic heterogeneity in schizophrenia, suggest that these dimensions may be good candidates to be used in the definition of affected in linkage studies. It may be that genetic heterogeneity is tied to the clinical heterogeneity that has been observed. We are currently in the process of (1) confirming that these clinical dimensions identified by others can be observed in the families and (2) determining how classification of affected individuals according to these dimensions influences linkage results. Multipoint analyses in the regions of interest will be conducted treating these clinical dimensions, as well as other variables such as season of birth and age at onset, as covariates.

Molecular analyses. In addition to what is described above, the molecular biologists have the following work ongoing or planned: (1) identify any potential candidate gene in narrowed regions and screen for mutations, (2) develop a yeast artificial chromosome (YAC) contig across the narrowed regions, (3) subclone YACs into cosmids, (4) identify genes through either exon trapping or cDNA screening, (5) screen genes for mutations, and (6) sequence the variations.

The goals which follow gene identification are to understand the gene function, to describe the mechanism responsible for the disease, to test the heterogeneity hypothesis, and to describe more etiologically homogeneous groups. Of course, it is our hope that success in this work will lead to the development of a new understanding of schizophrenia which will allow the development of new, more effective medications.

ACKNOWLEDGMENTS

The authors acknowledge the contribution of the patients and their families, Dr. William T. Carpenter, Jr. and the Maryland Psychiatric Research Center, Drs. Jurg Ott, Aravinda Chakravarti, and Swapan Nath. In addition, we are appreciative of the financial support obtained from Sandoz Pharmaceuticals and National Institute of Mental Health grants 1 R01 MH-45588 and 1 R01 35712 and National Institutes of Health grant DRR-OPD-GCRC #RR00722.

REFERENCES

American Psychiatric Association. 1987. *Diagnostic and statistical manual of mental disorders,* 3rd edition, revised. American Psychiatric Association, Washington, D.C.

———. 1994. *Diagnostic and statistical manual of mental disorders,* 4th edition. American Psychiatric Association, Washington, D.C.

Andreasen, N.C., J. Endicott, R.L. Spitzer, and G. Winokur. 1977. The family history method using diagnostic criteria. Reliability and validity. *Arch. Gen. Psychiatry* **34:** 1229.

Andreasen, N.C., S. Arndt, R. Alliger, D. Miller, and M. Flaum. 1995. Symptoms of schizophrenia. *Arch. Gen. Psychiatry* **52:** 341.

Antonarakis, S.E., J.L. Blouin, A.E. Pulver, P. Wolyniec, V.K. Lasseter, G. Nestadt, L. Kasch, R. Babb, H.H. Kazazian, B. Dombroski, et al. 1995. Schizophrenia susceptibility and chromosme 6p24-22. *Nat. Genet.* **11:** 235.

Arinami, T., M. Itokawa, H. Enguchi, H. Tagaya, S. Yano, H. Shimizu, H. Hamaguchi, and M. Toru. 1994. Association of dopamine D2 receptor molecular variant with schizophrenia (comments). *Lancet* **343:** 703.

Aschauer, H.N., G. Aschauer-Treiber, K.E. Isenberg, R.D. Todd, M.A. Knesevich, D.L. Garver, T. Reich, and C.R. Cloninger. 1990. No evidence for linkage between chromosome 5 markers and schizophrenia. *Hum. Hered.* **40:** 109.

Asherson, P., E. Parfitt, M. Sargeant, S. Tidmarsh, P. Buckland, C. Taylor, A. Clements, M. Gill, P. McGuffin, and M. Owen. 1992. No evidence for a pseudoautosomal locus in schizophrenia linkage analysis of mulitply affected families. *Br. J. Psychiatry* **161:** 63.

Barr, C.L., J.L. Kennedy, A.J. Pakstis, C.M. Castiglione, J.R. Kidd, L. Wetterberg, and K.K. Kidd. 1994. Linkage study of a susceptibility locus for schizophrenia in the pseudoautosomal region. *Schizophr. Bull.* **20:** 277.

Barr, C.L., J.L. Kennedy, A.J. Pakstis, L. Wetterburg, S.L. Beirut, C. Wadelius, J. Wahlstrom, L. Giuffra, L. Martinsson, J. Gelernter, J. Hallmayer, H.W. Moises, J. Kurth, L.L. Cavalli-Sforza, and K.K. Kidd. 1994. Progress in a genome scan for linkage in schizophrenia in a large Swedish kindred. *Am. J. Med. Genet.* **54:** 51.

Bassett, A.S. 1992. Chromosomal aberrations and schizophrenia autosomes. *Br. J. Psychiatry* **161:** 323.

Benes, F.M. 1993. Neurobiological investigations in cingulate cortex of schizophrenic brain. *Schizophr. Bull.* **19:** 537.

Benes, F.M., J. Davidson, and E.D. Bird. 1986. Quantitative cytoarchitectural studies of the cerebral cortex of schizophrenics. *Arch. Gen. Psychiatry* **43:** 31.

Black, D.W. and R. Fisher. 1992. Mortality in DSM-IIIR schizophrenia. *Schizophr. Res.* **7:** 109.

Bland, R.C. 1982. Predicting the outcome in schizophrenia. *Can. J. Psychiatry* **27:** 52.

Boyd, J.H., A. E. Pulver, and W. Stewart. 1986. Season of birth: Schizophrenia and bipolar disorder. *Schizophr. Bull.* **12:** 173.

Boyle, M.H., D.R. Offord, Y.A. Racine, and G. Catlin. 1991. Ontario child health study follow-up: Evaluation of sample loss. *J. Am. Acad. Child Adolesc. Psychiatry* **30:** 449.

Campion, D., T. D'Amato, H. Laklou, O. Sabate, M. Jay, M. Leboyer, A. Malafosse, P. Gorwood, M.C. Babron, D. Hillaire, F. Clerget-Darpoux, G. Waksman, and J. Mallet. 1992. Failure to replicate linkage between chromosome 5q11-q13 markers and schizophrenia in 28 families. *Psychiatry Res.* **4:** 171.

Cannon, T.D. and E. Marco. 1994. Structural brain abnormalities as indicators of vulnerability to schizophrenia. *Schizophr. Bull.* **20:** 89.

Cannon-Spoor, H.E., S.G. Potkin, and R.J. Wyatt. 1982. Measurement of premorbid adjustment in chronic schizophrenia. *Schizophr. Bull.* **8:** 470.

Collinge, J., L.E. Delisi, A. Boccio, E.C. Johnstone, A. Lane, C. Larkin, M. Leach, R. Lofthouse, F. Owen, M. Poulter, T. Shah, C. Walsh, and T.J. Crow. 1991. Evidence for a pseudo-autosomal locus for schizophrenia using the method of affected sibling pairs. *Br. J. Psychiatry*. **158:** 624.

Coon, H., J. Holik, M. Hoff, F. Reimherr, P. Wender, M. Myles-Worsley, M. Waldo, R. Freedman, and W. Byerley. 1994a. Analysis of chromosome 22 markers in nine schizophrenia pedigrees. *Am. J. Med. Genet.* **54:** 72.

Coon, H., S. Jensen, J. Holik, M. Hoff, M. Myles-Worsley, F. Reimherr, P. Wender, M. Waldo, R. Freedman, M. Leppert, and W. Byerley. 1994b. Genomic scan for genes predisposing to schizophrenia. *Am. J. Med. Genet.* **54:** 59.

Cottingham, R.W., Jr., R.M. Idury, and A. A. Schaffer. 1993. Faster sequential genetic linkage computations. *Am. J. Hum. Genet.* **53:** 252.

Crocq, M.A., R. Mant, P. Asherson, J. Williams, Y. Hode, A. Mayerova, D. Collier, L. Lannfelt, P. Sokoloff, J.C. Schwartz, M. Gill, J.P. Macher, P. McGuffin, and M.J. Owen. 1992. Association between schizophrenia and homozygosity at the dopamine D3 receptor gene (comments). *J. Med. Genet.* **29:** 858.

Crow, T.J., L.E. Delisi, R. Lofthouse, M. Poulter, T. Lehner, N. Bass, T. Shah, C. Walsh, A. Boccio-Smith, G. Shields, and J. Ott. 1994. An examination of linkage of schizophrenia and schizoaffective disorder to the pseudoautosomal region (Xp22.3) (comments). *Br. J. Psychiatry* **164:** 159.

Crowe, R.R., D.W. Black, R. Wesner, N.C. Andreasen, A. Cookman, and J. Roby. 1991. Lack of linkage to chromosome 5q11-q13 markers in six schizophrenia pedigrees. *Arch. Gen. Psychiatry* **48:** 357.

D'Amato, T., G. Waksman, M. Martinez, C. Laurent, P. Gorwood, D. Campion, M. Jay, C. Petit, C. Savoye, C. Bastard, M.C. Babron, F. Clerget-Darpoux, and J. Mallet. 1994. Pseudoautosomal region in schizophrenia: Linkage analysis of seven loci by sib-pair and lod-score methods. *Psychiatry Res.* **52:** 135.

D'Amato, T., D. Campion, P. Gorwood, M. Jay, O. Sabate, C. Petit, M. Abbar, A. Malafosse, M. Leboyer, D. Hillaire, F. Clerget-Darpoux, J. Feingold, G. Waksman, and J. Mallet. 1992. Evidence for a pseudoautosomal locus for schizophrenia. II. Replication of a non-random segregation of alleles at the DXYS14 locus. *Br. J. Psychiatry*. **161:** 59.

Dawson, E., J.F. Powell, P.C. Sham, M. Nothen, M.A. Crocq, P. Propping, J. Korner, M. Rietschel, J. Vanos, P. Wright, R.M. Murray, and M. Gill. 1995. An association study of a neurotrophin-3 (nt-3) gene polymorphism with schizophrenia. *Acta Psychiatr. Scand.* **92:** 425.

Delisi, L.E., U. Friedrich, J. Wahlstrom, A. Boccio-Smith, A. Forsman, K. Eklund, and T.J. Crow. 1994a. Schizophrenia and sex chromosome anomalies. *Schizophr. Bull.* **20:** 495.

Delisi, L.E., M. Devoto, R. Lofthouse, M. Poulter, A. Smith, G. Shields, N. Bass, G. Chen, A. Vita, C. Morganti, J. Ott, and T.J. Crow. 1994b. Search for linkage to schizophrenia on the X and Y chromosomes. *Am. J. Med. Genet.* **54:** 113.

Devlin, B. and N. Risch. 1995. A comparison of linkage disequilibrium measures for fine-scale mapping. *Genomics* **29:** 311.

Done, D.J., T.J. Crow, E.C. Johnstone, and A. Sacker. 1994. Childhood antecedents of schizophrenia and effective illness: Social adjustment at ages 7 and 11. *Br. Med. J.* **309:** 699.

Eaton, W.W. 1985. Epidemiology of schizophrenia. *Epidemiol. Rev.* **7:** 105.

———. 1991. Update on the epidemiology of schizophrenia. *Epidemiol. Rev.* **13:** 320.

Eaton, W.W., C. Hayward, and R. Ram. 1992. Schizophrenia and rheumatoid arthritis: A review. *Schizophr. Res.* **6:** 181.

Elston, R.C., E. Kringlen, and K.K. Namboodiri. 1973. Possible linkage relationships between certain blood groups and schizophrenia or other psychoses. *Behav. Genet.* **3:** 101.

Endicott, J., N. Andreasen, and R.L. Spitzer. 1975. *Family history research diagnostic criteria.* New York State Psychiatric Institute, New York.

Erlenmeyer-Kimling, L., B.A. Cornblatt, D. Rock, S. Roberts, M. Bell, and A. West. 1993. The New York high-risk project: Anhedonia, attentional deviance, and psychopathology. *Schizophr. Bull.* **19:** 141.

Fananas, L., P. Moral, M.A. Panadero, and J. Bertranpetit. 1992. Complement genetic markers in schizophrenia: C3, BF and C6 polymorphisms. *Hum. Hered.* **42:** 162.

Fananas, L., P. Moral, J. Tusquets, L. Marti, and J. Bertranpetit. 1990. Genetic markers in schizophrenia: ACPI, ESD, TF and GC polymorphisms. *Hum. Hered.* **40:** 136.

Fang, N., H. Coon, M. Hoff, M., J. Holik, D. Hadley, F. Reimherr, P. Wender, M. Myles-Worsley, M. Waldo, R. Freedman, and W. Byerley. 1995. Search for a schizophrenia susceptibility gene on chromosome 18. *Psychiatr. Genet.* **5:** 31.

Feighner, J.P., E. Robins, S.B. Guze, R.A. Woodruff, G. Winokur, and R. Munoz. 1972. Diagnostic criteria for use in psychiatric research. *Arch. Gen. Psychiatry* **26:** 57.

Fountain, J.W., M.R. Wallace, M.A. Bruce, B.R. Seizinger, A.G. Menon, J.F.Gusella, V.V. Michels, M.A. Schmidt, G.W. Dewald, and F.S. Collins. 1989. Physical mapping of a translocation breakpoint in neurofibromatosis. *Science* **244:**1085.

Garofalo, G., R.M. Ragusa, A. Argiolas, C. Scavuzzo, E. Spina, and C. Barletta. 1993. Evidence of chromosomal fragile sites in schizophrenic patients. *Ann. Genet.* **36:** 132.

Garver, D.L., T. Reich, K.E. Isenberg, and C.R. Cloninger. 1989. Schizophrenia and the question of genetic heterogeneity. *Schizophr. Bull.* **15:** 421.

Ghosh, S. 1995. Probability and complex genes. *Nat. Genet.* **9:** 223.

Gill, M., H. Vallada, C. Collier, P. Sham, P. Holmans, R. Murray, P. McGuffin, S. Nanko, M. Owen, S. Antonarakis, D. Housman, H. Kazazian, G. Nestadt, A.E. Pulver, R.E. Straub, C.J. MacLean, D. Walsh, K.S. Kendler, L. Delisi, M. Polymeropoulos, H. Coon, W. Byerley, R. Lofthouse, E. Gershon, L. Golden, and more than 22 others. 1996. A combined analysis of D22S278 marker alleles in affected sib-pairs support for a susceptibility locus for schizophrenia at chromosome 22q12. *Am. J. Med Genet.* **67:** 40.

Goldstein, J.M., M.T. Tsuang, and S.V. Faraone. 1989. Gender and schizophrenia: Implications for understanding the heterogeneity of the illness. *Psychiatry Res.* **28:** 243.

Gordon, C.T., D. Krasnewich, B. White, M. Lenane, and J.L. Rapoport. 1994. Brief report: Translocation involving chromosomes 1 and 7 in a boy with childhood-onset schizophrenia. *J. Autism Dev. Disorders* **24:** 537.

Gottesman, I.I. and J. Shields. 1982. *The epigenetic puzzle.* Cambridge University Press, New York.

Green, M.F., H.S. Bracha, P. Satz, and C.D. Christenson. 1994. Preliminary evidence for an association between minor physical anomalies and second trimester neurodevelopment in schizophrenia. *Psychiatry Res.* **53:** 119.

Griffon, N., M.A. Crocq, C. Pilon, M.P. Martres, A. Mayerova, G. Uyanik, E. Burgert, F. Duval, J.P. Macher, F. Javoy-Agid, C.A. Tamminga, J.C. Schwartz, and P. Sokoloff. 1996. Dopamine D3 receptor gene: Organization transcript variants, and polymorphism associated with schizophrenia. *Am. J. Med. Genet.* **67:** 63.

Gur, R.E. and G.D. Pearlson. 1993. Brain imaging in schizophrenia. A review. *Schizophr. Bull.* **19:** 337.

Gurling, H., G. Kalsi, A. Hui-Sui Chen, M. Green, R. Butler, T. Read, P. Murphy, D. Curtis, T. Sharma, H. Petursson, and J. Bryniolfsson. 1995. Schizophrenia susceptibility and chromosome 6p24-22. *Nat. Genet.* **11:** 234.

Gusella, J.F., N.S. Wexler, P.M. Conneally, S.L. Naylor, M.A. Anderson, R.E. Tanzi, P.C. Watkins, K. Ottina, M.R. Wallace, A.Y. Sakaguchi, A.B. Young, I. Shoulson, E. Bonilla, and J.B. Martin. 1983. A polymorphic DNA marker genetically linked to Huntington's disease. *Nature* **306:** 234.

Hattori, M. and S. Nanko. 1995. Association of neurotrophin-3 gene variant with severe forms of schizophrenia. *Biochem. Biophys. Res. Commun.* **209:** 513.

Holland, T. and C. Gosden. 1990. A balanced chromosomal translocation partially co-segregating with psychotic illness in a family. *Psychiatry Res.* **32:** 1.

Inayama, Y., H. Yoneda, T. Sakai, T. Ishida, Y. Nonomura, Y. Kono, R. Takahata, J. Koh, J. Sakai, A. Takai, Y. Inada, and H. Asaba. 1996. Positive association between a DNA sequence variant in the serotonin 2A receptor gene and schizophrenia. *Am. J. Med. Genet.* **67:** 103.

Itokawa, M., T. Arinami, N. Futamura, H. Hamaguchi, and M. Toru. 1993. A structural polymorphism of human dopamine D2 receptor, D2(Ser311→Cys). *Biochem. Biophys. Res. Commun.* **196:** 1369.

Jakob, H. and H. Beckmann 1986. Prenatal developmental disturbances in the limbic allocortex in schizophrenics. *J. Neural Transm.* **65:** 303.

Jones, P. and R.M. Murray. 1991. The genetics of schizophrenia is the genetics of neurodevelopment. *Br. J. Psychiatry* **158:** 615.

Jones, P., B. Rodgers, R. Murray, and M. Marmot. 1994. Child development risk factors for adult schizophrenia in the British 1946 birth cohort. *Lancet* **344:** 1398.

Kalsi, G., D. Curtis, J. Brynjolfsson, R. Butler, T. Sharma, P. Murphy, T. Read, H. Petursson, and H.M. Gurling. 1995. Investigation by linkage analysis of the XY pseudoautosomal region in the genetic susceptibility to schizophrenia. *Br. J. Psychiatry* **167:** 390.

Karayiorgou, M., M.A. Morris, B. Morrow, R.J. Shprintzen, R. Goldberg, J. Borrow, A. Gos, G. Nestadt, P.S. Wolyniec, V.K. Lasseter, H. Eisen, B. Childs, H.H. Kazazian, R. Kucherlapati, S.E. Antonarakis, A.E. Pulver, and D.E. Housman. 1995. Schizophrenia susceptibility associated with interstitial deletions of chromosome 22q11. *Proc. Natl. Acad. Sci.* **92:** 7612.

Katsanis, J., J. Ficken, W.G. Iacono, and M. Beiser. 1992. Season of birth and electrodermal activity in functional psychoses. *Biol. Psychiatry* **31:** 841.

Kendler, K.S. and S. Diehl. 1993. The genetics of schizophrenia: A current, genetic-epidemiologic perspective. *Schizophr. Bull.* **19:** 261.

Kendler, K.S., C.C. Masterson, R. Ungaro, and K.L. Davis. 1984. A family history study of schizophrenia-related personality disorders. *Am. J. Psychiatry* **41:** 424.

Kendler, K.S., M. McGuire, A. M. Gruenberg, A. O'Hare, M. Spellman, and D. Walsh. 1993. The Roscommon family study. III. Schizophrenia-related personality disorders in relatives. *Arch. Gen. Psychiatry* **50:** 781.

Kennedy, J.L., E.A. Billett, F.M. Macciardi, M. Verga, T.J. Parsons, H.Y. Meltzer, J. Lieberman, and J.A. Buchanan. 1995. Association study of dopamine d3 receptor gene and schizophrenia. *Am. J. Med. Genet.* **60:** 558.

Kennedy, J.L., L.A. Giuffra, H.W. Moises, L.L. Cavalli-Sforza, A.J. Pakstis, J.R. Kidd, C.M. Castiglione, B. Sjogren, L. Wetterberg, and K.K. Kidd. 1988. Evidence against linkage of schizophrenia to markers on chromosome 5 in a northern Swedish pedigree. *Nature* **336:** 166.

Keshavan, M.S., S. Anderson, and J.W. Pettegrew. 1994. Is schizophrenia due to excessive synaptic pruning in the prefrontal cortex? The Feinberg hypothesis revisited. *J.*

Psychiatr. Res. **28:** 239.

Kringlen, E. and G. Cramer. 1989. Offspring of monozygotic twins discordant for schizophrenia. *Arch. Gen. Psychiatry* **46:** 873.

Kruglyak, L. and E.S. Lander. 1995. Complete multipoint sib-pair analysis of qualitative and quantitative traits. *Am. J. Hum. Genet.* **57:** 439.

Kruglyak, L., M.J. Daly, M.P. Reeve-Daly, and E.S. Lander. 1996. Parametric and nonparametric linkage analysis: A unified multipoint approach. *Am. J. Hum. Genet.* **58:** 1347.

Kuokkanen, S., M. Sundvall, J.D. Terwilliger, P.J. Tienari, J. Wikstrom, R. Holmdahl, U. Pettersson, and L. Peltonen. 1996. A putative vulnerability locus to multiple sclerosis maps to 5p14-p12 in a region syntenic to the murine locus Eae2. *Nat. Genet.* **13:** 477.

Lasseter, V.K., A.E. Pulver, P.S. Wolyniec, G. Nestadt, D. Meyers, M. Karayiorgou, D. Housman, S. Antonarakis, H. Kazazian, L. Kasch, R. Babb, M. Kimberland, and B. Childs. 1995. Follow-up report of potential linkage for schizophrenia on chromosome 22q (part 3). *Am. J. Med. Genet.* **60:**172.

Lathrop, G.M. and J.M. Lalouel. 1984. Easy calculations of lod scores and genetic risks on small computers. *Am. J. Hum. Genet.* **36:** 460.

Lathrop, G.M., J.M. Lalouel, and R.L. White. 1986. Construction of human linkage maps: Likelihood calculations for multilocus linkage analysis. *Genet. Epidemiol.* **3:** 39.

Lathrop, G.M., J.M. Lalouel, C. Julier, and J. Ott. 1984. Strategies for multilocus linkage analysis in humans. *Proc. Natl. Acad. Sci.* **81:** 3443.

Levinson, D.F., D.B. Wildenauer, S.G. Schwab, M. Albus, J. Hallmayer, B. Lerer, W. Maier, D. Blackwood, W. Muir, D. St. Clair, S. Morris, H.W. Moises, L. Yang, H. Kristbjarnarson, T. Helgason, C. Wiese, D.A. Collier, P. Holmans, J. Daniels, M. Rees, P. Asherson, Q. Roberts, A. Cardno, M.J. Arranz, H. Vallada, et al. 1996. Additional support for schizophrenia linkage on chromosomes 6 and 8—A multicenter study. *Am. J. Med. Genet.* **67:** 580.

Lewis, S. 1989. Congenital risk factors for schizophrenia. *Psychol. Med.* **19:** 5.

Liang, K.Y. and A.E. Pulver. 1996. Analysis of case-control/family sampling design. *Genet. Epidemiol.* **13:** 253.

Lin, M.W., D. Curtis, N. Williams, M. Arranz, S. Nanko, D. Collier, P. McGuffin, R. Murray, M. Owen, M. Gill, and J. Powell. 1995. Suggestive evidence for linkage of schizophrenia to markers on chromosome 13q14.1-q32. *Psychr. Genet.* **5:** 117.

Lindsay, E.A., P. Rizzu, R. Antonacci, V. Jurecic, J. Delmas-Mata, C.C. Lee, U.J. Kim, P.J. Scambler, and A. Baldini. 1996. A transcription map in the CATCH22 critical region: Identification, mapping, and ordering of four novel transcripts expressed in heart. *Genomics* **32:** 104.

Lindsay, E.A., M.A. Morris, A. Gos, G. Nestadt, P.S. Wolyniec, V.K. Lasseter, R. Shprintzen, S.E. Antonarakis, A. Baldini, and A.E. Pulver. 1995. Schizophrenia and chromosomal deletions within 22q11.2. *Am. J. Hum. Genet.* **56:** 1502.

Lyon, M., C.E. Barr, T.D. Cannon, S.A. Mednick, and D. Shore. 1989. Fetal neural development and schizophrenia. *Schizophr. Bull.* **15:** 149.

Macciardi, F., J.L. Kennedy, L. Ruocco, L. Giuffra, P. Carrera, C. Marino, V. Rinaldi, E. Smeraldi, and M. Ferrari. 1992. A genetic linkage study of schizophrenia to chromosome 5 markers in a northern Italian population. *Biol. Psychiatry* **31:** 720.

Maier, W., F. Schmidt, S.G. Schwab, J. Hallmayer, J. Minges, M. Ackenheil, D. Lichtermann, and D.B. Wildenauer. 1995. Lack of linkage between schizophrenia and markers at the telomeric end of the pseudoautosomal region of the sex chromosomes. *Biol. Psychiatry* **37:** 344.

Malaspina, D., D. Warburton, X. Amador, M. Harris, and C.A. Kaufmann. 1992. Association of schizophrenia and partial trisomy of chromosome 5p. A case report. *Schizophr. Res.* **7:** 191.

Marsh, L., R.L. Suddath, N. Higgins, and D.R. Weinberger. 1994. Medial temporal lobe structures in schizophrenia: Relationship of size to duration of illness. *Schizophr. Res.* **11:** 225.

Maziade, M., M. Debraekeleer, P. Genest, D. Cliche, J.P. Fournier, Y. Garneau, C. Shriqui, M.A. Roy, L. Nicole, V. Raymond, and M. Vekemans. 1993. A balanced 2:18 translocation and familial schizophrenia: Falling short of an association. *Arch. Gen. Psychiatry* **50:** 73.

McGue, M. and I.I. Gottesman. 1991. The genetic epidemiology of schizophrenia and the design of linkage studies. *Eur. Arch. Psychiatry Clin. Neurosci.* **240:** 174.

McGuffin, P., M. Sargeant, G. Hetti, S. Tidmarsh, S. Whatley, and R.M. Marchbanks. 1990. Exclusion of a schizophrenia susceptibility gene from the chromosome 5q11-q13 region: New data and a reanalysis of previous reports. *Am. J. Hum. Genet.* **47:**524.

McNeil, T.F. 1995. Perinatal risk factors and schizophrenia: selective review and methodological concerns. *Epidemiol. Rev.* **17:** 107.

Moises, H.W., L. Yang, T. Li, B. Havsteen, R. Fimmers, M.P. Baur, X.H. Liu, and I.I. Gottesman. 1995a. Potential linkage disequilibrium between schizophrenia and locus D22S278 on the long arm of chromosome 22. *Am. J. Med. Genet.* **60:** 465.

Moises, H.W., L. Yang, H. Kristbjarnarson, C. Wiese, W. Byerley, F. Macciardi, V. Arolt, D. Blackwood, X. Liu, B. Sjogren, H.N. Auchauer, H.G. Hwu, K. Jang, W.J. Livesley, J.L. Kennedy, T. Zoega, O. Ivarsson, M.T. Bui, M.H. Yu, B. Havsteen, D. Commenges, J. Weissenbach, E. Schwinger, I.I. Gottesman, A.J. Pakstis, L. Wetterberg, K.K. Kidd, and T. Helgason. 1995b. An international two-stage genome-wide search for schizophrenia susceptibility genes. *Nat. Genet.* **11:** 321.

Murray, R.M. 1994. Neurodevelopmental schizophrenia: The rediscovery of dementia praecox. *Br. J. Psychiatry* **25:** 6.

Murray, R.M. and S.W. Lewis. 1987. Is schizophrenia a neurodevelopmental disorder? *Br. Med. J.* **285:** 681.

Murray, R.M. and E. O'Callaghan. 1991. Neurodevelopmental schizophrenia. *Schizophr. Monitor* **1:** 1.

Murray, R.M., A.M. Revellry, and P. McGuffin. 1986. Genetic vulnerability to schizophrenia. *Schizophr. Bull.* **9:** 3.

Nanko, S., H. Kunugi, T. Sasaki, R. Fukuda, T. Kawate, and H. Kazamatsuri. 1993. Pericentric region of chromosome 9 is a possible candidate region for linkage study of schizophrenia. *Biol. Psychiatry* **33:** 655.

Nanko, S., M. Hattori, S. Kuwata, T. Sasaki, R. Fukuda, X.Y. Dai, K. Yamaguchi, Y. Shibata, and H. Kazamatsuri. 1994. Neurotrophin-3 gene polymorphism associated with schizophrenia. *Acta Psychiatr. Scand.* **89:** 390.

Nimgaonkar, V.L., X.R. Zhang, J.G. Caldwell, R. Ganguli, and A. Chakravarti. 1993a. Association study of schizophrenia with dopamine D3 receptor gene polymorphisms: Probable effects of family history of schizophrenia? *Am. J. Med. Genet.* **48:** 214.

Nimgaonkar, V.L., R. Ganguli, W.A. Rudert, C. Vavassori,

B.S. Rabin, and M. Trucco. 1993b. A negative association of schizophrenia with an allele of the HLA DQB1 gene among African-Americans. *Schizophr. Res.* **8:** 199.

Nimgaonkar, V.L., W.A. Rudert, X.R. Zhang, W.F. Tsoi, M. Trucco, and N. Saha. 1995. Further evidence for an association between schizophrenia and the HLA DQB1 gene locus. *Schizophr. Res.* **18:** 43.

Okoro, C., R. Bell, P. Sham, S. Nanko, P. Asherson, M. Owen, M. Gill, P. McGuffin, R.M. Murray, and D. Collier. 1995. No evidence for linkage between the X-chromosome marker DXS7 and schizophrenia. *Am. J. Med. Genet.* **60:** 461.

Ott, J. 1991. *Analysis of human genetic linkage,* revised edition. The Johns Hopkins University Press, Baltimore.

Owen, M.J. 1992. Will schizophrenia become a graveyard for molecular geneticists? *Psychol. Med.* **22:** 289.

Palmour, R.M., S. Miller, A. Fielding, M. Vekemans, and F.R. Ervin. 1994. A contribution to the differential diagnosis of the "group of schizophrenias," Structural abnormality of chromosome 4. *J. Psychiatry Neruosci.* **19:** 270.

Parnas, J. 1985. Mates of schizophrenic mothers: A study of assortative mating from the American-Danish high-risk project. *Br. J. Psychiatry* **140:** 490.

———. 1988. Assortative mating in schizophrenia: Results from the Copenhagen high-risk study. *Psychiatry* **51:** 58.

Petty, R.G., P.E. Barta, G.D. Pearlson, I.K. McGilchrist, R.W. Lewis, A.Y. Tien, A. Pulver, D.D. Vaughn, M.F. Casanova, and R.E. Powers. 1995. Reversal of asymmetry of the planum temporale in schizophrenia. *Am. J. Psychiatry* **152:** 715.

Polymeropoulos, M.H., H. Coon, W. Byerley, E.S. Gershon, L. Goldin, T.J. Crow, J. Rubenstein, M. Hoff, J. Holik, A.M. Smith, G. Sheilds, N.J. Bass, M. Poulter, R. Lofthouse, A. Vita, C. Morganti, C.R. Merril, and L.E. DeLisi. 1994. Search for a schizophrenia susceptibility locus on human chromosome 22. *Am. J. Med. Genet.* **54:** 93.

Pulver, A.E. and S.J. Bale. 1989. Availability of schizophrenic patients and their families for genetic linkage studies: Findings from the Maryland epidemiology sample. *Genet. Epidemiol.* **6:** 671.

Pulver, A.E., K.Y. Liang, P.S. Wolyniec, J. McGrath, B.A. Melton, L. Adler, and B. Childs. 1992a. Season of birth of siblings of schizophrenic patients (comments). *Br. J. Psychiatry* **160:** 71.

Pulver, A.E., C.H. Brown, P. Wolyniec, J. McGrath, D. Tam, L. Adler, W.T. Carpenter, and B. Childs. 1990. Schizophrenia: Age at onset, gender and familial risk. *Acta Psychiatr. Scand.* **82:** 344.

Pulver, A.E., K.Y. Liang, C.H. Brown, P. Wolyniec, J. McGrath, L. Adler, D. Tam, W.T. Carpenter, and B. Childs. 1992b. Risk factors in schizophrenia season birth, gender, and familial risk. *Br. J. Psychiatry* **160:** 65.

Pulver, A.E., G. Nestadt, R. Goldberg, R.J. Shprintzen, M. Lamacz, P.S. Wolyniec, B. Morrow, M. Karayiorgou, S.E. Antonarakis, D. Housman, and R. Kucherlapati. 1994a. Psychotic illness in patients diagnosed with velo-cardio-facial syndrome and their relatives. *J. Nerv. Ment. Dis.* **182:** 476.

Pulver, A.E., V.K. Lasseter, L. Kasch, P. Wolyniec, G. Nestadt, J.L. Blouin, M. Kimberland, R. Babb, S. Vourlis, H. Chen, M. Lalioti, M.A. Morris, M. Karayiorgou, J. Ott, D. Meyers, S.E. Antonarakis, D. Housman, and H.H. Kazazian. 1995. Schizophrenia: A genome scan targets chromosomes 3p and 8p as potential sites of susceptibility genes. *Am. J. Med. Genet.* **60:** 252.

Pulver, A.E., M. Karayiorgou, P.S. Wolyniec, V.K. Lasseter, L. Kasch, G. Nestadt, S. Antonarakis, D. Housman, H.H. Kazazian, D. Meyers, J. Ott, M. Lamacz, K.Y. Liang, J. Hanfelt, G. Ullrich, N. DeMarchi, E. Ramu, P.R. McHugh, L. Adler, M. Thomas, W.T. Carpenter, T. Manschreck, C.T. Gordon, M. Kimberland, R. Babb, J. Puck, and B. Childs. 1994b. Sequential strategy to identify a susceptibility gene for schizophrenia: Report of potential linkage on chromosome 22q12-q13.1: Part 1. *Am. J. Med. Genet.* **54:** 36.

Pulver, A.E., M. Karayiorgou, V.K. Lasseter, P. Wolyniec, L. Kasch, S. Antonarakis, D. Housman, H.H. Kazazian, D. Meyers, G. Nestadt, J. Ott, K.Y. Liang, M. Lamacz, M. Thomas, B. Childs, S.R. Diehl, S. Wang, B. Murphy, C. Sun, F.A. O'Neill, L. Nie, P. Sham, J. Burke, B.W. Duke, F. Duke, and 29 others. 1994c. Follow-up of a report of a potential linkage for schizophrenia on chromosome 22q12-q13.1 (part 2). *Am. J. Med. Genet.* **54:** 44.

Rao, D.C., N.E. Morton, I.I. Gottesman, and R. Lew. 1981. Path analysis of qualitative data on pairs of relatives: Application to schizophrenia. *Hum. Hered.* **31:** 325.

Rimmer, J. and B. Jacobsen. 1976. Differential fertility of adopted schizophrenics and their half-siblings. *Acta Psychiatr. Scand.* **54:** 161.

Rios, R., F. Sole, C. Montes, A. Vicente, M.M. Perez, M. Valle, and F. Gascon. 1995. A new case of trisomy 5 as sole cytogenetic anomaly in acute myleoid leukemia. *Cancer Genet. Cytogenet.* **84:** 120.

Risch, N. and M. Baron. 1984. Segregation analysis of schizophrenia and related disorders. *Am. J. Hum. Genet.* **36:** 1039.

Roberts, G.W. 1991. Schizophrenia: A neuropathological perspective. *Br. J. Psychiatry* **158:** 8.

Ross, C.A. and G.D. Pearlson. 1996. Schizophrenia, the heteromodal association neocortex and development: Potential for a neurogenetic approach. *Trends Neurosci.* **19:** 171.

Sacchetti, E., A. Calzeroni, A. Vita, A. Terzi, F. Pollastro, and C.L. Cazzullo. 1992. The brain damage hypothesis of the seasonality of births in schizophrenia and major affective disorders: Evidence from computerised tomography. *Br. J. Psychiatry* **160:** 390.

Sacker, A., D.J. Done, T.J. Crow, and J. Golding. 1995. Antecedents of schizophrenia and affective illness. Obstetric complications (comments). *Br. J. Psychiatry* **166:** 734.

Saha, N., J.S.H. Tay, W.F. Tsoi, and E.H. Kua. 1990. Association of Duffy blood group with schizophrenia in Chinese (letter). *Genet. Epidemiol.* **7:** 303.

Sanders, A.R., D.E. Rincon-Limas, R. Chakraborty, B. Grandchamp, J.D. Hamilton, W.E. Fann, and P.I. Patel. 1992. Association between genetic variation at the porphobilinogen deaminase gene and schizophrenia. *Schizophr. Res.* **8:** 211.

Satsangi, J., M. Parkes, E. Louis, L. Hashimoto, N. Kato, K. Welsh, J.D. Terwilliger, G.M. Lathrop, J.I. Bell, and D.P. Jewell. 1996. Two stage genome-wide search in inflammatory bowel disease provides evidence for susceptibility loci on chromosomes 3, 7, and 12. *Nat. Genet.* **14:** 199.

Schaffer, A.A., S.K. Gupta, K. Shriram, and R.W. Cottingham. 1994. Avoiding recomputation in linkage analysis. *Hum. Hered.* **44:** 225.

Schwab, S.G., M. Albus, J. Hallmayer, S. Honig, M.

Borrmann, D. Lichtermann, R.P. Ebstein, M. Ackenheil, B. Lerer, N. Risch, W. Maier, and D.B. Wildenauer. 1995a. Evaluation of a susceptibility gene for schizophrenia on chromosome 6p by multipoint affected sib-pair linkage analysis. *Nat. Genet.* **11:** 325.

Schwab, S.G., B. Lerer, M. Albus, W. Maier, J. Hallmayer, R. Fimmers, D. Lichtermann, J. Minges, B. Bondy, M. Ackenheil, D. Altmark, D. Hasib, E. Gur, R.P. Ebstein, and D.B. Wildenauer. 1995b. Potential linkage for schizophrenia on chromosome 22Q12- Q13—A replication study. *Am. J. Med. Genet.* **60:** 436.

Sherrington, R., J. Brynjolfsson, H. Petursson, M. Potter, K. Dudleston, B. Barraclough, J. Wasmuth, M. Dobbs, and H. Gurling. 1988. Localization of a susceptibility locus for schizophrenia on chromosome 5. *Nature* **366:** 164.

Spielman, R.S., R.E. McGinnis, and W.J. Ewens. 1993. Transmission test for linkage disequilibrium: The insulin gene region and insulin-dependent diabetes mellitus (IDDM). *Am. J. Hum. Genet.* **52:** 506.

St. Clair, D., D. Blackwood, W. Muir, D. Baillie, A. Hubbard, A. Wright, and H.J. Evans. 1989. No linkage of chromosome 5q11-q13 markers to schizophrenia in Scottish families. *Nature* **339:** 305.

Straub, R.E., C.J. MacLean, F.A. O'Neill, J. Burke, B. Murphy, F. Duke, R. Shinkwin, B.T. Webb, J. Zhang, D. Walsh, and K.S. Kendler. 1995. A potential vulnerability locus for schizophrenia on chromosome 6p24-22: Evidence for genetic heterogeneity. *Nat. Genet.* **11:** 287.

Susser, E., R. Neugebauer, H.W. Hoek, A.S. Brown, S. Lin, D. Labovitz, and J.M. Gorman. 1996. Schizophrenia after prenatal famine. Further evidence. *Arch. Gen. Psychiatry* **53:** 25.

Taylor, M.A. 1992. Are schizophrenia and affective disorder related? A selective literature review. *Am. J. Psychiatry* **149:** 22.

Terwilliger, J.D. 1994.The available possibilities to analyze data of polygenic disease statistically. In *IV Workshop of the Nordic Genome Initiative,* August (Abstr.).

Tsuang, M.T. and S.V. Faraone. 1995. The case for heterogeneity in the etiology of schizophrenia. *Schizophr. Res.* **17:** 161.

Tsuang, M.T., M.W. Gilbertson, and S.V. Faraone. 1991. The genetics of schizophrenia current knowledge and future directions. *Schizophr. Res.* **4:** 157.

Wang, S., C.E. Sun, C.A. Walczak, J.S. Ziegle, B.R. Kipps, L.R. Goldin, and S.R. Diehl. 1995. Evidence for a susceptibility locus for schizophrenia on chromosome 6pter-p22. *Nat. Genet.* **10:** 41.

Wang, Z.W., D. Black, N. Andreasen, and R.R. Crowe. 1993. Pseudoautosomal locus for schizophrenia excluded in 12 pedigrees. *Arch. Gen. Psychiatry* **50:** 199.

Wei, J., C.N. Ramchand, and G.P. Hemmings. 1995. Association of polymorphic VNTR region in the first intron of the human TH gene with disturbances of the catecholamine pathway in schizophrenia. *Psychiatr. Genet.* **5:** 83.

Weinberger, D.R. 1987. Implications of normal brain development for the pathogenesis of schizophrenia. *Arch. Gen. Psychiatry* **44:** 660.

Wolyniec, P.S., A.E. Pulver, J.A. McGrath, and D. Tam. 1992. Schizophrenia: Gender and familial risk. *J. Psychiatr. Res.* **26:** 17.

Zamani, M.G., M. De Hert, M. Spaepen, M. Hermans, P. Marynen, J.J. Cassiman, and J. Peuskens. 1994. Study of the possible association of HLA class II, CD4, and CD3 polymorphisms with schizophrenia. *Am. J. Med. Genet.* **54:** 372.

Molecular Genetic Studies of Schizophrenia

P. McGuffin[1] and M.J. Owen[1,2]
Divisions of [1]Psychological Medicine and [2]Medical Genetics, University of Wales College of Medicine, Cardiff, United Kingdom

The familial basis of schizophrenia has hardly ever been in doubt. This has been true since Kraepelin produced the first comprehensive clinical description of the disorder, which he termed *dementia praecox*, almost exactly 100 years ago. The term *schizophrenia* was subsequently introduced by the Swiss psychiatrist Eugen Bleuler, but essentially both psychopathologists agreed that they were dealing with a hereditary condition. The evidence favoring a familial basis for schizophrenia has been well summarized by Gottesman (1991), who has reviewed Western European studies comprehensively, showing that the risk over a lifetime for a member of the general population is just under 1%. This increases to 3–4% in second-degree relatives and to around 10% in the first-degree relatives of schizophrenics. The risk also increases with the number of affected relatives, such that the lifetime risk for someone who has both a schizophrenic parent and sibling is about 16%. Such a pattern of findings tells us that we are not dealing with a regular Mendelian disorder. Rather, it suggests that multiple genes are involved and that these may not be acting in a simple additive fashion (Risch 1990).

Two types of natural experiment afforded by twin and adoption studies demonstrate that the aggregation of schizophrenia in families is influenced by genes. The consistent finding in all adoptee studies is that the adopted-away biological offspring of schizophrenic parents show an increased risk of the disorder. Similarly, so-called "adoptee-family studies," which compare the rates of schizophrenia in the biological relatives of adopted-away schizophrenics with adopted relatives or relatives of control adoptees, show that it is the genetic relatives of schizophrenics who are at an increased risk of themselves developing the disorder (McGuffin et al. 1995; for review, see Gottesman 1991).

There have been many twin studies of schizophrenia, all of which have shown the same pattern of findings with higher concordance in monozygotic than dizygotic twins. Two studies that used operational diagnostic criteria based on the Diagnostic and Statistical Manual 3rd Edition (DSM-III) or the 3rd Edition Revised (DSM-IIIR) (American Psychiatric Association 1980, 1987) found the same proband-wise concordance of 46% in monozygotic twins and markedly lower concordances of 10% (Farmer et al. 1987) or 4% (Onstad et al. 1991) in dizygotic twins.

Taking all of the evidence together from family, adoption, and twin studies, there is a consistent pattern of results favoring an important genetic contribution to schizophrenia, but not a simple Mendelian basis. Consequently, two important questions arise. The first is, How much does nature contribute to schizophrenia, and how much does nurture (and how do the two combine)? The second is, How can we actually locate and identify the genes involved?

The first of these questions can be answered by applying standard biometric models. Schizophrenia can be considered as a liability/threshold trait whereby liability to develop the disorder is continuously distributed in the population, but only those individuals whose liability at some point exceeds a certain threshold actually manifest the disease. Under this model, first put forward by Falconer (1965) as a general explanation of the transmission of familial disorders, liability is assumed to be contributed by multiple factors (genetic and environmental) so that the distribution tends to be normal. It is assumed that the relatives of affected individuals have a mean liability that is increased compared with the population mean and hence will more often lie beyond the threshold for being affected. Typically in biometric models, environmental factors are considered to have two component parts, shared environment that contributes to the aggregation of a trait within families, and non-shared, or residual, environment that does not (Neale and Cardon 1990; McGuffin et al. 1994). When such models have been applied to schizophrenia data, typically the finding is of a heritability (the proportion of variance in liability contributed by genes in a given population) of around 70% (McGue et al. 1985; McGuffin et al. 1994). Furthermore, it is usually possible to drop the shared environmental component from the model altogether. This increases heritability estimates and suggests that the familial clustering of schizophrenia may be explained entirely by genetic factors (McGuffin et al. 1994). Support for this conclusion comes from the results of adoption studies and findings on monozygotic twins reared apart which suggest that the environment in which an individual is raised has little or no effect on susceptibility to schizophrenia (Gottesman 1991). Thus, the findings from classic and quantitative genetics clearly point to an important genetic contribution to schizophrenia. However, such studies have been unable to define the mode of inheritance with any certainty, apart from excluding the possibility that schizophrenia is a single-gene disorder, or a collection of single-gene disorders. This has meant that attempts to locate and identify the genes involved have been fraught with difficulty.

LINKAGE AND POSITIONAL CLONING

The prospect of being able to carry out positional cloning in schizophrenia was at first sight highly attractive, given our ignorance about its pathophysiology. The process of detecting linkage in a disorder of unknown etiology progressing to identification of the disease gene and ultimately discovering the function of normal and aberrant gene products carries with it incremental benefits for predictive testing, diagnosis, and development of treatments. Thus far, positional cloning has proved to be highly successful in Mendelian diseases, but can the approach work in a complex disorder such as schizophrenia? There are several problems. The first is that conventional linkage analysis leading to accurate localization of disease genes requires precise knowledge about the mode of transmission. There is also a requirement for a gene of major effect operating and, optimally, it should be the same gene in all families. However, in schizophrenia there may be etiological heterogeneity and, as we have already noted, it seems likely that the majority of cases result from the interplay of several, perhaps many, genes.

Such difficulties are not peculiar to schizophrenia but are true of nearly all common familial diseases on which linkage analysis has been attempted. Problems are typically addressed by making a number of simplifying assumptions. First, it is assumed that genes of major effect are operating in at least some families, and this is usually taken to mean families in which multiple cases are found in two, three, or more generations. Second, it is postulated that, although there may be etiological heterogeneity in the disorder as a whole, each of those families that are found to contain multiple affecteds can be considered to be homogeneous. Third, it is assumed that even though no overall mode of transmission can be assumed with certainty, within multiply affected pedigrees it is safe to make approximate inferences (e.g., dominant inheritance with reduced penetrance).

This general approach has in fact been highly successful in identifying Mendelian subforms of common diseases such as Alzheimer's disease and breast cancer (McPherson et al. 1994; Sandbrink et al. 1996). In both of these examples, the major gene subforms are associated with early onset. In the case of breast cancer, it would appear that germ-line mutations in BRCA1 or BRCA2 are not involved in the etiology of late-onset cases; indeed, it would seem that late-onset breast cancer consists mainly of cases where inherited factors play a small role (McPherson et al. 1994). Similarly in Alzheimer's disease, late-onset cases tend to show a lower degree of familiality. Mutations in the APP gene are responsible for 15–20% of familial early-onset forms (Goate et al. 1991) but appear not to play a part in late-onset disease (Liddell et al. 1995). The majority of cases of early-onset dominant type Alzheimer's disease are not APP-related, and missense mutations in the presenilin-1 gene on chromosome 14 or the presenilin-2 gene on chromosome 1 are more common. It now seems that an intronic polymorphism in the presenilin-1 gene is also associated with the late-onset forms of the disease (Kehoe et al. 1996; Wragg et al. 1996).

All of this shows that making a set of simplifying assumptions about complex diseases can work. Nevertheless, the findings on schizophrenia have been less straightforward. Although families containing multiple affected members over several generations exist and have been identified by many different groups, none of these has so far been shown to result from the segregation of a single gene. Indeed, even in carefully chosen families, there are often "irregularities" such as skipped generations and a range of different phenotypes in addition to typical "cases" of schizophrenia. Moreover, there are no clear features such as early onset that allow such cases to be distinguished from schizophrenia as a whole. It is perhaps not surprising, therefore, that early optimism engendered by a report of a dominant gene with incomplete penetrance on chromosome 5q (Sherrington et al. 1988) was soon followed by disappointment when several other groups failed to replicate the finding (McGuffin et al. 1990).

Recent linkage results are reviewed in greater detail elsewhere in this volume and therefore are considered only briefly here. In our view, the most promising findings so far are those suggesting susceptibility loci on chromosomes 6, 8, 13, and 22.

The first finding of sustained interest came from a genome scan in 39 multiply affected families (Pulver et al. 1994a). Convincing evidence for linkage was not obtained, but a post-hoc analysis which maximized the LOD score by varying the genetic model suggested a susceptibility locus at 22q12-q13. The same group coordinated a four-center study aimed at replicating these findings, but the overall results were negative (Pulver et al. 1994b). However, a number of groups have also reported positive data from this region (Coon et al. 1994; Vallada et al. 1995). Subsequently, a group from the United Kingdom coordinated a meta-analysis of data from eleven centers using the more robust affected-sib-pairs approach, which suggested (p=0.001) a susceptibility loan linked to D22S278 (Schizophrenia Collaborative Linkage Group 1996). Two groups have subsequently attempted to pinpoint a chromosome 22 susceptibility locus with a greater accuracy using the transmission disequilibrium test and have reported the most significant results as being at the adjacent markers D22S278 (Moises et al. 1995a) and D22S283 (Vallada et al. 1995). Unfortunately, the weak association detected in the latter study was not statistically significant after correction for multiple testing. In the former study, transmission distortion was observed in pedigrees already showing allele sharing and may have resulted from linkage rather than association. Indeed, in a subsequent case-control study, we were unable to detect linkage disequilibrium between either D22S278 or D22S283 and schizophrenia (N.M. Williams et al. 1996).

The short arm of chromosome 6 was probably the most intensely studied part of the genome in the "premolecular" era of psychiatric genetic research, with many groups carrying out association studies of the HLA system as well as a smaller number performing linkage studies. The results overall gave no evidence of linkage, although some weak but fairly consistent associations emerged; particularly between HLAA9 and paranoid schizophrenia (McGuffin and Sturt 1986). Much more recently, Straub et al. (1995) published results of analyses of markers from chromosome 6p24-p22 in 265 Irish families multiply affected by schizophrenia which, allowing for heterogeneity, gave a maximum LOD score of 3.5 at D6S296. Multi-point analysis with this and other markers did not suggest linkage with HLA. Positive, but not highly significant, LOD scores were subsequently reported by three independent groups (Antonarakis et al. 1995; Schwab et al. 1995; Moises et al. 1995b) but not by others (Gurling et al. 1995; Mowry et al. 1995). The markers yielding strongest evidence for linkage differed somewhat between the four positive studies, but there was also a degree of overlap. Therefore, it seems likely that there is a susceptibility gene for schizophrenia at 6p24-p22 but that it is either of small overall effect or operating in only a small subset of families.

Rather weaker evidence has emerged that the short arm of chromosome 8 (Moises et al. 1995b; Pulver et al. 1995) may also contain a susceptibility gene, and we have reported preliminary evidence for linkage of schizophrenia to markers on chromosome 13q14-q32 (Lin et al. 1995) which is gaining support from other groups (see Pulver et al., this volume). Currently, attempts to replicate these findings are under way using a multicenter collaboration based on that assembled to study chromosome 22.

In summary, there appears to be emerging evidence from several different centers that positive results relating to chromosomes 6, 8, 13, and 22 cannot be explained purely by chance. However, for all four locations there is evidence of heterogeneity. Moreover, the evidence points to their being susceptibility loci, each of comparatively small effect and each neither necessary nor sufficient to cause schizophrenia. Thus far, schizophrenia would appear to be more like type 1 diabetes mellitus (Davies et al. 1994) than either Alzheimer's disease or breast cancer in being a common familial disorder where Mendelian subforms are either rare or nonexistent, but where the condition overall is substantially heritable and contributed to by multiple loci. The implications for further studies are therefore clear. These need to focus on methods capable of detecting genes of comparatively small effect independent of the mode of transmission. Consequently, there has been a shift away from attempting to study the cosegregation of markers and schizophrenia within large multiply affected pedigrees toward collection specifically of affected sib pairs and of samples for allelic association analyses. For the remainder of this paper we focus on the latter, with a particular emphasis on our own findings.

ASSOCIATION STUDIES

Providing that stratification can be excluded, the causes of allelic association between a marker and a disease are either pleiotropy or linkage disequilibrium. Pleiotropy is the phenomenon whereby a marker has two (or more) properties consisting of (1) being detectable as a polymorphism and (2) having a direct effect on a trait, such as susceptibility to a disease. Linkage disequilibrium results from a marker and a susceptibility locus being so tightly linked that the association between a particular allele and susceptibility to the disorder is maintained over many generations of recombination. In practice, linkage disequilibrium between two loci tends to occur if the distance between them is one centimorgan or less. Although it is theoretically possible, and may soon be practicably feasible, to carry out a systematic genome search with markers as closely spaced as this, for the present, allelic association studies have been restricted to attempts to "saturate" regions identified by linkage studies and to studies of candidate genes. In the latter case, there are clear attractions to studying those variations that affect protein structure or expression rather than relying on the maintenance of linkage disequilibrium (Sobell et al. 1992).

Abnormalities of dopaminergic neurotransmission have long been implicated in schizophrenia. It is now known that there are two families of dopamine receptors, classed as D1-like and D2-like, both of which are G-protein-coupled but have opposite effects on cAMP activity and differing pharmacological specificity (Sokoloff et al. 1992). Typical antipsychotic drugs have a high affinity for D2-like receptors, and much recent attention has focused on the members of the D2 family known as D3 and D4 that are largely expressed in limbic areas of the brain. In particular, studies on rat brain have shown that expression of the D3 receptor gene is up-regulated both by the administration of typical (e.g., haloperidol) and atypical neuroleptics (e.g., clozapine) (Buckland et al. 1992). In contrast, up-regulation of D1 receptors and the D2 receptor itself occurs only after the administration of typical neuroleptics (Buckland et al. 1993).

The human D3 receptor maps to chromosome 3q13.3 and has a polymorphic site in the first exon that gives rise to a glycine-to-serine substitution in the amino-terminal extracellular domain. This produces a *BalI* restriction site (Lannfelt et al. 1992). Two groups (our own in Cardiff, UK and another in Rouffach and

Paris, France) were independently able to demonstrate increased homozygosity at the *Bal*I D3 receptor polymorphism in schizophrenics compared with controls (Crocq et al. 1992). We were subsequently able to replicate this finding (Mant et al. 1994), and two other studies have provided partial support. Jonssen et al. (1993) found increased levels of homozygosity in schizophrenics who were good responders to neuroleptics, and Nimgaonkar et al. (1993) found a strong effect in schizophrenics with a family history of the disorder. In total, there have now been over 20 studies and, although many of these have shown small, nonsignificant or absent homozygosity effects in schizophrenia, a meta-analysis demonstrates a small excess of homozygotes of the 1-1 genotype associated with an odds ratio of 1.3 and significant heterogeneity (J. Williams et al., in prep.).

We have earlier mentioned that stratification needs to be excluded in allelic association studies. This refers to the phenomenon whereby there have been recent admixtures of populations such that a marker-disease association results simply from both the disease and a marker allele occurring at a higher frequency in one component of the population admixture than in another. Other than ensuring that studies are carried out on homogeneous populations with good ethnic matching between patients and controls, association studies can be carried out on family material consisting of affected individuals and both their parents. In such parent-offspring trios, comparing the frequency of transmitted with untransmitted alleles provides an internal control that is not affected by stratification. J. Williams et al. (in prep.) have performed a transmission test for linkage disequilibrium (Spielman et al. 1993) to family data from nine European centers and showed a significant distortion in the direction of homozygote transmission. Again, schizophrenia appeared more specifically to be associated with the 1-1 genotype with an odds ratio of approximately 2.

The functional significance of the glycine-to-serine change in exon 1 of the dopamine D3 receptor gene is still unknown. Possible explanations of the association with schizophrenia are either that the polymorphism itself confers the susceptibility or that it is in linkage disequilibrium with a different polymorphism in or near the D3 receptor gene. Asherson et al. (1996) have screened all six exons that make up the coding region of the gene using single-stranded conformational polymorphism analysis (SSCP). No other mutations were found that altered protein structure in a total of 36 schizophrenics and the same number of controls. Although no evidence of linkage was found in 24 multiply affected families, an excess of homozygotes was again observed among schizophrenics in a case-control comparison. When added to our earlier sample (Mant et al. 1994), the excess both of homozygotes overall and of the 1-1 genotype was significant with, as in some previous studies, most of the effect being contributed by males rather than females.

Because of their putative role as a principal site of therapeutic action of atypical neuroleptics such as clozapine, risperidone, and sertindole, recent attention has focused on the possible involvement of serotonin (5HT2) receptors in schizophrenia. A comparatively small-scale Japanese study suggested an association between the T102C polymorphism in the 5HT2a receptor gene and schizophrenia (Inayama et al. 1994), and in the UK, an association was reported between this marker and response to clozapine (Arranz et al. 1995). Our own group has been responsible for setting up a large European collaboration involving seven centers, the European Multicentre Association Study of Schizophrenia (EMASS), and we have examined the T102C polymorphism in 571 schizophrenic patients and 639 ethnically matched controls. This showed an association between schizophrenia and allele 2 that was highly significant but with a small odds ratio of only 1.3. Nevertheless, because the allele 2 is very common in European populations, the excess among schizophrenics corresponds to an attributable fraction of 0.35 (J. Williams et al. 1996).

The T102C polymorphism is "silent" in the sense of not changing the amino acid sequence of the protein. Although it is possible that it could still affect the secondary structure and stability of the mRNA (Arranz et al. 1995), another explanation is that it does not directly affect susceptibility to schizophrenia but is in linkage disequilibrium with some other functionally significant variant within the 5HT2a receptor gene. Erdmann et al. (1996) have carried out a mutation screen of the whole coding region and have reported two coding mutations, neither of which appears to show an allelic association with schizophrenia. Nevertheless, there may be other variants of pathogenetic significance in the promoter or other regulatory regions, and a search for these is in progress.

ANTICIPATION AND DYNAMIC MUTATIONS

Although pharmacological studies provide the most obvious candidate genes for molecular genetic studies of schizophrenia, less direct clues about what kinds of mutations are involved can be provided by patterns of disorder within families. In particular, the phenomenon of anticipation points to the involvement of trinucleotide repeat expansions. It has long been observed that for some inherited disorders there is a progressively earlier age at onset in successive generations, and this may be accompanied by increasing severity. Sir Frederick Mott (1910), director of the Neuropathological Laboratories at the Maudsley Hospital, first put forward what he called "the law of anticipation of the insane" and stated that "almost invariably in the case of insane parents and offspring, the offspring is affected earlier than the parent." The term was subsequently applied to neurological and other diseases, but the whole question of whether anticipation is a real phenomenon or whether it resulted from ascertainment biases was hotly disputed (Asherson et al. 1994). In particular, Penrose (1948) put forward a number of reasons why anticipation in myotonic dystrophy might really be artifactual. However, it is now known that the mutation involved in myotonic dystrophy consists of an expanded CTG repeat at the 3′ end of the gene (Brook et al. 1992), and increase in the size of this unstable mutation over generations is associated with earlier age of onset and a more severe form of the disorder. A number of other disorders, all of which affect the nervous system, have now been shown to involve trinucleotide repeat expansions. Although most of these diseases are very rare, one example, Huntington's disease, is reasonably common, and expansion of a CAG repeat explains variations in age of onset (Huntington's Disease Collaborative Research Group 1993).

Recent studies seeking to demonstrate anticipation in schizophrenia have shown lower average ages of onset in offspring than in parents in families multiply affected by the disorder. Although some have viewed this finding with a degree of skepticism (Asherson et al. 1994), others have been more sanguine (Bassett and Honer 1994). Consequently, studies have been mounted using repeat expansion detection (RED) analysis to compare findings in schizophrenics and controls. This has been carried out by our own group in Cardiff (O'Donovan et al. 1995) and by a collaboration in England involving London and Cambridge (Morris et al. 1995). Both studies show a maximum ligation product size that is greater in patients than controls; this has subsequently been replicated on an additional sample (O'Donovan et al. 1996). Although the patient/control differences are statistically significant in all three studies, all three show an overlap in the distribution of ligation product size between the patients and controls. Furthermore, the finding is not specific to schizophrenia, since both we (O'Donovan et al. 1995, 1996) and another group (Lindblad et al. 1995) find a similar effect in patients with bipolar disorder. Another puzzling finding is that there appears to be no consistent relationship between repeat size and age at onset of either schizophrenia or bipolar disorder, suggesting that a dynamic mutation is unlikely to account for much of the population variability in the age of onset of these disorders or to explain the apparent phenomenon of anticipation. Indeed, we have found that the unaffected parents of individuals with either bipolar disorder or schizophrenia carry repeats that are significantly larger than those of controls, but not significantly smaller than the affected offspring. This suggests that whatever is the nature of a CAG/CTG dynamic mutation in schizophrenia or bipolar disorder, it cannot on its own account for the transmission of these diseases, and it is of course uncertain as to whether there are different dynamic mutations in bipolar disorders and schizophrenia. Neither can RED analysis tell us whether there is just one or several different dynamic mutations in each disease. In summary, the evidence in favor of dynamic mutations in schizophrenia is persuasive, but, again, the genes containing such mutations appear, on their own, to have only a small effect.

CONCLUSIONS

Although the findings overall are complex and difficult to interpret, some consistent patterns are beginning to emerge in molecular genetic studies of schizophrenia. The results of linkage studies appear promising for susceptibility loci on chromosomes 6, 8, 13, and 22. It will be intriguing to see whether these are supported by large-scale collaborative studies that are nearing completion under the auspices of the European Science Foundation in Europe and the National Institutes of Mental Health in the United States. Although it is controversial, the dopamine D3 receptor gene's candidature as a susceptibility locus in schizophrenia appears to be holding up. The involvement of the 5HT2a receptor gene is of considerable interest and the search is on for functional variants in its promoter and regulatory regions. Although its identity is unknown, an anonymous gene or genes containing a CTG/CAG repeat seems likely to be involved in the etiology of schizophrenia or perhaps the major functional psychoses as a whole.

What is emerging is a disorder where multiple genes contribute to the liability, although each gene on its own has a comparatively small effect. This is precisely the model first put forward by Falconer to explain the transmission of common diseases and applied to schizophrenia almost 30 years ago by Gottesman and Shields (1967). However, what we are beginning to see is their statistical abstraction turning to a more tangible molecular reality. The main challenge now is how to convert tentative and suggestive findings of linkage into confident localizations to well-circumscribed regions. This will almost certainly require the use of large samples on the one hand of families containing affected relative pairs and on the other of unrelated individuals for linkage disequilibrium mapping. A second challenge will be to develop and refine methods to facilitate the genotyping of such large samples (Daniels et al. 1995). Finally, we need to develop methods to allow a large number of genes mapping to particular chromosomal regions to be screened for mutations.

ACKNOWLEDGMENTS

Our work has been supported by the MRC (UK), Glaxo Wellcome Research and Development, and the Welsh Scheme for Development of Health and Social Research.

REFERENCES

American Psychiatric Association. 1980. *Diagnostic and statistical manual (DSM-III)*, 3rd edition. American

Psychiatric Association, Washington, D.C.

American Psychiatric Association. 1987. *Diagnostic and statistical manual (DSM-IIIR)*, 3rd edition. American Psychiatric Association, Washington, D.C.

Antonarakis, S.E., J. Blouin, A.E. Pulver, P. Wolyniec, V.K. Lasseter, G. Nestadt, L. Kasch, R. Babb, H.H. Kazazian, B. Dombroski, M. Kimberland, J. Ott, D. Housman, M. Karayiorgou, and C.J. Maclean. 1995. Schizophrenia susceptibility and chromosome 6p24. *Nat. Genet.* **11:** 235.

Arranz, M.J., D. Collier, M. Sodhi, D. Ball, G. Roberts, J. Price, P. Sham, and R. Kerwin. 1995. Association between clozapine response and allelic variation in the 5HT2A receptor gene. *Lancet* **346:** 281.

Asherson, P., C. Walsh, J. Williams, M. Sargeant, C. Taylor, A. Clements, M. Gill, M. Owen, and P. McGuffin. 1994. Imprinting and anticipation. Are they relevant to genetic studies of schizophrenia? *Br. J. Psychiatry* **164:** 619.

Asherson, P., R. Mant, P. Holmans, J. Williams, A. Cardno, K. Murphy, L. Jones, D. Collier, P. McGuffin, and M.J. Owen. 1996. Linkage, association and mutational analysis of the dopamine D3 receptor gene in schizophrenia. *Mol. Psychiatry* **1:** 125.

Bassett, A.S. and G.H. Honer. 1994. Evidence for anticipation in schizophrenia. *Am. J. Genet.* **54:** 864.

Brook, J.D., M.E. McCurrach, H.G. Harley, A.J. Buckler, D. Church, H. Aburatani, K. Hunter, V.P. Stanton, J.P. Thirion, T. Hudson, R. Sohn, B. Zemelman, R.G. Snell, S.A. Rundle, S. Crow, J. Davies, P. Shelbourne, J. Buxton, C. Jones, V. Juvonen, K. Johnson, P.S. Harper, D.J. Shaw, and D.E. Housman. 1992. Molecular basis of myotonic dystrophy: Expansion of a trinucleotide (CTG) repeat at the 3′ end of a transcript encoding a protein kinase family member. *Cell* **68:** 799.

Buckland, P.R., M.C. O'Donovan, and P. McGuffin. 1992. Changes in dopamine D1, D2 and D3 receptor mRNA levels in rat brain following antipsychotic treatment. *Psychopharmacology* **106:** 479.

———. 1993. Clozapine and sulpiride upregulate dopamine D3 receptor mRNA levels. *Neuropharmacology* **32:** 901.

Coon, H., S.H. Jensen, J. Holik, M. Hoff, M. Myles-Worsley, F. Reimherr, P. Wender, W. Merilyne, R. Freedaman, M. Leppert, and W. Byerley. 1994. Genomic scan for genes predisposing to schizophrenia. *Am. J. Med. Genet.* **54:** 59.

Crocq, M.A., R. Mant, P. Asherson, J. Williams, Y. Hode, A. Mayerova, D. Collier, L. Lannfelt, P. Sokoloff, J.-C. Schwartz, M. Gill, J.-P. Macher, P. McGuffin, and M.J. Owen. 1992. Association between schizophrenia and homozygosity at the dopamine D3 receptor gene. *J. Med. Genet.* **29:** 858.

Daniels, J.K., N.M. Williams, R. Plomin, P. McGuffin, and M.J. Owen. 1995. Selective DNA pooling using automated technology: A rapid technique for allelic association studies in quantitative traits and complex diseases. *Psychiatr. Genet.* **153:** 268.

Davies, J.L., Y. Kawaguchi, S.T. Bennett, J.B. Copeman, H.J. Cordell, L.E. Pritchard, P.W. Reed, S.C.L. Gough, S.C. Jenkins, S.M. Palmer, K.M., Balfour, B.R. Rowe, M. Farrall, A.H. Barnett, S.C. Bain, and J.A. Todd. 1994. A genome-wide search for human type 1 diabetes susceptibility genes. *Nature* **371:** 132.

Erdmann, J., D. Shimron-Abarbanell, and M. Rietschel. 1996. Systematic screening for mutations in the human serotonin-2A (5HT2A) receptor gene: Identification of two naturally occurring receptor variants and association analysis in schizophrenia. *Hum. Gen.* **97:** 614.

Falconer, D.S. 1965. The inheritance of liability to certain diseases, estimated from the incidence among relatives. *Ann. Hum. Genet.* **29:** 51.

Farmer, A.E., P. McGuffin, and I.I. Gottesman. 1987. Twin concordance and DSM III schizophrenia: Scrutinizing the validity of the definition. *Arch. Gen. Psychiatry* **44:** 634.

Goate, A., M. Chartier-Harlin, M. Mullan, J. Brown, T. Crawford, L. Fidani, L. Giuffra, A. Haynes, N. Irving, L. James, R. Mant, P. Newton, K. Rooke, P. Roques, C. Talbot, M. Pericak-Vance, A. Roses, R. Williamson, M. Rossor, M. Owen, and J. Hardy. 1991. Segregation of a missense mutation in the amyloid precursor protein gene with familial Alzheimer's disease. *Nature* **349:** 704.

Gottesman, I.I. 1991. *Schizophrenia genesis.* W.H. Freeman, New York.

Gottesman, I.I. and J. Shields. 1967. A polygenic theory of schizophrenia. *Proc. Natl. Acad. Sci.* **1:** 199.

Gurling, H., G. Kalsi, A.H. Chen, M. Green, R. Butler, T. Read, P. Murphy, D. Curtis, T. Sharma, H. Petursson, and J. Brynjolfsson. 1995. Schizophrenia susceptibility and chromosome 6p24-22. *Nat. Genet.* **11:** 234.

Huntington's Disease Collaborative Research Group 1993. A novel gene containing a trinucleotide repeat that is expanded and unstable on Huntington's disease chromosomes. *Cell* **72:** 971.

Inayama, Y., H. Yoneda, T. Ishida, Y. Nonomura, Y. Kono, J. Koh, K. Kuroda, H. Higashi, H. Asaba, and T. Sakai. 1994. An association between schizophrenia and a serotonin receptor DNA marker (5HTR2). *Neuropsychopharmacology* **10:** 56.

Jonsson, E., L. Lannfelt, P. Sokoloff, J.C. Schwartz, and G. Sedrall. 1993. Lack of association between schizophrenia and alleles of the D3 receptor gene. *Acta. Psychiatr. Scand.* **87:** 345.

Kehoe, P., J. Williams, S. Lovestone, G. Wilcock, M.J. Owen, and the U.K. Alzheimer's Disease Collaborative Group. 1996. Presenilin 1 polymorphism and Alzheimer's disease. *Lancet* **347:** 1185.

Lannfelt, L., P. Sokoloff, M. Martres, C. Pilon, B. Giros, E. Jonsson, G. Sedvall, J.C. Schwartz, and R. Berger. 1992. Amino-acid substitution in the dopamine D3 receptor as a useful polymorphism for investigating psychiatric disorders. *Psychiatr. Genet.* **2:** 249.

Liddell, M.B., A.J. Bayer, and M.J. Owen. 1995. No evidence that common allelic variation in the amyloid precursor protein (APP) gene confers susceptibility to Alzheimer's disease. *Hum. Mol. Genet.* **4:** 853.(Abstr.)

Lin, M., D. Curtis, N. Williams, M. Arranz, S. Nanko, D. Collier, P. McGuffin, R. Murray, M. Owen, M. Gill, and J. Powell. 1995. Suggestive evidence for linkage of schizophrenia to markers on chromosome 13q14.1-q32. *Psychiatr. Genet.* **5:** 11.

Lindblad, K., P. Nylander, A. De Bruyn, D. Sourey, C. Zander, C. Engstrom, G. Holmgren, T. Hudson, J. Chotai, J. Mendlewicz, C. Van Broeckhoven, M. Schalling, and R. Adolfsson. 1995. Detection of expanded CAG repeats in bipolar affective disorder using the repeat expansion detection (RED) method. *Neurobiol. Dis.* **2:** 55.

Mant, R., J. Williams, P. Asherson, E. Parfitt, P. McGuffin, and M.J. Owen. 1994. Relationship between homozygosity at the dopamine D3 receptor gene and schizophrenia. *Am. J. Med. Genet.* **54:** 21.

McGue, M., I.I. Gottesman, and D.C. Rao. 1985. Resolving genetic models for the transmission of schizophrenia. *Genet. Epidemiol.* **2:** 99.

McGuffin, P. and E. Sturt. 1986. Genetic markers in schizophrenia. *Hum. Hered.* **16:** 461.

McGuffin, P., M.J. Owen, and A,E. Farmer. 1995. Genetic basis of schizophrenia. *Lancet* **346:** 678.

McGuffin, P., M.J. Owen, M.C. O'Donovan, A. Thapar, and I.I. Gottesman. 1994. *Seminars in psychiatric genetics.* Gaskell, London.

McGuffin, P., M. Sargeant, G. Hett, S. Tidmarsh, S. Whatley, and R.M. Marchbanks. 1990. Exclusion of a schizophrenia susceptibility gene from the chromosome 5q11-q13 region. New data and a reanalysis of previous reports. *Am. J. Hum. Genet.* **47:** 524.

McPherson, K., C.M. Steel, and J.M. Dixon. 1994. Breast cancer–Epidemiology, risk factors and genetics. *Br. Med. J.* **309:** 1003.

Moises, H.W., L. Yang, T. Li, B. Havsteen, R. Timmers, M.D. Baur, X. Liu, and I.I. Gottesman. 1995a. Potential linkage disequilibrium between schizophrenia and locus D22S278 on the long arm of chromosome 22. *Am. J. Med. Genet.* **60:** 465.

Moises, H.W., L. Yang, H. Kristbjarnarson, C. Wiese, W. Byerley, G. Macciardi, V. Arolt, D. Blackwood, X. Liu, B. Sjögren, H.N. Aschauer, H. Hwu, K. Jang, W.J. Livesley, J.L. Kennedy, T. Zoega, O. Ivarsson, M. Bui, M. Yu, B. Havsteen, D. Commenges, J. Weissenbach, E. Schwinger, I.I. Gottesman, A.J. Pakstis, L. Wetterburg, K.K. Kidd, and T. Helgason. 1995b. An international two-stage genome-wide search for schizophrenia susceptibility genes. *Nat. Genet.* **11:** 321.

Morris, A.G., E. Gaitonde, P.J. McKenna, J.D. Mollon, and D.M. Hunt. 1995. CAG repeat expansions and schizophrenia: Association with disease in females and with early age-at-onset. *Hum. Mol. Genet.* **4:** 1957.

Mott. F.W. 1910. Hereditary aspect of nervous and mental diseases. *Br. Med. J.* **2:** 1013.

Mowry, B.J., D.J. Mancarrow, D.P. Lennon, L.A. Sandkuijl, R.R. Crowe, J.M. Silverman, R.C. Mohs, L.J. Siever, J. Endicott, L. Sharpe, M.K. Walters, N.K. Hayward, and D.F. Levinson. 1995. Schizophrenia susceptibility and chromosome 6p24-22. *Nat. Genet.* **11:** 233.

Neale, M.C. and L.R. Cardon. 1990. *Methodology for genetic studies of twins and families.* Kluwer Academic, Dordrecht, The Netherlands.

Nimgaonkar, V.L., X.R. Zhang, J.G. Caldwell, R. Ganguli, and A. Chakravarti. 1993. Association study of schizophrenia with dopamine D3 receptor gene polymorphisms: Probable effects of family history of schizophrenia? *Am. J. Med. Genet.* **48:** 214.

O'Donovan, M.C., C. Guy, N. Craddock, K.C. Murphy, A.G. Cardno, L.A. Jones, M.J. Owen, and P. McGuffin. 1995. Expanded CAG repeats in schizophrenia and bipolar disorder. *Nat. Genet.* **10:** 380.

O'Donovan, M.C., C. Guy, N. Craddock, T. Bowen, P. McKeon, A. Macedo, W. Maier, D. Wildenauer, H.N. Aschauer, S. Sorbi, E. Feldman, L. Mynett-Johnson, E. Claffey, B. Nacimas, J. Valente, A. Douraco, E. Grassi, E. Lenzinger, A.M. Heiden, S. Moorhead, D. Harrison, J. Williams, P. McGuffin, and M.J. Owen. 1996. Confirmation of association between expanded CAG/CTG repeats and both schizophrenia and bipolar disorder. *Psychiatr. Med.* (in press).

Onstad, S., I. Skre, S. Torgersen, and E. Kringlen. 1991. Twin concordance for DSM-111-R schizophrenia. *Acta Psychiatr. Scand.* **83:** 395.

Penrose, L.S. 1948. The problem of anticipation in pedigrees of dystrophia myotonica. *Ann. Eugenics* **14:** 125.

Pulver, A.E., V.K. Lasseter, L. Kasch, P. Wolyniec, G. Nestadt, J.-L. Blouin, M. Kimberland, R. Babb, S. Vourlis, H. Chen, M. Lalioti, M.A. Morris, M. Karayiorgou, J. Ott, D. Meyers, S.E. Antonarakis, D. Housman, and H.H. Kazazian. 1995. Schizophrenia: A genome scan targets chromosome 3p and 8p as potential sites of susceptibility genes. *Am. J. Med. Genet.* **60:** 252.

Pulver, E.A., M. Karayiorgou, P. Wolyniec, V.K. Lasseter, L. Kasch, G. Nestadt, S. Antonarakis, D. Housman, H.H. Kazazian, D. Meyers, J. Ott, M. Lamacz, K. Liang, J. Hanfelt, G. Ullrich, N. DeMarchi, E. Ramu, P.R. McHugh, L. Adler, M. Thomas, W.T. Carpenter, T. Manschreck, C.T. Gordon, M. Kimberland, R. Babb, J. Puck, and B. Childs. 1994a. Sequential strategy to identify a susceptibility gene for schizophrenia: Report of potential linkage on chromosome 22q12-q13.1 (part 1). *Am. J. Med. Genet.* **54:** 36.

Pulver, A.E., M. Karayiorgou, V.K. Lasseter, P. Wolyniec, L. Kasch, S. Antonarakis, D. Housman, H.H. Kazazian, D. Meyers, G. Nestadt, J. Ott, K. Liang, M. Lamacz, M. Thomas, B. Childs, S.R. Diehl, S. Wang, B. Murphy, C. Sun, F.A. O'Neill, L. Nie, P. Sham, J. Burke, B.W. Dike, F. Duke, B.R. Kipps, J. Bray, W. Hunt, R. Shinkwin, M.N. Nuallain, Y. Su, C.J. Maclean, D. Walsh, K.S. Kendler, M. Gill, H. Vallada, R. Mant, P. Asherson, D. Collier, E. Parfitt, E. Roberts, S. Nanko, C. Walsh, J. Daniels, R. Murray, P. McGuffin, M. Owen, C. Laurent, J. Dumas, T. D'Amato, M. Jay, M. Martinez, D. Campion, and J. Mallet. 1994b. Sequential strategy to identify a susceptibility gene for schizophrenia: Report of a potential linkage on chromosome 22q12-q13.1 (part 2). *Am. J. Med. Genet.* **54:** 44.

Risch, N. 1990. Linkage strategies for genetically complex traits. III. The effect of marker polymorphism analysis on affected relative pairs. *Am. J. Hum. Genet.* **46:** 242.

Sandbrink, R., T. Hartmann, C.L. Masters, and K. Beyreuther. 1996. Genes contributing to Alzheimer's disease. *Mol. Psychiatry* **1:** 27.

Schizophrenia Collaborative Linkage Group. 1996. A combined analysis of D22S278 marker alleles in affected sib-pairs: Support for a susceptibility locus for schizophrenia at chromosome 22q12. *Am. J. Med. Genet.* **67:** 40.

Schwab, S.G., M. Albus, J. Hallnayer, S. Honig, M. Borrmann, D. Lichtermann, R.P. Ebstein, M. Ackenheil, B. Lerer, N. Risch, W. Maier, and D.R. Wildenauer. 1995. Evaluation of a susceptibility gene for schizophrenia on chromosome 6p by multipoint affected sib-pair linkage analysis. *Nat. Genet.* **11:** 325.

Sherrington, R., J. Brynjolfsson, H. Petursson, M. Potter, K. Dudleston, B. Barraclough, J. Wasmuth, M. Dobbs, and H. Gurling. 1988. Localization of a susceptibility locus for schizophrenia on chromosome 5. *Nature* **336:** 164.

Sobell, J.L., L.L. Heston, and S.S. Sommer. 1992. Delineation of genetic predisposition to multifactorial disease: A general approach on the threshold of feasibility. *Genomics* **12:** 1.

Sokoloff, P., L. Lannfeldt, M.P. Martres, B. Giros, M.L. Bouthenet, and J.C. Schwartz. 1992. The D3 dopamine receptor gene as a candidate gene for genetic linkage studies. In *Genetic research in psychiatry* (ed. J. Mendlewicz and H. Hippus), p. 135. Springer-Verlag, Berlin.

Spielman, R.S., R.E. McGinnis, and W.J. Ewenst. 1993. Transmission test for linkage disequilibrium: The insulin gene region and insulin-dependent diabetes mellitus (IDDM). *Am. J. Hum. Genet.* **52:** 506.

Straub, R.E., C.J. Maclean, F.A. O'Neill, J. Burke, B. Muphy, F. Duke, R. Shinkwin, B.T. Webb, J. Zhang, D. Walsh, and K.S. Kendler. 1995. A potential vulnerability locus for schizophrenia on chromosome 6p24-22: Evidence for genetic heterogeneity. *Nat. Genet.* **11:** 287.

Vallada, H., D. Curtis, P.C. Sham, R.M. Murray, P. McGuffin, S. Nanko, M. Gill, M. Owen, and D.A. Collier. 1995. Chromosome 22 markers demonstrate transmission disequilibrium with schizophrenia. *Psychiatr. Genet.* **5:** 127.

Williams, J., G. Spurlock, P. McGuffin, J. Mallet, M.M. Nothen, M. Gill, H.N. Aschauer, P. Nylander, F. Macciardi, and M.J. Owen. 1996. Association between schizophrenia and T102C polymorphism of the 5-hydroxytryptamine type 2a-receptor gene. *Lancet* **347:** 1294.

Williams, N.M., L.A. Jones, K.C. Murphy, A.G. Cardno, P. Asherson, J. Williams, P. McGuffin, and M.J. Owen. 1996. No evidence for allelic association between schizophrenia and markers D22S278 and D22S283. *Am. J. Med. Genet.* (in press).

Wragg, M., M. Hutton, C. Talbot, and the Alzheimer's Disease Collaborative Group. 1996. Genetic association between intronic polymorphism in presenilin-1 gene and late-onset Alzheimer's disease. *Lancet* **347:** 509.

Support for Schizophrenia Vulnerability Loci on Chromosomes 6p and 8p from Irish Families

R.E. STRAUB,[1] C.J. MACLEAN,[1,2] D. WALSH,[3] AND K.S. KENDLER[1,2]

Departments of [1]Psychiatry and [2]Human Genetics, Medical College of Virginia / Virginia Commonwealth University, Richmond, Virginia 23298; [3]The Health Research Board, Dublin, Ireland

Schizophrenia is a relatively common and frequently chronic and debilitating psychiatric disorder. Numerous twin, family, and adoption studies (Gottesman and Shields 1982; Kendler 1988; Kendler and Diehl 1993) suggest that genetic factors are of major etiologic importance. Several lines of evidence suggest that the mode of transmission is complex, perhaps including multiple genes and/or genetic heterogeneity, incomplete penetrance, and phenocopies (O'Rourke et al. 1982; Kendler and Diehl 1993; Prescott and Gottesman 1993; Cloninger 1994). To date, genetic linkage and association studies have not successfully identified the chromosomal location of vulnerability loci, and the non-replication of linkage and association findings in psychiatric disorders has been well chronicled (O'Donovan and Owen 1992; Cloninger 1994). Potential reasons for the difficulty of detection and confirmation of linkage have also been explored extensively (Elston 1994; Risch 1994; Suarez et al. 1994), and many authors have contributed their recommendations designed to overcome these difficulties (Baron 1990; Ott 1990; Risch 1990a,b; Kendler and Diehl 1993; Cloninger 1994). Given the complexities involved, it is unlikely that analysis of small numbers of pedigrees, using analytic methods designed for Mendelian disorders, will reveal the genetic etiology of this disorder. Indeed, the detection of linkage in a genetically complex trait such as schizophrenia may require large sample sizes (Martinez and Goldin 1989, 1990; Chen et al. 1992; Kendler and Diehl 1993; Suarez et al. 1994). Furthermore, standardized rules of ascertainment may improve chances of replication of positive results (Cloninger 1994).

When applied judiciously to samples of sufficient power, the complementary strategies of genetic linkage and association have met with some success in identifying genes in other complex disorders. The recent genome scans for insulin-dependent diabetes mellitus (Davies et al. 1994; Hashimoto et al. 1994) have yielded several new positive regions that are now targets for gene identification efforts and also have confirmed previously known loci. Likewise, studies in Alzheimer's disease (Tanzi et al. 1993), breast cancer (Easton et al. 1993), and tuberous sclerosis (European Chromosome 16 Tuberous Sclerosis Consortium 1993) have yielded multiple confirmed linkages and associations. Independent replication was essential to these successes, because some of the initial linkage findings were not striking. Because these diseases may resemble schizophrenia (e.g., genetically heterogeneous with incomplete penetrance), these advances provide justifiable optimism that when the same methodological rigor and molecular technologies are applied, we may expect some success in identifying vulnerability genes for schizophrenia.

Although no vulnerability genes have been unambiguously identified, several chromosomal regions and many candidate genes are currently under intensive scrutiny by a number of investigators. Initial positive linkage reports on chromosomes 6p (Straub et al. 1995; Wang et al. 1995) and 8p (Pulver et al. 1995) have been tentatively supported by a subsequent worldwide collaborative effort (Schizophrenia Linkage Collaborative Group for Chromosomes 3, 6 and 8 1996). However, the statistical evidence for each locus is only moderately convincing when evaluated by either traditional or recently proposed statistical criteria (Lander and Kruglyak 1995). Likewise, the potential linkage initially reported for 22q (Pulver et al. 1994) received only modest support during a collaborative follow-up (Gill et al. 1996). There is currently no consensus about how to interpret and utilize a pattern of multiple positive but non-significant linkage results (along with negative results), and therefore developing better strategies in this regard is an important goal.

The Irish Study of High Density Schizophrenia Families (ISHDSF) contains 1408 individuals in 265 pedigrees systematically ascertained from psychiatric facilities in Ireland and Northern Ireland. Using linkage analysis, we find strong support for the presence of loci influencing the susceptibility to schizophrenia in two chromosomal regions: 6p24-21 and 8p22-21. In this paper, we review our data only; an overview of the chromosome 6 findings by our group and other groups has been published previously (Straub et al. 1996).

METHODS

Pedigree ascertainment. ISHDSF is a collaborative project between the Medical College of Virginia; the Health Research Board, Dublin; and The Queen's University, Belfast. The linkage sample contained 1408 individuals from 265 systematically ascertained, multiplex schizophrenia pedigrees collected in Ireland and

Northern Ireland. Our entry "field" criteria were two or more first-, second-, or third-degree relatives who, according to the field psychiatrist, met DSM-III-R criteria for schizophrenia or poor-outcome schizoaffective disorder (PO-SAD) (Kendler et al. 1995). No exclusion criteria were used, so pedigrees were screened neither for bilineal descent of schizophrenia spectrum illness nor for the presence of other forms of psychopathology, such as bipolar illness. For inclusion into the linkage sample, each pedigree had to have two or more first-, second-, or third-degree relatives with a diagnosis of D1–D5 (see below), one or more of whom had a D1–D2 diagnosis. Of cases diagnosed with schizophrenia or schizoaffective disorder, 98.6% had psychiatric records.

Diagnostic assessment. The diagnostic instruments included the structured interview for DSM-III-R diagnosis (SCID) (Spitzer et al. 1992) for selected Axis I disorders (psychosis, major depression, mania, cyclothymia, dysthymia, alcohol abuse/dependence, panic disorder, and generalized anxiety disorder) and the structured interview for schizotypy (SIS) (Kendler et al. 1989) for putative schizophrenia spectrum personality disorders (schizotypal, paranoid, schizoid, and avoidant personality disorder). Diagnosis was made, using DSM-III-R criteria, based on all available information (personal history, hospital record, family history report) by individuals blind to knowledge of genotypes and to the psychopathology of relatives. Final diagnostic review was done by K.S.K. and D.W., whose agreement on diagnostic category was 74% (weighted κ: 0.94±0.05). The diagnostic categories are as follows:

Categories D1–D2 (narrow; 577 affecteds; 285 affected sib pairs): "core schizophrenic phenotypes"; schizophrenia, PO-SAD, and simple schizophrenia (Kendler et al. 1994).

Categories D1–D5 (intermediate; 700 affecteds; 420 affected sib pairs): a narrow definition of the schizophrenia spectrum including disorders which have been repeatedly shown to co-aggregate in pedigrees with narrowly defined schizophrenia (Kendler and Diehl 1993). This category adds to the narrow definition schizotypal personality disorder and all other nonaffective psychotic disorders (i.e., schizophreniform disorder, delusional disorder, atypical psychosis, and good-outcome SAD).

Categories D1–D8 (broad; 754 affecteds; 505 affected sib pairs): a broad definition of the schizophrenia spectrum. Includes all disorders that significantly aggregated in relatives of schizophrenic probands in the Roscommon family study (Kendler et al. 1993a,b,c), an epidemiological, controlled family study conducted in parallel in the west of Ireland. This category adds to the intermediate definition mood-incongruent and mood-congruent psychotic affective illness, and paranoid, avoidant, and schizoid personality disorder.

Categories D1–D9 (very broad; all psychiatric disorders; 961 affecteds): includes all other psychiatric disorders (e.g., nonpsychotic affective disorders, anxiety disorders, alcoholism, and other non-schizophrenia spectrum personality disorders).

Genotyping. DNA was extracted directly from blood, as well as from lymphoblastoid cell lines that were established by standard methods. Polymerase chain reaction (PCR) amplification and gel analysis of microsatellite markers were performed as described previously (Straub et al. 1993). To confirm familial relationships, we analyzed the data from 25 microsatellite markers simultaneously for allele sharing. All genotyping was done in the laboratory of Dr. Straub, by individuals blind to phenotype.

Linkage analysis. To calculate two-point (pairwise) LOD scores under the assumption of heterogeneity (hereafter termed H-LODs), the admixture test as implemented in the program MENDEL (Lange et al. 1988) was used, with modifications made by C.J.M. and L. Ploughman. We used four genetic models: dominant (Dom), additive on the penetrance scale (Pen), additive on the liability scale (Lia), and recessive (Rec). We only present the maximum LOD score for each marker; estimates of the recombination fractions (θ) and proportions of pedigrees segregating the disease locus (α) are available on request. The p values associated with H-LODs are greater than those seen with homogeneity LODs because the former require the estimation of an additional parameter (α). Parameters for the linkage analysis have been published previously (Straub et al. 1995).

Marker allele frequencies were calculated from at least 200 unrelated individuals. Based on prior epidemiological evidence that the prevalence of schizophrenia and other psychotic disorders in Ireland is approximately twice as great in males as in females (Kendler and Walsh 1995), penetrance values in females were set at 50% that of males. Selected H-LOD analyses were repeated assuming equal penetrances in the sexes; little change in results was seen. Finally, multipoint H-LODs and a nonparametric linkage (NPL) test were generated over the entire region using the GENEHUNTER (Kruglyak et al. 1996) (where results are expressed in LOD and normal deviate [z] units, respectively).

Those unfamiliar with linkage analysis may by puzzled at the multiplicity of tests described in this paper. LOD scores represent the traditional approach to linkage analysis used in classic medical genetic disorders (Morton 1956). The H-LOD test attempts to detect evidence for linkage in the presence of genetic heterogeneity by discounting evidence from the unlinked pedigrees (Smith 1963; Ott 1983). Nonparametric tests differ from H-LODs in not requiring a prior genetic model. Although lower in power, some consider these the methods of choice for linkage to complex disorders like schizophrenia (Lander and Schork 1994). Finally, two-point H-LODs utilize information only from a single genetic marker. We therefore present multipoint analyses that integrate evidence for linkage from all markers typed in a given region. We also examined evidence for linkage in these data using the C-test (MacLean et al. 1992) and extended sib-pair analysis (ESPA) (Sandkuijl 1989), and these data are presented elsewhere (Straub et al. 1995; Kendler et al. 1996).

RESULTS

Simulations of Statistical Power

We have examined the statistical power to detect linkage with LOD score analysis of the ISHDSF sample, assuming autosomal dominant transmission (see Methods section for parameters) and diagnostic category D1–D5. Using the LOD score calculated under heterogeneity (an admixture test), a vulnerability locus for schizophrenia segregating in 50% or more of the pedigrees in the ISHDSF can be detected more than 90% of the time. In contrast, if the most common major locus occurs in 10% or fewer of the pedigrees, our chances of detection are 10% or less. Power is still relatively good (67% at $\theta=0$ for LOD ≥ 3.7) when 30% of the pedigrees are linked. We have developed another measure of linkage, the C-test (MacLean et al. 1992), which is based on the sum of individual pedigree maximum LOD scores combined with a bootstrap method of estimating the null hypothesis distribution. Using the C-test, we found considerable power, even with the rigorous level of $p \leq 0.0001$, to detect linkage when only 20% of the pedigrees were linked.

Linkage Analysis: Chromosome 6

Markers and map of the region. Table 1 shows the marker characteristics and genetic map of the region, which was constructed using the genotyping data. The number of alleles and polymorphism information content (PIC) were those observed in the ISHDSF. Twenty markers spanning 36.8 cM (sex-averaged, Kosambi mapping function) were tested. This map constructed from the ISHDSF genotyping data agrees well with those from Genethon, the Cooperative Human Linkage Center, and a recent report (Volz et al. 1994). The largest gap in the sex-averaged map is 6.1 cM, between D6S470 and D6S443. D6S105 and D6S276 map distal to, D6S273 within, and D6S291 proximal to, the major histocompatibility (HLA) complex (Martin et al. 1995). All markers used were microsatellites of high heterozygosity, and since the locus information uniquely identifies specific microsatellite markers, we use those terms interchangeably.

Two-point LOD score results. Table 2 shows the maximum pairwise LOD scores, calculated under the assumption of heterogeneity using an admixture test (Smith 1963) as implemented by the program MEN-

Table 1. Chromosome 6p Markers and Genetic Map

				Distances (Kosambi cM)				
							sex average	
Region	Locus	Number of alleles	PIC	female	male	ratio	intermarker distance	map position
6	D6S477	13	0.79					0
6p24.2-p23	F13A1	10	0.68	1.4	2.4	0.6	1.9	1.9
6p24-p23	D6S309	11	0.82	3.1	3.2	0.9	3.2	5.1
6p24.2-p23	D6S277	14	0.77	0.3	2.3	0.1	1.3	6.4
6p24.2-p23	D6S263	17	0.80	0.2	0.1	2.0	0.2	6.6
6p24.2-p23	D6S296	23	0.83	0.9	0		0.4	7.0
6	D6S410	8	0.56	0.3	0		0.2	7.1
6p24.2-p23	D6S470	14	0.80	1.6	1.2	1.3	1.3	8.5
6p23	D6S443	8	0.61	9.9	2.3	4.3	6.1	14.6
6p23	D6S259	16	0.77	0.4	1.8	0.2	1.1	15.7
6p23	D6S260	22	0.89	1.5	0.8	1.9	1.1	16.8
6p23	D6S288	7	0.50	3.5	0		2.1	18.9
6p23	D6S274	17	0.84	1.4	1.3	1.1	1.0	19.9
6p22.3-p22.2	D6S285	9	0.67	1.8	1.3	1.4	1.7	21.6
6	D6S422	20	0.76	1.0	4.3	0.2	2.2	23.8
6p22.3-p21.3	D6S299	16	0.78	11.4	0		6.2	30.0
6p21.3	D6S276	18	0.76	0	0		0	30.0
6p22.2-21.3	D6S105	13	0.77	3.6	1.2	3.0	2.5	32.5
6p21.3	D6S273	8	0.73	2.3	2.1	1.1	2.1	34.6
6p21.3-21.2	D6S291	8	0.66	2.4	1.2	2.0	1.8	36.8

Cytogenetic locations are from the Genome Data Base (no locations were available for D6S477, D6S410, and D6S422). All other data, including the map constructed with the program CRI-MAP (Donis-Keller et al. 1987), are derived from ISHDSF genotyping data.

Table 2. Pairwise LOD Scores for Schizophrenia and Chromosome 6p Markers

	D1–D2				D1–D5				D1–D8				D1–D9			
Locus	Dom	Pen	Lia	Rec	Dom	Pen	Lia	Rec	Dom	Pen	Lia	Rec	Dom	Pen	Lia	Rec
D6S477	0.00	0.00	0.00	0.00	0.06	0.04	0.03	0.02	0.08	0.07	0.11	0.03	0.13	0.05	0.05	0.01
F13A1	0.17	0.29	0.22	0.11	0.58	0.82	1.11	0.90	1.13	1.54	0.21	0.80	0.16	0.30	0.50	0.56
D6S309	0.81	0.89	0.74	0.46	1.69	1.39	1.03	0.46	1.32	1.50	1.44	0.57	0.01	0.04	0.09	0.23
D6S277	0.67	0.72	0.73	0.58	1.45	1.39	1.12	0.25	1.04	1.20	1.14	0.32	0.04	0.22	0.18	0.21
D6S263	0.80	0.81	0.49	0.30	1.45	1.27	0.89	0.41	1.38	1.37	1.13	0.57	0.13	0.07	0.06	0.04
D6S296	0.93	1.18	1.15	1.06	2.40	2.70	2.94	2.05	2.81	3.51	3.32	1.89	0.92	1.27	1.44	0.91
D6S410	0.08	0.14	0.05	0.00	1.03	1.18	0.99	0.34	0.66	1.02	0.99	0.03	0.00	0.27	0.37	0.17
D6S470	1.15	1.18	0.69	0.37	1.88	1.72	1.40	0.51	2.08	2.19	2.23	0.89	0.61	0.65	0.63	0.66
D6S443	0.38	0.32	0.13	0.03	0.66	0.36	0.27	0.02	0.50	0.27	0.23	0.06	0.00	0.00	0.01	0.25
D6S259	0.49	0.67	0.35	0.13	0.69	0.78	0.80	0.38	0.90	0.97	1.04	0.54	1.39	1.04	0.94	0.91
D6S260	0.52	0.59	0.21	0.04	0.70	0.97	0.66	0.10	1.31	1.31	1.14	0.35	0.85	0.74	0.67	0.43
D6S288	0.03	0.01	0.01	0.00	0.52	0.40	0.59	0.62	0.34	0.19	0.19	0.22	0.00	0.00	0.05	0.38
D6S274	0.31	0.24	0.10	0.02	1.81	1.41	1.26	0.79	2.23	1.79	1.61	1.06	0.28	0.23	0.40	1.20
D6S285	0.30	0.31	0.19	0.12	1.47	1.45	1.83	1.37	1.78	1.78	1.78	0.92	1.63	1.37	1.69	1.31
D6S422	0.36	0.38	0.46	0.35	0.84	1.04	1.52	1.39	0.72	0.90	1.02	0.71	0.14	0.29	0.54	0.86
D6S299	0.15	0.07	0.06	0.04	0.34	0.27	0.31	0.29	0.30	0.33	0.54	1.07	0.10	0.34	0.68	0.75
D6S276	0.24	0.19	0.31	0.52	0.37	0.33	0.44	0.24	0.41	0.44	0.48	0.28	0.43	0.43	0.61	0.35
D6S105	0.41	0.31	0.07	0.12	0.24	0.20	0.16	0.13	0.27	0.27	0.33	0.26	0.21	0.09	0.09	0.03
D6S273	0.06	0.08	0.02	0.07	0.14	0.20	0.16	0.14	0.26	0.32	0.41	0.80	0.55	0.59	0.95	1.03
D6S291	0.92	0.97	0.99	1.03	0.63	0.66	0.57	0.43	0.43	0.61	0.75	0.98	0.66	0.86	0.88	0.85

The program MENDEL (Lange et al. 1988) was used to calculate LOD scores under the assumption of locus heterogeneity, which are presented as the maximum LOD scores at any recombination fraction. Diagnostic categories and genetic models are as described in the Methods section.

DEL (Lange et al. 1988). Four diagnostic models were used: D1–D2 (narrow), D1–D5 (intermediate), D1–D8 (broad), and D1–D9 (very broad). Under each diagnostic model, four different genetic models were used: Dom, Pen, Lia, and Rec. For a given diagnostic category, LOD scores were generally greatest under the Pen model. LOD scores under the Dom model were very similar to those under the Pen model, and Lia and Rec LOD scores were generally smaller. The largest LOD score was 3.51 (p=0.0002) with D6S296, under diagnostic category D1–D8 and the Pen genetic model, and this occurred at recombination fraction (θ)=0.004 and the proportion of linked pedigrees (α)=0.40. Results with diagnostic categories D1–D5 and D1–D8 were similar, but narrowing the disease definition (D1–D2) produced substantially smaller LOD scores, as did broadening the diagnostic category to include all psychiatric disorders (D1–D9).

Multipoint LOD scores. Figure 1 shows LOD scores calculated under the assumption of heterogeneity (H-LOD) from the multipoint program GENEHUNTER under diagnostic model D1–D8, under the four genetic models. We have placed marker D6S477, designated "A," at map position zero, and distal (tel) is to the left. Although there are multiple peaks, the primary peak occurs with model Pen at about 11 cM (max 2.74), which is between markers D6S470 and D6S443. The Dom and Pen models produce greater evidence for linkage than the Lia model, and there is little evidence for linkage under the Rec model.

Figure 2 shows GENEHUNTER results under the genetic model Pen for the four diagnostic models. The support for linkage is greatest under D1–D8 and D1–D5, with little support under D1–D2 and D1–D9.

Multipoint NPL results. Figure 3 shows the nonparametric results from GENEHUNTER, which are similar to the parametric results in that D1–D5 and D1–D8 are similar and D1–D2 and D1–D9 are similar and weaker. Compared to the H-LOD results, the peak (D1–D8, max 3.4) is slightly more distal, occurring at about 7 cM, at markers D6S296 and D6S410.

Estimation of α, proportion of pedigrees linked. The maximum likelihood estimation of α from the two-point LOD score calculation under heterogeneity (Table 2) generally ranges from 0.60 to 0.80 (data not shown). We think that these are likely to be overestimates, since simulations done at α=0.75 yielded LOD scores between 11 and 27, considerably greater than the maximum observed LOD score of 3.51. Simulations done at α=0.30 yielded LOD scores between 2.4 and 5.4, much closer to the observed LODs. Estimates of α from the GENEHUNTER program are shown in Table 3. Estimates from the two-point are much higher than those derived from multipoint data, which range from 0.14 to 0.25. We have also estimated α by two other methods (Straub et al. 1995). The first method uses the ESPA program (Sandkuijl 1989) results of shared versus not-shared alleles. The second uses the percentage of pedigrees demonstrating positive (>+0.1) LOD scores. Estimates of α from these two new methods vary considerably but are generally in the range of 0.15 to 0.30 (data not shown).

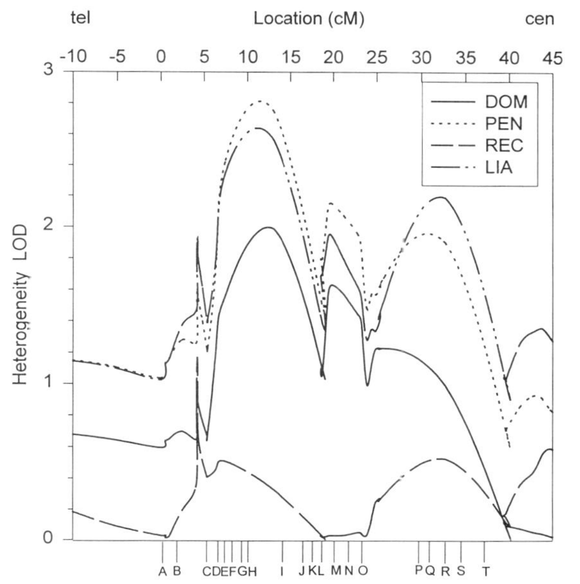

Figure 1. Multipoint heterogeneity LOD scores based on 20 markers in the 6p24-21 region under diagnostic model D1–D8 and all four genetic models. Marker A (D6S477) is arbitrarily set at map position zero. Calculations were performed by GENEHUNTER (Kruglyak et al. 1996), and results are expressed in LOD units. Right is distal (toward the telomere) and left is proximal (toward the centromere). Markers are designated as follows: A=D6S477, B=F13A1, C=D6S309, D=D6S277, E=D6S263, F=D6S296, G=D6S410, H=D6S470, I=D6S443, J=D6S259, K=D6S260, L=D6S288, M=D6S274, N=D6S285, O=D6S422, P=D6S299, Q=D6S276, R=D6S105, S=D6S273, T=D6S291.

Influence of unaffected individuals on LOD scores. To determine the effect of unaffected individuals on LOD scores, we performed an "affecteds only" analysis by setting the diagnosis of the unaffecteds to unknown. The results were similar to those above. For example, under the Pen model with diagnosis D1–D8, the maximum two-point LOD score for D6S296 was 3.47, for D6S470 it was 2.24, and for D6S285 it was 1.68.

Phenotypic analysis of "linked" pedigrees. A preliminary analysis of the distribution of diagnoses and selected symptom scales in the psychotic individuals did not suggest prominent differences between affected individuals from pedigrees with positive (LOD >+0.1) versus negative (LOD <–0.1) scores.

Linkage Analysis: Chromosome 8

Markers and map of the region. Characteristics of the 15 markers used in the 8p23-21 region are seen in Table 4. These were informative markers, with 6–16 alleles, and a mean (±S.D.) polymorphism information content of 0.68±0.13. The map covers 30 cM with an average inter-marker distance of 2.2±2.0 cM. The largest gap is 6.7 cM between D8S137 and D8S283.

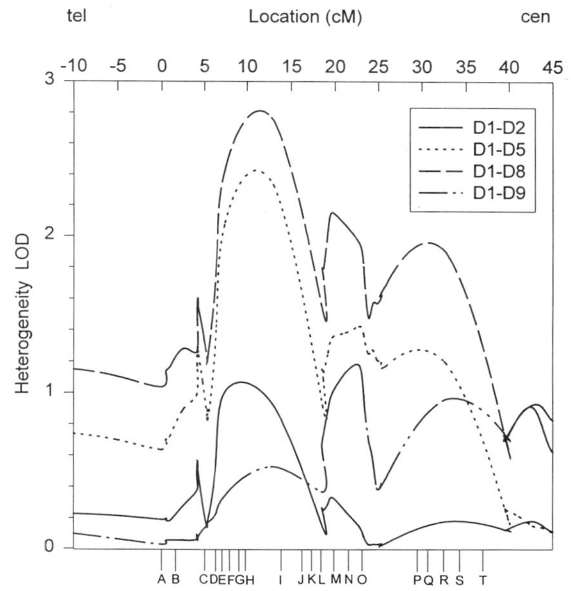

Figure 2. Multipoint heterogeneity LOD scores based on 20 markers in the 6p24-21 region for the narrow (D1–D2), intermediate (D1–D5), broad (D1–D8), and very broad (D1–D9) diagnostic models assuming the Pen genetic model. Map orientation and markers are as in Fig. 1.

Two-point LOD score results. Maximum pairwise H-LODs are presented in Table 5 for our four genetic and four diagnostic models. Positive evidence for linkage was seen across a range of diagnostic and ge-

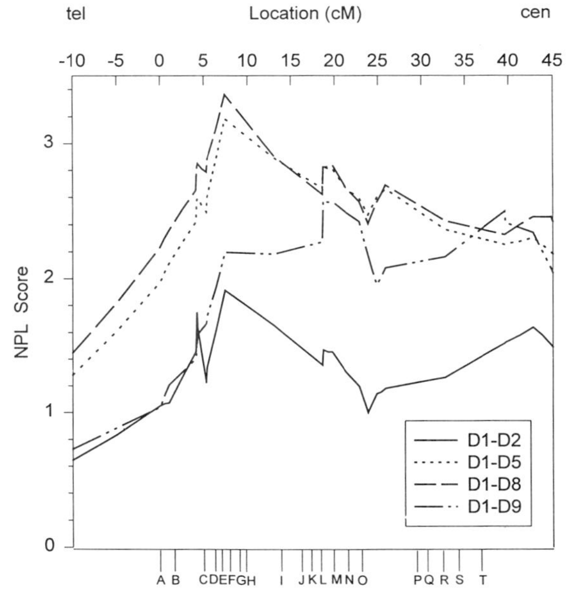

Figure 3. Multipoint NPL scores for the narrow (D1–D2), intermediate (D1–D5), broad (D1–D8), and very broad (D1–D9) diagnostic models. Calculations were performed by GENEHUNTER, and results are expressed as normal deviates (z-scores). Map orientation and markers are as in Fig. 1.

Table 3. Estimates of the Proportion of Families Segregating Disease Allele(s) on Chromosome 6p

	Proportion of families linked	
Locus	from two-point	from multipoint
D6S477	0.40	0.16
F13A1	0.80	0.18
D6S309	0.60	0.18
D6S277	0.80	0.20
D6S263	0.60	0.19
D6S296	0.80	0.18
D6S410	0.60	0.18
D6S470	0.80	0.25
D6S443	0.20	0.20
D6S259	0.30	0.21
D6S260	0.40	0.22
D6S288	0.30	0.21
D6S274	0.40	0.19
D6S285	0.80	0.19
D6S422	0.80	0.20
D6S299	0.15	0.20
D6S276	0.15	0.14
D6S105	0.30	0.14
D6S273	0.80	0.16
D6S291	0.60	0.16

Two-point values are from the program MENDEL, and multipoint values are from the program GENEHUNTER.

netic models. Unlike the evidence for linkage on chromosome 6, which was clearly strongest under diagnostic model D1–D8, the evidence is generally the same for D1–D8 and D1–D9, and for some markers, is actually greater with D1–D9 (especially D8S1731, D8S1715, and D8S133). The largest LOD score was 2.52 with D8S1715, under diagnostic category D1–D9 and the Rec genetic model.

Multipoint LOD scores. Figure 4 shows LOD scores calculated under the assumption of heterogeneity (H-LOD) from the multipoint program GENEHUNTER under diagnostic model D1–D8, under the four genetic models. The Dom genetic model produces by far the greatest evidence for linkage (unlike the two-point results), with a quite sharp peak at about 12 cM, near markers D8S1715 and D8S258, but this peak (2.34, p=0.002) has a broad shoulder extending another 10–15 cM proximal. Unlike the two-point results under diagnostic model D1–D8 shown in Table 5, the multipoint results under the Rec model are not positive.

Figure 5 depicts multipoint H-LODs for all four diagnostic models, assuming a dominant genetic model. The strongest evidence for linkage was found using D1–D8, and D1–D5 was similar, but D1–D9 was much weaker. These results differ considerably from the two-point results, where the LOD score under D1–D9 was usually greater than or equal to that under D1–D8.

Multipoint NPL results. NPL for all four diagnostic models is seen in Figure 6. In these analyses, the differences in evidence for linkage between diagnostic models was small. Two peaks were seen—one at about 3 cM near markers D8S511 and D8S1731 (max z=2.43, p=0.008) and the other at 15 cM near marker D8S298 (max z=2.51, p=0.006).

Estimation of α, proportion of pedigrees linked. As described above, we used four methods for estimating the proportion of linked pedigrees (α). As shown in Table 6, across the 15 markers, estimates from single-point and multipoint GENEHUNTER H-LOD scores were 0.25±0.16 and 0.11±0.02, respectively. Estimates

Table 4. Chromosome 8p Markers and Genetic Map

				Distances (Kosambi cM)				
							sex average	
Region	Locus	Number of alleles	PIC	female	male	ratio	intermarker distance	map position
8	D8S552	14	0.78					0
8pter-p23.1	D8S511	7	0.51	1.8	4.4	0.4	3.2	3.2
8	D8S1731	15	0.82	0.9	0		0.3	3.6
8p22	D8S261	12	0.73	5.2	4.4	1.2	4.9	8.4
8	D8S1715	15	0.42	5.2	1.8	2.9	3.2	11.6
8p22	D8S258	7	0.66	0.1	1.2	0.1	1.0	12.6
8	D8S282	13	0.66	0	2.2	0	1.3	13.9
8	D8S298	11	0.78	1.4	1.5	0.9	1.2	15.1
8p21.3-q11.1	D8S133	13	0.74	0.3	0		0.2	15.3
8	D8S1733	6	0.61	1.8	1.3	1.4	1.6	16.9
8p21.3-cen	D8S136	16	0.81	0	0.6	0.0	0.2	17.1
8	D8S1752	13	0.80	0.3	0.6	0.5	0.4	17.5
8	D8S1739	9	0.46	4.9	2.6	1.9	3.6	21.1
8p21.3-q11.1	D8S137	8	0.62	4.0	0		2.4	23.5
8	D8S283	14	0.80	9.7	4.4	2.2	6.7	30.2

Cytogenetic locations are from the Genome Data Base (no locations were available for some markers). All other data, including the map constructed with the program CRI-MAP (Donis-Keller et al. 1987), are derived from ISHDSF genotyping data.

Table 5. Pairwise LOD Scores for Schizophrenia and Chromosome 8p Markers

Locus	D1–D2				D1–D5				D1–D8				D1–D9			
	Dom	Pen	Lia	Rec	Dom	Pen	Lia	Rec	Dom	Pen	Lia	Rec	Dom	Pen	Lia	Rec
D8S552	0.85	0.92	0.74	0.81	0.28	0.37	0.47	0.38	0.52	0.46	0.44	0.57	0.32	0.35	0.19	0.00
D8S511	0.42	0.52	0.52	0.26	0.07	0.07	0.11	0.03	0.08	0.06	0.03	0.02	0.00	0.00	0.03	0.24
D8S1731	1.15	1.08	0.81	0.79	0.91	1.01	1.02	1.22	0.52	0.47	0.43	0.74	2.00	1.93	1.49	0.97
D8S261	0.30	0.29	0.42	0.78	0.07	0.14	0.19	0.26	0.00	0.02	0.05	0.34	0.62	0.45	0.46	0.63
D8S1715	0.38	0.53	0.31	0.15	0.33	0.66	0.67	0.23	0.20	0.63	0.73	0.36	1.63	2.36	2.20	2.52
D8S258	0.18	0.21	0.35	0.51	0.80	1.02	0.86	0.64	1.45	1.43	1.25	1.20	1.77	1.53	1.25	1.03
D8S282	0.46	0.78	0.88	1.07	0.02	0.34	0.39	0.21	0.23	0.62	0.92	0.82	0.31	0.60	0.62	0.58
D8S298	0.92	0.95	0.80	0.64	0.65	1.06	0.97	0.20	0.81	0.96	0.99	0.30	0.80	0.67	0.55	0.06
D8S133	0.23	0.47	0.68	0.78	1.04	1.64	1.57	1.45	0.58	0.74	1.02	1.08	1.43	1.79	1.98	2.08
D8S1733	0.35	0.44	0.29	0.27	0.03	0.21	0.13	0.00	0.06	0.14	0.09	0.00	0.39	0.36	0.35	0.01
D8S136	0.75	1.01	1.53	1.55	0.42	0.86	0.84	0.38	0.37	0.47	0.66	0.49	1.34	1.21	1.23	0.50
D8S1752	0.26	0.43	0.58	0.53	0.10	0.33	0.57	0.49	0.11	0.28	0.55	0.49	0.30	0.71	1.14	0.95
D8S1739	0.32	0.49	0.72	1.25	0.32	0.83	1.03	0.67	0.03	0.14	0.29	0.06	0.35	0.16	0.25	0.27
D8S137	0.13	0.13	0.13	0.18	0.25	0.16	0.21	0.19	0.26	0.16	0.19	0.09	0.44	0.16	0.08	0.03
D8S283	0.17	0.10	0.12	0.15	0.03	0.02	0.10	0.12	0.07	0.04	0.05	0.14	0.61	0.50	0.31	0.26

The program MENDEL (Lange et al. 1988) was used to calculate LOD scores under the assumption of locus heterogeneity, which are presented as the maximum LOD scores at any recombination fraction. Diagnostic categories and genetic models are as described in the Methods section.

of α derived from the ESPA program, and from the observed proportion of pedigrees with positive LOD scores, were 0.16±0.08 and 0.11±0.07, respectively. Taken together, the four methods suggest that the putative vulnerability locus on 8p is likely segregating in 10–25% of the pedigrees studied.

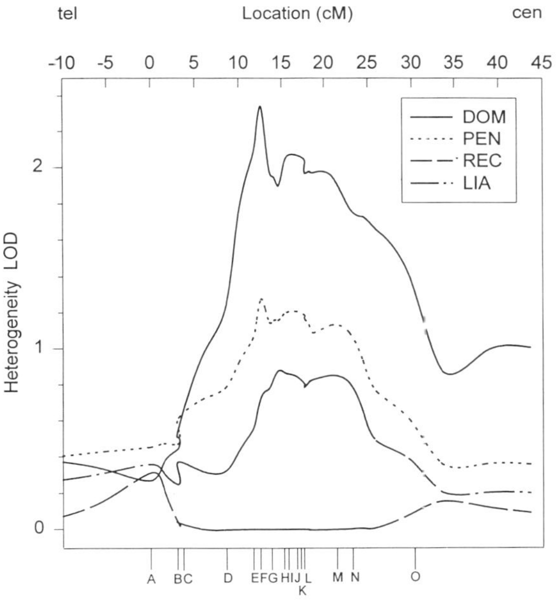

Figure 4. Multipoint heterogeneity LOD scores based on 15 markers in the 8p23-21 region under diagnostic model D1–D8 and all four genetic models. Marker A (D8S552) is arbitrarily set at map position zero. Calculations were performed by GENEHUNTER (Kruglyak et al. 1996), and results are expressed in LOD units. Right is distal (toward the telomere) and left is proximal (toward the centromere). Markers are designated as follows: A=D8S552, B=D8S511, C=D8S1731, D=D8S261, E=D8S1715, F=D8S258, G=D8S282, H=D8S298, I=D8S133, J=D8S1733, K=D8S136, L=D8S1752, M=D8S1739, N=D8S137, O=D8S283.

DISCUSSION

Evidence for linkage

Our results suggest that two chromosomal regions, 6p24-22 and 8p22-21, each contain a locus that in-

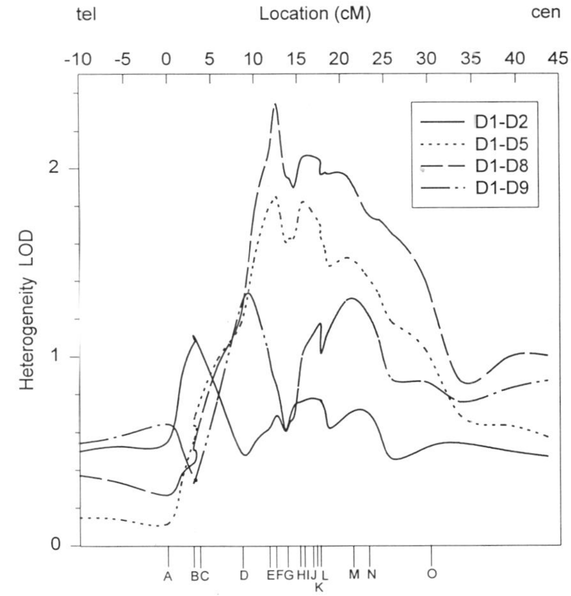

Figure 5. Multipoint heterogeneity LOD scores based on 15 markers in the 8p23-21 region for the narrow (D1–D2), intermediate (D1–D5), broad (D1–D8), and very broad (D1–D9) diagnostic models assuming the Dom genetic model. Map orientation and markers are as in Fig. 4.

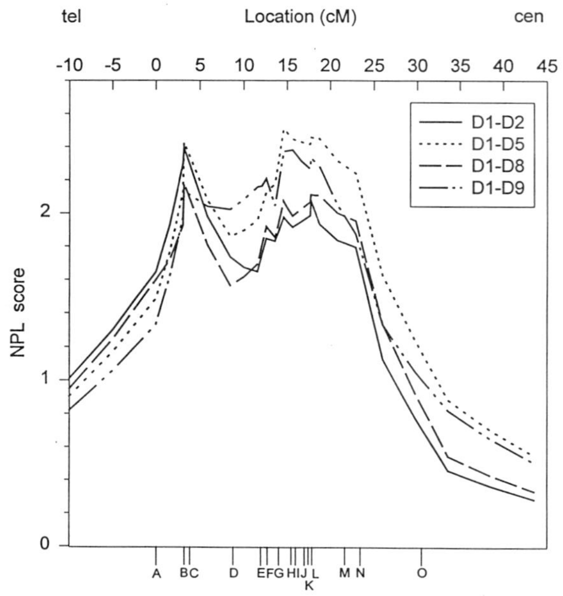

Figure 6. Multipoint NPL scores for the narrow (D1–D2), intermediate (D1–D5), broad (D1–D8), and very broad (D1–D9) diagnostic models. Calculations were performed by GENEHUNTER, and results are expressed as normal deviates (z-scores). Map orientation and markers are as in Fig. 4.

Table 6. Estimates of the Proportion of Families Segregating Disease Allele(s) on Chromosome 8p

	Proportion of families linked	
Locus	from two-point	from multipoint
D8S552	0.15	0.05
D8S511	0.10	0.07
D8S1731	0.15	0.08
D8S261	0.05	0.11
D8S1715	0.25	0.12
D8S258	0.60	0.13
D8S282	0.30	0.12
D8S298	0.40	0.12
D8S133	0.40	0.12
D8S1733	0.15	0.12
D8S136	0.40	0.12
D8S1752	0.20	0.12
D8S1739	0.15	0.12
D8S137	0.10	0.12
D8S283	0.40	0.10

Two-point values are from the program MENDEL, and multipoint values are from the program GENEHUNTER.

fluences the vulnerability to schizophrenia. These positive results are noteworthy because they were found with the largest schizophrenia sample currently being examined for genetic linkage, and they were observed over a range of genetic models and diagnostic categories. Unfortunately, the pairwise data provide little information about the mode of inheritance; for a given diagnostic category, LOD scores for dominant and recessive models were often similar. Furthermore, we do not know whether either of the putative loci is sufficient to cause schizophrenia in the linked pedigrees.

Statistical Significance

In complex disorders, extensive statistical work has not resolved the issue of the statistical significance of linkage results (Lander and Schork 1994). The traditional benchmark of a LOD score of 3 or, from nonparametric tests, a p value of less than 0.001, have become general guides in the *relative* evaluation of linkage results. Indeed, two previous studies in psychiatric genetics with very impressive statistics have yet to be supported by additional studies (Baron et al. 1987; Sherrington et al. 1988). Since the genetic architecture of schizophrenia is unknown, there is no firm theoretical basis to establish specific a priori thresholds of significance. Rather, *relatively* strong statistical evidence of linkage, especially when compared to data gathered during a genome scan, is probably best viewed as a tool to target specific genomic regions for further study using independent samples. Likewise, there is no consensus on specifically what does or does not constitute a valid independent replication of linkage.

Since LOD scores are most sensitive to misspecification of the mode of inheritance (Clerget-Darpoux et al. 1986), in order not to miss possible linkages we applied a battery of tests to the data from all markers tested. Here we used a total of 320 tests: 16 markers analyzed with five parametric tests (four LOD score calculations and the C-test) and one nonparametric test, at each of four diagnostic categories. We have not attempted to correct for multiple testing (Clerget-Darpoux et al. 1990; Weeks et al. 1990; Risch 1991; Lander and Schork 1994). Examination of the data demonstrates that the various tests are not independent, therefore a simple Bonferroni correction for the total number of tests would be inappropriate and likely to be too conservative. More importantly, for example, on chromosome 6, whether our highest LOD score was 3.51 (D6S296, Pen, D1–D8), or reduced due to the application of some correction factor, we would still have followed up these results in the same manner, i.e., to provide other investigators with a balanced and detailed account of our results, prior to publication, to facilitate replication studies.

We think that individual marker results are best evaluated in the context of results from the genome scan. Thus far, we have tested 223 markers, generally spaced at greater than 20-cM intervals elsewhere in the genome, and our findings with markers in these two regions were by far the strongest of any region examined in detail. Given that exclusion mapping is problematic in complex disorders, we do not attempt to estimate what percentage of the genome we have "excluded."

Genetic Heterogeneity

Since the average pedigree in our sample is small, it is difficult to determine specifically which pedigrees are "linked." For both regions, the estimates of the proportion of pedigrees linked produced by the admixture test usually ranged from 0.6 to 0.8, but our best estimate from two other methods is that the disease-associated allele(s) on chromosome 6 is segregating in roughly 15–30% of the pedigrees studied, and for chromosome 8 the range is slightly lower, about 10–25%. We note that although these are the best estimates we can currently generate, they are rather crude and predicated on the false assumption of simple genetic heterogeneity (the absence of multiple vulnerability genes contributing to disease in a single pedigree). Regardless of the actual proportion, we conclude that the data support the existence of genetic heterogeneity in schizophrenia.

Effect of Diagnoses

The potential effects of phenotypic ambiguities and new illness onset on linkage results are well known (Diehl and MacLean 1993). Since the results of "affecteds only" analysis were similar to the usual analysis where unaffecteds were considered unaffected, it appears that the information from unaffected individuals contributes little to the significance of the results. We have a large number of small pedigrees, containing 5.3 individuals on average, and we would not expect the results to be significantly altered by changes in diagnosis of a small number of individuals.

On chromosome 6, compared to both the intermediate (D1–D5) and broad (D1–D8) diagnostic categories, evidence for linkage lessened when the definition was narrowed to "core phenotypes" (D1–D2). This may be due to a loss of power because of a decreased number of affected individuals. Likewise, linkage evidence was weaker with the D1–D9 diagnostic category, which includes other psychiatric disorders *thought* to be unrelated genetically to schizophrenia (Kendler and Diehl 1993).

The two-point results on chromosome 8 are, unexpectedly, quite different. Expanding the diagnostic definition (from D1–D8 to D1–D9) to include as affected those individuals with anxiety disorders, alcoholism, and depression did not reduce the two-point evidence for linkage. For some markers, the evidence was actually greater under the expanded definition. Interestingly, this trend was not supported by the multipoint results, where the evidence under D1–D8 was stronger.

Location of the Putative Vulnerability Genes

Chromosome 6: Although there have been repeated suggestions of a relationship between HLA and schizophrenia, the evidence to date is weak (Goldin et al. 1987; Wright et al. 1993). There is no evidence in the ISHDSF linkage data that the putative locus is within the HLA region. The small LOD scores with D6S477 distally and D6S299 proximally suggest that these loci flank the putative disease locus. The strongest evidence for linkage comes from D6S296, but other markers also provide evidence of linkage, especially D6S470, D6S274, and D6S285. For most markers, the maximum LOD score occurs at large values of θ, which may be due to overestimation of map distances in the analysis of complex diseases, especially when the disease may be controlled by several genes acting epistatically (Risch and Giuffra 1992; Vieland et al. 1992). Simple comparison of the relative magnitudes of the pairwise LOD scores, therefore, is not sufficient to suggest a more precise location of the disease locus within this region of about 30 cM. Unfortunately, application of both parametric and nonparametric multipoint programs did not serve to narrow the region further.

Chromosome 8: As with chromosome 6, the pairwise LOD scores do not suggest the location of the putative gene. The parametric multipoint analysis shows a sharp peak at about 12 cM, but this is likely to be an artifact.

It is unlikely that additional markers analyzed with current linkage programs will narrow the region further, so we are testing a large number of markers for linkage disequilibrium. If disequilibrium is detectable, the target region should be reduced to the point where intensive sequencing and analysis of polymorphisms in positional candidate genes is justified.

THE FUTURE

It is not surprising that so far, these linkages have generated more questions than answers. Among the long list of things we do not yet know are: Which of the linkages represent real genes? Are these the genes of primary importance in schizophrenia? Are they necessary? Are they sufficient? Can they increase vulnerability alone or only in combinations? What are the most important combinations? More general questions include: Do the mutations produce defects in developmental pathways or neurotransmitter systems? How does having a missing or defective protein result in an elevated risk of disease? What environmental factors might interact with these genetic factors to affect onset and expression of the disease?

We are optimistic that at least some of the potential linkages represent real genes for schizophrenia, and that additional genes will be uncovered during the completion of the genome scan. When the target regions are narrowed satisfactorily, more complete gene sequences are available, and accurate localization of genes on the physical maps is accomplished, we will turn in earnest to the investigation of candidate genes, both functional and positional.

ACKNOWLEDGMENTS

This project was largely supported by grants MH-41953 and MH-45390 from the U.S. National Institute of Mental Health (NIMH). K.S.K. is supported by a research scientist award from NIMH (MH-01277). Data collection was conducted under the supervision of S. Humphries, M. Healy, and A. Finnerty. Additional interviews were conducted by M. Ni Nuallain, F. McMahon, J. Downing, T. Hebron, B. Hanratty, E. Crowe, M. Doherty, J. Bray, and L. Lowry. This project would not have been possible without the cooperation of the pedigrees themselves and the staffs of the many psychiatric hospitals and units in Ireland and Northern Ireland; their cooperation is gratefully acknowledged. We also acknowledge the assistance of S. Easter, C. L. Jackson, K. Williams, L. Thacker, B. Duke, R. McClelland, M. McGuire, A. O'Hare, and M.P. Spellman.

REFERENCES

Baron, M. 1990. Genetic linkage in mental illness. *Nature* **346:** 618.

Baron, M., N. Risch, R. Hamburger, B. Mandel, S. Kushner, M. Newman, D. Drumer, and R.H. Belmaker. 1987. Genetic linkage between X-chromosome markers and bipolar affective illness. *Nature* **326:** 289.

Chen, W.J., S.V. Faraone, and M.T. Tsuang. 1992. Linkage studies of schizophrenia: A simulation study of statistical power. *Genet. Epidemiol.* **9:** 123.

Clerget-Darpoux, F., M.-C. Babron, and C. Bonaïti-Pellié. 1990. Assessing the effect of multiple linkage tests in complex diseases. *Genet. Epidemiol.* **7:** 245.

Clerget-Darpoux, F., C. Bonaiti-Pellie, and J. Hochez. 1986. Effects of misspecifying genetic parameters in lod score analysis. *Biometrics* **42:** 393.

Cloninger, C.R. 1994. Turning point in the design of linkage studies of schizophrenia. *Am. J. Med. Genet.* **54:** 83.

Davies, J.L., Y. Kawaguchi, S.T. Bennett, J.B. Copeman, H.J. Cordell, L.E. Pritchard, P.W. Reed, S.C.L. Gough, S.C. Jenkins, S.M. Palmer, K.M. Balfour, B.R. Rowe, M. Farrall, A.H. Barnett, S.C. Bain, and J.A. Todd. 1994. A genome-wide search for human type 1 diabetes susceptibility genes. *Nature* **371:** 130.

Diehl, S.R., and C.J. MacLean. 1993. Better data analysis through data exploration (reply). *Am. J. Hum. Genet.* **53:** 776.

Donis-Keller, H., P. Green, C. Helms, S. Cartinhour, B. Weiffenbach, K. Stephens, T.P. Keith, D.W. Bowden, D.R. Smith, E.S. Lander, D. Botstein, G. Akots, K.S. Rediker, T. Gravius, V.A. Brown, M.B. Rising, C. Parker, J.A. Powers, D.E. Watt, E.R. Kauffman, A. Bricker, P. Phipps, H. Muller-Kahle, T.R. Fulton, S. Ng, J.W. Schumm, J.C. Braman, R.G. Knowlton, D.F. Barker, S.M. Crooks, S.E. Lincoln, M.J. Daly, and J. Abrahamson. 1987. A genetic linkage map of the human genome. *Cell* **51:** 319.

Easton, D.F., D.T. Bishop, D. Ford, G.P. Crockford, and Breast Cancer Linkage Consortium. 1993. Genetic linkage analysis in familial breast and ovarian cancer: Results from 214 families. *Am. J. Hum. Genet.* **52:** 678.

Elston, R.C. 1994. P values, power, and pitfalls in the linkage analysis of psychiatric disorders. In *Genetic approaches to mental disorders* (ed. E.S. Gershon, and C.R. Cloninger), p. 3. American Psychiatric Press, Washington, D.C.

European Chromosome 16 Tuberous Sclerosis Consortium. 1993. Identification and characterization of the tuberous sclerosis gene on chromosome 16. *Cell* **75:** 1305.

Gill, M., H. Vallada, D. Collier, P. Sham, P. Holmans, R. Murray, P. McGuffin, S. Nanko, M. Owen, S. Antonarakis, D. Housman, H. Kazazian, G. Nestadt, A.E. Pulver, R.E. Straub, C.J. MacLean, D. Walsh, K.S. Kendler, L. DeLisi, M. Polymeropoulos, H. Coon, W. Byerley, R. Lofthouse, and E. Gershon. 1996. A combined analysis of D22S278 marker alleles in affected sib-pairs: Support for a susceptibility locus for schizophrenia at chromosome 22q12. *Am. J. Med. Genet.* **67:** 40.

Goldin, L.R., L.E. DeLisi, and E.S. Gershon. 1987. Relationship of HLA to schizophrenia in 10 nuclear families. *Psychiatry. Res.* **20:** 69.

Gottesman, I.I. and J. Shields. 1982. *Schizophrenia: The epigenetic puzzle.* Cambridge University Press, New York.

Hashimoto, L., C. Habita, J.P. Beressi, M. Delepine, C. Besse, A. Cambon-Thomsen, I. Deschamps, J.I. Rotter, S. Djoulah, M.R. James, P. Froguel, J. Weissenbach, G.M. Lathrop, and C. Julier. 1994. Genetic mapping of a susceptibility locus for insulin-dependent diabetes mellitus on chromosome 11q. *Nature* **371:** 161.

Kendler, K.S. 1988. The genetics of schizophrenia: An overview. *Handb. Schizophr.* **3:** 437.

Kendler, K.S. and S.R. Diehl. 1993. The genetics of schizophrenia: A current, genetic-epidemiologic perspective. *Schizophr. Bull.* **19:** 261.

Kendler, K.S. and D.Walsh. 1995. Gender and schizophrenia. Results of an epidemiologically-based family study. *Br. J. Psychiatry* **167:** 184.

Kendler, K.S., J.A. Lieberman, and D. Walsh. 1989. The structured interview for schizotypy (SIS): A preliminary report. *Schizophr. Bull.* **15:** 559.

Kendler, K.S., M. McGuire, A.M. Gruenberg, and D. Walsh. 1994. An epidemiologic, clinical, and family study of simple schizophrenia in County Roscommon, Ireland. *Am. J. Psychiatry* **151:** 27.

———. 1995. Examining the validity of DSM-III-R schizoaffective disorder and its putative subtypes in the Roscommon family study. *Am. J. Psychiatry* **152:** 755..

Kendler, K.S., M. McGuire, A.M. Gruenberg, A. O'Hare, M. Spellman, and D. Walsh. 1993a. The Roscommon family study: I. Methods, diagnosis of probands, and risk of schizophrenia in relatives. *Arch. Gen. Psychiatry* **50:** 527.

———. 1993b. The Roscommon family study. III. Schizophrenia-related personality disorders in relatives. *Arch. Gen. Psychiatry* **50:** 781.

Kendler, K.S., M. McGuire, A.M. Gruenberg, M. Spellman, A. O'Hare, and D. Walsh. 1993c. The Roscommon family study: II. The risk of nonschizophrenic nonaffective psychoses in relatives. *Arch. Gen. Psychiatry* **50:** 645.

Kendler, K.S., C.J. MacLean, F.A. O'Neill, J. Burke, B. Murphy, F. Duke, R. Shinkwin, S.M. Easter, B.T. Webb, J. Zhang, D. Walsh, and R.E. Straub. 1996. Evidence for a schizophrenia vulnerability locus on chromosome 8p in the Irish study of high-density schizophrenia families. *Am. J. Psychiatry* **153:** 1534.

Kruglyak, L., M.J. Daly, M.P. Reeve-Daly, and E.S. Lander. 1996. Parametric and non-parametric linkage analysis: A unified multipoint approach. *Am. J. Hum. Genet.* **58:** 1347.

Lander, E. and L. Kruglyak. 1995. Genetic dissection of complex traits: Guidelines for interpreting and reporting linkage results. *Nat. Genet.* **11:** 241.

Lander, E.S. and N.J. Schork. 1994. Genetic dissection of complex traits. *Science* **265:** 2037.

Lange, K., D. Weeks, and M. Boehnke. 1988. Programs for pedigree analysis: MENDEL, FISHER, and dGENE. *Genet. Epidemiol.* **5:** 471.

MacLean, C.J., L.M. Ploughman, S.R. Diehl, and K.S. Kendler. 1992. A new test for linkage in the presence of locus heterogeneity. *Am. J. Hum. Genet.* **50:** 1259.

Martin, M., D. Mann, and M. Carrington. 1995. Recombination rates across the HLA complex: Use of microsatellites as a rapid screen for recombinant chromosomes. *Hum. Mol. Genet.* **4:** 423.

Martinez, M.M. and L.R. Goldin. 1989. The detection of linkage and heterogeneity in nuclear families for complex disorders: One versus two marker loci. *Am. J. Hum. Genet.* **44:** 552.

———. 1990. Power of the linkage test for a heterogeneous disorder due to two independent inherited causes: A simulation study. *Genet. Epidemiol.* **7:** 219.

Morton, N.E. 1956. The detection and estimation of linkage between the genes for elliptocytosis and the Rh blood type. *Am. J. Hum. Genet.* **8:** 80.

O'Donovan, M.C. and M.J. Owen. 1992. Advances and retreats in the molecular genetics of major mental illness. *Ann. Med.* **24:** 171.

O'Rourke, D.H., I.I. Gottesman, B.K. Suarez, J. Rice, and T. Reich. 1982. Refutation of the general single-locus model for the etiology of schizophrenia. *Am. J. Hum. Genet.* **34:** 630.

Ott, J. 1983. Linkage analysis and family classification under heterogeneity. *Ann. Hum. Genet.* **47:** 311.

———. 1990. Invited editorial: Cutting a Gordian knot in the linkage analysis of complex human traits. *Am. J. Hum. Genet.* **46:** 219.

Prescott, C.A. and I.I. Gottesman. 1993. Genetically mediated vulnerability to schizophrenia. [review]. *Psychiatr. Clin. North Am.* **16:** 245.

Pulver, A.E., M. Karayiorgou, P.S. Wolyniec, V.K. Lasseter, L. Kasch, G. Nestadt, S. Antonarakis, D. Housman, H.H. Kazazian, D. Meyers, J. Ott, M. Lamacz, K.-Y. Liang, J. Hanfelt, G. Ullrich, N. DeMarchi, E. Ramu, P.R. McHugh, L. Adler, M. Thomas, W.T. Carpenter, T. Manschreck, C.T. Gordon, M. Kimberland, R. Babb, J. Puck, and B. Childs. 1994. Sequential strategy to identify a susceptibility gene for schizophrenia: Report of potential linkage on chromosome 22q12-q13.1: Part 1. *Am. J. Med. Genet.* **54:** 36.

Pulver, A.E., V.K. Lasseter, L. Kasch, P. Wolyniec, G. Nestadt, J.-L. Blouin, M. Kimberland, R. Babb, S. Vourlis, H. Chen, M. Lalioti, M.A. Morris, M. Karayiorgou, J. Ott, D. Meyers, S.E. Antonarakis, D. Housman, and H.H. Kazazian. 1995. Schizophrenia: A genome scan targets chromosomes 3p and 8p as potential sites of susceptibility genes. *Am. J. Med. Genet.* **60:** 252.

Risch, N. 1990a. Linkage strategies for genetically complex traits. I. Multilocus models. *Am. J. Hum. Genet.* **46:** 222.

———. 1990b. Genetic linkage and complex diseases, with special reference to psychiatric disorders. *Genet. Epidemiol.* **7:** 3.

———. 1991. A note on multiple testing procedures in linkage analysis. *Am. J. Hum. Genet.* **48:** 1058.

———. 1994. Mapping genes for psychiatric disorders. In *Genetic approaches to mental disorders.* (ed. E.S. Gershon and C.R. Cloninger), p. 47. American Psychiatric Press, Washington, D.C.

Risch, N. and L. Giuffra. 1992. Model misspecification and multipoint linkage analysis. *Hum. Hered.* **42:** 77.

Sandkuijl, L.A. 1989. Analysis of affected sib pairs using information from extended families. *Prog. Clin. Biol. Res.* **329:** 117.

Schizophrenia Linkage Collaborative Group for Chromosomes 3, 6, and 8 (coordinated by D.F. Levinson). 1996. Additional support for schizophrenia linkage on chromosomes 6 and 8: A multicenter study. *Am. J. Med. Genet.* **67:** 580.

Sherrington, R., J. Brynjolfsson, H. Petursson, M. Potter, K. Dudleston, B. Barraclough, J. Wasmuth, M. Dobbs, and H. Gurling. 1988. Localization of a susceptibility locus for schizophrenia on chromosome 5. *Nature* **336:** 164.

Smith, C.A.B. 1963. Testing for heterogeneity of recombination fraction values in human genetics. *Ann. Hum. Genet.* **27:** 175.

Spitzer, R.L., J.B.W. Williams, M. Gibbon, and M.B. First. 1992. The structured clinical interview for *DSM-III-R* (SCID): I: History, rationale, and description. *Arch. Gen. Psychiatry* **49:** 624.

Straub, R.E., C.J. MacLean, and K.S. Kendler. 1996. The putative schizophrenia locus on chromosome 6p: A brief overview of the linkage studies. *Mol. Psychiatry* **1:** 89.

Straub, R.E., M.C. Speer, Y. Luo, K. Rojas, J. Overhauser, J. Ott, and T.C. Gilliam. 1993. A microsatellite genetic linkage map of human chromosome 18. *Genomics* **15:** 48.

Straub, R.E., C.J. MacLean, F.A. O'Neill, J. Burke, B. Murphy, F. Duke, R. Shinkwin, B.T. Webb, J. Zhang, D. Walsh, and K.S. Kendler. 1995. A potential vulnerability locus for schizophrenia on chromosome 6p24-22: Evidence for genetic heterogeneity. *Nat. Genet.* **11:** 287.

Suarez, B.K., C.L. Hampe, and P. Van Eerdewegh. 1994. Problems of replicating linkage claims in psychiatry. *Genetic approaches to mental disorders* (ed. E.S. Gershon and C.R. Cloninger), p. 23. American Psychiatric Press, Washington, D.C.

Tanzi, R., S. Gaston, A. Bush, D. Romano, W. Pettingell, J. Peppercorn, M. Paradis, S. Gurubhagavatula, B. Jenkins, and W. Wasco. 1993. Genetic heterogeneity of gene defects responsible for familial Alzheimer disease. *Genetica* **91:** 255.

Vieland, V.J., S.E. Hodge, and D.A. Greenberg. 1992. Adequacy of single-locus approximations for linkage analysis of oligogenic traits. *Genet. Epidemiol.* **9:** 45.

Volz, A., J.M. Boyle, H.M. Cann, R.W. Cottingham, H.T. Orr, and A. Ziegler. 1994. Report of the second international workshop on human chromosome 6. *Genomics* **21:** 464.

Wang, S., C. Sun, C.A. Walczak, J.S. Ziegle, B.R. Kipps, L.R. Goldin, and S.R. Diehl. 1995. Evidence for a susceptibility locus for schizophrenia on chromosome 6pter-6p22. *Nat. Genet.* **10:** 41.

Weeks, D.E., T. Lehner, E. Squires-Wheeler, C. Kaufmann, and J. Ott. 1990. Measuring the inflation of the lod score due to its maximization over model parameter values in human linkage analysis. *Genet. Epidemiol.* **7:** 237.

Wright, P., M. Gill, and R.M. Murray. 1993. Schizophrenia: Genetics and the maternal immune response to viral infection. *Am. J. Med. Genet.* **48:** 40.

Genotype and Phenotype Analysis at the 22q11 Schizophrenia Susceptibility Locus

M. KARAYIORGOU,[1] J.A. GOGOS,[1,2] B.L. GALKE,[1] J.A. JEFFERY,[3] G. NESTADT,[3] P.S. WOLYNIEC,[3] S.E. ANTONARAKIS,[4] H.H. KAZAZIAN,[5] D.E. HOUSMAN,[6] D.A. DRISCOLL,[7] AND A.E. PULVER[3]

[1]*The Rockefeller University, New York, New York 10021;* [2]*College of Physicians & Surgeons, Columbia University, Center for Neurobiology & Behavior, New York, New York 10032;* [3]*Department of Psychiatry & Behavioral Sciences, Johns Hopkins University School of Medicine, Baltimore, Maryland 21203;* [4]*Medical School and Division of Medical Genetics, Geneva University, Cantonal Hospital of Geneva, Switzerland 1211;* [5]*University of Pennsylvania Medical Center, Philadelphia, Pennsylvania 19104;* [6]*Center for Cancer Research, Massachusetts Institute of Technology, Cambridge, Massachusetts 02139;* [7]*Division of Human Genetics and Molecular Biology, Children's Hospital of Philadelphia, and Department of Obstetrics and Gynecology, University of Pennsylvania School of Medicine, Philadelphia, Pennsylvania 19104*

Schizophrenia is a common disorder with a lifetime prevalence of approximately 1%. The illness often develops in young adults who previously appeared normal, and it is characterized by a constellation of symptoms, including hallucinations and delusions (psychotic symptoms), severely inappropriate emotional responses, disordered thinking and concentration, erratic behavior, and social and occupational deterioration.

The etiology of the disease is unknown. Two main hypotheses have been formulated: the neurodevelopmental and the so-called "dopamine" hypothesis. According to the neurodevelopmental hypothesis, subtle developmental abnormalities occurring later during embryonic brain development (2nd or 3rd trimester) and affecting neuronal cell migration, organization, or myelination, are responsible for schizophrenia (LaFosse and Mednick 1991). Several lines of evidence seem to support this hypothesis, including, among others, observations of reduced density of neurons in the gray and superficial white matter, with increased density in the deeper white matter (Jakob and Beckmann 1986; Arnold et al. 1991; Benes et al. 1991; Akbarian et al. 1993a,b), as well as observations of higher frequencies among schizophrenia patients than among controls of minor physical anomalies similar to the ones found in patients with developmental disorders (such as malformed ears or palate) (Gualtieri et al. 1982; Guy et al. 1983; Green et al. 1989; Lane et al. 1993). There is also evidence for dysgenesis of corpus callosum (Swayze et al. 1990), as well as lost or reduced asymmetry in brains of schizophrenia patients (Rossi and Stratta 1995), which would also be consistent with a neurodevelopmental origin of the disease.

According to the dopamine hypothesis, schizophrenia is caused by overactivity of neurons containing or using dopamine (Goldstein and Deutch 1992). This hypothesis is supported by the fact that the drugs used to treat schizophrenia block dopamine receptor transmission, and agents that cause schizophrenia-like psychosis, such as PCP, crack, and amphetamines, increase dopamine levels. Mutational analysis of the cloned dopamine receptors suggests that the dysregulation is probably located downstream from the dopamine receptors, although recently, combined meta-analysis of data from several groups showed that a natural variation at codon 9 of D3 receptor (a Ser→Gly) might confer susceptibility to schizophrenia: Individuals homozygous for serine at codon 9 may have a moderately increased risk to develop schizophrenia (Shaikh et al. 1996).

Schizophrenia appears to have a significant genetic component. Studies have shown that the risk to develop the disease increases with the amount of gene sharing rather than with experience sharing (Gottesman 1991). For example, a twin brother of a schizophrenia patient (reared together or in separate families) and children with both parents suffering from schizophrenia have higher risks to develop the disease than do first-degree relatives, who in turn have higher risks than do second-degree relatives, and so on. In all of these cases, the risk is higher than the basic risk of 1% in the general population.

An interesting observation is that among monozygotic twins, if one suffers from schizophrenia, the other has only a 48% risk to develop the disease, instead of 100%. Both twins, however, transmit the disease to their offspring at the same risk. Clearly, influences from the environment also play an important role, but they are as difficult to define at this point as the genetics. Environmental influences could be specific stressors, obstetric complications, or viruses (some studies indicate a higher risk of schizophrenia among children born to mothers exposed to the influenza virus during the 2nd trimester of pregnancy [Machon et al. 1995; McGrath et al. 1995]). The environmental influences would, of course, act on a "fragile" genetic background.

The best way to describe schizophrenia genetically is as an oligogenic disease, with incomplete penetrance.

Efforts at localizing susceptibility genes have thus far provided promising leads: chromosomes 3 and 8 (Pulver et al. 1995; Moises et al. 1995b; our unpublished data), chromosome 6 (Antonarakis et al. 1995; Gurling et al. 1995; Moises et al. 1995b; Mowry et al. 1995; Schwab et al. 1995a; Straub et al. 1995), chromosome 13 (Lin et al. 1995; our unpublished data), and chromosome 22 (Pulver et al. 1994b; Coon et al. 1994a,b; Lasseter et al. 1995; Moises et al. 1995a,b; Schwab et al. 1995b; Vallada et al. 1995; Schizophrenia Collaborative Linkage Group [chromosome 22] 1996; our unpublished data). Precise localization, however, is somewhat ambiguous, and no gene has been narrowed down through linkage studies to a small genomic region, let alone identified by molecular methods.

MATERIALS AND METHODS

Fluorescence in situ hybridization (FISH). Metaphase chromosome spreads were prepared from the Epstein-Barr virus-transformed lymphoblastoid cell lines GM0980 and AP1268. Cosmid probes specific for loci D22S75 (N25) (ONCOR) and D22S66 (160b) were labeled by nick-translation with biotinylated-11-dUTP (Boehringer). Cosmid cos82, which maps to the long arm of chromosome 22, was used as a control probe. After preannealing of the probes with human Cot-1 DNA, hybridizations were performed at 37°C in 2x SSC, 10% dextran sulfate, and 50% deionized formamide, and slides were washed to a stringency of 0.1x SSC at 60°C. Signals were visualized with fluoresceinated avidin, and chromosomes were counterstained with DAPI. Fifteen metaphases were examined.

Diagnostic criteria. *Patient sample.* The majority of the schizophrenia patients (97%) are genetically unrelated individuals in the Maryland Epidemiologic Sample (MES). The MES is a systematic sample of patients with psychotic disorders who were admitted to one of 15 hospitals in the greater Baltimore area between 1983 and 1989. Diagnoses were assigned by psychiatrists using standard diagnostic criteria (DSM-III) and were based on a direct psychiatric examination and medical records. The remaining patients ($N = 4$) were identified through four independent families referred for study because of multiply affected relatives. These patients were evaluated and diagnosed in a similar manner to those in the MES. Ratings for clinical characteristics were based on the following: (1) *age at onset*: age at first psychotic symptoms, coded by a psychiatrist; (2) *history of learning problems*: based on patient report of having attended a special school or class for the learning disabled; (3) *obsessive-compulsive symptoms*: based on patient report and medical record review; and (4) *manic symptoms*: based on patient report and medical record review. Appropriate informed consent was obtained from all subjects.

Control sample. The controls are genetically unrelated individuals who were ascertained through (1) individuals donating a blood sample for human immunogenetics studies and (2) individuals donating a blood sample at a prenatal diagnostic center.

RESULTS AND DISCUSSION

Linkage studies suggest the presence of one or more loci contributing to schizophrenia susceptibility at 22q (Coon et al. 1994a,b; Pulver et al. 1994b; Lasseter et al. 1995; Moises et al. 1995a,b; Schwab et al. 1995b; Vallada et al. 1995; Schizophrenia Collaborative Linkage Group [chromosome 22] 1996; our unpublished data) within a broadly defined region extending from D22S276 (22q13) to CRYB2A and D22S941 (22q11). Two additional lines of evidence suggest the presence of a susceptibility locus at 22q11: (1) the higher than expected frequency of schizophrenia among velo-cardio-facial syndrome (VCFS) patients, a syndrome caused by 22q11 deletions (Shprintzen et al. 1992; Pulver et al. 1994a); in a pilot study, 4 of 14 adult VCFS patients evaluated for psychiatric illness were found to meet DSM-III-R criteria for schizophrenia (~28%, as compared to the 1% prevalence of schizophrenia in the general population) and (2) the identification of 22q11 deletions among about 2% of random schizophrenia patients (Karayiorgou et al. 1995); a subgroup of 100 patients diagnosed with DSM-III-R schizophrenia from the MES were examined by FISH for presence of the 22q11 deletion, and two were found to be deleted. The frequency of this deletion in the general population is estimated to be about 2 in 10,000. Most recently, we confirmed our initial observation by extending our search for 22q11 deletions in large numbers of schizophrenia patients and healthy controls using a polymerase chain reaction (PCR)-based approach we developed (M. Karayiorgou et al., in prep.).

Definition of the Deletion Boundaries

One of the first questions we asked upon identification of deletions in schizophrenia patients was whether the deletions harbored by the schizophrenia VCFS patients are more extensive than the ones harbored by the non-schizophrenia VCFS patients. We addressed this question by generating somatic cell hybrid cell lines. Hybrid clones that only segregated the deleted chromosome 22, along with the genomic DNA from a sample consisting of the two schizophrenia patients with the deletion from the MES, two VCFS patients who were also diagnosed with schizophrenia, and four VCFS patients who upon psychiatric examination were not found to have any signs of psychosis, were typed by PCR with 37 markers that cover the entire chromosome. We concluded from this experiment that there is no correlation between the extent of the deletion and the additional schizophrenia phenotype, since there was at least one schizophrenia patient (AP1037) with a smaller deletion, as indicated by the presence of two

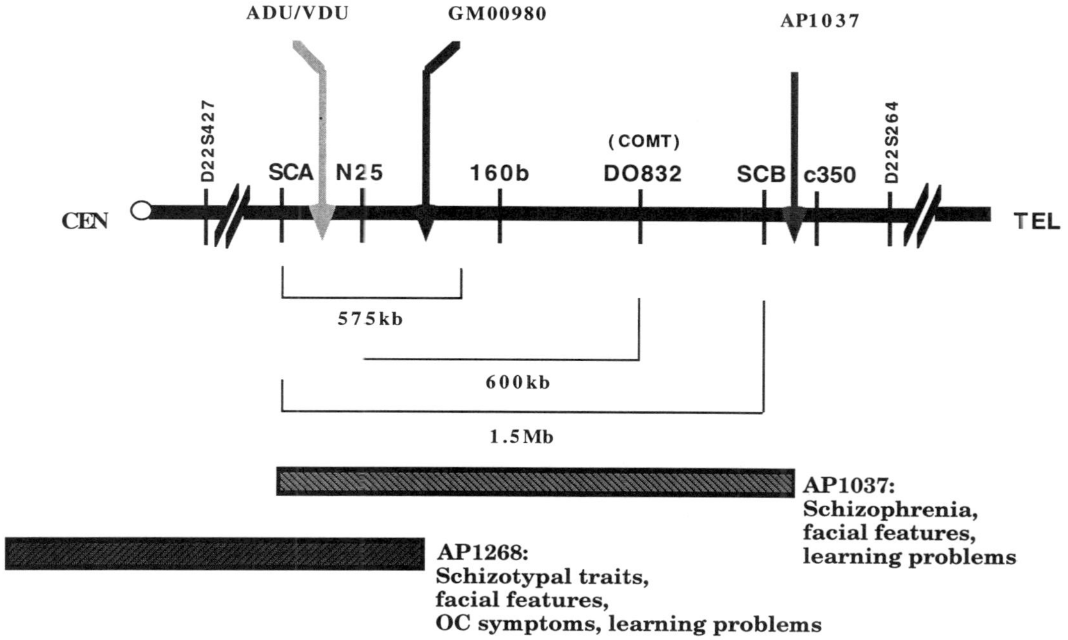

Figure 1. Map of the commonly deleted region on chromosome 22q11. Arrows indicate deletion, balanced, or unbalanced translocation breakpoints (AP1037, ADU/VDU, and GM0980, respectively). Patient AP1037 is a schizophrenia patient with a 22q11 deletion proximal to cosmid c350 (D22S695), flanked by markers D22S264 and D22S427 (described in detail in Karayiorgou et al. 1995). The distance between cosmids sc11.1A and sc11.1B (both included in the deletion) is about 1.5 Mb. This is the smallest deleted region described in association with schizophrenia so far, as well as the most commonly deleted region in DGS/VCFS. The ADU/VDU balanced translocation breakpoint of two (mother and daughter) DGS/VCFS patients, respectively, maps within the proximal 250 kb. Transcripts disrupted by this breakpoint are considered strong candidates for these syndromes. The gene for COMT maps on cosmid DO832, 600 kb distal to this region. Hatched bars indicate the deleted region for each patient.

copies of marker D22S264, which is included in the hemizygous deletions harbored by non-schizophrenia VCFS patients (Karayiorgou et al. 1995).

Patient AP1037 defines the shortest region of overlap for the schizophrenia critical region on chromosome 22q11 (Karayiorgou et al. 1995). This patient carries a hemizygous deletion flanked by markers D22S427 and D22S264 (the distal breakpoint is indicated in Fig. 1), a region estimated to be between 1.5 Mb and 2 Mb. Interestingly, this region contains the gene for catechol-*O*-*m*ethyl *t*ransferase (COMT) (Grossman et al. 1992), which is considered a strong candidate for the development of schizophrenia (Dunham et al. 1992; Propping and Nothen 1995) since it breaks down catecholamines, including the neurotransmitter dopamine.

Deletions of similar size are also found in 89% of cases with DiGeorge syndrome (DGS; MIM no. 188400[4]) (Driscoll et al. 1993) and about 76% of cases with VCFS (MIM no. 19243[4]) (Driscoll et al. 1993) (referred to as the "commonly deleted region"). The distal boundary of the shortest region of overlap (SRO) for DGS/VCFS is defined by the translocation breakpoint found in patient GM0980, a patient with DGS/VCFS features and an unbalanced 45,XX,-11,-22,+der(11)t(11;22)(q25;q11) karyotype. The breakpoint of this terminal deletion has been previously mapped between D22S75 (N25) and D22S66 (160b) (Li et al. 1994) and proximal to cosmid D0832 (D22S502), which contains the gene for COMT (Halford et al. 1993b). This result, along with results from overlap mapping of additional DGS/VCFS deletions, estimates the minimum size of the "critical region" involved in DGS/VCFS to be 300–575 kb (Halford et al. 1993b).

Patient AP1268 is the daughter of GM0980, a 28-year-old single white female. Direct psychiatric assessment by a psychiatrist blind to the study's objective revealed a history of persistent simple auditory hallucinations (i.e., hearing her name called), suspicions, odd beliefs, and paranoid ideas. Although she did not meet criteria for schizophrenia, her schizotypal traits and simple perceptual disturbances place her in the schizophrenia spectrum illnesses. In addition, she was diagnosed with a past history of persistent obsessive compulsive symptoms, which were distressing and ego dystonic (patient would feel at times that her hands were dirty and couldn't stop washing them to the point that they would blister; this would happen once per week over a period of 3 years). This finding is in accordance with the increased frequency of obsessive compulsive traits or symptoms previously observed among

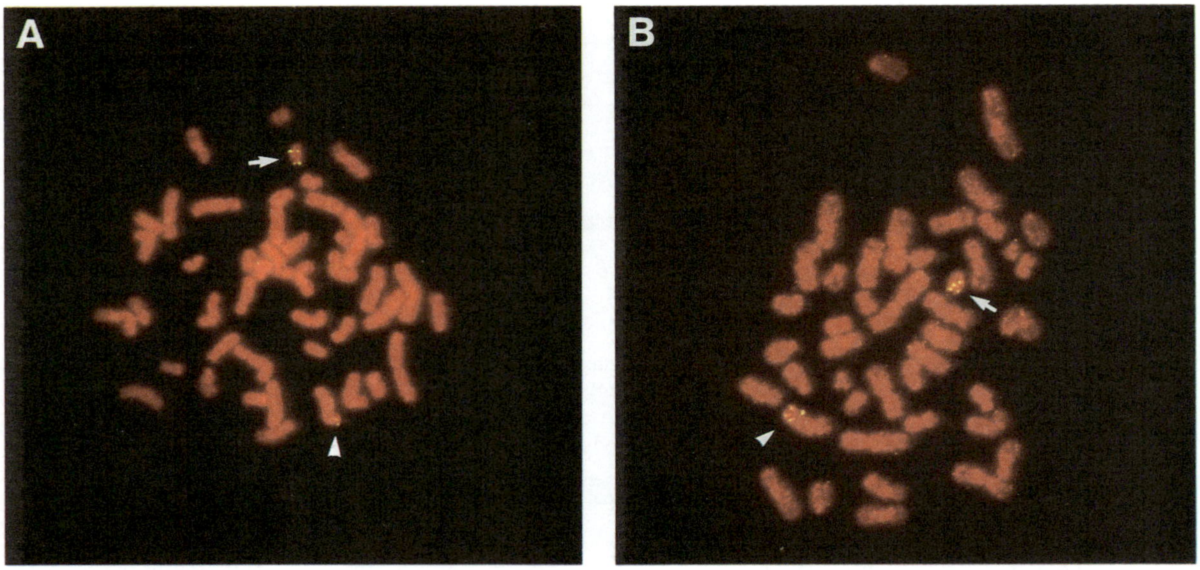

Figure 2. Fluorescence in situ hybridization with chromosome 22 cosmids. (*A*) Metaphase chromosomes from AP1268 hybridized with cosmids cos82 and N25. A hybridization signal for N25 is only present on the normal 22 (*arrow*) consistent with a deletion. Signal for cos82 is present on both the normal 22 and the der(11) (*arrowhead*). (*B*) Hybridization of cos82 and cosmid specific for locus D22S66 to metaphase chromosomes from AP1268. Signals are present for both cosmids on the normal 22 (*arrow*) and the der(11) (*arrowhead*). Hence, the translocation breakpoint lies proximal to locus D22S66.

schizophrenia patients with VCFS (Pulver et al. 1994a; also see below). The patient also had learning disabilities as a child and facial dysmorphologies consistent with VCFS (low-set ears) (see also below).

Cytogenetic analysis showed a 45,XX,-11,-22, +der(11)t(11;22)(q25;q11) karyotype like her mother (not shown). Comparison of mother/daughter breakpoints by FISH with cosmids for markers N25 (D22S75) and 160b (D22S66) suggested that the translocation breakpoints occur in the same region (Fig. 2) and result in deletion of 22pter→q11.2. Therefore, the breakpoint of AP1268 is proximal to the gene for COMT (Fig. 1) and this patient does not have a deletion of this gene. This was also confirmed using PCR-restriction fragment length polymorphism assays (not shown).

The presence of a more proximal distal breakpoint in this patient, who phenotypically did not meet the criteria for schizophrenia and was diagnosed with a schizophrenia spectrum disorder, suggests but does not prove that the proximal 300–575 kb of the extended deleted region have an important contribution to susceptibility to psychosis.

COMT as a Candidate Gene

Although this result would appear to exclude COMT from a major role in the development of the psychotic features in this patient, the underdeveloped nature of these features and the possibility of a long-range position effect of the translocation do not permit us to exclude a contribution from genes distal to the breakpoint (including COMT) to the development of 22q11-associated schizophrenia.

To study the role of COMT, we undertook a mutational analysis of the coding region, and the region surrounding splice donor and acceptor sites of COMT, using single-strand conformational polymorphism analysis (Glavac and Dean 1993) and chemical cleavage methodologies (Gogos et al. 1990). Our case-control sample consisted of 157 schizophrenics and 129 controls. Several DNA polymorphisms were identified (M. Karayiorgou et al., in prep.). One polymorphism caused an amino acid change in codon 158, from valine to methionine, creating an *Nla*III site. This was the only polymorphism identified within the coding region that caused an amino acid change, suggesting that it likely is the genetic cause underlying the high and low metabolizing activity of the COMT enzyme. Indeed, an exact correlation between low enzymatic activity and the presence of methionine in both alleles was observed (Lachman et al. 1996; M. Karayiorgou, unpubl.). The frequency of homozygotes for methionine (low metabolizers) in our control sample was about 22%, in agreement with previous estimations based on enzymatic assays (Weinshilboum and Raymond 1977), indicating that the frequency in our control sample is representative of the population frequency.

The identification of the genetic basis of high/low metabolizing alleles gave us the opportunity to test their frequency distribution in our case-control sample. No statistically significant differences in the frequency of low metabolizers or intermediate metabolizers (heterozygotes) between 157 schizophrenia patients and 129 controls were observed in our sample. In addition, no differences were observed in the distribution of the low metabolizing allele between hemizygously deleted VCFS patients who also develop schizophrenia, and hemizygously deleted VCFS patients who are free of psychosis (M. Karayiorgou et al., in prep.).

This gross analysis, however, did not provide information on a potential contribution of COMT to the manifestation of schizophrenia or the co-morbid conditions that are frequently observed among these patients. In addition, this analysis did not provide information regarding the possible relevance of COMT to the identification of distinct subtypes of schizophrenia. To address this, the distribution of the *Nla*III genotypes among the schizophrenia cases was examined in relation to a history of learning problems and a history of obsessive-compulsive symptoms, two variables chosen because they were observed consistently among schizophrenia patients with 22q11 deletions (Pulver et al. 1994a; Karayiorgou et al. 1995) and with increased frequency among schizophrenia patients in general (Insel and Akiskal 1986; Eisen and Rasmussen 1993; Pato et al. 1993; Nestadt et al. 1994; Berman et al. 1995; Moss et al. 1995). The distribution of the *Nla*III genotypes among the schizophrenia cases was also examined in relation to gender, age at onset, and a history of manic symptoms, since previous studies of this sample have demonstrated that these patient characteristics are associated with familial risk for schizophrenia (Pulver and Liang 1991; Wolyniec et al. 1992; Liang and Pulver 1996). For all variables tested, results were analyzed with the proportional odds model and, interestingly, indicated a statistically significant enrichment for homozygotes for the high activity (Val) allele among schizophrenia patients who also have obsessive-compulsive features (odds ratio: 2.34, with C.I. 1.01, 5.44, and p-value .0489) (M. Karayiorgou et al., in prep.).

Other Candidate Genes

As mentioned above, a region of 300–575 kb has been defined by deletion overlap mapping as the critical region for VCFS/DGS, and possibly schizophrenia. At least 16 genes have been identified within this region so far (Halford et al. 1993a,b; Demczuk et al. 1996; Gong et al. 1996; Sutherland et al. 1996). VCFS, which is a congenital malformation syndrome, presents in children with cleft palate; a typical facial dysmorphology characterized by low-set ears, broad squared nasal root, and epicanthal skinfolds; cardiac malformation, mostly of the conotruncal type; learning disabilities in almost all of the cases; as well as mild mental retardation in some of the cases (OMIM 1994). VCFS is phenotypically related to DGS and it has been hypothesized that the two syndromes may be etiologically the same (Scambler et al. 1992; Driscoll et al. 1993). Both are attributed to a microdeletion in the VCFS/DGS critical region on chromosome 22q11. Both syndromes affect multiple organ systems, derived from the third and fourth pharyngeal arches of the developing embryo.

Accordingly, based on the phenotype of the syndrome, some of the genes in the VCFS/DGS critical region are likely to be involved in neural crest cell migration and possibly in neuronal cell migration, as well. Given the possibility for a neurodevelopmental origin of schizophrenia, genes that could be involved in neuronal cell migration would be considered very strong candidates from the region.

Schizophrenia Phenotype and the 22q11 Locus

We examined if there are any common features among the schizophrenia patients with the 22q11 deletions. Based on the relatively small number of the patients we have identified so far, we have noticed that there is a high frequency of obsessive-compulsive features, facial dysmorphologies, and learning disabilities as children (Pulver et al. 1994a; our unpublished data). Interestingly, these variables are not exclusive to the schizophrenia patients with the 22q11 deletion, but they have been described in association with schizophrenia in general. For example, 20% of schizophrenia patients report obsessions and compulsions, features that are found in only 1–2% of the general population (Eisen and Rasmussen 1993; Berman et al. 1995). In addition (as mentioned in the introduction), there are several reports that individuals with schizophrenia are more likely than controls to have minor physical anomalies. Thus, these particular variables are not unique to the subset of schizophrenia patients with the deletion, but they are also seen in subsets of schizophrenia patients who have not been found to carry the deletion. It is then likely that the 22q11 region harbors genes that contribute to schizophrenia susceptibility in general. The deletion may be one way of interfering with the action of the gene or genes in the region, but there may be additional ways of mutating genes in the region (e.g., point mutations). On the basis of this assumption, we have undertaken an analysis of genes from this region in reference to schizophrenia. In addition to positional cloning approaches, we are also following the candidate gene approach, focusing initially on the genes located in the VCFS critical region. We are searching either for mutations present exclusively in schizophrenia patients, or for sequence variations present in higher frequencies among schizophrenia patients as a whole, in relation to healthy controls, or for sequence variations present in higher frequencies in subsets of schizophrenia patients. Obviously, in the absence of firm linkage, large numbers of patients and controls are necessary to attain statistical confidence, especially if the predisposing mutations are genetic variants also found at lower frequencies in healthy carriers.

CONCLUSION

We have previously demonstrated an association between 22q11 deletions and schizophrenia susceptibility (Karayiorgou et al. 1995 and unpubl.). Here, we describe a patient (AP1268) with a 22q11 deletion, the distal breakpoint of which is located more proximally than previously described. Since schizophrenia is a common disease (partly because of its genetic complexity), the psychotic and schizotypal features of patient AP1268 described here could still be fortuitous. If, however, these features are due to the 22q11 deletion, they would suggest that genes located within the deleted region (the proximal 300–575 kb of the commonly deleted 22q11 region) contribute to the development of psychosis. This is also the region harboring the gene or genes involved in the VCFS/DGS phenotype. More psychotic patients carrying unbalanced translocations or smaller deletions need to be identified.

The underdeveloped nature of psychotic symptoms of patient AP1268 could be explained by the well-established variable penetrance (often intrafamilial; Holder et al. 1993; McLean et al. 1993) observed in association with 22q11 deletions. An alternative explanation is that the deletion in this patient does not extend to include genes lying distally to cosmid 160b (D22S66), including the gene for COMT, as opposed to the 22q11-deleted schizophrenia patients identified so far (Karayiorgou et al. 1995).

Mutational analysis of the COMT gene did not identify mutations that would alter the coding sequence of the gene present exclusively, or in higher frequencies, among all schizophrenics. Although the level of expression of the COMT gene has not been studied and there are regions of the COMT gene we have not scanned for mutations (regulatory regions, 5′ UT, and part of 3′ UT), results from our mutational analysis argue against a major involvement of COMT in the development of schizophrenia. However, a statistically significant enrichment for homozygotes for the high-activity allele among schizophrenia patients who also have obsessive and compulsive features was observed (M. Karayiorgou et al., in prep.). This is a particularly interesting finding, since higher than expected frequencies of obsessive and compulsive features have been noted among the patients with the 22q11 deletion (Pulver et al. 1994a). Because the size of our sample of schizophrenia patients with obsessive-compulsive symptoms is relatively small ($N = 23$), these results need to be tested in larger samples and by other investigators. If confirmed, they can be interpreted in at least three ways: (1) Variation at codon 158 of the COMT gene (Val-158→Met) confers susceptibility to a subtype of schizophrenia; (2) the variation (Val-158→Met) is of no functional significance itself but indicates linkage disequilibrium between the high-activity COMT allele and alleles of a nearby locus predisposing to a subtype of schizophrenia; (3) the results signal indirectly another association. For example, it has been observed both in our sample (A. Pulver et al., unpubl.) and in other samples (Eisen and Rasmussen 1993; Berman et al. 1995) that schizophrenia patients who also have obsessions and compulsions have an earlier age at onset of schizophrenia. Based on this, the observed enrichment of homozygotes for the high-activity allele among schizophrenia patients who also have obsessions and compulsions may in fact indicate an underlying association between the low-activity allele and late onset of schizophrenia. Indeed, an enrichment for homozygotes for the low-activity allele was observed among the schizophrenia patients with age at onset 25 years and older, although analysis with the proportional odds model did not reach statistical significance.

Several chromosomal abnormalities have been described in association with schizophrenia (Bassett 1992). Most of them, however, are reports of isolated cases detected in karyotypic preparations, and none of them has satisfied two important criteria: (1) increased cases of schizophrenia among patients with a specific chromosomal abnormality and (2) increased numbers of a specific chromosomal abnormality among patients with schizophrenia. We have described the first case of a chromosomal abnormality in schizophrenia that satisfies both of these criteria (Karayiorgou et al. 1995). The value of such discoveries is manyfold and includes the following:

1. Potential to pinpoint a region to search for genes. This is very important for schizophrenia, since most involved loci are expected to harbor genes that only have minor effect, and therefore it is extremely hard in most cases either to identify or to narrow down the region of involvement through linkage studies alone.
2. Potential to develop easily scored genetic markers to study genotype/phenotype relations, even before specific genes are isolated (e.g., we are currently using a PCR-based protocol we developed, to screen for presence of the 22q11 deletion in other psychiatric samples, primarily samples of patients with affective disorder, to test the hypothesis of a genetic continuum between schizophrenia and affective disorder, as well as samples of patients with obsessive compulsive disorder).
3. Facilitation for generation of animal models (e.g., generation of long-range deletion in syntenic chromosomal region in mice using the cre-lox approach).
4. Opportunity to access dosage-sensitive genes involved in central nervous system function and dysfunction.

ACKNOWLEDGMENT

This work was supported by a grant from Sandoz Pharmaceuticals.

REFERENCES

Akbarian, S., A. Vinuela, J.J. Kim, S.G. Potkin, W.E. Bunney, and E.G. Jones. 1993a. Distorted distribution of nicotinamide-adenine dinucleotide phosphate-diaphorase neurons in temporal lobe of schizophrenics implies anomalous cortical development. *Arch. Gen. Psychiatry* **50:** 178.

Akbarian, S., W.E. Bunney, Jr., S.G. Potkin, S.B. Wigal, J.O. Hagman, C.A. Sandman, and E.G. Jones. 1993b. Altered distribution of nicotinamide-adenine dinucleotide phosphate-diaphorase cells in frontal lobe of schizophrenics implies disturbances of cortical development. *Arch. Gen. Psychiatry* **50:** 169.

Antonarakis, S.E., J.-L. Blouin, A.E. Pulver, P.S. Wolyniec, V.K. Lasseter, G. Nestadt, L. Kasch, R. Babb, H.H. Kazazian, B. Dombroski, M. Kimberland, J. Ott, D.E. Housman, M. Karayiorgou, and C.J. McLean. 1995. Schizophrenia susceptibility and chromosome 6p24-p22 (Letter to the Editor). *Nat. Genet.* **11:** 235.

Arnold, S.E., B.T. Hyman, G.W. van Hoesen, and A.R. Damasio. 1991. Some cytoarchitectural abnormalities of the entorhinal cortex in schizophrenia. *Arch. Gen. Psychiatry* **48:** 625.

Bassett, A.S. 1992. Chromosomal aberrations and schizophrenia. *Br. J. Psychiatry* **161:** 323.

Benes, F.M., J. McSparren, E.D. Bird, J.P. San Giovanni, and S.L. Vincent. 1991. Deficits in small interneurons in prefrontal and cingulate cortices of schizophrenic and schizoaffective patients. *Arch. Gen. Psychiatry* **48:** 996.

Berman, I., A. Kalinowski, S.M. Berman, J. Lengua, and A.I. Green. 1995. Obsessive and compulsive symptoms in chronic schizophrenia. *Compr. Psychiatry* **36:** 6.

Coon, H., J. Holik, M. Hoff, F. Reimherr, P. Wender, M. Myles-Worsley, M. Waldo, R. Freedman, and W. Byerley. 1994a. Analysis of chromosome 22 markers in nine schizophrenia pedigrees. *Am. J. Med. Genet.* **54:** 72.

Coon, H., S. Jensen, J. Holik, M. Hoff, M. Myles-Worsley, F. Reimherr, P. Wender, M. Waldo, R. Freedman, M. Leppert, and W. Byerley. 1994b. Genomic scan for genes predisposing to schizophrenia. *Am. J. Med. Genet.* **54:** 59.

Demczuk, S., G. Thomas, and A. Aurias. 1996. Isolation of a novel gene from the DiGeorge syndrome critical region with homology to *Drosophila* gdl and to human LAMC1 genes. *Hum. Mol. Genet.* **5:** 633.

Driscoll, D.A., J. Salvin, B. Sellinger, M.L. Budarf, D.M. McDonald-McGinn, E.H. Zackai, and B.S. Emanuel. 1993. Prevalence of 22q11 microdeletions in DiGeorge and velocardiofacial syndromes: Implications for genetic counselling and prenatal diagnosis. *J. Med. Genet.* **30:** 813.

Dunham, I., J. Collins, R. Wadey, and P. Scambler. 1992. Possible role for COMT in psychosis associated with velo-cardio-facial syndrome. *Lancet* **340:** 1361.

Eisen, J.L. and S.A. Rasmussen. 1993. Obsessive compulsive disorder with psychotic features. *J. Clin. Psychiatry* **54:** 373.

Glavac, D. and M. Dean. 1993. Optimization of the single-strand conformation polymorphism (SSCP) technique for detection of point mutations. *Hum. Mutat.* **2:** 404.

Gogos, J.A., M. Karayiorgou, H. Aburatani, and F.C. Kafatos. 1990. Detection of single base mismatches of thymine and cytosine residues by potassium permanganate and hydroxylamine in the presence of tetralkylammonium salts. *Nucleic Acids Res.* **18:** 6807.

Goldstein, M. and A.Y. Deutch. 1992. Dopaminergic mechanisms in the pathogenesis of schizophrenia. *FASEB J.* **6:** 2413.

Gong, W., B.S. Emanuel, J. Collins, D.H. Kim, Z. Wang, F. Chen, G. Zhang, B. Roe, and M.L. Budarf. 1996. A transcription map of the DiGeorge and velo-cardio-facial syndrome minimal critical region on 22q11. *Hum. Mol. Genet.* **5:** 789.

Gottesman, I.I. 1991. *Schizophrenia genesis: The origins of madness.* W.H. Freeman, New York.

Green, M.F., P. Satz, D.J. Gaier, S. Ganzell, and F. Kharabi. 1989. Minor physical anomalies in schizophrenia. *Schizophr. Bull.* **15:** 91.

Grossman, M.H., B.S. Emanuel, and M.L. Budarf. 1992. Chromosomal mapping of the human catechol-*O*-methyltransferase gene to 22q11.1→q11.2. *Genomics* **12:** 822.

Gualtieri, C.T., A. Adams, C.D. Shen, and D. Loiselle. 1982. Minor physical anomalies in alcoholic and schizophrenic adults and hyperactive and autistic children. *Am. J. Psychiatry* **139:** 640.

Gurling, H., G. Kalsi, A.H.-S. Chen, M. Green, R. Butler, T. Read, P. Murphy, D. Curtis, T. Sharma, H. Petursson, and J. Brynjolfsson. 1995. Schizophrenia susceptibility and chromosome 6p24-p22 (Letter to the Editor). *Nat. Genet.* **11:** 234.

Guy, J.D., M.V. Majorski, C.J. Wallace, and M.P. Guy. 1983. The incidence of minor physical anomalies in adult male schizophrenics. *Schizophr. Bull.* **9:** 571.

Halford, S., D.I. Wilson, S.C.M. Daw, C. Roberts, R. Wadey, S. Kamath, A. Wickremasinghe, J. Burn, J. Goodship, M.-G. Mattei, A.F.M. Moormon, and P.J. Scambler. 1993a. Isolation of a gene expressed during early embryogenesis from the region of 22q11 commonly deleted in DiGeorge syndrome. *Hum. Mol. Genet.* **2:** 1577.

Halford, S., R. Wadey, C. Roberts, S.C.M. Daw, J.A. Whiting, H. O'Donnell, I. Dunham, D. Bentley, E. Lindsay, A. Baldini, F. Francis, H. Lehrach, R. Williamson, D.I. Wilson, J. Goodship, I. Cross, J. Burn, and P.J. Scambler. 1993b. Isolation of a putative transcriptional regulator from the region of 22q11 deleted in DiGeorge syndrome, Shprintzen syndrome and familial congenital heart disease. *Hum. Mol. Genet.* **2:** 2099.

Holder, S.E., R.M. Winter, S. Kamath, and P.J. Scambler. 1993. Velocardiofacial syndrome in a mother and daughter: Variability of the clinical phenotype. *J. Med. Genet.* **30:** 825.

Insel, T.R. and H.S. Akiskal. 1986. Obsessive-compulsive disorder with psychotic features: A phenomenologic analysis. *Am. J. Psychiatry* **143:** 1527.

Jakob, H. and H. Beckmann. 1986. Parental developmental disturbances in the limbic allocortex in schizophrenics. *J. Neural Transm.* **65:** 303.

Karayiorgou, M., M.A. Morris, B. Morrow, R.J. Shprintzen, R. Goldberg, J. Borrow, A. Gos, G. Nestadt, P.S. Wolyniec, V.K. Lasseter, H. Eisen, B. Childs, H.H. Kazazian, R. Kucherlapati, S.E. Antonarakis, A.E. Pulver, and D.E. Housman. 1995. Schizophrenia susceptibility associated with interstitial deletions of chromosome 22q11. *Proc. Natl. Acad. Sci.* **92:** 7612.

Lachman, H.M., D.F. Papolos, T. Saito, Y.-M. Yu, C.L. Szumlanski, and R.M. Weinshilboum. 1996. Human catechol-O-methyltransferase pharmacogenetics: Description of a functional polymorphism and its potential application to neuropsychiatric disorders. *Pharmacogenetics* (in press).

LaFosse, M.J. and S.A. Mednick. 1991. A neurodevelopmental approach to schizophrenia research. In *Developmental neuropathology of schizophrenia* (ed. S.A. Mednick et al.), p. 211. Plenum Press, New York.

Lane, A., B. Cassidy, P. Murphy, N. Sheppard, R. Horgan, J. Keenan, J.L. Waddington, C. Larkin, and E. O'Callaghan. 1993. Minor physical anomalies in schizophrenia. *Ir. J. Med. Sci.* **162:** 27.

Lasseter, V.K., A.E. Pulver, P.S. Wolyniec, G. Nestadt, D. Meyers, M. Karayiorgou, D.E. Housman, S.E. Antonarakis, H.H. Kazazian, L. Kasch, R. Babb, M. Kimberland, and B. Childs. 1995. Follow-up report of potential linkage for schizophrenia on chromosome 22q: Part 3 (Letter to the Editor). *Am. J. Med. Genet.* **60:** 172.

Li, M., M.L. Budarf, B. Sellinger, M. Jaquez, R. Matalon, S. Ball, R.A. Pagon, S.S. Rosengren, B.S. Emanuel, and D.A. Driscoll. 1994. Narrowing the DiGeorge region (DGCR) using DGS-VCFS associated translocation breakpoints. *Am. J. Hum. Genet.* **55:** A10.

Liang, K.-Y. and A.E. Pulver. 1996. Analysis of case-control/family sampling design in psychiatric research. *Genet. Epidemiol.* (in press).

Lin, M.-W., D. Curtis, N. Williams, M. Arranz, S. Nanko, D. Collier, P. McGuffin, R. Murray, M. Owen, M. Gill, and J. Powell. 1995. Suggestive evidence for linkage of schizophrenia to markers on chromosome 13ql4.1-q32. *Psychiatr. Genet.* **5:** 117.

Machon, R.A., S.A. Mednick, and M.O. Huttunen. 1995. Fetal viral infection and adult schizophrenia: Empirical findings and interpretations. In *Neural development and schizophrenia* (ed. S.A. Mednick and J.M. Hollister), p. 191. Plenum Press, New York.

McGrath, J., D. Castle, and R. Murray. 1995. How can we judge whether or not prenatal exposure to influenza causes schizophrenia? In *Neural development and schizophrenia* (ed. by S.A. Mednick and J.M. Hollister), p.203. Plenum Press, New York.

McLean, S.D., H.M. Saal, N.B. Spinner, B.S. Emanuel, and D.A. Driscoll. 1993. Velo-cardio-facial syndrome: Intrafamilial variability of the phenotype. *Am. J. Dis. Child.* **147:** 1212.

Moises, H.W., L. Yang, T. Li, B. Havsteen, R. Fimmers, M.P. Baur, X. Liu, and I.I. Gottesman. 1995a. Potential linkage disequilibrium between schizophrenia and locus D22S278 on the long arm of chromosome 22. *Am. J. Med. Genet.* **60:** 465.

Moises, H.W., L. Yang, H. Kristbjarnarson, C. Wiese, W. Byerley, F. Macciardi, V. Arolt, D. Blackwood, X. Liu, B. Sjogren, H.N. Aschauer, H.-G. Hwu, K. Jang, W.J. Livesley, J.L. Kennedy, T. Zoega, O. Ivarsson, M.-T. Bui, M.-H. Yu, B. Havsteen, D. Commenges, J. Weissenbach, E. Schwinger, I.I. Gottesman, A.J. Pakstis, L. Wetterberg, K.K. Kidd, and T. Helgason. 1995b. An international two-stage genome-wide search for schizophrenia susceptibility genes. *Nat. Genet.* **11:** 321.

Moss, E., P.P. Wang, D.M. McDonald-McGinn, M. Gerdes, A.M. DaCosta, K.M. Christensen, D.A. Driscoll, B.S. Emanuel, M.L. Batshaw, and E.H. Zackai. 1995. Characteristic cognitive profile in patients with a 22q11 deletion: Verbal IQ exceeds nonverbal IQ. *Am. J. Hum. Genet.* **57:** (A91) (Abstr.).

Mowry, B.J., D.J. Nancarrow, D.P. Lennon, L.A. Sandkuijl, R.R. Crowe, J.M. Silverman, R.C. Mohs, L.J. Siever, J. Endicott, L. Sharpe, M.K. Walters, N.K. Hayward, and D.F. Levinson. 1995. Schizophrenia susceptibility and chromosome 6p24-22 (Letter to the Editor). *Nat. Genet.* **11:** 233.

Nestadt, G., J.F. Samuels, A.J. Romanoski, M.F. Folstein, and P.R. McHugh. 1994. Obsessions and compulsions in the community. *Acta Psychiatr. Scand.* **89:** 219.

Pato, M.T., F.G. Dowling, L. Jandorf, and C.N. Pato. 1993. Dual diagnosis: OCD and schizophrenia in the ECA study. In *Abstracts from the 146th Annual Meeting of the American Psychiatric Association*, San Francisco.

Propping, P. and M.M. Nothen. 1995. Schizophrenia: Genetic tools for unraveling the nature of a complex disorder. (Commentary). *Proc. Natl. Acad. Sci.* **92:** 7607.

Pulver, A.E. and K.-Y. Liang. 1991. Estimating effects of proband characteristics on familial risk: The association between age at onset and familial risk in the Maryland schizophrenia sample. *Genet. Epidemiol.* **8:** 339.

Pulver, A.E., G. Nestadt, R. Goldberg, R.J. Shprintzen, M. Lamacz, P.S. Wolyniec, B. Morrow, M. Karayiorgou, S.E. Antonarakis, D.E. Housman, and R. Kucherlapati. 1994a. Psychotic illness in patients diagnosed with velo-cardio-facial syndrome and their relatives. *J. Nerv. Ment. Dis.* **182:** 476.

Pulver, A.E., V.K. Lasseter, L. Kasch, P.S. Wolyniec, G. Nestadt, J.-L. Blouin, M. Kimberland, R. Babb, S. Vourlis, H. Chen, M. Lalioti, M.A. Morris, M. Karayiorgou, J. Ott, D. Meyers, S.E. Antonarakis, D.E. Housman, and H.H. Kazazian. 1995. Schizophrenia: A genome scan targets chromosomes 3p and 8p as potential sites for susceptibility genes. *Am. J. Med. Genet.* **60:** 252-260.

Pulver, A.E., M. Karayiorgou, P.S. Wolyniec, V.K. Lasseter, L. Kasch, G. Nestadt, S.E. Antonarakis, D.E. Housman, H.H. Kazazian, D. Meyers, J. Ott, M. Lamacz, K.-Y. Liang, J. Hanfelt, G. Ullrich, N. DeMarchi, R. Elango, P.R. McHugh, L. Adler, M. Thomas, W.T. Carpenter, T. Manschreck, C.T. Gordon, M. Kimberland, R. Babb, J. Puck, and B. Childs. 1994b. A sequential strategy to identify a susceptibility gene for schizophrenia: Report of potential linkage on chromosome 22q12-q13.1: Part 1. *Am. J. Med. Genet.* **54:** 36.

Rossi, A. and P. Stratta. 1995. Cerebral asymmetries in schizophrenia: Further evidence for a lateralization hypothesis. In *Neural development and schizophrenia* (ed. S.A. Mednick and J.M. Hollister), p. 71. Plenum Press, New York.

Scambler, P.J., D. Kelly, E. Lindsay, R. Williamson, R. Goldberg, R. Shprintzen, D.I. Wilson, J.A. Goodship, I.E. Cross, and J. Burn. 1992. Velo-cardio-facial syndrome associated with chromosome 22 deletions encompassing the DiGeorge locus. *Lancet* **339:** 1138.

Schizophrenia Collaborative Linkage Group (chromosome 22). 1996. A combined analysis of D22S278 marker alleles in affected sib-pairs: Support for a susceptibility locus for schizophrenia at 22q12. *Am. J. Med. Genet.* **67:** 40.

Schwab, S.G., M. Albus, J. Hallmayer, S. Honig, M. Borrmann, D. Lichtermann, R.P. Ebstein, M. Ackenheil, B. Lerer, N. Risch, W. Maier, and D.B.Wildenauer. 1995a. Evaluation of a susceptibility gene for schizophrenia on chromosome 6p by multipoint affected sib-pair linkage analysis. *Nat. Genet.* **11:** 325.

Schwab, S.G., B. Lerer, M. Albus, W. Maier, J. Hallmayer, R. Fimmers, D. Lichtermann, J. Minges, B. Bondy, M. Ackenheil, D. Altmark, D. Hasib, E. Gur, R.P. Ebstein, and D.B. Wildenauer. 1995b. Potential linkage for schizophrenia on chromosome 22q12-q13: A replication study. *Am. J. Med. Genet.* **60:** 436.

Shaikh, S., D.A. Collier, P.C. Sham, D. Ball, K. Aitchison, H. Vallada, I. Smith, M. Gill, and R.W. Kerwin. 1996. Allelic association between a Ser-9-Gly polymorphism in the dopamine D3 receptor gene and schizophrenia. *Hum. Genet.* **97:** 714.

Shprintzen, R.J., R. Goldberg, K.J. Golding-Kushner, and R.W. Marion. 1992. Late-onset psychosis in the velo-cardio-facial syndrome (Letter to the Editor). *Am. J. Med. Genet.* **42:** 141.

Straub, R.E., C.J. MacLean, F.A. O Neill, J. Burke, B. Murphy, F. Duke, R. Shinkwin, B.T. Webb, J. Zhang, D. Walsh, and K.S. Kendler. 1995. A potential vulnerability locus for schizophrenia on chromosome 6p24-22: Evidence for genetic heterogeneity. *Nat. Genet.* **11:** 287.

Sutherland, H.F., R. Wadey, J.M. McKie, C. Taylor, U. Atif, K.A. Johnstone, S. Halford, U.-J. Kim, J. Goodship, A. Baldini, and P.J. Scambler. 1996. Identification of a novel transcript disrupted by a balanced translocation associated with DiGeorge syndrome. *Am. J. Hum. Genet.* **59:** 23.

Swayze, V.W., N.C. Andreasen, J.C. Ehrhardt, W.T.C. Yuh, R.J. Alliger, and G.A. Cohen. 1990. Developmental abnormalities of the corpus callosum in schizophrenia. *Arch. Neurol.* **47:** 805.

Vallada, H.P., M. Gill, P. Sham, L.C.C. Lim, S. Nanko, P. Asherson, R.M. Murray, P. McGuffin, M. Owen, and D. Collier. 1995. Linkage studies on chromosome 22 in familial schizophrenia. *Am. J. Med. Genet.* **60:** 139.

Weinshilboum, R.M. and F.A. Raymond. 1977. Inheritance of low erythrocyte catechol-*O*-methyltransferase activity in man. *Am. J. Hum. Genet.* **29:** 125.

Wolyniec, P.S., A.E. Pulver, J.A. McGrath, and D. Tam. 1992. Schizophrenia: Gender and familial risk. *J. Psychiatr. Res.* **2:** 17.

Searching for Susceptibility Genes in Schizophrenia by Genetic Linkage Analysis

D.B. WILDENAUER,[1] J. HALLMAYER,[2] S.G. SCHWAB,[1] M. ALBUS,[3] G.N. ECKSTEIN,[1] P. ZILL,[4] S. HÖNIG,[4] M. STRAUSS,[4] M. BORRMANN,[3] D. LICHTERMANN,[5] R.P. EBSTEIN,[6] B. LERER,[7] N. RISCH,[8] AND W. MAIER[1]

[1]Department of Psychiatry, University of Bonn D-53105 Bonn, Germany; [2]Department of Psychiatry, University, Perth, Western Australia 6001; [3]Mental State Hospital, D-85529 Haar, Germany, [4] Department of Psychiatry, University of Munich, D-80336 München, Germany, [5]National Public Health Institute, Helsinki Finn-00300, Finland; [6]Sarah Herzog Hospital, Jerusalem 91351, Israel; [7]Department of Psychiatry, Hadassah-Hebrew University Medical Center, 91120 Jerusalem, Israel; [8]Department of Genetics, Stanford University, Stanford, California 94305

Schizophrenia is a devastating mental disease with severe impact on the affected individual as well as on family and social environment. Despite many years of research into possible structural and functional changes of the brain, the causes for schizophrenia have not been unraveled. It has been convincingly demonstrated that genetic factors play a major role in the etiology of this disease (Gottesman 1991).

During the last few years, linkage analysis combined with positional cloning strategies have led to the discovery of a large number of disease genes, not only in the case of monogenic inheritance, but also for diseases that are inherited in a more complex mode, such as diabetes and breast cancer. Therefore, it may be possible to also employ these methods successfully in the case of schizophrenia. However, schizophrenia presents several difficulties in applying these methods; for example, the mode of inheritance is unknown, the definition of the phenotype is controversial, and environmental factors seem to play an important role. Methods based on parametric maximum likelihood methodology require specification of the mode of inheritance and, therefore, estimation of disease gene frequencies may not be appropriate.

One possibility to overcome these problems is using affected sib-pair analysis (Penrose 1953; Risch 1990). In this analysis, one determines excess sharing of markers linked to a disease susceptibility locus in affected siblings identity by descent (ibd), allowing the detection of linkage without requiring assumptions about the mode of inheritance. In particular, in connection with the presently available highly polymorphic microsatellite markers, the approach can be used for scanning large chromosomal regions. The method has recently been successfully applied to analysis for susceptibility loci in insulin-dependent diabetes mellitus (Cordell and Todd 1995). Moreover, the method has also been used to implicate loci for behavioral traits like dyslexia (Cardon et al. 1994).

Several studies are currently under way with the aim to test for linkage between schizophrenia and markers spanning the whole human genome. Preliminary results by several groups suggested a susceptibility locus to be located on chromosome 6 (Antonarakis et al. 1995; Schwab et al. 1995a; Straub et al. 1995; Wang et al. 1995) and another on chromosome 22 (Lasseter et al. 1995; Pulver et al. 1994b). Statistical analysis with both parametric and nonparametric methods yielded significantly positive results in these regions.

METHODS

Ascertainment of pedigrees. Families with schizophrenia were selected systematically by asking patients hospitalized for schizophrenia or schizoaffective disorder (Research Diagnostic Criteria [RDC]; Spitzer et al. 1972) for affected relatives. The minimum criteria for including a family in the sample were one additional affected sibling with schizophrenia and the availability of both parents. This nuclear family was extended to other branches, when second- and third-degree relatives were affected and available. Lifetime diagnoses (RDC) were obtained based on best estimate diagnoses. These were derived from joining together the semi-structured clinical interview Schedule for Affective Disorders and Schizophrenia-Lifetime Version (SADS-La; Endicott and Spitzer 1978) family history information, and the medical records of the individual. Details of the diagnostic procedure are given elsewhere (Schwab et al. 1995b).

Genotyping. DNA was extracted from whole blood or immortalized lymphoblastoid cell lines using standard procedures. Amplification of microsatellite markers by PCR and detection of the electrophoretically separated products was carried out as described previously (Schwab et al. 1995a). Fluorescence technology was used for additional markers on chromosome 6 using an ABI Sequencer, Type 377. Genotypes were checked for compatibility with paternity without knowledge of the affection status.

Statistics. Two-point LOD scores were calculated between a putative disease locus and a marker locus using the FASTLINK (Cottingham et al. 1993; Schäffer et al. 1994) version 3 of MLINK of the program package LINKAGE (Lathrop and Lalouel 1984). Sib-pair analysis was carried out ibd. The observed distribution of shared to not-shared alleles was compared to 1/2 (independent segregation of marker alleles and disease). The mean test was used for calculating p values (Knapp et al. 1994a,b). Multipoint sib-pair analysis was carried out using the program ASPEX (Risch 1990; Schwab et al. 1995a).

RESULTS

Families with Schizophrenia

We have ascertained 59 pedigrees by screening consecutively admitted inpatients with schizophrenia or chronic schizoaffective disorder, mainly schizophrenia, as defined by the RDC criteria. In two areas of Germany (Mainz and Haar), 48 pedigrees were collected. In Israel, 11 families of Sephardic Jewish origin were recruited (details are given in Table 1). Full parental genotype information was available for 55 families. In 3 families the genotype of one missing parent was reconstructed by typing additional unaffected siblings; in one family the untyped parent could not be reconstructed. When all possible combinations formed from triplets, quadruplets, and the quintuplet were taken into account, the sample included 89 sib pairs.

For first analysis, the affection status was confined to the narrow defined, hard-core phenotype schizophrenia/chronic schizoaffective, since this should be the most likely one to contain a putative disease gene. There were also family members with other psychiatric diagnoses in our sample; i.e., members with major depression (23), bipolar I- (1), and bipolar II-disorder (1). These phenotypes were included for analysis of candidate genes or regions that may confer susceptibility to schizophrenia and affective disorders as well. Conditions like minor depression (18), personality disorder (4), and alcoholism (11) were not considered as affected, since there is no evidence for cosegregation with schizophrenia.

Genotyping

From these families, 383 DNA samples were available for genotyping. More than 300 restriction fragment length polymorphism and microsatellite markers have been analyzed in order to search for susceptibility genes. So far, we scanned chromosomes 1, 11, and 19 with markers spaced an average distance of 10 cM apart. No statistically significant positive LOD score could be detected in any of these chromosomes.

We also investigated polymorphic markers in or close to a variety of genes that may be considered as candidates for putative schizophrenia susceptibility genes. Examples are genes involved in signal transmission, brain development, and immune response. Given our results, none of the tested genes seems to transfer a higher susceptibility to schizophrenia, with the exception of GOLF (see below).

Finally, we carried out genotypings in regions that were communicated to us by other researchers in the field as possibly containing susceptibility genes, based on their linkage results. Three of these regions are of special interest, since in our family sample positive LOD scores were obtained.

Chromosome 22q12.13. Following up on a report on suggestive linkage for the marker IL2RB (Pulver et al. 1994b), we genotyped a number of markers located in an area of 20 cM on chromosome 22q12.13. Allele sharing was observed for several markers (Fig.1). Statistically significant p values were reached with the marker D22S280 ($p = 0.002$) and D22S422 ($p = 0.004$). Parametric two-point LOD score analysis revealed a value of 1.27 for the marker D22S304 and 1.13 for D22S27. A multipoint affected sib-pair analysis with 15 markers is shown in Figure 2. The area between the two markers D22S280 and D22S422 yielded a maximum LOD score of 2.03 (Fig. 2).

Table 1. Families with Schizophrenia Used in Linkage Analysis (Possible Sib-pair Combinations in Brackets)

	No. of families	Members total	Affected (total no.)	Affected/ family	Duplets	Triplets	Quadruplets	Quintuplets	Sib pairs (total no.)
Nuclear families	36	157	78	2.2	36	–	–	–	36
Extended families									
2 generation	8	72	18	2.25	5	3 (9)	–	–	14
3 generation	4	64	26	6.5	4	1 (3)	–	–	7
Families with Sephardic origin									
nuclear families	4	16	10	2.5	4	–	–	–	4
extended families	7	74	23	3.3	3	1 (3)	2 (12)	1 (10)	28
Total	59	383	155	2.6	52	5 (15)	2 (12)	1 (10)	89

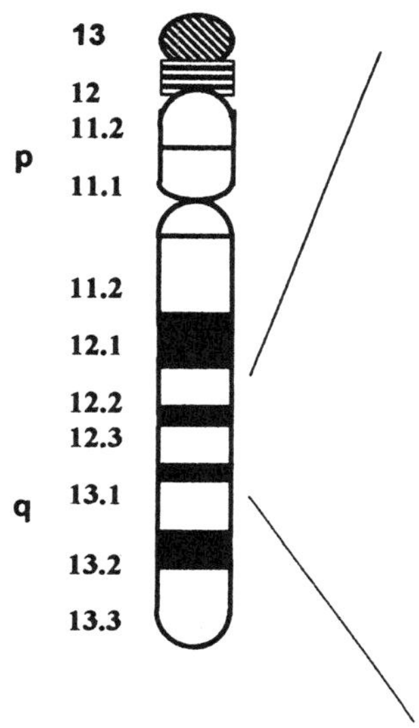

cM	Marker	Lod max (θ)	Alleles shared	Alleles not shared	p-value
	D22S275	0.20 (0.35)	75	80	-----
1					
0.5	D22S268	0.06 (0.35)	69	63	0.60
0.5	D22S528	-9.91 (0.00)	31	43	-----
	D22S273	1.13 (0.20)	76	58	0.12
2					
	D22S280	0.81 (0.25)	91	54	0.002
1					
	D22S422	0.89 (0.20)	95	60	0.004
	D22S281	0.24 (0.30)	65	61	0.73
1					
	D22S304	1.27 (0.15)	66	53	0.23
1					
	D22S424	-5.12 (0.00)	29	33	-----
1.5					
	D22S277	-17.38 (0.00)	78	70	0.51
	D22S278	0.56 (0.15)	58	55	0.78
	D22S283	0.37 (0.30)	78	70	0.51
3					
	D22S426	-9.83 (0.00)	43	38	0.58
4					
	D22S299	-7.25 (0.00)	73	75	-----

Figure 1. Chromosome 22: Two-point LOD scores (at the indicated recombination fraction) and allele-sharing data.

Chromosome 6p21-23. Evidence for a susceptibility gene for schizophrenia has been reported by Straub et al. (1995), Wang et al. (1995), and by us (Schwab et al. 1995a) on the short arm of chromosome 6. A maximum LOD score of 2.2 around the marker D6S285 has been obtained in our sample of 54 families by multipoint sib-pair analysis, but markers with positive LOD scores are spread over an area of more than 20 cM,

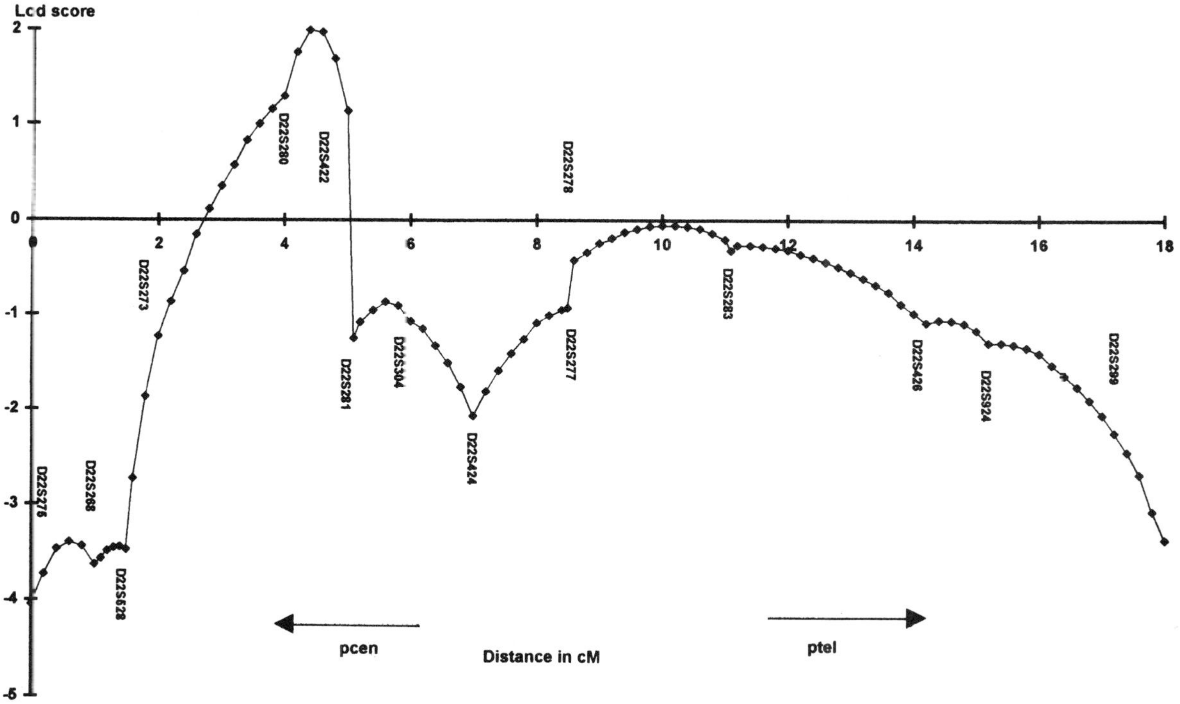

Figure 2. Chromosome 22: Multipoint affected sib-pair linkage analysis (distances according to published maps).

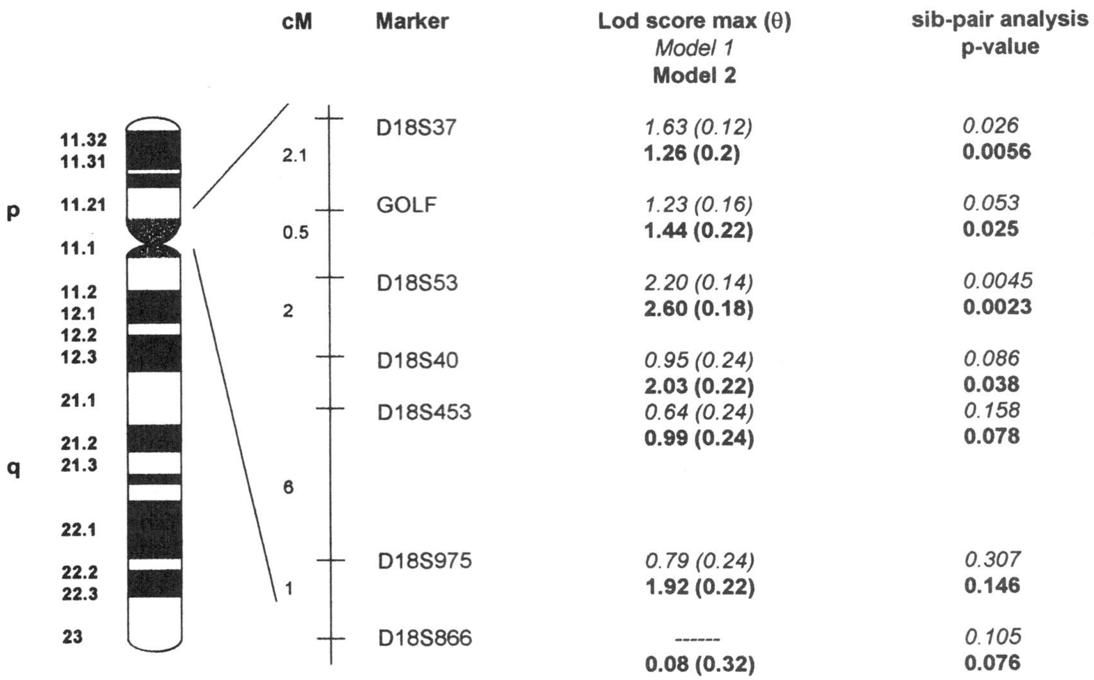

Figure 3. Chromosome 6: Multipoint affected sib-pair linkage analysis.

which cannot not be excluded from containing a susceptibility locus. In an attempt to narrow the region further, we typed 14 additional microsatellite markers within this region and extended the sample to 59 families, containing 89 sib-pair combinations (Table 1). A shift of the maximum LOD score (2.31 around marker D6S260) 5 cM distal to the marker D6S285 (Fig. 3) was obtained upon reevaluation by multipoint sib-pair analysis.

Chromosome 18p. While testing polymorphic short tandem repeats containing genes involved in signal transduction, we obtained a LOD score of 1.23 for the α subunit of the G protein GOLF, which is located on the short arm of chromosome 18. In close vicinity, the marker D18S53 has been reported by Berrettini et al. (1994) as potentially linked to a putative susceptibility gene for bipolar disorders. Additional markers flanking the region were typed. Two-point LOD score analyses were performed using narrow (schizophrenia, schizoaffective disorders = affected) and broad definition of the phenotype (including bipolar disorders and major depression). A LOD score of 2.46 was obtained for the marker D18S53 for the narrow disease model by affected-only analysis, and a LOD score of 2.65 for the wide disease model under the assumption of homogeneity (Fig. 4). Sib-pair analysis revealed a p value of 0.0045 for the narrow, and 0.0023 for the wide, disease model.

DISCUSSION

Although genetic causes for several neurodegenerative disorders like Alzheimer's disease or Huntington's chorea have already been uncovered, research in psychiatric disorders, e.g., schizophrenia and affective disorders, is still in the early stage of finding chromosomal regions where the disease causing dysfunction of the brain may have its origin.

Until recently, linkage analysis in schizophrenia has not been able to produce replicable evidence for linkage. Difficulties in ascertainment of multigeneration families with several affected members, unclear diagnostic boundaries, as well as misspecification of genetic parameters in statistical analysis, may have been the reason. In particular, ascertainment of a large number of affected siblings together with parents is difficult in psychiatric disorders due to lack of cooperation and a high rate of suicides. In addition, recruitment of parents is hampered by disrupted family life and broken home constellations, particularly in families with multiple schizophrenics.

The 59 families used in our work have been collected over several years in a systematic manner, in order to restrict ascertainment bias to a minimum. The sample comprises a mixture of small-sized "nuclear" families and medium-to-large pedigrees. All pedigrees contained a sibship of at least two siblings with the core phenotype schizophrenia or chronic schizoaffective disorder.

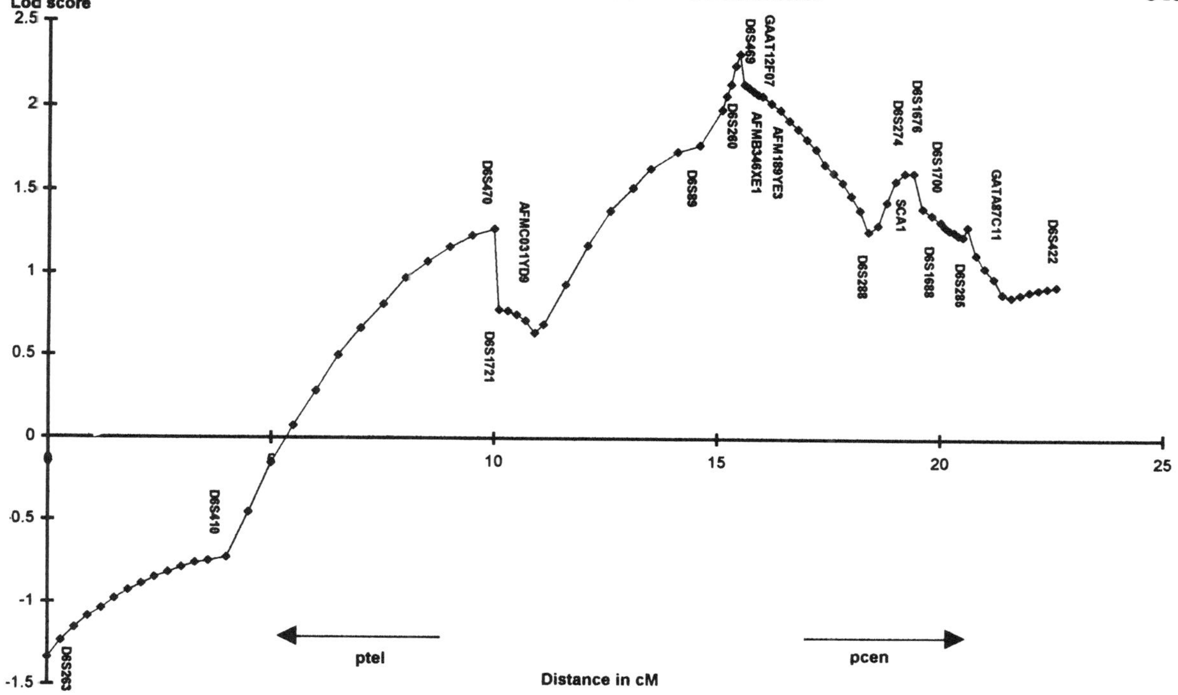

Figure 4. Chromosome 18: Two-point LOD scores (at the indicated recombination fractions) and allele-sharing data. (Model 1) Affected-only analysis with schizophrenia and chronic schizoaffective disorder; all others, phenotype unknown. (Model 2) Analysis with all affected phenotypes (schizophrenia, schizoaffective disorders, affective disorders); all others, phenotype unaffected.

Using this sample, we have been able to carry out the parametric classic two-point LOD score analysis and the nonparametric affected sib-pair method as well. For affected sib-pair analysis, we used only information obtained ibd, i.e., genetic information of both parents had to be available. Thus, we were able to determine unambiguously and independent from additional marker information the number of marker alleles shared ibd. Multipoint analysis across the whole region was carried out for the chromosome 22 and 6 area to increase the number of informative meioses (Schwab et al. 1995a).

Suggestive evidence was obtained in our pedigree sample for genes predisposing to schizophrenia in three chromosomal regions. Our maximum LOD score on chromosome 22 is close to the marker D22S278, for which supportive evidence ($p = 0.001$) was obtained in 296 sib pairs by the Schizophrenia Collaborative Linkage Group (chromosome 22) (1996), and is about 10 cM centromeric to the marker IL2RB, where maximum LOD score was reported originally by Pulver et al. (1994b). The region harboring the deletion responsible for the velo-cardio-facial syndrome, which is sometimes accompanied by schizophrenia (Pulver et al. 1994a), is 20–30 cM centromeric to the marker with maximum LOD score in our sample.

The strongest evidence for a susceptibilty locus has been obtained for chromosome 6p (Antonarakis et al. 1995; Schwab et al. 1995a; Straub et al. 1995; Wang et al. 1995). We report here the increase of number of families from 54 to 59 and LOD scores for an additional 14 markers. This was followed by a slight telomeric shift (5 cM) as well as a slight increase of the maximum LOD score. However, the interval likely to contain a susceptibility locus remains large. Since, in contrast to monogenic disorders, in complex disorders the identification of critical recombinations is impossible, a large number of sib pairs (200–1000) is needed to narrow the region on a statistical basis, a sample much larger than we have available to date.

Our finding on chromosome 18p is interesting in the light of the continuum hypothesis, which suggests that schizophrenia and affective psychosis may not be separate entities, but could be inherited along a genetic continuum (Crow 1986). The same markers D18S53 and D18S37, for which maximum LOD scores and statistically significant allele sharing were obtained in our analysis using a definition of the phenotype including both schizophrenia and affective psychoses, also provided the strongest evidence for a susceptibility locus for bipolar disorders in recent reports by Berrettini et al. (1994) and Stine et al. (1995).

In summary, we have reported supportive evidence for three chromosomal regions, where genes contributing to the etiology of schizophrenia may be located. One of the putative genes may also confer a higher susceptibility to affective psychoses. Existence of these genes is based at the moment solely on statistical evidence. Final proof has to come, of course, from identification of the genes and their products. Positional cloning of genes in a complex disorder such as schizophrenia might turn out to be an extremely difficult or even impossible task. Of paramount importance is to gather a large number of pedigrees with affected siblings in order to further narrow the region(s). Other methodologies such as association studies, linkage disequilibrium mapping, large-scale sequencing, and investigation of candidate genes might also contribute to the successful cloning of schizophrenia susceptibility genes.

ACKNOWLEDGMENTS

We express our gratitude to all patients and their family members—without their cooperation this work would not have been possible. This work was supported largely by grants from the Deutsche Forschungsgemeinschaft (M.A., W.M., D.B.W.) and from the German-Israeli Foundation for Scientific Research (B.L., R.P.E., D.B.W.). N.R. was supported by the National Institutes of Health grant HG-00348, and J.H. by the endowment fund of the Nancy Pritzker Laboratory, the Spunk Fund, and the Marianne Gerschel charitable acount.

REFERENCES

Antonarakis, S.E., J.-L. Blouin, A.E. Pulver, P. Wolyniec, V.K. Lasseter, G. Nestadt, L. Kasch, R. Babb, H.H. Kazazian, B. Dombroski, M. Kimberland, J. Ott, D. Housman, M. Karayiorgou, and C.J. MacLean. 1995. Schizophrenia susceptibility and chromosome 6p24-22. *Nat. Genet.* **11:** 325.

Berrettini, W.H., T.N. Ferraro, L.R. Goldin, D.E. Weeks, S. Detera-Wadleigh, J.I. Nurnberger, Jr., and E.S. Gershon. 1994. Chromosome 18 DNA markers and manic depressive illness: Evidence for a susceptibility gene. *Proc. Natl. Acad. Sci.* **91:** 5918.

Cardon, L.R., S.D. Smith, D.W. Fulker, U.J. Kimberling, B.F. Pennington, and J.C. DeFries. 1994. Quantitative trait locus for reading disability on chromosome 6. *Science* **266:** 276.

Cordell, H.J. and J.A. Todd. 1995. Multifactorial inheritance in type 1 diabetes. *Trends Genet.* **11:** 499.

Cottingham, R.W., R.M. Idury, and A.A. Schäffer. 1993. Faster sequential genetic linkage computations. *Am. J. Hum. Genet.* **53:** 252.

Crow, T.J. 1986. The continuum of psychosis and its implication for the structure of the gene. *Brit. J. Psychiatry* **149:** 419.

Endicott, J. and R.L. Spitzer. 1978. A diagnostic interview: The schedule for affective disorders and schizophrenia. *Arch. Gen. Psychiatry* **35:** 837.

Gottesman, I.I. 1991. *Schizophrenia genesis: The origin of madness.* W.H. Freeman, New York.

Knapp, M., S.A. Seuchter, and M.P. Baur. 1994a. Linkage analysis in nuclear families. 1. Optimality criteria for affected sib-pair tests. *Hum. Hered.* **44:** 37.

———. 1994b. Linkage analysis in nuclear families. 2. Relationship between affected sib-pair test and lod score analysis. *Hum. Hered.* **44:** 44.

Lasseter, V.K., A.E. Pulver, P.S. Wolnyiec, G. Nestadt, D. Mayers, M. Karayiorgou, S. Antonarakis, H. Kazazian, L. Kasch, R. Babb, M. Kimberland, and B. Childs. 1995. Follow-up report of potential linkage on chromosome 22q: Part 3. *Am. J. Med. Genet. Neuropsychiat. Genet.* **60:** 172.

Lathrop, G.M. and J.M. Lalouel. 1984. Easy calculation of lod scores and genetic risk on small computers. *Am. J. Hum. Genet.* **36:** 460.

Penrose, L.S. 1953. The general purpose sib-pair linkage test. *Ann. Eugenics* **18:** 120.

Pulver, A.E., G. Nestadt, R. Goldberg, R.J. Shprintzen, M. Lamacz, P.S. Wolyniec, B. Morrow, M. Karayiorgou, S.E. Antonarakis, D. Housman, and R. Kucherlapati. 1994a. Psychotic illness in patients diagnosed with velo-cardio-facial syndrome and their relatives. *J. Nerv. Ment. Dis.* **182:** 476.

Pulver, A.E., M. Karayiorgou, P.S. Wolyniec, V.K. Lasseter, L. Kasch, G. Nestadt, S. Antonarakis, D. Housman, H.H. Kazazian, D. Meyers, J. Ott, M. Lamacz, K.A. Liang, J. Hansfeldt, G. Ullrich, N. DeMarchi, E. Ramu, P.R. McHugh, L. Adler, M. Thomas, W.T. Carpenter, T. Manschreck, C.T. Gordon, M. Kimberland, M. Babb, J. Puck, and B. Childs. 1994b. Sequential strategy to identify a susceptibility gene for schizophrenia: Report of potential linkage on chromosome 22q12-q13.1: Part 1. *Am. J. Med. Genet. Neuropsychiatr. Genet.* **54:** 36.

Risch, N. 1990. Linkage strategies for genetically complex traits. II. The power of affected relative pairs. *Am. J. Hum. Genet.* **46:** 229.

Schäffer, A.A., S.K. Gupta, K. Shriram, and R.W. Cottingham. 1994. Avoiding recomputation in linkage analysis. *Hum. Hered.* **44:** 225.

Schizophrenia Collaborative Linkage Group (chromosome 22). 1996. A combined analysis of D22S278 marker alleles in affected sib-pairs: Support for a suceptibility locus for schizophrenia at chromosome 22q12. *Am. J. Med. Genet. Neuropsychiatr. Genet.* **67:** 40.

Schwab, S.G., M. Albus, J. Hallmayer, S. Hönig, M. Borrman, D. Lichtermann, R.P. Ebstein, M. Ackenheil, B. Lerer, N. Risch, W. Maier, and D.B. Wildenauer. 1995a. Evaluation of a susceptibility gene for schizophrenia on chromosome 6p by multipoint affected sib-pair linkage analysis. *Nat. Genet.* **11:** 325.

Schwab, S.G., B. Lerer, M. Albus, W. Maier, J. Hallmayer, R. Fimmers, D. Lichtermann, J. Minges, B. Bondy, M. Ackenheil, D. Altmark, D. Hasib, E. Gur, R.P. Ebstein, and D.B. Wildenauer. 1995b. Potential linkage for schizophrenia on chromosome 22q12-13: A replication study. *Am. J. Med. Genet. Neuropsychiatr. Genet.* **60:** 436.

Spitzer, R.L., J. Endicott, and E. Robins. 1972. *Research diagnostic criteria (RDC) for a selected group of functional disorders*, 3rd edition. New York State Department of Mental Hygiene Biometrics Research, New York.

Stine, O.C., J. Xu, R. Koskela, F.J. McMahon, M. Gschwend, C. Friddle, C.D. Clark, M.G. McInnis, S.G. Simpson, T.S. Breschel, E. Vishio, K. Raskin, H. Feilotter, E. Chen, S. Shen, S. Folstein, D.A. Meyers, D. Botstein, T.G. Marr, and J.R. DePaulo. 1995. Evidence for linkage of bipolar disorder to chromosome 18 with a parent-of-origin effect. *Am. J. Hum. Genet.* **57:** 1384.

Straub, R.E., C.J. MacLean, F.A. O'Neil, J. Burke, B. Murphy, F. Duke, R. Shinkwin, B.T. Webb, J. Zhang, D. Walsh, and K.S. Kendler. 1995. A potential vulnerability locus for schizophrenia on chromosome 6p24-22: Evidence for genetic heterogeneity. *Nat. Genet.* **11:** 287.

Wang, S., C. Sun, C.A. Walczak, J.S. Ziegle, B.R. Kipps, L.R. Goldin, and S.R. Diehl. 1995. Evidence for a susceptibility locus for schizophrenia on chromosome 6pter-p22. *Nat. Genet.* **10:** 41.

Summary: Function and Dysfunction of the Nervous System

Z.W. Hall
National Institute of Neurological Disorders and Stroke, National Institutes of Health, Bethesda, Maryland 20892

Like its predecessors, the 61st Cold Spring Harbor Symposium signified both symbol and substance in its choice of subject: symbolic in its pronouncement that a new topic, *Function and Dysfunction in the Nervous System*, has now entered the hallowed canon of Cold Spring Harbor Symposia; substantive in that the 61st Symposium brought together in a new and exciting way several lines of brain research that are not commonly combined. The significance of the 61st Symposium can be readily recognized by placing it within the context of previous Cold Spring Harbor Symposia on the nervous system, whose changing emphases have marked the progress of our field. The Symposia of 1952 and 1965 (*The Neuron* and *Sensory Receptors*, respectively) focused on single cells; the interactions between nerve cells formed the chief theme of the Symposium of 1975 (*The Synapse*); the symposium entitled *Molecular Neurobiology* in 1983 recognized the impact of modern molecular biology on the neurosciences; and the title of the Symposium of 1990 (*The Brain*) quietly asserted that the entire brain was now ripe for the rigors of quantitative biology. Against this background, the almost coy title of the 61st Symposium gave only the barest hint of its bold excursion into new territory. Many of the questions that have so dominated our past discussions at Cold Spring Harbor, e.g., the mechanisms of signaling in the nervous system or how the connectivity of the nervous system arises during development, were only peripherally represented at the 61st Symposium, which gave center stage to questions of sensory perception, of memory and learning, and of neurological and psychiatric disease. The change was clearly seen in our choice of experimental animals. Although past meetings swarmed with squid, crayfish, sea slugs, and frogs, mammals dominated in 1996. Indeed, apart from a stray fruit fly or worm and the occasional contaminating yeast, the 61st Symposium focused almost entirely on mice and men. Whereas the dominance of mice is readily explained by the power of molecular genetics in generating "knock-out and knock-in" animals, the prominence of humans as experimental subjects arises from two sources, both major themes of the Symposium: first, our increasing ability to link human behavior to biology; and second, our increasing success in attacking the problems of human brain disease.

All authors cited here without dates refer to papers in this volume.

The breadth of these themes and the recent success of experimental science in these areas gave an air of excitement and discovery to the week. Eighty-six speakers and 94 posters produced an abundance of new data and new ideas, testifying to the intense intellectual activity of the meeting. The graceful setting, good food, and unobtrusively efficient organization by the Cold Spring Harbor staff ensured the dominance of science. We are grateful to Bruce Stillman and Jim Watson for their choice of theme and participants, and to the staff at Cold Spring Harbor Laboratory who were responsible for making the week extraordinarily pleasant as well as scientifically exciting.

BRAIN DISEASE

Genetic Diseases of the Brain

Molecular genetics is the major tool of modern biology, transforming every field that it touches. Its impact has been nowhere greater than on diseases of the brain, in part because these diseases have been so intractable to other methods of analysis. Estimates suggest that half of all human genes are expressed in the brain, and that approximately one-third of all genetic diseases involve the brain. More than 60 human genes have already been identified whose defects result in brain disease, and several hundred more are thought to be awaiting discovery. An observation by Huda Zoghbi (Orr and Zoghbi) at the meeting illustrates the impact of molecular genetics on neurology. She pointed out that prior to the clarification resulting from cloning of the responsible genes, neurologists had made more than 50 attempts to classify the cerebellar ataxias, as they tried to pick out common nosological threads from the bewildering variety of symptoms presented by individual patients. Classification by molecular genetics now settles the issue.

When a new disease gene is discovered, the result is decisive and its impact often dramatic, generating new tools and new ideas. The strong evolutionary conservation of gene sequence and function coupled with the ability to move genes from organism to organism means that even distant biological systems can be quickly brought to bear on problems of human disease. A striking example of the relevance of distant organisms is provided by the discovery in yeast of proteins that appear to propagate conformational changes in a way that resembles the changes propagated by infectious prion proteins in the human spongiform encephalopathies (Wickner et al.).

The large number of genes related to brain disease that have now been identified means that the general pathway by which progress is made is clear, even as the particular results continue to surprise us. Various stepping stones along this pathway were well represented at the meeting. For convenience we divide them into four steps: Find the gene; discover its function; make a mouse; and treat the disease.

Find the gene. The first step in investigating a genetic trait is to recognize its pattern of heritability. An unexpected and interesting non-neurological example on the inheritance of handedness was presented by Amar Klar (Klar). Although handedness has been previously considered to be a polygenic trait or one with variable penetrance, Klar postulates that it is specified by a single gene with two alleles, one of which is associated exclusively with right-handedness, and the other with random handedness (i.e., equal frequency of both left and right). This strikingly simple hypothesis clarifies a confusing picture on the inheritance of handedness, including the discordance among monozygotic twins. The stage is now set for a search for linkage.

As numerous examples at the meeting demonstrated, discovery of a disease gene by positional cloning is usually straightforward if the gene is inherited in Mendelian fashion. For disorders in which inheritance is more complex, the initial step of establishing linkage is likely to be difficult. This is illustrated by the major psychiatric disorders, schizophrenia and manic-depressive illness, which clearly have a genetic component, but in which linkage has been difficult to establish. In the case of schizophrenia, several genome scans with multicenter analysis of particular regions have led to the identification of major regions of interest on chromosomes 6, 22, and 8, with others possibly on chromosomes 13 and 18 (Pulver et al.; McGuffin and Owen; Wildenauer et al.; Straub et al.). The involvement of chromosome 22 is further indicated by the increased susceptibility to schizophrenia associated with deletions in the 22q11 region (Karayiorgou et al.). Although the general agreement on loci that has been reached between different groups is encouraging, no genes have yet been identified. The evidence so far suggests that there is not a major locus for schizophrenia, but a variety of susceptibility genes of relatively modest effect; even in subpopulations, no single gene appears to be either necessary or sufficient.

In the case of bipolar manic-depressive illness, linkage to several loci, including regions on chromosomes 18 and 21q, has been detected and independently confirmed (DePaulo and McMahon). Although both schizophrenia and affective disorders are thought to arise from alterations in amine systems, attempts to demonstrate the involvement of specific candidate genes have so far yielded relatively little. One potentially interesting observation is the association of a particular expanded repeat in the first intron of the human serotonin transporter gene with an increased frequency of affective disorder (Harmar et al.).

In the case of both schizophrenia and inherited affective disorders, the sobering conclusion is that much work remains to be done in identifying the genes involved, involving perhaps thousands of patients. The increasing progress and power of genetic technology, however, assures us that if linkage is found, the gene can be discovered. As techniques of high-throughput sequencing of the genome and of recognizing expressed sequences improve, the identification of important genes in other genetically complex disorders of the brain, such as stroke, epilepsy, autism, Tourette's syndrome, obsessive-compulsive disorder, or Parkinson's disease, will become an increasingly easier task. In several of these cases, such as epilepsy, for example, significant progress has already been made, both with respect to the human genes, and with genes in spontaneous mouse mutants (Noebels et al.).

Investigate the gene's function. Once the gene is found, the next stage is to understand what its protein product does and how it causes disease. In this phase of the narrative, the tools suddenly change: The sequencers, the statistical methods, and the gene-hunter programs are moved to the back shelf, and the equipment for antibody production, immunocytochemistry, and yeast two-hybrid analysis is moved to the front of the bench. Sometimes the gene is known and its identification has immediate conceptual impact. The discovery that defects in the enzyme superoxide dismutase can cause familial amyotrophic lateral sclerosis (ALS) (Siddique), for example, immediately underlined the importance of oxidative damage in the pathogenesis of the disease. In other cases, the discovered gene may be already known, but its relation to the disease may be obscure, as in the case of the androgen receptor in spinobulbar muscular atrophy (Fischbeck et al.). Finally, there are cases in which the gene product is totally unknown. These are potentially the most powerful discoveries, because they can provide new clues to both the disease and the basic biology of brain function.

Alzheimer's disease is such an example. Four genes are presently known in which mutations or polymorphisms are associated with an increased incidence of Alzheimer's disease. The first to be discovered was the gene for the β-amyloid precursor protein (βAPP), in which six different missense mutations have been identified that lead to early onset of the disease (Clark et al.). In transfected cells, all of these mutations lead to increased secretion of the amyloid β protein (Aβ), the major constitutent of the amyloid plaques which are the pathological hallmark of Alzheimer's disease. The discovery that mutations in the βAPP gene could cause Alzheimer's disease was a key factor in establishing the importance of β amyloid as a pathogenic agent rather than a by-product of the disease. Two more recently described genes responsible for familial early-onset Alzheimer's disease that encode the related proteins, presenilin 1 and 2 (St. George-Hyslop et al.), offer further clues to the pathogenesis of the disease. One effect of disease-associated mutations in the presenilin genes is to increase secretion of the longer form (Aβ42) compared to the shorter form (Aβ40) of the Aβ peptide (Selkoe; St. George-Hyslop et al.). Because both increased secretion of the Aβ peptide, and an increased proportion of the longer form, predispose to Aβ aggregation and plaque formation, a satisfying unifying hypothesis emerges in which the common defect in all forms of the disease is the increased deposition of amyloid to form plaques. Perhaps because the hypothesis is so appealing, we should be particularly cautious about accepting it until experimental support for it is very solid.

The normal functions of βAPP and the presenilins are unknown. In neurons, βAPP is targeted to axonal surface membranes and later becomes redistributed into dendrites as well (Tienari et al.). The presenilins are associated predominantly with internal membranes of the endoplasmic reticulum and the Golgi and are thought to play a role in intracellular membrane trafficking. Curiously, the presenilins appear in immunoprecipitations as cleaved amino- and carboxy-terminal peptides (Selkoe; St. George-Hyslop et al.). Whether these are the biologically active forms or represent degradation products remains to be determined.

The fourth gene related to Alzheimer's disease is the ApoE gene, in which one allele, apoE4, is associated with increased susceptibility, and another, apoE2, with decreased risk. Although the function of ApoE in serum transport of cholesterol is well known, the mechanism by which different alleles of the gene influence the onset of Alzheimer's disease is unclear. ApoE4 is present in amyloid plaques, and some evidence suggests that the different forms of the protein vary in their ability to promote Aβ aggregation.

An apparently unrelated, but interesting and important, advance in the investigation of Alzheimer's disease concerns the origin of the paired helical filaments, found in Alzheimer's disease as in some other types of neurodegenerative disease. The predominant protein in the filaments is the microtubule-associated protein tau. Tau, isolated from paired helical filaments, shows both increased phosphorylation at normally phosphorylated sites and new phosphorylation at novel sites, suggesting that the primary event in paired helical filament formation may be the abnormal phosphorylation of tau. Recent results, however, suggest that the initiating event may not be increased phosphorylation, but rather the association of microtubules with intracellular heparan sulfate (Goedert et al.). Interestingly, intracellular heparan sulfate appears to be increased in Alzheimer's disease, an observation that offers a possible insight into the neuropathology of the disease. Whether the formation of the paired helical filaments is responsible for cellular injury or is simply a response to it remains unknown.

A second instructive example of the progress from genetics to disease mechanisms is offered by the CAG repeat diseases—Huntington's disease, dentatorubro-pallidoluysial atrophy (DRPLA or Smith's disease), spinocerebellar atrophy type I and type III (Machado-Joseph disease), and spinobulbar muscular atrophy (Kennedy's disease). In each of these gain-of-function diseases, the protein encoded by the defective gene contains an expanded polyglutamine tract (Gusella et al.; Orr and Zoghbi; Fischbeck et al.; Sadou et al.). Recent investigations have focused on possible protein-protein interactions mediated by the expanded polyglutamine tracts that might be the cause of these diseases. Several interacting proteins have been identified by various techniques, and it remains to be seen which, if any, of the interactions so far identified in the test tube is responsible for the resulting neuronal degeneration. Perhaps the leading candidate at the moment is GAPDH, which has been shown to bind to the expanded, but not the normal, forms of huntingtin and ataxin-1, which are the proteins affected in Huntington's disease and spinocerebellar atrophy, respectively. GAPDH also binds to the protein product of the DRPLA gene and to the androgen receptor, which is altered in spinobulbar muscular atrophy. A serum has been obtained that is specific for proteins containing expanded, but not normal, repeats and will be useful in future investigations (Sadou et al.).

The idea that a common mechanism might underlie the pathology seen in all four of these diseases is intriguing, although it leaves open the question of the cellular specificity observed in each case. The cellular specificity, which is puzzling in view of the common biochemical mechanism that is postulated, should perhaps not be overemphasized, since as Gusella pointed out (Gusella et al.), there is considerable overlap in the affected populations of cells for these diseases, especially when late or severe cases are considered.

Other genes in the larger family of trinucleotide repeat disorders have different nucleotide repeats that are outside the coding region, and thus different mechanisms of pathogenesis must be sought. In the case of fragile X, the nucleotide expansion occurs in the 5′-untranslated region of a gene that encodes an RNA-binding ribosomal protein. Expansion of a CGG repeat results in abnormal methylation that silences transcription of the gene (Eberhart and Warren; Q. Liu et al.). In the case of myotonic dystrophy, the repeat occurs in the 3′-untranslated region of the mRNA, causing it to bind to a protein that may function in the nuclear export of mRNA (Caskey et al.).

How do the gene alterations responsible for these diseases arise? Little is known about the origins of the trinucleotide repeat diseases. A fascinating story emerges, however, from the study of two demyelinating peripheral neuropathies, Charcot-Marie-Tooth disease 1A (CMT 1A) and hereditary neuropathy with pressure palsy (HNPP) (Warner et al.). Both of these disorders appear to arise from a recombinational hot spot that is apparently the inherited remains of an ancient transposon embedded within the genome. Increased recombination at this site can result in the tandem duplication of a 1.5-Mb DNA segment, yielding CMT 1A, or in a reciprocal 1.5-Mb deletion, associated with HNPP. Curiously, these rearrangements occur preferentially on the paternally inherited chromosome. The net effect of the rearrangement is to change the gene dosage, resulting in overexpression or underexpression of a gene within the segment, most likely the gene encoding PMP22, a peripheral myelin protein of unknown function.

Make a mouse. Perhaps the most important single tool that can result from cloning a disease gene is a mouse model of the disease. A mouse that reproduces the disease allows investigation of the normal function of the gene, how the altered gene leads to pathogenesis, and, ultimately, of therapeutic strategies. Three examples of mouse models were described at the meeting that illustrate their usefulness in different ways.

The first example is the familial amyotrophic lateral sclerosis (FALS) mouse. In a subgroup of patients with FALS, the disease has been shown to arise from mutations in the gene encoding superoxide dismutase (SOD). Expression of these mutated human genes results in a mouse that develops a disease of motor weakness whose neuropathology and symptoms closely replicate those seen in the human disease (Williamson et al.; D. Price et al.). Because these mice have a normal, endogenous SOD and their phenotype is entirely different from that of an SOD –/– mouse, the disease is clearly not due to a loss of function of SOD, but to a gain of function which is deleterious. Current experiments focus on the hypothesis that the mutations produce an altered enzyme specificity, resulting in the production of increased levels of free radicals or in an abnormal profile of the different free radical species.

The second example is offered by the CAG trinucleotide repeat diseases, for which the SCA1 mouse is the first successful disease model. In this case, human ataxin with an expanded glutamine repeat is expressed specifically in Purkinje cells by putting the altered gene under a cell-specific promoter. The resulting mouse shows progressive neurological deficits, including ataxia, that are reminiscent of the human disease (Orr and Zoghbi). This represents an important advance, as it is the first of the CAG trinucleotide repeat diseases to be reproduced in a mouse. Attempts to produce a genetically altered mouse with Huntington's disease have so far been unsuccessful (MacDonald et al.). The null mouse for Huntington's does not survive past embryonic day 8, and attempts to produce heterozygotes, expressing both the mouse and the human gene, have so far failed, as they show either no phenotype or severe birth defects with lethality.

The spongiform encephalopathies caused by prions provide the third example of the usefulness of transgenic mice in investigation of disease. Recent experiments have shown that transgenic mice null for the normal prion protein (PrPx) do not develop symptoms of scrapie after inoculation with infectious prion protein (PrPsc) and produce no increase in infectious particles (Prusiner; Weissmann et al.). Both of these normal responses are restored by transgenes encoding PrPx. These experiments establish the key role of the normal prion protein in the pathogenesis of the disease and provide crucial evidence for the idea that scrapie, and by implication other spongiform encephalopathies, arise by conversion of the normal protein into an infectious agent (Prusiner; Weissmann et al.). By expressing transgenes encoding altered prion proteins or prion proteins from different species, the requirements for the conversion can be established. In other experiments, tissue with normal prion protein expression was grafted into null mice, which were then infected contralaterally with scrapie prions. The finding that only the grafted tissue becomes pathological suggests that the damage caused by prions is cell-autonomous (Weissmann et al.). In a number of recent cases reported in young adults in Great Britain, the pathology differs from typical cases of Creutzfeld-Jakob disease in showing numerous large PrP-containing amyloid plaques throughout the cerebral cortex, basal ganglia, and cerebellum (Ironside et al.). The relation of these diseases to bovine spongiform encephalopathy remains uncertain.

Although experiments in mice will continue to be invaluable in understanding inherited neurodegenerative diseases, more extensive investigations on cells in culture will be essential if we are to understand the cellular mechanisms by which damage is produced. Experiments on transfected neuroblastoma cells expressing expanded-repeat versions of the protein huntingtin show that they have reduced survival in the presence of cAMP, which may be useful in understanding Huntington's disease (Sadou et al.). Another series of experiments on ScN2A cells suggests that the altered form of PrP produces changes in signaling related to membrane processes (DeArmond et al.). These experiments are a first step, but much more work in this area will be needed.

Treat the disease. The ultimate aim of research on disease, of course, is to generate treatments that will prevent, slow, or reverse the disease process. In none of the cases discussed above is a treatment currently available. For a number of diseases of the nervous system, disease results from a toxic gain of function. In the case of ALS, of the trinucleotide diseases, of familial Alzheimer's disease due to mutations in the APP gene, and of the prion diseases, pathology results when a protein exerts a deleterious effect. The task of therapy is thus not to replace a function, but to find out what the mutated protein is doing to damage the cell, and how to interfere with that process. The good news is that in most cases the defect is small. These are, after all, often adult-onset diseases, which means that the cells have been able to live and function a very long time despite the altered gene. What this likely means is that some process is only slightly awry, and that only over many years do the consequences of this marginal misfunction accumulate to cause cellular injury and death. If the process is only slightly askew, then only a small perturbation may be necessary to prevent the development and progression of the pathology. The bad news is, of course, that the effects of a small perturbation over many years may be difficult to detect, offering a strenuous challenge to clinical research. Imagine the difficulties of a trial, for example, to test the effect of a drug that slows the progress of Alzheimer's disease over a period of five years. In addition to the length of time and the number of patients involved, the difficulties also include the devising of suitable biological markers for the disease that can serve as end points for clinical trials.

In any case, what we need to know are the pathways by which the altered proteins cause pathology and the ways in which cells respond to injury. We will then need to design drugs that will interfere with the offending processes and that will enhance the pathways that ameliorate the effect. Structural biology is likely to become a crucial tool in this effort, as protein-protein interactions will be the key to understancing these pathways; what will be needed are molecules designed to weaken or strengthen these interactions.

Neuronal Death and Injury

A major theme that appeared in various contexts during the meeting is the question of how neurons are injured and how they die. This theme was sounded with respect to AIDS, where neuronal damage appears to arise not from viral infection of neurons, but from the effects of viral products or cytokines that are produced by infected macrophages and microglia (R. Price); with respect to the neurodegenerative diseases (Alzheimer's disease, Huntington's disease, Parkinson's disease, and ALS), in which specific classes of neurons in adults die for unknown reasons; with respect to the CGA trinucleotide diseases, in which an expanded polyglutamine tract causes neurons to die; with respect to prion disease, in which a misfolded protein apparently causes neuronal death; and with respect to ischemic and excitotoxic cell death. Although in none of these cases is the molecular mechanism known, a number of common themes link studies in these areas, suggesting that common mechanisms may be at work.

Several lines of evidence point to the role of oxidative damage. Perhaps the best example is FALS, in which an enzyme responsible for inactivating oxygen free radicals, SOD, is mutated (Siddique). A second mechanism that may be common to many cases of cellular injury is the activation of proteases that are associated with cell death pathways. Neuronal damage can also be caused by prolonged exposure to excitatory amino acids, produced as the result of ischemic, hypoglycemic, or traumatic insult. Two new agents that appear to play a role in excitotoxic cell death were described at the meeting. Strickland (Strickland et al.) reported experiments indicating that tissue plasminogen activator (tPA) plays a role in excitotoxic cell death produced either by kainate injection into the hippocampus or after experimental cerebral ischemia. Animals null for tPA, or for its substrate plasminogen, were resistant to neuronal degeneration produced either by kainate injection into the hippocampus or by experimentally produced focal ischemia. Protease inhibitors given acutely produced the same results. A second agent that may play an important role in excitatory cell death is zinc. Zinc is stored in synaptic vesicles and secreted during synaptic activity. Although at low concentrations zinc attenuates the activation of NMDA receptors, at higher concentrations it enters cells and appears to be associated with neuronal degeneration (Choi). A third agent that is likely to be important in regulating cell injury in several different contexts is NO. Experiments by Enikolopov (Peunova et al.) have shown that in cultured PC12 cells, NO protects against apoptosis. It apparently does so by inducing members of the Bcl-2 family that regulate the cell death pathway. These results could explain an earlier observation that NOS-positive neurons, originally identified on the basis of the diaphorase activity of NOS, are resistant to cell death.

BEHAVIOR AND THE BRAIN

If the first notable theme of the meeting was human disease, the second was surely the complex properties and behaviors of the brain. The mammalian brain, which a generation ago some thought too complex for serious scientific investigation, is now squarely in the sights of modern neuroscientists. One of the major factors sparking the upsurge in brain studies is the development of powerful noninvasive imaging techniques that allow the functioning human brain to be visualized, thus showing us a new anatomy of the nervous system. The coupling of functional brain imaging with increasingly sophisticated behavioral tasks has proved a particularly potent combination, opening such elusive areas as planning, intention, and the importance of emotion to memory (Cahill et al.) to new biological investigation. For many of these studies, the unique language abilities of humans makes them the organism of choice for investigation. Subjects can be instructed, and their responses conveyed, by verbal means. In fact, the new imaging techniques have revitalized, and opened to new investigation, the anatomical basis of human language itself. The combination of imaging and well-designed behavioral tasks has revised and extended the century-old models of Broca and Wernicke, based on the study of subjects with clinical lesions (Raichle).

In other mammals, notably nonhuman primates and rodents, the increased sophistication of neuropsychological testing and training has enlarged the span of behavioral research. There has probably never been a Cold Spring Harbor Symposium in which so much behavioral research was presented. We heard about sophisticated language tasks, symmetry testing, Morris water mazes (which now are found in the laboratory of every self-respecting molecular neurobiologist interested in memory and learning), passive avoidance tests, Barnes platform mazes, and delayed non-match-to-sample tests, all surely novel topics for Cold Spring Harbor.

Much of the new enthusiasm for behavior arises from the possibilities of genetics. The earlier studies on *Drosophila* of Seymour Benzer and his colleagues introduced genetics as a systematic tool for linking behavior to biology. Although progress in the biology of behavior in simple organisms such as *Drosophila* and *Caenorhabditis elegans* continues (see, e.g., Tully et al.; Chou et al.), the development of techniques for genetically altering mice has led to a resurgence of interest in using mice to study behavior. One of the most exciting reports at the meeting demonstrated the success of a genetic screen in mice to isolate mutants with alterations in their circadian rhythms (King and Takahashi). After mutagenesis with ethylnitrosourea, screening of as few as 2000 mice is believed to cover over 90% of the genome in looking for dominant mutations in the F_1 generation. With this encouraging example, the isolation of other mouse mutants deficient in particular behaviors should soon follow.

Circadian Rhythms

One of the simplest and most highly conserved aspects of behavior, seen in organisms ranging from *Neurospora* to humans, is the diurnal rhythm. In higher animals, circadian oscillations in behavior originate in the brain. In mammals, a single nucleus, the suprachiasmatic nucleus, acts as the circadian clock, receiving input about light from the eye, and through its output, generating the rhythm that is transmitted to effector systems. There is now general agreement that the oscillator is cell-autonomous and not mediated by synaptic circuits. Thus, isolated cells maintain a circadian rhythm. Recently, rapid progress has been made in *Drosophila*, where genetics had identified several of the elements involved. Two genes, *per* and *tim*, have been identified as closely associated with the clock. The proteins encoded by these genes cycle with the circadian oscillator, as do their mRNAs, but with a phase lag. Experiments show that the two proteins are associated in a complex that is believed to regulate transcription of the respective genes through an autoregulatory feedback loop (Young et al.; Rosbash et al.). Whether the mechanism of transcriptional inhibition by the *tim-per* complex is direct or through one or more intermediate factors is not yet known. The cycle also involves regulation of protein phosphorylation and degradation; the precise roles that these play and their molecular mechanisms remain for future investigation.

Surprisingly, although the general properties of the circadian rhythms in *Drosophila* and mammals are similar, genes that are homologous to *per* and *tim* have not been found in mammals. The recent discovery of a mouse clock gene mutation, obtained by mutagenesis followed by a behavioral screen (King and Takahashi), should result in rapid identification of the particular gene involved and its comparison with *per* and *tim*; from the phenotype conferred by the mutation, the mammalian gene appears to be an ortholog of those found in *Drosophila* and in *Neurospora*.

Sensations, Perceptions, and Plasticity

One mark of the change in our field is that the hegemony of the visual system within the world of sensory physiology appears finally to have been breached. Indeed, this Symposium was marked by the prominence of the nose, mediating feeding, sex, and aversive behaviors, among others. Much of the excitement in olfaction arises from the recent identification of a large family of approximately 1000 genes encoding seven-transmembrane proteins that appear to act as mammalian olfactory receptor molecules (Mombaerts et al.; Buck). Each gene is expressed in only a small number of olfactory receptor neurons, and each neuron may express only one of these genes. The group of sensory neurons expressing each receptor gene is confined to one of four large zones in the olfactory epithelium, within which they are apparently randomly distributed. Axons from the group of neurons expressing the same gene all then converge to a small number of bilaterally symmetric glomeruli in the olfactory bulb. How such a topographic map is established in the olfactory bulb is unknown. Because olfactory receptors are expressed before synaptic contact is made, a retrograde mechanism seems unlikely; the most intriguing suggestion is that the olfactory receptors themselves might play a role in establishing correct synaptic connections, although what the ligand might be in this case is unclear. A second, unrelated class of seven-transmembrane receptors, isolated by single-cell analysis, appears to mediate olfaction in the vomeronasal organ, an anatomically distinct organ of olfaction responsible for the activation of innate reproductive and social behaviors by pheromones (Mombaerts et al.).

Although the large number of mammalian odorant receptor genes and their pattern of expression argue strongly that they are the primary receptors to which odorous molecules bind, a direct demonstration of this role still has not been achieved, nor has a particular behavioral response in mammals been associated with a single receptor. A functional receptor that mediates a specific odorant response has been identified in *C. elegans* (Chou et al.). Both loss-of-function and gain-of-function experiments demonstrate that a gene encoding a member of the seven-transmembrane family of receptors mediates the worm's response to the odorant diacetyl. The gene is part of a large family of related genes in *C. elegans*, many of which have been shown to be expressed in chemosensory cells. Interestingly, in *C. elegans*, the evidence is clear that a single cell has several distinct types of receptor molecules which appear to share a single signaling pathway. Although in mammals each odorant is thought to activate several sensory neurons, expressing different olfactory receptor molecules, in the case of diacetyl a single receptor residing in a single chemosensory cell appears to mediate the response of the organism to low concentrations of the chemical.

The activation of odorant receptors in the mammalian olfactory epithelium is thought to stimulate a specific G protein, G_{olf}, which stimulates adenylyl cyclase II, leading to an increase in cAMP and the opening of a cyclic nucleotide-gated cation channel (Reed). Recent experiments suggest that the related chemosensory system of taste also utilizes a G-protein-linked pathway of sensory transduction to mediate the detection of bitter and sweet tastants. Both transducin and gustducin, a taste-specific G protein similar to transducin, are found in taste receptor cells, where they can be activated by a bitter tastant; both also activate a taste-specific phosphodiesterase similar to that seen in photoreceptors (Wong et al.). Transgenic mice that are null for gustducin show altered responses to both bitter and sweet tastants. Although receptors for bitter and sweet tastants have not been isolated, the demonstration that G proteins are activated by a specific tastant strongly suggests that they are seven-transmembrane domain receptors.

Bringing odor and taste into the world of G-protein receptor-mediated sensory responses means that the next great challenge within the field of sensory transduction is to understand the molecular basis of the transduction of mechanical signals. Hearing and vestibular function depend on channels whose opening and closing are controlled by mechanical tension through the tip link (Gillespie et al.). Given the small number of channels and their apparent lack of homology with known channels, their isolation will be a daunting task. Success has been recently achieved, however, in identifying candidate myosin components of the molecular motor used to adjust the tension exerted on the channels through the tip links, thus setting the dynamic range of the channels (Gillespie et al.).

In addition to progress in unraveling the molecular mechanisms of sensation, important advances are now being made in understanding the higher-level mechanisms for processing sensory information that underlie our conscious sense of the external world, that is, our perceptions. Psychophysical studies have made clear for some time that the nervous system not only receives and analyzes complex information from the external world, but imposes its own order upon it. What is most notable about recent work is our increasing ability to relate conscious awareness of sensory events to neural substrates. One source of insight has been the analysis of human subjects with specific brain lesions (Koch and Braun). Another arises from physiological experiments in trained primates. Thus, monkeys can be trained to respond to an array of moving dots that have the appearance of transparent surfaces moving past each other in such a fashion as to give the impression of a rotating cylinder. When the animals are given ambiguous information such that the direction of rotation of the cylinder is uncertain, they respond approximately half of the time with one direction and half with the other. Physiological recording from behaving animals shows that cells in the medial temporal area can be found whose firing rates are correlated with the perceived direction of movement (Andersen et al.). These neurons represent perception rather than simple sensation; their activity depends on what the monkey perceives rather than on the stimulus alone.

The cellular mechanism underlying a different kind of perception is seen in another experiment in which discrete linear segments can be aligned in the visual field so that a continuous line is seen, a familiar psychophysical "illusion." Recording from pyramidal cells in layer VI of monkey visual cortex shows that cells that respond to similar orientations are connected by horizontal collaterals. Activation of one cell lowers the electrical threshold of others of similar orientation preference (Gilbert et al.), thus providing a possible explanation for the generation of a continuous line from separate segments.

Perceptions can be altered by lesions in the nervous system, as vividly illustrated by the Dorcas Cummings Lecturer, Dr. V.S. Ramachandran, who described several unusual patients who are unable to recognize faces (prosopagnosia), or who recognize familiar faces, but are unable to score their emotional significance (Capgras syndrome), or who seem unable to acknowledge that a previously functioning limb is now paralyzed (anosagnosia). Careful description and behavioral testing coupled with precise delineation of the lesions involved offers an unusual window into the higher functions of the brain. This is most strikingly illustrated by the reorganization of perceptions in those with amputated upper limbs, who now perceive stimuli to either the regions near the stump or to the face as coming from the phantom limb. These results can be explained by the reorganization of cortical representation, as shown by magnetoencephalographic studies (Ramachandran). As a result of the amputation, the area of cortex that previously represented the amputated lower arm is now invaded by enlargement of the two adjacent cortical representations of the upper arm and face.

These results on human patients fit neatly into a

previous series of investigations in primates showing that cortical sensory and motor maps are not stable in the adult, but change depending on their relative use (Merzenich et al.). In each case, areas of the cortex that undergo continued use expand their functional representations into neighboring areas. Within the expanded areas, the receptive fields of the cortical neurons become smaller and more refined. The expansions in representation can occur across a distance of a centimeter or more (Ramachandran), and they can occur with a rapidity that makes it unlikely that axonal sprouting is the cause. A major challenge is to discover the precise cellular mechanisms that underlie these changes.

Other examples of reorganization after injury were offered by experiments showing that after partial ablation of the retina (Gilbert et al.) and amblyopia (Kiorpes and Movshon), cortical changes occur to restore the perceptual "gaps" that otherwise might occur. Investigation of the remarkable plasticity of the adult brain not only gives insight into brain function, but also is clinically important as a mechanism of recovery from stroke and from traumatic brain or spinal cord injury. If ways were known to stimulate and promote these mechanisms, recovery in adults might be enhanced. We know that in children, dramatic reorganizations are possible; children who have undergone hemispherectomy, for example, often show remarkable functional recovery. Experiments in which the alteration of sensory input to children with learning disorders improves their learning abilities give encouragement to efforts to understand and use the innate plasticity of the brain in treating disabilities of many types.

Learning and Memory: Global Aspects

The ability of the adult brain to reorganize itself as the result of experience is the biological basis of learning and memory. One of the most satisfying developments of recent years has been the increasing establishment of connections between studies of learning and memory carried out at different levels of investigation. Studies have flourished at all levels. Neuropsychological studies have been invigorated by the ability to define the lesions in patients through imaging; improvements in slice and electrophysiological recording technology have allowed ever-more sophisticated investigation of the mechanisms involved in synaptic plasticity; genetic investigations have continued in flies, and, with the advent of "knockout" and "knock-in" mice, in mammals; and the molecular biology of memory, barely more than a hopeful term a decade ago, is now a full-blown field of investigation. The intense research activity on memory and learning has revealed its variety: Separate mechanisms may mediate memory in the amygdala, the hippocampus, and the striatum (Squire and Zola); or CA1 and CA3 in the hippocampus (Nakanishi et al.); or even on apical versus basal dendrites of the same cell (Mayford et al.). Nevertheless, amid the profusion of different types and mechanisms of memory, glimmers of order and simplification are seen. There is emerging and widespread agreement about the types of memory in the temporal domain, extending not only to different brain regions, but also to different organisms. At the molecular level, the emergence of the transcriptional factor CREB as a central positive and negative regulator of long-term memory in flies, *Aplysia*, and mammals has served to emphasize the fundamentally conservative nature of the molecular mechanisms subserving memory.

Neuropsychological studies in humans have continued to emphasize one of the main points of the pioneering studies of Brenda Milner on H.M. in the 1950s, namely, that memory is distinct from other cognitive functions (Squire and Zola). Furthermore, by studying patients with different brain lesions, it has been possible to identify regions of the brain associated with different types of learning. Lesions in the medial-temporal lobe, including not only the hippocampus and associated structures, but also the parahippocampal, perirhinal, and entorhinal cortices, do not affect short-term memory but do disrupt long-term memory. The medial-temporal lobe is not thought to be the storage site for long-term memory, but lesions there produce temporally graded retrograde amnesia, suggesting that these structures direct the consolidation of memories in the neocortex, the site of storage. Importantly, medial-temporal lobe damage appears to be specific for declarative or explicit memory; nondeclarative (skill or implicit learning) memory is not affected (Squire and Zola).

A different kind of memory is encoded in the amygdala. The amygdala is essential for aversive or fear conditioning, whereby animals learn to associate specific stimuli with aversive responses. The amygdala receives input from both thalamus and cortex, and projects to the hypothalamus and midbrain, which mediate the physiological components of the aversive response. Recent electrophysiological studies of the amygdala allow links to be made between behavior and electrical signaling (Quirk et al.). Aversive conditioning is accompanied by a change in the responsiveness of neurons in the lateral nucleus of the amygdala, the first relay station for sensory input. The lateral nucleus receives inputs from several different modalities (visual, auditory, olfactory, somatosensory), making it a suitable site for associative plasticity, and blockade of NMDA receptors here prevents fear conditioning. Because the latency of the conditioned changes in the amygdala is shorter than those in the cortex, the conditioning pathway is likely to lead directly from thalamic nuclei.

Further definition of local circuits within the amygdala will be required to understand how this nucleus functions in the consolidation of aversive memories, but the ability to measure physiological changes in a behaviorally defined context seems a powerful advantage for this system. Although most work at the cellular level has focused on the hippocampus, our incomplete understanding of the behavioral correlates of cellular changes in the hippocampus has been a limiting factor. Some progress has been made in understanding the role of the hippocampus in memory of place, but declarative memory, by its very nature, is less accessible in animals than in humans. Eichenbaum (Eichenbaum et al.) reported neuropsychological and electrophysiological experiments using olfactory learning in rats to show the role of the hippocampal system in supporting a flexible system of associations that is formally equivalent to what is seen in declarative memory in humans.

The most complete picture that we have of the different types of memory and their relationships is based on studies of a conditioned aversive response in *Drosophila* (Tully et al.). Here the combination of carefully designed behavioral tests and the use of genetic mutants has revealed four overlapping, but separable, memory processes that differ in their temporal, pharmacological, and behavioral properties. Taken together, they can account for the entire time course of Pavlovian olfactory learning in *Drosophila*.

The overlapping phases of short-term and middle-term memory precede long-term memory and are necessary for it. A fourth component, anesthesia-resistant memory, also arises from short-term and middle-term memory but is not required for long-term memory. Of these forms of memory, the only one that ultimately persists is long-term memory. The properties of the memory components and their characteristic time courses depend on the complex interplay of positive and negative regulatory factors, and offer an explanation for the familiar and well-established observation that spaced training is more effective than massed training ("cramming") in producing long-term learning. Although formal dissection of the memory process into its components does not require knowledge of its biochemical mechanism, part of the power of genetics is that identification of the genes involved leads directly to biochemical mechanisms. In this case, a single pathway, the cAMP pathway, appears to be involved. Translation of the kinetic components of memory into the half-lives of components of the pathway appears to be well on its way.

Learning and Memory: Cellular and Molecular Mechanisms

Although the work in *Drosophila* leads to conclusions about the forms of memory and its biochemical mechanisms, we have little information about the specific synapses involved and how changes in intracellular second messengers and gene transcription in particular cells are translated into changes in synaptic function. Currently, the most active system in which answers to these questions are being sought is the rodent hippocampus, where the molecular mechanisms of LTP and LTD are being pursued. Transgenic mice, in which particular genes are "knocked out" or are overexpressed, are one of the most promising tools in these investigations. These have the advantage of allowing changes in cellular properties to be linked to changes in behavior.

At the meeting, we heard about changes in cellular plasticity in transgenic mice with altered expression of CaM kinase (Mayford et al.; Tonegawa et al.); nitric oxide synthase isoforms (Mayford et al.); BDNF (Griesbeck et al.); cholinergic receptors (Changeux et al.); glutamate receptors (Silva et al.; Nakanishi et al.; Tonegawa et al.); and neurofibromatosis-1 GAP protein (Silva et al.). As several of the investigators stressed, however, interpreting the effects of transgenic manipulations is not always straightforward. One problem is genetic background. Berrettini's experiments on opiate addiction in mice (Ferraro and Berrettini) remind us of the range of behaviorial variation in different mouse strains. A second problem is the difficulty of disentangling the direct functional effects of an alteration in gene expression from its developmental effects. Thus, genetic changes may trigger secondary effects during development aimed at compensating them, or they may change the course of a particular developmental pathway for other reasons. Finally, the interconnectedness of the brain means that a change in one region may have as its primary cause changes in other regions to which it is connected by anatomical or hormonal pathways.

Fortunately, progress in addressing these problems is being made. Tissue-specific promoters can allow restriction of genetic changes to particular regions of the brain, e.g., the CA1 region of the hippocampus (Tonegawa et al.), and conditional gene expression, via a tetracycline-sensitive promoter, for example (Mayford et al.; Tonegawa et al.), allow acute effects to be observed in isolation from possible developmental changes. One of the most important advances is the increasing sophistication and completeness of the behavioral and cellular tests given to animals with altered gene expression. The deficits in spatial learning exhibited by CAMKII mutants are more compelling given their normal performance on a version of the task with a visible platform, just as the deficient passive avoidance of mice lacking specific nicotinic receptor subtypes is more revealing given their normal performance on spatial learning tests (Changeux et al.). At the cellular level, the significance of reduced LTD in mGluR2 mutants is enhanced by demonstration of normal LTP at the same synapse (Nakanishi et al.). Reversal of particular defects by specific interventions also buttresses the argument for their specificity. Perhaps most notable in this regard was the demonstration that LTP in BDNF knockout mice could be reversed by adenovirus-mediated BDNF gene transfer in tissue slices (Griesbeck et al.).

DEVELOPMENT

One of the major sub-themes that emerged from the meeting was the relationship between mechanisms of plasticity in the adult and during development. This theme was perhaps most clearly apparent for the neurotrophins, whose classic role as target-derived growth factors suddenly seems too restrictive to account for the increasing number of processes in which they seem to be involved. The essential role of neurotrophins in plasticity was made clear by the finding that BDNF-deficient mice show impaired LTP (Griesbeck et al.). BDNF also appears to play a role in cortical dendrite formation (Riddle et al.). In cultured cortical slices, BDNF stimulates dendritic outgrowth; moreover, normal outgrowth in the slices is truncated by addition of a soluble form of trkB, the receptor for BDNF. Interestingly, the stimulation of dendritic growth by BDNF requires electrical activity, possibly through a calcium-dependent mechanism. Thus, blockers of NMDA receptors or of voltage-gated calcium channels blunt the effect of BDNF. The source of endogenous BDNF in these experiments is unknown, but one could imagine a model in which BDNF is released by axons and taken up into dendrites, thus reversing the classic paradigm. The BDNF that is taken up may form signaling endosomes, such as those described for uptake via nerve terminals (Beattie et al.). The requirement for electrical activity shown in these experiments links dendritic growth to function, and to a large body of evidence on the role of activity in shaping synaptic connections.

The importance of electrical activity was demonstrated in another developmental context by experiments that examined the mechanisms of synapse formation in the *Xenopus* retinotectal system (Cline et al.). An attractive feature of this system is that there is a rostrocaudal gradient of synaptic maturation in the tectum which allows synapses at different stages of development to be seen in a single preparation. A striking feature of synaptic maturation in the tectum is that the complement of glutamate receptors appears to change. The newest synapses have largely NMDA receptors, whereas older synapses have both NMDA and AMPA receptors. The increase in functional AMPA receptors observed during development is activity-dependent and appears to involve calcium and CAMKII. The proposed developmental sequence has a striking resemblance to the mechanisms of postsynaptic plasticity that have been suggested for LTP at CA1 synapses in the hippocampus. In both cases, electrical stimulation is postulated to increase synaptic strength by increasing the number of functional AMPA receptors. Calcium, acting through CAMKII, appears to be involved in both cases.

In other work on developing synapses, Yancopoulos and colleagues (Glass et al.) showed that a receptor tyrosine kinase that is localized to the adult neuromuscular junction is a key component in synaptic differentiation at the neuromuscular junction. Mice that lack the MuSK kinase are strikingly similar to those lacking agrin, the synaptic organizing factor released by motor nerves. In both cases, the number of nerve-associated AChR clusters in the muscle is stongly reduced. Although direct binding of agrin to MuSK has not been shown, the results suggest that MuSK is an essential component of the agrin receptor and that other components remain to be identified. Agrin is known to cause tyrosine phosphorylation of the AChR, but the role of MuSK in this phosphorylation is unclear. In C2 myotubes, the AChR is complexed with both src and fyn, two members of the src protein tyrosine kinase family, but experiments suggest that src is responsible for AChR phosphorylation (Wang et al.). Fischbach (Rosen et al.) described how another neurally released factor, ARIA, which is member of the neuregulin family, acts on a receptor tyrosine kinase. These observations on agrin and ARIA provide a point of entry into the hitherto unknown intracellular signaling cascades that mediate synaptic differentiation.

For the neurotrophins, although the discovery of the trk receptors shifted much of the experimental activity away from the biology to the intracellular signaling pathways, the functional role of p75, the first neurotrophin receptor to be characterized, has remained unclear. Recent experiments suggest that it may play a role in mediating cell death. These experiments (Carter et al.) make clear that p75 can act independently of trk receptors and that the activation of p75 can result in increased expression of the transcription facor NF-κB. p75 thus appears to mediate a response similar to that of the related receptors for TNF-α, which act through the MADD pathway to kill cells. Finally, in at least one instance in the developing nervous system, namely in the retina, the interaction of NGF with p75 appears to mediate cell death.

CONCLUSION

The 61st Cold Spring Harbor Symposium was a rich feast of neuroscience at the end of the twentieth century. The topics discussed and the questions asked would have astounded our predecessors of 45 years ago. The genetic basis of schizophrenia, and the single-cell neurobiological correlates of perception, to name but two examples, are problems that were literally off the known and charted waters of neuroscience at that time. The central problem, of understanding how the brain works, has, of course, not changed. What has changed are the tools that allow us to obtain hard answers from complex biological systems. As we look ahead, we cannot possibly imagine what tools our successors in the next century will have and what their specific achievements will be. Perhaps we can pose a more modest aim, however, by asking ourselves what new frontiers will be acknowledged by the title of the next Cold Spring Harbor Symposium on the brain. I can think of two that I would like to see: *Mind and*

Brain; and *New Treatments for Neurological and Psychiatric Disorders.* I hope to see you there.

ACKNOWLEDGMENTS

I am grateful to Drs. Robert Zalutsky and Story Landis of the National Institute of Neurological Disorders and Stroke, for helpful discussions and for comments on the manuscript.

Author Index

Subject Index

D

Q

R

S